&Govoni &Hayes

DRUGS AND NURSING IMPLICATIONS

Govoni & Hayes

Margaret T. Shannon, R.N., Ph.D.
Director, Division of Nursing
Our Lady of Holy Cross College
New Orleans, Louisiana

Billie Ann Wilson, R.N., Ph.D.
Director, Nursing Program
Loyola University
New Orleans, Louisiana

with
Carolyn L. Stang, Pharm.D.
Assistant Pharmacy Director
   for Clinical Services
Evanston Hospital
Evanston, Illinois

DRUGS AND NURSING IMPLICATIONS

7th Edition

APPLETON & LANGE
Norwalk, Connecticut

0-8385-1779-X

Copyright © 1992 by Appleton & Lange
Simon & Schuster Business and Professional Group
Copyright © 1971, 1978, 1982 by Appleton-Century-Crofts.
Copyright © 1965 by Meredith Publishing Company.

92 93 94 95 96 / 10 9 8 7 6 5 4 3 2

Prentice Hall International (UK) Limited, *London*
Prentice Hall of Australia Pty. Limited, *Sydney*
Prentice Hall Canada, Inc., *Toronto*
Prentice Hall Hispanoamericana, S.A., *Mexico*
Prentice Hall of India Private Limited, *New Delhi*
Prentice Hall of Japan, Inc., *Tokyo*
Simon & Schuster Asia Pte. Ltd., *Singapore*
Editora Prentice Hall do Brasil Ltda., *Rio de Janeiro*
Prentice Hall, *Englewood Cliffs, New Jersey*

Library of Congress Catalog Card Number: 92-053127

Editor in Chief: Barbara Ellen Norwitz
Production: CRACOM Corporation
Designer: Diane M. Beasley

PRINTED IN THE UNITED STATES OF AMERICA

To

Alvin, Theresa, Ellen, and Michael,

without whom this edition would not have been possible

◆

CONTENTS

PREFACE

The seventh edition of *Drugs and Nursing Implications* remains true to the commitment of previous editions to provide nurses with a comprehensive drug reference. Each drug monograph has been carefully developed to provide the nurse with all the current information needed to make appropriate decisions regarding drug administration. This edition, however, has been extensively revised to make it easier to use and more consistent with the nursing process approach to patient/client care.

We recognize that decision making relative to pharmacotherapeutics is a complex and intrinsically cyclic process. For example, assessments are made both prior to and following drug administration. These assessments provide data for (1) evaluation of the therapeutic efficacy of the drug, (2) evaluation of the efficacy of nursing interventions, (3) decisions regarding continuation or modification of nursing interventions, and (4) development of new nursing diagnoses with related nursing interventions. Thus, nursing diagnoses may change as a result of an achieved therapeutic effect, therapeutic failure, manifestation of an adverse/side effect, or a demonstrated learning need.

Because the decision-making process related to drug administration is a cyclic one, the Nursing Implications section of each monograph is formatted in a straightforward manner, with sections on administration, assessment and drug effects, and patient and family education. From these sections the reader can easily identify information pertinent to an individual patient situation and readily incorporate it into the nursing process.

One of the many new features of the seventh edition is the inclusion of seven chapters on pharmacotherapeutics and the role of the nurse in drug administration. These chapters provide information essential for each nurse to know. Two other significant changes to the seventh edition are related to prototype drugs and IV drug administration information.

Prototype drugs are considered representative of all drugs in their particular drug classification. In general, all drugs in the class will have similar actions, uses, side effects, and nursing implications as the prototype drug. Thus learning about the vast number of drugs available can be simplified by focusing on the prototype representative of each class.

The prototype drugs were placed in the alphabetical listing in previous editions. In this edition the prototype drugs have been placed in a separate section and arranged by pharmacologic and therapeutic classification similar to the classification scheme used by the American Hospital Formulary Service (AHFS). This arrangement of the prototype drugs by pharmacologic and therapeutic category enables the nurse to identify different classes of drugs that have similar therapeutic implications or that primarily affect the same physiologic system. This arrangement allows for a more logical physiologic approach to learning about drugs. Throughout this book most drugs are keyed to a prototype drug. If no prototype is indicated, the drug has a unique pharmacologic action and cannot meaningfully be placed in a class with a single representative agent. A summary of the prototype classifications and their representative drugs is listed inside the front and back covers for easy reference.

New to this edition is comprehensive information regarding administration of IV drugs. Each IV drug monograph contains directions related to drug reconstitution, dilution, method of administration, rate of infusion, and nursing assessment and interventions specific to the IV form of the drug. Thus the seventh edition eliminates the need for additional resources related to administration of IV drugs.

With the addition of chapters on pharmacotherapeutics and the role of the nurse in drug administration, the emphasis on prototypes as representatives of drug classes, the inclusion of comprehensive IV drug information, and extensively developed drug monographs, this book becomes a comprehensive resource for drug administration that can be used also as a basic pharmacology text.

We believe that the changes incorporated into this edition will be welcomed by nurses, student nurses, and other health-care professionals who have come to rely on *Drugs and Nursing Implications* as the definitive resource for drug administration.

Margaret T. Shannon
Billie Ann Wilson

ACKNOWLEDGMENTS

The authors wish to acknowledge the contributions of the following individuals to this work: Michelle Alexander, RN; Gerry Hickey, RN, BS Pharmacy, BSN; Linda McCuistion, RN, MN; Debra Theriot, RN, BS Biology, BSN; Gail Wilson, RN, BSN.

The authors wish to express their appreciation to Barbara Norwitz, Editor in Chief, Appleton & Lange, and to Mary Espenschied, CRACOM Corporation, for the assistance they provided in the development and preparation of this edition.

Finally the authors wish to express their appreciation to all their past and present nursing students who have provided the inspiration for this work. It is for these individuals and all who strive for excellence in patient care that the revision of the work was undertaken.

HOW TO USE THIS BOOK

Introductory chapters have been provided as a resource for those seeking essential information about pharmacotherapeutics and the nurse's role in drug administration. The reader is directed to carefully review this material and refer to it when specific information is needed relative to some facet of drug administration.

A glossary of Clinical Conditions and Associated Signs & Symptoms related to drug use has been provided in Chapter 3. Throughout the book the reader is referred back to this glossary for specific clinical manifestations of conditions associated with drug use, such as hypokalemia and Cushing's syndrome.

Any given drug can be known by a variety of names. First it will have a formal chemical name that describes its chemical structure. Early in development the pharmaceutical manufacturer may assign the drug a code name, which is much easier to use than the formal chemical name. If the drug looks promising and the manufacturer anticipates marketing the drug, a "nonproprietary" or *generic* name is given to the drug. The generic name then becomes the official name for the drug in the United States. The manufacturer then assigns a "proprietary" name that is trademarked by the individual manufacturer. This name is known as the *trade* or *brand* name of the drug. The trade name is used by the manufacturer to market the drug to physicians and pharmacists. Because a single drug can be made by several different pharmaceutical manufacturers, the generic name is the preferred name when learning about drugs. The generic name can also help identify a drug's pharmacologic class and prototype.

The drugs are listed in the alphabetical section of the book by *generic* name. Each drug is indexed by both its generic and trade name. Combination drugs will not be found in the alphabetical section of this book since they are referenced solely by trade name. An appendix of commonly used combination drugs with their generic components has been provided so that each component may be located separately in the alphabetical section. When a combination drug is noted in the index, the reader will be referred to the appendix.

Generic names for all drugs discussed in the book are listed in the alphabetical section, and the reader will be referred to a specific page in the prototype section, Section II, if the drug is a prototype for a class of drugs. If the drug is not a prototype but belongs to a class for which a prototype has been designated, the reader will note that the prototype drug is identified above the generic name for the drug. The reader should review all the information provided in each drug monograph, as well as the information provided under the prototype for the class. Individual drug monographs contain the following information:

Generic and Trade Names and Classifications The generic name is given followed in parentheses by its phonetic spelling. Common trade names are listed followed by the drug classifications.

Pregnancy Category Drugs may be categorized as category A, B, C, D, or X according to risk-benefit ratio for the mother and fetus, with A being the lowest and X the highest risk. If the FDA pregnancy category is known, it will be indicated. Refer to the appendix for a more complete description of pregnancy categories.

Schedule   Controlled substances, such as narcotics, are classified as belonging to one of five schedules I to V according to abuse potential, with I having the highest and V the lowest potential for abuse. Refer to the appendix for a more complete description of each schedule.

Actions/Pharmacodynamics   This entry describes the mechanism by which the specific drug produces physiologic and biochemical changes at the cell, tissue, or organ level.

Uses   The therapeutic applications of each drug are described in terms of normal use and unlabeled use. An unlabeled use is literally one that does not appear on the drug label or in the manufacturer's literature on the use of the drug. The unlabeled use is, nevertheless, an accepted use for the drug.

Route & Dosage   Route is specified as SC, IM, IV, PO, PR, nasal, ophthalmic, vaginal, topical, aural, and intrathecal; doses are listed separately for adult and child and according to use.

Pharmacokinetics   This section lists information about onset, peak, and duration of drug action. It also lists the mechanism of metabolism and elimination when known.

Contraindications & Precautions   Many drugs are contraindicated and therefore should not be used in specific pathophysiologic conditions, during pregnancy, or with particular drugs or food. In other cases the drug should be used with great caution because of a greater than average risk or untoward effects.

Adverse/Side Effects   Virtually all drugs have adverse/side effects that may be bothersome to some individuals but not to others. In this entry, adverse/side effects are listed according to systems or organs with the most common printed in italics and those that are life-threatening underlined.

Diagnostic Test Interferences   This entry describes the effect of the drug on various diagnostic tests and alerts the nurse to possible misinterpretations of test results.

Drug Interactions   Individual drugs, drug classes, and foods that interact with the drug under discussion are listed. Drugs may interact to inhibit or enhance one another; thus drug interactions may improve the therapeutic response, lead to therapeutic failure, or produce specific untoward reactions. Only drugs that have been shown to cause clinically significant interactions with the drug under discussion are listed.

Incompatibilities   Solutions and drug additives physically incompatible with the drug under discussion are listed. Therefore these solutions and drug additives should not be mixed in solution with the drug.

Nursing Implications   Nursing implications are listed under three headings: Administration, Assessment & Drug Effects, and Patient & Family Education. Before administering a drug, the nurse should read all three sections to determine (1) the appropriate administration techniques, (2) the assessments that should be made before and after administration of the drug and indicators of drug effectiveness, and (3) essential patient or family education related to the drug.

BASIC PHARMACOLOGY

NURSE'S ROLE IN DRUG ADMINISTRATION

NURSING PROCESS APPLIED TO DRUG ADMINISTRATION

The nursing process is a formal, structured process that is used as a framework to guide patient care practices and drug administration in a wide variety of contemporary nursing practice settings. This process includes patient assessment, nursing diagnosis, planning, intervention, and evaluation.

In the *assessment* phase the nurse develops a client data base using information from both the personal history and the physical assessment. The nurse must pay particular attention to the history of past and current illness, the drugs used to treat those conditions, and the patient's response to those medications. Additionally the nurse must assess the patient's psychological response to the current diagnosis and social-cultural influences on the patient's compliance with drug therapy. For example, does the patient have access to a pharmacy and sufficient financial resources to fill prescriptions, or does the drug therapy threaten a cultural health care practice?

The *nursing diagnosis* is a statement that reflects the summary and analysis of available data, delineating the concern or problem area that nursing care can address. Nursing diagno-

sis statements reflect a variety of actual or potential concerns, and each problem or concern is addressed through a separate nursing diagnosis. Some commonly used nursing diagnoses related to medication administration are knowledge deficit, noncompliance, alterations in comfort, and ineffective coping.

The *planning* phase of the nursing process allows the nurse and the patient or family to jointly establish clear and specific goals. These goals should be measurable, as evidenced by specific behaviors: for example, the patient will be able to identify each of his or her cardiac medications and state the anticipated effects of each medication within 1 week.

The *intervention* phase of the nursing process includes correct and timely administration of medications, as well as the initiation of the teaching process to help the individual reach the set goals. Nurses must be creative teachers. They should assess the individual's learning style and design interventions to meet identified learning needs.

In the *evaluation* phase the nurse refers to the initial assessment and goals of care to determine whether the interventions resulted in attainment of the goals. For example, in evaluating the outcome of drug teaching, the nurse should ascertain the patient's understanding of correct dosage, administration techniques, and reportable adverse effects.

THERAPEUTIC AIM OF DRUG THERAPY

The aim of drug therapy is to modify an existing physiological function. The most common mechanisms by which drugs act to modify physiological functions fall into the following categories: replacing a function (for example, insulin), enhancing a function (for example, bronchodilation with theophylline), impeding a function (for example, decreasing heart rate and blood pressure with propranolol), destroying tissues (for example, chemotherapy with radioactive iodine), and destroying an infection or infestation (for example, destroying bacterial infection with penicillin).

MAJOR DRUG CLASSIFICATIONS AND PROTOTYPES

Learning the actions, interactions, doses, and adverse effects of hundreds of drugs would be nearly impossible. Fortunately, therapeutic agents are classified into a number of different types based on similar therapeutic action or mechanism of action. The classifications in this book are based on the Pharmacologic-Therapeutic Classification of the American Hospital Formulary Service (AHFS). For each of these drug classifications, prototypes can be identified that are representative of the entire class of drugs. If the actions of the prototype drug can be learned, the characteristics of the other drugs in that class may be inferred. Learning about the prototype provides a basic framework on which to build a further understanding of the similarities and dissimilarities of the drugs in a class.

MEDICATION ORDERS

Components of a Legal Medication Order

Nurses administer medications in accordance with the physician's orders. The essential components of a legal medication order include the following:

1. Date on an outpatient prescription; date and time on an inpatient order.
2. Patient name for an outpatient; patient identification number for an inpatient.
3. Drug name (generic or trade) and strength of dose.
4. Frequency of dose and duration of therapy, if applicable. It is assumed that a medication ordered in a hospital is to be administered continuously until otherwise specified or until the order expires according to hospital policy.
5. Physician's full signature, with the physician's name printed below if the signature is illegible. Outpatient prescriptions should have the physician's state licensing number and Drug Enforcement Administration (DEA) identification number.
6. Outpatient prescriptions also have sections for specifying number of refills permitted.

In summary, the essential parts of the legal medication order include the clear delineation of patient name, name of drug, dose of drug, frequency and duration of administration, physician's signature, and date of the order being written. The nurse is legally responsible for interpreting each of these components before administering the drug. This information directs the nurse in the calculation, preparation, and administration of the medication. If the nurse cannot read the physician's orders or if the order seems erroneous, he or she must question the order before giving the drug. When in doubt, the nurse should call the physician who ordered the drug for clarification.

Generic and Trade Names

All drugs may be identified by both generic and trade names. The generic, or nonproprietary, name derives from the chemical substance from which the drug is made. This name has been approved by the Food and Drug Administration (FDA). The trade, or proprietary, name of a drug is the name a particular pharmaceutical company has chosen to market its version of the drug. If a physician wants a particular trade name drug dispensed, the words "dispense as written" should appear on the prescription.

Not all forms of a drug may have the same effective rate of absorption (referred to as bioavailability). When the generic drug has a low solubility or a high proportion of inert ingredients to active drug content, it may have a lower bioavailability than another manufacturer's product. When a patient complains that a medication doesn't work anymore, the reason may be that a generic formulation has been substituted that has a lower bioavailability for that individual.

Scheduled and prn Medication

Scheduled medications are to be administered at set intervals within a 24-hour period. Orders for these medications indicate the frequency as number of times in a day or specified times during the day. Abbreviations commonly used in prescriptions include the following:

a.c. = before meals	q = every
b.i.d. = twice a day	q.d. = every day
h = hour	q.i.d. = four times a day
h.s. = hour of sleep	q.o.d. = every other day
p.c. = after meals	s = second
prn = as necessary	t.i.d. = three times a day

An order for a drug to be given every 6 hours or q6h may not reflect the same drug administration times as a drug ordered q.i.d. which asks that the drug be administered four times in a day. The nurse has the responsibility to clarify an order with a physician if the nurse believes that a different dosing schedule would be more beneficial. For example, a diuretic ordered on a b.i.d. schedule may be given late enough in the evening to cause the patient to awaken from sleep to void. In consultation with the physician the nurse may administer the last dose earlier, thus eliminating the necessity for the patient to void during the night.

A prn order refers to a medication that may be given as circumstances indicate or as needed. The nurse is given some latitude in interpreting the patient's status when deciding when to give the medication. The types of medication most frequently ordered prn are analgesics, antiemetics, and laxatives. The guidelines for prn orders are the same as those for scheduled drugs but may have a range of doses and times of administration. For example, a patient may have an order for meperidine 50 to 100 mg IM q4–6h. The nursing assessment determines when and at what dose prn drugs are administered.

Stat Orders

A stat order is one that should be executed immediately. Drugs ordered in this manner should receive the utmost priority. Stat drugs often have the effect of modifying a serious physiological response, and delay in administration could jeopardize the patient. Common clinical examples include stat antihypertensives for a patient with extremely high blood pressure and stat nitroglycerin for a patient experiencing severe chest pain. Stat drugs are often administered by the intravenous route so that the drug reaches its target site quickly. Administration of a stat medication should be followed by frequent assessment and evaluation to determine if the desired effect has been achieved.

NURSES' LEGAL RESPONSIBILITIES

"Five Rights" of Medical Administration

At all times the nurse is legally responsible for correctly administering medication to the patients in the nurse's care. The legal responsibilities of the nurse are often summarized in the five rights of medication administration:

1. *Right Patient:* Always double-check the patient's name band. The nurse cannot assume that a patient answering in the affirmative when a name is called really is the stated person.
2. *Right Drug:* Check both drug name and correctness of therapy. Many medications have similar sounding names or spelling, for example, Zantac and Xanax, cefotaxime and ceftazidime.
3. *Right Route:* Ask if the drug should be given by this route, how else this drug can be given, and whether this is the correct route for this patient.
4. *Right Time:* Ask if this is the correct time for administration and when the last dose was given. Confirm that the schedule for drug doses is consistent with maintaining therapeutic levels and minimizing toxicity. Consider any physiological factors (for example, advanced age, hepatic disease) that could alter the dose or dosing schedule.
5. *Right Dose:* Ask what the recommended dose for this drug is, if this dose is appropriate for this patient, and whether there are laboratory results or therapeutic serum levels that could alter the drug dose.

Documentation of Medication Administration

Correct and complete documentation is an imperative step in the cycle of drug administration. Documentation includes the precise time of administration, the initials of the nurse responsible for administration, and the site of administration for parenteral doses. The nurse's full signature and title should be recorded on the medication administration record for that date and shift. Correct documentation in medication records can improve patient care. For example, it can ensure that a patient does not receive several intramuscular injections of pain medication in the same site.

COMMON MEDICATION ERRORS

The most common medication errors stem from inadequate attention to the five rights of medication administration. Common errors include the following:

1. *Wrong patient:* Administering a medication to the roommate of the intended patient because of inattentiveness to patient identification armbands.
2. *Wrong drug:* Picking a medication that appears to be the needed medication without double checking the actual name of the drug. For example, NPH insulin is administered when the order specifies regular insulin.
3. *Wrong route:* A common error with regard to route is the misadministration of an unusual oral form of a drug. For example, a chewable tablet is handed to the patient, who swallows it whole, or conversely a sustained action form of a medication is chewed or crushed.
4. *Wrong time:* Errors in timing of medication most commonly occur when a patient receives most of his or her medication at the same time of the day but has one scheduled at a different time. A possible error is that all medications are given at the same time or the one individually scheduled is inadvertently overlooked.
5. *Wrong dose:* An error in dose calculation may be due to a calculation error or to inattentiveness to unit dose medications (for example, a 25 mg dose is given in lieu of a 12.5 mg dose). If unsure of the drug dose calculation, the nurse should have colleagues verify the calculation.

Other common errors of medication administration include not verifying an illegibly written order and incorrectly transcribing a medication order given over the telephone.

WITHHOLDING ORDERED MEDICATIONS

Medications may be withheld for a variety of reasons. The nurse caring for the patient is responsible for conveying to the physician and other health care workers the reason for withholding the ordered drug. Patients may refuse their medications; the drug may be on a temporary hold awaiting a test, or parameters may be set describing when to hold a given medication, such as a specific blood pressure or heart rate. Each institution has its own method of documenting a withheld drug. The nurse must be aware of situations that require his or her clinical judgment to withhold a medication pending notification of the physician caring for the patient. Frequently the decision to delay or hold a medication is based on the nurse's physical assessment or interpretation of some laboratory data. Many medications require close assessment and monitoring of laboratory data to evaluate the effectiveness of the therapy. The nurse is responsible for knowing which drugs require additional laboratory data as a basis for clinical judgment.

CONTROLLED SUBSTANCES

The Controlled Substance Act of 1970 provides legal control of addictive and habituating drugs by both the Food and Drug Administration (FDA) and the Drug Enforcement Agency (DEA). Nurses must be aware of the implications for nursing practice regarding the classification for these drugs and the requirements for documentation and storage of the drugs. The five levels of classification (schedules 1 through V) are listed in Appendix A. Pharmacists are required to label controlled drugs by placing the letter "C" and the Roman numeral for the schedule in the upper right corner of the prescription blank.

NEEDED DRUG INFORMATION

The nurse who is faced with an order for the administration of an unfamiliar drug is legally responsible for developing an understanding of the medication in question. Beyond developing familiarity with the drug, the nurse must be able to translate available data into appropriate teaching for the patient for whom the drug is intended.

Actions/Pharmacodynamics and Uses

When evaluating information regarding a new drug, the nurse should compare the data describing the action (pharmacodynamics) of the drug within the body (see Chapter 5), as well as clinical descriptions of when it is used or indicated, with the clinical situation of the patient. The nurse should evaluate if this is indeed the correct drug for this patient and this condition.

Labeled vs Unlabeled Indications Drug indications listed in the manufacturer's package insert are often referred to as "FDA-approved" or simply "approved" indications or uses. However, drugs are often used appropriately for indications not listed in the manufacturer's package insert. These are best referred to as "unlabeled" indications.

FDA-approved indications are based on data supplied by the manufacturer demonstrating that adequate and well-controlled trials support these uses and that the drug is documented to be safe and effective at the time it is marketed. Only FDA-approved indications will be found in references such as the *Physicians' Desk Reference (PDR)*.

The FDA does not approve or disapprove of how a drug is used by a physician once the drug is marketed. An unlabeled indication may or may not be appropriate or rational, depending on accepted medical practice and reports in the medical literature. The physician uses professional judgment in assessing the potential efficacy of a drug when it is used for an unlabeled indication.

Orphan Drugs In 1983, President Reagan signed the Orphan Drug Act. This act allowed for special grants and tax breaks to support research for products or indications that showed promise as treatments for rare diseases or for products that could not be patented.

The act defines a rare disease or condition as "any disease or condition which (a) affects less than 200,000 persons in the United States or (b) affects more than 200,000 persons in the United States and for which there is no reasonable expectation that the cost of developing and making available in the United States a drug for such disease or condition will be recovered from sales in the United States of such drug." "Orphan" products can include drugs, biologics, medical devices, foods for medical purposes, and veterinary products that are useful in treating rare diseases but lack commercial sponsors and thus are often unavailable to patients because of limited commercial interest.

Contraindications & Precautions

The nurse must determine the relative and absolute contraindications to administration of the drug and determine if any of these conditions are present in the patient's physical examination or health and illness history. If absolute contraindications are present, it is the nurse's responsibility to investigate further with the physician the advisability of administering the drug.

In addition to contraindications, precautions are listed for many drugs. Precautions alert the nurse to those physiological and psychological conditions that may predispose a patient to negative, undesirable drug effects. When such conditions exist in the patient, the nurse must carefully assess and evaluate the patient response to drug therapy.

Therapeutic and Adverse/Side Effects

In evaluating a new drug therapy the nurse must be aware of the potential side effects of the medication. The nurse is responsible for knowing normal laboratory data and discriminating between anticipated and potentially adverse effects. The importance of a thorough assessment as part of the nursing process is evident in this situation. The nurse must have a baseline evaluation of the patient's physical status to be able to recognize subtle changes in status.

Drug Usage for Pregnant Patients

The thorough assessment of a woman of childbearing age should include a question regarding the possibility that she is pregnant, especially before a new drug regimen is started. The nurse would be remiss not to ask questions about reproductive cycles during a physical examination and health history.

Most drug effects on the fetus occur in the first trimester, although drugs can affect the fetus throughout its development. The nurse is expected to have a working understanding of the classification system used to describe the effects of the drug on the fetus and to be able to translate that information to a patient. For the FDA-assigned classification system to identify pregnancy-associated risk with different drug therapies, see Appendix C.

TECHNIQUES OF DRUG ADMINISTRATION

In this chapter the various drug forms are described and the administration techniques appropriate to different routes are discussed.

DRUG FORMS

Drugs are manufactured in a variety of forms, each intended to be administered by a specific route. Knowledge of the various drug forms is essential to ensure that the correct route and proper administration techniques are used.

Oral drugs may be given as solids or liquids. Solid preparations include tablets, capsules, caplets, enteric coated tablets, sustained release tablets, troches, lozenges, pastilles, and buccal and sublingual tablets. Liquid preparations include solutions, elixirs, suspensions, syrups, and gargles. Most often, the medications that require reconstitution from a dry to a liquid form are administered parenterally.

Solids

Tablets A tablet is a compounded form in which the drug is mixed with a binding agent to hold the tablet together before administration. Disintegrating agents may be added to help break up the tablet in the gastrointestinal tract. If the dose is small, an inert agent may be used to form the drug into a size suitable for administration. Most tablets are designed to be swallowed whole. Some tablets are scored, allowing them to be cut into fractions. However, dose forms that deliver the correct quantity are preferable because cutting a tablet may lead to an imprecise dose. Chewable tablets are designed to be chewed before swallowing. Chewing enhances the uptake of the drug in the stomach.

Capsules A capsule is a modified tablet in which the medication in powder form is encased in a two-part gelatin capsule. In the stomach the gelatin breaks down, releasing the medication. The capsule may be pulled apart and the contents mixed with fluids for administration through enteral tubes.

Caplets Caplets are a relatively new form of medication preparation frequently found in over-the-counter (OTC) medications. They are compounded like tablets, with the addition of a solid gelatin coating. Caplets are marketed as easy to swallow and provide another form of tamper resistance for OTC preparations.

Buccal Medications Buccal medications are designed to be absorbed by the mucous membrane of the mouth. They are placed in the buccal pocket in the superior-posterior aspect of the internal cheek next to the molars. The medication must be allowed to dissolve completely before the patient drinks or eats.

Sublingual Medications Sublingual medications are tiny, concentrated tablets that dissolve quickly when placed under the tongue. They deliver drugs to the venous system quickly and efficiently. The patient must not chew or swallow the tablet, and it must dissolve completely.

Troches, Lozenges, and Pastilles Troches, lozenges, and pastilles are similar preparations designed to dissolve in the mouth. Generally they are used to distribute antiseptic, anesthetic, antibiotic, or antifungal medications to the mouth and posterior oropharynx.

Enteric Coating Some tablets are enteric coated. An enteric coating has a two-fold protective mechanism: it either allows the drug to pass through the acidic *pH* of the stomach or protects the stomach from the irritation.

Time Release Capsules Time release capsules deliver a drug dose over an extended time. The medication in the capsule is further enclosed in a smaller casing that dissolves slowly, releasing the drug in the body.

Sustained Release Medications Sustained release drugs have a prolonged action because of their slow release in the body. These drugs generally maintain a steady medication level in the bloodstream and enhance patient compliance with drug therapy by decreasing frequency of doses. The nurse must be especially careful to note that long-duration medications often have the same name as their shorter acting forms and are designated with abbreviations such as "SR" for sustained release or "XL" for extra long acting.

Liquids

Solutions Oral drugs may be dissolved in a liquid, usually water, which may be colored and flavored to enhance palatability. Drugs given in-travenously may be dissolved in a variety of liquids including normal saline, 5% dextrose, and lactated Ringer's solutions.

Elixirs Elixirs are clear liquid preparations of drugs that contain water, variable alcohol content, and glycerine or other sweetening agents.

Suspensions Drug particles or powders may be suspended in a liquid. These preparations must be shaken vigorously to distribute the drug particles evenly throughout the medium. Dose size can vary substantially depending on the degree of drug distribution in the liquid.

Syrups Some medications are based in a sugar syrup, often to disguise the taste of the drug.

Gargles Gargles are solutions of the medications used in troches and lozenges. They frequently are warmed to a tepid degree (49C [120F]) to prevent scalding of the oral mucosa. These preparations are designed to be gargled and expectorated.

Reconstitution of Dry Drug Forms

Some medications are supplied in a dry form to which liquid is added at the time of administration. Antibiotics and steroids are two examples of drugs that may be reconstituted from a dry to a liquid form. Most reconstituted medications are administered parenterally. Some medications given by the oral route also require reconstitution; an example is powdered Metamucil, a bulk-forming laxative. The parenteral medications to be reconstituted usually require a given volume of a specific diluent solution to equal a prescribed dose of milligrams per milliliter. The nurse must be careful to add the correct volume and correct diluent solution. Frequently the nurse must wait for the powdered drug to dissolve into solution. No particulate matter should be visible before administration.

ROUTES OF ADMINISTRATION

Routes of medication administration fall into three broad classifications: enteral, cutaneous, and parenteral. The most frequently used route is *enteral administration,* in which the drug enters the bloodstream through the gastrointestinal tract. Drugs given enterally are given by mouth (orally), by rectum, by nasogastric tube, or by tube placement in the stomach or jejunum. *Cutaneous administration* methods deliver the drug through a skin or modified skin surface and include topical (dermatologic); inhalation; eye, ear, and nose; and vaginal medications. *Parenteral administration* is commonly used to mean a modified vascular access, in which medication is diffused to the bloodstream following an intradermal, subcutaneous, or intramuscular injection, and intravenous administration, in which the medication is introduced directly into the bloodstream.

Enteral Administration

Oral Administration
Oral administration of drugs requires an alert, cooperative patient with an intact swallowing reflex. Ideally the head of the patient's bed should be elevated at least 30 degrees. Allowing the patient at least 120 ml (4 oz) of fluid (if not contraindicated) should ensure that the drug reaches the stomach. The nurse must stay with the patient during the swallow

ing of the drug to ensure complete administration and to prevent aspiration of drugs or liquids. On occasion the nurse may have to modify administration techniques to meet patient needs and preferences. For example, drugs can be crushed to be administered with applesauce or some other thickening agent. Time release, sustained release, and enteric coated medications are unsuitable for crushing, breaking, or chewing, since these actions defeat the purpose of the form. In general, liquid preparations should not be mixed and solid forms should not be dissolved in liquid forms before administration.

Rectal Administration
Drugs administered rectally are usually in a solid glycerine suppository form or in a liquid enema form. This route is limited to medications that do not irritate the delicate tissue of the rectum. Absorption of a drug by this route is altered by fecal content of the rectum, erratic blood flow to the tissue, and expulsion of the medication.

Administration is best achieved with the patient in a left lateral side-lying position. The nurse should always wear gloves to give rectal medications. The tapered end of the water-based lubricated suppository is placed one finger length into the rectum to pass the anal sphincter (Fig. 2-1). The patient should be in-

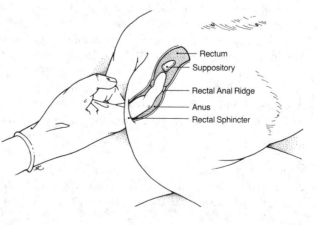

◆ **FIGURE 2–1** After donning a clean glove, insert rectal suppository beyond the anal-rectal ridge to ensure it is retained. (From Smith S and Duell D: Clinical Nursing Skills, ed 3. Norwalk, Conn: Appleton & Lange, 1992.)

Rectum
Suppository
Rectal Anal Ridge
Anus
Rectal Sphincter

structed to take deep breaths during the insertion of the suppository or enema to decrease sphincter tone. The patient should also be told to hold the drug for at least 30 minutes unless the drug given is a cathartic or laxative agent.

Enteral Tubes Administration of medication via nasogastric or percutaneous gastric tube requires vigilant nursing care. Patients should be positioned in Fowler's or semi-Fowler's position to protect the patient from reflux aspiration. Before each episode of medication administration the nurse should ascertain placement of the tube by either withdrawal of gastric contents or insufflation of 20 ml of air and auscultation of a "swoosh" sound over the gastric region. The nurse should be aware, however, that it may not be possible to reliably determine the placement of small-bore feeding tubes by any technique other than radiography.

Medications should be administered in solution form when available. Tablets must be crushed into a fine powder and made into a solution or suspension for administration. The nurse should flush the enteric tube of medication residue after administering the solution. If the medication is to remain in the stomach for full effect, positioning the patient on the left side may decrease passage into the duodenum. If the medication is to be absorbed in the gastrointestinal tract, positioning the patient on the right side may enhance the passage of the medication into the duodenum.

Small-bore tubes are narrow, small French feeding tubes that cause less irritation to the mucosa of the nares and oropharynx than the larger bore tubes more commonly used for decompression of the stomach. One difficulty of drug administration with a small-bore tube is that crushed medications easily become lodged in the inner lumen of the tube, occluding the lumen. Medications to be administered down a small-bore tube should be in liquid form. Drug administration with a small-bore feeding tube

requires vigilant nursing care to maintain the potency of the tube.

Cutaneous Administration

Topical Dermatologic, or topical, drug administration techniques include a variety of options. One of these is long-acting patches that release small quantities of medication such as scopolamine, nitroglycerin, and estrogen through the skin. Fever enhances the release and uptake of the drug and may necessitate removal of the patch. Sites of application can be rotated to minimize local skin reactions to the adhesives used on the patches. Ordinarily, hairy areas are avoided, since patch-to-skin contact will be compromised. Other dermatologic preparations include petroleum-based ointments, water-based creams, and powders. When applying dermatologic preparations the nurse must use gloves or tongue depressors to remove creams and ointments from their containers to avoid contaminating the storage vessel. Topical drugs should be applied in thin layers unless otherwise specified.

Inhalation Inhalation is the most difficult means of administration, especially for older patients and children. Many patients have difficulty coordinating their respiratory patterns for the use of inhalers, and the metered dose is lost to the atmosphere. In addition, several pieces of therapeutic equipment are involved in aerosolizing medications. The nurse is responsible for understanding and teaching appropriate techniques of inhalation therapy, as well as for evaluating the patient's ability to use the equipment and the patient's physiological response.

Eye, Ear, and Nose *Ophthalmic solutions* and ointments should be applied after all exudate has been cleared. The nurse or patient should wash hands before administering eye medications. For eye drop application the patient should gaze upward while the conjunctival sac is gently pulled out and the medication instilled into

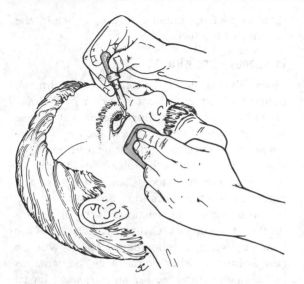

◆ **FIGURE 2–2**   Drop eye medication in the center of lower conjunctival sac. (From Smith S and Duell D: Clinical Nursing Skills, ed 3. Norwalk, Conn: Appleton & Lange, 1992.)

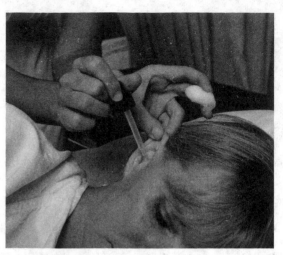

◆ **FIGURE 2–3**   Lift pinna upward and back to administer medication into ear canal. (From Smith S and Duell D: Clinical Nursing Skills, ed 3. Norwalk, Conn: Appleton & Lange, 1992.)

the sac (Fig. 2-2). Generally a 1 cm ribbon of ointment is applied to the lower conjunctival sac. Pressing on the lacrimal duct for 30–60 seconds decreases tearing and decreases systemic absorption of the drug. Ointments are applied in a thin ribbon along the inside margin of the conjunctiva. The patient should keep the eyes shut for 2 minutes to enhance absorption of the drug. Patients should be warned that their vision will be fuzzy for several minutes following the application of ointment.

Aural means pertaining to the ear. Medications given by the aural route should be warmed to body temperature to prevent activation of the vestibular system, possibly causing a sensation of dizziness. For administration to an adult, the external pinna should be pulled back and upward for instillation of ear drops (Fig. 2-3). For a child the pinna should be pulled down and out to help straighten the ear canal. The patient should lie on his or her side with the affected ear uppermost, so that the drug can reach the eardrum. If cotton balls are needed to keep the medication in the ear, they should be presoaked in the medication to avoid wicking the drug away from the eardrum. Gentle massage of the preauricular area may help the passage of the solution down the ear canal.

Nasal sprays and drops are administered to the nostrils and mucous membranes. The patient should blow his or her nose gently before administration. Ideally the patient should be positioned with the head reclined so that the medication can make contact with the tissue of the nasopharynx (Fig. 2-4). The dropper is never placed more than 1 cm (1/3 in) into the naris.

Vaginal Administration   Vaginal medications can be administered in douches, creams, or suppositories (Fig. 2-5). Douche fluids should be warmed prior to administration.

Parenteral Administration

Parenteral administration refers not only to administration beyond the gastrointestinal tract

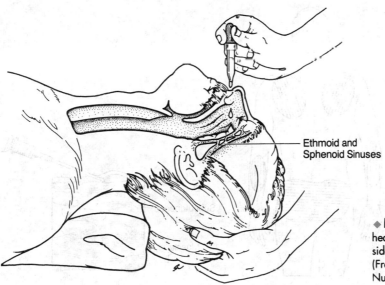

Ethmoid and
Sphenoid Sinuses

◆ **FIGURE 2–4**   Instruct patient to tilt head backwards and place dropper inside nares when instilling nose drops. (From Smith S and Duell D: Clinical Nursing Skills, ed 3. Norwalk, Conn: Appleton & Lange, 1992.)

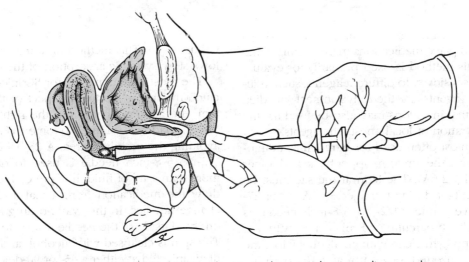

◆ **FIGURE 2–5**   Insert vaginal suppositories at least two inches using glove or applicator as shown. (From Smith S and Duell D: Clinical Nursing Skills, ed 3. Norwalk, Conn: Appleton & Lange, 1992.)

but also to administration via a needle into a body space. These methods include intradermal, subcutaneous, intramuscular, and intravenous administration. Intrathecal and epidural administrations are performed in hospitals but are not common means of drug administration. Intracardiac, intrasynovial, and intraarterial infusion and extracorporeal and isolated perfusion techniques are rarely performed methods of administration that are usually carried out by a physician and are not discussed in this text.

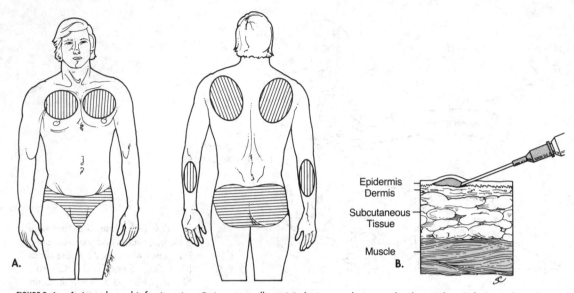

Epidermis
Dermis

Subcutaneous
Tissue

Muscle

A.
B.

◆ FIGURE 2–6   **A.** Intradermal infection sites. **B.** Insert needle at 15-degree angle just under the epidermis for intradermal injection. (From Smith S and Duell D: Clinical Nursing Skills, ed 3. Norwalk, Conn: Appleton & Lange, 1992.)

Intradermal   Intradermal administration of drugs is used to place medications in the dermis of the skin. This method is used primarily for evaluations of sensitivity to different agents, such as allergenic agents in the environment or diet. Intradermal injections may also be used for the administration of local anesthetic agents.

Sites most often used for intradermal administration are the forearm, upper back, and upper chest (Fig. 2-6A). The skin at the site must be stretched taut during the injection. A 26- or 27-gauge (very fine), 1/2- to 5/8-inch needle is used with a tuberculin or 1 ml syringe. After the area is sponged clean with an alcohol wipe, the needle is inserted, bevel up, at a 10- to 15-degree angle until the needle just enters the skin (Fig. 2-6B). Ordinarily, intradermal injections are limited to 0.5 ml or less. This amount should cause the formation of a small bleb. The needle should be withdrawn quickly, and the patient should be cautioned not to rub the site.

Subcutaneous   The subcutaneous (SC or SQ) method of drug administration deposits the medication in a pocket of vascular subcutaneous tissue. This method of administration allows slow systemic absorption of the drug.

The most common sites for SC injections include the lateral posterior aspect of the upper arm, the anterior thigh, and the right and left lower quadrants of the abdomen (Fig. 2-7A), avoiding the umbilical area. A 23- to 25-gauge, 1/2- to 5/8-inch needle is used to deliver no more than 1 ml of fluid. It is preferable to withdraw the medication from a vial and then to change needles. In this way no drug is present on the outside of the needle to irritate the skin. The skin is cleansed with alcohol, and the needle is injected at either a 45- or 90-degree angle (Fig. 2-7B), depending on the amount of subcutaneous tissue. A commonly used technique is to pinch 5 cm (2 in) of skin together in one of the selected sites and to inject the medication at a 45-degree angle into the pocket formed between the pinched-up tissue and the muscle mass below. When the needle is in the skin, the plunger is aspirated for blood. If no blood is present, the injection is deposited, but if blood

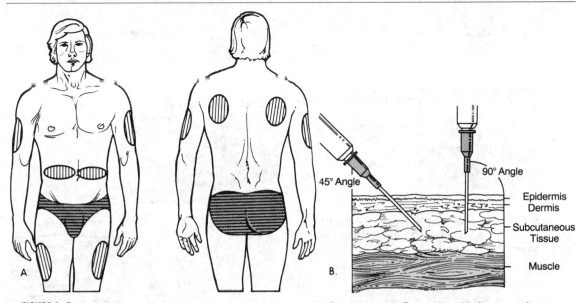

◆ **FIGURE 2–7** **A.** Rotate sites for subcutaneous injections given routinely. **B.** Insert needle at 45- or 90-degree angle into tissue for subcutaneous injection. (From Smith S and Duell D: Clinical Nursing Skills, ed 3. Norwalk, Conn: Appleton & Lange, 1992.)

is present, the needle should be withdrawn. The drugs most commonly administered by the SC route are insulin and heparin.

Intramuscular The intramuscular (IM) method of drug administration is used most commonly for immunizations and the administration of antibiotics and analgesic medications. The most common sites in adults are the deltoid muscle of the arm, anterior and lateral aspects of the thigh, and the dorsal and ventrogluteal sites, on the hip.

Within general guidelines the needle size used for an IM injection is at the nurse's discretion. The needle length must be proportionate to the size of the patient. For an average, 70 kg patient a 1 1/2-inch needle is used. Needle sizes range from a 1-inch needle for a child or a frail elderly person with a small muscle mass to a 2-inch needle for an obese patient. The gauge of the needle depends on the size of the patient and the viscosity of the medication to be administered. Average gauges for IM injections range from 20 to 22; a 19-gauge needle may be

used for thick solutions. An IM injection is suitable for a dose volume of up to 3 ml at one site. Beyond this volume the patient has increased pain at the injection site, and the drug is poorly absorbed.

As with an SC injection, after the dose is drawn up, the needle should be changed to prevent skin irritation. The nurse may also pull a small air bubble (0.2 to 0.3 ml) into the syringe; this helps to clear the needle of the medication once injected and to decrease the backflow of the drug along the needle track. The nurse should place the needle at a 90-degree angle to the skin (Fig. 2-8A) and use a dartlike action to embed the needle in the muscle tissue. Slow insertion of an IM needle is usually painful. Once the needle is in the muscle, the nurse must aspirate back on the plunger to be certain that the needle has not inadvertently been placed in a blood vessel. If blood is noted, the nurse should pull the needle out, prepare a new dose with new equipment, and select a new site for administration. When the needle is properly inserted, 1 to 2 cm (1/4 to 1/2 in) of

15

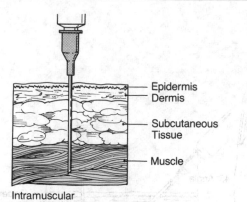

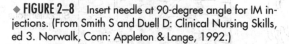

Epidermis
Dermis

Subcutaneous
Tissue

Muscle

Intramuscular

◆ **FIGURE 2–8** Insert needle at 90-degree angle for IM injections. (From Smith S and Duell D: Clinical Nursing Skills, ed 3. Norwalk, Conn: Appleton & Lange, 1992.)

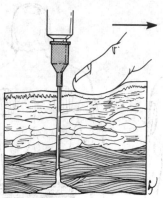

Z-Track Injection

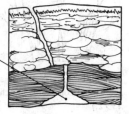

Medication

the needle should remain visible. In the rare event of the needle's snapping, there must be access to the needle for withdrawal using forceps.

Another technique for IM administration is called *Z track* (Fig. 2-9). This technique laterally displaces tissues by a small amount when the needle is "darted" into place. When the needle is quickly withdrawn, the tissue is released and it slides back into place, trapping the medication. This method is often used to administer analgesic agents, since it prevents seepage of the drug out along the needle track.

The muscle mass sites should be as relaxed as possible during the administration of an IM injection. The sites of IM administration are described in the following discussions.

◆ **FIGURE 2–9** Z-track is used to prevent seepage of drug out along needle track to skin. (From Smith S and Duell D: Clinical Nursing Skills, ed 3. Norwalk, Conn: Appleton & Lange, 1992.)

Arm (Deltoid) The deltoid is the large muscle mass of the upper arm (Fig. 2-10). The landmark for this site is the acromion process of the scapula on the posterior portion of the shoulder. It is helpful to imagine the deltoid muscle as shaped like an inverted teardrop. The injection site should be in the upper portion of the muscle. Measuring two to three fingerbreadths below the acromion process on the lateral mid-

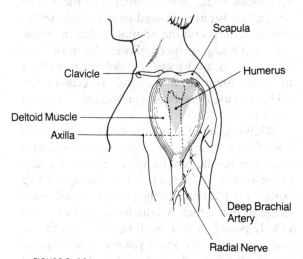

Scapula

Clavicle

Humerus

Deltoid Muscle

Axilla

Deep Brachial Artery

Radial Nerve

◆ **FIGURE 2–10** Administer IM or subcutaneous injection in deltoid area. Use shaded area as a guide for injection site. (From Smith S and Duell D: Clinical Nursing Skills, ed 3. Norwalk, Conn: Appleton & Lange, 1992.)

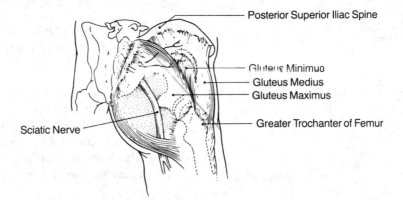

— Posterior Superior Iliac Spine

— Gluteus Minimus
— Gluteus Medius
— Gluteus Maximus

— Greater Trochanter of Femur

Sciatic Nerve —

◆ **FIGURE 2–11**   *Place injection above and outside diagonal line. (From Smith S and Duell D: Clinical Nursing Skills, ed 3. Norwalk, Conn: Appleton & Lange, 1992.)*

line of the arm gives the correct position for administration. When possible, the injection should be given in the nondominant arm.

Hip (Dorsogluteal)   The site for a dorsogluteal muscle injection is found by imagining a line from the posterior iliac spine and the greater trochanter (Fig. 2-11). The posterior iliac spine is palpated where the spine and pelvis meet and the sacral region begins. The medication should be administered above the imaginary line at the midpoint.

Hip (Ventrogluteal)   With the heel of the hand placed on the greater trochanter of the femur (Fig. 2-12) and the thumb directed toward the umbilicus, the position of the anterior-superior iliac spine is marked with the index finger. The middle finger is used to trace the curvature of the iliac crest. The area at the base of the space between the index and middle finger is the correct site for administration of a ventrogluteal injection.

Thigh (Vastus Lateralis and Rectus Femoris Muscles)   The vastus lateralis and rectus femoris muscles are defined in the adult by measuring a hand's width below the greater trochanter and above

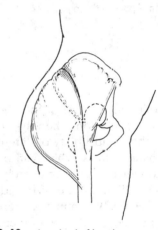

◆ **FIGURE 2–12**   *Place heel of hand over greater trocanter. (From Smith S and Duell D: Clinical Nursing Skills, ed 3. Norwalk, Conn: Appleton & Lange, 1992.)*

the knee (Fig. 2-13). The rectus femoris is the most anterior muscle mass, and the vastus lateralis is the most lateral leg muscle.

Intravenous   Intravenous (IV) administration is the most direct route of entry of a drug into the body. It can also be the most dangerous route. Because the drug does not undergo an extended absorption period, its effects are rapid.

17

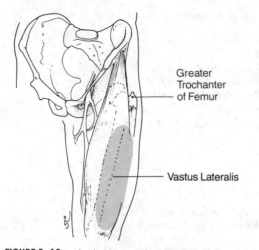

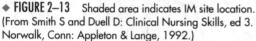

◆ FIGURE 2–13 Shaded area indicates IM site location. (From Smith S and Duell D: Clinical Nursing Skills, ed 3. Norwalk, Conn: Appleton & Lange, 1992.)

Since many drugs can erode and irritate vessel walls, the nurse must be attentive to solutions and dilutions of drugs and the recommended rates of infusion. The nurse must also be aware of the compatibility of different drugs and solutions and know which can be infused together and which require an entirely separate and dedicated IV line. The size and type of catheter chosen for IV administration reflect the anticipated durations and type of therapy to be administered. Generally the smaller bore catheters are less irritating to vessel walls. Institutional policies provide recommendations for the care of the IV catheter, specify the frequency of changing sites, and offer guidelines for drug administration via the IV route.

IV Push In an IV push (also referred to as direct IV) the medication is administered rapidly over several minutes. The dose given by direct IV is usually small. A rule of thumb is to administer no more than 1 mg/min, but the rate should always be checked for each drug being administered.

IV Intermittent In an intermittent IV administration (also referred to as IV piggyback) the medication is infused on a set schedule based on the physician order. At the completion of the infusion the nurse must flush the IV line to prevent backflow and clotting of blood in the catheter. In a piggyback administration the patient may receive a continuous infusion of fluid to which the piggyback medication is added, or a heparin lock may be used for access.

IV Continuous Medication may be infused at a constant rate in a set volume of fluid to maintain a therapeutic drug level.

IV Central The more central the access to the body core, as in the subclavian or internal and external jugular vessels, the greater the potential for life-threatening infection. These central lines are usually reserved for patients who have limited venous access and may be critically ill.

IV Peripheral The most common access sites for the IV route are the veins of the hands and forearms. The vein is accessed either by inserting a needle directly into the vessel or by slipping a plastic catheter over a needlelike guide wire. The introduction of a catheter into a vessel can cause irritation and inflammation. The nurse must carefully assess the integrity of the dressing covering the IV access and monitor the site for the symptoms of phlebitis, such as soreness to light touch, swelling, and redness. Many institutions do not permit the use of lower extremity veins because of the risk of thrombophlebitis with subsequent clot development at the site and further risk of pulmonary embolism.

Insertion of IV Catheter General guidelines for insertion of the IV catheter include wrapping a tourniquet above the anticipated entry site to get the vessel to swell. Skin preparation is completed to cleanse the skin of microorganisms before the IV puncture. The nurse must stabilize the blood vessel before advancing the needle through the skin and into the vessel. Once the vein has been penetrated, the IV access needle or catheter must be flushed to prevent clotting of blood if it is not connected to a continuous IV infusion. Follow institutional policy for the appropriate flushing solution (either heparin or saline or a combination thereof). It is imperative that the IV line be secured to the skin using some type of an occlusive dressing, according to institutional protocol.

3

ASSESSMENT & DRUG EFFECTS

PATIENT ASSESSMENT

Health care providers use psychosocial and biophysical parameters to assess a patient's need for and response to drug therapy. Among the most important biophysical parameters are the following.

Cardiovascular Status   Cardiovascular status is assessed through evaluation of blood pressure; cardiac rate and rhythm; presence or absence of chest pain; presence and strength of the peripheral pulses; color, temperature, and turgor of the skin; and presence of edema. Laboratory work may include cardiac enzymes, digitalis level, electrolytes, serum concentrations of cardiac-related drugs, and complete blood count.

Respiratory Status   Evaluation of respiratory rate, rhythm, and effort; lung sounds, especially listening for the presence and location of adventitious sounds; dyspnea; need for supplemental oxygen; use of accessory muscles; cyanosis; clubbing; cough; sputum production; and smoking history constitute the respiratory assessment. Laboratory work may include arterial blood gases or pulse oximeter values.

Renal Status   Presence of flank pain, adequacy of urine output (30 ml/h), color and clarity of urine, and specific gravity of urine are assessed. Renal function can be compromised by inadequate cardiac function. Laboratory work includes blood urea nitrogen (BUN) and creatinine levels, specific gravity, culture and sensitivity testing, measurement of protein and electrolytes.

Central Nervous System Status   Assessment of the CNS includes level of cognitive functioning in comparison to baseline level of alertness and orientation, often assessed via the Glasgow Coma Scale; intactness of the cranial nerves; and motion and sensation in the extremities. The CNS is influenced by both cardiac and respiratory status, and conversely both systems are affected by the CNS. Laboratory work may include blood levels of glucose, metabolic toxins, oxygen, and carbon dioxide; and an analysis of the cerebrospinal fluid (CSF) and culture and sensitivity testing of the CSF.

Laboratory Studies   Measurement of electrolytes, BUN, creatinine, and glucose can be specific to an organ system or can be used to interpret overall fluid and electrolyte status. Another common laboratory study is the complete blood count (CBC), which includes a hematocrit (count of red blood cells) and a white blood cell count (WBC) (a measure of the body's response to infection). Laboratory values are usually evaluated over a period of time to see trends. Each laboratory value must be considered in the context of what could be anticipated for the patient in view of his or her clinical picture, the physical assessment, and drug therapies.

ASSESSMENT OF THERAPEUTIC DRUG EFFECTS

Therapeutic effects are the signs indicating that a drug is doing what is anticipated or expected. During drug therapy the patient must be monitored for these effects. The patient must also be taught what to expect as an adequate therapeutic response.

ASSESSMENT OF ADVERSE/SIDE EFFECTS

Common side effects are physiological responses to a drug that may be part of the drug's action in the body but that are unwanted by the patient. Such effects can be anticipated with many medications. It is difficult to design a drug that has a single physiological application. Unwanted effects of drug therapy tend to be annoying, mild to moderately unpleasant, and dose related. These effects commonly include GI distress (nausea, constipation, diarrhea), mild skin irritations, or a slightly more profound effect of the drug than anticipated for the dose.

There are also clinical situations in which a drug is administered because of one of the anticipated side effects. Narcotics have the side effect, usually unwanted, of slowing GI motility and causing constipation. Therefore a narcotic may be given to slow peristalsis. Patients who experience anaphylaxis or a severe reaction to a drug within minutes of its administration must be treated quickly with removal of the drug from the body, administration of an antidote, if one is available, and physiological support through the crisis period. Other adverse effects are more insidious. Among those that should be

observed for are hypersensitivity, cardiotoxicity, respiratory depression, nephrotoxicity, CNS stimulation or depression, fluid and electrolyte imbalance, and endocrine dysfunction.

Drug Hypersensitivity   A drug hypersensitivity occurs when a patient has an allergic or exaggerated response to a medication. An allergic response may be manifested by pruritus, urticaria, rash, or potentially fatal anaphylaxis. With an exaggerated response the pharmacological effect is amplified at a normal dose range. This sensitivity may be managed by decreasing the dose of the drug. A clinical example of this type of hypersensitivity reaction is the profound hypotension resulting from the application of 1 cm (1/2 in) of topical nitroglycerin for chest pain management in the hospital. The nurse is legally responsible for evaluating the patient's response to every medication. When a patient has a hypersensitivity reaction, the medication should be withheld pending notification of the physician.

Cardiotoxicity   Cardiotoxicity, a deleterious effect on the heart's functioning as a result of drug therapy, is commonly manifested by alterations in the conduction system through the heart. Some cardiotoxic drugs damage cardiac tissue rather than influencing the conduction system, but the mechanism by which this injury occurs is poorly understood and is the subject of intense research.

Respiratory Depression   Opioid analgesic agents are the most common cause of respiratory depression in all age groups. The respiratory depression is mediated through the effect of the drug on the brainstem respiratory mechanism and is dose related. A degree of respiratory depression can be overcome by the use of various sensory stimuli. Opiates slow the respiratory rate, leading to hypoventilation and a relative rise in alveolar carbon dioxide. This increase in carbon dioxide may be well tolerated in a patient with no underlying disease but can have devastating effects on a patient with increased intracranial pressure (ICP), chronic obstructive pulmonary disease (COPD), or asthma.

Nephrotoxicity Nephrotoxicity is a potential problem with several classes of drugs including aminoglycosides, antineoplastics, and immunosuppressants.

Nephrotoxicity can decrease renal function, thus decreasing drug excretion. Decreased drug excretion will result in accumulation of a drug in the body with other possible toxic effects. Signs and symptoms suggestive of nephrotoxicity are hematuria, oliguria, and rising BUN and creatinine values.

CNS Depression and Excitation The CNS can be affected by a number of drug classes and physiological conditions. The most common adverse effects are excessive depression with sedation or, conversely, excessive stimulation and agitation. Of importance is the fact that drugs that have CNS depressant effects in adults may cause CNS excitation in children and elderly patients.

Fluid and Electrolyte Imbalances Clinical manifestations of fluid and electrolyte imbalances are most often seen in patients receiving diuretic therapy. It is important to know whether the diuretic is a potassium-sparing or potassium-wasting type. Patients need to be educated about the importance of potassium replacement to prevent hyperkalemia or hypokalemia and consequent life-threatening arrhythmias. In addition, patients must be advised not to replace large urinary losses primarily with free water.

Endocrine Dysfunction Long-term, high-dose adrenal corticosteroid therapy suppresses the patient's production of adrenal steroids. To discontinue corticosteroid therapy the dose of the drug must be gradually tapered to allow the hypothalamus, pituitary gland, and adrenal system

(HPA axis) time to begin producing these steroids. While on long-term, high-dose therapy the patient is at risk for a variety of nontherapeutic effects, such as hyperglycemia, fat deposition in the trunk and face, muscle wasting in the extremities, peptic ulcers, pancreatitis, severe mood changes, osteoporosis, and an increased susceptibility to infection.

CLINICAL CONDITIONS ASSOCIATED WITH DRUG THERAPY

When assessing patients the nurse should always attempt to correlate assessment findings with the patient's health status and therapeutic medication regimen. Critical to this process is an understanding of the significance of various signs and symptoms and knowledge of the clinical conditions these might represent.

In some cases, observed signs and symptoms are manifestations of anticipated side effects of medications. In other cases the observed findings indicate therapeutic failure or development of serious adverse effects of medication.

Throughout this book reference is made to a wide variety of clinical conditions associated with medication therapy. Each of these conditions is characterized by observable signs and symptoms. To assist the nurse in arriving at a judgment regarding observed findings, an extensive glossary of clinical conditions and associated signs and symptoms is provided at the end of this chapter.

VARIABLES AFFECTING DRUG ACTION

The nurse must consider variables that affect the fate of drugs once they enter the body. Each patient has characteristics that can potentially alter the effects of a drug in his or her body. The consideration of which drugs will have an altered course is especially important when patients take several potent drugs concurrently for extended periods.

Route & Dosage

The method of administration of the drug alters its rate of absorption and subsequent availability within the body tissues. The most common routes of administration are oral, IM, SC, and IV. These methods of administration produce different degrees of drug availability in the body and have vastly different rates of drug distribution and onset of action.

Oral Administration The most common route for administration of drugs is the oral route. Despite the ease of administration and relative cost savings of this method, it is affected by the greatest number of variables. Drug absorption may be influenced by gastric and intestinal pH, motility of the stomach and small intestine, blood supply to the stomach, presence or absence of food, and lipid or water solubility of the drug.

Other factors that alter the availability are binding agents, which hold pills or capsules together, and disintegrators, which absorb fluids in the stomach to break the medication apart. The formulation of the medication can vary among manufacturers, altering the availability of the medication as it enters the bloodstream.

IM and SC Administration Drugs administered by intramuscular (IM) or subcutaneous (SC) injection, commonly referred to as parenteral administration, enter the bloodstream by diffusion. Absorption into the bloodstream depends on the relative speed of blood flow through the tissue. The rate is slow for SC injections and moderate for IM injections. Absorption from both IM and SC injections can be accelerated by applying heat or massage to increase blood flow to the area. Conversely, absorption may be impaired by the application of ice or the concomitant injection of epinephrine, both of which constrict blood vessels and slow uptake into the blood. Conversely a method of prolonging the effect of an IM injection is to place the drug in a depot solution that is absorbed slowly.

IV Administration The intravenous (IV) route delivers the drug directly to the bloodstream, ensuring prompt onset of action. This route allows the most complete absorption and the most rapid onset of action. Potential difficulties with IV administration are toxic effects of the drug because of a high degree of absorption and thrombophlebitis, or irritation to the vein, at the site of administration.

Dosage Dose of the drug also affects its action within the body. Generally, the larger the dose, the greater the action within the body, up to a level that will produce adverse effects. Most drugs can be administered in a range of therapeutic doses, depending on the characteristics of the patient receiving the drug.

Patient Characteristics

Age An understanding of how drug administration changes across the life span must incorporate an understanding of physiological variations at different ages, as well as developmental aspects that alter responses to drugs.

Pediatric Considerations Pediatric patients generally include children under 12 years of age. Calculations of drug doses for children are based on age, weight, and subsequent determination of body surface area (BSA) using nomograms (see Appendix B). Most drugs approved for use in children have recommended single or daily doses (mg/kg/dose or mg/kg/d) based on milligrams per kilogram of body weight or square meters of BSA.

Adult Considerations From a pharmacological view-point, adulthood begins at age 12. In this text, "adult" dosages are meant for persons 12 years of age and older. Elderly adults (those over 65) normally have a decreased glomerular filtration rate, cardiac index, maximal breathing capacity, and hepatic blood flow. In addition, the body develops a higher percentage of fat and a lower percentage of total body water. These physiological changes mean that a greater proportion of lipid-soluble drugs may accumulate in the body fat, a higher plasma concentration of water-soluble drugs may be noted as total body water decreases, and drug metabolism by the liver and excretion by the kidney may be diminished.

Body Weight Total body weight and the normal proportions of body water, lean body mass, and body fat, which are estimated according to age and sex, are the basis for most drug doses. Patients who have experienced profound weight loss and are significantly below their ideal body weight may require alterations of their total drug dose.

A patient who is obese may have altered blood flow through adipose tissue and the skin, which impairs the absorption and distribution of medications delivered by IM, SC, or topical routes. Lipid-bound drugs can build up to toxic concentrations in the adipose tissue, and the patient must be monitored closely for effects of such medications.

Pathologic Conditions Preexisting pathologic conditions often necessitate changes in medication therapies to accommodate the underlying disease. Liver and kidney dysfunction are two disorders that commonly require medication alteration because they prolong drug action and thus increase potential for toxicity. The extent or severity of disease should be the primary determinant of the drug dose. The nurse must watch closely for the earliest signs of adverse drug effects in patients with an underlying renal or hepatic disorder. Timely reporting of these effects will assist the physician in altering drug doses appropriately.

Drug Interactions

The concurrent administration of other drugs, foods, and alcohol can alter drug action. The more drugs administered, the higher the likelihood of interaction. The mechanisms of interaction may alter absorption, distribution, metabolism, or excretion of the drug. Because of the potential for interaction, the nurse must understand the mechanism of action of each drug being administered. Many drugs have specific properties that lead to drug interactions, such as being highly plasma bound, inducing or inhibiting hepatic enzyme production, and altering GI absorption or motility.

Whether the interaction of one drug with another or the interaction of food with a drug will cause an adverse reaction depends on (1) the presence of factors (for example, disease, impaired organ function, drug dose) that predispose the patient to adverse effects and (2) the nurse's awareness of the need for appropriate monitoring and prevention. Some of the common drug-drug and drug-food interactions are described in the following discussions.

Drug Interactions The following classes of drugs are frequently involved in drug interactions because of one or more of their properties:

- *Antacids:* adsorb other drugs; increase gastric pH and emptying times and slow delivery of drugs to the absorptive sites in the duodenum; alter urinary pH
- *Anticoagulants:* bind to plasma proteins, thus displacing other drugs into the plasma and increasing their concentration.
- *Barbiturates:* increase production of hepatic drug-metabolizing enzymes; potentiate other central nervous system (CNS) depressants
- *Monoamine Oxidase (MAO) Inhibitors:* store norepinephine, so that displacement of these stores by other drugs may cause hypertensive episode; have an intrinsic hypoglycemic effect
- *Nonsteroidal Antiinflammatory Drugs (NSAIDs):* prostaglandin inhibition may alter renal function; inhibit platelet function, which may increase likelihood of bleeding.

- *Potassium-wasting Diuretics:* alter renal excretion of potassium and other substances excreted by the kidneys
- *Salicylates:* interfere with renal excretion of drugs; alter urine pH; may displace other drugs from plasma binding sites; in large doses have an intrinsic hypoglycemic effect

Drug-Food Interactions Drug interactions with foods are varied and can increase or decrease drug absorption and inhibit the mechanism of action of the drug. Further, some drugs stimulate or depress the appetite or alter taste sensation or uptake of glucose, minerals, vitamins, and electrolytes.

Some classes of drugs that depress appetite are amphetamines, some antibiotics, carbonic anhydrase inhibitors, and cardiac glycosides (digitalis) preparations. Appetite stimulants include antidepressants, major and minor tranquilizers, steroid hormones, and tetrahydrocannabinol (THC, or marijuana). Drugs that alter taste sensation include numerous chemotherapeutic agents, antibiotics, phenytoin, and chlorphenir-amine maleate, a common ingredient in over-the-counter cold and allergy products.

Foods may be contraindicated, relatively contraindicated, or actually encouraged with some medications. Many drugs have guidelines for administration that include food-specific interactions, and it is the nurse's responsibility to apply those guidelines during the administration of medications.

GLOSSARY OF CLINICAL CONDITIONS AND ASSOCIATED SIGNS AND SYMPTOMS

acute dystonia an extrapyramidal symptom manifested by abnormal posturing, grimacing, spastic torticollis (neck torsion), and oculogyric (eyeball movement) crisis.

agranulocytosis a sudden drop in leukocyte count; often followed by a severe infection manifested by high fever, chills, prostration, and ulcerations of mucous membrane such as in the mouth, rectum, or vagina.

akathisia an extrapyramidal symptom manifested by a compelling need to move or pace, without specific pattern, and an inability to be still.

anaphylactoid reaction an excessive allergic response manifested by wheezing, chills, generalized pruritic urticaria, diaphoresis, sense of uneasiness, agitation, flushing, palpitations, coughing, difficulty breathing, cardiovascular collapse.

anticholinergic actions inhibition of parasympathetic response manifested by dry mouth, decreased peristalsis, constipation, blurred vision, urinary retention.

blood dyscrasia a pathological condition manifested by fever, sore mouth or throat, unexplained fatigue, easy bruising or bleeding.

bradycardia slowing of the heart, which may result in light-headedness, syncope, fatigue.

cardiotoxicity impairment of cardiac function manifested by one or more of the following: hypotension, arrhythmias, precordial pain, dyspnea, electrocardiogram (ECG) abnormalities, cardiac dilation, congestive failure.

cholinergic response stimulation of the parasympathetic response manifested by lacrimation, diaphoresis, salivation, abdominal cramps, diarrhea, nausea, vomiting.

circulatory overload excessive vascular volume manifested by increased central venous pressure (CVP), elevated blood pressure, tachycardia, distended neck veins, peripheral edema, dyspnea, cough, pulmonary rales.

CNS stimulation excitement of the CNS manifested by hyperactivity, excitement, nervousness, insomnia, tachycardia.

CNS toxicity impairment of CNS function manifested by ataxia, tremor, incoordination, paresthesias, numbness, impairment of pain or touch sensation, drowsiness, confusion, headache, anxiety, tremors, behavior changes.

congestive heart failure (CHF) impaired pumping ability of the heart manifested by paroxysmal nocturnal dyspnea, cough, fatigue or dyspnea on exertion, tachycardia, peripheral or pulmonary edema, weight gain.

Cushing's syndrome fatty swellings in the interscapular area (buffalo hump) and in the facial area (moon face), distension of the abdomen, ecchymoses following even minor trauma, impotence, amenorrhea, high blood pressure, general weakness, loss of muscle mass, osteoporosis, psychosis.

dehydration decreased intracellular or extracellular fluid manifested by elevated temperature, dry skin and mucous membranes, decrease tissue turgor, sunken eyes, furrowed tongue, low blood pressure, diminished or irregular pulse, muscle or ab-dominal cramps, thick secretions, hard feces and impaction, scant urinary output, urine specific gravity above 1.030, elevated hemoglobin.

disulfiram-type reaction an Antabuse-type reaction manifested by facial flushing, pounding headache, sweating, slurred speech, abdominal cramps, nausea, vomiting, tachycardia, fever, palpitations, drop in blood pressure, dyspnea, sense of chest constriction; symptoms may last up to 24 hours.

heat stroke a life-threatening condition manifested by absence of sweating; red, dry, hot skin; dilated pupils; dyspnea; full bounding pulse; temperature above 40C (105F); mental confusion.

hepatic toxicity impairment of liver function manifested by jaundice, dark urine, pruritus, light colored stools, eosinophilia, itchy skin or rash; per-sistently high elevations of alanine amino-transferase (ALT) and aspartate aminotransferase (AST).

hyperammonemia elevated level of ammonia or ammonium in the blood manifested by lethargy, decreased appetite, vomiting, asterixis (flapping tremor), weak pulse, irritability, decreased responsiveness, seizures.

hypercalcemia elevated serum calcium manifested by deep bone and flank pain, renal calculi, anorexia, nausea, vomiting, thirst, constipation, muscle hypotonicity, pathologic fracture, bradycardia, lethargy, psychosis.

hyperglycemia elevated blood glucose manifested by flushed, dry skin; low blood pressure and elevated pulse; tachypnea, Kussmaul's respirations; polyuria, polydipsia; polyphagia; lethargy and drowsiness.

hyperkalemia excessive potassium in blood, which may produce life-threatening cardiac arrhythmias, including bradycardia and heart block, unusual fatigue, weakness or heaviness of limbs, general muscle weakness, muscle cramps, paresthesias, flaccid paralysis of extremities, shortness of breath, nervousness, confusion, diarrhea, GI distress.

hypermagnesemia excessive magnesium in blood, which may produce cathartic effect, profound thirst, flushing, sedation, confusion, depressed deep tendon reflexes (DTRs), muscle weakness, hypotension, depressed respirations.

hypernatremia excessive sodium in blood, which may produce confusion, neuromuscular excitability, muscle weakness, seizures, thirst, dry and flushed skin, dry mucous membranes, pyrexia, agitation, oliguria or anuria.

hypersensitivity reactions excessive and abnormal sensitivity to given agent manifested by urticaria, pruritus, wheezing, edema, redness, anaphylaxis.

hyperthyroidism excessive secretion of the thyroid glands, which increases basal metabolic rate, resulting in warm, flushed, moist skin; tachycardia, exophthalmos, infrequent lid blinking, lid edema, weight loss in spite of increased appetite, frequent urination, menstrual irregularity, breathlessness, hypoventilation, congestive heart failure, excessive sweating.

hyperuricemia excessive uric acid in blood, resulting in pain in flank, stomach, or joints, and changes in intake and output ratio and pattern.

hypocalcemia abnormally low blood calcium, which may result in depression, psychosis, hyper-reflexia, diarrhea, cardiac arrhythmias, hypotension, muscle spasms, paresthesias of feet, fingers, tongue, positive Chvostek's sign; severe deficiency (tetany): carpopedal spasms, spasms of face muscle, laryngospasm, generalized convulsions.

hypoglycemia abnormally low glucose level in the blood, which may result in acute fatigue, restlessness, malaise, marked irritability and weakness, cold sweats, excessive hunger, headache, dizziness, confusion, slurred speech, loss of consciousness, death.

hypokalemia abnormally low level of potassium in blood, which may result in malaise, fatigue, paresthesia, depressed reflexes, muscle weakness and cramps, rapid, irregular pulse, arrhythmias, hypotension, vomiting, paralytic ileus, mental confusion, depression, delayed thought process, abdominal distension, polyuria, shallow breathing and shortness of breath.

hypomagnesemia abnormally low level of magnesium in blood, resulting in nausea, vomiting, cardiac arrhythmias; neuromuscular symptoms: tetany, positive Chvostek's and Trousseau's signs, seizures, tremors, ataxia, vertigo, nystagmus, muscular fasciculations.

hypophosphatemia abnormally low level of phosphates in blood, resulting in muscle weakness, anorexia, malaise, absent deep tendon reflexes, bone pain, paresthesias, tremors, negative calcium balance, osteomalacia, osteoporosis.

hypothyroidism condition due to deficiency of thyroid hormone that lowers basal metabolic rate and may result in periorbital edema, lethargy, puffy hands and feet, cool, pale skin, vertigo, nocturnal cramps, decreased GI motility, constipation, hypotension, slow pulse, depressed muscular activity, enlarged thyroid gland.

hypoxia insufficient oxygenation in the blood manifested by dyspnea, tachypnea, headache, restlessness, cyanosis, tachycardia, dysrhythmias, confusion, decreased level of consciousness, euphoria or delirium.

jaundice excessive bilirubin in the blood manifested by yellow sclera or skin, dark urine, clay colored stools, pruritus.

leukopenia abnormal decrease in number of white blood cells, usually below 5000 per cubic millimeter, resulting in fever, chills, sore mouth or throat, unexplained fatigue.

metabolic acidosis a decrease in pH value of the extracellular fluid caused by either an increase in hydrogen ions or a decrease in bicarbonate ions. It may result in one or more of the following: lethargy, headache, weakness, abdominal pain, nausea, vomiting, dyspnea, hyperpnea progressing to Kussmaul breathing; dehydration, thirst, weakness, flushed face, full bounding pulse, progressive drowsiness, mental confusion, combativeness.

metabolic alkalosis an increase in the pH value of the extracellular fluid caused by either a loss of acid from the body (e.g., through vomiting) or an increased level of bicarbonate ion (e.g., through ingestion of sodium bicarbonate). It may result in muscle weakness, irritability, confusion, muscle twitching, slow and shallow respirations, convulsive seizures.

myopathy any disease or abnormal condition of striated muscles manifested by muscle weakness, myalgia, diaphoresis, fever, reddish brown urine (myoglobinuria), or oliguria.

nephrotoxicity an impairment of the nephrons of the kidney manifested by one or more of the following: oliguria, urinary frequency, hematuria, cloudy urine, rising BUN and serum creatinine, fever, graft tenderness or enlargement.

neuroleptic malignant syndrome (NMS) a potentially fatal complication associated with antipsychotic drugs manifested by hyperpyrexia, altered mental status, muscle rigidity, irregular pulse, fluctuating BP, diaphoresis, and tachycardia.

ototoxicity an impairment of the ear manifested by one or more of the following: headache, dizziness or vertigo, nausea, and vomiting with motion, ataxia, nystagmus.

paralytic ileus paralysis of the intestinal wall of the ileum manifested by one or more of the following: abdominal distension, constipation, absent bowel sounds usually associated with nausea, vomiting, and epigastric pain.

pseudomembranous enterocolitis life-threatening superinfection characterized by severe diarrhea and fever.

pseudoparkinsonism an extrapyramidal symptom manifested by slowing of volitional movement (akinesia), mask facies, rigidity and tremor at rest, especially upper extremities, pill rolling motion.

pulmonary edema excessive fluid in the lung tissue manifesting one or more of the following: shortness of breath, cyanosis, persistent productive cough (frothy sputum may be blood tinged), expiratory rales, restlessness, anxiety, increased heart rate, sense of chest pressure.

renal insufficiency reduced capacity of the kidney to perform its functions as manifested by one or more of the following: dysuria, oliguria, hematuria, swelling of lower legs and feet.

superinfection a new infection by an organism different from the initial infection being treated by antimicrobial therapy manifested by one or more of the following: black, hairy tongue; glossitis, stomatitis; anal itching; loose, foul-smelling stools; vaginal itching or discharge; sudden fever; cough.

tardive dyskinesia an extrapyramidal symptom manifested by involuntary rhythmic, bizarre movements of face, jaw, mouth, tongue, and sometimes extremities.

thrombophlebitis inflammation of a vein associated with thrombus formation manifested by one or more of the following: arm or leg pain, tenderness or swelling, warmth, Homan's sign, prominence of superficial veins.

urinary tract infection invasion of microorganisms into the urinary tract system as manifested by one or more of the following: fever, polyuria, urgency, frequency, flank pain.

vasovagal symptoms a transient vascular and neurogenic reaction marked by pallor, nausea, vomiting, bradycardia, and rapid fall in arterial blood pressure.

water intoxication (dilutional hyponatremia) less than normal concentration of sodium in the blood resulting from excess extracellular and intracellular fluid and producing one or more of the following: lethargy, confusion, headache, decreased skin turgor, tremors, convulsions, coma, anorexia, nausea, vomiting, diarrhea, sternal fingerprinting, weight gain, edema, full bounding pulse, jugular vein distension, rales, signs and symptoms of pulmonary edema.

PATIENT & FAMILY EDUCATION

Patient education has become one of the most challenging components of nursing care. Within the past 10 years the patient has become a more educated consumer of health care, and the volume of therapeutic drug therapies has dramatically expanded. Nurses in all settings find themselves in the role of teacher, explaining medication therapies and helping patients manage their own medication regimens.

Thorough assessment, creative planning, and teaching to meet the learning needs of patients on medication therapies are essential to achieve optimum results from drug therapy. This part of the nurse's role can be frustrating, but it may also be one of the most rewarding aspects of the nurse's professional responsibilities.

The nursing process provides an effective tool for successful patient education. The nursing process is a way of analyzing, organizing, and structuring time and resources to meet the patient's learning needs.

PRINCIPLES OF TEACHING

Assessment of Learning Needs

In the assessment phase the nurse must gather data about the learner to analyze that individual's learning needs. The information gathered helps determine the teaching plan. The nurse and patient must be able to agree on the desired outcome of the teaching session by writing or verbalizing a goal statement.

When the goal statement is stated in behavioral terms, the next step in the process, evaluation of the goal, is simplified. Such a goal statement or behavioral objective describes the changes in learner or patient behaviors by describing what the learner will know (cognitive), be able to do (psychomotor), and value or believe (affective).

Subsequent evaluation is directed toward determining how well the patient achieved the stated goal. When the patient is unable to fully achieve the goal as stated, the nurse again begins the assessment phase to determine what impeded the patient from reaching the goal.

When planning patient education about drug therapies, the nurse most often uses teaching strategies that focus on goals stated in terms of what the patient or learner will know (cognitive) about the drug or be able to do (psychomotor) with the drug.

Patient and Family Readiness

The nurse must be able to assess both the patient and the family for their readiness to learn. The learning process may be enhanced or impeded by a number of factors, including the patient's physiological and psychological status, timing of teaching, and environmental influences.

Physiological Status   Assessing the patient's physiological status may be as simple as checking physical abilities such as visual acuity to read the medication bottle or coordination and strength to open a child safety lid on a prescription bottle. Other physical conditions may impair or deplete the patient's energy level, for example, a debilitating illness, an instability of vital signs, or chronic pain.

Timing and Environmental Influences Time is often a limited resource. Nurses must be flexible and creative to make use of the limited time available for medication teaching. Teaching should begin at the administration of the first dose of a drug. Many institutions use a flowsheet to document the type and time of teaching so that the nurse can continue to follow the teaching plan. Organization of the content should reflect the critical components, including the most vital information for the patient to know about this medication at this time. The nurse can use positive feedback to reinforce the points that have already been learned. This enhances motivation and drug regimen compliance. Patient teaching should be completed without rushing the individual. Patients must be allowed to learn at their own pace. If the interaction with the nurse is cut short and the patient's understanding is limited, the teaching may have to be continued in another session or with a referral to another agency.

The ideal environment for learning has good lighting and ventilation, comfortable temperature and furniture, low noise levels, and a degree of privacy. The setting need not be complex or sophisticated but must be free of distractions.

Language used both in one-to-one teaching situations and in printed patient education materials must be at a level suitable for patient understanding and in a type size the patient can read. If the patient cannot read, an audiocassette of instructions may be made as an adjunct teaching tool. The language used should be simple and succinct, and any analogies should be completely clear. The nurse should build on previous knowledge by asking the patient to explain what he or she currently knows about medication Y, then offer to continue to the next step of understanding.

Maintaining attention and participation can be challenging. Teaching periods should be short and to the point. The nurse should watch for behavioral cues of waning participation, for example, a change in facial expression, altered eye contact, or barrier body language, such as arms folded and looking away.

Cultural Implications Culture should always be considered in planning the total nursing care of a patient. When preparing to teach a patient about medications and drug therapies, the nurse must consider the patient's cultural background and ethnicity. Cultural and ethnic awareness and sensitivity can help the nurse assist the patient to integrate previously learned health behaviors with new therapies. It is especially important to consider the patient's and family's definitions of health and illness and the impact of the current illness on his or her roles and responsibilities. When teaching patients about their medication, the nurse must take into account cultural beliefs and practices that could supplement and enhance the prescribed medication therapy. Many cultural groups have specific beliefs regarding nutrition and activity during illness, which should be explored. Common cultural concerns to be considered in health and illness include the patient's perception of pain, adaptation to chronic illness, a family's response to the birth of a child, and preparation for the death of an elder.

APPROPRIATE DRUG INFORMATION

The nurse is responsible for determining that the patient understands the purpose of the drug. After a teaching session the patient should be able to state the intended purpose of each drug in his or her own words.

How the patient and significant others are taught about the anticipated therapeutic response and expected side effects that should be reported to health care providers depends on the nurse's assessment of the patient's and family's cognitive abilities. This teaching should emphasize the wanted or anticipated effects of the therapy.

The patient should be able to identify the most important side effects of the medication. Again, the nurse is responsible for determining the most important and relevant side effects and for educating the patient to understand, recognize, and report those side effects. Part of this process is encouraging the patient to participate in follow-up visits with the health care providers.

Effects to Report

Along with teaching which side effects to recognize comes the issue of teaching which effects to report. The nurse must individualize this information based on a thorough assessment. Patients should be told to report any uncomfortable or unpleasant effect so that it can be evaluated and relieved if possible. They must also be taught to recognize signs and symptoms of threatening but perhaps not uncomfortable side effects of each drug they are taking.

Dosage and Administration Information

Correct dosing must be included in patient teaching. The nurse must be particularly aware of the individual's ability to calculate doses, especially when the dose is not available in a convenient form. Instructions should include convenient methods of measuring or tracking doses, such as standard measuring spoons for home use, diagrams of how many pills to take, or syringes or medicine cups taped at the appropriate level of the dose.

Compliance with route and times of administration can be difficult for patients. Multiple drug therapies with frequent doses are the most challenging for patients to comply with and nurses to teach. Patients rely on the nurse's understanding of various medications to help them plan a daily schedule. General guidelines for teaching include associating medication doses with routine daily events, such as awakening time, meals, and bedtime. It is the nurse's responsibility to assess the flexibility of the patient's schedule and the medication.

Considering the patient's normal routine, the nurse may suggest that the patient take the medication immediately before retiring and keep the morning dose at the bedside with fluid to take the drug on arising in the morning. Another technique for medication regimens is use of a check-off calendar for the day and time of medications. Some clients may require diagramed clock faces and other symbols to take medications on time. Small medicine containers are also available at minimal cost as a reminder system. Patients can be taught to stock these containers using a master plan for the day's medications.

Describing the route of the medication administration is a critical element of patient teaching. Nurses are often so familiar with medical abbreviations and the administration of medications that they overlook this step of patient teaching. The nurse should have the patient perform a return demonstration of the drug administration before completion of the teaching episode or before discharge from the health care setting.

When to Withhold a Drug

Unless the patient has reached a high level of cognitive understanding about the drug regimen or has been given specific instruction on when to withhold a dose, he or she should be advised to consult health care providers before changing the dose schedule. A patient who is taught when to withhold a drug should also be taught the ramifications of withholding doses and whom to notify.

5

PHARMACODYNAMICS

The biochemical and physiological effects of a drug and its mechanism of action at the cellular level are referred to as the *pharmacodynamic* effects of the drug. An understanding of the pharmacodynamics of a given drug or class of drugs helps the nurse anticipate patient response to a drug, both therapeutically and adversely, and predict potential drug interactions.

Most drugs interact at a specific site or receptor on the cell's outer membrane, thus altering that cell's normal function. A few drugs pass through the cell membrane and act directly on intracellular components.

Drugs that mimic at least some of the effects of an endogenous substance are referred to as *agonists*. Agonist drugs initiate or augment a physiologic reaction. Drugs that block a cellular receptor, preventing the binding and subsequent effect of an endogenous substance, are referred to as *antagonists*.

Drugs alter cellular function by a variety of mechanisms. The drug may bind to a receptor on the cell surface that controls a series of intracellular reactions, resulting in the final physiological effect. Epinephrine and similar adrenergic agonists can bind to a receptor site on the cardiac muscle cell surface that stimulates the enzyme adenyl cyclase to convert adenosine triphosphate (ATP) to cyclic adenosine mono-

phosphate (cAMP) within the cell. The cAMP then stimulates the intracellular proteins responsible for increasing the rate and force of myocardial contractility. Similarly, an adrenergic antagonist, such as propranolol, can attach to the same surface receptor and inhibit the stimulation of the enzyme, thus preventing the increase in heart rate and contractility.

Other drugs may attach to receptors on the cell surface that regulate cell membrane permeability to various substrates. For example, the contraction of cardiac muscle is dependent on the flow of calcium ions across the cell's membrane, which is regulated by specific calcium-dependent channels. The calcium channel antagonist verapamil inhibits the flow of ions through these channels, thereby decreasing the contractility of the cardiac muscle.

Some drugs do penetrate the cell's outer membrane and act directly on intracellular components. Most antineoplastic agents act intracellularly by directly disrupting the cell's ability to replicate. Alkylating agents, such as cyclophosphamide, cross-link cellular DNA, preventing the formation of RNA needed for cell division. Although these agents bind preferentially to rapidly dividing cells, they also inhibit the replication of normal healthy cells.

Pharmaceutical agonists and antagonists may

31

be extremely specific for a particular receptor site, or they may interact with a wide variety of sites. Epinephrine, for example, is an endogenous neurotransmitter secreted by the adrenal gland. It binds to a variety of receptors on smooth and cardiac muscle. By binding to and stimulating alpha-adrenergic receptors located on vascular smooth muscle, epinephrine causes vasoconstriction. Stimulation of $beta_1$-adrenergic receptors found on cardiac muscle causes increased heart rate and force of contraction. Stimulation of $beta_2$-adrenergic receptors located in the lungs and pancreas will cause bronchodilation and increased secretion of insulin respectively.

The administration of exogenous epinephrine (Adrenalin) will stimulate *all* three types of adrenergic receptors. However, there may be circumstances where it is desirable only to stimulate or inhibit one of the three types of adrenergic receptors. Drugs have been developed that preferentially stimulate or inhibit only one or two of these adrenergic receptors. Methoxamine is a selective alpha-adrenergic agonist that can cause vasoconstriction without causing tachycardia. Isoproterenol, a nonselective beta agonist, primarily stimulates the $beta_1$- and $beta_2$-adrenergic receptors, causing bronchodilation and increasing heart rate and cardiac contractility with little effect on vascular smooth muscle. A selective $beta_2$-adrenergic agonist, such as albuterol, will cause bronchodilation with minimal effect on heart rate.

The pharmacodynamic effects of a drug depend not only on the binding to a particular receptor site but also on the concentration of the drug at the receptor site. The relationship between drug concentration and magnitude of subsequent action is known as the *dose-response relationship*. It is this relationship that will determine the minimum effective dose of a drug and the maximum dose that does not cause unacceptable toxicity. The efficacy of a drug is dependent on delivering an amount of a drug to the receptor site adequate to compete with or displace an endogenous or exogenous substrate. The drug must be capable of physically reaching the site of action by passing through various physiological barriers (i.e., the gastrointestinal tract or blood-brain barrier). The drug also must bind a sufficient number of the receptors to alter the physiological response.

The amount of drug needed to produce a given response will vary widely, even among drugs in the same chemical and therapeutic class. The affinity of a drug for a receptor site is often referred to as its potency. More "potent" drugs have a greater affinity for the receptor site and thus require smaller doses to obtain the same physiological response as less potent agents. The more potent drugs will cause adverse effects at lower doses as well.

The dose-response relationship is often referred to as the *therapeutic range* of a drug. The therapeutic range describes those drug concentrations below which the desired effect will not be achieved and above which unacceptable toxicity will occur. Drugs with a wide therapeutic range, such as ampicillin, allow for a wide range of doses that may improve efficacy without increasing the risk of certain dose-dependent adverse reactions. On the other hand, drugs like digoxin have a very narrow therapeutic range between efficacy and toxicity. A certain amount of digoxin is needed to increase the contractility of the heart. However, only slightly more drug in the body will cause serious toxicity. Drugs with a narrow therapeutic range are often monitored and adjusted with the use of serum drug levels.

Just as endogenous hormones and neurotransmitters regulate a variety of physiological functions, drugs too rarely cause a single physiological response. The concentration of drug needed to stimulate the desired reaction at one site may be adequate at a different receptor site to cause an undesired response. Although the primary site of action of amitriptyline, a tricyclic antidepressant, is the CNS, it also inhibits the cholinergic response of the bladder to the need to void, resulting in urinary retention. Similarly, drugs designed to interact with only specific types of receptors may loose this specificity at higher concentrations. At low doses the selective beta$_1$-adrenergic antagonist atenolol blocks only the beta$_1$-adrenergic receptors on the heart with no effect on the beta$_2$ receptors of the lung. However, at the higher end of its dosing range, atenolol also blocks the beta$_2$ receptors, causing bronchoconstriction in susceptible individuals.

Pharmacodynamics describe how the drug works in the body. An understanding of the mechanisms of action and dose-response relationships assists the practitioner in selecting the appropriate drug and dose for a particular disease state. These same principles also assist in anticipating adverse drug reactions and drug interactions.

6

PHARMACOKINETICS

Pharmacokinetics is the study of the relationship between the dose of a drug and the drug's concentration in biologic fluids. It examines the absorption, distribution, metabolism, and elimination of drugs in the body.

ABSORPTION

The amount of a drug that reaches the intended site of action is dependent on the physical and chemical properties of the drug. These properties also will determine the potential route(s) of administration for that drug. The rate and extent of drug absorption from any administration site into the systemic circulation is referred to as the drug's *bioavailability*. Drugs administered by the intravenous (IV) route are 100% bioavailable; that is, all the administered drug reaches the systemic circulation. The entire amount of a drug administered by the oral or rectal route may or may not reach the systemic circulation intact. Bioavailability is expressed as a percentage of the administered dose that reaches the systemic circulation. A drug's onset of action and time to peak serum levels are reflected in its *rate* of absorption from the administration site. However, it is the *extent* of drug absorption from the site of administration that will affect the overall activity of the drug.

The rate and extent of oral drug absorption is affected by the chemical stability of a drug in the acidic environment of the stomach, its solubility at stomach and intestinal pH, and its transit time through the gastrointestinal (GI) tract. Theophylline, a bronchodilator, is completely absorbed from the GI tract. The same amount of drug will reach the systemic circulation whether administered orally or intravenously. On the other hand, less of an orally administered dose of penicillin will reach the systemic circulation compared to an equivalent IV dose because of its poor stability in stomach acid. Similar concerns regarding solubility and stability will affect drug absorption from intramuscular (IM), subcutaneous (SC), rectal, and other routes of administration.

The presence or absence of food in the stomach can affect the absorption of some orally administered drugs. Food stimulates acid secretion, which can increase the breakdown of acid-labile drugs. Food can alter the rate of absorption (i.e., time to maximal levels or effect) but not always the total extent, or amount, of drug absorbed. A delay in the time to onset or peak activity usually is not significant for drugs administered for chronic conditions (e.g., hypertension, rheumatoid arthritis). The delay may be relevant in acute situations such as

Food may decrease the extent of drug absorption by forming insoluble complexes with the drug. Dairy products form an insoluble complex with tetracycline, thus decreasing its absorption. Food also can increase the absorption of some drugs. A fatty meal enhances the absorption of the antifungal antibiotic griseofulvin.

The amount of an orally or rectally administered drug reaching the systemic circulation also can be affected by *first pass metabolism.* First pass metabolism refers to the hepatic or gut wall metabolism of a drug that occurs after absorption but before the drug reaches the systemic circulation. The mesenteric vasculature surrounding the GI tract flows directly to the liver. If the drug undergoes extensive hepatic metabolism, significant amounts of the drug can be inactivated on this "first pass" through the liver. Propranolol is an example of a drug with significant first pass metabolism. It takes 10–40 mg of propranolol orally to provide the same effects as 1 mg intravenously. Some drugs are specifically designed to be activated on this first pass through the liver. These drugs are called *prodrugs.* Enalapril, a prodrug, is metabolized to its active form, enalaprilat, in the liver. Although enalaprilat may be given IV, it is unstable administered orally. Therefore oral administration requires the use of a prodrug. Drugs administered parenterally (IV, IM, SC), topically, and sublingually avoid first pass metabolism by the liver.

An additional factor that affects absorption is the dosage form or formulation of the drug. Formulation (e.g., tablet, capsule, liquid) can affect the drug's dissolution and thus the rate and extent of absorption. Liquid formulations may be absorbed more quickly than solid dosage forms, since they do not need to dissolve first into an absorbable size. Digoxin, for example, is 100% absorbed IV, but only 70% of the oral tablet reaches the systemic circulation. The bioavailability of the elixir and liquid-filled capsules (Lanoxicaps) increases to 90% because of improved solubility and dissolution. This illustrates how the same dose of digoxin can produce different serum levels, depending on the dosage form and route of administration used.

Solid dosage forms can be formulated to dissolve rapidly or very slowly. Dosage forms specifically designed to release the drug over a prolonged period of time are called sustained, extended, or controlled release. The letters "SR," "CR," and "XL" or terms such as "Duratab" or "Extentab," associated with the brand name of a drug, usually designate a sustained release formulation. Most sustained release products should not be cut, crushed, or opened. This will destroy the sustained release properties of the formulation, leading to unexpected toxicity from a rapid bolus of the drug or shorter duration of action. There are a few sustained release products specifically designed to be split or opened. Certain theophylline sustained release tablets may be broken in half (but not crushed), or theophylline capsules may be opened and sprinkled on food. It is best to check with a pharmacist before altering any sustained release dosage form.

Drugs may also be given special coatings to protect them from the low pH of the stomach. These enteric coated products are designed to dissolve in the higher pH of the small intestine. Enteric coating may be used to protect acid-labile drugs, such as omeprazole, from being destroyed in the stomach or may be used to protect the stomach from extremely irritating drugs such as aspirin. As with sustained release formulations, enteric coated drugs should not be crushed or split.

Formulation can affect the absorption of parenterally administered drugs as well. Regular insulin, for example, is a very rapid acting insulin with a short duration of action. By suspending the insulin in other substances, the longer acting NPH and lente insulins are created. *Depot* formulations of parenteral products combine the active drug in different vehicles (peanut oil, propylene glycol) or with suspending agents to retard its absorption from the IM or SC injection site. These long acting suspensions and depot formulations should not be administered IV because of the risk of embolization.

DISTRIBUTION

Once the drug has reached the systemic circulation, it must be distributed to its ultimate site of action. It may have to pass from the intravascular space into various extravascular fluids and tissues. Electrochemical properties of the drug, molecular size, protein binding, and the presence of active transport systems will determine the extent of drug distribution to different tissues (liver, kidney, bone, breast milk) and across specialized barriers (blood-brain barrier, placenta, abscess wall). Some drugs may distribute extensively into a wide variety of tissues and are said to have a large volume of distribution. Other drugs may be limited to the intravascular space and have a relatively small volume of distribution.

The extent to which a drug is bound to plasma proteins, especially albumin, can significantly affect the distribution of the drug. Only nonbound drug is free to diffuse across tissue membranes to the site of action. Protein-bound drug is not pharmacologically active. Alterations in protein binding can have a major effect on the activity of highly protein bound drugs (>90% bound to plasma proteins). If two highly bound drugs are given together, they will compete for the finite number of protein-binding sites, resulting in increased levels of free active drug. Similarly, a decrease in the number of protein-binding sites (i.e., hypoalbuminemia) can result in increased levels of free active drug.

METABOLISM

Most drugs undergo some form of *biotransformation* or *metabolism* in the body. The goal of the biotransformation is to modify the drug so that it can be inactivated, eliminated, or trans-formed into a more active form. Many drugs need to be metabolized to an inactive form that is more easily excreted in the urine or bile. Some drugs may be metabolized to pharmacologically active or partially active metabolites. The antiarrhythmic drug procainamide is metabolized in the liver to *n*-acetyl procainamide (NAPA), which has significant antiarrhythmic activity.

The primary site of drug metabolism is the liver. Hepatic enzyme systems perform hundreds of reactions that may be classified as phase I (preparatory) reactions or phase II (conjugation) reactions. Phase I reactions allow the drug to be more easily processed by the phase II enzyme systems. Phase II reactions produce very polar compounds that can be excreted in the urine. Drugs may undergo one or both types of reactions.

The functioning of hepatic enzymes is affected by many factors. Age can have a significant influence on the liver's ability to metabolize drugs. Neonates cannot conjugate drugs efficiently because these enzyme systems have not fully matured. Therefore neonates are more susceptible to toxicity from drugs inactivated by phase II reactions (e.g., acetaminophen, chloramphenicol). Elderly patients have a decreased ability to perform phase I reactions. Their systems may have more difficulty inactivating drugs that rely on this type of metabolism such as benzodiazepines (diazepam) and phenothiazines (chlorpromazine). Social habits can affect hepatic enzyme systems. Alcohol and smoking can increase the metabolism of some drugs by increasing the metabolic activity of certain enzymes. Disease states such as cirrhosis and hepatitis and conditions that affect liver blood flow (e.g., congestive heart failure) can significantly alter drug metabolism. Even the drugs themselves can alter their own metabolism or the metabolism of concurrently administered drugs. Drugs such as rifampin that can increase the activity of hepatic enzymes are called *enzyme inducers*. Enzyme induction increases the rate of drug metabolism, resulting in lower serum drug levels and shorter duration of action. Drugs can also compete for or *inhibit* hepatic enzyme activity, resulting in increased serum drug levels and prolonged duration of action.

The liver is not the only site of drug metabolism. Catecholamines, such as norepinephrine or dopamine, are metabolized in the plasma and tissues by the enzymes catechol-o-methyl transferase (COMT) and monoamine oxidase (MAO). Other drugs may be metabolized by enzymes found primarily in the kidneys or lungs. Finally, some drugs are not metabolized at all and may be excreted totally intact. Most antibiotics are excreted by the kidneys unchanged. Knowing if, where, and how a drug is metabolized will help the clinician understand alterations in patient response to drugs and help predict certain drug interactions.

ELIMINATION

What goes into the body must eventually come out. Renal excretion is the primary route of elimination for most drugs. Drugs can be excreted renally by glomerular filtration or active secretion into the renal tubules. As with hepatic metabolism, competition for elimination pathways, resulting in prolonged drug activity, can occur in patients receiving multiple drugs. This is especially true of drugs eliminated by renal tubular secretion. Probenecid competes with penicillin and cephalosporin antibiotics for the same tubular secretion sites. This interaction is often used therapeutically to prolong the activity of the antibiotic.

Renal function declines as part of normal aging and can be adversely affected by a number of diseases and toxic substances (including drugs). It is important to have some assessment of a patient's renal function before initiating drug therapy. The usual recommended dosage ranges are based on patients with normal renal function. Lower doses are often needed in elderly patients or patients with varying degrees of renal insufficiency to avoid drug accumulation and toxicity. Serum creatinine is commonly used as an estimate of a patient's renal function. Creatinine is a breakdown product of muscle metabolism that is produced at a constant rate and is filtered through the glomerulus. Because muscle mass generally decreases with increasing age and is proportional to patient weight, renal function estimates need to consider patient age and weight along with serum creatinine. Elderly patients can have decreased renal function even though the measured serum creatinine is within normal limits. This is because of their decreased muscle mass and thus production of creatinine. The patient's creatinine clearance (Cl_{cr}) is a better estimate of renal function than serum creatinine alone. Creatinine clearance can be measured by a 24-hour urine collection or estimated using various equations and nomograms that factor in age and weight.

Other routes of elimination include the biliary tract, lungs, and sweat glands. The biliary tract may be the primary route of elimination for some drugs or may be a secondary route, especially if the primary route of elimination becomes impaired. Drugs excreted through the biliary tract may be deposited in the feces for elimination or may be reabsorbed in the intestines for further distribution or recycling. The reabsorption of drugs excreted into the GI tract is called *enterohepatic circulation*.

Drugs may be eliminated from the body by a single or multiple pathways. The sum of all routes of elimination is referred to as the *total body clearance*.

Half-life is another term used to describe drug elimination. It is the time required for the serum concentration of a drug to decrease by 50%. Half-life is useful in selecting an optimal dosing interval. Drugs dosed at intervals less than their half-life will accumulate in the body, often to toxic levels. Drugs with long half-lives may be able to be dosed once or twice a day. Half-life also can be used to predict when the drug will reach a constant serum level or be totally eliminated from the body.

The state of equilibrium between the amount of drug entering the body and the amount of drug being eliminated from the body is called *steady state*. The steady state concentration reflects the maximum accumulation of the drug and thus its pharmacological effect at a given dosage regimen. Serum concentrations of the drug will remain constant at this point unless the dose or dosing interval is changed. The time it takes for a drug to reach steady state is dependent on the drug's half-life. If a drug is dosed at intervals approximating its half-life, it will attain steady state concentrations after the fourth or fifth dose. For example, if a drug with a half-life of 5 hours is dosed every 6 hours, it will reach 87.5% of its steady state concentration (and maximum effect) after 3 doses and 95% of its steady state concentration after 5 doses or approximately 30 hours. Prior to steady state, the drug will continue to accumulate, resulting in progressively higher serum levels. Similarly, a drug with a half-life of 24 hours will not reach steady state or maximal effect for at least 5 days. Large initial doses or *loading doses* may be given for drugs with very long half-lives to shorten the time required to reach a steady state concentration. Digoxin is a drug with a half-life of approximately 1.5 days. Patients will often be loaded or "digitalized" with 1 mg of digoxin over 24 hours and then started on a maintenance dose of 0.125 mg or 0.25 mg every 24 hours. The loading dose will give the patient a therapeutic level within 24 to 48 hours rather than 1 to 2 weeks without the loading dose. Anytime the dose or dosing interval of a drug is changed, it will take approximately 5 half-lives on the new regimen to achieve the full effect of the change.

Conversely, the half-life of a drug can be used to estimate the amount of time necessary to completely eliminate the drug from the body. Since 50% of the remaining drug will be removed each half-life, an interval of 5 half-lives must lapse after the last dose is administered for more than 95% of the drug to be eliminated from the body.

An understanding of the pharmacokinetics of a drug helps the clinician anticipate the onset of action and maximum effect of the drug and the potential drug interactions. Knowledge of both the pharmacokinetics and pharmacodynamics of a drug assists the clinician in making appropriate dosage adjustments in patients in hope of avoiding potential adverse reactions.

CHAPTER

7

DOSAGE CALCULATIONS

To give the right dose of a medication, the nurse must be able to calculate drug dosages. This requires that the nurse be knowledgeable about common units of measurement and equivalents among systems. The commonly used systems of measurement are the metric system, the apothecary system, and the household system. The metric system is the system of measurement most frequently used. Commonly used equivalents within and among the three systems of measurement are shown in Appendix B.

It is important to remember that with the apothecary and household systems, several different equivalents can often be used to solve the same problem. Because of the lack of precision of these systems, different equivalents may yield somewhat different answers. These answers, while different, would all be considered correct.

A comprehensive presentation of dosage calculation using the method illustrated in this chapter, dimensional analysis, is presented in *A Unified Approach to Dosage Calculation* (1991) by B. A. Wilson and M. T. Shannon published by Appleton & Lange. The text teaches you this new problem-solving skill and how to apply it to all types of clinical calculations. With this clearly explained, consistent approach a nurse will be able to calculate dosages for all medications without having to memorize multiple formulas.

A UNIFIED APPROACH TO DOSAGE CALCULATION

The safest method of dosage calculation is a common sense method used in physical science called *dimensional analysis*. In dimensional analysis, like units are canceled from the numerator and the denominator of a ratio leaving the desired units of the answer. Dimensional analysis is used to solve the following basic problem for illustration:

Sample Problem   How many kilograms are in 4 pounds?

Question:	x kg = 4 lb
Conversion factor:	2.2 lb = 1 kg *or*
	$\dfrac{1 \text{ kg}}{2.2 \text{ lb}}$ *or* $\dfrac{2.2 \text{ lb}}{1 \text{ kg}}$
Solution:	x kg = 4 l̶b̶ $\times \dfrac{1 \text{ kg}}{2.2 \text{ l̶b̶}}$
Answer:	x kg = 1.82 kg

The same method of problem solving, dimensional analysis, will be used to solve the remaining examples in this chapter. This one method can be used to solve all types of dosage calculations involving tablets, liquids by mouth, injections, and intravenous medications.

CALCULATING DOSAGES OF NONPARENTERAL MEDICATIONS

Calculated doses for nonparenteral medications such as pills, capsules, and unscored tablets or suppositories should be rounded to the nearest whole number. Calculated doses of scored tablets should be rounded to the nearest half or quarter, depending on how the tablet is scored. With problems involving oral liquid medications it is generally accurate enough to round to one decimal place. Medications for infants and small children may require a greater degree of accuracy.

Example 1   How many tablets would you administer if the doctor ordered 2 mg of lorazepam? Available are 0.5 mg tablets.

Step 1   Convert the doctor's order in milligrams to the correct number of tablets for administration by stating the order as an equation in the following form:

$$x \text{ tab} = 2 \text{ mg}$$

Step 2   Identify the proper equivalents from the problem or a system of measurement needed to convert milligrams to tablets.

Needed equivalent: 1 tab = 0.5 mg

$$\frac{1 \text{ tab}}{0.5 \text{ mg}} \quad or \quad \frac{0.5 \text{ mg}}{1 \text{ tab}}$$

Step 3   Set up the equation so that the unwanted label (mg) is in both the numerator and denominator; the milligram label cancels out and leaves only the desired label (tab) on both sides of the equal sign.

$$x \text{ tab} = 2 \text{ m\!g} \times \frac{1 \text{ tab}}{0.5 \text{ m\!g}}$$

Step 4   Perform the mathematical calculations.

$$x \text{ tab} = 2 \times \frac{1 \text{ tab}}{0.5}$$

Answer: x tab = 4 tablets

Example 2   The order is to give 0.12 g of secobarbital by suppository. On hand are 1-grain suppositories. How many suppositories will you give?
Needed Equivalents: 1000 mg = 1 g; 60 mg = 1 grain; 1 supp = 1 grain

$$x \text{ supp} = 0.12 \text{ g\!/} \times \frac{1000 \text{ m\!g}}{1 \text{ g\!/}} \times \frac{1 \text{ grain}}{60 \text{ m\!g}} \times \frac{1 \text{ supp}}{1 \text{ grain}}$$

Answer: x supp = 1.8 supp
Therefore, give 2 suppositories.

CALCULATING DOSAGES OF PARENTERAL MEDICATIONS

Intramuscular Administration

Parenteral medications are defined as injected medications absorbed by a route other than the gastrointestinal tract. Parenteral medication routes include intradermal, subcutaneous, intramuscular, and intravenous. Parenteral medications are measured with syringes marked to the nearest tenth or hundredth of a cubic centimeter (cc), depending on which type of syringe is used. (Note that 1 cc equals 1 ml.) Consequently, for consistency the answers to these problems are expressed to the nearest hundredth decimal place.

Example 3   The order is to give carbenicillin IM 800 mg q6h. The vial states that the concentration of the medication is 1 g/2.5 cc. How many cubic centimeters should you give?
Needed equivalents: 1 g = 1000 mg; 2.5 cc = 1 g

$$x \text{ cc} = 800 \text{ mg} \times \frac{1 \text{ g\!/}}{1000 \text{ m\!g}} \times \frac{2.5 \text{ cc}}{1 \text{ g\!/}}$$

Answer: x cc = 2 cc
Therefore, give 2 cc.

Reconstitution of a Dry Powder

Medications that become unstable in solution over time are often manufactured as dry powders. An appropriate diluent, such as sterile water or normal saline, must be added to these medications prior to administration. The process of adding the diluent is referred to as reconstitution of the medication.

In the solving of problems with reconstituted medications, the amount of diluent is never used. Only the concentration resulting from the addition of the diluent is used.

Example 4   The order is to give 350 mg of oxacillin q4h IM. Directions for reconstitution of the 1 g vial state, "Add 5.7 ml of sterile water. Each 1.5 ml will then contain 250 mg of medication." How many milliliters will you give?
Needed equivalent: 1.5 ml = 250 mg

$$x \text{ ml} = 350 \text{ mg} \times \frac{1.5 \text{ ml}}{250 \text{ mg}}$$

Answer: x ml = 2.1 ml
Therefore, give 2.1 ml.

Intravenous Fluids

Intravenous (IV) infusion rates can be calculated in terms of the number of drops per minute (gtts/min) or the number of cubic centimeter per hour (cc/h) needed to administer the fluid ordered by the physician. When rates are calculated in drops per minute, it is necessary to know how many drops per cubic centimeter (drop factor) are delivered by the IV tubing. The drop factor varies with the manufacturer.

Example 5   The order is to infuse 1000 cc of Ringer's lactate solution over the next 8 h. Determine the rate in drops per minute using an infusion set with a drop factor of 15 gtts/cc.
Needed equivalents: 1000 cc = 8 h; 15 gtts = 1 cc; 1 h = 60 min

$$x \frac{\text{gtts}}{\text{min}} = \frac{1000 \text{ cc}}{8 \text{ h}} \times \frac{15 \text{ gtts}}{1 \text{ cc}} \times \frac{1 \text{ h}}{60 \text{ min}}$$

Answer:

$$x \frac{\text{gtts}}{\text{min}} = \frac{31.3 \text{ gtts}}{\text{min}}$$

The answer must be a whole number. Therefore

$$x \frac{\text{gtts}}{\text{min}} = \frac{31 \text{ gtts}}{\text{min}}$$

Therefore the rate is 31 gtts/min.

Answers for drops per minute and cubic centimeters per hour of an IV infusion are expressed as whole numbers, since decimal numbers are not clinically feasible.

Intravenous Medications

Intravenous medications may be given by continuous or intermittent infusion. The physician usually indicates the type and amount of medication to be given at specific intervals, relying on the nurse to follow the manufacturer's recommendations for dilution and rate of administration.

Intermittent Infusion of IV Medications   The manufacturer recommends a range of dilutions and a range of infusion times for intermittent infusion of IV medications (IV piggyback). The nurse selects both a dilution and infusion time appropriate to the patient's physical condition.

Example 6   The order is to give 6 million U of penicillin G q4h IV piggyback. The medication is to be dissolved in 150 cc of IV fluid, and the recommended infusion time is 1 1/2 h. Using a drop factor of 10 gtts/cc, determine the rate in drops per minute.
Needed equivalents: 150 cc = 1.5 h; 10 gtts = 1 cc; 1 h = 60 min

$$\frac{x \text{ gtts}}{\text{min}} = \frac{150 \text{ cc}}{1.5 \text{ h}} \times \frac{10 \text{ gtts}}{1 \text{ cc}} \times \frac{1 \text{ h}}{60 \text{ min}}$$

Answer:

$$\frac{x \text{ gtts}}{\text{min}} = \frac{16.7 \text{ gtts}}{\text{min}}$$

Therefore the rate is 17 gtts/min.

Continuous Infusion of IV Medications

Rates for medications administered continuously are calculated according to the manner in which the physician orders the medication. When the rate of infusion is ordered in terms such as milligrams per hour, micrograms per minute, or units per hour, the method of calculation used must include both the specified rate of infusion and the concentration of the medication in the IV solution.

Example 7 The order is to give heparin 1200 U/h. The concentration of the IV is 30,000 U of heparin per 1000 cc of solution. Using tubing with a drop factor of 60 gtts/cc, determine the rate in drops per minute and cubic centimeters per hour.

Step 1 Find drops per minute
Needed equivalents: 1200 U = 1 h; 1000 cc = 30,000 U; 1 h = 60 min; 60 gtts = 1 cc.

$$\frac{x \text{ gtts}}{\text{min}} = \frac{1200 \text{ U}}{1 \text{ h}} \times \frac{1000 \text{ cc}}{30,000 \text{ U}} \times \frac{60 \text{ gtts}}{1 \text{ cc}} \times \frac{1 \text{ h}}{60 \text{ min}}$$

Answer:

$$\frac{x \text{ gtts}}{\text{min}} = \frac{40 \text{ gtts}}{\text{min}}$$

Therefore the rate is 40 gtts/min.

Step 2 Find cubic centimeters per hour.
Needed equivalents: 1200 U = 1 h; 1000 cc = 30,000 U

$$\frac{x \text{ cc}}{\text{h}} = \frac{1200 \text{ U}}{1 \text{ h}} \times \frac{1000 \text{ cc}}{30,000 \text{ U}}$$

Answer:

$$\frac{x \text{ cc}}{\text{h}} = \frac{40 \text{ cc}}{\text{h}}$$

Therefore the rate is 40 cc/h.

Example 8 The physician has ordered a continuous infusion of theophylline at a rate of 25 mg/h. The concentration of theophylline is 500 mg/500 cc. Using a drop factor of 20 gtts/cc, determine the rate of the IV in drops per minute and cubic centimeters per hour.

Step 1 Find drops per minute
Needed equivalents: 500 cc = 500 mg; 20 gtts = 1 cc; 1 h = 60 min

$$\frac{x \text{ gtts}}{\text{min}} = \frac{25 \text{ mg}}{1 \text{ h}} \times \frac{500 \text{ cc}}{500 \text{ mg}} \times \frac{20 \text{ gtts}}{1 \text{ cc}} \times \frac{1 \text{ h}}{60 \text{ min}}$$

Answer:

$$\frac{x \text{ gtts}}{\text{min}} = \frac{8.3 \text{ gtts}}{\text{min}}$$

Therefore the rate is 8 gtts/min.

Step 2 Find cubic centimeters per hour
Needed equivalent: 500 cc = 500 mg

$$\frac{x \text{ cc}}{\text{h}} = \frac{25 \text{ mg}}{1 \text{ h}} \times \frac{500 \text{ cc}}{500 \text{ mg}}$$

Answer:

$$\frac{x \text{ cc}}{\text{h}} = \frac{25 \text{ cc}}{\text{h}}$$

Therefore the rate is 25 cc/h.

Calculation of Dosage Being Administered

Given the concentration of an IV solution and the cubic centimeters per hour being delivered, the nurse should know how to calculate the amount of medication the patient is receiving per minute or per hour.

Example 9 The order is to give heparin 25,000 U in 1000 cc of IV fluid at a rate of 40 cc/h. Determine how many units per hour the patient is receiving.
Needed equivalent: 25,000 U = 1000 cc

$$\frac{x \text{ U}}{h} = \frac{40 \text{ cc}}{h} \times \frac{25{,}000 \text{ U}}{1000 \text{ cc}}$$

Answer:

$$\frac{x \text{ U}}{h} = \frac{1000 \text{ U}}{h}$$

Therefore the patient is receiving 1000 U/h.

Example 10 The patient is to receive theophylline at a rate of 20 cc/h. The concentration of the medication is 500 mg/1000 cc of IV fluid. Determine how many milligrams per hour the patient is receiving.
Needed equivalent: 500 mg = 1000 cc

$$\frac{x \text{ mg}}{h} = \frac{20 \text{ cc}}{h} \times \frac{500 \text{ mg}}{1000 \text{ cc}}$$

Answer:

$$\frac{x \text{ mg}}{h} = \frac{10 \text{ mg}}{h}$$

Therefore the patient is receiving 10 mg/h.

Example 11 The order is oxytocin 5 U/500 cc of IV fluid at 66 cc/h. Determine how many milliunits per hour the patient is receiving.
Needed equivalents: 5 U = 500 cc; 1000 mU = 1 U; 1 h = 60 min

$$\frac{x \text{ mU}}{min} = \frac{66 \text{ cc}}{h} \times \frac{5 \text{ U}}{500 \text{ cc}} \times \frac{1000 \text{ mU}}{1 \text{ U}} \times \frac{1 \text{ h}}{60 \text{ min}}$$

Answer:

$$\frac{x \text{ mU}}{min} = \frac{11 \text{ mU}}{min}$$

Therefore the patient is receiving 11 mU/min.

CALCULATION OF DOSAGES BASED ON BODY SURFACE AREA

Child's Dosage

When a child's body surface area (BSA) in square meters is known or calculated using a nomogram (see Appendix B), a safe dose for the child may be determined from the adult dose using the following formula:

$$\text{Estimated child dose} = \text{Adult dose} \times \frac{\text{Child's BSA}}{1.73 \text{ m}^2}$$

Example 12 The usual adult dosage for cephalexin is 500 mg PO q6h. The elixir form contains 125 mg/5 cc. Determine the safe dose for a child whose body surface area is 0.36 m².

Estimated child dose:

$$x \text{ mg} = 500 \text{ mg} \times \frac{0.36 \text{ m}^2}{1.73 \text{ m}^2}$$

$$x \text{ mg} = 104 \text{ mg}$$

The volume of Keflex needed per dose:
Needed equivalent: 5 cc = 125 mg

$$x \text{ cc} = 104 \text{ mg} \times \frac{5 \text{ cc}}{125 \text{ mg}}$$

Answer:

$$x \text{ cc} = 4.16 \text{ cc}$$

Therefore, administer 4.16 cc.

Dosage of Chemotherapeutic Medications for Adults

When the BSA of an adult is known or determined by using a nomogram, the appropriate dosage of chemotherapeutic drugs can be determined.

Example 13 The order is to give 150 mg of procarbazine hydrochloride orally every day for 10 d to an adult. The adult's BSA is 1.10 m². The manufacturer's recommended dosage range PO is 50–200 mg/m²/d and not to exceed 300 mg/d. Determine the maximum and minimum recommended doses. Is the doctor's order within the safe range for this drug? Note: mg/m²/d is expressed as

$$\frac{mg}{m^2 \times d}$$

A. Minimum recommended daily dose

$$\frac{x \text{ mg}}{d} = 1.10 \text{ m}^2 \times \frac{50 \text{ mg}}{m^2 \times d}$$

Answer:

$$\frac{x \text{ mg}}{d} = 55 \text{ mg}$$

Therefore the minimum daily dose is 55 mg.

B. Maximum recommended daily dose

$$\frac{x \text{ mg}}{d} = 1.10 \text{ m}^2 \times \frac{200 \text{ mg}}{m^2 \times d}$$

Answer:

$$\frac{x \text{ mg}}{d} = 220 \text{ mg}$$

Therefore the maximum daily dose is 220 mg.

Conclusion: Consequently the doctor's order of 150 mg *does not* exceed the maximum recommended daily dose.

SECTION

II

PROTOTYPE DRUGS

ANTIGOUT AGENT

COLCHICINE
(kol´chi-seen)
Trade name: Novocolchine
Classifications: ANTIGOUT; ORPHAN DRUG
Pregnancy: Category C

ACTIONS/PHARMACODYNAMICS Alkaloid of the autumn crocus *Colchicum autumnale* with antimitotic and indirect antiinflammatory properties. Binds to microtubular protein, thereby arresting spindle formation in metaphase, and interfering with movement of mobile cells. Selective action in gouty arthritis believed to be related to inhibition of microtubule formation in leukocytes, thus interfering with their migration and phagocytosis in gouty joints. Lactic acid produced by phagocytosis is reduced, and crystal deposition fostered by acid pH is decreased. The net effect is inhibition of inflammation and reduction of pain and swelling. Colchicine is nonanalgesic and nonuricosuric. Direct action on bone marrow produces temporary leukopenia, later replaced by leukocytosis. Stimulates prostaglandin synthesis, which may be one of the reasons for GI side effects. Tends to increase fecal excretion of sodium, potassium, fat, nitrogen, and carotene and in large doses may reduce serum cholesterol and interfere with absorption of vitamin B_{12}. Tolerance to colchicine does not develop.

USES Prophylactically for recurrent gouty arthritis and for acute gout, either as single agent or in combination with a uricosuric such as probenecid, allopurinol, or sulfinpyrazone. **Unlabeled use:** sarcoid arthritis, chondrocalcinosis (pseudogout), arthritis associated with erythema nodosum, leukemia, adenocarcinoma, acute calcific tendonitis, familial Mediterranean fever, multiple sclerosis, primary biliary cirrhosis, mycosis fungoides, and in experimental studies of normal and abnormal cell division. **Orphan drug:** proposed use to arrest progression of neurologic disability caused by chronic progressive multiple sclerosis.

PHARMACOKINETICS Absorption: rapidly absorbed from GI tract. **Peak:** 0.5–2 h; may have multiple peaks because of enterohepatic cycling. **Distribution:** widely distributed; concentrates in leukocytes, kidney, liver, spleen, and intestinal tract. **Metabolism:**

partially metabolized in liver. **Elimination:** primarily excreted in feces; 10–20% excreted in urine in 24 h.

ROUTE & DOSAGE

Acute Gouty Attack

Adult	PO	0.5–1.2 mg followed by 0.5–0.6 mg q1–2h until pain relief or intolerable GI symptoms (max 4 mg/attack)
	IV	2 mg followed by 0.5 mg q6h until relief or intolerable GI symptoms (max 4 mg/attack)

Prophylaxis

Adult	PO	0.5 or 0.6 mg every night or every other night as needed (up to 1.8 mg/d may be needed for severe cases)
	IV	0.5–1 mg 1–2 times/d

Surgical Patients

Adult	PO	0.5 or 0.6 mg t.i.d. starting 3 d before surgery and continuing for 3 d after surgery

CONTRAINDICATIONS & PRECAUTIONS Contraindicated in: blood dyscrasias; severe GI, renal, hepatic, or cardiac disease; use of IV colchicine in patients with both renal and hepatic dysfunction. Severe local irritation can result from SC or IM use. Safe use during pregnancy (category C), in nursing mothers, and in children not established. **Cautious use in:** elderly and debilitated patients, early manifestations of GI, renal, hepatic, or cardiac disease.

ADVERSE/SIDE EFFECTS Dose-related. **CNS:** mental confusion, peripheral neuritis, syndrome of muscle weakness (accompanied by elevated serum creatine kinase).**GI:** *nausea, vomiting, diarrhea, abdominal pain,* anorexia, hemorrhagic gastroenteritis, steatorrhea, hepatotoxicity, pancreatitis. **Hematologic:** neutropenia, bone marrow depression, thrombocytopenia, agranulocytosis, aplastic anemia. **Renal:** azotemia, proteinuria, hematuria, oliguria.

DIAGNOSTIC TEST INTERFERENCES Possible interference with *urinary steroid (17-OHCS)* determinations when done by modifications of Reddy, Jenkins, Thorn procedure. False-positive *urine tests for RBCs and hemoglobin* reported.

DRUG INTERACTIONS May decrease intestinal absorption of vitamin B_{12}.

NURSING IMPLICATIONS

Administration

- Administer oral drug with milk or food to reduce possibility of GI upset.
- **IV** *preparation:* Do not dilute colchicine with 5% dextrose injection or other fluids that may change pH of colchicine solution, since a precipitate may form. Dilute with 0.9% NaCl injection that does not contain a bacteriostatic agent. Discard turbid solutions.
- Injection should be made over 2–5 min by direct IV or into tubing of free-flowing IV with compatible fluid.
- Care must be taken to prevent extravasation of IV colchicine because severe tissue irritation including nerve damage can result.
- Since acute gout can be precipitated by even minor surgical procedures, the patient is usually given colchicine before and after surgery.
- To avoid cumulative toxicity, a given course of colchicine therapy for acute gout is generally not repeated within 3 d.
- Preserved in tight, light-resistant containers preferably between 15 and 30C (59 and 86F), unless otherwise directed by manufacturer.

Assessment & Drug Effects

- Baseline and periodic determinations of serum uric acid and creatinine are advised, as well as CBC, including Hgb, serum electrolytes, and urinalysis.
- Side effects (dose-related) are most likely to occur during the initial course of treatment. A latent period of several hours between drug administration and onset of toxic symptoms is usual.
- Early signs of colchicine toxicity include weakness, abdominal discomfort, anorexia, nausea, vomiting, and diarrhea, regardless of administration route. Report to physician. To avoid more serious toxicity, drug should be discontinued promptly until symptoms subside.
- Monitor I&O (during acute gouty attack). High fluid intake promotes excretion and reduces danger of crystal formation in kidneys and ureters.
- Keep physician informed of patient's progress. Drug should be stopped when pain of acute gout is relieved. Therapeutic response: articular pain and swelling generally subside within 8–12 h and usually disappear in 24–72 h after PO therapy, and 6–12 h after IV administration.

Patient & Family Education

- Patients taking colchicine at home should be advised to withhold drug and report to the physician the onset of GI symptoms or signs of bone marrow depression (nausea, sore throat, bleeding gums, sore mouth, fever, fatigue, malaise, unusual bleeding or bruising).
- Patients with gout should be instructed to keep colchicine at hand at all times so they can start therapy or increase dosage, as prescribed by physician, at the first suggestion of an acute attack.
- Physician may prescribe sodium bicarbonate, or sodium or potassium citrate, to maintain alkaline urine and thus prevent formation of urate stones.
- Fermented beverages such as beer, ale, and wine may precipitate gouty attack and therefore should be avoided. The physician may allow distilled alcoholic beverages in moderation.

ANTIHISTAMINE (H$_1$-RECEPTOR ANTAGONIST)

DIPHENHYDRAMINE HYDROCHLORIDE

(dye-fen-hye´dra-meen)

Trade names: Allerdryl, Belix, Ben-Allergin, Bena-D, Benadryl, Benahist, Benaphen, Benoject, Benylin, Compoz, Diahist, Dihydrex, Diphen, Diphenacen, Fenylhist, Hyrexin, Insomnal, Nordryl, Nytol with DPH, Sleep-Eze 3, Sominex Formula 2, Tusstat, Twilite, Valdrene, Wehdryl

Classifications: ANTIHISTAMINE; H$_1$-RECEPTOR ANTAGONIST; AUTONOMIC NERVOUS SYSTEM AGENT; ANTICHOLINERGIC (PARASYMPATHOLYTIC); ANTIPARKINSONISM AGENT; GI AGENT; ANTIEMETIC; ANTITUSSIVE

Pregnancy: Category C

ACTIONS/PHARMACODYNAMICS Ethanolamine antihistamine with significant anticholinergic activity. High incidence of drowsiness, but GI side effects are minor. Competes for H$_1$-receptor sites on effector cells, thus blocking histamine release. (Histamine promotes capillary permeability and edema formation and constriction of respiratory, GI, and vascular smooth muscle.) Effects in parkinsonism and drug-induced extrapyramidal symptoms are apparently related to its ability to suppress central cholinergic activity and to prolong action of dopamine by inhibiting its reuptake and storage. Does not inhibit gastric secretion but has strong antiemetic effect. Also has prominent sedative and

Common side effects in *italic*; life-threatening effects <u>underlined</u>; generic names in **bold**; classifications in SMALL CAPS

47

anticholinergic activity and demonstrates central antitussive action and some local anesthetic properties.

USES Temporary symptomatic relief of various allergic conditions and to treat or prevent motion sickness, vertigo, and reactions to blood or plasma in susceptible patients. Also used in anaphylaxis as adjunct to epinephrine and other standard measures after acute symptoms have been controlled; in treatment of parkinsonism and drug-induced extrapyramidal reactions; as a nonnarcotic cough suppressant; as a sedative-hypnotic; and for treatment of intractable insomnia.

ROUTE & DOSAGE

Allergy Symptoms, Antiparkinsonism, Motion Sickness, Nighttime Sedation

Adult	PO	25–50mg t.i.d. or q.i.d. (max 300 mg/d)
	IV/IM	10–50 mg q4–6h (max 400 mg/d)
Child	PO/IV/IM	6–12 y: 12.5 –25 mg q4–6h (max 300 mg/24 h)
		2–6 y: 6.25 mg q4–6h (max 300 mg/2 h)

Nonproductive Cough

Adult	PO	25 mg q4–6h (max 100 mg/d)
Child	PO	6–12 y: 12.5 mg q4–6h (max 50 mg/24 h)
		2–6 y: 6.25 mg q4–6h (max 25 mg/24 h)

PHARMACOKINETICS Absorption: readily absorbed from GI tract but only 40–60% reaches systemic circulation. **Onset:** 15–30 min. **Peak:** 1–4 h. **Duration:** 4–7 h. **Distribution:** crosses placenta; distributed into breast milk. **Metabolism:** metabolized in liver; some degradation in lung and kidney. **Elimination:** mostly excreted in urine within 24 h.

CONTRAINDICATIONS & PRECAUTIONS

Contraindicated in: hypersensitivity to antihistamines of similar structure; lower respiratory tract symptoms (including acute asthma); narrow-angle glaucoma; prostatic hypertrophy, bladder neck obstruction; GI obstruction or stenosis; pregnancy (category C), nursing mothers, prematures, and newborns; use as nighttime sleep aid in children < age 12. **Cautious use in:** history of asthma; convulsive disorders; increased IOP; hyperthyroidism; hypertension, cardiovascular

disease; diabetes mellitus; elderly patients, infants, and young children.

ADVERSE/SIDE EFFECTS CNS: *drowsiness,* dizziness, headache, fatigue, disturbed coordination, tingling, heaviness and weakness of hands, tremors, euphoria, nervousness, restlessness, insomnia; confusion; (especially in children): hallucinations, excitement, fever, ataxia, athetosis, convulsions, coma; toxic encephalopathy with excessive topical applications. **CV:** palpitation, *tachycardia,* mild hypotension or hypertension, <u>cardiovascular collapse</u>. **ENT:** tinnitus, acute labyrinthitis, vertigo, dry nose, throat, nasal stuffiness. **Eye:** blurred vision, diplopia, photosensitivity, dry eyes. **GI** *dry mouth,* nausea, epigastric distress, anorexia, vomiting, constipation or diarrhea. **GU:** urinary frequency or retention, dysuria. **Hematologic:** leukopenia, <u>agranulocytosis</u>, hemolytic anemia. **Hypersensitivity:** skin rash, urticaria, photosensitivity, <u>anaphylactic shock</u>. **Respiratory:** thickened bronchial secretions, wheezing, sensation of chest tightness.

DIAGNOSTIC TEST INTERFERENCES In common with other antihistamines, diphenhydramine should be discontinued 4 d prior to ***skin testing*** procedures for allergy because it may obscure otherwise positive reactions.

DRUG INTERACTIONS Alcohol and other CNS DEPRESSANTS, MAO INHIBITORS compound CNS depression.

NURSING IMPLICATIONS

Administration

- GI side effects may be lessened by administration of drug with food or milk.
- When diphenhydramine is used for motion sickness, the first dose is given 30 min before exposure to motion. For duration of exposure, it is given before meals and on retiring.
- Administer IM injection deep into large muscle mass; alternate injection sites. Avoid perivascular or SC injections of the drug because of its irritating effects. Hypersensitivity reactions (including anaphylactic shock) are more likely to occur with parenteral injections than with PO administration.
- ***IV injection:*** IV diphenhydramine may be given by direct IV undiluted at a rate of 25 mg or a fraction thereof over 1 min.
- Store in tightly covered containers at 15–30C (59–86F) unless otherwise directed by manufacturer. Store injection and elixir formulations in light-resistant containers protected from light.

Common side effects in *italic*; life-threatening effects <u>underlined</u>; generic names in **bold**; classifications in SMALL CAPS

- Elixir or syrup formulations are used for relief of cough.

Assessment & Drug Effects
- Patients with blood pressure problems who are receiving the drug parenterally should be closely observed, with BP being monitored.
- Drowsiness is most prominent during the first few days of therapy and often disappears with continued therapy. Elderly patients are especially likely to manifest dizziness, sedation, and hypotension. Side rails and supervision of ambulation may be advisable for some patients.
- Patients receiving long-term therapy should have periodic blood counts.

Patient & Family Education
- Patients using topical diphenhydramine, should be warned to avoid excessive applications to skin eruptions. Toxic encephalopathy has been associated with improper topical use.
- Warn the patient about possible additive CNS depressant effects with concurrent use of alcohol and other CNS depressants.
- Caution the patient against activities requiring alertness and coordination until drug response has been evaluated.
- The drug has an atropinelike drying effect (thickens bronchial secretions) that may make expectoration difficult. Advise patient to increase fluid intake if not contraindicated.
- Antihistamines have no therapeutic effect on the common cold. Their continued popularity stems from their drying effect.

ANTIPRURITIC

HYDROXYZINE HYDROCHLORIDE
(hye-drox´i-zeen)
Trade names: Atarax, Atozine, Durrax, E-Vista, Hyzine-50, Orgatrax, Quiess, Vistaril Intramuscular, Vistacon, Vistaject

HYDROXYZINE PAMOATE
Trade names: Hy-Pam, Vamate, Vistaril Oral
Classifications: ANTIHISTAMINE; ANTIPRURITIC; CNS AGENT; ANXIOLYTIC; GI AGENT; ANTIEMETIC
Pregnancy: Category C

ACTIONS/PHARMACODYNAMICS Piperazine derivative structurally and pharmacologically related to other cyclizines (e.g., buclizine, chlorcyclizine). In common with such agents, it causes CNS depression and has anticholinergic, antiemetic, bronchodilator, and antihistaminic activity. Its tranquilizing (ataractic) effect is produced primarily by depression of hypothalamus and brain-stem reticular formation, rather than cortical areas. Also has skeletal muscle relaxant effect and mild antisecretory and analgesic activity.

USES Emotional or psychoneurotic states characterized by anxiety, tension, or psychomotor agitation; to relieve anxiety, control nausea and emesis, and reduce narcotic requirements before or after surgery or delivery. Also used in management of pruritus due to allergic conditions, e.g., chronic urticaria, atopic and contact dermatoses, and in treatment of acute and chronic alcoholism with withdrawal symptoms or delirium tremens.

ROUTE & DOSAGE

Anxiety

Adult	PO	25–100 mg t.i.d. or q.i.d.
	IM	25–100 mg q4–6h
Child	PO	<6 y: 50 mg/d in divided doses
		>6 y: 50 mg/d in divided doses
	IM	1.1 mg/kg q4–6h

Pruritus

Adult	PO	25 mg t.i.d. or q.i.d.
	IM	25 mg q4–6h
Child	PO	>6 y: 50–100 mg/d in divided doses
		<6 y: 50 mg/d in divided doses
	IM	1.1 mg/kg q4–6h

Nausea

Adult	IM	25–100 mg q4–6h
Child	IM	1.1 mg/kg q4–6h

PHARMACOKINETICS Absorption: readily absorbed from GI tract. **Onset:** 15–30 min PO. **Duration:** 4–6 h. **Distribution:** not known if it crosses placenta or is distributed into breast milk. **Metabolism:** metabolized in liver. **Elimination:** probably excreted in bile.

CONTRAINDICATIONS & PRECAUTIONS Contraindicated in: known hypersensitivity to hydroxyzine; use as sole treatment in psychoses or depression. Safe use during early pregnancy (category C) or

Common side effects in *italic*; life-threatening effects underlined; generic names in **bold**; classifications in SMALL CAPS

49

in nursing mothers not established. **Cautious use in:** history of allergies; the elderly.

ADVERSE/SIDE EFFECTS *Drowsiness* (usually transitory), sedation, dizziness, injection site reactions, hypotension, *dry mouth,* headache; rarely: involuntary motor activity, tremor, convulsions. **Hypersensitivity:** urticaria, dyspnea, chest tightness, wheezing, erythematous macular eruptions, erythema multiforme. **Other:** Phlebitis, hemolysis, thrombosis, digital gangrene from inadvertant IV or intraarterial injection.

DIAGNOSTIC TEST INTERFERENCES Possibility of false-positive **urinary 17-hydroxycorticosteroid** determinations (modified Glenn-Nelson technique).

DRUG INTERACTIONS Alcohol and CNS DEPRESSANTS add to CNS depression; TRICYCLIC ANTIDEPRESSANTS and other ANTICHOLINERGICS have additive anticholinergic effects; may inhibit pressor effects of **epinephrine.**

INCOMPATIBILITIES Solution/additive: aminophylline, amobarbital, chloramphenicol, dimenhydrinate, penicillin G, pentobarbital, phenobarbital.

NURSING IMPLICATIONS

Administration

▪ Tablets may be crushed before administration and taken with fluid of patient's choice. Capsule may be emptied and contents swallowed with water or mixed with food. Liquid formulations are available.

▪ *IM administration* should be made deep into body of a relatively large muscle. The Z-track technique of injection may be used to prevent SC infiltration. In adults the preferred site is the upper outer quadrant of buttock or the midlateral thigh. In children the recommended site is the midlateral muscle of thigh. *Infants and small children:* periphery of upper outer quadrant of gluteal region should be used only if necessary (e.g., in burn patient with limited injection sites). The deltoid muscle should be used only if well developed; avoid lower and mid-third of arm to prevent radial nerve injury.

▪ Hydroxyzine must not be administered by SC, intraarterial, or IV injections. Inadvertent injection by these routes may cause painful site, tissue damage, and may lead to thrombosis or phlebitis.

▪ Protect hydroxyzine from light. Store at 15–30C (59–86F) unless otherwise specified.

Assessment & Drug Effects

▪ Drowsiness may occur and usually disappears with continued therapy or following reduction of dosage.

▪ Dry mouth is uncomfortable and sets the stage for potential loss of taste and other serious clinical problems. If patient is on high dosage of hydroxyzine, monitor condition of oral membranes daily.

▪ Usefulness of hydroxyzine should be reevaluated periodically. Effectiveness of use beyond 4 mo should be reassessed on basis of individual's response to the drug.

▪ When CNS depressants are prescribed concomitantly, dosage of the depressant is reduced up to 50%.

Patient & Family Education

▪ Forewarn the patient about the possibility of drowsiness and dizziness, and caution against driving or performing hazardous tasks requiring mental alertness and physical coordination during hydroxyzine therapy.

▪ Alcohol and hydroxyzine should not be taken at the same time. Concomitant use enhances the effects of both agents.

▪ Patient should be advised that if she becomes pregnant during therapy or intends to become pregnant, she should communicate with her physician about the desirability of discontinuing the drug.

▪ Dry mouth may be relieved by frequent warm water rinses, increasing fluid intake, and by use of a salivary substitute (e.g., Moi-stir, Xero-Lube) if necessary. Avoid frequent use of commercial mouth rinses; they can change normal flora of the mouth and permit onset of a superinfection.

▪ Urge patient to give scrupulous care to teeth. Avoid irritation or abrasion of gums and other oral tissues.

▪ Advise patient to consult physician before self-dosing with OTC medications.

ANTIVERTIGO AGENT

MECLIZINE HYDROCHLORIDE
(mek´li-zeen)
Trade names: Antivert, Antrizine, Bonamine, Bonine, Dizmiss, Motion Cure, Ru-Vert-M, Whevert
Classifications: ANTIHISTAMINE; ANTIVERTIGO AGENT; H_1-RECEPTOR ANTAGONIST; GI AGENT; ANTIEMETIC
Pregnancy: Category B

ACTIONS/PHARMACODYNAMICS Long-acting piperazine antihistamine, structurally and pharmacologically related to cyclizine compounds. Has marked effect in blocking histamine-induced vasopressive response but only slight anticholinergic action. In common with similar agents, also exhibits CNS depression, antispasmodic, antiemetic, and local anesthetic activity. Has marked depressant action on labyrinthine excitability and on conduction in vestibular-cerebellar pathways.

USES Management of nausea, vomiting, and dizziness associated with motion sickness and in vertigo associated with diseases affecting vestibular system.

ROUTE & DOSAGE

Motion Sickness

Adult	PO	25–50 mg 1 h before travel, may repeat q24h if necessary for duration of journey

Vertigo

Adult	PO	25–100 mg/d in divided doses

PHARMACOKINETICS Absorption: readily absorbed from GI tract. **Onset:** 1 h. **Duration:** 8–24 h. **Distribution:** crosses placenta. **Elimination:** half-life: 6 h; excreted primarily in feces.

CONTRAINDICATIONS & PRECAUTIONS Contraindicated in: pregnancy (category B); and pediatric age group. **Cautious use in:** angle-closure glaucoma, prostatic hypertrophy.

ADVERSE/SIDE EFFECTS *Drowsiness,* dry mouth, blurred vision, fatigue.

NURSING IMPLICATIONS

Administration
- Drug may be given without regard to meals.

Assessment & Drug Effects
- Since drug may cause drowsiness, supervision of ambulation, particularly with the elderly, may be warranted.
- When meclizine is prescribed for vertigo, assess effectiveness of drug and inform physician, as dosage adjustment may be required.

Patient & Family Education
- Forewarn patients about side effects such as drowsiness, and advise patients not to drive a car or engage in other hazardous activities until their reactions to the drug are known.
- Caution patients that the sedative action may be additive to that of alcohol, barbiturates, narcotic analgesics, or other CNS depressants.
- When meclizine is prescribed for motion sickness, instruct patient to take it 1 h before departure.

AMEBICIDE

EMETINE HYDROCHLORIDE
(em´e-teen)
Classifications: ANTIINFECTIVE; AMEBICIDE
Pregnancy: Category X

ACTIONS/PHARMACODYNAMICS Natural or synthetic alkaloid of ipecac with direct lethal action on *Entamoeba histolytica* in tissues. More effective against motile forms (trophozoites) than cysts. Causes degeneration of nucleus and cytoplasm of amebae and eradicates parasites, possibly by interfering with multiplication of trophozoites. Also has adrenergic and neuromuscular blocking activities and expectorant, diaphoretic, and emetic actions but is not used clinically for these effects.

USES In combination with other amebicides in management of acute fulminating amebic dysentery (intestinal amebiasis) or for acute exacerbations of chronic amebic dysentery. Highly effective in treatment of extraintestinal amebiasis (amebic abscess, amebic hepatitis). **Unlabeled use:** irrigation solution (emetine in NaCl injection) used at site of amebic abscess (after pus aspiration); malaria (caused by *Plasmodium falciparum*).

PHARMACOKINETICS Absorption: erratic oral absorption; therefore is given IM. **Distribution:** highest concentrations in lung, kidney, and spleen. **Elimination:** appears in urine 20–40 min after injection; still present in urine 40–60 d after discontinued.

CONTRAINDICATIONS & PRECAUTIONS Contraindicated in: patients who have received a

Common side effects in *italic*; life-threatening effects underlined; generic names in **bold**; classifications in SMALL CAPS

51

ROUTE & DOSAGE

Amebic Dysentery

Adult	IM/Deep SC	1 mg/kg b.i.d. (morning & evening) for 3–10 d (max 65 mg/kg or 650 mg in 10 d)
Child	IM/Deep SC	<8 y: 1 mg/kg b.i.d. for 4+ d (max 10 mg/d) > 8 y: 1 mg/kg b.i.d. for 4+ d (max 20 mg/d)

Hepatic Amebiasis or Abscess

Adult	IM/Deep SC	1 mg/kg b.i.d. (morning & evening) for up to 10 d (max 65 mg/kg or 650 mg in 10 d); do not repeat in <6 wk

course of emetine 6–8 wk previously; treatment of mild symptoms or carriers of amebiasis; heart or kidney disease; pregnancy (category X); children except those with severe dysentery not controlled by other amebicides. Safe use in nursing mothers not established. **Cautious use in:** debilitated or elderly patients; hypotension; patients about to have surgery.

ADVERSE/SIDE EFFECTS CNS: skeletal muscle weakness, tenderness, stiffness, pain; tremors, peripheral neuropathy, loss of sense of taste. **CV (cardiotoxicity):** hypotension, tachycardia, arrhythmias, myocarditis, *pericarditis,* precordial pain, dyspnea, ECG abnormalities, gallop rhythm, cardiac dilatation, CHF. **GI:** *diarrhea;* abdominal cramps; *nausea and vomiting associated with dizziness, faintness, headache,* epigastric burning and pain. **Other:** large doses: acute lesions in heart, *liver,* kidney, intestinal tract, skeletal muscle; *injection site reactions (frequent):* aching, tenderness, and local muscle weakness; eczematous, urticarial, or purpuric lesions; necrosis, cellulitis, abscess, decrease in serum potassium, thrombocytopenia.

DRUG INTERACTIONS Not established.

NURSING IMPLICATIONS

Administration

- Emetine is administered by deep SC or IM injection. Aspirate carefully after needle is introduced. *IV injection is dangerous and is specifically contraindicated.*

- Emetine is very irritating to tissues. Wash hands thoroughly after handling drug.
- Emetine for treatment of acute fulminating amebic dysentery is administered only long enough to control symptoms (usually 3–5 d). For extraintestinal amebiasis (amebic hepatitis or abscess) it is generally given for 10 d; another amebicide should be given simultaneously or as an immediate follow-up to guarantee eradication of *E. histolytica* from primary lesions in intestines.
- Protect drug from light.

Assessment & Drug Effects

- Emetine is a potent drug. Patients should be hospitalized and on absolute bed rest during therapy and for several days thereafter. Tachycardia may occur in patients permitted to ambulate. It is also advisable for patients to remain sedentary for several weeks after drug is terminated.
- Make a record of injection sites and observe these sites daily. Muscle ache and tenderness at area of injection occur frequently.
- Toxic action may be cumulative. The patient should be closely observed and advised to report any unusual symptom, no matter how minor it may seem.
- Emetine is potentially toxic to the heart. An ECG should be taken before emetine is initiated, as well as after the fifth dose, on completion of therapy, and 1 wk later. ECG changes usually appear about 7 d after drug is administered; they are generally reversible. Report their appearance immediately.
- Pulse (rate and quality) and BP should be recorded at least 3 times daily. Tachycardia frequently precedes appearance of ECG abnormalities.
- ECG alterations may persist in some patients 2 mo or more after discontinuation of drug. Some patients experience dyspnea until drug is stopped.
- Emetine should be discontinued on the appearance of tachycardia, a precipitous fall in BP, marked weakness or other neuromuscular symptoms, and severe GI effects. These adverse reactions should be reported promptly.
- Monitor neuromuscular function, especially of neck and extremities (most likely involved). Report immediately any signs of weakness and complaints of fatigue, listlessness, muscular stiffness, tenderness, or pain. These symptoms usually appear before more serious symptoms and thus may serve as guides to avoid overdosage.
- Monitor I & O. Report oliguria or change in I & O ratio.
- Record number, unusual odor, and consistency of

stools. Suspect emetine-induced reaction if stools increase in number following improvement of diarrhea.

Patient & Family Education
- Advise patients to remain sedentary and to restrict activity for several weeks after completion of drug therapy to prevent development of tachycardia.
- Advise patients to immediately report weakness, fatigue, listlessness, muscle stiffness, tenderness, or pain.

ANTHELMINTIC

MEBENDAZOLE
(me-ben´da-zole)
Trade name: Vermox
Classifications: ANTIINFECTIVE; ANTHELMINTIC

ACTIONS/PHARMACODYNAMICS Carbamate with unusually broad spectrum of anthelmintic activity. Mechanism of action not known. Inhibits formation of worm's microtubules and inhibits glucose and other nutrient uptake by susceptible helminths.

USES Treatment of *Trichuris trichiura* (whipworm), *Enterobius vermicularis* (pinworm), *Ascaris lumbricoides* (roundworm), *Ancylostoma duodenale* (common hookworm), *Necator americanus* (American hookworm) in single or mixed infections. **Unlabeled use:** beef, dwarf, and pork tapeworm and threadworm infections.

ROUTE & DOSAGE

Enterobiasis

Adult	PO	100 mg as single dose
Child	PO	100 mg as single dose

Other Infestations

Adult	PO	100 mg b.i.d. × 3 d
Child	PO	100 mg b.i.d. × 3 d

PHARMACOKINETICS Absorption: minimal absorption from GI tract (2–10% of oral dose). **Metabolism:** metabolized to inactive metabolite. **Elimination:** half-life: 3–9 h; primarily eliminated in feces.

CONTRAINDICATIONS & PRECAUTIONS Contraindicated in: safe use during pregnancy (category C), in nursing women, and in children <2 y not established.

ADVERSE/SIDE EFFECTS Transient abdominal pain, diarrhea, dizziness, fever (possibly due to tissue necrosis in cysts).

NURSING IMPLICATIONS

Administration
- May be given without regard to food. Food in GI tract reportedly does not affect drug action.
- Commercial chewable tablet may be chewed, crushed, mixed with food, or swallowed whole.

Assessment & Drug Effects
- If cure does not occur within 3 wk after initiation of therapy, second course of treatment is advised.
- Because pinworms are readily transmitted from person to person, all family members should be examined and treated simultaneously.

Patient & Family Education
- Emphasize importance of washing hands thoroughly after toilet and before eating. Disinfect toilet facilities daily.
- Keep hands away from mouth; keep fingernails short.
- Handle bedding carefully without shaking it to avoid dispersing ova into the air.
- Advise patient to change underclothing, bedclothes, towels, and facecloths daily and to bathe frequently, preferably by showering. Infected person should sleep alone.

ANTIBIOTIC: AMINOGLYCOSIDE

GENTAMICIN SULFATE
(jen-ta-mye sin)
Trade names: Garamycin, Garamycin Ophthalmic, Genoptic, Gentacidin
Classifications: ANTIINFECTIVE; AMINOGLYCOSIDE ANTIBIOTIC
Pregnancy: Category C

ACTIONS/PHARMACODYNAMICS Broad-spectrum aminoglycoside antibiotic derived from

Common side effects in *italic*; life-threatening effects <u>underlined</u>; generic names in **bold**; classifications in SMALL CAPS

53

Micromonospora purpu.rea, an actinomycete. Action is usually bactericidal. Appears to act by binding directly and irreversibly to bacterial 30s ribosomal subunits, thereby inhibiting protein biosynthesis. Active against a wide variety of gram-negative bacteria, including *Citrobacter, Escherichia coli, Enterobacter, Klebsiella, Proteus* (including indole-positive and indole-negative strains), *Pseudomonas aeruginosa*, and *Serratia* sp. Also effective against certain gram-positive organisms, particularly penicillin-sensitive and some methicillin-resistant strains of *Staphylococcus aureus*. Cross-resistance and allergenicity with other members of the aminoglycoside group have been demonstrated. Has neuromuscular blocking action, in common with other aminoglycoside antibiotics.

USES Parenteral use restricted to treatment of serious infections of GI, respiratory, and urinary tracts, CNS, bone, skin, and soft tissue (including burns) when other less toxic antimicrobial agents are ineffective or are contraindicated. Has been used in combination with other antibiotics. Also used topically for primary and secondary skin infections and for superficial infections of external eye and its adnexa. **Unlabeled use:** prophylaxis of bacterial endocarditis in patients undergoing operative procedures or instrumentation.

ROUTE & DOSAGE

Moderate to Severe Infection

Adult	IV/IM	1.5–2 mg/kg loading dose followed by 3–5 mg/kg/d in 2–3 divided doses
	Topical	1–2 drops of solution in eye q4h up to 2 drops q1h or small amount of ointment b.i.d. or t.i.d.
Child	IV/IM	6–7.5 mg/kg/d in 3–4 divided doses
Neonate	IV/IM	2.5 mg/kg q12h

Acute Pelvic Inflammatory Disease

Adult	IV/IM	2 mg/kg followed by 1.5 mg/kg q8h

Prophylaxis of Bacterial Endocarditis

Adult	IV/IM	1.5 mg/kg 30 min before procedure; may repeat in 8 h
Child	IV/IM	<27 kg: 2 mg/kg 30 min before procedure; may repeat in 8 h

PHARMACOKINETICS Absorption: well absorbed from IM site. **Peak:** 30–90 min IM. **Distribution:** widely distributed in body fluids, including ascitic, peritoneal, pleural, synovial, and abscess fluids; poor CNS penetration; concentrates in kidney and inner ear; crosses placenta. **Metabolism:** not metabolized. **Elimination:** half-life: 2–4 h; excreted unchanged in urine; small amounts accumulate in kidney and are eliminated over 10–20 d; small amount excreted in breast milk.

CONTRAINDICATIONS & PRECAUTIONS Contraindicated in: history of hypersensitivity to or toxic reaction with any aminoglycoside antibiotic. Safe use during pregnancy (category C) and in nursing mothers not established. **Cautious use in:** impaired renal function; history of eighth cranial (acoustic) nerve impairment; preexisting vertigo or dizziness or tinnitus; dehydration, fever; use in the elderly, prematures, neonates, and infants; obesity, neuromuscular disorders: myasthenia gravis, parkinsonian syndrome; hypocalcemia, heart failure, topical applications to widespread areas.

ADVERSE/SIDE EFFECTS CNS: ototoxicity (vestibular disturbances, impaired hearing), optic neuritis, peripheral neuritis, paresthesias (numbness, tingling of skin), headache, lethargy, tremors, muscle cramps and twitching, convulsions, neuromuscular blockade: skeletal muscle weakness, apnea, respiratory paralysis (high doses); acute organic brain syndrome, pseudotumor cerebri (rare); arachnoiditis (intrathecal use). **GI:** anorexia, nausea, vomiting, weight loss, increased salivation; proctitis, enterocolitis (rare). **Hematologic:** increased or decreased reticulocyte counts; granulocytopenia, agranulocytosis, thrombocytopenia (fever, bleeding tendency), thrombocytopenic purpura, anemia. **Hypersensitivity:** rash, pruritus, urticaria, exfoliative dermatitis, eosinophilia, burning sensation of skin, drug fever, joint pains, laryngeal edema, anaphylaxis. **Renal:** <u>Nephrotoxicity:</u> proteinuria, cells or casts in urine, oliguria, hematuria, unusual thirst, rising BUN, nonprotein nitrogen, serum creatinine; *decreased creatinine clearance*, renal damage. **Topical and ophthalmic:** photosensitivity, sensitization, erythema, pruritus; burning, stinging, and lacrimation (ophthalmic formulation). **Other:** transient increase in AST (SGOT), ALT (SGPT), and serum LDH and bilirubin; hepatomegaly, splenomegaly; loss of hair and eyebrows; pulmonary fibrosis, hypotension or hypertension; local irritation and pain following IM use; thrombophlebitis, abscess, superinfections, syndrome of hypocalcemia (tetany, weakness, hypokalemia, hypomagnesemia).

DRUG INTERACTIONS Amphotericin B, capre-

omycin, cisplatin, methoxyflurane, polymyxin B, vancomycin, increase risk of nephrotoxicity. **Ethacrynic acid** and **furosemide** may increase risk of ototoxicity. GENERAL ANESTHETICS and NEUROMUSCULAR BLOCKING AGENTS (e.g., **succinylcholine**) potentiate neuromuscular blockade. **Indomethacin** may increase gentamicin levels in neonates.

INCOMPATIBILITIES Solution/additive: fat emulsion, TPN, **amphotericin B, ampicillin, carbenicillin,** CEPHALOSPORINS, **cytarabine, heparin. Y-site:** **furosemide, iodipamide.**

NURSING IMPLICATIONS

Administration
Parenteral
- For administration by intermittent IV infusion to adults, a single dose of gentamicin is diluted with 50–200 ml of 0.9% NaCl or 5% dextrose injection and infused over 30 min–2 h. For pediatric patients, amount of infusion fluid may be proportionately smaller depending on patient's needs but should be sufficient to be infused over the same time period as for adults.
- Gentamicin is stable for 24 h at room temperature in 0.9% NaCl or 5% dextrose injection, or other IV fluids recommended by manufacturer.
- Note that commercial IV piggyback preparations and gentamicin for intrathecal use contain no preservatives and therefore must be used promptly once opened. Any unused portion should be discarded.
- Gentamicin for IV or IM administration is clear and colorless or slightly yellow. Gentamicin for intrathecal use is a clear and colorless solution. Do not use solutions that are discolored or that contain particulate matter.
- Culture and susceptibility tests should be performed initially (before first dose) and periodically during continued therapy. Therapy may begin pending test results.

Ophthalmic
- Ask patient to close eyes gently and not to blink. Immediately apply pressure to inner canthus for 1 min after instillation.
- After administration of ophthalmic ointment, instruct patient to keep eyes closed for 1–2 min to assure medication contact. Caution patient that vision will be blurred for a few minutes.

Topical
- Wash affected area with mild soap and water, rinse, and dry thoroughly, unless otherwise prescribed by physician. Gently apply small amount of medication to lesions. Cover with sterile gauze if desired.
- Topical applications, particularly gentamicin cream preparations, should not be made to large denuded body surfaces because systemic absorption and toxicity are possible.
- In treatment of impetigo contagiosa, individual crusts should first be removed (gently) to allow topical medication to contact infected site. Removal may be facilitated by soaking crusts with warm soap and water or by application of wet compresses. Consult physician regarding specific procedure.
- Store gentamicin preparations between 2–30C (36–86F) unless otherwise directed by manufacturer.

Assessment & Drug Effects
Parenteral
- Most infections respond to therapy within 24–48 h. Gentamicin is generally continued for 7–10 d. If improvement does not occur in 3–5 d, susceptibility tests should be repeated and therapy reevaluated.
- Baseline weight, vital signs, and tests of renal function and vestibular and auditory function should be determined before therapy and at regular intervals during treatment. Vestibular and auditory function should be checked again 3–4 wk after drug is discontinued (the time that deafness is most likely to occur).
- Creatinine clearance and serum drug concentrations should be determined at frequent intervals, particularly for patients with impaired renal function, infants (renal immaturity), the elderly, and patients receiving high doses or therapy beyond 10 d, patients with fever or extensive burns, edema, obesity.
- I&O should be monitored. Because urine drug concentrations generally are high, patient is kept well hydrated during therapy to prevent chemical irritation of renal tubules. Report oliguria, unusual appearance of urine, change in I&O ratio or pattern, and presence of edema (prolongs elimination time).
- Ototoxic effect (see Signs & Symptoms, chap 3) is greatest on the vestibular branch of eighth cranial (acoustic) nerve (symptoms: headache, dizziness or vertigo, nausea, and vomiting with motion, ataxia, nystagmus). However, damage to the auditory branch (tinnitus, roaring noises, sensation of fullness in ears, hearing impairment) may also occur. Generally, conversational hearing range is not affected. Prompt reporting is critical to prevent permanent damage.
- Generally, dosages are adjusted to maintain peak

Common side effects in *italic*; life-threatening effects underlined; generic names in **bold**; classifications in SMALL CAPS

55

serum gentamicin concentrations of 4–10 µg/ml, and trough concentrations of 1–2 µg/ml. Peak concentrations above 12 µg/ml and trough concentrations above 2 µg/ml are associated with toxicity.

- Blood specimens for peak serum gentamicin concentrations are generally drawn 30 min–1 h after IM administration, and 30 min after completion of a 30–60 min IV infusion. For trough levels, blood specimens are drawn just before the next IM or IV dose. Blood should be collected in nonheparinized tubes.

- Be alert for signs of bacterial overgrowth (opportunistic infections) with resistant or nonsusceptible organisms (diarrhea, anogenital itching, vaginal discharge, stomatitis, glossitis).

Patient & Family Education

- Caution patients using topical applications to: (1) avoid excessive exposure to sunlight because of danger of photosensitivity; (2) withhold medication and notify physician if condition fails to improve within 1 wk, worsens, or signs of irritation or sensitivity occur; and (3) apply medication as directed and only for length of time prescribed (overuse can result in superinfections).

ANTIBIOTIC: ANTIFUNGAL

AMPHOTERICIN B

(am-foe-ter´i-sin)
Trade name: Fungizone
Classifications: ANTIINFECTIVE; ANTIFUNGAL ANTIBIOTIC
Pregnancy: Category B

ACTIONS/PHARMACODYNAMICS Fungistatic antibiotic produced by *Streptomyces nodosus*. Fungicidal at higher concentrations, depending on sensitivity of fungus. Exerts antifungal action on both resting and growing cells at least in part by selectively binding to sterols in fungus cell membrane. This action increases membrane permeability, thus allowing leakage of potassium and other intracellular constituents. Because it may also bind somewhat to human cytoplasmic sterols, it can have severe adverse effects. Antifungal action decreases at low pH.

USES Used intravenously for a wide spectrum of potentially fatal systemic fungal (mycotic) infections including aspergillosis, blastomycosis, coccidioidomycosis, cryptococcosis, disseminated candidiasis,

histoplasmosis, paracoccidioidomycosis, sporotrichosis, and others. Has been used to potentiate antifungal effects of flucytosine (Ancobon) and to provide anticandidal prophylaxis in certain susceptible patients receiving immunosuppressive therapy. Used topically for cutaneous and mucocutaneous infections caused by *Candida* (Monilia). **Unlabeled use:** treatment of candiduria, fungal endocarditis, meningitis, septicemia; fungal infections of urinary bladder and urinary tract; amebic meningoencephalitis, and paracoccidioidomycosis.

ROUTE & DOSAGE

All Systemic Indications

Adult	IV	An IV test dose of 1 mg dissolved in 20 ml of D5W by slow infusion (over 10–30 min) is recommended to lessen the risk of an anaphylactic reaction *Initial dose:* 250 µg/kg/d IV infused over 4–6 h in a single dose, adjusted daily in increments of 250 µg/kg/d, or faster if tolerated, up to 1.0 mg/kg/d or 1.5 mg/kg/d q.o.d.; a total daily dosage of 1.5 mg/kg should not be exceeded; usual daily dose is about 50 mg/d except in severe infections
Child	IV	Same as for adult except that the *minimum dilution* of amphotericin B in pediatric patients (≤17 y) is 0.1 mg/ml in D5W administered over 2–6 h

Candiduria (Bladder Irrigation)

Adult	50 mg/1000 ml sterile water instilled continuously into the bladder via a 3-way closed drainage catheter system at a rate of 1000 ml/24 h

PHARMACOKINETICS Peak effect: 1–2 h after IV infusion. **Duration:** 20 h. **Distribution:** minimal amounts enter CNS, eye, bile, pleural, pericardial, synovial, or amniotic fluids; similar plasma and urine concentrations. **Elimination:** half-life: 24–48 h; excreted renally; can be detected in blood up to 4 wk and in urine for 4–8 wk after discontinuing therapy.

CONTRAINDICATIONS & PRECAUTIONS
Contraindicated in: hypersensitivity to amphotericin. **Cautious use in:** severe bone marrow depression or renal function impairment. Safe use during preg-

nancy (category B) and in nursing mothers not established.

ADVERSE/SIDE EFFECTS CNS: headache, sedation, muscle pain, arthralgia, weakness. **CV: CHF. ENT (ototoxicity):** tinnitus, vertigo, loss of hearing. **GI:** nausea, vomiting, diarrhea, epigastric cramps, anorexia, weight loss. **Hematologic:** anemia, thrombocytopenia, *leukocytosis.* **Metabolic:** *hypokalemia, hypomagnesemia.* **Hypersensitivity:** pruritus, urticaria, skin rashes, fever, dyspnea, anaphylaxis. **Renal:** nephrotoxicity, urine with low specific gravity. **Topical:** dry skin, erythema, pruritus, burning sensation; allergic contact dermatitis, exacerbation of lesions. **Other:** *fever, chills,* pain; arthralgias, thrombophlebitis (IV site), superinfections.

DRUG INTERACTIONS AMINOGLYCOSIDES, **capreomycin, cisplatin, carboplatin, colistin, cyclosporine, mechlorethamine, furosemide, vancomycin** increase the possibility of nephrotoxicity; CORTICOSTEROIDS potentiate hypokalemia; with DIGITALIS GLYCOSIDES, hypokalemia increases the risk of digitalis toxicity.

INCOMPATIBILITIES Solution/Additive: Any **saline**-containing solution (precipitate will form), PARENTERAL NUTRITION SOLUTIONS, **calcium chloride, calcium gluconate, cimetidine, edetate calcium disodium, metaraminol, methyldopa, polymyxin, potassium chloride, ranitidine, verapamil. Y-site:** AMINOGLYCOSIDES, PENICILLINS, PHENOTHIAZINES, **clindamycin, cotrimoxazole, diphenhydramine, dopamine, dobutamine, heparin** (flush lines with D5W not NS), **lidocaine, procaine, tetracycline, vitamins.**

NURSING IMPLICATIONS

Administration

- Check with physician regarding IV flow rate. Generally the drug is administered slowly over 6 h. Rapid infusion can cause cardiovascular collapse. If a reaction occurs, interrupt therapy and report promptly to physician.
- Intensity of adverse reactions may be reduced by reduction of dosage or by administering drug on alternate days. Some physicians prescribe prophylactic use (e.g., 1 h before infusion) of aspirin or acetaminophen, antiemetics, antihistamines, and corticosteroids.
- Commonly causes local inflammatory reaction or thrombosis at injection site, particularly if extravasation occurs. Risk of thrombophlebitis associated with IV infusion may be reduced by using scalp vein needle in the most distal vein possible, by alternating veins, by addition of heparin or hydrocortisone (as prescribed) to the infusion, and by alternate day dosage schedule.
- Frequently check IV site for leakage. It is more likely to occur in the *elderly* patient because loss of tissue elasticity with aging may promote extravasation around the needle.

Preparation of IV Solution

- Keep dry powder refrigerated between 2–8C (36–46F) and protected from light. Avoid freezing.
- Reconstitute 50 mg vial only with 10 ml of sterile water for injection without preservatives or bacteriostatic agent to produce a concentration of 5 mg/ml. Follow manufacturer's directions.
- Reconstituted preparation is stable for 24 h at room temperature protected from light and for 1 wk under refrigeration. Discard any solution before this time if it is cloudy or contains a precipitate.
- For IV infusion each 1 mg of the reconstituted amphotericin B is further diluted with 10 ml of 5% dextrose injection having a pH above 4.2 (coagulation occurs at pH less than 5). Solutions prepared for IV infusion have a concentration of 100 µg/ml and must be used promptly.
- If in-line filter is used, the mean pore diameter should be no less than 1 µm, to avoid reducing concentration of amphotericin B delivered.
- Manufacturer recommends protecting aqueous solutions of amphotericin B from light during IV infusion. Follow agency policy.

Topical Application

- Do not cover with plastic wrap, plastic cloth, rubber, or other occlusive dressings. Ask physician to specify when and how lesions are to be washed.
- Topical treatment should be discontinued promptly if signs of hypersensitivity, irritation, or worsening of lesions occurs.
- Store topical forms in well-closed containers at room temperature, 15–30C (59–86F), unless otherwise directed.

Assessment & Drug Effects

- Prior to systemic therapy, diagnosis is confirmed by positive cultures or histologic studies.
- During initial IV therapy, monitor TPR and BP and observe patient closely for adverse effects. If a test dose (1 mg over 20–30 min) is given, monitor vital signs every 30 min for at least 4 h. Febrile reactions (fever, chills, headache, nausea) occur in 20–90% of patients, usually 1–2 h after beginning infusion, and subside within 4 h after drug is discontinued. The severity of this reaction usually decreases with

Common side effects in *italic*; life-threatening effects underlined; generic names in **bold**; classifications in SMALL CAPS

57

continued therapy. Keep physician informed.

- The appearance of mild erythema surrounding skin lesions may be an indication to reduce frequency of topical application. Consult with physician.
- Renal and hematologic status should be determined before therapy. During dosage regulation period, CBC, serum electrolytes (especially K, Mg, Na, Ca), and renal function tests (e.g., BUN, serum creatinine, creatinine clearance) including urinalysis are performed 2 or 3 times weekly, then at least weekly during therapy. Liver function tests are also done periodically throughout therapy.
- Adequate hydration and adjustment of daily dose reportedly are possible means of avoiding or minimizing nephrotoxicity. Consult physician for guidelines.
- Monitor I&O and weight. Report immediately oliguria, any change in I&O ratio and pattern, or appearance of urine, e.g., sediment, pink or cloudy urine (hematuria), abnormal renal function tests, unusual weight gain or loss. Generally, renal damage is reversible if drug is discontinued when first signs of renal dysfunction appear.
- If BUN exceeds 40 mg/dl or serum creatinine rises above 3 mg/dl, withhold drug and report to physician. Dosage should be reduced or drug discontinued until renal function improves.
- Hypokalemia occurs commonly and occasionally can be life threatening. Potassium supplementation is usually necessary. Monitor laboratory reports and observe for and report immediately the onset of possible signs of hypokalemia (see chap 3).
- The drug is potentially ototoxic. Report promptly any evidence of hearing loss or complaints of tinnitus, vertigo, or unsteady gait. Tinnitus may not be a complaint in the elderly or in the very young. Other signs of ototoxicity (i.e., vertigo or hearing loss) are more reliably reported in these age groups.

Patient & Family Education
- Notify physician if improvement does not occur within 1–2 wk or if lesions appear to worsen.
- Nail infections (onychomycoses) usually require several months or longer.
- Towels and clothing in contact with affected areas should be washed after each treatment.
- Topical cream slightly discolors the skin. Generally, lotion and ointment do not stain skin when rubbed in, but nail lesions may be stained.
- To remove cream or lotion from fabric, wash with soap and water. Ointment can be removed from fabric with a standard cleaning fluid.

ANTIBIOTIC: CEPHALOSPORIN, FIRST GENERATION

CEPHALOTHIN SODIUM
(sef-a´loe-thin)
Trade names: Keflin, Seffin
Classifications: ANTIINFECTIVE; BETA-LACTAM ANTIBIOTIC; FIRST GENERATION CEPHALOSPORIN
Pregnancy: Category B

ACTIONS/PHARMACODYNAMICS Semisynthetic first generation cephalosporin is derived from cephalosporin C, fermentation product of the fungus *Cephalosporium acremonium*. Drug structure characterized by a ß-lactam ring (like the penicillin structure). First generation cephalosporins are characterized by the most narrow gram-negative antibacterial spectrum and by the greatest antibacterial activity against gram-positive bacteria when compared to second and third generation agents. *Bactericidal action:* preferentially binds to one or more of the penicillin-binding proteins (PBP) located on cell walls of susceptible organisms. This inhibits third and final stage of bacterial wall synthesis, thus killing the bacterium. Active against gram-positive organisms including staphylococci, *Streptococcus pneumoniae*, beta-hemolytic streptococci, *Streptococcus faecalis;* and against gram-negative microbes including *Escherichia coli, Klebsiella* sp, *Proteus mirabilis;* variable activity on *Salmonella* sp, *Haemophilus influenzae, Shigella* sp, *Bacteroides fragilis,* and anaerobes.

USES Severe infections of respiratory, GI, and GU tracts; bone and joint infections, skin and soft tissue infections; and for septicemia, endocarditis, meningitis. Also used for perioperative prophylaxis in patients with high risk of infection. Used in intraperitoneal dialysis procedures. **Unlabeled use:** treatment of ventriculitis in hydrocephalic children.

PHARMACOKINETICS Peak levels: 30 min after IM; 15 min after IV. **Distribution:** poor CNS penetration except with inflamed meninges; penetrates aqueous humor and other body fluids; crosses placenta. **Elimination:** half-life: 30–60 min; 52–75% excreted unchanged in urine in 24 h; small amount excreted in breast milk.

ROUTE & DOSAGE

Moderate to Severe Infections

Adult	IV/IM	250 mg–2 g q4–6h, up to 2 g q4h (max 12 g/d)
Child	IV/IM	80–160 mg/kg/d in 4–6 divided doses

Surgical Prophylaxis

Adult	IV/IM	1–2 g 30–60 min before surgery, then q6h for 24 h
Child	IV/IM	20–30 mg/kg 30–60 min before surgery, then q6h for 24 h

CONTRAINDICATIONS & PRECAUTIONS Contraindicated in: hypersensitivity to cephalosporin. Safety for use during pregnancy (category B) not determined. Cautious use in: history of allergies to other β-lactams; impaired renal or hepatic function, patient on sodium restriction; nursing mothers; concomitant use of high doses of heparin; GI disease, especially colitis.

ADVERSE/SIDE EFFECTS CNS: dizziness, vertigo, headache, fatigue, malaise. GI: dysgeusia, glossitis, *nausea, vomiting,* anorexia, abdominal cramps, *diarrhea,* flatulence, pseudomembranous enterocolitis. Hematologic: neutropenia, leukopenia, pancytopenia, agranulocytosis, thrombocytopenia, hypoprothrombinemia, hemolytic anemia, positive direct Coombs' test. Hepatic: transient rise in ALT, AST, LDH, total bilirubin, and alkaline phosphatase. Hypersensitivity: morbilliform rash, pruritus, urticaria, serum sickness–like reactions, anaphylactic shock, eosinophilia, drug fever. Other: superinfections, especially *Pseudomonas* or *Candida;* local reactions: pain, induration, slough, abscess (IM site); thrombophlebitis (IV site).

DIAGNOSTIC TEST INTERFERENCES Most cephalosporins cause false-positive (black-brown or green-brown color) *urine glucose* reaction with copper reduction reagents, e.g., Benedict's or Clinitest, but not with enzymatic glucose oxidase reagents, e.g., Clinistix, Tes-Tape. With high doses, falsely elevated *serum and urine creatinine* (with Jaffe reaction) reported. False-positive direct Coombs' test (may interfere with *cross-matching procedures* and *hematologic studies*), false-positive *urinary protein* (sulfosalicylic acid method), and falsely elevated *urinary 17-ketosteroids* (Zimmerman reaction) have also been reported.

DRUG INTERACTIONS Probenecid decreases renal elimination.

INCOMPATIBILITIES Solution/additive: AMINOGLYCOSIDES, aminophylline, bleomycin, cimetidine, colistimethate, cytarabine, diphenhydramine, dopamine, methylprednisolone, calcium chloride, calcium gluceptate, calcium gluconate, erythromycin, TETRACYCLINES, penicillin G, phenobarbital, polymyxin B, metoclopramide. Y-site: AMINOGLYCOSIDES, cytarabine, erythromycin, TETRACYCLINES, polymyxin B, metoclopramide.

NURSING IMPLICATIONS

Administration

- **Reconstitution of IV solutions:** dilute each 1 g with at least 10 ml sterile water for injection. Reconstituted solution may be further diluted with IV solution recommended by manufacturer.
- IV cephalothin may be given by direct IV at a rate of 1 g over 3–5 min or by intermittent infusion.
- Risk of phlebitis may be reduced by use of a small needle in a large vein for IV administration.
- IM injection is prepared by adding 4 ml sterile water for injection to each gram of cephalothin (resultant solution: 500 mg/2.2 ml). If vial contents do not completely dissolve, add more diluent (0.2–0.4 ml), and warm vial slightly.
- IM injection causes intense pain and induration. If cephalothin IM is prescribed, administer injection deep into large muscle mass such as gluteus maximus or lateral aspect of thigh. Rotate injection sites.
- Solutions for IM and intermittent IV infusion (may be stored at room temperature) should be administered within 12 h after reconstitution. Replace freshly prepared solution every 24 h in prolonged treatment with IV infusion.
- Slight discoloration of solution may occur, especially when stored at room temperature; however, this does not affect potency.
- Refrigeration protects potency for 96 h after reconstitution.

Assessment & Drug Effects

- Culture and sensitivity tests should be performed before and during therapy. Therapy may be started pending test results.
- Before therapy is initiated, determine history of hypersensitivity to cephalosporins or penicillins, other allergies, particularly to drugs.
- Observe IV sites for evidence of inflammatory reaction. IV infusions of doses larger than 6 g/d for > 3 d can result in thrombophlebitis.
- Report falling urinary output or change in I&O ratio. Patients with renal dysfunction and those re-

Common side effects in *italic*; life-threatening effects underlined; generic names in **bold**; classifications in SMALL CAPS

59

ceiving high doses in the presence of dehydration are particularly susceptible to nephrotoxic reactions.

- Superinfections caused by overgrowth of nonsusceptible organisms may occur, particularly during prolonged use of cephalosporins.
- Antibiotic-associated pseudomembranous enterocolitis is a life-threatening superinfection caused by *Clostridium difficile;* may occur in 4–9 d or as long as 6 wk after cephalothin is discontinued. Most apt to occur in the chronically ill or debilitated elderly patient, especially if undergoing abdominal surgery or if in an intensive care unit.
- If diarrhea occurs, check for fever. Report diarrhea and fever promptly.
- Periodic hematologic studies including PT and PTT and evaluations of renal and hepatic functions are recommended in patients receiving high doses and during prolonged therapy.
- If an unexplained fever develops, check temperature twice daily. If temperature remains high, suspect drug-induced fever. Discuss with physician.

Patient & Family Education

- Report early signs of superinfections (see chap 3).
- Report loose stools or diarrhea promptly.
- Yogurt or buttermilk, 120 ml (4 oz) of either (if allowed), may serve as a prophylactic against intestinal superinfection by helping to maintain normal intestinal flora.
- Signs and symptoms of hypersensitivity reaction (see chap 3) should be reported promptly. Drug should be discontinued.
- Advise patient to report signs of hemostatic defects (ecchymoses, petechiae, nose bleeds).

ANTIBIOTIC: CEPHALOSPORIN, SECOND GENERATION

CEFONICID SODIUM

(se-fon´i-sid)
Trade name: Monocid
Classifications: ANTIINFECTIVE; BETA-LACTAM ANTIBIOTIC; SECOND GENERATION CEPHALOSPORIN
Pregnancy: Category B

ACTIONS/PHARMACODYNAMICS Semisynthetic, second generation cephalosporin antibiotic with drug structure characterized by a ß-lactam ring

(like the penicillin structure); generally resistant to hydrolysis by ß-lactamases. Preferentially binds to one or more of the penicillin-binding proteins (PBP) located on cell walls of susceptible organisms. This inhibits third and final stage of bacterial wall synthesis, thus killing the bacterium. Second generation cephalosporins are usually active against the organisms susceptible to first generation cephalosporins. In addition they are active against Haemophilus influenzae, Providencia sp, Clostridium sp, Peptococcus sp, and against some strains of Citrobacter, Enterobacter, Serratia, Neisseria, Proteus, Escherichia coli, and Klebsiella that are resistant to first generation cephalosporins. Second generation agents are generally inactive against enterococci, methicillin-resistant staphylococci, Acinetobacter, Listeria monocytogenes, and Pseudomonas. Partial cross-allergenicity between penicillins and cephalosporins has been reported; also, tolerance to cefonicid's bactericidal effects has been displayed in some strains of gram-positive cocci including Staphylococcus aureus and group B streptococci. Cefonicid has not been associated with hemostatic defects.

USES Moderate to severe infections such as septicemia, infections of lower respiratory tract, bones and joints, skin and skin structures, and urinary tract (UTI). Also used for perioperative prophylaxis. **Unlabeled use:** uncomplicated gonorrhea.

ROUTE & DOSAGE

Moderate to Severe Infections

Adult	IV/IM	1 g q24h, up to 2 g/24 h

Surgical Prophylaxis

Adult	IV/IM	1 g 60 min before surgery

PHARMACOKINETICS Peak levels: 1 h after IM; 5 min after IV. **Distribution:** poor CNS penetration even with inflamed meninges; crosses placenta. **Metabolism:** not metabolized. **Elimination:** half-life: 3.5–5.8 h; 90–99% excreted unchanged in urine within 24 h; small amount excreted in breast milk.

CONTRAINDICATIONS & PRECAUTIONS Contraindicated in: hypersensitivity to cephalosporins and related antibiotics; severely impaired renal or hepatic function. Safe use during pregnancy (category B) and in children not established. **Cautious use in:** nursing mothers, patient with history of delayed-type reaction to penicillins or other drugs; GI disease, especially colitis.

Common side effects in *italic*; life-threatening effects <u>underlined</u>; generic names in **bold**; classifications in SMALL CAPS

ADVERSE/SIDE EFFECTS GI: Nausea, vomiting, *diarrhea*, pseudomembranous enterocolitis. **Hematologic:** elevations of: BUN, serum creatinine, liver function tests: alkaline phosphatase, AST, ALT, LDH; elevated platelet counts, leukopenia, neutropenia positive Coombs' test, eosinophilia, anemia. **Hypersensitivity:** fever, rash, pruritus, erythema, myalgia, anaphylactoid reaction. **Other:** pain with IM injection; burning sensation, phlebitis (IV administration), flulike syndrome, superinfections (by *Candida, Pseudomonas, Enterobacter* sp).

DIAGNOSTIC TEST INTERFERENCES A false-positive reaction for ***urine glucose*** may occur with copper sulfate reduction reagents, e.g., Benedict's or Clinitest; tests based on glucose oxidase reactions are apparently not affected, e.g., TesTape, Clinistix, Diastix.

DRUG INTERACTIONS Probenecid decreases renal elimination.

INCOMPATIBILITIES Solution/additive: AMINOGLYCOSIDES. **Y-site:** AMINOGLYCOSIDES.

NURSING IMPLICATIONS

Administration

- *Single dose IM or direct (bolus) IV injection:* reconstitute with sterile water for injection and shake well to assure complete dissolution of drug; 500 mg of drug to 2 ml diluent gives about 220 mg/ml; 1 g drug to 2.5 ml diluent gives about 325 mg/ml. After reconstitution, inspect for particulate matter; if present, discard solution.
- *IV infusion:* dilute reconstituted cefonicid in 50–100 ml 0.9% NaCl injection, Ringer's injection, or other diluent suggested by manufacturer.
- Direct (bolus) IV injections of reconstituted solution should be made slowly over 3–5 min. Injection may be made directly or through IV tubing if patient is receiving a compatible parenteral fluid recommended by manufacturer. Examine IV site daily for evidence of inflammation.
- IM injections should be made deeply into large muscle mass. Pain and discomfort at IM site occurs commonly. If dose is 2 g, give 1/2 dose in different large muscle masses. Rotate injection sites.
- When cefonicid is given for prophylaxis during ce-

sarean section, it is administered only after umbilical cord has been clamped.
- After reconstitution or dilution, solutions are stable for 24 h at room temperature or 72 h if refrigerated 5C (41F). Slight yellowing does not indicate loss of potency.

Assessment & Drug Effects

- Culture and susceptibility tests should be performed before and periodically during therapy, if indicated. Therapy may be initiated before test results are available.
- Before therapy begins, determine history of hypersensitivity to cephalosporins, penicillins, or other drugs.
- Although cephalosporins may be used in individuals with history of hypersensitivity to penicillin, they should not be used if individual has experienced an immediate reaction to penicillin, such as bronchospasm, urticaria, angioedema.
- Monitor I&O ratio and pattern, particularly in patients with impaired renal function, patients > 50 y, or who are receiving high doses.
- Monitor temperature. Report temperature alterations and the onset of flulike symptoms (chills, malaise).
- Superinfections caused by overgrowth of nonsusceptible organisms may occur, particularly during prolonged use of cephalosporins.
- Antibiotic-associated pseudomembranous enterocolitis is a life-threatening superinfection caused by *Clostridium difficile;* may occur in 4–9 d or as long as 6 wk after cephalothin is discontinued. Most apt to occur in the chronically ill or debilitated elderly patient, especially if undergoing abdominal surgery or if in an intensive care unit.
- If diarrhea occurs, check for fever. Report diarrhea and fever promptly.
- Periodic hematologic studies including PT and PTT and evaluations of renal and hepatic functions are recommended in patients receiving high doses and during prolonged therapy.

Patient & Family Education

- Superinfections caused by overgrowth of nonsusceptible organisms may occur, particularly during prolonged use of cephalosporins. Report early signs and symptoms (see chap 3) promptly.
- Instruct patient to report loose stools or diarrhea.
- Yogurt or buttermilk, 120 ml (4 oz) of either (if allowed), may serve as a prophylactic against intestinal superinfection by helping to maintain normal intestinal flora.

Common side effects in *italic*; life-threatening effects underlined; generic names in **bold**; classifications in SMALL CAPS

61

ANTIBIOTIC: CEPHALOSPORIN, THIRD GENERATION

CEFOTAXIME SODIUM

(sef-oh-taks´eem)

Trade name: Claforan

Classifications: ANTIINFECTIVE; BETA-LACTAM ANTIBIOTIC; CEPHALOSPORIN, THIRD GENERATION

Pregnancy: Category B

for gonococcal ophthalmia caused by PPNG in adults, children, and neonates.

ROUTE & DOSAGE

Moderate to Severe Infections

Adult	IV/IM	1–2 g q8–12h, up to 2 g q4h (max 12 g/d)
Child	IV/IM	≤1 wk: 50 mg/kg q12h
		1–4 wk: 50 mg/kg q8h
		1 mo–12 y: 50–180 mg/kg/d in 4–6 divided doses

Surgical Prophylaxis

Adult	IV/IM	1 g 30–90 min before surgery

ACTIONS/PHARMACODYNAMICS Broadspectrum semisynthetic third generation cephalosporin antibiotic. Preferentially binds to one or more of the penicillin-binding proteins (PBP) located on cell walls of susceptible organisms. This inhibits third and final stage of bacterial cell wall synthesis, thus killing the bacterium. Generally active against a wide variety of gram-negative bacteria including most of the Enterobacteriaceae. Also active against some organisms resistant to first and second generation cephalosporins and currently available aminoglycoside antibiotics and penicillins, e.g., *Escherichia coli, Klebsiella pneumoniae,* and *Serratia marcescens.* Other susceptible organisms: *Bacteroides fragilis, Morganella morganii, Proteus mirabilis, Salmonella, Shigella, Haemophilus influenzae, Neisseria gonorrhoeae,* groups A and B streptococci, *Staphylococcus aureus, Bacteroides, Eubacterium, Peptostreptococcus,* and *Peptococcus.* Inhibits some strains of *Clostridium,* but *C. difficile* is resistant to the drug, as is *Listeria monocytogenes.* Partial cross-allergenicity between penicillins and cephalosporins has been reported. Cefotaxime and the aminoglycosides are potentially incompatible.

USES Serious infections of lower respiratory tract, skin and skin structures, bones and joints, CNS (including meningitis and ventriculitis), gynecologic and GU tract infections, including uncomplicated gonococcal infections caused by penicillinase-producing *Neisseria gonorrhoeae* (PPNG). Also used to treat bacteremia or septicemia, intraabdominal infections, and for perioperative prophylaxis. **Unlabeled uses:** currently recommended by CDC for treatment of disseminated gonococcal infections (gonococcal arthritis-dermatitis syndrome) and as drug of choice

PHARMACOKINETICS Peak levels: 30 min after IM; 5 min after IV. **Distribution:** CNS penetration except with inflamed meninges; also penetrates aqueous humor, ascitic and prostatic fluids; crosses placenta. **Metabolism:** partially metabolized in liver to active metabolites. **Elimination:** half-life: 1 h; 50–60% excreted unchanged in urine in 24 h; small amount excreted in breast milk.

CONTRAINDICATIONS & PRECAUTIONS Contraindicated in: hypersensitivity to cephalosporins and other ß-lactam antibiotics. Safe use during pregnancy (category B) not established. **Cautious use in:** history of type I hypersensitivity reactions to penicillins; history of allergy to other ß-lactams; renal impairment; history of colitis or other GI disease; nursing mothers.

ADVERSE/SIDE EFFECTS GI: nausea, vomiting, *diarrhea,* abdominal pain, colitis, pseudomembranous colitis, anorexia. **Hematologic:** transient leukopenia, granulocytopenia, thrombocytopenia, neutropenia, eosinophilia, positive direct Coombs' test, transient increases in BUN and serum creatinine concentrations. **Hypersensitivity:** rash, pruritus, fever. **Other:** nocturnal perspiration; *IV site reactions:* inflammatory reaction, phlebitis, thrombophlebitis; *IM site:* pain, induration, and tenderness. Also, superinfections, transient increases in serum AST, ALT, LDH, bilirubin, alkaline phosphatase concentrations.

DIAGNOSTIC TEST INTERFERENCES May cause falsely elevated *serum* or *urine creatinine* values (Jaffe reaction). False-positive reactions for *urine glucose* have not been reported using copper sulfate reduction methods, e.g., Benedict's, Clinitest;

Common side effects in *italic*; life-threatening effects underlined; generic names in **bold**; classifications in SMALL CAPS

however, since it has occurred with other cephalosporins, it may be advisable to use glucose oxidase tests (Clinistix, Tes-Tape, Diastix). Positive direct antiglobulin (Coombs') test results may interfere with hematologic studies and cross matching procedures.

DRUG INTERACTIONS Probenecid decreases renal elimination; **alcohol** produces disulfiram reaction.

INCOMPATIBILITIES Solution/additive: AMINOGLYCOSIDES, **aminophylline, sodium bicarbonate. Y-site:** AMINOGLYCOSIDES, **doxapram, aminophylline, sodium bicarbonate.**

NURSING IMPLICATIONS

Administration

- Follow manufacturer's suggestions concerning appropriate diluents. **IM injections:** add 3 ml diluent to vial containing 1 g drug providing a solution of approximately 300 mg cefotaxime/ml. Administer IM injection deeply into large muscle mass (e.g., upper outer quadrant of gluteus maximus). Aspirate to avoid inadvertent injection into blood vessel. If IM dose is 2 g, divide dose and administer into 2 different sites.
- **IV infusion:** add 50 or 100 ml diluent to 1 or 2 g drug. Generally intermittent IV infusion is infused over 20–30 min, preferably via butterfly or scalp vein–type needles.
- **IV injection:** add 10 ml diluent to vial with 1 or 2 g drug providing a solution containing 95 or 180 mg cefotaxime/ml, respectively. Inject directly into vein over 3–5 min period or slowly into tubing of freely flowing compatible IV solution.
- Do not admix cefotaxime with sodium bicarbonate or any fluid with a pH > 7.5 or with an aminoglycoside.
- Risk of phlebitis may be reduced by use of a small needle in a large vein.
- Cefotaxime therapy should continue for at least 48–72 h after patient becomes afebrile or other signs of infection have disappeared. Therapy for group A beta-hemolytic streptococci should be continued for a minimum of 10 d to reduce risk of glomerulonephritis and rheumatic fever.
- Storage. **Dry powder:** preferably at 15–30C (59–86F), unless otherwise directed by manufacturer. Protect from excessive light. **Reconstituted solutions:** may be stored in original containers for 24 h at room temperature at 15–30C (59–86F); for 10 days under refrigeration at 5C (41F) or less, or for at least 13 wk in frozen state.

Assessment & Drug Effects

- Culture and susceptibility tests should be performed before initiation of therapy and periodically during therapy, if indicated. Therapy may be instituted pending test results.
- Before therapy is initiated, determine previous hypersensitivity reactions to cephalosporins, penicillins, and history of other allergies, particularly to drugs.
- Report change in I&O ratio and pattern in patients with impaired renal function or with chronic UTI or who are receiving high dosages or an aminoglycoside concomitantly. Renal status (serum creatinine, creatinine clearance, BUN) should be evaluated at regular intervals during therapy and for several months after drug has been discontinued.
- Superinfection due to overgrowth of nonsusceptible organisms may occur, particularly with prolonged therapy.
- Report onset of diarrhea promptly. Check for fever. If diarrhea is mild, discontinuation of cefotaxime may be sufficient.
- If diarrhea is severe, suspect antibiotic-associated pseudomembranous colitis, a life-threatening superinfection (may occur in 4–9 d or as long as 6 wk after cephalosporin therapy is discontinued). Chronically ill or debilitated elderly patients undergoing abdominal surgery or those in an intensive care unit are most vulnerable.
- Periodic hematologic studies (including PT and PTT) and evaluation of renal and hepatic functions are recommended with high doses or prolonged therapy.

Patient & Family Education

- Superinfections caused by overgrowth of nonsusceptible organisms may occur, particularly during prolonged use. Report early signs and symptoms promptly.
- Yogurt or buttermilk, 120 ml (4 oz) of either (if allowed), may serve as a prophylactic against intestinal superinfection by helping to maintain normal intestinal flora.
- Report loose stools or diarrhea.

ANTIBIOTIC: CLINDAMYCIN

CLINDAMYCIN HYDROCHLORIDE

(klin-da-mye´sin)
Trade name: Cleocin Hydrochloride

CLINDAMYCIN PALMITATE HYDROCHLORIDE

Trade name: Cleocin Pediatric

CLINDAMYCIN PHOSPHATE

Trade names: Cleocin Phosphate, Cleocin T,
Dalacin C
Classifications: ANTIINFECTIVE; ANTIBIOTIC;
SKIN AGENT; ANTIACNE
Pregnancy: Category B

ACTIONS/PHARMACODYNAMICS Semisynthetic derivative of lincomycin with which it shares neuromuscular blocking properties and other actions. Reported to have greater degree of antibacterial activity in vitro, better absorption, and lower incidence of GI side effects than lincomycin. Suppresses protein synthesis by binding to 50 S subunits of bacterial ribosomes, and therefore inhibits other antibiotics (e.g., erythromycin) that act at this site. Particularly effective against susceptible strains of anaerobic streptococci, *Bacteroides* (especially *B. fragilis*), *Fusobacterium, Actinomyces israelii, Peptococcus,* and *Clostridium* sp. Also effective against aerobic gram-positive cocci, including *Staphylococcus aureus, Staphylococcus epidermidis,* streptococci (except *S. faecalis*), and pneumococci.

USES Serious infections when less toxic alternatives are inappropriate. Topical applications are used in treatment of acne vulgaris. **Unlabeled uses:** in combination with pyrimethamine for toxoplasmosis in patients with AIDS.

ROUTE & DOSAGE

Moderate to Severe Infections

Adult	PO	150–450 mg q6h
	IM/IV	300–900 mg q6–8h (max 2700 mg/d)
Child	PO	8–25 mg/kg/d q6–8h
	IM/IV	15–40 mg/kg/d q6–8h

Acne Vulgaris

Adult	Topical	Apply to affected areas b.i.d.

PHARMACOKINETICS Absorption: approximately 90% absorbed from GI tract; 10% of topical application is absorbed through skin. **Peak:** 45–60 min PO; 3 h IM. **Duration:** 6 h PO; 8–12 h IM. **Distribution:** widely distributed except for CNS; crosses placenta; distributed into breast milk. **Metabolism:** metabolized in liver. **Elimination:** half-life: 2–3 h; excreted in urine and feces.

CONTRAINDICATIONS & PRECAUTIONS Contraindicated in: history of hypersensitivity to clindamycin or lincomycin; history of regional enteritis, ulcerative colitis, or antibiotic-associated colitis. Safe use during pregnancy (category B) and in nursing mothers not established. Not recommended for infants <1 mo. **Cautious use in:** history of GI disease, renal or hepatic disease; atopic individuals (history of eczema, asthma, hay fever); older patients.

ADVERSE/SIDE EFFECTS GI: *diarrhea,* abdominal pain, flatulence, bloating, *nausea, vomiting,* <u>pseudomembranous colitis</u>; esophageal irritation, loss of taste, medicinal taste (high IV doses). **Hematologic:** leukopenia, eosinophilia, <u>agranulocytosis</u>, thrombocytopenia. **Hepatic:** jaundice, abnormal liver function tests. **Hypersensitivity:** *skin rashes,* urticaria, pruritus, fever, serum sickness. **Skin:** dryness, contact dermatitis, gram-negative folliculitis, irritation, oily skin. **Other:** sensitization, swelling of face (following topical use); hypotension (following IM), cardiac arrest (rapid IV), generalized myalgia, superinfections, proctitis, vaginitis. **Local reactions:** pain, induration, sterile abscess (following IM injections); thrombophlebitis (IV infusion).

DIAGNOSTIC TEST INTERFERENCES Clindamycin may cause increases in *serum alkaline phosphatase, bilirubin, creatine phosphokinase* (CPK) from muscle irritation following IM injection; *AST, ALT.*

DRUG INTERACTIONS Chloramphenicol, erythromycin possibly are mutually antagonistic to clindamycin; neuromuscular blocking action enhanced by NEUROMUSCULAR BLOCKING AGENTS **(atracurium, tubocurarine, pancuronium).**

INCOMPATIBILITIES Solution/Additive: ceftriaxone, ranitidine, tobramycin.

Common side effects in *italic*; life-threatening effects <u>underlined</u>; generic names in **bold**; classifications in SMALL CAPS

NURSING IMPLICATIONS

Administration

- Determine history of any previous sensitivities to drugs or other allergens.
- Administer clindamycin capsules with a full (240 ml [8 oz]) glass of water to prevent esophagitis.
- Absorption of oral clindamycin is not significantly affected by food or gastric acid, although peak serum levels may be somewhat delayed.
- Note expiration date of oral solution; retains potency for 14 d at room temperature. Do not refrigerate, as chilling causes thickening and thus makes pouring it difficult.
- Deep IM injection is recommended. Rotate injection sites and observe daily for evidence of inflammatory reaction. Single IM doses should not exceed 600 mg.
- IV clindamycin is never given as a bolus dose. The infusion should not exceed 1200 mg in 1 h. Prescribed continuous flow rate is slow to minimize risk of cardiac arrhythmias.
- Follow manufacturer's directions for reconstituting the parenteral drug, for storage time, compatible IV fluids, and IV infusion rates. Reportedly, local reactions following IV administration can be minimized by avoiding prolonged use of indwelling catheters.
- Store in tight containers at 15–30C (59–86F) unless otherwise directed.

Assessment & Drug Effects

- Culture and susceptibility testing should be performed initially and periodically during therapy.
- Monitor BP and pulse in patients receiving drug parenterally. Hypotension has occurred following IM injection. Advise patient to remain recumbent following drug administration until BP has stabilized.
- Severe diarrhea and colitis, including pseudomembranous colitis, have been associated with oral (highest incidence), parenteral, and topical clindamycin. Report immediately the onset of watery diarrhea, with or without fever; passage of tarry or bloody stools, pus, intestinal tissue, or mucus; abdominal cramps, or ileus. Symptoms may appear within a few days to 2 wk after therapy is begun or up to several weeks following cessation of therapy.
- Elderly and bedridden patients are at a higher risk of developing severe colitis and therefore should be closely observed.
- Be alert to signs of superinfection (see chap 3).
- Be alert for signs of anaphylactoid reactions (see chap 3), which require immediate attention.

Patient & Family Education

- Instruct patient to take drug for the full course of therapy as prescribed.
- Instruct patient to report loose stools or diarrhea promptly.
- Drug therapy is stopped if patient develops significant diarrhea (more than 5 loose stools daily).
- Antiperistaltic agents may prolong and worsen diarrhea by delaying removal of toxins from colon. Advise patient not to self-medicate with antidiarrheal preparations.
- Patients using topical preparation for acne should be instructed to discontinue other acne preparations unless otherwise directed by physician. Advise patient to keep medication away from eyes.
- Since 10% absorption of topical medication is possible, instruct patient to report the onset of systemic reactions to physician.

ANTIBIOTIC: ERYTHROMYCIN

ERYTHROMYCIN

(er-ith-roe-mye´sin)
Trade names: Akne-Mycin Ery-Tab, Apo-Erythro Base, A/T/S, E-Mycin, Eryc, EryDerm, Erythrocin, Erythromid, Erythromycin Base, Ilotycin, Novorythro, Robimycin, RP-Mycin, Staticin, T-Stat
Classifications: ANTIINFECTIVE; ERYTHROMYCIN ANTIBIOTIC; SKIN AGENT; ANTIACNE
Pregnancy: Category B

ACTIONS/PHARMACODYNAMICS Macrolide antibiotic produced by a strain of *Streptomyces erythreus.* Considered one of the safest antibiotics in use today. Bacteriostatic or bactericidal, depending on nature of organism and drug concentration used. Antibacterial spectrum is similar to but broader than that of penicillin; commonly used as penicillin substitute in hypersensitive patients for infections not requiring high antibiotic blood levels. More active against gram-positive than gram-negative bacteria. Effectiveness against *Chlamydia trachomatis* is basis for its topical use in prophylaxis of neonatal inclusion conjunctivitis. Acts by inhibiting protein synthesis of sensitive microorganisms. Resistant mutants are especially frequent among staphylococci.

USES Pneumococcal pneumonia, *Mycoplasma pneumoniae* (primary atypical pneumonia), acute

Common side effects in *italic*; life-threatening effects underlined; generic names in **bold**; classifications in SMALL CAPS

65

pelvic inflammatory disease caused by *Neisseria gonorrhoeae* in females sensitive to penicillin, infections caused by susceptible strains of staphylococci, streptococci, and certain strains of *Haemophilus influenzae*. Also used in intestinal amebiasis, Legionnaires disease, uncomplicated urethral, endocervical, and rectal infections caused by *Chlamydia trachomatis*, for prophylaxis of ophthalmia neonatorum caused by *N. gonorrhoeae*, *C. trachomatis*, and for chlamydial conjunctivitis in neonates. Considered an acceptable alternative to penicillin for treatment of streptococcal pharyngitis, for prophylaxis of rheumatic fever and bacterial endocarditis, for treatment of diphtheria as adjunct to antitoxin and for carrier state, and as alternate choice in treatment of primary syphilis in patients allergic to penicillins. **Topical applications:** pyodermas, acne vulgaris, and external ocular infections, including neonatal chlamydial conjunctivitis and gonococcal ophthalmia.

ROUTE & DOSAGE

Moderate to Severe Infections

Adult	PO	250–500 mg q6h; 333 mg q8h
	IV	250–1000 mg q6h
Child	PO	30–50 mg/kg/d divided q6h
	IV	15–20 mg/kg/d in 4 divided doses
	Topical	Apply ointment to infected eye 1 or more times/d

Prophylaxis for Streptococcal Infections

Adult	IV	250 mg b.i.d. *or* 1 g/1 h before procedure, then 500 mg q6h for 8 doses
Child	IV	20 mg/kg 1 h before procedure, then 10 mg/kg q6h for 8 doses

Chlamydia trachomatis Infections

Adult	PO	500 mg q.i.d. *or* 666 mg q8h
Child	Topical	Apply 0.5–1 cm ribbon in lower conjunctival sacs shortly after birth

PHARMACOKINETICS Absorption: erythromycin base is acid labile; most erythromycins are absorbed in small intestine. **Peak:** 1–4 h PO. **Distribution:** widely distributed to most body tissues; low concentrations in CSF; concentrates in liver and bile; crosses placenta. **Metabolism:** partially metabolized in liver. **Elimination:** half-life: 1.5–2 h; primarily excreted in bile; excreted in breast milk.

CONTRAINDICATIONS & PRECAUTIONS Contraindicated in: hypersensitivity to erythromycins. Safe use during pregnancy not established. **Cautious use in:** impaired hepatic function.

ADVERSE/SIDE EFFECTS GI: *nausea, vomiting, abdominal cramping,* diarrhea, heartburn, anorexia. **Hypersensitivity reactions:** fever, eosinophilia, urticaria, skin eruptions, fixed drug eruption, anaphylaxis. **CNS:** ototoxicity: reversible bilateral hearing loss, tinnitus, vertigo. **Other:** superinfections by nonsusceptible bacteria, yeasts, or fungi. **Topical:** erythema, desquamation, burning, tenderness, dryness or oiliness, pruritus.

DIAGNOSTIC TEST INTERFERENCES False elevations of **urinary catecholamines, urinary steroids,** and AST (SGOT), ALT (SGPT) (by colorimetric methods).

DRUG INTERACTIONS Serum levels and toxicities of **carbamazepine, cyclosporine, digoxin, theophylline, triazolam, warfarin** increased. **Ergotamine** may increase peripheral vasospasm.

INCOMPATIBILITIES Solution/additive: amino-phylline, TETRACYCLINES, **pentobarbital, secobarbital, streptomycin, heparin, cephalothin, colistimethate, metaraminol, metoclopramide**, vitamin B complex with C, **ampicillin**.

NURSING IMPLICATIONS

Administration

- Activity of erythromycin may be decreased in acid medium and by the presence of food in the stomach. Administered preferably on an empty stomach 1 h before or 3 h after meals. Do not give with, or immediately before or after, fruit juices, and advise patient not to crush or chew tablets.
- Enteric-coated tablets may be given without regard to meals.
- When switching from tablet to a PO liquid preparation, dosing may require adjustment.
- Before receiving erythromycin for gonorrhea, patients suspected of having syphilis should have microscopic examination for *Treponema pallidum* and monthly serologic tests for a minimum of 4 mo.
- In treatment of primary syphilis, spinal fluid should be examined before treatment and as part of follow-up after therapy.
- *Prophylaxis: neonatal eye infection:* ribbon of ointment approximately 0.5–1 cm long is placed into lower conjunctival sac of neonate shortly after birth. Use a new tube of erythromycin for each neonate.

Common side effects in *italic*; life-threatening effects underlined; generic names in **bold**; classifications in SMALL CAPS

- **For topical applications to skin:** Consult physician about procedure to use for cleaning affected area prior to each application.
- Ointment preparation for skin problems should not be used in eyes or in external ear if eardrum is perforated. Drug should be discontinued if signs of sensitivity or irritation appear.
- For treatment of eye infections, use only preparations labeled for ophthalmic use.
- Store in tightly capped containers preferably between 15–30C (59–86F) unless otherwise directed by manufacturer.

Assessment & Drug Effects

- GI symptoms after PO administration are dose related. Report their onset to physician. If symptoms persist after dosage reduction, physician may prescribe drug to be given with meals in spite of impaired absorption.
- Pseudomembranous colitis, (see chap 3), a potentially life-threatening condition, may occur during or after antibiotic therapy.
- Observe for symptoms of superinfection by overgrowth of nonsusceptible bacteria or fungi. Emergence of resistant staphylococcal strains is highly predictable during prolonged therapy.
- Hepatic function tests should be performed periodically during prolonged drug regimens.
- Hepatotoxicity is believed to be a hypersensitivity reaction. Premonitory signs and symptoms may include abdominal pain, nausea, vomiting, fever, leukocytosis, and eosinophilia Jaundice may or may not be present.
- Symptoms of hepatotoxicity may appear a few days after initiation of drug but usually occur after 1–2 wk of continuous therapy. Symptoms are reversible with prompt discontinuation of erythromycin.
- Ototoxicity can occur with all forms of erythromycin. The reaction appears to develop most frequently in patients receiving 4 g/d or more, the elderly, female patients, and patients with renal or hepatic dysfunction. It is reversible with prompt discontinuation of drug.

Patient & Family Education

- Watch for signs and symptoms of superinfection (see Chapter 3). Report immediately.
- Observe for signs and symptoms of pseudomembranous colitis (see Chapter 3), which may occur even after drug is discontinued. Report immediately.
- Advise patient to report any ototoxic effects including dizziness, vertigo, nausea, tinnitus, roaring noises, hearing impairment (see Chapter 3).

ANTIBIOTIC: OTHER BETA-LACTAM

IMIPENEM CILASTATIN SODIUM

(i-mi-pen´em) (sye-lo-stat´in)
Trade name: Primaxin
Classifications: ANTIINFECTIVE; BETA-LACTAM ANTIBIOTIC
Pregnancy: Category C

ACTIONS/PHARMACODYNAMICS Fixed combination of imipenem, a beta-lactam antibiotic, and cilastatin, an inhibitor of dipeptidase inactivation of imipenem. Concomitant use prevents renal metabolism of imipenem, resulting in its higher urinary concentrations and decreased imipenem-induced proximal renal tubular necrosis. Action of imipenem: inhibition of mucopeptide synthesis in bacterial cell walls leading to cell death. Also may have a postantibiotic inhibitory effect. After exposure of susceptible organisms to imipenem these organisms do not immediately resume growth after drug is removed. Has the greatest microbiologic spectrum of any beta-lactam antibiotic, surpassing that of all the third-generation cephalosporins. Has high degree of stability in presence of beta-lactamases and is bactericidal against 90% or more of the clinically important bacterial pathogens. Acts synergistically with aminoglycoside antibiotics against some isolates of *Pseudomonas aeruginosa.* Infections resistant to cephalosporins, penicillins, and aminoglycosides have responded to treatment with this combination. Partial cross-allergenicity among penicillins and other beta-lactams has been reported.

USES Treatment of serious infections caused by susceptible organisms in the urinary tract, lower respiratory tract, bones and joints, skin and skin structures; also intraabdominal, gynecologic, and mixed infections; bacterial septicemia and endocarditis.

ROUTE & DOSAGE

Serious Infections

Adult	IV	250–500 mg infused over 20–30 min q6–8h; up to 1 g infused over 40–60 min q6h
	IM	500 or 750 mg q12h
Child	IV	15–25 mg/kg q6h
	IM	15–25 mg/kg q12h

Common side effects in *italic*; life-threatening effects underlined; generic names in **bold**; classifications in SMALL CAPS

67

PHARMACOKINETICS **Distribution:** widely distributed; limited concentrations in CSF; crosses placenta; in breast milk. **Elimination:** half-life: 1 h; 70% of dose excreted in urine within 10 h.

CONTRAINDICATIONS & PRECAUTIONS Contraindicated in: hypersensitivity to any component of product, multiple allergens. Safe use in pregnancy (category C) or in children <12 y not established. **Cautious use in:** nursing mothers, patient with CNS disorders (e.g., seizures, brain lesions, history of recent head injury); renal impairment; patients with history of penicillin allergies.

ADVERSE/SIDE EFFECTS CNS: seizures, dizziness, confusion, somnolence, encephalopathy, myoclonus, tremors, paresthesia, headache. **CV:** (rare): palpitation, hypotension, tachycardia. **GI:** *nausea, vomiting,* diarrhea, pseudomembranous colitis, hemorrhagic colitis, gastroenteritis, abdominal pain, glossitis, tongue papillae hypertrophy, heartburn. **Hypersensitivity:** rash, fever, chills, dyspnea, pruritus. **Respiratory:** chest discomfort, hyperventilation, dyspnea. **Skin:** rash, pruritus, urticaria, candidiasis, flushing, increased sweating, skin texture change, facial edema. **Other:** hyponatremia, hyperkalemia, transient hearing loss, tinnitus (rare); weakness, oliguria/anuria, polyuria, polyarthralgia; *phlebitis and pain at injection site.* Altered laboratory findings: increased WBC, AST, ALT, alkaline phosphatase, BUN, LDH, creatinine; decreased Hgb, Hct, eosinophilia. Causal relationship not established: increase or decrease in platelets, positive Coombs' test, abnormal PT, superinfections.

DRUG INTERACTIONS aztreonam, cephalosporins, penicillins may antagonize the antibacterial effects.

INCOMPATIBILITIES **Solution/additive:** Ringer's lactate, stable in dextrose-containing solutions for only 4 h.

NURSING IMPLICATIONS

Administration

▪ Follow manufacturer's recommendation for preparation of infusion solution. Dilute each dose with 10 ml of D5W, NS, or other compatible infusion solution. After reconstitution the resulting solution contains 2.5 mg/ml, or 5 mg/ml. Agitate the solution until clear. Color should range from colorless to yellow. Further dilute with 100 ml of selected infusion solution.

▪ *Caution:* imipenem-cilastatin is not intended for direct or bolus injection. Administer each 500 mg or fraction thereof over 20–30 min.

▪ Nausea appears to be related to infusion rate, and if it presents during infusion, slow the rate. Occurs most frequently with 1-g doses.

▪ If aminoglycoside is administered concomitantly, do not admix, but administer from separate containers through same IV tubing. Inspect solution visually before administration for particulate matter. Do not administer if particulate matter is present.

▪ Stability of IV solutions depends on diluent used for reconstitution. Consult manufacturer's recommendations. Most IV solutions retain potency for 4 h at 15–30C (59–86F) or for 24 h if refrigerated at 4C (39F). Avoid freezing.

▪ Administer IM suspension by deep injection into the gluteal muscle with a 21–gauge, 2–inch needle. Aspiration is necessary to avoid inadvertent injection into a blood vessel.

▪ Use reconstituted IM injection within 1 h after preparation.

▪ *Caution:* IM solution should not be given IV, and IV solution should not be given IM.

Assessment & Drug Effects

▪ A careful history should be elicited to determine previous hypersensitivity reaction to beta-lactam antibiotics (penicillins and cephalosporins) or to other allergens.

▪ When allergic reaction occurs (hives, wheezing, rash, pruritus), discontinue drug and notify physician.

▪ Monitor closely patients most vulnerable to CNS adverse effects: patient with history of seizures, recent head injury or other CNS disorders; the elderly; patients on high dosage, undergoing hemodialysis, or taking drugs that lower seizure threshold.

▪ If focal tremors, myoclonus, or seizures occur, call physician. Dosage modification may prevent seizure recurrence.

▪ Inspect patient's mouth on a regular basis to detect superinfection (see Signs & Symptoms, chap 3).

▪ If patient develops mild diarrhea during treatment, discontinuation of drug may be sufficient. If diarrhea is severe and accompanied by abdominal pain and fever, pseudomembranous colitis (see Chapter 3) should be ruled out. Call physician promptly.

▪ The sodium content derived from cilastatin sodium and sodium bicarbonate buffer in the fixed combination is about 0.8 mEq (18.4 mg) in the 250 mg dose. This should be considered in patient on restricted sodium intake.

Common side effects in *italic;* life-threatening effects underlined; generic names in **bold**; classifications in SMALL CAPS

- Laboratory evaluation of renal, hematologic, and hepatic systems should be scheduled periodically during prolonged therapy with this drug. Urge patient to keep appointments.
- Hypotension or hyperventilation symptoms may suggest onset of a hypersensitivity episode; they are rarely associated with infusion rate.

Patient & Family Education
- Instruct patient to immediately report pruritus or symptoms of respiratory distress.
- Instruct patient to report loose stools or diarrhea promptly.
- Instruct patient to report pain or discomfort at IV infusion site since phlebitis occurs in approximately 3% of patients.

ANTIBIOTIC: PENICILLIN, AMINOPENICILLIN

AMPICILLIN
(am-pi-sill´in)
Trade names: Amcap, Amcill, Ampicin, Ampilean, D-Amp, Novo-Ampicillin, Omnipen, Penbritin, Pfizerpen-A, Polycillin, Principen, SK-Ampicillin, Supen, Totacillin

AMPICILLIN SODIUM
Trade names: Omnipen-N, Polycillin N, SK-Ampicillin-N, Totacillin-N
Classifications: ANTIINFECTIVE; BETA-LACTAM ANTIBIOTIC; AMINOPENICILLIN
Pregnancy: Category B

ACTIONS/PHARMACODYNAMICS A broad-spectrum semisynthetic aminopenicillin, ampicillin is relatively stable in gastric acid, is highly bactericidal even at low concentrations, but is inactivated by penicillinase (beta-lactamase). Resembles penicillin G in its activity against gram-positive microorganisms such as alpha- and beta-hemolytic streptococci, *Diplococcus pneumoniae,* non-penicillinase-producing staphylococci, and *Listeria*. Major advantage over penicillin G is enhanced action against most strains of enterococci and several gram-negative strains including *Escherichia coli, Neisseria gonorrhoeae, N. meningitidis, Haemophilus influenzae, Proteus*

mirabilis, Salmonella (including *typhosa*), and *Shigella*. Inactive against *Mycoplasma,* rickettsiae, fungi, and viruses.

USES Infections of GU, respiratory, and GI tracts and skin and soft tissues; also gonococcal infections, bacterial meningitis, otitis media, sinusitis, and septicemia and for prophylaxis of bacterial endocarditis. Used parenterally only for moderately severe to severe infections.

ROUTE & DOSAGE

Systemic Infections

Adult	PO	250–500 mg q6h
	IM/IV	250 mg–2 g q6h
Child	PO	25–50 mg/kg/d divided q6h
	IM/IV	25–100 mg/kg/d divided q6h

Meningitis

Adult	IV	150–200 mg/kg/d divided q4–6h
Child	IV	Same as for adult

Gonorrhea

Adult	PO	3.5 g with 1 g probenecid ×1
	IM/IV	500 mg q8–12h

PHARMACOKINETICS Absorption: oral dose is 50% absorbed. **Peak effect:** 5 min IV, 1 h IM, 2 h PO. **Duration:** 6–8 h. **Distribution:** most body tissues; high CNS concentrations only with inflamed meninges; crosses the placenta. **Metabolism:** minimal hepatic metabolism. **Elimination:** half-life 1–1.8 h; 90% excreted in urine; excreted into breast milk.

CONTRAINDICATIONS & PRECAUTIONS Contraindicated in: hypersensitivity to penicillin derivatives. Safe use during pregnancy (category B) not established. **Cautious use in:** history of severe reactions to cephalosporins, infectious mononucleosis.

ADVERSE/SIDE EFFECTS Similar to those for penicillin G. **CNS (with high doses):** convulsive seizures. **GI:** *diarrhea,* nausea, vomiting, pseudomembranous colitis. **Hypersensitivity:** pruritus, urticaria, eosinophilia, hemolytic anemia, thrombocytopenia, leukopenia, agranulocytosis, interstitial nephritis, anaphylactoid reaction. **Other:** severe pain (following IM); phlebitis (following IV); *rash;* superinfections.

DIAGNOSTIC TEST INTERFERENCES Elevated *CPK* levels may result from local skeletal muscle injury following IM injection. *Urine glucose:* high

Common side effects in *italic*; life-threatening effects underlined; generic names in **bold**; classifications in SMALL CAPS

69

urine drug concentrations can result in false-positive test results with Clinitest or Benedict's (enzymatic glucose oxidase methods, e.g., Clinistix, Diastix, TesTape are not affected). *SGOT(AST)* may be elevated (significance not known).

DRUG INTERACTIONS Allopurinol increases incidence of rash. Effectiveness of the AMINOGLYCOSIDES may be impaired in patients with severe end-stage renal disease. **Chloramphenicol, erythromycin**, and **tetracycline** may reduce bactericidal effects of ampicillin; this interaction is primarily significant when low doses of ampicillin are used. Ampicillin may interfere with the contraceptive action of ORAL CONTRACEPTIVES. Female patients should be advised to consider nonhormonal contraception while on antibiotics. **Drug–food interactions:** food may decrease absorption of ampicillin, so it should be taken 1 h before or 2 h after meals.

INCOMPATIBILITIES Solution/additive: any dextrose-containing solution, including parenteral nutrition solutions. **Y-site: clindamycin, erythromycin**, AMINOGLYCOSIDES, **lidocaine, verapamil.**

NURSING IMPLICATIONS

Administration
- Before therapy begins, determine previous hypersensitivity reactions to penicillins, cephalosporins, and other allergens.
- Culture and sensitivity tests should be done initially and periodically during therapy. Therapy may be initiated before results are known.
- Food hampers rate and extent of absorption. Maximum absorption is achieved if it is taken with a full glass of water on an empty stomach (at least 1 h before or 2 h after meals).
- May be reconstituted with sterile or bacteriostatic water for injection. Follow manufacturer's directions for amount of diluent to use. Solutions for IM or direct IV should be administered within 1 h after preparation.
- For IV infusion, the reconstituted solution must be added to suitable IV fluid. Solutions containing dextrose can inactivate ampicillin.
- Administration of drug by direct IV should be done slowly, over at least 10–15 min. Rapid administration can result in seizures.
- Contact dermatitis occurs frequently in sensitized individuals. Those who must handle ampicillin repeatedly are advised to wear disposable gloves.
- Solutions are stable for 14 d under refrigeration. Do not freeze; store in tightly covered containers. Date

and time of reconstitution and discard date should appear on container; medication should be dispensed with a calibrated measuring device. Shake well before using.
- Capsules and unopened vials are stored between 15 and 30C (59 and 86F) unless otherwise directed. Keep oral preparations tightly covered.

Assessment & Drug Effects
- Note that the sodium content must be taken into consideration in patients on sodium restriction.
- Inspect skin daily and instruct patient to do the same. The appearance of a rash should be carefully evaluated to differentiate an ampicillin rash (nonallergenic) from a hypersensitivity reaction. Report promptly to physician if it appears.
- *Ampicillin rash* characteristically is dull red, macular or maculopapular, and mildly pruritic. It generally begins on light-exposed or pressure areas such as knees, elbows, palms, and soles and may spread in a symmetric pattern over most of body. The rash usually develops after 5–14 d of treatment, but occasionally appears on first day of therapy or after therapy has stopped. It disappears within 1 wk after discontinuation of drug therapy.
- The incidence of ampicillin rash is higher in patients with infectious mononucleosis or other viral infections, *Salmonella* infections, lymphocytic leukemia, or hyperuricemia or in patients taking allopurinol.
- Baseline and periodic assessments of renal, hepatic, and hematologic functions are advised, particularly during prolonged or high-dose therapy.

Patient & Family Education
- Because ampicillin rash is believed to be nonallergenic, its appearance is not an absolute contraindication to future therapy.
- Advise patient to report diarrhea and not to self-medicate. A detailed report should be given to the physician regarding onset, duration, character of stools, associated symptoms, and patient's temperature and weight to help rule out the possibility of drug-induced, potentially fatal pseudomembranous colitis (see chap 3).
- Superinfections (see Chapter 3) are more likely to occur with broad-spectrum derivatives of penicillin, such as ampicillin. Instruct patient to report the onset of black, hairy tongue; oral lesions (stomatitis, glossitis); rectal or vaginal itching; vaginal discharge; loose, foul-smelling stools; or unusual odor to urine.
- Instruct patient to take medication around the clock, not to miss a dose, and to continue taking

medication until it is all gone (usually 10 d) unless otherwise directed by physician or pharmacist.

- If no improvement is noted within a few days after therapy is started, physician should be notified.

- Treatment for most infections is continued 48–72 h beyond the time that patient becomes asymptomatic or negative cultures are obtained.

ANTIBIOTIC: PENICILLIN, NATURAL

PENICILLIN G POTASSIUM

Trade names: Crystapen, Megacillin, Novopen-G, P-50, Pentids, Pfizarpen

PENICILLIN G SODIUM

Classifications: ANTIINFECTIVE; BETA-LACTAM ANTIBIOTIC; NATURAL PENICILLIN
Pregnancy: Category B

ACTIONS/PHARMACODYNAMICS Acid-labile, penicillinase-sensitive, natural penicillin derived from cultures of *Penicillium notatum* or related molds. Antimicrobial spectrum is relatively narrow compared to that of the semisynthetic penicillins. Bactericidal at therapeutic serum levels; bacteriostatic at lower concentrations. Acts by interfering with synthesis of mucopeptides essential to formation and integrity of bacterial cell wall. Effective primarily on immature cell walls of rapidly growing and dividing cells; minimally effective or ineffective on dormant or mature organisms. Action is inhibited by penicillinase; therefore penicillin G is ineffective against many strains of *Staphylococcus aureus*. Highly active against gram-positive cocci (e.g., non-penicillinase-producing *Staphylococcus, Streptococcus* groups A, C, G, H, L, M, and *Streptococcus pneumoniae*); and gram-negative cocci (*Neisseria gonorrhoeae, N. meningitidis*). Also effective against gram-positive bacilli (*Bacillus anthracis, Clostridium* species including gas gangrene and tetanus, and certain species of *Corynebacterium, Erysipelothrix,* and *Listeria*); gram-negative bacilli (*Fusobacterium, Pasteurella, Streptobacillus,* and *Bacteroides* species). Parenteral penicillin G is effective against some strains of *Salmonella* and *Shigella* and Spirochetes (*Treponema pallidum, T. pertenue, Leptospira*). The penicillins are not active against fungi, plasmodia, amebae, rickettsiae, and viruses. In large doses, peni-

cillin G is capable of inhibiting platelet aggregation and may also act as a CNS irritant.

USES Moderate to severe systemic infections caused by penicillin sensitive microorganisms: actinomycosis, anthrax, diphtheria (carrier state), empyema, erysipelas, gas gangrene, gonorrheal infections, leptospirosis, mastoiditis, meningitis, acute osteomyelitis, otitis media, pinta, pneumonia, rat-bite fever, sinus infections; certain staphylococcal infections; streptococcal infections, including scarlet fever; syphilis (all stages), tetanus, urinary tract infections, Vincent's gingivostomatitis, yaws. Also used as prophylaxis in patients with rheumatic or congenital heart disease. Since oral preparations are absorbed erratically and thus must be given in comparatively high doses, this route is generally used only for mild or stabilized infections or long-term prophylaxis.

ROUTE & DOSAGE

Moderate to Severe Infections		
Adult	PO	1.6–3.2 million U divided q6h
	IV/IM	1.2–24 million U divided q4h
Child	PO	25,000–100,000 U/kg divided q6h
	IV/IM	25,000–300,000 U/kg divided q4h

PHARMACOKINETICS Absorption: 15–30% of PO dose absorbed; very acid labile. **Peak:** 30–60 min PO; 15–30 min IM. **Distribution:** widely distributed; good CSF concentrations with inflamed meninges; crosses placenta; distributed in breast milk. **Metabolism:** 16–30% metabolized. **Elimination:** half-life: 0.4–0.9 h; 60% excreted in urine within 6 h.

CONTRAINDICATIONS & PRECAUTIONS
Contraindicated in: hypersensitivity to any of the penicillins or cephalosporins; administration of oral drug to patients with severe infections, nausea, vomiting, hypermotility, gastric dilatation, cardiospasm. Use of penicillin G sodium in patients on sodium restriction; safe use during pregnancy (category B) or in nursing mothers not established. **Cautious use in:** history of or suspected atopy or allergy (asthma, eczema, hay fever, hives); history of allergy to cephalosporins; renal or hepatic dysfunction, myasthenia gravis, epilepsy, neonates, young infants. Use in nursing mothers may lead to sensitization of infants.

ADVERSE/SIDE EFFECTS Electrolyte imbalance: hyperkalemia (penicillin G potassium); hypokalemia, alkalosis, hypernatremia, CHF (penicillin G sodium). **Hypersensitivity: (1) immediate** (usually occurs within

Common side effects in *italic*; life-threatening effects <u>underlined</u>; generic names in **bold**; classifications in SMALL CAPS

71

2–30 min after drug administration): localized ana-phylaxis: itchy palms or axilla or generalized pruritus or urticaria, flushed skin, coughing, sneezing, feeling of uneasiness; systemic anaphylaxis: fever, vomiting, diarrhea, severe abdominal cramps, widespread in-crease in capillary permeability and vasodilation with resulting edema (mouth, tongue, pharynx, larynx), laryngospasm, bronchospasm, hypotension, circula-tory collapse, cardiac arrhythmias, cardiac arrest. **(2) Accelerated** (occurs in 1–72 h): malaise, fever, *ur-ticaria,* erythema or other skin reactions and (less commonly) angioneurotic and laryngeal edema, asthma. **(3) Delayed or late** (develops after 72 h): serum sickness (fever, malaise, pruritus, urticaria, lym-phadenopathy, arthralgia, angioedema of face and extremities, neuritis prostration, eosinophilia). *Skin rashes* ranging from urticaria to exfoliative dermatitis, Stevens-Johnson syndrome, fixed-drug eruptions, contact dermatitis; hemolytic anemia, granulocytope-nia, neutropenia, leukopenia, thrombocytopenia, SLE-like syndrome, interstitial nephritis, Loeffler's syndrome, vasculitis. **Injection site reactions:** pain, in-flammation, abscess, phlebitis, thrombophlebitis. **Superinfections**: especially with *Candida* and gram-negative bacteria (e.g., *Proteus, Pseudomonas*). **Toxicity:** bone marrow depression, granulocytopenia, hepatitis (infrequent), neuromuscular irritability: twitching, lethargy, confusion, stupor, hyperreflexia, multifocal myoclonus, localized or generalized seizures, coma. **With oral therapy:** nausea, vomiting, epigastric distress, diarrhea, flatulence, dark discol-oration of tongue, sore mouth or tongue. **Other:** in-creased bleeding time, Jarisch-Herxheimer reaction (syphilis), drug fever.

DIAGNOSTIC TEST INTERFERENCES *Blood grouping and compatibility tests:* possible inter-ference associated with penicillin doses greater than 20 million units daily. *Urine glucose:* massive doses of penicillin may cause false-positive test results with Benedict's solution and possibly Clinitest but not with glucose oxidase methods, e.g., Clinistix, Diastix, TesTape. *Urine protein:* massive doses of penicillin can produce false-positive results when turbidity measures are used (e.g., acetic acid and heat, sulfo-salicylic acid); Ames reagent reportedly not affected. *Urinary PSP excretion tests:* false decrease in uri-nary excretion of PSP. *Urinary steroids:* large IV doses of penicillin may interfere with accurate mea-surement of urinary 17-OHCS (Glenn-Nelson tech-nique not affected).

DRUG INTERACTIONS Probenecid decreases renal elimination; penicillin G may decrease efficacy of ORAL CONTRACEPTIVES; **colestipol** decreases peni-cillin absorption; POTASSIUM-SPARING DIURETICS may cause hyperkalemia with penicillin G potassium. **Drug-food interactions:** food increases breakdown in stomach.

INCOMPATIBILITIES Solution/additive: dextran 40, fat emulsion, aminophylline, amphotericin B, cephalothin, chlorpromazine, dopamine, hy-droxyzine, metaraminol, TETRACYCLINES, **pento-barbital, prochlorperazine, promazine, sodium bicarbonate, thiopental, metoclopramide.**

NURSING IMPLICATIONS

Administration
General
- Patient should be informed that he or she is going to receive penicillin therapy.
- Note whether physician has prescribed penicillin G potassium or sodium.
- At least 10 d of continuous treatment is recom-mended for streptococcal infections to prevent possible sequelae such as rheumatic fever.
- The stability of penicillin G is affected by changes in pH (most stable at pH 6.0–7.0), and therefore it is physically incompatible with many drugs.
- Store penicillin G tablets at room temperature in tightly closed containers. Avoid excessive heat. Store oral suspensions and syrups in refrigerator and discard unused portions after 14 d. The dry powder (for parenteral use) may be stored at room temperature. After reconstitution (initial dilution), solutions may be stored for 1 wk under refrigera-tion. Intravenous infusion solutions containing penicillin G are stable at room temperature for at least 24 h.

Oral Administration
- Oral penicillin G should be taken on an empty stomach, at least 1 h before or 2 h after meals to re-duce possibility of destruction by gastric acid and delay in absorption by food.
- Administer with a full glass of water. Instruct pa-tient to avoid acidic beverages 1 h before and after taking oral penicillin G.

Parenteral Administration (IM & IV)
- See manufacturer's labeling for directions on preparation of initial dilution. Loosen powder by tapping vial against palm of hand. Holding vial hor-izontally, rotate it while directing stream of diluent against wall of vial. Shake vial vigorously until powder is completely dissolved. (For IV adminis-tration, the initial dilution should be further diluted with 0.9% NaCl or 5% dextrose for IV use.)

Common side effects in *italic*; life-threatening effects underlined; generic names in **bold**; classifications in SMALL CAPS

- Carefully select IM site. Accidental injection into or near a nerve can cause irritation with severe pain and dysfunction. IM injection is made deep into a large muscle mass. Inject slowly. Rotate injection sites.
- IV penicillin G is given by continuous infusion. In high doses, IV penicillin G should be administered slowly to avoid electrolyte imbalance from potassium or sodium content. Physician will prescribe specific flow rate.

Assessment & Drug Effects

- Culture and sensitivity tests should be done prior to initiation of therapy; however, treatment may be started before results are known.
- Hypersensitivity reactions are more likely to occur with parenteral penicillin but may also occur with the oral drug. Skin rash is the most common type allergic reaction and should be reported promptly to physician.
- Before treatment with penicillin is initiated, an exact history should be obtained of patient's previous exposure and sensitivity to penicillins and cephalosporins and other allergic reactions of any kind.
- Observe all patients closely for at least 30 min following administration of parenteral penicillin. The rapid appearance of a red flare or wheal at the IM or IV injection site is a possible sign of sensitivity. Report to physician. Also suspect an allergic reaction if patient becomes irritable, has nausea and vomiting, breathing difficulty, or sudden fever.
- Reactions to penicillin may be rapid in onset or may not appear for days or weeks. Symptoms usually disappear fairly quickly once drug is stopped, but in some patients may persist for 5 d or more and require hospitalization for treatment.
- Allergy to penicillin is unpredictable. It has occurred in patients with a negative history of penicillin allergy and also in patients with no known prior contact with penicillin (sensitization may have occurred from penicillin used commercially in foods and beverages).
- Neuromuscular irritability occurs most commonly in patients receiving parenteral penicillin in excess of 20 million U/d who have renal insufficiency, hyponatremia, or underlying CNS disease, notably myasthenia gravis or epilepsy. Seizure precautions are indicated. Symptoms usually begin with twitching, especially of face and extremities.
- Monitor I&O, particularly in patients receiving high parenteral doses. Report oliguria, hematuria, and changes in I&O ratio. Consult physician regarding optimum fluid intake. Dehydration increases the concentration of drug in kidneys and can cause renal irritation and damage.
- Neonates, young infants, the elderly, and patients with impaired renal function receiving high-dose penicillin therapy should be closely observed for signs of toxicity. Urinary excretion of penicillin is significantly delayed in these patients.
- Patients on high-dose therapy should be closely observed for evidence of bleeding, and bleeding time should be monitored. (In high doses, penicillin interferes with platelet aggregation.)
- Patients receiving prolonged treatment should have renal, hepatic, and hematologic systems evaluated at regular intervals. Additionally, electrolyte balance and cardiovascular status should be checked periodically in patients receiving high parenteral doses.
- Cultures should be taken following completion of treatment to determine need for further medication.

Patient & Family Education

- Inform patients that hypersensitivity reaction may be delayed. Advise them to immediately report urticaria, pruritus, fever, malaise, and other signs of a delayed reaction (see adverse/side effects).
- When used for infection, penicillin is to be taken around the clock (i.e., t.i.d. means q8h, q.i.d. means q6h, etc.) Instruct patient not to miss any doses and to continue taking the medication until it is all gone, unless otherwise directed by the physician.
- Measure liquid dosage form with specially marked measuring device. Household teaspoons vary in measure and therefore are not advised.
- Some patients receiving penicillin for treatment of syphilis develop Jarisch-Herxheimer reaction. This reaction resembles penicillin allergy but is thought to be due to the toxic products released from spirochetes killed by penicillin. It occurs 8–24 h following treatment with penicillin and is characterized by headache, chills, fever, myalgia, arthralgia, malaise, and worsening of syphilitic skin lesions. Advise patient to notify physician if these symptoms appear. The reaction is usually self-limiting.
- Advise patient to check with physician if symptoms do not improve within a few days or if they get worse.
- Instruct patient to report signs and symptoms of superinfection (see Signs & Symptoms, chap 3).
- Patients with diabetes who are receiving massive doses of penicillin should be advised of the possibility of obtaining false-positive urine glucose test results.

Common side effects in *italic*; life-threatening effects <u>underlined</u>; generic names in **bold**; classifications in SMALL CAPS

73

- Impress on patient importance of medical follow-up; present evidence suggests that glomerulonephritis, a possible complication of streptococcal infection, may not be prevented by penicillin.

ANTIBIOTIC: TETRACYCLINE

TETRACYCLINE HYDROCHLORIDE
(tet-ra-sye´kleen)

Trade names: Achromycin, Achromycin V, Nor-Tet, Novotetra, Panmycin, Retet, Robitet, SK-Tetracycline, Sumycin, Tetra-C, Tetracap, Tetracyn, Tetralan, Tetram, Topicycline

Classifications: ANTIINFECTIVE; TETRACYCLINE ANTIBIOTIC; SKIN AGENT; ANTIACNE

Pregnancy: Category D

Note: Tetracycline hydrochloride, ophthalmic, is discussed on p 990.

ACTIONS/PHARMACODYNAMICS Broad spectrum antibiotic derived from *Streptomyces aureofaciens* or produced semisynthetically from oxytetracycline. Effective against a variety of gram-positive and gram-negative bacteria and against most chlamydiae, mycoplasmas, rickettsiae, and certain protozoa (e.g., amebae). Tetracyclines usually are bacteriostatic but may be bactericidal in high concentrations; it is believed they affect multiplying microorganisms. Mechanism of antimicrobial action not fully understood. Appears to act by selectively binding to bacterial 30S ribosomal subunits of susceptible organisms. This position prevents access of transfer RNA to acceptor sites on messenger RNA-ribosome complex, with resultant inhibition of protein synthesis. Transient increases in BUN are believed to be caused by an antianabolic action. Exerts antiacne action by suppressing growth of *Proprionibacterium acnes* within sebaceous follicles, thereby reducing free fatty acid content in sebum. Free fatty acids are thought to be produced by breakdown of triglycerides by lipases liberated from *P. acne* and are believed to be largely responsible for inflammatory skin lesions (papules, pustules, cysts) and comedones of acne. Evidence suggests that topical tetracycline may be as effective as the oral preparation for treatment of mild to moderate acne; moderate to severe acne may require oral and topical tetracycline. Indiscriminate use, including widespread incorporation of tetracyclines in animal feed to increase their growth rate, has produced tetracycline-resistant organisms. Cross-resistance betweeen tetracyclines has been exhibited.

USES Chlamydial infections (e.g., lymphogranuloma venereum, psittacosis, trachoma, inclusion conjunctivitis, nongonococcal urethritis); mycoplasmal infections (e.g., *Mycoplama pneumoniae*); rickettsial infections (e.g., Q fever, Rocky Mt Spotted fever, typhus); spirochetal infections: relapsing fever (*Borrelia*), leptospirosis, syphilis (penicillin-hypersensitive patients); amebiases; uncommon gram-negative bacterial infections (e.g., brucellosis, shigellosis, cholera, gonorrhea [penicillin-hypersensitive patients], granuloma inguinale, tularemia); gram-positive infections (e.g., tetanus). Also used orally and topically (solution) for inflammatory acne vulgaris; topical ointment is used for superficial skin infections. (See **tetracycline hydrochloride, ophthalmic**, for ophthalmic uses.) **Unlabeled use:** actinomycosis, acute exacerbations of chronic bronchitis; Lyme disease; pericardial effusion (metastatic); acute PID; sexually transmitted epididymoorchitis; with quinine for multidrug-resistant strains of *Plasmodium falciparum* malaria; antiinfective prophylaxis for rape victims; recurrent cystic thyroid nodules; melioidosis; and as fluorescence test for malignancy.

ROUTE & DOSAGE

Systemic Infection

Adult	PO	250–500 mg b.i.d.–q.i.d. (1–2 g/d)
	IM	250 mg once/d *or* 300 mg/d in 2–3 divided doses
Child	PO	>8 y: 25–50 mg/kg/d in 2–4 divided doses
	IM	>8 y: 15–25 mg/kg/d in 2–3 divided doses (max 250 mg/injection)

Acne

Adult	PO	500–1000 mg/d in 4 divided doses
	Topical	Apply to cleansed areas twice daily
Child	PO	>8 y: Same as for adult
	Topical	Same as for adult

PHARMACOKINETICS **Absorption:** 75–80% of dose absorbed orally. **Peak:** 2–4 h. **Distribution:** widely distributed, preferentially binds to rapid growing tissues; crosses placenta; enters breast milk. **Metabolism:** not metabolized; enterohepatic cycling. **Elimination:**

Common side effects in *italic*; life-threatening effects <u>underlined</u>; generic names in **bold**; classifications in SMALL CAPS

half-life: 6–12 h; 50–60% excreted in urine within 72 h.

CONTRAINDICATIONS & PRECAUTIONS Contraindicated In: hypersensitivity to tetracyclines or to any ingredient in the formulation; severe renal or hepatic impairment, common bile duct obstruction; use during tooth development (last half of pregnancy) (category D), during infancy and childhood to the 8th year, and in nursing women. Safe use of topical tetracycline preparations in children <11 y not established. **Cautious use in:** history of renal or hepatic dysfunction; myasthenia gravis; history of allergy, asthma, hay fever, urticaria; undernourished patients.

ADVERSE/SIDE EFFECTS CNS: headache, intracranial hypertension (rare). **Eye:** pigmentation of conjunctiva due to drug deposit; transient myopia (rare). **GI:** reported mostly for oral administration, but also may occur with parenteral tetracycline: *nausea, vomiting,* epigastric distress, heartburn (pyrosis), *diarrhea,* bulky loose stools, steatorrhea, *abdominal discomfort, flatulence,* dry mouth; dysphagia, retrosternal pain, esophagitis, esophageal ulceration (oral administration). **Hematologic:** (infrequent): neutropenia, thrombocytopenia, toxic granulation of granulocytes, leukocytosis, decreased leukocyte ascorbic acid, atypical lymphocytes; positive antinuclear antibodies; hypokalemia, folate deficiency with megaloblastic anemia; acute hemolytic anemia. **Hepatic:** particularly patients with impaired renal or hepatic function: abnormally high liver function test values, decrease in serum cholesterol, fatty degeneration of liver (jaundice, increasing nitrogen retention [azotemia], hyperphosphatemia, acidosis, irreversible shock). **Hypersensitivity:** (uncommon): urticaria, angioedema, pruritus, skin rashes, erythema multiforme, exfoliative dermatitis, drug fever, *photosensitivity,* eosinophilia, asthma, serumlike reaction (fever, headache, arthralgia), anaphylaxis, anaphylactic purpura. **Renal:** (particularly in patients with renal disease): increase in BUN/serum creatinine, renal impairment even with therapeutic doses; Fanconi-like syndrome (outdated tetracyclines). Characterized by polyuria, polydipsia, nausea, vomiting, glycosuria, proteinuria acidosis, aminoaciduria. **Skin:** dermatitis, *phototoxicity:* discoloration of nails, onycholysis (loosening of nails); cheilosis; fixed drug eruptions particularly on genitalia; thrombocytopenic purpura. With topical applications: skin irritation, dry scaly skin, transient stinging or burning sensation, slight yellowing of skin at application site, acute contact dermatitis. **Superinfections:** vulvovaginitis, pruritus vulvae or ani (possibly hypersensitivity), foul-smelling stools or vaginal discharge, stomatitis, glossitis; black hairy tongue (lingua nigra), pharyngitis, laryngitis, dysphagia, diarrhea: staphylococcal enterocolitis, pseudomembranous colitis (rare); gram-negative folliculitis (long-term therapy). **Other:** decrease in serum levels of B complex vitamins and ascorbic acid; pancreatitis, microscopic brown-black discoloration of thyroid gland; pericarditis, exacerbation of systemic lupus erythematosus (possibly hypersensitivity); exacerbation of myasthenia gravis; local reactions: pain and irritation (IM site), thrombophlebitis (IV site); Jarisch-Herxheimer reaction (see Nursing Implications).

DIAGNOSTIC TEST INTERFERENCES Tetracyclines may cause false increases in *urinary catecholamines* (by fluorometric methods), and false decreases in *urinary urobilinogen.* Parenteral tetracyclines containing ascorbic acid reportedly may produce false-positive *urinary glucose* determinations by copper reduction methods (e.g., Benedict's reagent, Clinitest); tetracyclines may cause false-negative results with glucose oxidase methods (e.g., Clinistix, TesTape).

DRUG INTERACTIONS ANTACIDS, **calcium,** and **magnesium** bind tetracycline in gut and decrease absorption. ORAL ANTICOAGULANTS potentiate hypoprothrombinemia. ANTIDIARRHEAL AGENTS with kaolin and pectin may decrease absorption. Effectiveness of ORAL CONTRACEPTIVES decreased. **Methoxyflurane** may produce fatal nephrotoxicity. **Drug-food interactions:** dairy products and iron supplements decrease tetracycline absorption.

NURSING IMPLICATIONS

Administration for All Routes

- Check expiration date for all tetracyclines. Fanconi-like syndrome (renal tubular dysfunction) and also a LE-like syndrome have been attributed to outdated tetracycline preparations.
- Tetracyclines decompose with age, exposure to light, and when improperly stored under conditions of extreme humidity, heat, or cold. The resultant product may be toxic. Tetracycline preparations should be stored in tightly covered containers, in a dry place, protected from light preferably between 15–30C (59–86F), unless otherwise directed by manufacturer.
- Tetracyclines are generally avoided during pregnancy (particularly the last half), in nursing women, or in children < 8 y because they bind to calcium in developing bones and teeth. The net result is permanent yellow-gray-brown discoloration

Common side effects in *italic;* life-threatening effects underlined; generic names in **bold;** classifications in SMALL CAPS

75

of deciduous and permanent teeth, enamel hypoplasia, and retardation of skeletal development and bone growth.

Administration: Intramuscular

- IM tetracycline preparations are not to be given IV. Commerically prepared IM solution contains procaine HCl and therefore is not appropriate for IV administration.
- If IM tetracycline is prescribed, ask patient if he or she is allergic to any of the "caine" local anesthetics. (Tetracycline for IM use contains 40 mg procaine HCl per vial.)
- *Preparation of IM tetracycline:* Powder for IM injection is reconstituted by adding 2 ml sterile water for injection or 0.9% NaCl injection to 100- or 250-mg vial. Resultant solution may be stored at room temperature but should be discarded after 24 h. (Directions may vary with manufacturer.)
- Administer IM injection deep into body of a relatively large muscle mass, e.g., gluteus maximus or midlateral thigh. Alternate injection sites and observe daily for irritation and swelling.
- IM administration of tetracycline is generally not prescribed because it causes local irritation and is extremely painful. Additionally, serum levels produced by IM tetracyclines are lower than equivalent oral doses.

Administration: Oral

- Instruct to take oral tetracyclines on an empty stomach at least 1 h before or 2 h after meals (food, milk, and milk products can reduce absorption by 50% or more). To reduce possibilitiy of esophageal or gastric irritation, advise to (1) take each dose with a full glass (240 ml) of water, (2) remain standing for about 90 s after taking medication, and (3) avoid taking drug within 1 h of lying down.
- Shake oral suspension well before pouring to assure uniform distribution of drug. Preparation should be dispensed with a calibrated liquid measure.
- If patient is having GI symptoms (e.g., nausea, vomiting, anorexia) physician may prescribe taking oral tetracycline with food, (exception: not foods high in calcium such as milk or milk products). If symptoms persist, drug should be discontinued.
- If patient is bedridden or has difficulty swallowing pills, consult physician about ordering the oral suspension formulation.

Assessment & Drug Effects

- Culture and sensitivity tests are recommended prior to first dose and periodically to confirm susceptibility of infecting organism to tetracycline.

- Initial and periodic studies of renal, hepatic, and hematopoietic function should be performed, particularly during high-dose, long-term therapy.
- GI symptoms (e.g., nausea, vomiting, diarrhea) are generally dose-dependent, occurring mostly in patients receiving 2 g/d or more and in patients on prolonged therapy. These symptoms are associated chiefly with oral tetracycline but may occur also with parenteral preparations. GI symptoms that appear during the first few days of therapy probably are caused by direct drug irritation. Report to physician. Frequently, symptoms can be controlled by reducing dosage or by administration of oral drug with compatible foods.
- Be alert to evidence of superinfections (see Chapter 3). Regularly inspect tongue and mucous membrane of mouth for candidiasis (thrush). Suspect superinfection if patient complains of irritation or soreness of mouth, tongue, throat, vagina, or anus or persistent itching of any area, diarrhea, or foul-smelling excreta or discharge.
- Superinfections occur most frequently in patients who are receiving prolonged tetracycline therapy, who are debilitated, or who have diabetes, leukemia, systemic LE, or lymphoma. Women taking oral contraceptives reportedly are more susceptible to vaginal candidiasis. Tetracycline should be discontinued if superinfection develops.
- Follow-up cultures should be obtained from all gonococcal infection sites 3–7 d after completion of tetracycline therapy to verify eradication of infection.
- Monitor I&O in patients receiving parenteral tetracycline. Report oliguria or any changes in appearance of urine or in I&O.
- Hepatotoxicity (sometimes associated with pancreatitis) occurs most frequently in patients receiving other hepatotoxic drugs or who have a history of renal or hepatic impairment. Periodic hepatic and renal function tests and serum tetracycline levels are recommended in these high-risk patients. Serum tetracycline concentrations should not be allowed to exceed 15 µg/ml.
- Patients with renal or hepatic impairment usually require lower and less frequent doses and careful monitoring of renal and hepatic function. Serum tetracycline levels should be closely monitored.

Patient & Family Education

- Instruct to report the onset of diarrhea to physician. It is important to determine whether diarrhea is due to irritating drug effect or to superinfections or pseudomembranous colitis (caused by overgrowth of toxin-producing bacteria: *Clostridia difficile*) (see Chapter 3). The latter two conditions can be life threatening and require immediate discontinuation of tetracycline and prompt initiation of symptomatic and supportive therapy.

- The incidence of superinfection (see chap 3) may be reduced by meticulous care of mouth, skin, and perineal area. Encourage patient to rinse mouth of food debris after eating; advise daily flossing and use of a soft-bristled toothbrush. Instruct patient to wash hands several times a day, particularly after each bowel movement, and before eating.

- Warn to avoid direct exposure to sunlight while taking tetracycline and for a few days after therapy is terminated to reduce possibility of photosensitivity reaction. The reaction appears like an exaggerated sunburn. It starts within a few minutes to hours following sun exposure and may begin with paresthesias (tingling, burning sensation). Symptoms may persist 1 or 2 d after drug is discontinued. Some experience loosening of nails and nail discoloration. Sunscreen agents provide only limited protection.

- Patients on long-term therapy should be advised to report immediately the onset of severe headache or visual disturbances. These are possible symptoms of increased intracranial pressure and necessitate prompt discontinuation of tetracycline to prevent irreversible loss of vision.

- Tetracycline therapy for brucellosis or spirochetal infections may cause a Jarisch-Herxheimer reaction. Symptoms are believed to be caused by release of endotoxins from phagocytized organisms. The reaction is usually mild and appears abruptly within 6–24 h after initiation of therapy. It is manifested by malaise, fever, chills, headache, adenopathy, leukocytosis, exacerbation of skin lesions, arthralgia, transient hypotension. Treatment is symptomatic; recovery generally occurs within 24 h.

- Esophagitis and esophageal ulceration have been associated with bedtime administration of tetracycline capsules or tablets with insufficient fluid, particularly to patients with hiatal hernia or esophageal problems. Sudden onset of painful or difficult swallowing (dysphagia) should be reported immediately to physician.

- Avoid contact of topical medication with eyes, nose, or mouth. Warn patient that tetracycline may stain clothing.

- Clean affected skin area with soap and water; rinse and dry well before application of topical tetracycline, unless otherwise directed.

- Some patients experience stinging and burning sensation with topical applications. Advise to report symptoms to physician if they become pronounced or persist or if infection worsens.

- Skin treated with topical drug will exhibit bright yellow to green fluorescence under ultraviolet light and "black light."

- Topicycline contains a sulfite that can cause an allergic reaction (itching, wheezing, anaphylaxis) in susceptible persons, e.g., asthmatics or atopic (allergic) individuals.

- Most patients respond to acne therapy in 2–8 wk, but maximal results may not be apparent for up to 12 wk of therapy.

ANTILEPROSY (SULFONE) AGENT

DAPSONE
(dap´sone)
Trade names: Avlosulfon, DDS
Classifications: ANTIINFECTIVE; ANTILEPROSY (SULFONE) AGENT
Pregnancy: Category C

ACTIONS/PHARMACODYNAMICS Sulfone derivative chemically related to sulfonamides, with bacteriostatic and bactericidal activity similar to that group. Spectrum of activity includes *Mycobacterium leprae* (Hansen's bacillus), *Mycobacterium tuberculosis*, and limited activity against *Pneumocystis carinii* and *Plasmodium*. Interferes with bacterial cell growth by competitive inhibition of folic acid synthesis by susceptible organisms. (Mammalian cells cannot synthesize folic acid and therefore are unaffected by this inhibition.) Mechanism of action in dermatitis herpetiformis is unknown. Drug is effective against dapsone-sensitive multibacillary (borderline, borderline lepromatous, or lepromatous) leprosy, and dapsone-sensitive paucibacillary (indeterminate, tuberculoid, or borderline tuberculoid) leprosy. Resistant strains of initially susceptible *M. leprae* develop slowly in a stepwise fashion over periods of 5–24 y. Recently, however, reports of dapsone-resistant organisms have increased, involving *M. leprae* recovered from newly diagnosed cases of leprosy in patients who have not had prior treatment with dapsone. Carcinogenicity in small animals has been reported. With prior arrangement, drug sensitivity determination is available without charge from USPHS.

Common side effects in *italic*; life-threatening effects underlined; generic names in **bold**; classifications in SMALL CAPS

77

USES Drug of choice for treatment of all forms of leprosy (unless organism is shown to be dapsone resistant). Used in dapsone-sensitive multibacillary leprosy (with clofazimine and rifampin) and in dapsone-sensitive paucibacillary leprosy (with rifampin, clofazimine, or ethionamide). Also used prophylactically in contacts of patients with all forms of leprosy except tuberculoid and indeterminate leprosy. Used for treatment of dermatitis herpetiformis. **Unlabeled use:** chemoprophylaxis of malaria (with pyrimethamine), systemic and discoid lupus erythematosus, pemphigus vulgaris, dermatosis (especially those associated with bullous eruptions, mucocutaneous lesion, inflammation or pustules); rheumatoid arthritis, allergic vasculitis; treatment of initial episodes of *P. carinii* pneumonia (with trimethoprim) in limited number of adults with AIDS.

ROUTE & DOSAGE

Tuberculoid and Indeterminate-type Leprosy

Adult   PO   100 mg/d (with 6 mo of rifampin 600 mg/d) for a minimum of 3 y

Lepromatous and Boderline Lepromatous Leprosy

Adult   PO   100 mg/d for ≥ 10 y

Dermatitis Herpetiformis

Adult   PO   50 mg/d; may be increased to 300 mg/d if necessary (max 500 mg/d)

Prophylaxis for Close Contacts of Patient with Multibacillary Leprosy

Adult   PO   50 mg/d
Child   PO   6–12 y: 25 mg/d
                  2–5 y: 25 mg 3 times/wk
                  6–23 mo: 12 mg 3 times/wk
                  <6 mo: 6 mg 3 times/wk

PHARMACOKINETICS Absorption: rapidly and nearly completely absorbed from GI tract. **Peak:** 2–8 h. **Distribution:** distributed to all body tissues; high concentrations in kidney, liver, muscle, and skin; crosses placenta; distributed into breast milk. **Metabolism:** metabolized in liver. **Elimination:** half-life: 20–30 h; 70–85% excreted in urine; remainder excreted in feces; traces of drug may be found in body for 3 wk after discontinuation of repeated doses.

CONTRAINDICATIONS & PRECAUTIONS Contraindicated in: hypersensitivity to sulfones or its derivatives; advanced renal amyloidosis, anemia, methemoglobin reductase deficiency. Safe use during pregnancy (category C) and by nursing mothers not established. **Cautious use in:** chronic renal, hepatic,

pulmonary, or cardiovascular disease, refractory anemias, albuminuria, G6PD deficiency.

ADVERSE/SIDE EFFECTS CNS: headache, nervousness, insomnia, vertigo, peripheral neuropathy (with high doses); paresthesia, muscle weakness. **GI:** anorexia, nausea, vomiting, abdominal pain; toxic hepatitis, cholestatic jaundice (reversible with discontinuation of drug therapy); increased ALT, AST, LDH; hyperbilirubinemia. **Hematologic:** in patient with or without G6PD deficiency; *dose-related hemolysis,* Heinz body formation, *methemoglobinemia with cyanosis,* hemolytic anemia; aplastic anemia (rare), leukopenia, agranulocytosis. **Hypersensitivity:** cutaneous reactions (especially bullous multibilliform and scarlatiniform reactions); erythema multiforme, exfoliative dermatitis, toxic epidermal necrolysis, allergic rhinitis, urticaria. **Renal:** albuminuria, nephrotic syndrome, renal papillary necrosis. **Skin:** drug-induced lupus erythematosus, phototoxicity. **Other:** tachycardia, blurred vision, tinnitus, fever, male infertility, infectious mononucleosis–like syndrome; *reactional states.* Sulfone syndrome: fever, malaise, exfoliative dermatitis, hepatic necrosis with jaundice, lymphadenopathy, methemoglobinemia, anemia.

DRUG INTERACTIONS Activated charcoal decreases dapsone absorption and enterohepatic circulation; **pyrimethamine, trimethoprim** increase risk of adverse hematologic reactions; **rifampin** decreases dapsone levels 7–10 fold.

NURSING IMPLICATIONS

Administration
- Administer with food to reduce possibility of GI distress.
- In some cases the physician considers that the benefits of continuing dapsone therapy for leprosy in the pregnant woman outweigh the potential risks to the fetus; most physicians believe the drug should be used during pregnancy only when clearly needed.
- Preserve in tightly covered, light-resistant containers at 15–30C (59–86F). Drug discoloration apparently does not indicate a chemical change.

Assessment & Drug Effects
- CBC are performed before initiation of therapy, weekly during the first month of therapy, at monthly intervals for at least 6 mo, and semiannually thereafter.
- Periodic determinations of dapsone blood levels are recommended.

- Nearly all patients demonstrate hemolysis. Manufacturer states that Hgb level is generally decreased by 1–2 g/dl; reticulocytes increase by 2–12%; RBC life span is shortened; and methemoglobinemia occurs in most patients receiving dapsone. Unless hemolysis or methemoglobinemia is severe, drug is not discontinued.
- Therapeutic effects in leprosy may not appear until after 3–6 mo of therapy. Skin lesions respond well; recovery from nerve involvement is usually limited.
- Monitor temperature during first few weeks of therapy. If fever is frequent or severe, leprosy reactional state should be ruled out. Reduction of or interruption of therapy may be sufficient.
- Suspect methemoglobinemia if patient appears cyanotic and mucous membranes have a brownish hue. Report to physician. Usually, discontinuation of therapy is not required unless anoxemia is present.
- Patients who complain of malaise, fever, chills, anorexia, nausea, and vomiting and have jaundice should have liver function tests performed. Dapsone therapy should be suspended until etiology is identified.
- Lepromatous eye lesions sometimes develop or progress during treatment, since the drug does not appreciably penetrate ocular tissues.
- Leprosy is transmitted by active skin lesions or nasal discharge of infected persons, but only susceptible people develop the disease. Reportedly most people have partial or complete resistance to leprosy.

Patient & Family Education

- Report to physician if symptoms of leprosy do not improve within 3 mo or if they get worse. Bacterial resistance to dapsone may be suspected.
- The appearance of a rash with bullous lesions around elbows and other joints should be reported promptly. Drug-induced or worsening of skin lesions require withdrawal of dapsone.
- Caution patient to report promptly if symptoms of peripheral neuropathy with motor loss (muscle weakness) develop. A particular area in which such weakness develops is in the base of thumbs; patient complains of difficulty in writing. The drug should be withdrawn. Complete recovery may occur, but it usually takes many months, even years.
- Optimum duration of therapy has not been determined. The World Health Organization recommends continuing treatment for lepromatous leprosy at least 10 y and perhaps for life.

ANTIMALARIAL

CHLOROQUINE HYDROCHLORIDE
(klor´oh-kwin)
Trade name: Aralen Hydrochloride

CHLOROQUINE PHOSPHATE
Trade name: Aralen Phosphate
Classifications: ANTIINFECTIVE; ANTIMALARIAL
Pregnancy: Category C

ACTIONS/PHARMACODYNAMICS Synthetic 4-aminoquinoline derivative and blood schizonticidal agent. Antimalarial activity is believed to be based on ability to form complexes with DNA of parasite, thereby inhibiting replication and transcription to RNA and nucleic acid synthesis. Highly active against asexual erythrocytic forms of the four species of *Plasmodium: P. vivax, P. malariae, P. ovale,* and most strains of *P. falciparum* (the most virulent affecting humans). Action mechanism is unknown. Acts as a suppressive agent in patient with vivax or malariae malaria; terminates acute attacks and increases intervals between treatment and relapse of malaria. Eliminates gametocytes (sexual forms of the organism) of *P. vivax,* but not *P. falciparum;* therefore, abolishes the acute attack of *P. falciparum* malaria but does not prevent the infection. Chloroquine-resistant strains have been reported. Also acts as a tissue amebicide, has antiinflammatory action, antihistamine, and antiserotonic properties; and inhibits prostaglandin F_2 synthesis. Demonstrates affinity for melanin-bearing cells, which may explain certain adverse effects related to eyes, ears, and skin.

USES Suppression and treatment of malaria caused by *P. malariae, P. ovale, P. vivax,* and susceptible forms of *P. falciparum,* and in the treatment of extraintestinal amebiasis. Concomitant therapy with primaquine is necessary for radical cure of vivax and malariae malarias. **Unlabeled uses:** discoid and systemic lupus erythematosus, porphyria cutanea tarda, solar urticaria, polymorphous light eruptions, and in rheumatoid arthritis (as second-line therapy).

PHARMACOKINETICS Absorption: rapidly and almost completely absorbed. **Peak:** 1–2 h. **Distribution:** widely distributed; concentrates in lungs, liver, erythrocytes, eyes, skin, and kidneys; crosses placenta. **Metabolism:** partially metabolized in liver to active metabolites. **Elimination:** half-life: 70–120 h; eliminated in urine; excreted in breast milk.

ROUTE & DOSAGE

Doses are expressed in terms of chloroquine base: 500 mg tablet = 300 mg base; 50 mg injection = 40 mg base.

Acute Malaria

Adult	PO	600 mg base followed by 300 mg base at 6, 24, and 48 h
	IM	200 mg base q6h prn; not to exceed 800 mg base/24 h
Child	PO	10 mg base/kg; then 5 mg base/kg at 6, 24, and 48 h
	IM	5 mg base/kg q12h

Malaria Suppression

Adult	PO	300 mg base the same day each week starting 2 wk before exposure and continuing for 4–6 wk after leaving the area of exposure (max 300 mg base/wk)
Child	PO	5 mg base/kg the same day each week starting 2 wk before exposure and continuing for 4–6 wk after leaving the area of exposure (max 300 mg base/wk)

Extraintestinal Amebiasis

Adult	PO	600 mg base/d for 2 d; then 300 mg base/d for 2–3 wk
Child	PO	10 mg base/kg/d for 2–3 wk

Rheumatoid Arthritis, SLE

Adult	PO	150 mg base/d with evening meal

CONTRAINDICATIONS & PRECAUTIONS

Contraindicated in: hypersensitivity to 4-aminoquinolines, psoriasis; porphyria, renal disease, 4-aminoquinoline-induced retinal or visual field changes; long-term therapy in children. Safe use during pregnancy (category C), in nursing women, and women of childbearing potential not established. **Cautious use in:** impaired hepatic function, alcoholism, eczema, patients with G6PD deficiency, infants and children, hematologic, GI, and neurologic disorders.

ADVERSE/SIDE EFFECTS

CNS: mild transient headache, fatigue, irritability, confusion, psychic stimulation, psychoses, nightmares, skeletal muscle weakness, paresthesias, reduced reflexes, vertigo.

CV: hypotension; ECG changes. **Ear:** ototoxicity (rare), tinnitus, impaired hearing, auditory nerve damage. **Eye:** (usually reversible): blurred vision, disturbances of accommodation, night blindness, scotomas, visual field defects, photophobia, corneal edema, opacity or deposits. **GI:** *diarrhea,* abdominal cramps, *nausea,* vomiting, anorexia. **Hematologic:** anemia, leukopenia, thrombocytopenia, agranulocytosis, hemolytic anemia. **Other:** bleaching of scalp, eyebrows, body hair, and freckles, pruritus, patchy alopecia (reversible), slight weight loss, myalgia, lymphedema of upper limbs, acute intermittent porphyria.

DRUG INTERACTIONS Aluminum- and **magnesium**-containing ANTACIDS and LAXATIVES decrease chloroquine absorption, so separate administration by at least 4 h; chloroquine may interfere with response to **rabies vaccine**.

NURSING IMPLICATIONS

Administration

- GI side effects may be minimized by administering PO drug immediately before or after meals.
- Children are extremely susceptible to overdosage of chloroquine (especially the parenteral formulation) and other 4-aminoquinoline compounds. PO administration should begin as soon as possible. Long-term therapy is not recommended in children.
- Store in tightly closed container preferably between 15–30C (59–86F), unless otherwise directed by manufacturer.

Assessment & Drug Effects

- CBC and ECG are advised before initiation of therapy and periodically thereafter in patients on long-term therapy.
- A test for G6PD deficiency is recommended for American blacks and individuals of Mediterranean ancestry before therapy.
- Retinopathy (generally irreversible) can be progressive even after termination of therapy. Patient may be asymptomatic or complain of night blindness, scotomas, visual field changes, blurred vision, or difficulty in focusing. Chloroquine should be discontinued immediately.
- Patients on long-term therapy should be questioned regularly about skeletal muscle weakness, and periodic tests should be made of muscle strength and deep tendon reflexes. Positive signs are indications to terminate therapy.

Patient & Family Education

- Report promptly visual or hearing disturbances, muscle weakness, or loss of balance, symptoms of blood dyscrasia (fever, sore mouth or throat, unexplained fatigue, easy bruising or bleeding).
- Use of dark glasses in sunlight or bright light may provide comfort (because of photophobia) and reduce risk of ocular damage.
- Therapeutic effects in rheumatoid arthritis do not generally occur until after several weeks of therapy. Chloroquine can cause dizziness. Therefore, advise patient to avoid driving or other potentially hazardous activities until reaction to drug is known.
- May cause rusty yellow or brown discoloration of urine.

ANTITRICHOMONAL

METRONIDAZOLE
(me-troe-ni´da-zole)

Trade names: Flagyl I.V., Flagyl I.V. RTU, Metizol, Metric 21, Metro I.V., Protostat
Classifications: ANTIINFECTIVE; ANTITRICHOMONAL; AMEBICIDE
Pregnancy: Category B

ACTIONS/PHARMACODYNAMICS Synthetic compound with direct trichomonicidal and amebecidal activity against *Trichomonas vaginalis* (causes a venereal disease), *Entamoeba histolytica,* and *Giardia lamblia*. Also exhibits antibacterial activity against obligate anaerobic bacteria, gram-negative anaerobic bacilli, and clostridia. Microaerophilic streptococci and most aerobic bacteria are resistant. Metronidazole enters bacterial cells more readily under anaerobic conditions; after reduction in the cell, it binds to and degrades DNA. Frequency of postoperative infection and non-spore-forming anaerobic infections reported to be decreased with prophylactic use of the drug before and up to 7 d after surgery.

USES Asymptomatic and symptomatic trichomoniasis in females and males; acute intestinal amebiasis and amebic liver abscess; preoperative prophylaxis in colorectal surgery, elective hysterectomy or vaginal repair, and emergency appendectomy. IV metronidazole is used for the treatment of serious infections caused by susceptible anaerobic bacteria in intraabdominal infections, skin infections, gynecologic infections, septicemia, and for both pre- and postoperative prophylaxis. **Unlabeled use:** treatment of pseudomembranous colitis, Crohn's disease.

ROUTE & DOSAGE

Trichomoniasis, Giardiasis, *Gardnerella*

Adult	PO	2 g once; or 250 mg t.i.d. or 500 mg b.i.d. for 7 d
Child	PO	15 mg/kg/d in 3 divided doses for 7–10 d
Infant	PO	10–30 mg/kg/d for 5–8 d

Amebiasis

Adult	PO	500–750 mg t.i.d.
Child	PO	35–50 mg/kg/d in 3 divided doses

Anaerobic Infections

Adult	PO	7.5 mg/kg q6h (max 4 g/d)
	IV	15 mg/kg loading dose, then 7.5 mg/kg q6h (max 4 g/d)

Pseudomembranous Colitis

Adult	PO	250–500 mg t.i.d.
	IV	250–500 mg t.i.d. or q.i.d.

PHARMACOKINETICS Absorption: 80% of dose absorbed from GI tract. **Peak:** 1–3 h. **Distribution:** widely distributed to most body tissues, including CSF, bone, cerebral and hepatic abscesses; crosses placenta; distributed in breast milk. **Metabolism:** 30–60% metabolized in liver. **Elimination:** half-life: 6–8 h; 77% excreted in urine; 14% excreted in feces within 24 h.

CONTRAINDICATIONS & PRECAUTIONS
Contraindicated in: blood dyscrasias, active CNS disease, first trimester of pregnancy (category B), nursing mothers. **Cautious use in:** coexistent candidiasis; second and third trimesters of pregnancy; alcoholism; hepatic disease.

ADVERSE/SIDE EFFECTS Allergic: rash, urticaria, pruritus, flushing. **CNS:** vertigo, headache, ataxia, incoordination (rare), confusion, irritability, depression, restlessness, weakness, fatigue, drowsiness, insomnia, sensory neuropathy, paresthesias. **GI:** *nausea,* vomiting, anorexia, epigastric distress, abdominal cramps, diarrhea, constipation, dry mouth, metallic or bitter taste. **GU:** polyuria, dysuria, pyuria, incontinence, cystitis, decreased libido, dyspareunia, dryness of vagina and vulva, sense of pelvic pressure.

Common side effects in *italic*; life-threatening effects underlined; generic names in **bold**; classifications in SMALL CAPS

Other: moderate neutropenia, leukopenia; nasal congestion, fever, fleeting joint pains, ECG changes (flattening of T wave); overgrowth of *Candida;* proctitis.

DIAGNOSTIC TEST INTERFERENCES Metronidazole may interfere with certain chemical analyses for AST, resulting in decreased values.

DRUG INTERACTIONS ORAL ANTICOAGULANTS potentiate hypoprothrombinemia; **alcohol** may elicit disulfiram reaction; **disulfiram** causes acute psychosis; **phenobarbital** increases metronidazole metabolism; may increase **lithium** levels; **fluorouracil, azothiaprine** may cause transient neutropenia.

INCOMPATIBILITIES Solution/additive: TPN, **aztreonam, dopamine.**

NURSING IMPLICATIONS

Administration

- Tablets may be crushed before ingestion if patient cannot swallow them whole.
- Administer oral preparation immediately before, with, or immediately after meals or with food or milk to reduce GI distress.
- Lower than normal doses should be given in the presence of hepatic disease.
- Therapy instituted during the second or third trimester of pregnancy should be over a 7 d period. The 2 g PO dose (1 d) produces a high serum level that may reach fetal circulation.

Parenteral Administration

- Do not give direct IV bolus injection because of low pH of reconstituted product.
- Sequence for preparing solution (important): (a) reconstitution with 4.4 ml sterile water or NS, (b) dilution in IV solution to yield 8 mg/ml in NS, D5W, or lactated Ringer's for infusion, (c) pH neutralization with approximately 5 mEq sodium bicarbonate injection for each 500 mg of Flagyl I.V. used.
- Administer IV solution slowly at a rate of one dose per hour.
- Flagyl I.V. RTU does not require mixing, diluting or neutralizing. Each container contains 14 mEq of sodium.
- Avoid use of aluminum-containing equipment when manipulating IV product (including syringes equipped with aluminum needles or hubs).
- Do not mix IV metronidazole with any other drug.
- CO_2 will be generated when neutralized with sodium bicarbonate; release of pressure within container may be necessary.

- Precipitation occurs if neutralized solution is refrigerated. Use diluted and neutralized solution within 24 h of preparation.
- Storage and stability: Reconstituted Flagyl I.V. is chemically stable for 96 h when stored below 30C (86F) in room light. Diluted and neutralized IV solutions containing Flagyl I.V. should be used within 24 h of mixing. Flagyl I.V. RTU should be stored at 15–30C (59–86F); protect from light during storage.

Assessment & Drug Effects

- Presence of trichomonads should be confirmed by wet smear or by cultures before start of therapy for trichomoniasis and before a course of retreatment.
- Total and differential leukocyte counts are recommended before, during, and after therapy, especially if a second course is necessary.
- Therapy should be discontinued immediately if symptoms of CNS toxicity (see Chapter 3) develop. Monitor especially for seizures and peripheral neuropathy (e.g., numbness and paresthesia of extremities).
- Monitor for signs of sodium retention, especially in patients on corticosteroid therapy or with a history of CHF.
- Patients on lithium should be monitored for elevated lithium levels.
- Candidiasis may appear or become more prominent with metronidazole therapy. Report to physician promptly.
- Repeated feces examinations, usually up to 3 mo, are necessary to assure that amebae have been eliminated.

Patient & Family Education

- Dosage regimens are individualized sometimes on the basis of anticipated compliance. Caution the patient to adhere closely to the established regimen without schedule interruption or changing the dose.
- During therapy for trichomoniasis it is recommended that the patient refrain from intercourse unless the male partner wears a condom to prevent reinfection.
- Sexual partners should receive concurrent treatment. Asymptomatic trichomoniasis in the male is a frequent source of reinfection of the female.
- Warn patient that ingestion of alcohol during metronidazole therapy may induce a disulfiram-type reaction (see Signs & Symptoms, chap 3). Alcohol or alcohol-containing medications should be avoided for at least 48 h after treatment is completed.
- Inform patient that urine may appear dark or red-

dish brown (especially with higher than recommended doses). This appears to have no clinical significance.

- Advise patient to report symptoms of candidal overgrowth: furry tongue, color changes of tongue, glossitis, stomatitis; vaginitis, curdlike, milky vaginal discharge; proctitis. Treatment with a candicidal agent may be indicated.
- The 7 d regimen for trichomoniasis reportedly has a higher cure rate than the single day schedule. In addition, with the extended treatment period, reinfection of the female may be minimized long enough to treat sexual contacts.

ANTITUBERCULOSIS AGENT

ISONIAZID (ISONICOTINIC ACID HYDRAZIDE)

(eye-soe-nye´a-zid)

Trade names: INH, Isotamine, Laniazid, Nydrazid, PMS Isoniazid, Rimifon, Teebaconin
Classifications: ANTIINFECTIVE; ANTITUBERCULOSIS AGENT
Pregnancy: Category C

ACTIONS/PHARMACODYNAMICS Hydrazide of isonicotinic acid with highly specific action against *Mycobacterium tuberculosis*. Exerts bacteriostatic action against actively growing (i.e., undergoing cell division) tubercle bacilli; may be bactericidal in higher concentrations. Postulated to act by interfering with biosynthesis of bacterial proteins, nucleic acid, and lipids. Reported to have some MAO-inhibiting properties and to act as a competitive antagonist of pyridoxine (vitamin B_6). Also may cause alterations in vitamin D metabolism.

USES Treatment of all forms of active tuberculosis caused by susceptible organisms and as preventive in high-risk persons (e.g., household members, persons with positive tuberculin skin test reactions). May be used alone or with other tuberculostatic agents. **Unlabeled use:** treatment of atypical mycobacterial infections; tuberculous meningitis; action tremor in multiple sclerosis.

PHARMACOKINETICS Absorption: readily absorbed from GI tract; food may reduce rate and extent of absorption. **Peak:** 1–2 h. **Distribution:** distributed to all body tissues and fluids including the CNS; crosses placenta. **Metabolism:** inactivated by acetyla-

tion in liver. **Elimination:** half-life: 1–4 h; 75–96% excreted in urine in 24 h; excreted in breast milk.

ROUTE & DOSAGE

Treatment

Adult	PO/IM	5 mg/kg up to 300 mg/d
Child	PO/IM	10–20 mg/kg up to 300–500 mg/d

Preventive Therapy

Adult	PO	300 mg/d
Child	PO	10 mg/kg up to 300 mg/d or 15 mg/kg 3 times/wk

CONTRAINDICATIONS & PRECAUTIONS Contraindicated in: history of isoniazid-associated hypersensitivity reactions, including hepatic injury; acute liver damage of any etiology; pregnancy (category C) unless risk is warranted. **Cautious use in:** chronic liver disease; renal dysfunction; history of convulsive disorders; chronic alcoholism; persons over 35 y.

ADVERSE/SIDE EFFECTS Usually dose related. **CNS:** *paresthesias, peripheral neuropathy,* headache, unusual tiredness or weakness, tinnitus, dizziness, vertigo, ataxia, somnolence, excessive dreaming, insomnia, amnesia, euphoria, toxic psychosis, changes in affect and behavior, depression, impaired memory, hyperreflexia, muscle twitching, slurred speech, hallucinations, convulsions. **Eye:** blurred vision, visual disturbances, optic neuritis, atrophy. **GI:** nausea, vomiting, epigastric distress, dry mouth, constipation. **Hematologic:** <u>agranulocytosis</u>, hemolytic or <u>aplastic anemia</u>, thrombocytopenia, eosinophilia, methemoglobinemia. **Hepatotoxicity:** elevated AST, ALT; bilirubinemia, jaundice, hepatitis. **Hypersensitivity:** fever, chills, skin eruptions (morbiliform, maculopapular, purpuric, urticarial), lymphadenitis, vasculitis. **Metabolic/endocrine:** decreased vitamin B_{12} absorption, pyridoxine (vitamin B_6) deficiency, pellagra, gynecomastia, hyperglycemia, glycosuria, hyperkalemia, hypophosphatemia, hypocalcemia, acetonuria, metabolic acidosis, proteinuria. **Other:** dyspnea, urinary retention (males), drug-related fever, rheumatic and lupus erythematosus–like syndromes, irritation at injection site.

DIAGNOSTIC TEST INTERFERENCES Isoniazid may produce false-positive results using *copper sulfate tests,* e.g., *Benedict's solution, Clinitest,* but not with glucose oxidase methods (e.g., Clinstix, Dextrostix, TesTape).

Common side effects in *italic*; life-threatening effects <u>underlined</u>; generic names in **bold**; classifications in SMALL CAPS

83

DRUG INTERACTIONS Cycloserine, ethion-amide enhance CNS toxicity; may increase **pheny-toin** levels, resulting in toxicity; ALUMINUM-CONTAINING ANTACIDS decrease GI absorption; **disulfiram** may cause coordination difficulties or psychotic reactions; **alcohol** increases risk of hepatotoxicity. **Drug-Food:** food decreases rate and extent of isoniazid absorption; should be taken 1 h before meals.

NURSING IMPLICATIONS

Administration

- PO isoniazid is best taken on an empty stomach at least 1 h before or 2 h after meals as food interferes with its absorption. However, if GI irritation occurs, drug may be taken with meals.
- Isoniazid in solution tends to crystallize at low temperatures; if this occurs, solution should be allowed to warm to room temperature to redissolve crystals before use.
- Local transient pain may follow IM injections. Massage injection site following drug administration. Rotate injection sites.
- Preserved in tightly closed, light-resistant containers at 15–30C (59–86F), unless otherwise directed by manufacturer.

Assessment & Drug Effects

- Appropriate susceptibility tests should be performed before initiation of therapy and periodically thereafter to detect possible bacterial resistance.
- Therapeutic effects usually become evident within the first 2–3 wk of therapy. Over 90% of patients receiving optimal therapy have negative sputum by the sixth month.
- Eye examinations are recommended initially and whenever visual symptoms appear. Early cessation of therapy usually results in resolution of ocular reactions.
- Inactivation of the drug is genetically determined and affects plasma drug concentration. Slow inactivation leads to high plasma drug levels and increased risk of toxicity and is found among Egyptians, Jews, Scandinavians, and other Caucasians, and in approximately 50% of blacks.
- Isoniazid-induced pyridoxine (vitamin B_6) depletion causes neurotoxic effects. B_6 supplementation (10–50 mg) usually accompanies isoniazid use.
- Peripheral neuritis, the most common toxic effect, is usually preceded by paresthesias of feet and hands (numbness, tingling, burning). Patients particularly susceptible include alcoholics and patients with liver disease, malnourished patients, diabetics, slow inactivators, pregnant women, and the elderly.

- Monitor BP during period of dosage adjustment. Some patients experience orthostatic hypotension; therefore, caution against rapid positional changes. Supervision of ambulation may be indicated, particularly in the elderly.
- Diabetic patients should be observed for loss of diabetes control. Both true glycosuria and false-positive Benedict's tests have been reported.
- Isoniazid hepatitis (sometimes fatal) usually develops during the first 3–6 mo of treatment, but it may occur at any time during drug therapy. It is much more frequent in patients 35 y or older, especially in those who ingest alcohol daily.
- Continuation of isoniazid therapy after the onset of hepatic dysfunction increases risk of severe liver damage.
- Patients should be carefully interviewed and examined at monthly intervals for early detection of signs and symptoms of hepatotoxicity (see Chapter 3). By the time overt signs (dark urine, jaundice or scleral icterus) appear, patient has already developed hepatitis.
- Check weight at least twice weekly under standard conditions.

Patient & Family Education

- Warn patient that concurrent ingestion of tyramine-containing foods (e.g., aged cheeses, smoked fish) may cause palpitation, flushing, and blood pressure elevation.
- Warn patient that histamine-containing foods (e.g., skipjack, tuna, sauerkraut juice, yeast extracts) may cause exaggerated drug response (headache, hypotension, palpitation, sweating, itching, flushing, diarrhea).
- Instruct patient to withhold medication and report promptly to physician if signs and symptoms of hepatotoxicity develop. Some physicians order monthly liver function tests throughout therapy.
- Advise patient to avoid or at least to reduce alcohol intake while on isoniazid therapy because of increased risk of hepatotoxicity.
- Hypersensitivity reaction should be reported immediately and all drugs withheld. Generally, it occurs within 3–7 wk after initiation of therapy.
- Isoniazid may produce a sense of euphoria, which tempts the patient to do more than he or she should. Stress the importance of planned rest periods.
- In general, isoniazid therapy is continued for 6 mo–2 y for original treatment of active tuberculosis. When used for preventive therapy, isoniazid is usually continued for 12 mo. Duration of treatment is

Common side effects in *italic*; life-threatening effects <u>underlined</u>; generic names in **bold**; classifications in SMALL CAPS

generally shorter when both isoniazid and rifampin are used.

- Niacin (vitamin B$_3$) and folate stores are decreased during isoniazid therapy. Folates are found in a wide variety of foods.

ANTIVIRAL

ACYCLOVIR

(ay-sye´-kloe-ver)
Trade names: Acycloguanosine, Zovirax

ACYCLOVIR SODIUM

Classifications: ANTIINFECTIVE; ANTIVIRAL
Pregnancy: Category C

ACTIONS/PHARMACODYNAMICS Synthetic acyclic purine nucleoside analog, derived from guanine. Reduces viral shedding and formation of new lesions and speeds healing time. Acyclovir triphosphate preferentially interferes with DNA synthesis of herpes simplex virus types 1 and 2 (HSV-1 and HSV-2) and varicella-zoster virus, thereby inhibiting viral replication. Demonstrates antiviral activity against herpes virus simiae (B virus), Epstein-Barr (infectious mononucleosis), varicella-zoster and cytomegalovirus. Does not eradicate the latent herpes virus.

USES Parenterally for treatment of initial and recurrent mucosal and cutaneous herpes simplex virus (HSV-1 and HSV-2) infections in immunocompromised adults and children and for severe initial episodes of herpes genitalis in immunocompetent (normal immune system) patients. Used orally for treatment of initial episodes of genital herpes, for management of selected patients with severe recurrent episodes, and for prophylaxis to reduce frequency and severity of recurrent infections. Used topically for initial episodes of herpes genitalis and in non-life-threatening mucocutaneous herpes simplex virus infections in immunocompromised patients. **Unlabeled use:** for treatment of eczema herpeticum caused by HSV localized and disseminated herpes zoster and varicella-zoster (chickenpox).

PHARMACOKINETICS Absorption: oral dose is 15–30% absorbed. **Peak Effect:** 1.5–2 h after oral dose. **Distribution:** distributes into most tissues with lower levels in the CNS; crosses placenta. **Metabolism:** drug is primarily excreted unchanged. **Elimination:** half-life: 2.5–5 h; renally eliminated; also excreted in breast milk.

ROUTE & DOSAGE

Genital Herpes Simplex

Adult	PO	200 mg q4h 5 times/d
	IV	5 mg/kg q8h
Child	IV	<12 y: 250 mg/m² q8h

Prophylaxis for Genital Herpes Simplex

Adult	PO	200 mg 2–5 times/d or
		400 mg b.i.d.

Herpes Zoster

Adult	PO	800 mg q4h 5 times/d

Herpes Simplex Encephalitis

Adult	IV	10 mg/kg q8h
Child	IV	10 mg/kg q8h

Dosing Adjustment for Renal Insufficiency (All Indications)

Creatinine Clearance	25–50 ml/min same dose q12h
	10–25 ml/min same dose q24h

CONTRAINDICATIONS & PRECAUTIONS Contraindicated in: rapid or bolus injection of acyclovir—infuse over 1 h. Safe use during pregnancy (category C) and in children not established. **Cautious use in:** nursing mother, renal insufficiency, dehydration.

ADVERSE/SIDE EFFECTS (generally minimal and infrequent): **CNS:** *headache,* light-headedness, lethargy, fatigue, tremors, confusion, seizures, dizziness. **GI:** *nausea, vomiting, diarrhea.* **Renal:** glomerulonephritis, renal tubular damage, acute renal failure. **Skin:** rash, urticaria, pruritus, burning, stinging sensation, irritation, sensitization. **Other:** inflammation or phlebitis at IV injection site, sloughing (with extravasation); fever, muscle cramps, arthralgia, menstrual abnormalities, edema.

DRUG INTERACTIONS Probenecid decreases acyclovir elimination; **zidovudine** may cause increased drowsiness and lethargy.

INCOMPATIBILITIES Solution/Additive: bacteriostatic water for injection, albumin, hetastarch, **dopamine, dobutamine.**

Common side effects in *italic*; life-threatening effects <u>underlined</u>; generic names in **bold**; classifications in SMALL CAPS

85

NURSING IMPLICATIONS

Administration

Parenteral

- Reconstituted first by adding 10 ml sterile water for injection to 500 mg vial (provides concentration of 50 mg/ml). Note: solutions containing benzyl alcohol are toxic to neonates. Shake well to assure complete dissolution of drug. This solution should be used within 12 h.
- To reduce risk of renal injury and phlebitis, final concentration should be 7 mg/ml or less. Once prepared, diluted solution should be used within 24 h.
- Manufacturer approves use of standard commercially available electrolyte and glucose solutions for infusion solution; incompatible with blood products and protein-containing solutions.
- Intended for IV infusion only and must be administered over a period of at least 1 h to prevent renal tubular damage. Rapid or bolus IV and IM or SC administration must be avoided.
- Monitor IV flow rate carefully; infusion pump or microdrip infusion set preferred. Usual rate of administration is a single dose over 60 min. Observe infusion site during and for a few days following infusion.
- Keep patient adequately hydrated during first 2 h after infusion to maintain sufficient urinary flow and thus prevent precipitation of drug in renal tubules.
- Consult physician about amount and length of time oral fluids need to be pushed after IV drug treatment.
- Refrigeration of reconstituted solution may cause precipitation; however, crystals will redissolve at room temperature.
- Store acyclovir powder and reconstituted solutions at controlled room temperature preferably at 15–30C (59–86F) unless otherwise directed by manufacturer.

Oral

- Absorption of oral acyclovir is not affected by food.
- Store capsules in tight, light-resistant containers at 15–30C (59–86F) unless otherwise directed.

Topical

- Thorough hand washing is needed before and after treatment of lesions and after handling and disposition of secretions. Virus is killed by soap and water.
- Use liquid soap for hand washing to prevent cross-contamination.
- Apply topical preparation with finger cot or surgical glove to prevent further self-infection as well as spread of virus to others. Use sufficient ointment to completely cover lesions.
- Store at 15–25C (59–78F) unless otherwise directed.

Assessment & Drug Effects

- Monitor I&O ratio and pattern, especially after IV administration. Note: unusual tiredness and weakness suggest poor hydration as well as early renal failure.
- Baseline and periodic renal function studies should be done. This is particularly important with IV administration. Elevations of BUN and serum creatinine and decreases in creatinine clearance indicate need for dosage adjustment, discontinuation of drug, or correction of fluid and electrolyte balance.
- Prophylactic use of the oral drug will require careful monitoring for possible long-term side effects and for viral resistance to acyclovir and is generally given for no longer than 6 mo pending complete evaluation of the benefits and dangers of prolonged use of acyclovir.
- Notify physician if local reactions to topical drug are pronounced or annoying and if no improvement is noted within 1 wk.
- Pregnant patients should be followed closely to detect reinfection.
- Patients with history of neurologic problems, drug related or otherwise, are reportedly more prone to manifest acyclovir-induced neurologic symptoms.
- Immunocompromised patients receiving prolonged or repeated therapy have developed drug resistance.

Patient & Family Education

- Therapy is most effective when started as soon as possible after onset of signs and symptoms.
- Even after the HSV infection is controlled, latent virus can be activated by such stimuli as stress, trauma, fever, exposure to sunlight, sexual intercourse, menstruation, treatment with immunosuppressive drugs.
- Warn patient to refrain from sexual intercourse if either partner has signs or symptoms of herpes infection.
- Acyclovir is not a cure for herpetic infections. HSV-1 virus (cold sore or fever blister) remains latent for patient's lifetime and may emerge intermittently to cause symptoms.
- Caution not to exceed recommended dosage, frequency of drug administration, or specified duration of therapy. Urge patient to contact physician if relief is not obtained or side effects appear.
- Women with genital herpes reportedly are at a high risk level for developing cervical cancer. Urge pa-

Common side effects in *italic*; life-threatening effects <u>underlined</u>; generic names in **bold**; classifications in SMALL CAPS

tient to have periodic Papanicolaou (Pap) smears to detect early cervical changes.

- Caution patient not to exceed recommended dosage, frequency of drug administration, or specified duration of therapy. Urge patient to consult physician if relief is not obtained or side effects appear.

Topical Application

- Cleanse affected areas with soap and water 3 or 4 times daily; dry well. Hair dryer may be helpful. Wear loose fitting clothing and absorbent (e.g., cotton) underclothing.
- Avoid drug contact in or around eyes. Any unexplained eye symptoms (e.g., redness, pain) should be reported immediately. Untreated infection can lead to corneal keratitis and blindness.
- Avoid use of OTC emollient creams or ointments unless specifically prescribed by physician. These agents tend to delay healing and may even spread lesions.
- Topical applications do not prevent transmission to other individuals and do not prevent recurrence.

QUINOLONE

CIPROFLOXACIN HYDROCHLORIDE

(ci-pro-flox´a-cin)
Trade name: Cipro
Classification: ANTIINFECTIVE; QUINOLONE
Pregnancy: Category X

ACTIONS/PHARMACODYNAMICS Synthetic quinolone that is a broad spectrum bactericidal agent. Inhibits DNA-gyrase, an enzyme necessary for bacterial DNA replication and some aspects of transcription, repair, recombination, and transposition. Effective against many gram-positive and gram-negative organisms including *Citrobacter diversus, Enterobacter cloacae, Enterobacter aerogenes, Escherichia coli, Haemophilus influenzae, Klebsiella pneumoniae, Neisseria gonorrhoeae, Proteus mirabilis, Proteus vulgaris, Pseudomonas aeruginosa, Serratia marcescens, Staphylococcus aureus, Staphylococcus pyogenes, Shigella,* and *Salmonella.* Less active against gram-positive than gram-negative bacteria, although active against many gram-positive aerobic bacteria, including penicillinase-producing, non-penicillinase-producing, and methicillin-resistant staphylococci. However many strains of strepto-

cocci are relatively resistant to the drug. Inactive against most anaerobic bacteria. Resistant to some strains of methicillin-resistant *S. aureus* (MRSA).

USES UTIs, lower respiratory tract infections, skin and skin structure infections, bone and joint infections, and GI infection or infectious diarrhea.

ROUTE & DOSAGE

UTI

Adult	PO	250 mg q12h
	IV	200 mg q12h, infused over 60 min

Moderate to Severe Systemic Infection

Adult	PO	500–750 mg q12h
	IV	200–400 mg q12h, infused over 60 min

PHARMACOKINETICS Absorption: 60–80% absorbed from GI tract. **Peak:** 1–2 h. **Distribution:** widely distributed including prostate, lung, and bone; crosses placenta; distributed into breast milk. **Elimination:** half-life: 3.5–4 h; excreted primarily in urine with some biliary excretion.

CONTRAINDICATIONS & PRECAUTIONS Contraindicated in: known hypersensitivity to ciprofloxacin or other quinolones, pregnant women (category X), nursing mothers, and children. **Cautious use in:** known or suspected CNS disorders (i.e., severe cerebral arteriosclerosis or seizure disorders), patients receiving theophylline derivatives or caffeine, severe renal impairment and crystalluria during ciprofloxacin therapy, and patients on coumarin therapy.

ADVERSE/SIDE EFFECTS CNS: headache, *vertigo, malaise,* seizures (especially with rapid IV infusion). **GI:** *nausea, vomiting, diarrhea, cramps, gas.* **Skin:** *rash,* transient increases in liver transaminases, alkaline phosphatase, lactic dehydrogenase, and eosinophilia count, *phlebitis, pain, burning, pruritus,* and *erythema* at infusion site.

DIAGNOSTIC TEST INTERFERENCES Ciprofloxacin does not interfere with urinary glucose determinations using cupric sulfate solution or with glucose ovadase tests.

DRUG INTERACTIONS May increase **theophylline** levels 15–30%; ANTACIDS, **sulcralfate, iron** decrease absorption of ciprofloxacin.

Common side effects in *italic*; life-threatening effects <u>underlined</u>; generic names in **bold**; classifications in SMALL CAPS

87

NURSING IMPLICATIONS

Administration

- IV ciprofloxacin must be diluted before administration in NS or D5W to a final concentration of 1–2 mg/ml. Appropriate dilutions are 200 mg in 100 ml and 400 mg in 200 ml.
- Properly diluted IV ciprofloxacin solution should be infused slowly over 60 min.
- Discontinue other IV infusion while infusing ciprofloxacin or infuse through another site.
- Administration of an antacid should not be concomitant with or within 4 h of the ciprofloxacin dose.
- For patients with renal impairment, dose is lowered according to creatinine clearance.
- Reconstituted IV solution is stable for 14 d refrigerated.

Assessment & Drug Effects

- Culture and sensitivity tests should be done prior to initial dose. Treatment may be implemented pending results.
- Urine pH should be less than 6.8, especially in the elderly and patients receiving high dosages of ciprofloxacin, to reduce the risk of crystalluria.
- Patients should be well hydrated; monitor I&O and assess for signs and symptoms of crystalluria.
- Monitor plasma theophylline concentrations, since drug may interfere with half-life.
- Administration with theophylline derivatives or caffeine can cause CNS stimulation.
- Assess for signs and symptoms of GI irritation (e.g., nausea, diarrhea, vomiting, abdominal discomfort) in clients receiving high dosages and in the elderly.
- Monitor PT in patients receiving coumarin therapy.
- Assess for signs and symptoms of superinfections (see chap 3).

Patient & Family Education

- Advise fluid intake of 2–3 L/d if not contraindicated.
- Instruct patient not to exceed the recommended dosage.
- Instruct patient to restrict caffeine and advise of the effects (e.g., nervousness, insomnia, anxiety, tachycardia).
- Instruct patient of potential adverse effects of taking a theophylline derivative and of the need to report possible toxicity.
- Instruct patient to report nausea, diarrhea, vomiting, and abdominal pain or discomfort.
- Inform patient that drug may cause lightheadedness and that caution should be taken with hazardous activities until reaction to drug is known.

SULFONAMIDE

SULFISOXAZOLE

(sul-fi-sox´a-zole)
Trade names: Gantrisin, Gulfasin, Lipo Gantrisin, SK-Soxazole
Classifications: ANTIINFECTIVE; SULFONAMIDE
Pregnancy: Categories B and D (if near term)

ACTIONS/PHARMACODYNAMICS Short-acting derivative of sulfanilamide. In common with other sulfonamides, has broad antimicrobial spectrum against both gram-positive and gram-negative organisms. Bacteriostatic action believed to be by competitive inhibition of p-aminobenzoic acid (PABA), thereby interfering with folic acid biosynthesis required for bacterial growth. Increase in resistant organisms is a limitation to usefulness of sulfonamides; cross-resistance to other sulfonamides is possible. Since sulfisoxazole and its derivatives are highly soluble in alkaline urine and slightly acidic urine and are excreted rapidly, the risk of crystalluria is small.

USES Acute, recurrent, and chronic urinary tract infections and chancroid; adjunctive therapy in trachoma, chloroquine-resistant strains of malaria, acute otitis media due to *Haemophilus influenzae,* and meningococcal and *H. influenzae* meningitis. Ophthalmic preparations used in treatment of conjunctivitis, corneal ulcer, and other superficial eye infections and as adjunct to systemic sulfonamide therapy for trachoma. Topical vaginal preparation used for *H. vaginalis* vaginitis.

ROUTE & DOSAGE

Infection by Susceptible Organisms

Adult	PO	2–4 g initially, followed by 4–8 g/d in 4–6 divided doses
	Vaginal	1 applicator full 1–2 times/d
Child	PO	75 mg/kg initially, followed by 150 mg/kg/d in 4–6 divided doses (max 6 g/d)

PHARMACOKINETICS Absorption: readily absorbed from GI tract. **Peak:** 2–4 h. **Distribution:** distributed in extracellular space; crosses blood-brain barrier and placenta; detected in breast milk. **Metabolism:** metabolized in liver. **Elimination:** half-life: 4.6–7.8 h; 95% excreted in urine in 24 h.

CONTRAINDICATIONS & PRECAUTIONS Contraindicated in: history of hypersensitivity to sulfonamides, salicylates, or chemically related drugs; use in treatment of group A beta-hemolytic streptococcal infections; infants <2 mo of age (except in treatment of congenital toxoplasmosis), pregnancy (category B); category D if near term, nursing mothers; porphyria; advanced renal or hepatic disease; intestinal and urinary obstruction. **Cautious use in:** impaired renal or liver function; severe allergy; bronchial asthma; blood dyscrasias; patients with G6PD deficiency.

ADVERSE/SIDE EFFECTS Low toxicity level but may include the following: **CNS:** headache, peripheral neuritis, peripheral neuropathy, tinnitus, hearing loss, vertigo, insomnia, drowsiness, mental depression, acute psychosis, ataxia, convulsions, kernicterus (newborns). **GI:** *nausea, vomiting, diarrhea,* abdominal pains, hepatitis, jaundice, pancreatitis, stomatitis, impaired folic acid absorption. **Hematologic:** acute hemolytic anemia (especially in patients with G6PD deficiency), aplastic anemia, methemoglobinemia, agranulocytosis, thrombocytopenia, leukopenia, eosinophilia, hypoprothrombinemia. **Hypersensitivity:** headache, *fever,* chills, arthralgia, malaise, pruritus, urticaria, conjunctival or scleral infection, rash, erythema multiforme including *Stevens-Johnson syndrome, exfoliative dermatitis,* allergic myocarditis, serum sickness, anaphylactoid reactions, photosensitivity, vascular lesions. **Renal:** *crystalluria,* hematuria, proteinuria, anuria, toxic nephrosis. **Other:** conjunctivitis, goiter, hypoglycemia, diuresis, overgrowth of nonsusceptible organisms, LE phenomenon, retardation of corneal healing (ophthalmic ointment), alopecia, reduction in sperm count, lymphadenopathy, local reaction following IM injection, fixed drug eruptions.

DIAGNOSTIC TEST INTERFERENCES Sulfonamides may interfere with *BSP* retention and *PSP* excretion tests and may affect results of *thyroid function* tests (*I-131* may be decreased for about 7 d). Large doses of sulfonamides reportedly may produce false-positive *urine glucose* determinations with copper reduction methods (e.g., Benedict's and Clinitest). Sulfonamides may produce false-positive results for *urinary protein* (with sulfosalicylic acid test) and may interfere with *urine urobilinogen* determinations using Ehrlich's reagent or Urobilistix. Follow-up cultures are unreliable unless *p*-aminobenzoic acid is added to culture medium.

DRUG INTERACTIONS PABA-CONTAINING LOCAL ANESTHETICS may antagonize sulfa's effects; ORAL ANTICOAGULANTS potentiate hypoprothrombinemia; may potentiate sulfonylurea-induced hypoglycemia.

NURSING IMPLICATIONS

Administration

- Tablet may be crushed before administration and taken with full glass of water or other fluid.
- Administration with food appears to delay but reportedly does not reduce amount of drug absorbed.
- Preserve in tight, light-resistant containers. Store at 15–30C (59–86F).

Assessment & Drug Effects

- Monitor I&O. Report oliguria and changes in I&O ratio. Fluid intake should be adequate to support urinary output of at least 1500 ml/d to prevent crystalluria and stone formation.
- Since a fall in urinary pH (more acidic) increases risk of crystalluria, daily check of urine pH with Nitrazine paper or Labstix is advisable.
- Report increasing urine acidity. If urine is highly acidic, physician may prescribe a urinary alkalinizer.
- Monitor temperature. Sudden appearance of fever may signify sensitization (serum sickness) or hemolytic anemia (frequent in patients with G6PD deficiency, which is most common among black males and Mediterranean ethnic groups). These reactions generally develop within 10 d after start of drug. Agranulocytosis may develop after 10 d–6 wk of therapy.
- Fever with sore throat, malaise, unusual fatigue, joint pains, pallor, bleeding tendencies, rash, and jaundice are early manifestations of blood dyscrasias or hypersensitivity reactions. Report them immediately.
- Skin lesions, papular or vesiculobullous lesions, especially on sun-exposed areas, Stevens-Johnson syndrome (severe erythema multiforme) may be preceded by high fever, severe headache, stomatitis, conjunctivitis, rhinitis, urticaria, balanitis (inflammation of penis or clitoris). Termination of drug therapy is indicated.
- Frequent kidney function tests and urinalyses are recommended; complete blood tests and hepatic function tests are advised, especially in patients receiving sulfonamides for longer than 2 wk.

Common side effects in *italic*; life-threatening effects underlined; generic names in **bold**; classifications in SMALL CAPS

89

- Diabetic patients receiving oral hypoglycemic agents should be closely observed for hypoglycemic reactions. Determinations of blood glucose levels are advised before and shortly after initiation of sulfonamide therapy.

Patient & Family Education

- The patient should understand clearly that the established dosage regimen must be followed: patient should not omit, increase, interrupt, or decrease dose. The full course of treatment should be completed.
- Caution patients not to take OTC medications without consulting physician. Many analgesic mixtures contain aspirin in combination with *p*-aminobenzoic acid. Inform patients that excessive doses of vitamin C acidify urine and therefore should be avoided (to prevent crystalluria).
- Advise patients using topical applications to stop treatment if local irritation or sensitivity reaction develops and to report to physician. Patient should be informed that sensitization to topical application precludes future systemic use of sulfonamides.
- Oral contraceptives may be unreliable while patient is receiving a sulfonamide. Advise an alternate method of contraception. Breakthrough bleeding should be considered evidence of an interaction.
- Advise patients to avoid exposure to ultraviolet light and excessive sunlight to prevent photosensitivity reaction during therapy and for several months after treatment is discontinued.
- Advise patient to inform dentist or new physician of taking a sulfonamide.

URINARY TRACT ANTIINFECTIVE

TRIMETHOPRIM
(trye-meth´oh-prim)
Trade names: Proloprim, Trimpex
Classification: URINARY TRACT ANTIINFECTIVE
Pregnancy: Category C

ACTIONS/PHARMACODYNAMICS Antiinfective and folic acid antagonist with slow bactericidal action. Binds to and reversibly blocks enzyme reduction of folic acid to its active metabolite tetrahydrofolic acid, thus preventing bacterial synthesis of thymidine, an essential nucleoside in DNA. This binding and interference with cell growth is 1000 times stronger in bacterial than in mammalian cells.

Most pathogens causing urinary tract infection (UTI) are in normal vaginal and fecal flora. Trimethoprim concentration in vaginal secretions is higher than in serum, and sufficient amounts of the drug are excreted in feces to reduce or eliminate susceptible fecal organisms. Thus, drug is effective against most common UTI pathogens, including *Escherichia coli, Enterobacter* species, *Klebsiella pneumoniae, Proteus mirabilis*, most strains of *Haemophilus influenzae, Streptococcus pneumoniae, Streptococcus pyogenes, Staphylococcus* organisms (including *S. saprophyticus*). Not effective against *Bacteroides, Lactobacillus* species, *Chlamydia* or *Pneumocystis carinii, Pseudomonas aeruginosa*. Resistant strains of Enterobacteriaceae (*E. coli* and *Klebsiella* and *Proteus* species) may develop during therapy. Emergence of trimethoprim-resistant organisms occurs more frequently when drug is used alone than when used in combination therapy. Efficacy as treatment of UTI appears to match that of amoxicillin, ampicillin, co-trimoxazole, nitrofurantoin, or sulfisoxazole.

USES Initial episodes of acute uncomplicated UTIs. **Unlabeled use:** treatment and prophylaxis of chronic and recurrent UTI in both men and women; treatment in conjunction with dapsone of initial episodes of *Pneumocystis carinii* pneumonia; treatment of traveler's diarrhea.

ROUTE & DOSAGE

Urinary Tract Infection
Adult   PO   100 mg b.i.d. or 200 mg once/d

Travelers Diarrhea
Adult   PO   200 mg b.i.d.

PHARMACOKINETICS Absorption: almost completely absorbed from GI tract. **Peak:** 1–4 h. **Distribution:** widely distributed, including lung, saliva, middle ear fluid, bile, bone, CSF; crosses placenta; appears in breast milk. **Metabolism:** metabolized in liver. **Elimination:** half-life: 8–11 h; 80% excreted in urine unchanged.

CONTRAINDICATIONS & PRECAUTIONS Contraindicated in: megaloblastic anemia secondary to folate deficiency; creatinine clearance <15 ml/min, impaired renal or hepatic function, possible folate deficiency; pregnancy (category C), nursing mothers, children with fragile X chromosome associated with mental retardation. Safe use in infants < 2 mo old and efficacy in children < 12 y old has not been established.

Common side effects in *italic*; life-threatening effects <u>underlined</u>; generic names in **bold**; classifications in SMALL CAPS

ADVERSE/SIDE EFFECTS GI: epigastric discomfort, nausea, vomiting, glossitis, abnormal taste sensation. **Hematologic:** thrombocytopenia (rare), neutropenia, *megaloblastic anemia*, methemoglobinemia, leukopenia. **Skin:** rash, pruritus, exfoliative dermatitis, photosensitivity (phototoxic) (rare). **Other:** fever, increased serum transaminases (ALT, AST), bilirubin, creatinine, BUN.

DIAGNOSTIC TEST INTERFERENCES Interferes with serum **methotrexate assays** that use a competitive binding protein technique with a bacterial dehydrofolate reductase as the binding protein. May cause falsely elevated creatinine values when Jaffe reaction is used.

DRUG INTERACTIONS May inhibit **phenytoin** metabolism, causing increased levels.

NURSING IMPLICATIONS

Administration

- Administer with 240 ml (8 oz) of fluid if not contraindicated.
- Store at 15–30C (59–86F) in dry, light-protected place.

Assessment & Drug Effects

- Culture and susceptibility tests are conducted before trimethoprim therapy is initiated; however, therapy may be started before test results have been received.
- Recurrent infection after terminating prophylactic treatment of UTI may occur even after 6 mo of therapy. A possible reason may be noncompliance. Reenforce necessity to adhere to established drug regimen.
- Periodic urine cultures are recommended. Follow-up cultures may be ordered at end of treatment to verify elimination of causative organism.
- Monitor creatinine clearance tests.
- Assess urinary pattern during treatment. Altered pattern (frequency, urgency, nocturia, retention, polyuria) may reflect emerging drug resistance, necessitating change of drug regimen. Periodically check for bladder distension.
- Trimethoprim may worsen the psychomotor regression associated with mental retardation because of potential drug-induced folate deficiency.
- Elderly, malnourished, alcoholic, pregnant, or debilitated patients are especially susceptible to the hematologic toxic effects. Changes in temperature pattern and I&O ratio pattern should be recognized and reported.

- Drug-induced rash, a common side effect, is usually maculopapular, pruritic, or morbilliform and appears 7–14 d after start of therapy with daily doses of 200 mg or less.
- *Overdose symptoms:* nausea, vomiting, diarrhea, mental depression, confusion, facial swelling, elevated serum transaminases.

Patient & Family Education

- Uncomplicated UTIs usually respond to treatment if patient takes all of prescribed medication.
- Discuss fluid intake pattern with the patient. Frequently the elderly self-limit fluids; therefore teaching should focus on fluid intake as an important adjunct to drug therapy.
- Usually the adult patient should attempt to maintain fluid intake of 2000–3000 ml/d (if not contraindicated) to help flush out urinary bacteria.
- Before full drug effects are experienced, patient may have pain and discomfort with voiding, which can be relieved by a urinary analgesic. Pain and hematuria should be reported immediately.
- Tell patient not to postpone voiding even though increases in fluid intake may cause more frequent urination.
- Caution against use of douches or sprays during treatment periods, and stress careful perineal hygiene to prevent reinfection.
- Symptoms of a hematologic disorder (fever, sore throat, pallor, purpura, ecchymosis) should be reported promptly.
- If severe traveler's diarrhea does not respond to 3–5 d therapy with trimethoprim (i.e., persistence of symptoms of severe nausea, abdominal pain, diarrhea with mucus or blood, and dehydration), patient should consult a physician.

ALKYLATING AGENT

CYCLOPHOSPHAMIDE
(sye-kloe-foss'fa-mide)
Trade names: Cytoxan, Neosar, Procytox
Classifications: ANTINEOPLASTIC; ALKYLATING AGENT; IMMUNOSUPPRESSANT
Pregnancy: Category C

ACTIONS/PHARMACODYNAMICS Cell-cycle-nonspecific alkylating agent chemically related to the nitrogen mustards. Action mechanism unknown but

Common side effects in *italic*; life-threatening effects underlined; generic names in **bold**; classifications in SMALL CAPS

91

thought to be the result of cross-linkage of DNA strands, thereby blocking synthesis of DNA, RNA, and protein. Has pronounced immunosuppressive activity and is a highly toxic drug; thus therapeutic effects are usually accompanied by some evidence of toxicity. Thought to stimulate release of antidiuretic hormone (vasopressin) with resulting nonacute hyponatremia. Associated with increased risk of secondary malignancies that may be detected several years after cyclophosphamide has been discontinued. Parenteral use of drug in combination therapy before conception has been associated with cardiac and lymph abnormalities in the infant. Advantages over other nitrogen mustards include effectiveness of oral preparations and the possibility of giving fractional doses over long periods of time.

USES As single agent or in combination with other chemotherapeutic agents in treatment of malignant lymphoma, multiple myeloma, leukemias, mycosis fungoides (advanced disease), neuroblastoma, adenocarcinoma of ovary, carcinoma of breast, or malignant neoplasms of lung. **Unlabeled use:** to prevent rejection in homotransplantation; to treat severe rheumatoid arthritis, multiple sclerosis, systemic lupus erythematosus, Wegener's granulomatosis, nephrotic syndrome.

ROUTE & DOSAGE

Neoplasm

Adult	PO	Initial: 1–5 mg/kg/d Maintenance: 1–5 mg/kg q7–10d
	IV	Initial: 40–50 mg/kg in divided doses over 2–5 d up to 100 mg/kg
		Maintenance: 10–15 mg/kg q7–10d or 3–5 mg twice weekly
Child	PO	Initial: 2–8 mg/kg or 60–250 mg/m² Maintenence: 2–5 mg/kg or 50–150 mg/m² twice weekly
	IV	Initial: 2–8 mg/kg or 60–250 mg/m²

PHARMACOKINETICS Absorption: readily absorbed from GI tract. **Peak:** 1 h PO. **Distribution:** widely distributed, including brain, breast milk; crosses placenta. **Metabolism:** metabolized in liver. **Elimination:** half-life: 4–6 h; excreted in urine as active metabolites and unchanged drug.

CONTRAINDICATIONS & PRECAUTIONS

Contraindicated in: men and women in childbearing years; serious infections (including chickenpox, herpes zoster); live virus vaccines; myelosuppression; pregnancy (category C), nursing mothers. **Cautious use**

in: history of radiation or cytotoxic drug therapy; hepatic and renal impairment, recent history of steroid therapy; bone marrow infiltration with tumor cells; history of urate calculi and gout; patients with leukopenia, thrombocytopenia.

ADVERSE/SIDE EFFECTS GI: *nausea, vomiting,* mucositis, *anorexia,* hepatotoxicity, diarrhea. **GU:** sterile hemorrhagic and nonhemorrhagic cystitis, bladder fibrosis, nephrotoxicity. **Metabolic:** severe hyperkalemia, SIADH, hyponatremia, weight gain (but without edema) or weight loss, hyperuricemia. **Myelosuppression:** leukopenia, *neutropenia,* acute myeloid leukemia, anemia, thrombophlebitis, interference with normal healing. **Pulmonary:** pulmonary emboli and edema, pneumonitis, interstitial pulmonary fibrosis. **Skin:** *alopecia* (reversible), transverse ridging of nails, pigmentation of nail beds and skin (reversible), nonspecific dermatitis. **Other:** transient dizziness, fatigue, facial flushing, diaphoresis, drug fever, anaphylaxis, secondary neoplasia.

DIAGNOSTIC TEST INTERFERENCES Cyclophosphamide suppresses positive reactions to **Candida, mumps, trichophytons,** and **tuberculin PPD skin tests. Papanicolaou (PAP)** smear may be falsely positive.

DRUG INTERACTIONS Succinylcholine, prolonged neuromuscular blocking activity; **doxorubicin** may increase cardiac toxicity.

NURSING IMPLICATIONS

Administration

- Administer PO drug on empty stomach. If nausea and vomiting are severe, however, it may be taken with food. An antiemetic medication may be prescribed to be given before the drug.
- Store cyclophosphamide PO solution in refrigerator at 2–8C (36–46F), and use within 14 d.
- *IV solution:* To reconstitute, add sterile water for injection or bacteriostatic water for injection (paraben-preserved only) to vial and shake vigorously to dissolve (5 ml to 100 mg vial). Should be used within 24 h if stored at room temperature, or within 6 d if refrigerated.
- Usually extravasation does not cause local irritation; however, it should be avoided.
- Administering cyclophosphamide late in the evening with a sedative may help the patient tolerate nausea.
- Store at temperature between 2 and 30C (36 and

86F) unless otherwise recommended by the manufacturer.

Assessment & Drug Effects

- Total and differential leukocyte count, platelet count, and hematocrit are determined initially and at least 2 times per week during maintenance period. Baseline and periodic determinations of liver and kidney function and serum electrolytes also should be made. Microscopic urine examinations are recommended after large IV doses.
- Thrombocytopenia is rare, but if it occurs (count of 100,000/mm³ or lower), watch for signs of unexplained bleeding or easy bruising. If count continues to descend, drug will be discontinued.
- Ordinarily a leukopenia of 3000–4000 mm³ can be maintained without risk of serious complications.
- Marked leukopenia is the most serious side effect. It can be fatal. Nadir may occur in 2–8 d after first dose but may be as late as 1 mo after a series of several daily doses. Leukopenia usually reverses 7–10 d after therapy is discontinued.
- Check leukocyte count. During severe leukopenic period, protect patient from infection and trauma and from visitors and medical personnel who have colds or other infections.
- Report onset of unexplained chills, sore throat, tachycardia. Monitor temperature carefully and report an elevation immediately. The development of fever in a neutropenic patient (granulocyte count < 1000) is a medical emergency because sepsis can develop quickly in these patients.
- During period of neutropenia, purulent drainage may become serosanguineous because there are not enough WBC to create pus. Because of suppressed immune mechanisms, wound healing may be prolonged or incomplete. Observe and report character of wound drainage.
- If a pattern of nausea and vomiting can be detected, an attempt should be make to plan the treatment, meals, and antiemetic so as not to confront patient with food or start therapy when nausea is at its peak.
- I&O ratio and pattern should be monitored. Since the drug is a chemical irritant, PO and IV fluid intake is generally increased to help prevent renal irritation and hemorrhagic cystitis. Have patient void frequently, especially after each dose and just before retiring to bed. Paradoxically, in patients with SIADH (a rare side effect) fluid intake may have to be restricted. Consult physician.
- Because patients are usually well hydrated as part of the therapy, watch for symptoms of water intoxication or dilutional hyponatremia. Should this condition occur, fluid intake will be reduced. Report to physician.
- Promptly report hematuria or dysuria. Drug schedule is usually interrupted and fluids are forced. Alert patient to the fact that hematuria may resolve spontaneously, or it may persist several months. In some cases it has been serious enough to require transfusions.
- Record body weight at least twice weekly (basis for dose determination). Alert physician to sudden change or slow, steady weight gain or loss over a period of time that appears inconsistent with caloric intake.
- Diarrhea may signal onset of hyperkalemia, particularly if accompanied by colicky pain, nausea, bradycardia, and skeletal muscle weakness. These symptoms warrant prompt reporting to physician.
- Hyperuricemia occurs commonly during early treatment period in patients with leukemias or lymphoma. Report edema of lower legs and feet; joint, flank, or stomach pain.
- Before institution of cyclophosphamide therapy, observe and report the signs of hepatotoxicity (frothy dark urine, light-colored stools, jaundice, pruritus) that are most apt to appear in the patient with liver impairment.
- The immunosuppressive property of cyclophosphamide makes the patient particularly susceptible to varicella-zoster infections (chickenpox, herpes zoster). Particular care should be taken to screen young visitors.
- Report any sign of overgrowth with opportunistic organisms, especially in patient receiving corticosteroids or who has recently been on steroid therapy.
- Report fever, dyspnea, and nonproductive cough. Pulmonary toxicity is not common, but the already debilitated patient is particularly susceptible.

Patient & Family Education

- Urge patient to adhere to dosage regimen and not to omit, increase, decrease, or delay doses. If for any reason drug cannot be taken, notify physician.
- Alopecia occurs in about 33% of patients on cyclophosphamide therapy. Hair loss may be noted 3 wk after therapy begins; regrowth (often differs in texture and color) usually starts 5–6 wk after drug is withdrawn and may occur while patient is on maintenance doses.
- Because of mutagenic potential, adequate means of contraception should be employed during and for at least 4 mo after termination of drug treatment. Breastfeeding should be discontinued before cyclophosphamide therapy is initiated.

Common side effects in *italic*; life-threatening effects <u>underlined</u>; generic names in **bold**; classifications in SMALL CAPS

93

■ Amenorrhea may last up to 1 y after cessation of therapy in 10–30% of women.

ANTIMETABOLITE

FLUOROURACIL

(flure-oh-yoor´a-sil)

Trade names: Adrucil, Efudex, 5-Fluorouracil (5-FU), Fluoroplex

Classifications: ANTINEOPLASTIC; ANTIMETABOLITE

Pregnancy: Category D

ACTIONS/PHARMACODYNAMICS Pyrimidine antagonist and cell-cycle specific. Blocks action of enzymes essential to normal DNA and RNA synthesis and may become incorporated in RNA to form a fraudulent molecule; unbalanced growth and death of cell follow. Has higher affinity for tumor tissue than healthy tissue. Highly toxic, especially to proliferative cells in neoplasms, bone marrow, and intestinal mucosa. Low therapeutic index with high potential for severe hematologic toxicity. Both local and systemic administration increase skin pigmentation. Is not intended as adjuvant to surgery or for prophylaxis.

USES Systemically as single agent and in combination with other antineoplastics for palliative treatment of carefully selected patients with inoperable neoplasms of breast, colon or rectum, stomach, pancreas, urinary bladder, ovary, cervix, liver. Also topically for solar or actinic keratoses and superficial basal cell carcinoma. **Unlabeled uses:** to induce repigmentation in vitiligo; actinic cheilitis, malignant effusions, mucosal leukoplakia.

ROUTE & DOSAGE

Carcinoma

Adult	IV	12 mg/kg/d for 4 consecutive days up to 800 mg *or* until toxicity develops *or* 12 d therapy; may repeat at 1 mo intervals; if toxicity occurs, 15 mg/kg once weekly can be given until toxicity subsides

Actinic and Solar Keratosis

Adult	Topical	Apply cream b.i.d. for 2–4 wk

Superficial Basal Cell Carcinoma

Adult	Topical	Apply 5% cream b.i.d. for 3–6 wk

PHARMACOKINETICS Distribution: distributed to tumor, intestinal mucosa, bone marrow, liver, and CSF; probably crosses placenta. **Metabolism:** rapidly metabolized in liver. **Elimination:** half-life: 16 min; 15% excreted in urine, 60–80% excreted through lungs as carbon dioxide.

CONTRAINDICATIONS & PRECAUTIONS Contraindicated in: poor nutritional status; myelosuppression. Safe use during pregnancy (category D) and in nursing women not established. **Cautious use in:** major surgery during previous month; history of high-dose pelvic irradiation, metastatic cell infiltration of bone marrow, previous use of alkylating agents; men and women in childbearing ages; hepatic and renal impairment.

ADVERSE/SIDE EFFECTS CNS: euphoria, insomnia, acute cerebellar syndrome (dysmetria, nystagmus, ataxia, severe mental deterioration); pustular contact hypersensitivity. **CV** (cardiotoxicity): mild angina to crushing central chest pain with ECG changes. **GI:** anorexia, *nausea, vomiting, stomatitis,* esophagopharyngitis, medicinal taste, *diarrhea,* proctitis, paralytic ileus, GI hemorrhage. **Hematologic:** anemia, <u>leukopenia</u>, thrombocytopenia, eosinophilia, hemolytic-uremic syndrome. **Hypersensitivity:** pustular contact eruption, edema of face, eyes, tongue, legs. **Skin:** SLE-like dermatitis, *alopecia,* nail changes or loss (rare); photosensitivity, erythema, increased pigmentation, skin dryness and fissuring, pruritic maculopapular rash. **Topical:** local pain, pruritus, hyperpigmentation, burning at site of application, dermatitis, suppuration, swelling, scarring, toxic granulation. **Other:** nephrotoxicity, epistaxis, photophobia, lacrimation.

DIAGNOSTIC TEST INTERFERENCES Fluorouracil may increase excretion of *5-hydroxyindoleacetic acid (5-HIAA)* and decrease *plasma albumin* (because of drug-induced protein malabsorption).

INCOMPATIBILITIES Solution/Additive: **Cytarabine, diazepam, doxorubicin, droperidol.** Y-Site: droperidol.

NURSING IMPLICATIONS

Administration

■ Fluorouracil IV is to be administered under the direct supervision of a physician experienced in cancer chemotherapy.

Common side effects in *italic*; life-threatening effects <u>underlined</u>; generic names in **bold**; classifications in SMALL CAPS

- Dose is determined by actual weight unless patient is obese, in which case ideal weight is used.
- Avoid skin exposure while handling drug.
- Currently recommended procedure for safe handling of injectable fluorouracil: double-glove with latex surgeon's gloves, and change the double set after every 30 min of exposure. If a drug spill occurs, gloves should be changed immediately after it is cleaned up.
- This drug may be given without dilution by direct IV injection over 1–2 min.
- Inspect injection site frequently; avoid extravasation. If it occurs, stop infusion and restart in another vein. Ice compresses may reduce danger of local tissue damage from infiltrated solution.
- Fluorouracil solution is normally colorless to faint yellow. Slight discoloration during storage does not appear to affect potency or safety. Discard dark yellow solution. If a precipitate forms, redissolve drug by heating to 60C (140F) and shake vigorously. Allow to cool to body temperature before administration.
- Consult physician about preparation of lesion before application of topical drug.
- Use nonmetallic applicator or gloved fingers to apply topical drug. If unprotected fingers are used, wash hands thoroughly.
- Occlusive dressings with topical drug may cause an inflammatory reaction on adjacent healthy tissue and are therefore not recommended. A porous gauze dressing used for cosmetic purposes does not cause inflammation.
- Second-degree burns from contact of plastic eyeglass frames with treated skin have been reported. The frames appear to act like an occlusive dressing. Risk of burns or irritation may be reduced by (1) advising patient not to use other creams, ointments, moisturizers while they are being treated with fluorouracil, (2) treating skin that contacts frames only at night when glasses are not worn, and (3) using the lowest effective strength of topical preparation.
- Store drugs at 15–30C (59–86F) unless otherwise directed. Protect from light and freezing.

Assessment & Drug Effects
- Total and differential leukocyte counts should be determined before each dose is administered. Drug should be discontinued if leukopenia occurs (WBC <3500/mm^3) or if patient develops thrombocytopenia (platelet count <100,000/mm^3). Baseline and periodic checks of hematocrit and liver and kidney function test are also advised.
- Commonly, leukopenic nadir is reached 9–14 d after initial dose but may be delayed as long as 20 d. Usually count is in normal range by thirtieth day. Monitor blood counts as indicators for design of patient care.
- During leukopenic period (WBC <3500/mm^3) patient should be in protective isolation.
- During thrombocytopenic period (day 7–17), watch for and report signs of abnormal bleeding from any source; inspect skin for ecchymotic and petechial areas. Protect patient from trauma.
- Report disorientation or confusion; drug should be withdrawn immediately. Symptoms may occur earlier in each subsequent course of treatment and increase in severity.
- Establish a reference data base for body weight, I&O ratio and pattern, food preferences and dietary habits, bowel habits, and condition of mouth.
- Antiemetics may be ordered before and after drug administration to alleviate nausea and vomiting. Monitor carefully if vomiting is intractable and report to physician.
- Indications for drug discontinuation: severe stomatitis, leukopenia (WBC < 3500/mm^3 or rapidly decreasing count), intractable vomiting, diarrhea, thrombocytopenia (platelets < 100,000/mm^3), hemorrhage from any site.
- A dose sufficient to create mild toxicity (anorexia, vomiting) may be necessary to produce antineoplastic effects.
- Stomatitis, a reliable early sign of toxicity, often precedes the leukopenic period by days. Inspect patient's mouth daily. Promptly report cracked lips, xerostomia, white patches, and erythema of buccal membranes.
- Report development of maculopapular rash, which usually responds to symptomatic treatment and is reversible.
- Inspect pressure areas daily (coccyx region, elbows, heels). Danger of skin breakdown is greatly increased in a patient with immunosuppression, myelosuppression, and poor nutritional status.
- A skin lesion treated with topical fluorouracil heals without scarring within 1–2 mo after cessation of therapy. **Expected response of lesion to topical 5-FU:** erythema followed in sequence by vesiculation, erosion, ulceration, necrosis, epithelialization. Applications of drug are continued until ulcerative stage is reached (2–6 wk after initial applications) and then discontinued.
- Systemic toxicity may follow use of topical drug on large ulcerated area. Report symptoms promptly.
- If skin area treated with topical medication fails to respond to treatment, a biopsy is usually done to rule out frank neoplastic disease.

Common side effects in *italic*; life-threatening effects underlined; generic names in **bold**; classifications in SMALL CAPS

95

Patient & Family Education

- Inform the patient of the importance of prompt reporting of the first *signs of toxicity:* anorexia, vomiting, nausea, stomatitis, diarrhea, GI bleeding.
- Periodic checks on liver and kidney function will be scheduled. Urge the ambulatory patient to keep appointments for clinical evaluation.
- Caution patient not to change dosage regimen, i.e., not to increase, or omit doses or change dosage intervals.
- Caution patient to avoid exposure to sunlight or to ultraviolet lamp treatments. Protect exposed skin; if it is necessary to go outdoors, apply sun-screen lotion (SPF 12 or above). Avoid midday exposure. Photosensitivity usually subsides 2–3 mo after last dose.
- Photophobia and lacrimation are frequent side effects. If these effects are bothersome, report to physician. Dark glasses may be helpful.
- If patient manifests difficulty in maintaining balance while ambulating, report symptom to physician promptly.
- Prepare patient for alopecia, an expected transient toxic effect. Discuss plans for cosmetic substitution if patient desires; new hair growth usually begins within 6–8 wk.
- Contraception is advisable during 5-FU treatment. Advise patient to report to physican if she suspects pregnancy.

NITROGEN MUSTARD

MECHLORETHAMINE HYDROCHLORIDE
(me-klor-eth´a-meen)
Trade name: Mustargen
Classifications: ANTINEOPLASTIC; NITROGEN MUSTARD; ALKYLATING AGENT
Pregnancy: Category D

ACTIONS/PHARMACODYNAMICS Analogue of mustard gas and standard of reference for nitrogen mustards. Forms highly reactive carbonium ion, which causes cross-linking and abnormal base-pairing in DNA, thereby interfering with DNA replication and RNA and protein synthesis. Cell-cycle nonspecific, i.e., highly toxic to rapidly proliferating cells at any time during cell cycle. Actions simulate those of x-ray therapy, but nitrogen mustards produce more acute tissue damage and more rapid recovery. Has strong myelosuppressive and weak immunosuppressive activity and is a powerful vesicant. Therapy may be associated with incidence of a second malignant tumor, particularly if mechlorethamine is combined with radiation therapy or with other antineoplastics.

USES Generally confined to nonterminal stages of neoplastic disease. Employed as single agent or in combination with other agents in palliative treatment of Hodgkin's disease (stages III and IV), lymphosarcoma, mycosis fungoides, polycythemia vera, bronchogenic carcinoma, chronic myelocytic or chronic lymphocytic leukemia. Also for intrapleural, intrapericardial and intraperitoneal palliative treatment of metastatic carcinoma resulting in effusion.

ROUTE & DOSAGE

Advanced Hodgkin's Disease

Adult	IV	6 mg/m² on day 1 and 8 of a 28 d cycle

Other Neoplasms

Adult	IV	0.4 mg/kg given as a single dose *or* in divided doses of 0.1–0.2 mg/kg/d; may repeat course in 3–6 wk

PHARMACOKINETICS Metabolism: rapid transformation to metabolites. **Elimination:** not detectable in blood within a few minutes; <0.01% excreted in urine.

CONTRAINDICATIONS & PRECAUTIONS Contraindicated in: pregnancy at least until third trimester, lactation; myelosuppression; infectious granuloma, known infectious diseases, acute herpes zoster; intracavitary use with other systemic bone marrow suppressants. **Cautious use in:** bone marrow infiltration with malignant cells, chronic lymphocytic leukemia, men or women in childbearing age, use with x-ray treatment or other chemotherapy in alternating courses.

ADVERSE/SIDE EFFECTS CNS: neurotoxicity: vertigo, tinnitus, diminished hearing, headache, drowsiness, peripheral neuropathy, lightheadedness, paresthesias, cerebral deterioration, coma. **GI:** stomatitis, xerostomia, anorexia, *nausea, vomiting,* diarrhea, peptic ulcer, jaundice. **Hematopoietic:** leukopenia, *thrombocytopenia,* lymphocytopenia, agranulocytosis, *anemia,* hyperheparinemia. **Reproductive:** delayed catamenia, oligomenorrhea, amenorrhea, azoospermia, impaired spermatogenesis, total germinal aplasia, chromosomal abnormalities. **Skin:** pruritus, hyperpigmentation, maculopapular skin eruptions (rare), herpes zoster, alopecia. **Other:** hyperuricemia, weakness, fever, hypersensitivity reactions. *With extravasation: painful inflammatory reaction, tissue sloughing, thrombosis, thrombophlebitis.*

DRUG INTERACTIONS Mechlorethamine (nitrogen mustards) may reduce effectiveness of ANTIGOUT AGENTS by raising serum uric acid levels; dosage adjustments may be necessary.

NURSING IMPLICATIONS

Administration

- Surgical gloves should be worn to protect skin during preparation and administration of solution. Avoid inhalation of vapors and dust and contact of drug with eyes and skin.
- If drug contacts the skin, flush contaminated area immediately with copious amounts of water for at least 15 min, followed by 2% sodium thiosulfate solution. Irritation may appear after a latent period.
- If eye contact occurs, irrigate immediately with copious amounts of 0.9% NaCl, followed by ophthalmologic examination as soon as possible.
- Prepare mechlorethamine solution immediately before administration by adding 10 ml sterile water for injection or 0.9% NaCl injection to drug vial. With needle still in rubber stopper, shake vial several times to hasten dissolving. Solution will contain 1 mg mechlorethamine per 1 ml of solution.
- Do not use discolored solution or contents of vial in which there are drops of moisture.
- If direct IV injection is to be made, needle used to withdraw dose should be discarded and a fresh needle used to administer medication.
- Reconstituted solution may be injected over 3–5 min directly into any suitable vein. However, to reduce risk of severe infections from extravasation or high concentration of the drug, injection is made preferably directly into tubing or sidearm of freely flowing IV infusion. Some clinicians flush vein with running IV solution for 2–5 min to clear tubing of any remaining drug.
- If drug extravasates, prompt subcutaneous or intradermal injection with isotonic sodium thiosulfate solution (1/6 molar) and application of ice compresses intermittently for a 6–12 h period may reduce local tissue damage and discomfort. Tissue induration and tenderness may persist 4–6 wk, and tissue may slough.
- Give drug preferably early in the day to prevent interference with sleep by side effects.
- Intracavitary administration is preceded by removal of most of the fluid in the cavity to be treated.

- Intrapleural or intrapericardial injection of nitrogen mustard is given directly through the thoracentesis needle.
- Intraperitoneal injection is given through a rubber catheter inserted into the paracentesis trocar or through an 18-gauge needle inserted in another site.
- Immediately after intracavitary administration, change the patient's position (prone, supine, right side, left side, knee-chest) q5–10min for 1 h, to assure full contact of drug with all parts of the cavity. Paracentesis may be done 24–36 h later to remove any remaining fluid.
- Rubber gloves, tubing, glassware, etc. used in the preparation and administration of mechlorethamine should be soaked in an aqueous solution of equal volumes of sodium thiosulfate 5% and sodium bicarbonate 5% for 45 min for neutralization.
- Any unused injection solution and mechlorethamine vials should also be treated (neutralized) with an equal volume of sodium thiosulfate and sodium bicarbonate solution for 45 min before disposal.

Assessment & Drug Effects

- Begin flow chart with established baseline data relative to body weight, I&O ratio and pattern, and blood picture as reference for design of drug and nursing care regimens.
- Mechlorethamine dosage is determined on basis of ideal dry body weight, i.e., unaugmented by edema or ascites. Record daily weight. Alert physician to sudden or slow, steady weight gain.
- Pain is rare with intrapleural injection, but transient cardiac irregularities may occur. Monitor cardiac function during and after treatment until cardiac status is stable.
- Pain is common with intraperitoneal injection and usually is associated with nausea, vomiting, and diarrhea lasting 2–3 d.
- Nausea and vomiting may occur 1–3 h after drug injection; vomiting usually subsides within 8 h, but nausea may persist. Attempt to schedule treatments, other drugs, and meals so as to avoid peak times of nausea.
- Prolonged vomiting and diarrhea can produce **signs of blood volume depletion:** decreased skin turgor, shrunken and dry tongue, postural hypotension, weakness, confusion. Carefully monitor and record patient's fluid losses.
- Myelosuppressive symptoms appear by the fourth day after treatment begins and are maximal by tenth day. Generally, lymphocytopenia begins within 24 h and is maximum in 6–8 d. Significant granulocytopenia usually occurs within 6–8 d, is

Common side effects in *italic*; life-threatening effects <u>underlined</u>; generic names in **bold**; classifications in SMALL CAPS

97

maximum between 14–25 d, with recovery complete within 2 wk of its nadir.

- Thrombocytopenia usually manifests 6–8 d after a treatment. Petechiae, ecchymoses, or abnormal bleeding from intestinal and buccal membranes should be reported immediately. During period of thrombocytopenia, injections, use of a rectal thermometer or rectal tube, and other invasive procedures should be kept to a minimum.
- Report symptoms of unexplained fever, chills, sore throat, tachycardia, and mucosal ulceration, as they may signal onset of agranulocytosis (see Signs & Symptoms, chap 3).
- Symptoms of depression of leukopenic system may be evident up to 50 d or more from the start of therapy.
- Profound immunosuppression places patient at risk for infections, poor healing, and lowered defense mechanisms for combating stress. Prevent exposure of patient to persons with infection, especially upper respiratory tract infections, and plan nursing interventions to keep patient's expenditure of energy at a minimum.
- Herpes zoster may be precipitated by mechlorethamine treatment and usually necessitates withdrawal of the drug. It occurs commonly in patients with lymphoma.
- Rapid neoplastic cell and leukocyte destruction leads to elevated serum uric acid (hyperuricemia; see Signs & Symptoms, chap 3) and potential renal urate calculi.
- Preventive measures against incidence of hyperuricemia include increased fluid intake, alkalinizing of urine, and administration of allopurinol.
- Establish baselines for oral care by inspecting oral cavity before chemotherapy begins. Note and record state of hydration of oral mucosa, condition of gingiva, teeth, tongue, mucosa, and lips. If prosthetic devices do not fit properly, record.
- If patient has correctable oral problems, they should be treated before antineoplastic therapy is begun. Institute corrective measures to minimize possibility of irritation or infection after immunosuppression and myelosuppression have been established. Facilitate consultation with a dentist if necessary.

Patient & Family Education
- Laboratory studies of peripheral blood are essential guides for determining when to give another course of therapy. Urge patient to keep appointments for clinical evaluation.
- Explain the significance of thrombocytopenia with the development of bleeding tendencies and advise patient to report any signs of bleeding immediately.

- Warn patient to use caution to prevent falls or other traumatic injuries, especially during periods of thrombocytopenia.
- Encourage patient to increase fluid intake up to 3000 ml/d if allowed to minimize risk of renal stones. Urge prompt reporting of symptoms including flank or joint pain, swelling of lower legs and feet, changes in voiding pattern.
- Azoospermia and amenorrhea after a course of therapy may be irreversible. Occasionally spermatogenesis may return in patients in remission several years after intensive chemotherapy. This should be discussed with patient before therapy is started.
- High doses and regional infusion of mechlorethamine increase incidence of tinnitus and deafness. Alert patient to report symptoms promptly.
- Discuss the problem of alopecia (reversible) with the patient. If desired, facilitate cosmetic substitution.
- As oral complications increase because of drug-induced cell destruction, the following guidelines are useful: discontinue flossing when platelet count decreases to between 15,000 and 10,000; discontinue brushing when count is between 10,000 and 5000. Maintain oral hygiene with wet cotton swabs and gentle stream of warm water. Consult physician about oral antiseptic and anesthetic agent.
- Apply thin film of petroleum jelly to cracked, dry lips. Avoid use of lemon and glycerin swabs, which irritate membranes, change consistency of saliva, and may promote decalcification of teeth.
- Continuous meticulous oral hygiene measures are important to prevent oral infection from superinfection or trauma, to relieve discomfort, and to prevent demineralization of tooth surfaces because of saliva deprivation.
- Brush teeth using soft-bristled toothbrush (softened with warm water); if gums are painful, use moistened cotton covered finger or rubber tip on toothbrush. Use fluoride toothpaste or medication at least once a day.
- Cleansing before and after meals is important. Encourage patient to floss teeth gently with waxed floss before brushing, at least once daily. Do it for patient if necessary.
- In presence of ulcerations or dysphagia, avoid hot or cold foods and drinks; avoid spicy, sour, dry, rough or chunky foods as well as smoking and alcoholic beverages.
- Xerostomia may be relieved by use of a saliva substitute (available OTC) such as Xero-Lube, Moi-Stir, Orex, Salivart.

Common side effects in *italic*; life-threatening effects underlined; generic names in **bold**; classifications in SMALL CAPS

ANTITUSSIVE

BENZONATATE
(ben-zoe´na-tate)
Trade name: Tessalon
Classification: ANTITUSSIVE
Pregnancy: Category C

ACTIONS/PHARMACODYNAMICS Nonnarcotic antitussive chemically related to **tetracaine.** Antitussive activity reported to be somewhat less effective than that of **codeine.** Suppresses mediation of cough reflex by exerting selective topical anesthetic action on stretch receptors in respiratory passages, lungs, and pleura. Also suppresses cough reflex transmission at level of medulla. Does not inhibit respiratory center at recommended doses.

USES Decreases frequency and intensity of nonproductive cough in acute and chronic respiratory conditions. Also used in bronchoscopy, thoracentesis, and other procedures when coughing must be avoided.

ROUTE & DOSAGE

Antitussive

Adult	PO	100 mg t.i.d. prn up to 600 mg/d
Child	PO	<10 y: 8 mg/kg/d in 3–6 divided doses

PHARMACOKINETICS Onset: 15–20 min.
Duration: 3–8 h.

CONTRAINDICATIONS & PRECAUTIONS Contraindicated in: safe use during pregnancy (category C) and lactation not established.

ADVERSE/SIDE EFFECTS Low incidence. **CNS:** drowsiness, sedation headache, mild dizziness. **GI:** constipation, nausea. **Skin:** skin rash, pruritus. **Other:** transitory rise in blood pressure, nasal congestion, chilly sensation, burning sensation of eyes, numbness or tightness of chest.

NURSING IMPLICATIONS

Administration
- Oral medication is supplied in soft capsules called Perles.
- Perles must be swallowed whole.
- Store in airtight containers protected from light.

Assessment & Drug Effects
- Auscultate lungs anteriorly and posteriorly at scheduled intervals.
- Observe character and frequency of coughing and volume and quality of sputum. Keep physician informed.

Patient & Family Education
- Instruct patient not to chew oral preparation (Perle) and not to allow it to dissolve in mouth. It should be swallowed whole. If it dissolves, mouth, tongue, and pharynx will be anesthetized. Also it is unpleasant to taste.
- Objective of treatment with an antitussive agent is to reduce overactive nonproductive coughing but not to suppress the cough completely.

EXPECTORANT

GUAIFENESIN
(gwye-fen´e-sin)
Trade names: Amonidrin, Anti-Tuss, Breonesin, Colrex, Dilyn, Gee-Gee, GG-Cen, Glyceryl Guaiacolate, Glycotuss, Glytuss, Guaituss, Hytuss, Malotuss, Mytussin, Nortussin, Resyl, Robitussin
Classification: EXPECTORANT
Pregnancy: Category C

ACTIONS/PHARMACODYNAMICS Enhances reflex outflow of respiratory tract fluids by irritation of gastric mucosa and aids in expectoration by reducing adhesiveness and surface tension of secretions.

USES To combat dry, nonproductive cough associated with colds and bronchitis. A common ingredient in cough mixtures.

ROUTE & DOSAGE

Cough

Adult	PO	200–400 mg q4h up to 2.4 g/d
Child	PO	6–11 y: 100–200 mg q4h up to 1.2 g/d
		2–5 y: 50–100 mg q4h up to 600 mg/d

ADVERSE/SIDE EFFECTS Low incidence: GI upset, nausea, drowsiness.

Common side effects in *italic*; life-threatening effects underlined;
generic names in **bold**; classifications in SMALL CAPS

99

DIAGNOSTIC TEST INTERFERENCES Guaifenesin may produce color interferences with certain laboratory determinations of urinary 5-hydroxyindoleacetic acid *(5-HIAA)* and vanillylmandelic acid *(VMA).*

DRUG INTERACTIONS By inhibiting platelet function, guaifenesin may increase risk of hemorrhage in patients receiving **heparin** therapy.

NURSING IMPLICATIONS

Administration
- Drug is most effective when taken q4h around the clock or during waking hours.
- Carefully observe maximum daily doses for adults and children.
- Follow dose with a full glass of water if not contraindicated.

Assessment & Drug Effects
- Persistent cough may indicate a serious condition requiring further diagnostic work.
- Monitor effectiveness of drug. If high fever, rash, or headaches develop, notify physician.

Patient & Family Education
- Increase in fluid intake will also help to loosen mucus. Encourage patient to drink at least 8 glasses of fluid daily.
- Instruct patient to contact physician if cough persists beyond 1 wk.
- Advise patient to contact physician if high fever, rash or headache develops.

MUCOLYTIC

ACETYLCYSTEINE
(a-se-til-sis´tay-een)
Trade names: Airbron, Mucomyst, Mucosol, *N*-Acetylcysteine
Classification: MUCOLYTIC; ANTIDOTE
Pregnancy: Category B

ACTIONS/PHARMACODYNAMICS Derivative of naturally occurring amino acid L-cysteine. Probably acts by disrupting disulfide linkages of mucoproteins in purulent and nonpurulent secretions, thereby lowering viscosity and facilitating their removal. Maximal mucolytic activity occurs at pH 7–9. Acetylcysteine is a precursor of hepatic glutathione, which normally inactivates a hepatotoxic metabolite of acetaminophen.

USES Adjuvant therapy in patients with abnormal, viscid, or inspissated mucous secretions in acute and chronic bronchopulmonary diseases, and in pulmonary complications of cystic fibrosis and surgery, tracheostomy, and atelectasis. Also used in diagnostic bronchial studies and as an antidote for acetaminophen poisoning. **Unlabeled use:** as an ophthalmic solution for treatment of dry eye (keratoconjunctivitis sicca). As an enema to treat bowel obstruction due to meconium ileus.

ROUTE & DOSAGE

Mucolytic

Adult	Inhalation	1–10 ml of 20% solution q4–6h *or* 2–20 ml of 10% solution q4–6h
	Direct instillation	1–2 ml of 10–20% solution q1–4h
Child	Inhalation	Same as for adult
	Direct instillation	Same as for adult

Acetaminophen Toxicity

Adult	PO	140 mg/kg followed by 70 mg/kg q4h for 17 doses (use a 5% solution)
Child	PO	Same as for adult

PHARMACOKINETICS Onset: 1 min after inhalation or instillation. **Peak:** 5–10 min. **Metabolism:** deacetylated in liver to cysteine and subsequently metabolized.

CONTRAINDICATIONS & PRECAUTIONS Contraindicated in: hypersensitivity to acetylcysteine; patients at risk of gastric hemorrhage. Safe use during pregnancy (category B) and in nursing mothers not established. **Cautious use in:** patients with asthma, the elderly, debilitated patients with severe respiratory insufficiency.

ADVERSE/SIDE EFFECTS CNS: dizziness, drowsiness. **GI:** nausea, *vomiting,* stomatitis. **Respiratory:** bronchospasm, rhinorrhea, burning sensation in upper respiratory passages, epistaxis. **Hepatoxicity:** urticaria.

NURSING IMPLICATIONS

Administration

- The 20% solution may be diluted with NS or water for injection. The 10% solution may be used undiluted.
- May be given by direct instillation into tracheostomy (1–2 ml of 10–20% solution).
- Treatments commonly administered when patient arises, before meals, and prior to retiring at night.
- For maximum effect, instruct patient to clear airway, if possible, by coughing productively prior to aerosol administration.
- Bronchospasm is most likely to occur in patients with asthma, and it may happen unpredictably. If it occurs, drug should be discontinued immediately.
- Once opened, vial can be stored in refrigerator to retard oxidation; use within 96 h. However, dilutions should be freshly prepared and used within 1 h; does not contain an antimicrobial agent. A light purple color apparently does not significantly impair its mucolytic effectiveness.
- Unopened vial should be stored at 15–30C (59–86F), unless otherwise directed.

Assessment & Drug Effects

- Have suction apparatus immediately available. Increased volume of respiratory tract fluid may be liberated; suction or endotracheal aspiration may be necessary to establish and maintain an open airway. Elderly and debilitated patients require close monitoring to prevent aspiration of excessive secretions.
- Unpleasant odor of drug (rotten egg odor of hydrogen sulfide) and excess volume of liquefied bronchial secretions may cause nausea and possibly vomiting, particularly when face mask is used. Odor becomes less noticeable with continued inhalation.

Patient & Family Educaton

- Instruct patient to immediately report difficulty with clearing the airway or any other respiratory distress.
- Advise patient to report nausea, as an antiemetic may be indicated.

ADRENERGIC AGONIST, ALPHA (SYMPATHOMIMETIC)

METHOXAMINE HYDROCHLORIDE

(meth-ox´a-meen)

Trade name: Vasoxyl

Classifications: AUTONOMIC NERVOUS SYSTEM AGENT; ALPHA-ADRENERGIC AGONIST (SYMPATHOMIMETIC)

Pregnancy: Category C

ACTIONS/PHARMACODYNAMICS Direct-acting sympathomimetic amine pharmacologically related to phenylephrine. Acts almost exclusively on alpha-adrenergic receptors. Pressor action is due primarily to direct peripheral vasoconstriction, which in turn causes rise in arterial BP. Has no direct effect on heart but tends to slow ventricular rate by vagal stimulation in response to elevated BP. Large doses may produce bradycardia. Markedly reduces renal blood flow. CNS-stimulating action. True tachyphylaxis not reported.

USES To support, restore, or maintain BP during anesthesia and to terminate some episodes of paroxysmal supraventricular tachycardia.

ROUTE & DOSAGE

Hypotension During Anesthesia

Adult	IM	5–20 mg
	IV	3–5 mg
Child	IM	0.25 mg/kg
	IV	0.08 mg/kg

Paroxysmal Supraventricular Tachycardia

Adult	IM	10–20 mg
	IV	5–15 mg over 3–5min

PHARMOCOKINETICS Onset: immediately after IV. **Peak:** 0.5–2 min IV; 15–20 min IM. **Duration:** 5–15 min IV; 60–90 min IM. **Metabolism:** unknown. **Elimination:** unknown.

CONTRAINDICATIONS & PRECAUTIONS

Contraindicated in: severe coronary or cardiovascular disease; hypovolemia, in combination with local anesthetics for tissue infiltration; within 2 wk of MAO inhibitors; pregnancy: category C. **Cautious use in:** history of hypertension or hyperthyroidism; following use of ergot alkaloids.

Common side effects in *italic*; life-threatening effects underlined; generic names in **bold**; classifications in SMALL CAPS

101

ADVERSE/SIDE EFFECTS Paresthesias, feeling of coldness (particularly with high dosage), restlessness, nervousness, high blood pressure, projectile vomiting, severe headache, pilomotor erection (gooseflesh), urinary urgency, bradycardia.

DRUG INTERACTIONS Phentolamine and PHENOTHIAZINES block vasopressor response. BETA BLOCKERS may increase amount of methoxamine available to receptor sites. **Atropine** blocks reflex bradycardia and enhances vasopressor effects. MAO INHIBITORS, **vasopressin**, and ERGOT ALKALOIDS may cause hypertensive crisis.

NURSING IMPLICATIONS

Administration
- Administer undiluted by direct IV at a rate of 5 mg/min if systolic BP is less than 60 mm Hg.
- May be diluted in 250 ml 5% dextrose and infused at rate needed to maintain blood pressure.
- Supplemental IM dose may be administered after emergency IV infusion.
- *Antidote for extravasation:* Area should be infiltrated as soon as possible with 10–15 ml normal saline solution containing 5–10 mg phentolamine.
- Protect drug from light.

Assessment & Drug Effects
- Patients should be under close supervision.
- Monitor vital signs. Report any increase in BP above level prescribed by physician; report slowing of heart rate.
- Be alert for sudden changes in blood pressure and pulse after drug has been discontinued.
- Monitor intake and output. Urinary frequency with retention is a possibility. Report oliguria or change in I&O ratio.
- Methoxamine injection contains a bisulfite, an allergen for some patients.

Patient & Family Education
- Instruct patient to report headache, which may be severe. This adverse effect may require analgesia for relief.
- Instruct patient to report nausea, since it may be accompanied by projectile vomiting.

ADRENERGIC AGONIST, ALPHA AND BETA (SYMPATHOMIMETIC)

EPINEPHRINE
(ep-i-nef´rin)
Trade names: Bronkaid Mist, Epinephrine Pediatric, EpiPen Auto-Injector, Primatene Mist Suspension

EPINEPHRINE BITARTRATE
Trade names: AsthmaHaler, Bronkaid Mist Suspension, Bronitin Mist Suspension, Epitrate, Medihaler-Epi, Primatene Mist Suspension

EPINEPHRINE HYDROCHLORIDE
Trade names: Adrenalin Chloride, Bronkaid Mistometer, Dysne-Inhal, Epifrin, Glaucon, SusPhrine

EPINEPHRINE, RACEMIC
Trade names: AsthmaNefrin, Dey-Dose Epinephrine, microNefrin, S-2 Inhalant, Vaponefrin

EPINEPHRYL BORATE
(ep-i-nef´rill bor´ate)
Trade names: Epinal, Eppy/N
Classifications: AUTONOMIC NERVOUS SYSTEM AGENT; ALPHA- AND BETA-ADRENERGIC AGONIST; BRONCHODILATOR; RESPIRATORY SMOOTH MUSCLE RELAXANT
Pregnancy: Category C

ACTIONS/PHARMACODYNAMICS Naturally occurring catecholamine obtained from animal adrenal glands; also prepared synthetically. Acts directly on both alpha and beta receptors; the most potent activator of alpha receptors. Imitates all actions of sympathetic nervous system except those on arteries of the face and sweat glands. Strengthens myocardial contraction; increases systolic but may decrease diastolic blood pressure; increases cardiac rate and cardiac output. In common with other adrenergic agonists, stimulates the enzyme adenyl cyclase and consequently enhances synthesis of cyclic AMP (cAMP), which mediates bronchial smooth muscle relaxation. Also constricts bronchial arterioles and inhibits histamine release, thus reducing congestion and edema and increasing tidal volume and vital capacity. Constricts arterioles, particularly in skin, mucous membranes and kidneys, but dilates skeletal muscle blood vessels. Raises blood sugar by promoting conversion of glycogen reserves in liver to glucose and inhibits insulin release in pancreas. Relaxes uterine smooth musculature and inhibits uterine contractions. CNS stimulation believed to result from peripheral effects. Topical application to the eye lowers intraocular pressure, possibly by decreasing aqueous humor formation and by increasing facility of aqueous outflow; produces brief mydriasis and slight relaxation of ciliary muscle. Has only slight effect on normal eye and reportedly is more effective in light-colored eyes than in dark eyes.

USES Temporary relief of bronchospasm, acute asthmatic attack, mucosal congestion, hypersensitivity and anaphylactic reactions, syncope due to heart block or carotid sinus hypersensitivity, and to restore cardiac rhythm in cardiac arrest. Ophthalmic preparation is used in management of simple (open-angle) glaucoma, generally as an adjunct to topical miotics and oral carbonic anhydrase inhibitors; also used as ophthalmic decongestant. Relaxes myometrium and inhibits uterine contractions; prolongs action and delays systemic absorption of local and intraspinal anesthetics. Used topically to control superficial bleeding.

PHARMACOKINETICS Absorption: inactivated in GI tract. **Onset:** 3–5 min, 1 h on conjunctiva. **Peak:** 20 min, 4–8 h on conjunctiva. **Duration:** 12–24 h topically. **Distribution:** widely distributed; does not cross blood-brain barrier; crosses placenta. **Metabolism:** metabolized in tissue and liver by monoamine oxidase (MAO) and catecholamine-methyltransferase (COMT). **Elimination:** small amount excreted unchanged in urine; excreted in breast milk.

CONTRAINDICATIONS & PRECAUTIONS Contraindicated in: hypersensitivity to sympathomimetic amines; narrow-angle glaucoma; hemorrhagic, traumatic, or cardiogenic shock; cardiac dilatation, cerebral arteriosclerosis, coronary insufficiency, arrhythmias, organic heart or brain disease; during second stage of labor; for local anesthesia of fingers, toes, ears, nose, genitalia. Safe use during pregnancy (category C), in nursing women, and in children not established. **Cautious use in:** elderly or debilitated patients; prostatic hypertrophy; hypertension; diabetes mellitus; hyperthyroidism; Parkinson's disease; tuber-

ROUTE & DOSAGE

Anaphylaxis

Adult	SC	0.1–0.5 ml of 1:1000 q10–15min prn
	IV	0.1–0.25 ml of 1:1000 q10–15min
Child	SC	0.01 ml/kg of 1:1000 q10–15min prn
	IV	0.01 ml/kg of 1:1000 q10–15min

Cardiac Arrest

Adult	IV	0.1–1 mg (1–10 ml of 1:10,000) q5min as needed
	Intracardiac	0.1–1 mg
Child	IV	0.01 mg/kg (0.1 ml/kg of 1:10,000) q5min as needed
	Intracardiac	0.05–0.1 mg/kg

Asthma

Adult	SC	0.1–0.5 ml of 1:1000 q20min–4h
	Inhalation	1 inhalation q4h prn
Child	SC	0.01 ml/kg of 1:1000 q20min–4h
	Inhalation	1 inhalation q4h prn

Glaucoma

Adult	Topical	1–2 drops 0.25–2% solution 1/d or b.i.d.
Child	Topical	Same as for adult

Ocular Mydriasis, Hemostasis

Adult	Topical	1–2 drops 0.1% ophthalmic or 0.1% nasal solution
Child	Topical	Same as for adult

Topical Hemostatic

Adult	Topical	1:50,000–1:1000 applied topically; or 1:500,000–1:50,000 mixed with a local anesthetic
Child	Topical	Same as for adult

culosis; psychoneurosis; in patients with long-standing bronchial asthma and emphysema with degenerative heart disease; in children <6 y of age.

ADVERSE/SIDE EFFECTS Nasal use: *burning, stinging,* dryness of nasal mucosa, sneezing, rebound congestion. **Ophthalmic use:** *transient stinging or burning of eyes,* lacrimation, browache, headache,

Common side effects in *italic*; life-threatening effects underlined; generic names in **bold**; classifications in SMALL CAPS

103

rebound conjunctival hyperemia, allergy, iritis; with prolonged use: melanin-like deposits on lids, conjunctiva, and cornea; corneal edema; loss of lashes (reversible); maculopathy with central scotoma in aphakic patients (reversible). **Systemic reactions:** *nervousness,* restlessness, sleeplessness, fear, anxiety, *tremors,* severe headache, cerebrovascular accident, weakness, dizziness, syncope, pallor, nausea, vomiting, sweating, dyspnea, precordial pain, *palpitations,* hypertension, <u>MI</u>, tachyarrhythmias including <u>ventricular fibrillation</u>; bronchial and <u>pulmonary edema</u>, urinary retention, <u>tissue necrosis</u>, metabolic acidoses, elevated serum lactic acid, transient elevations of blood glucose, altered state of perception and thought, psychosis.

DRUG INTERACTIONS May increase hypotension in circulatory collapse or hypotension caused by PHENOTHIAZINES. Additive toxicities with other SYMPATHOMIMETICS **(phenylpropanolamine).** ALPHA AND BETA ADRENERGIC BLOCKING AGENTS (e.g., **ergotamine, propranolol**) antagonize effects of epinephrine. GENERAL ANESTHETICS increase cardiac irritability.

INCOMPATIBILITIES Solution/additive: sodium bicarbonate, **aminophylline, cephapirin, hyaluronidase, mephentermine, warfarin. Y-site:** sodium bicarbonate, **aminophylline.**

NURSING IMPLICATIONS

Administration
Parenteral

- A tuberculin syringe may assure greater accuracy in measurement of parenteral doses.
- Medication errors associated with epinephrine have resulted in fatalities. Be certain to check type of solution prescribed, concentration, dosage, and route.
- Epinephrine injection should be protected from exposure to light at all times. Do not remove ampul or vial from carton until ready to use.
- Before withdrawing epinephrine suspension into syringe, shake vial or ampul thoroughly to disperse particles; then inject promptly.
- Carefully aspirate before injecting epinephrine. Inadvertent IV injection of usual SC or IM doses can result in sudden hypertension and possibly cerebral hemorrhage.
- Drug absorption (and action) can be hastened by massaging the injection site.
- Vascular constriction from repeated injections may

cause tissue necrosis. Rotate injection sites and observe for signs of blanching.

- If IM route is prescribed, injection into buttocks should be avoided. Epinephrine-induced vasoconstriction favors growth of anaerobic *Clostridium welchii,* which may be present in feces and on buttocks.
- For IV use in cardiac resuscitation, if the 1:1000 1 ml ampules are used, the dose should be further diluted with 10 ml of sodium chloride injection.
- As a maintenance dose, dilute in 500 ml 5% dextrose.
- Give each 1 mg over 1 min or longer; may be given more rapidly in cardiac arrest.

Inhalation

- Treatment should start with first symptoms of bronchospasm. The least number of inhalations that provide relief should be used. To prevent excessive dosage, at least 1 or 2 min should elapse before taking additional inhalations of epinephrine. Caution patient that overuse or too frequent use can have severe adverse effects.
- Patient should be in an upright position when aerosol preparation is used. The reclining position can result in overdosage by producing large droplets instead of fine spray.
- Instruct patient to rinse mouth and throat with water immediately after inhalation to avoid swallowing residual drug (may cause epigastric pain and systemic effects from the propellant in the aerosol preparation) and to prevent dryness of oropharyngeal membranes.
- If patient is also taking isoproterenol, it should not be used concurrently with epinephrine. A 4h interval should elapse before a change is made from one drug to the other.

Topical

- Nose drops should be instilled with head in lateral, head-low position to prevent entry of drug into throat. Discuss with physician.
- Instruct patient to rinse nose dropper or spray tip with hot water after each use to prevent contamination of solution with nasal secretions.

Ophthalmic

- It is generally advisable to remove soft contact lenses before instilling eye drops.
- To prevent excessive systemic absorption, instruct patient to apply gentle finger pressure against nasolacrimal duct immediately after drug is instilled for at least 1 or 2 min following instillation.
- When separate solutions of epinephrine and a topical miotic are used, the miotic should be instilled 2–10 min prior to epinephrine because of the conjunctival sac's limited capacity.

Common side effects in *italic*; life-threatening effects <u>underlined</u>; generic names in **bold**; classifications in SMALL CAPS

Assessment & Drug Effects

Parenteral

- Following IV administration monitor BP, pulse, respirations, and urinary output and observe patient closely. Epinephrine may widen pulse pressure. If disturbances in cardiac rhythm occur, withhold epinephrine and notify physician immediately. Keep physician informed of any changes in intake-output ratio.
- Patients receiving epinephrine IV should be on cardiac monitor. Have full crash cart immediately available.
- When epinephrine is administered IV, blood pressure should be checked repeatedly during first 5 min, then checked q3–5min until stabilized.
- Advise patient to report to physician if symptoms are not relieved in 20 min or if they become worse following inhalation.

Inhalation

- Advise patient to report to physician if symptoms are not relieved in 20 min or if they become worse following inhalation.
- Advise patient to report bronchial irritation, nervousness, or sleeplessness. Dosage should be reduced.

Patient & Family Education

- Forewarn patient that intranasal application may sting slightly.
- Inform patient that intranasal applications frequently cause rebound congestion. Caution to use medication as prescribed and to inform physician if drug is not effective. In general, nose drops should not be used for longer than 3 or 4 d.
- Ophthalmic preparation may cause mydriasis, with blurred vision and sensitivity to light in some patients being treated for glaucoma. Drug is usually administered at bedtime or following prescribed miotic to minimize these symptoms.
- Inform patient that transitory stinging may follow initial ophthalmic administration and that headache and browache occur frequently at first but usually subside with continued use. Advise patient to report to physician if symptoms persist.
- Patient should be instructed to discontinue epinephrine eye drops and to consult a physician if signs of hypersensitivity develop (edema of lids, itching, discharge, crusting eyelids).
- Patients hypersensitive to insect stings should be taught how to self-administer epinephrine. Advise these patients not to go barefoot outside and to avoid bright colors and perfume.
- Patients subject to acute asthmatic attacks and responsible family members should be taught how to administer epinephrine subcutaneously. Medication and equipment should be available for home emergency. Confer with physician.
- Inhalation epinephrine reduces bronchial secretions and thus may make mucous plugs more difficult to dislodge. Physician may prescribe bronchial hygiene program, including percussion and postural drainage, planned coughing and deep breathing exercises, and adequate hydration (3000–4000 ml) to facilitate expectoration. Spirometric measurements may be used to assess response to therapy.
- Tolerance can occur with repeated or prolonged use. Caution the patient to report tolerance to physician; continued use of epinephrine in the presence of tolerance can be dangerous.
- Epinephrine may increase blood glucose levels. Patients with diabetes may experience loss of diabetes control.
- Instruct patient to take medication only as prescribed and to report the onset of systemic effects of epinephrine.
- Discard discolored or precipitated solutions.

ADRENERGIC AGONIST, BETA (SYMPATHOMIMETIC)

ISOPROTERENOL HYDROCHLORIDE

(eye-soe-proe-ter´e-nole)
Trade names: Aerolone, Arm-a Med Isoproterenol, Dey-Dose Isoproterenol, Dispos-a-Med Isoproterenol, Isuprel, Vapo-Iso

ISOPROTERENOL SULFATE

Trade name: Medihaler-Iso
Classifications: AUTONOMIC NERVOUS SYSTEM AGENT; BETA-ADRENERGIC AGONIST (SYMPATHOMIMETIC); BRONCHODILATOR; RESPIRATORY SMOOTH MUSCLE RELAXANT
Pregnancy: Category C

ACTIONS/PHARMACODYNAMICS Synthetic sympathomimetic amine. Acts directly on $beta_1$-adrenergic receptors with little or no effect on alpha-adrenoceptors. Action mechanism: activates adenyl cyclase, enzyme that catalyzes conversion of cytoplasmic ATP to cAMP. Resulting increase in cAMP levels causes relaxation of bronchial, GI, and uterine smooth muscle and prevents the release of histamine and slow-reacting substance of anaphylaxis. Drug in-

Common side effects in *italic*; life-threatening effects <u>underlined</u>; generic names in **bold**; classifications in SMALL CAPS

105

duced stimulation of beta$_1$-adrenergic receptors results in increased cardiac output and work by increasing strength of cardiac contraction and, to a slight degree, rate of contraction. Produces slight increase in systolic BP and decrease in diastolic pressure. Reduces total peripheral resistance and increases venous return to the heart by mobilizing blood from vascular reservoirs. Peripheral and coronary vasodilating drug effects may aid tissue perfusion. Stimulation of beta$_2$-adrenoceptors relaxes bronchospasm and, by increasing ciliary motion, facilitates expectoration of pulmonary secretions. May dilate trachea and main bronchi past the resting diameter. Increases hepatic glycogenolysis but, unlike epinephrine, stimulates insulin secretion and thus rarely produces hyperglycemia. Can also cause central excitation, but this is rarely significant. Tolerance to isoproterenol may develop (especially with prolonged use or too frequent use); rebound bronchospasm may occur after drug effects end. In advanced cardiac life support (ACLS) isoproterenol is a temporary measure until pacemaker therapy begins. Use in cardiac arrest debatable.

USES Bronchodilator in treatment of bronchial asthma and reversible bronchospasm induced by anesthesia. Also used as cardiac stimulant in cardiac arrest, carotid sinus hypersensitivity, cardiogenic and bacteremic shock, Adams-Stokes syndrome, or ventricular arrhythmias. Used in treatment of shock that persists after replacement of blood volume. **Unlabeled use:** treatment of status asthmaticus in children.

PHARMACOKINETICS Absorption: rapidly absorbed from oral inhalation, or parenteral administration. **Onset:** immediate. **Duration:** 1 h oral inhalation; 2 h SC. **Metabolism:** action terminated by tissue uptake and metabolized by COMT in liver, lungs, and other tissues. **Elimination:** 40–50% excreted in urine unchanged.

CONTRAINDICATIONS & PRECAUTIONS Contraindicated in: preexisting cardiac arrhythmias associated with tachycardia; tachycardia caused by digitalis intoxication, central hyperexcitability, cardiogenic shock secondary to coronary artery occlusion and MI; simultaneous administration with epinephrine. Safe use during pregnancy (category C), and by nursing mothers not established. **Cautious use in:** sensitivity to sympathomimetic amines, elderly and debilitated patients, hypertension, coronary insufficiency and other cardiovascular disorders, renal dysfunction, hyperthyroidism, diabetes, prostatic hypertrophy, glaucoma, tuberculosis, during anesthesia by cyclopropane.

ROUTE & DOSAGE

Bronchospasms

Adult	Metered Dose Inhaler	1–2 inhalations 4–6 times/d; no more than 6 inhalations in any hour during a 24 h period
Child	Metered Dose Inhaler	Same as for adult
Adult	Compressed Air or IPPB	0.5 ml of 0.5% solution diluted to 2–2.5 ml with water or saline up to 5 times/d
	IV	0.01–0.02 mg prn
Child	Compressed Air or IPPB	0.5 ml of 0.5% solution diluted to 2–2.5 ml with water or saline over 10–20 min up to 5 times/d

Cardiac Arrhythmias/Cardiac Resuscitation

Adult	IV	0.02–0.06 mg bolus, followed by 5μg/min infusion
	SC	0.15–0.2 mg prn
Child	IV	2.5 μg/min or 0.1μg/kg/min by continuous infusion

ADVERSE/SIDE EFFECTS CNS: headache, mild tremors, nervousness, anxiety, lightheadedness, vertigo, insomnia, excitement, weakness, fatigue. **CV:** flushing, palpitations, tachycardia, unstable BP, paradoxic Adams-Stokes seizures (rare), anginal pain, ventricular arrhythmias. **GI:** nausea, vomiting, swelling of parotids (prolonged use), bad taste, buccal ulcerations (sublingual administration). **Other:** severe prolonged asthma attack, sweating, bronchial irritation and edema (particularly with inhalations of powder); hyperglycemia. **Overdosage:** (especially after excessive use of aerosols): *tachycardia,* palpitations, nervousness, nausea, vomiting.

DRUG INTERACTIONS Epinephrine and other SYMPATHOMIMETIC AMINES increase effects and cause cardiac toxicity. HALOGENATED GENERAL ANESTHETICS exacerbate arrhythmias. BETA BLOCKERS antagonize effects.

INCOMPATIBILITIES Solution/additive: sodium bicarbonate, **aminophylline**.

NURSING IMPLICATIONS

Administration
Parenteral
- **IV injection:** dilute 1 ml of 1:5000 solution to 10 ml with sodium chloride or 5% dextrose injection to produce a 1:50,000 solution.

Common side effects in *italic*; life-threatening effects underlined; generic names in **bold**; classifications in SMALL CAPS

- **IV infusion:** dilute 10 ml 1:5000 solution in 500 ml 5% dextrose to produce a 1:250,000 solution.
- Microdrip or constant-infusion pump is recommended to prevent sudden influx of large amounts of drug.
- IV infusion rate should be prescribed by physician, with specific guidelines for regulating flow or terminating infusion in relation to heart rate, premature beats, ECG changes, precordial distress, BP, central venous pressure (CVP), and urine flow. Infusion rate is generally decreased or infusion may be temporarily discontinued if heart rate exceeds 110 bpm, because of the danger of precipitating arrhythmias.
- IV adminstration is regulated by continuous ECG monitoring. Patient must be observed and response to therapy must be monitored continuously noting heart rate, ECG pattern, BP and central venous pressure as well as (for patients with shock) urine volume, blood pH, and PCO_2 levels.
- Isoproterenol solutions lose potency with standing, and solutions gradually become pink to brownish pink from exposure to air, light, heat, or contact with metal or alkali. Discard if precipitate or discoloration is present.
- Incidence of arrhythmias is high, particularly when drug is administered IV to patients with cardiogenic shock or ischemic heart disease, digitalized patients, or to those with electrolyte imbalance. Check pulse before and during IV administration. Rate > 110 usually indicates need to slow infusion rate or discontinue infusion. Consult physician for guidelines.
- Facilities for administration of oxygen mixtures and respiratory assistance should be immediately available during IV administration.

Sublingual Tablet
- Patient should be forewarned of potential transient facial flushing, palpitation, and precordial discomfort. (Systemic effects reported to occur more frequently by this route than by inhalation.) Instruct patient to allow tablet to dissolve under tongue, without sucking, and not to swallow saliva (may cause epigastric pain) until drug has been completely absorbed. Sublingual tablet may be administered rectally, if prescribed.
- Prolonged use of sublingual tablets may damage teeth, possibly because of drug acidity. Advise patient to rinse mouth with water after medication has been completely absorbed and between doses.

Oral Inhalation
- Note that dosage and recommended method of inhaling may vary with type of inhaler and formulation used. Patient should be carefully instructed in use of equipment and cautioned to take the lowest effective dose necessary to obtain relief.
- Treatment should start with first symptoms of bronchospasm.

Metered Dose Inhaler (MDI): Instructions for Use
- Shake MDI thoroughly to activate.
- Breathe out through nose expelling as much air from lungs as possible.
- Close lips and teeth around open end of mouthpiece placed well into mouth aimed at back of throat.
- Inhale deeply while pressing down on canister to activate spray mechanism.
- Try to hold breath for 10 s; then slowly exhale through nose or pursed lips.
- Wait 2 full min before starting a second inhalation, if it is necessary.

Metered Powder Inhaler: Instructions for Use
- Caution patient not to take forced deep breaths but to breathe with normal force and depth. Observe patient closely for exaggerated systemic drug action (tachycardia, palpitation, nausea, vomiting). Patients requiring more than 3 aerosol treatments within 24 h should be under close medical supervision.

Intermittent Positive Pressure Breathing (IPPB) (follow IPPB manufacturer's instructions)
- Patient will sit erect in chair or, if not able, lie in semi-Fowler's position.
- Instruct patient to *allow machine to do the work* (deliver medication into air passages and breath for the patient).
- Dentures should be left in place.
- Treatment usually lasts 15–20 min and may be repeated up to 5 times/d if necessary.
- Rinse mouth immediately after inhalation therapy to prevent dryness and throat irritation.

General
- Store in tight, light-resistant containers preferably between 15–30C (59–86F) unless otherwise directed.

Assessment & Drug Effects
- Since drug action increases strength, rate and work of heart, arrhythmias from ischemia may develop.
- Tolerance to bronchodilating effect and cardiac stimulant effect may develop with prolonged use.
- Parotid swelling after prolonged use has been reported. Drug should be discontinued if this occurs.
- Rebound bronchospasm may occur when effects of drug end. Once tolerance has developed, continued use can result in serious adverse effects.

Patient & Family Education
- Caution patients to take medication as prescribed;

i.e., they should not increase, decrease, or omit doses or change intervals between doses. Advise patients to report to physician if treatment fails to give satisfactory relief.

- Inform patient taking repeated doses of isoproterenol (as well as responsible family members) about adverse effects, and advise them to report onset of such reactions to physician.

- Inform patient that saliva and sputum may appear pink after inhalation treatment.

ADRENERGIC ANTAGONIST, ALPHA (SYMPATHOLYTIC)

PRAZOSIN HYDROCHLORIDE

(pra´zoe-sin)

Trade name: Minipress

Classifications: AUTONOMIC NERVOUS SYSTEM AGENT; ALPHA-ADRENERGIC ANTAGONIST (BLOCKING AGENT, SYMPATHOLYTIC); CARDIOVASCULAR AGENT; ANTIHYPERTENSIVE, VASODILATOR

Pregnancy: Category C

ACTIONS/PHARMACODYNAMICS Quinazoline alpha$_1$-adrenergic blocking agent. Action: by selective competitive inhibition of alpha$_1$-adrenoceptors produces vasodilation in both resistance (arterioles) and capacitance (veins) vessels with the result that both peripheral vascular resistance and blood pressure are reduced. Lowers blood pressure in supine and standing positions with most pronounced effect on diastolic pressure. Has minor effect on heart rate and cardiac output in the supine position and does not increase plasma renin activity. Tolerance to antihypertensive effect rarely occurs. Considered a step 2 drug in the stepped-care approach to antihypertensive drug therapy, reserved for the patient who has failed to respond to diet, exercise, weight reduction, or therapy with a step 1 drug. Effective when used concomitantly with a beta-adrenergic blocking agent and a thiazide diuretic. Infrequently used in monotherapy because of its tendency to support sodium and water retention resulting in increased plasma volume.

USES Treatment of hypertension. **Unlabeled use:** severe refractory congestive heart failure, Raynaud's disease or phenomenon, ergotamine-induced peripheral ischemia, pheochromocytoma, benign prostatic hypertrophy.

ROUTE & DOSAGE

Hypertension

Adult	PO	Start with 1 mg h.s.; then 1 mg b.i.d. or t.i.d.; may increase to 20 mg/d in divided doses

PHARMACOKINETICS Absorption: approximately 60% of oral dose reaches the systemic circulation. **Onset:** 2 h. **Peak:** 2–4 h. **Duration:** <24 h. **Distribution:** widely distributed, including into breast milk. **Metabolism:** extensively metabolized in liver. **Elimination:** half-life: 2–4 h; 6–10% excreted in urine, the rest in bile and feces.

CONTRAINDICATIONS & PRECAUTIONS Contraindicated in: safe use during pregnancy (category C), in nursing mothers, and in children not established. **Cautious use in:** chronic renal failure; hypertensive patient with cerebral thrombosis; men with sickle cell trait.

ADVERSE/SIDE EFFECTS CNS: *dizziness, headache, drowsiness*, nervousness, vertigo, depression, paresthesia, insomnia. **CV:** edema, dyspnea, syncope *first-dose phenomenon*, postural hypotension, *palpitations*, tachycardia, angina. **Eye; Ear:** blurred vision, tinnitus, reddened sclerae. **GI:** dry mouth, *nausea*, vomiting, diarrhea, constipation, abdominal discomfort, pain. **GU:** urinary frequency, incontinence, priapism (especially in men with sickle cell anemia), impotence. **Skin:** rash, pruritus, alopecia, lichen planus. **Other:** diaphoresis, epistaxis, nasal congestion, arthralgia, transient leukopenia, increased serum uric acid, and BUN.

DRUG INTERACTIONS DIURETICS and other HYPOTENSIVE AGENTS increase hypotensive effects.

NURSING IMPLICATIONS

Administration

- The initial dose of prazosin should be taken at bedtime to reduce possibility of side effects such as postural hypotension and syncope. However, if first dose is taken during the day, patient should be advised not to drive a car for about 4 h after drug ingestion.

- Food may delay absorption but does not affect extent of absorption. Taking drug with food may reduce incidence of faintness and dizziness.

- Store prazosin capsules at 15–30C (59–86F) in tightly closed container away from strong light. Do not freeze.

Assessment & Drug Effects

- First-dose phenomenon (rare side effect: 0.15% of patients) is characterized by a precipitous decline in BP, bradycardia, and consciousness disturbances (syncope) within 90–120 min after the initial dose of prazosin. Recovery is usually within several hours. Preexisting low plasma volume (from diuretic therapy or salt restriction), beta-adrenergic therapy, and recent stroke appear to increase the risk of this phenomenon.
- Monitor blood pressure. If it falls precipitously with first dose, notify physician promptly.
- Full therapeutic effect of prazosin may not be achieved until 4–6 wk of therapy.

Patient & Family Education

- During early phase of prazosin treatment, advise patient to avoid situations that would result in injury should syncope occur. In most cases, effect does not recur after initial period of therapy; however, it may occur during acute febrile episodes, when prazosin dose is increased, or when another antihypertensive drug is added to the medication regimen.
- Postural hypotension can pose a problem with ambulation. Advise patient to make position and direction changes slowly and in stages. Dangle legs and move ankles a minute or so before standing when arising in the morning or after a nap.
- Caution patient who is experiencing light-headedness, dizziness, a sense of impending loss of consciousness, or blurred vision to lie down immediately. Attempting to stand or ambulate may result in a fall.
- Until reaction to prazosin therapy is known (i.e., potential development of side effects), patient should not undertake any activity that might become a hazard in the presence of dizziness, syncope, or weakness.
- Advise to take drug at same time(s) each day. Encourage patient who has been taught to monitor own BP to keep a daily record noting BP and time taken, when medication was taken, which arm was used, position (i.e., standing, sitting) and time of day. Take this record to physician for reference at checkup appointment.
- Encourage male patients to promptly report priapism or impotence. A change in the drug regimen usually reverses these difficulties. Since acute episodes of priapism followed by impotence spontaneously occur in men with sickle cell anemia, another antihypertensive should be selected. In these patients, drug-induced priapism is frequently irreversible.

- Advise not to take OTC medications, especially those that may contain an adrenergic agent (e.g., remedies for coughs, colds, allergy), until a physician has been consulted.
- Side effects usually disappear with continuation of therapy, but dosage reduction may be necessary.

ADRENERGIC ANTAGONIST, BETA (SYMPATHOLYTIC)

PROPRANOLOL HYDROCHLORIDE

(proe-pran´oh-lole)

Trade names: Apo-Propranolol, Detensol, Inderal, Inderal LA, PMS Propranolol
Classifications: AUTONOMIC NERVOUS SYSTEM AGENT; BETA-ADRENERGIC ANTAGONIST (BLOCKING AGENT, SYMPATHOLYTIC); CARDIOVASCULAR AGENT; ANTIARRHYTHMIC; ANTIHYPERTENSIVE
Pregnancy: Category C

ACTIONS/PHARMACODYNAMICS Nonselective beta blocker of both cardiac (beta$_1$) and bronchial (beta$_2$) adrenoreceptors which competes with epinephrine and norepinephrine for available beta-receptor sites. Blocks cardiac effects of beta-adrenergic stimulation; as a result, reduces heart rate, myocardial irritability (class II antiarrhythmic) and force of contraction, depresses automaticity of sinus node and ectopic pacemaker, and decreases AV and intraventricular conduction velocity. In higher doses, exerts direct quinidine-like effects which depress cardiac function. Propranolol also blocks bronchodilator effect of catecholamines and reduces plasma levels of free fatty acids, and tends to promote retention of sodium; therefore, a diuretic is frequently given concurrently. Inhibition of epinephrine, the result of beta-adrenergic blockade, prevents premonitory signs of hypoglycemia in the diabetic and may also augment hypoglycemia by interfering with catecholamine-induced glycogenolysis. Propranolol may also block insulin release from pancreas with resulting hyperglycemia. Lowers both supine and standing blood pressures in hypertensive patients. Hypotensive effect (i.e., lowered systolic and diastolic blood pressure) is associated with decreased cardiac output, suppressed renin activity, as well as beta-blockade. Increases exercise tolerance by blocking sympathetic effects of exertion and decreases myocardial oxygen requirements in patients with frequent angi-

Common side effects in *italic*; life-threatening effects underlined; generic names in **bold**; classifications in SMALL CAPS

109

nal attacks. Also decreases platelet aggregability. Mechanism of antimigraine action unknown but thought to be related to inhibition of cerebral vasodilation and arteriolar spasms.

USES Management of cardiac arrhythmias, myocardial infarction, tachyarrhythmias associated with digitalis intoxication, anesthesia, and thyrotoxicosis, hypertrophic subaortic stenosis, angina pectoris due to coronary atherosclerosis, pheochromocytoma, hereditary essential tremor; also treatment of hypertension alone, but generally with a thiazide or other antihypertensive as step 1 agent. Available in fixed-dose combination with **hydrochlorothiazide** (Inderide). **Unlabeled use:** anxiety states, migraine prophylaxis, essential tremors, schizophrenia, tardive dyskinesia, acute panic symptoms (e.g., stage fright), recurrent GI bleeding in cirrhotic patients, treatment of aggression and rage.

ROUTE & DOSAGE

Hypertension

Adult	PO	40 mg b.i.d.; usually need 160–480 mg/d in divided doses
Child	PO	1 mg/kg/d in 2 divided doses (1–5 mg/kg/d)

Angina

Adult	PO	10–20 mg b.i.d. or t.i.d.; may need 160–320 mg/d in divided doses

Arrhythmias

Adult	PO	10–30 mg t.i.d. or q.i.d.
	IV	0.5–3 mg q4h prn
Child	PO	1–4 mg/kg/d in 4 divided doses (max 16 mg/kg/d)
	IV	10–20 µg/kg/min over 10 min

Acute MI

Adult	PO	180–240 mg/d in divided doses

Migraine Prophylaxis

Adult	PO	80 mg/d in divided doses; may need 160–240 mg/d

PHARMACOKINETICS Absorption: completely absorbed from GI tract but undergoes extensive first-pass metabolism. **Peak:** 60–90 min immediate release; 6 h sustained release; 5 min IV. **Distribution:** widely distributed including CNS, placenta, and breast milk. **Metabolism:** almost completely metabolized in liver.

Elimination: half-life: 2.3 h; 90–95% excreted in urine as metabolites; 1–4% excreted in feces.

CONTRAINDICATIONS & PRECAUTIONS

Contraindicated in: greater than first-degree heart block; CHF, right ventricular failure secondary to pulmonary hypertension; sinus bradycardia, cardiogenic shock, significant aortic or mitral valvular disease; bronchial asthma or bronchospasm, severe COPD, allergic rhinitis during pollen season; concurrent use with adrenergic-augmenting psychotropic drugs or within 2 wk of MAO inhibition therapy. Safe use during pregnancy (category C), in nursing mothers, and in children not established. **Cautious use in:** peripheral arterial insufficiency; history of systemic insect sting reaction; patients prone to nonallergenic bronchospasm (e.g., chronic bronchitis, emphysema); major surgery; renal or hepatic impairment; diabetes mellitus; patients prone to hypoglycemia; myasthenia gravis; Wolff-Parkinson-White syndrome.

ADVERSE/SIDE EFFECTS Allergic: erythematous, psoriasis-like eruptions, pruritus, fever, pharyngitis, respiratory distress. **CNS:** drug-induced psychosis, sleep disturbances, depression, *confusion,* agitation, giddiness, light-headedness, *fatigue,* vertigo, syncope, weakness, *drowsiness,* insomnia, vivid dreams, visual hallucinations, delusions, reversible organic brain syndrome. **CV:** palpitation, profound *bradycardia,* AV heart block, cardiac standstill, hypotension, angina pectoris, tachyarrhythmia, acute CHF, peripheral arterial insufficiency resembling Raynaud's disease, myotonia, paresthesia of hands. **Eye; Ear:** dry eyes (gritty sensation), visual disturbances, conjunctivitis, tinnitus, hearing loss, nasal stuffiness. **GI:** dry mouth, cheilostomatitis, nausea, vomiting, heartburn, diarrhea, constipation, flatulence, abdominal cramps, mesenteric arterial thrombosis, ischemic colitis. **Hematologic:** transient eosinophilia, thrombocytopenic or nonthrombocytopenic purpura, <u>agranulocytosis</u>, hypoglycemia, hyperglycemia (rare); hypocalcemia (patients with hyperthyroidism). **Respiratory:** dyspnea, <u>laryngospasm</u>, bronchospasm. **Skin:** reversible alopecia, hyperkeratoses of scalp, palms, feet; nail changes, dry skin. **Other:** brown discoloration of tongue (rare), pancreatitis, weight gain, impotence or decreased libido, Peyronie's disease (rare), LE-like reaction, cold extremities, leg fatigue, arthralgia.

DIAGNOSTIC TEST INTERFERENCES BETA-ADRENERGIC BLOCKERS may produce false-negative test results in exercise tolerance ECG tests, and ele-

Common side effects in *italic*; life-threatening effects <u>underlined</u>; generic names in **bold**; classifications in SMALL CAPS

vations in: **serum potassium, peripheral platelet count, serum uric acid, serum transaminase, alkaline phosphatase, lactate dehydrogenase, serum creatinine, BUN**, and an increase or decrease in **blood glucose** levels in diabetic patients.

DRUG INTERACTIONS PHENOTHIAZINES have additive hypotensive effects. BETA-ADRENERGIC AGONISTS (e.g., **albuterol**) antagonize effects. **Atropine** and TRICYCLIC ANTIDEPRESSANTS block bradycardia. DIURETICS and other HYPOTENSIVE AGENTS increase hypotension. High doses of **tubocurarine** may potentiate neuromuscular blockade. **Cimetidine** decreases clearance, increases effects. ANTACIDS may decrease absorption.

NURSING IMPLICATIONS

Administration

- For direct IV give each 1 mg over 1 min either undiluted or diluted in 10 ml of 5% dextrose.
- For intermittent infusion, further dilute in 50 ml of normal saline solution and give over 15–20 min.
- Manufacturer recommends giving oral propranolol before meals and at bedtime. Food enhances bioavailability of propranolol. Advise patient to be consistent with regard to taking propranolol with food or on an empty stomach to minimize variations in absorption.
- Tablet may be crushed before administration and taken with fluid of patient's choice.
- Retitration may be necessary when patient is switched from Inderal to Inderal LA (sustained-release capsule). It is not a simple mg-for-mg substitution. Blood pressure monitoring until drug effectiveness is demonstrated will be necessary.
- Because propranolol impairs reflex responses of the heart, manufacturer recommends that it be withdrawn gradually 48 h before major surgery, with exception of patients with pheochromocytoma. (However, many clinicians prefer to continue the beta blocker at lower doses.)
- When propranolol is to be discontinued, dosage is reduced gradually over a period of 1–2 wk and patient is closely monitored.
- Preserve in tightly closed, light-resistant containers at 15–30C (59–86F).

Assessment & Drug Effects

- Take apical pulse and BP before administering drug.
- Withhold drug if heart rate < 60 bpm or systolic BP ≤ 90 mm Hg.
- Careful medical history and physical examination are essential to rule out allergies, asthma, and other obstructive pulmonary disease. Propranolol can cause bronchiolar constriction even in normal subjects.
- Apical pulse, respiration, BP, and circulation to extremities should be closely monitored throughout period of dosage adjustment. Consult physician regarding acceptable parameters.
- For patients being treated for hypertension, checking blood pressure near end of dosage interval or before administration of next dose is a way of evaluating if control is adequate or whether more frequent dosage intervals are indicated.
- Bradycardia is the most common adverse cardiac effect especially in patients with **digitalis** intoxication and Wolff-Parkinson-White syndrome.
- When propranolol is administered IV, ECG, BP, and pulmonary wedge pressure must be carefully monitored. Reduction in sympathetic stimulation caused by beta blocking action can result in cardiac standstill.
- Adverse reactions generally occur most frequently following IV administration; however, incidence is also high following oral use in the elderly and in patients with impaired renal function. Reactions may or may not be dose related and commonly occur soon after therapy is initiated.
- I & O ratio and daily weight are significant indexes for detecting fluid retention and developing heart failure.
- Plasma volume may increase with consequent risk of CHF if dietary sodium is not restricted in patients receiving propranolol without concomitant diuretic therapy. Consult physician regarding allowable salt intake.
- Because of beta blocking action, usual rise in pulse rate may not occur in response to stress situations, such as fever or following vigorous exercise.
- In patients taking propranolol for angina pectoris, exercise performance studies and ECGs are recommended before therapy to establish baseline data, and during therapy to determine dosage requirements and need to continue treatment. Therapy is not continued unless there is reduced pain and increased work capacity.
- Fasting for more than 12 h may induce hypoglycemic effects fostered by propranolol.
- Caution to avoid prolonged exposure of extremities to cold. If patient complains of cold, painful, or tender feet or hands, examine them carefully for evidence of impaired circulation. Peripheral pulses may still be present even though circulation is impaired.

- When propranolol is given for prolonged periods, periodic determinations should be made of hematologic, renal, hepatic, and cardiac function.

Patient & Family Education

- Patient receiving propranolol at home should be informed about usual pulse rate and should be instructed to take radial pulse before each dose. Advise patient to report to physician if it is slower than base level or becomes irregular. (Consult physician for parameters.)
- Propranolol suppresses clinical signs of hypoglycemia (e.g., BP changes, increased pulse rate) and may prolong hypoglycemia. Patient should be alert to other signs of possible hypoglycemia not affected by propranolol such as excessive sweating, hunger, fatigue, inability to concentrate. Instruct patient to report these easily overlooked and tolerated symptoms.
- Stress importance of compliance and warn patient not to alter established regimen, i.e., not to omit, increase, or decrease dosage or change dosage interval.
- Abrupt discontinuation of propranolol can precipitate withdrawal syndrome: tremulousness, sweating, severe headache, malaise, palpitation, rebound hypertension, MI and life-threatening arrhythmias (in patients with angina pectoris).
- Normotensive patients on prolonged therapy should be cautioned that propranolol may cause mild hypotension (experienced as dizziness or lightheadedness). Advise to make position changes slowly and to avoid prolonged standing and to notify physician if these symptoms persist.
- Since propranolol may cause dizziness and lightheadedness, caution to avoid driving and other potentially hazardous activities until reaction to drug is known.
- Smoking increases hepatic metabolism of propranolol, leading to unpredictable or diminished drug effects. Advise to stop smoking; but if it continues, more frequent monitoring for clinical effects of the drug is indicated.
- Advise to consult physician before self-medicating with OTC drugs.
- Instruct patient to inform dentist, surgeon, or ophthalmologist (propranolol lowers normal and elevated intraocular pressure) that he or she is taking propranolol.

ADRENERGIC ANTAGONIST (SYMPATHOLYTIC): ERGOT ALKALOID

ERGOTAMINE TARTRATE

(er-got´a-meen)
Trade names: Ergomar, Ergostat, Gynergen, Medihaler Ergotamine, Wigrettes
Classifications: AUTONOMIC NERVOUS SYSTEM AGENT; ALPHA-ADRENERGIC ANTAGONIST (SYMPATHOLYTIC); ERGOT ALKALOID
Pregnancy: Category X

ACTIONS/PHARMACODYNAMICS Natural amino acid alkaloid of ergot. Alpha-adrenergic blocking agent with direct stimulating action on cranial and peripheral vascular smooth muscles and depressant effect on central vasomotor centers. In vascular headache, exerts vasoconstrictive action on previously dilated cerebral vessels, reduces amplitude of arterial pulsations, and antagonizes effects of serotonin (implicated in cause of vascular headaches). Does not demonstrate intrinsic sedative or analgesic actions. By unknown mechanism, ergotamine activity can damage vascular endothelium, with subsequent occlusion, thrombosis, and gangrene. Large doses may induce slight elevation of BP and diminish arterial blood flow sufficiently to cause tissue ischemia. Myometrium stimulation (oxytocic effect) becomes more prominent with dose increases and as uterine sensitivity to ergot develops during adolescence and pregnancy. Small doses given in third stage of labor promote strong uterine response without significant side effects. Stimulates chemoreceptor trigger zone (CTZ) and therefore may cause nausea and vomiting. May inhibit prolactin secretion.

USES As single agent or in combination with caffeine to prevent or abort migraine, cluster headache (histamine cephalalgia), and other vascular headaches. Not recommended for migraine prophylaxis because of the possibility of adverse effects.

PHARMACOKINETICS Absorption: variable absorption orally. **Peak:** 0.5–3 h. **Distribution:** crosses blood-brain barrier. **Metabolism:** extensive first-pass metabolism in liver. **Elimination:** half-life: 2.7 h initial phase, 21 h terminal phase; 96% eliminated in feces; excreted in breast milk.

ROUTE & DOSAGE

Vascular Headaches

Adult	PO	1–2 mg followed by 1–2 mg q30min until headache abates or until max of 6 mg/24h or 10 mg/wk
	Inhalation	1 inhalation (360 µg) q5min to a max of 6 inhalations in 24h or 15/wk
	PR	2 mg qh to a max of 4 mg/24h or 10 mg/wk

CONTRAINDICATIONS & PRECAUTIONS

Contraindicated in: hypersensitivity; pregnancy (category X), use in children; sepsis; obliterative vascular disease, thromboembolic disease; prolonged use of excessive dosage; hepatic and renal disease; severe pruritus; marked arteriosclerosis, history of MI, coronary artery disease, hypertension; infectious states; anemia, and malnutrition. **Cautious use in:** lactation, elderly patients.

ADVERSE/SIDE EFFECTS

Acute ergotism: *nausea, vomiting,* diarrhea, abdominal pain, unquenchable thirst, paresthesias, pain (spasms) of facial muscles, tongue, limbs and lumbar region with difficulty in walking; delirium, paresthesias, convulsive seizures, rapid or weak or irregular pulse, confusion, itching and cold skin; (occasionally): gangrene of nose, digits, ears. **Chronic ergotism:** intermittent claudication, muscle pains, *weakness,* numbness, coldness and cyanosis of digits (Raynaud's phenomenon). **Other:** complete absence of medium- and large-vessel pulsations in extremities; precordial distress and pain; angina pectoris, transient bradycardia or tachycardia; elevated or lowered BP; depression; drowsiness; mixed miosis (rare); kidney failure; fibrotic changes (long-term therapy), partial necrosis of tongue, disagreeable aftertaste.

DRUG INTERACTIONS

With high doses of BETA-ADRENERGIC BLOCKERS, possibility of additive vasoconstrictor effects; **erythromycin, troleandomycin** may cause severe peripheral vasospasm.

NURSING IMPLICATIONS

Administration

- Since degree of pain relief is proportional to rapidity of treatment, drug therapy should begin as soon after onset of migraine attack as possible, preferably during migraine prodrome (scintillating scotomas, visual field defects, nausea, paresthesias usually on side opposite to that of the migraine).
- Sublingual tablets should not be chewed or swallowed. They should be allowed to completely dissolve.
- Metered dose nebulizers administer an exact dose and are safe if used as directed. Review instructions with patient.
- Preserve in light-resistant container preferably between 15–30C (59–86F) unless otherwise directed by manufacturer.

Assessment & Drug Effects

- Nausea and vomiting are adverse reactions that occur in about 10% of patients after they take ergotamine. Patient may need an antiemetic. Consult with physician.
- Extended use of ergotamine may result in dependence with the need to increase the dose to obtain relief from vascular headache.
- Carefully monitor patients with PVD for development of peripheral ischemia.
- Patients receiving high ergotamine doses for prolonged periods may experience increased frequency of headaches, fatigue, and depression. Discontinuation of the drug in these patients results in severe withdrawal headache that may last a few days.
- ***Overdose symptoms:*** nausea, vomiting, weakness and pain in legs, numbness and tingling in fingers and toes, tachycardia or bradycardia, hypertension or hypotension, and localized edema.

Patient & Family Education

- If migraine attacks occur more frequently or are not relieved, advise patient to report this to physician.
- Advise patient to lie down in a quiet, dark room for 2–3 h after drug administration.
- Instruct patient to report claudication, muscle pain or weakness of extremities, cold or numb digits, irregular heartbeat, nausea, or vomiting. Carefully protect extremities from exposure to cold temperatures; provide warmth, but not heat, to ischemic areas.
- Warn the woman of childbearing age to avoid use of ergotamine if she suspects she is pregnant because of its oxytocic effect.
- Warn patients not to increase dosage without consulting physician; overdosage is the chief cause of untoward effects from the drug.
- Avoid self-dosing with OTC drugs without advice of physician.

Common side effects in *italic*; life-threatening effects underlined; generic names in **bold**; classifications in SMALL CAPS

113

ANTICHOLINERGIC (PARASYMPATHOLYTIC): ANTIPARKINSONISM AGENT

LEVODOPA (L-DOPA)

(lee-voe-doe´pa)
Trade names: Dopar, Larodopa
Classifications: AUTONOMIC NERVOUS SYSTEM AGENT; ANTICHOLINERGIC (PARASYMPATHOLYTIC); ANTIPARKINSONISM AGENT
Pregnancy: Category C

ACTIONS/PHARMACODYNAMICS Metabolic precursor of dopamine, a catecholamine neurotransmitter. Unlike dopamine, levodopa readily crosses the blood-brain barrier. Precise mechanism of action unknown. Levodopa restores dopamine levels in extrapyramidal centers (believed to be depleted in parkinsonism). Cardiac stimulation may be produced by action of dopamine on beta-adrenergic receptors. Also may augment secretion of growth hormone, which in turn is postulated to affect glucose utilization.

USES Idiopathic Parkinson's disease, postencephalitic and arteriosclerotic parkinsonism, and parkinsonism symptoms associated with manganese and carbon monoxide poisoning. **Unlabeled use:** to relieve pain of herpes zoster (shingles); hepatic coma (caused by cirrhosis or fulminating hepatitis), bone pain in metastatic breast carcinoma; adjunctive therapy in CHF.

ROUTE & DOSAGE

Parkinson's Disease

Adult	PO	500 mg to 1 g daily in 2 or more equally divided doses; may be increased by 100–750 mg q3–7d to maximal response or 8 g/d; if used in combination with carbidopa, decrease levodopa dose by 75–80%

PHARMACOKINETICS Absorption: rapidly and well absorbed from GI tract; lower absorption if taken with food. **Peak:** 1–3 h. **Distribution:** widely distributed in body. **Metabolism:** most of drug is decarboxylated to dopamine in lumen of GI tract, liver, and serum. **Elimination:** half-life: 1 h; 80–85% of dose excreted in urine in 24 h.

CONTRAINDICATIONS & PRECAUTIONS
Contraindicated in: known hypersensitivity to levodopa; narrow-angle glaucoma patients with suspicious pigmented lesion or history of melanoma; acute psychoses, severe psychoneurosis, within 2 wk of use of MAO inhibitors. Safe use during pregnancy (category C), in nursing mothers, and in children < 12 y not established. **Cautious use in:** cardiovascular, renal, hepatic, or endocrine disease, history of MI with residual arrhythmias; peptic ulcer; convulsions: psychiatric disorders; chronic wide-angle glaucoma; diabetes; pulmonary diseases, bronchial asthma; patients receiving antihypertensive drugs.

ADVERSE/SIDE EFFECTS Altered laboratory values: elevated BUN, AST, ALT, alkaline phosphatase, LDH, bilirubin, protein-bound iodine, serum level of growth hormone; decreased glucose tolerance; hypokalemia, decreased WBC, Hgb, Hct. **CV:** *orthostatic hypotension;* palpitations, tachycardia, hypertension, phlebitis. **Eye:** *blepharospasm,* diplopia, blurred vision, dilated pupils, oculogyric crises (rare). **GI:** *anorexia, nausea, vomiting,* abdominal distress, flatulence, dry mouth, dysphagia, sialorrhea; burning sensation of tongue, bitter taste, diarrhea or constipation; duodenal ulcer (rarely), GI bleeding. **Hematologic:** hemolytic anemia, <u>agranulocytosis</u>, reduced hemoglobin and hematocrit, leukopenia. **Neuropsychiatric** (frequent): *choreiform and involuntary movements,* increased hand tremor, bradykinetic episodes (on–off phenomena), trismus, grinding of teeth (bruxism), ataxia, muscle twitching, numbness, weakness, fatigue, headache, opisthotonos, confusion, agitation, anxiety, euphoria, insomnia, nightmares; (less frequent): psychotic episodes with paranoid delusions or hallucinations, severe depression, including suicidal tendencies, hypomania; convulsions (rare). **Other:** rhinorrhea, flushing, skin rashes, dark sweat or urine, increased sweating, bizarre breathing patterns; urinary retention or incontinence, increased sexual drive, priapism, postmenopausal bleeding, weight gain or loss, edema; hiccups (rarely), loss of hair, and <u>malignant melanoma</u>; hepatotoxicity.

DIAGNOSTIC TEST INTERFERENCES *Urine glucose:* false-negative tests may result with use of glucose oxidase methods (e.g., Clinistix, Tes-Tape) and false-positive results with the copper reduction method (e.g., Clinitest), especially in patients receiving large doses. It is reported that Clinistix and Tes-Tape may be used if reading is taken at margin of wet and dry tape. *Urinary ketones:* there is possibility

Common side effects in *italic*; life-threatening effects <u>underlined</u>; generic names in **bold**; classifications in SMALL CAPS

of false-positive tests by dip-sticks, e.g., Acetest (equivocal), Ketostix, Labstix; *Serum and urinary uric acid:* false elevations by colorimetric methods, but not with uricase; *Urinary protein:* false increases by Lowry method; *Urinary VMA:* false decreases by Pisano method; *Urinary catecholamine:* false increases by Hingerty method. *PKU urine test:* interference.

DRUG INTERACTIONS MAO INHIBITORS may precipitate hypertensive crisis; TRICYCLIC ANTIDEPRESSANTS augment postural hypotension; PHENOTHIAZINES, **haloperidol** may antagonize the therapeutic effects of levodopa; **pyridoxine** can reverse effects of levodopa; ANTICHOLINERGICS may exacerbate abnormal involuntary movements; **methyldopa** may increase toxic CNS effects; HALOGENATED GENERAL ANESTHETICS increase risk of arrhythmias. **Drug-food interactions:** food decreases the rate and extent of levodopa absorption.

NURSING IMPLICATIONS

Administration

- Ingestion of levodopa with meals, especially if high in protein, appears to interfere with plasma-to-CNS transport of the drug. Administration of drug between meals and with low protein snack (if desired) may decrease fluctuations in clinical response.
- Store in tight, light-resistant containers preferably between 15–30C (59–86F) unless otherwise directed by manufacturer.

Assessment & Drug Effects

- Monitor vital signs, particularly during period of dosage adjustment. Report alterations in blood pressure, pulse, and respiratory rate and rhythm.
- Orthostatic hypotension is usually asymptomatic, but some patients experience dizziness and syncope. Caution patient to make positional changes slowly, particularly from recumbent to upright position, and to dangle legs a few minutes before standing. Supervision of ambulation is indicated. Tolerance to this effect usually develops within a few months of therapy. Support stockings may help some patients. Consult physician.
- Rate of dosage increase is determined primarily by patient's tolerance and response to levodopa. Make accurate observations and report promptly adverse reactions (generally dose related and reversible) and therapeutic effects.
- Therapeutic effects: significant improvement usu-

ally appears during second or third week of therapy, but it may not occur for 6 mo or more in some patients. Therapeutic effect on Parkinson's disease appears to decline after 6–8 y of therapy.

- All patients should be closely monitored for behavior changes.
- Patients with chronic wide-angle glaucoma should be monitored during therapy for changes in intraocular pressure.
- Patients with diabetes should be observed carefully for alterations in diabetes control. Frequent monitoring of blood sugar is advised.
- All patients on extended therapy should be checked periodically for symptoms of diabetes and acromegaly and for functioning of hematopoietic, hepatic, and renal systems.
- About 80% of patients on full therapeutic doses for ≥1 y develop abnormal involuntary movements such as facial grimacing, exaggerated chewing, protrusion of tongue, rhythmic opening and closing of mouth, bobbing of head, jerky arm and leg movements, and exaggerated respiration. Symptoms tend to increase if dosage is not reduced.
- Muscle twitching and spasmodic winking (blepharospasm) are early signs of overdosage; report them promptly.
- Chronic management may be accompanied by the on-off phenomenon: rapid unpredictable swings in intensity of motor symptoms of parkinsonism evidenced by increase in bradykinesia (attacks of "leg freezing" or slow body movement). The patient is unable to perform ADL such as walking during the "off" periods as opposed to independent ability during "on" periods. Attacks develop within minutes, last 1–3 h, usually appear at same time of day, and are due to excessive drug levels. The phenomenon may be precipitated by emotional stress.
- Solicit help of family members to establish a baseline profile of the patient's disabilities. This information is essential for accurate differentiation between desired response to therapy and drug-induced neuropsychiatric adverse reactions.

Patient & Family Education

- Pyridoxine (vitamin B$_6$) may need to be limited: 5 mg or more daily may reverse therapeutic effects of levodopa.
- Food sources of pyridoxine include wheat germ, green vegetables, banana, whole grain cereals, muscular and glandular meats (especially liver), legumes. Discuss dietary practices.
- Caution patient not to take OTC preparations or fortified cereals unless approved by physician.

Multivitamins, antinauseants, and fortified cereals usually contain vitamin B$_6$.

- Elevation of mood and sense of well-being may precede objective improvement. Stress the importance of resuming activities gradually and observing safety precautions to avoid injury. The patient with a history of cardiac problems should be cautioned against overactivity.

- Urge patient to maintain prescribed drug regimen. Sudden withdrawal of medication can lead to parkinsonism crisis (with return of marked rigidity, akinesia, tremor, hyperpyrexia) or to neuroleptic malignant syndrome.

- Inform patients that a metabolite of levodopa may cause urine to darken on standing and may also cause sweat to be dark-colored.

ANTICHOLINERGIC (PARASYMPATHOLYTIC): ANTIMUSCARINIC, ANTISPASMODIC

ATROPINE SULFATE
(a´troe-peen)

Trade names: Atropisol, Buf-Opto Atropine, Dey-Dose, Isopto Atropine, S.M.P. Atropine

Classifications: AUTONOMIC NERVOUS SYSTEM AGENT; ANTICHOLINERGIC (PARASYMPATHOLYTIC); ANTIMUSCARINIC; ANTISPASMODIC; CYCLOPEGIC; MYDRIATIC

Pregnancy: Category C

ACTIONS/PHARMACODYNAMICS This naturally occurring alkaloid and tertiary amine derived from *Atropa belladonna* and other members of the plant Solanaceae selectively blocks all muscarinic responses to acetylcholine (ACh), whether excitatory or inhibitory. Forms strong drug-receptor binding at postganglionic neuroeffector sites in smooth muscle, cardiac muscle, SA and AV nodes, and exocrine glands, thereby blocking action of ACh, and antagonizes action of serotonin, norepinephrine, and histamine. Blocks vagal impulses to heart with resulting decrease in AV conduction time, increase in heart rate and cardiac output, and shortened PR interval. Vasodilates small blood vessels with little effect on blood pressure. Selective depression of CNS relieves rigidity and tremor of Parkinson's syndrome. Toxic doses stimulate the CNS; still larger doses depress the CNS. Reduces amplitude, tone, and frequency of smooth muscle contractions in stomach, intestinal tract, ureters, urinary bladder, gallbladder, and bile ducts. Antisecretory action (vagolytic effect) suppresses sweating, lacrimation, salivation, and secretions from nose, mouth, pharynx, and bronchi. Conventional doses of atropine have little effect on gastric, pancreatic, or hepatic secretions. Atropine is a potent bronchodilator when bronchoconstriction has been induced by parasympathomimetics; also relieves histamine-induced bronchoconstriction but not as effectively as epinephrine or isoproterenol does. Produces mydriasis (dilation of pupils) and cycloplegia (paralysis of accommodation) by blocking responses of iris sphincter muscle and ciliary muscle of lens to cholinergic stimulation; effects are produced with systemic or local administration. Usually does not elevate intraocular pressure except in patients with angle-closure glaucoma.

USES Adjunct in symptomatic treatment of GI disorders (e.g., peptic ulcer, pylorospasm, GI hypermotility, irritable bowel syndrome) and spastic disorders of biliary tract. Relaxes upper GI tract and colon during hypotonic radiography. **Ophthalmic use:** to produce mydriasis and cycloplegia before refraction and for treatment of anterior uveitis and iritis. **Preoperative use:** to suppress salivation, perspiration, and respiratory tract secretions; to reduce incidence of laryngospasm, reflex bradycardia arrhythmia, and hypotension during general anesthesia. **Cardiac uses:** for sinus bradycardia or asystole during CPR or that is induced by drugs or toxic substances (e.g., pilocarpine, beta-adrenergic blockers, organophosphate pesticides, and *Amanita* mushroom poisoning); for management of selected patients with symptomatic sinus bradycardia and associated hypotension and ventricular irritability; for diagnosis of sinus node dysfunction and in evaluation of coronary artery disease during atrial pacing; for management of chronic symptomatic sinus node dysfunction. **Other uses:** oral inhalation for short-term treatment and prevention of bronchospasms associated with asthma, bronchitis, and COPD and as drying agent in upper respiratory infection. Adjunctive therapy for hypermotility of GU tract.

PHARMACOKINETICS Absorption: well absorbed from all administration sites. **Peak effect:** 30 min IM, 2–4 min IV, 1–2 h SC, 1.5–4 h inhalation, 30–40 min topical. **Duration:** inhibition of salivation 4 h; mydriasis 7–14 d. **Distribution:** distributed in most body tissues; crosses blood-brain barrier and placenta. **Metabolism:** metabolized in liver. **Elimination:** half-life 2–3 h; 77–94% excreted in urine in 24 h.

ROUTE & DOSAGE

Preanesthesia

Adult	IV/IM/SC	0.2–1 mg 30–60 min before surgery
Child	SC	3–6 kg: 0.1 mg 30–60 min before surgery
		7–9 kg: 0.2 mg 30–60 min before surgery
		12–16 kg: 0.3 mg 30–60 min before surgery

Arrhythmias

Adult	IV/IM	0.5–1 mg q1–2 h prn to a max of 2 mg
Child	IV/IM	0.01–0.03 mg/kg for 1–2 doses

Organophosphate Antidote

Adult	IV/IM	1–2 mg q5–60min until muscarinic signs and symptoms subside (may need up to 50 mg)
Child	IV/IM	0.05 mg/kg q10–30 min until muscarinic signs and symptoms subside

COPD

Adult	Nebulizer	0.025 mg/kg diluted with 3–5 ml saline, administered via nebulizer 3–4 times daily (max 2.5 mg/d)
Child	Nebulizer	0.05 mg/kg diluted with 3–5 ml saline, administered via nebulizer 3–4 times daily

Uveitis

Adult	Ophthalmic	1–2 drops of solution or small amount of ointment in eye up to t.i.d.
Child	Ophthalmic	Same as for adult

Cycloplegia

Adult	Ophthalmic	1 drop of solution or small amount of ointment in eye 1 h before the procedure
Child	Ophthalmic	1–2 drops in eye b.i.d. for 1–3 d prior to procedure or a small amount of ointment in conjunctival sac t.i.d. for 1–3 d prior to procedure with last dose applied several hours before the procedure

CONTRAINDICATIONS & PRECAUTIONS

Contraindicated in: hypersensitivity to belladonna alkaloids; synechiae; angle-closure glaucoma; parotitis; obstructive uropathy, e.g., bladder neck obstruction caused by prostatic hypertrophy; intestinal atony, paralytic ileus, obstructive diseases of GI tract, severe ulcerative colitis, toxic megacolon; tachycardia secondary to cardiac insufficiency or thyrotoxicosis; acute hemorrhage; myasthenia gravis. Safe use during pregnancy (category C) and in nursing women not established. **Cautious use in:** myocardial infarction, hypertension, hypotension; coronary artery disease, CHF, tachyarrhythmias; gastric ulcer, GI infections, hiatal hernia with reflux esophagitis; hyperthyroidism; chronic lung disease; hepatic or renal disease; the elderly; debilitated patients; children under 6 y of age; Down syndrome; autonomic neuropathy, spastic paralysis, brain damage in children; patients exposed to high environmental temperatures; patients with fever.

ADVERSE/SIDE EFFECTS CNS: headache, ataxia, dizziness, excitement, irritability, convulsions, drowsiness, fatigue, weakness; mental depression, confusion, disorientation, hallucinations. **CV:** hypertension or hypotension, ventricular tachycardia, palpitation, paradoxical bradycardia, AV dissociation, atrial or <u>ventricular fibrillation</u>. **Eye:** mydriasis, blurred vision, photophobia, increased intraocular pressure, cycloplegia, eye dryness, local redness. **GI:** dry mouth with thirst, dysphagia, loss of taste, nausea, vomiting, constipation, delayed gastric emptying, antral stasis, paralytic ileus. **GU:** urinary hesitancy and retention, dysuria, impotence. **Skin:** flushed, dry skin; anhidrosis, rash, urticaria, contact dermatitis, allergic conjunctivitis, fixed-drug eruption.

DIAGNOSTIC TEST INTERFERENCES _Upper GI series:_ findings may require qualification because of anticholinergic effects of atropine (reduced gastric motility and delayed gastric emptying). **_PSP excretion test:_** atropine may decrease urinary excretion of PSP (phenolsulfonphthalein).

DRUG INTERACTIONS Amantadine, ANTIHISTAMINES, TRICYCLIC ANTIDEPRESSANTS, **quinidine, disopyramide, procainamide** add to anticholinergic effects. **Levodopa** effects decreased. **Methotrimeprazine** may precipitate extrapyramidal effects. PHENOTHIAZINES' antipsychotic effects decreased (decreased absorption).

NURSING IMPLICATIONS

Administration

- IV atropine is given by direct IV undiluted or diluted in up to 10 ml of sterile water. Administer 1 mg or fraction thereof over 1 min.

- Smaller doses of atropine are indicated for the elderly.
- Wash hands after administering eye drops. Anisocoria (unequal pupil size, blurred vision) has occurred in nurses and physicians from rubbing their eyes with atropine-contaminated fingers.
- Protect in airtight, light-resistant containers at room temperature, preferably 15–30C (59–86F) unless otherwise directed by manufacturer.

Assessment & Drug Effects

- Monitor vital signs. Pulse is a sensitive indicator of patient's response to atropine. Be alert to changes in quality, rate, and rhythm of pulse and respiration and to changes in blood pressure and temperature.
- Initial paradoxic bradycardia following IV atropine usually lasts only 1–2 min; it most likely occurs when IV is administered slowly (more than 1 min) or when small doses (less than 0.5 mg) are used. Postural hypotension occurs when patient ambulates too soon after parenteral administration.
- Atropine may contribute to the problem of urinary retention. Palpate lower abdomen for distension. Monitor I&O, especially in older patients and in patients who have had surgery. Have patient void before giving atropine.
- If constipation is a problem, check for abdominal distension and auscultate for bowel sounds.
- Geriatric and debilitated patients sometimes manifest drowsiness or CNS stimulation (excitement, agitation, confusion) with usual doses of atropine or other belladonna alkaloids. In addition to dosage adjustment, side rails and supervision of ambulation may be indicated.
- Infants, small children, and the elderly are especially prone to developing "atropine fever" (hyperpyrexia due to suppression of perspiration and heat loss), which increases the risk of heatstroke.
- Intraocular tension and depth of anterior chamber should be determined before and during therapy with ophthalmic preparations to avoid glaucoma attacks. Note that ophthalmic solutions and ointments are available in various strengths.
- Frequent and continued use of eye preparations, as well as overdosage, can have systemic effects. Studies reveal that over one half of atropine deaths have resulted from systemic absorption following ocular administration in infants and children.
- Onset of mydriatic action may be slower and duration longer in persons with dark eyes.
- Infants, children with spastic paralysis, brain damage, or Down syndrome (mongolism), and blonde, blue-eyed individuals appear to be highly sensitive to the effects of atropine and related drugs.

- Patients receiving atropine via inhalation sometimes manifest mild CNS stimulation with doses in excess of 5 mg and mental depression and other mental disturbances with larger doses.

Patient & Family Education

- Urge patient to keep dentist appointments. Since saliva is a natural mouthwash, teeth are much more vulnerable to decay when salivation is suppressed.
- The following measures may help to relieve dry mouth: maintain adequate hydration; small, frequent mouth rinses with tepid water; meticulous mouth and dental hygiene; gum chewing or sucking hard, sour candy (sugarless).
- Prepare for visual acuity to be impaired for several days and to protect eyes from bright light by wearing dark glasses while pupils are dilated.
- In addition to causing drowsiness, sensitivity to light and blurring of near vision, atropine will temporarily impair ability to judge distance. Avoid driving and other activities requiring visual acuity and mental alertness.
- Ophthalmic preparations should be discontinued if eye pain, conjunctivitis, palpitation, rapid pulse, or dizziness occurs. Report symptoms promptly to physician.

CHOLINERGIC (PARASYMPATHOMIMETIC): CHOLINESTERASE INHIBITOR

NEOSTIGMINE BROMIDE

(nee-oh-stig´meen)
Trade name: Prostigmin Bromide

NEOSTIGMINE METHYLSULFATE

Trade names: Prostigmin, Prostigmin Methylsulfate
Classifications: AUTONOMIC NERVOUS SYSTEM AGENT; CHOLINERGIC (PARASYMPATHOMIMETIC); CHOLINESTERASE INHIBITOR
Pregnancy: Category C

ACTIONS/PHARMACODYNAMICS Synthetic quaternary ammonium analog of physostigmine, but less likely to cause disturbing side effects. Produces reversible cholinesterase inhibition or inactivation and thus allows intensified and prolonged effect of

Common side effects in *italic*; life-threatening effects <u>underlined</u>;
generic names in **bold**; classifications in SMALL CAPS

acetylcholine at cholinergic synapses (basis for use in myasthenia gravis). Also produces generalized cholinergic response, including miosis, increased tonus of intestinal and skeletal muscles, constriction of bronchi and ureters, slower pulse rate, and stimulation of salivary and sweat glands. Has direct stimulant action on voluntary muscle fibers and possibly on autonomic ganglia and CNS neurons. Use in amenorrhea or as pregnancy test is based on premise that delayed menstruation may be due to diminished vascular responsiveness to acetylcholine.

USES To prevent and treat postoperative abdominal distension and urinary retention; for symptomatic control of and sometimes for differential diagnosis of myasthenia gravis; and to reverse the effects of non-depolarizing muscle relaxants, e.g., tubocurarine.

ROUTE & DOSAGE

Diagnosis of Myasthenia Gravis

Adult	IM	0.022 mg/kg; may increase to 0.031 mg/kg if first test is inconclusive
Child	IM	0.025–0.04 mg/kg

Treatment of Myasthenia Gravis

Adult	PO	15–375 mg/d in 3–6 divided doses
	IM/IV	0.5–2.5 mg
Child	PO	7.5–15 mg t.i.d. or q.i.d. or 0.333 mg/kg or 10 mg/m² 6 times/d
Neonate	PO	1–4 mg q2–3h
	IM	0.03 mg/kg q2–4h

Reversal of Nondepolarizing Neuromuscular Blockade

Adult	IV	0.5–2.5 mg slowly
Neonate	IV	0.04 mg/kg

Postoperative Distension and Urinary Retention

Adult	IM	0.25 mg q4–6h for 2–3 d

PHARMACOKINETICS Absorption: poorly absorbed from GI tract (1–2%). **Onset:** 10–30 min IM or IV; 2–4 h PO. **Peak:** 20–30 min IM or IV; 1–2 h PO. **Distribution:** not reported to cross placenta or appear in breast milk. **Metabolism:** hydrolyzed by cholinesterases; also metabolized in liver. **Elimination:** half-life: 50–90 min; 80% of drug and metabolites excreted in urine within 24 h.

CONTRAINDICATIONS & PRECAUTIONS

Contraindicated in: hypersensitivity to neostigmine, cholinergics, or bromides; bradycardia, hypotension; mechanical obstruction of intestinal or urinary tract; peritonitis. Pregnancy (category C); lactation; administration with other cholinergic drugs. **Cautious use in:** recent ileorectal anastomoses, epilepsy, bronchial asthma; bradycardia, recent coronary occlusion; vagotonia; hyperthyroidism; cardiac arrhythmias; peptic ulcer.

ADVERSE/SIDE EFFECTS Muscarinic effects: *nausea,* vomiting, eructation, epigastric discomfort, abdominal cramps, diarrhea, involuntary or difficult defecation or micturition, *increased salivation* and bronchial secretions, tightness in chest, sneezing, cough, dyspnea, diaphoresis, lacrimation, miosis, blurred vision, bradycardia, hypotension. **Nicotinic effects:** muscle cramps, *fasciculations,* twitching, pallor, elevated BP, fatigability, generalized weakness, respiratory depression, paralysis. **Overdosage:** CNS stimulation, agitation, fear, <u>death</u>.

DRUG INTERACTIONS Succinylcholine decamethonium may prolong phase I block or reverse phase II block; neostigmine antagonizes effects of **tubocurarine, atracurium, vecuronium, pancuronium; procainamide, quinidine, atropine** antagonize effects of neostigmine.

NURSING IMPLICATIONS

Administration

- Read labels of solutions carefully before administration. Injection is available in three concentrations: 1:1000 (1 mg/ml); 1:2000 (0.5 mg/ml); 1:4000 (0.25 mg/ml).
- *IV injection:* IV neostigmine methylsulfate may be given by direct IV undiluted at a rate of 0.5 mg or a fraction thereof over 1 min.
- Note that size of oral dose is considerably larger than that of parenteral dose because drug is poorly absorbed when taken orally (15 mg of oral drug is approximately equivalent to 0.5 mg of parenteral form).
- Regulation of dosage interval is extremely difficult; dosage must be adjusted for each patient to deal with unpredictable exacerbations and remissions.

Assessment & Drug Effects

- Check pulse before giving drug to bradycardic patients. If below 80/min, consult physician. Atropine will be ordered to restore heart rate.
- For treatment of myasthenia gravis: monitor pulse, respiration, and BP during period of dosage adjustment.

Common side effects in *italic*; life-threatening effects <u>underlined</u>; generic names in **bold**; classifications in SMALL CAPS

119

- Report promptly and record accurately the onset of myasthenic symptoms and drug side effects in relation to last dose in order to assist physician in determining lowest effective dosage schedule.
- GI (muscarinic) side effects occur especially during early therapy and may be reduced by taking drug with milk or food. Physician may prescribe atropine or other anticholinergic agent to suppress side effects (*note:* these drugs may mask toxic symptoms of neostigmine).
- In myasthenic patients the time that muscular weakness appears may indicate whether patient is in cholinergic or myasthenic crisis. Weakness that appears approximately 1 h after drug administration suggests **cholinergic crisis (overdose)** and is treated by prompt withdrawal of neostigmine and immediate administration of atropine. Weakness that occurs 3 h or more after drug administration is more likely to be due to **myasthenic crisis (underdose or drug resistance)** and is treated by more intensive anticholinesterase therapy.
- Signs and symptoms of myasthenia gravis that may be relieved by neostigmine: lid ptosis; diplopia; drooping facies; difficulty in chewing, swallowing, breathing, or coughing; weakness of neck, limbs, and trunk muscles. Record drug effect and duration of action.
- Manifestations of neostigmine overdosage often appear first in muscles of neck and those involved in chewing and swallowing, with muscles of shoulder girdle and upper extremities affected next.
- When neostigmine is used as antidote for tubocurarine or other nondepolarizing neuromuscular blocking agents (usually preceded by atropine), monitor respiration, maintain airway or assisted ventilation, and give oxygen as indicated. Respiratory assistance is continued until recovery of respiration and neuromuscular transmission is assured.
- When neostigmine is used to relieve urinary retention, report to physician if patient does not urinate within 1 h after first dose.

Patient & Family Education
- Frequently, drug therapy is required both day and night, with larger portions of total dose being given at times of greater fatigue, as in the late afternoon and at mealtimes.
- Encourage patient to keep a diary of "peaks and valleys" of muscle strength.
- Patient and responsible family members should be taught to keep an accurate record for physician of patient's response to drug, as well as how to recognize side effects, how to modify dosage regimen according to patient's changing needs, or how to administer atropine if necessary.

- Patients should be aware that certain factors may require an increase in size or frequency of dose (e.g., physical or emotional stress, infection, menstruation, surgery), whereas remission requires a decrease in dosage.
- Some patients become refractory to neostigmine after prolonged use and require change in dosage or medication.

DIRECT-ACTING CHOLINERGIC (PARASYMPATHOMIMETIC)

BETHANECHOL CHLORIDE
(be-than´e-kole)
Trade names: Duvoid, Myotonachol, Urabeth, Urecholine
Classification: AUTONOMIC NERVOUS SYSTEM AGENT; DIRECT ACTING CHOLINERGIC (PARASYMPATHOMIMETIC)
Pregnancy: Category C

ACTIONS/PHARMACODYNAMICS Synthetic choline ester with effects similar to those of acetylcholine (ACh). Acts directly on postsynaptic receptors, and since it is not hydrolyzed by cholinesterase, its actions are more prolonged than those of ACh. Produces muscarinic effects primarily on GI tract and urinary bladder. Increases tone and peristaltic activity of esophagus, stomach, and intestines; contracts detrusor muscle of urinary bladder, usually enough to initiate micturition. Directly binds to and activates cholinergic receptors. Activity is chiefly muscarinic; nicotinic actions are minimal in usual doses.

USES Acute postoperative and postpartum nonobstructive (functional) urinary retention, and for neurogenic atony of urinary bladder with retention. **Unlabeled use:** in selected cases of adynamic ileus, gastric atony and retention, reflux esophagitis, congenital megacolon, familial dysautonomia; for prevention and treatment of bladder and salivary gland inhibition induced by tricyclic antidepressants, and for prophylaxis and treatment of phenothiazine-induced bladder dysfunction.

PHARMACOKINETICS Absorption: well absorbed PO. **Onset:** 30 min PO; 5–15 min SC. **Peak:** 60–90 min PO; 15–30 min SC. **Duration:** 1–6 h PO; 2 h SC.

Common side effects in *italic*; life-threatening effects underlined; generic names in **bold**; classifications in SMALL CAPS

Distribution: does not cross blood-brain barrier. **Metabolism:** unknown. **Elimination:** unknown.

ROUTE & DOSAGE

Urinary Retention

Adult	PO	10–50 mg b.i.d. to q.i.d. (max 120 mg/d)
	SC	2.5–5 mg t.i.d. or q.i.d. prn
Child	PO	0.2 mg/kg or 0.6 mg/m² t.i.d.

CONTRAINDICATIONS & PRECAUTIONS

Contraindicated in: COPD, history of or active bronchial asthma; hyperthyroidism; recent urinary bladder surgery, cystitis, bacteriuria, urinary bladder neck or intestinal obstruction, peptic ulcer, recent GI surgery, peritonitis, marked vagotonia, pronounced vasomotor instability, AV conduction defects, severe bradycardia, hypotension or hypertension, coronary artery disease, recent MI, epilepsy, parkinsonism. Safe use during pregnancy (category C), in nursing women, and in children <8 y not established. Do not give IM or IV.

ADVERSE/SIDE EFFECTS Dose-related. **CV:** hypotension with dizziness, faintness, flushing, orthostatic hypotension (large doses); mild reflex tachycardia, atrial fibrillation (hyperthyroid patients), transient complete heart block. **Eye:** blurred vision, miosis, lacrimation. **GI:** nausea, vomiting, abdominal cramps, diarrhea, borborygmi, belching, salivation, fecal incontinence (large doses), urge to defecate (or urinate). **Respiratory:** acute asthmatic attack, dyspnea (large doses). **Other:** increased sweating, malaise, headache, substernal pain or pressure, hypothermia.

DIAGNOSTIC TEST INTERFERENCES Bethanechol may cause increases in *serum amylase* and *serum lipase*, by stimulating pancreatic secretions, and may increase *AST, serum bilirubin,* and *BSP retention* by causing spasms in sphincter of Oddi.

DRUG INTERACTIONS **Ambenonium, neostigmine,** other CHOLINESTERASE INHIBITORS compound cholinergic effects and toxicity; **mecamylamine** may cause abdominal symptoms and hypotension; **procainamide, quinidine, atropine, epinephrine** antagonize effects of bethanechol.

NURSING IMPLICATIONS

Administration

- Bethanechol (PO) should be given on an empty stomach (1 h before or at least 2 h after meals) to lessen possibility of nausea and vomiting, unless otherwise advised by physician.
- Bethanechol may be prescribed with meals following bilateral vagotomy in patients with gastric atony. The drug is given orally in incomplete gastric retention, and SC if retention is complete.
- *To determine minimum effective PO dose:* physician may prescribe initial test dose of 5–10 mg repeated at hourly intervals to a maximum of 30 mg, unless satisfactory response or disturbing side effects intervene. Alternatively, 10 mg followed at 6 h intervals by 25 mg then 50 mg, until desired response obtained.
- *To determine minimum effective SC dose:* physician may prescribe initial test dose of 2.5 mg repeated at 15 to 30 min intervals to a maximum of 4 doses, unless satisfactory response or disturbing side effects intervene.
- Sterile solution of bethanechol is intended for subcutaneous use only. After inserting needle, aspirate carefully before injecting drug to avoid inadvertent entry into a blood vessel. Life-threatening symptoms of cholinergic stimulation can occur if it is given IM or IV.
- *Antidote:* Syringe containing atropine sulfate (specific antidote) should be ready for instantaneous use to abolish severe side effects, 0.6–1.2 mg for adults administered IM, slow IV, or SC; and 0.01 mg/kg for infants and children repeated every 2 h, if necessary. Specific directions for administering antidote should be prescribed by physician.
- Store at 15–30C (59–86F), unless otherwise directed.

Assessment & Drug Effects

- Adverse effects are most commonly associated with subcutaneous administration, and high PO doses. Monitor BP and pulse in these patients. Observe patient for at least 1 h following SC administration. Report early signs of overdosage: salivation, sweating, flushing, abdominal cramps, nausea.
- Monitor I&O. Observe and record patient's response to bethanechol, and report any failure of the drug to relieve the particular condition for which it was prescribed.
- Monitor respiratory status. Promptly report dyspnea or any other indication of respiratory distress.
- Since drug may cause dizziness and blurred vision, supervision of ambulation may be indicated.

Common side effects in *italic;* life-threatening effects underlined; generic names in **bold**; classifications in SMALL CAPS

121

Patient & Family Education

- Orthostatic hypotension is a possible side effect. Therefore, caution patient to make position changes slowly and in stages, particularly from recumbent to upright posture, not to stand still for prolonged periods, to avoid hot baths or showers, and to sit or lie down at first indication of faintness.
- Because bethanechol may cause dizziness and faintness, caution patient to avoid driving or other potentially hazardous activities until reaction to drug has been determined.
- Inform patient that drug may cause blurred vision. Advise appropriate caution.

SKELETAL MUSCLE RELAXANT, CENTRAL ACTING

CYCLOBENZAPRINE HYDROCHLORIDE

(sye-kloe-ben´za-preen)

Trade name: Flexeril
Classification: AUTONOMIC NERVOUS SYSTEM AGENT; CENTRAL-ACTING SKELETAL MUSCLE RELAXANT
Pregnancy: Category B

ACTIONS/PHARMACODYNAMICS Structurally and pharmacologically related to tricyclic antidepressants. Relieves skeletal muscle spasm of local origin without interfering with muscle function. Believed to act primarily within CNS at brainstem; some action at spinal cord level is also probable. Depresses tonic somatic motor activity, although both gamma and alpha motoneurons are affected. In common with other tricyclic compounds, it increases circulating norepinephrine by blocking its synaptic reuptake. Also has sedative effects and potent central and peripheral anticholinergic (atropinelike) activity.

USES Short-term adjunct to rest and physical therapy for relief of muscle spasm associated with acute musculoskeletal conditions. Not effective in treatment of spasticity associated with cerebral palsy or cerebral or cord disease.

PHARMACOKINETICS Absorption: well absorbed from GI tract with some first pass elimination in liver. **Onset:** 1 h. **Peak:** 3–8 h. **Duration:** 12–24 h. **Distribution:** highly protein bound (93%). **Metabolism:** metabolized in liver to inactive metabolites. **Elimination:** half-life: 1–3 d; slowly excreted in urine with some elimination in feces; may be excreted in breast milk.

ROUTE & DOSAGE

Muscle Spasm

Adult	PO	20–40 mg/d in 2–4 divided doses; max 60 mg/d

CONTRAINDICATIONS & PRECAUTIONS Contraindicated in: acute recovery phase of MI, patients with cardiac arrhythmias, heart block or conduction disturbances, CHF, hyperthyroidism. Use for periods longer than 2 or 3 wk not recommended by manufacturer. Safe use during pregnancy (category B), in nursing mothers, and children < 15 y not established. **Cautious use in:** patients receiving anticholinergic medications; prostatic hypertrophy, history of urinary retention, angle closure glaucoma; increased IOP, seizures; cardiovascular disease; hepatic impairment; elderly, debilitated patients; history of psychiatric illness.

ADVERSE/SIDE EFFECTS CNS: *drowsiness, dizziness,* weakness, fatigue, asthenia, paresthesias, tremors, muscle twitching, insomnia, euphoria, disorientation, mania, ataxia. **CV:** tachycardia, syncope, palpitation, vasodilation, chest pain, orthostatic hypotension, dyspnea; with high doses, possibility of severe arrhythmias. **GI:** *dry mouth,* indigestion, unpleasant taste, coated tongue, tongue discoloration, vomiting, anorexia, abdominal pain, flatulence, diarrhea, paralytic ileus. **GU:** increased or decreased libido, impotence. **Hypersensitivity:** pruritus, urticaria, skin rash, edema of tongue and face. **Other:** sweating, myalgia, hepatitis, alopecia. Shares toxic potential of tricyclic antidepressants.

DRUG INTERACTIONS Alcohol, BARBITURATES, other CNS DEPRESSANTS enhance CNS depression; potentiates anticholinergic effects of **phenothiazine** and other ANTHICHOLINERGICS; MAO INHIBITORS may precipitate hypertensive crisis — use with extreme caution.

NURSING IMPLICATIONS

Administration

- Do not administer drug if patient is receiving an MAO inhibitor (e.g., furazolidone, isocarboxazid, pargyline, tranylcypromine).
- Cyclobenzaprine is intended for short-term (2 or 3 wk) treatment because risk-benefit associated with prolonged use is not known.

Common side effects in *italic*; life-threatening effects underlined; generic names in **bold**; classifications in SMALL CAPS

- Store in tightly closed container, preferably at 15–30C (59–86F) unless otherwise directed by manufacturer.

Assessment & Drug Effects

Because of risk of drowsiness and dizziness, supervision of ambulation may be indicated, especially in the elderly.

- Withhold drug and notify physician if signs of hypersensitivity, e.g., pruritus, urticaria, rash, appear.

Patient & Family Education

- Forewarn patient about side effects of drowsiness and dizziness. Advise patient to avoid driving and other potentially hazardous activities until reaction to drug is known.
- Caution patient to avoid alcohol and other CNS depressants (unless otherwise directed by physician) because cyclobenzaprine enhances their effects.
- Advise patient that dry mouth may be relieved by increasing total fluid intake (if not contraindicated).
- Keep physician informed of therapeutic effectiveness. Spasmolytic effect usually begins within 1 or 2 d and may be manifested by lessening of pain and tenderness, increase in range of motion, and ability to perform ADL.

SKELETAL MUSCLE RELAXANT, DEPOLARIZING

SUCCINYLCHOLINE CHLORIDE

(suk-sin-ill-koe´leen)

Trade names: Anectine, Quelicin, Sucostrin, Sux-Cert, Incert

Classification: AUTONOMIC NERVOUS SYSTEM AGENT; DEPOLARIZING SKELETAL MUSCLE RELAXANT

Pregnancy: Category C

ACTIONS/PHARMACODYNAMICS Synthetic, ultrashort-acting depolarizing neuromuscular blocking agent with high affinity for acetylcholine (ACh) receptor sites. Initial transient contractions and fasciculations are followed by sustained flaccid skeletal muscle paralysis produced by state of accommodation that develops in adjacent excitable muscle membranes. Rapidly hydrolyzed by plasma pseudocholinesterase. May increase vagal tone initially, particularly in children and with high doses, and sub-

sequently produce mild sympathetic stimulation. IOP may increase slightly and may persist after onset of complete paralysis. Reported to have histamine-releasing properties. Has no known effect on consciousness or pain threshold.

USES To produce skeletal muscle relaxation as adjunct to anesthesia; to facilitate intubation and endoscopy, to increase pulmonary compliance in assisted or controlled respiration, and to reduce intensity of muscle contractions in pharmacologically induced or electroshock convulsions.

ROUTE & DOSAGE

Surgical and Anesthetic Procedures

Adult	IV	0.3–1.1 mg/kg administered over 10–30 s; may give additional doses prn
	IM	2.5–4 mg/kg up to 150 mg
Child	IV	1–2 mg/kg administered over 10–30 s; may give additional doses prn
	IM	2.5–4 mg/kg up to 150 mg

Prolonged Muscle Relaxation

Adult	IV	0.5–10 mg/min by continuous infusion

PHARMACOKINETICS Onset: 0.5–1 min IV; 2–3 min IM. **Duration:** 2–3 min IV; 10–30 min IM. **Distribution:** crosses placenta in small amounts. **Metabolism:** metabolized in plasma by pseudocholinesterases. **Elimination:** excreted in urine.

CONTRAINDICATIONS & PRECAUTIONS
Contraindicated in: hypersensitivity to succinylcholine; family history of malignant hyperthermia. Safe use in pregnancy (category C) not established. **Cautious use in:** during delivery by cesarean section; renal, hepatic, pulmonary, metabolic, or cardiovascular disorders; dehydration, electrolyte imbalance, patients taking digitalis, severe burns or trauma, fractures, spinal cord injuries, degenerative or dystrophic neuromuscular diseases, low plasma pseudocholinesterase levels (recessive genetic trait, but often associated with severe liver disease, severe anemia, dehydration, marked changes in body temperature, exposure to neurotoxic insecticides, certain drugs); collagen diseases, porphyria, intraocular surgery, glaucoma.

ADVERSE/SIDE EFFECTS CNS: *muscle fasciculations,* profound and prolonged muscle relaxation, muscle pain. **CV:** *bradycardia,* tachycardia, hypotension, hypertension, arrhythmias, sinus arrest.

Common side effects in *italic*; life-threatening effects <u>underlined</u>; generic names in **bold**; classifications in SMALL CAPS

123

Respiratory: _respiratory depression,_ bronchospasm, hypoxia, apnea. **Other:** malignant hyperthermia, increased IOP, excessive salivation, enlarged salivary glands, myoglobinemia, hyperkalemia; hypersensitivity reactions (rare); decreased tone and motility of GI tract (large doses).

DRUG INTERACTIONS Aminoglycosides, colistin, cyclophosphamide, cyclopropane, echothiophate iodide, halothane, lidocaine, MAGNESIUM SALTS, **methotrimeprazine,** NARCOTIC ANALGESICS, ORGANO-PHOSPHAMIDE INSECTICIDES, MAO INHIBITORS, PHENOTHI-AZINES, **procaine, procainamide, quinidine, quinine, propranolol** may prolong neuromuscular blockade; DIGITALIS GLYCOSIDES may increase risk of cardiac arrhythmias.

INCOMPATIBILITIES Solution/Additive: sodium bicarbonate, thiopental.

NURSING IMPLICATIONS

Administration
- Only freshly prepared solutions should be used; succinylcholine hydrolyzes rapidly with consequent loss of potency.
- Primarily administered by anesthesiologist or under direct observation.
- Initial small test dose may be given to determine individual drug sensitivity and recovery time.
- IV succinylcholine chloride may be given by direct IV undiluted over 10–30 seconds.
- IV succinylcholine chloride may be diluted, 1 g in 1L of D5W or NS, and given by intermittent or continuous infusion at a rate not to exceed 10 mg/min.
- IM injections are made deeply, preferably high into deltoid muscle.
- Expiration date and storage before and after reconstitution varies with the manufacturer.

Assessment & Drug Effects
- Baseline serum electrolyte determinations advised. Electrolyte imbalance (particularly potassium, calcium, magnesium) can potentiate effects of neuromuscular blocking agents.
- Transient apnea usually occurs at time of maximal drug effect (1–2 min); spontaneous respiration should return in a few seconds or, at most, 3 or 4 min.
- Facilities for emergency endotracheal intubation, artificial respiration, and assisted or controlled respiration with oxygen should be immediately available. A nerve stimulator may be used to assess nature and degree of neuromuscular blockade.

- Selective muscle paralysis following drug administration develops in the following sequence: levator eyelid muscles, mastication, limbs, abdomen, glottis, intercostals, diaphragm. Recovery generally occurs in reverse order.
- Tachyphylaxis (reduced response) may occur after repeated doses.
- Adverse effects are primarily extensions of pharmacologic actions.
- Monitor vital signs and keep airway clear of secretions.

Patient & Family Education
- Patient may experience postprocedural muscle stiffness and pain (caused by initial fasciculations following injection) for as long as 24–30 h.
- Inform patient that hoarseness and sore throat are common even when pharyngeal airway has not been used.
- Instruct to report residual muscle weakness.

SKELETAL MUSCLE RELAXANT, NONDEPOLARIZING

TUBOCURARINE CHLORIDE
(too-boe-kyoo-ar´een)
Trade name: Tubarine
Classifications: AUTONOMIC NERVOUS SYSTEM AGENT; NONDEPOLARIZING SKELETAL MUSCLE RELAXANT
Pregnancy: Category C

ACTIONS/PHARMACODYNAMICS Curare alkaloid, nondepolarizing neuromuscular blocking agent extracted from the plant _Chondodendron tomentosum._ Produces skeletal muscle relaxation or paralysis by competing with acetylcholine at cholinergic receptor sites on skeletal muscle endplate and thus blocks nerve impulse transmission. Also has histamine-releasing and ganglionic blocking properties. Has no known effect on intellectual functions, consciousness, or pain threshold.

USES To induce skeletal muscle relaxation as adjunct to general anesthesia, to facilitate management of mechanical ventilation, to reduce intensity of muscle contractions in tetanus and in pharmacologically or electrically induced convulsions, to treat spastic states in children, and for diagnosis of myasthenia gravis when conventional tests have been inconclusive.

ROUTE & DOSAGE

Adjunct to General Anesthesia

Adult   IV   6–9 mg followed by 3–4.5 mg in 3–5 min if necessary

Electroshock

Adult   IV   0.165 mg/kg administered slowly IV

Diagnosis of Myasthenia Gravis

Adult   IV   0.004–0.033 mg/kg

PHARMACOKINETICS Peak: 2–5 min. **Duration:** 20–30 min if used alone. **Metabolism:** demethylated in liver. **Elimination:** half-life: 1–3 h; 33–75% excreted in urine within 24 h; 11% excreted in bile; crosses placenta.

CONTRAINDICATIONS & PRECAUTIONS

Contraindicated in: hypersensitivity to curare preparations; when histamine release is a hazard; hyperthermia; electrolyte imbalance; acidosis; neuromuscular disease; renal disease. Safe use during pregnancy (category C) not established. **Cautious use in:** impaired cardiovascular, renal, hepatic, pulmonary, or endocrine function; hypotension; carcinomatosis; thyroid disorders; collagen diseases; porphyria; familial periodic paralysis; history of allergies; myasthenia gravis; elderly or debilitated patients.

ADVERSE/SIDE EFFECTS Slight dizziness, feeling of warmth, profound and prolonged muscle weakness and flaccidity, respiratory depression, hypoxia, apnea, increased bronchial and salivary secretions, bronchospasm, decreased GI motility, *hypotension,* circulatory collapse, malignant hyperthermia, hypersensitivity reactions.

DRUG INTERACTIONS SKELETAL MUSCLE RELAXANTS, INHALED ANESTHETICS, AMINOGLYCOSIDES, **polymyxin B, clindamycin, quinidine, quinine, procainamide**, DIURETICS, **amphotericin B** may potentiate neuromuscular blockade.

INCOMPATIBILITIES Solution/Additive: Trimethaphan.

NURSING IMPLICATIONS

Administration

- Primarily administered by anesthesiologist or under direct observation.
- May be given undiluted (3mg/ml) by direct IV over 60–90 seconds.
- Solutions of drug should not be used if more than faintly discolored.
- Tubocurarine is incompatible with solutions that have a high pH such as barbiturates; therefore, do not mix in same syringe.

Assessment & Drug Effects

- Baseline tests of renal function and determinations of serum electrolytes are generally done before drug administration. Electrolyte imbalance (particularly potassium and magnesium) can potentiate the effects of nondepolarizing neuromuscular blocking agents.
- Monitor BP, vital signs, and airway until assured of patient's recovery from drug effects. Ganglionic blockade (hypotension) and histamine liberation (increased salivation, bronchospasm) and neuromuscular blockade (respiratory depression) are known effects of tubocurarine.
- Selective muscle paralysis following drug administration occurs in the following sequence: jaw muscles, levator eyelid muscles and other muscles of head and neck, limbs, intercostals and diaphragm, abdomen, trunk. Facial and diaphragm muscles are first to recover, followed in order by legs, arms, shoulder girdle, trunk, larynx, hands, feet, pharynx. Muscle function is usually restored within 90 min.
- Measure and record I&O ratio during day of drug administration. Renal dysfunction will prolong drug action. Peristaltic action may be suppressed. Check for bowel sounds.

Patient & Family Education

- Tubocurarine is retained in the body long after effects of neuromuscular blockade appear to have dissipated. Instruct patient to report residual muscle weakness.

BLOOD DERIVATIVE, PLASMA VOLUME EXPANDER *(side tab)*

BLOOD DERIVATIVE, PLASMA VOLUME EXPANDER

NORMAL SERUM ALBUMIN, HUMAN

(al-byoo´min)

Trade names: Albuconn, Albuminar, Albutein, Buminate, Plasbumin

Classifications: BLOOD DERIVATIVE; PLASMA VOLUME EXPANDER

Pregnancy: Category C

ACTIONS/PHARMACODYNAMICS Obtained by fractionating pooled venous and placental human plasma, which is then sterilized by filtration and heat to minimize possibility of transmitting hepatitis B virus or HIV. Risk of sensitization is reduced because it lacks cellular elements and contains no coagulation factors, Rh factor, or blood group antibodies. Expands volume of circulating blood by osmotically shifting tissue fluid into general circulation. Normally, albumin accounts for 70–80% of the colloidal osmotic pressure of plasma. In well-hydrated patients, each volume of the 25% solution draws about 3.5 volumes of interstitial fluid into the circulation within 15 min. Supplied in two strengths: 5% (approximately isotonic and isosmotic with normal human plasma), and 25% (equivalent to 5 volumes of 5% albumin in producing hemodilution). Both strengths now contain 130–160 mEq of sodium per liter.

USES To restore plasma volume and maintain cardiac output in hypovolemic shock; for prevention and treatment of cerebral edema; as adjunct in exchange transfusion for hyperbilirubinemia and erythroblastosis fetalis; to increase plasma protein level in treatment of hypoproteinemia; and to promote diuresis in refractory edema. Also used for blood dilution prior to or during cardiopulmonary bypass procedures. Has been used as adjunct in treatment of adult respiratory distress syndrome (ARDS).

CONTRAINDICATIONS & PRECAUTIONS Contraindicated in: severe anemia, cardiac failure, patients with normal or increased intravascular volume. Safe use during pregnancy (category C) not established. **Cautious use in:** low cardiac reserve, pulmonary disease, absence of albumin deficiency; hepatic or renal failure, dehydration, hypertension, restricted sodium intake.

ROUTE & DOSAGE

Emergency Volume Replacement

Adult   IV   25 g; may repeat in 15–30 min if necessary (max 250 g)

Colloidal Volume Replacement (Nonemergency)

Child   IV   12.5 g; may repeat in 15–30 min if necessary

Hyperbilirubinemia, Erythroblastosis Fetalis

Child   IV   1 g/kg of 25% solution 1–2 h before transfusion

Hypoproteinemia Prophylaxis in Neonates

Child   IV   1.4–1.8 ml/kg of 25% solution

ADVERSE/SIDE EFFECTS Possibly due to allergy or to protein overload: fever, chills, urticaria, rash, flushing, circulatory overload, pulmonary edema (with rapid infusion); hypotension, hypertension, dyspnea, tachycardia, nausea, vomiting, increased salivation, headache, back pain.

DIAGNOSTIC TEST INTERFERENCES False rise in *alkaline phosphatase* when albumin is obtained partially from pooled placental plasma (levels reportedly decline over period of weeks).

INCOMPATIBILITIES Solution/additive: verapamil.

NURSING IMPLICATIONS

Administration

- May be administered without regard to blood typing and cross-matching.
- Solutions that show a sediment or appear turbid should not be used.
- In general, 5% solution is used for hypovolemic patients, whereas more concentrated 25% solution is used when fluid (and sodium) intake must be restricted as in hypoproteinemia accompanied by peripheral edema, cerebral edema, and in pediatric patients.
- Normal serum albumin, 5%, is infused without further dilution. Normal serum albumin, 25%, may be infused undiluted or diluted in NS or D5W (with sodium restriction). Specific flow rate should be ordered by physician.
- *Administration rate for hypovolemic shock:* initially administered as rapidly as necessary to restore blood volume. As blood volume approaches normal, rate should be reduced to avoid circulatory overload and pulmonary edema; 5% concentration is admin-

Common side effects in *italic*; life-threatening effects <u>underlined</u>; generic names in **bold**; classifications in SMALL CAPS

istered undiluted at rate not exceeding 2–4 ml/min. 25% concentration is given undiluted or diluted in 5% dextrose or 0.9% NaCl injection (as prescribed), no faster than 1 ml/min.

- **Administration rate for patients with normal blood volumes** 5% albumin human solution not to exceed 5–10 ml/min; 25% solution not to exceed 2 or 3 ml/min. Usual rate for children is 1/4–1/2 the adult rate.
- May be administered in combination or in conjunction with sterile water for injection, dextrose, sodium lactate, or NaCl injections, whole blood or plasma. Consult pharmacist for compatible IV infusion fluids.
- Once container is opened, solution should be used within 4 h, since it contains no preservatives or antimicrobials. Discard unused portion.
- Store at room temperature, but not exceeding 37C (98.6F).

Assessment & Drug Effects

- Monitor BP, pulse and respiration, and IV albumin flow rate. Flow rate adjustments may be required to avoid too rapid a rise in BP.
- Laboratory parameters used to monitor dosage of albumin include *plasma albumin (normal):* 3.5–5 g/dl; *total serum protein (normal):* 6–8.4 g/dl; Hgb; Hct; and serum electrolytes.
- Observe closely for signs of circulatory overload and pulmonary edema (see Signs & Symptoms, chap 3). If signs and symptoms appear, slow infusion rate just sufficiently to keep vein open, and report immediately to physician.
- With injuries or surgery, as BP rises, observe for bleeding points that failed to bleed at lower BP.
- Monitor I&O ratio and pattern. Report changes in urinary output. Increase in colloidal osmotic pressure usually causes diuresis, which may persist 3–20 h.
- When albumin is given to patients with cerebral edema, fluids are generally withheld completely during succeeding 8 h.

Patient & Family Education

- Instruct patient to immediately report chills, nausea, headache, or back pain.

ANTICOAGULANT

WARFARIN SODIUM

(war´far-in)
Trade names: Coufarin, Coumadin Sodium, Panwarfin, Warfilone, Warnerin
Classifications: BLOOD FORMER; ORAL ANTICOAGULANT
Pregnancy: Category D

ACTIONS/PHARMACODYNAMICS Indirectly interferes with blood clotting by depressing hepatic synthesis of vitamin K–dependent coagulation factors: II (prothrombin), VII (proconvertin), IX (Christmas factor or plasma thromboplastin component), and X (Stuart-Prower factor). Deters further extension of existing thrombi and prevents new clots from forming. Has no effect on already synthesized circulating coagulation factors or on circulating thrombi. Does not reverse ischemic tissue damage and has no effect on platelets. Unlike heparin, action is cumulative and more prolonged. Warfarin is not cross allergenic with other coumarin derivatives. Some patients have an inherited resistance to warfarin and other oral anticoagulants (an autosomal dominant derivative) and thus require larger than usual doses to achieve therapeutic effects.

USES Prophylaxis and treatment of deep venous thrombosis and its extension, pulmonary embolism; treatment of atrial fibrillation with embolization. Also used as adjunct in treatment of coronary occlusion, cerebral transient ischemic attacks (TIAs), and as a prophylactic in patients with prosthetic cardiac valves. Used extensively as rodenticide.

ROUTE & DOSAGE

Adult	PO/IV	10–15 mg/d for 2–5 d, then 2–10 mg once/d with dose adjusted to maintain a PT 1.2–2 times control

PHARMACOKINETICS Absorption: well absorbed from GI tract. **Onset:** 2–7 d. **Peak:** 0.5–3 d. **Distribution:** 97% protein bound; crosses placenta. **Metabolism:** metabolized in liver. **Elimination:** half-life: 0.5–3 d; excreted in urine and bile.

CONTRAINDICATIONS & PRECAUTIONS
Contraindicated in: hemorrhagic tendencies: vitamin C

Common side effects in *italic*; life-threatening effects underlined; generic names in **bold**; classifications in SMALL CAPS

127

or K deficiency, hemophilia, coagulation factor deficiencies, dyscrasias; active bleeding; open wounds, active peptic ulcer, visceral carcinoma, esophageal varices, malabsorption syndromes; hypertension (diastolic BP >110 mm Hg), cerebral vascular disease; pregnancy (category D); pericarditis with acute MI; severe hepatic or renal disease; continuous tube drainage of any orifice; subacute bacterial endocarditis; recent surgery of brain, spinal cord, or eye; regional or lumbar block anesthesia; threatened abortion; unreliable patients. **Cautious use in:** alcoholism, allergic disorders, during menstruation, nursing mother, elderly, debilitated patients; *endogenous factors that may increase prothrombin time response (enhance anticoagulant effect):* carcinoma, CHF, collagen diseases, hepatic and renal insufficiency, diarrhea, fever, pancreatic disorders, malnutrition, vitamin K deficiency, alcoholism; *endogenous factors that may decrease prothrombin time response (decrease anticoagulant response):* edema, hypothyroidism, hyperlipidemia, hypercholesterolemia, chronic alcoholism, hereditary resistance to coumarin therapy.

ADVERSE/SIDE EFFECTS Major or minor hemorrhage from any tissue or organ. **GI:** anorexia, nausea, vomiting, abdominal cramps, diarrhea, steatorrhea, stomatitis. **Hypersensitivity:** dermatitis, urticaria, pruritus, fever, anaphylaxis (rare). **Other:** increased serum transaminase levels, hepatitis, jaundice, priapism (rare), burning sensation of feet, transient hair loss. With prolonged use of high doses: myalgia, bone pain, osteoporosis. **Overdosage:** internal or external bleeding, paralytic ileus; skin necrosis of toes (purple toes syndrome), tip of nose, buttocks, thighs, calves, female breast, abdomen, and other fat-rich areas.

DIAGNOSTIC TEST INTERFERENCES Warfarin (coumarins) may cause alkaline urine to be red-orange; may enhance *uric acid* excretion, cause elevation of *serum transaminases,* and may increase *lactic dehydrogenase* activity.

DRUG INTERACTIONS In addition to the drugs listed opposite, many other drugs have been reported to alter the expected response to warfarin; however, clinical importance of these reports has not been substantiated. The addition or withdrawal of any drug to an established drug regimen should be made cautiously, with more frequent PT determinations than usual and with careful observation of the patient and dose adjustment as indicated.

Drugs that May Enhance Anticoagulant Effect	
Acetohexamide	HEPATOTOXIC DRUGS
Acetaminophen	**Influenza vaccine**
Alcohol (acute intoxication)*	**Isoniazid**
ALKYLATING AGENTS	MAO INHIBITORS
Allopurinol	**Meclofenamate**
AMINOGLYCOSIDES	**Mefenamic acid**
AMINOSALICYLIC ACID	**Methyldopa**
Amiodarone	**Methylphenidate**
ANABOLIC STEROIDS†	**Metronidazole**†
ANTIBIOTICS (ORAL)	**Mineral oil**
ANTIMETABOLITES	**Miconazole**
ANTIPLATELET DRUGS	**Nalidixic acid**
Aspirin	**Neomycin** (oral)
Asparaginase	NSAIDS
BROMELAINS	**Plicamycin**
Chloral hydrate*,†	Potassium products
Chloramphenicol	PROLONGED NARCOTICS
Chlorpropamide	**Propoxyphene**
Chymotrypsin	**Propylthiouracil**
Cimetidine	PYRAZOLONES†
Cincophen	**Quinidine**
Clofibrate	**Quinine**
Co-trimoxazole	SALICYLATES†
Danazol	**Streptokinase**†
Dextran	**Sulindac**
Dextrothyroxine†	SULFONAMIDES
Diazoxide	SULFONYLUREAS
Dietary deficiencies	TCAS
Disulfiram†	TETRACYCLINES
DIURETICS*	**Tolbutamide**
Drugs affecting blood elements	THIAZIDES
	THYROID DRUGS
Erythromycin	**Urokinase**
Ethacrynic acid	Vitamin E
Glucagon	
Guanethidine	

Drugs that May Reduce Anticoagulant Effect	
Alcohol (chronic alcoholism)*,†	**Glutethimide**†
BARBITURATES†	**Griseofulvin**
Carbamazepine	LAXATIVES
Chloral hydrate*,†	**Mercaptopurine**
Cholestyramine†	ORAL CONTRACEPTIVES
CORTICOSTEROIDS	(containing ESTROGENS)†
Corticotropin	**Rifampin**
DIURETICS	**Spironolactone**
Ethchlorvynol	Vitamin C
	Vitamin K (dietary)

*Increased or decreased response.
†Avoid concurrent use if possible.

Common side effects in *italic*; life-threatening effects underlined; generic names in **bold**; classifications in SMALL CAPS

INCOMPATIBILITIES Solution/Additive: ammonium chloride, 5% dextrose, Ringer's lactate, AMINOGLYCOSIDES, **ascorbic acid, epinephrine, metaraminol, oxytocin, promazine, tetracycline, vancomycin, vitamin B complex with C.**

NURSING IMPLICATIONS

Administration

- Tablet may be crushed before administration and taken with fluid of patient's choice.
- For IV administration add 2 ml of supplied diluent to 50 mg of warfarin powder. Administer immediately by direct IV at a rate of 25 mg (1ml)/min.
- In an emergency, sodium heparin may be administered initially along with warfarin (both may be given in same syringe). Since heparin may affect PT, blood sample should be drawn just prior to next heparin dose, at least 5 h after last IV injection, or 24 h after last SC dose.
- *Antidote:* In the event of bleeding, anticoagulant effect usually is reversed by omitting 1 or more doses of warfarin and by administration of specific antidote phytonadione (vitamin K_1) 2.5–10 mg orally. Physician may advise patient to carry vitamin K_1 at all times but not to take it until after consultation If bleeding persists or progresses to a severe level, vitamin K_1 5–25 mg IV is given, or a fresh whole blood transfusion may be necessary.
- Protect all preparations from light and moisture (tablets). Discard discolored or precipitated solutions.

Assessment & Drug Effects

- PT should be determined before initiation of therapy and then daily until maintenance dosage is established.
- Start flow chart indicating prothrombin activity data, control values, administered anticoagulant doses.
- Usual aim of therapy is to adjust dose so as to maintain PT at 1 1/2–2 1/2 times the control (12–15 s), or 15–35% of normal prothrombin activity.
- When patient is receiving maintenance dosage, PT determinations may be prescribed at 1–4-week intervals depending on patient's response. Periodic urinalyses, stool guaiac, and liver function tests are also usually performed. Optimum time to draw blood sample: 12–18 h after last dose.
- Since so many drugs interfere with the activity of anticoagulant drugs, a careful medication history should be obtained before start of therapy and whenever altered responses to therapy require interpretation.
- Elderly, psychotic, or alcoholic patients require close monitoring because they present serious noncompliance problems.
- Continued anticoagulant therapy is not advised in the absence of laboratory facilities or patient compliance.
- Patients with greatest risk of hemorrhage include those whose PT is difficult to regulate, who have an aortic valve prosthesis, or who are receiving long-term anticoagulant therapy and the elderly and debilitated.
- Suspect skin necrosis (local gangrene) and report to physician immediately if area is painful and skin appears purple-black surrounded by redness. Lesions usually occur within 3 d after initiation of therapy. Incidence is high in elderly, obese patients.

Patient & Family Education

- Inform patient that bleeding can occur even though PT is within therapeutic range. Advise patient to withhold dose and to notify physician immediately if bleeding or signs of bleeding appear: hematuria, bright red or black tarry stools, hematemesis, gingival bleeding with toothbrushing, ecchymoses, petechiae (often occur in ankle areas), epistaxis, bloody sputum, chest pain (hemopericardium), abdominal or lumbar pain or swelling (retroperitoneal bleeding), menorrhagia, pelvic pain, severe or continuous headache, faintness or dizziness (intracranial bleeding); prolonged oozing from any minor injury (e.g., nicks from shaving).
- Instruct patient and family to withhold dose and to report immediately any symptoms of hepatitis (dark urine, itchy skin, jaundice, abdominal pain, light stools) or hypersensitivity reaction.
- Instruct patient to avoid brand interchange, to take drug at same time each day, and not to alter dose.
- Menstrual flow is generally normal but may be slightly increased or prolonged. Advise patient to notify physician if there is an unusual increase in bleeding. PT should be checked at least monthly in menstruating women.
- Smoking increases metabolism and therefore may increase dose requirement. Patient should stop smoking or at least greatly modify amount of smoking during anticoagulant therapy.
- Influenza vaccine decreases hepatic metabolism of warfarin, leading to augmented anticoagulant effect as evidenced by hemorrhage. Patient is at risk of

bleeding for up to 1 mo after receiving the vaccine.
- PT may be lengthened (enhanced anticoagulant effect) by fever, prolonged hot weather, malnutrition, diarrhea.
- PT may be shortened by a high-fat diet, sudden increase in vitamin K–rich foods (cabbage, cauliflower, broccoli, asparagus, lettuce, turnip greens, onions, spinach, kale, fish, liver), coffee or green tea (caffeine), or by tube feedings with high vitamin K content.
- Urge patient to maintain a well-balanced diet and to avoid excess intake of alcohol.
- Advise patient to inform dentist or any new physician about anticoagulant therapy and duration of treatment.
- Instruct patient to use a soft toothbrush and to floss teeth gently with waxed floss. Also advise use of electric razor for shaving.
- If patient becomes pregnant while on anticoagulant therapy, she should be informed of the potential risk of congenital malformations.
- Warn patient against taking any other drug unless specifically approved by physician or pharmacist. Anticoagulant action is affected by many prescription drugs as well as commonly used OTC preparations: e.g., antacids, antihistamines, **aspirin**, mineral oil, oral contraceptives or vitamin C (in large doses).
- Patient should carry on his or her person medical identification card or jewelry, such as Medic Alert, that notes medications and physician's name, address, and telephone number. (May be purchased in a pharmacy.)

HEMATOPOIETIC GROWTH FACTOR

EPOETIN ALFA (HUMAN RECOMBINANT ERYTHROPOIETIN)

(e-po-e-tin)
Trade names: Epogen, Procrit
Classifications: BLOOD FORMER; HEMATOPOIETIC GROWTH FACTOR; HORMONE
Pregnancy: Category C

ACTIONS/PHARMACODYNAMICS Erythropoietin is a glycoprotein that stimulates RBC production. It is produced in the kidney and stimulates bone marrow production of RBCs (erythropoiesis). Hypoxia and anemia generally increase the production of erythropoietin.

USES Elevates the hematocrit of patients with anemia secondary to chronic renal failure (CRF)—patients may or may not be on dialysis; other anemias related to malignancies and AIDS.

ROUTE & DOSAGE

Anemia

Adult	SC/IV	3–500 U/kg/dose 3 times/wk; usually start with 50–100 U/kg/dose until target Hct range of 30–33% (max 36%) is reached; Hct should not increase by more than 4 points in any 2 wk period; rapid increase in Hct increases the risk of serious adverse reactions (hypertension, seizures); may increase dose if Hct has not increased 5–6 points after 8 wk of therapy; reduce dose after target range is reached or the Hct increases by > 4 points in any 2 wk period; dose usually increased or decreased by 25 U/kg increments.
Child	SC	150 U/kg/dose 3 times/wk initially; when Hct increased to 35%, decrease dose by 25 U/kg/dose until Hct reaches 40%

PHARMACOKINETICS Onset: 7–14 d. **Metabolism:** metabolized in serum. **Elimination:** half-life: 4–13 h; minimal recovery in urine.

CONTRAINDICATIONS & PRECAUTIONS Contraindicated in: uncontrolled hypertension and known hypersensitivity to mammalian cell–derived products and albumin (human). **Cautious use in:** pregnancy (category C) and nursing mothers. Safety and effectiveness in children has not been established.

ADVERSE/SIDE EFFECTS CNS: seizures, *headache*. **CV:** *hypertension*. **GI:** nausea, diarrhea. **Hematologic:** *iron deficiency*, thrombocytosis, *clotting of AV fistula*. **Other:** sweating, bone pain, arthralgias.

NURSING IMPLICATIONS

Administration
- Do not shake solution. Shaking may denature the glycoprotein, rendering it biologically inactive.
- Prior to use visually inspect solution for particulate

matter. Do not use if solution is discolored or if it contains particulate matter.

- Use only one dose per vial, and do not reenter vial.
- Do not give with any other drug solution.
- May be given undiluted by direct IV as a bolus dose.
- Discard any unused portion of the vial. It contains no preservatives.
- Store at 2–8C (36–46F). Do not freeze or shake.

Assessment & Drug Effects

- Prior to initiation of therapy the patient's iron stores, including transferrin and serum ferritin, should be evaluated.
- BP should be adequately controlled prior to initiation of therapy and must be closely monitored and controlled during therapy. Hypertension is a side effect that must be controlled.
- Patients with uncontrolled hypertension should not be treated with this drug.
- BP may rise during early therapy as the Hct increases. Notify physician of a rapid rise in Hct (> 4 points in 2 wk). Dosage will need to be reduced because of risk of serious hypertension.
- Monitor for hypertensive encephalopathy in patients with CRF during period of increasing Hct.
- The potential for seizures exists during periods of rapid Hct increase (> 4 points in 2 wk). Monitor for premonitory neurological symptoms, i.e., aura, and report their appearance promptly.
- The risk of thrombotic events, e.g., MI, CVA, TIA, is increased, especially for patients with CRF. Monitor for them closely.
- Patients may require additional heparin during dialysis to prevent clotting of the vascular access or artificial kidney. Monitor APTT closely.
- Hct should be determined twice weekly until it is stabilized in the target range (30–33%) and the maintenance dose of epoetin alpha has been determined. Hct should then be monitored at regular intervals.
- A CBC with differential and platelet count should be performed regularly.
- Monitor BUN, creatinine, phosphorus, and potassium regularly.
- Monitor for signs and symptoms of hyperkalemia (see chap 3). Report them promptly.
- Epoetin alfa has caused polycythemia in cases where the Hct was not carefully monitored with appropriate dosage adjustments.
- Supplemental iron may be required to increase and maintain transferrin saturation to levels that will adequately support Epogen-stimulated erythropoiesis.

Patient & Family Education

- Stress the importance of complying with antihypertensive medication and dietary restrictions.
- During the first 90 d of therapy, patients should not drive or be involved in other hazardous activity because of possible seizure activity.
- As Hct increases, there is an improved sense of well-being and quality of life. The importance of compliance with dietary and dialysis prescriptions should be reinforced.
- Inform patient that headache is a common adverse effect. It should be reported if it is severe or persistent, as it may indicate developing hypertension.
- Stress importance of keeping all follow-up appointments.

HEMOSTATIC

AMINOCAPROIC ACID

(a-mee-noe-ka-proe´ik)
Trade names: Amicar, EACA (epsilon-aminocaproic acid)
Classifications: BLOOD FORMER & COAGULATOR; HEMOSTATIC
Pregnancy: Category C

ACTIONS/PHARMACODYNAMICS   Synthetic hemostatic with specific antifibrinolysis action. Acts principally by inhibiting plasminogen activator substance; to a lesser degree slightly inhibits activity of plasmin (fibrinolysin), which is concerned with destruction of clots. Does not control bleeding caused by loss of vascular integrity.

USES To control excessive bleeding resulting from systemic hyperfibrinolysis, a pathologic condition that may accompany heart surgery, portocaval shunt, abruptio placentae, aplastic anemia, and carcinoma of lung, prostate, cervix, and stomach. Also used in urinary fibrinolysis associated with severe trauma, anoxia, shock, urologic surgery, and neoplastic diseases of GU tract. **Unlabeled use:** to prevent hemorrhage in hemophiliacs undergoing dental extraction; as a specific antidote for streptokinase or urokinase toxicity; to prevent recurrence of subarachnoid hemorrhage, especially when surgery is delayed; for management of amegakaryocytic thrombocytopenia; and to prevent or abort hereditary angioedema episodes.

Common side effects in *italic*; life-threatening effects underlined; generic names in **bold**; classifications in SMALL CAPS

131

ROUTE & DOSAGE

Hemostatic

Adult	PO/IV	4–5 g during first hour; then 1–1.25 g qh for 8 h or until bleeding is controlled (max 30 g/24h)
Child	PO/IV	100 mg/kg during first hour; then 33.3 mg/kg qh (max 18 g/m²/24 h)

PHARMACOKINETICS Absorption: rapidly absorbed from GI tract. **Peak:** 2 h. **Distribution:** readily penetrates RBCs and other body cells. **Elimination:** 80% excreted as unmetabolized drug in 12 h.

CONTRAINDICATIONS & PRECAUTIONS Contraindicated in: severe renal impairment; active disseminated intravascular clotting (DIC); upper urinary tract bleeding. Safe use during pregnancy (category C) not established. **Cautious use in:** cardiac, renal, or hepatic disease; history of pulmonary embolus, or other thrombotic diseases.

ADVERSE/SIDE EFFECTS CNS: dizziness, malaise, headache, seizures. **CV:** faintness, orthostatic hypotension; dysrhythmias; thrombophlebitis, thromboses. **ENT:** tinnitus, nasal congestion. **Eye:** conjunctival erythema. **GI:** nausea, vomiting, cramps, diarrhea, anorexia. **GU:** diuresis, dysuria, urinary frequency, oliguria, reddish-brown urine (myoglobinuria), acute renal failure. **Gynecologic:** prolonged menstruation with cramping. **Skin:** rash.

DIAGNOSTIC TEST INTERFERENCES *Serum potassium* may be elevated (especially in patients with impaired renal function).

DRUG INTERACTIONS ESTROGENS, ORAL CONTRACEPTIVES may cause hypercoagulation.

NURSING IMPLICATIONS

Administration

- If oral therapy is prescribed, note that patient may have to take as many as 10 tablets or 4 tsp for a 5 g dose during the first hour of treatment. (Each tablet contains 500 mg; syrup contains 250 mg/ml.)
- Parenteral aminocaproic acid should always be diluted before use. Each 4 ml (1g) of prepared solution is diluted with 50 ml of NS, 5% dextrose in water or saline, or Ringer's.
- Physician will order specific IV flow rate. Usual rate of administration is 5 g or a fraction thereof over first hour (5 g/250 ml); each additional gram over 1 h.

- Rapid administration should be avoided to prevent hypotension, faintness, and bradycardia or other arrhythmias.
- Check IV site at frequent intervals for extravasation. Observe for signs of thrombophlebitis (see Signs & Symptoms, chap 3).
- Store in tightly closed containers at 15–30C (59–86F) unless otherwise directed. Avoid freezing.

Assessment & Drug Effects

- Monitor vital signs and I&O. Record response to aminocaproic therapy and keep physician informed.
- Report possible signs of **myopathy:** muscle weakness, myalgia, diaphoresis, fever, reddish-brown urine (myoglobinuria), oliguria. Drug should be discontinued promptly.
- Patients receiving prolonged therapy should have routine laboratory measurements of creatine phosphokinase activity and urinalyses for early detection of myopathy.
- Be alert to and report signs of **thrombotic complications:** arm or leg pain, tenderness or swelling, Homan's sign, prominence of superficial veins, chest pain, breathlessness, dyspnea.

Patient & Family Education

- Instruct patient to report difficulty urinating or reddish brown urine.
- Report arm or leg pain, chest pain, or difficulty breathing.

IRON PREPARATION

FERROUS SULFATE

Trade names: Feosol, Fer-In-Sol, Fer-Iron, Fero-Gradumet, Ferospace, Ferralyn, Ferra-TD, Fesofor, Hematinic, Mol-Iron, Novoferrosulfa, Slow-Fe
Classifications: BLOOD FORMER; IRON PREPARATION
Pregnancy: Category A

ACTIONS/PHARMACODYNAMICS Standard iron preparation against which other oral iron preparations are usually measured. Reportedly the cheapest form of supplemental iron and as effective as other more expensive iron salts. Corrects erythropoietic abnormalities induced by iron deficiency but does not stimulate erythropoiesis. May reverse gastric, esophageal, and other tissue changes caused by lack of iron. Ferrous sulfate contains 200 mg/g elemental iron; ferrous sulfate exsiccated contains 300 mg/g elemental iron.

USES To correct simple iron deficiency and to treat iron deficiency (microcytic, hypochromic) anemias. Also may be used prophylactically during periods of increased iron needs, as in infancy, childhood, and pregnancy.

ROUTE & DOSAGE

Iron Deficiency

Adult	PO	750–1500 mg/d in 1–3 divided doses
Child	PO	6–12 y: 600 mg/d in divided doses
		<6 y: 75–225 mg/d in divided doses

Iron Supplement

Pregnancy	PO	300–600 mg/d in divided doses
Infants	PO	1 mg/kg/d for 3 y up to 15 mg/d
Low birth weight	PO	2 mg/kg/d up to 15 mg/d

PHARMACOKINETICS Absorption: 5–10% absorbed in healthy individuals; 10–30% absorbed in iron-deficiency; food decreases amount absorbed. **Distribution:** transported by transferrin to bone marrow, where it is incorporated into hemoglobin; crosses placenta. **Elimination:** most of iron released from hemoglobin is reused in body; small amounts are lost in desquamation of skin, GI mucosa, nails, and hair; 12–30 mg/mo lost through menstruation.

CONTRAINDICATIONS & PRECAUTIONS

Contraindicated in: peptic ulcer, regional enteritis, ulcerative colitis; hemolytic anemias (in absence of iron deficiency), hemochromatosis, hemosiderosis, patients receiving repeated transfusions, pyridoxine-responsive anemia; cirrhosis of liver; pregnancy (category A).

ADVERSE/SIDE EFFECTS Generally minimal: **GI:** *nausea, heartburn,* anorexia, *constipation,* diarrhea, epigastric pain, abdominal distress, *black stools.* **Metabolic:** iron-overload hemosiderosis (rare). **Other:** yellow-brown discoloration of eyes and teeth (liquid forms.) **Large chronic doses in infants:** rickets (due to interference with phosphorus absorption). **Massive overdosage:** lethargy, drowsiness, nausea, vomiting, abdominal pain, diarrhea, local corrosion of stomach and small intestines, pallor or cyanosis, metabolic acidosis, <u>shock, cardiovascular collapse</u>, convulsions, <u>liver necrosis</u>, coma, renal failure, <u>death</u>.

DIAGNOSTIC TEST INTERFERENCES By coloring feces black, large iron doses may cause false-positive tests for ***occult blood with orthotoluidine*** (Hematest, Occultest, Labstix); ***guaiac reagent benzidine test*** is reportedly not affected.

DRUG INTERACTIONS ANTACIDS decrease iron absorption; iron decreases absorption of TETRACYCLINES, **ciprofloxacin, ofloxacin; chloramphenicol** may delay iron's effects; iron may decrease absorption of **penicillamine. Drug-food interactions:** food decreases absorption of iron; ascorbic acid (vitamin C) may increase iron absorption.

NURSING IMPLICATIONS

Administration

- PO iron preparations are best absorbed when taken on an empty stomach (i.e., between meals). However, to minimize gastric distress it may be necessary to administer the drug with or immediately after meals; or the physician may prescribe smaller doses.
- Because iron is potentially corrosive, tablets or capsules should not be taken within 1 h of bedtime, and adequate liquid should accompany ingestion of medication to assure passage into stomach.
- If the patient experiences difficulty in swallowing tablet or capsule, consult physician about prescribing a liquid formulation or a less corrosive form, such as ferrous gluconate.
- In general, liquid preparations should be well diluted and administered through a straw or placed on the back of tongue with a dropper to prevent staining of teeth and to mask taste. Instruct the patient to rinse mouth with clear water immediately after ingestion. Staining of teeth may be minimized by brushing teeth at bedtime with sodium bicarbonate (baking soda).
- Feosol elixir may be mixed with water, but it is not compatible with milk, fruit juice, or wine vehicles. However, the preparation Fer-In-Sol (drops) may be given in water or in fruit or vegetable juice, according to manufacturer.
- Preserve in tightly closed containers. Protect from moisture. Do not use discolored tablets. Store at 15–30C (59–86F).

Common side effects in *italic*; life-threatening effects <u>underlined</u>; generic names in **bold**; classifications in SMALL CAPS

133

Assessment & Drug Effects

- A complete health history should be recorded to determine dietary iron intake, adequacy of diet in general, possible drug-induced causes of anemia, e.g., aspirin, quinidine, phenylbutazone, among others. Other possible causes that should be investigated include abnormal menstrual blood loss, occult blood loss, and reduced iron absorption and utilization.
- Most iron deficiency anemia in patients ≥ 45 y is due to occult bleeding as from an undetected GI mass, rather than from an inadequate diet.
- Simple iron deficiency may be asymptomatic, but it is usually associated with ill-defined symptoms, such as anorexia, easy fatigability, headache, dizziness, tinnitus, and sensitivity to cold. Pagophagia (craving for ice) may be a symptom of iron deficiency anemia. As iron depletion becomes more severe, signs and symptoms may include dyspnea on exertion, palpitation, menstrual disturbances, decreased libido, waxy pallor, paresthesias, epithelial changes including itchy skin, brittleness of hair and nails and ridging, flattening, or concavity of nails, and Plummer-Vinson syndrome (severe anemia): dysphagia, stomatitis, atrophic glossitis.
- Hemoglobin and reticulocyte values should be monitored during therapy. In the absence of satisfactory response after 3 wk of drug treatment, possible reasons for failure warrant investigation.
- Therapeutic response may be experienced within 48 h as a sense of well-being, increased vigor, improved appetite, and decreased irritability (in children). Reticulocyte response begins in about 4 d; it usually peaks in 7–10 d (reticulocytosis) and returns to normal after 2 or 3 wk. Hemoglobin generally increases by 2 g/dl and hematocrit by 6% in 3 wk.
- Iron therapy is usually continued for 2–3 mo after the hemoglobin level has returned to normal (roughly twice the period required to normalize hemoglobin concentration).
- As a general rule, iron should not be administered for longer than 6 mo except in repeated pregnancies, persistent bleeding, or menorrhagia.

Patient & Family Education

- Instruct patient not to crush tablet or empty contents of capsule before administration.
- Ascorbic acid increases absorption of iron. Consuming citrus fruit or tomato juice with iron preparation (except the elixir) may increase its availability.
- Iron absorption may be inhibited if the iron preparation is taken with milk, eggs, or caffeine beverages.
- *Foods high in iron content:* organ meats, brewer's yeast, wheat germ, egg yolk, dried beans, dried fruits, oysters, most muscle meats, fish, fowl, nutrient added breakfast cereals, green vegetables, dark molasses.
- Inform patient that iron preparations cause dark green or black stools. Advise patient to report constipation or diarrhea. These symptoms may be relieved by adjustments in dosage or diet or by change to another iron preparation.

THROMBOLYTIC ENZYME

STREPTOKINASE

(strep-toe-kye′nase)
Trade names: Kabikinase, Streptase
Classifications: BLOOD FORMER; THROMBOLYTIC ENZYME
Pregnancy: Category A

ACTIONS/PHARMACODYNAMICS Derivative of the purified filtrates of beta-hemolytic streptococci. Promotes thrombolysis by activating the conversion of plasminogen to plasmin, the enzyme that degrades fibrin, fibrinogen, and other procoagulant proteins into soluble fragments. This fibrinolytic activity is effective both outside and within the formed thrombus/embolus. Decreases blood and plasma viscosity and erythrocyte aggregation tendency, thus increasing perfusion of collateral blood vessels. Bacterial source bestows strong antigenic properties: support of antibody formation and high potential for allergic reactions. Use has been associated with altered platelet function. Streptokinase (SK) activity is expressed in international units (U): 1 U equals amount of drug required to activate enough blood plasminogen to lyse a standard fibrin clot within 10 min under standard conditions.

USES Acute extensive deep venous thrombosis, acute arterial thrombosis or embolism, acute pulmonary embolus, coronary artery thrombosis, MI, and arteriovenous cannula occlusion.

PHARMACOKINETICS Metabolism: rapidly cleared from circulation by antibodies. **Elimination:** half-life: 83 min; does not cross placenta, but antibodies do.

Common side effects in *italic*; life-threatening effects <u>underlined</u>; generic names in **bold**; classifications in SMALL CAPS

ROUTE & DOSAGE

Coronary Artery Thrombosis, MI

Adult   IV   1.5 million IU infused over 60 min
        IC*   15,000–20,000 IU bolus, followed by
            2000–4000 IU/min for 60 min

Deep Vein Thrombosis, Pulmonary Embolism, Arterial Embolism

Adult   IV   250,000 IU over 30 min loading dose,
           then 100,000 IU/h for 48–72 h

Occluded Cannula

Adult   IV   250,000 IU in 2 ml over 25–35 min;
           clamp for 2 h, then aspirate cannula.

*Intracoronary.

CONTRAINDICATIONS & PRECAUTIONS Contraindicated in:
active internal bleeding; very recent cardiopulmonary resuscitation; recent (within 2 mo) intraspinal, intracranial, intraarterial procedures; intracranial neoplasm; CVA, severe uncontrolled hypertension; history of allergic response to SK, recent streptococcal infection; obstetrical delivery; diabetic hemorrhagic retinopathy; ulcerative colitis, diverticulitis; any condition in which bleeding presents a hazard or would be difficult to manage because of location; pregnancy (category A); safe use during lactation or in children, not established. **Cautious use in:** patient with preexisting hemostatic deficits; conditions accompanied by risk of cerebral embolism; septic thrombophlebitis; uremia, hepatic failure.

ADVERSE/SIDE EFFECTS Allergic: *major* (12%)
(bronchospasm, periorbital swelling, angioneurotic edema, anaphylaxis); *mild* (urticaria, itching, headache, musculoskeletal pain, flushing, nausea, pyrexia). **Hematologic:** phlebitis, *bleeding or oozing at sites of percutaneous trauma;* prolonged systemic hypocoagulability; spontaneous bleeding (GU, GI, retroperitoneal); unstable blood pressure; reperfusion atrial or ventricular dysrhythmias, acute CVA or MI (causal relationship not established).

DIAGNOSTIC TEST INTERFERENCES Streptokinase promotes increases in *TT, APTT,* and *PT.*

DRUG INTERACTIONS ANTICOAGULANTS increase
risk of bleeding; **aminocaproic acid** reverses the action of streptokinase.

NURSING IMPLICATIONS

Administration

- The patient is frequently premedicated with a corticosteroid that can be repeated during the treatment to minimize pyrogenic or allergic reaction.
- Heparin is contraindicated during IV infusion of SK but may be continued during intracoronary administration. After SK infusion and when thrombin time (TT) has decreased to less than twice normal control value (usually 4 h after discontinuation of therapy), anticoagulation therapy is restarted.
- SK is reconstituted with 5 ml 0.9% NaCl injection (preferred) or 5 ml 5% dextrose injection. Roll or tilt vial; avoid shaking to prevent foaming or increase in flocculation. Reconstituted solution may be carefully diluted again, avoiding shaking or agitation of the solution. Slight flocculation does not interfere with drug action; discard solution with large amount of flocculant.
- For rate of IV administration refer to route & dosage table.
- Observe infusion site frequently. If phlebitis occurs, it can usually be controlled by diluting the infusion solution.
- Reconstituted solution should be stored at 2–4C (36–39F). Discard after 24 h. Store unopened vials at 15–30C (59–86F).

Assessment & Drug Effects

- Thrombi more than 7 d old respond poorly to SK therapy; therefore IV infusion is started as soon as possible after the thrombotic event.
- Before SK treatment is started, heparin is discontinued and baseline control levels are established for thrombin time (TT), activated partial thromboplastin time (APTT), prothrombin time (PT), Hct, and platelet count. Treatment is delayed until TT and APTT are less than 2 times the normal control level.
- Spontaneous bleeding occurs about twice as often with SK as with heparin. Protect patient from invasive procedures: IM injections are contraindicated. Also prevent undue manipulation during thrombolytic therapy to prevent bruising.
- During treatment with SK, TT is generally kept at about 2 times or more baseline value and checked q3–4h.
- Monitor for excessive bleeding q15min for the first hour of therapy, q30min for second to eighth hour, then q8h.
- Patient is at risk for postthrombolytic bleeding for 2–4 d after intracoronary SK treatment. Continue monitoring vital signs until laboratory tests confirm anticoagulant control.

- Report signs of potential serious bleeding; gum bleeding, epistaxis, hematoma, spontaneous ecchymoses, oozing at catheter site, increased pulse, pain from internal bleeding. SK infusion should be interrupted, then resumed when bleeding stops.
- Report promptly symptoms of a major allergic reaction; therapy will be discontinued and emergency treatment instituted. Minor symptoms (e.g., itching, nausea) respond to concurrent antihistamine or corticosteroid treatment or both without interruption of SK administration.
- Check pulse frequently. Be alert to changes in cardiac rhythm, especially during intracoronary instillation. Dysrhythmias signal need to stop therapy at once.
- Monitor BP. Mild changes can be expected, but report substantial changes (greater than ± 25 mm Hg). Therapy may be discontinued.
- Check patient's temperature during treatment. A slight elevation, 0.8C (1.5F), perhaps with chills, occurs in about one third of the patients. An elevation to 40C (104F) or more requires symptomatic treatment.
- If an analgesic-antipyretic is indicated, avoid giving aspirin because of its antiplatelet action.

Patient & Family Education
- Instruct patient to immediately report symptoms of hypersensitivity, e.g., dyspnea, urticaria, pruritus.

BRONCHODILATOR (RESPIRATORY SMOOTH MUSCLE RELAXANT)

THEOPHYLLINE
(thee-off′i-lin)
Trade names: Bronkodyl, Duraphyl, Elixicon, Elixophyllin, Lanophyllin, PMS Theophylline, Pulmopylline, Quibron-T, Respbid, Slo-Bid, Slo-Phyllin, Somophyllin, Somophyllin-12, Sustaire, Theo-Dur, Theo-24, Theolair, Theolixir, Theon, Theophyl, Theospan, Uniphyl, and others

THEOPHYLLINE SODIUM GLYCINATE
Trade names: Acet-Am, Synophylate
Classifications: BRONCHODILATOR (RESPIRATORY SMOOTH MUSCLE RELAXANT); CNS AGENT; RESPIRATORY & CEREBRAL STIMULANT; XANTHINE
Pregnancy: Category C

ACTIONS/PHARMACODYNAMICS Methyl xanthine derivative with pharmacologic actions qualitatively similar to those of other xanthines, e.g., caffeine, theobromine; occurs naturally in tea. Relaxes smooth muscle by direct action, particularly of bronchi and pulmonary vessels, and stimulates medullary respiratory center with resulting increase in vital capacity. Also relaxes smooth muscles of biliary and GI tracts. Stimulates myocardium, thereby increasing force of contractions and cardiac output, and stimulates all levels of CNS, but to a lesser degree than caffeine. Produces mild diuresis by increasing renal blood flow and by inhibiting sodium and chloride reabsorption at proximal tubule. At cellular level, xanthines block phosphodiesterase, thereby promoting cyclic AMP accumulation. Cyclic AMP excess promotes catecholamine stimulation of lipolysis, glycogenolysis, and gluconeogenesis and induces release of epinephrine from adrenal medulla cells. Unlike sympathomimetic agents, tolerance to bronchodilator effects of theophylline derivatives rarely develops.

USES Prophylaxis and symptomatic relief of bronchial asthma, as well as bronchospasm associated with chronic bronchitis and emphysema. Also used for emergency treatment of paroxysmal cardiac dyspnea and edema of CHF. **Unlabeled use:** treatment of apnea and bradycardia of prematures and to reduce severe bronchospasm associated with cystic fibrosis and acute descending respiratory infection. Theophylline sodium glycinate is a mixture of sodium theophylline and aminoacetic (glycine). Contains 45–47% theophylline. Similar actions, uses, adverse reactions, and precautions as other theophylline derivatives but claimed to produce less gastric irritation.

PHARMACOKINETICS Absorption: most products are 100% absorbed from GI tract. **Peak:** IV 30 min; uncoated tablet 1 h; sustained release 4–6 h. **Duration:** 4–8 h; varies with age, smoking, and liver function. **Distribution:** crosses placenta. **Metabolism:** extensively metabolized in liver. **Elimination:** parent drug and metabolites excreted by kidneys; excreted in breast milk.

CONTRAINDICATIONS & PRECAUTIONS Contraindicated in: hypersensitivity to xanthines; coronary artery disease or angina pectoris when myocardial stimulation might be harmful; severe renal or liver impairment. Safe use during pregnancy (category C)

Common side effects in *italic*; life-threatening effects <u>underlined</u>; generic names in **bold**; classifications in SMALL CAPS

ROUTE & DOSAGE

Bronchospasm (all doses based on ideal body weight)
Loading Dose

Adult/Child	PO/IV	5 mg/kg loading dose

*Maintenance Dose**

Adult nonsmoker	PO/IV	0.4 mg/kg/h
Adult smoker	PO/IV	0.6 mg/kg/h
Adult with CHF or Cirrhosis	PO/IV	0.2 mg/kg/h
Child	PO/IV	10–12 y: 0.6 mg/kg/h
Child	PO/IV	1–9 y: 0.8 mg/kg/h
Infant	PO/IV	6–11 mo: 0.7 mg/kg/h
Infant	PO/IV	2–6 mo: 0.4 mg/kg/h
Neonate	PO/IV	0.13 mg/kg/h

*IV by continuous infusion; PO divided q6h (immediate release divided q8–12h sustained release)

and lactation not established. **Cautious use in:** children; compromised cardiac or circulatory function, hypertension; hyperthyroidism; peptic ulcer; prostatic hypertrophy; glaucoma; diabetes mellitus; the elderly and neonates.

ADVERSE/SIDE EFFECTS CNS: (stimulation): irritability, restlessness, insomnia, dizziness, headache, tremor, hyperexcitability, muscle twitching, drug-induced seizures. **CV:** palpitation, *tachycardia*, extrasystoles, flushing, marked hypotension, circulatory failure. **GI:** *nausea*, vomiting, anorexia, epigastric or abdominal pain, diarrhea, activation of peptic ulcer. **Renal:** transient urinary frequency, albuminuria, kidney irritation. **Respiratory:** tachypnea, respiratory arrest. **Other:** fever, dehydration, possibility of increased urinary catecholamine excretion.

DIAGNOSTIC TEST INTERFERENCES False-positive elevations of *serum uric acid* (Bittner or colorimetric methods). *Probenecid* may cause false high serum theophylline readings, and spectrophotometric methods of determining *serum theophylline* are affected by a furosemide, sulfathiazole, phenylbutazone, probenecid, theobromine.

DRUG INTERACTIONS Increases **lithium** excretion, lowering lithium levels; **cimetidine,** high-dose **allopurinol** (600 mg/d), **ciprofloxacin, eryth-**romycin, **troleandomycin** can significantly increase theophylline levels.

INCOMPATIBILITIES Solution/Additive: amikacin, bleomycin, CEPHALOSPORINS, **chlorpromazine, clindamycin, codeine phosphate, dimenhydrinate, dobutamine, dopamine, doxapram, doxorubicin, epinephrine, hydralazine, hydroxyzine, insulin, isoproterenol, levorphanol, meperidine, methadone, methylprednisolone, morphine, nafcillin, norepinephrine, oxytetracycline, papaverine, penicillin G, pentazocine, procaine, prochlorperazine, promazine, promethazine, tetracycline, verapamil, vitamin B complex with C. Y-Site:** amiodarone, codeine phosphate, clindamycin, PHENOTHIAZINES (**chlorpromazine, prochlorperazine,** etc), **epinephrine, dobutamine, dopamine, levorphanol, meperidine, methadone, morphine, norepinephrine, verapamil.**

NURSING IMPLICATIONS

Administration

- Oral preparations should preferably be administered with a full glass of water and may be given after meals to minimize gastric irritation. Food and antacids delay but do not reduce extent of absorption.
- Sustained-release forms and enteric coated tablets must be swallowed whole. Chewable tablets must be chewed thoroughly before swallowing. Slow-release theophylline Sprinkle granules can be taken on an empty stomach or mixed with applesauce or water.
- Timing of dose is critical. Be certain patient understands the necessity to adhere to the proper intervals between doses.
- IV solution of 100% theophylline is available in D5W in concentrations of 4 mg/ml, 2 mg/ml, 1.6 mg/ml, 0.8 mg/ml, and 0.4 mg/ml. Administer at a rate not to exceed 20 mg/min.
- IV theophylline ethylenediamine solution with a concentration of 25 mg/ml may be given undiluted by direct IV at a rate of 20 mg/min or diluted in up to 200 ml of D5W and infused over 30 min.

Assessment & Drug Effects

- Therapeutic theophylline plasma level ranges from 10–20 µg/ml (a narrow therapeutic range). Levels exceeding 20 µg/ml are associated with toxicity. Theophylline saliva levels (sometimes used when

Common side effects in *italic*; life-threatening effects underlined; generic names in **bold**; classifications in SMALL CAPS

137

CARDIOVASCULAR AGENTS

proximately 60% of simultaneous plasma levels.

- Once-a-day administration may not adequately control asthmatic patients, smokers, or children. These patients need to have regular frequent serum concentration tests in the beginning of therapy to prevent toxicity.
- Cigarette smoking induces hepatic microsomal enzyme activity, decreasing serum half-life and increasing body clearance of theophylline. This effect requires close monitoring of drug level in the heavy smoker. An increase of dosage from 50–100% is usual in heavy smokers.
- During early therapy, dizziness is a relatively common side effect in the elderly. Take necessary safety precautions and forewarn patient of this possibility.
- Monitor vital signs and I&O. Improvement in quality of pulse and respiration and diuresis are expected clinical effects.
- Observe and report early signs of possible toxicity: anorexia, nausea, vomiting, dizziness, shakiness, restlessness, abdominal discomfort, irritability, palpitation, tachycardia, marked hypotension, cardiac arrhythmias, seizures.
- If theophylline is given to a patient with severe cardiac disease, monitor for tachycardia. Conversely, theophylline toxicity may be masked in patients with tachycardia.
- Plasma clearance of xanthines may be reduced in patients with heart failure, renal or hepatic dysfunction, alcoholism, high fever. Dosage regulation must be closely monitored particularly in these patients.
- Overdose with prolonged release preparation necessitates observing patient for a longer period of time than if conventional formulation had been ingested. Continued slow absorption leads to high plasma concentrations for a prolonged period.
- In the neonate of a mother using this drug, slight tachycardia, jitteriness, and apnea have been observed.
- Theophylline metabolism in the infant <6 mo and in prematures is prolonged as is the half-life; therefore close monitoring for side effects is especially crucial in this age group.

Patient & Family Education
- Take medication at the same time every day.
- Charcoal-broiled foods (high in polycyclic carbon content) may increase theophylline elimination and reduce the half-life as much as 50%.
- Limit caffeine intake, which may increase incidence of adverse effects.
- Inform patient that cigarette smoking may significantly lower theophylline plasma concentration.
- A low-carbohydrate, high-protein diet increases theophylline elimination, and a high-carbohydrate, low-protein diet decreases it.
- Urge patient to drink adequate fluids (at least 2000 ml/d) to decrease viscosity of airway secretions.
- Warn patient to avoid self-dosing with OTC medications, especially cough suppressants, which may cause retention of secretions and CNS depression.
- Since theophylline is distributed into breast milk it may be advisable for the infant to be nursed just before mother takes the drug.

ANGIOTENSIN-CONVERTING ENZYME INHIBITOR

CAPTOPRIL
(kap´toe-pril)
Trade name: Capoten
Classifications: CARDIOVASCULAR AGENT; ANGIOTENSIN-CONVERTING ENZYME INHIBITOR; ANTIHYPERTENSIVE; VASODILATOR
Pregnancy: Category C

ACTIONS/PHARMACODYNAMICS   Lowers blood pressure (renovascular and essential) by specific inhibition of the angiotensin-converting enzyme (ACE). This interrupts conversion sequences initiated by renin that lead to formation of angiotensin II, a potent endogenous vasoconstrictor. ACE inhibition alters hemodynamics without compensatory reflex tachycardia or changes in cardiac output (except in patient with CHF). Peripheral vascular resistance is lowered by vasodilation, but vascular bed perfusion in brain, heart, and peripheral circulation is preserved. Inhibition of ACE also leads to decreased circulating aldosterone, a secretory response to angiotensin II stimulation. (Aldosterone, an adrenal cortex hormone, promotes sodium and fluid retention.) Reduced circulating aldosterone (drug-induced) is associated with a potassium-sparing effect. Captopril may interfere with degradation of bradykinin (a potent vasodilator) and increase plasma levels of a prostaglandin E_2 metabolite with vasodilator properties. In heart failure, captopril administration is followed by a fall in CVP and pulmonary wedge pressure; hypotensive action appears to be unrelated to plasma renin levels.

Common side effects in *italic*; life-threatening effects underlined; generic names in **bold**; classifications in SMALL CAPS

USES First line monotherapy and stepped-care approach to antihypertensive therapy of all forms of hypertension as step 1, 2, 3, or 4 agent. It is also used in conjunction with digitalis and diuretics in treatment of CHF. **Unlabeled use:** idiopathic edema.

ROUTE & DOSAGE

Hypertension

Adult	PO	6.25–25 mg t.i.d.; may increase to 50 mg t.i.d. (max 450 mg/d)

Congestive Heart Failure

Adult	PO	6.25–12.5 mg t.i.d.; may increase to 50 mg t.i.d. (max 450 mg/d)

PHARMACOKINETICS Absorption: 60–75% absorbed; food may decrease absorption 25–40%. **Onset:** 15 min. **Peak:** 1–2 h. **Duration:** 6–12 h. **Distribution:** distributed to all tissues except CNS; crosses placenta. **Metabolism:** some liver metabolism. **Elimination:** excreted primarily in urine; excreted in breast milk.

CONTRAINDICATIONS & PRECAUTIONS Contraindicated in: pregnancy (category C); safe use in nursing mothers and children not established. **Cautious use in:** impaired renal function, patient with solitary kidney; collagen-vascular diseases (scleroderma, SLE); patients receiving IMMUNOSUPPRESSANTS or other drugs that cause leukopenia or agranulocytosis; coronary or cerebrovascular disease; severe salt/volume depletion.

ADVERSE/SIDE EFFECTS CNS: headache, dizziness, paresthesias, insomnia, fatigue. **CV:** slight increase in heart rate, first dose hypotension, dizziness, fainting. **GI:** nausea, vomiting, GI distress, abdominal pain, constipation, diarrhea, dry mouth, loss of appetite, reversible "scalded mouth sensation" (loss of taste perception, persistent salt or metallic taste); weight loss. **Hematologic:** hyponatremia (patient with CHF), hyperkalemia, neutropenia, <u>agranulocytosis</u>, pancytopenia. **Hypersensitivity:** serum sickness-like reaction, arthralgia, skin eruptions. **Hepatic:** azotemia, impaired renal function, nephrotic syndrome, membranous glomerulonephritis. **Skin:** *maculopapular rash*, alopecia, urticaria, pruritus, angioedema, photosensitivity. **Other:** positive antinuclear antibody (ANA) titers, *cough*.

DIAGNOSTIC TEST INTERFERENCES In some patients, elevated ***urine protein levels*** may persist even after captopril has been discontinued.

Possibility of transient elevations of ***BUN*** and ***serum creatinine***, slight increase in ***serum potassium***, and ***serum prolactin***, increases in ***liver enzymes***, and false-positive ***urine acetone*** (using sodium nitroprusside reagent). Captopril may decrease ***fasting blood sugar*** in the nondiabetic and cause hypoglycemia in the diabetic patient controlled with antidiabetic drug therapy.

DRUG INTERACTIONS NITRATES, DIURETICS, and ANTIHYPERTENSIVES enhance hypotensive effects. **Aspirin** and other NSAID's may antagonize hypotensive effects. POTASSIUM-SPARING DIURETICS (**spironolactone, amiloride**) increase potassium levels. **Probenecid** decreases elimination and increases effects. **Drug-food interactions:** Food decreases absorption; take 30–60 min before meals.

NURSING IMPLICATIONS
Administration
- A sudden exaggerated hypotensive response may occur within 1–3 h of first dose, especially in those with high BP or on a diuretic and restricted salt intake.
- Best administered 1 h before meals. Food reduces absorption by 30–40%. Tablet may have a slight sulfurous odor.
- Store in light-resistant containers at no more than 30C (86F) unless otherwise directed.

Assessment & Drug Effects
- A sudden exaggerated hypotensive response may occur within 1–3 h of first dose, especially in those with high BP or on a diuretic and restricted salt intake.
- Bed rest and BP monitoring are advised for the first 3 h after the initial dose.
- At least 2 wk of therapy may be required before full therapeutic effects are achieved.
- Baseline urinary protein levels should be established before initiation of therapy and checked at monthly intervals for the first 8 mo of treatment and then periodically thereafter.
- Proteinuria occurs in 1–2% of patients and may reach levels as high as 1 g/d. (Normal value: <150 mg/24 h.)
- WBC and differential counts are recommended before therapy is begun and at approximately 2-wk intervals for the first 3 mo of therapy and then periodically thereafter.

Patient & Family Education
- Report to physician without delay the onset of unexplained fever, unusual fatigue, sore mouth or throat, easy bruising or bleeding (pathognomonic of agranulocytosis).

Common side effects in *italic*; life-threatening effects <u>underlined</u>; generic names in **bold**; classifications in SMALL CAPS

139

- Mild skin eruptions are most likely to appear during the first 4 wk of therapy and may be accompanied by fever and eosinophilia.
- Patient should consult physician promptly if vomiting or diarrhea occur.
- Darkening or crumbling of nailbeds may occur but is reversible with dosage reduction.
- Taste impairment occurs in 5–10% of patients and generally reverses in 2–3 mo even with continued therapy.
- Use OTC medications only with approval of the physician. Inform surgeon or dentist that captopril is being taken. Alert diabetic patient that captopril may produce hypoglycemia. Monitor blood glucose closely during first few weeks of therapy.

ANTIARRHYTHMIC

PROCAINAMIDE HYDROCHLORIDE

(proe-kane-a´mide)

Trade names: Procamide SR, Procan, Promine, Pronestyl, Pronestyl SR, Rhythmin, Sub-Quin
Classifications: CARDIOVASCULAR AGENT; ANTIARRHYTHMIC
Pregnancy: Category C

ACTIONS/PHARMACODYNAMICS Amide analog of procaine hydrochloride with cardiac actions similar to those of quinine. Class Ia antiarrhythmic agent. Depresses excitability of myocardium to electrical stimulation, reduces conduction velocity in atria, ventricles, and His-Purkinje system. Increases duration of refractory period, especially in the atria. Produces slight change in contractility of cardiac muscle and cardiac output; suppresses automaticity of His-Purkinje ventricular muscle. May have anticholinergic properties. Produces peripheral vasodilaton and hypotension, especially with IV use. Larger doses induce AV block and ventricular extrasystoles that may proceed to ventricular fibrillation. Local anesthetic properties are equal to but more sustained than those of procaine, and CNS stimulation is less than that of procaine. Prolonged administration often leads to development of positive antinuclear antibodies (ANA) in about 50% of patients.

USES Prophylactically to maintain normal sinus rhythm following conversion of atrial flutter or fibrillation by other methods. Also to prevent recurrence of paroxysmal atrial fibrillation and tachycardia, paroxysmal AV junctional rhythm, ventricular tachycardia, ventricular and atrial premature contractions. Also cardiac arrhythmias associated with surgery and anesthesia. **Unlabeled use:** malignant hyperthermia.

ROUTE & DOSAGE

Arrhythmias

Adult	PO	1 g followed by 250–500 mg q3h *or* 500 mg–1 g q6h sustained release
	IM	0.5–1 g q4–6h until able to take PO
	IV	100 mg q5min at a rate of 25–50 mg/min until arrhythmia is controlled or 1 g given, then 2–6 mg/min
Child	PO	40–60 mg/kg/d divided q4–6h
	IV	3–6 mg/kg q10–30min (max 100 mg/dose), then 0.02–0.08 mg/kg/min

PHARMACOKINETICS Absorption: 75–95% absorbed from GI tract. **Peak**: 15–60 min IM; 30–60 min PO. **Duration**: 3 h; 8 h with sustained release. **Distribution**: distributed to CSF, liver, spleen, kidney, brain, and heart; crosses placenta; distributed into breast milk. **Metabolism**: metabolized in liver to *N*-acetylprocainamide (NAPA), an active metabolite (30–60% metabolized to NAPA). **Elimination**: half-life: 3 h procainamide, 6 h NAPA; excreted in urine.

CONTRAINDICATIONS & PRECAUTIONS Contraindicated in: myasthenia gravis; hypersensitivity to procainamide or procaine; blood dyscrasias; complete AV block, second and third degree AV block unassisted by pacemaker. **Cautious use in:** patient who has undergone electrical reversion to sinus rhythm; hypotension, cardiac enlargement, CHF, MI, coronary occlusion, ventricular dysrhythmia from digitalis intoxication, hepatic or renal insufficiency, electrolyte imbalance, bronchial asthma, history of SLE. Safe use in pregnancy (category C) or in nursing mothers not established.

ADVERSE/SIDE EFFECTS CNS: dizziness, mental depression, psychosis with hallucinations. **CV**: severe hypotension, pericarditis, ventricular fibrillation, AV block, tachycardia, flushing. **GI** (mostly PO): bitter taste, nausea, vomiting, diarrhea, anorexia. **Hematologic**: agranulocytosis with repeated use; thrombocytopenia. **Hypersensitivity**: fever, muscle and joint pain, angioneurotic edema, maculopapular rash, pruritus, eosinophilia, rarely: generalized or digital vasculitis, proximal myopathy, and Sjögren's syndrome. **Other**: *SLE-like syndrome (50% of patients on large doses for*

Common side effects in *italic*; life-threatening effects underlined; generic names in **bold**; classifications in SMALL CAPS

1 y): polyarthralgias, pleuritic pain, pleural effusion, erythema, skin rash, myalgia, fever.

DIAGNOSTIC TEST INTERFERENCES Procainamide increases the plasma levels of *alkaline phosphatase, bilirubin, lactic dehydrogenase and AST.* It may also alter results of the *edrophonium test.*

DRUG INTERACTIONS Other ANTIARRHYTHMICS add to therapeutic and toxic effects; ANTICHOLINERGIC AGENTS compound anticholinergic effects; ANTIHYPERTENSIVES add to hypotensive effects; **cimetidine** may increase procainamide and NAPA levels with increase in toxicity.

INCOMPATIBILITIES Solution/Additive: **bretylium, ethacrynate.**

NURSING IMPLICATIONS

Administration

- Procainamide administration by IV infusion pump requires constant monitoring to maintain desired flow rate. Keep patient in supine position. Be alert to signs of too rapid administration of drug—*speed shock:* irregular pulse, tight feeling in chest, flushed face, headache, loss of consciousness, shock, cardiac arrest.
- When procainamide is given direct IV, dilute each 100 mg with 10 ml of D5W or sterile water for injection.
- When procainamide is given by IV infusion, add 1 g of procainamide to 250–500 ml of D5W solution. Yields 4 mg/ml in 250 ml or 2 mg/ml in 500 ml.
- IV dosage over a period of several hours is controlled by assessment of procainamide plasma levels. *Effective nontoxic therapeutic level:* 3–10 µg/ml (8–16 µg/ml is potentially toxic, and toxicity is common at plasma levels > 16 µg/ml).
- Oral preparation is best taken on empty stomach 1 h before or 2 h after meals with a full glass of water to enhance absorption. If drug causes gastric distress, administer with food.
- Immediate-release (but not sustained-release) tablet may be crushed if patient is unable to swallow it whole.
- Sustained-release tablet must be swallowed whole. It has a wax matrix that is not absorbed but appears in the stool.
- Apical radial pulses should be checked before each dose of procainamide during period of adjustment to the oral route.
- First PO dose should be given at least 4 h after last IV dose.
- Procainamide solution is stable for 24 h at room temperature and for 7 d under refrigeration at 2–8C (36–46F). Avoid freezing the solution. Refrigeration will retard color changes in solution. Slight yellowing does not alter drug potency, but discard solution if it is markedly discolored or precipitated.
- Store tablets in dark, airtight containers. Procainamide is hygroscopic; therefore do not store in bathroom medicine cabinet or in refrigerator where moisture levels are high.

Assessment & Drug Effects

- Patients at particular risk for adverse effects are those with severe heart, hepatic, or renal disease and hypotension.
- Monitor the patient's ECG and BP continuously during IV drug administration.
- IV drug is temporarily discontinued when (1) arrhythmia is interrupted, (2) severe toxic effects are present, (3) QRS complex is excessively widened (greater than 50%), (4) PR interval is prolonged, or (5) BP drops 15 mm Hg or more. Obtain rhythm strip and notify physician.
- A complication of procainamide infusion given to treat atrial dysrhythmia is the onset of ventricular tachycardia (a lethal arrhythmia) evidenced by increased rate to as high as 200 bpm.
- Ventricular dysrhythmias are usually abolished within a few minutes after IV dose and within an hour after PO or IM administration.
- Digitalization may have preceded procainamide in patients with atrial arrhythmias. Cardiotonic glycosides may induce sufficient increase in atrial contraction to dislodge atrial mural emboli, with subsequent pulmonary embolism. Report promptly complaints of chest pain, dyspnea, and anxiety.
- Therapeutic procainamide blood levels are reached in approximately 24 h if kidney function is normal but are delayed in presence of renal impairment.

Patient & Family Education

- Advise patient to monitor and report immediately *evidence of kidney dysfunction:* changes in I&O ratio and body weight, local edema (tight shoes or rings). Encourage keeping a record of weekly weight for comparison purposes. If weight gain of 1 kg (2 lb) or more is accompanied by local edema, patient should notify the physician.
- Instruct patient on maintenance doses to record and report date, time, and duration of *fibrillation episodes:* lightheadedness, giddiness, weakness, or syncope.
- Instruct patient to keep a record of pulse rates. Report changes in rate or quality.
- Instruct patient to report to the physician *signs of reduced procainamide control:* weakness, irregular pulse, unexplained fatiguability, anxiety.

Common side effects in *italic*; life-threatening effects underlined; generic names in **bold**; classifications in SMALL CAPS

- Before discharge, work with patient to design a 24 h dosing schedule for all prescribed drugs that will best fit into ADL at home.
- At no time should a dose be doubled or an interval changed because a previous dose was missed. Procainamide should be taken at evenly spaced intervals around the clock unless otherwise prescribed.

ANTILIPEMIC: BILE ACID SEQUESTRANT

CHOLESTYRAMINE RESIN
(koe-less-tear´a-meen)
Trade names: Cholybar, Questran, Questran Light
Classifications: CARDIOVASCULAR AGENT; ANTILIPEMIC; BILE ACID SEQUESTRANT; ANTIPRURITIC
Pregnancy: Category C

ACTIONS/PHARMACODYNAMICS Quaternary ammonium anion-exchange resin used for its cholesterol-lowering effect. Adsorbs and combines with intestinal bile acids in exchange for chloride ions to form an insoluble, nonabsorbable complex that is excreted in the feces. As a result, bile salts are continually (but not entirely) prevented from reentry to the enterohepatic circulation. Increased fecal loss of bile acids leads to lowered serum total cholesterol by decrease in low density lipoprotein (LDL) cholesterol and in reduction of bile acid deposit in dermal tissues, presumably the reason why cholestyramine relieves itching. LDL is the main component of serum cholesterol and reportedly is involved in development of atherosclerosis. Serum triglyceride levels may increase or remain unchanged. Sequestration of bile acids may interfere with absorption of calcium, dietary fat, and fat-soluble vitamins A, D, and K. As an anion-exchange resin, cholestyramine may have a strong affinity for selected drugs given concomitantly.

USES As adjunct to diet therapy in management of patients with primary hypercholesterolemia (type IIa hyperlipedemia) with a significant risk of atherosclerotic heart disease and MI; for relief of pruritus secondary to partial biliary stasis. **Unlabeled use:** to control diarrhea caused by excess bile acids in colon; for hyperoxaluria.

ROUTE & DOSAGE

Hypercholesterolemia

Adult	PO	4 g b.i.d. to q.i.d. a.c. and h.s.; may need up to 24 g/d
Child	PO	8–16 g/d in 2–3 divided doses a.c. and h.s.

Hyperlipoproteinemia

Adult	PO	4–8 g b.i.d. to q.i.d. a.c. and h.s. (≤ 32 g/d)

Pruritus

Adult	PO	4 g b.i.d. to q.i.d. a.c. and h.s. (≤ 16 g/d)

PHARMACOKINETICS Absorption: not absorbed from GI tract. **Elimination:** excreted in feces as insoluble complex.

CONTRAINDICATIONS & PRECAUTIONS Contraindicated in: complete biliary obstruction, hypersensitivity to bile acid sequestrants. Safe use by pregnant women, nursing mothers, and children ≤ 6 y not established. **Cautious use in:** bleeding disorders; hemorrhoids; impaired GI function, peptic ulcer, malabsorption states (e.g., steatorrhea); phenylketonuria (Questran Light only).

ADVERSE/SIDE EFFECTS CNS: headache, anxiety, dizziness, fatigue, tinnitus, syncope, drowsiness, femoral nerve pain, paresthesia. **CV:** claudication, arteritis, thrombophlebitis, myocardial infarction, angina. **Eye:** arcus juvenilis, uveitis. **GI:** *constipation,* fecal impaction, hemorrhoids, abdominal pain and distension, flatulence, bloating sensation, belching, nausea, vomiting, heartburn, anorexia, diarrhea, steatorrhea. **Hypersensitivity:** urticaria, dermatitis, asthma, shortness of breath. **Musculoskeletal:** backache, muscle and joint pains, arthritis, osteoporosis. **Renal:** hematuria, dysuria, burnt odor to urine, diuresis. **Other:** weight loss or gain, increased libido, swollen glands, edema, gingival bleeding, iron, calcium, vitamin A, D, and K deficiencies (from poor absorption); hypoprothrombinemia, hyperchloremic acidosis, decreased erythrocyte folate levels, rash, irritations of skin, tongue, and perianal areas.

DIAGNOSTIC TEST INTERFERENCES Cholestyramine therapy may be accompanied by increased serum *AST, phosphorus, chloride,* and *alkaline phosphatase* levels; decreased *serum calcium, sodium,* and *potassium* levels.

DRUG INTERACTIONS Decreases the absorption of ORAL ANTICOAGULANTS, **digoxin,** TETRACYCLINES, **penicillins, phenobarbital,** THYROID HORMONES, THIAZIDE DIURETICS, IRON SALTS, FAT-SOLUBLE VITAMINS **(A, D, E, K)** from the GI tract—administer cholestyramine 1 h before or 2 h after these drugs.

NURSING IMPLICATIONS

Administration

- Place contents of one packet or one level scoopful on surface of at least 120 to 180 ml (4–6 oz) of water or other preferred liquid. Permit drug to hydrate by standing without stirring 1–2 min, twirling glass occasionally; then stir until suspension is uniform. Rinse glass with small amount of liquid and have patient drink remainder to ensure entire dose is taken. Administer before meals.
- Water, highly flavored liquids, or other noncarbonated drinks, thin soups, diluted pulpy fruit juices, or fruits with high moisture content such as applesauce or crushed pineapple disguise taste somewhat and may encourage compliance.
- Always dissolve cholestyramine before administration; it is irritating to mucous membranes and may cause esophageal impaction if administered dry.
- Color may vary with different batches, but this does not affect drug action. Has a slight aminelike odor and a disagreeable taste; in solution its consistency is sandy or gritty.
- Store in tightly closed container at 15–30C (59–86F) unless otherwise specified.

Assessment & Drug Effects

- Long-term use of cholestyramine resin can increase bleeding tendency. Be alert to early symptoms of hypoprothrombinemia (petechiae, ecchymoses, abnormal bleeding from mucous membranes, tarry stools) and report their occurrence promptly.
- Preexisting constipation may be worsened in the elderly, women, and in those taking >24 g/d.
- Supplemental vitamins A and D and folic acid may be required by patient on long-term therapy.
- Serum cholesterol levels are reduced within 24–48 h after treatment starts and may continue to decline for a year. After withdrawal of cholestyramine, cholesterol levels usually return to baseline level in about 2 to 4 wk.
- If response is unsatisfactory after 3 mo of treatment, drug is usually withdrawn.
- Periodic erythrocyte folate levels are recommended, particularly in children.

Patient & Family Education

- Report constipation immediately to physician.
- High bulk diet with adequate fluid intake is an essential adjunct to cholestyramine treatment and generally resolves the problems of constipation and bloating sensation.
- Warn patient not to omit doses. Sudden withdrawal can promote uninhibited absorption of other drugs taken concomitantly, leading to toxicity or overdosage.
- Usually GI side effects subside after the first month of drug therapy.
- The following symptoms may be drug-induced and should be reported promptly: severe gastric distress with nausea and vomiting, unusual weight loss, black stools, severe hemorrhoids (GI bleeding), sudden back pain.

ANTILIPEMIC: LIPID-LOWERING AGENT

LOVASTATIN

(loe-vah-stat´in)
Trade names: Mevacor, Mevinolin
Classifications: CARDIOVASCULAR AGENT; ANTILIPEMIC; LIPID-LOWERING AGENT
Pregnancy: Category X

ACTIONS/PHARMACODYNAMICS Fungal metabolite derived from *Aspergillus terreus;* reduces plasma cholesterol levels by interfering with body's ability to produce its own cholesterol. Mevolanic acid, a metabolite of lovastatin, inhibits synthesis of the hepatic reductase 3-hydroxy-3-methylglutaryl coenzyme A (HMG-CoA), which is essential to hepatic production of cholesterol. This cholesterol-lowering effect triggers induction of low-density lipoprotein (LDL) receptors, which promote removal of LDL and very low density lipoprotein (VLDL) remnants (precursors of LDL) from plasma. Lovastatin therapy also results in an increase in plasma high-density lipoprotein (HDL) concentrations. (HDLs collect excess cholesterol from body cells and transport it to liver for excretion.) Although cholesterol is the precursor of steroid hormones, lovastatin appears to have little effect on steroidogenesis. Lovastatin action is enhanced by its concomitant administration with a bile acid sequestrant (e.g., cholestyramine).

Common side effects in *italic*; life-threatening effects <u>underlined</u>; generic names in **bold**; classifications in SMALL CAPS

143

USES Adjunct to diet for treatment of primary moderate hypercholesterolemia (types IIa and IIb) when diet and other nonpharmacologic measures have failed to reduce elevated total LDL cholesterol levels. Lovastatin is less effective in treatment of homozygous familial hypercholesterolemia than primary hypercholesterolemia, possibly because in these persons LDL receptors are not functional.

ROUTE & DOSAGE

Hypercholesterolemia

Adult   PO   20–40 mg 1–2 times/d

PHARMACOKINETICS Absorption: approximately 30% absorbed from GI tract; extensive first pass metabolism. **Onset:** 2 wk. **Peak:** 4–6 wk. **Distribution:** crosses blood-brain barrier and placenta; distributed into breast milk. **Metabolism:** metabolized in liver to active metabolites. **Elimination:** 83% excreted in feces; 10% excreted in urine.

CONTRAINDICATIONS & PRECAUTIONS

Contraindicated in: active liver disease, unexplained elevations of serum transaminases. Safe use in pregnancy (category X) or by nursing mothers and children not established. **Cautious use in:** patient who consumes substantial quantities of alcohol; history of liver disease; patient with risk factor predisposing to development of renal failure secondary to rhabdomyolysis.

ADVERSE/SIDE EFFECTS Drug is generally well tolerated. **CNS:** dizziness, mild transient headache, insomnia, fatigue. **Eye:** lenticular opacities (without change in visual acuity), blurred vision. **GI:** dyspepsia, dysgeusia, heartburn, nausea, constipation, diarrhea, flatus, abdominal pain and cramps. **Hematologic:** increases in serum transaminases, elevated creatine phosphokinase (CPK). **Skin:** rash, pruritus.

DRUG INTERACTIONS cyclosporine, erythromycin, gemfibrozil increase risk of myopathy and rhabdomyolysis.

NURSING IMPLICATIONS

Administration

- Administer lovastatin with meals.
- Store tablets at 5–30C (41–86F) in light-resistant, tightly closed container.

Assessment & Drug Effects

- Blood cholesterol levels are monitored periodcally.
- Liver function tests are performed q4–6wk during first 15 mo of therapy.
- Drug-induced increases in serum transaminases, usually not associated with jaundice or other clinical signs or symptoms, return to normal when drug is discontinued. If these values rise and remain at 3 times upper level of normal, drug will be discontinued and liver biopsy considered.

Patient & Family Education

- Caution patient not to interrupt, increase, decrease, or omit dosage without advice of physician.
- Patient should promptly report muscle tenderness or pain, especially if accompanied by fever or malaise. If CPK is elevated or if myositis is diagnosed, drug will be discontinued.
- Alcohol should be avoided or at least reduced.
- Be certain that patients understand that lovastatin is not a substitute for, but an addition to, diet therapy.

CALCIUM CHANNEL BLOCKER

VERAPAMIL HYDROCHLORIDE

(ver-ap´a-mill)
Trade names: Calan, Calan SR, Isoptin, Isoptin Oral, Isoptin Parenteral, Isoptin SR, Veralens
Classifications: CARDIOVASCULAR AGENT; CALCIUM CHANNEL BLOCKER; ANTIARRHYTHMIC; VASODILATOR
Pregnancy: Category C

ACTIONS/PHARMACODYNAMICS Inhibits calcium ion influx through slow channels into cell of myocardial and arterial smooth muscle (both coronary and peripheral blood vessels). As a result, intracellular calcium remains at subthreshold levels insufficient to stimulate cell excitation and contraction. Verapamil dilates coronary arteries and arterioles and inhibits coronary artery spasm; thus myocardial oxygen delivery is increased (antianginal effect). Decreases and slows SA and AV node conduction (antiarrhythmic effect) without effect on normal arterial action potential or intraventricular conduction. By vasodilation of peripheral arterioles, drug decreases total peripheral vascular resistance and reduces arterial BP at rest. May slightly decrease heart rate. Does not alter total serum calcium levels.

Common side effects in *italic*; life-threatening effects underlined; generic names in **bold**; classifications in SMALL CAPS

USES Supraventricular tachyarrhythmias; Prinzmetal's (variant) angina, chronic stable angina; unstable, crescendo or preinfarctive angina and essential hypertension. **Unlabeled use:** paroxysmal supraventricular tachycardia; prophylaxis of migraine headache; and as alternate therapy in manic depression.

ROUTE & DOSAGE

Angina

Adult	PO	80 mg q6–8h; may increase up to 320–480 mg/d in divided doses

Hypertension

Adult	PO	40–80 mg t.i.d. *or* 90–240 mg sustained release 1–2 times/d up to 480 mg/d

Supraventricular Tachycardia

Adult	PO	240–480 mg/d in divided doses
	IV	5–10 mg IV push; may repeat in 15–30 min if needed
Child	IV	<1 y: 0.1–0.2 mg/kg
	IV	1–15 y: 2–5 mg/kg

PHARMACOKINETICS Absorption: 90% absorbed, but only 25–30% reaches systemic circulation (first pass metabolism). **Peak:** 1–2 h PO; 4–8 h extended release; 5 min IV. **Distribution:** widely distributed, including CNS; crosses placenta; present in breast milk. **Metabolism:** metabolized in liver. **Elimination:** half-life: 2–8 h; 70% excreted in urine; 16% in feces.

CONTRAINDICATIONS & PRECAUTIONS Contraindicated in: severe hypotension (diastolic <90 mm Hg), cardiogenic shock, cardiomegaly, digitalis toxicity, second- or third-degree AV block; Wolff-Parkinson-White syndrome including atrial flutter and fibrillation; accessory AV pathway, left ventricular dysfunction, severe CHF, sinus node disease, sick sinus syndrome (except in patient with functioning ventricular pacemaker). Safe use during pregnancy (category C), in nursing mothers, or in children (oral) not established. **Cautious use in:** Duchenne's muscular dystrophy; hepatic and renal impairment; MI followed by coronary occlusion, aortic stenosis.

ADVERSE/SIDE EFFECTS CNS: dizziness, vertigo, *headache,* fatigue, sleep disturbances, depression, syncope. **CV:** *hypotension,* congestive heart failure, bradycardia, severe tachycardia, peripheral edema, <u>AV block</u>. **Eye, ear:** blurred vision, equilibrium disturbances. **GI:** nausea, abdominal discomfort, *constipation.* **Hematologic:** inhibition of platelet function,

elevated liver enzymes. **Other:** pruritus, flushing, pulmonary edema, muscle fatigue, diaphoresis, scalp hair loss.

DIAGNOSTIC TEST INTERFERENCES Verapamil may cause elevations of serum *AST, ALT, alkaline phosphatase.*

DRUG INTERACTIONS BETA-BLOCKERS increase risk of CHF, bradycardia, or heart block; significantly increased levels of **digoxin** and **carbamazepine** and toxicity; potentiates hypotensive effects of HYPOTENSIVE AGENTS; levels of **lithium** and **cyclosporine** may be increased, increasing their toxicity; **calcium salts** (IV) may antagonize verapamil effects.

INCOMPATIBILITIES Solution/Additive: albumin, aminophylline, amphotericin B, hydralazine, cotrimazole. Y-Site: ampicillin, mezlocillin, nafcillin, oxacillin, sodium bicarbonate.

NURSING IMPLICATIONS

Administration

- Administer oral dose with food to reduce gastric irritation.
- Abrupt withdrawal of verapamil may increase and extend duration of pain in the angina patient.
- *IV injection:* IV verapamil may be given by direct IV diluted in 5 ml of sterile water for injection at a rate of 10 mg/min.
- Inspect parenteral drug preparation before administration. Solution should be clear and colorless.
- Store at 15–30C (59–86F) and protect from light.

Assessment & Drug Effects

- Establish baseline data before treatment is started: BP, pulse, and laboratory evaluations of hepatic and renal function.
- Transient asymptomatic hypotension may accompany IV bolus. Instruct patient to remain in recumbent position for at least 1 h after dose is given to diminish subjective effects of hypotension.
- If IV verapamil is given concurrently with digitalis, monitor for AV block or excessive bradycardia.
- Monitor I&O ratio during IV and early oral maintenance therapy. Renal function impairment prolongs duration of action, increasing potential for toxicity and incidence of side effects. Advise patient to report gradual weight gain and evidence of edema (tight rings on fingers, ankle swelling).
- The incidence of adverse reactions is highest with IV administration, in the elderly, in patients with impaired renal function and patients of small

Common side effects in *italic*; life-threatening effects <u>underlined</u>; generic names in **bold**; classifications in SMALL CAPS

145

stature. Drug action may be prolonged in these patients. Continuous ECG monitoring during IV administration is essential.

- During early treatment for hypertension, check BP shortly before administration of next dose to evaluate degree of control.
- Verapamil should decrease angina frequency, nitroglycerin consumption, and episodes of ST segment deviation.

Patient & Family Education

- Patient receiving verapamil at home should be informed about usual pulse rate and should be instructed to take radial pulse before each dose. An irregular pulse or one slower than base level should be reported.
- Caution patient to take drug exactly as prescribed.
- Warn patient to adhere to established guidelines for exercise program.
- Caution against driving or operating dangerous equipment until patient's response to verapamil is established. Dizziness (experienced as lightheadedness) during early treatment period is common.
- Advise patient to decrease caffeine-containing beverage intake (i.e., coffee, tea, chocolate).
- Until tolerance to reduced BP is established, advise patient to change positions slowly from recumbent to standing to prevent falls because of vertigo.
- Instruct patient to report easy bruising, petechiae, unexplained bleeding.
- Advise patient not to use OTC drugs, especially aspirin, unless they are specifically prescribed.

CARDIAC GLYCOSIDE

DIGOXIN
(di-jox´in)
Trade names: Lanoxicaps, Lanoxin
Classifications: CARDIOVASCULAR AGENT; CARDIAC GLYCOSIDE; ANTIARRHYTHMIC
Pregnancy: Category A

ACTIONS/PHARMACODYNAMICS Widely used glycoside of *Digitalis lanata*. Acts by increasing the force and velocity of myocardial systolic contraction (positive inotropic effect). It also decreases conduction velocity through the atrioventricular node. Action is more prompt and less prolonged than that of digitalis and digitoxin. Also, it is less likely to give

rise to cumulative effects because it is more readily absorbed and exchanged in the body and is rather rapidly excreted in urine.

USES Rapid digitalization and for maintenance therapy in CHF, atrial fibrillation, atrial flutter, paroxysmal atrial tachycardia.

ROUTE & DOSAGE

Digitalizing Dose

Adult	PO	10–15 µg/kg (1 mg) in divided doses over 24–48 h
	IV	10–15 µg/kg (1 mg) in divided doses over 24 h
Child	PO/IV	>10 y: 10–15 µg/kg (1.5–2 mg)
		2–10 y: 20–40 µg/kg
		<2 y: 40–60 µg/kg
		Neonate (term): 30–50 µg/kg
		Premature: 20 µg/kg

Maintenance Dose

Adult	PO/IV	0.1–0.375 mg/d
Child	PO/IV	>10 y: 0.125–0.25 mg/d
		2–10 y: 6–7.5 µg/kg/d
		<2 y: 7.5–9 µg/kg/d
		Neonate (term): 6–7.5 µg/kg/d
		Premature: 3.75 µg/kg/d

PHARMACOKINETICS Absorption: 70% PO tablets; 90% PO liquid and capsules. **Onset:** 1–2 h PO; 5–30 min IV. **Peak:** 6–8 h PO; 1–5 h IV. **Duration:** 3–4 d in fully digitalized patient. **Distribution:** widely distributed; tissue levels significantly higher than plasma levels; crosses placenta. **Metabolism:** approximately 14% in liver. **Elimination:** half-life: 34–44 h; 80–90% excreted by kidneys; may appear in breast milk.

CONTRAINDICATIONS & PRECAUTIONS Contraindicated in: digitalis hypersensitivity, ventricular fibrillation, ventricular tachycardia unless due to CHF. Full digitalizing dose not given if patient has received digoxin during previous week or if slowly excreted cardiotonic glycoside has been given during previous 2 wk. **Cautious use in:** renal insufficiency, hypokalemia, advanced heart disease, acute MI, incomplete AV block, cor pulmonale; hypothyroidism; lung disease; pregnancy (category A), nursing women, premature and immature infants, children, elderly or debilitated patients.

ADVERSE/SIDE EFFECTS CNS: fatigue, muscle weakness, headache, facial neuralgia, mental depression, paresthesias, hallucinations, confusion, drowsiness, agitation, dizziness. **CV:** arrhythmias, hypotension, AV block. **Eye:** visual disturbances. **GI:** anorexia, nausea, vomiting, diarrhea. **Other:** diaphoresis, recurrent malaise, dysphagia.

DRUG INTERACTIONS ANTACIDS, **cholestyramine, colistipol** decrease digoxin absorption; DIURETICS, CORTICOSTEROIDS, **amphotericin B,** LAXATIVES, **sodium polystyrene sulfonate** may cause hypokalemia, increasing the risk of digoxin toxicity; **calcium IV** may increase risk of arrhythmias if administered together with digoxin; **quinidine, verapamil, amiodarone, flecainide** significantly increase digoxin levels, and digoxin dose should be decreased by 50%; **erythromycin** may increase digoxin levels; **succinylcholine** may potentiate arrhythmogenic effects.

INCOMPATIBILITIES Solution/Additive: **dobutamine, doxapram.**

NURSING IMPLICATIONS

Administration
- Digoxin may be given without regard to food. Administration after food may slightly delay rate of absorption but total amount absorbed is not affected.
- Tablet may be crushed and mixed with fluid or food if patient cannot swallow it whole.
- When patient is controlled on maintenance doses, generally radial pulse is taken for 1 full min before drug administration.
- *IV injection:* Direct IV injection of digoxin may be administered undiluted or diluted in 4 ml of sterile water, D5W, or NaCl 0.9% (if prescribed). Administer each direct IV dose over at least 5 min.
- Infiltration of parenteral drug into subcutaneous tissue can cause local irritation and sloughing.

Assessment & Drug Effects
- Be familiar with patient's baseline data (e.g., quality of peripheral pulses, blood pressure, clinical symptoms, serum electrolytes, creatinine clearance) as a foundation for making assessments.
- Before administering digoxin, check laboratory reports for serum levels of digoxin, potassium, mag-

nesium, and calcium. Notify physician of abnormal values.
- Before administering digoxin, take apical pulse for 1 full min noting rate, rhythm, and quality. If changes are noted, withhold digoxin, take rhythm strip if patient is on ECG monitor, notify physician promptly.
- Monitor for signs and symptoms of digoxin toxicity.
- Although a fall in ventricular rate to 60/min in adults (70/min in children) is one criterion for withholding medication, any change in pulse rate or rhythm should be interpreted as a sign of digitalis intoxication and should be reported promptly.
- In children, cardiac arrhythmias are usually reliable signs of early toxicity. Early indicators in adults (anorexia, nausea, vomiting, diarrhea, visual disturbances) are rarely initial signs in children.
- *Therapeutic range of serum digoxin:* 0.8–2 ng/ml; *toxic levels:* >2 ng/ml. Blood samples for determining plasma digoxin levels should be drawn at least 5–6 h after daily dose and preferably just before next scheduled daily dose.
- Monitor I&O ratio during digitalization, particularly in patients with impaired renal function, and for edema daily and auscultate chest for rales.
- Concurrent antibiotic-digoxin therapy could precipitate toxicity because of altered intestinal flora. Monitor serum digoxin levels closely.
- Patient should be closely observed when being transferred from one preparation (tablet, elixir, or parenteral) to another; e.g., when tablet is replaced by elixir potential for toxicity increases since ≥ 30% of drug is absorbed.

Patient & Family Education
- When digoxin is prescribed for atrial fibrillation, advise patient to report to physician if pulse falls below 60 or rises above 110 or if patient detects skipped beats or other changes in rhythm.
- Instruct patient to suspect toxicity and report to physician if any of the following occur: anorexia, nausea, vomiting, diarrhea, or visual disturbances
- Instruct patient to weigh each day under standard conditions. Report weight gain > 1 kg (2 lb)/d.
- Instruct patient to take digoxin precisely as prescribed, not to skip or double a dose or change dose intervals, and to take it at same time each day.
- Caution patient not to take OTC medications, especially those for coughs, colds, allergy, GI upset, or obesity without prior approval of physician.
- Patient should continue with brand originally prescribed unless otherwise directed by physician.

Common side effects in *italic*; life-threatening effects <u>underlined</u>; generic names in **bold**; classifications in SMALL CAPS

147

CENTRAL-ACTING ANTIHYPERTENSIVE

METHYLDOPA
(meth-ill-doe´pa)

Trade names: Aldomet, Apo-Methyldopa, Dopamet, Medimet, Novomedopa

METHYLDOPATE HYDROCHLORIDE
(meth-ill-doe´pate)

Trade name: Aldomet Ester HCl Injection
Classifications: CARDIOVASCULAR AGENT; CENTRAL-ACTING ANTIHYPERTENSIVE; AUTONOMIC NERVOUS SYSTEM AGENT; ALPHA-ADRENERGIC AGONIST (SYMPATHOMIMETIC)
Pregnancy: Category C

ACTIONS/PHARMACODYNAMICS Structurally related to catecholamines and their precursors. Exact mechanism of action unknown; metabolic product of the drug appears to act on both CNS and peripheral vasculature by displacing norepinephrine from its storage sites. Has weak neurotransmitter properties; inhibits decarboxylation of dopa, thereby reducing concentration of dopamine, a precursor of norepinephrine; also inhibits the precursor of serotonin. Lowers standing and supine BP, and unlike adrenergic blockers, it is not so prone to produce orthostatic hypotension, diurnal blood pressure variations, or exercise hypertension. Reduces renal vascular resistance; maintains cardiac output without acceleration, but may slow heart rate; tends to support sodium and water retention. Although it has sedative effect, it also increases REM sleep.

USES Step 2 agent in stepped care approach in treatment of sustained moderate to severe hypertension, particularly in patients with renal dysfunction. Also used in selected patients with carcinoid disease. Parenteral form has been used for treatment of hypertensive crises but is not preferred because of its slow onset of action.

PHARMACOKINETICS Absorption: about 50% absorbed from GI tract. **Peak:** 4–6 h. **Duration:** 24 h PO; 10–16 h IV. **Distribution:** crosses placenta, distributed into breast milk. **Metabolism:** metabolized in liver and GI tract. **Elimination:** half-life: 1.7 h; excreted primarily in urine.

ROUTE & DOSAGE

Hypertension

Adult	PO	250 mg b.i.d. or t.i.d.; may be increased up to 3 g/d in divided doses
	IV	250–500 mg q6h given over 30–60 min, up to 1 g q6h
Child	PO	10–65 mg/kg/d in 2–4 divided doses (max 3 g/d)
	IV	20–65 mg/kg/d in 4 divided doses

CONTRAINDICATIONS & PRECAUTIONS
Contraindicated in: active hepatic disease (hepatitis, cirrhosis), pheochromocytoma, blood dyscrasias. Safe use during pregnancy (category C) not established. **Cautious use in:** history of impaired liver or renal function or disease; angina pectoris, history of mental depression, young or elderly patients.

ADVERSE/SIDE EFFECTS Allergic: *fever,* skin eruptions, ulcerations of soles of feet, flulike symptoms, lymphadenopathy, eosinophilia. **CNS:** *sedation, drowsiness,* sluggishness, headache, weakness, fatigue, dizziness, vertigo, paresthesias, Bell's palsy, *decrease in mental acuity,* inability to concentrate, amnesia-like syndrome, involuntary choreoathetotic movements, parkinsonism, mild psychoses, depression, nightmares. **CV:** orthostatic hypotension, syncope (carotid sinus hypersensitivity), aggravation of angina pectoris, bradycardia, myocarditis, edema, weight gain *(sodium and water retention),* paradoxic hypertensive reaction (especially with IV administration). **GI:** diarrhea, constipation, abdominal distension, malabsorption syndrome, nausea, vomiting, dry mouth, sore or black tongue, sialadenitis. **Hematologic:** *positive direct Coombs' test* (common especially in blacks), hemolytic anemia (rare), granulocytopenia, agranulocytosis. **Hepatotoxicity** (believed to be allergic reaction): abnormal liver function tests, hepatic necrosis (rare), jaundice, hepatitis. **Other:** *nasal stuffiness,* gynecomastia, lactation, *decreased libido, impotence,* hypothermia (large doses), positive tests for lupus and rheumatoid factors, granulomatous skin lesions, pancreatitis.

DRUG INTERACTIONS AMPHETAMINES, TRICYCLIC ANTIDEPRESSANTS, PHENOTHIAZINES may attenuate antihypertensive response; methyldopa may inhibit effectiveness of **ephedrine; haloperidol** may exacerbate psychiatric symptoms; with **levodopa,** additive hypotension, increased CNS toxicity, especially psychosis; increases risk of **lithium** toxicity; **methotrimeprazine** causes excessive hypotension; MAO

INHIBITORS may cause hallucinations; **phenoxybenzamine** may cause urinary incontinence.

INCOMPATIBILITIES Solution/additive: amphotericin B, methohexital, verapamil. Y-site: fat emulsion.

DIAGNOSTIC TEST INTERFERENCES Methyldopa may interfere with **serum creatinine** measurements using alkaline picrate method, **AST** by colorimetric methods, and **uric acid** measurements by phosphotungstate method (with high methyldopa blood levels); it may produce false elevations of **urinary catecholamines** and increase in **serum amylase** in methyldopa-induced sialadenitis.

NURSING IMPLICATIONS

Administration
- IV methyldopa may be given diluted in 100–200 ml of D5W. Administer over 30–60 min.
- To minimize daytime sedation, physician may prescribe dosage increases to be made in the evening. Some patients maintain adequate BP control with a single evening dose.

Assessment & Drug Effects
- During IV infusion of methyldopate, check BP and pulse at least q30min until stabilized, and observe for adequacy of urinary output.
- During period of dosage adjustment, physician may request BP to be taken at regular intervals in lying, sitting, and standing positions.
- Transient sedation, drowsiness, mental depression, weakness, and headache commonly occur during first 24–72 h of therapy or whenever dosage is increased. Symptoms tend to disappear with continuation of therapy or dosage reduction.
- Elderly patients and patients with impaired renal function are particularly likely to manifest orthostatic hypotension with dizziness and light-headedness during period of dosage adjustment. Supervision of ambulation is advisable.
- Monitor I&O. Report oliguria and changes in I&O ratio. Weigh patient daily under standard conditions, and check for edema because methyldopa favors sodium and water retention.
- Baseline and regularly scheduled blood counts and liver function tests are advised during first 6–12 wk of therapy or if patient develops unexplained fever.
- Be alert to and report symptoms of mental depression (e.g., anorexia, insomnia, inattention to personal hygiene, withdrawal). Drug-induced depression may persist after drug is withdrawn.

- Rising BP indicating tolerance to drug effect may occur during week 2 or 3 of therapy.

Patient & Family Education
- Caution patient that hot baths and showers, prolonged standing in one position, and strenuous exercise may enhance orthostatic hypotension. Instruct patient to make position changes slowly, particularly from recumbent to upright posture and to dangle legs a few minutes before standing.
- Caution patient that methyldopa may affect ability to perform activities requiring concentrated mental effort, especially during first few days of therapy or whenever dosage is increased; patient should avoid potentially hazardous tasks such as driving a car until reaction to drug is known.
- Advise patient not to take OTC medications unless approved by physician.

NITRATE VASODILATOR

NITROGLYCERIN
(nye-troe-gli′ser-in)
Trade names: Deponit, Minitran, Nitro-Bid, Nitro-Bid IV, Nitrocap, Nitrodisc, Nitro-Dur, Nitrogard, Nitrogard-SR, Nitroglyn, Nitrol, Nitrolingual, Nitrong, Nitrong SR, Nitrospan, Nitrostat, Nitrostat I.V., Nitro-T.D., Transderm-Nitro, Tridil
Classifications: CARDIOVASCULAR AGENT; NITRATE VASODILATOR
Pregnancy: Category C

ACTIONS/PHARMACODYNAMICS Organic nitrate and potent venodilator with antianginal, antiischemic, and antihypertensive effects. Relaxes vascular smooth muscle by unknown mechanism, resulting in dose-related dilation of both venous (predominant) and arterial blood vessels. Postcapillary vessel and large vein dilation promotes peripheral pooling of blood, reduction of peripheral resistance, and decreased venous return to the heart. Both left ventricular preload and afterload are reduced and myocardial oxygen consumption or demand is decreased. Therapeutic doses may reduce systolic, diastolic, and mean BP; heart rate is usually slightly increased. Collateral circulation in patients with MI is improved,

Common side effects in *italic*; life-threatening effects <u>underlined</u>;
generic names in **bold**; classifications in SMALL CAPS

149

and blood flow to ischemic areas is increased. Cross tolerance with other nitrates may occur.

USES Prophylaxis, treatment, and management of angina pectoris. IV nitroglycerin is used to control BP in perioperative hypertension, CHF associated with acute MI; to produce controlled hypotension during surgical procedures, and to treat angina pectoris in patient who has not responded to nitrate or beta-blocker therapy. **Unlabeled use:** sublingual and topical nitroglycerin: to reduce cardiac workload in patients with acute MI and in CHF; ointment: in adjunctive treatment of Raynaud's disease.

ROUTE & DOSAGE

Angina

Adult	SL	1–2 sprays (0.4–0.8 mg) *or a* 0.15–0.6 mg tablet q3–5min as needed to a max of 3 doses in 15 min
	PO	1.3–9 mg q8–12h
	IV	Start with 5 µg/min and titrate q3–5min until desired response
	Topical	Apply a transdermal unit once q24h *or* leave on for 10–12 h; then remove and have a 10–12 h nitrate-free interval Apply 1.5–5 cm (1/2–2 in) of ointment q4–6h

PHARMACOKINETICS Absorption: significant loss to first pass metabolism after oral dosing. **Onset:** 2 min SL; 3 min PO; 30 min ointment. **Duration:** 30 min SL; 3–5 h PO; 3–6 h ointment. **Distribution:** widely distributed; not known if distributes to breast milk. **Metabolism:** extensively metabolized in liver. **Elimination:** half-life: 1–4 min; inactive metabolites excreted in urine.

CONTRAINDICATIONS & PRECAUTIONS Contraindicated in: hypersensitivity, idiosyncrasy, or tolerance to nitrates; severe anemia; head trauma, increased ICP; glaucoma (sustained release forms). Also (IV nitroglycerin): hypotension, uncorrected hypovolemia, constrictive pericarditis, pericardial tamponade. Safe use during pregnancy (category C), in nursing mothers, or in children not established. **Cautious use in:** severe hepatic or renal disease, conditions that cause dry mouth, early MI.

ADVERSE/SIDE EFFECTS CNS: *headache (50%),* apprehension, blurred vision, weakness, vertigo, dizziness, faintness. **CV:** *postural hypotension,* palpitations, tachycardia (sometimes with paradoxical bradycardia), increase in angina, syncope, and <u>circulatory collapse</u>. **GI:** nausea, vomiting, involuntary passing of urine and feces, abdominal pain, dry mouth. **Hematologic:** methemoglobinemia (high doses). **Skin:** cutaneous vasodilation with flushing, rash, exfoliative dermatitis, contact dermatitis with transdermal patch; topical allergic reactions with ointment: pruritic eczematous eruptions, <u>anaphylactoid reaction</u> characterized by oral mucosal and conjunctival edema. **Other:** muscle twitching, pallor, perspiration, cold sweat; local sensation in oral cavity at point of dissolution of sublingual forms.

DIAGNOSTIC TEST INTERFERENCES Nitroglycerin may cause increases in determinations of *urinary catecholamines* and *VMA;* may interfere with the Zlatkis-Zak color reaction, causing a false report of decreased *serum cholesterol*.

DRUG INTERACTIONS Alcohol, ANTIHYPERTENSIVE AGENTS compound hypotensive effects; IV nitroglycerin may antagonize **heparin** anticoagulation.

INCOMPATIBILITIES Solution/Additive: 5% dextrose, hydralazine, phenytoin.

NURSING IMPLICATIONS

Administration

- Drug forms appropriate for angina prophylaxis include ointment, transdermal unit, translingual spray, transmucosal tablet, and oral sustained release forms. Drug forms appropriate for acute angina include sublingual tablet, translingual spray, or transmucosal tablet.

Sublingual Tablet

- Instruct patient to sit or lie down upon first indication of oncoming anginal pain and to place tablet under tongue or in buccal pouch (hypotensive effect of drug is intensified in the upright position).
- Instruct patient to allow tablet to dissolve naturally and not to swallow until drug is entirely dissolved. Advise patient with dry mouth to take a sip of water or place 1 ml saline under the tongue before taking the nitroglycerin tablet.
- If pain is not relieved after 1 tablet, additional tablets may be taken at 5 min intervals, but not more than 3 tablets should be taken in a 15 min period. Taking more tablets than necessary can further decrease coronary blood flow by producing systemic hypotension.
- For hospitalized patient, tablets should be kept at bedside. Allocate a specific number (usually 10

tablets) in an appropriate container, label, and make sure patient knows location and use. Request patient to report all attacks. Count tablets daily.

Extend Release Buccal Tablet

- Tablet is placed between lip and gum above incisors or between cheek and gum allowing slow dissolution over 3–5 h.
- Inform patient that touching tongue to tablet or drinking hot fluids hastens tablet dissolution, which can lead to decreased duration of medication effect and onset of anginal pain.
- Tablet should not be chewed or swallowed.

Sustained Release Tablet or Capsule

- Should be taken on an empty stomach (1 h before or 2 h after meals), with a full glass of water, and swallowed whole.
- Sustained release form helps to prevent anginal attacks; it is not intended for immediate relief of angina.

Translingual Spray

- Do not shake cannister. Spray preferably on or under tongue. Do not inhale spray.
- May be repeated q5min for a maximum of 3 metered doses.
- Wait at least 10 seconds before swallowing.

Transdermal Ointment

- Using dose-determining applicator (patch) supplied with package, squeeze prescribed dose onto the applicator. Place patch with ointment-side down onto desired site. Using applicator spread ointment in a thin, uniform layer to premarked 5.5 by 9 cm (2 1/4 by 3 1/2 in) square nonhairy skin surface. (Areas commonly used: chest, abdomen, anterior thigh, forearm.) Cover with transparent wrap and secure with tape. Avoid getting ointment on fingers.
- Rotate application sites to prevent dermal inflammation and sensitization. Remove ointment from previously used sites before reapplication.
- Keep ointment container tightly closed and store in cool place.

Transdermal Unit

- Transdermal unit is applied at the same time each day, preferably to skin site free of hair and not subject to excessive movement. Avoid abraded, irritated, or scarred skin. Clip hair if necessary.
- Change application site each time to prevent skin irritation and sensitization.

Intravenous Solution

- Must be diluted in 5% dextrose injection or 0.9% NaCl injection prior to infusion.
- Use only glass bottles and manufacturer-supplied IV tubing. Regular IV tubing can absorb 40–80% of nitroglycerin.

- IV nitroglycerin, properly diluted, is administered by continuous infusion regulated exactly by an infusion pump.
- Initial rate is 5 µg/min, titrated in 5 µg/min increments q3–5 min until desired response is achieved.
- IV dosage titration requires careful and continuous hemodynamic monitoring.
- IV nitroglycerin is available in differing concentrations. Be attentive to the dilution, dosage, and directions for administration on each vial or ampul.
- Check to see if patient has transdermal patch or ointment in place before starting IV infusion. The patch (or ointment) is usually removed to prevent overdosage. When there is to be a switch from IV to transdermal nitroglycerin, the IV infusion rate is reduced by 50% with simultaneous application of 5 or 10 mg/24 h transdermal patch.
- Stable for at least 48 h when stored at controlled room temperature between 15–30C (59–86F) and mixed and stored in a glass container.
- Use only glass containers for storage of reconstituted IV solution. Polyvinyl chloride (PVC) plastic can absorb nitroglycerin and therefore should not be used. Non-polyvinyl-chloride (non-PVC) sets are recommended or provided by manufacturer.

Assessment & Drug Effects

- IV nitroglycerin should be administered with extreme caution to patients with hypotension or hypovolemia since the IV drug may precipitate a severe hypotensive state.
- IV nitroglycerin solution contains a substantial amount of ethanol as diluent. Ethanol intoxication can develop with high doses of IV nitroglycerin (vomiting, lethargy, coma, breath smells of alcohol). Monitor patient closely for change in levels of consciousness and for dysrhythmias. If intoxication occurs, infusion should be stopped promptly; patient recovers immediately with discontinuation of drug administration.
- At particular risk of intoxication with IV nitroglycerine is the patient with impaired hepatic metabolism with ischemic heart disease, cardiac dysfunction, or the alcohol-sensitive patient.
- During an acute angina attack, remain with patient monitoring vital signs and assessing for worsening of angina. If relief has not been obtained following the third dose of sublingual or translingual nitroglycerin, notify physician immediately.
- Moisture on sublingual tissue is required for dissolution of sublingual tablet. However, because chest pain typically leads to dry mouth, a patient may be unresponsive to sublingual nitroglycerin.
- Approximately 50% of all patients experience mild

Common side effects in *italic*; life-threatening effects underlined; generic names in **bold**; classifications in SMALL CAPS

to severe headaches following nitroglycerin. Assess patient and consult as needed with physician about analgesics and dosage adjustment.

- Transient headache usually lasts about 5 min after sublingual administration and seldom longer than 20 min. Assess degree of severity.
- Postural hypotension may occur even with small doses of nitroglycerin. Patient may complain of dizziness or weakness due to postural hypotension. Supervision of ambulation may be indicated especially with the elderly or debilitated patient.
- Before initiation of treatment with transdermal preparations take baseline BP and heart rate, with patient in sitting position.
- One hour after transdermal (ointment or unit) medication has been applied, check BP and pulse again with patient in sitting position. Report measurements to physician.
- Assess for and report blurred vision or dry mouth.
- Assess for and report the following topical reactions to drug administration: contact dermatitis from the transdermal patch; pruritus and erythema from the ointment.
- Any local burning or tingling from the sublingual form has no clinical significance.
- *Overdose symptoms:* hypotension, tachycardia; warm, flushed skin becoming cold and cyanotic; headache, palpitations, confusion, nausea, vomiting, moderate fever, and paralysis. Tissue hypoxia leads to coma, convulsions, cardiovascular collapse. Death can occur from asphyxia.

Patient & Family Education

- Advise patient using sublingual tablet that as soon as pain is completely relieved, any remaining tablet may be expelled from mouth, especially if patient is experiencing unpleasant side effects such as headache. Advise patient to relax for 15–20 min after taking tablet to prevent dizziness or faintness.
- Advise patient that pain not relieved by 3 sublingual tablets over a 15 min period may indicate acute MI or severe coronary insufficiency. Advise patient to contact physician immediately or have someone take patient directly to emergency room.
- Sublingual tablets may be taken prophylactically 5–10 min prior to exercise or other stimulus known to trigger anginal (drug effect lasts 30–60 min).
- Instruct patient to keep record for physician of number of angina attacks, amount of medication required for relief of each attack, and possible precipitating factors.
- Instruct patient using transdermal unit that contact with water, e.g., bathing, swimming, does not affect the unit.

- If faintness, dizziness, or flushing occurs following application of transdermal unit or ointment advise patient to remove unit immediately from skin and notify physician.
- Sublingual formulation can be administered while transdermal unit or ointment is in place.
- Advise patient to report blurred vision or dry mouth. Both warrant discontinuation of drug.
- Dizziness, lightheadedness, and syncope (due to postural hypotension) occur most frequently in the elderly. Recovery may be hastened by head-low position, deep breathing, and movements of extremities. Advise patient to make position changes slowly and to avoid prolonged standing.
- Inform patient that severe postural hypotension (sharp drop in BP), vertigo, flushing, or pallor may occur if alcohol is ingested too soon after taking nitroglycerin.
- Advise patient to report any increase in frequency, duration, or severity of anginal attack.
- Withdrawal following prolonged use must be gradual to prevent precipitating anginal attack.

NONNITRATE VASODILATOR

HYDRALAZINE HYDROCHLORIDE
(hye-dral´a-zeen)
Trade names: Alazine, Apresoline, Dralzine
Classifications: CARDIOVASCULAR AGENT; NONNITRATE VASODILATOR; ANTIHYPERTENSIVE
Pregnancy: Category C

ACTIONS/PHARMACODYNAMICS The only phthalazine used clinically in North America. Reduces BP mainly by direct effect on vascular smooth muscles of arterial-resistance vessels, resulting in vasodilation; has little effect on venous-capacitance vessels. Diastolic reponse is often greater than systolic Vasodilation reduces peripheral resistance and substantially improves cardiac output, renal and cerebral blood flow. Hypotensive effect may be limited by sympathetic reflexes, which increase heart rate, stroke volume, and cardiac output. Postural hypotensive effect is reportedly less than that produced by ganglionic blocking agents. Usually increases plasma renin activity.

USES Most commonly in stepped-care approach to treat moderate to severe hypertension (step 3 agent).

Common side effects in *italic*; life-threatening effects underlined; generic names in **bold**; classifications in SMALL CAPS

Also in early malignant hypertension and resistant hypertension that persists after sympathectomy. **Unlabeled uses:** conjunctively with cardiac glycosides and other vasodilators in short-term treatment of acute CHF; unexplained pulmonary hypertension.

ROUTE & DOSAGE

Hypertension

Adult	PO	10–50 mg q.i.d.
	IM	10–50 mg q4–6h
	IV	10–20 mg q4–6h
Child	PO	3–7.5 mg/kg/d in 4 divided doses
	IM/IV	1.7–3.5 mg/kg/d in 4 divided doses

PHARMACOKINETICS Absorption: readily absorbed from GI tract. **Onset:** 20–30 min. **Peak:** 2 h. **Duration:** 2–6 h. **Distribution:** crosses placenta; distributed into breast milk. **Metabolism:** metabolized in intestinal wall and liver. **Elimination:** half-life: 2–8 h; 90% rapidly excreted in urine; 10% excreted in feces.

CONTRAINDICATIONS & PRECAUTIONS Contraindicated in: coronary artery disease, mitral valvular rheumatic heart disease, MI, tachycardia, SLE. Safe use during pregnancy (category C) or in nursing mothers not established. **Cautious use in:** cerebrovascular accident, advanced renal impairment, use with MAO inhibitors.

ADVERSE/SIDE EFFECTS CNS: *headache,* dizziness, peripheral neuritis (pyridoxine deficiency), paresthesias, tremors, psychotic reactions (depression, anxiety, disorientation). **CV:** *palpitation,* angina, *tachycardia,* flushing, orthostatic hypotension, paradoxical pressor response, arrhythmias, <u>profound shock</u> (overdosage). **Eye:** lacrimation, conjunctivitis. **GI:** anorexia, nausea, vomiting, diarrhea, constipation, abdominal pain, paralytic ileus. **GU:** difficulty in urination, glomerulonephritis, impotence (rare). **Hematologic:** reduced hemoglobin and RBCs, anemia (immune hemolysis), leukopenia, <u>agranulocytosis</u>, purpura. **Hypersensitivity:** rash, urticaria, pruritus, fever, chills, arthralgia, eosinophilia, cholangitis, hepatitis, obstructive jaundice. **Other:** nasal congestion, muscle cramps, lymphadenopathy, splenomegaly; sweating, rheumatoid or SLE-like syndrome, neutrophilic dermatosis, fixed drug eruption, sodium and fluid retention (edema) with long-term therapy.

DRUG INTERACTIONS BETA-BLOCKERS and other ANTIHYPERTENSIVE AGENTS compound hypotensive effects.

INCOMPATIBILITIES Solution/Additive: aminophylline, ampicillin, chlorothiazide, edetate calcium disodium, hydrocortisone, mephentermine, methohexital, nitroglycerin, phenobarbital, verapamil

DIAGNOSTIC TEST INTERFERENCES Positive *direct Coombs' tests* in patients with hydralazine-induced SLE. Hydralazine interferes with urinary *17-OHCS* determinations *(modified Glenn-Nelson technique).*

NURSING IMPLICATIONS

Administration

- Bioavailability of hydralazine is increased by taking it with food. (Food reduces first pass metabolism of drug in the intestinal wall). It is advisable to be consistent in taking drug either with meals or on an empty stomach to minimize fluctuations in plasma drug levels. Consult physician.
- Most patients receiving parenteral hydralazine are transferred to oral form within 24–48 h.
- Administer undiluted solution by direct IV. Give each 10 mg or fraction thereof over 1 min.
- Do not add hydralazine to IV solutions. It may be given through a Y tube or three-way stopcock of infusion set.
- IV use recommended only when the oral route is not feasible.
- Discontinuation of hydralazine should be accomplished gradually to avoid sudden rise in BP and acute heart failure. Patients should be informed of the dangers of abrupt withdrawal.
- Store at 15–30C (59–86F) in tight, light-resistant containers unless otherwise directed. Avoid freezing.

Assessment & Drug Effects

- LE cell preparation and antinuclear antibody titer determinations are advised before initiation of therapy and periodically during prolonged therapy.
- Baseline and periodic determinations should also be made of BUN, creatinine clearance, uric acid, serum potassium, blood glucose, and ECG.
- BP and heart rate should be closely monitored in patients receiving parenteral hydralazine. Check every 5 min until it is stabilized at desired level, then every 15 min thereafter throughout hypertensive crisis.
- I&O should be monitored when drug is given parenterally and in those with renal dysfunction. Output may be increased in some patients because of improved renal blood flow.

Common side effects in *italic*; life-threatening effects <u>underlined</u>; generic names in **bold**; classifications in SMALL CAPS

153

Patient & Family Education

- Instruct patient to monitor weight and check for edema and to report sudden gain or apparent slow increase in weight and the onset of edema. Sodium retention has occurred with long-term use.
- Some patients experience headache and palpitations within 2–4 h after first PO dose. Symptoms usually subside spontaneously. Advise patient to inform physician of adverse reactions; most can be controlled.
- Because of the possibility of postural hypotension, caution patient to make position changes slowly and to avoid standing still, hot baths/showers, strenuous exercise, and excessive alcohol intake.
- Caution patient to lie down or sit down (in head-low position) if faintness or dizziness occurs. Patients who engage in potentially hazardous activities such as driving should be advised of the possibility of these symptoms.
- Hydralazine, 100 mg, contains tartrazine, which may cause an allergic reaction in some patients, frequently in those who also have aspirin hypersensitivity.

RAUWOLFIA ALKALOID

RESERPINE
(re-ser´peen)

Trade names: Serpalan, Serpasil, Serpate, Sk-Reserpine, and others

Classifications: CARDIOVASCULAR AGENT; RAUWOLFIA ALKALOID; ANTIHYPERTENSIVE; CNS AGENT; PSYCHOTHERAPEUTIC; ANTIPSYCHOTIC (TRANQUILIZER)

Pregnancy: Category D

ACTIONS/PHARMACODYNAMICS Principal alkaloid of *Rauwolfia serpentina* (Indian snakeroot). Interferes with binding of 5-hydroxytryptamine (serotonin) at receptor sites, decreases synthesis of norepinephrine by depleting dopamine (their precursor), and competitively inhibits their reuptake in storage granules. Causes depletion of these biogenic amines (norepinephrine, serotonin) in CNS, peripheral nervous system, heart, and other organs and tissues. Sympathetic inhibitory action is reflected in small but persistent decrease in BP, frequently associated with bradycardia, and reduced cardiac output. Usually does not cause orthostatic hypotension, and has no marked effect on renal blood flow. Central effect results in tranquilization and sedation similar to that produced by chlorpromazine.

USES Mild essential hypertension and as adjunctive therapy with other antihypertensive agents in the more severe forms of hypertension. Also used in agitated psychotic states, primarily in patients intolerant to phenothiazines or patients who also require antihypertensive medication. **Unlabeled use:** to reduce vasospastic attacks in Raynaud's phenomenon and other peripheral vascular disorders, and for short-term symptomatic treatment of thyrotoxicosis.

ROUTE & DOSAGE

Hypertension

Adult	PO	0.5 mg/d initially; reduced to 0.1–0.25 mg/d

PHARMACOKINETICS Peak: 2 h. **Distribution:** widely distributed, especially to adipose tissue; crosses blood-brain barrier and placenta; distributed in breast milk. **Metabolism:** extensively metabolized to inactive compounds. **Elimination:** half-life: 4.5 and 11.3 h; slowly excreted, 60% in feces within 96 h and 10% in urine.

CONTRAINDICATIONS & PRECAUTIONS
Contraindicated in: hypersensitivity to rauwolfia alkaloids; history of mental depression; acute peptic ulcer, ulcerative colitis; patients receiving electroconvulsive therapy; within 7–14 days of MAO inhibitor therapy. Safe use during pregnancy (Category D) and in nursing mothers not established. **Cautious use in:** renal insufficiency; cardiac arrhythmias; cardiac damage; cerebrovascular accident; epilepsy; bronchitis; asthma; elderly patients, debilitated patients; gallstones; obesity; chronic sinusitis; parkinsonism; pheochromocytoma.

ADVERSE/SIDE EFFECTS CNS: *drowsiness,* sedation, *lethargy,* mental depression, nervousness, anxiety, nightmares, increased dreaming, headache, dizziness, increased appetite, dull sensorium; prolonged use of large doses: CNS stimulation (parkinsonian syndrome): tremors, muscle rigidity; <u>respiratory depression</u>, convulsions, hypothermia. **CV:** bradycardia, *edema,* CHF (rare), orthostatic hypotension, increased AV conduction time (prolonged therapy); anginalike symptoms, arrhythmias. **ENT:** *nasal congestion,* epistaxis, lacrimation, blurred vision; miosis, ptosis, conjunctival congestion (acute toxicity); causal relationship not established: glaucoma, uveitis, optic atrophy, deafness. **GI:** dry mouth or excessive salivation, nausea, vomiting, abdominal cramps, diarrhea, reactivation of peptic ulcer (hypersecretion), heartburn, biliary colic, decreased carbohydrate tolerance. **Hematologic:** thrombocytopenic purpura, anemia, prolonged BT. **Hypersensitivity:** pruritus, rash, asthma. **Reproductive:** menstrual irregularities, breast engorgement, galactorrhea, gynecomastia, feminization (males), impaired sexual function, impotence. **Other:** muscle aches, dysuria, fixed-drug eruptions.

DIAGNOSTIC TEST INTERFERENCES Possibility of elevated *blood glucose* values; however, it is also reported that reserpine may decrease thiazide-induced hyperglycemia. Increase in *serum prolactin* with chronic administration of rauwolfia alkaloids; overdoses may cause initial increase in excretion of *urinary catecholamines;* decreases with chronic administration. Large doses may cause initial rise in *urinary 5 HIAA* excretion. Initial IM doses may increase *urinary VMA* excretion followed by decrease by end of third day of therapy (with oral or parenteral administration). Possible interference with *urinary steroid* colorimetric determinations: *17-OHCS* and *17-KS.*

DRUG INTERACTIONS Diuretics, other HYPOTENSIVE AGENTS compound hypotensive effects; CARDIAC GLYCOSIDES **(digoxin)** may increase risk of arrhythmias; MAO INHIBITORS may cause excitation and hypertension; CNS DEPRESSANTS compound depression; may decrease response to **levodopa.**

NURSING IMPLICATIONS

Administration

- Reserpine is administered with meals or with milk or other food to minimize possibility of gastric irritation (drug increases gastric secretions).
- Advise patient to take drug at the same time each day, not to skip or double doses, and not to stop therapy without advice of physician.
- Preserve in tight, light-resistant containers, preferably at 15–30C (59–86F), unless otherwise directed by manufacturer.

Assessment & Drug Effects

- Take BP and pulse at intervals prescribed by physician. Both should be taken before each parenteral dose. Compare readings with baseline determinations and keep physician informed. (Note: drop in BP may be accompanied by bradycardia.)
- Postural hypotension occurs rarely with usual PO doses but is not uncommon in patients receiving large parenteral doses. Supervise ambulation as indicated.
- Monitor I&O especially in patients with impaired renal function. Report changes in I&O ratio and pattern.
- Full therapeutic effect of oral drug for hypertension may not occur until 2–3 wk of therapy, and effects may persist for as long as 4–6 wk after drug is discontinued.
- Special precautions should be observed when reserpine is prescribed for the elderly and the obese patient (half-life is reportedly prolonged in obese patients). Anticipate increased incidence of adverse/side effects.
- Mental depression is a serious side effect and may be severe. It occurs most commonly in high dosage regimens, e.g., 0.5–1 mg/d or more; may not appear until 2–8 mo of therapy and may last for several months after drug is withdrawn.
- Because rauwolfia alkaloids are cumulative and have a long duration of action, dosage adjustments when necessary are usually made at 7–14 d intervals.
- Rauwolfia alkaloids tend to lower the threshold for convulsions. Patients with epilepsy should be monitored for possible need of adjustment in anticonvulsant dosage.
- Rauwolfia alkaloids should be discontinued 1 wk before electroconvulsive therapy.

Patient & Family Education

- Since drowsiness, sedation, and dizziness are possible side effects, caution patient to avoid driving and other potentially hazardous activities until reaction to drug has been determined.
- Counsel patient regarding possible side effects and importance of prompt reporting. Untoward effects are usually minimal with proper dosage and adequate supervision.
- Instruct patient and responsible family members to report the following possible beginning symptoms of depression: early morning insomnia, anorexia, inability to concentrate, despondency, self-deprecation, attitude of detachment, mood swings, or impotence. Hospitalization may be necessary.
- Instruct patient to report symptoms of dizziness, lightheadedness to physician. Advise patient to make position changes slowly, particularly from recumbent to upright posture, and to lie down or sit down (head-low position) if patient feels faint. Also advise patient not to take hot showers or hot tub baths, and not to stand still for prolonged periods.
- Advise patient to check for edema and to record weight daily. Distinction must be made between

Common side effects in *italic*; life-threatening effects <u>underlined</u>; generic names in **bold**; classifications in SMALL CAPS

155

weight gain from edema and that from increased appetite. Consult physician about gain of 1–2 kg (3–5 lb) in 1 wk.

- Advise patient not to take OTC medications without prior approval of physician or pharmacist. Many preparations for coughs and colds contain adrenergic agents that affect the actions of rauwolfia alkaloids.
- Since reserpine decreases carbohydrate tolerance, diabetics should monitor blood glucose carefully and notify physician of hyperglycemic symptoms (see chap 3).

ANALGESIC, ANTIPYRETIC: NARCOTIC (OPIATE) AGONIST

MORPHINE SULFATE

(mor´feen)
Trade names: Astramorph PF, Duramorph, Epimorph, Morphitec, M.O.S., MSIR, MS Contin, Roxanol, RMS, Statex
Classifications: CNS AGENT; ANTIPYRETIC; ANALGESIC; NARCOTIC (OPIATE) AGONIST
Pregnancy: Category B
Controlled substance: Schedule II

ACTIONS/PHARMACODYNAMICS A natural opium alkaloid with agonist activity through binding with the same receptors as endogenous opioid peptides (enkephalins or endorphins). Both agonist and peptide decrease neurotransmitter release, an action thought to be related to interference with calcium entry into neurons. Narcotic agonist effects are identified with 3 types of receptors: analgesia at supraspinal level, euphoria, respiratory depression and physical dependence (mu receptor); analgesia at spinal level, sedation and miosis (kappa); and dysphoric, hallucinogenic and cardiac stimulant effects (sigma). Secondary pharmacologic effects include CNS: CTZ stimulation, depressed cough reflex, pupillary constriction even in total darkness; CV: inhibition of baroreceptors (possibly leading to orthostatic hypotension and fainting); GI: reduced gastric motility and secretions resulting in delayed digestion; inhibition of peristalsis leading to constipation; GU: increased tone of bladder smooth muscle and sphincter resulting in urinary retention. Has abuse potential: psychological dependence, and physical tolerance and dependence may develop with repeated uncon-

trolled use; however, most patients receiving narcotic analgesics under medical supervision do not develop dependence syndromes.

USES Symptomatic relief of severe acute and chronic pain after nonnarcotic analgesics have failed and as preanesthetic medication; also used to relieve dyspnea of acute left ventricular failure and pulmonary edema and pain of MI.

ROUTE & DOSAGE

Pain Relief

Adult	PO	10–30 mg q4h prn *or* 15–30 mg extended release q8–12h; increase dose prn for pain relief
	IV	2.5–15 mg q4h *or* 0.8–10 mg/h by continuous infusion; dose may be increased prn to control pain *or* 5–10 mg given epidurally q24h
	IM/SC	5–20 mg q4h
	PR	10–20 mg q4h prn
Child	IV	0.05–0.1 mg/kg q4h *or* 0.025–2.6 mg/kg/h by continuous infusion
	IM/SC	0.1–0.2 mg/kg q4h (no more than 15 mg/dose)

PHARMACOKINETICS Absorption: variably absorbed from GI tract. **Peak:** 60 min PO; 20–60 min PR; 50–90 min SC; 30–60 min IM; 20 min IV. **Duration:** up to 7 h. **Distribution:** crosses blood-brain barrier and placenta; distributed in breast milk. **Metabolism:** metabolized primarily in liver. **Elimination:** 90% of drug and metabolites excreted in urine in 24 h; 7–10% excreted in bile.

CONTRAINDICATIONS & PRECAUTIONS Contraindicated in: hypersensitivity to opiates; increased intracranial pressure, convulsive disorders; acute alcoholism; acute bronchial asthma, chronic pulmonary diseases, severe respiratory depression; chemical-irritant-induced pulmonary edema; prostatic hypertrophy; diarrhea caused by poisoning until the toxic material has been eliminated; undiagnosed acute abdominal conditions; following biliary tract surgery and surgical anastomosis; pancreatitis; acute ulcerative colitis; severe liver or renal insufficiency; Addison's disease, hypothyroidism; during labor for delivery of a premature infant, in premature infants. Safe use during pregnancy (category B; D in long-term use or when high dose used) not established. **Cautious use in:** toxic psychosis; cardiac arrhythmias, cardiovascular disease; emphysema;

kyphoscoliosis; cor pulmonale; severe obesity; reduced blood volume; very old, very young, or debilitated patients; labor.

ADVERSE/SIDE EFFECTS Allergic: *pruritus*, rash, urticaria, hemorrhagic urticaria (rare), anaphylactoid reaction (rare), edema. **CNS:** respiratory depression, euphoria, insomnia, disorientation, visual disturbances, dysphoria, paradoxic CNS stimulation (restlessness, tremor, delirium, insomnia), convulsions (infants and children); decreased cough reflex, drowsiness, dizziness, miosis. **CV:** bradycardia, palpitations, syncope; flushing of face, neck, and upper thorax; orthostatic hypotension. **GI:** *constipation*, anorexia, dry mouth, biliary colic, *nausea*, vomiting, elevated transaminase levels. **GU:** urinary retention or urgency, dysuria, oliguria, reduced libido or potency (prolonged use). **Other:** sweating, prolonged labor and respiratory depression of newborn, precipitation of porphyria. **Overdosage:** severe respiratory depression (as low as 2–4/min) or arrest; pulmonary edema, deep sleep, coma; skeletal muscle flaccidity; cold, clammy skin; hypotension, bradycardia, cardiac arrest, marked miosis, hypothermia.

DIAGNOSTIC TEST INTERFERENCES False-positive **urine glucose** determinations may occur using Benedict's solution. **Plasma amylase** and **lipase** determinations may be falsely positive for 24 h after use of morphine; transaminase levels may be elevated.

DRUG INTERACTIONS CNS DEPRESSANTS, SEDATIVES, BARBITURATES, **alcohol**, BENZODIAZEPINES, and TRICYCLIC ANTIDEPRESSANTS potentiate CNS depressant effects. Use MAO INHIBITORS cautiously; they may precipitate hypertensive crisis. PHENOTHIAZINES may antagonize analgesia.

INCOMPATIBILITIES Solution/additive: aminophylline, amobarbital, chlorothiazide, heparin, meperidine, methicillin, phenobarbital, phenytoin, sodium bicarbonate, thiopental, pentobarbital. Y-site: minocycline, tetracycline.

NURSING IMPLICATIONS

Administration

- Before administering the drug, note respiratory rate, depth, and rhythm and size of pupils. Respirations of 12/min or below and miosis are signs of toxicity. Withhold drug and report to physician.
- Narcotic agonist analgesics should be given in

smallest effective dose and for the shortest time compatible with patient's needs. Dosage for elderly or debilitated patients: lower than for adult.

- The extended release tablet should not be broken in half, crushed, or chewed.
- **Oral solution:** dilute in approximately 30 ml or more of fluid or semisolid food. A calibrated dropper comes with the bottle. Read labels carefully when using liquid preparation; available solutions: 20 mg/ml; 100 mg/ml.
- May be given by direct IV, diluted in 5 ml of sterile water for injection, over 4–5 min.
- Morphine is physically and chemically incompatible with many solutions. Do not mix with other drugs without the advice of a pharmacist.
- When narcotic analgesic therapy is started, a fixed, individualized schedule provides effective management because blood levels can be maintained and peaks of pain can be prevented; usually a 4 h interval is adequate.
- Fullest analgesic effect is achieved if drug is administered before patient experiences intense pain (morphine relieves continuous dull pain more effectively than sharp intermittent pain, which generally requires higher doses).
- Patient scheduled for pain relief surgical procedure should not receive extended release tablet within 24 h of surgery.
- Store at 15–30C (59–86F). Avoid freezing. Suppositories should be refrigerated. Protect all formulations from light.

Assessment & Drug Effects

- Observe patient closely to be certain pain relief is achieved. During the first 2 or 3 d of effective pain relief, patient may sleep many hours. This could be misinterpreted as excessive dosing rather than the first sign of relief in a pain-exhausted patient. If respiratory and other vital functions are within normal parameters, delay attempts to reduce dose for at least 3 d after it has been started. Record relief of pain (preferably in patient's own words) and duration of analgesia for reference when dosage modification is being considered.
- Elevated pulse or respiratory rate, restlessness, anorexia, or drawn facial expression may indicate need for analgesia.
- Differentiate among restlessness as a sign of pain and the need for medication, restlessness associated with hypoxia, and restlessness caused by morphine-induced CNS stimulation (a paradoxic reaction that is particularly common in women and elderly patients).

Common side effects in *italic*; life-threatening effects underlined; generic names in **bold**; classifications in SMALL CAPS

157

- Respiratory depression can be severe for as long as 24 h after epidural or intrathecal administration.
- Patients in particular jeopardy for severe respiratory depression after epidural or intrathecal injection: the elderly or debilitated or those who have decreased respiratory reserve (e.g., emphysema, severe obesity, kyphoscoliosis).
- Patient monitoring for respiratory depression should be continued for at least 24 h after each epidural or intrathecal dose.
- Monitor vital signs at regular intervals. Morphine-induced respiratory depression may occur even with small doses, and it increases progressively with higher doses (generally reaching maximum within 90 min following SC, 30 min after IM, and 7 min after IV administration).
- Narcotic analgesics also depress cough and sigh reflexes and thus may induce atelectasis, especially in postoperative patients. Purposefully encourage changes in position, deep breathing, and coughing (unless contraindicated) at regularly scheduled intervals.
- Nausea and orthostatic hypotension (with lightheadedness and dizziness) most often occur in ambulatory patients or when a supine patient assumes the head-up position or in patients not experiencing severe pain.
- Closely observe the patient with increased intracranial pressure or with head injury. Morphine effects may obscure neurologic signs of further increase in intracranial pressure.
- Monitor I&O ratio and pattern. Report oliguria or urinary retention. Morphine may dull perception of bladder stimuli; therefore, encourage the patient to void at least q4h. Palpate lower abdomen to detect bladder distension.
- Check for abdominal distension and intestinal peristaltic sounds after administration of extended release tablet. If paralytic ileus develops, stop use of tablet.
- Morphine-induced constipation can be a serious side effect and should not go untreated. Concomitant administration of a stool softener combined with a peristaltic stimulant, e.g., **senna with docusate** (Senokot), is effective prophylaxis. Encourage patient to drink ample fluids. Do not allow patient to go more than 2 d without a bowel movement.
- Abrupt withdrawal of drug in the presence of physical dependence initiates the *abstinence syndrome*. Usually withdrawal symptoms ("cold turkey") develop at time the next dose would ordinarily be given. Symptoms gradually intensify reaching a maximum in 36–72 h and subside over 5–10 d.

Patient & Family Education
- Patient should avoid alcohol and other CNS depressants while receiving morphine. Advise against use of any OTC drug unless it has been approved by the physician.
- Caution not to smoke or ambulate without assistance after receiving the drug. Bed side rails are advisable.
- Since morphine may cause drowsiness, dizziness, or blurred vision, patient should be cautioned to avoid tasks requiring alertness (e.g., driving a car) until drug response is known.

ANALGESIC, ANTIPYRETIC: NONNARCOTIC

ACETAMINOPHEN
(a-seat-a-mee′noe-fen)
Trade names: A'Cenol, Acephen, Anacin-3, Anuphen, APAP, Atasol, Campain, Datril Extra Strength, Dolanex, Halenol, Liquiprim, Panadol, Pedric, Robigesic, Rounox, Tapar, Tempra, Tylenol, Valadol
Classifications: CNS AGENT; NONNARCOTIC ANALGESIC, ANTIPYRETIC
Pregnancy: Category B

ACTIONS/PHARMACODYNAMICS Unlike aspirin, acetaminophen has little effect on platelet junction, does not affect bleeding time, and generally produces no gastric bleeding. Produces analgesia by unknown mechanism, perhaps by action on peripheral nervous system. Reduces fever by direct action on hypothalamus heat-regulating center with consequent peripheral vasodilation, sweating, and dissipation of heat.

USES Fever reduction. Temporary relief of mild to moderate pain. Generally as substitute for aspirin when the latter is not tolerated or is contraindicated.

PHARMACOKINETICS Absorption: rapid and almost complete absorption from GI tract; less complete absorption from rectal suppository. **Peak effect:** 0.5–2 h. **Duration:** 3–4 h. **Distribution:** well distributed in all body fluids; crosses placenta. **Metabolism:** extensively metabolized in liver. **Elimination:** half-life: 1–3 h; 90–100% of drug excreted as metabolites in urine; excreted in breast milk.

CONTRAINDICATIONS & PRECAUTIONS Hypersensitivity to acetaminophen or phenacetin. **Contraindicated in:** children <3 y, unless directed by a physician; repeated administration to patients with anemia or hepatic disease. Safe use during pregnancy (category B) or in nursing women not established. **Cautious use in:** arthritic or rheumatoid conditions affecting children <12 y; alcoholism; malnutrition; thrombocytopenia.

ROUTE & DOSAGE

Adult	PO	325–650 mg q4–6h (max 4 g/d)
	PR	650 mg q4–6h (max 4 g/d)
Child	PO	0–3 mo: 40 mg q4–6h
		4–11 mo: 80 mg q4–6h
		1–2 y: 120 mg q4–6h
		2–3 y: 160 mg q4–6h
		4–5 y: 240 mg q4–6h
		6–8 y: 320 mg q4–6h
		9–10 y: 400 mg q4–6h
		11–12 y: 480 mg q4–6h
	PR	2–5 y: 120 mg q4–6h (max 720 mg/d)
		6–12 y: 325 mg q4–6h (max 2.6 g/d)

ADVERSE/SIDE EFFECTS Negligible with recommended dosage; rash. **Acute poisoning:** anorexia, nausea, vomiting, dizziness, lethargy, diaphoresis, chills, epigastric or abdominal pain, diarrhea. Onset of hepatotoxicity: elevation of serum transaminases (ALT, AST) and bilirubin. Hypoglycemia, hepatic coma, acute renal failure, seizures, delirium. **Chronic ingestion:** neutropenia, pancytopenia, leukopenia, thrombocytopenic purpura. *Hepatotoxicity in alcoholics:* renal damage.

DIAGNOSTIC TEST INTERFERENCES Acetaminophen may cause (1) false increases in *urinary 5-HIAA* (5-hydroxyindoleacetic acid) by-product of serotonin; (2) false decreases in *blood glucose* (by glucose oxidase–peroxidase procedure); (3) false increases in *urinary glucose* (with certain instruments in glucose analyses); and (4) false increases in *serum uric acid* (with phosphotungstate method).

DRUG INTERACTIONS Cholestyramine may decrease acetaminophen absorption. With chronic coadministration, BARBITURATES, **carbamazepine, phenytoin, and rifampin** may increase potential for chronic hepatotoxicity. Chronic excessive ingestion of **alcohol** will increase risk of hepatotoxicity.

NURSING IMPLICATIONS

Administration

- May be crushed and taken with fluid of patient's choice. Chewable tablets should be thoroughly chewed and wetted before they are swallowed.
- Coadministration with a high-carbohydrate meal may significantly retard absorption rate.
- Store in light-resistant containers at room temperature, preferably between 15–30C (59–86F), unless otherwise directed.

Assessment & Drug Effects

- With high doses or long-term therapy, periodic tests of hepatic, renal, and hematopoietic function are advised.
- Individuals with poor nutrition or who have ingested alcohol over prolonged periods are prone to hepatotoxicity even from moderate acetaminophen doses.
- High abuse potential; psychological dependence can occur. Withdrawal following long-term use has been associated with restlessness and excitement in some patients.
- Most poisonings result from suicide attempts or accidental ingestion.

Patient & Family Education

- Caution patient about taking other medications containing acetaminophen without medical advice.
- Overdosing and chronic use can cause liver damage and other toxic effects.
- Should not be used for self-medication of pain for more than 10 d in adults or 5 d in children, without consulting a physician. It should not be used for fever persisting longer than 3 d and never for fever over 39.5C (103F) or for recurrent fever without medical direction. No more than 5 doses in 24 h should be given to children unless prescribed by physician.

Common side effects in *italic*; life-threatening effects underlined; generic names in **bold**; classifications in SMALL CAPS

159

ANALGESIC, ANTIPYRETIC: NONSTEROIDAL ANTIINFLAMMATORY DRUG (NSAID)

IBUPROFEN

(eye-byoo´proe-fen)

Trade names: Advil, Amersol, Apsifen, Brufen, Haltran, Ifen, Ibuprin, Medipren, Motrin, Nuprin, Pamprin-IB, Rufen, Trendar

Classifications: CNS AGENT; NONNARCOTIC ANALGESIC; ANTIPYRETIC; NSAID

Pregnancy: Category B

ACTIONS/PHARMACODYNAMICS Prototype of the propionic acid NSAIDs with nonsteroidal anti-inflammatory activity and significant antipyretic and analgesic properties. Comparable to aspirin in analgesic action, but higher doses are required for antiinflammatory effect; also reported to cause fewer GI symptoms than aspirin in equieffective doses. Blocks prostaglandin synthesis by inhibiting cyclooxygenase, the enzyme that converts arachidonic acid to precursors of prostaglandins (cyclic endoperoxidases). Ibuprofen activity also includes modulation of T-cell function, inhibition of inflammatory cell chemotaxis, decreased release of superoxide radicals, or increased scavenging of these compounds at inflammatory sites. Inhibits platelet aggregation and prolongs bleeding time but does not affect prothrombin or whole blood clotting times. Has no uricosuric action, glucocorticoid- or adrenocorticoid-stimulating properties. Cross-sensitivity with aspirin and other nonsteroidal antiinflammatory drugs has been reported.

USES Chronic, symptomatic rheumatoid arthritis and osteoarthritis; relief of mild to moderate pain; primary dysmenorrhea, reduction of fever. **Unlabeled use:** gout, juvenile rheumatoid arthritis, psoriatic arthritis, ankylosing spondylitis, vascular headache.

PHARMACOKINETICS Absorption: 80% absorbed from GI tract. **Onset:** 1 h antipyretic effect. **Peak:** 1–2 h. **Duration:** 6–8 h. **Metabolism:** metabolized in liver. **Elimination:** half-life: 2–4 h; excreted primarily in urine; some biliary excretion.

CONTRAINDICATIONS & PRECAUTIONS Contraindicated in: patient in whom urticaria, severe rhinitis, bronchospasm, angioedema, nasal polyps are precipitated by aspirin or other NSAIDs; active peptic ulcer, bleeding abnormalities. Safe use during pregnancy (category B), by nursing mothers, or by children < 6 mo not established. **Cautious use in:** hypertension, history of GI ulceration, impaired hepatic or renal function, chronic renal failure, cardiac decompensation, patients with SLE.

ROUTE & DOSAGE

Inflammatory Disease

Adult	PO	400–800 mg t.i.d. or q.i.d. (max 3200 mg/d)
Child	PO	< 20 kg: up to 400 mg/d in divided doses
		20–30 kg: up to 600 mg/d in divided doses
		30–40 kg: up to 800 mg/d in divided doses

Mild to Moderate Pain, Dysmenorrhea

Adult	PO	400 mg q4–6h up to 1200 mg/d

Fever

Adult	PO	200–400 mg t.i.d. or q.i.d. (max 1200 mg/d)
Child	PO	6 mo–12 y: 5–10 mg/kg q4–6h up to 40 mg/kg/d

ADVERSE/SIDE EFFECTS CNS: headache, dizziness, light-headedness, anxiety, emotional lability, paresthesias, hallucinations, fatigue, malaise, drowsiness, anxiety, confusion, depression, aseptic meningitis. **CV:** arrhythmias (causal relationship not established); hypertension, palpitation, congestive heart failure (patient with marginal cardiac function); peripheral edema. **Eye/Ear:** amblyopia (blurred vision, decreased visual acuity, scotomas, changes in color vision); nystagmus, visual-field defects; tinnitus, impaired hearing. **GI:** dry mouth, gingival ulcerations, dyspepsia, *heartburn, nausea,* vomiting, anorexia, diarrhea, constipation, bloating, flatulence, epigastric or abdominal discomfort or pain, GI ulceration, *occult blood loss.* **Hematologic:** thrombocytopenia, neutropenia, hemolytic or <u>aplastic anemia</u>, leukopenia; decreased Hgb, Hct; transitory rise in AST, ALT, serum alkaline phosphatase; rise in (Ivy) bleeding time. **Renal:** acute renal failure, polyuria, azotemia, cystitis, hematuria, nephrotoxicity, decreased creatinine clearance. **Skin:** maculopapular and vesicobullous skin eruptions, erythema multiforme, pruritus, rectal itching, acne. **Other:** sore throat, epistaxis, flushing, fluid retention with edema, Stevens-Johnson syndrome, <u>toxic hepatitis</u>, hypersensitivity

Common side effects in *italic*; life-threatening effects <u>underlined</u>; generic names in **bold**; classifications in SMALL CAPS

reactions, <u>anaphylaxis</u>, bronchospasm, serum sickness, SLE, angioedema.

DRUG INTERACTIONS ORAL ANTICOAGULANTS, **heparin** may prolong bleeding time; may increase **lithium** toxicity.

NURSING IMPLICATIONS

Administration

- Absorption rate is slower and drug plasma level is reduced when ibuprofen is administered with food; therefore it is usually given on an empty stomach, e.g., 1 h before or 2 h after meals.
- If GI intolerance occurs, ibuprofen may be taken with meals or milk.
- Tablet may be crushed if patient is unable to swallow it whole and mixed with food or liquid before swallowing.
- Do not administer to child <12 y without advice of physician.
- Store preferably at 15–30C (59–86F) in tightly closed, light-resistant container unless otherwise directed by manufacturer.

Assessment & Drug Effects

- Patients with history of cardiac decompensation should be observed closely for evidence of fluid retention and edema.
- Baseline and periodic evaluations of Hgb, renal and hepatic function, and auditory and ophthalmologic examinations are recommended in patients receiving prolonged or high dose therapy.
- Side effects appear to be dose related. Physician will rely on accurate observation and reporting to estimate lowest effective dosage level.
- ***Symptoms of acute toxicity in children:*** apnea, cyanosis, response only to painful stimuli, dizziness, nystagmus.
- As with other NSAIDs, the antipyretic and antiinflammatory effects of ibuprofen may mask usual signs and symptoms of infection or other diseases.

Patient & Family Education

- Instruct patient to report immediately passage of dark tarry stools, "coffee ground" emesis, frankly bloody emesis, or other GI distress.
- Advise patient to report immediately to physician the onset of skin rash, pruritus, jaundice.
- Instruct patient to report immediately blood or protein in urine.
- Inform patients about possible CNS effects (lightheadedness, dizziness, drowsiness), and caution them to avoid dangerous activities until reaction to the drug has been determined.

- Patient who experiences any visual disturbances (e.g., amblyopia including blurred vision) should have ophthalmoscopic evaluation. Symptoms usually gradually disappear when drug is withdrawn.
- Optimum therapeutic response generally occurs within 2 wk (e.g., relief of pain, stiffness, or swelling; or improved joint flexion and strength). When satisfactory response occurs, dosage should be reviewed by physician and adjusted as required.
- Patient should be cautioned to report any unexplained bleeding (e.g., epistaxis, menorrhagia).
- Avoid self-medication with ibuprofen if taking prescribed drugs or if being treated for a serious condition without consulting physician.
- Avoid taking aspirin or acetaminophen concurrently with ibuprofen.
- Avoid taking ibuprofen if there is a history of a severe allergic reaction (asthma, urticaria, shock) to aspirin or another NSAID.
- Inform patient that alcohol and NSAIDs may increase risk of GI ulceration and bleeding tendencies and, therefore, should be avoided, unless otherwise advised by physician.
- Advise patient to inform dentist or surgeon that drug is being taken.

ANALGESIC, ANTIPYRETIC: SALICYLATE

ASPIRIN (ACETYLSALICYLIC ACID)

Trade names: Alka-Seltzer, Ancasal, A.S.A., Aspergum, Astrin, Bayer, Bayer Children's, Cosprin, Easprin, Ecotrin, Empirin, Encaprin, Entrophen, Hipirin, Measurin, Novasen, St Joseph Children's, Supasa, Triaphen-10, ZORprin
Classifications: CNS AGENT; SALICYLATE ANALGESIC, ANTIPYRETIC; NSAID
Pregnancy: Category D

ACTIONS/PHARMACODYNAMICS The acetyl portion of the aspirin molecule is responsible for certain actions such as inhibition of platelet aggregation that other salicylates (which are nonacetylated) do not exhibit. Major actions appear to be associated primarily with inhibiting the formation of prostaglandins involved in the production of inflammation, pain, and fever. **Antiinflammatory action:** aspirin and other salicylates irreversibly acetylate and inactivate cyclooxygenase, an enzyme required for prostaglandin

Common side effects in *italic*; life-threatening effects <u>underlined</u>; generic names in **bold**; classifications in SMALL CAPS

161

synthesis. Prostaglandins directly contribute to the inflammatory process, e.g., by releasing lysosomal substances and increasing lymphocyte activation and formation of autoantibodies. As an antiinflammatory agent, aspirin appears to be involved in enhancing antigen removal and in reducing the spread of inflammation in ground substances. These antiinflammatory actions also contribute to analgesic effects. **Analgesic action:** principally peripheral with limited action in the CNS, possibly on the hypothalamus; results in relief of mild to moderate pain. **Antipyretic action:** in addition to inhibiting prostaglandin synthesis, aspirin lowers body temperature in fever by indirectly causing centrally mediated peripheral vasodilation and sweating. **Antiplatelet action:** aspirin (but not other salicylates) powerfully inhibits platelet aggregation by irreversibly inhibiting platelet cyclooxygenase, an enzyme necessary for synthesis of thromboxane A_2 (TXA_2), which induces platelet aggregation. Measurable antiplatelet effect may persist 3–8 d. High serum salicylate concentrations can impair hepatic synthesis of blood coagulation factors VII, IX, and X, possibly by inhibiting action of vitamin K. **Antithrombotic action:** is believed to be limited to males, but studies are continuing to evaluate the effectiveness of aspirin in low doses in preventing first or subsequent heart attacks and thromboembolic disorders in both sexes. **Uricosuric effect:** is enhanced by high doses of aspirin (over 5 g/d) and is suppressed by usual analgesic doses (less than 2 g/d). **Hypocholesterolemic and hypoglycemic effects:** achieved with large doses. Chronic use does not lead to tolerance or addiction.

USES To relieve pain of low to moderate intensity. Also for various inflammatory conditions, such as acute rheumatic fever, systemic LE, rheumatoid arthritis, osteoarthritis, bursitis, and calcific tendonitis, and to reduce fever in selected febrile conditions. Used to reduce recurrence of TIA due to fibrin platelet emboli and risk of stroke in men; to prevent recurrence of MI; as prophylaxis against MI in men with unstable angina. **Unlabeled use:** as prophylactic against thromboembolism; to prevent cataract and progression of diabetic retinopathy; and to control symptoms related to gluten sensitivity.

PHARMACOKINETICS Absorption: 80–100% absorbed (depending on formulation), primarily in stomach and upper small intestine. **Peak levels:** 15 min to 2 h. **Distribution:** widely distributed in most body tissues; crosses placenta. **Metabolism:** asprin is hydrolyzed to salicylate in GI mucosa, plasma, and erythrocytes; salicylate is metabolized in liver.

Elimination: half-life: aspirin 15–20 min; salicylate 2–18 h (dose dependent); 50% of dose is eliminated in the urine in 2–4 h (low doses) or 15–30 h (high doses). Excreted in breast milk.

ROUTE & DOSAGE

Analgesic/Antipyretic

Adult	PO/PR	350–650 mg q4h; max 4 g/d
Child	PO/PR	40–65 mg/kg/d in 4–6 divided doses; max 3.6 g/d

Arthritic Conditions

Adult	PO	3.6–5.4 g/d in 4–6 divided doses
Child	PO	90–100 mg/kg/d in 4–6 divided doses; max 130 mg/kg/d

Thromboembolic Disorders

Adult	PO	325–650 mg 1 or 2 times/d

TIA Prophylaxis

Adult	PO	650 mg b.i.d.

MI Prophylaxis

Adult	PO	80–325 mg/d

CONTRAINDICATIONS & PRECAUTIONS Contraindicated in: history of hypersensitivity to salicylates including methyl salicylate (oil of wintergreen); sensitivity to other NSAIDs; patients with "aspirin triad" (aspirin sensitivity, nasal polyps, asthma); chronic rhinitis; chronic urticaria; history of GI ulceration, bleeding, or other problems; hypoprothrombinemia, vitamin K deficiency, hemophilia, or other bleeding disorders; CHF. Do not use aspirin during pregnancy (category D), especially in third trimester, in nursing mothers, and in prematures, neonates, and children under 2 y, except under advice and supervision of physician; do not use in children and teenagers with chickenpox or influenza-like illnesses (because of possible association with Reye's syndrome). **Cautious use in:** otic diseases; gout; children with fever accompanied by dehydration; hyperthyroidism; cardiac disease; renal or hepatic impairment; G6PD deficiency; anemia; preoperatively; Hodgkin's disease.

ADVERSE/SIDE EFFECTS CNS: dizziness, confusion, drowsiness. **ENT:** tinnitus, hearing loss. **GI:** *nausea*, vomiting, diarrhea, anorexia, *heartburn, stomach pains*, ulceration, occult bleeding, GI bleeding. **Hematologic:** thrombocytopenia, <u>agranulocytosis</u>,

Common side effects in *italic*; life-threatening effects <u>underlined</u>; generic names in **bold**; classifications in SMALL CAPS

leukopenia, neutropenia, hemolytic anemia. **Hypersensitivity:** urticaria, bronchospasm, <u>anaphylactic shock</u>, laryngeal edema. **Skin:** petechiae, easy bruising, rash. **Other:** sweating, thirst, hypoglycemia, impaired renal function, iron deficiency anemia, prolonged bleeding time, prolonged pregnancy and labor with increased bleeding, hepatotoxity.

DIAGNOSTIC TEST INTERFERENCES *Bleeding time* is prolonged 3–8 d (life of exposed platelets) following a single 325 mg (5 grains) dose of aspirin. Large doses of salicylates equivalent to 5 g or more of aspirin per day may cause prolonged *prothrombin time* by decreasing prothrombin production); interference with *pregnancy tests* (using mouse or rabbit); decreases in *serum cholesterol, potassium, PBI, T_3 and T_4 concentrations* and an increase in *T_3 resin uptake. Serum uric acid* may increase when plasma salicylate levels are below 10 and decrease when above 15 mg/dl using colorimetric methods. *Urine 5-HIAA:* aspirin may interfere with tests using fluorescent methods. *Urine ketones:* salicylates interfere with Gerhardt test (reaction with ferric chloride produces a reddish color that persists after boiling). *Urine glucose:* moderate to large doses of salicylates equivalent to an aspirin dosage ≥ 2.4 g/d may produce false-negative results with glucose oxidase methods (e.g., Clinistix, TesTape) and false-positive results with copper reduction methods (Benedict's solution, Clinitest). Urinary *PSP excretion* may be reduced by salicylates. Salicylates may cause *urine VMA* to be falsely elevated (by most tests), or reduced (by Pisano method). Salicylates may interfere with or cause false decreases in plasma theophylline levels using Schack and Waxler method. High plasma salicylate levels may cause abnormalities in *liver function tests*.

DRUG INTERACTIONS **Aminosalicylic acid** increases risk of salicylate toxicity. **Ammonium chloride** and other ACIDIFYING AGENTS decrease renal elimination and increase risk of salicylate toxicity. ANTICOAGULANTS increase risk of bleeding. ORAL HYPOGLYCEMIC AGENTS increase hypoglycemic activity with aspirin doses >2 g/d. CARBONIC ANHYDRASE INHIBITORS enhance salicylate toxicity. CORTICOSTEROIDS add to ulcerogenic effects. **Methotrexate** toxicity is increased. Low doses of salicylates may antagonize uricosuric effects of **probenecid** and **sulfinpyrazone.**

NURSING IMPLICATIONS

Administration

- Gastic irritation may be minimized by administering with a full glass of water (240 ml), milk, food, or antacids. Enteric coated tablets dissolve too quickly if administered with milk; also they should not be crushed or chewed.
- Schedule aspirin administration at least 30 min before physical therapy or other planned exercise to keep discomfort at a minimum.
- For treatment of rheumatic diseases, physician may prescribe daily dose increase of 1 or 2 tablets per day on basis of serum salicylate concentrations or until therapeutic response occurs (usually within 3–5 d after beginning regular dosing) or symptoms of toxicity (salicylism) intervene. Symptoms of toxicity are often eliminated after dosage reduction of as little as 325 mg (5 grains or 1 tablet).
- Store preferably between 15 and 30C (59 and 86F) in airtight container and a dry environment unless otherwise directed by manufacturer. Store suppositories in a cool place or refrigerate but do not freeze.

Assessment & Drug Effects

- Serum salicylate concentration associated with analgesia and antipyresis: 30–100 μg/ml. Therapeutic range for rheumatic disease is 250–300 μg/ml; for antiinflammatory action: 150–300 μg/ml; for antiplatelet action: 100 μg/ml. Symptoms of toxicity generally occur with serum salicylate levels over 300 μg/ml.
- Previous nonreaction to salicylates does not guarantee future safety. Some individuals develop an acute and specific intolerance to aspirin, although they may have taken it for years without incident. The reaction is nonimmunologic; symptoms usually occur 15 min to 3 h after ingestion: profuse rhinorrhea, erythema, nausea, vomiting, intestinal cramps, diarrhea.
- Patients with asthma, nasal polyps, perennial vasomotor rhinitis, hay fever, or chronic urticaria demonstrate a high frequency of salicylate hypersensitivity.
- In adults a sensation of fullness in the ears, tinnitus, and decreased or muffled hearing are the most frequent symptoms associated with chronic salicylate overdosage.
- Potential for toxicity is high in elderly chronic aspirin users because they have less serum protein to bind salicylate and also are less able to excrete it.
- Children tend to manifest salicylate toxicity by hyperventilation, agitation, mental confusion, or other

Common side effects in *italic*; life-threatening effects <u>underlined</u>; generic names in **bold**; classifications in SMALL CAPS

163

behavioral changes, drowsiness, lethargy, sweating, and constipation.

- In children, and infants particularly, salicylate toxicity is enhanced by the dehydration that frequently accompanies fever or illness. Monitor these patients closely.
- Children on high doses of aspirin are particularly prone to develop hypoglycemia (see Chapter 3). Monitor the diabetic child carefully for indicated need of insulin adjustment. See also Diagnostic Test Interferences.
- Because of the possible association of aspirin usage with Reye's syndrome, do not give aspirin to children or teenagers with symptoms of varicella (chickenpox) or influenza-like illnesses before consulting a physician.

Patient & Family Education

- GI disturbances may be reduced by use of enteric-coated tablets or extended release tablets.
- Buffered aspirin preparations in an effervescent vehicle, e.g., Alka-Seltzer, are more rapidly absorbed than plain aspirin and reportedly cause less GI irritation and bleeding. Alka-Seltzer, however, has a high sodium content (approximately 24 mEq of sodium per 32 mg tablet).
- Buffered aspirin or aspirin administered with an antacid may be better tolerated than conventional tablets.
- When aspirin is prescribed for dysmenorrhea, explain that for best results aspirin should be taken 1 or 2 d before menses (to reduce prostaglandin-induced uterine contractions). Patients having heavy menstrual blood loss should be advised to take another analgesic, such as acetaminophen, instead of aspirin.
- To reduce risk of bleeding, aspirin therapy is usually discontinued about 1 wk before surgery. Patients undergoing oral surgery should be advised not to take aspirin-containing gum or gargles and not to chew aspirin products for at least 1 wk following surgery. Prolonged contact with aspirin can cause hemorrhage and injury to oral tissues.
- Chronic administration of high-dose aspirin during the last 3 mo of pregnancy can prolong pregnancy and labor, increase maternal bleeding before and after delivery, and cause weight increase and hemorrhage in the neonate.
- Discontinue use with onset of ringing or buzzing in the ears, impaired hearing, dizziness, or GI discomfort or bleeding and report to physician. Hearing impairment resulting from salicylate overdosage can generally be reversed within 24 h by reducing the dose.

- In general, adults should not use aspirin for self-medication of pain beyond 5 d without consulting a physician. In adults or children, aspirin should not be used longer than 3 d for fever and never for fever over 39.5C (103F) or 38.9C (102F) if patient is over 60 or for recurrent fever without medical direction. Consult physician before using aspirin for any fever accompanied by rash, severe headache, stiff neck, marked irritability, or confusion (all possible symptoms of meningitis).
- Caution patient on large doses of aspirin to avoid alcohol. See Drug Interactions.
- Prolonged use of high salicylate doses can lead to iron-deficiency anemia, especially in women. Average blood loss with daily use of several aspirin tablets is reportedly 2–6 ml; 10% of patients on chronic high doses may lose as much as 80 ml/d.
- Observe and report signs of bleeding (e.g., petechiae, ecchymoses, bleeding gums, bloody or black stools, cloudy or bloody urine) and symptoms of salicylism.
- Maintain adequate fluid intake (consult physician for guidelines) to prevent salicylate crystalluria.
- Avoid other medications containing aspirin unless directed by physician, because of danger of overdosing. (There are more than 500 OTC aspirin-containing compounds.)
- Most aspirin tablets develop a hard shell with age, a change that lengthens disintegration time, increases risk of GI irritation, and delays onset of therapeutic action. Advise patient not to buy aspirin in large quantities.
- Aspirin tablets rapidly hydrolyze on exposure to heat, moisture, and air. Instruct patient to smell tablet before taking it. If a vinegarlike (acetic acid) odor is detected, discard all tablets.

ANESTHETIC, GENERAL

THIOPENTAL SODIUM

(thye-oh-pen´tal)
Trade name: Pentothal
Classifications: CNS AGENT; GENERAL ANESTHETIC; BARBITURATE SEDATIVE-HYPNOTIC
Pregnancy: Category C
Controlled substance: Schedule III

ACTIONS/PHARMACODYNAMICS Ultra-short-acting barbiturate that induces brief general anesthesia without analgesia by depression of CNS. Induction is not unpleasant; loss of consciousness is rapid. Depression of respiratory function is potent and may be prolonged in patient with myasthenia gravis. Reduction in cardiac output (myocardial depression), and peripheral vasodilation frequently accompany anesthesia. Reduces perfusion pressure to kidney, leading to decreased urine output but without renal damage. Rapid redistribution of agent out of brain reduces anesthesia level and increases reflex airway hyperactivity to mechanical stimulation. Muscle relaxation is slight (uterine muscle is unaffected), and relexes are poorly controlled. Since analgesia is slight, thiopental is seldom used alone except for brief minor procedures. For most general anesthetic procedures, concomitant use of a skeletal relaxant, a narcotic agonist analgesic, and an inhalation agent (e.g., nitrous oxide) for maintenance of anesthesia is common.

USES To induce hypnosis and anesthesia prior to or as supplement to other anesthetic agents or as sole agent for brief (15 min) operative procedures. Also used as an anticonvulsant and sedative-hypnotic and for narcoanalysis and narcosynthesis in psychiatric disorders.

ROUTE & DOSAGE

Induction

Adult	IV	Test dose of 25–75 mg; then 50–75 mg at 20–40 s intervals; an additional 50 mg may be given if needed
Child	IV	3–5 mg/kg initially, followed by 1 mg/kg if needed

Convulsions

Adult	IV	75–125 mg

Narcoanalysis

Adult	IV	100 mg/min until confusion occurs

PHARMACOKINETICS **Onset:** 30–60 s. **Duration:** 10–30 min. **Distribution:** distributed into muscle and liver; crosses placenta. **Metabolism:** metabolized in liver. **Elimination:** half-life: 12 min; excreted in urine.

CONTRAINDICATIONS & PRECAUTIONS **Absolute contraindications:** hypersensitivity to barbiturates, history of paradoxic excitation, absence of suitable veins for IV administration, status asthmaticus, acute intermittent or other hepatic porphyrias. Safe use during pregnancy (category C), in nursing women, and in children not established. **Cautious use**

in: coronary artery disease, hypotension, shock; conditions that may potentiate or prolong hypnotic effect including excessive premedication, hepatic or renal dysfunction, myxedema, Addison's disease, severe anemia, increased BUN; increased intracranial pressure; myasthenia gravis; asthma and other respiratory diseases.

ADVERSE/SIDE EFFECTS CNS: headache, retrograde amnesia, emergence delirium, prolonged somnolence and recovery. **CV:** myocardial depression, arrhythmias, circulatory depression. **GI:** nausea, vomiting, regurgitation of gastric contents. **Rectal:** irritation, cramping, rectal bleeding, diarrhea. **Respiratory:** respiratory depression with apnea; hiccups, sneezing, coughing, bronchospasm, laryngospasm. **Other:** hypersensitivity reactions, anaphylaxis (rare), hypothermia, thrombosis and sloughing (with extravasation); salivation, shivering, skeletal muscle hyperactivity.

DIAGNOSTIC TEST INTERFERENCES *Thiopental* may cause decrease in ^{123}I and ^{131}I *thyroidal uptake* test results.

DRUG INTERACTIONS CNS DEPRESSANTS potentiate CNS and respiratory depression. PHENOTHIAZINES increase risk of hypotension. **Probenecid** may prolong anesthesia.

INCOMPATIBILITIES **Solution/additive:** DEXTROSE-RINGER'S COMBINATIONS, **10% dextrose, amikacin, cephapirin, codeine phosphate, dimenhydrinate, diphenhydramine, ephedrine, fibrinolysin, hydromorphone, insulin, levorphanol, meperidine, metaraminol, methadone, morphine, norepinephrine, penicillin G, prochlorperazine, promazine, promethazine, succinylcholine, tetracycline, benzquinamide, chlopromazine, doxapram, glycopyrrolate, sodium bicarbonate.**

NURSING IMPLICATIONS

Administration

- Reconstitute with one of the following diluents: sterile water, normal saline, or 5% dextrose for injection; sterile water is not used for injection if concentration is <2%; such a solution causes hemolysis.
- Solution should be freshly prepared and used promptly. If a precipitate is present, discard solution. Unused portions should be discarded within 24 h.
- Test dose may be given to assess unusual sensitiv-

Common side effects in *italic*; life-threatening effects underlined; generic names in **bold**; classifications in SMALL CAPS

165

ity to thiopental. Following administration, patient should be observed for at least 1 min for unexpected deep anesthesia or respiratory depression.

- Administer slowly by direct IV to avoid overdose.
- If intraarterial injection or extravasation occurs, the site will require particular attention to prevent arteritis, neuritis, and skin slough. An intraarterial injection usually causes extreme pain before patient loses consciousness. Consult physician.
- Store at room temperature 15–30C (59–86F). Avoid excessive heat; protect from freezing.

Assessment & Drug Effects

- Monitor vital signs q3–5min before, during, and after anesthetic administration until recovery and into postoperative period, if necessary.
- Hypovolemia, cranial trauma, or premedication with opioids increases potential for apnea and symptoms of myocardial depression (decreased cardiac output and arterial pressure). Report increases in pulse rate or drop in blood pressure.
- Shivering, excitement, muscle twitching may develop during recovery period from thiopental anesthesia if patient is in pain.

Patient & Family Education

- Inform patient that onset of drug effect is rapid, with loss of consciousness within 30–60 seconds.

ANESTHETIC, LOCAL (ESTER-TYPE)

PROCAINE HYDROCHLORIDE
(proe´kane)
Trade name: Novocain
Classifications: CNS AGENT; LOCAL ANESTHETIC (ESTER-TYPE)
Pregnancy: Category C

ACTIONS/PHARMACODYNAMICS Ester of benzoic acid with local anesthetic properties. Decreases sodium flux into nerve cell (possibly by competing with calcium ions for membrane sites that control permeability to sodium). Thus depresses initial depolarization and prevents propagation and conduction of the nerve impulse. This local anesthetic action produces loss of sensation and motor activity in circumscribed areas of the body close to the injection or application site. Generally, a local vasoconstrictor (e.g., epinephrine) is added to the in-

jection solution to minimize systemic absorption, promote local hemostasis, and prolong local anesthetic action. Lacks surface anesthetic activity.

USES Spinal anesthesia and epidural and peripheral nerve block by injection and infiltration methods.

ROUTE & DOSAGE

Spinal Anesthesia

Adult	SC	10% solution diluted with 0.9% NaCl at 1 ml/5 s

Infiltration Anesthesia/Peripheral Nerve Block

Adult	SC	0.25–0.5% solution

PHARMACOKINETICS Absorption: rapidly absorbed from injection site. **Onset:** 2–5 min. **Duration:** 1 h. **Metabolism:** hydrolyzed by plasma pseudocholinesterases. **Elimination:** 80% of metabolites excreted in urine; half-life: 7.7 min.

CONTRAINDICATIONS & PRECAUTIONS Contraindicated in: known hypersensitivity to procaine or to other drugs of similar chemical structure, to PABA, and to parabens; generalized septicemia, inflammation, or sepsis at proposed injection site; cerebrospinal diseases (e.g., meningitis, syphilis); heart block, hypotension, hypertension; bowel pathology, GI hemorrhage. Safe use in early pregnancy (category C) has not been established. **Cautious use in:** debilitated, elderly, or acutely ill patients; obstetric delivery; increased intraabdominal pressure; known drug allergies and sensitivities, dysrhythmias; shock.

ADVERSE/SIDE EFFECTS CNS: excitatory: anxiety, nervousness, dizziness, tinnitus, circumoral paresthesia, blurred vision, tremors, drowsiness, sedation, convulsions, respiratory arrest. **CV:** myocardial depression, arrhythmias including bradycardia (also fetal bradycardia); hypotension. **GI:** nausea, vomiting. **Skin:** cutaneous lesions of delayed onset, urticaria, pruritus, angioneurotic edema, sweating, syncope, anaphylactoid reaction. **Other: With caudal or epidural anesthesia:** urinary retention, fecal or urinary incontinence, loss of perineal sensation and sexual function, slowing of labor and increased incidence of forceps delivery, headache, backache, high or total spinal block. **With spinal anesthesia:** postspinal headache, arachnoiditis, palsies, spinal nerve paralysis, meningism.

INCOMPATIBILITIES Solution/additive: aminophylline, amobarbital, chlorothiazide, magnesium sulfate, phenobarbital, phenytoin, secobarbital, sodium bicarbonate.

NURSING IMPLICATIONS

Administration

▪ Reconstitution of solution: to prepare 60 ml of a 0.5% solution (5 mg/ml), dilute 30 ml of 1% solution with 30 ml sterile distilled water. Add 0.5–1 ml epinephrine 1:1000/100 ml anesthetic solution for vasoconstrictive effect (1:200,000–1:100,000).

▪ Do not use solutions that are cloudy, discolored, or that contain crystals. Discard unused portion of solutions not containing a preservative. Avoid use of solution with preservative for spinal, epidural, or caudal block.

▪ Injection should be slow with frequent aspirations to avoid inadvertent intravascular administration, which can lead to a systemic reaction.

▪ When used as spinal anesthetic, procaine is injected into the subarachnoid space, usually in interspace between L2 and L5.

▪ Store at 10–30C (59–86F). Avoid freezing.

Assessment & Drug Effects

▪ Reactions during dental procedure are usually mild, transient and produced by epinephrine added to local anesthetic (headache, palpitation, tachycardia, hypertension, dizziness).

▪ Procaine with epinephrine should be used with caution in body areas with limited blood supply (fingers, toes, ears, nose). If used, inspect particular area for evidence of reduced perfusion (vasospasm): pale, cold, sensitive skin.

▪ Hypotension is the most important complication of spinal anesthesia. Risk period is during first 30 min after induction and is intensified by changes in position that promote decreased venous return, or by preexisting hypertension, pregnancy, old age, or hypovolemia.

▪ Hypersensitivities and anaphylactic reactions are not usually dose related.

Patient & Family Education

▪ Inform patient that there will be temporary loss of sensation in the area of the injection.

▪ Caution patient given drug for dental procedure that hot liquids or foods should not be consumed until sensation returns.

ANTICONVULSANT: BARBITURATE

PHENOBARBITAL
(fee-noe-bare´bi-tal)
Trade names: Barbita, Gardenal, Luminal, Solfoton

PHENOBARBITAL SODIUM
Trade names: Luminal Sodium
Classifications: CNS AGENT; BARBITURATE ANTICONVULSANT; SEDATIVE-HYPNOTIC
Pregnancy: Category D
Controlled substance: Schedule IV

ACTIONS/PHARMACODYNAMICS Long-acting barbiturate. Sedative and hypnotic effects of barbiturates appear to be due primarily to interference with impulse transmission of cerebral cortex by inhibition of reticular activating system (concerned with both sleep and arousal mechanisms). Initially, barbiturates suppress REM sleep, but with chronic therapy REM sleep returns to normal. Has no analgesic properties, and small doses may increase reaction to painful stimuli. CNS depression may range from mild sedation to coma, depending on dosage, route of administration, degree of nervous system excitability, and drug tolerance. Phenobarbital limits spread of seizure activity by increasing threshold for motor cortex stimuli. Anticonvulsant action of phenobarbital is shared by mephobarbital, but not other barbiturates, and is reportedly unrelated to sedative effect. Phenobarbital lowers serum bilirubin levels by inducing production of glucuronyl transferase; also increases excretion and flow of bile salts. Barbiturates are habit forming. Tolerance and physical and psychological dependence may occur, especially with long-term use. Use in the elderly is generally being replaced by shorter-acting agents.

USES Long-term management of tonic-clonic (grand mal) seizures and partial seizures; status epilepticus, eclampsia, febrile convulsions in young children. Also used as a sedative in anxiety or tension states; in pediatrics as preoperative and postoperative sedation and to treat pylorospasm in infants. **Unlabeled uses:** treatment and prevention of hyperbilirubinemia in neonates and in the management of chronic cholestasis; benzodiazepine withdrawal.

Common side effects in *italic*; life-threatening effects <u>underlined</u>; generic names in **bold**; classifications in SMALL CAPS

167

ROUTE & DOSAGE

Anticonvulsant

Adult	PO	100–300 mg/d
	IV/IM	200–600 mg up to 20 mg/kg
Child	PO	3–5 mg/kg or 125 mg/m²/d
	IV/IM	100–400 mg up to 20 mg/kg

Sedative

Adult	PO	30–120 mg/d
	IV/IM	100–200 mg/d
Child	PO	6 mg/kg/d or 180 mg/m² in 3 divided doses
	IV/IM	16–100 mg/d (1–3 mg/kg)

PHARMACOKINETICS Absorption: 70–90% absorbed slowly from GI tract. **Peak:** 8–12 h PO; 30 min IV. **Duration:** 4–6 h IV. **Distribution:** 20–45% protein bound; crosses placenta; enters breast milk. **Metabolism:** oxidized in liver to inactivated metabolites. **Elimination:** half-life: 2–6 d; excreted in urine.

CONTRAINDICATIONS & PRECAUTIONS Contraindicated in: sensitivity to barbiturates, manifest hepatic or familial history of porphyria; severe respiratory or renal disease; history of previous addiction to sedative hypnotics; uncontrolled pain; pregnancy (particularly early pregnancy) (category D), nursing mothers, timed-release formulation for children <12 y of age. **Cautious use in:** impaired hepatic, renal, cardiac, or respiratory function; history of allergies; elderly or debilitated patients; patients with fever; hyperthyroidism; diabetes mellitus, or severe anemia; during labor and delivery, lactation; patient with borderline hypoadrenal function.

ADVERSE/SIDE EFFECTS CNS: *somnolence,* nightmares, insomnia, "hangover," headache, anxiety, thinking abnormalities, dizziness, nystagmus, irritability, paradoxic excitement and exacerbation of hyperkinetic behavior (in children); confusion or depression or marked excitement (elderly or debilitated patients); ataxia. **CV:** bradycardia, syncope, hypotension. **GI:** nausea, vomiting, constipation, diarrhea, epigastric pain. **Hypersensitivity:** rash, angioneurotic edema, fever, serum sickness, urticaria; hypoventilation, apnea, laryngospasm, bronchospasm, circulatory collapse. **Injection site** (extravasation): thrombosis, gangrene transient pain, tenderness, redness. **IV:** coughing, hiccuping, laryngospasm. **Skin:** mild maculopapular, morbilliform rash; exfoliative dermatitis (rare), erythema multiforme, Stevens-Johnson syndrome. **Other:** liver damage, megaloblastic anemia, hypocalcemia, osteomalacia, rickets, myalgic, neuralgic, arthritic pain (rare); agranulocytosis, thrombocytopenia, folic acid deficiency, vitamin D deficiency. **Overdosage:** respiratory depression, CNS depression, coma, death.

DIAGNOSTIC TEST INTERFERENCES Barbiturates may affect ***bromsulphalein*** retention tests (by enhancing hepatic uptake and excretion of dye) and increase ***serum phosphatase.***

DRUG INTERACTIONS Alcohol, CNS DEPRESSANTS compound CNS depression; phenobarbital may decrease absorption and increase metabolism of ORAL ANTICOAGULANTS; increases metabolism of CORTICOSTEROIDS, ORAL CONTRACEPTIVES, ANTICONVULSANTS, **digitoxin,** possibly decreasing their effects; ANTIDEPRESSANTS potentiate adverse effects of phenobarbital; **griseofulvin** decreases absorption of phenobarbital.

INCOMPATIBILITIES Solution/Additive: **benzquinamide, cephalothin, chlorpromazine, codeine phosphate, ephedrine, hydralazine, hydrocortisone sodium succinate, hydroxyzine, insulin, levorphanol, meperidine, methadone, morphine, norepi-nephrine,** TETRACYCLINES, **procaine, prochlorperazine, promazine, promethazine, ranitidine, streptomycin, vancomycin.**

NURSING IMPLICATIONS

Administration

- Commercially prepared solutions for injection (sodium phenobarbital) may be diluted with most IV infusion solutions. If not absolutely clear, discard.
- ***Preparation of IV solution:*** slowly introduce sterile water for injection into ampule with sterile syringe. Use at least 10 ml of diluent. Rotate ampule to hasten dissolving drug (may take several minutes). If solution not clear in 5 min or if a precipitate remains, discard.
- IV administration rate: no greater than 60 mg/min. Administer reconstituted IV solution no later than 30 min after preparation.
- Keep patient under constant observation when drug is administered IV, and record vital signs at least every hour or more often if indicated.
- Extravasation of IV phenobarbital may cause necrotic tissue changes that may necessitate skin grafting. Frequently check the injection site.
- Administer IM deep into large muscle mass; volume should not exceed 5 ml at any one site.

Common side effects in *italic*; life-threatening effects underlined; generic names in **bold**; classifications in SMALL CAPS

Patients receiving large doses should be closely observed for at least 30 min to assure that narcosis is not excessive.

- When administering oral barbiturates, observe that patient actually swallows the pill and does not "cheek" it.
- If patient cannot swallow pill, it may be crushed before administration, then mixed with a fluid or with food. (Do not permit patient to swallow dry crushed drug.)
- Store at 15–30C (59–86F) unless otherwise directed by manufacturer.

Assessment & Drug Effects

- Therapeutic serum concentrations of 15–40 $\mu g/ml$ produce anticonvulsant activity in most patients. These values are usually attained after 2 or 3 wk of therapy with a dose of 100–200 mg/d.
- Serum concentrations >50 $\mu g/ml$ may cause coma; concentrations >80 $\mu g/ml$ are potentially lethal.
- Phenobarbital and other long-acting barbiturates may be cumulative in action. Doses in excess of 400 mg/d for more than 90 d are likely to cause some degree of physical dependence.
- Barbiturates do not have analgesic action, and they may be expected to produce restlessness when given to patients in pain.
- The elderly or debilitated patient and children sometimes have parodoxical response to barbiturate therapy: i.e., irritability, marked excitement (inappropriate tearfulness and aggression in children), depression, and confusion. Be alert to unexpected responses and report promptly. Protect the elderly patient from falling, irrational behavior, and effects of depression (anorexia, social withdrawal).
- Hepatic function and hematology tests and determinations of serum folate and vitamin D levels are advised during prolonged therapy.
- Barbiturates increase the metabolism of many drugs, leading to decreased pharmacologic effects of those drugs. Whenever a barbiturate is added to an established regimen of another drug, close observation for changes in effectiveness of the first drug is essential, at least during early phase of barbiturate use.
- Barbiturates decrease or reduce pharmacologic effects of the following drugs (groups): anticoagulants (coumarins), carbamazepine, corticosteroids, digitoxin, doxycycline, estradiol, griseofulvin, oral contraceptives, quinidine, phenothiazines, tricyclic antidepressants. See drug interactions for more information.
- Monitor for and report *chronic toxicity symptoms*:

ataxia, slurred speech, irritability, poor judgment, slight dysarthria, nystagmus on vertical gaze, confusion, insomnia, somatic complaints.

- ***Acute toxicity (serum concentration >80 $\mu g/ml$) symptoms:*** profound CNS depression, respiratory depression that may progress to Cheyne-Stokes respirations, hypoventilation, cyanosis; cold, clammy skin; hypothermia, pupils constricted (but may be dilated in severe intoxication), shock, oliguria, tachycardia, hypotension, respiration arrest, circulatory collapse, death.

Patient & Family Education

- Patients receiving anticonvulsant therapy may experience drowsiness during first few weeks of treatment, but this usually diminishes with continued use of the barbiturate.
- Caution patient to avoid potentially hazardous activities requiring mental alertness such as driving a car or operating machinery, until response to drug is known.
- Alcohol in any amount given with a barbiturate may severely impair judgment and abilities; it should not be consumed by a patient on barbiturate therapy.
- Phenobarbital increases vitamin D metabolism, leading to subtherapeutic levels and possibly onset of osteomalacia, or rickets (long-term therapy). Advise patient to increase vitamin D fortified foods (e.g., milk products). A vitamin D supplement may be prescribed.
- Long-term therapy may result in nutritional folate (B_9) deficiency. Laboratory confirmation is the basis for urging patient to maintain adequate dietary folate intake: fresh vegetables (especially green leafy), fresh fruits, whole grains, liver. A supplement of folic acid may be prescribed.
- Large doses over extended time may cause vitamin B_{12} deficiency.
- Caution patient to adhere to drug regimen; i.e., intervals between doses should not be changed and doses should not be increased or decreased without advice.
- Warn patient not to stop taking drug abruptly because of danger of withdrawal symptoms (8–12 h after last dose), which can be fatal. Early symptoms include apprehension, hand and finger tremors, weakness, dizziness, disturbed vision, nausea, vomiting, sweating, orthostatic hypotension, insomnia. More severe symptoms may develop 2–8 d after withdrawal: delirium, convulsion, status epilepticus (patient with epilepsy). Withdrawal symptoms may occur after a course of therapy with

Common side effects in *italic*; life-threatening effects <u>underlined</u>; generic names in **bold**; classifications in SMALL CAPS

169

600–800 mg/d for 35 d and may last up to 15 d after abrupt cessation of drug therapy.

- Instruct patients on prolonged therapy to report to physician the onset of fever, sore throat or mouth, malaise, easy bruising or bleeding, petechiae, jaundice, rash.
- Advise patients taking barbiturates at home not to keep drug on bedside table or in a readily accessible place. Patients have been known to forget having taken the drug and in half-wakened conditions have accidentally overdosed themselves.
- It is important that pregnancy be avoided in patients receiving barbiturates (reportedly teratogenic). Patients on prolonged therapy should consider alternative methods of contraception in addition to or instead of oral contraceptives to prevent unplanned pregnancy. The neonate born of mother who received barbiturate therapy throughout the last trimester may show withdrawal symptoms for 1–14 d after birth. Symptoms resemble congenital opiate withdrawal symptoms: hyperactivity, restlessness, tremor, hyperreflexia, disturbed sleep.

ANTICONVULSANT: BENZODIAZEPINE

DIAZEPAM

(dye-az´e-pam)

Trade names: Apo-Diazepam, Diazemuls, E-Pam, Meral, Meval, Neo-Calme, Novodipam, Rival, Serenack, Stress-Pam, Valium, Valrelease, Vivol

Classifications: CNS AGENT; BENZODIAZEPINE ANTICONVULSANT; ANXIOLYTIC

Pregnancy: Category D

ACTIONS/PHARMACODYNAMICS Psychotherapeutic agent related to chlordiazepoxide; reportedly superior in antianxiety and anticonvulsant activity, with somewhat shorter duration of action. Like chlordiazepoxide, appears to act at both limbic and subcortical levels of CNS. Shortens REM and stage 4 sleep but increases total sleeptime. Causes transient analgesia after IV administration.

USES Drug of choice for status epilepticus. Management of anxiety disorders, for short-term relief of anxiety symptoms, to allay anxiety and tension prior to surgery, cardioversion and endoscopic procedures, as an amnesic, and treatment for restless legs.

Also used to alleviate acute withdrawal symptoms of alcoholism, voiding problems in the elderly, and adjunctively for relief of skeletal muscle spasm associated with cerebral palsy, paraplegia, athetosis, stiffman syndrome, tetanus.

ROUTE & DOSAGE

Status Epilepticus

Adult	IM/IV	5–10 mg; repeat if needed at 10–15 min intervals up to 30 mg; repeat if needed q2–4h
Child	IM/IV	<5 y: 0.2–0.5 mg slowly q2–5min up to 5 mg
		>5 y: 1 mg slowly q2–5min up to 10 mg; repeat if needed q2–4 h

Anxiety, Muscle Spasm, Convulsions, Alcohol Withdrawal

Adult	PO	2–10 mg b.i.d. to q.i.d. *or* 15–30 mg/d sustained release
	IM/IV	2–10 mg; repeat if needed in 3–4 h
Child	PO	>6 mo: 1–2.5 mg b.i.d. or t.i.d.

PHARMACOKINETICS Absorption: readily absorbed from GI tract; erratic IM absorption. **Onset:** 30–60 min PO; 15–30 min IM; 1–5 min IV. **Peak:** 1–2 h PO. **Duration:** 15 min–1 h IV; up to 3 h PO. **Distribution:** crosses blood-brain barrier and placenta; distributed into breast milk. **Metabolism:** metabolized in liver to active metabolites. **Elimination:** half-life: 20–50 h; excreted primarily in urine.

CONTRAINDICATIONS & PRECAUTIONS Contraindicated in: *Injectable form:* shock, coma, acute alcohol intoxication, depressed vital signs, obstetrical patients, infants ≤30 d of age. *Tablet form:* children <6 mo of age, acute narrow-angle glaucoma, untreated open-angle glaucoma, during or within 14 d of MAO inhibitor therapy. Safe use during pregnancy (category D) and lactation, not established. **Cautious use in:** epilepsy, psychoses, mental depression; myasthenia gravis; impaired hepatic or renal function; drug abuse, addiction-prone individuals. Injectable diazepam used with extreme caution in the elderly, the very ill, and patients with COPD.

ADVERSE/SIDE EFFECTS CNS: *drowsiness*, fatigue, ataxia, confusion, paradoxic rage, dizziness, vertigo, amnesia, vivid dreams, headache, slurred speech, tremor, muscle weakness; EEG changes, tardive dyskinesia. **CV:** hypotension, tachycardia, edema, cardiovascular collapse. **Eye:** blurred vision, diplopia, nystagmus. **GI:** xerostomia, nausea, constipation. **GU:** incontinence, urinary retention, gyneco-

Common side effects in *italic*; life-threatening effects underlined; generic names in **bold**; classifications in SMALL CAPS

mastia (prolonged use), changes in libido, menstrual irregularities. **Other:** hiccups, coughing, throat and chest pain, <u>laryngospasm</u>, ovulation failure, neutropenia, hepatic dysfunction including jaundice; pain, venous thrombosis, phlebitis at injection site.

DRUG INTERACTIONS Alcohol, CNS DEPRESSANTS, ANTICONVULSANTS potentiate CNS depression; **cimetidine** increases diazepam plasma levels, increases toxicity; may decrease antiparkinson effects of **levodopa;** may increase **phenytoin** levels; smoking decreases sedative and antianxiety effects.

INCOMPATIBILITIES Solution/Additive: bleomycin, benzquinamide, dobutamine, doxapram, doxorubicin, fluorouracil, glycopyrrolate, heparin, nalbuphone. **Y-Site:** heparin, potassium chloride, vitamin B complex with C.

NURSING IMPLICATIONS

Administration

- Tablet may be crushed before administration and taken with fluid or mixed with food.
- Supervise oral ingestion to assure drug is swallowed.
- Avoid IV infusion of diazepam; it may precipitate in IV fluids. Also diazepam interacts with plastic IV administration sets and containers with significant reduction in availability of drug.
- *IV injection:* To prevent swelling, irritation, venous thrombosis, phlebitis, give direct IV by injecting drug slowly, taking at least 1 min for each 5 mg (1 ml) given to adults and taking at least 3 min to inject 0.25 mg/kg body weight of children.
- If injection cannot be made directly into vein, manufacturer suggests making injection slowly through infusion tubing as close as possible to vein insertion. Check needle site frequently to prevent extravasation.
- Avoid small veins and intraarterial administration.
- IM administration should be made deep into large muscle mass. Inject slowly. Rotate injection sites.
- When diazepam is used with a narcotic analgesic, the narcotic dose is reduced by at least one third and given in small increments. In some cases, especially in the elderly, the narcotic is unnecessary.
- Abrupt discontinuation of diazepam should generally be avoided. Doses should be tapered to termination.
- Preserved in tight, light-resistant containers at

15–30C (59–86F), unless otherwise specified by manufacturer.

Assessment & Drug Effects

- Most adverse reactions are dose related. Physician will rely on accurate observations and reporting of patient's response to the drug to determine lowest effective maintenance dose.
- Maximum effect may require 1–2 wk; patient tolerance to therapeutic effects may develop after 4 wk of treatment.
- Suicidal tendencies may be present in anxiety states accompanied by depression. Observe necessary preventive precautions.
- When diazepam is given parenterally, hypotension, muscular weakness, tachycardia, and respiratory depression may occur. Observe patient closely and monitor vital signs.
- Periodic blood cell counts and liver function tests are recommended during prolonged therapy.
- Adverse reactions such as drowsiness, ataxia, constipation and urinary retention are more likely to occur in the elderly and debilitated or in those receiving larger doses. Dosage adjustment may be necessary. Supervise ambulation.
- Monitor I&O ratio, including bowel elimination.
- Smoking increases metabolism of diazepam; therefore clinical effectiveness is lowered. Heavy smokers may need a higher dose than the nonsmoker.
- Psychic and physical dependence may occur in patients on long-term high dosage therapy, in those with histories of alcohol or drug addiction, or in those who self-medicate.

Patient & Family Education

- Alcohol and other CNS depressants should be avoided during therapy with diazepam, unless otherwise advised by physician. Concomitant use of these agents can cause severe drowsiness, respiratory depression, and apnea.
- Because of possible sedation, activities requiring mental alertness and precision should be avoided until reaction to diazepam has been evaluated.
- The patient should be advised that if she becomes pregnant during therapy or intends to become pregnant she should communicate with her physician regarding desirability of discontinuing drug.
- Caution patient to take drug as prescribed and not to change dose or dose intervals.
- Patient should check with physician before taking any OTC drug while on diazepam therapy.

Common side effects in *italic*; life-threatening effects <u>underlined</u>; generic names in **bold**; classifications in SMALL CAPS

171

ANTICONVULSANT: HYDANTOIN

PHENYTOIN
(fen´i-toy-in)
Trade names: Dilantin-125, Dilantin-30 Pediatric, Dilantin Infatab

PHENYTOIN SODIUM EXTENDED
Trade name: Dilantin Kapseals

PHENYTOIN SODIUM PROMPT
Trade names: Dilantin, Diphenylan Sodium
Classifications: CNS AGENT; HYDANTOIN ANTI-CONVULSANT; CARDIOVASCULAR AGENT; ANTIARRHYTHMIC
Pregnancy: Category D

ACTIONS/PHARMACODYNAMICS Hydantoin derivative chemically related to phenobarbital. Precise mechanism of anticonvulsant action not known, but drug use is accompanied by reduced voltage, frequency, and spread of electrical discharges within the motor cortex, resulting in seizure activity inhibition. Unlike phenobarbital, phenytoin has little hypnotic action and has limited ability to modify threshold in electroconvulsive seizures. Has class IB antiarrhythmic properties similar to those of lidocaine and tocainamide (also class IB agents); in abnormal tissue causes slight increase in AV conduction velocity depressed by digitalis glycosides, prolongs effective refractory period, suppresses ventricular pacemaker automaticity, and may slow conduction or cause complete block in abnormal ventricular fibers. Shortens action potential duration and improves resting potential. Membrane stabilizing effect on pancreas may inhibit effective insulin release. Induces hepatic microsomal enzymes and therefore affects the metabolism of many other drugs. Like other hydantoin derivatives, increases metabolic inactivation of vitamin D and has antifolate properties.

USES To control tonic-clonic (grand mal) seizures, psychomotor and nonepileptic seizures (e.g., Reye's syndrome, after head trauma). Also used to prevent or treat seizures occurring during or after neurosurgery. Is not effective for absence seizures. **Unlabeled use:** Antiarrhythmic agent (phenytoin IV)

especially in treatment of digitalis-induced arrhythmias; treatment of trigeminal neuralgia (tic douloureux).

ROUTE & DOSAGE

Anticonvulsant

Adult	PO	15–18 mg/kg or 1 g loading dose; then 300 mg/d in 1–3 divided doses; may be gradually increased by 100 mg/wk until seizures are controlled
	IV	15–18 mg/kg or 1 g loading dose; then 100 mg t.i.d.
Child	PO/IV	500–600 mg loading dose; then 5 mg/kg or 250 mg/m² in 2–3 divided doses

PHARMACOKINETICS Absorption: completely absorbed from GI tract. **Peak:** 1.5–3 h prompt release; 4–12 h extended release. **Distribution:** 95% protein bound; crosses placenta; small amount in breast milk. **Metabolism:** oxidized in liver to inactive metabolites. **Elimination:** half-life: 22 h; metabolites excreted by kidneys.

CONTRAINDICATIONS & PRECAUTIONS
Contraindicated in: hypersensitivity to hydantoin products, rash, seizures due to hypoglycemia, sinus bradycardia, complete or incomplete heart block, Adams-Stokes syndrome. **Cautious use in:** impaired hepatic or renal function; alcoholism; blood dyscrasias; hypotension, heart block, bradycardia, severe myocardial insufficiency, impending or frank heart failure; elderly, debilitated, gravely ill patients; pancreatic adenoma; pregnancy (category D), nursing mothers; diabetes mellitus, hyperglycemia; respiratory depression; acute intermittent porphyria.

ADVERSE/SIDE EFFECTS CNS:
Usually dose-related: nystagmus, *drowsiness,* ataxia, dizziness, mental confusion, tremors, insomnia, headache, seizures. **CV:** bradycardia, hypotension, cardiovascular collapse, ventricular fibrillation, phlebitis. **Eye:** photophobia, conjunctivitis, diplopia, blurred vision. **GI:** *gingival hyperplasia,* nausea, vomiting, constipation, epigastric pain, dysphagia, loss of taste, weight loss, hepatitis, liver necrosis. **Hematologic:** thrombocytopenia, leukopenia, leukocytosis, agranulocytosis, pancytopenia, eosinophilia; megaloblastic, hemolytic, or aplastic anemias. **Metabolic:** fever, hyperglycemia, glycosuria, weight gain, edema, transient increase in serum thyrotropic (TSH) level. **Skin:** alopecia, hirsutism (especially in young female); rash: scarlatini-

Common side effects in *italic*; life-threatening effects underlined; generic names in **bold**; classifications in SMALL CAPS

form, maculopapular, urticarial, morbilliform; (may be fatal): bullous, exfoliative, or purpuric dermatitis; Stevens-Johnson syndrome, <u>toxic epidermal necrolysis</u>, keratosis, neonatal hemorrhage. **Other:** acute renal failure, osteomalacia or rickets associated with hypocalcemia and elevated alkaline phosphatase activity; acute pneumonitis, pulmonary fibrosis; periarteritis nodosum, acute systemic lupus erythematosus, craniofacial abnormalities (with enlargement of lips); Peyronie's disease, lymphadenopathy.

DIAGNOSTIC TEST INTERFERENCES Phenytoin (hydantoins) may produce lower than normal values for *dexamethasone* or *metyrapone* tests; may increase serum levels of *glucose, BSP,* and *alkaline phosphatase* and may decrease *PBI* and *urinary steroid* levels.

DRUG INTERACTIONS Alcohol decreases phenytoin effects; OTHER ANTICONVULSANTS may increase or decrease phenytoin levels; phenytoin may decrease absorption and increase metabolism of ORAL ANTICOAGULANTS; phenytoin increases metabolism of CORTICOSTEROIDS and ORAL CONTRACEPTIVES, thus decreasing their effectiveness; **amiodarone, chloramphenicol,** and **omeprazole** increase phenytoin levels; ANTITUBERCULOSIS AGENTS decrease phenytoin levels. **Drug-food interactions:** Folic acid, calcium, and vitamin D absorption may be decreased by phenytoin; phenytoin absorption may be decreased by enteral nutrition supplements.

INCOMPATIBILITIES Solution/additive: 5% dextrose, **amikacin, aminophylline, bretylium, cephapirin, codeine phosphate, dobutamine, insulin, levorphanol, lidocaine, lincomycin, meperidine, metaraminol, methadone, morphine, nitroglycerin, norepinephrine, pentobarbital, procaine, secobarbital, streptomycin. Y-site: amikacin, bretylium, dobutamine, lidocaine, heparin, potassium chloride, vitamin B complex with C.**

NURSING IMPLICATIONS

Administration

- If patient cannot take a whole tablet, it may be crushed before administration. Drug should be mixed with food (e.g., applesauce) or fluid; have patient swallow a fluid first; then follow with the diluted or mixed drug along with a full glass of water, milk, or with food. This drug is strongly alkaline, and should not be swallowed without prior

preparation to prevent esophageal and gastric direct contact.

- Shake suspension vigorously before pouring to ensure uniform distribution of drug. Suspension is available in two concentrations; 125 mg/5 ml and 30 mg/5 ml and is dispensed in bottles or individual unit dose foil pouches.
- Prompt release capsules and chewable tablets are not intended for once-a-day dosage since drug is too quickly bioavailable and can therefore lead to toxic serum levels.
- Extended-release capsules only are used for once-a-day dosage regimens.
- Two chewable tablets are not dose-exchangeable for one 100 mg capsule of phenytoin sodium: capsules contain 92 mg, but tablet contains 50 mg.
- Solubility of phenytoin is pH dependent; therefore, to prevent precipitation, avoid mixing it with other drugs or adding to any infusion solution.
- A slightly yellowed injectable solution may be used safely. Precipitation may be caused by refrigeration, but slow warming to room temperature restores clarity. Do not administer unclear solution.
- During IV phenytoin administration, observe injection site frequently to prevent infiltration. Local soft tissue irritation may be serious, leading to erosion of tissues. The elderly woman, especially with peripheral vascular disease, seems to be at high risk.
- Administer 50 mg or fraction thereof over 1 min (25 mg/min in elderly or when used as antiarrhythmic). Usually phenytoin is not given as a continuous infusion.
- To minimize local venous irritation, each IV injection is followed with an injection of sterile saline through the same in-place catheter or needle.
- To reduce side effects with IV administration, lower doses than the usual adult range are given to geriatric, severely ill, debilitated patients or those with liver damage, and the flow rate is reduced to 50 mg over a 2–3-min period.
- Store phenytoin at 15–30C (59–86F) in tightly closed container. Protect from light.

Assessment & Drug Effects

- *Therapeutic serum concentration:* 10–20 µg/ml; *Toxic level:* 30–50 µg/ml; *Lethal level:* 100 µg/ml. Steady state therapeutic levels are not achieved for at least 7–10 d.
- Margin between toxic and therapeutic IV dose is relatively small. Continuously monitor vital signs and symptoms during IV infusion and for an hour afterward. Watch for respiratory depression. If patient is elderly or has cardiac disease, constant observation and a cardiac monitor are necessary.

- Observe patient closely for neurologic side effects. Have on hand oxygen, **atropine,** vasopressor, assisted ventilation, seizure precaution equipment (mouth gag, nonmetal airway, suction apparatus).
- Gingival hyperplasia appears most commonly in children and adolescents and never occurs in edentulous patients. Adjustment of phenytoin dosage for patients on insulin or of sulfonylurea dosage may be necessary.
- Patients on prolonged therapy should have adequate intake of vitamin D–containing foods and sufficient exposure to sunlight.
- Periodic checks are indicated for decrease in serum calcium levels. Particularly susceptible: black children, patients receiving other anticonvulsants concurrently, who are inactive, have limited exposure to sun, or whose dietary intake is inadequate.
- Observe patient for symptoms of folic acid deficiency: neuropathy, mental dysfunction.
- Serum concentration of magnesium may be decreased by phenytoin therapy. Be alert to symptoms of hypomagnesemia (see Chapter 3); neuromuscular symptoms: tetany, positive Chvostek's and Trousseau's signs, seizures, tremors, ataxia, vertigo, nystagmus, muscular fasciculations.

Patient & Family Education
- Inform patient that drug may make urine pink or red to red-brown.
- Phenytoin can unmask a low thyroid reserve. Advise patient on long-term therapy to report symptoms of fatigue, dry skin, deepening voice.
- Caution patient to report promptly onset of liver dysfunction as evidenced by jaundice. Since phenytoin is largely metabolized in the liver, impairment of liver function leads to increased serum levels and toxicity. Early recognition of a toxic reaction may save the patient's life.
- Caution patient not to alter prescribed drug regimen. Abrupt drug discontinuation may precipitate seizures and status epilepticus.
- Advise patient not to request change in drug brand when refilling prescription. Differences can alter phenytoin serum levels.
- Warn patient about the effects of alcohol: alcohol intake may increase phenytoin serum levels, leading to phenytoin toxicity. Dosage for chronic alcoholics needs to be higher.
- Phenytoin should be discontinued immediately if a measleslike skin rash appears.
- If patient is receiving phenytoin to prevent major seizures, it probably will not be stopped during pregnancy because of the risk of precipitated status epilepticus with attendant hypoxia, a danger to both mother and fetus.
- Influenza vaccine during phenytoin treatment may increase seizure activity. Patient should be alerted in case a change in dose is necessary.

ANTICONVULSANT: SUCCINIMIDE

ETHOSUXIMIDE
(eth-oh-sux´i-mide)
Trade Name: Zarontin
Classifications: CNS AGENT; SUCCINIMIDE ANTICONVULSANT
Pregnancy: Category C

ACTIONS/PHARMACODYNAMICS Succinimide anticonvulsant. Reduces frequency of epileptiform attacks, apparently by depressing motor cortex and elevating CNS threshold to stimuli. Usually ineffective in management of psychomotor or major motor seizures.

USES Management of absence (petit mal) seizures, myoclonic seizures, and akinetic epilepsy. May be administered with other anticonvulsants when other forms of epilepsy coexist with petit mal.

ROUTE & DOSAGE

Absence Seizures

Adult	PO	250 mg b.i.d.; may increase q4–7d prn (max 1.5 g/d)
Child	PO	6–12 y: Same as for adult
		3–6 y: 250 mg/d; may increase q4–7d prn (max 1 g/d)

PHARMACOKINETICS Absorption: readily absorbed from GI tract. **Peak:** 4 h; steady state: 4–7 d. **Metabolism:** metabolized in liver. **Elimination:** half-life: 30 h in children, 60 h in adults; excreted slowly in urine; small amounts excreted in bile and feces.

CONTRAINDICATIONS & PRECAUTIONS Contraindicated in: hypersensitivity to succinimides; severe liver or renal disease; use alone in mixed types of epilepsy (may increase frequency of grand mal seizures). Safe use during pregnancy (category C), in nursing mothers, and in children <3 y not established.

ADVERSE/SIDE EFFECTS CNS: drowsiness, hiccups, ataxia, dizziness, headache, euphoria, restlessness, irritability, anxiety, hyperactivity, aggressiveness, depression, inability to concentrate, fatigue, muscle weakness, lethargy, confusion, sleep disturbances, night terrors, hypochondriacal behavior; rarely: psychosis, increased depression with overt suicidal intentions, auditory hallucinations. **Eye:** blurred vision, myopia, photophobia, periorbital edema. **GI:** nausea, vomiting, *anorexia, epigastric distress,* abdominal pain, *weight loss,* diarrhea, constipation, swelling of the tongue. **GU:** increased libido, vaginal bleeding, renal dysfunction potential. **Hematologic:** eosinophilia, leukopenia, thrombocytopenia, <u>agranulocytosis, pancytopenia, aplastic anemia</u>, positive direct Coombs' test. **Skin:** hirsutism, alopecia, erythema multiforme, Stevens-Johnson syndrome, pruritic erythematous skin eruptions, urticaria, <u>exfoliative dermatitis</u>, SLE. **Other:** hyperemia, gingival hyperplasia.

DRUG INTERACTIONS Carbamazepine decreases ethosuximide levels; **isoniazid** significantly increases ethosuximide levels; levels of both **phenobarbital** and ethosuximide may be altered with increased seizure frequency.

NURSING IMPLICATIONS

Administration

- May be taken with food if GI distress occurs.
- Store capsules in tight containers, and syrup in light-resistant containers at 15–30C (59–86F); avoid freezing.

Assessment & Drug Effects

- Baseline and periodic hematologic studies and tests of liver and renal function should be made.
- GI symptoms, drowsiness, ataxia, dizziness, and other neurologic side effects occur frequently and indicate the need for dosage adjustment.
- Close observation is required during the period of dosage adjustment and whenever other medications are added to or eliminated from the drug regimen. *Therapeutic serum levels:* 40–80 μg/ml.
- Behavioral changes are most likely to occur in the patient with a prior history of psychiatric disturbances. Close supervision is indicated. Drug should be withdrawn slowly if these symptoms appear.

Patient & Family Education

- Abrupt withdrawal of ethosuximide (whether used alone or in combination therapy) may precipitate seizures or petit mal status. Caution patient to discontinue drug only under physician supervision.
- May impair mental and physical abilities; caution the patient to avoid driving a motor vehicle and other hazardous activities.
- Caution the patient and responsible family members to report any unusual sign or symptoms promptly to the physician.
- Instruct patient to monitor weight on a weekly basis. Anorexia and weight loss should be reported to physician and may indicate need to reduce dosage.
- Instruct the patient to carry a wallet identification card or jewelry (e.g., Medic Alert) indicating that patient has epilepsy, is taking medication, and the physician's name and telephone number.

ANXIOLYTIC, SEDATIVE-HYPNOTIC: BARBITURATE

SECOBARBITAL

(see-koe-bar´bi-tal)
Trade names: Novosecobarb, Seconal

SECOBARBITAL SODIUM

Trade name: Seconal Sodium
Classifications: CNS AGENT; ANXIOLYTIC; SEDATIVE-HYPNOTIC; BARBITURATE
Pregnancy: Category C
Controlled substance: Schedule II

ACTIONS/PHARMACODYNAMICS: Short-acting barbiturate with CNS depressant effects and anticonvulsant action similar to that of phenobarbital.

USES Hypnotic for simple insomnia and preoperatively to provide basal hypnosis for general, spinal, or regional anesthesia. Effective in the emergency control of acute convulsive conditions (e.g., tetanus, toxic reactions to poisons) and in the management of acute agitated behavior.

PHARMACOKINETICS Absorption: 90% absorbed from GI tract. **Onset:** 15–30 min PO; 7–10 min IM; 1–3 min IV. **Duration:** 1–4 h PO; 15 min IV. **Distribution:** crosses placenta; distributed into breast milk. **Metabolism:** metabolized in liver. **Elimination:** half-life: 30 h; excreted in urine.

Common side effects in *italic*; life-threatening effects <u>underlined</u>; generic names in **bold**; classifications in SMALL CAPS

175

ROUTE & DOSAGE

Sedative

Adult	PO	100–300 mg/d in 3 divided doses
Child	PO/PR*	4–6 mg/kg/d in 3 divided doses

Preoperative Sedative

Adult	PO	100–300 mg 1–2 h before surgery
Child	PO	50–100 mg 1–2 h before surgery
	PR*	>3 y: 60–120 mg 1–2 h before surgery
		6 mo–3 y: 60 mg 1–2 h before surgery
		< 6 mo: 30–60 mg 1–2 h before surgery
	IM	4–5 mg/kg 1–2 h before surgery

Hypnotic

Adult	PO/IM	100–200 mg
Child	IM	3–5 mg/kg

Acute Convulsive Episode

Adult	IM	5.5 mg/kg repeated q3–4h if needed
	IV	5.5 mg/kg repeated q3–4h if needed; infuse at ≤50 mg/15 s
Child	IM	3–5 mg/kg

Adjunct to Spinal Anesthesia

Adult	IV	50–100 mg (max 250 mg/dose), infused at ≤ 50 mg/15 s
Child	PR*	> 40 kg: 5 mg/kg
		< 40 kg: 4 mg/kg

*Make the rectal solution by diluting the IV with lukewarm tap water to a concentration of 10–15 mg/ml and administer rectally following a cleansing enema.

CONTRAINDICATIONS & PRECAUTIONS Contraindicated in: history of sensitivity to barbiturates; pregnancy category C; parturition, fetal immaturity, uncontrolled pain. Use of sterile injection containing polyethylene glycol vehicle in patients with renal insufficiency. **Cautious use in:** pregnant women with toxemia or history of bleeding.

ADVERSE/SIDE EFFECTS Drowsiness, lethargy, hangover, paradoxical excitement in the elderly patient; respiratory depression, laryngospasm, fall in BP (with rapid IV).

DRUG INTERACTIONS Phenmetrazine antagonizes effects of secobarbital; CNS DEPRESSANTS, **alcohol,** SEDATIVES compound CNS depression; MAO INHIBITORS cause excessive CNS depression; **methoxyflurane** increases risk of nephrotoxicity.

INCOMPATIBILITIES Solution/Additive: **benzquinamide, codeine, cimetidine, ephedrine, erythromycin, glycopyrrolate, hydrocortisone, insulin, levorphanol, methadone, norepinephrine, pentazocine, phenytoin, procaine, sodium bicarbonate, streptomycin, tetracycline, vancomycin. Y-site: cimetidine, glycopyrrolate.**

NURSING IMPLICATIONS

Administration

- Discard parenteral solutions that are not clear or that contain a precipitate.
- Aqueous solutions of secobarbital sodium for injection are not stable; they must be freshly prepared and used within 30 min after container is opened. Reconstitute secobarbital sodium powder with sterile water for injection (incompatible with bacteriostatic water for injection or lactated Ringer's injection). Following addition of water, rotate ampul; do not shake it. Several minutes are required to dissolve drug completely. If solution is not completely clear within 5 min, do not use. Consult package literature for details.
- Secobarbital sodium injection in aqueous polyethylene glycol vehicle is more stable than aqueous solution. It should be refrigerated (2–8C, 36–46F). May be diluted with sterile water for injection, 0.9% NaCl, or Ringer's injection (not lactated). Consult package literature for details.
- Administer IM injection deep into large muscle mass. Carefully aspirate before injecting drug to avoid inadvertent entry into blood vessel.
- IV secobarbital may be administered by direct IV at a rate of 50 mg or a fraction thereof over 30–60 seconds.

Assessment & Drug Effects

- Patients receiving drug IV must be kept under constant observation. Monitor BP, pulse, and respiration q3–5 min.
- Following IM injection of large hypnotic dose, observe patient closely for 20–30 min to assure that hypnosis is not excessive.
- When secobarbital is administered to pregnant patient, fetal heart beat should be closely monitored. Report slowing or irregularities.
- If patient cannot swallow pill, it may be crushed before administration, then mixed with a fluid or with food. (Do not permit patient to swallow dry crushed drug.)

Common side effects in *italic*; life-threatening effects underlined; generic names in **bold**; classifications in SMALL CAPS

- The elderly or debilitated patient and children sometimes have paradoxical response to barbiturate therapy, i.e., irritability, marked excitement (inappropriate tearfulness and aggression in children), depression and confusion. Be alert to unexpected responses and report promptly. Protect the elderly patient from falling, irrational behavior, and effects of depression (anorexia, social withdrawal).
- Although it is uncommon, the patient may become irritable, uncooperative, and restive after a subhypnotic dose of a short-acting barbiturate.
- Barbiturates do not have analgesic action, and they may be expected to produce restlessness when given to patients in pain.
- Alcohol in any amount given with a barbiturate may severely impair judgment and abilities; it should not be consumed by a patient on barbiturate therapy.
- Long-term therapy may result in nutritional folate (B$_9$) and vitamin D deficiency.
- Hepatic function and hematology tests and determinations of serum folate and vitamin D levels are advised during prolonged therapy.
- Barbiturates increase the metabolism of many drugs, leading to decreased pharmacologic effects of those drugs. Whenever a barbiturate is added to an established regimen of another drug, close observation for changes in effectiveness of the first drug is essential, at least during early phase of barbiturate use.
- *Chronic toxicity (dependence; drug abuse):* behavior simulates that of the chronic alcoholic: desire or need to continue taking the drug without physician's knowledge; self-limited abstinence periods; patient begins to see a number of physicians, never admitting to multiple prescriptions. Symptoms: ataxia, slurred speech, irritability, poor judgment, slight dysarthria, nystagmus on vertical gaze, confusion, insomnia, somatic complaints.
- *Acute toxicity (intoxication):* profound CNS depression, respiratory depression that may progress to Cheyne-Stokes respirations, hypoventilation, cyanosis; cold, clammy skin; hypothermia, pupils constricted (but may be dilated in severe intoxication), shock, oliguria, tachycardia, hypotension, respiration arrest, circulatory collapse, death. Frequently, pressure sores are on skin surfaces pressured by the unconscious patient's body weight; these may develop within 4 h after drug ingestion.

Patient & Family Education
- Following drug administration an ambulatory patient should be adivsed to avoid driving a car or other potentially hazardous activities for the remainder of day.
- Advise patients taking barbiturates at home not to keep drug on bedside table or in a readily accessible place. Patients have been known to forget having taken the drug, and in half-wakened conditions have accidentally overdosed themselves.
- It is important that pregnancy be avoided in patients receiving barbiturates (reportedly teratogenic). Patients on prolonged therapy should consider alternative methods of contraception in addition or instead of oral contraceptives to prevent unplanned pregnancy. The neonate born of a mother who received barbiturate therapy throughout the last trimester may show withdrawal symptoms for 1–14 d after birth. Symptoms resemble congenital opiate withdrawal symptoms: hyperactivity, restlessness, tremor, hyperreflexia, disturbed sleep.
- Instruct patients on prolonged therapy to report to physician the onset of fever, sore throat or mouth, malaise, easy bruising or bleeding, petechiae, jaundice, rash.

ANXIOLYTIC, SEDATIVE-HYPNOTIC: BENZODIAZEPINE

LORAZEPAM
(lor-a´ze-pam)
Trade names: Ativan, Alzapam
Classifications: CNS AGENT; BENZODIAZEPINE; ANXIOLYTIC, SEDATIVE-HYPNOTIC
Pregnancy: Category D
Controlled substance: Schedule IV

ACTIONS/PHARMACODYNAMICS Most potent of the available benzodiazepines. Effects (anxiolytic, sedative, hypnotic, and skeletal muscle relaxant) are mediated by the inhibitory neurotransmitter GABA (gamma aminobutyric acid). Action sites: thalamic, hypothalamic, and limbic levels of CNS. Limitations and interactions similar to those of chlordiazepoxide.

USES Management of anxiety disorders, and for short-term relief of symptoms of anxiety. Also used for preanesthetic medication to produce sedation and

Common side effects in *italic*; life-threatening effects underlined; generic names in **bold**; classifications in SMALL CAPS

177

to reduce anxiety and recall of events related to day of surgery. **Unlabeled use:** for management of status epilepticus, chemotherapy-induced nausea and vomiting.

ROUTE & DOSAGE

Antianxiety

Adult	PO	2–6 mg/d in divided doses (max 10 mg/d)

Insomnia

Adult	PO	2–4 mg at bedtime

Premedication

Adult	IM	2–4 mg (0.05 mg/kg) at least 2 h before surgery
	IV	0.044 mg/kg up to 2 mg 15–20 min before surgery

PHARMACOKINETICS Absorption: readily absorbed from GI tract. **Onset:** 1–5 min IV; 15–30 min IM. **Peak:** 60–90 min IM; 2 h PO. **Duration:** 12–24 h. **Distribution:** crosses placenta; distributed into breast milk. **Metabolism:** not metabolized in liver. **Elimination:** half-life: 10–20 h; excreted in urine.

CONTRAINDICATIONS & PRECAUTIONS Contraindicated in: known sensitivity to benzodiazepines; acute narrow-angle glaucoma; primary depressive disorders or psychosis; children <12 y (PO preparation); coma, shock, acute alcohol intoxication; pregnancy (category D), and nursing mothers. **Cautious use in:** renal or hepatic impairment; organic brain syndrome; myasthenia gravis; narrow-angle glaucoma; suicidal tendency; GI disorders; elderly and debilitated patients; limited pulmonary reserve.

ADVERSE/SIDE EFFECTS Usually disappear with continued medication or with reduced dosage. **CNS:** anterograde amnesia, *drowsiness, sedation,* dizziness, weakness, unsteadiness, disorientation, depression, sleep disturbance, restlessness, confusion, hallucinations. **CV:** hypertension or hypotension. **Eye:** blurred vision, diplopia. **Ear:** depressed hearing. **GI:** nausea, vomiting, abdominal discomfort, anorexia.

DRUG INTERACTIONS Alcohol, CNS DEPRESSANTS, ANTICONVULSANTS potentiate CNS depression; **cimetidine** increases lorazepam plasma levels, increases toxicity; lorazepam may decrease antiparkinsonism effects of **levodopa;** may increase **phenytoin** levels; smoking decreases sedative and antianxiety effects.

INCOMPATIBILITIES Y-Site: ondansetron.

NURSING IMPLICATIONS

Administration

- IM lorazepam is injected undiluted, deep into a large muscle mass.
- Prepare lorazepam for IV administration immediately before use. Dilute with an equal volume of sterile water, D5W, or NS. Do not use a discolored solution or one that has a precipitate.
- *IV injection:* diluted drug is injected directly into vein or into IV infusion tubing at rate not to exceed 2 mg/min and with repeated aspiration to confirm IV entry. Extreme precautions should be taken to prevent intraarterial injection and perivascular extravasation.
- Inadvertent intraarterial injection may produce arteriospasm resulting in gangrene that may require amputation.
- Patients >50 y may have more profound and prolonged sedation with IV lorazepam. Usually an initial dose of 2 mg should not be exceeded.
- When lorazepam is given as a preoperative medication, the narcotic analgesic should be administered at the usual preoperative time.
- When higher oral dosage is required, the evening dose should be increased before the daytime doses.
- Keep parenteral preparation in refrigerator; do not freeze. Store tablets at 15–30C (59–86F) unless manufacturer specifies otherwise.

Assessment & Drug Effects

- Equipment for maintaining patent airway should be immediately available before IV administration. Partial airway obstruction has occurred in the lorazepam-medicated patient undergoing regional anesthesia.
- IM or IV lorazepam injection of 2–4 mg is usually followed by a depth of drowsiness or sleepiness that permits patient to respond to simple instructions whether patient appears to be asleep or awake.
- Supervise ambulation of elderly patient for at least 8 h after lorazepam injection to prevent falling and injury.
- Periodic blood counts and liver function tests are

Common side effects in *italic*; life-threatening effects underlined; generic names in **bold**; classifications in SMALL CAPS

recommended for the patient on long-term therapy.

- Closely supervise patient who exhibits depression with anxiety; the possibility of suicide exists, particularly when there is apparent improvement in mood.

Patient & Family Education

- Most patients will have difficulty recalling perioperative events. This *retrograde amnesia* is optimum within 2 h after IM administration and 15–20 min after IV injection. Full recall and recognition may not return for about 8 h. Inform patient of this possibility.
- If a narcotic analgesic, another tranquilizer, or sedative is given with injectable lorazepam, lack of recall may extend for as long as 48 h.
- Advise patients to refrain from any hazardous activity, including dangerous sports and driving a car, for a least 24–48 h after receiving IM injection of lorazepam. If patients are on PO drug therapy, patients should not drive until the sedative action of lorazepam has diminished.
- Advise patient to avoid large volume intake of coffee. Anxiolytic effects of lorazepam can significantly be altered by 500 mg caffeine (1 cup of coffee contains 125–250 mg caffeine).
- Alcoholic beverages should not be consumed for at least 24–48 h after an injection and should be avoided when patient is on an oral regimen.
- Habituation and dependence may be developed with use of this drug.
- If daytime psychomotor function is impaired, see physician; change in regimen or drug may be needed.
- Regimen termination should be done gradually over a period of several days. Warn patient on long-term therapy not to stop the drug abruptly because symptoms similar to those of barbiturate and alcohol withdrawal may be induced: feelings of panic, tonic-clonic seizures, tremors, abdominal and muscle cramps, sweating, vomiting.
- Advise patient not to self-medicate with OTC drugs unless the physician approves.
- Tell the patient that if she becomes pregnant or wishes to become pregnant, she should discuss drug continuation with her physician.

ANXIOLYTIC, SEDATIVE-HYPNOTIC: CARBAMATE

MEPROBAMATE
(me-proe-ba´mate)
Trade names: Equanil, Meprospan, Miltown, Neuramate, Neurate
Classifications: CNS AGENT; PSYCHOTHERAPEUTIC; CARBAMATE ANXIOLYTIC, SEDATIVE-HYPNOTIC
Pregnancy: Category D
Controlled substance: Schedule IV

ACTIONS/PHARMACODYNAMICS Propanediol carbamate derivative structurally and pharmacologically related to carisoprodol. CNS depressant actions similar to those of barbiturates. Acts on multiple sites in CNS and appears to block corticothalamic impulses. Has no effect on medulla, reticular activating system, or autonomic nervous system. Skeletal muscle relaxant effect is probably related to sedative rather than to direct action. Hypnotic doses suppress REM sleep.

USES To relieve anxiety and tension of psychoneurotic states and as adjunct in disease states associated with anxiety and tension. Also used to promote sleep in anxious, tense patients.

ROUTE & DOSAGE

Sedative

Adult	PO	1.2–1.6 g/d in 3–4 divided doses (max 2.4 g/d)
Child	PO	100–200 mg b.i.d. or t.i.d.

Hypnotic

Adult	PO	400–800 mg
Child	PO	200 mg

PHARMACOKINETICS Absorption: well absorbed from GI tract. **Peak:** 1–3 h. **Onset:** 1 h. **Distribution:** uniformly distributed throughout body; crosses placenta. **Metabolism:** rapidly metabolized in liver. **Elimination:** half-life: 10–11 h; renally excreted; excreted in breast milk.

CONTRAINDICATIONS & PRECAUTIONS Contraindicated in: history of hypersensitivity to meprobamate or related carbamates such as carisoprodol and

---

Common side effects in *italic*; life-threatening effects underlined; generic names in **bold**; classifications in SMALL CAPS

tybamate; history of acute intermittent porphyria; pregnancy (category D), nursing women, children <6 y. **Cautious use in:** impaired renal or hepatic function; convulsive disorders; history of alcoholism or drug abuse; patients with suicidal tendencies.

ADVERSE/SIDE EFFECTS Allergy or idiosyncrasy: itchy, urticarial, or erythematous maculopapular rash; exfoliative dermatitis, petechiae, purpura, ecchymoses, eosinophilia, peripheral edema, angioneurotic edema, adenopathy, fever, chills, proctitis, bronchospasm, oliguria, anuria, Stevens-Johnson syndrome; anaphylaxis. **CNS:** *drowsiness and ataxia,* dizziness, vertigo, slurred speech, headache, weakness, paresthesias, impaired visual accommodation, paradoxic euphoria and rage reactions, seizures in epileptics, panic reaction, rapid EEG activity. **CV:** hypotensive crisis, syncope, palpitation, tachycardia, arrhythmias, transient ECG changes. **GI:** anorexia, nausea, vomiting, diarrhea. **Hematologic:** aplastic anemia (rare): leukopenia, agranulocytosis, thrombocytopenia. **Other:** exacerbation of acute intermittent porphyria, grand mal attack, respiratory depression, and circulatory collapse (toxic doses).

DIAGNOSTIC TEST INTERFERENCES Meprobamate may cause falsely high *urinary steroid* determinations. *Phentolamine* tests may be falsely positive; meprobamate should be withdrawn at least 24 h and preferably 48–72 h before the test.

DRUG INTERACTIONS Alcohol and other CNS DEPRESSANTS potentiate CNS depression.

NURSING IMPLICATIONS

Administration
- May be administered with food to minimize gastric distress.
- Treatment of meprobamate physical dependence consists of gradual drug withdrawal over 1–2 wk to prevent onset of withdrawal symptoms.
- Store drug at 15–30C (59–86F), unless otherwise specified by manufacturer.

Assessment & Drug Effects
- The elderly and debilitated patients are prone to oversedation and to the hypotensive effects of meprobamate, especially during early therapy. Generally, lower doses are prescribed and dose increases are made gradually.
- Caution patient to make position changes slowly, especially from recumbent to upright, and to dangle legs for a few minutes before standing. Supervise ambulation, if necessary.

- Hypnotic doses may cause increased motor activity during sleep. Side rails are advisable.
- If daytime psychomotor function is impaired, consult physician. A change in regimen or drug may be indicated.
- Continued effectiveness of response to meprobamate should be assessed at the end of 4 mo.
- Psychic or physical dependence may occur with long-term use of high doses.
- Sudden withdrawal in physically dependent patients may precipitate preexisting symptoms or withdrawal reactions within 12–48 h: vomiting, ataxia, muscle twitching, mental confusion, hallucinations, convulsions, trembling, sleep disturbances, increased dreaming, nightmares, insomnia. Symptoms usually subside within 12–48 h.
- *Therapeutic blood level range:* 0.5–2 mg/dl. Blood levels of 3–10 mg/dl usually correspond with symptoms of mild to moderate overdosage (e.g., slurred speech, ataxia, stupor, light coma); levels of 10–20 mg/dl correspond with deep coma, hypotension, respiratory depression, heart failure, and frequently lead to death. Levels above 20 mg/dl are usually lethal.

Patient & Family Education
- Warn patient that tolerance to alcohol will be lowered.
- Caution patient to avoid driving a car or engaging in other hazardous activities until drug response has been determined.
- Patients should be instructed to report immediately an onset of skin rash, sore throat, fever, bruising, unexplained bleeding.
- Instruct patient to take drug as prescribed.

PSYCHOTHERAPEUTIC: ANTIDEPRESSANT, BICYCLIC

FLUOXETINE HYDROCHLORIDE

(flu´-ox-e-tine)
Trade name: Prozac
Classifications: CNS AGENT; PSYCHOTHERAPEUTIC; BICYCLIC ANTIDEPRESSANT
Pregnancy: Category B

ACTIONS/PHARMACODYNAMICS A phenylpropylamine derivative oral antidepressant chemically unrelated to tricyclic, tetracyclic, or other available antidepressants. Antidepressant effect is presumed to be linked to its inhibition of CNS presynaptic neuronal uptake of serotonin.

USES Depression. **Unlabeled uses:** obesity, bulimia nervosa, obsessive compulsive disorders.

ROUTE & DOSAGE

Depression

Adult	PO	20 mg/d in AM; may increase to max of 80 mg/d

PHARMACOKINETICS Absorption: 60–80% absorbed from GI tract. **Onset:** 1–3 wk. **Peak:** 4–8 h. **Distribution:** widely distributed, including CNS. **Metabolism:** metabolized in liver to active metabolite, norfluoxetine. **Elimination:** half-life: fluoxetine 2–3 d, norfluoxetine 7–9 d; > 80% excreted in urine; 12% in feces.

CONTRAINDICATIONS & PRECAUTIONS Contraindicated in: hypersensitivity. **Cautious use in:** hepatic and renal impairment, anorexia, hyponatremia, diabetes, and patients with history of suicidal ideations. Elderly may require dose adjustments. Safety in pregnancy (category B), lactation, and in children not established.

ADVERSE/SIDE EFFECTS CNS: *headache, nervousness, anxiety, insomnia,* drowsiness, fatigue, tremor, dizziness, hypomania, mania. **CV:** palpitations, hot flushes, chest pain. **GI:** *nausea, diarrhea,* anorexia, dyspepsia, increased appetite, dry mouth. **Skin:** rash, pruritus, sweating, hypersensitivity reactions. **Other:** blurred vision, myalgias, arthralgias, flu-like syndrome, hyponatremia, sexual dysfunction, menstrual irregularities.

DRUG INTERACTIONS Concurrent use of **tryptophan** may cause agitation, restlessness, and GI distress; no data available on concurrent use of MAO INHIBITORS— use cautiously; increases half-life of **diazepam**; may increase toxicity of TRICYCLIC ANTIDEPRESSANTS.

NURSING IMPLICATIONS

Administration

- Administer single dose in AM. Any additional doses should be administered at noon.
- Provide suicidal or potentially suicidal patient with small quantities of prescription medication.

Assessment & Drug Effects

- Use with caution in elderly patient and patient with impaired renal or hepatic function (may need lower dose).
- Use with caution in anorexic patient, since weight loss is a possible side effect.
- Monitor for signs and symptoms of anaphylactoid reaction (see chap 3). Report them immediately.
- Monitor for signs of improved affect. Requires approximately 2–3 wk for therapeutic effects to be felt.
- Weigh weekly to monitor weight loss, particularly in the elderly or nutritionally compromised patient. Report significant weight loss to physician.
- Observe for and promptly report rash or urticaria and signs and symptoms of fever, leukocytosis, arthralgias, carpal tunnel syndrome, edema, respiratory distress, and proteinuria. Drug may have to be discontinued or adjunctive therapy instituted with steroids or antihistamines.
- Observe for dizziness and drowsiness and employ safety measures (up with assistance, side rails, etc.) as indicated.
- Observe for and report increased anxiety, nervousness, or insomnia; modification of drug dose may be needed.
- Observe for seizures in patients with a history of seizures. Use appropriate safety precautions.
- Closely supervise patients who are high suicide risks, especially during initial therapy.
- Carefully monitor patients with hepatic or renal impairment for signs of toxicity (e.g., agitation, restlessness, nausea, vomiting, seizures).
- Monitor serum sodium level for development of hyponatremia, especially in patients who are taking diuretics or are otherwise hypovolemic.
- Monitor diabetics for loss of control; hypoglycemia has occurred during initiation of therapy, and hyperglycemia during drug withdrawal.

Patient & Family Education

- Instruct patient to take medication in AM for single dose or AM and noon for divided doses to prevent insomnia.
- Instruct patient that therapeutic effects may take from several days to 5 wk to develop fully.
- Advise patient to notify physician of intent to become pregnant or if breast feeding.
- Instruct patient that a rash could be one sign of a serious group of adverse effects and to notify physician if noted.
- Caution patients, particularly the elderly, to exercise safety precautions and to avoid hazardous tasks if dizziness noted.

Common side effects in *italic*; life-threatening effects <u>underlined</u>; generic names in **bold**; classifications in SMALL CAPS

181

- Instruct patients to consult physician if they are taking any other medications or if any new medications are prescribed.
- Advise patients to consult with physician before they take OTC drugs.
- Advise diabetics of possible loss of diabetic control and need for careful monitoring.
- Advise those with history of seizures of possible increase in seizure activity.

PSYCHOTHERAPEUTIC: ANTIDEPRESSANT, MONOAMINE OXIDASE INHIBITOR

PHENELZINE SULFATE

(fen´el-zeen)
Trade name: Nardil
Classifications: CNS AGENT; PSYCHOTHERAPEUTIC; MAO INHIBITOR ANTIDEPRESSANT
Pregnancy: Category C

ACTIONS/PHARMACODYNAMICS Potent hydrazine MAO inhibitor with amphetamine-like pharmacologic properties. Precise mode of action not known. Antidepressant and diverse effects believed to be due to irreversible inhibition of MAO (mitochondrial enzyme involved in degradation and excretion of sympathomimetic amines), thereby permitting increased concentrations of endogenous epinephrine, norepinephrine, serotonin, and dopamine within presynaptic neurons and at receptor sites. Also thought to inhibit hepatic microsomal drug-metabolizing enzymes; thus may intensify and prolong the effects of many drugs. Termination of drug action depends on regeneration of MAO, which occurs 2–3 wk after discontinuation of therapy. Exerts paradoxic hypotensive effect (apparently by ganglionic blocking action), suppresses REM sleep, and may decrease serum cholinesterase. MAO inhibitor has unpredictable effect on convulsive threshold in epilepsy.

USES Management of endogenous depression, depressive phase of manic-depressive psychosis, and severe exogenous (reactive) depression not responsive to more commonly used therapy.

PHARMACOKINETICS Absorption: readily absorbed from GI tract. **Onset:** 2 wk. **Metabolism:** rapidly metabolized. **Elimination:** half-life: unknown; 79% of metabolites excreted in urine in 96 h.

ROUTE & DOSAGE

Depression

Adult	PO	15 mg t.i.d.; rapidly increased to at least 60 mg/d; may need up to 90 mg/d

CONTRAINDICATIONS & PRECAUTIONS
Contraindicated in: hypersensitivity to MAO inhibitors; pheochromocytoma; hyperthyroidism; CHF, cardiovascular or cerebrovascular disease; impaired renal function, hypernatremia; atonic colitis; glaucoma; history of frequent or severe headaches; history of liver disease, abnormal liver function tests; elderly or debilitated patients; paranoid schizophrenia. Safe use during pregnancy (category C) and lactation and in children < 16 y of age not established. **Cautious use in:** epilepsy; pyloric stenosis; diabetes; depression accompanying alcoholism or drug addiction; manic-depressive states; agitated patients; suicidal tendencies; chronic brain syndromes; history of angina pectoris.

ADVERSE/SIDE EFFECTS Constipation, *dry mouth,* dizziness or vertigo, headache, *orthostatic hypotension,* drowsiness or *insomnia,* weakness, fatigue, *nausea,* vomiting, *anorexia,* weight gain, edema, tremors, twitching, hyperreflexia, mania, hypomania, confusion, memory impairment, blurred vision, hyperhidrosis, skin rash. <u>Hypertensive crisis:</u> intense occipital headache, palpitation, marked hypertension, stiff neck, nausea, vomiting, sweating, fever, photophobia, dilated pupils, bradycardia or tachycardia, constricting chest pain, intracranial bleeding. **Less common:** glaucoma, nystagmus, incontinence, dysuria, urinary frequency or retention, transient impotence, galactorrhea, gynecomastia, black tongue, hypernatremia, transient respiratory and cardiovascular depression, jaundice, delirium, hallucinations, euphoria, acute anxiety reaction, akathisia, ataxia, toxic precipitation of schizophrenia, convulsions, peripheral neuropathy, photosensitivity, normocytic and normochromic anemia, leukopenia. **Severe overdosage:** faintness, hypotension or hypertension, hyperactivity, marked agitation, anxiety, seizures, trismus, opisthotonos, <u>respiratory depression, coma, circulatory collapse.</u>

DIAGNOSTIC TEST INTERFERENCES Phenelzine may cause a slight false increase in **serum bilirubin.**

DRUG INTERACTIONS TRICYCLIC ANTIDEPRES-SANTS may cause hyperpyrexia, seizures; **fluoxetine** may cause hyperthermia, diaphoresis, tremors, seizures, delirium; SYMPATHOMIMETIC AGENTS (e.g., **amphetamine, phenylephrine, phenylpropa nolamine, guanethidine,** and **reserpine** may cause hypertensive crisis; CNS DEPRESSANTS have additive CNS depressive effects; OPIATE ANALGESICS (especially **meperidine**) may cause hypertensive crisis and circulatory collapse; **buspirone,** hypertension; GENERAL ANESTHETICS, prolonged hypotensive and CNS depressant effects; hypertension, headache, hyperexcitability reported with **dopamine, methyldopa, levodopa, tryptophan; metrizamide** may increase risk of seizures; HYPOTENSIVE AGENTS and DIURETICS have additive hypotensive effects. **Drug-food interactions:** aged meats or aged cheeses, protein extracts, sour cream, alcohol, anchovies, liver, sausages, overripe figs, bananas, avocados, chocolate, soy sauce, bean curd, natural yogurt, fava beans—tyramine-containing foods—may precipitate hypertensive crisis.

NURSING IMPLICATIONS

Administration

- MAO inhibitors should be discontinued at least 10 d before elective surgery to allow time for recovery of MAO before anesthetics are given.
- Rapid withdrawal of MAO inhibitors should be avoided, particularly after high dosage, since a rebound effect may occur (headache, excitability, hallucinations, and possibly depression).
- Preserve in tightly covered containers away from heat and light.

Assessment & Drug Effects

- Before initiation of phenelzine treatment, it is advisable to evaluate patient's BP in standing and recumbent positions. Baseline blood cell counts and liver function tests should also be performed.
- Many adverse reactions associated with MAO inhibitors are dose-related. Physician will rely on accurate observations and prompt reporting of patient's response to therapy to determine spacing and lowest effective dosage.
- In titrating initial dosages, BP and pulse should be monitored between doses, and patient should be closely observed for evidence of adverse drug effects. Thereafter, monitor at regular intervals throughout therapy.
- Monitor I&O ratio and pattern until dosage is stabilized to identify indirect indices of edema and urinary dysfunction. Report changes and abnor-

malities; impaired renal function increases the possibility of toxicity from cumulative effects.

- Hypomania (exaggeration of motility, feelings, and ideas) may occur as depression improves. This reaction may also appear at higher than recommended doses or with long-term therapy. Report immediately.
- Observe for and report therapeutic effectiveness of drug: improvement in sleep pattern, appetite, physical activity, interest in self and surroundings, as well as lessening of anxiety and bodily complaints.
- Patient with diabetes should be closely observed for signs of hypoglycemia (see chap 3). Reduced dosage of insulin or oral antidiabetic drug may be necessary.
- Patients on prolonged therapy should be checked periodically for altered color perception, visual fields, and fundi. Changes in red-green vision may be the first indication of eye damage.
- Periodic hematologic studies and liver function tests are recommended during prolonged therapy and high dosage.

Patient & Family Education

- If no therapeutic response occurs after 3 or 4 wk, drug is usually discontinued. Maximum antidepressant effects generally appear in 2–6 wk and persist several weeks after drug withdrawal.
- Advise patient to avoid self-medication. OTC preparations containing dextromethorphan, sympathomimetic agents, or antihistamines (e.g., cough, cold, and hay fever remedies, appetite suppressants) can precipitate severe hypertensive reactions if taken during therapy or within 2–3 wk after discontinuation of an MAO inhibitor.
- Headache and palpitation, prodromal symptoms of hypertensive crisis, indicate need to discontinue drug therapy. Instruct patient to report immediately the onset of these symptoms or any other unusual effects.
- Ingestion of foods and beverages containing tyramine or tryptophan or drugs containing pressor agents can result in severe hypertensive reactions.
- Foods that must be avoided include red wine, particularly Chianti; some beers; cheese (except cottage, ricotta, cream); smoked or pickled fish (herring); beef or chicken liver, summer (dry) sausage; fava or broad bean pods; yeast vitamin supplements. Questionable foods are ripe avocado, ripe fresh banana, sour cream, yogurt, soy sauce.
- Advise against excessive drinking of caffeine beverages: coffee, tea, cocoa, or cola.
- Provide patient and responsible family members with a list of foods and beverages that may cause

Common side effects in *italic*; life-threatening effects <u>underlined</u>; generic names in **bold**; classifications in SMALL CAPS

183

hypertensive reactions. These substances should be avoided during drug therapy and for at least 2–3 wk after therapy has been discontinued.

■ Elastic stockings and elevation of legs when sitting may minimize hypotensive effects of drug (discuss with physician).

■ Instruct patient to make position changes slowly, especially from recumbent to upright posture, and to dangle legs over bed a few minutes before ambulating. Also caution against standing still for prolonged periods. Patient should avoid hot showers and baths (resulting vasodilatation may potentiate hypotension) and should lie down immediately if feeling lightheaded or faint.

■ Instruct patient to check weight 2 or 3 times per week and report unusual gain.

■ Instruct patient to report jaundice. Hepatotoxicity is believed to be a hypersensitivity reaction unrelated to dosage or duration of therapy.

■ MAO inhibitors may suppress anginal pain that would otherwise serve as a warning sign of myocardial ischemia. Caution patient to avoid overexertion while receiving drug therapy.

PSYCHOTHERAPEUTIC: ANTIDEPRESSANT, TRICYCLIC

IMIPRAMINE HYDROCHLORIDE
(im-ip′ra-meen)

Trade names: Impril, Janimine, Novopramine, SK-Pramine, Tipramine, Tofranil

IMIPRAMINE PAMOATE

Trade name: Tofranil-PM
Classifications: CNS AGENT; PSYCHOTHERAPEUTIC; TRICYCLIC ANTIDEPRESSANT
Pregnancy: Category C

ACTIONS/PHARMACODYNAMICS Tricyclic antidepressant (TCA) and tertiary amine, structurally related to the phenothiazines. In contrast with phenothiazines, which act on dopamine receptors, TCAs potentiate both norepinephrine and serotonin in the CNS by blocking their reuptake by presynaptic neurons. The resulting increase in the availability of these biogenic amines is thought to be the basis for antidepressant effects. Exhibits anticholinergic, antihistaminic, hypotensive, sedative, mild analgesic,

and peripheral vasodilator effects. Decreases number of awakenings from sleep, markedly reduces time in REM sleep, and increases stage 4 sleep. Prolongs myocardial repolarization time and may produce quinidinelike conduction abnormalities (arrhythmias, heart block) that can be life threatening with overdosage. Relief of nocturnal enuresis is perhaps due to anticholinergic activity and to nervous system stimulation, resulting in earlier arousal to sensation of full bladder.

USES Endogenous depression and occasionally for reactive depression. Imipramine is the only TCA used as temporary adjuvant treatment of enuresis in children > 6 y. **Unlabeled uses:** Certain syndromes that mimic or overlap diagnostically with depression: alcoholism, cocaine withdrawal; attention deficit disorder with or without hyperactivity (children > 6 y and adolescents); with amphetamines or methylphenidate for narcolepsy; phobic anxiety syndromes such as panic disorders and agoraphobia; obsessive-compulsive neurosis; chronic intractable pain.

ROUTE & DOSAGE

Depression

Adult	PO	75–100 mg/d (up to 300 mg/d) in 1 or more divided doses
	IM	50–100 mg/d in divided doses
Child	PO	1.5 mg/kg/d; may increase by 1 mg/kg/d q3–4d to a max of 5 mg/kg/d

Enuresis in Childhood

Child	PO	25 mg 1 h before bedtime; <12 y: may increase to 50 mg nightly (max dose 2.5 mg/kg)
		> 12 y: may increase to 75 mg nightly; (max dose 2.5 mg/kg)

PHARMACOKINETICS: **Absorption:** Completely absorbed from GI tract. **Peak:** 1–2 h PO; 30 min IM. **Metabolism:** metabolized to the active metabolite desipramine in liver. **Elimination:** half-life: 8–16 h; primarily excreted in urine, small amount in feces; crosses placenta; may be secreted in breast milk.

CONTRAINDICATIONS & PRECAUTIONS Contraindicated in: hypersensitivity to tricyclic drugs; acute recovery period after MI, defects in bundle-branch conduction; severe renal or hepatic impairment; use of hydrochloride in children < 12 y except to treat enuresis; use of pamoate in children of any age. Safe

Common side effects in *italic*; life-threatening effects <u>underlined</u>; generic names in **bold**; classifications in SMALL CAPS

use during pregnancy (category D) and in nursing mothers not established. **Cautious use in:** children, adolescents, the elderly; respiratory difficulties; cardiovascular, hepatic, or GI diseases; blood disorders; increased intraocular pressure, narrow-angle glaucoma, schizophrenia, hypomania in manic episodes, patient with suicidal tendency, seizure disorders; prostatic hypertrophy, urinary retention; alcoholism, hyperthyroidism; electroshock therapy.

ADVERSE/SIDE EFFECTS CNS: *sedation, drowsiness,* dizziness, headache, fatigue, numbness, tingling (paresthesias) of extremities; incoordination, ataxia, tremors, peripheral neuropathy, extrapyramidal symptoms (including parkinsonism effects and tardive dyskinesia); lowered seizure threshold, altered EEG patterns, delirium, disturbed concentration, confusion, hallucinations, anxiety, nervousness, insomnia, vivid dreams, restlessness, agitation, shift to hypomania, mania; exacerbation of psychoses; hyperpyrexia. **CV:** *orthostatic hypotension,* mild sinus tachycardia; *arrhythmias,* hypertension or hypotension, palpitation, MI, CHF, *heart block,* ECG changes, stroke, flushing, cold cyanotic hands and feet (peripheral vasospasm). **Endocrine:** testicular swelling, gynecomastia (men), galactorrhea and breast enlargement (women), increased or decreased libido, ejaculatory and erectile disturbances, delayed or absent orgasm (male and female); elevation or depression of blood glucose levels. **ENT:** nasal congestion, tinnitus. **Eye:** *blurred vision,* disturbances of accommodation, *slight mydriasis,* nystagmus, aggravation of glaucoma (rare). **GI:** *dry mouth* (and dental caries), constipation, heartburn, excessive appetite, craving for sweets, weight gain, nausea, vomiting, diarrhea, slowed gastric emptying time, flatulence, abdominal cramps, esophageal reflux, anorexia, stomatitis, increased salivation, black tongue, peculiar taste, paralytic ileus. **GU:** *urinary retention,* delayed micturition, nocturia, paradoxic urinary frequency. **Hematologic:** bone marrow depression; agranulocytosis, eosinophilia, thrombocytopenia. **Hypersensitivity:** skin rash, erythema, petechiae, urticaria, pruritus, photosensitivity, angioedema (face, tongue, generalized); drug fever. **Other:** excessive perspiration, cholestatic jaundice, precipitation of acute intermittent porphyria; dyspnea, changes in heat and cold tolerance, hair loss, syndrome of inappropriate antidiuretic hormone secretion (SIADH).

DIAGNOSTIC TEST INTERFERENCES Imipramine elevates *serum bilirubin, alkaline phosphatase* and may increase or decrease *blood glu-*cose. It decreases *urinary 5-HIAA* and *VMA* excretion and may falsely increase excretion of *urinary catecholamines.*

DRUG INTERACTIONS MAO INHIBITORS may precipitate hyperpyretic crisis, tachycardia, or seizures; ANTIHYPERTENSIVE AGENTS potentiate orthostatic hypotension; CNS DEPRESSANTS, **alcohol** add to CNS depression; **norepinephrine** and other SYMPATHOMIMETICS may increase cardiac toxicity; **cimetidine** decreases hepatic metabolism, thus increasing imipramine levels; **methylphenidate** inhibits metabolism of imipramine and thus may increase its toxicity.

NURSING IMPLICATIONS

Administration

- Administer with or immediately after food to reduce gastric irritation. Single daily dose can be given before bedtime if dizziness and drowsiness are bothersome or dangerous during the day. If insomnia and stimulation are problems, drug can be administered in the AM. Check with physician.
- Crystals may form in some ampuls of injectable imipramine. To dissolve them, immerse intact ampul in warm water for about 1 min.
- Because of long serum half-life, dose adjustments are not made more frequently than q4d.
- Monitor BP and pulse rate for tachycardia and other arrhythmias. Withhold drug and notify physician if systolic BP falls more than 20 mm Hg or if there is a sudden increase in pulse rate.

Assessment & Drug Effects

- During long-term therapy, periodic assessment of hepatic, renal, cardiac, and hematologic status should be made.
- Elderly patients with preexisting cardiac disturbances and patients receiving high doses require close monitoring of cardiac conduction status (ECG, Holter monitor), supine and standing BP, and plasma TCA concentrations at regular intervals during therapy.
- Orthostatic hypotension tends to be mild in normotensive individuals but may be marked in pretreatment hypertensive or cardiac patients.
- Accurate early reporting to physician about patient's response to drug therapy is essential to prevent serious adverse effects.
- Dose sensitivity and side effects are most likely to occur in adolescents and the elderly. A lower initial dose should be used for these patients.

Common side effects in *italic*; life-threatening effects underlined; generic names in **bold**; classifications in SMALL CAPS

- During the first 2 wk of therapy, elderly patients sometimes develop **confusional reaction:** restlessness, disturbed sleep, forgetfulness. Symptoms last 3–20 d. Report them to physician.
- Elderly patients taking TCAs may gain weight because they tend to develop a greatly increased appetite and a craving for sweets. These symptoms are not correlated with clinical improvement of depression. Weight control measures may be indicated.
- Weigh patient under standard conditions at least biweekly: a gain of 0.5–1.0 kg (1 1/2–2 lb) within 2–3 d and frank edema should be reported.
- Monitor I&O ratio and bowel elimination, at least until maintenance dosage is stabilized, to detect urinary retention or frequency, constipation, or paralytic ileus.
- Signs of therapeutic effectiveness of TCAs may not occur for 2 wk or more after initiation of imipramine.
- A trial of therapy with adequate dose is not judged a failure for at least 1 mo. If there is no improvement, drug is discontinued. With apparent improvement, maintenance dosage can be instituted. *Therapeutic plasma TCA level:* 150–300 mg/ml.
- Report promptly early signs of agranulocytosis (see Signs & Symptoms, chap 3).
- Report **signs of cholestatic jaundice:** flulike symptoms, yellow skin or sclerae, dark urine, light-colored stools, pruritus.
- Observe patient with history of glaucoma. The onset of a severe headache, halos around light, dilated pupils, eye pain, nausea, and vomiting may signal an acute attack. Notify physician promptly.
- *Extrapyramidal symptoms* (tremors, twitching, ataxia, incoordination, hyperreflexia, drooling) may occur in patients receiving large doses and especially in the elderly. Notify physician if they are noted.
- Promptly report appearance of **psychogenic reactions:** transition from depression to hypomania or mania, hallucinations, delusion (especially apt to occur in patients with organic brain damage or history of psychosis). TCA therapy will be discontinued.
- Hyperglycemia or hypoglycemia (see Signs & Symptoms, chap 3) may occur in some patients. Diabetic patients should be monitored, particularly during early therapy.
- Frequently inspect oral mucosa, especially gingival surfaces under dentures. Dry mouth may cause poor adhesion of dentures and interfere with speech, mastication, and swallowing and can cause reduction in food and liquid intake. Dry mouth is a known factor in noncompliance. Alert physician.

- Some products (Janimine, Tofranil) contain tartrazine, which can cause an allergic reaction in susceptible patients. Frequently these individuals also have aspirin hypersensitivity.
- Overdose onset may be sudden. Monitoring should focus on the following potential **signs of toxicity:** QRS prolongation (to 100 ms or greater), arrhythmias, hypotension, respiratory depression, altered level of consciousness, seizures. Coma may be accompanied by warm skin, dilated pupils, and tachycardia (atropine syndrome) and hypertension and hyperreflexia.

Patient & Family Education

- Instruct patient to change position slowly and in stages, especially from recumbency to upright posture and to dangle legs over bed for a few minutes before ambulation.
- In some patients, effectiveness decreases with continued drug administration. Counsel parent to inform physician if this occurs.
- Caution responsible family members not to allow child to self-medicate.
- TCA metabolism may be increased by smoking, thus changing dose requirements. Some patients on TCA therapy experience complete recovery within 4–6 wk; others may require drug therapy for several years or for life. Advise appropriately.
- Advise patient not to use OTC drugs while on a TCA unless physician approves. Many preparations contain sympathomimetic amines, which in combination with imipramine could precipitate severe hypertension in some patients.
- Warn patient to avoid hazardous tasks such as driving a motor vehicle or operating machinery until drug response is known.
- Exposure to strong sunlight should be avoided because of potential photosensitivity. Advise use of sunscreen lotion with sun protection factor (SPF) of 12–15 if allowed.
- When patient is discharged from medical management, instruct patient and responsible family members not to double or skip doses or change dose interval.

Common side effects in *italic*; life-threatening effects underlined; generic names in **bold**; classifications in SMALL CAPS

PSYCHOTHERAPEUTIC: ANTIMANIC

LITHIUM CARBONATE

(li´thee-um)

Trade names: Carbolith, Duralith, Eskalith, Eskalith CR, Lithane, Lithizine, Lithobid, Lithonate, Lithotabs

LITHIUM CITRATE

Trade name: Cibalith-S
Classifications: CNS AGENT; PSYCHOTHERAPEUTIC; ANTIMANIC
Pregnancy: Category D

ACTIONS/PHARMACODYNAMICS The lithium ion behaves in the body much like the sodium ion; but its exact mechanism of action is unclear. Competes with various physiologically important cations: Na, K, Ca, Mg; therefore it affects cell membranes, body water, and neurotransmitters. At the synapse it accelerates catecholamine destruction, inhibits the release of neurotransmitters, and decreases sensitivity of postsynaptic receptors. Thus neurotransmitter overactivity assumed to occur in mania is corrected. Has antidepressant and antimanic effects. Alters renal function by decreasing renal concentrating ability and water reabsorption. Initial increase in sodium and potassium excretion returns to pretreatment levels after 1 wk of continuous therapy. Other possible effects: blocks some of the behavior manifestations of drug-induced mania (amphetamines, cocaine); may alter calcium, magnesium, and parathyroid hormone homeostasis; blocks release of thyroxine and triiodothyronine; produces neutrophilia and may enhance lymphocyte activity. Increases or decreases glucose tolerance, decreases sensitivity to insulin, and reduces intestinal absorption of water and glucose.

USES Control and prophylaxis of acute mania and the acute manic phase of mixed bipolar disorder. **Unlabeled uses:** acute and recurrent depression (unipolar affective disorder), schizophrenic disorders, disorders of impulse control, alcohol dependence, antineoplastic drug–induced neutropenia, aplastic anemia, SIADH, cyclic neutropenia.

PHARMACOKINETICS Absorption: readily absorbed from GI tract. **Peak:** 0.5–3 h carbonate; 15–60 min citrate. **Distribution:** crosses blood-brain barrier and placenta; distributed into breast milk. **Metabolism:** not metabolized. **Elimination:** half-life: 20–27 h; 95% excreted in urine, 1% in feces, 4–5% in sweat.

ROUTE & DOSAGE

Mania

Adult	PO	*Initial:* 600 mg t.i.d. *or* 900 mg sustained-release b.i.d. *or* 30 ml (48 mEq) of solution t.i.d.
		Maintenance: 300 mg t.i.d. or q.i.d. *or* 15–20 ml (24–32 mEq) solution in 2–4 divided doses (max 2.4 g/d)
Child	PO	15–60 mg/kg/d in divided doses

CONTRAINDICATIONS & PRECAUTIONS Contraindicated in: significant cardiovascular or renal disease, brain damage, severe debilitation, dehydration or sodium depletion; patients on low salt diet or receiving diuretics; pregnancy, especially first trimester (category D), nursing mothers, children <12 y. **Cautious use in:** elderly patients; thyroid disease; epilepsy; concomitant use with haloperidol and other antipsychotics; parkinsonism; diabetes mellitus; severe infections; urinary retention.

ADVERSE/SIDE EFFECTS CNS: dizziness, *headache, lethargy,* drowsiness, *fatigue,* slurred speech, psychomotor retardation, giddiness, incontinence, restlessness, seizures, confusion, blackout spells, disorientation, *recent memory loss,* stupor, coma, EEG changes. **CV:** arrhythmias, hypotension, vasculitis, peripheral circulatory collapse, ECG changes. **EENT:** impaired vision, transient scotomas, tinnitus. **Endocrine:** diffuse thyroid enlargement, hypothyroidism, *nephrogenic diabetes insipidus,* transient hyperglycemia, glycosuria, hyponatremia. **GI:** *nausea, vomiting, anorexia, abdominal pain, diarrhea, dry mouth,* metallic taste. **Neuromuscular:** *fine hand tremors,* coarse tremors, choreoathetotic movements; fasciculations, clonic movements, incoordination including ataxia, *muscle weakness,* hyperreflexia, encephalopathic syndrome (weakness, lethargy, fever, tremors, confusion, extrapyramidal symptoms). **Skin:** (thought to be toxicity rather than allergy): pruritus, maculopapular rash, hyperkeratosis, chronic folliculitis, transient acneiform papules (face, neck, intertriginous areas), anesthesia of skin, cutaneous ulcers, drying and thinning of hair, allergic vasculitis. **Other:** *reversible leukocytosis* (14,000 to 18,000/mm^3), albuminuria, oliguria, urinary incontinence, polyuria, polydipsia, increased uric acid ex-

Common side effects in *italic*; life-threatening effects underlined; generic names in **bold**; classifications in SMALL CAPS

187

cretion, edema, weight gain (common) or loss, exacerbation of psoriasis; flulike symptoms.

DRUG INTERACTIONS Carbamazepine, haloperidol, PHENOTHIAZINES increase risk of neurotoxicity, extrapyramidal effects, and tardive dyskinesias; DIURETICS, NSAIDS, **methyldopa, probenecid,** TETRACYCLINES decrease renal clearance of lithium, increasing pharmacologic and toxic effects; THEOPHYLLINES, **urea, sodium bicarbonate, sodium or potassium citrate** increase renal clearance of lithium, decreasing its pharmacologic effects.

NURSING IMPLICATIONS

Administration
- GI symptoms may be minimized by taking drug with meals.
- ***Dose control:*** (1) Generally dosage regimen is designed to maintain serum lithium levels of 1.0–1.5 mEq/L in acute mania and 0.6–1.6 mEq/L during maintenance treatment. (2) Blood sample for determining serum lithium level is drawn prior to next dose (8–12 h after last dose) when lithium level is fairly stable. (3) If serum lithium is above 1.5 mEq/L or if a clinical event has decreased patient's tolerance to lithium (e.g., persistent vomiting or diarrhea, excessive sweating in hot weather, change in I&O ratio, intercurrent infection, fever, noncompliance), consult physician before administering next dose. (4) Timing of blood study and an accurate analysis of patient's condition will determine if next dose is to be changed or delayed.
- Store at 15–30C (59–86F) unless otherwise directed and protect from light and moisture.

Assessment & Drug Effects
- Transient nausea and general discomfort appear to coincide with peak rise in serum lithium levels. Report persistent symptoms. Dosage may be adjusted to provide levels without high peaks.
- Hospitalization is usually a necessity during initial treatment stage to permit daily serum lithium determinations until therapeutic dose is established.
- Weigh patient daily; check ankles, tibiae, and wrists for edema. Report changes in I&O ratio, sudden weight gain, or edema.
- Polydipsia and polyuria, apparently not dose-related, are common early side effects, particularly in the elderly. Symptoms may lessen but then reappear after several months or even years of maintenance.
- Onset of therapeutic effects usually is preceded by a lag of 1–2 wk. If drug control is not apparent within 1–3 wk, drug is usually withdrawn.

- Therapeutic response to lithium therapy is evidenced by changed facial affect, improved posture, assumption of self-care, improved ability to concentrate, improved sleep pattern. Keep physician informed of progress.
- Early signs of lithium intoxication may occur several days after starting therapy and when lithium levels are between 1.5–2.0 mEq/L: vomiting, diarrhea, lack of coordination, drowsiness, muscular weakness, slurred speech. Withhold one dose, call physician. Drug should not be stopped abruptly.
- When lithium levels are above 2.0 mEq/L, symptoms may include ataxia, blurred vision, giddiness, tinnitus, muscle twitching or coarse tremors, and a large output of dilute urine.
- The encephalopathic syndrome may be induced when lithium is given concomitantly with haloperidol or with other antipsychotic medication, particularly in the elderly. Promptly report to the physician early signs of extrapyramidal reactions.
- The fine tremor of hand or jaw, polyuria, mild thirst, transient mild nausea, and general discomfort that may occur in early treatment of mania sometimes persist throughout therapy. Usually, however, symptoms subside with temporary reduction of dose. If symptoms persist, drug is withdrawn. Keep physician informed of all presenting signs and symptoms.
- Diffuse thyroid enlargement, generally without change in thyroid function, has occurred in some patients (mostly women) after 5 mo–2 y of lithium therapy. Laboratory studies of thyroid hormone and periodic palpation of the thyroid gland should be a part of preventive therapy. Be alert to and report symptoms of hypothyroidism (see chap 3). Symptoms are reversible when lithium is discontinued and supplemental thyroid is provided.
- Neonates born of mothers who took lithium during pregnancy may have high serum lithium level manifested by flaccidity, poor reflexes, cardiac dysrhythmia, and chronic twitching.
- Note that Lithane contains tartrazine, which may cause an allergic-type reaction in susceptible patients. It is frequently seen in persons who also have aspirin hypersensitivity.
- The elderly require special monitoring to prevent toxicity, which may occur at serum levels ordinarily tolerated by other patients. Ability to excrete lithium decreases with aging; thus a smaller dose than usual may give desired control.

Patient & Family Education
- Instruct patient to be alert to increased output of dilute urine and persistent thirst. Chronic lithium

therapy may be associated with diminished renal concentrating ability occasionally presenting as nephrogenic diabetes insipidus (with polydypsia and polyuria). Dose reduction may be indicated.

- Teach patient to establish and adhere to a schedule for testing renal function by periodic evaluations of urine specific gravity (**normal:** 1.005–1.025).
- Because dehydration is a possibility, advise patient to contact physician if diarrhea or fever develops. Avoid practices that may encourage dehydration: hot environment, excessive caffeine beverages (diuresis).
- Urge patient to drink plenty of liquids (2–3 L/d) during stabilization period and at least 1–1 1/2 L/d during remainder of therapy.
- 6–10 g salt intake (average American) is required to keep serum lithium in the therapeutic range.
- Normal dietary salt intake can be inadvertently compromised by lack of understanding. Caution patient to avoid self-prescribed low-salt regimen, self-dosing with Rolaids, Soda-mints, or other sodium antacids, high sodium foods (e.g., prepared meats and diet soda). Also warn against "crash" diets or diet pills that reduce appetite and food, salt, and fluid intake.
- Reduced intake of fluid and sodium can accelerate lithium retention with subsequent toxicity. Conversely, marked increase in sodium intake can increase lithium excretion and reduce drug effect.
- Lithium may impair both physical and mental ability. Caution against any activity demanding alertness (e.g., driving a car) until clinical response to drug has been established.
- Contraceptive measures should be used during lithium therapy but if the patient becomes pregnant she should be informed of the potential risks to the fetus. If therapy is continued, serum lithium levels must be closely monitored to prevent toxicity. Renal clearance of lithium increases during pregnancy but reverts to lower rate immediately after delivery; dose, therefore, will be reduced to prevent toxicity.
- Warn patient not to switch brands of lithium carbonate. Because of varying fillers, a different brand may introduce a change in dose requirement.
- Urge patient to adhere to established dosage regimen, i.e., not to change or omit doses and not to change dose intervals.
- Clinical follow-up and regular checks on serum lithium levels are essential if treatment is to be safe and effective. Emphasize importance to family and patient of keeping all appointments for clinic visits.

PSYCHOTHERAPEUTIC: ANTIPSYCHOTIC (TRANQUILIZER), BUTYROPHENONE

HALOPERIDOL
(ha-loe-per´i-dole)
Trade names: Haldol, Peridol

HALOPERIDOL DECANOATE

Trade name: Haldol
Classifications: CNS AGENT; PSYCHOTHERAPEUTIC; BUTYROPHENONE; ANTIPSYCHOTIC (TRANQUILIZER)
Pregnancy: Category C

ACTIONS/PHARMACODYNAMICS Potent, long-acting butyrophenone derivative with pharmacologic actions similar to those of piperazine phenothiazines but with higher incidence of extrapyramidal effects and less hypotensive and relatively low sedative activity. Exerts strong anti-emetic effect and impairs central thermoregulation. Produces weak central anticholinergic effects and transient orthostatic hypotension. Actions thought to be related to competitive blockade of postsynaptic dopamine receptors in the brain.

USES Management of manifestations of psychotic disorders and for control of tics and vocal utterances of Gilles de la Tourette's syndrome; for treatment of agitated states in acute and chronic psychoses. Used for short-term treatment of hyperactive children and for severe behavior problems in children of combative, explosive hyperexcitability. **Unlabeled use:** cancer chemotherapy as an antiemetic in doses smaller than those required for antipsychotic effects; treatment of autism; alcohol dependence; chorea.

PHARMACOKINETICS Absorption: well absorbed from GI tract; 60% reaches systemic circulation. **Onset:** 30–45 min IM. **Peak:** 2–6 h PO; 10–20 min IM; 6–7 d decanoate. **Distribution:** distributes mainly to liver with lower concentration in brain, lung, kidney, spleen, heart. **Metabolism:** metabolized in liver. **Elimination:** half-life: 13–35 h; 40% excreted in urine within 5 d; 15% eliminated in feces; excreted in breast milk.

Common side effects in *italic*; life-threatening effects underlined; generic names in **bold**; classifications in SMALL CAPS

189

ROUTE & DOSAGE

Psychosis

Adult	PO	0.2–5 mg b.i.d. or t.i.d.
	IM	2–5 mg repeated q4h prn
Child	PO	0.5 mg/d in 2–3 divided doses; may be increased by 0.5 mg q5–7d to 0.05–0.15 mg/kg/d

Severe Psychosis

Adult	PO	3–5 mg b.i.d. or t.i.d.; may need up to 100 mg/d
	IM	2–5 mg; may repeat qh prn; decanoate can be administered q4wk
Child	PO	0.05–0.15 mg/kg/d in 2–3 divided doses

Tourette's Disorder

Adult	PO	0.2–5 mg b.i.d. or t.i.d.
Child	PO	0.05–0.075 mg/kg/d in 2–3 divided doses

CONTRAINDICATIONS & PRECAUTIONS Contraindicated in: Parkinson's disease, parkinsonism, seizure disorders, coma; alcoholism; severe mental depression, CNS depression; thyrotoxicosis. Safe use during pregnancy (category C), in nursing mothers, and in children <3 y not established. **Cautious use in:** elderly or debilitated patients, urinary retention, glaucoma, severe cardiovascular disorders; patients receiving anticonvulsant, anticoagulant, or lithium therapy.

ADVERSE/SIDE EFFECTS CNS: *extrapyramidal reactions:* parkinsonian symptoms, dystonia, akathisia, tardive dyskinesia (after long-term use); insomnia, restlessness, anxiety, euphoria, agitation, drowsiness, mental depression, lethargy, fatigue, weakness, tremor, ataxia, headache, confusion, vertigo; neuroleptic malignant syndrome, hyperthermia, grand mal seizures, exacerbation of psychotic symptoms. **CV:** tachycardia, ECG changes, hypotension, hypertension (with overdosage). **Endocrine:** menstrual irregularities, galactorrhea, lactation, gynecomastia, impotence, increased libido, hyponatremia, hyperglycemia, hypoglycemia. **Eyes:** blurred vision. **GI:** dry mouth, anorexia, nausea, vomiting, constipation, diarrhea, hypersalivation. **GU:** urinary retention, priapism. **Hematologic:** mild and usually transient leukopenia, leukocytosis, anemia, tendency toward lymphomonocytosis, agranulocytosis (rare). **Respiratory:** laryngospasm, bronchospasm, increased depth of respiration, bronchopneumonia, respiratory depression. **Skin:** diaphoresis, maculopapular and ac-

neiform rash, alopecia; (rarely), photosensitivity. **Other:** cholestatic jaundice, variations in liver function tests, decreased serum cholesterol.

DRUG INTERACTIONS CNS DEPRESSANTS, OPIATES, **alcohol** increase CNS depression; may antagonize activity of ORAL ANTICOAGULANTS; ANTICHOLINERGICS may increase intraocular pressure; **methyldopa** may precipitate dementia.

NURSING IMPLICATIONS

Administration

- Haloperidol tablets may be taken with a full glass (240 ml) of water or with food or milk.
- Haloperidol PO concentrate may form a precipitate when mixed with coffee or tea. Avoid these beverages as diluents and administer oral form either undiluted or with some other fluid.
- Haloperidol should be administered by deep IM injection into the gluteus. A 5 cm (2 in) long, 21-gauge needle is recommended. Do not exceed 3 ml per injection site.
- Although orthostatic hypotension is not common, take necessary safety precautions. Have patient recumbent at time of parenteral administration and for about 1 h after injection.
- Dosing regimen should be tapered when therapy is to be discontinued. Abrupt termination of treatment can initiate extrapyramidal symptoms.
- Store in light-resistant container at 15–30C (59–86F), unless otherwise specified by manufacturer. Discard darkened solutions; slight yellowing does not affect potency, however.

Assessment & Drug Effects

- Because of long half-life of haloperidol, therapeutic effects are slow to develop in early therapy or when established dosing regimen is changed.
- Monitor patient's mental status daily: appearance and general behavior, thought content, affect and mood, sensorium.
- Target symptoms expected to decrease with successful haloperidol treatment include hallucinations, insomnia, hostility, agitation, and delusions.
- "Therapeutic window" effect (point at which increased dose or concentration actually decreases therapeutic response) may occur after long period of high doses. Close observation is imperative when doses are changed.
- Monitor BP and muscle tone for the hospitalized patient. Establish baseline measurements before treatment is initiated. It is reported that a high diastolic reading at the beginning of therapy may be predictive of susceptibility to neuroleptic malignant

syndrome. The condition is more common in the young, in males, in nonschizophrenic psychiatric patients, and in patients taking lithium concomitantly.

- **Neuroleptic malignant syndrome (NMS)** reportedly occurs more frequently than formerly recognized. The syndrome is potentially fatal but can be reversible if recognized and treated early. NMS resembles a severe form of parkinsonian muscle rigidity, autonomic instability (labile BP, increased TPR, diaphoresis), altered mental status. It can progress to coma, acute respiratory or renal failure, and cardiovascular collapse.
- Symptoms of NMS can appear suddenly after initiation of therapy or after months or years of taking neuroleptic (antipsychotic) medication. Treatment: stop drug immediately; give intensive symptomatic and supportive care.
- Patients <40 y appear to be more susceptible than older patients to parkinsonism (akinesia, tremor, rigidity, excessive salivation, hyperreflexia).
- Risk of tardive dyskinesia appears to be greater in women receiving high doses and the elderly. It can occur after long-term therapy and even after therapy is discontinued. The syndrome is characterized by involuntary dyskinetic motions: rhythmic, wormlike movements of tongue, puffing of cheeks, chewing, mouth puckering, tongue protrusion. Drug should be stopped as soon as possible; the syndrome is potentially irreversible.
- Extrapyramidal (neuromuscular) reactions occur frequently during first few days of treatment. Symptoms are usually dose related and are controlled by dosage reduction or concomitant administration of antiparkinson drugs. Discontinuation of therapy may be necessary. Reactions appear to be more prominent in younger patients.
- Be alert for behavioral changes in patients who are concurrently receiving antiparkinson drugs.
- Haloperidol is administered cautiously to patients receiving anticonvulsant medication because it may lower the convulsant threshold. The established dose of the anticonvulsant is not changed.
- When haloperidol is used to control mania or cyclic disorders, the patient should be closely observed for rapid mood shift to depression. Depression may represent a drug side effect or reversion from a manic state.
- Periodic blood studies and liver function tests are advised in patients on prolonged therapy.
- Haldol tablets (1, 5, and 10 mg) contain tartrazine, which can cause an allergic reaction in certain individuals. It is frequently seen in persons who also have aspirin sensitivity.

Patient & Family Education
- Avoid use of alcohol during therapy.
- Advise patient not to drive a car or engage in other activities requiring mental alertness and physical coordination until drug response is known.
- Xerostomia may promote dental problems. Discuss oral hygiene with patient. Encourage adequate fluid intake.
- Caution patient that drug can cause a photosensitivity reaction and therefore to avoid overexposure to sun or sunlamp and to use a suncreen.

PSYCHOTHERAPEUTIC: ANTIPSYCHOTIC (TRANQUILIZER), PHENOTHIAZINE

CHLORPROMAZINE

CHLORPROMAZINE HYDROCHLORIDE

(klor-proe´ma-zeen)
Trade names: Chlorpromanyl, Clorazine, Largactil, Novochlorpromazine, Ormazine, Promapar, Promaz, Sonazine, Thorazine, Thor-Prom
Classifications: CNS AGENT; PSYCHOTHERAPEUTIC; PHENOTHIAZINE ANTIPSYCHOTIC (TRANQUILIZER); GI AGENT; ANTIEMETIC
Pregnancy: Category C

ACTIONS/PHARMACODYNAMICS Phenothiazine derivative with actions at all levels of CNS. Mechanism that produces strong antipsychotic effects is unclear, but thought to be related to blockade of postsynaptic dopamine receptors in the brain. Actions on hypothalamus and reticular formation produce strong sedation, hypotension, and depressed temperature regulation. Has strong alpha adrenergic blocking action and weak anticholinergic effects. Directly depresses the heart; may increase coronary blood flow. Exerts quinidinelike antiarrhythmic action. Also produces skeletal muscle relaxation, weak anorexiant, antihistaminic, and antipruritic effects; lowers convulsive threshold and depresses cough reflex. Antiemetic effect by suppression of the chemoreceptor trigger zone (CTZ). Inhibitory effect on dopamine reuptake, may be the basis for moderate extrapyramidal symptoms.

Common side effects in *italic*; life-threatening effects <u>underlined</u>; generic names in **bold**; classifications in SMALL CAPS

191

Antipsychotic drugs are sometimes called neuroleptics (or tranquilizers) because they tend to reduce initiative and interest in environment, decrease displays of emotions or affect, suppress spontaneous movements and complex behavior, and decrease psychotic symptoms. Spinal reflexes and unconditioned nociceptive-avoidance behaviors remain intact.

USES To control manic phase of manic-depressive illness, for symptomatic management of psychotic disorders, including schizophrenia, in management of severe nausea and vomiting, to control excessive anxiety and agitation before surgery, and for treatment of severe behavior problems in children, e.g., attention deficit disorder. Also used for treatment of acute intermittent porphyria, intractable hiccups, and as adjunct in treatment of tetanus.

ROUTE & DOSAGE

Psychotic Disorders, Agitation

Adult	PO	25–100 mg t.i.d. or q.i.d.; may need up to 1000 mg/d
	IM/IV	25–50 mg up to 600 mg q4–6h
Child	PO	>6 mo: 0.55 mg/kg q4–6h prn up to 500 mg/d
	PR	>6 mo: 1.1 mg/kg q6–8h
	IM/IV	>6 mo: 0.55 mg/kg q6–8h

Nausea and Vomiting

Adult	PO	10–25 mg q4–6h prn
	PR	50–100 mg q6–8h
	IM/IV	25–50 mg q3–4h prn
Child	PO	>6 mo: 0.55 mg/kg q4–6h prn up to 500 mg/d
	PR	>6 mo: 1.1 mg/kg q6–8h
	IM/IV	>6 mo: 0.55 mg/kg q6–8h

Intractable Hiccups

Adult	PO/IM/IV	25–50 mg t.i.d. or q.i.d.

PHARMACOKINETICS Absorption: rapid absorption with considerable first pass metabolism in liver; rapid absorption after IM. **Onset:** 30–60 min. **Peak:** 2–4 h PO; 15–20 min IM. **Duration:** 4–6 h. **Distribution:** widely distributed; accumulates in brain; crosses placenta. **Metabolism:** metabolized in liver. **Elimination:** half-life: biphasic 2 and 30 h; excreted in urine as metabolites; excreted in breast milk.

CONTRAINDICATIONS & PRECAUTIONS

Contraindicated in: hypersensitivity to phenothiazine derivatives; withdrawal states from alcohol; comatose states, brain damage, bone marrow depression, Reye's syndrome; children < 6 mo. Safe use during pregnancy (category C), and in nursing mothers not established. **Cautious use in:** agitated states accompanied by depression, seizure disorders, respiratory impairment due to infection or COPD; glaucoma, diabetes, hypertensive disease, peptic ulcer, prostatic hypertrophy; thyroid, cardiovascular, and hepatic disorders; patients exposed to extreme heat or organophosphate insecticides; previously detected breast cancer.

ADVERSE/SIDE EFFECTS Usually dose related. **CNS:** *sedation, drowsiness,* dizziness, restlessness, neuroleptic malignant syndrome, tardive dyskinesias, tumor, syncope, headache, weakness, insomnia, reduced REM sleep, bizarre dreams, cerebral edema, convulsive seizures, hypothermia, inability to sweat, depressed cough reflex, *extrapyramidal symptoms,* EEG changes. **CV:** orthostatic hypotension, hypertension, palpitation, tachycardia, bradycardia, ECG changes (usually reversible): prolonged QT and PR intervals, blunting of T waves, ST depression. **Eye:** blurred vision, lenticular opacities, mydriasis, photophobia. **GI:** dry mouth; constipation, adynamic ileus, cholestatic jaundice, aggravation of peptic ulcer, dyspepsia, increased appetite. **GU:** anovulation, infertility, pseudopregnancy, menstrual irregularity, gynecomastia, galactorrhea, priapism, inhibition of ejaculation, reduced libido, urinary retention and frequency. **Hematologic:** agranulocytosis, thrombocytopenic purpura, pancytopenia (rare). **Respiratory:** nasal congestion, laryngospasm, bronchospasm, respiratory depression, depressed cough reflex. **Skin/hypersensitivity:** fixed-drug eruption, urticaria, reduced perspiration, contact dermatitis, exfoliative dermatitis, photosensitivity, eczema, anaphylactoid reactions, hypersensitivity vasculitis; hirsutism (long-term therapy). **Other:** weight gain, hypoglycemia, hyperglycemia, glycosuria (high doses), enlargement of parotid glands, idiopathic edema, muscle necrosis (following IM), SLE-like syndrome, sudden unexplained death.

DIAGNOSTIC TEST INTERFERENCES Chlorpromazine (phenothiazines) may increase **cephalin flocculation**, and possibly other **liver function tests;** also may increase **PBI.** False-positive result may occur for **amylase, 5-hydroxyindole acetic acid, porphobilinogens, urobilinogen** (Ehrlich's reagent), and **urine bilirubin** (Bili-Labstix). False-positive or false-negative **pregnancy test** results possibly caused by a metabolite of phenothiazines, which discolors urine depending on test used.

Common side effects in *italic*; life-threatening effects underlined; generic names in **bold**; classifications in SMALL CAPS

DRUG INTERACTIONS Alcohol, CNS DEPRESSANTS increase CNS depression; ANTACIDS, ANTIDIARRHEALS decrease absorption—space administration 2 h before or after administration of chlorpromazine; **phenobarbital** increases metabolism of phenobarbital; GENERAL ANESTHETICS increase excitation and hypotension; antagonizes antihypertensive action of **guanethidine; phenylpropanolamine** poses possibility of sudden death; TRICYCLIC ANTIDEPRESSANTS intensify hypotensive and anticholinergic effects; ANTICONVULSANTS decrease seizure threshold—may need to increase anticonvulsant dose.

INCOMPATIBILITIES Solution/additive: aminophylline, amphotericin B, ampicillin, chloramphenicol, chlorothiazide, cimetidine, dimenhydrinate, heparin, methacillin, methohexital, penicillin G, pentobarbital, phenobarbital, ranitidine, thiopental. **Y-site:** aminophylline, amphotericin B, ampicillin, chloramphenicol, chlorothiazide, methacillin, methohexital, penicillin G, phenobarbital, thiopental.

NURSING IMPLICATIONS

Administration

- Watch to see that oral drug is swallowed and not hoarded. Suicide attempt is a constant possibility in depressed patients, particularly when they are improving.
- Chlorpromazine concentrate should be mixed just before administration in at least 1/2 glass juice, milk, water, coffee, tea, carbonated beverage, or with semisolid food.
- Maintenance therapy is usually administered as a single dose at bedtime.
- Avoid parenteral drug contact with skin, eyes, and clothing because of its potential for causing contact dermatitis.
- Inject IM preparations slowly and deep into upper outer quadrant of buttock; massage site well. Avoid SC injection; it may cause tissue irritation and nodule formation. If irritation is a problem, consult physician about diluting medication with normal saline or 2% procaine. Rotate injection sites.
- The patient should remain recumbent for at least 1/2 h after parenteral administration. Observe closely. Hypotensive reactions may require head-low position and pressor drugs, e.g., phenylephrine (Neo-Synephrine), norepinephrine (Levophed). Epinephrine and other pressor agents are contraindicated since they may cause sudden paradoxical drop in BP.
- Avoid injecting undiluted chlorpromazine into a vein. Each 25 mg should be diluted with 24 ml of NS to produce a concentration of 1 mg/ml. May be further diluted in up to 1000 ml of NS for continuous infusion.
- IV chlorpromazine may be given by direct IV diluted in 24 ml of NS. Administer 1 mg or fraction thereof over 2 min.
- A specific flow rate should be ordered for the IV infusion. Usual rate: 1–2 mg/min. Monitor BP.
- Lemon yellow color of parenteral preparation does not alter potency; if otherwise colored or markedly discolored, solution should be discarded.
- All forms are stored preferably between 15–30C (59–86F) protected from light, unless otherwise specified by the manufacturer. Avoid freezing.

Assessment & Drug Effects

- Before initiating treatment, establish baseline BP (in standing and recumbent positions), pulse, and respiratory capacity values.
- Hypotensive reactions, dizziness, and sedation are common during early therapy, particularly in patients on high doses and in the elderly receiving parenteral doses. Patients usually develop tolerance to these side effects; however, lower doses or longer intervals between doses may be required.
- Be alert for signs of neuroleptic malignant syndrome (see chap 3). Report immediately.
- Smoking increases metabolism of phenothiazines, resulting in shortened half-life and more rapid clearance of drug. Higher dosage in smokers may be required. Advise patient to stop or at least reduce smoking, if possible.
- Monitor I&O ratio and pattern. Urinary retention due to mental depression and compromised renal function may occur. If serum creatinine becomes elevated, therapy should be discontinued.
- Note that chlorpromazine can suppress the cough reflex. Be alert to danger of bronchopneumonia, which may occur in the severely depressed patient, especially the elderly.
- Support hose and elevation of legs when sitting may minimize drug-induced hypotension (discuss with physician). Supervise ambulation.
- May affect temperature regulating mechanism.
- Antiemetic effect of chlorpromazine may obscure signs of overdosage of other drugs or other causes of nausea and vomiting.
- Be alert to complaints of diminished visual acuity, reduced night vision, photophobia, and a perceived brownish discoloration of objects. Patient may be more comfortable with dark glasses.
- Diabetics or prediabetics on long-term, high-dose therapy should be monitored for reduced glucose

---

Common side effects in *italic*; life-threatening effects <u>underlined</u>; generic names in **bold**; classifications in SMALL CAPS

tolerance and loss of diabetes control. Urine and blood glucose should be checked regularly.

- Early manifestations of agranulocytosis (see Signs & Symptoms, chap 3) are most likely to occur within first 4–10 wk of therapy, particularly in women and the elderly. Blood studies should be instituted promptly.
- CBC, liver function tests, urinalysis, ocular examinations, EEG (in patients > 50 y) are recommended before and periodically during prolonged therapy.

Patient & Family Education

- Take chlorpromazine with food or a full glass of water or milk (240 ml) to reduce possibility of gastric irritation.
- Some patients fail to experience improvement until 7 or 8 wk into therapy and therefore may not realize the importance of medication compliance. Stress necessity of keeping appointments for follow-up evaluation of dosage regimen.
- Urge patient on home therapy not to alter dosing regimen; tell patient not to give the drug to another person.
- May cause pink to red-brown discoloration of urine.
- Photosensitivity associated with chlorpromazine therapy is a phototoxic reaction. Severity of response depends on amount of exposure and drug dose. Exposed skin areas have appearance of an exaggerated sunburn. If reaction occurs, report to physician. Patient should wear protective clothing and sun screen lotion with SPF above 12 when outdoors, even on dark days.
- Oral candidiasis occurs frequently in patients receiving phenothiazines. Emphasize meticulous oral hygiene.
- Extrapyramidal symptoms occur most often in patients on high dosage, the pediatric patient with severe dehydration and acute infection, the elderly, and women. These symptoms are frightening to the uninformed. Be sure patient and family members understand the importance of prompt reporting. Usually symptoms disappear with dosage adjustment.
- Chlorpromazine may impair mental and physical abilities, especially during early therapy. Caution patient against driving a car or undertaking activities requiring precision and mental alertness until drug response is known.
- Abrupt withdrawal of drug or deliberate dose skipping, especially after prolonged therapy with large doses, can cause onset of extrapyramidal symptoms (see Chapter 3) and severe GI disturbances. Urge patient to adhere to dosage regimen without

changes. When treatment is to be discontinued, dosage must be tapered off gradually over a period of several weeks.

RESPIRATORY AND CEREBRAL STIMULANT: AMPHETAMINE

AMPHETAMINE SULFATE

(am-fet´a-meen)
Trade name: Racemic Amphetamine Sulfate
Classifications: CNS AGENT; RESPIRATORY AND CEREBRAL STIMULANT; AMPHETAMINE; ANOREXIANT
Pregnancy: Category C
Controlled substance: Schedule II

ACTIONS/PHARMACODYNAMICS Indirect-acting synthetic sympathomimetic amine (noncatecholamine) with peripheral alpha- and beta-adrenergic activity. Chemically and pharmacologically related to ephedrine. Marked stimulant effect on CNS thought to be due to action on cerebral cortex and possibly the reticular activating system. Acts indirectly on adrenergic receptors by increasing synaptic release of norepinephrine and dopamine in brain and by blocking reuptake at presynaptic membranes. CNS stimulation results in increased motor activity, diminished sense of fatigue, alertness, wakefulness, and mood elevation. In hyperkinetic children it exerts a paradoxic sedative effect by unclear mechanism. Peripheral actions produce mydriasis without cycloplegia, nasal decongestion, mild bronchodilation and respiratory stimulation, vasoconstriction, increased systolic and diastolic blood pressures, and decreased urinary bladder tone coupled with sphincter constriction. Anorexigenic effect thought to result from direct inhibition of lateral hypothalamic appetite center, as well as mood elevation.

USES Narcolepsy, attention deficit disorder in children (hyperkinetic behavioral syndrome, and minimal brain dysfunction). Use as short-term adjunct to control exogenous obesity not generally recommended because of its potential for abuse. **Unlabeled uses:** in combination with other drugs for treatment-resistant depression.

PHARMACOKINETICS Absorption: rapid. **Peak effect:** 1–5 h. **Duration:** up to 10 h. **Distribution:** all tissues,

Common side effects in *italic*; life-threatening effects underlined; generic names in **bold**; classifications in SMALL CAPS

especially CNS. **Metabolism:** metabolized in liver. **Elimination:** half-life: 10–30 h; renal elimination; excreted in breast milk.

ROUTE & DOSAGE

Narcolepsy
Adult	PO	5–60 mg/d divided q4–6h in 2–3 doses
Child	PO	>12 y: 10 mg/d; may increase by 10 mg at weekly intervals
		6–12 y: 5 mg/d; may increase by 5 mg at weekly intervals

Attention Deficit Disorder
Child	PO	6 y: 5 mg 1–2 times/d; may increase by 5 mg at weekly intervals (max 40 mg/d)
		3–5 y: 2.5 mg 1–2 times/d; may increase by 2.5 mg at weekly intervals

Obesity
Adult	PO	5–10 mg 1 h before meals

CONTRAINDICATIONS & PRECAUTIONS Contraindicated in: hypersensitivity to sympathomimetic amines; history of drug abuse; severe agitation; hyperthyroidism; diabetes mellitus, moderate to severe hypertension, advanced arteriosclerosis, angina pectoris or other cardiovascular disorders; Gilles de la Tourette disorder; glaucoma; during or within 14 d after treatment with MAOIs. Safe use during pregnancy (category C) and in nursing mothers not established. **Cautious use in:** mild hypertension.

ADVERSE/SIDE EFFECTS Allergy: urticaria. **CNS:** *irritability,* psychosis, *restlessness,* nervousness, headache, *insomnia,* weakness, *euphoria,* dysphoria, drowsiness, trembling hyperactive reflexes. **CV:** *palpitation,* elevated BP; *tachycardia,* vasculitis. Endocrine (with high doses): impotence, change in libido. **GI:** dry mouth, anorexia, unusual weight loss, nausea, vomiting, diarrhea, or constipation.

DIAGNOSTIC TEST INTERFERENCES Elevations in *serum thyroxine* (T_4) levels with high amphetamine doses.

DRUG INTERACTIONS Acetazolamide, sodium bicarbonate decrease amphetamine elimination; **ammonium chloride, ascorbic acid** increase amphetamine elimination; effects of both amphetamine and BARBITURATE may be antagonized if given together; **furazolidone** may increase BP effects of amphetamines, and interaction may persist for several weeks after furazolidone is discontinued; **guanethidine, guanadryl** antagonize antihypertensive effects; because MAO INHIBITORS, **selegiline** can precipitate hypertensive crisis (fatalities reported), do not administer amphetamines during or within 14 d of these drugs; PHENOTHIAZINES may inhibit mood elevating effects of amphetamines; TRICYCLIC ANTIDEPRESSANTS enhance amphetamine effects through increased norepinephrine release; BETA-AGONISTS increase cardiovascular adverse effects.

NURSING IMPLICATIONS

Administration
- The last dose should be administered no later than 6 h before patient retires to avoid insomnia.
- As an anorexigenic, drug is administered on an empty stomach 30–60 min before meal.
- Store at 15–30C (59–86F) unless otherwise directed.

Assessment & Drug Effects
- Tolerance to the mood elevating effects commonly occurs within a few weeks. When clinical effectiveness appears to be waning, evaluation is indicated, not a dose increase.
- Insulin dose in diabetes may require adjustment. Monitor closely.
- Effect of amphetamines on growth in children is not known. Close monitoring is advised.
- Response to the drug is more variable in children than in adults. Acute toxicity has occurred over a wide range of dosage.

Patient & Family Education
- Keep physician informed of clinical response and persistent or bothersome side effects. Amphetamine exerts a stimulating effect that masks fatigue. After the exhilaration has disappeared, fatigue and depression are usually greater than before, and a longer period of rest is needed.
- Drug may impair ability to engage in hazardous activities such as operating an automobile or machinery.
- To relieve mouth dryness: frequent rinses with clear water, especially after eating; increase fluid intake, if allowed; sugarless chewing gum.
- Meticulous oral hygiene is required, as decreased saliva encourages demineralization of tooth surfaces and mucosal erosion. Gentle brushing of tongue surface helps to reduce halitosis. Use of a commercially avilable oral lubricant, such as Moi-Stir or Xero-Lube, can relieve soft tissue problems and reduce the potential of caries.

Common side effects in *italic*; life-threatening effects underlined; generic names in **bold**; classifications in SMALL CAPS

195

- Tolerance to the anorexiant effect usually occurs within a few weeks. As effect lessens (appetite increases), dose increase is not indicated.
- Caffeine-containing beverages should be avoided, as caffeine increases amphetamine-like and related amine effects.
- Following prolonged administration of high doses, amphetamine should gradually be withdrawn. Abrupt withdrawal may result in lethargy, profound depression, or other psychotic manifestations that may persist for several weeks.
- Tolerance almost invariably develops to the euphoric and anorexigenic effects of amphetamines. Drug should be discontinued when tolerance develops. Generally, tolerance does not occur when amphetamine is used for attention deficit disorders or narcolepsy.
- Amphetamines have a high abuse potential because of their excitatory and euphoric effects.

RESPIRATORY & CEREBRAL STIMULANT: ANOREXIANT

DIETHYLPROPION HYDROCHLORIDE

(dye-eth-il-proe´pee-on)
Trade names: Nobesine, Propion, Regibon, Tenuate, Tenuate Dospan, Tepanil
Classifications: CNS AGENT; RESPIRATORY & CEREBRAL STIMULANT; ANOREXIANT; AMPHETAMINE
Pregnancy: Category B
Controlled substance: Schedule IV

ACTIONS/PHARMACODYNAMICS Sympathomimetic amine and amphetamine cogener. Has lower incidence of amphetamine-type adverse effects but reportedly is less effective as an appetite suppressant. Anorexigenic action probably secondary to direct (CNS) stimulation of appetite control center in hypothalamus and limbic regions. Also produces mild psychic stimulation and vasopressor effects.

USES Used solely in management of exogenous obesity as short-term (a few weeks) adjunct in a regimen of weight reduction based on caloric restriction.

PHARMACOKINETICS Absorption: Readily absorbed from GI tract. **Duration:** 4 h, regular tablets; 10–14 h, sustained release. **Elimination:** half-life: 4–6 h; excreted in urine.

ROUTE & DOSAGE

Obesity

Adult	PO	25 mg t.i.d. 30–60 min a.c. or 75 mg sustained release qd midmorning

CONTRAINDICATIONS & PRECAUTIONS Contraindicated in: known hypersensitivity or idiosyncrasy to sympathomimetic amines; severe hypertension, advanced arteriosclerosis; hyperthyroidism; glaucoma; agitated states, history of drug abuse. Safe use during pregnancy (category B) and in children < 12 not established. **Cautious use in:** hypertension, arrhythmias, symptomatic cardiovascular disease; epilepsy; diabetes mellitus.

ADVERSE/SIDE EFFECTS CNS: mild euphoria, restlessness, *nervousness,* dizziness, headache, irritability, hyperactivity, insomnia, drowsiness, mood changes, lethargy. **CV:** palpitation, tachycardia, precordial pain, rise in BP. **GI:** nausea, vomiting, diarrhea, constipation, dry mouth, unpleasant taste. **Hypersensitivity:** urticaria, rash, erythema. **Other:** muscle pain, dyspnea, hair loss, blurred vision, severe dermatoses (chronic intoxication); polyuria, dysuria, increased sweating, impotence, changes in libido, gynecomastia, menstrual irregularities, bone marrow depression, increase in convulsive episodes in patients with epilepsy.

DRUG INTERACTIONS Acetazolamide, sodium bicarbonate decrease diethylpropion elimination; **ammonium chloride, ascorbic acid** increase diethylpropion elimination; a BARBITURATE and diethylpropion taken together may antagonize the effects of both drugs; **furazolidone** may increase blood pressure effects of amphetamines, and interaction may persist for several weeks after discontinuation of furazolidone; **guanethidine, guanadryl** antagonize antihypertensive effects; MAO INHIBITORS, **selegiline** can cause hypertensive crisis (fatalities reported)—amphetamines should not be administered at the same time as or within 14 days of these drugs; PHENOTHIAZINES may inhibit mood elevating effects of amphetamines; TRICYCLIC ANTIDEPRESSANTS enhance amphetamine effects by increasing norepinephrine release; BETA AGONISTS increase cardiovascular adverse effects.

NURSING IMPLICATIONS

Administration

- Administer on an empty stomach, 1/2–1 h before meals.

Common side effects in *italic*; life-threatening effects underlined; generic names in **bold**; classifications in SMALL CAPS

- Additional dose sometimes prescribed in mid-evening to control nighttime hunger. Rarely causes insomnia except in high doses.
- Dosage should be carefully titrated in patients with diabetes.
- Store between 15 and 30C (59 and 86F) in well-closed container unless otherwise specified.

Assessment & Drug Effects
- Patients with epilepsy should be observed closely for reduction in seizure control.
- Anorexigenic effect seldom lasts more than a few weeks. If tolerance develops, drug should be discontinued.
- Varying degrees of psychologic and rarely physical dependence can occur. Drugs related to amphetamines are frequently misused by emotionally unstable individuals.

Patient & Family Education
- Sustained-release tablets should be swallowed whole and not chewed.
- Avoid driving a car or other hazardous activities until reaction to drug is determined.

RESPIRATORY AND CEREBRAL STIMULANT: XANTHINE

CAFFEINE
(kaf-een´)
Trade names: Caffedrine, Dexitac, NoDoz, Quick Pep, S-250, Tirend, Vivarin

CAFFEINE AND SODIUM BENZOATE

CITRATED CAFFEINE

Classifications: CNS AGENT; RESPIRATORY AND CEREBRAL STIMULANT; XANTHINE
Pregnancy: Category C

ACTIONS/PHARMACODYNAMICS Methylxanthine with actions similar to those of other xanthines (e.g., theophylline). Chief action is thought to be related to inhibition of the enzyme phosphodiesterase, which results in higher concentrations of cyclic AMP. Another possible mechanism is inhibition of central cell surface receptors for adenosine. Releases epinephrine and norepinephrine from adrenal medulla, producing CNS stimulation. Small doses improve psychic and sensory awareness and reduce drowsiness and fatigue by stimulating cerebral cortex. Higher doses stimulate medullary, respiratory, vasomotor, and vagal centers. Produces smooth muscle relaxation (especially bronchi) and dilation of coronary, pulmonary, and systemic blood vessels by direct action on vascular musculature. Mild diuretic action may result from increase in renal blood flow and glomerular filtration rate and decrease in renal tubular reabsorption of sodium and water. Increases contractile force of heart and cardiac output by direct stimulation of myocardium. Also stimulates secretion of gastric acid and digestive enzymes. Relief of headache is perhaps due to mild cerebral vasoconstriction action and increased vascular tone.

USES Orally as a mild CNS stimulant to aid in staying awake and restoring mental alertness, and as an adjunct in narcotic and nonnarcotic analgesia. Used parenterally as an emergency stimulant in acute circulatory failure, as a diuretic, and to relieve spinal puncture headache. **Unlabeled use:** topical treatment of atopic dermatitis, and neonatal apnea.

ROUTE & DOSAGE

Mental Stimulant

Adult	PO	100–200 mg q3–4h prn

Circulatory Stimulant

Adult	IM	200–500 mg prn

Spinal Puncture Headaches

Adult	IV	500 mg over 1 h; may repeat × 1 dose

Neonatal Apnea

Child	PO/IV	20 mg/kg as a loading dose, followed by a maintenance dose 2–3 d later of 5–10 mg/kg 1–2 times/d

PHARMACOKINETICS Absorption: rapidly absorbed. **Peak:** 15–45 min. **Distribution:** widely distributed throughout body; crosses blood brain barrier and placenta. **Metabolism:** metabolized in liver. **Elimination:** half-life: 3–5 h in adults, 36–144 h in neonates; excreted in urine as metabolites; excreted in breast milk in small amounts.

CONTRAINDICATIONS & PRECAUTIONS Contraindicated in: acute MI, symptomatic cardiac arrhythmias, palpitations; peptic ulcer; insomnia, panic attacks. Safe use during pregnancy (category C), in nursing women, and in children not established.

Common side effects in *italic*; life-threatening effects underlined; generic names in **bold**; classifications in SMALL CAPS

197

ELECTROLYTIC & WATER BALANCE AGENTS

Cautious use in: diabetes mellitus; hiatus hernia; hypertension with heart disease.

ADVERSE/SIDE EFFECTS CNS: *nervousness, insomnia,* restlessness, irritability, confusion, agitation, fasciculations, delirium, twitching, tremors, clonic convulsions, respiratory depression and arrest. **CV:** tingling of face, flushing, palpitation, rapid heart beat, tachycardia or bradycardia, ventricular ectopic beats, hypotension. **GI:** nausea, vomiting; epigastric discomfort, gastric irritation (oral form), diarrhea, hematemesis, kernicterus (neonates). **Other:** scintillating scotomas, tinnitus, increased urination, marked diuresis, hyperglycemia, tachypnea, increase in blood cholesterol.

DIAGNOSTIC TEST INTERFERENCES Caffeine reportedly may interfere with diagnosis of pheochromocytoma or neuroblastoma by increasing urinary excretion of **catecholamines, VMA,** and **5-HIAA** and may cause false positive increases in **serum urate** (by **Bittner method**).

DRUG INTERACTIONS Caffeine may increase effects of **cimetidine** by inhibiting its metabolism; caffeine increases cardiovascular stimulating effects of BETA-ADRENERGIC AGONISTS; possibly increases **theophylline** toxicity.

NURSING IMPLICATIONS

Administration

- IV caffeine may be administered undiluted by direct IV at a rate of 250 mg or a fraction thereof over 1 min when used in an emergency situation.
- With neonates, caffeine without sodium benzoate is ordinarily used.
- Caffeine should be administered slowly by IV route to neonates. Check with physician regarding preferred rate.
- IV caffeine given to adults for spinal puncture headache is administered at a rate of 500 mg over 1 h by infusion.
- Timed-release preparations should be administered not less than 6 h before bedtime.

Assessment & Drug Effects

- Large doses may cause intensification rather than reversal of severe drug-induced depressions. Monitor vital signs closely.
- Children are more susceptible than adults to the CNS effects of caffeine and therefore should be closely observed following administration.
- Monitor blood glucose levels in diabetics, as caffeine may elevate serum level.

Patient & Family Education

- Caffeine usually restricted with ulcers because caffeine stimulates gastric secretions. Patients who insist on drinking coffee should be advised to drink it with meals, well diluted, and with milk.
- Patients with diabetes should be advised that caffeine in large amounts may impair glucose tolerance.
- Advise patients who consume large amounts of caffeine that headache, dizziness, anxiety, irritability, nervousness, and muscle tension may result from excessive use, as well as from abrupt withdrawal of coffee (or oral caffeine) in heavy users. Withdrawal symptoms usually occur 12–18 h following last coffee intake.

DIURETIC, LOOP

FUROSEMIDE
(fur-oh´se-mide)
Trade names: Fumide, Furomide, Lasix, Luramide
Classifications: ELECTROLYTIC & WATER BALANCE AGENT; LOOP DIURETIC
Pregnancy: Category C

ACTIONS/PHARMACODYNAMICS Rapid-acting potent sulfonamide "loop" diuretic and antihypertensive with pharmac ologice effects and uses almost identical to those of ethacrynic acid. Exact mode of action not clearly defined. As with ethacrynic acid, urinary pH falls after administration, but in some patients bicarbonate excretion may temporarily increase the pH. Renal vascular resistance decreases, and renal blood flow may increase during drug administration. Inhibits reabsorption of sodium and chloride primarily in loop of Henle and also in proximal and distal renal tubules. Enhances excretion of potassium, hydrogen, calcium, magne sium, ammonium, bicarbonate, and possibly phosphate. Reportedly less ototoxic than ethacrynic acid.

USES Treatment of edema associated with CHF, cirrhosis of liver, and renal disease, including nephrotic syndrome. May be used for management of hypertension, alone or in combination with other antihypertensive agents, and for treatment of hypercalcemia. Has been used concomitantly with mannitol

Common side effects in *italic*; life-threatening effects underlined; generic names in **bold**; classifications in SMALL CAPS

for treatment of severe cerebral edema, particularly in meningitis.

ROUTE & DOSAGE

Edema

Adult	PO	20–80 mg in 1 or more divided doses up to 600 mg/d if needed
	IV/IM	20–40 mg in 1 or more divided doses up to 600 mg/d
Child	PO	2 mg/kg; may be increased by 1–2 mg/kg q6–8h up to a max of 6mg/kg/dose
	IV/IM	1 ng/kg; may be increased by 1mg/kg q2h if needed up to a max of 6 mg/kg/dose

Hypertension

Adult	PO	10–40 mg b.i.d. (max 480 mg/d

PHARMACOKINETICS Absorption: 60 of oral dose absorbed from GI tract. **Peak:** 60–70 min PO; 20–60 min IV. **Onset:** 30–60 min PO; 5 min IV. **Duration:** 2 h. **Distribution:** crosses placenta. **Metabolism:** small amount metabolized in liver. **Elimination:** half-life: 30 min; rapidly excreted in urine; 50% of oral dose and 80% of IV dose excreted within 24 h; excreted in breastmilk.

CONTRAINDICATIONS & PRECAUTIONS

Contraindicated in: history of hypersensitivity to furosemide or sulfonamides; increasing oliguria, anuria, fluid and electrolyte depletion states; hepatic coma; pregnancy (category C). **Cautious use in:** infants, elderly patients; hepatic cirrhosis, nephrotic syndrome; cardiogenic shock associated with acute MI; history of SLE, history of gout; patients receiving digitalis glycosides or potassium-depleting steroids.

ADVERSE/SIDE EFFECTS CV:
postural hypotension, dizziness with excessive diuresis, acute hypotensive episodes, circulatory collapse, thromboembolic episodes. **Fluid and electrolyte imbalance:** hypovolemia, dehydration, hyponatremia, *hypokalemia*, hypochloremia metabolic alkalosis, hypomagnesemia, hypocalcemia (tetany), hyperammonemia. **GI:** nausea, vomiting, oral and gastric burning, anorexia, diarrhea, constipation, abdominal cramping, acute pancreatitis, jaundice. **GU:** flank and loin pain, allergic interstitial nephritis, irreversible renal failure, bladder pressure or spasm, urinary frequency. **Hematologic:** anemia, leukopenia, aplastic anemia (rare), thrombocytopenic purpura, agranulocytosis (rare). **Ototoxicity:** tinnitus, vertigo, feeling of fullness in ears, hearing loss (rarely permanent). **Skin:** pruritus, urticaria, exfoliative dermatitis, erythema multiforme (rare), purpura, photosensitivity, porphyria cutanea tarde, necrotizing angiitis (vasculitis). **Other:** hyperglycemia, glycosuria, elevated BUN, hyperuricemia, acute gout (rare), increased perspiration; paresthesias; blurred vision, activation of SLE, muscle spasms, weakness; thrombophlebitis, pain at IM injection site.

DIAGNOSTIC TEST INTERFERENCES
Furosemide may cause elevations in *BUN, serum amylase, cholesterol, triglycerides, uric acid* and *blood glucose* levels, and may decrease *serum calcium, magnesium, potassium,* and *sodium* levels.

DRUG INTERACTIONS
OTHER DIURETICS enhance diuretic effects; with **digoxin,** increased risk of toxicity because of hypokalemia; NONDEPOLARIZING NEUROMUSCULAR BLOCKING AGENTS (e.g., **tubocurarine)** prolong neuromuscular blockage; CORTICO-STEROIDS, **amphotericin B** potentiate hypokalemia; decreased **lithium** elimination and increased toxicity; SULFONYLUREAS, **insulin** blunt hypoglycemic effects; NSAIDs may attenuate diuretic effects.

INCOMPATIBILITIES
Solution/Additive: dobutamine, doxapram, doxorubicin, droperidol, gentamicin; metoclopramide, netilmicin. **Y-Site:** doxorubicin, droperidol, gentamicin, metoclopramide, netilmicin, vinblastine, vincristine.

NURSING IMPLICATIONS

Administration
- May be taken with food or milk to reduce possibility of gastric irritation.
- Schedule doses to avoid nocturia and sleep disturbance (e.g., a single dose is generally administered in the morning; twice-a-day doses may be prescribed for 8 AM and 2 PM).
- Intermittent dosage schedule is frequently used to allow time for natural correction of electrolyte and acid-base imbalance (e.g., drug is given for 2–4 consecutive days each week).
- Slight discoloration of tablets reportedly does not alter potency; however, yellow or otherwise discolored injection solutions should be discarded.
- *IV injection:* IV furosemide may be given by direct IV undiluted at a rate of 20 mg or a fraction thereof over 1 min. With high doses a rate of 4 mg/min is recommended to decrease risk of ototoxicity.
- Protect syringes from light once they are removed from package.
- Infusion solutions in which furosemide has been

Common side effects in *italic*; life-threatening effects underlined; generic names in **bold**; classifications in SMALL CAPS

199

mixed should be used within 24 h. Reportedly compatible with D5W, NaCl 0.9%, and Ringer's injection, lactated.

- Store tablets and parenteral solution at controlled room temperature, preferably at 15–30C (59–86F) unless otherwise directed. Protect from light.
- Store oral solution in refrigerator, preferably at 2–8C (36–46F). Protect from light and freezing.

Assessment & Drug Effects

- Patients receiving the drug parenterally should be observed carefully, and BP and vital signs closely monitored. Sudden death from cardiac arrest has been reported.
- Close observation of the elderly patient is particularly essential during period of brisk diuresis. Sudden alteration in fluid and electrolyte balance may precipitate adverse reactions: anorexia, nausea, vomiting, thirst, dry mouth, confusion, weakness, fatigue, lightheadedness, dizziness, perspiration, muscle cramps, bladder spasm, and urinary frequency. Report these symptoms to physician.
- Monitor for signs and symptoms of hypokalemia (see chap 3).
- Monitor I&O ratio and pattern. Report decrease or unusual increase in output. Excessive diuresis can result in dehydration and hypovolemia, circulatory collapse, and hypotension.
- Weith patient daily under standard conditions.
- Monitor BP during periods of diuresis and through period of dosage adjustment.
- Excessive dehydration is most likely to occur in the elderly, in those with chronic cardiac disease on prolonged salt restriction, or in those receiving sympatholytic agents.
- Frequent determinations should be made of blood count, serum and urine electrolytes, CO_2, BUN, blood sugar, and uric acid during first few months of therapy and periodically thereafter.

Patient & Family Education

- Consult physician regarding allowable salt and fluid intake.
- To reduce or prevent potassium depletion, daily ingestion of potassium-rich foods (e.g., bananas, oranges, peaches, dried dates) maybe prescribed.
- Instruct patient regarding signs and symptoms of hypokalemia (see chap 3). Advise patient to report muscle cramps or weakness.
- Patients receiving high doses or other antihypertensive drugs concurrently are subject to episodes of postural hypotension usually experienced as light-headedness, dizziness, weakness, lethargy. Caution patient to make position changes slowly.

Also advise against prolonged standing, hot baths or showers, and strenuous exercise in hot weather.
- Instruct patient to avoid replacing fluid losses with large amounts of free water.
- Advise against prolonged exposure to direct sun.
- Furosemide may cause hyperglycemia. Diabetics and patients with decompensated hepatic cirrhosis require careful urine and blood glucose monitoring.

DIURETIC, OSMOTIC

MANNITOL
(man´i-tole)
Trade name: Osmitrol
Classifications: ELECTROLYTIC & WATER BALANCE AGENT; OSMOTIC DIURETIC
Pregnancy: Category C

ACTIONS/PHARMACODYNAMICS Prepared commercially by reduction of dextrose. Induces diuresis by raising osmotic pressure of glomerular filtrate, thereby inhibiting tubular reabsorption of water and solutes. In large doses, may increase rate of electrolyte excretion, particularly sodium, chloride, and potassium. Reduces elevated intraocular and cerebrospinal pressures by increasing plasma osmolality, thus inducing diffusion of water from these fluids back into plasma and extravascular space.

USES To promote diuresis in prevention and treatment of oliguric phase of acute renal failure following cardiovascular surgery, severe traumatic injury, surgery in presence of severe jaundice, hemolytic transfusion reaction. Also used to reduce elevated intraocular (IOP) and intracranial pressure (ICP), to measure glomerular filtration rate (GFR), to promote excretion of toxic substances, to relieve symptoms of pulmonary edema, and as irrigating solution in transurethral prostatic reaction to minimize hemolytic effects of water. Commercially available in combination with sorbitol for urogenital irrigation.

PHARMACOKINETICS Onset: 1–3 h diuresis; 30–60 min IOP; 15 min ICP. **Duration:** 4–6 h IOP; 3–8 h IC P. **Distribution:** confined to extracellular space; does not cross blood-brain barrier except with very high plasma levels in the presence of acidosis. **Meta-**

Common side effects in *italic*; life-threatening effects underlined; generic names in **bold**; classifications in SMALL CAPS

bolism: small quantity metabolized to glycogen in liver. **Elimination:** half-life: 100 min; rapidly excreted by kidneys.

ROUTE & DOSAGE

Acute Renal Failure

Adult   IV   **Test dose:** 0.2 g/kg or 12.5 g as a 15–20% solution over 3–5 min
Positive response: 30–50 ml of urine over next 2–3 h, may repeat test dose 1 time; if still negative, do not use
Treatment: 50–100 g as 15–20% solution over 90 min to several hours

Edema, Ascites

Adult   IV   100 g as a 10–20% solution over 2–6 h

Elevated IOP or ICP

Adult   IV   1.5–2 mg/kg as a 15–25% solution over 30–60 min

Acute Chemical Toxicity

Adult   IV   100–200 g depending on urine output

Measurement of GFR

Adult   IV   100 ml of 20% solution diluted with 180 ml NaCl injection infused at a rate of 20 ml/min

CONTRAINDICATIONS & PRECAUTIONS Contraindicated in: anuria; marked pulmonary edema or CHF; metabolic edema; organic CNS disease, intracranial bleeding; shock, severe dehydration, history of allergy. Safe use during pregnancy (category C) and in children

ADVERSE/SIDE EFFECTS CNS: headache, tremor, convulsions, dizziness, transient muscle rigidity. **CV:** edema, CHF, anginalike pain, hypotension, hypertension, thrombophlebitis. **Eye:** blurred vision. **GI:** dry mouth, nausea, vomiting. **GU:** marked diuresis, urinary retention, nephrosis, uricosuria. **Metabolic:** *fluid and electrolyte imbalance,* especially <u>hyponatremia</u>; dehydration, acidosis. **Other:** arm pain, back ache; with extravasation: local edema, skin necrosis; chills, fever, allergic reactions.

NURSING IMPLICATIONS

Administration

- IV infusion flow rate (prescribed by physician) is generally adjusted to maintain urine flow of at least 30–50 ml/h. See route & dosage for specific rates.

- A test dose is given to patients with marked oliguria to check adequacy of renal function. Response is considered satisfactory if urine flow of at least 30–50 ml/h is produced over 2–3 h after drug administration.
- Parenteral mannitol may crystalize when exposed to low temperatures. If crystallization occurs, place bottle in hot water bath (appr oximately 50C) and periodically shake vigorously. Cool to body temperature before administration. Do not use solution if crystals ca nnot be completely dissolved.
- Concentrations higher than 15% have a greater tendency to crystallize. Administration set with an in-line IV filter should be used w hen infusing concentrations of 15% or above.
- Mannitol should not be added to whole blood transfusion. However, if blood must be given simultaneously, at least 20 mEq of NaCl sho uld be added to each liter of mannitol solution to avoid pseudoagglutination.
- Store preferably at 15–30C (59–86F) unless otherwise directed. Avoid freezing.

Assessment & Drug Effects

- Patients receiving urologic irrigations of mannitol should be observed closely for systemic reactions.
- Care should be taken to avoid extravasation. Observe injection site for signs of inflammation or edema.
- Serum and urine electrolytes (particularly sodium, potassium, and chloride), CVP, and renal function should be closely monitored during therapy.
- I&O must be a ccurately measured and recorded to achieve proper fluid balance.
- Monitor allowable PO fluid intake volume.
- Monitor vital signs and carefully note possible indications of fluid and electrolyte imbalance (e.g., thirst, muscle cramps or weakness, paresthesias, and signs of CHF.
- Be alert to the possibility that a rebound increase in ICP sometimes occurs about 12 h after drug administration. Patient may complain of headache or confusion.
- Take accurate daily weight.

Patient & Family Education

- Advise patient to report any of the following: thirst, muscle cramps or weakness, paresthesia, dyspnea, or headache.
- Instruct family members to immediately report any evidence of confusion.

DIURETIC, POTASSIUM-SPARING

SPIRONOLACTONE
(speer-on-oh-lak´tone)
Trade names: Aldactone, Novospiroton, Sincomen
Classifications: ELECTROLYTIC & WATER BALANCE AGENT; POTASSIUM-SPARING DIURETIC; SYNTHETIC HORMONE
Pregnancy: Category D

ACTIONS/PHARMACODYNAMICS Steroidal compound and specific pharmacologic antagonist of aldosterone. Presumably acts by competing with aldosterone for cellular receptor sites in distal renal tubule. Promotes sodium and chloride (and water) excretion without concomitant loss of potassium. Diuretic effect reportedly not associated with hyperuricemia or hyperglycemia. Activity depends on presence of endogenous or exogenous aldosterone. Lowers systolic and diastolic pressures in hypertensive patients by unknown mechanism. Potentially mutagenic and tumorigenic.

USES Clinical conditions associated with augmented aldosterone production, as in essential hypertension, refractory edema due to CHF, hepatic cirrhosis, nephrotic syndrome, and idiopathic edema. May be used to potentiate actions of other diuretics and antihypertensive agents or for its potassium-sparing effect. Also used for treatment of (and as presumptive test for) primary aldosteronism. **Unlabeled use:** hirsutism in women with polycystic ovary syndrome or idiopathic hirsutism; adjunct in treatment of myasthenia gravis and familial periodic paralysis.

PHARMACOKINETICS Absorption: approximately 73% absorbed from GI tract. **Onset:** gradual. **Peak:** 2–3 d; max effect may take up to 2 wk. **Duration:** 2–3 d or more. **Distribution:** crosses placenta, distributed into breast milk. **Metabolism:** metabolized in liver and kidneys to active metabolites. **Elimination:** half-life: 1.3–2.4 h parent compound, 18–23 h metabolites, 40–57% excreted in urine, 35–40% in bile.

CONTRAINDICATIONS & PRECAUTIONS Contraindicated in: anuria, acute renal insufficiency, progressing impairment of renal function, hyperkalemia. Safe use during pregnancy (category D) and lactation not established. **Cautious use in:** BUN of 40 mg/dl or greater, hepatic disease.

ROUTE & DOSAGE

Edema

Adult	PO	25–200 mg/d in divided doses; continued for at least 5 d; dose adjusted to optimal response; if no response, a thiazide or loop diuretic may be added
Child	PO	3.3 mg/kg/d in single or divided doses; continued for at least 5 d; dose adjusted to optimal response

Hypertension

Adult	PO	25–100 mg/d in single or divided doses; continued for at least 2 wk; dose adjusted to optimal response

Primary Aldosteronism: Diagnosis

Adult	PO	Short test: 400 mg/d for 4 d
		Long test: 400 mg/d for 3–4 wk

Primary Aldosteronism: Treatment

Adult	PO	100–400 mg/d in divided doses

ADVERSE/SIDE EFFECTS CNS: lethargy, mental confusion, fatigue (with rapid weight loss), headache, drowsiness, ataxia. **Endocrine:** gynecomastia (both sexes), inability to achieve or maintain erection, androgenic effects (hirsutism, irregular menses, deepening of voice); parathyroid changes, decreased glucose tolerance. **GI:** abdominal cramps, nausea, vomiting, anorexia, diarrhea. **Skin:** maculopapular or erythematous rash, urticaria. **Other:** fluid and electrolyte imbalance (particularly hyperkalemia and hyponatremia); elevated BUN, mild acidosis, drug fever, agranulocytosis, SLE, hypertension (postsympathectomy patient), hyperuricemia, gout.

DIAGNOSTIC TEST INTERFERENCES Spironolactone may produce marked increases in *plasma cortisol* determinations by *Mattingly fluorometric* method; these may persist for several days after termination of drug (spironolactone metabolite produces fluorescence). There is the possibility of false elevations in measurements of *digoxin serum levels* by *RIA* procedures.

DRUG INTERACTIONS Combinations of spironolactone and acidifying doses of **ammonium chloride** may produce systemic acidosis; use these combinations with caution. Diuretic effect of spiro-

Common side effects in *italic*; life-threatening effects <u>underlined</u>; generic names in **bold**; classifications in SMALL CAPS

nolactone may be antagonized by **aspirin** and other SALICYLATES (possibly by competing for same receptor sites). Patients receiving spironolactone and **digitoxin** or similar CARDIAC GLYCOSIDES concurrently should be monitored for decreased effect of cardiac glycoside (spironolactone shortens its half-life, possibly by acting as enzyme inducing agent). Hyperkalemia may result with POTASSIUM SUPPLEMENTS (spironolactone conserves potassium).

NURSING IMPLICATIONS

Administration

- Administer with food to enhance absorption.
- Tablet may be crushed before administration and taken with fluid of patient's choice.
- Preserve in tight, light-resistant containers. Suspension is stable for 1 mo under refrigeration.

Assessment & Drug Effects

- Check blood pressure before initiation of therapy and at regular intervals throughout therapy.
- Serum electrolytes should be monitored, especially during early therapy. Be alert for signs of fluid and electrolyte imbalance.
- Monitor daily I&O and check for edema. Report lack of diuretic response or development of edema; both may indicate tolerance to drug.
- Weigh patient under standard conditions before therapy begins and daily throughout therapy. Weight is a useful index of need for dosage adjustment. For patients with ascites, physician may want measurements of abdominal girth.
- Observe for and report immediately the onset of mental changes, lethargy, or stupor in patients with hepatic disease.
- Adverse reactions are generally reversible with discontinuation of drug. Gynecomastia appears to be related to dosage level and duration of therapy; it may persist in some after drug is stopped.

Patient & Family Education

- Inform patient that maximal diuretic effect may not occur until third day of therapy and that diuresis may continue for 2 or 3 d after drug is withdrawn.
- Instruct patient to report signs of hyponatremia (see chap 3), most likely to occur in patients with severe cirrhosis.
- Instruct patient to avoid replacing fluid losses with large amounts of free water (can result in dilutional hyponatremia).
- Generally, patient should avoid excessive intake of high-potassium foods and salt substitutes.

DIURETIC, THIAZIDE

HYDROCHLOROTHIAZIDE

(hye-droe-klor-oh-thye´a-zide)
Trade names: Apo-Hydro, Aquazide H, Chlorzide, Diaqua, Diu-Scrip, Esidrix, Hydro-Chlor, HydroDiuril, Hydromal, Hydro-T, Hydro-Z, Oretic, SK-Hydrochlorothiazide, Thiuretic, HCTZ, Urozide, Zide
Classifications: ELECTROLYTIC & WATER BALANCE AGENT; THIAZIDE DIURETIC; CARDIOVASCULAR AGENT; ANTIHYPERTENSIVE
Pregnancy: Category B

ACTIONS/PHARMACODYNAMICS Benzothiadiazine (thiazide) derivative. Similar to chlorothiazide. Action mechanism unclear; diuretic action is associated with drug interference with transport of sodium ions across renal tubular epithelium. This enhances excretion of sodium, chloride, potassium, bicarbonates, and water. **Action site:** cortical dilution segment of nephron. **Other actions:** hypotensive action (direct arteriolar dilation), elevated plasma renin activity, and precipitation of diabetes in the prediabetic patient.

USES Adjunct in treatment of edema associated with CHF, hepatic cirrhosis, renal failure, and in the stepped-care management of hypertension (step 1 and 2 agent). **Unlabeled use:** nephrogenic diabetes insipidus, hypercalciuria, and treatment of electrolyte disturbances associated with renal tubular acidosis.

ROUTE & DOSAGE

Edema

Adult	PO	25–200 mg/d in 1–3 divided doses

Hypertension

Adult	PO	12.5–100 mg/d in 1–2 divided doses
Child	PO	2.2 mg/kg/d in 2 divided doses

PHARMACOKINETICS Absorption: incompletely absorbed. **Onset:** 2 h. **Peak:** 4 h. **Duration:** 6–12 h. **Distribution:** distributed throughout extracellular tissue; concentrates in kidney; crosses placenta; distributed in breast milk. **Metabolism:** does not appear to be metabolized. **Elimination:** half-life: 45–120 min; excreted in urine.

Common side effects in *italic*; life-threatening effects underlined; generic names in **bold**; classifications in SMALL CAPS

203

CONTRAINDICATIONS & PRECAUTIONS Contraindicated in: hypersensitivity to thiazides or other sulfonamides; anuria, pregnancy (category B), lactation. **Cautious use in:** bronchial asthma, allergy; hepatic cirrhosis; renal dysfunction; history of gout, SLE; diabetes mellitus; the elderly.

ADVERSE/SIDE EFFECTS CNS: mood changes, unusual tiredness or weakness, dizziness, lightheadedness, paresthesias. **CV:** irregular heartbeat, weak pulse, orthostatic hypotension. **GI:** dry mouth, increased thirst, nausea, vomiting, anorexia, diarrhea, pancreatitis, jaundice. **Hematologic:** <u>agranulocytosis</u>, thrombocytopenia, <u>aplastic anemia</u>, leukopenia. **Metabolic:** *hyperglycemia*, glycosuria, *hyperuricemia*, *hypokalemia*. **Other:** hypersensitivity reactions, photosensitivity, blurred vision, yellow vision (xanthopsia), muscle spasm.

DIAGNOSTIC TEST INTERFERENCES Falsely decreased value in ***total urinary estrogen*** by ***spectrophotometric assay.*** See chlorothiazide, p 430.

DRUG INTERACTIONS Amphotericin B, CORTICOSTEROIDS increase hypokalemic effects; SULFONYLUREAS, **insulin** may antagonize hypoglycemic effects; **cholestyramine, colistipol** decrease thiazide absorption; **diazoxide** intensifies hypoglycemic and hypotensive effects; increased potassium and magnesium loss may cause **digoxin** toxicity; decreases **lithium** excretion and increases toxicity; increases risk of NSAID-induced renal failure and may attenuate diuresis.

NURSING IMPLICATIONS

Administration

- May be taken with food or milk to reduce GI upset.
- Schedule doses to avoid nocturia and interrupted sleep. Administer PO drug early in AM after eating to prevent gastric irritation. If given in 2 doses, schedule second dose no later than 3 PM.
- Store tablets in tightly closed container at 15–30C (59–86F) unless otherwise directed.

Assessment & Drug Effects

- Antihypertensive effects may be noted in 3–4 d; maximal effects may require 3–4 wk.
- Baseline and periodic determinations of serum electrolytes, blood counts, BUN, blood glucose, uric acid, CO_2, are recommended.
- Check BP before initiation of therapy and at regular intervals.
- Closely monitor for development of hypokalemia, which increases the risk of digoxin toxicity.

- Monitor I&O and check for edema.
- Be aware that drug may cause hyperglycemia and loss of glycemic control in diabetics.
- Drug may cause orthostatic hypotension, dizziness.
- Prolonged therapy requires periodic hematologic studies.

Patient & Family Education

- Advise patient to consult physician before using OTC drugs. Many contain large amounts of sodium as well as potassium.
- Instruct patient to monitor weight daily.
- Avoid calcium supplements; may result in hypercalcemia. Discuss with physician.
- Drug causes impaired glucose tolerance. Advise the diabetic patient to monitor blood glucose closely.
- Report signs of hypokalemia (see chap 3) to physician.
- Instruct patient with orthostatic hypotension to change positions slowly, to avoid hot baths or showers, extended exposure to sunlight, and sitting or standing still for long periods.
- Warn patient about possibility of photosensitivity reaction—usually occurs 10–14 d after initial sun exposure.

REPLACEMENT SOLUTION

CALCIUM GLUCONATE
(gloo´koe-nate)
Trade name: Kalcinate
Classifications: ELECTROLYTIC & WATER BALANCE AGENT; REPLACEMENT SOLUTION

ACTIONS/PHARMACODYNAMICS Calcium is an essential element for regulating the excitation threshold of nerves and muscles, for blood clotting mechanisms, cardiac function (rhythm, tonicity, contractility), maintenance of renal function, for body skeleton and teeth. Also plays a role in regulating storage and release of neurotransmitters and hormones; regulating amino acid uptake and absorption of vitamin B_{12}; gastrin secretion, and in maintaining structural and functional integrity of cell membranes and capillaries. Calcium gluconate acts like digitalis on heart, increasing cardiac muscle tone and force of systolic contractions (positive inotropic effect).

Common side effects in *italic*; life-threatening effects <u>underlined</u>; generic names in **bold**; classifications in SMALL CAPS

USES Negative calcium balance (as in neonatal tetany, hypoparathyroidism, vitamin D deficiency, alkalosis). Also to overcome cardiac toxicity of hyperkalemia, for cardiopulmonary resuscitation, to prevent hypocalcemia during transfusion of citrated blood. Also as antidote for magnesium sulfate, for acute symptoms of lead colic, to decrease capillary permeability in sensitivity reactions, and to relieve muscle cramps from insect bites or stings. Oral calcium may be used to maintain normal calcium balance during pregnancy, lactation, and childhood growth and to prevent primary osteoporosis. Also in osteoporosis, osteomalacia, chronic hypoparathyroidism, rickets, and as adjunct in treatment of myasthenia gravis and Eaton-Lambert syndrome. **Unlabeled use:** to antagonize aminoglycoside-induced neuromuscular blockage, and as "calcium challenge" to diagnose Zollinger-Ellison syndrome and medullary thyroid carcinoma.

PHARMACOKINETICS Absorption: approximately 1/3 of dose absorbed from small intestine. **Onset:** immediately after IV. **Distribution:** crosses placenta. **Elimination:** primarily excreted in feces; small amounts excreted in urine, pancreatic juice, saliva, and breast milk.

ROUTE & DOSAGE

All doses are in terms of *elemental calcium*. 1 g calcium gluconate = 90 mg (4.5 mEq) elemental calcium

Supplement for Osteoporosis

Adult	PO	1–2 g b.i.d. to q.i.d.
	IV	7 mEq q1–3d
Child	PO	45–65 mg/kg/d in divided doses
	IV	1–7 mEq q1–3d
Neonate	PO	50–150 mg/kg/d (max 1 g)
	IV	1 mEq q1–3d

Hypocalcemic Tetany

Adult	IV	4.5–16 mEq prn
Child	IV	0.5–0.7 mEq/kg t.i.d. or q.i.d.
Neonate	IV	2.4 mEq/kg/d in divided doses

CPR

Adult	IV	2.3–3.7 mEq × 1

Hyperkalemia with Cardiac Toxicity

Adult	IV	2.25–14 mEq q1–2min

Exchange Transfusions with Citrated Blood

Adult	IV	1.35 mEq for each 100 ml of blood
Neonate	IV	0.45 mEq for each 100 ml of blood

CONTRAINDICATIONS & PRECAUTIONS Contraindicated in: ventricular fibrillation, metastatic bone disease, injection into myocardium; administration by SC or IM routes; renal calculi, hypercalcemia, predisposition to hypercalcemia (hyperparathyroidism, certain malignancies). **Cautious use in:** digitalized patients, renal or cardiac insufficiency, sarcoidosis, history of lithiasis, immobilized patients.

ADVERSE/SIDE EFFECTS *Hypercalcemia.* **IV injection:** tingling sensations, calcium (chalky) taste. **Rapid IV:** sense of oppression or "heat waves" (vasodilation), hypotension, bradycardia and other arrhythmias, syncope, <u>cardiac arrest</u>. **Local reactions:** tissue irritation, burning, cellulitis, soft tissue calcification, necrosis and sloughing (following IV extravasation). **PO preparation:** constipation, increased gastric acid secretion.

DIAGNOSTIC TEST INTERFERENCES IV calcium may cause false decreases in ***serum and urine magnesium*** (by Titan yellow method) and transient elevations of ***plasma 11-OHCS*** levels by Glenn-Nelson technique. Values usually return to control levels after 60 min; ***urinary steroid*** values (17-OHCS) may be decreased.

DRUG INTERACTIONS May enhance inotropic and toxic effects of **digoxin; magnesium** may compete for GI absorption; decreases absorption of TETRACYCLINES, QUINOLONES **(ciprofloxacin)**; antagonizes the effects of **verapamil** and possibly other CALCIUM CHANNEL BLOCKERS.

NURSING IMPLICATIONS

Administration

- Oral calcium preparations are best utilized when administered 2–3 h after meals.
- IV calcium should be administered slowly through a small-bore needle into a large vein to avoid possibility of extravasation and resultant necrosis. If calcium is administered to children, scalp veins should be avoided.
- Most often physician will prescribe a specific IV flow rate. High concentrations of calcium suddenly reaching the heart can cause fatal cardiac arrest.
- *IV injection:* IV solution may be given undiluted direct IV at a rate of 0.5 ml or a fraction thereof over 1 min.
- *IV infusion:* IV solution may be diluted in 1 L of NS and given over 12–24 h.
- Direct IV injection may be accompanied by cutaneous burning sensations and peripheral vasodila-

Common side effects in *italic*; life-threatening effects <u>underlined</u>; generic names in **bold**; classifications in SMALL CAPS

205

tion, with moderate fall in BP. Injection should be stopped if patient complains of any discomfort. Patient should be advised to remain in bed for 15–30 min or more following injection, depending on response.

Assessment & Drug Effects
- During IV administration, ECG is monitored to detect evidence of hypercalcemia: decreased QT interval associated with inverted T wave.
- Observe IV site closely. Extravasation may result in tissue irritation and necrosis.
- Monitor for hypocalcemia and hypercalcemia (see Signs & Symptoms, chap 3).
- In sustained therapy, frequent determinations should be made of calcium and phosphorus (tend to vary inversely) and magnesium. Deficiencies in other ions, particularly magnesium, frequently coexist with calcium ion depletion.

Patient & Family Education
- Instruct patients regarding signs and symptoms of hypercalcemia (see chap 3) and advise them to report any promptly.
- Inform patient that milk and milk products are best sources of calcium (and phosphorus). Other good sources include dark green vegetables, soy beans, tofu, and canned fish with bones.
- Advise patient that calcium absorption can also be inhibited by zinc-rich foods: nuts, seeds, sprouts, legumes, soy products (tofu).
- Advise patient to check with physician before self-medicating with a calcium supplement.

CARBONIC ANHYDRASE INHIBITOR

ACETAZOLAMIDE
(a-set-a-zole´a-mide)
Trade names: Acetazolam, Ak-Zol, Apo-Acetazolamide, Cetazol, Dazamide, Diamox, Diamox Sequels, Hydrazol

ACETAZOLAMIDE SODIUM
Trade name: Diamox Parenteral
Classifications: EYE PREPARATION: CARBONIC ANHYDRASE INHIBITOR; LOOP DIURETIC; CNS AGENT; ANTICONVULSANT
Pregnancy: Category C

ACTIONS/PHARMACODYNAMICS Diuretic effect is due to inhibition of carbonic anhydrase activity in proximal renal tubule, preventing formation of carbonic acid. Absence or reduced hydrogen ion inhibits renal tubular reabsorption of sodium, thereby promoting bicarbonate elimination along with that of potassium and water. Net result is alkaline diuresis with conservation of chloride and ammonia. After 3 or 4 d of continuous inhibition, mild metabolic acidosis develops with concomitant reduction in diuresis. Inhibition of carbonic anhydrase in eye reduces rate of aqueous humor formation with consequent lowering of intraocular pressure. This effect is independent of systemic acid-base balance and diuretic action. Mechanism of anticonvulsant action unknown but is thought to involve inhibition of CNS carbonic anhydrase, which retards abnormal paroxysmal discharge from CNS neurons.

USES Seizures: absence or petit mal, generalized tonic-clonic (grand mal), and focal; reduction of intraocular pressure in open-angle glaucoma and secondary glaucoma; preoperative treatment of acute closed-angle glaucoma; drug-induced edema and as adjunct in treatment of edema due to congestive heart failure; acute high-altitude sickness. **Unlabeled use:** to prevent uric acid or cystine renal calculi; to treat acute pancreatitis, premenstrual syndrome (PMS), metabolic alkalosis, and hypokalemic and hyperkalemic forms of familial periodic paralysis; to increase secretion of phenobarbital or lithium.

PHARMACOKINETICS Absorption: well absorbed from GI tract. **Onset:** 1 h regular release; 2 h sustained release; 2 min IV. **Peak effect:** 2–4 h reg; 8–18 h sustained; 0.25 min IV. **Duration:** 8–12 h reg; 18–24 h sustained; 4–5 h IV. **Distribution:** distributed throughout body, concentrating in RBCs, plasma, and kidneys; crosses placenta. **Elimination:** half-life: 2.4–5.8 h; excreted primarily in urine.

CONTRAINDICATIONS & PRECAUTIONS Contraindicated in: hypersensitivity to sulfonamides and derivatives (e.g., thiazides), marked renal and hepatic dysfunction; Addison's disease or other types of adrenocortical insufficiency; hyponatremia, hypokalemia, hyperchloremic acidosis; prolonged administration to patients with hyphema or chronic noncongestive angle-closure glaucoma. Safe use during pregnancy (category C) or in nursing mothers not established. **Cautious use in:** history of hypercalciuria; diabetes mellitus, gout, patients receiving digitalis, obstructive pulmonary disease, respiratory acidosis.

ROUTE & DOSAGE

Glaucoma

Adult	PO	250 mg 1–4 times/d; 500 mg sustained release b.i.d.
	IM/IV	500 mg, may repeat in 2–4 h
Child	PO	8–30 mg/kg/d in 3 doses
	IM/IV	5–10 mg/kg q6h

Epilepsy

Adult	PO	8–30 mg/kg/d in 1–4 doses
Child	PO	Same as for adult

Edema

Adult	PO	250–375 mg every AM (5 mg/kg)
Child	PO/IM/IV	5 mg/kg or 150 mg/m² every AM

High Altitude Sickness

Adult	PO	250 mg q8–12h *or* 500 mg sustained release q12–24h, starting 24–48 h before climb and continuing for 48 h at high altitude

ADVERSE/SIDE EFFECTS CNS: paresthesias, sedation, malaise, disorientation, depression, fatigue, muscle weakness, flaccid paralysis. **GI:** anorexia, nausea, vomiting, weight loss, dry mouth, thirst, diarrhea. **Hematologic/electrolyte imbalance (as for other sulfonamides):** bone marrow depression with agranulocytosis, thrombocytopenic purpura, hemolytic anemia, aplastic anemia, leukopenia, pancytopenia; increased serum bilirubin. Increased excretion of calcium, potassium, magnesium, and sodium; metabolic acidosis; hyperglycemia; hyperuricemia. **Renal:** glycosuria, urinary frequency, polyuria, dysuria, hematuria, crystalluria. **Other:** exacerbation of gout, hepatic dysfunction.

DIAGNOSTIC TEST INTERFERENCES False-positive **urinary protein** determinations; falsely high values for **urine urobilinogen;** depressed **iodine uptake** values (exception: hypothyroidism).

DRUG INTERACTIONS Renal excretion of AMPHETAMINES, **ephedrine, flecainide, quinidine, procainamide,** TRICYCLIC ANTIDEPRESSANTS may be decreased, thereby enhancing or prolonging their effects. Renal excretion of **lithium** is increased. Excretion of **phenobarbital** may be increased. **Amphotericin B** and CORTICOSTEROIDS may accelerate potassium loss. DIGITALIS GLYCOSIDES may predispose persons with hypokalemia to digitalis toxicity; puts patients on high doses of SALICYLATES at high risk for salicylate toxicity.

NURSING IMPLICATIONS

Administration

- May be taken with food or meals to minimize GI upset.
- Tablet (not sustained release form) may be softened in 2 tsp of hot water and added to 2 tsp of honey or syrup to disguise bitter taste. Avoid syrups containing alcohol or glycerin. Alternatively, tablet(s) may be crushed and suspended in syrup (250–500 mg/5 ml syrup). The drug does not dissolve in fruit juices. Prepare just before administration.
- Diuretic dose administered in morning to avoid interrupted sleep.
- IV acetazolamide may be given by direct IV with each 500 mg diluted in 5 ml of sterile water for injection. Administer at a rate of 500 mg or fraction thereof over 1 min.
- Acetazolamide may be added to compatible IV fluids and administered as a continuous infusion over 4–8 h.
- Parenteral solution use within 24 h of reconstitution is strongly recommended by manufacturer. (Each 500 mg vial should be reconstituted with at least 5 ml sterile water for injection before use.)
- Store oral preparations at 15–30C (59–86F) unless otherwise directed.

Assessment & Drug Effects

- Observe for mild to severe metabolic acidosis.
- Monitor I&O and body weight.
- Weigh under standard conditions before drug therapy is initiated and daily thereafter.
- Potassium loss tends to be greatest during early therapy.
- Observe for and advise patient to report signs of hypokalemia or metabolic acidosis.
- Blood pH, blood gases, urinalysis, CBC, and serum electrolyte determinations are recommended initially and at periodic intervals during prolonged drug therapy or during concomitant therapy with other diuretics or digitalis.

Patient & Family Education

- Do not accept brand interchange unless approved by physician.
- Adequate fluid intake (1.5–2.5 L/24 h) should be maintained to reduce risk of kidney stones.
- Report numbness, tingling, burning, and other paresthesias, drowsiness, and visual problems.

Common side effects in *italic*; life-threatening effects underlined; generic names in **bold**; classifications in SMALL CAPS

207

- Report sore throat or mouth, unusual bleeding, fever, skin or renal problems.
- When acetazolamide is given in high doses or for prolonged periods, patient may need potassium-rich diet and potassium supplement.

CYCLOPLEGIC

CYCLOPENTOLATE HYDROCHLORIDE
(sye-kloe-pen´toe-late)
Trade names: Ak-Pentolate, Cyclogyl, Mydplegic
Classifications: EYE PREPARATION; CYCLOPLEGIC; MYDRIATIC; AUTONOMIC NERVOUS SYSTEM AGENT; ANTICHOLINERGIC (PARASYMPATHOLYTIC)
Pregnancy: Category C

ACTIONS/PHARMACODYNAMICS Tertiary amine antimuscarinic compound with systemic side effects and CNS toxicity, similar to those of atropine. Acts by blocking response of iris sphincter muscle and muscle of accommodation in ciliary body to cholinergic stimulation with resulting dilation (mydriasis) and paralysis of accommodation (cycloplegia). Binds to melanin in pupil; thus highly pigmented eyes (brown eyes) may be less responsive to cycloplegic and mydriatic actions.

USES To produce mydriasis and cycloplegia as an aid in refraction and for diagnostic ophthalmoscopic procedures. Unlabeled use: for prophylaxis of posterior synechiae.

ROUTE & DOSAGE

Cycloplegic Refraction

Adult	Topical	1 drop of 1% solution in sye 40–50 min before procedure, followed by 1 drop in 5 min; may need 2% solution in patients with darkly pigmented eyes.
Child	Topical	1 drop of 0.5–1% solution in eye 40–50 min before procedure, followed by 1 drop in 5 min; may need 2% solution in patients with darkly pigmented eyes.

PHARMACOKINETICS Peak: 25–75 min. **Duration:** 24 h.

CONTRAINDICATIONS & PRECAUTIONS Contraindicated in: narrow-angle glaucoma, excessively increased intraocular pressure. Safe use during pregnancy (category C) and in nursing women not established. **Cautious use in:** elderly patients, brain damage (in children), Down's syndrome (mongolism), spastic paralysis in children; blue-eyed individuals.

ADVERSE/SIDE EFFECTS (Systemic absorption) **CNS:** psychotic reaction, behavior disturbances, ataxia, incoherent speech, restlessness, hallucinations, somnolence, disorientation, failure to recognize people, grand mal seizures. **Eye:** blurred vision, temporary burning sensation on instillation, eye dryness, photophobia, conjunctivitis, contact dermatitis, increased intraocular pressure. **GI:** abdominal distension, vomiting, adynamic ileus.

NURSING IMPLICATIONS

Administration
- Systemic absorption may be minimized by depressing lacrimal sac (inner canthus) for 1 or 2 min after instillation of drug. This is especially advisable in children and when the 2% solution is used.
- Store in well-closed containers preferably at 15–30C (59–86F) unless otherwise directed by manufacturer.

Assessment & Drug Effects
- Tonometric examination before drop instillation is advised in patients past middle age and in patients with increased intraocular pressure.
- Observe patient closely for 30 min after instillation of drops for signs of systemic absorption (see adverse/side effects).
- Carefully monitor patients with seizure disorders, since systemic absorption may precipitate a seizure.

Patient & Family Education
- Drug will cause disabling blurring of vision; advise against driving and other potentially hazardous activities until reaction to drug is known.
- Wearing dark glasses may relieve sensitivity to light (photophobia). If symptom persists for > 36 h after drug is discontinued, notify physician.

Common side effects in *italic*; life-threatening effects underlined; generic names in **bold**; classifications in SMALL CAPS

MIOTIC (ANTIGLAUCOMA AGENT)

PILOCARPINE HYDROCHLORIDE
(pye-loe-kar′peen)

Trade names: Adsorbocarpine, Akarpine, Almocarpine, Isopto Carpine, Minims Pilocarpine, Miocarpine, Ocusert, Pilo, Pilocar, Pilokair

Classifications: EYE PREPARATION; MIOTIC (ANTIGLAUCOMA AGENT); AUTONOMIC NERVOUS SYSTEM AGENT; DIRECT-ACTING CHOLINERGIC (PARASYMPATHOMIMETIC)

Pregnancy: Category C

ROUTE & DOSAGE

Acute Glaucoma

Adult	Topical	1 drop of 1–2% solution in affected eye q5–10min for 3–6 doses, then 1 drop q1–3h until IOP is reduced
Child	Topical	Same as for adult

Chronic Glaucoma

Adult	Topical	1 drop of 0.5–4% solution in affected eye q4–12h or 1 ocular system (Ocusert) q7d
Child	Topical	Same as for adult

Miotic

Adult	Topical	1 drop of 1% solution in affected eye
Child	Topical	Same as for adult

ACTIONS/PHARMACODYNAMICS Tertiary amine derived from chief alkaloid of *Pilocarpus jaborandi*. Acts directly on cholinergic receptor sites, thus mimicking acetylcholine. Induces miosis, spasm of accommodation, and fall in intraocular pressure (IOP) that may be preceded by a transitory rise. Decrease in IOP results from stimulation of ciliary and pupillary sphincter muscles, which pull iris away from filtration angle, thus facilitating outflow of aqueous humor. Also decreases production of aqueous humor.

USES Open-angle and angle-closure glaucomas; to reduce IOP and to protect the lens during surgery and laser iridotomy; to counteract effects of mydriatics and cycloplegics following surgery or ophthalmoscopic examination.

PHARMACOKINETICS **Absorption:** penetrates cornea rapidly. **Onset:** miosis: 10–30 min; IOP reduction: 60 min. **Peak:** miosis: 30 min; IOP reduction: 75 min. **Duration:** miosis: 4–8 h; IOP reduction: 4–14 h (7 d with Ocusert).

CONTRAINDICATIONS & PRECAUTIONS **Contraindicated in:** secondary glaucoma, acute iritis, acute inflammatory disease of anterior segment of eye. Safe use during pregnancy (category C), and in nursing mothers has not been established. **Cautious use in:** bronchial asthma; hypertension. **Ocular therapeutic system:** not used in acute infectious conjunctivitis, keratitis, retinal detachment, or when intense miosis is required.

ADVERSE/SIDE EFFECTS Generally well tolerated. Ciliary spasm with browache, twitching of eyelids, eye pain with change in eye focus, miosis, *diminished vision in poorly illuminated areas,* blurred vision, reduced visual acuity, sensitivity. **Infrequent:** contact allergy, lacrimation, follicular conjunctivitis, conjunctival irritation, cataract, retinal detachment. **Systemic:** nausea, vomiting, abdominal cramps, diarrhea, epigastric distress, salivation, bronchospasm, tachycardia, tremors, increased sweating.

DRUG INTERACTIONS The actions of pilocarpine and **carbachol** are additive when used concomitantly.

NURSING IMPLICATIONS

Administration
- During acute phase, physician may prescribe instillation of drug into unaffected eye also, to prevent bilateral attack of acute glaucoma.
- During instillation of eye drops, care should be taken to prevent contamination of dropper tip and solution and to avoid touching eyelids or surrounding area with the dropper tip.
- Immediately after instillation of drops, apply gentle digital pressure to periphery of nasolacrimal drainage system for 1–2 min to prevent delivery of drug to nasal mucosa and general circulation. Excess solution around eye or on hands should be removed immediately with a tissue.

Assessment & Drug Effects

- Hourly tonometric tests may be done during early treatment with pilocarpine because drug may cause an initial transitory increase in IOP.
- Brow pain and myopia tend to be more prominent in younger patients and generally disappear with continued use of drug.

Patient & Family Education

- The patient should understand that therapy for glaucoma is prolonged and that adherence to established regimen is crucial to prevent blindness.
- Since drug causes blurred vision and difficulty in focusing, caution patient to avoid hazardous activities such as driving a car or operating machinery until vision clears.
- Inform patient to withhold medication if symptoms of irritation or sensitization persist and to report to physician.

Ocular Therapeutic System (Ocusert)

- Releases 20 μg/h for 7 d. The unit is placed in the eye cul-de-sac, where it remains for a week. Slow release of drug provides a nonfluctuating concentration of pilocarpine in the ciliary body and iris.
- The 20 μg/h system produces reduction in IOP about equal to that produced by topical application of 28 mg pilocarpine as a 2% solution q6h.
- Induced myopia, miosis, and spasm of accommodation is less than that produced by eyedrops. However, since transient blurring and dimness of vision may occur following Ocusert insertion, have patient do so at bedtime; myopia will be at a stable level in the AM.
- Several hours after Ocusert insertion, induced myopia decreases to a low base level that persists for the life of the therapeutic system.
- Conjunctival irritation with mild erythema and increase in mucus secretion may accompany early use of Ocusert. Usually these symptoms subside, but if they do not, notify physician.
- If the system contacts an unclean surface, wash it with cool tap water before replacing it into cul-de-sac.
- If retention of the system is a problem, the superior conjunctival cul-de-sac may be a preferred site for insertion. This location is also preferred during sleep.
- Ocusert may be transferred from the lower conjunctival sac to the superior sac by closing eyelids, rolling the eye toward the nose and, with gentle digital pressure through the closed eyelid, directly moving the system. Avoid moving it over the colored part of the eye.
- If an unexpected increase in drug action occurs (sudden miosis, ciliary spasm, decreased visual acuity), the system should be removed and replaced with a new one.
- If system ruptures, is deformed or grossly contaminated, discard and replace with another.
- Instruct patient to check for presence of Ocusert before retiring at night and upon rising. If the ocular system slips out during sleep, its effect continues for a short time.
- While IOP increases immediately with removal of Ocusert, it does not reach uncontrolled levels for 2–3 d.
- Information about inserting the ocular system is included in the drug package. Review these directions carefully with patient and ask for demonstration to test patient's ability to adjust, insert, and remove the system.
- Advise patient to keep follow-up appointments.
- Store ocular system form at 2–8C (35–46F); avoid freezing. Store solutions in tight, light-resistant containers.

MYDRIATIC

HOMATROPINE HYDROBROMIDE

(hoe-ma´troe-peen)
Trade names: AK-Homatropine, Homatrine, Homatrocel, Isopto Homatropine
Classifications: EYE PREPARATION; MYDRIATIC; CYCLOPLEGIC; AUTONOMIC NERVOUS SYSTEM AGENT; ANTICHOLINERGIC (PARASYMPATHOLYTIC)
Pregnancy: Category C

ACTIONS/PHARMACODYNAMICS Synthetic alkaloid with actions, contraindications, precautions, and adverse reactions similar to those of atropine (p 116). Blocks responses of sphincter and ciliary muscles of iris to cholinergic stimulation. Resulting mydriatic and cycloplegic actions occur more rapidly and are less prolonged than with atropine. Cycloplegia is usually incomplete unless applications are made repeatedly.

USES Mydriatic for ocular examination and as cycloplegic to measure errors of refraction. Also inflammatory conditions of uveal tract, ciliary spasm, as a cycloplegic and mydriatic in preoperative and postoperative conditions, and as an optical aid in select patients with axial lens opacities.

ROUTE & DOSAGE

Cycloplegic Refraction

Adult   Topical   1–2 drops of 2% or 5% solution in eye repeated in 5–10 min if necessary

Ocular Inflammation

Adult   Topical   1–2 drops of 2% or 5% solution in eye up to q3-4h

PHARMACOKINETICS Peak: 30–90 min. **Duration:** 6 h to 4 d.

CONTRAINDICATIONS & PRECAUTIONS
Contraindicated in: primary (narrow-angle) glaucoma or predisposition to glaucoma; children <6 y. **Cautious use in:** increased IOP, infants, children, the elderly or debilitated; hypertension; hyperthyroidism; diabetes; cardiac disease.

ADVERSE/SIDE EFFECTS Increased IOP, *blurred vision, photophobia*. **Prolonged use:** local irritation, congestion, edema, eczema, follicular conjunctivitis. **Excessive dosage:** symptoms of atropine poisoning (flushing, dry skin, mouth, nose; decreased sweating; fever, rash, rapid, irregular pulse; abdominal and bladder distension; hallucinations, confusion).

DRUG INTERACTIONS None established.

NURSING IMPLICATIONS

Administration
- Systemic absorption may be minimized by applying pressure against inner canthus of eye (lacrimal duct) during and for 1 or 2 min after instillation, particularly when stronger solutions are used.
- Recommended dosage should not be exceeded.
- Store drug at 15–30C (59–86F); protect from light and avoid freezing.

Assessment & Drug Effects
- Determinations of IOP and width of anterior chamber angle (gonioscopy) are advised before and during drug use, particularly if therapy is prolonged. Drug may increase IOP even in the normal eye.
- Photophobia associated with mydriasis may require patient to wear dark glasses.
- Since drug causes blurred vision, supervision of ambulation may be indicated, especially in the elderly.

Patient & Family Education
- Instruct patient in proper technique of eye drop instillation.
- Instruct patient not to rub or squeeze lids together after instillation of drops.
- Advise the patient to report immediately the onset of eye pain, changes in visual acuity, rapid pulse, or dizziness.
- Advise the patient to report dryness of mouth.
- Since the drug produces blurred vision, advise patient against driving and hazardous activities.
- If photophobia or blurred vision persist longer than 3 days after drug is discontinued, inform physician.

VASOCONSTRICTOR, DECONGESTANT

NAPHAZOLINE HYDROCHLORIDE
(naf-az´oh-leen)
Trade names: Ak-Con, Albalon, Allerest, Clear Eyes, Comfort, Degest-2, Muro's Opcon, Nafazair, Naphcon, Privine, VasoClear, Vasocon
Classifications: EENT PREPARATION; VASOCONSTRICTOR; DECONGESTANT; AUTONOMIC NERVOUS SYSTEM AGENT; ALPHA-ADRENERGIC AGONIST (SYMPATHOMIMETIC)
Pregnancy: Category C

ACTIONS/PHARMACODYNAMICS Direct-acting imidazoline derivative with marked alpha-adrenergic activity. Produces rapid and prolonged vasoconstriction of arterioles, thereby decreasing fluid exudation and mucosal engorgement. Differs from other sympathomimetic amines in that systemic absorption may cause CNS depression rather than stimulation.

USES Topically, as nasal decongestant and ocular vasoconstrictor.

PHARMACOKINETICS Onset: within 10 min. **Duration:** 2–6 h.

CONTRAINDICATIONS & PRECAUTIONS Contraindicated in: Narrow-angle glaucoma; concomitant use with MAO inhibitors or tricyclic antidepressants. Safe use during pregnancy (category C), in infants, and children not established. **Cautious use in:** hypertension, cardiac irregularities, advanced arteriosclerosis; diabetes; hyperthyroidism; elderly patients.

ROUTE & DOSAGE

Congestion

Adult	Nasal	2 drops or sprays of 0.05% solution in each nostril q3–6h for no more than 3–5 d
	Ophthalmic	1–3 drops of 0.1% solution q3–4h prn or 1–2 drops of a 0.01–0.03% solution q4h prn
Child	Nasal	1–2 drops or sprays of 0.025% solution q3–6h for no more than 3–5 d

ADVERSE/SIDE EFFECTS Nasal use: transient stinging or burning, dryness of nasal mucosa, hypersensitivity reactions. **Ophthalmic use:** pupillary dilation, increased intraocular pressure, rebound redness of the eye, headache, hypertension, nausea, weakness, sweating. **Overdosage:** drowsiness, hypothermia, bradycardia, shocklike hypotension, coma.

NURSING IMPLICATIONS

Administration

- Instill nasal spray with patient in upright position. If administered in reclining position, a stream rather than a spray may be ejected, with possibility of systemic reaction.
- When nose drops are instilled, the amount of drug swallowed can be minimized by taking care not to direct the flow toward nasopharynx and by proper positioning of patient. Position used depends on condition being treated. Consult physician. *Parkinson position:* patient supine, head over edge of bed and turned to affected side (used for treating nasal passages and frontal and maxillary sinuses). *Proetz position:* patient supine, with head hanging straight back over edge of bed (used to treat ethmoid and sphenoid sinuses). Both positions can also be accomplished by placing pillow under patient's shoulders.
- Following nasal instillation of spray, rinse dropper or spray top in hot water to prevent contamination of solution.
- Preserve in tight container preferably at 15–30C (59–86F) unless otherwise specified by manufacturer. Protect from freezing.

Assessment & Drug Effects

- Rebound congestion and chemical rhinitis can occur with frequent and continued use.
- Periodically monitor BP for development or worsening of hypertension, especially with ophthalmic route.
- **Overdose:** bradycardia and hypotension can result. Report promptly.

Patient & Family Education

- Advise patient not to exceed prescribed regimen. Explain that systemic effects can result from swallowing excessive medication.
- If nasal congestion is not relieved after 5 d, advise patient to discontinue medication and to contact physician.
- To prevent contamination of eye solution, care should be taken not to touch eyelid or surrounding area with dropper tip.

ANTACID, ADSORBENT

ALUMINUM HYDROXIDE [AL(OH)$_3$]

Trade names: ALternaGEL, Alu-Cap, Alugel, Alu-Tab, Amphojel, Dialume
Classifications: GI AGENT; ANTACID; ADSORBENT
Pregnancy: Category C

ACTIONS/PHARMACODYNAMICS Nonsystemic antacid with moderate neutralizing action. Decreases rate of gastric emptying and has demulcent, adsorbent, and mild astringent properties. Reduces acid concentration and pepsin activity by raising pH of gastric and intraesophageal secretions. Does not reduce gastric acid output. Reacts with gastric acid to form aluminum chloride; believed to be responsible for astringent and constipating effects. Chloride is reabsorbed in small intestines, thus preserving systemic acid-base balance. Neutralizing capacity of liquid suspension is reported to surpass that of dried gel because particle size is much smaller. Lowers serum phosphate by binding dietary phosphorus to form insoluble aluminum phosphate, which is excreted in feces. This prevents formation of urinary phosphatic calculi by decreasing excretion of phosphates in urine. Its phosphate-binding capacity is not as great as that of aluminum carbonate.

USES Symptomatic relief of gastric hyperacidity associated with gastritis, esophageal reflux, and hiatal hernia; adjunct in treatment of gastric and duodenal ulcer. Also has been used in management of hyperphosphatemia of renal failure and in treatment of phosphatic urinary calculi. More commonly used in combination with other antacids.

ROUTE & DOSAGE

Antacid

Adult   PO   600 mg t.i.d. or q.i.d.

PHARMACOKINETICS Absorption: minimal absorption. **Peak effect:** slow onset. **Duration:** 2 h when taken with food; 3 h when taken 1 h after food. **Elimination:** excreted in feces as insoluble phosphates.

CONTRAINDICATIONS & PRECAUTIONS Contraindicated in: prolonged use of high doses in presence of low serum phosphate. Pregnancy: category C. **Cautious use in:** renal impairment; gastric outlet obstruction; elderly patients; decreased bowel activity (e.g., patients receiving anticholinergic, antidiarrheal, or antispasmodic agents); patients who are dehydrated or on fluid restriction.

ADVERSE/SIDE EFFECTS *Constipation,* fecal impaction, intestinal obstruction, hypophosphatemia, dialysis dementia (thought to be due to aluminum intoxication), hypomagnesemia.

DRUG INTERACTIONS Aluminum will decrease absorption of **chloroquine, cimetidine, ciprofloxacin, digoxin, isoniazid,** IRON SALTS, NSAIDs, **norfloxacin, ofloxacin, phenytoin, phenothiazines, quinidine, tetracycline, thyroxine. Sodium polystyrene sulfonate** may cause systemic alkalosis.

NURSING IMPLICATIONS

Administration

- Instruct patient to chew tablet until it is thoroughly wetted before swallowing it (undissolved particles increase risk of developing intestinal concretions). **For antacid use:** follow well-chewed tablet with one-half glass of water or milk; follow liquid preparation (suspension) with sip of water to assure passage into stomach. **For phosphate lowering:** follow tablet, capsule, or suspension with full glass of water or fruit juice.
- For healing an active peptic ulcer, some physicians prescribe antacid 1 and 3 h after meals and at bed-

time. Others alternate antacid and meals on a 2 h schedule and advise patients to take an extra antacid dose when discomfort is felt.

- Store between 15 and 30C (59 and 86F) in tightly closed container.

Assessment & Drug Effects

- Note number and consistency of stools. Constipation occurs commonly and is dose related. Intestinal obstruction from fecal concretions has been reported.
- Serum calcium and phosphorus levels should be determined at periodic intervals with prolonged high-dose therapy or impaired renal function.

Patient & Family Education

- Patients receiving large doses of antacids for prolonged periods and who eat a diet low in phosphorus can develop hypophosphatemia within 2 wk of continuous antacid use. The elderly patient in a poor nutritional state is at high risk.
- Since frequency of meals may vary in the elderly particularly, help patient design a diet-antacid regimen that will protect the gastric mucosa.
- Antacid may cause stools to appear speckled or whitish.
- Pain is used as a clinical guide for adjusting dosage. Keep physician informed. Pain that persists beyond 72 h may signify serious complications.
- Length of antacid therapy for patients with duodenal ulcer is usually 4–6 wk, and for gastric ulcers until healing has taken place.
- Caution individuals who self-medicate with antacids to seek medical help if indigestion is accompanied by shortness of breath, sweating, or chest pain, if stools are dark or tarry, or if symptoms are recurrent.
- A person should seek medical advice and supervision if self-prescribed antacid use exceeds 2 wk.

ANTIDIARRHEAL

DIPHENOXYLATE HYDROCHLORIDE WITH ATROPINE SULFATE
(dye-fen-ox´i-late)
Trade names: Diphenatol, Lofene, Lomanate, Lomotil, Lonox, Lo-Trol, Low-Quel, Nor-Mil
Classifications: GI AGENT; ANTIDIARRHEAL
Pregnancy: Category C
Controlled substance: Schedule V

ACTIONS/PHARMACODYNAMICS Diphenoxylate is a synthetic narcotic structurally related to meperidine. Commer-cially available only with atropine sulfate, added in subtherapeutic doses to discourage deliberate overdosage. Inhibits mucosal receptors responsible for peristaltic reflex, thereby reducing GI motility. Has little or no analgesic activity or risk of dependence, except in high doses.

USES Adjunct in symptomatic management of diarrhea.

ROUTE & DOSAGE

Diarrhea

Adult	PO	1–2 tablets or 1–2 teaspoonfuls (5 ml) 3–4 times/d (each tablet or 5 ml contains 2.5 mg diphenoxylate HCl and 0.025 mg atropine sulfate)
Child	PO	2–12 y: 0.3–0.4 mg/kg/d of liquid in divided doses

PHARMACOKINETICS Absorption: readily absorbed from GI tract. **Onset:** 45–60 min. **Peak:** 2 h. **Duration:** 3–4 h. **Distribution:** distributed into breast milk. **Metabolism:** rapidly metabolized to active and inactive metabolites in liver. **Elimination:** half-life: 4.4 h; excreted slowly through bile into feces; small amount excreted in urine.

CONTRAINDICATIONS & PRECAUTIONS

Contraindicated in: hypersensitivity to diphenoxylate or atropine; severe dehydration or electrolyte imbalance, advanced liver disease, obstructive jaundice, diarrhea caused by pseudomembranous enterocolitis associated with use of broad-spectrum antibiotics; diarrhea associated with organisms that penetrate intestinal mucosa; diarrhea induced by poisons until toxic material is eliminated from GI tract; glaucoma; children < 2 y of age. Safe use during pregnancy (category C) or in nursing women not established. **Cautious use in:** advanced hepatic disease, abnormal liver function tests; renal function impairment, patients receiving addicting drugs, addiction-prone individuals or those whose history suggests drug abuse; ulcerative colitis; young children (particularly patients with Down's syndrome).

ADVERSE/SIDE EFFECTS CNS: headache, sedation, drowsiness, dizziness, lethargy, numbness of extremities; restlessness, euphoria, mental depression, weakness, general malaise. **CV:** flushing, palpitation, tachycardia. **Eye:** nystagmus, mydriasis, blurred vision, miosis (toxicity). **GI:** nausea, vomiting, anorexia, dry mouth, abdominal discomfort or distension, paralytic ileus, toxic megacolon. **Hypersensitivity:** pruritus, angioneurotic edema, giant urticaria, rash. **Other:** urinary retention, swelling of gums.

DRUG INTERACTIONS MAO INHIBITORS may precipitate hypertensive crisis; **alcohol** and other CNS DEPRESSANTS may enhance CNS effects; also see **atropine,** p 116.

NURSING IMPLICATIONS

Administration
- If necessary, tablet may be crushed and taken with fluid of patient's choice.
- Dosage should be reduced as soon as initial control of symptoms occurs.
- Drug should be withheld in presence of severe dehydration or electrolyte imbalance until appropriate corrective therapy has been initiated.
- Treatment is generally continued for 24–36 h before it is considered ineffective.
- Addiction to diphenoxylate is possible at high dosages and with prolonged use.
- Store in tightly covered, light-resistant container, preferably between 15 and 30C (59 and 86F), unless otherwise directed by manufacturer.

Assessment & Drug Effects
- Report signs of atropine poisoning (atropinism): dry mouth, flushing, hyperthermia, tachycardia, urinary retention; may occur even with recommended doses in children, particularly those with Down's syndrome.
- Dehydration occurs more rapidly in the younger child and may further influence variability of response to diphenoxylate and predispose patient to delayed toxic effects. Close monitoring is essential.
- Observe for and report abdominal distension. Distention is an ominous sign in patients with ulcerative colitis.
- Monitor for signs and symptoms of dehydration (see Chapter 3).
- Estimation of fluid loss can be made by careful measurements of body weight and I&O.
- Monitor frequency and consistency of stools.

Patient & Family Education
- Counsel patient to take medication only as directed by physician.

Common side effects in *italic*; life-threatening effects underlined; generic names in **bold**; classifications in SMALL CAPS

- Instruct patient to notify physician if diarrhea persists or if fever, bloody stools, palpitation, or other adverse reactions occur.
- Since drug can cause dizziness and drowsiness, advise patient to use caution when driving or performing other activities requiring coordination and alertness.

ANTIEMETIC

PROCHLORPERAZINE
(proe-klor-per´a-zeen)
Trade name: Compazine

PROCHLORPERAZINE EDISYLATE
Trade name: Compazine

PROCHLORPERAZINE MALEATE
Trade names: Chlorazine, Chlorpazine, Compazine, Stemetil
Classifications: GI AGENT; ANTIEMETIC; PSYCHOTHERAPEUTIC; PHENOTHIAZINE ANTIPSYCHOTIC
Pregnancy: Category C

ACTIONS/PHARMACODYNAMICS Piperazine phenothiazine derivative with similar actions, contraindications, and interactions as chlorpromazine. Has greater extrapyramidal effects and antiemetic potency but fewer sedative, hypotensive, and anticholinergic effects than chlorpromazine. Not as effective in treatment for vertigo or motion sickness.

USES Management of manifestations of psychotic disorders, of excessive anxiety, tension, and agitation, and to control severe nausea and vomiting.

PHARMACOKINETICS Absorption: readily absorbed from GI tract. **Onset:** 30–40 min PO; 60 min PR; 10–20 min IM. **Duration:** 3–4 h PO; 10–12 h sustained release PO; 3–4 h PR; up to 12 h IM. **Distribution:** crosses placenta; distributed into breast milk. **Metabolism:** metabolized in liver. **Elimination:** excreted in urine.

ROUTE & DOSAGE

Severe Nausea, Vomiting, Anxiety, Psychotic Disorders

Adult:	PO	5–10 mg t.i.d. or q.i.d.; sustained release: 10–15 mg q12h;
	IM	5–10 mg q3–4h; up to 40 mg/d
	IV	2.5–10 mg q6–8h; max 40 mg/d
	PR	25 mg b.i.d.
Child:	PO	2.5 mg 1–3 times/d or 5 mg b.i.d.; max 15 mg/d
	IM	0.13 mg/kg q3–4h
	PR	2.5 mg b.i.d. or t.i.d. up to 20–25 mg/d

CONTRAINDICATIONS & PRECAUTIONS
Contraindicated in: hypersensitivity to phenothiazines; bone marrow depression; comatose or severely depressed states; children < 9 kg (20 lb) or 2 y of age; pediatric surgery; short-term vomiting in children or vomiting of unknown etiology; Reye's syndrome or other encephalopathies; history of dyskinetic reactions or epilepsy. Pregnancy category C. **Cautious use in:** patient with previously diagnosed breast cancer, children with acute illness or dehydration.

ADVERSE/SIDE EFFECTS *Drowsiness,* dizziness, hypotension, contact dermatitis, photosensitivity, galactorrhea, amenorrhea, blurred vision, cholestatic jaundice, leukopenia, agranulocytosis, *extrapyramidal reactions (akathesia, dystonia or parkinsonism),* persistent tardive dyskinesia, acute catatonia.

DRUG INTERACTIONS Alcohol, CNS DEPRESSANTS increase CNS depression; ANTACIDS, ANTIDIARRHEALS decrease absorption—administer 2 h apart; **phenobarbital** increases metabolism of prochlorperazine; GENERAL ANESTHETICS increase excitation and hypotension; antagonizes antihypertensive action of **guanethidine; phenylpropanolamine** poses possibility of sudden death; TRICYCLIC ANTIDEPRESSANTS intensify hypotensive and anticholinergic effects; decreases seizure threshold—ANTICONVULSANT dosage may need to be increased.

INCOMPATIBILITIES Solution/Additive: aminophylline, amphotericin B, ampicillin, calcium glucepate, calcium gluconate, cephalothin, chloramphenicol, chlorothiazide, hydrocortisone, methohexital, penicillin G sodium, phenobarbital, sodium bicarbonate, dimenhydrinate, hydromorphone, midazolam, pentobarbital, thiopental.

Common side effects in *italic*; life-threatening effects underlined; generic names in **bold**; classifications in SMALL CAPS

215

NURSING IMPLICATIONS

Administration

- Strength of liquid formulations: syrup: 5 mg/5 ml; PO concentrate: 10 mg/ml. Do not confuse the preparations.
- Note dosage of pediatric suppository. Do not confuse 2.5 mg for 25 mg (adult dose size).
- Oral concentrate is not to be administered to children.
- To ensure stability and palatability of oral concentrate add prescribed dose to 60 ml or more of diluent just prior to administration. Suggested diluents: tomato or fruit juice, carbonated drinks, water, semisolid foods (e.g., puddings, soups).
- IM injection in adults should be made deep into the upper outer quadrant of the buttock. Do not mix IM solution in the same syringe with other agents. Follow agency policy regarding IM injection site for children.
- Give direct IV by diluting in D5W, NS, or other compatible diluent to a concentration of 1 mg/ml and give at a maximum rate of 5 mg/min.
- Avoid skin contact with oral concentrate or injection solution because of possibility of contact dermatitis.
- Minimum effective dosage is advised. Keep physician informed of patient's response to drug therapy.
- Dosage for elderly, emaciated patients and for children should be advanced slowly.
- Slight yellowing does not appear to alter potency; however, markedly discolored solutions should be discarded. Protect drug from light; do not freeze. Store at temperature between 15 and 30C (59 and 86F) unless otherwise instructed by manufacturer.

Assessment & Drug Effects

- Postoperative patients who have received prochlorperazine may have depressed cough reflex and should be carefully positioned to prevent aspiration of vomitus.
- Monitor I&O ratio and elimination pattern. Depressed patients frequently cut back on fluid intake and do not seek help for constipation.
- Most elderly and emaciated patients and children, especially those with dehydration or acute illness, appear to be particularly susceptible to extrapyramidal effects. Be alert to onset of symptoms: in early therapy watch for pseudoparkinson's and acute dyskinesia. After 1–2 mo, be alert to akathisia.
- Keep in mind that the antiemetic effect may mask toxicity of other drugs or make it difficult to diagnose conditions with a primary symptom of nausea, such as intestinal obstruction and increased intracranial pressure.
- It has been reported that although patient is not responsive during acute catatonia (side effect), everything that happens during the episode can be recalled. Approach patient accordingly.
- Exposure to high environmental temperature, to sun's rays, or to a high fever associated with serious illness places this patient at risk for heat stroke. Be alert to signs: red, dry, hot skin, full bounding pulse, dilated pupils, dyspnea, confusion, temperature over 40.6C (105F), elevated BP. Inform physician and institute measures to reduce body temperature rapidly.

Patient & Family Education

- Counsel patient to take drug as prescribed and not to alter dose or schedule. Consult physician before stopping the medication.
- Since drug may impair mental and physical abilities, especially during first few days of therapy, caution patient to avoid hazardous activities such as driving a car until response to drug is known.
- This drug may color urine reddish brown. It also may cause the sun-exposed skin to turn gray-blue.
- Advise patient to protect skin from direct sun's rays and to use a sunscreen lotion (SPF > 12) to prevent photosensitivity reaction.
- Instruct patient to withhold dose and report to the physician if the following symptoms persist more than a few hours: tremor, involuntary twitching, exaggerated restlessness. Other reportable symptoms include light-colored stools, changes in vision, sore throat, fever, rash.

ANTISECRETORY (H_2-RECEPTOR ANTAGONIST)

CIMETIDINE

(sye-met´i-deen)
Trade names: Novocimetine, Peptol, Tagamet
Classifications: GI AGENT; ANTISECRETORY (H_2-RECEPTOR ANTAGONIST); ANTIHISTAMINE
Pregnancy: Category B

ACTIONS/PHARMACODYNAMICS

Enzyme inhibitor structurally similar to histamine. Belongs to the antihistamine group with high selectivity for histamine H_2-receptors on parietal cells (minimal effect on H_1-receptors). By reversible competitive inhibition of histamine at the H_2-receptor sites suppresses all phases of daytime and nocturnal basal gastric acid secretion. Indirectly reduces pepsin secretion. Blocks secretion stimulated physiologically by histamine and pentagastrin and by food, muscarinic agonists, caffeine, and insulin. Inhibits cytochrome P-450 oxidase system, which affects metabolism of other drugs such as warfarin, phenobarbital and theophylline. Also blocks synthesis and release of parathyroid hormone and associated hypercalcemia in patients with primary hyperparathyroidism. Demonstrates weak antiandrogenic and neurologic effects. Is not a cholinergic. Has no effect on lower esophageal sphincter pressure, gastric motility or emptying, biliary or pancreatic secretion. It has been suggested, but not established, that cimetidine therapy may predispose the patient to gastric carcinoma.

USES

Short-term treatment of active duodenal ulcer and prevention of ulcer recurrence (at reduced dosage) after it is healed. Also used for short-term treatment of active benign gastric ulcer and for pathologic hypersecretory conditions such as Zollinger-Ellison syndrome. **Unlabeled use:** prophylaxis of stress-induced ulcers, upper GI bleeding, and aspiration pneumonitis; gastroesophageal reflux, chronic urticaria, acetaminophen toxicity.

PHARMACOKINETICS

Absorption: 70% of oral dose absorbed from GI tract. **Peak:** 1–1.5 h. **Distribution:** widely distributed; crosses blood-brain barrier and placenta. **Metabolism:** metabolized in liver. **Elimination:** half-life: 2 h; most of drug excreted in urine in 24 h; excreted in breast milk.

CONTRAINDICATIONS & PRECAUTIONS

Contraindicated in: known hypersensitivity to cimetidine. Safe use in nursing mothers, during pregnancy (category B), or in children <16 y not established. **Cautious use in:** elderly or critically ill patients; impaired renal or hepatic function; organic brain syndrome.

ADVERSE/SIDE EFFECTS

CNS: drowsiness, dizziness, light-headedness, depression, headache, reversible confusional states, paranoid psychosis, symptoms of brainstem dysfunction (e.g., ataxic gait, diplopia, peripheral neuropathy). **CV (rare):** cardiac arrhythmias and cardiac arrest after rapid IV bolus dose. **GI:** mild transient diarrhea; severe diarrhea, constipation, abdominal discomfort. **Gynecologic:** gynecomastia and breast soreness, galactorrhea, reversible impotence. **Hematologic:** increased prothrombin time; rare: neutropenia, leukopenia, thrombocytopenia, aplastic anemia. **Musculoskeletal:** exacerbation of joint symptoms in patients with preexisting arthritis. **Other:** rash, Stevens-Johnson syndrome, reversible alopecia, fever; slight increase in serum uric acid, BUN, creatinine; transient pain at IM site; hypospermia.

DIAGNOSTIC TEST INTERFERENCES

Cimetidine may cause false-positive *hemoccult test for gastric bleeding* if test is performed within 15 min of oral cimetidine administration.

DRUG INTERACTIONS

Cimetidine decreases the hepatic metabolism of **warfarin, phenobarbital, phenytoin, diazepam, propranolol, lidocaine, theophylline,** thus increasing their activity and toxicity; ANTACIDS may decrease absorption of cimetidine.

INCOMPATIBILITIES

Solution/additive: amphotericin B, cefamandole, cephalothin, atropine, cefazolin, chlorpromazine, pentobarbital, secobarbital.

ROUTE & DOSAGE

Duodenal Ulcer

Adult	PO	300 mg q.i.d. or 400 mg b.i.d. or 800 mg h.s.
	IM/IV	300 mg q6–8h
Child	PO/IM/IV	20–40 mg/kg/d in 4 divided doses

Duodenal Ulcer, Maintenance Therapy

Adult	PO	400 mg h.s.

Gastric Ulcer

Adult	PO	300 mg q.i.d. with meals and h.s.
	IM/IV	300 mg q6–8h

Pathologic Hypersecretory Disease

Adult	PO	300 mg q.i.d. with meals and h.s.; may increase up to 2400 mg/d
	IM/IV	300 mg q6–8h; may increase up to 2400 mg/d

Common side effects in *italic*; life-threatening effects underlined; generic names in **bold**; classifications in SMALL CAPS

217

NURSING IMPLICATIONS

Administration

- Oral form may be taken with meals. Absorption may be decreased by antacids but is unaffected by food.
- Administration of antacid to control acute ulcer pain should be at least 1 h before or 1 h after food and cimetidine.
- Oral administration is substituted for IV therapy when bleeding has been controlled for at least 48 h.
- A moderate (i.e., less than 60%) level of 24 h acid suppression is provided by doses of 800 mg h.s., 400 mg b.i.d., or 300 mg q.i.d. However, the 800 mg dose-effect is limited to nocturnal acid suppression with no effect on daytime gastric secretion.
- *Intermittent IV injection:* dilute 300 mg in at least 50 ml 5% dextrose injection or other compatible IV solution and infuse over 15–20 min.
- *IV injection:* dilute in 0.9% NaCl injection or other compatible IV solution to a total volume of 20 ml and inject within not less than 2 min.
- Parenteral solutions are stable for 48 h at room temperature when added to commonly used IV solutions for dilution. Follow manufacturer's directions.
- Store all forms of cimetidine at 15–30C (59–86F) protected from light unless otherwise directed by manufacturer.

Assessment & Drug Effects

- Ulcer healing may occur within the first 2 wk of therapy but generally requires at least 4 wk in most patients. Short-term (i.e., 8 wk) therapy of active duodenal ulcer does not prevent ulcer recurrence when drug is discontinued.
- Monitor pulse of patient during first few days of drug regimen. Bradycardia after PO as well as IV administration should be reported. Pulse usually returns to normal within 24 h after drug discontinuation.
- Monitor I&O ratio and pattern, particularly in the elderly, severely ill, and in patients with impaired renal function.
- Adynamic ileus has been reported in patients receiving cimetidine to prevent and treat stress ulcers. Report loss of bowel sounds, absence of bowel movement or flatus, vomiting, crampy pain, abdominal distension.
- Periodic evaluations of blood count and renal and hepatic function are advised during therapy.
- Be alert to onset of confusional states, particularly in the elderly or severely ill patient. Symptoms oc-

cur within 2–3 d after first dose. Report immediately: drug should be withdrawn. Symptoms usually resolve within 3–4 d after therapy is discontinued.
- If patient complains of severe headache, check BP and report an elevation to the physician.
- Ingestion of tyramine-rich foods (cheddar cheese, beef-extract, yogurt, aged meats, soy sauce, Chianti wine) can lead to transient hypertension and severe headache (MAOI-like reaction), especially if patient is elderly and has hepatic impairment. Cimetidine interference with liver metabolism can lead to excess in circulation of tyramine.
- Cimetidine impairs absorption of protein-bound vitamin B_{12}; therefore patient who takes cimetidine in divided doses to continuously suppress acid gastric secretion is at risk for vitamin B_{12} deficiency. (No risk for patient who takes drug at bedtime to suppress nocturnal acid production.)

Patient & Family Education

- Be certain that patient is aware of the importance of taking cimetidine exactly as prescribed. Sudden discontinuation of therapy reportedly has caused perforation of chronic peptic ulcer.
- Urge patient to seek advice about self-medication with any OTC drug.
- Mild bilateral gynecomastia and breast soreness may occur after ≥ 1 mo of therapy. It may disappear spontaneously or remain throughout therapy. Instruct patient to report this symptom to physician.
- Caution patient to promptly report recurrence of gastric pain or bleeding (black, tarry stools or "coffee ground" vomitus) and to notify physician if diarrhea continues more than 1 d.
- Caution patient to avoid driving and other potentially hazardous activities until reaction to drug is known.
- Impress on patient and responsible family member(s) that duodenal or gastric ulcer is a chronic, recurrent condition that requires long-term maintenance drug therapy.
- Therapy for active duodenal ulcer is continued until healing is demonstrated by endoscopy (usually 4–6 wk, but not to exceed 8 wk).
- Maintenance therapy at reduced dosage after healing of active duodenal ulcer appears to limit recurrence, particularly if patient understands importance of other antiulcer therapeutic measures: no smoking, life-style that promotes reduced stress.

BULK LAXATIVE

PSYLLIUM HYDROPHILIC MUCILOID

(sill´i-um)

Trade names: Hydrocil, Instant, Karasil, Konsyl, Metamucil, Modane Bulk, Novomucilax, Prodiem Plain, Pro-Lax, Reguloid, Serutan, Siblin, Syllact, V-Lax
Classifications: GI AGENT; BULK LAXATIVE
Pregnancy: Category C

ACTIONS/PHARMACODYNAMICS Highly refined colloid of blond psyllium seed (*Plantago ovata*) with equal amount of dextrose added as dispersing agent. On contact with water, produces bland, lubricating, gelatinous bulk, which promotes peristalsis and natural elimination. Contains negligible amounts of sodium and about 14 calories per dose (instant-mix effervescent form is flavored and contains 0.25 g sodium and 43 calories per dose). Reportedly, chronic use may reduce plasma cholesterol, possibly by interfering with reabsorption of bile acids.

USES Chronic atonic or spastic constipation and constipation associated with rectal disorders or anorectal surgery.

ROUTE & DOSAGE

Constipation or Diarrhea

Adult	PO	1–2 rounded tsp or 1 packet 1–3 times/d prn
Child	PO	≥ 6 y: 1 tsp in water h.s.

PHARMACOKINETICS Absorption: not absorbed from GI tract. **Onset:** 12–24 h. **Peak:** 1–3 d.

CONTRAINDICATIONS & PRECAUTIONS Contraindicated in: esophageal and intestinal obstruction, fecal impaction, undiagnosed abdominal pain. Pregnancy category C.

ADVERSE/SIDE EFFECTS Eosinophilia, *nausea and vomiting, diarrhea,* with excessive use; GI tract strictures when drug used in dry form, abdominal cramps.

DRUG INTERACTIONS Psyllium may decrease absorption and clinical effects of ANTIBIOTICS, **warfarin, digoxin, nitrofurantoin,** SALICYLATES.

NURSING IMPLICATIONS

Administration

- Fill an ordinary 8 oz (240 ml) water glass with cool water, milk, fruit juice, or other liquid; sprinkle powder into liquid; stir briskly; and drink immediately (if effervescent form is used, add liquid to powder). Granules should not be chewed.
- Best results are obtained if each dose is followed by an additional glass of liquid.
- Be cautious with elderly patient who may aspirate the drug.

Assessment & Drug Effects

- If patient complains of retrosternal pain after taking the drug, report this promptly to physician. The drug may be lodged as a gelatinous mass (because of poor mixing) in the esophagus.
- When psyllium is used as either a bulk laxative or to treat diarrhea, the expected effect is formed stools.
- Laxative effect usually occurs within 12–24 h. Administration for 2 or 3 d may be needed to establish regularity.
- Assess for complaints of abdominal fullness. Smaller, more frequent doses spaced throughout the day may be indicated to relieve discomfort of abdominal fullness.

Patient & Family Education

- Inform patient that drug works to relieve both diarrhea and constipation by restoring a more normal moisture level to stool.
- Inform patient that drug may reduce appetite if it is taken before meals.
- Note sugar and sodium content of preparation if patient is on low-sodium or low-calorie diet. Some preparations contain natural sugars, whereas others contain artificial sweeteners.
- Instruct patients on restricted calorie diets to read the number of calories per dose, which can vary from 1 to approximately 100 calories.
- Instruct patient about prevention of constipation (e.g., proper hydration, increased fiber in diet, regulation of bowel pattern).

Common side effects in *italic*; life-threatening effects <u>underlined</u>; generic names in **bold**; classifications in SMALL CAPS

219

SALINE CATHARTIC

MAGNESIUM HYDROXIDE

Trade names: Magnesia, Magnesia Magma, Milk of Magnesia, M.O.M.
Classifications: GI AGENT; SALINE CATHARTIC; ANTACID
Pregnancy: Category B

ACTIONS/PHARMACODYNAMICS Milk of Magnesia is an aqueous suspension of magnesium hydroxide with rapid and long-acting neutralizing action. Although classified as nonsystemic antacid, 5–10% of the magnesium may be absorbed to produce alkaline urine. Also may cause slight acid rebound. Acts as antacid in low doses and as mild saline laxative at higher doses. Reacts with hydrochloric acid in stomach to form magnesium chloride, which has neutralizing action. Magnesium chloride causes osmotic retention of fluid, which distends colon, resulting in mechanical stimulation of peristaltic activity. Each milliliter of magnesium hydroxide contains about 2.4–2.9 mEq of magnesium and reportedly is capable of neutralizing approximately 2.7 mEq of gastric acid.

USES Short-term treatment of occasional constipation, for relief of GI symptoms associated with hyperacidity, and as adjunct in treatment of peptic ulcer. Also has been used in treatment of poisoning by mineral acids and arsenic, and as mouthwash to neutralize acidity.

ROUTE & DOSAGE

Laxative

Adult	PO	2.4–4.8 g (30–60 ml)/d in 1 or more divided doses
Child	PO	6–11 y: 1.2–2.4 g (15–30 ml)/d in 1 or more divided doses
		2–5 y: 0.4–1.2 g (5–15 ml)/d in 1 or more divided doses

PHARMACOKINETICS Absorption: 15–30% of magnesium is absorbed. **Onset:** 3–6 h. **Distribution:** small amounts of magnesium distributed in saliva and breast milk. **Elimination:** excreted in feces; some renal excretion.

CONTRAINDICATIONS & PRECAUTIONS Contraindicated in: abdominal pain, nausea, vomiting, diarrhea, severe renal dysfunction, fecal impaction, intestinal obstruction or perforation, rectal bleeding, colostomy, ileostomy. Safe use during pregnancy (category B) and in children < 2 y not established.

ADVERSE/SIDE EFFECTS Excessive dosage: nausea, vomiting, abdominal cramps, *diarrhea,* alkalinization of urine, dehydration. **Hypermagnesemia:** weakness, nausea, vomiting, lethargy, mental depression, hyporeflexia, hypotension, bradycardia, complete heart block and other ECG abnormalities, respiratory depression, coma. **Prolonged use:** rectal concretions (rare), electrolyte imbalance.

DRUG INTERACTIONS Milk of Magnesia decreases absorption of **chlordiazepoxide, dicumarol, digoxin, isoniazid.**

NURSING IMPLICATIONS

Administration

- Shake bottle well before pouring to assure administration of suspension.
- For antacid action, usually given 20–60 min before meals and at bedtime. Mix suspension with water or follow with sufficient water to assure that it reaches the stomach.
- When intended for antacid use, laxative effect of Milk of Magnesia can be minimized by coadministering it or alternating it with an antacid with constipating effects, e.g., calcium carbonate or aluminum hydroxide. Consult physician.
- For laxative effect, follow the drug with at least a full glass of water to enhance drug action. Administer in the morning or at bedtime. Most effective when taken on an empty stomach.
- Store at room temperature in tightly covered container. Slowly absorbs carbon dioxide on exposure to air. Avoid freezing.

Assessment & Drug Effects

- Evaluate the patient's continued need for drug. Prolonged and frequent use of laxative doses may lead to dependence. Additionally, even therapeutic doses can raise urinary pH and thereby predispose susceptible patients to urinary infection and urolithiasis.
- Monitor signs of elevated serum magnesium concentrations, which may cause bradycardia and other symptoms of hypermagnesemia (see chap 3).

Patient & Family Education

- Inform patient that the cause of persistent or recurrent constipation or gastric distress should be investigated by a physician.
- Correct patient's misconceptions about constipation. The omission of one day's evacuation is not constipation and will not cause accumulation of poisons in the body.

STIMULANT LAXATIVE

BISACODYL

(bis-a-koe´dill)

Trade names: Apo-Bisacodyl Bisacolax, Bisco-Lax, Dacodyl, Deficol, Dulcolax, Fleet Bisacodyl, Laxit, Theralax
Classification: GI AGENT; STIMULANT LAXATIVE
Pregnancy: Category C

ACTIONS/PHARMACODYNAMICS Diphenylmethane laxative structurally related to phenolphthalein. Induces peristaltic contractions by direct stimulation of sensory nerve endings in the colonic wall. Bisacodyl also expands intestinal fluid volume by increasing epithelial permeability.

USES Temporary relief of acute constipation and for evacuation of colon before surgery, proctoscopic, sigmoidoscopic, and radiologic examinations. Also used to cleanse colon before delivery and to relieve constipation in patients with spinal cord damage.

ROUTE & DOSAGE

Laxative

Adult	PO	5–15 mg prn up to 30 mg for special procedures
	PR	10 mg prn
Child	PO	≥ 6 y: 5–10 mg prn
	PR	≥ 2 y: 10 mg
		< 2 y: 5 mg

PHARMACOKINETICS Absorption: 5–15% absorbed from GI tract. **Onset:** 6–8 h PO; 15–60 min PR.

Metabolism: metabolized in liver. **Elimination:** excreted in urine, bile, and breast milk.

CONTRAINDICATIONS & PRECAUTIONS Contraindicated in: acute surgical abdomen, nausea, vomiting, abdominal cramps, intestinal obstruction, fecal impaction; use of rectal suppository in presence of anal or rectal fissures, ulcerated hemorrhoids, proctitis. **Cautious use in:** pregnancy (category C).

ADVERSE/SIDE EFFECTS Systemic effects not reported. Rarely: mild cramping, nausea, vertigo, diarrhea, fluid and electrolyte disturbances (especially potassium and calcium).

DRUG INTERACTIONS ANTACIDS will cause early dissolution of enteric coated tablets, resulting in abdominal cramping.

NURSING IMPLICATIONS

Administration

- In view of action time, administer PO drug in the evening or before breakfast. Suppository may be inserted at time bowel movement is desired.
- Tablets are enteric coated; therefore, to avoid gastric irritation, they should be swallowed whole and not cut, crushed, or chewed. Preferably taken with a full glass (240 ml) of water or other liquid.
- Tablets should not be taken within 1 h of antacids or milk. These substances may cause premature dissolution of enteric coating, with release of drug in stomach resulting in gastric irritation and loss of cathartic action.
- *Administration of rectal suppository:* Moisten suppository with water-soluble lubricant or plain water to facilitate insertion. Spread buttocks, and gently insert into anus, rounded end first, using forefinger to advance it beyond the internal sphincter (about 5 cm [2 in] or length of forefinger). Have patient hold it for 10–20 min and to defecate when urge is felt.
- Bisacodyl tablets and suppositories are preserved in tightly closed containers at temperatures not exceeding 30C (86F).

Assessment & Drug Effects

- Bisacodyl usually produces 1 or 2 soft formed stools. Periodically evaluate patient's need for continued use of bisacodyl.
- Because of OTC availability, laxative abuse, especially among the elderly, is widespread.
- Indiscriminate use of laxatives or dietary fiber can lead to changes in intestinal bacterial flora and to decreased absorption of vitamin K, drugs, and nu-

Common side effects in *italic*; life-threatening effects underlined; generic names in **bold**; classifications in SMALL CAPS

221

trients, because of decreased transit time in the intestine.

Patient & Family Education

- Instruct patient not to take bisacodyl within 1 h of taking antacids or milk.
- Inform the habitual laxative user that a normal pattern for elimination varies from 3 bowel movements a day to 3 a week, depending on a self-established functionally effective schedule.
- High fiber in the diet is frequently prescribed as a supplement and eventual substitute for laxative use. Examples of high fiber foods: fruits, vegetables, bran.
- High-fiber foods should be added slowly to regular diet to avoid gas and diarrhea, and fluid intake should be adequate (at least 6–8 glasses/d).

STOOL SOFTENER

DOCUSATE CALCIUM (DIOCTYL CALCIUM SULFOSUCCINATE)

(dok´yoo-sate)
Trade names: DCS, PMS-Docusate Calcium, Pro-Cal-Sof, Surfak

DOCUSATE POTASSIUM

Trade names: Dialose, Diocto-k, Kasof

DOCUSATE SODIUM

Trade names: Colace, Dio-Sul, Disonate, DGSS, D-S-S, Duosol, Lax-gel, Laxinate 100, Modane Soft, Pro-Sof, Regulax, Regutol
Classifications: GI AGENT; STOOL SOFTENER
Pregnancy: Category C

ACTIONS/PHARMACODYNAMICS Anionic surface-active agent with emulsifying and wetting properties. Detergent action lowers surface tension, permitting water and fats to penetrate and soften stools for easier passage. Action is also thought to be related to its ability to increase cyclic adenosine monophosphate (cAMP) in colonic mucosal cells, thereby stimulating secretion of intestinal fluid.

USES Prophylactically in patients who should avoid straining during defecation and for treatment of constipation associated with hard, dry stools (e.g., following anorectal surgery, MI).

ROUTE & DOSAGE

Stool Softener

Adult	PO	50–500 mg/d
	PR	50–100 mg added to enema fluid
Child	PO	6–12 y: 40–120 mg/d
		3–6 y: 20–60 mg/d
		< 3 y: 10–40 mg/d

CONTRAINDICATIONS & PRECAUTIONS Contraindicated in: atonic constipation, nausea, vomiting, abdominal pain, fecal impaction, structural anomalies of colon and rectum, intestinal obstruction or perforation; use of docusate sodium in patients on sodium restriction; use of docusate potassium in patients with renal dysfunction; concomitant use of mineral oil; pregnancy (category C).

ADVERSE/SIDE EFFECTS Rare: occasional mild abdominal cramps, *diarrhea*, nausea, bitter taste, throat irritation (liquid preparation), rash.

DRUG INTERACTIONS Docusate will increase systemic absorption of **mineral oil.**

NURSING IMPLICATIONS

Administration

- Administer with a full glass of water if allowed.
- FDA Panel on Laxatives recommends against daily use of docusate for > 1 wk.
- Store in tightly covered containers. Syrup formulations should be stored in tight, light-resistant containers at 15–30C (59–86F) unless directed otherwise.

Assessment & Drug Effects

- Assess effectiveness of drug. Report continued straining during defecation to physician.
- If diarrhea develops, withhold drug and notify physician.
- Effect on stools is usually apparent 1–3 d after first dose.

Patient & Family Education

- Advise patient to take sufficient liquid with each dose and to increase fluid intake during the day, if allowed. Oral liquid (not syrup) may be administered in milk, fruit juice, or infant formula to mask bitter taste.

- Docusate enhances systemic absorption of mineral oil; therefore, concomitant use is not recommended.
- Docusate should not be administered for prolonged periods in lieu of proper dietary management or treatment of underlying causes of constipation.

GOLD COMPOUND

AUROTHIOGLUCOSE

(aur-oh-thye-oh-gloo´kose)
Trade names: Gold thioglucose, Solganal
Classifications: GOLD COMPOUND ANTIINFLAMMATORY
Pregnancy: Category C

ACTIONS/PHARMACODYNAMICS Slow-acting parenteral preparation of approximately 50% gold. Available commercially as a suspension in anhydrous vegetable oils to delay absorption and prolong action. Major clinical effect is suppression of joint inflammation in early arthritic disease. Has no effect on reparative process, but studies suggest that it may significantly slow or arrest disease progression. Mechanism of antiinflammatory action not clearly understood. Gold uptake by macrophages with subsequent inhibition of migration and phagocytic action, thereby suppressing immune responsiveness, may be principal mechanism.

USES Adjunctive treatment of both adult and juvenile active rheumatoid arthritis. Generally used when adequate trial with salicylates or other NSAIDs has not been satisfactory. **Unlabeled use:** psoriatic arthritis, Felty's syndrome, pemphigus, nondisseminated LE.

ROUTE & DOSAGE

Rheumatoid Arthritis

Adult	IM	10 mg 1st wk, 25 mg 2nd and 3rd wk, then 50 mg/wk to a cumulative dose of 1 g; if improvement occurs, continue at 25–50 mg q2–3wk, then q3–4wk indefinitely or until side effects occur
Child	IM	6–12 y: 1mg/kg/wk (max 25 mg) for 20 wk; if improvement, continue at 1 mg/kg (max 25 mg) q2–4wk

PHARMACOKINETICS Absorption: slowly and irregularly absorbed from IM site. **Peak:** 4–6 h. **Distribution:** widely distributed, especially to synovial fluid; does not cross blood-brain barrier; crosses placenta. **Metabolism:** unknown. **Elimination:** half-life: 3–27 d; 50–90% of dose ultimately excreted in urine; 10–50% in feces; excreted in breast milk.

CONTRAINDICATIONS & PRECAUTIONS
Contraindicated in: Gold allergy or history of severe toxicity from previous therapy with gold or other heavy metals; severe debilitation; uncontrolled diabetes mellitus; renal or hepatic insufficiency, history of hepatitis; uncontrolled CHF; marked hypertension; tuberculosis; severe anemia, hemorrhagic diathesis, agranulocytosis or other blood dyscrasias; disseminated LE, Sjögren's syndrome, recent radiation therapy; colitis; urticaria, eczema, history of exfoliative dermatitis. Safe use during pregnancy (category C), in nursing women, and in children under 6 y not established. **Cautious use in:** elderly patients; history of drug allergy or hypersensitivity; history of blood dyscrasias; history of renal or hepatic disease; compromised cerebral or cardiovascular circulation; presence of skin rash.

ADVERSE/SIDE EFFECTS Eye: iritis, keratitis, corneal ulcer; gold deposits in eye. **GI:** nausea, vomiting, abdominal cramps, anorexia, metallic taste, glossitis, gingivitis, diarrhea. **Hematologic:** eosinophilia, agranulocytosis, thrombocytopenia, leukopenia, granulocytopenia, panmyelopathy, aplastic anemia. **Hypersensitivity:** anaphylactic shock, syncope, bradycardia, thickening of tongue, dysphagia, dyspnea. **Renal:** nephrotic syndrome, proteinuria, hematuria. **Skin:** *pruritus, urticaria, erythema,* "gold dermatitis," fixed-drug eruptions, exfoliative dermatitis with alopecia and nail shedding; Stevens-Johnson syndrome, photosensitivity reactions. **Other:** hepatitis, immunologic destruction of synovial fluid, exacerbation of arthralgia (temporary), fever, local irritation at injection site, vaginitis, proteinuria, nephrotic syndrome, pulmonary fibrosis, interstitial pneumonitis.

DIAGNOSTIC TEST INTERFERENCES Low *PBI* (by *chloric acid method)*; test interference may persist for several weeks after gold therapy is discontinued.

DRUG INTERACTIONS ANTIMALARIALS, IMMUNOSUPPRESSANTS, **penicillamine, phenylbutazone** increase risk of blood dyscrasias.

Common side effects in *italic*; life-threatening effects underlined; generic names in **bold**; classifications in SMALL CAPS

223

NURSING IMPLICATIONS

Administration

- Administered only to carefully selected patients who can be under constant supervision of a physician thoroughly familiar with parenteral gold therapy.
- Hold vial horizontally and shake vigorously to ensure uniform suspension. Heating vial to body temperature (by placing in a warm-water bath) facilitates drug withdrawal.
- Aurothioglucose must not be injected intravenously. Needle and syringe must be dry when dose is prepared.
- Administer drug by deep IM injection (preferably intragluteally). An 18- or 20-gauge, 1 1/2-inch needle is recommended (for obese patients a 2-inch needle may be preferable). Patient should be lying down when drug is administered.
- Patient should remain recumbent for 10 min after injection to overcome possible nitritoid reaction. Observe patient for 20—30 min after injection for hypersensitivity reactions.
- Gold therapy is contraindicated following a severe reaction but may be attempted at reduced initial dosage schedule and careful monitoring after a mild reaction.
- Store in light-resistant containers at 15–30C (59–86F) unless otherwise directed. Protect from freezing and light.

Assessment & Drug Effects

- Baseline renal and hepatic function tests, CBC, and urinalysis should be done before initiation of therapy. Thereafter, urinalysis (for protein and sediment) should be performed before each injection. CBC (including Hgb, RBC, WBC and differential, platelet counts) should be determined before every second injection throughout therapy.
- Pregnancy should be ruled out before gold treatment begins. Women of childbearing age should be warned about the potential hazards of becoming pregnant during therapy and counseled about the use of birth control.
- Therapeutic effectiveness may not be apparent before 6–8 wk of gold therapy.
- During early treatment, some patients complain of exacerbation of joint pain after injection. It usually subsides after the first few injections.
- Interview and examine patient before each injection to detect early signs and symptoms suggestive of gold toxicity. Beginning toxicity generally involves skin and mucous membranes anywhere in body. Inspect skin carefully and use tongue blade

and flashlight to examine mouth and throat. The following are suggestive of *gold reaction* and should be reported promptly: itching (often precedes dermatitis and eosinophilia), bruising or bleeding, tenderness, metallic taste (frequently precedes sore mouth, tongue, or throat), gray-blue discoloration of skin and mucous membranes, diarrhea or loose stools, indigestion, unexplained malaise; signs of hepatotoxicity (yellow sclerae and skin, clay-colored stools, dark urine, pruritus).
- A rapid improvement in joint pain and mobility also may signify that patient is approaching toxic tissue levels. Interruption of therapy, at least temporarily, is indicated.
- Precipitous decline in platelets or counts <100,000/mm^3, or leukocytes <4000/mm^3, granulocytes <1500/mm^3, eosinophils >5%, rapid fall in Hgb value, and presence of proteinuria or hematuria are all indications to withhold therapy pending further studies.

Patient & Family Education

- Before initiation of treatment, patient should be well informed regarding dangers associated with gold therapy and requirements for compliance in receiving scheduled doses, keeping laboratory appointments, and for prompt reporting of adverse effects.
- Provide patient with a list of possible adverse effects that should be reported. If therapy is interrupted at the onset of gold toxicity, serious reactions can be avoided. Note that elderly patients are particularly sensitive to the effects of gold therapy, and some patients appear to have a genetic predisposition to gold toxicity.
- Adverse reactions are most likely to occur during second and third month of therapy or when cumulative aurothioglucose dose is 300–500 mg. However, they may appear at any time during therapy or several months after treatment has been discontinued (gold is slowly eliminated from body).
- Instruct patient to report any unusual color or odor to urine, or change in I&O ratio and pattern.
- Advise patient to report early signs of infection that may indicate onset of agranulocytosis (unusual fatigue or weakness, malaise, chills, fever, sore throat); possible signs of reduced platelets (thrombocytopenia): unexplained bleeding, e.g., bleeding gums, nosebleeds, dark urine (hematuria), black stools, petechiae, purpura, easy bruising. Also instruct patient to report signs of hepatotoxicity (see Signs & Symptoms, chap 3).
- Be alert to vulnerability of patient to secondary infection because of the possible immunosuppres-

Common side effects in *italic*; life-threatening effects underlined; generic names in **bold**; classifications in SMALL CAPS

sive effect of gold. Caution patient to avoid contact with persons who have colds or recent vaccination or who have been exposed recently to communicable disease.

- Inform patient that the necessity to increase the amount of aspirin or other prescribed NSAID for analgesia is a significant indication of diminishing response to gold therapy and therefore should be reported to physician.
- Since gray to blue pigmentation (chrysiasis) may occur on light-exposed skin areas, caution patient to minimize exposure to sunlight and artificial ultraviolet light.
- *Symptomatic treatment of stomatitis:* Advise careful oral hygiene. Use a soft toothbrush or finger covered with moistened cotton or moistened gauze. Rub gently. Floss carefully with waxed dental floss once daily. Rinse mouth frequently with warm water, tea, or saline (if allowed). Caution against overuse of commercial mouth washes especially those that are bactericidal. Many contain alcohol which enhances drying and irritation and can change mouth flora.

ADRENAL CORTICOSTEROID: GLUCOCORTICOID

PREDNISONE
(pred´ni-sone)
Trade names: Apo-Prednisone, Colisone, Deltasone, Meticorten, Orasone, Panasol, Prednicen-M, Sterapred, Winpred
Classifications: SYNTHETIC HORMONE; ADRENAL CORTICOSTEROID; GLUCOCORTICOID; ANTIINFLAMMATORY; IMMUNOSUPPRESSANT
Pregnancy: Category C

ACTIONS/PHARMACODYNAMICS Immediate-acting synthetic analog of hydrocortisone. Effect depends on biotransformation to prednisolone, a conversion that may be impaired in patient with liver dysfunction. Has less mineralocorticoid activity than hydrocortisone, but sodium (therefore fluid) retention and potassium depletion can occur. Shares contraindications and precautions and adverse/side effects with fludrocortisone, p 227. On weight basis 5 mg prednisone is equivalent to 5 mg prednisolone, 20 mg hydrocortisone, and 25 mg cortisone. Safe use

by pregnant women (category C), children, or during lactation not established.

USES May be used as a single agent or conjunctively with antineoplastics in cancer therapy; also used in treatment of myasthenia gravis and inflammatory conditions and as an immunosuppressant.

ROUTE & DOSAGE

Antiinflammatory

Adult	PO	5–60 mg/d in single or divided doses
Child	PO	0.1–0.15 mg/kg/d in single or divided doses

PHARMACOKINETICS Absorption: readily absorbed from GI tract. **Peak:** 1–2 h. **Duration:** 1–1.5 d. **Distribution:** crosses placenta; distributed into breast milk. **Metabolism:** metabolized in liver. **Elimination:** half-life: 3.5 h; hypothalamus-pituitary axis suppression: 24–36 h; excreted in urine.

DRUG INTERACTIONS BARBITURATES, **phenytoin, rifampin** increase steroid metabolism—increased doses of prednisone may be needed; **amphotericin B,** DIURETICS increase potassium loss; **ambenonium, neostigmine, pyridostigmine** may cause severe muscle weakness in patients with myasthenia gravis; may inhibit antibody response to VACCINES, TOXOIDS.

NURSING IMPLICATIONS

Administration

- Before administration, tablet may be crushed and then taken with fluid of patient's choice.
- Oral drug may be taken at mealtimes or with a snack to reduce gastric irritation.
- The initial suppressive dosing regimen should be brief, especially if alternate-day therapy is anticipated. Usually 4–10 d is sufficient for satisfactory clinical response in many allergic and collagen diseases.
- Alternate-day therapy (ADT, i.e., single dose administered every other day) is used when long-term PO glucocorticoid treatment is anticipated. ADT may be advised to keep daily dose at minimal levels and to reduce degree of "steroid rebound" with withdrawal.
- Cortisol plasma levels are maximal between 2 and 8 AM and minimal between 4 PM and midnight (*normal:* 7–28 µg/dl in AM and below 10 µg/dl at 8 PM). Exogenous corticosteroids suppress adrenal cortex activity less when given in the morning. To mini-

Common side effects in *italic*; life-threatening effects underlined; generic names in **bold**; classifications in SMALL CAPS

225

mize HPA axis suppression, replacement steroid should be given before 9 AM.

- Dose adjustment may be required if patient is subjected to severe stress (serious infection, surgery, or injury) or if a remission or disease exacerbation occurs.
- To prevent withdrawal symptoms and permit adrenals to recover from drug-induced partial atrophy, doses are gradually reduced by scheduled decrements (various regimens).
- Protect drug from light and air in tightly closed dark container.
- Store at temperature between 15–30C (59–86F).

Assessment & Drug Effects

- Establish baseline and continuing data regarding BP, I&O ratio and pattern, weight, and sleep pattern. Start flow chart as reference for planning individualized pharmacotherapeutic patient care.
- Check and record BP during dose stabilization period at least 2 times daily. Report an ascending pattern.
- Urine specimens every 24 h for studies of 17-KS may be prescribed to rule out Cushing's syndrome. *Normal 17-KS values:* men, 10–25 mg/24 h; women < 50 y; 5–15 mg/24 h; women > 50 y; 4–8 mg/24 h.
- During long-term therapy, patient should be monitored for evidence of HPA axis suppression by determining plasma cortisol levels at weekly intervals.
- Two-hour postprandial blood glucose, serum potassium, chest x-ray, and routine laboratory studies are performed at regular intervals during long-term steroid therapy.
- The elderly patient and the patient with low serum albumin are especially susceptible to adverse/side effects because of excess circulating free glucocorticoids.
- If patient has a history of diabetes mellitus, urine should be tested for glycosuria daily. Report positive findings; dietary and antidiabetic medication dose adjustments may be indicated.
- Be alert to signs of hypocalcemia (see chap 3). Patients with hypocalcemia have increased requirements for pyridoxine (vitamin B_6), vitamins C and D, and folates.
- Be alert to possibility of masked infection and delayed healing (antiinflammatory and immunosuppressive actions). Prednisone suppresses early classic signs of inflammation that are diagnostically important: capillary dilation (heat, redness), phagocytosis (pus formation), swelling (pain), fibrin deposition (clot formation). When patient is on an extended therapy regimen, incidence of oral *Candida* infection is high. Inspect mouth daily for

symptoms: white patches, black furry tongue, painful membranes and tongue.

- Exaggerated sense of well-being and analgesic effects may encourage patient to increase physical activity even if acute disease process still exists. Discuss with physician and work with patient and family to plan reasonable and safe range of activities and daily living.
- Compression and spontaneous fractures of long bones and vertebrae present hazards, particularly in long-term corticosteroid treatment of rheumatoid arthritis or diabetes, in immobilized patients, and the elderly. Supervise getting out of bed or chair. Report persistent backache or chest pain (possible symptoms of vertebral or rib fracture). Patient's mattress should be firm or supported by a bedboard.
- Be aware of previous history of psychotic tendencies. Watch for changes in mood and behavior, emotional stability, sleep pattern, or psychomotor activity, especially with long-term therapy, that may signal onset of recurrence. Report symptoms to physician.
- If a patient is receiving aspirin concomitantly with a corticosteroid, salicylism may be induced when the corticosteroid dosage is decreased or discontinued.
- Ordinarily long-term corticosteroid therapy is not interrupted when patient undergoes major surgery, but dosage may be increased.
- Abrupt discontinuation of corticosteroids after long-term therapy may result in ***withdrawal syndrome*** (myalgia, fever, arthralgia, malaise) and ***hypocorticism*** (anorexia, vomiting, nausea, fatigue, dizziness, hypotension, hypoglycemia, myalgia, arthralgia).
- If during withdrawal the disease flares up, a dosage increase followed by a more gradual withdrawal may be necessary.
- Patient is supervised about 1 y after withdrawal from systemic corticosteroids or until HPA axis function is restored. During period of HPA axis suppression, severe stress (trauma, surgery, infections) may induce symptoms of adrenal insufficiency necessitating reinstitution of corticosteroid treatment.

Patient & Family Education

- Counsel patient to take drug as prescribed and not to alter dosing regimen or stop medication without consulting physician. Additionally, patient should not give any of the drug to another person.
- Inform patient that a slight weight gain with improved appetite is expected, but after dosage is sta-

bilized, a sudden slow but steady weight increase (2 kg [5 lb]) wk) should be reported.

- Encourage patient to avoid alcohol and caffeine (secretagogues); may contribute to steroid-ulcer development in long term therapy.
- Dyspepsia with hyperacidity should not be ignored. Encourage patient to report symptoms to physician and not to self-medicate to find relief.
- Warn patient not to use aspirin or other OTC drugs unless they are prescribed specifically by the physician.
- Warn patient to report slow healing, any vague feeling of being sick without clear etiologic definition, or return of pretreatment symptoms.
- The immunocompromised patient should be fastidious about personal hygiene, give special attention to foot care, and be particularly cautious about bruising or abrading the skin.
- Single doses of corticosteroids or use for a short period (> 1 wk) does not produce withdrawal symptoms when drug is discontinued, even with moderately large doses.
- Patient or family should be advised to tell a dentist or new physician about recent prolonged corticosteroid treatment.
- Advise patient receiving corticosteroid to carry a medical identification card or jewelry with recorded diagnosis, drug therapy, and name of physician.
- Urge patient to adhere to scheduled appointments for regimen reevaluation.

ADRENAL CORTICOSTEROID: MINERALOCORTICOID

FLUDROCORTISONE ACETATE

(floo-droe-kor´ti-sone)
Trade name: Florinef Acetate
Classifications: SYNTHETIC HORMONE; ADRENAL CORTICOSTEROID; MINERALOCORTICOID
Pregnancy: Category C

ACTIONS/PHARMACODYNAMICS Long-acting synthetic steroid with potent mineralocorticoid and moderate glucocorticoid activity. Small doses produce marked sodium retention, increased urinary potassium excretion, and elevated BP. If protein intake is inadequate, fludrocortisone induces negative nitrogen balance.

USES Partial replacement therapy for adrenocortical insufficiency and for treatment of salt-losing forms of congenital adrenogenital syndrome. **Unlabeled use:** to increase systolic and diastolic blood pressure in patients with severe hypotension secondary to diabetes mellitus or to levodopa therapy.

ROUTE & DOSAGE

Adrenocortical Insufficiency

Adult	PO	0.1 mg/d; dose may range from 0.1 mg 3 times/wk to 0.2 mg/d
Child	PO	Same as for adult

Salt-losing Adrenogenital Syndrome

Adult	PO	0.1–0.2 mg/d
Child	PO	Same as for adult

PHARMACOKINETICS Absorption: readily absorbed from GI tract. **Peak:** 1.7 h. **Metabolism:** metabolized in liver. **Elimination:** half-life: 3.5 h.

CONTRAINDICATIONS & PRECAUTIONS Contraindicated in: hypersensitivity to glucocorticoids, idiopathic thrombocytopenic purpura, psychoses, acute glomerulonephritis, viral or bacterial diseases of skin, infections not controlled by antibiotics, active or latent amebiasis, hypercorticism (Cushing's syndrome), smallpox vaccination or other immunologic procedures. (Topical steroids contraindicated in presence of varicella, vaccinia, on surfaces with compromised circulation, and in children < 2y.) Safe use in nursing mothers, during pregnancy (category C) not established. **Cautious use in:** children, diabetes mellitus; chronic, active hepatitis positive for hepatitis B surface antigen; hyperlipidemia; cirrhosis; stromal herpes simplex; glaucoma, tuberculosis of eye; osteoporosis; convulsive disorders; hypothyroidism; diverticulitis, nonspecific ulcerative colitis, fresh intestinal anastomoses, active or latent peptic ulcer, gastritis, esophagitis; thromboembolic disorders; CHF, metastatic carcinoma; hypertension, renal insufficiency; history of allergies; active or arrested tuberculosis; systemic fungal infection; myasthenia gravis.

ADVERSE/SIDE EFFECTS Dose and treatment-duration dependent. **CNS:** vertigo, headache, nystagmus, ataxia (rare), increased intracranial pressure with papilledema (usually after discontinuation of medication), mental disturbances, aggravation of pre-existing psychiatric conditions, insomnia. **CV:** syncopal episodes, thrombophlebitis, thromboembolism or

Common side effects in *italic*; life-threatening effects underlined; generic names in **bold**; classifications in SMALL CAPS

227

fat embolism, palpitation, tachycardia, necrotizing angiitis. **Endocrine:** suppressed linear growth in children, decreased glucose tolerance; hyperglycemia, manifestations of latent diabetes mellitus; hypocorticism; amenorrhea and other menstrual difficulties. **Eye:** posterior subcapsular cataracts (especially in children), glaucoma, exophthalmos, increased intraocular pressure with optic nerve damage, perforation of the globe, fungal infection of the cornea, decreased or blurred vision. **Fluid and electrolyte disturbances:** hypocalcemia; *sodium and fluid retention;* hypokalemia and hypokalemic alkalosis; CHF, hypertension. **GI:** *nausea,* increased appetite, ulcerative esophagitis, pancreatitis, abdominal distension, peptic ulcer with perforation and hemorrhage, melena. **Hematologic:** thrombocytopenia. **Musculoskeletal (long-term use):** osteoporosis, compression fractures, muscle wasting and weakness, tendon rupture, aseptic necrosis of femoral and humeral heads. **Skin:** skin thinning and atrophy, *acne, impaired wound healing;* petechiae, ecchymosis, easy bruising; suppression of skin test reaction; hypopigmentation or hyperpigmentation, hirsutism, acneiform eruptions, subcutaneous fat atrophy; allergic dermatitis, urticaria, angioneurotic edema, increased sweating. **Other:** negative nitrogen balance, anaphylactoid or hypersensitivity reactions; aggravation or masking of infections; malaise, hiccups, hoarseness, dry mouth, sore throat (with inhalation therapy), weight gain, obesity; increased or decreased motility and number of sperm, decreased serum concentration of vitamins A and C; urinary frequency and urgency, enuresis. **Overdose:** anxiety, mental confusion, depression, hyperglycemia, hypokalemia, hypernatremia, polycythemia, hypertension, edema, GI cramping or bleeding, ecchymoses, "moon" facies. **With parenteral therapy:** IV site: pain, irritation, necrosis, atrophy, sterile abscess; Charcot-like arthropathy following intraarticular use; burning and tingling in perineal area (after IV injection).

DRUG INTERACTIONS The antidiabetic effects of **insulin** and SULFONYLUREAS may be diminished; **amphotericin B,** DIURETICS may increase potassium loss; **warfarin** may decrease prothrombin time; **indomethacin, ibuprofen** can potentiate the pressor effect of fludrocortisone; ANABOLIC STEROIDS increase risk of edema and acne; **rifampin** may increase the hepatic metabolism of fludrocortisone.

NURSING IMPLICATIONS

Administration

- Concomitant oral cortisone or hydrocortisone therapy may be advisable to provide substitute therapy approximating normal adrenal activity.

- Store in airtight containers at 15–30C (59–86F). Protect from light.

Assessment & Drug Effects

- Monitor for signs of hypokalemia (see chap 3) and hyperkalemic metabolic alkalosis (see chap 3).
- Periodic checking of serum electrolyte levels is usual during prolonged therapy. Supplemental calcium and potassium chloride, as well as restricted salt intake, may be necessary during long-term therapy.
- Monitor weight and I&O ratio to observe onset of fluid accumulation, especially if patient is on unrestricted salt intake and without potassium supplement. Report weight gain of 2 kg (5 lb)/wk.
- Monitor and record BP daily. If transient hypertension develops as a consequence of therapy, report to physician. Usually the dose will be reduced to 0.05 mg/d.
- During period of dosage adjustment, BP should be checked q4–6h and weight at least every other day.
- The patient may become hypoglycemic during the dose regulation period if without food more than 4–5 h. Schedule laboratory tests so as to prevent long periods without nourishment.
- *Signs of overdosage (hypercorticism):* psychosis, excess weight gain, edema, congestive heart failure, ravenous appetite, severe insomnia, increase in BP.
- *Signs of insufficient dosage (hypocorticism):* loss of weight and appetite, nausea, vomiting, diarrhea, muscular weakness, increased fatigue, hypotension.

Patient & Family Education

- Instruct patient to report signs of hypokalemia (see chap 3).
- Alert patient to *signs of potassium depletion associated with high sodium intake:* muscle weakness, paresthesias, circumoral numbness; fatigue, anorexia, nausea, mental depression, polyuria, delirium, diminished reflexes, arrhythmias, cardiac failure, ileus, ECG changes.
- Patient may be advised to eat foods with high potassium content. Consult with physician and dietician. A potassium supplement may be necessary.
- Sodium intake may or may not require regulation, depending on individual needs and clinical situation. Teach the patient that salt intake is a significant regulator of drug efficacy. Signs of edema should be reported immediately.
- Instruct patient to weigh daily under standard conditions and to report steady weight gain.
- Intercurrent infection, trauma, or unexpected stress of any kind should be reported promptly by patient on maintenance therapy.

- Advise patient to wear or carry medical identification card or jewelry stating drug being used and physician's identity.

See hydrocortisone, p 255, for additional nursing implications.

ANDROGEN/ANABOLIC STEROID

TESTOSTERONE

(tess-toss´ter-one)

Trade names: Andro 100, Androlan, Andronaq-50, Histerone, Malogen, Testaqua, Testoject-50

Classifications: SYNTHETIC HORMONE; ANDROGEN/ANABOLIC STEROID; ANTINEOPLASTIC

Pregnancy: Category X

Controlled substance: Schedule III

ACTIONS/PHARMACODYNAMICS Synthetic steroid compound with both androgenic and anabolic activity (1:1). Controls development and maintenance of secondary sexual characteristics. **Androgenic activity:** responsible for the growth spurt of the adolescent and for growth termination by epiphyseal closure. In males and some females reduces excretion of phosphorus, nitrogen, potassium, sodium, and chloride. Increases erythropoiesis, possibly by stimulating production of renal or extrarenal erythropoietin, and promotes vascularization and darkening of skin. Antagonizes effects of estrogen excess on female breast and endometrium. **Anabolic activity:** increases protein metabolism and decreases its catabolism. Large doses suppress spermatogenesis, thereby causing testicular atrophy. Unlike other androgens, testosterone and its esters do not produce cholestatic hepatitis or creatinuria.

USES Androgen replacement therapy, delayed puberty (male), palliation of female mammary cancer (1–5 y postmenopausal), and to treat postpartum breast engorgement. Available in fixed combination with estrogens in many preparations.

PHARMACOKINETICS Absorption: cypionate and **enanthate** are slowly absorbed from lipid tissue. **Duration:** 2–4 wk **cypionate** and **enanthate. Distribution:** 98% bound to sex hormone–binding globulin. **Metabolism:** primarily metabolized in liver. **Elimination:** half-life: 10–100 min; 90% excreted in urine, 6% in feces.

ROUTE & DOSAGE

Male Hypogonadism

Adult   IM   10–25 mg 2–3 times/wk

Inoperable Breast Cancer

Adult   IM   50–100 mg short-acting testosterone 3 times/wk

Postpartum Breast Engorgement

Adult   IM   25–50 mg/d for 3–4 d

CONTRAINDICATIONS & PRECAUTIONS Contraindicated in: hypersensitivity or toxic reactions to androgens; serious cardiac, hepatic, or renal disease; pregnancy (category X), (possibility of virilization of external genitalia of female fetus); in nursing mothers; hypercalcemia; known or suspected prostatic or breast cancer in male; benign prostatic hypertrophy with obstruction; patients easily stimulated sexually; elderly, asthenic males who may react adversely to androgenic overstimulation; conditions aggravated by fluid retention; hypertension. **Cautious use in:** cardiac, hepatic, and renal disease; prepubertal males, geriatric patients, acute intermittent porphyria.

ADVERSE/SIDE EFFECTS CNS: excitation, insomnia. **CV:** skin flushing and vascularization. **GI:** nausea, vomiting, anorexia, diarrhea, gastric pain, jaundice. **Hematologic:** leukopenia. **Metabolic:** hypercalcemia, hypercholesterolemia, *sodium and water retention (especially in elderly) with edema.* **Renal:** renal calculi (especially in the immobilized patient), bladder irritability. **Reproductive:** *increased libido.* **Skin:** *acne,* injection site irritation and sloughing. **Other:** hypersensitivity to testosterone, <u>anaphylactoid reaction</u> (rare), precipitation of acute intermittent porphyria. Androgenic: (virilization) female: suppression of ovulation, lactation, or menstruation; hoarseness or deepening of voice (often irreversible); hirsutism; oily skin; clitoral enlargement; regression of breasts; male-pattern baldness (in disseminated breast cancer). Male: prepubertal: premature epiphyseal closure, phallic enlargement, priapism. Postpubertal: testicular atrophy, decreased ejaculatory volume, azoospermia, oligospermia (after prolonged administration or excessive dosage), impotence, epididymitis, priapism, *gynecomastia.* Hypoestrogenic: female: flushing, sweating; vaginitis with pruritus, drying, bleeding; menstrual irregularities.

Common side effects in *italic*; life-threatening effects <u>underlined</u>; generic names in **bold**; classifications in SMALL CAPS

DIAGNOSTIC TEST INTERFERENCES Testosterone alters *glucose tolerance* tests; decreases *thyroxine-binding globulin concentration* (resulting in decreased total T_4 serum levels and increased resin of T_3 and T_4). Increases *creatinine* and *creatinine* excretion (lasting up to 2 wk after therapy is discontinued) and alters response to *metyrapone test.* It suppresses *clotting factors II, V, VII, X* and decreases excretion of *17-ketosteroids*. May increase or decrease *serum cholesterol.*

DRUG INTERACTIONS ORAL ANTICOAGULANTS may potentiate hypoprothrombinemia. May decrease **insulin** requirements.

NURSING IMPLICATIONS

Administration

- IM injections should be made deep into gluteal musculature. A wet syringe or needle may cloud the solution, but potency of material reportedly is unaffected.
- Store IM formulations prepared in oil at room temperature. Warming and shaking vial will redisperse precipitated crystals.
- Store at 15–30C (59–86F).

Assessment & Drug Effects

- Check I&O and weigh patient daily during dose adjustment period. Weight gain (due to sodium and water retention) suggests need for decreased dosage. When dosage is stabilized, urge patient to check weight at least twice weekly and to report increases, particularly if accompanied by edema in dependent areas. Dose adjustment and diuretic therapy may be started.
- Periodic serum cholesterol and calcium determinations as well as cardiac and liver function tests should be performed throughout testosterone therapy.
- Improvement from testosterone therapy is slow. Therapeutic response in patients with breast cancer is usually apparent within 3 mo after regimen begins. If signs of disease progression appear, therapy should be terminated. In patients with metastatic breast cancer, hypercalcemia usually indicates progression of bone metastasis.
- If serum calcium rises above 14 mg/dl, androgenic therapy is terminated.
- Promptly report signs and symptoms of hypercalcemia (see Chapter 3). The immobilized patient is particularly prone to develop hypercalcemia. Treatment includes withdrawing testosterone. Calcium, phosphate, and BUN levels should be checked daily.

- Testosterone-induced anabolic action enhances hypoglycemia (hyperinsulinism). Instruct diabetic to report sweating, tremor, anxiety, vertigo. Dosage adjustment of antidiabetic agent may be required.
- Observe the patient who is on concomitant anticoagulant treatment for signs of overdosage (e.g., ecchymoses, petechiae). Report promptly to physician; anticoagulant dose may need to be reduced.
- Prepubertal or adolescent males should be monitored throughout therapy to avoid precocious sexual development and premature epiphyseal closure. Skeletal stimulation may continue 6 mo beyond termination of therapy.

Patient & Family Education

- Instruct male to report priapism (sustained and often painful erections occurring especially in early replacement therapy), reduced ejaculatory volume, and gynecomastia. The symptoms indicate necessity for temporary withdrawal or discontinuation of testosterone therapy.
- Instruct to notify physician promptly if pregnancy is suspected or planned. Masculinization of the fetus is most likely to occur if testosterone (androgen) therapy is provided during first trimester of pregnancy.
- At dosage required to treat carcinoma, androgens may cause virilism in women. Advise them to report increase in libido (early sign of toxicity), growth of facial hair, deepening of voice, male-pattern baldness. The onset of hoarseness can easily be overlooked unless its significance as an early and possibly irreversible sign of virilism is appreciated. Reevaluation of treatment plan is indicated.

ANTIDIABETIC: INSULIN

INSULIN INJECTION

(in´su-lin)

Trade names: Humulin R, Novolin R, Regular Insulin, Regular Iletin I, Beef Regular Iletin II, Pork Regular Iletin II, Regular Purified Pork Insulin, Velosulin, Velosulin Human

Classifications: SYNTHETIC HORMONE; INSULIN ANTIDIABETIC

Pregnancy: Category B

ACTIONS/PHARMACODYNAMICS Short-acting, clear, colorless solution of exogenous unmodified insulin extracted from beta cells in beef or pork pancreas (as labeled) or synthesized by recombinant DNA technology (human). Enhances transmembrane passage of glucose across cell membranes of most body cells and by unknown mechanism may itself enter the cell to activate selected intermediary metabolic processes. Promotes conversion of glucose to glycogen, inhibits fatty acid mobilization from fat depots, promotes triglyceride synthesis, stimulates protein production, and promotes intracellular shift of potassium and magnesium. In the diabetic, insulin temporarily restores proper utilization of glucose and fat, thereby preventing glycosuria, diabetic ketoacidosis, and coma. Insulin injection is the only form of insulin that can be given IV.

USES Emergency treatment of diabetic ketoacidosis or coma, to initiate therapy in patient with insulin-dependent diabetes mellitus (type I, IDDM), and in combination with intermediate-acting or long-acting insulin to provide better control of blood glucose concentrations in the diabetic patient. Used IV to stimulate growth hormone secretion (glucose counterregulatory hormone) to evaluate pituitary growth hormone reserve in patient with known or suspected growth hormone deficiency. Other uses include promotion of intracellular shift of potassium in treatment of hyperkalemia (IV); to induce hypoglycemic shock as therapy in psychiatry.

PHARMACOKINETICS Absorption: rapidly absorbed from IM and SC injections. **Onset:** 0.5–1 h. **Peak:** 2–3 h. **Duration:** 5–7 h. **Distribution:** throughout extracellular fluids. **Metabolism:** metabolized primarily in liver with some metabolism in kidneys. **Elimination:** half-life: biological, up to 13 h; < 2% excreted in urine.

ROUTE & DOSAGE

Diabetes Mellitus

Adult	SC	5–10 U 15–30 min a.c. and h.s.; dose adjustments based on blood glucose determinations
Child	SC	2–4 U 15–30 min a.c. and h.s.; dose adjustments based on blood glucose determinations

Ketoacidosis

Adult	IV	2.4–7.2 U loading dose; followed by 2.4–7.2 U/h continuous infusion
Child	IV	0.1 U/kg load; followed by 0.1 U/h continuous infusion

CONTRAINDICATIONS & PRECAUTIONS
Contraindicated in: Hypersensitivity to insulin animal protein.

ADVERSE/SIDE EFFECTS Hypersensitivity (usually occurs when insulin is at peak action point): localized allergic reactions at injection site; generalized urticaria or bullae, lymphadenopathy, anaphylaxis rare. **Hypoglycemia (hyperinsulinism):** *profuse sweating,* hunger, headache, *nausea, tremulousness,* tremors, *palpitation,* tachycardia, weakness, fatigue, nystagmus, circumoral pallor; numb mouth, tongue, and other paresthesias; visual disturbances (diplopia, blurred vision, mydriasis), staring expression, confusion, personality changes, ataxia, incoherent speech, apprehension, irritability, inability to concentrate, personality changes, uncontrolled yawning, loss of consciousness, delirium, hypothermia, convulsions, Babinski reflex, coma. (Urine glucose tests will be negative). **Other:** posthypoglycemia or rebound hyperglycemia (Somogyi effect), lipoatrophy and lipohypertrophy of injection sites; insulin resistance. **Overdosage:** psychic disturbances, i.e., aphasia, personality changes, maniacal behavior.

DIAGNOSTIC TEST INTERFERENCES Large doses of insulin may increase urinary excretion of **VMA.** Insulin can cause alterations in ***thyroid function tests*** and ***liver function test*** and may decrease ***serum potassium*** and ***serum calcium***.

DRUG INTERACTIONS Alcohol, ANABOLIC STEROIDS, MAO INHIBITORS, **guanethidine,** SALICYLATES may potentiate hypoglycemic effects; **dextrothyroxine,** CORTICOSTEROIDS, **epinephrine** may antagonize hypoglycemic effects; **furosemide,** THIAZIDE DIURETICS increase serum glucose levels; **propranolol** and other BETA-BLOCKERS may mask symptoms of hypoglycemic reaction.

INCOMPATIBILITIES Solution/Additive: aminophylline, amobarbital, chlorothiazide, cytarabine, dobutamine, pentobarbital, phenobarbital, phenytoin, secobarbital, sodium bicarbonate, thiopental. Y-site: dobutamine.

NURSING IMPLICATIONS

Administration
- Insulin Injection (variously called "regular," "neutral," "plain," "ordinary," "unmodified," or just "in-

Common side effects in *italic*; life-threatening effects underlined; generic names in **bold**; classifications in SMALL CAPS

231

sulin") should not be confused with the modified insulins.

- Regular insulin (beef or pork) is often mixed with intermediate acting insulins (as prescribed by physician) to attain good control. Regular insulin (human) should not be mixed with any other insulin.
- Insulins should not be mixed unless prescribed by physician. In general, regular insulin is drawn up into syringe first to avoid contaminating the bottle with the second insulin.
- Any change in the strength (e.g., U–40, U–100), brand (manufacturer), purity, type (regular, etc.), species (beef, pork, human), or sequence of mixing two kinds of insulin is made by the physician only, since a simultaneous change in dosage may be necessary.
- Always use a syringe that corresponds with strength of insulin to be administered. Standardized color code for cap and syringe markings are red for U–40, orange for U–100.
- Regular insulin is generally administered 15–30 min before a meal so that peak action will coincide with postprandial hyperglycemia.
- Avoid injection of cold insulin; it can lead to lipodystrophy, reduced rate of absorption, and local reactions.
- Inject insulin into area that has a substantial layer of fat and is free of large blood vessels and nerves.
- Commonly used injection sites: upper arms, thighs, abdomen (avoid area over urinary bladder and 2 in [5 cm] around navel), buttocks, and upper back (if fat is loose enough to pick up). Rotate sites.
- Available injection sites are lost when lipodystrophy (seen predominantly in women and children) or hypertrophy or thickening develops. Lipodystrophy has been associated with inadequate rotation of injection sites, use of cold insulin, and a lipogenic effect of insulin. Injection of highly purified pork insulin or human insulin directly into lesions corrects the lipodystrophy.
- Allow approximately 1 in (2.5 cm) between injection sites and avoid reuse of a site for 6–8 wk, if possible. Maintain an injection record or chart to assure systematic site rotation.
- IV regular insulin may be given by direct IV undiluted. Administer 50 U or a fraction thereof over 1 min.
- When insulin is administered by continuous infusion, rate must be ordered by physician.
- Regular insulin may be adsorbed into the container or tubing when added to an IV infusion solution. Amount lost is variable and depends on concentration of insulin, infusion system, contact duration,

and flow rate. In general, the less the concentration of insulin in the solution and the slower the rate of flow, the greater the percentage adsorbed. Monitor patient response closely.
- In general, dosage is adjusted to maintain postprandial blood glucose below 160 mg/dl.
- Insulin is stable at room temperature up to 1 mo. Avoid exposure to direct sunlight or to temperature extremes (safe range is wide: 5–38C [40–100F]). Refrigerate but do not freeze stock supply. Insulin tolerates temperatures above 38C with less harm than freezing.

Assessment & Drug Effects
- Frequency of blood glucose and urine glucose monitoring is determined by the type of insulin regimen and health status of the patient.
- Usually urine test for ketones is not done routinely in stabilized diabetics. It is checked routinely in new, unstable, and juvenile diabetes and if patient has lost weight, exercises vigorously, or has an illness and whenever urine contains glucose or the blood glucose is elevated.
- Presence of acetone without sugar in the urine usually signifies insufficient carbohydrate intake. Acetone with sugar may indicate onset of ketoacidosis. Notify physician promptly.
- Monitor for hypoglycemia (see Signs & Symptoms, chap 3) at time of peak action of insulin. Onset of hypoglycemia (blood sugar: 50–40 mg/dl) may be rapid and sudden. Restlessness and diaphoresis during sleep are suggestive of a hypoglycemic reaction.
- During treatment for ketoacidosis with IV insulin, check BP, I&O ratio, and urine glucose and ketones every hour.
- Patients with severe hypoglycemia may receive glucagon, epinephrine, or IV glucose 10–50%. As soon as patient is fully conscious, oral carbohydrate, (e.g., dilute corn syrup or orange juice with sugar, Gatorade, or Pedialyte) should be given to prevent secondary hypoglycemia.
- Morning hyperglycemia may be caused by (1) a simple waning of circulating insulin, (2) the Somogyi phenomenon, or (3) the "dawn" phenomenon. **Dawn phenomenon:** in normal individuals an increase in circulating insulin during the 3–7 AM period is associated with surges in growth hormone. In the diabetic there may be a greater-than-normal secretion of growth hormone, which predisposes to development of hyperglycemia. **Somogyi phenomenon:** Hypoglycemia caused by insulin excess stimulates release of glucose counter-

Common side effects in *italic*; life-threatening effects underlined; generic names in **bold**; classifications in SMALL CAPS

regulatory hormones, which cause hyperglycemia. Suspect Somogyi phenomenon if evening blood or urine glucose levels are low followed by morning hyperglycemia.

- With simple waning of insulin, blood glucose values increase progressively through the night; with the Somogyi phenomenon, blood glucose levels usually decrease to the hypoglycemic or near-hypoglycemic range around 3 AM, then rise by 7 or 8 AM. In the dawn phenomenon, blood glucose values usually do not increase until after 3 AM.
- Dawn phenomenon and waning insulin are treated by increasing overnight insulin coverage. Somogyi phenomenon is treated by reducing dose of insulin that is active overnight or increasing prebedtime snack.
- After delivery, maternal insulin requirements usually are less than prepregnant dosage. Observe postpartum patient closely for hypoglycemia. Insulin requirement gradually returns to prepregnancy level within 1–6 wk.

Patient & Family Education

- For self-injection of an arm, suggest that patient press back of upper arm against a chair back so that tissue is "bunched up," making needle insertion easier.
- If patient is engaged in active sports, it has been suggested that injection of insulin be made into the abdomen rather than into a muscle that will be heavily taxed.

Special Points on Adverse Reactions:

- Local reactions at injection site sometimes develop 1–3 wk after therapy starts. Symptoms may last several hours to days but usually disappear with continued use. Advise patient to report symptoms.
- During early period of dosage regulation, some patients experience visual difficulties. Advise patient to delay changing prescription lenses until vision stabilizes (usually 3–6 wk).
- Hypoglycemic reaction (insulin shock) can result from excess insulin, insufficient food intake, vomiting, diarrhea, unaccustomed exercise, infection, illness, nervous or emotional tension, or overindulgence in alcohol.
- Hypoglycemic reaction is an emergency situation, since prolonged hypoglycemia can cause irreversible brain damage. Instruct patient and responsible family members to respond promptly to beginning symptoms of hypoglycemia. Advise patient to take 4 oz (120 ml) of any fruit juice or regular carbonated beverage (1.5–3 oz [45–90 ml] for child) followed by a meal of longer-acting carbohydrate

or protein food. Failure to show signs of recovery within 30 min indicates necessity for emergency treatment.

- Since severe hypoglycemia may develop suddenly, physician may advise patient to keep a supply of glucagon on hand for home emergency use.
- Advise patient to carry some form of fast-acting carbohydrate (e.g., lump sugar, Life-Savers or other candy) at all times to treat hypoglycemia.
- Loss of diabetes control (hyperglycemia or hypoglycemia) occurs commonly at the beginning of a menstrual period. Advise patient to do blood tests regularly during this time and to adjust insulin dosage accordingly, as prescribed by physician.
- *Diabetic ketoacidosis* is a medical emergency that appears over a period of weeks in controlled diabetics or in a few hours in noncontrolled patients. Blood sugar levels may rise as high as 300–800 mg/dl or higher. Precipitating factors: omission of insulin, improperly balanced diet, overeating, failure to increase insulin dosage during times of increased need, such as rapid growth in juveniles, fever, infection, emotional stress, surgery, trauma, and pregnancy.
- Inform patient and family of signs and symptoms of diabetic ketoacidosis (see p 235).
- In the event of an illness, advise patient to continue taking insulin, to go to bed, and to drink liberally (every hour if possible) of noncaloric liquids. Do not force liquids if nauseated or vomiting. Consult physician for insulin regulation if unable to eat prescribed diet.
- Because women in third trimester of pregnancy and nursing mothers may have lactose in urine, cupric sulfate reagents such as Clinitest should not be used. Glucose oxidase reagents, e.g., Chemstrip uG, Chemstrip uGK, Clinistix, Diastix, Tes-Tape, may be used.
- During lactation, frequent blood glucose determinations are advised. Both Benedict's test and Clinitest (urine tests based in copper sulfate reduction) give positive readings for lactose; therefore they should not be used during this period. Greater reliance will be placed on blood glucose analyses and on urine tests based on glucose oxidase, e.g., Chemstrip uG, Clinistix, Tes-Tape.
- Caution patients to avoid OTC medications (which may have high sugar content) unless approved by physician. Aspirin or ascorbic acid in large doses may cause positive urine glucose test.
- When the patient plans to travel, advise carrying ample insulin, at least 2 or 3 syringes and needles, and an adequate supply of emergency carbohydrate in hand luggage or handbag.

Common side effects in *italic*; life-threatening effects <u>underlined</u>; generic names in **bold**; classifications in SMALL CAPS

233

- Insulin absorption is decreased during the first 30 min after smoking. This interaction combined with a known increase in catecholamine release during smoking may have significant clinical effects. A heavy smoker may require up to 30% more insulin than the nonsmoker.
- In the event of unavoidable insulin shortage, advise patient to reduce dosage temporarily, decrease food intake by one-third of usual quantity, and drink generous amounts of liquids with little or no caloric value (water, coffee, tea, clear soup, broth).

ANTIDIABETIC: SULFONYLUREA

TOLBUTAMIDE
(tole-byoo´ta-mide)
Trade names: Mobenol, Novobutamide, Orinase, Tolbutone

TOLBUTAMIDE SODIUM
Trade name: Orinase Diagnostic
Classifications: SYNTHETIC HORMONE;
SULFONYLUREA ANTIDIABETIC
Pregnancy: Category C

ACTIONS/PHARMACODYNAMICS Short-acting sulfonylurea compound chemically related to sulfonamides, but without antiinfective activity. Lowers blood glucose concentration by stimulating pancreatic beta cells to synthesize and release insulin. No action demonstrated if functional beta cells are absent. During long-term use it is proposed that extrapancreatic effects (increased number of insulin receptors on cell membranes, decreased hepatic uptake of insulin, and increased peripheral utilization of insulin) also contribute to hypoglycemic effect of sulfonylurea drugs. Responsiveness to blood glucose–lowering effects with long-term therapy may decline in some patients. Alternatively, patient who has become poorly responsive to other sulfonylureas may be responsive to tolbutamide. May be mildly goitrogenic without producing clinical hypothyroidism or thyroid enlargement. It has not been established that long-term cardiovascular or neural complications of diabetes can be prevented by the sulfonylureas.

USES Management of mild to moderately severe, stable non-insulin-dependent diabetes (type II, NIDDM) that is not controlled by diet and weight reduction alone. Also used in treatment of patients who are unresponsive to other sulfonylureas and adjunctively with insulin to stabilize certain cases of labile diabetes. Used as diagnostic agent to rule out pancreatic islet cell adenoma or diabetes.

ROUTE & DOSAGE

Diabetes

Adult	PO	250 mg to 3 g/d in 1–2 divided doses

PHARMACOKINETICS Absorption: readily absorbed from GI tract. **Peak:** 3–5 h. **Distribution:** distributed into extracellular fluids. **Metabolism:** principally metabolized in liver. **Elimination:** half-life: 7 h; 75–85% excreted in urine; some elimination in feces.

CONTRAINDICATIONS & PRECAUTIONS
Contraindicated in: hypersensitivity to sulfonylureas or to sulfonamides, history of repeated episodes of diabetic ketoacidosis (with or without coma), type I (IDDM) diabetes; as sole therapy; diabetic coma; severe stress, infection, trauma, or major surgery; severe renal insufficiency, hepatic or endocrine disease. Safe use during pregnancy (category C) or use in children not established. **Cautious use in:** cardiac, thyroid, pituitary, or adrenal dysfunction; history of peptic ulcer; alcoholism; the elderly, debilitated, malnourished, or uncooperative patient.

ADVERSE/SIDE EFFECTS GI: cholestatic jaundice (rare); (dose related): nausea, epigastric fullness, heartburn, anorexia, constipation, diarrhea. **Hematologic:** agranulocytosis, thrombocytopenia, leukopenia, hemolytic anemia, aplastic anemia, pancytopenia. **Metabolic:** hepatic porphyria, disulfiram-like reactions, SIADH. **Skin:** allergic skin reactions: pruritus, erythema, urticaria, morbilliform or maculopapular eruptions; porphyria cutanea tarda, photosensitivity. **Other:** taste alterations, headache, vertigo (rare). **Overdosage:** Hypoglycemia without loss of consciousness or neurologic symptoms: unusual fatigue, tremulousness, hunger, drowsiness, GI distress, sweating, anxiety, headache; severe: visual disturbances, ataxia, paresthesias, confusion, tachycardia, seizures, coma.

DIAGNOSTIC TEST INTERFERENCES The sulfonylureas may produce abnormal *thyroid function*

Common side effects in *italic*; life-threatening effects underlined; generic names in **bold**; classifications in SMALL CAPS

test results, and reduced ***RAI uptake*** (after long-term administration). A tolbutamide metabolite may cause false-positive ***urinary protein*** values when turbidity procedures are used (such as heat and acetic acid or sulfosalicylic acid); Ames reagent strips reportedly not affected.

DRUG INTERACTIONS Phenylbutazone increases hypoglycemic effects; THIAZIDE DIURETICS may attenuate hypoglycemic effects; **alcohol** may produce disulfiram reaction; BETA-BLOCKERS may mask symptoms of a hypoglycemic reaction.

NURSING IMPLICATIONS

Administration
- Total dose may be taken before breakfast but preferably in divided doses after meals.
- Tablet may be crushed and taken with full glass of water if patient desires.
- Because of danger of nocturnal hypoglycemia, tolbutamide should not be taken at bedtime unless specifically prescribed.
- Transfer from insulin to tolbutamide (sulfonylurea) is best controlled in the hospital. For patients receiving 20 U or less of insulin daily, insulin may be stopped abruptly; oral drug is usually started at maintenance dose.
- For patients receiving 20–40 U of insulin daily, tolbutamide is started at maintenance level, with concurrent 30–50% reduction in insulin dose. Further daily decrease of insulin is done gradually.
- For patients taking more than 40 U of insulin daily, tolbutamide is initiated at maintenance level in conjunction with a 20% reduction in insulin on first day followed by cautious decremental adjustments of insulin to omission.
- If tolbutamide is used during pregnancy, it is discontinued at least 2 wk before the expected delivery date to prevent prolonged severe hypoglycemia (4–10 d) in the neonate.
- Store below 40C (104F), preferably between 15–30C (59–86F), in well-closed container; avoid freezing.

Assessment & Drug Effects
- During initial period of therapy, patient should be under close medical supervision until dosage is established. One or 2 wk of therapy may be required before full therapeutic effect is achieved.
- Elderly patients may be hyperresponsive to oral antidiabetic therapy; thus the initial dose should be low and given before breakfast. If blood and urine glucose tests are negative during first 24 h of therapy, initial dose may be continued on a daily basis.
- If a patient stabilized on tolbutamide is exposed to stress (e.g., infection, surgery), loss of blood glucose control may occur. Tolbutamide may be discontinued and replaced by insulin.
- Detection of a hypoglycemic reaction in a diabetic patient also receiving a beta-blocker, especially if elderly, is difficult. Monitor closely during adjustment period, watching for symptoms of impending hypoglycemia (see chap 3).
- Hypoglycemic symptoms may be especially vague in the elderly; therefore, check out nondefinitive vague complaints. Observe patient carefully, especially 2–3 h after eating, check urine for sugar and ketone bodies and capillary blood glucose.
- Repetitive complaints of headache and weakness a few hours after eating may signal incipient hypoglycemia. Report to physician.
- The potential for hypoglycemia in nursing infants presents the necessity to decide whether to discontinue nursing or to temporarily transfer to insulin (if diet alone is inadequate for blood sugar control).
- Pruritus and rash, frequently reported side effects, may clear spontaneously; however, if they persist, drug will be discontinued.
- Effectiveness of any hypoglycemic agent declines over time. This phenomenon is called secondary (drug) failure.
- Patients most prone to secondary failure may be underweight, erratic in their meal schedules, careless about dosage, or they may have developed drug resistance.

Patient & Family Education
- Impress on the patient and family that oral antidiabetic drug therapy controls diabetes but will never cure it.
- The patient or family member should fully understand that the physician must be informed promptly of **symptoms of hyperglycemia and ketoacidosis:** flushed, dry skin, weight loss, fatigue, Kussmaul respiration, double or blurred vision, soft eyeballs, irritability, fruity smelling breath, abdominal cramps, nausea, vomiting, diarrhea, dyspnea, polydipsia, polyphagia, polyuria, headache, hypotension, weak and rapid pulse, positive ketonuria and glycosuria. Report symptoms promptly so that emergency antidiabetic therapy can be instituted.
- Hypoglycemia is frequently caused by overdosage

Common side effects in *italic*; life-threatening effects underlined; generic names in **bold**; classifications in SMALL CAPS

235

of hypoglycemic drug, inadequate or irregular food intake, nausea, vomiting, diarrhea, and added exercise without caloric supplement or dose adjustment. Its occurrence indicates need for immediate reevaluation of patient's diet, medication regimen, and compliance. It is most likely to appear in patients > 50 y of age. Report to physician.

- Teach patient that undereating is as hazardous as overeating. Warn that a self-directed weight-loss regimen or skipped meals interfere with drug control of diabetes.
- Urge patient to report promptly any illness. The physician may want to evaluate need for insulin.
- Instruct patient to avoid self-medication with OTC drugs unless approved or prescribed by physician.
- Alcohol, even in moderate amounts, can precipitate a disulfiram-type reaction (see Signs & Symptoms, chap 3). The patient should be aware of becoming hypoglycemic after ingesting alcohol; an observer may mistakenly think he or she is inebriated, and therefore patient may be deprived of necessary emergency treatment.
- Because of potential photosensitivity (especially in the alcoholic), it may be wise for the patient to protect exposed skin areas from the sun with a sunscreen lotion (SPF 12–15).
- Advise patient to report promptly signs of hepatic toxicity, renal insufficiency, or blood dyscrasia (see chap 3).
- Advise patient to weigh self at least weekly and to report a progressive gain, especially if edema is present. These signs indicate the necessity to discontinue tolbutamide.
- When a drug that affects the hypoglycemic action of sulfonylureas (see Drug Interaction) is withdrawn or added to the tolbutamide regimen, the patient should be alerted to the added danger of loss of control (hyperglycemia). Urine tests and blood glucose tests and test for ketone bodies should be carefully monitored and possibly increased in frequency for several days to determine if antidiabetic drug dose adjustment is indicated.
- Patients using oral contraceptives should be advised to use another form of birth control.
- Advise patient who wishes to become pregnant that a transfer to insulin for blood glucose control is recommended by many clinicians.
- Instruct the patient to carry medical identification card or jewelry at all times (available from most drug stores). Card information should include patient and physician's names and addresses, diagnosis, medication, and dose being taken.

ESTROGEN

ESTRADIOL
(ess-tra-dye´ole)
Trade names: Estrace, Estraderm

ESTRADIOL CYPIONATE
Trade names: Depo-Estradiol Cypionate, Depogen, Dura-Est rin, Estro-Cyp, Estroject-LA, and others

ESTRADIOL VALERATE
Trade names: Delestrogen, Dioval, Duragen-10, Estraval, Femogex, Gynogen LA, Valergen
Classifications: HORMONE; ESTROGEN
Pregnancy: Category X

ACTIONS/PHARMACODYNAMICS Natural or synthetic steroid hormone secreted principally by the ovarian follicles, and also by the adrenals, corpus luteum, placenta, and testes. Estrogen binds to a specific intracellular receptor, forming a complex that stimulates synthesis of proteins responsible for estrogenic effects. Action of these estrogen-protein complexes is not clear, but their presence in estrogen-responsive tissues (female genital organs, breasts, pituitary, and hypothalamus) facilitates the palliative response to estrogenic treatment in women with metastatic breast cancer. In general, estradiol (estrogens) effects simulate those produced by the endogenous hormone: maintenance of normal maturation and secondary sex characteristics of the female. Promotes endometrial lining development, but prolonged exposure leads to abnormal endometrial hyperplasia, a condition usually associated with an abnormal bleeding pattern. Conversely, estrogen-stimulated endometrium suddenly deprived of estrogen may bleed within 48–72 h. Estradiol is weakly anabolic and may induce sodium and water retention and edema. Opposes bone resorption without stimulating bone growth; thus estrogen replacement is probably effective therapy for estrogen deficiency-induced osteoporosis. Other effects: decreases intestinal motility; enhances coagulability of blood; increases plasminogen levels, and decreases platelet adhesiveness. Effect on plasma lipids: may increase HDL and plasma triglycerides, slightly reduce LDL,

Common side effects in *italic*; life-threatening effects <u>underlined</u>; generic names in **bold**; classifications in SMALL CAPS

and reduce elevated plasma cholesterol levels. Reduces pituitary release of gonadotropins (LH and FSH), resulting in inhibition of lactation and ovulation and reduction of sebaceous secretion. May mask onset of climacteric. Men receiving estrogens are more prone than nonusers to nonfatal MI, pulmonary embolism, and thrombosis. There is no evidence that estrogen therapy for postmenopausal women increases risk of breast cancer. Combination estrogen-progestin therapy removes the risk in healthy postmenopausal woman of thrombosis or hypercoagulation.

USES Natural or surgical menopausal symptoms, kraurosis vulvae, atrophic vaginitis, primary ovarian failure, female hypogonadism, castration. Used adjunctively with diet, calcium and physical therapy to prevent and treat postmenopausal osteoporosis; also for palliation in advanced prostatic carcinoma and inoperable metastic breast cancer in women at least 5 y after menopause. Combined with progestins in many oral contraceptive formulations.

ROUTE & DOSAGE

Menopause, Atrophic Vaginitis, Kraurosis Vulvae, Female Hypogonadism, Female Castration, Primary Ovarian Failure

Adult	PO	1–2 mg/d in a cyclic regimen
	Topical	2–4 g *vaginal cream* intravaginally once/d for 1–2 wk, then 1–2 g/d for 1–2 wk, then 1 g 1–3 times/wk; *transdermal patch* twice weekly in a cyclic regimen
	IM	1–5 mg once q3–4wk (cypionate); 10–25 mg once q4wk (valerate)

Metastatic Breast Cancer

Adult	PO	10 mg t.i.d.

Prostatic Cancer

Adult	PO	1–2 mg t.i.d.
	IM	30 mg once q1–2 wk (valerate)

Postpartum Breast Engorgement

Adult	IM	10–25 mg at end of first stage of labor (valerate)

PHARMACOKINETICS Absorption: rapid absorption from GI tract; readily absorbed through skin and mucous membranes; slow absorption from IM injections. **Distribution:** distributed throughout body tissues, especially in adipose tissue; crosses placenta. **Metabolism:** metabolized primarily in liver. **Elimination:** excreted in urine; excreted in breast milk.

CONTRAINDICATIONS & PRECAUTIONS Contraindicated in: known or suspected pregnancy (category X), estrogenic-dependent neoplasms, breast cancer (except in selected patients being treated for metastatic disease). History of thromboembolic disorders; active arterial thrombosis or thrombophlebitis; undiagnosed abnormal genital bleeding; history of cholestatic disease; thyroid dysfunction; blood dyscrasias. **Cautious use in:** adolescents with incomplete bone growth; endometriosis, lactation; hypertension, cardiac insufficiency; diseases of calcium and phosphate metabolism (metabolic bone disease); cerebrovascular disease; mental depression; benign breast disease, family history of breast or genital tract neoplasm; diabetes mellitus; gallbladder disease; pre-existing leiomyoma, abnormal mammogram, history of idiopathic jaundice of pregnancy; varicosities; asthma; epilepsy; migraine headaches; hepatic or renal dysfunction; jaundice, acute intermittent porphyria, pyridoxine deficiency.

ADVERSE/SIDE EFFECTS CNS: headache, migraine, dizziness, metal depression, chorea, convulsions. **CV:** thromboembolic disorders, hypertension. **Eye:** intolerance to contact lenses, worsening of myopia or astigmatism, scotomas. **GI:** *nausea,* vomiting, anorexia, increased appetite, diarrhea, abdominal cramps or pain, constipation, bloating, colitis, acute pancreatitis, cholestatic jaundice, benign hepatoadenoma. **GU:** mastodynia, breast secretion, spotting, changes in menstrual flow, dysmenorrhea, amenorrhea, cervical erosion, altered cervical secretions, premenstrual-like syndrome, vaginal candidiasis, endometrial cystic hyperplasia, reactivation of endometriosis, increased size of preexisting fibromyomats, cystitislike syndrome, hemolytic uremic syndrome; in men: gynecomastia, testicular atrophy, feminization, impotence (reversible). **Metabolic:** reduced carbohydrate tolerance, hyperglycemia, hypercalcemia, folic acid deficiency, fluid retention. **Skin:** dermatitis, pruritus, seborrhea, oily skin, acne; photosensitivity, chloasma, loss of scalp hair, hirsutism. **Other:** pain and postinjection flare at injection site; sterile abscess; leg cramps, weight changes, acute intermittent porphyria, change in libido.

DIAGNOSTIC TEST INTERFERENCES Estradiol reduces response of ***metyrapone*** test and excretion

Common side effects in *italic*; life-threatening effects <u>underlined</u>; generic names in **bold**; classifications in SMALL CAPS

237

of *pregnanediol. Increases: BSP* retention, norepinephrine-induced *platelet aggregability, hydrocortisone, PBI, T₄, sodium, thyroxine-binding globulin* (TBG), *prothrombin and factors VII, VIII, IX* and *X; serum triglyceride,* and *phospholipid* concentrations, *renin* substrate. *Decreases: antithrombin III, pyridoxine* and *serum folate* concentrations, serum *cholesterol,* values for the *T₃ resin uptake* test, *glucose tolerance.* May cause false-positive test for *LE cells* or *antinuclear antibodies* (ANA).

DRUG INTERACTIONS BARBITURATES, **phenytoin, rifampin** decrease estrogen effect by increasing its metabolism; ORAL ANTICOAGULANTS may decrease hypoprothrombinemic effects.

NURSING IMPLICATIONS

Administration

- To avoid overstimulation of estrogen-activated tissues and to mimic natural menses, estrogens are usually administered on a cyclic dosage regimen: 3 wk on and 1 wk off medication. This schedule may not be used, however, for male or hysterectomized patients.
- Take PO medication with or immediately after solid food to reduce nausea.
- For administration of intravaginal or transdermal drug forms, see specific information under patient & family education.
- Protect tablets from light and moisture in well-closed container. Store at 15–30C (59–86F) and protect from freezing, unless otherwise directed by manufacturer.

Assessment & Drug Effects

- Nausea, frequently at breakfast time, seldom interferes with eating or causes weight loss and usually disappears after 1 or 2 wk of drug use.
- Spotting or breakthrough bleeding occurring when a barbiturate and estradiol are taken concurrently indicates reduced availability of the estrogen.
- Estrogen stimulation in women sterilized because of endometriosis may cause serious bleeding in remaining foci of endometrial tissues. Report unexplained and sudden pain.
- Because estradiol decreases free thyroxine, patient on therapy for a nonfunctioning thyroid may need an increase in thyroid replacement agent while also receiving an estrogen.
- Patients with cardiac or renal dysfunction or hypertension should be monitored carefully. Check BP on a regular basis.

- Severe hypercalcemia (> 15 mg/dl) may be caused by estradiol therapy in patients with breast cancer and bone metastasis.
- Intravaginal estrogen cream is readily absorbed and reaches blood levels approaching those of parenteral or orally administered estrogen. Systemic hyperestrogenic effects may result from overdosage of intravaginal cream or from overexposure of abraded skin surfaces of hands to estrogen.
- Estrogen treatment is usually interrupted at least 4 wk before surgery that may be associated with a prolonged period of immobilization or with vascular complications.

Patient & Family Education

- Emphasize need for compliance with established dosage schedule. It should not be altered unless physician prescribes a change.
- Urge patient to read the patient package insert (PPI) carefully; then discuss it with patient to assure her complete understanding of estrogen therapy.
- Patient should promptly report intermittent bleeding to physician.
- Advise patient to determine weight under standard conditions 1 or 2 times/wk and to report sudden weight gain or other signs of fluid retention.
- Teach patient how to elicit **Homan's sign:** pain in calf and popliteal region with forced dorsiflexion of foot (early sign of thrombosis).
- Instruct patient to report a positive Homan's sign and the following symptoms of thromboembolic disorders immediately: tenderness, swelling, and redness in extremity; sudden, severe headache or chest pain; slurring of speech; change in vision; tenderness, pain, sudden shortness of breath. If physician is not available, patient should go to the nearest hospital emergency room.
- Advise diabetic users to report positive urine or blood glucose tests promptly.
- Urge decreased caffeine intake, since estrogen depresses caffeine metabolism.
- Teach self-examination of breasts, emphasizing a monthly schedule.
- Estrogen users sometimes sunburn more easily and develop brown, blotchy spots on exposed skin (reversible with termination of therapy).
- Long-term or high-dosage therapy with estrogens is reduced or terminated gradually.
- Reassure male patients that estrogen-induced feminization and impotence are reversible with termination of therapy.
- Estrogen-primed or -stimulated endometrium may bleed 48–72 h after dose is discontinued. In cyclic therapy, estradiol is resumed on schedule before drug-induced vaginal bleeding stops.

Common side effects in *italic*; life-threatening effects underlined; generic names in **bold**; classifications in SMALL CAPS

- Withdrawal bleeding may occur even after oophorectomy and after menopause.

Intravaginal Application

- Instruct patient to insert calibrated dosage applicator approximately 5 cm (2 in), directing it slightly back toward sacrum. Instill medication by pushing plunger. Patient should remain in recumbent position about 30 min to prevent losing the medication. Observe perineal area before each administration: if mucosa is red, swollen, or excoriated or if there is a change in vaginal discharge, report to physician.
- Instruct patient to wash her hands well before and after the application. Also tell her not to use tampons while on vaginal cream therapy.

Transdermal Application

- If oral estrogens are being taken, start treatment 1 wk after withdrawal of PO therapy, or sooner if symptoms reappear.
- Cleanse and dry selected skin area on trunk of body, preferably the abdomen. Avoid application to the breasts, to an irritated, abrased, oily area, or to the waistline.
- Place adhesive side down on skin and press firmly in place with palm of the hand for 10 seconds.
- If system falls off, the same system may be reapplied, or if necessary, a new one can be applied. Return to original treatment schedule.
- Rotate application site with an interval of at least 1 wk between applications to a particular site.

PITUITARY (ANTIDIURETIC)

VASOPRESSIN INJECTION

(vay-soe-press´in)
Trade name: Pitressin

VASOPRESSIN TANNATE

Trade name: Pitressin Tannate
Classifications: HORMONE; PITUITARY; ANTIDIURETIC
Pregnancy: Category X

ACTIONS/PHARMACODYNAMICS Polypeptide hormone extracted from animal posterior pituitaries. Possesses pressor and antidiuretic (ADH) principles, but is relatively free of oxytocic properties. Produces concentrated urine by increasing tubular reabsorption of water (ADH activity), thus preserving up to 90% water. May increase sodium and decrease potassium reabsorption but plays no causative role in edema formation. In doses greater than those required for ADH effects, directly stimulates smooth-muscle contraction (especially in small arterioles and capillaries), thereby decreasing blood flow to splanchnic, coronary, GI, pancreatic, skin, and muscular systems. Small doses may produce anginal pain; large doses may precipitate MI, decrease heart rate and cardiac output, and increase pulmonary arterial pressure and BP. Pressor effects on GI system promote increased peristalsis (especially in large bowel), increased GI sphincter pressure, and decreased gastric secretion without effect on gastric acid concentration. Also contracts smooth muscle of gallbladder and urinary bladder; in large doses may stimulate uterine contraction. Promotes release of growth hormone, FSH, and corticotropin. The tannate (in peanut oil) is preferred for chronic therapy; intranasal aqueous vasopressin is effective for daily maintenance of mild diabetes insipidus.

USES Antidiuretic to treat diabetes insipidus, to dispel gas shadows in abdominal roentgenography, and as prevention and treatment of postoperative abdominal distension. Also given to treat transient polyuria due to ADH deficiency (related to head injuries or to neurosurgery). **Unlabeled use:** test for differential diagnosis of nephrogenic, psychogenic, and neurohypophyseal diabetes insipidus; test to elevate ability of kidney to concentrate urine, and provocative test for pituitary release of corticotropin and growth hormone; emergency and adjunct pressor agent in the control of massive GI hemorrhage (e.g., esophageal varices).

PHARMACOKINETICS Duration: 2–8 h in aqueous solution, 48–72 h in oil, 30–60 min IV infusion. **Distribution:** extracelluar fluid. **Metabolism:** metabolized in liver and kidneys. **Elimination:** half-life: 10–20 min; excreted in urine.

CONTRAINDICATIONS & PRECAUTIONS Contraindicated in: chronic nephritis accompanied by nitrogen retention; ischemic heart disease, PVCs, advanced arteriosclerosis; during first stage of labor. **Cautious use in:** epilepsy; migraine; asthma; heart failure, angina pectoris; any state in which rapid addition to extracellular fluid may be hazardous; vascular disease; preoperative and postoperative polyuric pa-

Common side effects in *italic*; life-threatening effects <u>underlined</u>; generic names in **bold**; classifications in SMALL CAPS

239

tients, renal disease; goiter with cardiac complications; elderly patients, children; pregnancy (category X).

ROUTE & DOSAGE

Diabetes Insipidus

Adult	IM/SC	5–10 U aqueous solution 2–4 times/d (5–60 U/d) or 1.25–2.5 U in oil q2–3d
	Intranasal	Apply to cotton plegit or intranasal spray
Child	IM/SC	2.5–10 U aqueous solution 2–4 times/d

Abdominal Distension, Abdominal Radiographic Procedures

Adult	IM/SC	5 U with 5–10 U q3–4h prn or 5–15 U 2 h and 30 min prior to procedure

GI Hemorrhage

Adult	IV	0.1–1 U/ml in D5W or NS at 0.2–0.4 U/min up to 0.9 U/min

ADVERSE/SIDE EFFECTS Infrequent with low doses. **Hypersensitivity:** rash, urticaria, <u>anaphylaxis</u>; *tremor,* sweating, bronchoconstriction, *circumoral and facial pallor,* angioneurotic edema, *eructations, passage of gas, nausea, vomiting, pounding in head,* anginal (in patient with coronary vascular disease), <u>cardiac arrest</u>, uterine cramps, *water intoxication* (especially with tannate). **Intraarterial infusion:** cardiac arrhythmia, pulmonary edema, bradycardia, gangrene at injection site. **Intranasal:** congestion, rhinorrhea, irritation, mucosal ulceration and pruritus, headache, conjunctivitis, heartburn, postnasal drip, abdominal cramps, increased bowel movements secondary to excessive use. **Large doses:** blanching of skin, abdominal cramps, nausea (almost spontaneously reversible), hypertension, bradycardia, minor arrhythmias, premature atrial contraction, heart block, <u>peripheral vascular collapse</u>, coronary insufficiency, <u>MI</u>.

DIAGNOSTIC TEST INTERFERENCES. Vasopressin increases *plasma cortisol* levels.

DRUG INTERACTIONS Alcohol, **demeclocycline, epinephrine, heparin, lithium, phenytoin** may decrease antidiuretic effects of vasopressin; **guanethidine, neostigmine** increase vasopressor actions; **chlorpropamide, clofibrate, carbamazepine,** THIAZIDE DIURETICS may increase antidiuretic activity.

NURSING IMPLICATIONS

Administration

- Vasopressin tannate should never be administered IV. Before withdrawing drug for IM administration, warm ampul to body temperature and shake vigorously to disperse active principle.
- Intraarterial infusion constricts the splanchnic and peripheral vasculature and may cause gangrene in the peripheral entry vessel. Inspect infusion site and catheter at hourly intervals for blanching of skin. If noted, stop infusion stat and question physician about immediate local treatment (immediate flushing of catheter with a vasodilator has been prescribed). If vasopressin is to be continued, it should be administered via central venous catheter.
- The tannate injection is often painful, and allergic reactions may develop. It is preferred for use in chronic therapy because of its longer duration of action.
- Administration of 1 or 2 glasses of water with vasopressin tannate may reduce side effects and improve therapeutic response.
- Vasopressin aqueous injection may be given by continuous IV diluted with NS or D5W (0.1–1 U/ml) at a rate titrated to patient's response.
- *Vasopressin test* (rarely used) to determine functional ability of kidney to concentrate urine: give vasopressin 5–10 U IM; measure specific gravity 1 and 2 h later (results are equivalent to those resulting from 18 h of water deprivation). Normal response: urine osmolality 600 mmol/kg or greater; specific gravity greater than 1.020. In diabetes-insipidus-like syndromes, urine remains hypoosmotic relative to plasma.

Assessment & Drug Effects

- Infants and children are more susceptible to volume disturbances (such as sudden reversal of polyuria) than adults are. Monitor closely.
- At beginning of therapy, establish baseline data of BP, weight, I&O pattern and ratio. Monitor both BP and weight throughout therapy. Report sudden changes in pattern to physician.
- Be alert to the fact that even small doses of vasopressin may precipitate MI or coronary insufficiency, especially in elderly patients. Emergency equipment and drugs (antiarrhythmics) should be readily available.
- Dose used to stimulate diuresis has little effect on BP.
- Check patient's alertness and orientation frequently during therapy. Lethargy and confusion associated

Common side effects in *italic*; life-threatening effects <u>underlined</u>; generic names in **bold**; classifications in SMALL CAPS

with headache may signal onset of water intoxication, which, although insidious in rate of development, can lead to convulsions and terminal coma.

- If water intoxication (see Signs & Symptoms, chap 3) occurs, vasopressin is withdrawn and fluid intake is restricted until specific gravity is at least 1.015 and polyuria occurs. With severe overhydration, osmotic diuresis is effected by drug therapy (e.g., mannitol, alone or in conjunction with furosemide).
- Urine output, specific gravity and serum osmolality are monitored while patient is hospitalized.

Patient & Family Education
- Polyuria and thirst of diabetes insipidus are usually controlled for 36–48 h with a single dose of the tannate.
- Patient with vascular disease and diabetes insipidus may receive small doses of vasopressin. Patient should be prepared for possibility of anginal attack and should have available a coronary vasodilator (e.g., nitroglycerin). Such pain should be reported to the physician.
- At home, patient must measure and record data related to polydipsia and polyuria. Teach patient to determine specific gravity and how to keep an accurate record of output. Patient should understand that intense thirst should diminish with treatment and that undisturbed normal sleep should be restored.
- Patient should avoid hypertonic fluids (e.g., undiluted syrups), since these increase urine volume.

PROGESTIN

PROGESTERONE
(proe-jess´ter-one)
Trade names: Gesterol 50, Progestaject, Progestasert
Classifications: HORMONE; PROGESTIN
Pregnancy: Category X

ACTIONS/PHARMACODYNAMICS Steroid hormone synthesized and released by testes, ovary, adrenal cortex, and placenta. Has estrogenic, anabolic, and androgenic activity. Physiologic precursor to estrogens, androgens, and adrenocortical steroids. Transforms endometrium from proliferative to secretory state; suppresses pituitary gonadotropin secretion, thereby blocking follicular maturation and ovulation. Acting with estrogen, promotes mammary gland development without causing lactation and increases body temperature 1F at time of ovulation (thermogenic action). Stimulates endocervical secretion of glycogen and thick mucus. Relaxes estrogen-primed myometrium and prohibits spontaneous contraction of uterus. Sudden drop in blood levels of progestin (and estradiol) causes "withdrawal bleeding" from endometrium. Intrauterine placement of progesterone (intrauterine progesterone contraceptive system) hypothetically inhibits sperm capacitation or survival, alters uterine milieu so as to prevent nidation, and suppresses endometrial proliferation (antiestrogenic effect).

USES Secondary amenorrhea, functional uterine bleeding, endometriosis, and premenstrual syndrome. As an intrauterine agent (Progestasert) and in combination with estrogens provides fertility control. Largely supplanted by new progestins, which have longer action and oral effectiveness.

ROUTE & DOSAGE

Amenorrhea

Adult	IM	5–10 mg for 6–8 consecutive days

Uterine Bleeding

Adult	IM	5–10 mg/d for 6 d

Premenstrual Syndrome

Adult	PR	200–400 mg/d

Intrauterine Contraceptive

Adult	Intrauterine	Insert in uterus for 1 y

PHARMACOKINETICS Absorption: rapid absorption from IM site. **Metabolism:** extensively metabolized in liver. **Elimination:** half-life: 5 min; excreted primarily in urine; excreted in breast milk.

CONTRAINDICATIONS & PRECAUTIONS Contraindicated in: hypersensitivity to progestins, known or suspected breast or genital malignancy; use as a pregnancy test; thrombophlebitis, thromboembolic disorders; cerebral apoplexy (or its history), severely impaired liver function or disease, undiagnosed vaginal bleeding, missed abortion, use during first 4 mo of pregnancy (category X), nursing mother. Progestasert: pregnancy or suspicion of pregnancy. **Cautious use in:** anemia, diagnostic test for pregnancy; diabetes

Common side effects in *italic*; life-threatening effects <u>underlined</u>; generic names in **bold**; classifications in SMALL CAPS

241

mellitus, history of psychic depression; persons susceptible to acute intermittent porphyria or with conditions that may be aggravated by fluid retention (asthma, seizure disorders, cardiac or renal function, migraine); impaired liver function, previous ectopic pregnancy, presence or history of salpingitis, venereal disease, unresolved abnormal Pap smear, genital bleeding of unknown etiology, previous pelvic surgery.

ADVERSE/SIDE EFFECTS CNS: migraine headache, dizziness, lethargy, mental depression, somnolence, insomnia. **CV:** thromboembolic disorders, pulmonary embolism. **Eye:** change in vision, proptosis, diplopia, papilledema, retinal vascular lesions. **GI:** hepatic disease, cholestatic jaundice; *nausea,* vomiting, abdominal cramps. **GU:** gynecomastia, galactorrhea, vaginal candidiasis, chloasma, cervical erosion and changes in secretions, *breakthrough bleeding,* dysmenorrhea, amenorrhea, pruritus valvae. **Metabolic:** hyperglycemia, decreased libido, transient increase in sodium and chloride excretion, pyrexia. **Skin:** *acne,* pruritus, allergic rash, photosensitivity, urticaria, hirsutism, alopecia. **Other:** *edema, weight changes;* pain at injection site; fatigue.

DIAGNOSTIC TEST INTERFERENCES Progestins may decrease levels of *urinary pregnanediol,* and increase levels of *serum alkaline phosphatase, plasma amino acids, urinary nitrogen,* and *coagulation factors VII, VIII, IX* and *X.* They also decrease *glucose tolerance* (may cause false-positive *urine glucose* tests) and lower *HDL* (high density lipoprotein) levels.

NURSING IMPLICATIONS

Administration
- Immerse vial in warm water momentarily to redissolve crystals and to facilitate aspiration of drug into syringe.
- Inject deeply IM. Injection site may be irritated. Inspect used sites carefully and rotate areas systematically.
- Store drug at 15–30C (59–86F) unless otherwise specified by manufacturer. Protect from freezing and light.

Assessment & Drug Effects
- A physical examination with special reference to pelvic organs, breasts, hepatic function, and a Pap test should precede therapy with a progestin and should be performed q6–12mo while patient is taking the drug.
- Baseline data for comparative value about patient's

weight, I&O ratio, BP, and pulse should be recorded at onset of progestin therapy. Deviations should be reported promptly.
- Monitor weight. Report a steady gain to physician.
- Progestins can affect endocrine and hepatic function tests. An interval of up to 60 d following cessation of therapy may be necessary before laboratory results can be considered definitive.
- In susceptible patients, progestins reportedly may precipitate attack of **acute intermittent porphyria:** common manifestations include severe, colicky abdominal pain, vomiting, distension, diarrhea, constipation.

Patient & Family Education
- Caution patient to avoid exposure to UV light and prolonged periods of time in the sun. Photosensitivity severity is related to both time of exposure and dose. A phototoxic drug reaction usually looks like an exaggerated sunburn but may also produce acute eczematous or urticarial reactions. The reaction can occur within 5–18 h after exposure to sun and is maximal by 36–72 h.
- Advise use of a sunscreen lotion (SPF > 12) that contains para-amino-benzoic acid (PABA) on exposed skin surfaces whenever patient goes outdoors, even on dark days.
- Advise patient to inform physician promptly if any of the following occur: sudden severe headache or vomiting, dizziness or fainting, numbness in an arm or leg, pain in calves accompanied by swelling, warmth, and redness; acute chest pain or dyspnea.
- Caution patient to report promptly unexplained sudden or gradual, partial or complete loss of vision, ptosis, or diplopia. The progestin should be discontinued and appropriate diagnostic and therapeutic measure instituted.
- Instruct a diabetic user of progestin or progestin combination drug to monitor clinical signs of loss of diabetes control. If blood glucose tests become positive or if hypoglycemic symptoms occur, the physician should be consulted.
- Instruct patient to notify physician if she suspects pregnancy while receiving progestational therapy. She should be apprised of the potential risk to the fetus from exposure to progestin.

Intrauterine Progesterone Contraceptive System (Progestasert)
- During the first 2 mo of Progestasert use, another method of birth control (foam or condom) should be used.
- Advise patient to return to the physician within 3 mo after insertion of the system for evaluation of its placement and efficacy; thereafter unless untoward

symptoms present, an annual visit for evaluation and replacement should be expected.

- Spotting, cramping, and discomfort during first 3 mo can be relieved by nonnarcotic analgesics.
- Regular cyclic pattern of ovulation continues while Progestasert is in place.
- The menstrual period during Progestasert use is frequently heavier and longer than usual. If increased menstrual bleeding continues, however, patient should consult her physician.
- The Progestasert threads should be checked frequently during first few months and after menstruation (times when expulsion is most likely to occur). If patient cannot feel threads, she should go to physician for an examination and prescription for another method of birth control.
- Warn against pulling on threads for any reason. If the IUD is partially expelled, it should be removed; however, the user should not try to remove it herself nor allow her partner to attempt to do so.
- Instruct patient to consult with physician if a period is missed and pregnancy is suspected. The device should be removed during pregnancy.
- Fever, acute pelvic pain and tenderness, unusual bleeding, severe cramping are symptoms that indicate infection. Report to the physician for immediate treatment.
- To prevent pregnancy, the system must be replaced 1 y after insertion. Pelvic examination must be done. Pap smear, breast examination, Hct evaluation should be done.

THYROID AGENT: ANTITHYROID

PROPYLTHIOURACIL

(proe-pill-thye-oh-yoor´a-sill)
Trade names: Propyl-Thyracil, PTU
Classifications: SYNTHETIC HORMONE; ANTITHYROID AGENT
Pregnancy: Category D

ACTIONS/PHARMACODYNAMICS

Relatively nontoxic thioamide. Interferes with organification of iodine and blocks synthesis of thyroxine (T_4) and triiodothyronine (T_3). Does not interfere with release and utilization of stored thyroid; thus antithyroid action is delayed days and weeks until preformed T_3 and T_4 are degraded. Drug-induced hormone reduction results in compensatory release of thyrotropin (TSH), which causes marked hyperplasia and vascularization of thyroid gland. With good adherence to drug regimen, chemical euthyroidism can be achieved 6–12 wk after start of thioamide therapy.

USES Hyperthyroidism, iodine-induced thyrotoxicosis, and hyperthyroidism associated with thyroiditis; to establish euthyroidism prior to surgery or radioactive iodine treatment; palliative control of toxic nodular goiter.

ROUTE & DOSAGE

Hyperthyroidism

Adult	PO	300–450 mg/d divided q8h; may need 600–1200 mg/d initially
Child	PO	>10 y: 150–300 mg/d or 150 mg/m²/d
		6–10 y: 50–150 mg/d
		Neonates: 5–10 mg/kg/d

Thyrotoxic Crisis

Adult	PO	200 mg q4–6h until full control achieved

PHARMACOKINETICS Absorption: rapidly absorbed from GI tract. **Peak:** 1–1.5 h. **Distribution:** appears to concentrate in thyroid gland; crosses placenta; some distribution into breast milk. **Metabolism:** rapidly metabolized to inactive metabolites. **Elimination:** half-life: 1–2 h; 35% excreted in urine within 24 h.

CONTRAINDICATIONS & PRECAUTIONS Contraindicated in: last trimester of pregnancy (category D), nursing mothers, concurrent administration of sulfonamides or coal tar derivatives such as aminopyrine or antipyrine. **Cautious use in:** infection; concomitant administration of anticoagulants or other drugs known to cause agranulocytosis; bone marrow depression; impaired hepatic function.

ADVERSE/SIDE EFFECTS CNS: ototoxicity (rare), *paresthesias, headache, vertigo, drowsiness, neuritis.* **GI:** *nausea, vomiting, diarrhea, dyspepsia,* loss of taste, sialoadenitis, hepatitis. **Hematologic:** myelosuppression, lymphadenopathy, periarteritis, hypoprothrombinemia, thrombocytopenia, leukopenia, agranulocytosis. **Hypothyroidism** (goitrogenic): enlarged thyroid, reduced GI motility, periorbital edema, puffy hands and feet, bradycardia, cool and pale skin, worsening of ophthalmopathy, sleepiness, fatigue, mental depression, dizziness, vertigo, sensitivity to cold, paresthesias, nocturnal muscle cramps, changes in menstrual periods, unusual weight gain. **Skin:** *skin rash, urticaria, pruritus,* hyperpigmentation, lightening of hair color, abnormal hair loss. **Other:**

drug fever, lupuslike syndrome, arthralgia, myalgia, hypersensitivity vasculitis.

DIAGNOSTIC TEST INTERFERENCES Propylthiouracil may elevate *prothrombin time* and serum *alkaline phosphatase, AST, ALT* levels.

NURSING IMPLICATIONS

Administration
- Administer PTU at the same time each day with relation to meals. Food may alter drug response by changing absorption rate.
- If drug is being used to improve thyroid state before radioactive iodine (RAI) treatment, PTU should be discontinued 3 or 4 d before treatment to prevent interference with RAI uptake. PTU therapy may be resumed if necessary 3–5 d after the RAI administration.
- Store drug in light-resistant container at 15–30C (59–86F).

Assessment & Drug Effects
- About 10% of patients with hyperthyroidism have leukopenia <4000 cells/mm³ and relative granulopenia.
- Objective signs of clinical response to PTU (usually within 2 or 3 wk): significant weight gain, reduced pulse rate, reduced serum T_4.
- When thyroid gland is greatly enlarged, satisfactory euthyroid state may be delayed for several months.
- Long-term PTU therapy is usually monitored by follow-up examinations and hematologic studies q2–3mo. As soon as patient is euthyroid, thyroid hormone (especially T_3) may be added to regimen to prevent goitrogenic-induced hypothyroidism and to suppress TSH production.
- Be alert to signs of hypoprothrombinemia: ecchymoses, purpura, petechiae, unexplained bleeding. Warn ambulatory patients to report these signs promptly.
- Important diagnostic signs of excess dosage: contraction of a muscle bundle when pricked, mental depression, hard and nonpitting edema, and need for high thermostat setting and extra blankets in winter (cold intolerance).
- Urticaria may occur (3–7% of patients) during weeks 2 to 8 of treatment. Switching to another thioamide is usual if rash is severe.

Patient & Family Education
- Generally duration of therapy covers a period of 6 mo to several years, followed by remission in 25% of patients. Medication is then stopped in the hope that natural remission will occur.

- If surgery fails to render patient euthyroid, PTU treatment may be reinstituted.
- To prevent hypothyroidism in mother, thyroid may be given concomitantly with PTU throughout pregnancy and after delivery with little effect on fetus.
- Postpartum patients receiving PTU should not nurse their babies. Exacerbation of hyperthyroidism 3–4 mo postpartum in the mother is common; PTU therapy can be reinstituted.
- Advise patient to report severe skin rash or swelling of cervical lymph nodes. Therapy may be discontinued.
- Warn patient to report sore throat, fever, and rash immediately (most apt to occur in first few months of treatment). Drug will be discontinued and hematologic studies initiated. If agranulocytosis is diagnosed, patient may be given broad-spectrum antibiotics and placed on reverse isolation.
- Advise patients to avoid use of OTC drugs for asthma, coryza, or cough treatment without checking with the physician. Iodides sometimes included in such preparations are contraindicated.
- Teach patient how to take pulse accurately. Advise daily check.
- Clinical response is monitored through changes in weight and pulse. Advise patient to chart weight 2 or 3 times weekly. Continued tachycardia, diarrhea, fever, irritability, listlessness, vomiting, weakness, should be reported as signs of inadequate therapy or thyrotoxicosis.
- Instruct patient in remission to continue monitoring and recording weight and pulse rate. Patient should report onset of tremor, anxiety state, gradual ascending pulse rate, and loss of weight to the physician (signs of hormone deficiency).
- Urge patient not to alter drug regimen: not to increase, decrease, or omit doses nor change administration intervals.
- Check with physician about use of iodized salt and inclusion of seafood in the diet.

THYROID AGENT: THYROID

LEVOTHYROXINE SODIUM (T_4)
(lee-voe-thye-rox´een)
Trade names: Eltroxin, Levothroid, Noroxine, Synthroid, Synthrox, Syroxine
Classifications: SYNTHETIC HORMONE; THYROID
Pregnancy: Category A

ACTIONS/PHARMACODYNAMICS Synthetically prepared monosodium salt and levo isomer of thyroxine, with similar actions and uses: 0.1 mg is equivalent to 65 mg desiccated thyroid and is about 600 times more potent. Thyroxine, principal component of thyroid gland secretions, determines normal thyroid function. Drug action not clearly understood, but principal effect is increase in the metabolic rate of all body tissues.

USES Specific replacement therapy for diminished or absent thyroid function resulting from primary or secondary atrophy of gland, surgery, excessive radiation or antithyroid drugs, congenital defect. Administered orally for hypothyroid state; administered IV for myxedematous coma or other thyroid dysfunctions demanding rapid replacement, as well as in failure to respond to oral therapy.

ROUTE & DOSAGE

Thyroid Replacement

Adult	PO	25–50 µg/d, gradually increased by 50–100 µg q1–4wk to usual dose of 100–400 µg/d
	IV	1/2 of usual PO dose
Child	PO	0–6 mo: 8–10 µg/kg/d or 25–50 µg/d
		6–12 mo: 6–8 µg/kg/d or 50–75 µg/d
		1–5 y: 5–6 µg/kg/d or 75–100 µg/d
		6–12 y: 4–5 µg/kd/d or 100–150 µg/d
		>12 y: 2–3 µg/kg/d or >150 µg/d
	IV	1/2 of usual PO dose

Myxedema Coma

Adult	IV	250–500 µg IV stat; then 100–300 µg after 24 h if needed; then 50–200 µg/d until patient is stable and can take drug PO

PHARMACOKINETICS Absorption: variable and incompletely absorbed from GI tract (50–80%). **Peak:** 3–4 wk. **Duration:** 1–3 wk. **Distribution:** gradually released into tissue cells. **Elimination:** half-life: 6–7 d.

CONTRAINDICATIONS & PRECAUTIONS Contraindicated in: hypersensitivity to levothyroxine; thyrotoxicosis, severe cardiovascular conditions, adrenal insufficiency. Pregnancy (category A). **Cautious use in:** angina pectoris, hypertension, impaired renal function.

ADVERSE/SIDE EFFECTS CNS: irritability, nervousness, *insomnia,* headache (pseudotumor cerebri in children), tremors, craniosynostosis (excessive doses in children). **CV:** palpitations, tachycardia, arrhythmias, angina pectoris, hypertension. **GI:** nausea, diarrhea, change in appetite. **Other:** menstrual irregularities, weight loss, heat intolerance, sweating, fever, leg cramps, temporary hair loss (children).

DRUG INTERACTIONS Cholestyramine, colestipol decrease absorption of levothyroxine; **epinephrine, norepinephrine** increase risk of cardiac insufficiency; ORAL ANTICOAGULANTS may potentiate hypoprothrombinemia.

NURSING IMPLICATIONS

Administration

- Administered as single dose, preferably before breakfast, to prevent insomnia. Food interferes with absorption of levothyroxine.
- Maintenance dosage for the elderly may be 25% lower than for heavier and younger adults.
- There is great urgency in achieving full thyroid replacement in infants or children because of the critical importance of the hormone in sustaining growth and development; therefore doses are generally higher than adult doses.
- Parenteral preparation should be reconstituted with NaCl injection immediately before administration. Shake vial until solution is clear. Discard unused portion.
- IV solution prepared by adding supplied diluent (5 ml NS without preservatives) to 0.5 mg of powder. Resulting concentration is 0.1 mg/ml.
- IV solution is administered by direct IV at a rate of 0.1 mg or a fraction thereof over 1 min.
- *Transfer from levothyroxine to liothyronine:* discontinue levothyroxine before starting small dose of liothyronine. *Transfer from liothyronine to levothyroxine:* start levothyroxine; then, after several days, discontinue liothyronine.
- Store in tight, light-resistant container at 15–30C (59–86F).

Assessment & Drug Effects

- Assess for therapeutic effectiveness, which includes diuresis, loss of weight and puffiness, increased sense of well-being and activity tolerance, and rise of T_3 and T_4 serum levels toward normal.
- Pulse rate is an important index of drug effectiveness. During dose adjustment, count the pulse before each dose. If rate is > 100, consult physician.

Common side effects in *italic*; life-threatening effects <u>underlined</u>; generic names in **bold**; classifications in SMALL CAPS

245

- Monitor for adverse effects during early adjustment. If metabolism increases too rapidly, especially in elderly and heart disease patients, symptoms of angina or cardiac failure may appear.
- Levothyroxine may aggravate severity of previously obscured symptoms of diabetes mellitus, Addison's disease, or diabetes insipidus. Therapy for these disorders may require adjustment.
- Therapy with levothyroxine results in euthyroidism and a return to normal of laboratory values.
- Baseline and periodic tests of thyroid function and of bone age, growth, and psychomotor function in children are recommended.
- Some children have partial hair loss after a few months; it returns even with continued therapy.
- Closely monitor prothrombin time and assess for evidence of bleeding if patient is receiving concurrent anticoagulant therapy.
- A decrease in anticoagulant dosage may be needed 1–4 wk after concurrent levothyroxine is started.
- Note that Synthroid 0.1 and 0.3 mg tablets contain tartrazine, which may cause an allergic-type reaction in certain patients. It is frequently seen in persons who also have aspirin hypersensitivity.

Patient & Family Education
- Inform patient that thyroid replacement therapy is usually life long.
- When patient is euthyroid, teach him or her how to self-monitor pulse rate. Instruct patient to notify physician if rate begins to increase or if rhythm changes are noted.
- Instruct patient to immediately report signs of toxicity (e.g., chest pain, palpitations, nervousness).
- Tell patient that differences in bioequivalence exist among brands and to accept no change.
- Caution patient to avoid OTC medications unless approved by physician.

IMMUNOMODULATOR

INTERFERON ALFA-2A

(in-ter-feer´on)
Trade names: Roferon-A Injection
Classifications: IMMUNOMODULATOR; ANTINEO-PLASTIC; ANTIVIRAL; ORPHAN DRUG
Pregnancy: Category C

ACTIONS/PHARMACODYNAMICS Interferon (IFN) alfa-2A, one of 4 types of alpha interferon, is a highly purified protein and natural product of human leukocytes within 4–6 h after viral stimulation. Also produced by recombinant DNA technology (rIFN-A) from a genetically engineered strain of *Escherichia coli* (contains the gene for a human alpha interferon). Has a broad spectrum of antiviral, cytotoxic, and immunomodulating activity (i.e., favorably adjusts immune system to better combat foreign invasion of antigens and viruses). *Antiviral action:* reprograms virus-infected cells to inhibit various stages of virus replication. *Antitumor action:* suppresses cell proliferation. *Immunomodulating action:* enhances phagocytic activity of macrophages and augments specific cytotoxicity of lymphocytes for target cells. IFN is species specific but not virus specific; it partially inhibits viral replication and is immediately produced at site of viral entry by any cell; thus, the immune system and the interferon system of defense are complementary. Antibodies to human leukocyte interferon may occur spontaneously in patient who has never received exogenous interferon.

USES To induce hairy-cell leukemia remission in splenectomized and nonsplenectomized patients; treatment of hepatitis C. **Unlabeled use:** chronic hepatitis B virus infection, solid tumors, human papilloma virus (HPV)-associated diseases, malignant melanoma, AIDS-associated Kaposi's sarcoma. **Orphan drug:** Proposed use treatment of Kaposi's sarcoma in AIDS patients.

PHARMACOKINETICS Absorption: well absorbed after IM or SC injection. **Peak:** 15–60 min IV; 1–8 h IM. **Distribution:** widely distributed, concentrating in spleen, kidney, liver, and lung. **Metabolism:** metabolized principally in kidney. **Elimination:** half-life: 5.1 h.

CONTRAINDICATIONS & PRECAUTIONS Contraindicated in: hypersensitivity to alpha interferons or any component of product and to mouse immunoglobulin. Safe use during pregnancy (category C), by nursing mothers, or by children < 18 y not established. **Cautious use in:** cardiac disease or history of cardiac illness, severe cardiac, renal, or hepatic disease; seizure disorders, compromised CNS function; myelosuppression; chickenpox (existing or recent, including recent exposure), herpes zoster.

ADVERSE/SIDE EFFECTS *Flulike syndrome (fever, chills, myalgia, headache).* **CNS:** *fatigue,* dizzi-

ROUTE & DOSAGE

Hairy Cell Leukemia

Adult   SC/IM   3 million U/d for 16–24 wk; may be reduced to 3 times/wk for maintenance therapy

AIDS-related Kaposi's Sarcoma

Adult   SC/IM   36 million U/d for 10–12 wk; may then be reduced to 3 times/wk

Genital and Anal Warts

Adult   Intralesional   1 million U injected in each lesion 3 times/wk on alternate days for 3 wk

Chronic Viral Hepatitis

Adult   SC/IM   1–3 million U/d for 1 wk, then 3 times/wk for 1–6 mo

ness, weakness, confusion, paresthesias, leth-argy, psychosis, depression, nervousness, gait disturbances, psychomotor retardation, aphasia, forgetfulness, amnesia, sedation, sleep disturbances, anxiety, claustrophobia, loss of libido. **CV:** hypotension, edema, hypertension, pulmonary edema, arrhythmias, chest pain, MI, CHF, palpitations, syncope, hot flushes, Raynaud's phenomenon. **GI:** nausea, vomiting, diarrhea, anorexia with weight loss, abdominal fullness, hypermotility, stomatitis, xerostomia, change in taste, oropharyngeal candidiasis, excessive salivation. **Hematologic:** leukopenia, neutropenia, thrombocytopenia, coagulopathy, myelosuppression. **Skin:** rash, dry skin, pruritus, partial alopecia (eyelash growth increases), urticaria, reactivation of herpes labialis, diaphoresis. **Other:** dryness or inflammation of oropharynx, transient impotence, arthralgia, renal toxicity, proteinuria, mild to moderate hepatotoxicity, visual disturbances, conjunctivitis.

DIAGNOSTIC TEST INTERFERENCES Decreased Hgb, Hct; elevated fasting blood sugar, serum phosphorus, serum creatinine, AST, ALT, alkaline phosphatase, LDH; hypocalcemia.

NURSING IMPLICATIONS

Administration

- IFN should be administered under the guidance of a qualified physician.
- After reconstitution, solutions must be used within 30 d. Inspect solution for particulate matter and discoloration before administration.

- SC administration is recommended especially for patient who is at risk for bleeding (platelet count less than 50,000).
- IFN is best administered in the morning to permit daytime hours for accurate assessment of toxicity. Consistency in time of dose administration each day is important.
- Store sterile powder and its accompanying diluent, reconstituted solution, and injectable solution in refrigerator at 2–8C (36–46F). Do not freeze or shake solution.

Assessment & Drug Effects

- Establish baseline data before therapy begins: CBC, peripheral and bone marrow hairy cells; liver and renal function. Monitor monthly during treatment period.
- Monitor I&O ratio and pattern. Patient should be well hydrated during early stages of treatment. Encourage increased intake to at least 2500 ml if tolerated. Keep physician informed of patient's fluid intake.
- Be aware of potential side effects. If detected early, most are reversible.
- Flulike syndrome (fever, chills) occurs in most patients 2–6 h after a dose of IFN (may be controlled by acetaminophen). Anorexia may persist after such an episode. Symptoms tend to lessen with continued therapy.
- Monitor laboratory reports and be alert to **symptoms of coagulopathy:** ecchymoses, petechiae, unexplained bleeding. (Mean time to nadir: white blood count: 22 d; platelets: 17 d.)
- Monitor BP and vital signs. If there is a history of heart disease or if patient is in advanced stages of cancer, monitor cardiac function, especially if acute self-limiting toxicities (fever, chills) occur during IFN therapy. The elderly are particularly susceptible to cardiotoxicity.
- CNS adverse reactions are usually mild, although dose limiting; they are reversible within a few days to 3 wk after dose reduction or discontinuation. The neurologic side effect of gait difficulty becomes a greater hazard when accompanied by dizziness and hypotension. Protect patient from falling and supervise ambulation.
- Nausea and vomiting are usually controlled by an antiemetic.
- IFN myelosuppression supports delayed healing and increases potential for oral superinfection with Candida albicans. If stomatitis (sore mouth with ulceration), gingivitis, or white patches on oropharyngeal membrane surfaces are evidenced, alert physician.

- During blood nadir period, protect patient from infection. All caregivers should be conscientious about hand washing; visitors or caregivers with colds and anyone who has been recently vaccinated should not have contact with the patient.

Patient & Family Education

- The patient should be informed of the risks of severe and even fatal adverse reactions as well as the benefits from IFN therapy.
- Drug may be self-administered after therapy is well established and effectiveness of patient teaching has been evaluated. Read patient information sheet about IFN with patient before his or her discharge from agency.
- Fatigue, a common side effect, affects patient's activity. Rest periods should be provided for the child in school, and the teacher notified of this need. Advise adults to pace their activity so as to conserve energy expenditure; they may not be able to return to work.
- Careful periodic neuropsychiatric monitoring of patient is recommended. Urge patient on home therapy to keep scheduled evaluation visits.
- Urge prompt reporting if symptoms of infection develop (sore throat, fever, vomiting, diarrhea).
- If IFN is being given to a fertile, nonpregnant woman, she should be using effective contraception.
- Caution patient not to change brands of interferon alfa without first consulting the physician (because of risk of dosage change).

IMMUNOSUPPRESSANT

CYCLOSPORINE

(sye´kloe-spor-een)
Trade name: Sandimmune
Classification: IMMUNOSUPPRESSANT
Pregnancy: Category C

ACTIONS/PHARMACODYNAMICS Immunosuppressant agent derived from extract of a soil fungus. Action in reducing transplant rejection appears to be due to selective and reversible inhibition of helper T-lymphocytes (which normally stimulate antibody function). This creates an imbalance in favor of suppressor T-lymphocytes (which inhibit antibody production); thus immune response is subdued. Unlike other immunosuppressive agents, it does not cause clinically significant bone marrow suppression. Believed to have antimalarial and antischistosomal, as well as antifungal, activity.

USES In conjunction with adrenal corticosteroids to prevent organ rejection after kidney, liver, and heart transplants (allografts). Has had limited use in pancreas, bone marrow, and heart/lung transplantations. Also used for treatment of chronic transplant rejection in patients previously treated with other immunosuppressants. **Unlabeled use:** Sjögren's syndrome to prevent rejection of heart–lung and pancreatic transplants.

ROUTE & DOSAGE

Prevention of Organ Rejection

Adult	PO	14–18 mg/kg beginning 4–12 h before transplantation and continued for 1–2 wk after surgery; then gradual reduction by 5%/wk; *maintenance:* 5–10 mg/kg/d
	IV	5–6 mg/kg beginning 4–12 h before transplantation and continued after surgery until patient can take oral
Child	PO	Same as for adult
	IV	Same as for adult

PHARMACOKINETICS Absorption: variably and incompletely absorbed (30%). **Peak:** 3–4 h. **Distribution:** widely distributed; 33–47% distributed to plasma; 41–50% to RBCs; crosses placenta; distributed into breast milk. **Metabolism:** extensively metabolized in liver, including significant first pass metabolism; considerable enterohepatic circulation. **Elimination:** half-life: 19–27 h; primarily eliminated in bile and feces; 6% excreted in urine.

CONTRAINDICATIONS & PRECAUTIONS Contraindicated in: hypersensitivity to cyclosporine or to ingredients in commercially available formulations, e.g., Cremophor (polyoxyl 35 castor oil); recent contact with or bout of chickenpox, herpes zoster; administration of live virus vaccines, to patient or family members. Safe use during pregnancy (category C), in nursing women, and in children not established. **Cautious use in:** renal, hepatic, pancreatic, or bowel dysfunction; hyperkalemia; hypertension; infection; malabsorption problems (e.g., liver transplant patients).

ADVERSE/SIDE EFFECTS CNS: *tremor,* convulsions, headache, paresthesias, hyperesthesia, flush-

Common side effects in *italic*; life-threatening effects underlined; generic names in **bold**; classifications in SMALL CAPS

ing, night sweats, insomnia, visual hallucinations, confusion, anxiety, flat affect, depression, lethargy, weakness, paraparesis, ataxia, amnesia. **CV:** *hypertension,* MI (rare). **ENT:** sinusitis, tinnitus, hearing loss, sore throat. **GI:** gingival hyperplasia, diarrhea, *nausea, vomiting,* abdominal discomfort, anorexia, gastritis, constipation. **Hematologic:** leukopenia, anemia, thrombocytopenia, *hypermagnesemia, hyperkalemia,* hyperuricemia, *decreased serum bicarbonate,* hyperglycemia. **Renal:** urinary retention, frequency, nephrotoxicity (oliguria). **Skin:** *hirsutism,* acne, oily skin, flushing. **Other:** lymphoma, gynecomastia, chest pain, leg cramps, edema, fever, chills, weight loss.

DIAGNOSTIC TEST INTERFERENCES *Hyperlipidemia* and abnormalities in *electrophoresis* reported; believed to be due to polyoxyl 35 castor oil (Cremophor) in IV cyclosporine.

DRUG INTERACTIONS AMINOGLYCOSIDES, **danazol, diltiazem, doxycycline, erythromycin, ketoconazole, methylprednisolone, metoclopramide, nicardipine,** NSAIDS, **prednisolone, verapamil** may increase cyclosporine levels; **carbamazepine, isoniazid, octreotide, phenobarbital, phenytoin, rifampin** may decrease cyclosporine levels; **acyclovir,** AMINOGLYCOSIDES, **amphotericin B, cimetidine, erythromycin, ketoconazole, melphalan, ranitidine, cotrimoxazole, trimethoprim** may increase risk of nephrotoxicity; POTASSIUM-SPARING DIURETICS, ACE INHIBITORS **(captopril, enalapril)** may potentiate hyperkalemia.

NURSING IMPLICATIONS

Administration

- Before use, inspect concentrate for injection and diluted parenteral preparations for particulate matter and discoloration. Cyclosporine parenteral concentrate must be diluted immediately before administration: dilute each ml in 20–100 ml of 0.9% NaCl or 5% dextrose injection.
- Administer IV solution by slow infusion over approximately 2–6 h, as prescribed by physician. Rapid IV can result in nephrotoxicity.
- Store preferably at 15–30C (59–86F) in well-closed containers. Do not refrigerate. Protect ampuls from light. Once opened, PO solution should be dated and contents used within 2 mo.

Assessment & Drug Effects

- Patients receiving the drug parenterally should be observed continuously for at least 30 min after start of IV infusion and at frequent intervals thereafter to detect allergic or other adverse reactions.
- Hypersensitivity reactions have been associated with Cremophor emulsifying agent in the parenteral formulation but not with the PO solution, which does not contain this ingredient.
- Monitor I&O ratio and pattern. Nephrotoxicity has been reported in about one third of transplant patients. It has occurred in mild forms as late as 2–3 mo after transplantation. In severe form it can be irreversible, and therefore early recognition is critical.
- Report signs and symptoms suggestive of nephrotoxicity (see Signs & Symptoms, chap 3). Laboratory values respond to dosage reduction.
- Signs of rejection in patients with renal transplant can be almost indistinguishable from nephrotoxicity.
- **Indicators of graft rejection:** low blood or plasma cyclosporine concentrations occurring with rapid rise in serum creatinine, fever, graft tenderness or enlargement. Laboratory values do not respond to dosage reduction.
- Monitor vital signs. Be alert to indicators of local or systemic infection that can be fungal, viral, or bacterial. Also report significant rise in BP.
- Lymph glands and breasts should be gently palpated at periodic intervals (consult physician) to detect abnormalities. Patients who have received T-cell globulin appear to be particularly prone to complications.
- Periodic tests should be made of neurologic function. Neurotoxic effects generally occur over 13–195 days after initiation of cyclosporine therapy. Signs and symptoms are reportedly fully reversible with dosage reduction or discontinuation of drug.
- Baseline and periodic tests are advised for (1) renal function (BUN, serum creatinine), (2) liver function (AST, ALT, serum amylase, bilirubin, and alkaline phosphatase), and (3) serum potassium.
- Blood or plasma drug concentrations should be monitored at regular intervals, particularly in patients receiving the drug orally for prolonged periods, as drug absorption is erratic.

Patient & Family Education

- Use the specially calibrated pipette provided to measure dose.
- Medication may be taken with meals to reduce nausea or GI irritation.
- Palatability of oral solution may be enhanced by mixing it with milk, chocolate milk, or orange juice, preferably at room temperature. Mix in a glass rather than a plastic container. Stir well, drink im-

mediately, and rinse glass with small quantity of diluent to assure getting entire dose.

- Take medication at same time each day to maintain therapeutic blood levels.
- Keep scheduled follow-up appointments.
- If possible, patient should see a dentist before start of cyclosporine treatment. Advise patient to practice good oral hygiene. Inspect mouth daily for white patches, sores, swollen gums.
- Reassure patient that hirsutism is reversible with discontinuation of drug.

OXYTOCIC

OXYTOCIN INJECTION
(ox-i-toe´sin)
Trade names: Pitocin, Syntocinon, Syntocinon Nasal Spray
Classification: OXYTOCIC

ACTIONS/PHARMACODYNAMICS Synthetic, water-soluble polypeptide consisting of eight amino acids, identical pharmacologically to the oxytocic principle of posterior pituitary. Oxytocic activity: 10 USP posterior pituitary U/ml. By direct action on myofibrils, produces phasic contractions characteristic of normal delivery. Promotes milk ejection (letdown) reflex in nursing mother, thereby increasing flow (not volume) of milk; also facilitates flow of milk during period of breast engorgement. Uterine sensitivity to oxytocin increases during gestation period and peaks sharply before parturition. Exerts slight intrinsic ADH-like effect in large doses. Not used for elective induction of labor.

USES To initiate or improve uterine contraction at term only in carefully selected patients and only after cervix is dilated and presentation of fetus has occurred; used to stimulate letdown reflex in nursing mother and to relieve pain from breast engorgement. Uses include management of inevitable, incomplete, or missed abortion; stimulation of uterine contractions during third stage of labor; stimulation to overcome uterine inertia; control of postpartum hemorrhage and promotion of postpartum uterine involution. Also used to induce labor in cases of maternal diabetes, preeclampsia, eclampsia, and erythroblastosis fetalis.

ROUTE & DOSAGE

Antepartum

Adult	IV	Start at 1 mU/min; may increase by 1 mU/min q15min up to a max of 20 mU/min

Postpartum

Adult	IV	Infuse a total of 10 U at a rate of 20–40 mU/min after delivery

To Promote Milk Ejection

Adult	Nasal	1 spray or 1 drop in 1 or both nostrils 2–3 min before nursing or pumping

PHARMACOKINETICS Absorption: destroyed in GI tract. **Onset:** immediately IV; few minutes nasal. **Duration:** 1 h IV; 20 min nasal. **Distribution:** distributed throughout extracellular fluid; small amount may cross placenta. **Metabolism:** rapidly destroyed in liver and kidneys. **Elimination:** half-life: 3–5 min; small amounts excreted unchanged in urine.

CONTRAINDICATIONS & PRECAUTIONS
Contraindicated in: hypersensitivity to oxytocin, significant cephalopelvic disproportion, unfavorable fetal position or presentations that are undeliverable without conversion before delivery, obstetric emergencies in which benefit-to-risk ratio for mother or fetus favors surgical intervention, fetal distress in which delivery is not imminent, prematurity, placenta previa, prolonged use in severe toxemia or uterine inertia, hypertonic uterine patterns, previous surgery of uterus or cervix including cesarean section, conditions predisposing to thromboplastin or amniotic fluid embolism (dead fetus, abruptio placentae), grand multiparity, invasive cervical carcinoma, primipara > 35 y of age, past history of uterine sepsis or of traumatic delivery, intranasal route during labor, simultaneous administration of drug by two routes. **Cautious use in:** concomitant use with cyclopropane anesthesia or vasoconstrictive drugs.

ADVERSE/SIDE EFFECTS Fetus: bradycardia and
other arrhythmias, hypoxia, intracranial hemorrhage, trauma from too rapid propulsion through pelvis, neonatal jaundice, death. **Mother:** hypersensitivity leading to uterine hypertonicity, tetanic contractions, uterine rupture, anaphylactic reactions, postpartum hemorrhage, cardiac arrhythmias, pelvic hematoma, nausea, vomiting, hypertensive episodes, subarachnoid hemorrhage, increased blood flow, fatal afibrinogenemia, ADH effects leading to severe water in-

Common side effects in *italic*; life-threatening effects underlined; generic names in **bold**; classifications in SMALL CAPS

toxication and hyponatremia, hypotension, ECG changes, PVCs, anxiety, dyspnea, precordial pain, edema, cyanosis or redness of skin, <u>cardiovascular spasm and collapse</u>. *Citrate:* parabuccal irritation.

DRUG INTERACTIONS VASOCONSTRICTORS cause severe hypertension; **cyclopropane anesthesia** causes hypotension, maternal bradycardia, arrhythmias.

INCOMPATIBILITIES Solution/additive: **Fibrinolysin, warfarin.**

NURSING IMPLICATIONS

Administration

- Oxytocin administration should be supervised by persons having thorough knowledge of the drug and the skill to identify complications. A qualified physician should be immediately available to manage complications.
- Time of administration of oxytocin in relation to delivery of baby or placenta varies with physician's preference. The nurse should have a clear understanding of when drug is to be administered with respect to progress of labor. Infusion flow rates are established by physician. Accurate control of infusion is critical.
- Oxytocin should never be administered by more than one route at a time.
- When diluting oxytocin for IV infusion, rotate bottle gently to distribute medicine throughout solution.
- **Preparation of IV solution:** For inducing labor, add 10 U (1 ml) of oxytocin to 1 L of D5W or NS to give 10 mU/ml. For postpartum bleeding, add 10–40 U of oxytocin to 1 L of D5W or NS to give 10–40 mU/ml.
- Administer properly diluted IV solution by continuous infusion only. See recommended rates (mU/min) in route & dosage table.
- During delivery, IM oxytocin is most easily injected deep into deltoid muscle. Massage injection site to assist quick absorption.
- Unless otherwise directed by manufacturer, store oxytocin solution in refrigerator but do not freeze.

Assessment & Drug Effects

- Before instituting treatment, start flow charts to record maternal BP and other vital signs, I&O ratio, weight, strength, duration, and frequency of contractions, as well as fetal heart tone and rate.
- During infusion period, monitor fetal heart rate and maternal BP and pulse at least q15min; evaluate tonus of myometrium during and between contractions and record on flow chart. Report change in rate and rhythm immediately.
- If contractions are prolonged (occurring at less than 2 min intervals) and if monitor records contractions about 50 mm Hg or if contractions last 90 seconds or longer, stop infusion to prevent fetal anoxia, turn patient on her side, and notify physician. Stimulation will wane rapidly within 2–3 min. Oxygen administration may be necessary.
- If local or regional (caudal, spinal) anesthesia is being given to the patient receiving oxytocin, be alert to the possibility of hypertensive crisis: sudden intense occipital headache, palpitation, marked hypertension, stiff neck, nausea, vomiting, sweating, fever, photophobia, dilated pupils, bradycardia or tachycardia, constricting chest pain.
- Monitor I&O during labor. If patient is receiving drug by prolonged IV infusion, watch for symptoms of water intoxication (drowsiness, listlessness, headache, confusion, anuria, weight gain). Report changes in alertness and orientation and changes in I&O ratio, i.e., marked decrease in output with excessive intake.
- The fundus should be checked frequently during the first few postpartum hours and several times daily thereafter.
- Incidence of hypersensitivity or allergic reactions is higher when oxytocin is given by IM or IV injection rather than by IV infusion (diluted solution).

Patient & Family Education

- Inform patient of purpose and anticipated effect of oxytocin.
- Instruct patient to report sudden, severe headache immediately.

PROSTAGLANDIN

DINOPROSTONE (PGE$_2$, PROSTAGLANDIN E$_2$)
(dye-noe-prost´one)
Trade name: Prostin E$_2$
Classifications: PROSTAGLANDIN; OXYTOCIC

ACTIONS/PHARMACODYNAMICS Synthetically prepared member of the prostaglandin E$_2$ series that appears to act directly on myometrium and on gastrointestinal, bronchial, and vascular smooth mus-

Common side effects in *italic*; life-threatening effects <u>underlined</u>;
generic names in **bold**; classifications in SMALL CAPS

251

cle. Stimulation of gravid uterus in early weeks of gestation is more potent than that of oxytocin. Contractions are qualitatively similar to those that occur during term labor. Vaginal administration has the advantages of concentrated drug action on the target tissue and of being noninvasive. Dinoprostone can produce uterine contractions when given orally, intramuscularly, intravenously, or intraamniotically and extraamniotically, but use of these routes is investigational in the United States. Has high success rate when used as abortifacient before twentieth week and for stimulation of labor in cases of intrauterine fetal death. In addition to oxytocic action, dinoprostone enhances edema formation and pain-producing actions of bradykinin and other autocoids associated with the inflammatory process. May have teratogenic potential.

USES To terminate pregnancy from twelfth week through second trimester as calculated from first day of last regular menstrual period; to evacuate uterine content in management of missed abortion or intrauterine fetal death up to 28 wk gestational age, and to manage benign hydatidiform mole. **Unlabeled use:** cervical ripening prior to labor induction.

ROUTE & DOSAGE

Evacuation of Uterus

Adult	Intravaginal	Insert suppository high in vagina; repeat q2–5h until abortion occurs or membranes rupture; max total dose 240 mg

PHARMACOKINETICS Absorption: slowly absorbed from vagina. **Onset:** 10 min. **Duration:** 2–3 h. **Distribution:** widely distributed in body. **Metabolism:** rapidly metabolized in lungs, kidneys, spleen, and other tissues. **Elimination:** excreted mainly in urine; some excreted in feces.

CONTRAINDICATIONS & PRECAUTIONS

Contraindicated in: acute pelvic inflammatory disease, history of pelvic surgery, uterine fibroids, cervical stenosis, active cardiac, pulmonary, renal, or hepatic disease. **Cautious use in:** history of hypertension, hypotension, asthma, epilepsy, anemia, diabetes mellitus; jaundice, history of hepatic, renal, or cardiovascular disease; cervicitis, acute vaginitis, infected endocervical lesion.

ADVERSE/SIDE EFFECTS CNS: headache, tremor, tension. **CV:** transient hypotension, flushing, cardiac arrhythmias, myocardial infarction. **Eye:** eye pain, blurred vision. **GI:** *nausea, vomiting, diarrhea.* **Musculoskeletal:** paresthesias, backache, joint inflammation or pain, arthralgia, stiff neck, nocturnal leg cramps, muscle cramps or pain. **Reproductive:** vaginal pain, endometritis, vaginitis, vulvitis, vaginismus, breast tenderness, uterine rupture. **Respiratory:** dyspnea, cough, hiccups. **Other:** chills, *fever,* dehydration, diaphoresis, rash, skin discoloration, urine retention.

DRUG INTERACTIONS OXYTOCICS used with extreme caution.

NURSING IMPLICATIONS

Administration

- Dinoprostone is to be used only by trained personnel in hospital settings with intensive care and operating room facilities.
- Antiemetic and antidiarrheal medication may be prescribed before dinoprostone to minimize GI side effects.
- Patient should remain in supine position for 10 min after administration of dinoprostone suppository to prevent expulsion and enhance absorption.
- Failure to pass the placenta within 1 h after fetus is delivered may require use of an oxytocic or curettage.
- Store suppositories in freezer at temperature not exceeding –20C (–4F) unless otherwise specified by manufacturer.

Assessment & Drug Effects

- Although rupture of the membranes is not a contraindication to use of dinoprostone, be aware that profuse bleeding may result in expulsion of the suppository. Observe patient carefully, after insertion of the drug.
- Monitor uterine contractions and observe for and report excessive vaginal bleeding and cramping pain. Keep pad count. Save all clots and tissues for physician inspection and laboratory analysis.
- In most patients, abortion usually occurs within 30 h. (When used in conjunction with oxytocin, time may be shortened to 12–14 h.)
- Monitor vital signs. Fever is a physiologic response of the hypothalamus to use of dinoprostone and occurs within 15–45 min after insertion of suppository. Temperature returns to normal within 2–6 h after discontinuation of medication.
- Monitor and record vital signs for about 3 d after discontinuation of dinoprostone administration.

Common side effects in *italic;* life-threatening effects underlined; generic names in **bold**; classifications in SMALL CAPS

Chills, shivering, or fever greater than 2F (signs of retained placenta) above normal may signal onset of sepsis and should be reported.

- Dinoprostone-induced fever usually occurs 1–16 h following drug administration. It is self-limiting and defervesces after drug is stopped; lochia is not foul smelling and fundus is not tender.
- Observe patient closely during entire period of drug action: report wheezing, chest pain, dyspnea, and significant changes in BP and pulse to the physician.

Patient & Family Education

- Advise patient to continue taking her temperature (late afternoon) for a few days after discharge. Advise her to contact physician with onset of fever, bleeding, abdominal cramps, abnormal or foul-smelling vaginal discharge.
- Douches, tampons, intercourse, and tub baths should be avoided for at least 2 wk. Clarify with physician.
- In some women, ovulation may be established as early as 2 wk after abortion. Patient should be advised about appropriate contraception.
- If patient has had a joint disorder, dinoprostone may exacerbate pain and limitation because of its effect on the inflammatory process.

ANTIACNE (RETINOID)

ISOTRETINOIN (13-CIS-RETINOIC ACID)

(eye-soe-tret´i-noyn)
Trade name: Accutane
Classifications: SKIN & MUCOUS MEMBRANE AGENT; ANTIACNE; RETINOID
Pregnancy: Category X

ACTIONS/PHARMACODYNAMICS Highly toxic metabolite of retinol (vitamin A). Principal actions: regulation of cell (e.g., epithelial) differentiation and proliferation and of altered lipid composition on skin surface. Decreases sebum secretion by reducing sebaceous gland size; inhibits gland cell differentiation; blocks follicular keratinization. Composition of liquid sebum is changed during treatment but is restored to pretreatment composition at end of therapy. Prolonged clinical remissions in many patients may be secondary to additional action mechanisms: antiinflammatory, antibacterial, antineoplastic. Shares with other retinoids immunoadjuvant activity, which leads to increased production and cytotoxic effects of lymphocytes. Female patients with severe facial acne seem to respond to treatment better than males, especially if the latter have trunk acne. Reportedly teratogenic.

USES Treatment of severe recalcitrant cystic or conglobate acne in patient unresponsive to conventional treatment, including systemic antibiotics. **Unlabeled uses:** lamellar ichthyosis, oral leukoplakia, hyperkeratosis, acne rosacea, scarring gram-negative folliculitis; adjuvant therapy of basal cell carcinoma of lung and cutaneous T-cell lymphoma (mycosis fungoides); and psoriasis.

ROUTE & DOSAGE

Cystic Acne

Adult	PO	0.5–1mg/kg/d in 2 divided doses; max recommended dose 2 mg/kg/d

Disorders of Keratinization

Adult	PO	up to 4 mg/kg/d in divided doses

PHARMACOKINETICS Absorption: rapid absorption after slow dissolution in GI tract; 25% of administered drug reaches systemic circulation. **Peak:** 3.2 h. **Distribution:** not fully understood; appears in liver, ureters, adrenals, ovaries and lacrimal glands. **Metabolism:** metabolized in liver; enterohepatically cycled. **Elimination:** half-life: 10–20 h; excreted in urine and feces in equal amounts.

CONTRAINDICATIONS & PRECAUTIONS Contraindicated in: pregnancy (category X); sensitivity to parabens (preservatives in the formulation), nursing mothers. **Cautious use in:** coronary artery disease; diabetes mellitus; obesity; alcoholism; rheumatologic disorders; history of pancreatitis, hepatitis; retinal disease; elevated triglycerides.

ADVERSE/SIDE EFFECTS Most are dose-related, i.e., occurring at doses >1 mg/kg/d; reversible with termination of therapy. **CNS:** lethargy, headache, insomnia, fatigue, paresthesias, dizziness, visual disturbances, pseudotumor cerebri. **Eye:** reduced night vision, dry eyes, papilledema, eye irritation, *conjunctivitis*, corneal opacities. **GI:** dry mouth,

Common side effects in *italic*; life-threatening effects underlined; generic names in **bold**; classifications in SMALL CAPS

253

anorexia, nausea, vomiting, abdominal pain, nonspecific GI symptoms, acute hepatotoxic reactions, inflammatory bowel disease including regional ileitis, mild GI bleeding, weight loss, inflammation and bleeding of gums. **GU:** WBC in urine, proteinuria, hematuria, abnormal menses. **Hematologic:** (casual relationship not established): leukopenia, elevated platelet count, decreased RBCs, elevated sedimentation rate. **Musculoskeletal:** arthralgia; acute arthritis, bone, joint, and muscle pain and stiffness; chest pain, skeletal hyperostosis (especially in athletic people and with prolonged therapy). **Skin:** *cheilitis*, skin fragility, dry skin, pruritus, peeling of face, palms, and soles; photosensitivity (photoallergic and phototoxic), erythema, skin infections, petechiae, nail brittleness, rash, thinning of hair, erythema nodosum; hypopigmentation or hyperpigmentation (rare); urticaria, exaggerated healing response (painful exuberant granulation tissue with crusting). **Other:** epistaxis, *dry nose*, mild bleeding and bruising, disseminated herpes simplex, edema, respiratory infections; acute pancreatitis; hyperglycemia, increased AST, ALT; hyperuricemia, *increased serum concentrations of triglycerides by 50–70%*, serum cholesterol by 15–20%, VLDL cholesterol by 50–60%, LDL cholesterol by 15–20%.

DRUG INTERACTIONS VITAMIN A SUPPLEMENTS increase toxicity.

NURSING IMPLICATIONS

Administration
- Take isotretinoin with or shortly after meals.
- Patients who have acne principally on chest and back and patients who weigh more than 70 kg may need a dose at higher end of dose range.
- Formerly used topical antiacne medication should be discontinued before isotretinoin therapy is begun.
- After 2 wk of treatment, regimen is reassessed and dose adjusted as warranted.
- A single course of therapy provides adequate control in many patients. If a second course is necessary, it is delayed at least 8 wk because improvement may continue without the drug.
- Isotretinoin is photosensitive. Store in tight, light-resistant container at 15–30C (59–86F). Capsules remain stable for 2 y.

Assessment & Drug Effects
- Baseline control values for blood lipids should be determined at outset of treatment with isotre-tinoin,

then at 2 wk, 1 mo, and every month thereafter throughout course of therapy. If patient has consumed alcohol, test should be delayed for 36 h (alcohol increases serum triglyceride).
- Liver function tests are performed at 2- or 3-wk intervals for 6 mo and then once a month thereafter during treatment. Signs of liver dysfunction (jaundice, pruritus, dark urine) should be reported promptly.
- Blood glucose should be closely monitored in diabetic and diabetic-prone patients.
- Persistence of hypertriglyceridemia (levels above 500–800 mg/dl) despite a reduced dose indicates necessity to stop drug to prevent onset of acute pancreatitis.
- Monitor serum lipid levels; advise an appropriate diet (low cholesterol, low saturated fat, increased polyunsaturated fat).
- During the first few weeks, transient exacerbations of acne may occur. Urge patient to maintain drug regimen, however, since recurring symptoms may signify response of deep unseen lesions to the drug.
- If visual disturbances occur along with nausea, vomiting, and headache, instruct to discontinue the medication at once and report to the physician to rule out benign intracranial hypertension. Patient should be screened for papilledema. If papilledema is present, isotretinoin should be discontinued.
- Visual disturbances may also signify development of corneal opacities, which should be ruled out by ophthalmic examination. If corneal opacities are present, drug will be discontinued. Urge patient to return for a follow-up examination in 6 wk; usually the opacities have resolved during that period.

Patient & Family Education
- Be certain that the patient fully understands that serious fetal abnormalities can be produced by this drug if it is continued through pregnancy.
- Pregnancy should be ruled out by pregnancy test within 2 wk of starting treatment. Patient should use a reliable contraceptive at least 1 mo before and throughout treatment and for 1 mo after therapy has been discontinued.
- Patients should be advised not to donate blood for transfusions for at least 30 days after isotretinoin is discontinued.
- Weight reduction and restriction of alcohol and dietary fat intake are prophylactic against development of hypertriglyceridemia.
- Advise not to self-medicate with multivitamins,

which usually contain vitamin A. Toxicity of isotretinoin is enhanced by vitamin A supplements.

- Protect face from extremes in weather (e.g., wind, cold) to decrease compounding of drug-induced dry skin and mucous membranes.
- Warn to avoid or minimize exposure of the treated skin to sun or sunlamps. Photosensitivity (photoallergic and phototoxic) potential is high. The risk of skin cancer may be increased by this drug.
- Sun screens provide protection against ultraviolet radiation; advise to use a sunscreen (SPF 15 or more) and to wear protective clothing when outdoors.
- Report abdominal pain, rectal bleeding, or severe diarrhea, possible symptoms of drug-induced inflammatory bowel disease. Drug treatment will be discontinued.
- Dry mouth and cheilitis (inflamed, chapped lips), frequent side effects of isotretinoin, are distressing and are potential preconditions conducive to infections. Urge patient to keep lips moist and softened (use thin layer of lubricant such as petroleum jelly) and to rinse mouth with water as necessary for comfort. Commercial rinses should be avoided because of alcohol or other mucosal irritant components.
- Advise to report joint pain, such as pain in the great toe (symptom of gout and hyperuricemia).
- Caution not to share drug with friend because it is associated with side effects that necessitate medical supervision.

ANTIINFLAMMATORY

HYDROCORTISONE (CORTISOL)

(hye-droe-kor´ti-sone)

Trade names: Aeroseb-HC, Cetacort, Cortaid, Cort-Dome, Cortof, Cortenema, Cortril, DermaCort, Dermolate, Hydrocortone, Hytone, Proctocort, Synacort

HYDROCORTISONE ACETATE

Trade names: Biosone, CaldeCort, Carmol HC, Colifoam, Cortaid, Cortamed, Cort-Dome, Cortef Acetate, Cortifoam, Epifoam, Hydrocortone Acetate

HYDROCORTISONE CYPIONATE

Trade name: Cortef Fluid

HYDROCORTISONE SODIUM PHOSPHATE

Trade names: Efcortesol, Hydrocortone Phosphate

HYDROCORTISONE SODIUM SUCCINATE

Trade names: A-hydroCort, Solu-Cortef

HYROCORTISONE VALERATE

Trade name: Westcort

Classifications: SKIN & MUCOUS MEMBRANE AGENT; ANTIINFLAMMATORY; ANTIACNE; SYNTHETIC HORMONE; ADRENAL CORTICOSTEROID; GLUCOCORTICOID; MINERALOCORTICOID; IMMUNOSUPPRESSANT

Pregnancy: Category C

ACTIONS/PHARMACODYNAMICS Short-acting synthetic steroid with both glucocorticoid and mineralocorticoid properties that affect nearly all systems of the body. Action mechanism: crosses cell membrane and complexes with specific cytoplasmic receptors. These induce DNA transcribed synthesis of specific enzymes responsible for systemic effects of corticosteroids. **Antiinflammatory (glucocorticoid) action:** stabilizes leukocyte lysosomal membranes; inhibits phagocytosis and release of allergic substances (e.g.,

Common side effects in *italic*; life-threatening effects <u>underlined</u>; generic names in **bold**; classifications in SMALL CAPS

255

bradykinin, histamine); suppresses fibroblast formation and collagen deposition (which prevents wound healing); reduces capillary dilation and permeability; and increases responsiveness of cardiovascular system to circulating catecholamines. **Immunosuppressive action:** modifies immune response to various stimuli; reduces antibody titers; and suppresses cell-mediated hypersensitivity reactions. **Mineralocorticoid action:** promotes sodium retention, but under certain circumstances (e.g., sodium loading), enhances sodium excretion; promotes potassium excretion; and increases glomerular filtration rate (GFR). **Metabolic action:** promotes hepatic gluconeogenesis, protein catabolism, redistribution of body fat, and lipolysis. Interrupts or retards normal linear growth in children. Prolonged therapy may result in suppressed functions of the hypothalamic-pituitary-adrenal (HPA) axis.

USES Replacement therapy in adrenocortical insufficiency; to reduce serum calcium in hypercalcemia, to suppress undesirable inflammatory or immune responses, to produce temporary remission in nonadrenal disease, and to block ACTH production in diagnostic tests. Use as antiinflammatory or immunosuppressive agent largely replaced by synthetic glucocorticoids that have minimal mineralocorticoid activity.

ROUTE & DOSAGE

Adrenal Insufficiency, Antiinflammatory

Adult	PO	10–320 mg/d in 3–4 divided doses
	IM/IV	15–800 mg/d in 3–4 divided doses up to 2 g/d
Child	PO	0.56–8 mg/kg/d in 3–4 divided doses
	IM/IV	0.16–1 mg/kg 1–2 times/d

Intraarticular, Intralesional (Acetate Salt)

Adult	IM	5–50 mg q3–5d for bursae; once q1–4wk for joints

Antiinflammatory Agent

Adult	Topical	Apply a small amount to the affected area 1–4 times/d
	PR	Insert 1% cream, 10% foam, 10–25 mg suppository, or 100 mg enema nightly

PHARMACOKINETICS Absorption: readily absorbed from GI tract and IM injection site. **Onset:** 1–2 h PO; immediately IV; 3–5 d PR. **Peak:** 1 h PO; 4–8 h IM. **Duration:** 1–1.5 d PO/IM; 0.5–4 wk intraarticular. **Distribution:** distributed primarily to muscles, liver, skin, intestines, kidneys; crosses placenta. **Metabolism:** hepatically metabolized. **Elimination:** half-life: 1.5–2 h; HPA suppression 8–12 h; metabolites excreted in urine; excreted in breast milk.

CONTRAINDICATIONS & PRECAUTIONS

Contraindicated in: hypersensitivity to glucocorticoids, idiopathic thrombocytopenic purpura, psychoses, acute glomerulonephritis, viral or bacterial diseases of skin, infections not controlled by antibiotics, active or latent amebiasis, hypercorticism (Cushing's syndrome), smallpox vaccination or other immunologic procedures. (Topical steroids contraindicated in presence of varicella, vaccinia, on surfaces with compromised circulation, and in children <2 y). Safe use in nursing mothers, during pregnancy (category C) not established. **Cautious use in:** children, diabetes mellitus; chronic, active hepatitis positive for hepatitis B surface antigen; hyperlipidemia; cirrhosis; stromal herpes simplex; glaucoma, tuberculosis of eye; osteoporosis; convulsive disorders; hypothyroidism; diverticulitis, nonspecific ulcerative colitis, fresh intestinal anastomoses, active or latent peptic ulcer, gastritis, esophagitis; thromboembolic disorders; CHF, metastatic carcinoma; hypertension, renal insufficiency; history of allergies; active or arrested tuberculosis; systemic fungal infection; myasthenia gravis.

ADVERSE/SIDE EFFECTS Dose and treatment-duration dependent. **CNS:** vertigo, headache, nystagmus, ataxia (rare), increased intracranial pressure with papilledema (usually after discontinuation of medication), mental disturbances, aggravation of pre-existing psychiatric conditions, insomnia. **CV:** syncopal episodes, thrombophlebitis, thromboembolism or fat embolism, palpitation, tachycardia, necrotizing angiitis. **Endocrine:** suppressed linear growth in children, decreased glucose tolerance; hyperglycemia, manifestations of latent diabetes mellitus; hypocorticism; amenorrhea and other menstrual difficulties. **Eye:** posterior subcapsular cataracts (especially in children), glaucoma, exophthalmos, increased intraocular pressure with optic nerve damage, perforation of the globe, fungal infection of the cornea, decreased or blurred vision. **Fluid and electrolyte disturbances:** hypocalcemia; *sodium and fluid retention;* hypokalemia and hypokalemic alkalosis; CHF, hypertension. **GI:** *nausea,* increased appetite, ulcerative esophagitis, pancreatitis, abdominal distension, peptic ulcer with perforation and hemorrhage, melena. **Hematologic:** thrombocytopenia. **Musculoskeletal (long-term use):** osteoporosis, compression fractures, muscle wasting and weakness, tendon rupture, aseptic necrosis of femoral and humeral heads. **Skin:** skin thinning and atrophy, *acne, impaired wound healing;* petechiae, ecchymosis, easy bruisings; suppression of skin test reaction; hypopigmentation or hyperpigmentation, hirsutism, acneiform eruptions, subcutaneous fat atrophy; allergic dermatitis, urticaria, angioneurotic edema, increased sweating. **Other:** negative nitrogen balance, anaphylactoid or hypersensitivity reactions; aggravation or masking of infections; malaise, hiccups, hoarseness, dry mouth, sore throat (with inhalation therapy), weight gain, obesity; increased or decreased motility and number of sperm, decreased serum concentration of vitamins A and C; urinary frequency and urgency, enuresis. **Overdose:** anxiety, mental confusion, depression, hyperglycemia, hypokalemia, hypernatremia, polycythemia, hypertension, edema, GI cramping or bleeding, ecchymoses, "moon" facies. **With parenteral therapy: IV site:** pain, irritation, necrosis, atrophy, sterile abscess; Charcot-like arthropathy following intraarticular use; burning and tingling in perineal area (after IV injection).

DIAGNOSTIC TEST INTERFERENCES Hydrocortisone (corticosteroids) may increase serum *cholesterol, blood glucose,* serum *sodium, uric acid* (in acute leukemia) and *calcium* (in bone metastasis). It may decrease serum *calcium, potassium, PBI, thyroxin (T₄), triiodothyronine (T₃)* and reduce *thyroid I 131* uptake. It increases *urine glucose* level and *calcium* excretion; decreases *urine 17-OHCS* and *17-KS* levels. May produce false-negative results with nitroblue tetrazolium test for systemic bacterial infection and may suppress reactions to skin tests.

DRUG INTERACTIONS BARBITURATES, **phenytoin, rifampin** may increase hepatic metabolism, thus decreasing cortisone levels; ESTROGENS potentiate the effects of hydrocortisone; NSAIDs compound ulcerogenic effects; **cholestyramine, colistipol** decrease hydrocortisone absorption; DIURETICS, **amphotericin B** exacerbate hypokalemia; ANTICHOLINESTERASE AGENTS (e.g., **neostigmine**) may produce severe weakness; immune response to VACCINES and TOXOIDS may be decreased.

INCOMPATIBILITIES Solution/Additive: amobarbital, ampicillin, bleomycin, colistimethate, dimenhydrinate, doxapram, doxorubicin, ephedrine, heparin, hydralazine, metaraminol, methicillin, nafcillin, pentobarbital, phenobarbital, prochlorperazine, promethazine, secobarbital, TETRACYCLINES. **Y-site: ergotamine, phenytoin.**

NURSING IMPLICATIONS

Administration

- Oral drug may be taken at mealtimes or with a (low-salt) snack to reduce gastric irritation.
- Counsel patient to take drug as prescribed and not to alter dosing regimen or stop medication without consulting physician.
- Inject IM preparation deep into upper outer quadrant of buttock to avoid local atrophy. Avoid using deltoid muscle. Rotate injection site.
- Avoid SC injection; may produce sterile abscess or pseudoatrophy with persistent depression of overlying dermis lasting several weeks or months.
- *IV injection:* IV hydrocortisone may be given by direct IV undiluted or diluted in NS or D5W. Administer at a rate of 25 mg or a fraction thereof over 1 min.
- Solutions that have been diluted for IV infusion should be administered within 24h of dilution.
- Cortisol plasma levels are maximal between 2 and 8 AM and minimal between 4 PM and midnight (*normal:* 7–28 g/dl in AM and below 10 g/dl at 8 PM). Exogenous corticosteroids suppress adrenal cortex activity less when given in the morning. To minimize HPA axis suppression, replacement steroid should be given before 9 AM.
- The retention enema preparation Cortenema produces the same systemic effects as other formulations of hydrocortisone. Administer preferably after a bowel movement. Advise patient to lie on left side at least 30 min, but if given at bedtime, the enema should be retained at least 1 h or all night if possible. This route is usually used for 21 d, then withdrawn gradually if intestinal symptoms do not abate. Report rectal infection or irritation.

Occlusive Dressing

- A light film of the topical preparation should be massaged into affected area gently and thoroughly until it disappears. If an occlusive dressing is to be used, apply medication sparingly, rub until it disappears, and then reapply, leaving a thin coat over lesion. Completely cover area with transparent plastic or other occlusive device or vehicle. Consult physician about frequency of dressing change.
- Occlusive vehicles or transparent plastic enhance absorption. Avoid covering a weeping or exudative lesion.
- Rates of penetration of topical corticosteroid differ in various anatomic sites: thus comparatively small doses are used on face, scalp, scrotum, axilia, and groin. Usually occlusive dressings are not applied to these areas.
- An occlusive dressing increases percutaneous penetration as much as 10%. Discomfort and warmth

---

may be troublesome. Inspect skin carefully between applications for ecchymotic, petechial, and purpuric signs, maceration, secondary infection, skin atrophy, striae or miliaria; if present, stop medication and notify physician.

- Store medication at 15–30C (59–86F) unless otherwise directed by manufacturer. Protect drug from light and freezing.

Assessment & Drug Effects

- Establish baseline and continuing data regarding BP and I&O ratio and pattern, weight, and sleep pattern.
- Check and record BP during dose stabilization period at least 2 times daily. Report an ascending pattern.
- During long-term therapy, patient should be monitored for evidence of HPA axis suppression by determining plasma cortisol levels at weekly intervals.
- Two-hour postprandial blood glucose, serum potassium, chest x-ray, and routine laboratory studies are performed at regular intervals during long-term steroid therapy.
- The elderly and the patient with low serum albumin are especially susceptible to adverse or side effects because of excess circulating free glucocorticoids.
- If patient has a history of diabetes mellitus, urine should be tested for glycosuria daily. Report positive findings.
- Be alert to signs of hypocalcemia (see Chapter 3). Patients with hypocalcemia have increased requirements for pyridoxine (vitamin B_6), vitamins C and D, and folates.
- Ophthalmoscopic examinations including tonometry are recommended every 2–3 mo, especially if patient is receiving ophthalmic steroid therapy.
- Compression and spontaneous fractures of long bones and vertebrae present hazards, particularly in long-term corticosteroid treatment of rheumatoid arthritis or diabetes, in immobilized patients, and in the elderly. Supervise getting out of bed or chair. Report persistent backache or chest pain (possible symptoms of vertebral or rib fracture). Patient's mattress should be firm or supported by a bedboard.
- Be aware of previous history of psychotic tendencies. Watch for changes in mood and behavior, emotional instability, sleep pattern, or psychomotor activity, especially with long-term therapy, that may signal onset of recurrence. Report symptoms to physician.
- Be alert to possibility of masked infection and delayed healing (antiinflammatory and immunosuppressive actions). Hydrocortisone suppresses early classic signs of inflammation: capillary dilation (heat, redness), phagocytosis (pus formation), swelling (pain), fibrin deposition (clot formation).

- If a patient is receiving aspirin concomitantly with a corticosteroid, salicylism may be induced when the corticosteroid dosage is decreased or discontinued.
- Dose adjustment may be required if patient is subjected to severe stress (serious infection, surgery, or injury) or if a remission or disease exacerbation occurs.
- Single doses of corticosteroids or use for a short period (<1 wk) do not produce withdrawal symptoms when discontinued, even with moderately large doses. Precautions should be taken, however, when a patient is transferred from systemic to PO or nasal inhalation therapy and when long-term therapy is being discontinued.
- Abrupt discontinuation of corticosteroids after long-term therapy may result in **withdrawal syndrome** (myalgia, fever, arthralgia, malaise) and **hypocorticism** (anorexia, vomiting, nausea, fatigue, dizziness, hypotension, hypoglycemia, myalgia, arthralgia).

Patient & Family Education

- Inform patient taht a slight weight hgain with improved appetite is expected, but after dosage is stabilized, a sudden slow but steady weight increase (2 kg [5 lb]/wk) should be reported.
- Encourage patient to avoid alcohol and caffeine, which may contribut to steroid-ulcer development in long-term therapy.
- Dyspepsia with hyperacidity should not be ignored. Encourage patient to report symptoms to physician and not to self-medicate to find relief.
- Warn patient not to use aspirin or other OTC drugs unless prescribed specifically by the physician.
- With hydrocortisone treatment, abosorption of calcium and vitamin D is decreased and protein catabolism is promoted. A high protein, calcium, and vitamin D diet may be prescribed to reduce risk of corticosteroid-induced osteoporosis.
- Warn patient to report slow healing, any vague feeling of being sick, or return to pretreatment symptoms.
- Exaggerated sense of well-being and analgesic effects (painless joints) may encourage patient to increase physical activity even if acute disease process still exists. Discuss with physician and work with patient and family to plan reasonable and safe range of ADL.

- When corticosteroid is given for rheumatoid arthritis, complete relief is not sought because of the hazards of continuous treatment. A regimen of rest, physical therapy, and salicylates continues during steroid therapy.
- Instruct patient to report promptly if initial therapeutic response is followed by relapse. Contact sensitivity of sensitivity to corticosteroid impurities may develop. The medication will be changed in kind or dose.
- To prevent withdrawal symptoms, advise patient not to abruptly discontinue drug: doses are gradually reduced.
- If during withdrawal the disease flares up, a dosage increase followed by a more gradual withdrawal may be necessary. Advise patient to report exacerbation of disease during drug withdrawal.
- Patient or family should be advised to tell a dentist or new physician about recently prolonged corticosteroid treatment.
- Advise patient receiving corticosteroid to carry a medical identification card or jewelery with recorded diagnosis, drug therapy, and name of physician.

Topical Applications (Hydrocortisone and Its Esters)

- Warn patient not to self-dose with OTC topical preparations of a corticosteroid more than / d. They should not be used for children <2 y. If symptoms do not abate, consult physician.
- Usually topical preparations are applied to hydrated skin, i.e., after a shower or bath when skin is damp or wet. Cleansing and application of prescribed preparation should be done with extreme gentleness because of fragility, easy bruisability and poor healing skin.
- Hazard of systemic toxicity is higher in small children because of the greater ratio of skin surface area to body weight. Apply sparingly. Although adrenal suppression from topical therapy infrequently occurs, whole-body applications of potent corticosteroid, occlusion, and stress may present a hazard. Replacement therapy before surgery may be given to prevent adrenal crisis.
- Urge patient on long-term therapy with topical corticosterone to check shelf-life date.
- Since absorption of corticosteroid through abraded skin is greater than through normal skin, a healed area can simulate sudden withdrawal of medication by causing withdrawal symptoms with continued application.

ANTIPSORIATIC

ANTHRALIN
(an'thra-lin)
Trade names: Anthra-Derm, Anthraforte, Anthranol, Dithranol, Drithocreme, Dritho-Scalp, Lasan
Classifications: SKIN AGENT; ANTIPSORIATIC
Pregnancy: Category C

ACTIONS/PHARMACODYNAMICS Inhibits nucleic protein synthesis, which decreases rate of mitosis and proliferation of epidermal cells in psoriasis. Time required for epidermal cell to migrate from basal layer of epidermis to surface and be cast off in psoriasis is 3–4 d as compared to 26–28 d for normal skin.

USES Topical treatment of quiescent or chronic plaque psoriasis. **Unlabeled use:** topical treatment of alopecia areata.

ROUTE & DOSAGE

Psoriasis

Adult	Topical	Apply sparingly to affected areas 1–2 times/d

PHARMACOKINETICS **Absorption:** low absorption through intact skin.

CONTRAINDICATIONS & PRECAUTIONS **Contraindicated in:** applications to acute psoriasis eruptions or where inflammation is present, pregnancy (category C), nursing mothers, and children. Do not apply to genitalia, face, or intertriginous and flexural areas. **Cautious use in:** erythema, renal disease.

ADVERSE/SIDE EFFECTS Sensitivity reactions, erythema of adjacent normal skin, possible renal irritation, folliculitis, temporary discoloration of gray or white hair, fingernails, and skin; increased sedimentation rate; hyperuricemia.

NURSING IMPLICATIONS

Administration
- Make a preliminary test for sensitivity on a small area of skin. Red-haired and other fair-skinned individuals are especially sensitive to the drug.

Common side effects in *italic*; life-threatening effects <u>underlined</u>; generic names in **bold**; classifications in SMALL CAPS

259

- Usually applied at bedtime and should remain on skin for length of time specified by physician (time varies from 10–20 min to 8–12 h).
- Apply thin coat to affected sites only. Neighboring uninvolved skin should be protected with petrolatum.
- Use only on quiescent or chronic patches. Avoid uninvolved skin, acute eruptions, or inflamed skin. Wear a finger cot or plastic gloves (anthralin discolors skin and fingernails), and wash hands thoroughly after completing treatment.
- Treated part should be covered with gauze, stockinette, old underwear, or old pajamas. Discuss with physician.
- Avoid getting anthralin (a powerful ocular irritant) into the eyes or on mucous membranes. Do not apply to face, intertriginous areas, or to genitalia unless directed to do so by physician.
- *Scalp treatment:* comb hair to remove scales. Apply medication sparingly only to affected areas of scalp. Cover pillow with plastic to avoid staining. Scalp is shampooed at end of prescribed contact period. May temporarily discolor gray or white hair.
- Preserve in tightly covered containers, preferably between 15–30C (59–86F), and protect from light unless otherwise directed by manufacturer.

Assessment & Drug Effects

- Erythema on normal skin may indicate the need to reduce frequency or strength of medication or to temporarily withdraw anthralin.
- Treatment should be discontinued if lesions appear to be spreading or with onset of skin irritation or pustular folliculitis.
- Weekly urine tests are recommended to determine evidence of renal irritation. Note: alkaline urine may take on a brown stain.

Patient & Family Education

- Continued applications, particularly of ointments, without intermittent cleansing permit accumulation of moisture, dead cells, and other tissue waste products, which may cause maceration. Consult physician.
- Warmed mineral oil is commonly used for removing ointment from skin. Removal should be followed by bathing. Cream formulations are removed by bathing.
- Manufacturer advises removing any medication from bath, shower, sink, or other equipment by rinsing immediately with hot water to prevent discoloration and by using suitable cleanser to remove any residual surface deposits.

PEDICULICIDE

PERMETHRIN
(per-meth´rin)
Trade name: Nix
Classifications: SKIN AGENT; PEDICULICIDE
Pregnancy: Category B

ACTIONS/PHARMACODYNAMICS   Synthetic pyrethroid with pediculocidal and ovidical activity against *Pediculus humanus* var. *capitis* (head louse). Permethrin inhibits sodium ion influx through nerve cell membrane channels, resulting in delayed repolarization of the action potential and paralysis of the pest. Since lice are completely dependent on blood for survival, they die within 24–48 h if unable to burrow into the skin. Drug is also active against ticks, mites, and fleas. For unknown reasons, head louse infestations are rarely seen in American blacks.

USES Pediculosis capitis.

ROUTE & DOSAGE

Head Lice

Adult	Topical	Apply sufficient volume to clean wet hair to saturate the hair and scalp; leave on 10 min; then rinse hair thoroughly
Child	Topical	> 2 y: Same as for adult

PHARMACOKINETICS Absorption: <2% of amount applied is absorbed through intact skin. **Metabolism:** rapidly hydrolyzed to inactive metabolites. **Elimination:** excreted primarily in urine.

CONTRAINDICATIONS & PRECAUTIONS Contraindicated in: hypersensitivity to pyrethrins, crysanthemums, sulfites, or other preservatives or dyes; acute inflammation of the scalp; pregnancy (category B). Safe use in nursing mothers and children < 2 y of age or in the elderly not documented.

ADVERSE/SIDE EFFECTS (On scalp): *pruritus, transient tingling,* burning, stinging, numbness; erythema, edema, rash.

NURSING IMPLICATIONS

Administration

- Drug action results from topical application of the formulation. It is not a shampoo. Scalp as well as hair should be saturated by the lotion.

- Prior to treatment with permethrin, use regular shampoo, thoroughly rinse and towel-dry hair and scalp. Shake lotion well before application. One container holds enough for at least one treatment, but two containers may be necessary if patient has long hair. Do not retain left-over medicine.

- Following 10 min exposure to the medication, hair and scalp should be thoroughly rinsed and dried with a clean towel. Head lice are usually eliminated with one treatment.

- Store drug away from heat at 15–25C (59–77F) and direct light. Avoid freezing.

Assessment & Drug Effects

- If patient is known to be sensitive to any pyrethrin or pyrethroid, therapy should not be attempted, or if a reaction occurs, treatment should be stopped.

Patient & Family Education

- When hair is dry, patient may want to comb it with a fine-tooth comb (furnished with medication) to remove dead lice and remaining nits or nit shells. While not a therapeutic requirement, this combing has cosmetic value.

- Permethrin remains on hair shaft up to 14 d; therefore recurrence of infestation rarely occurs (<1%).

- Instruct patient or parent to inspect hair shafts daily for at least 1 wk to determine drug effectiveness. If live lice are observed after 7 d, contact physician. A renewed prescription for a second treatment may be ordered. Signs of inadequate treatment: pruritis, erythema, excoriation, infected scalp areas.

- Regular shampooing may be resumed after treatment; residual deposit of drug on hair is not reduced.

- Permethrin is usually irritating to the eyes and mucosa. Flush well with water if medicine accidentally gets into eyes.

PSORALEN

METHOXSALEN

(meth-ox´a-len)
Trade names: 8-MOP, Oxsoralen, UltraMOP
Classifications: SKIN AGENT; PSORALEN
Pregnancy: Category C

ACTIONS/PHARMACODYNAMICS A psoralen derivative with strong photosensitizing effects: used with ultraviolet-A light (UVA) in therapeutic regimens called PUVA ([P]-psoralen). After photoactivation by long wavelength UVA, methoxsalen combines with epidermal cell DNA, causing photo-damage (cytotoxic action) and inhibition of the rapid and uncontrolled epidermal cell turnover characteristic of psoriasis, and an inflammatory reaction with erythema. Methoxsalen is also strongly melanogenic. Skin color depends on melanin, product of melanocytes in the basal layer of epidermis. UVA energizes the intracellular oxidation of tyrosine to melanin precursor dihydroxyphenylalanine; methoxsalen enhances the reaction. Repigmentation induced by PUVA appears to be the result of several mechanisms including increased synthesis of melanin, increased number and hypertrophy of functioning melanocytes, and stimulation of migration of melanocytes up the follicles to repopulate the epidermis. Long-term effects of PUVA treatment include increased risk of cutaneous cancer. The safe total cumulative dose of UVA in PUVA therapy over a period of time has not been established.

USES With controlled exposure to UVA to repigment vitiliginous skin and for symptomatic treatment of severe disabling psoriasis that is refractory to other forms of therapy. **Unlabeled use:** (PUVA therapy) mycosis fungoides.

PHARMOKINETICS Absorption: variably absorbed from GI tract. **Peak:** 2 h. **Duration:** 8–10 h. **Distribution:** preferentially taken up by epidermal cells; distributes into lens of eye. **Elimination:** half-life: 0.75–2.4 h; 80–90% excreted in urine within 8 h.

CONTRAINDICATIONS & PRECAUTIONS Contraindicated in: sunburn, sensitivity (or its history) to psoralens, diseases associated with photosensitivity (e.g., LE, albinism, melanoma or its history), invasive squamous cell cancer, cataract, aphakia, previous exposure to arsenic or ionizing radiation, pregnancy (category C); safe use (oral) in children not established. **Cautious use in:** hepatic insufficiency, GI disease, chronic infection, treatment with known photosensitizing agents; immunosuppressed patient, cardiovascular disease, nursing mothers; safe use (lotion) in children < 12 y not established.

ADVERSE/SIDE EFFECTS CNS: nervousness, dizziness, headache, mental depression or excitation, vertigo, insomnia. **Eye:** cataract formation, ocular damage. **GI:** cheilitis, *nausea* and other GI distur-

Common side effects in *italic*; life-threatening effects underlined;
generic names in **bold**; classifications in SMALL CAPS

261

ROUTE & DOSAGE

Idiopathic Vitiligo

Adult   Topical   Apply lotion 1–2 h before exposure to UV light once/wk

Psoriasis

Adult   PO   Administer 1.5–2 h before exposure to UV light 2–3 times/wk

<30 kg: 10 mg

30–50 kg: 20 mg

51–65 kg: 30 mg

66–80 kg: 40 mg

81–90 kg: 50 mg

91–115 kg: 60 mg

>115 kg: 70 mg

bances, toxic hepatitis. **Skin:** phototoxic effects: <u>severe edema and erythema</u>, *pruritus,* painful blisters; <u>burning</u>, peeling, thinning, freckling, and accelerated aging of skin; hyper- or hypopigmentation; severe skin pain (lasting 1–2 mo). Also: <u>malignant melanoma</u> (rare), cell carcinoma, cutaneous neuritis, photoallergic contact dermatitis (with topical use), exacerbation of latent photosensitive dermatoses. **Other:** transient loss of muscular coordination, edema, leg cramps, systemic immune effects; acute myeloid leukemia, preleukemia, drug fever.

DRUG INTERACTIONS *Anthralin, coal tar, griseofulvin,* PHENOTHIAZINES, *naladixic acid,* SULFONAMIDES, BACTERIOSTATIC SOAPS, TETRACYCLINES, THIAZIDES compound photosensitizing effects. **Drug-food interactions:** food will increase peak and extent of absorption.

NURSING IMPLICATIONS

Administration

- Methoxsalen (PUVA therapy) should be under the complete control of a physician with special competence and experience in photochemotherapy.
- To prevent GI distress, oral doses are best administered with milk or food.
- Maintain a consistent time relationship between food-drug ingestion. Food digestion and absorption appear to affect drug serum levels.
- Methoxsalen is always administered on an alternate day schedule because the full extent of a phototoxic reaction may be delayed for ≤ 48 h.

- Only small (less than 10 cm²), well-defined areas are treated with lotion. Systemic treatment is used for large areas.
- The lotion is applied with cotton swabs, allowed to dry 1–2 min, then reapplied. Borders of the lesion should be protected with petrolatum and sunscreen lotion to prevent hyperpigmentation.
- Finger cots or gloves should be used to apply lotion to prevent photosensitization and burned skin.
- Store lotion and capsules in light-resistant containers at 15–30C (59–86F) unless otherwise directed by manufacturer.

Assessment & Drug Effects

- A pretreatment ophthalmologic exam is performed to rule out cataract; it should be repeated periodically during treatment and at yearly intervals thereafter. UVA exposure to a drug-loaded lens leads to drug-protein binding and cataract formation.
- CBC, renal and hepatic function tests, and antinuclear antibody tests are monitored during PO psoralen therapy.
- Fair-skinned patients appear to be at greatest risk for photochemotherapeutic toxicity from PUVA therapy (see adverse/side effects).
- Repigmentation is more rapid on fleshy areas, i.e., face, abdomen, buttocks, than on hands or feet.
- Effective repigmentation may require 6–9 mo of treatment; periodic treatment usually is necessary to retain pigmentation. If, after 3 mo of treatment, there is no apparent response, methoxsalen is discontinued.

Patient & Family Education

- Sunlight is sometimes used as the UV light source with the exposure time factor well controlled by prescription.
- After drug ingestion and UVA exposure, additional exposure to UV light (direct or indirect) should be avoided for at least 8 h.
- After topical application, the initial sunlight exposure is limited to 1 min, with subsequent gradual and incremental exposures by prescription. The patient should fully understand the intended schedule.
- After topical methoxsalen application and UVA exposure, the patient should not expose skin to additional UV light for 24–48 h.
- If sunlight cannot be avoided after the treatment, sunscreen lotion (with SPF 15 or higher) and protective clothing (hat, golves) should cover all exposed areas including lips, to prevent burning or blistering.

- Sunscreen lotions containing benzophenone (e.g., Solbar) appear to give best protection from drug-induced phototoxicity.
- During PUVA therapy, sunscreen lotion is applied to the skin for about one third of the initial exposure time until there is sufficient tanning. It should not be applied to psoriatic areas before the treatment.
- Sunbathing is contraindicated for at least 48 h after PUVA treatment. Sunburn and photochemotherapy are additive in the production of burning and erythema.
- Wraparound UVA opaque goggles are worn during PUVA treatment. After treatment, wraparound sunglasses with UVA-absorbing properties must be worn both indoors and outdoors during daylight hours for 24 h.
- Warn patient not to substitute prescription sunglasses or photosensitive darkening glasses; they may actually increase danger of cataract formation.
- Instruct patient to alert physician to appearance of new psoriatic areas, to flares, or to regressed cleared skin areas should they occur during treatment and maintenance periods.

SCABICIDE

LINDANE
(lin´dane)

Trade names: Gamabenzene, G-Well, Kwell, Kwildane, Scabene
Classifications: SKIN AGENT; SCABICIDE; PEDICULICIDE; ANTIINFECTIVE
Pregnancy: Category C

ACTIONS/PHARMACODYNAMICS Benzene hydrocarbon originally developed as an agricultural insecticide. Has ectoparasitic and ovicidal activity against the two variants of *Pediculus humanus* — *Pediculus capitis* (head louse) and *Pediculus pubis* (crab louse) — and the arthropod *Sarcoptes scabiei* (scabies). Action of drug follows its direct absorption by parasites and ova (nits). Drug absorption through the exoskeleton stimulates the nervous system, resulting in seizures and death. Resistance to lindane may develop in *P. capitis,* but evidence of resistance in *S. scabiei* is inconclusive. Carcinogenesis or tu-

morogenesis has not been documented. Lindane is not prophylactic for pediculosis.

USES To treat head and crab lice and scabies infestations and to eradicate their ova.

ROUTE & DOSAGE

Adult	Topical	Apply to all body areas except the face; leave lotion on 8–12 h; then rinse off; leave shampoo on 5 min; then rinse thoroughly; do not repeat in < 1 wk
Child	Topical	same as for adult

PHARMACOKINETICS Absorption: slowly and incompletely absorbed through intact skin; maximum absorption from face, scalp, axillae. **Distribution:** stored in body fat. **Metabolism:** metabolized in liver. **Elimination:** excreted in urine and feces.

CONTRAINDICATIONS & PRECAUTIONS Contraindicated in: premature neonates, patient with known seizure disorders; application to eyes, face, mucous membranes, urethral meatus, open cuts or raw, weeping surfaces; prolonged or excessive applications or simultaneous application of creams, ointments, oils. Use during pregnancy (category B) or by nursing mothers not recommended by CDC. **Cautious use in:** children < 10 y.

ADVERSE/SIDE EFFECTS Occur in < 0.001% of patients. **Chronic exposure to vapors:** fatal aplastic anemia and other hematologic problems. **CNS:** CNS stimulation (usually after accidental ingestion or misuse of product): restlessness, dizziness, tremors, convulsions. **Inhalation:** headache, nausea, vomiting, irritation of ENT. **Skin:** eczematous eruptions.

NURSING IMPLICATIONS

Administration

- To reduce percutaneous absorption, all skin lotions and creams and oil-based hair dressings should be completely removed, and skin should be allowed to dry and cool before application of lindane.
- *Cream or lotion:* Shake container well. *Scabies:* Apply thin film of formulation from neck down over entire body surface including soles of feet. Scabies rarely affects head of adults or child, but may infest infant's scalp. Avoid face and urethral meatus. Pay particular attention to intertriginous areas (finger webs and other body creases and folds), wrists, elbows, and belt line. Rub drug in; allow skin to dry

Common side effects in *italic*; life-threatening effects underlined; generic names in **bold**; classifications in SMALL CAPS

263

and cool after application. After 8–12 h remove medication by bath or shower. Reapplication is rarely necessary, unless living mites can be demonstrated. **Crab lice:** Apply thin film of drug to hair and skin of pubic area and, if infected, to thighs, trunk, axillary areas. Leave in place 8–12 h and follow with bath or shower. Observation of living lice after 7 d indicates the need for reapplication.

- **Shampoo: Head lice:** Apply quantity sufficient to wet hair and skin (30/ml [1 oz] for short, 45 ml [1 1/2 oz] for medium, and 60 ml [2 oz] for long hair). Work drug thoroughly onto hair shafts and scalp and allow to remain in place 4 min. (Initially, nits are found at shaft-scalp junction). Add small amounts of water sufficient to make a thick lather; then rinse well with water; dry with clean towel. Pay particular attention to areas above and behind ears and occipital region. Use fine-tooth comb or tweezers to remove remaining nit shells. If necessary, treatment may be repeated after 7 d but not more than twice in 1 wk. **Crab lice:** See above. Repeat treatment after 7 d only if live lice can be demonstrated.
- The care giver should wear plastic disposable or rubber gloves when applying lindane, especially if she is pregnant or if she is applying medication to more than one patient, to avoid prolonged skin contact.
- Store drug at 15–30C (59–86F) in tight container away from direct light and heat. Protect from freezing.

Assessment & Drug Effects

- Microscopic confirmation of scabies mites is recommended before treatment if diagnosis is in doubt.
- Case-finding efforts should include not only the sex partner but also other family members and close-contact persons. Suspect scabies if a person complains of nocturnal itching (classic symptom).

- Both scabies and *P. pubis* infestation are sexually transmitted diseases. The sex partner should be identified and treated simultaneously. The patient with crab lice should be examined for venereal disease.
- Recurring limited infestations of scabies may indicate a domestic animal source (e.g., cat, dog, cattle, poultry). Recurrence of any of the discussed infestations may indicate inadequate disinfection of fomites.
- Burrows made by scabies mites (may or may not be visible) appear as grayish black straight or S-shaped lines with a papule containing the mite at one end and surrounded by a mild erythematous area.

Patient & Family Education

- Instruct patient on proper application of medication.
- Lindane is highly toxic drug if topical applications are excessive or if swallowed or inhaled. Caution patients to keep it out of reach of children.
- Lindane shampoo is an effective disinfectant for personal items such as combs, crushes. Clothing and bedding should be boiled or dry-cleaned.
- Penetration of the skin with scabies mites causes an intolerable itching that may persist 2–3 wk after they have been killed by medication. If patients are uninformed about this, they may think treatment has failed and use lindane more freely and for a longer period than prescribed. Abuse can cause an itch-scratch cycle and drug overdosage from increased percutaneous absorption.
- Instruct patient to discontinue medication and report to a physician if signs of irritation, sensitization, or itching occur.
- Caution against applying medication to face, mouth, open skin lesions, or to eyelashes; avoid contact with eyes. If accidental eye contact occurs, flush with water.

SECTION

III

ALPHABETICAL GENERIC DRUG LIST

ABSORBABLE GELATIN SPONGE

Trade name: Gelfoam
Classifications: BLOOD COAGULATOR;
HEMOSTATIC

ACTIONS/PHARMACODYNAMICS This sterile, water-insoluble, nonantigenic sponge is capable of absorbing many times its weight in blood and provides an absorbable matrix into which clot forms and granulation tissue may grow. It is not for brisk arterial bleeding. It is entirely absorbed in 4–6 wk when implanted in tissue. When applied to bleeding areas of skin or nasal, rectal, or vaginal mucosa, it completely liquefies in 2–5 d.

USES Adjunct to control bleeding and capillary oozing in highly vascular areas that are difficult to suture. **Unlabeled use:** Aid in healing of wounds and decubitus ulcers.

ROUTE & DOSAGE

Hemostasis: use sterile technique. Cut to desired size (minimal amount is applied to cover area).

Dry application: compress piece(s) before application to bleeding surface. After application, hold in place with moderate pressure for 10–15 s.

Moist application: immerse piece(s) in either sterile isotonic saline or thrombin solution. Sponge should swell to original size and shape. Wet piece may be blotted with gauze before it is applied to bleeding point. Hold in place for 10–15 s with cotton pledget or gauze; remove pledget carefully with a few drops of sterile water so as not to disturb gelatin sponge.

Decubitus ulcer: after debridement, gelatin sponge is placed aseptically in ulcer and covered with dry, sterile dressing. Dressing may be changed daily, but gelatin sponge should not be disturbed; new sponges may be added as required. If infection develops, sponge should be removed.

CONTRAINDICATIONS & PRECAUTIONS Contraindicated in: frank infection; postpartum hemorrhage or menorrhagia; as sole hemostatic agent in patients with blood dyscrasias; closure of skin edges. **Cautious use in:** closed tissue spaces. Avoid overpacking.

NURSING IMPLICATIONS

Administration

- Use contents as soon as possible after opening package. Discard unused portions.
- Manufacturer cautions not to resterilize product because absorption time may be affected.
- Since gelatin sponge is completely absorbed, there is not need to remove it.

Assessment & Drug Effects

- Since gelatin sponge absorbs fluid and expands, report to physician if patient complains of pain or discomfort.
- Be alert to *signs of infection:* malaise, fever, tenderness, redness, swelling. Report immediately.

Prototype: propranolol, p 109

ACEBUTOLOL HYDROCHLORIDE

(a-se-byoo´toe-lole)
Trade name: Sectral
Classifications: AUTONOMIC NERVOUS SYSTEM AGENT; BETA-ADRENERGIC ANTAGONIST (BLOCKING AGENT, SYMPATHOLYTIC); CARDIOVASCULAR AGENT; ANTIHYPERTENSIVE; ANTIARRHYTHMIC
Pregnancy: Category B

ACTIONS/PHARMACODYNAMICS Beta$_1$-selective adrenergic blocking agent with mild intrinsic sympathomimetic activity (partial beta-agonist activity). Exhibits antiarrhythmic activity (class II antiarrhythmic agent). At low dosage inhibits response to adrenergic stimuli by competitively blocking beta$_1$-adrenergic receptors (cardiac) while having limited effect on beta$_2$-adrenergic receptors on vascular and bronchial smooth muscles. Selectivity diminishes with high doses, resulting in both beta$_1$- and beta$_2$-adrenoceptor blocking action. Produces negative chronotropic and inotropic activity; i.e., decreases exercise-induced heart rate, inhibits reflex orthostatic tachycardia, and decreases cardiac output at rest or during exercise. Decreases both systolic and diastolic BP at rest and during exercise. Antiarrhythmic activity is related to slowed conduction through AV node, resulting in increased AV node refractoriness; has limited effect on SA node. On a weight basis, displays 10–30% greater blocking activity than propranolol does.

USES Mild to moderate hypertension. Stepped-care approach to antihypertensive therapy as step 1 or

Common side effects in *italic*; life-threatening effects underlined; generic names in **bold**; classifications in SMALL CAPS

step 2 drug. Management of recurrent stable ventricular arrhythmias. **Unlabeled use:** Supraventricular arrhythmias, chronic stable angina pectoris.

ROUTE & DOSAGE

Hypertension

Adult	PO	400–800 mg/d in 1–2 divided doses (max 1200 mg/d)

Ventricular Arrhythmias

Adult	PO	200 mg b.i.d. increased to 600–1200 mg/d

Angina Pectoris

Adult	PO	300–400 mg t.i.d.

In Renal Impairment

Creatinine clearance	<50 ml/min: reduce dose by 50%
Creatinine clearance	<25 ml/min: reduce dose by 75%

PHARMACOKINETICS Absorption: well absorbed after PO administration; undergoes extensive first-pass metabolism in liver with an average bioavailability of 40%. (In geriatric patients, bioavailability increases twofold.) **Peak:** 3 h. **Distribution:** minimally into CSF; crosses placenta; is excreted in breast milk. **Metabolism:** metabolized in liver to diacetolol with activity equipotent to parent compound. **Elimination:** half-life: acebutolol 3–4 h, metabolite 8–13 h; 50–60% excreted via bile into feces, and 30–40% excreted in urine.

CONTRAINDICATIONS & PRECAUTIONS Contraindicated in: overt CHF, second or third degree AV block, severe bradycardia, cardiogenic shock. Safety during pregnancy (category B), lactation, or in children <12 y not established. **Cautious use in:** impaired cardiac function, well-compensated CHF, mesenteric or peripheral vascular disease; patients undergoing major surgery involving general anesthesia; renal or hepatic impairment; labile diabetes mellitus; hyperthyroidism; bronchospastic disease (asthma, emphysema); avoid abrupt withdrawal.

ADVERSE/SIDE EFFECTS CNS: *fatigue,* dizziness, insomnia, drowsiness, confusion, fainting, decreased libido. **CV:** *bradycardia,* hypotension, CHF. **GI:** nausea, *diarrhea, constipation,* flatulence. **Respiratory:** bronchospasm, pulmonary edema, dyspnea. **Sensitivity reactions:** antinuclear antibodies (ANA) (10–30% of patients). **Other:** back or joint pain, <u>agranulocytosis</u>, impotence, hypoglycemia (may mask symptoms of a hypoglycemic reaction).

DRUG INTERACTIONS OTHER HYPOTENSIVE AGENTS, DIURETICS increase hypotensive effect; with **albuterol, metaproterenol, terbutaline,** or **pirbuterol** there is mutual antagonism with acebutolol; NSAIDS blunt hypotensive effect; decreases hypoglycemic effect of **glyburide;** increases bradycardia and sinus arrest with **amiodarone.**

DIAGNOSTIC TEST INTERFERENCES See **propranolol,** p 109.

NURSING IMPLICATIONS

Administration
- Check apical pulse before administration. If slower than 60 bpm, consult physician.
- Store at 15–30C (59–86F).

Assessment & Drug Effects
- Monitor BP and cardiac status throughout therapy. Report bradycardia and hypertension to physician.
- Monitor I&O ratio and pattern. Report changes to physician, e.g., dysuria, nocturia, oliguria, weight change.
- Monitor for Signs & Symptoms of CHF, especially peripheral edema, dyspnea, activity intolerance. (See other Signs & Symptoms, chap 3.)
- In long-term therapy, incidence of drug-induced positive ANA titer is high, especially in women and in the elderly. Complaints about persistent lupus-like symptoms (myalgia, arthritis, arthralgia) suggest ANA sensitivity and should be reported to the physician. Discontinuation of drug therapy usually reverses symptoms.
- If patient is also receiving a catecholamine-depleting drug (e.g., reserpine), observe for marked bradycardia or hypotension. Acebutolol prevents compensatory tachycardia; therefore patient may experience vertigo, syncope, or orthostatic changes in BP.

Patient & Family Education
- Teach patients how to check their pulse before they take medication. Advise patient to notify physician if pulse is below 60.
- Warn patient that CNS adverse effects are the most common, e.g., insomnia, drowsiness, confusion.
- Warn patient not to drive or operate equipment requiring alertness and manual skills until response to drug is known.
- Caution patient not to increase, decrease, omit, or discontinue drug regimen without advice from the physician.
- Abrupt withdrawal may exacerbate angina or pre-

Common side effects in *italic*; life-threatening effects <u>underlined</u>; generic names in **bold**; classifications in SMALL CAPS

267

cipitate MI in patient with heart disease or thyroid storm in patient with thyrotoxicosis.

- Contact physician promptly at the first signs or symptoms of CHF (see Signs & Symptoms, chap 3).
- Advise diabetics that drug may mask symptoms of hypoglycemia (see Signs & Symptoms, chap 3) and may potentiate insulin-induced hypoglycemia.
- Avoid use with OTC oral cold preparations and topical nasal decongestants containing alpha-adrenergic agonists (e.g., phenylephrine). An exaggerated hypertensive reaction is a potential hazard.
- Following gradual withdrawal over 2 wk patient should temporarily limit physical activity.

ACETAMINOPHEN

See CENTRAL NERVOUS SYSTEM AGENT, NONNARCOTIC ANALGESIC, ANTIPYRETIC prototype, p 158.

ACETAZOLAMIDE

See EYE, EAR, NOSE, AND THROAT PREPARATIONS, CARBONIC ANHYDRASE INHIBITOR prototype, p 206.

Prototype: tolbutamide, p 234

ACETOHEXAMIDE

(a-seat-oh-hex´a-mide)
Trade names: Dimelor, Dymelor
Classifications: HORMONE; SULFONYLUREA ANTIDIABETIC
Pregnancy: Category C

ACTIONS/PHARMACODYNAMICS Promotes increased effectiveness of endogenous insulin. More potent and has longer action than tolbutamide, but actions, uses, precautions, and adverse reactions are similar. Lowers blood glucose by stimulating pancreatic beta cells to secrete insulin. With prolonged administration, hypoglycemic activity appears to be enhanced by extra-pancreatic effects: principally, increased peripheral sensitivity to insulin and reduc-

tion in liver glucose production. Also has moderate uricosuric effect, probably due to its primary metabolite, hydroxyhexamide.

USES Mild to moderately severe stable type II diabetes, NIDDM (noninsulin dependent diabetes mellitus). Also reduces insulin requirements in select patients with type I diabetes, IDDM (insulin dependent diabetes mellitus). Preferred by some clinicians for patients who also have gout.

ROUTE & DOSAGE

Glycemic Control

Adult	PO	250 mg/d before breakfast; may be increased by 250–500 mg q5–7d (max 1.5 g/d); doses >1 g should be given before breakfast and dinner.

PHARMACOKINETICS Absorption: rapidly absorbed from GI tract. **Onset:** 1 h. **Peak:** 2–4 h. **Duration:** 12–24 h. **Distribution:** breast milk. **Metabolism:** metabolized in liver to active metabolite. **Elimination:** half-life 5–6 h; 80–95% eliminated in urine; 15% in bile.

CONTRAINDICATIONS & PRECAUTIONS Contraindicated in: hypersensitivity to sulfonylureas; severe impairment of hepatic, renal, thyroid or other endocrine function; as sole therapy for IDDM and in diabetes complicated by ketosis, acidosis, coma, infection, trauma, hyperglycemia, and glycosuria associated with primary renal disease. Safe use during pregnancy (category C), in nursing mothers, and in children not established. **Cautious use in:** renal insufficiency, history of hepatic porphyria.

ADVERSE/SIDE EFFECTS Generally dose-related. **GI:** nausea, vomiting, epigastric fullness, anorexia, stomach pain or discomfort, heartburn, diarrhea. **Hematologic:** agranulocytosis, leukopenia, pancytopenia, thrombocytopenia, aplastic anemia, severe hypoglycemia. **Hypersensitivity:** erythema, urticaria, pruritus, rash, photosensitivity. **Other:** headache, dizziness.

DIAGNOSTIC TEST INTERFERENCES *Serum uric acid* levels may be appreciably reduced.

DRUG INTERACTIONS Alcohol may elicit disulfiram reaction; **warfarin, aspirin** and other SALICYLATES, **chloramphenicol, clofibrate, fenfluramine, guanethidine,** MAO INHIBITORS, **oxytetracycline, phenylbutazone, probenecid, sulfinpyrazone,** and SULFONAMIDES may enhance hypoglycemic effects; with **diazoxide** there is mutual antagonism and effects of both drugs are reduced; THIAZIDE DIURETICS may exacerbate hyperglycemia, resulting in need for increased acetohexamide doses; **phenytoin** may decrease effects of acetohexamide; BETA-ADRENERGIC BLOCKERS may mask symptoms of hypoglycemia.

NURSING IMPLICATIONS

Administration
- Administer daily dose before breakfast.
- Doses in excess of 1 g are normally divided and given before breakfast and dinner.
- Store at 15–30C (59–86F) unless otherwise directed.

Assessment & Drug Effects
- Blood and urine glucose concentrations should be closely monitored during first 24 h after therapy is initiated.
- The elderly, malnourished, and debilitated patients and those with impaired hepatic or renal function or adrenal or pituitary insufficiency require close monitoring because they have a tendency to develop an exaggerated hypoglycemic response to acetohexamide, which may be difficult to recognize.
- Patients are usually given at least a 7 d trial period to determine therapeutic response. Favorable response is indicated by reduction in diabetes hyperglycemia symptoms (see chap 3).
- Monitor for signs and symptoms of hypoglycemia (see chap 3), which indicate a need for dosage adjustment.
- Periodic tests of liver function are recommended, i.e., bilirubin, cholesterol, AST, ALT.
- Dermatologic reactions tend to be transient and frequently subside even with continuation of therapy. However, if they persist or are severe, discontinuation of drug may be necessary.

Patient & Family Education
- Patient should ingest some form of sugar such as orange juice, sugar cube, table sugar (dissolved in water), corn syrup, or honey if symptoms of hypoglycemia develop, and seek medical assistance.
- During conversion from one antidiabetic agent to another, patient should check urine for glucose and ketones (acetone) at least 3 times a day and report to physician as directed. Blood glucose monitoring may also be prescribed.
- Caution patient not to take any other medication unless approved or prescribed by physician.
- Alcoholic beverages may produce a disulfiram-type reaction (see Signs & Symptoms, chap 3).

- Advise patient to avoid prolonged direct exposure to sun to prevent photosensitivity reaction.

Prototype: bethanechol, p 120

ACETYLCHOLINE CHLORIDE
(a-se-teel-koe´leen)
Trade name: Miochol
Classifications: AUTONOMIC NERVOUS SYSTEM AGENT; DIRECT ACTING CHOLINERGIC (PARASYMPATHOMIMETIC); MIOTIC
Pregnancy: Category C

ACTIONS/PHARMACODYNAMICS Quaternary ammonium compound. Acts directly on postjunctional effector cells of eye to produce intense miosis by stimulating contraction of iris sphincter muscles.

USES To obtain rapid and complete miosis after delivery of lens in cataract surgery; also in penetrating keratoplasty, iridectomy, and other surgical procedures of anterior segment.

ROUTE & DOSAGE

Miosis

Adult	Topical	0.5–2 ml 1% solution instilled into anterior chamber of eye

PHARMACOKINETICS Onset: 10 s. **Duration:** 10 min. **Metabolism:** rapidly hydrolyzed to cholic and acetic acid.

ADVERSE/SIDE EFFECTS Low toxicity. With systemic absorption: transient hypotension, bradycardia. Also reported: temporary lens opacities and iris atrophy following use of hypertonic solutions.

NURSING IMPLICATIONS

Administration
- Immediately before use, dust cap, peel off label, and immerse in 70% ethanol or other sterilizing solution for 30 min or more. Stream of gas, e.g., ethylene oxide, should not be used (forms formic acid).
- Using aseptic technique, rubber stopper is pressed down sufficiently to dislodge center rubber plug seal, thus releasing solvent (sterile water) from upper chamber.
- Shake vial gently to dissolve and mix drug in lower

Common side effects in *italic*; life-threatening effects <u>underlined</u>; generic names in **bold**; classifications in SMALL CAPS

chamber. If center rubber plug seal does not go down or is down, do not use vial.

- After plunger-stopper is cleansed with 70% alcohol or other suitable germicide, desired dose is drawn into dry sterile syringe with sterile new 18- to 20-gauge needle. Needle is replaced with suitable atraumatic cannula for intraocular instillation.
- As solution is unstable, it should be reconstituted immediately before use. Discard unused portion.
- Pilocarpine 2% or physostigmine 0.25% (long-acting miotics) may be prescribed topically before dressing is applied to maintain miosis.
- Systemic reactions are treated with intravenous atropine 0.6–0.8 mg.

Assessment & Drug Effects
- Monitor hypotension and bradycardia, which are transient and normally disappear rapidly.

ACETYLCYSTEINE
See MUCOLYTIC prototype, p 100.

ACYCLOVIR
See ANTIINFECTIVES, ANTIVIRAL prototype, p 85.

Prototype: procainamide, p 140

ADENOSINE
(a-den´o-sin)
Trade name: Adenocard
Classifications: CARDIOVASCULAR AGENT; ANTIARRHYTHMIC
Pregnancy: Category C

ACTIONS/PHARMACODYNAMICS Slows conduction through the atrioventricular (AV) and sinoatrial (SA) nodes. Can interrupt the reentry pathways through the AV node. Depresses left ventricular function, but effect is transient due to short half-life.

USES Conversion to sinus rhythm of paroxysmal supraventricular tachycardia (PSVT) including PSVT

associated with accessory bypass tracts (Wolff-Parkinson-White syndrome). **Unlabeled use:** afterload-reducing agent in low output states; to prevent graft occlusion following aortocoronary bypass surgery; to produce controlled hypotension during cerebral aneurysm surgery; "chemical" stress test.

ROUTE & DOSAGE

Supraventricular Tachycardia

Adult	IV	6 mg rapid IV bolus (over 1–2 s); may repeat in 1–2 min with 12 mg IV push × 2 (total of 3 doses); max recommended dose is 12 mg; injection should be given directly into the vein or as proximal as possible in the IV line and followed by a rapid saline flush

PHARMACOKINETICS Absorption: rapid uptake by erythrocytes and vascular endothelial cells after IV administration. **Onset:** 20–30 s. **Metabolism:** Rapid uptake into cells; degraded by deamination to inosine, hypoxanthine, and adenosine monophosphate. **Elimination:** half-life: 10 s; route of elimination unknown.

CONTRAINDICATIONS & PRECAUTIONS Contraindicated in: AV block, preexisting second and third degree block or sick sinus rhythm without pacemaker, since a heart block may result. Also contraindicated in atrial flutter, atrial fibrillation and ventricular tachycardia because the drug is ineffective. **Cautious use in:** asthmatics, pregnancy (category C), hepatic and renal failure.

ADVERSE/SIDE EFFECTS *Transient facial flushing,* transient dyspnea, atrial fibrillation or flutter, irritability in children.

DRUG INTERACTIONS Dipyridamole can potentiate the effects of adenosine; **theophylline** will block the electrophysiologic effects of adenosine; **carbamazepine** may increase risk of heart block.

NURSING IMPLICATIONS

Administration
- For rapid bolus IV, administer directly into vein. If given by IV line, administer as proximal as possible, and follow with a rapid saline flush.
- Must be given as a rapid bolus IV over 1–2 s.
- The solution must be clear at time of use. Since it contains no preservatives, discard used portion.
- If high level block develops after one dose, do not repeat dose.

- Emergency resuscitation drugs and equipment must always be available during administration.
- Store at room temperature 15–30C (59–86F). Do not refrigerate, as crystallization may occur. If crystals do form, dissolve by warming to room temperature.

Assessment & Drug Effects
- Because of the short half-life (10 s), adverse side effects are generally self-limiting.
- Use a hemodynamic monitoring system during administration.
- Monitor BP and heart rate q15–30s for several minutes after administration.
- An ECG is recommended to confirm efficiency of adenosine.
- Potential for bronchospasms in asthma patients is thought to exist. Monitor carefully.
- At the time of conversion to normal sinus rhythm, PVCs, PACs, sinus bradycardia, and sinus tachycardia, as well as various degrees of AV block, are seen on the ECG. These usually last only a few seconds and resolve without intervention.

Patient & Family Education
- Inform patient that facial flushing may occur.

Prototype: isoproterenol, p 105

ALBUTEROL
(al-byoo´ter-ole)

Trade names: Proventil, Proventil Repetabs, Salbutamol, Ventolin, Ventolin Rotocaps

Classifications: AUTONOMIC NERVOUS SYSTEM AGENT; BETA-ADRENERGIC AGONIST (SYMPATHOMIMETIC); BRONCHODILATOR (RESPIRATORY SMOOTH MUSCLE RELAXANT)

Pregnancy: Category C

ACTIONS/PHARMACODYNAMICS Synthetic sympathomimetic amine and moderately selective beta$_2$ adrenergic agonist with comparatively long action. Has more prominent effect on beta$_2$ receptors (particularly smooth muscles of bronchi, uterus, and vascular supply to skeletal muscles than on beta$_1$ (heart) receptors. Minimal or no effect on alpha-adrenergic receptors. Acts by stimulating conversion of intracellular ATP (adenosine triphosphate) to cAMP (cyclic adenosine monophosphate), a mediator of cell responses including beta-adrenergic activity. Inhibits histamine release by mast cells. Produces bronchodilation, regardless of administration route, by relaxing smooth muscles of bronchial tree. This decreases airway resistance, facilitates mucus drainage, and increases vital capacity. As effective as isoproterenol and metaproterenol, but produces more prolonged bronchodilation with little direct cardiac stimulation. Can cause some peripheral vasodilation.

USES To relieve bronchospasm associated with acute or chronic asthma, bronchitis, or other reversible obstructive airway diseases. Also used to prevent exercise-induced bronchospasm. **Unlabeled use:** as adjunct in treatment of refractory heart failure and to stimulate intracellular transport of potassium in hyperkalemic familial periodic paralysis.

ROUTE & DOSAGE

Bronchospasm

Adult	PO	2–4 mg 3–4 times/d
		4–8 mg sustained release 2 times/d
	Inhaled:	1–2 inhalations q4–6h
Child	PO	6–12 y: 2 mg 3–4 times/d
		2–6 y: 0.1 mg/kg 3 times/d
	Inhaled:	6–12 y: 1–2 inhalations q4–6h

PHARMACOKINETICS Onset: inhaled: 5–15 min; PO 30 min. **Peak effect:** inhaled: 0.5–2 h; PO 2.5 h. **Duration:** inhaled: 3–6 h; PO 4–6 h (8–12 h with sustained release). **Metabolism:** metabolized in liver; may cross the placenta. **Elimination:** half-life 2.75 h; 76% of dose eliminated in urine in 3 d.

CONTRAINDICATIONS & PRECAUTIONS Contraindicated in: safe use not established during pregnancy (category C) and in nursing mothers; use of albuterol aerosol or tablets in children <12 y, and use of oral syrup in children <2 y. **Cautious use in:** cardiovascular disease, hypertension, hyperthyroidism, diabetes mellitus, hypersensitivity to sympathomimetic amines or to fluorocarbon propellant used in inhalation aerosols.

ADVERSE/SIDE EFFECTS CNS: *tremor*, anxiety, nervousness, restlessness, convulsions, weakness, headache, hallucinations. **CV:** palpitation, hypertension, hypotension, bradycardia, reflex tachycardia. **Eye:** blurred vision, dilated pupils. **GI:** nausea, vomiting. **Other:** muscle cramps, hyperglycemia in diabetics, hoarseness, hypersensitivity reaction.

Common side effects in *italic*; life-threatening effects underlined; generic names in **bold**; classifications in SMALL CAPS

271

A

DIAGNOSTIC TEST INTERFERENCES Transient small increases in *plasma glucose* may occur.

DRUG INTERACTIONS With **epinephrine,** other SYMPATHOMIMETIC BRONCHODILATORS, possible additive effects; MAO INHIBITORS, TRICYCLIC ANTIDEPRESSANTS potentiate action on vascular system; BETA-ADRENERGIC BLOCKERS antagonize the effects of both drugs.

NURSING IMPLICATIONS

Administration

- Tablets and syrup should be stored between 2 and 30C (36 and 86F) in tight, light-resistant container.
- Store canisters between 15 and 30C (59 and 86F) away from heat and direct sunlight.

Assessment & Drug Effects

- Most common adverse effect associated with oral drug is fine tremor in fingers, which may interfere with precision handwork. Keep physician informed of any unusual symptoms.
- Children 2–6 y old appear to be more prone to experience CNS stimulation (hyperactivity, excitement, nervousness, insomnia), tachycardia, GI symptoms. Report promptly to physician.
- If drug-induced insomnia is a problem, consult physician about giving last albuterol dose several hours before bedtime.

Patient & Family Education

- Patient should receive explicit directions for correct use of medication and inhaler. Periodically check adequacy of patient's technique. Avoid contact of drug with eyes.
- If patient is also receiving beclomethasone (Vanceril) inhalation treatments, albuterol should be administered 20–30 min before, to allow deeper penetration of beclomethasone into lungs, unless otherwise directed by physician.
- Caution patient not to increase number or frequency of inhalations without advice of physician.
- Significant subjective improvement in pulmonary function should occur within 60–90 min after drug administration. Advise patient to notify physician if albuterol fails to provide relief, as this can signify worsening of pulmonary function. Reevaluation of patient's condition and therapy may be indicated.
- Since albuterol can cause dizziness or vertigo, caution patient to take necessary precautions.
- Emphasize dangers of self-prescribed OTC drugs without physician approval. Many medications (e.g., cold remedies) contain sympathomimetics that may intensify albuterol action.

Prototype: hydrocortisone, p 255

ALCLOMETASONE DIPROPRIONATE
(al-clo-met´a-sone)
Trade names: Alclovate
Classifications: SKIN AGENT; ANTIINFLAMMATORY; SYNTHETIC HORMONE; ADRENAL CORTICOSTEROID
Pregnancy: Category C

ACTIONS/PHARMACODYNAMICS Alclometasone dipropionate is a synthetic corticosteroid with topical antiinflammatory activity.

USES As a topical corticosteroid, the drug is used for the relief of the inflammatory and pruritic manifestations of corticosteroid-responsive dermatoses.

ROUTE & DOSAGE

Antiinflammatory

Adult	Topical	0.05% cream or ointment applied sparingly b.i.d. or t.i.d.; may use occlusive dressing for resistant dermatoses.

PHARMACOKINETICS Absorption: minimal absorption through intact skin.

CONTRAINDICATIONS & PRECAUTIONS Contraindicated in: hypersensitivity to drug or other corticosteroids or to any ingredient in the formulation. Should not be used in the treatment of acne, rosacea, or perioral dermatitis.

ADVERSE/SIDE EFFECTS Itching, burning, erythema, dryness, irritation, skin cracking and fissure.

NURSING IMPLICATIONS

Administration

- Apply a thin coat of cream on clean, dry skin.
- Avoid application near eyes.
- Do not use an occlusive dressing in presence of infection or draining lesions.
- Continue treatment for a few days after clearing of lesions to prevent recurrence.

Assessment & Drug Effects

- Systemic absorption is especially likely with occlusive dressings, prolonged treatment, application to large surface area, and when used on children.
- When risk of systemic absorption is high, monitor for indications of Cushing's syndrome (see Signs & Symptoms, chap 3).

Patient & Family Education

- Stop drug and notify physician if skin ulceration, hypersensitivity, or infection occur.
- Report any signs of local adverse reactions to physicians.
- Do not apply to face unless directed by physician.
- Treated skin should not be bandaged unless directed by physician.
- Do not use tight-fitting diapers or plastic pants on child being treated in diaper area.

Prototype: morphine, p 156

ALFENTANIL HYDROCHLORIDE
(al-fen´ta-nill)
Trade name: Alfenta
Classifications: CNS AGENT; NARCOTIC (OPIATE) AGONIST ANALGESIC; GENERAL ANESTHETIC
Pregnancy: Category C
Controlled substance: Schedule II

ACTIONS/PHARMACODYNAMICS Narcotic agonist analgesic with rapid onset and short duration of action. Brief duration is advantageous for short surgical procedures but necessitates incremental injections or continuous infusion for long operations. CNS effects of alfentanil appear to be related to interaction of drug with opiate receptors. Suppresses increase in plasma concentrations of stress response hormones (antidiuretic hormone and growth hormone), although clinical significance of this action during surgery is unclear. Tolerance to analgesic effects of alfentanil infusion has not been observed.

USES Major component of balanced anesthesia; analgesic, analgesic supplement, and primary anesthetic for induction of anesthesia when endotracheal and mechanical ventilation are required.

PHARMACOKINETICS Onset: 2 min. **Duration:** injection 30 min; continuous infusion 45 min. **Distribution:** crosses placenta. **Metabolism:** completely

metabolized in liver. **Elimination:** half-life: 46–213 min; excreted in breast milk.

ROUTE & DOSAGE

Anesthesia Induction

Adult	IV	8–20 μg/kg for surgery lasting ≤ 30 min; maintenance anesthesia can be maintained with incremental doses of 3–5 μg/kg *or* a continuous infusion of 0.5–1 μg/kg/min (total dose of 8–40 μg/kg)

CONTRAINDICATIONS & PRECAUTIONS Contraindicated in: safe use during pregnancy (category C), in children <12 y, or during lactation not established. **Cautious use in:** elderly, history of pulmonary disease.

ADVERSE/SIDE EFFECTS CV: hypotension, hypertension, tachycardia, bradycardia. **GI:** *nausea,* vomiting, anorexia, constipation, cramps. **Respiratory:** apnea, respiratory depression, dyspnea. **Other:** dizziness; thoracic muscle rigidity; pruritus, euphoria, drowsiness, flushing, rash, diaphoresis; extremities feel heavy and warm.

DRUG INTERACTIONS BETA-ADRENERGIC BLOCKERS increase incidence of bradycardia; CNS DEPRESSANTS such as BARBITURATES, TRANQUILIZERS, NEUROMUSCULAR BLOCKING AGENTS, OPIATES, and INHALATION GENERAL ANESTHETICS may enhance the cardiovascular and CNS effects of alfentanil both in magnitude and duration when administered with alfentanil; enhancement or prolongation of postoperative respiratory depression also may result from concomitant administration of any of these agents with alfentanil.

NURSING IMPLICATIONS

Administration

- Alfentanil has been administered by devices for patient-controlled analgesia.
- ***Preparation of solution:*** compatibility has been demonstrated in solution (concentration range: 25–80 μg/ml) with diluents: normal saline, 5% dextrose in normal saline, D5W, and lactated Ringer's.
- Alfentanil is available in concentrations of 500 μg (as HCl) per milliliter. When 20 ml of alfentanil is added to 230 ml of compatible IV solution, the resulting concentration is 40 μg/ml.
- Store at 15–30C (59–86F). Avoid freezing.

Common side effects in *italic*; life-threatening effects <u>underlined</u>; generic names in **bold**; classifications in SMALL CAPS

Assessment & Drug Effects

- If a narcotic antagonist has been administered to overcome residual effects of alfentanil, observe patient frequently for symptoms of increased sympathetic stimulation (arrhythmias) and for evidence of depressed postoperative analgesia (tachycardia, pain, pupillary dilation, spontaneous muscle movement).
- Monitor vital signs at regular intervals during recovery period: check for bradycardia, especially if patient is also taking a beta-blocker.
- When alfentanil is used as a postoperative analgesic, many patients experience dizziness, sedation, nausea and vomiting.
- Adequacy of spontaneous ventilation must be evaluated carefully during postoperative period. Monitor chest wall movement and quality of respirations.
- Drug's narcotic effects wear off quickly with neglible residual effects.

Patient & Family Education

- If drug is used for patient-controlled analgesia, instruct patient to report unpleasant side effects.

Prototype: colchicine, p 46

ALLOPURINOL

(al-oh-pure´i-nole)
Trade names: Lopurin, Zurinol, Zyloprim
Classification: ANTIGOUT AGENT
Pregnancy: Category C

ACTIONS/PHARMACODYNAMICS In contrast to uricosuric agents, which act by increasing renal excretion of uric acid, allopurinol reduces endogenous uric acid by selectively inhibiting action of xanthine oxidase, enzyme responsible for converting hypo-xanthine to xanthine and xanthine to uric acid (end product of purine catabolism). Thus, urate pool is decreased by the lowering of both serum and urinary uric acid levels, and hyperuricosuria is prevented. Has no analgesic, antiinflammatory, or uricosuric actions; therefore not useful for acute gouty attack and may actually aggravate and prolong it. May inhibit hepatic microsomal enzymes and thus affect metabolism of certain drugs. Unlike uricosuric agents, action is not antagonized by salicylates.

USES To control primary hyperuricemia that accompanies severe gout and to prevent possibility of flare-up of acute gouty attack; to prevent recurrent calcium oxalate stones; prophylactically to reduce severity of hyperuricemia associated with antineoplastic and radiation therapies, both of which greatly increase plasma uric acid levels by promoting nucleic acid degradation. **Unlabeled use:** to reduce hyperuricemia secondary to Lesch-Nyhan syndrome, polycythemia vera, G6PD deficiency, sarcoidosis, and therapy with thiazides or ethambutol.

ROUTE & DOSAGE

Hyperuricemia

Adult	PO	100 mg/d; may increase by 100 mg/wk (max 800 mg/d); doses >300 mg/d should be divided

Secondary Hyperuricemia

Adult	PO	200–800 mg/d for 2–3 d or longer; doses >300 mg/d should be divided
Child	PO	6–10 y: 100 mg t.i.d. <6 y: 50 mg t.i.d.

PHARMACOKINETICS Absorption: 80–90% absorbed from GI tract. **Onset:** 24–48 h. **Peak:** 2–6 h. **Metabolism:** 75–80% metabolizes to the active metabolite oxypurinol. **Elimination:** half-life: 1–3 h (half-life of oxypurinol: 18–30 h); slowly excreted in urine; excreted in breast milk.

CONTRAINDICATIONS & PRECAUTIONS Contraindicated in: hypersensitivity to allopurinol; as initial treatment for acute gouty attacks; idiopathic hemochromatosis (or those with family history); children (except those with hyperuricemia secondary to neoplastic disease and chemotherapy). Safe use during pregnancy (category C) and in nursing mothers not established. **Cautious use in:** impaired hepatic or renal function, history of peptic ulcer, lower GI tract disease, bone marrow depression.

ADVERSE/SIDE EFFECTS CNS: drowsiness, headache, vertigo. **GI:** nausea, vomiting, diarrhea, abdominal discomfort, indigestion, malaise. **Hematologic:** agranulocytosis, aplastic anemia, transient leukopenia or leukocytosis, bone marrow depression, pancytopenia, thrombocytopenia. **Skin:** urticaria or pruritus, pruritic maculopapular rash, toxic epidermal necrolysis. **Other:** hepatotoxicity, xanthine renal calculi.

DIAGNOSTIC TEST INTERFERENCES Possibility of elevated blood levels of *alkaline phos-*

Common side effects in *italic*; life-threatening effects underlined; generic names in **bold**; classifications in SMALL CAPS

phatase and *serum transaminases* (AST, ALT), and decreased blood *Hct, Hgb, leukocytes.*

DRUG INTERACTIONS Alcohol may inhibit renal excretion of uric acid; **ampicillin, amoxicillin** increase risk of skin rash; enhances anticoagulant effect of **warfarin;** toxicity from **azathioprine, mercaptopurine, cyclophosphamide** increased; increases hypoglycemic effects of **chlorpropamide;** THIAZIDES increase risk of allopurinol toxicity and hypersensitivity (especially with impaired renal function).

NURSING IMPLICATIONS

Administration

- Best tolerated when taken following meals; tablet may be crushed and taken with fluid or mixed with food.
- When used with antineoplastic therapy, allopurinol should be prescribed 1 or 2 d before chemotherapy begins.
- Store at 15–30C (59–86F) in a tightly closed container.

Assessment & Drug Effects

- Baseline CBC and liver and kidney function tests should be performed before therapy is initiated and then monthly, particularly during first few months of therapy.
- Aim of therapy is to lower serum urate level gradually to about 6 mg/dl. Serum uric acid levels should be evaluated at least every 1–2 wk to check adequacy of dosage. A sudden decrease in serum uric acid can precipitate an acute gouty attack.
- Acute gouty attacks are most likely during first 6 wk of therapy, possibly because of mobilization of urates from tissue deposits. Concurrent prophylactic therapy with colchicine may be prescribed, for the first 3–6 mo of therapy.
- Monitor I&O ratio and pattern. Decreased renal function causes drug accumulation.
- Urinary pH should be checked at regular intervals. Excessive alkalinity can make uric acid stones more difficult to dissolve.
- The elderly and patients with renal disorders tend to have a higher than usual incidence of renal stones and drug toxicity including dermatologic (hypersensitivity) problems.
- A life-threatening toxicity syndrome has occurred 2–4 wk after initiation of therapy, commonly in patients with impaired renal function, and is generally accompanied by malaise, fever, and aching, a diffuse erythematous, desquamating rash, hepatic dysfunction, eosinophilia, and worsening of renal function. Report immediately to physician the onset of rash or fever. Drug should be withdrawn.
- Therapeutic response is indicated by normal serum and urinary uric acid levels (usually by 1–3 wk), gradual decrease in size of tophi, absence of new tophaceous deposits (after approximately 6 mo), with consequent relief of joint pain and increased joint mobility.

Patient & Family Education

- It is advisable to maintain fluid intake sufficient to produce urinary output of at least 2000 ml/d (fluid intake of at least 3000 ml/d). Instruct patient to report diminishing urinary output, cloudy urine, unusual color or odor to urine, pain or discomfort on urination.
- Instruct patient to report promptly the onset of itching or rash, especially if ampicillin is prescribed concurrently.
- A skin rash, which may appear after 1–5 wk (and reportedly even after 2 y) of therapy, is the most common adverse reaction and is an indication to stop drug therapy.
- Physician may advise patient to limit high purine foods, e.g., organ meats (e.g., kidney, liver), anchovies, sardines, salmon, meat soups, gravies, dried peas and beans, asparagus, cauliflower, mushrooms, spinach, peppers.
- For treatment of oxalate stones, advise patient to abstain from high oxalate foods: tea, chocolate, rhubarb, spinach, nuts, beets, figs, peppers.
- Advise patient to minimize exposure and to shield eyes from ultraviolet or sunlight. Ultraviolet light may stimulate the development of cataracts. Patients should be examined periodically for lens changes.
- Caution patient to avoid driving or performing other complex tasks until reaction to drug has been evaluated.
- Allopurinol is generally continued indefinitely; patient should remain under medical supervision. The drug can cause severe adverse reactions.

ALPHA₁-PROTEINASE INHIBITOR (HUMAN)

(pro´ten-ase)
Trade name: Prolastin
Classification: ENZYME INHIBITOR
Pregnancy: Category C

ACTIONS/PHARMACODYNAMICS Alpha₁-proteinase inhibitor (α_1-PI; α_1-antitrypsin) is extracted

Common side effects in *italic*; life-threatening effects underlined; generic names in **bold**; classifications in SMALL CAPS

275

from plasma and used in patients with panacinar emphysema who have α_1-antitrypsin deficiency. α_1-Antitrypsin deficiency is a chronic, hereditary, and usually fatal autosomal recessive disorder that results in a slowly progressive, panacinar emphysema. It is believed to be due to a chemical imbalance of elastase and its primary inhibitor, α_1-PI. As a result, elastin structures of the alveoli are destroyed by elastase.

USES Indicated for chronic replacement therapy in patients with α_1-antitrypsin deficiency and demonstrable panacinar emphysema.

ROUTE & DOSAGE

Adult	IV	60 mg/kg once weekly administered at a rate of ≥0.08 ml/kg/min

PHARMACOKINETICS Distribution: crosses placenta; distributed into breast milk. **Metabolism:** undergoes catabolism in the intravascular space; approximately 33% is catabolized per day, with estimated production levels of 34 mg/kg/d. **Elimination:** half-life: 4.5–5.2 d.

CONTRAINDICATIONS & PRECAUTIONS Contraindicated in: individuals with selective IgA deficiencies. **Cautious use in:** patients with significant heart disease or other conditions that may be aggravated with slight increases in plasma volume. During pregnancy use only when clearly needed and when the potential benefits outweigh the potential hazards to the fetus. Safety and efficacy in children has not been established.

ADVERSE/SIDE EFFECTS Hematologic: leukocytosis. **CNS:** dizziness, fever (may be delayed). **Other:** Hepatitis B if not immunized

NURSING IMPLICATIONS

Administration
- Reconstitute with sterile water for injection supplied by manufacturer to yield a concentration of 20 mg/ml.
- Administer within 3 h after reconstitution. Give alone, without mixing with other agents. If necessary, it may be diluted with normal saline.
- Administer properly diluted drug by direct IV injection at rate of at least 0.08 ml/kg/min.
- Administration by intermittent or continuous infusion not recommended.

- Hepatitis B vaccine should be administered prior to utilizing this drug.
- Refrigerate unreconstituted drug at 2–8C (35–46F). Do not refrigerate after reconstitution. Discard unused solution.

Assessment & Drug Effects
- Monitor serum α_1-PI level. Minimum serum concentration level should be 80 mg/ml.
- Assess respiratory status (rate, dyspnea, lung sounds) prior to any therapy.
- Caution should be used in patients at risk for circulatory overload.

Patient & Family Education
- Advise patient to avoid smoking and notify physician of any changes in respiratory pattern.

Prototype: lorazepam, p 177

ALPRAZOLAM
(al-pray´zoe-lam)
Trade name: Xanax
Classifications: CNS AGENT; BENZODIAZEPINE ANXIOLYTIC, SEDATIVE-HYPNOTIC
Pregnancy: Category D
Controlled substance: Schedule IV

ACTIONS/PHARMACODYNAMICS CNS depressant. Mode of action not known but appears to act at the limbic, thalamic, and hypothalamic levels of the CNS. Compared to most drugs of this class, the possibility of drug accumulation is minimal; duration of activity is relatively short, and it is associated with significantly less drowsiness. Has antidepressant as well as anxiolytic actions.

USES Management of anxiety disorders or for short-term relief of anxiety symptoms. Also used as adjunct in management of anxiety associated with depression and agitation and for panic disorders, such as agoraphobia.

ROUTE & DOSAGE

Anxiety Disorders

Adult	PO	0.25–0.5 mg t.i.d. (max 4 mg/d)

Panic Attacks

Adult	PO	1–2 mg t.i.d. (max 8 mg/d)

Common side effects in *italic*; life-threatening effects underlined; generic names in **bold**; classifications in SMALL CAPS

PHARMACOKINETICS **Absorption:** rapidly absorbed. **Peak:** 1–2 h. **Distribution:** crosses placenta. **Metabolism:** oxidized in liver to inactive metabolites. **Elimination:** half-life: 12–15 h; renal elimination.

CONTRAINDICATIONS & PRECAUTIONS **Contraindicated in:** sensitivity to benzodiazepines; acute narrow angle glaucoma; pulmonary disease; use alone in primary depression or psychotic disorders; during pregnancy (category D), in nursing mothers and children <18 y. **Cautious use in:** impaired renal or hepatic function; history of alcoholism; geriatric and debilitated patients. Effectiveness for long-term treatment (>4 mo) not established.

ADVERSE/SIDE EFFECTS **CNS:** *drowsiness, sedation,* light-headedness, dizziness, syncope, depression, headache, confusion, insomnia, nervousness, fatigue, clumsiness, unsteadiness, rigidity, tremor, restlessness, paradoxical excitement, hallucinations, muscle spasticity. **CV:** tachycardia, hypotension, ECG changes. **Skin:** itching. **Other:** blurred vision, dyspnea, slurred speech.

DRUG INTERACTIONS **Alcohol** and other CNS DEPRESSANTS, ANTICONVULSANTS, ANTIHISTAMINES, BARBITURATES, NARCOTIC ANALGESICS, BENZODIAZEPINES compound CNS depressant effects; **cimetidine, disulfiram** increase alprazolam effects (decreased metabolism); ORAL CONTRACEPTIVES may increase or decrease alprazolam effects.

NURSING IMPLICATIONS

Administration

- May be administered without regard to meals.
- Store in light-resistant containers at 15–30C (59–86F), unless otherwise directed.

Assessment & Drug Effects

- Patients receiving continuing therapy should have periodic blood counts, urinalyses, and blood chemistry studies.
- Drowsiness and sedation are the most common side effects. Monitor especially the elderly or debilitated, who may require supervised ambulation or side rails.

Patient & Family Education

- Adverse reactions, which may occur during early high dose therapy, usually disappear with continuing therapy. Advise patient to keep physician informed; dosage adjustments may be indicated.

Instruct patient to make position changes slowly and in stages.

- Alprazolam potentiates effects of alcoholic beverages and other CNS depressants; caution patient not to use them or OTC medications containing antihistamines (sleep aids, cold, hayfever or allergy remedies) without consulting physician.
- Advise patient to avoid driving and other potentially hazardous activities until reaction to drug is determined.
- Following continuous use, dosage should be tapered off before drug is stopped. Abrupt discontinuation of drug may cause **withdrawal symptoms:** nausea, vomiting, abdominal and muscle cramps, sweating, confusion, tremors, convulsions.

Prototype: dinoprostone, p 251

ALPROSTADIL (PGE$_1$)
(al-pross′ta-dil)
Trade name: Prostin VR Pediatric
Classification: PROSTAGLANDIN

ACTIONS/PHARMACODYNAMICS Actions include vasodilation, inhibition of platelet aggregation, and stimulation of intestinal and uterine smooth muscles. Preserves ductal patency by relaxing smooth muscle of ductus arteriosus. This results in improved oxygenation of blood and perfusion of lower body of neonates with congenital cardiac anomalies. In high doses, lowers BP by reducing peripheral resistance. Heart rate and cardiac output may rise reflexly.

USES Temporary measure to maintain patency of ductus arteriosus in infants with ductal-dependent congenital heart defects until corrective surgery can be performed.

ROUTE & DOSAGE

Maintain Patency of Ductus Arteriosus		
Child	IV/Intraarterial/Intraaortic	0.05–0.1 µg/kg/min; may increase gradually to max of 0.4 µg/kg/min if necessary

PHARMACOKINETICS **Onset:** 15 min to 3 h. **Metabolism:** rapidly metabolized in lungs. **Elimination:** half-life: 5–10 min; metabolites excreted through kidneys.

Common side effects in *italic*; life-threatening effects underlined;
generic names in **bold**; classifications in SMALL CAPS

277

A

CONTRAINDICATIONS & PRECAUTIONS Contraindicated in: respiratory distress syndrome (hyaline membrane disease). **Cautious use in:** bleeding tendencies.

ADVERSE/SIDE EFFECTS CNS: *fever,* seizures; lethargy. **CV:** *flushing,* bradycardia, hypotension, tachycardia; CHF, ventricular fibrillation, shock. **GI:** diarrhea, gastric regurgitation. **Hematologic:** disseminated intravascular coagulation (DIC), thrombocytopenia. **Renal (infrequent):** oliguria, anuria, hematuria. **Respiratory:** apnea. **Other:** rash on face and arms, alopecia.

NURSING IMPLICATIONS

Administration

- Infusion solution is prepared by diluting 500 μg alprostadil with NaCl or dextrose injection to volume appropriate for pump delivery system. Prepare fresh solution q24h. Discard unused portions.
- A 500 μg ampule diluted in 250 ml yields a concentration of 2 μg/ml.
- May be infused at rate of 0.05–0.1 μg/kg/min up to a maximum of 0.4 μg/kg/min.
- Infusion rate should be reduced immediately if arterial pressure drops significantly or if fever occurs. If apnea or bradycardia occurs, infusion should be discontinued promptly.
- Flushing (peripheral arterial vasodilation) is usually controlled by repositioning catheter (by qualified personnel).
- Prolonged infusion not recommended because it increases risk of ductal rupture, by contributing to its fragility, and increases risk of damage to pulmonary artery and aorta.
- Store at 2–8C (36–46F) unless otherwise directed by manufacturer. Protect from freezing.

Assessment & Drug Effects

- Arterial pressure is measured intermittently throughout infusion by umbilical cord catheter, auscultation, or with Doppler transducer.
- Cardiovascular and CNS symptoms, including apnea, reportedly occur more frequently in neonates weighing less than 2 kg (4.4 lb) at birth, during first hour of drug infusion.
- Monitor intermittently throughout the infusion (1) arterial pressure, (2) arterial blood gases PO_2 and PCO_2, (3) arterial blood pH, (4) ECG, (5) heart rate, (6) BP, (7) respiratory rate, and (8) rectal temperature.
- With aortic arch abnormalities, also monitor for systemic BP, pulmonary artery and descending aorta pressures, return of palpable femoral pulse, and urinary output.
- Therapeutic response in infants with cyanotic heart disease (restricted pulmonary blood flow) is indicated by increase in blood oxygenation (PO_2), usually evident within 30 min. **Normal PO_2 for neonates;** 60–70 mm Hg.
- Therapeutic response in infants with restricted systemic blood flow is indicated by increased pH in those with acidosis; increased systemic BP and urinary output, return of palpable pulses, and decreased ratio of pulmonary artery to aortic pressure.

Prototype: streptokinase, p 134

ALTEPLASE RECOMBINANT (t-PA)

(al´te-plase)
Trade names: Actilyse, Activase
Classifications: BLOOD FORMER; THROMBOLYTIC ENZYME
Pregnancy: Category C

ACTIONS/PHARMACODYNAMICS This recombinant DNA–derived form of human tissue–type plasminogen activator (t-PA) is a thrombolytic agent. In contrast to anticoagulants, which prevent propagation of thrombi, t-PA and plasminogen activators such as streptokinase promote thrombolysis by hydrolyzing the arginine-valine peptide bond in plasminogen to form the active proteolytic enzyme plasmin. Plasmin is capable of degrading fibrin, fibrinogen, and factors V, VIII, and XII.

USES Indicated in selective cases of acute MI, preferably within 6 h of attack for recanalization of the coronary artery. **Unlabeled use:** in limited number of cases for lysis of acute pulmonary emboli and lysis of arterial occlusions in peripheral vessels and bypass vessels.

ROUTE & DOSAGE

Acute MI

Adult	IV	60 mg over first hour, with 6–10 mg infused over first 1–2 min; then 20 mg/h over next 2 h (100 mg over 3 h)

PHARMACOKINETICS Peak: 5–10 min after infusion completed. **Duration:** baseline values restored in

3 h. **Metabolism:** metabolized in liver. **Elimination:** half-life: 26.5 min; excreted in urine.

CONTRAINDICATIONS & PRECAUTIONS Con-
traindicated in: active internal bleeding, history of cerebrovascular accident, recent (within 2 mo) intracranial or interspinal surgery or trauma, intercranial neoplasm, arteriovenous malformation, bleeding disorders, and severe uncontrolled hypertension. **Cautious use in:** pregnancy (category C), recent major surgery (within 10 d), cerebral vascular disease, recent GI or GU bleeding, recent trauma, hypertension, >75 y, hemorrhagic ophthalmic conditions, current use of oral anticoagulants.

ADVERSE/SIDE EFFECTS Hematologic: internal and superficial bleeding (cerebral, retroperitoneal, GU, GI).

NURSING IMPLICATIONS

Administration

- IV infusion of alteplase should be started as soon as possible after the thrombolytic event, preferably within 6 h.
- **Reconstitution:** do not use a vial if vacuum has been broken. Dilute contents of vial with sterile water for injection supplied by manufacturer. Use a large-bore needle (e.g., 18 gauge). Slight foaming is usual. Resulting concentration is 1 mg/ml.
- Drug may be administered as reconstituted (1 mg/ml) or further diluted with an equal volume of NS or D5W to yield 0.5 mg/ml.
- For **acute MI:** administer 60% of total dose in the first hour with 6–10 mg given as a bolus dose over 1–2 min and remainder of first dose infused over hour 1. Follow with second dose (20% of total) over hour 2, and third dose (20% of total) over hour 3.
- For **pulmonary embolism:** administer entire dose over a 2 h period.
- For **patients weighing <65 kg:** calculate dose using 1.25 mg/kg over 3 h.
- Do not exceed a total dose of 100 mg. Higher doses have been associated with intracranial bleeding.
- Follow infusion of drug by flushing IV tubing with 30–50 ml of NS or D5W.
- If serious bleeding in a critical location (intracranial, GI, retroperitoneal, pericardial) occurs, immediately discontinue alteplase and any concomitant heparin therapy.
- Reconstituted drug is stable for 8 h in above solutions at room temperature (2–30C; 36–86F). Since there are no preservatives, discard any unused solution after that time.

- While patient is receiving this medication, do not allow patient out of bed.

Assessment & Drug Effects

- Before administration, coagulation tests need to be done including APTT, bleeding time, PT, TT.
- Blood for Hct, Hgb, and platelet count should be drawn before administration for baseline values in case of bleeding.
- Check vital signs frequently. Be alert to changes in cardiac rhythm. Dysrhythmias signal need to stop therapy at once.
- Monitor for excess bleeding q15min for the first hour of therapy, q30min for second to eighth hour, then q8h.
- Monitor neurological checks throughout drug infusion q30min and qh for the first 8 h after infusion.
- Spontaneous bleeding occurs twice as often with alteplase as with heparin. Protect patient from invasive procedures: IM injections are contraindicated. Also prevent physical manipulation of patient during thrombolytic therapy to prevent bruising.
- Report **signs of bleeding:** gum bleeding, epistaxis, hematoma, spontaneous ecchymoses, oozing at catheter site, increased pain from internal bleeding. The alteplase infusion should be interrupted, then resumed when bleeding stops.
- If blood gas determination is needed, select the radial rather than the femoral artery because of greater ease in applying a pressure dressing to control oozing. Pressure to puncture sites, if necessary, should be maintained for up to 30 min.
- Inquire about pregnancy, recent delivery, recent surgery of any type, as these increase the risk of bleeding.
- Patient is at risk for postthrombolytic bleeding for 2–4 d after intracoronary alteplase treatment. Continue monitoring vital signs until laboratory reports confirm anticoagulant control.
- Hct should be drawn following drug administration to detect possible blood loss.

Patient & Family Education

- Patient should report immediately a sudden severe headache.
- Patient should report blood in urine and bloody or tarry stools.
- Patient should report if there is any sign of bleeding or oozing from cuts or places of injection.
- While receiving this medicine, patient should move around as little as possible and not get out of bed when alone.
- To help prevent serious bleeding, advise patient to

Common side effects in *italic*; life-threatening effects <u>underlined</u>; generic names in **bold**; classifications in SMALL CAPS

279

follow instructions given by physician very carefully.

▪ Instruct patient to report any unusual or allergic reactions to alteplase, anistreplase, streptokinase, or urokinase. Also report allergy to any other substances such as food, preservatives, or dyes.

ALUMINUM ACETATE SOLUTION

Trade names: Acid Mantie, Bluboro, Burow's Solution, Modified Burow's Solution, Domeboro, Otic Domeboro, Pedi-Boro
Classifications: SKIN & MUCOUS MEMBRANE AGENT; ANTIINFLAMMATORY; ANTIPRURITIC

ACTIONS/PHARMACODYNAMICS Modified Burow's solution contains aluminum sulfate and calcium acetate. Has antiinflammatory, antipruritic, mild astringent, and antiseptic properties. Reportedly maintains protective acidity of skin.

USES Mildly irritated or inflamed skin and mucous membranes. Also has been used as astringent gargle, as irrigating solution to remove tissue debris, and for soaks, douche, and sitz bath.

ROUTE & DOSAGE

Wet Dressings
Adult   Topical   1:10–1:40 solution applied for 15–30 min q4–8h

Gargle
Adult   Topical   1:10 solution

Otic Preparation
Adult   Topical   4–6 drops instilled slowly along wall of external ear q2–3h

---

DRUG INTERACTIONS Enzyme activity of **topical collagenase** inhibited by aluminum acetate solution.

NURSING IMPLICATIONS

Administration
▪ Following instillation of otic preparation (e.g., Otic Domeboro), have patient maintain position with affected ear uppermost for about 2 min. If physician prescribes an ear wick, solution may be added to wick as often as directed.
▪ For wet dressings, warm or cold solution (as or-

dered) may be carefully poured on dressing at prescribed intervals. May be bandaged lightly and loosely, but do not cover with plastic or other occlusive material without consulting the physician.
▪ Protect eyes from solution.
▪ Burow's and modified Burow's solutions have limited compatibility with vitamin A, neomycin, and other water-soluble antibiotics.
▪ The activity of products containing benzalkonium chloride, e.g., Buro-Sol, is antagonized by soap and soap substitutes such as pHisoHex and pHisoDerm. If these agents have been used, skin should be rinsed thoroughly prior to treatment.
▪ Store drug below 30C (86F). Avoid freezing.

Assessment & Drug Effects
▪ Use should be discontinued if irritation or extension of inflammatory condition occurs.

Patient & Family Education
▪ Instruct patient in proper technique of administration.

Prototype: aluminum hydroxide, p 212

ALUMINUM CARBONATE, BASIC

Trade name: Basaljel
Classifications: GI AGENT; ANTACID
Pregnancy: Category C

ACTIONS/PHARMACODYNAMICS Nonsystemic antacid with actions, uses, contraindications, and adverse reactions similar to those of aluminum hydroxide. (Acid neutralizing capacity is 13 or 14 mEq for tablet, capsule, and suspension, and 22 mEq for extra strength suspension.) Demonstrates greatest phosphate-binding capacity of all aluminum-containing antacids. Lowers serum phosphate by binding dietary and GI phosphates to form insoluble, nonabsorbable aluminum phosphate, which is excreted in feces. This prevents formation of phosphatic urinary calculi by decreasing excretion of phosphate in urine.

USES Primarily in conjunction with a low phosphate diet to reduce hyperphosphatemia in patients with renal insufficiency and for prophylaxis and treatment of phosphatic renal calculi. Also used as an antacid.

PHARMACOKINETICS Absorption: minimal absorption. **Peak:** slow onset. **Elimination:** excreted in feces as insoluble phosphates.

Common side effects in *italic*; life-threatening effects underlined; generic names in **bold**; classifications in SMALL CAPS

ROUTE & DOSAGE

Antacid

Adult   PO   5–10 ml of regular suspension, *or* 2.5–5 ml of extra strength suspension, or 2 capsules or tablets q2h

Phosphate Lowering

Adult   PO   10–30 ml of regular suspension, *or* 5–15 ml of extra strength suspension, or 2–6 capsules or tablets 1h p.c. and h.s.

CONTRAINDICATIONS & PRECAUTIONS Contraindicated in: patients on fluid restriction or who are dehydrated; decreased bowel motility (e.g., patients receiving anticholinergics, antidiarrheals, antispasmodics), intestinal obstruction. Pregnancy: category C. **Cautious use in:** elderly patients; impaired renal function; patients on sodium restriction.

ADVERSE/SIDE EFFECTS Constipation, fecal impaction, intestinal obstruction, hypophosphatemia, transient hypercalciuria, calcium and vitamin A deficiency.

DRUG INTERACTIONS Aluminum will decrease the absorption of **chloroquine, cimetidine, ciprofloxacin, digoxin, isoniazid, iron salts,** NONSTEROIDAL ANTIINFLAMMATORY DRUGS, **norfloxacin, ofloxacin, phenytoin,** PHENOTHIAZINES, **quinidine, tetracycline, thyroxine.**

NURSING IMPLICATIONS

Administration

- Antacid dose may be followed by a little water to assure passage into stomach; it is generally given between meals and at bedtime.
- For serum phosphate lowering or prevention of phosphate stones, mix dose in a full glass of water or fruit juice. Usually given 1 h p.c.
- Aluminum carbonate contains CO_2. On exposure to air, CO_2 is lost; therefore, keep container tightly covered.
- Store in a tight container at 15–30C (59–86F) unless otherwise directed by manufacturer.

Assessment & Drug Effects

- If used to control urinary calculi, measure and record I&O, and strain all urine. Monitor for evidence of bleeding and infection: fever, chills, dysuria, and hematuria.
- Excessive doses for prolonged periods can lead to hypophosphatemia (see Signs & Symptoms, chap 3). In general, hypophosphatemia is a problem only in patients who are also on a low phosphate diet or who have sustained diarrhea.
- Periodic determinations should be made of urinary pH and serum calcium, phosphates, and other electrolytes in patients on long-term therapy.
- Note number and consistency of stools; intestinal obstruction from fecal concretions is a possibility.

Patient & Family Education

- Physician will prescribe a high fluid intake for the patient with urinary calculi. The amount prescribed is variable. Some sources suggest 10 or more glasses of fluid daily; some recommend daily intake in excess of 3000 ml; others advise sufficient liquids to produce a daily urinary output at least 2000–3000 ml or more.
- A moderate acid ash diet may be used to acidify the urine to discourage phosphate calculi formation. *High acid ash foods:* eggs, meat, fish, poultry, corn, lentils, breads, pasta, bacon, cranberry juice, plums, prunes. Ascorbic acid also has been used to acidify urine. Low phosphorus diet may be used to treat hyperphosphatemia. Restrictions may be placed on the following **high phosphorus foods:** milk and selected milk products, eggs, fish, lean meat, carbonated beverages, fruits, instant beverages sold as powders.
- Patients on sodium restriction should be advised about sodium content of the various forms of aluminum carbonate.

ALUMINUM HYDROXIDE

See GASTROINTESTINAL AGENT, ANTACID, ADSORBENT prototype, p 212.

Prototype: aluminum hydroxide, p 212

ALUMINUM PHOSPHATE

Trade name: Phosphaljel
Classification: ANTACID
Pregnancy: Category C

ACTIONS/PHARMACODYNAMICS Slow-acting nonsystemic antacid with properties similar to those of aluminum hydroxide but does not increase fecal

Common side effects in *italic*; life-threatening effects <u>underlined</u>; generic names in **bold**; classifications in SMALL CAPS

281

excretion of phosphate. Has one fourth the acid neutralizing capacity of aluminum hydroxide.

USES Antacid in preference to aluminum hydroxide gel when a high phosphorus diet cannot be maintained or to reverse hypophosphatemia induced by aluminum hydroxide, or in patients with diarrhea or pancreatic insufficiency.

ROUTE & DOSAGE

Antacid
Adult   PO   600 mg t.i.d. or q.i.d.

PHARMACOKINETICS Absorption: minimal absorption. **Peak:** slow onset. **Duration:** 2 h when taken with food; 3 h when taken 1 h after food. **Elimination:** excreted in feces as insoluble phosphates.

CONTRAINDICATIONS & PRECAUTIONS Contraindicated in: high dose therapy in patients with impaired renal function or who are on sodium-restricted diets. **Cautious use in:** pregnancy (category C).

ADVERSE/SIDE EFFECTS Constipation, hyperphosphatemia, intestinal obstruction.

DRUG INTERACTIONS Aluminum will decrease the absorption of **chloroquine, cimetidine, ciprofloxacin, digoxin, isoniazid, iron salts,** NONSTEROIDAL ANTIINFLAMMATORY DRUGS, **norfloxacin, ofloxacin, phenytoin,** PHENOTHIAZINES, **quinidine, tetracycline, thyroxine.**

NURSING IMPLICATIONS

Administration
- Antacid dose is generally given between meals (2 h p.c.) and at bedtime.
- May be given undiluted and followed by sufficient liquid to assure passage into stomach.

Assessment & Drug Effects
- Monitor I&O ratio and pattern and serum phosphate levels in patients receiving prolonged therapy.
- If serum phosphate level is elevated (normal: 2.5–4.5 mg/dl), a low phosphate diet may be prescribed (e.g., decreased intake of milk and dairy products).
- Note number and consistency of stools. If constipation is a problem, physician may prescribe concurrent therapy with a magnesium antacid, or administration of a laxative or stool softener as needed.

Patient & Family Education
- Instruct patient to increase fiber in diet and fluid intake (if not contraindicated) if constipation is a problem.
- Advise use of a stool softener as needed to relieve constipation.

Prototype: acyclovir, p 85

AMANTADINE HYDROCHLORIDE
(a-man´ta-deen)
Trade name: Symmetrel
Classifications: ANTIINFECTIVE; ANTIVIRAL; AUTONOMIC NERVOUS SYSTEM AGENT; ANTICHOLINERGIC (PARASYMPATHOLYTIC); ANTIPARKINSONISM AGENT
Pregnancy: Category C

ACTIONS/PHARMACODYNAMICS Synthetic primary amine with virostatic action. Believed to act by inhibiting penetration of host cell by virus or by preventing uncoating of viral nucleic acid. Because it does not suppress antibody formation, it can be administered for interim protection in combination with influenza A virus vaccine until antibody titer is adequate or to augment prophylaxis in a previously vaccinated individual. Active against several strains of influenza A virus; not effective against influenza B infections. Has mild anticholinergic activity. Mechanism of action in parkinsonism not understood, but may be related to release of dopamine and other catecholamines from neuronal storage sites and also to anticholinergic effects. Reportedly less effective than levodopa, but produces more rapid clinical response and causes fewer adverse reactions.

USES In initial therapy or as adjunct with anticholinergic drugs or levodopa in treatment of all forms of parkinsonism (arteriosclerotic, idiopathic, postencephalitic) and for relief of drug-induced extrapyramidal reactions, and symptomatic parkinsonism caused by carbon monoxide poisoning. Also used for prophylaxis and symptomatic treatment of influenza A infections. **Unlabeled use:** primary enuresis, pseudosclerosis, neuroleptic malignant syndrome (NMS), management of cocaine dependency and withdrawal.

PHARMACOKINETICS Absorption: readily and almost completely absorbed from GI tract. **Onset:** within 48 h. **Peak:** 1–4 h. **Distribution:** distributed to saliva, nasal secretions, breast milk, placenta, CSF. **Metabolism:** not metabolized. **Elimination:** half-life: 9–37 h (prolonged in renal insufficiency); 90% excreted unchanged in urine.

ROUTE & DOSAGE

Influenza A

Adult	PO	200 mg once/d or 100 mg q12h
Child	PO	1–9y: 4.4–8.8 mg/kg in 2–3 equal doses (max 150 mg/d)

Parkinsonism

Adult	PO	100 mg 1–2 times/d; start with 100 mg/d if patient is on other antiparkinsonism medications

Drug-induced Extrapyramidal Symptoms

Adult	PO	100 mg b.i.d., up to 400 mg/d if needed

CONTRAINDICATIONS & PRECAUTIONS Contraindicated in: safe use during pregnancy (category C), in nursing mothers, and in children <1 y not established. **Cautious use in:** history of epilepsy or other types of seizures; CHF, peripheral edema, orthostatic hypotension; recurrent eczematoid dermatitis; psychoses, severe psychoneuroses; hepatic disease; renal impairment; elderly patients with cerebral arteriosclerosis.

ADVERSE/SIDE EFFECTS Usually dose related. **CNS:** *dizziness, light-headedness,* headache, ataxia, irritability, anxiety, *nervousness, difficulty in concentrating,* mood or other mental changes, confusion, visual and auditory hallucinations, *insomnia,* nightmares, convulsions. **CV:** orthostatic hypotension, peripheral edema, dyspnea, CHF. **Eye:** blurring or loss of vision. **GI:** anorexia, *nausea,* vomiting, dry mouth. **Hematologic:** leukopenia.

DRUG INTERACTIONS Alcohol enhances CNS effects; may potentiate effects of ANTICHOLINERGICS.

NURSING IMPLICATIONS

Administration

- **Influenza prophylaxis:** drug is begun as soon as exposure to infected persons is anticipated and continued for at least 10 d.
- If insomnia is a problem, medication should be scheduled several hours before bedtime. Suggest that patient limit number of daytime naps.
- May be swallowed with water, milk, or taken with food.

- Use supplied calibrated device for measuring syrup formulation.
- May be used in conjunction with influenza A vaccine (generally in high-risk patients who have not been vaccinated previously) until protective antibodies develop (10–21 d) after vaccine administration.
- Store in tightly closed container preferably at 15–30C (59–86F) unless otherwise directed by manufacturer. Avoid freezing.

Assessment & Drug Effects

- Since drug may cause dizziness and lightheadedness, supervision of ambulation and side rails may be indicated.
- Monitor for mental status changes; nervousness, difficulty concentrating, or insomnia may indicate need for dosage adjustment.
- Patients with history of seizures should be monitored closely for loss of seizure control.
- Establish a baseline profile of the patient's disabilities for accurate differentiation between disease symptoms (e.g., dementia) and drug-induced neuropsychiatric adverse reactions.
- Closely observe for toxicity with doses above 200 mg/d. Monitor vital signs for at least 3 or 4 d after increases in dosage.
- Patients with cerebrovascular disease or impaired renal function are more prone to develop symptoms of toxicity. Monitor particularly when dosage adjustments are made.
- Monitor urinary output and pH, serum electrolytes, vital signs.
- Livedo reticularis occurs most frequently in women receiving drug for 1 mo or longer for parkinsonism. It is a diffuse, rose-colored mottling of skin, usually confined to lower extremities, but it may also appear on arms and is preceded by or accompanied by ankle edema. Condition may be more noticeable when patient stands or is exposed to cold; color fades when legs are elevated. Appears within 1 mo–1 y after initiation of drug therapy and may subside with continued therapy, but disappears gradually in 2–12 wk after drug is discontinued.
- Patients with parkinsonism may show reduction of salivation, akinesia, and rigidity within 4–48 h after initiation of therapy. Generally, drug has little effect on tremors. If significant improvement is not noted within 1–2 wk, drug is usually discontinued.
- **Parkinsonism, extrapyramidal reactions:** CNS and psychic disturbances are most likely to appear within 1 d to a few days after initiation of drug therapy, or after dosage has been increased. Symptoms tend to subside when drug is given in two divided doses.

Common side effects in *italic*; life-threatening effects underlined; generic names in **bold**; classifications in SMALL CAPS

283

Patient & Family Education

- To be effective in treatment of influenza, must be administered preferably within 24 h but no later than 48 h after onset of symptoms and should be continued for 24–48 h after symptoms disappear. Advise patient to report to physician if there is no improvement within this time.

- Because orthostatic hypotension may be a problem, caution patient not to go to sleep in a sitting position, and advise elderly male patients particularly to sit down to urinate, especially at night.

- Advise patient to make all position changes slowly, particularly from recumbent to upright position, and to dangle legs a few minutes before standing. Caution patient to lie down immediately if faint or dizzy.

- Onset of shortness of breath, peripheral edema, significant weight gain, dizziness, inability to concentrate, and other changes in mental status, dysuria, and eye symptoms should be reported to physician.

- Activities requiring mental alertness such as driving a car should be avoided until patient's response to the drug has been evaluated.

- Maximum therapeutic response generally occurs within 2 wk–3 mo. Effectiveness sometimes wanes after 6–8 wk of treatment. Report to physician.

- Abrupt discontinuation of therapy for parkinsonism may precipitate within 1–3d a *parkinsonian crisis:* severe akinesia, rigidity, tremor. Warn patient to adhere to established dosage regimen.

- In other patients, abrupt withdrawal can result in *neuroleptic malignant syndrome:* low grade fever and symptoms similar to parkinsonian crisis.

Prototype: neostigmine, p 118

AMBENONIUM CHLORIDE

(am-be-noe´nee-um)

Trade name: Mytelase
Classifications: AUTONOMIC NERVOUS SYSTEM AGENT; CHOLINERGIC (PARASYMPATHOMIMETIC); CHOLINESTERASE INHIBITOR
Pregnancy: Category C

ACTIONS/PHARMACODYNAMICS   Synthetic quaternary ammonium compound. Indirect acting and a slowly reversible cholinesterase inhibitor approximately six times more potent than neostigmine

but similar with respect to uses, contraindications, and adverse reactions. Inhibits destruction of acetylcholine (ACh) by cholinesterase, thereby prolonging effects of ACh (neurotransmitter) at postsynaptic receptor sites. Produces fewer severe cholinergic (muscarinic) effects than neostigmine, but has more prolonged duration of action and possibly greater tendency to accumulate. Has direct stimulant effect on striated muscles.

USES Symptomatic treatment of myasthenia gravis for patients who cannot tolerate neostigmine bromide or pyridostigmine bromide because of bromide sensitivity. Has been used in conjunction with corticosteroids, ephedrine sulfate, and potassium chloride to increase muscle strength.

ROUTE & DOSAGE

Myasthenia Gravis

Adult	PO	2.5–5 mg t.i.d. or q.i.d.; may increase q1–2d to 50–75 mg t.i.d. or q.i.d. if necessary
Child	PO	0.3 mg/kg/d in 3–4 divided doses; may need up to 1.5 mg/kg/d in 3–4 divided doses

PHARMACOKINETICS Absorption: poorly absorbed from GI tract. **Onset:** 20–30 min. **Duration:** 3–8h. **Metabolism:** unknown. **Elimination:** unknown.

CONTRAINDICATIONS & PRECAUTIONS Contraindicated in: intestinal or urinary tract obstruction; patients receiving mecamylamine. Safe use during pregnancy (category C) and in nursing women not established. **Cautious use in:** epilepsy, bradycardia, cardiac arrhythmias, recent coronary occlusion; bronchial asthma; hyperthyroidism; vagotonia; peptic ulcer, megacolon.

ADVERSE/SIDE EFFECTS Exaggerated cholinergic (muscarinic) effects. **CNS:** muscle cramps, headache, confusion, dizziness, incoordination, fasciculations, agitation, restlessness, muscle weakness, paralysis, slurred speech, convulsions, respiratory depression. **CV:** bradycardia. **GI:** nausea, vomiting, diarrhea, abdominal cramps, excessive salivation. **Eye :** blurred vision, lacrimation. **Respiratory:** bronchospasm, increased bronchial secretions, dyspnea. **Other:** diaphoresis.

DRUG INTERACTIONS Demecarium and other CHOLINESTERASE INHIBITORS possibly compound toxicity; **mecamylamine, succinylcholine, pro-**

cainamide, quinidine, AMINOGLYCOSIDES increase neuromuscular blocking effects with possibility of respiratory depression; **atropine** antagonizes effects of ambenonium.

NURSING IMPLICATIONS

Administration

- Administration with food or milk may minimize muscarinic side effects.
- In general, medication schedule is planned so that larger doses are given when patient experiences the most fatigue or muscle weakness. Patients who have difficulty in eating may benefit by taking drug 30 to 45 min before meals.
- Store preferably at 15–30C (59–86F) unless otherwise directed.

Assessment & Drug Effects

- Hazards of cumulative effects and overdosage are high; therefore atropine sulfate should always be immediately available to treat severe cholinergic reactions.
- Monitor vital signs during dosage adjustment periods.
- Monitor for *manifestations of inadequate ventilation:* unusual apprehension, restlessness, rapid pulse and respirations, rising BP.
- Dosage requirements may vary according to disease exacerbations and remissions and stress-provoking factors. The effects of a given dosage change may not appear for several days because of cumulative action. If a dosage increase produces no effect, physician may reduce dose to previous level. Record drug effect and duration of drug action. Keep physician informed.
- It is important to record time that adverse symptoms appear. When muscle weakness occurs within 1 h after drug administration, suspect overdosage. *Other signs of overdosage:* headache, weakness of muscles of neck, chewing, and swallowing, increased salivation. Weakness that begins 3 h or more after drug administration is probably due to underdosage or drug resistance.

Patient & Family Education

- Patients and responsible family members should be taught to recognize adverse effects, how to modify the doses accordingly, and when and how atropine should be taken.
- Patients on long-term therapy may become refractory to drug. Responsiveness usually returns when dosage is reduced or drug is withdrawn for several days.
- Advise patient to carry card or jewelry indicating medical diagnosis and medication(s) being taken.

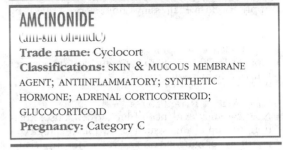

Prototype: hydrocortisone, p 255

AMCINONIDE

(am-sin´oh-nide)
Trade name: Cyclocort
Classifications: SKIN & MUCOUS MEMBRANE AGENT; ANTIINFLAMMATORY; SYNTHETIC HORMONE; ADRENAL CORTICOSTEROID; GLUCOCORTICOID
Pregnancy: Category C

ACTIONS/PHARMACODYNAMICS Synthetic fluorinated topical agent. Has vasoconstrictor, antipruritic, and antiinflammatory actions equal to those produced by betamethasone and triamcinolone.

USES Adjunctively in treatment and relief of inflammatory and pruritic manifestations of corticoid-responsive dermatoses such as psoriasis and eczematous and contact dermatitis.

ROUTE & DOSAGE

Antiinflammatory

Adult	Topical	Apply a thin film b.i.d. or t.i.d.

CONTRAINDICATIONS & PRECAUTIONS Contraindicated in: history of hypersensitivity to corticosteroids; ophthalmic use; markedly impaired circulation; systemic or local viral infection, fungal infection, tuberculosis of skin. Safe use during pregnancy (category C) or in nursing mothers not established. **Cautious use in:** children. Application over large areas of the body, skin infections, on the face.

ADVERSE/SIDE EFFECTS Most frequently with occlusive dressings. Burning, itching, irritation, dryness, folliculitis, hypertrichosis, perioral dermatitis, patchy hypopigmentation, allergic contact dermatitis, *skin maceration, skin atrophy,* striae, miliaria, secondary infection.

NURSING IMPLICATIONS

Administration

- Cleanse area to be treated before applying cream to reduce risk of infection. Unless otherwise directed, use tepid water.
- Apply a thin film of medication to cleansed affected

Common side effects in *italic*; life-threatening effects <u>underlined</u>; generic names in **bold**; classifications in SMALL CAPS

285

areas and rub in gently and thoroughly until it disappears. Do not use in or near the eyes.
- Do not bandage or otherwise cover treated area or apply occlusive dressing unless prescribed by physician.
- Occlusive dressings should not be used if lesions are exudative, weeping, or infected.
- Store at 15–30C (59–86F) in tightly closed container unless otherwise directed.

Assessment & Drug Effects
- Note carefully evidence of limited response, irritation, or skin changes such as atrophy, telangiectasis, or hypopigmentation and report to physician.
- Systemic absorption, which could lead to growth retardation (in children) and adrenal suppression, may occur with use of topical corticosteroid on large skin areas for prolonged periods and particularly if occlusive dressings are used.
- Report evidence of intercurrent infection, which will require prompt control by adjunctive treatment. Question physician about continuation of amcinonide therapy during antifungal or antimicrobial treatment.

Patient & Family Education
- Instruct patient on correct application of medication and appropriate use of bandage or other occlusive dressing.
- Advise patient to avoid exposure of treated areas to sunlight. Severe sunburn may occur, especially when occlusive dressings have been used.

Prototype: gentamicin, p 53

AMIKACIN SULFATE
(am-i-kay´sin)

Trade name: Amikin
Classifications: ANTIINFECTIVE; AMINOGLYCOSIDE ANTIBIOTIC
Pregnancy: Category C

ACTIONS/PHARMACODYNAMICS Semisynthetic derivative of kanamycin with broad range of antimicrobial activity that includes many strains resistant to other aminoglycosides. Pharmacologic properties essentially the same as those of gentamicin. Unlike other aminoglycoside antibiotics, resists destruction by bacterial enzymes (except acetyltransferase and an adenylating enzyme). Like other aminoglycosides, appears to inhibit protein synthesis in bacterial cell and is usually bactericidal. Effective against a wide variety of gram-negative bacteria including *Escherichia coli, Enterobacter, Klebsiella pneumoniae*, most strains of *Pseudomonas aeruginosa*, and many strains of *Proteus* species, *Serratia, Providencia stuartii, Citrobacter freundii, Acinetobacter*. Also effective against penicillinase and non-penicillinase-producing *Staphylococcus* species, and against *Mycobacterium tuberculosis* and atypical mycobacteria.

USES Primarily for short-term treatment of serious infections of respiratory tract, bones, joints, skin, and soft tissue, CNS (including meningitis), peritonitis burns, recurrent urinary tract infections (UTI). **Unlabeled use:** intrathecal or intraventricular administration, in conjunction with IM or IV dosage.

ROUTE & DOSAGE

Moderate to Severe Infections (All Doses Based on Ideal Body Weight)

Adult	IV/IM	5–7.5 mg/kg loading dose; then 7.5 mg/kg q12h
Child	IV/IM	5–7.5 mg/kg loading dose; then 5 mg/kg q8h or 7.5 mg/kg q12h
Neonate	IV/IM	10 mg/kg loading dose; then 7.5 mg/kg q12h

Uncomplicated UTI

Adult	IV/IM	250 mg q12h

PHARMACOKINETICS Peak: 30 min IV; 45 min to 2 h IM. **Distribution:** does not cross blood-brain barrier; crosses placenta; accumulates in renal cortex. **Elimination:** half-life: 2–3 h in adults, 4–8 h in neonates; 94–98% excreted renally in 24 h, remainder in 10–30 d.

CONTRAINDICATIONS & PRECAUTIONS Contraindicated in: history of hypersensitivity or toxic reaction with an aminoglycoside antibiotic. Safe use during pregnancy (category C), in nursing mothers, neonates and infants, or use for period exceeding 14 d not determined. **Cautious use in:** impaired renal function; eighth cranial (auditory) nerve impairment; preexisting vertigo or dizziness, tinnitus, or dehydration, fever; the elderly, prematures, neonates and infants; myasthenia gravis; parkinsonism; hypocalcemia.

Common side effects in *italic*; life-threatening effects <u>underlined</u>; generic names in **bold**; classifications in SMALL CAPS

ADVERSE/SIDE EFFECTS CNS: neurotoxicity: drowsiness, unsteady gait, weakness, clumsiness, paresthesias, tremors, convulsions. **ENT:** *ototoxicity: auditory:* high frequency hearing loss, complete hearing loss (occasionally permanent), tinnitus; ringing or buzzing in ears, *vestibular:* dizziness, ataxia. **GI:** nausea, vomiting. **Hematologic: (infrequent):** anemia, leukopenia, granulocytopenia, thrombocytopenia. **Hypersensitivity:** skin rash, urticaria, pruritus, redness. **Renal:** oliguria, urinary frequency, hematuria, tubular necrosis, azotemia. **Other:** unusual thirst, superinfections, peripheral neuritis, hepatotoxicity, hypokalemia, hypomagnesemia.

DRUG INTERACTIONS ANESTHETICS, SKELETAL MUSCLE RELAXANTS have additive neuromuscular blocking effects; **acyclovir, amphotericin B, bacitracin, capreomycin, cephalosporins, colistin, cisplatin, carboplatin, methoxyflurane, polymyxin B, vancomycin, furosemide, ethacrynic acid** increase risk of ototoxicity and nephrotoxicity.

INCOMPATIBILITIES Solution/additive: amino-phylline, amphotericin B, CEPHALOSPORINS, **chlor-othiazide, erythromycin, heparin, oxytetracycline,** PENICILLINS, **phenytoin, thiopental, vitamin B complex with C, warfarin. Y-Site: amphotericin B, heparin, phenytoin, thiopental.**

NURSING IMPLICATIONS

Administration

- To prepare IV solution, add contents of 500 mg vial to 100 or 200 ml 5% dextrose or 0.9% NaCl injection or other diluent recommended by manufacturer. For pediatric patients, volume of diluent depends on patient need.
- Administer a single adult dose over at least 30–60 min by IV infusion. Increase infusion time to 1–2 h for infants.
- Monitor drip rate carefully. A rapid rise in serum amikacin level can cause respiratory depression (neuromuscular blockade) and other signs of toxicity.
- Manufacturer recommends that no other drug be combined with amikacin.
- Color of solution may vary from colorless to light straw color or very pale yellow. Discard solutions that appear discolored or that contain particulate matter.
- Store at 15–30C (59–86F) unless otherwise directed.

Assessment & Drug Effects

- Culture and susceptibility tests should be performed before initial dose.
- Tests of renal function and vestibulocochlear nerve function should be performed before therapy and at regular intervals during therapy; should be closely monitored in the elderly, in patients with history of ear problems, patients with renal impairment, or during high dose or prolonged therapy.
- Blood for peak amikacin levels is drawn about 1 h after IM administration. If drug is administered by IV infusion, time for drawing blood depends on IV infusion rate. In general, blood is drawn immediately after completion of a 1 h infusion or 30 min following completion of a 30 min infusion. Trough levels are drawn immediately before the next IM or IV dose.
- Periodic measurements of peak and trough serum amikacin levels in addition to serum creatinine or creatinine clearance (generally preferred) are advised, especially in the presence of impaired renal function, in neonates, and in the elderly.
- Peak serum amikacin concentrations above 30–35 µg/ml are not recommended; trough levels should not exceed 5 µg/ml. Prolonged high trough or peak levels are associated with toxicity.
- Amikacin serum levels are reportedly lower in patients with fever.
- Ototoxicity primarily involves the cochlear (auditory) branch. High frequency deafness usually appears first and can be detected only by audiometer.
- Observe for and question about auditory symptoms (tinnitus, roaring noises, sensation of fullness in ears, hearing loss) and vestibular disturbances (dizziness or vertigo, nystagmus, ataxia).
- Monitor and report any changes in I&O, oliguria, hematuria, or cloudy urine. Keeping patient well hydrated reduces risk of nephrotoxicity. Consult physician regarding optimum fluid intake.
- Increasing serum creatinine and BUN, decreasing urine specific gravity and creatinine clearance, and presence of albumin and casts, WBC, and RBC in urine are indicators of declining renal function.
- If treatment is more than 10 d, daily tests of renal function and weekly audiograms and vestibular tests are strongly advised.
- Be on the alert for symptoms of respiratory tract infections and other symptoms indicative of superinfections. Notify physician should they occur.

Common side effects in *italic*; life-threatening effects underlined; generic names in **bold**; classifications in SMALL CAPS

287

A

Prototype: spironolactone, p 202

AMILORIDE HYDROCHLORIDE
(a-mill´oh-ride)
Trade name: Midamor
Classifications: WATER BALANCE AGENT;
POTASSIUM SPARING DIURETIC
Pregnancy: Category B

ACTIONS/PHARMACODYNAMICS Potassium-sparing diuretic with mild diuretic and antihypertensive actions. Induces urinary excretion of sodium, e.g., bicarbonates, and calcium and reduces excretion of potassium and hydrogen ions by direct action on distal renal tubules. Potassium-sparing action results in rise of total body concentration of potassium; reduction in hydrogen ions causes moderate increase in urinary pH. Effect on serum uric acid is reportedly variable and requires further study. Diuretic action is independent of aldosterone and carbonic anhydrase.

USES Potassium-sparing effect in prevention or treatment of diuretic-induced hypokalemia in patients with CHF, hepatic cirrhosis, or hypertension. Also used in management of primary hyperaldosteronism. Usually combined with a potassium-wasting (kaliuretic) diuretic such as a thiazide or loop diuretic. **Unlabeled uses:** with hydrochlorothiazide for recurrent calcium nephrolithiasis, lithium-induced polyuria.

ROUTE & DOSAGE

Diuretic

Adult	PO	5 mg/d; may increase up to 20 mg/d in 1–2 divided doses

PHARMACOKINETICS Absorption: 50% absorbed from GI tract. **Onset:** 2 h. **Peak:** 6–10 h. **Duration:** 24 h. **Elimination:** half-life: 6–9 h; 20–50% excreted unchanged in urine, 40% in feces.

CONTRAINDICATIONS & PRECAUTIONS Contraindicated in: elevated serum potassium (>5.5 mEq/L), concomitant use of other potassium-sparing diuretics; anuria, acute or chronic renal insufficiency; evidence of diabetic nephropathy; type I (insulin-dependent) diabetes mellitus; metabolic or respiratory acidosis; hepatic function impairment. Safe use in pregnancy (category B), nursing mothers, and chil-

dren not established. **Cautious use in:** debilitated patients; diet-controlled or uncontrolled diabetes mellitus; cardiopulmonary disease; the elderly.

ADVERSE/SIDE EFFECTS Generally well tolerated. **CNS:** *headache,* dizziness, nervousness, confusion, paresthesias, drowsiness. **CV:** cardiac arrhythmias. **Electrolyte imbalance/hematologic:** hyperkalemia, hyponatremia, leukopenia, neutropenia, aplastic anemia, positive Coombs' test. **ENT:** tinnitus, nasal congestion. **Eye:** visual disturbances, increased intraocular pressure. **GI:** *diarrhea* or constipation, anorexia, *nausea,* vomiting, abdominal cramps, dry mouth, thirst. **GU:** polyuria, dysuria, bladder spasms, urinary frequency. **Gynecologic:** impotence, decreased libido. **Respiratory:** dyspnea, shortness of breath. **Skin:** rash, pruritus, photosensitivity reactions. **Other:** weakness, fatigue, muscle cramps, photosensitivity.

DIAGNOSTIC TEST INTERFERENCES Manufacturer advises discontinuing amiloride in patients with diabetes mellitus at least 3 d before ***glucose tolerance*** tests.

DRUG INTERACTIONS Blood from blood banks, ACE INHIBITORS (e.g., **captopril**), **spironolactone, triamterene,** POTASSIUM SUPPLEMENTS may cause hyperkalemia with cardiac arrhythmias; possibility of increased **lithium** toxicity (decreased renal elimination); possibility of altered **digoxin** response; NSAID'S may attenuate antihypertensive effects. **Drug-food interactions:** POTASSIUM-CONTAINING SALT SUBSTITUTES increase risk of hyperkalemia.

NURSING IMPLICATIONS

Administration

- Once-a-day dose should be given in the morning.
- Administered preferably with food to reduce possibility of gastric distress.
- Store at 15–30C (59–86F) in a tightly closed container unless otherwise directed.

Assessment & Drug Effects

- Serum potassium levels should be monitored for all patients, particularly when therapy is initiated, whenever dosage adjustments are made, and during any illness that may affect kidney function.
- Monitor for signs and symptoms of hyperkalemia and hyponatremia (see chap 3).
- Hyperkalemia occurs in about 10% of patients receiving amiloride. Serum potassium can rise suddenly and without warning.

Common side effects in *italic*; life-threatening effects <u>underlined</u>; generic names in **bold**; classifications in SMALL CAPS

- Hyperkalemia is more common in the elderly and in patients with diabetes or renal disease.
- Intermittent evaluations of BUN, creatinine, and ECG are advised for patients with renal or hepatic dysfunction, diabetes mellitus, or who are elderly or debilitated.

Patient & Family Education

- Generally taken in the morning to avoid interrupting nighttime sleep. Advise patient to take amiloride at the same time each day.
- Teach patients signs and symptoms of hypokalemia and hyponatremia (see chap 3) and instruct them to report any immediately.
- Potassium supplements, salt substitutes, high intake of dietary potassium are contraindicated. Exception: these measures may be prescribed for patients with severe or refractory hypokalemia.
- Because amiloride can cause visual disturbances and dizziness, particularly during early therapy, advise patient to be cautious when driving or performing other potentially hazardous tasks.

AMINO ACID, ESSENTIAL, INJECTION

Trade names: Aminosyn-RF, Nephramine, RenAmin
Classification: CALORIC AGENT

ACTIONS/PHARMACODYNAMICS Contains only essential amino acids prepared to be diluted with hypertonic dextrose solution and administered by central vein. By supplying patient with sufficient essential amino acids and calories, excess nitrogen in patient's body can be used up in manufacture of nonessential acids for anabolism. Since the mixture reduces rate of blood urea production and minimizes serum potassium, magnesium, and phosphorus imbalances, it is appropriate for use in patients with potentially reversible renal decompensation when oral nutrition is not possible or impractical. See Amino Acid Solution for adverse reactions and for information concerning TPN (total parenteral nutrition or hyperalimentation).

ROUTE & DOSAGE

Parenteral Nutrition

Adult	IV	250–500 ml/d mixed with an appropriate amount of dextrose, electrolytes, and vitamins

CONTRAINDICATIONS & PRECAUTIONS Contraindicated in: severe uncorrected electrolyte and acid-base imbalances; hyperammonemia; decreased circulating blood volume; inborn errors of amino acid metabolism. **Cautious use in:** pediatric patients, especially low-birth-weight infants.

ADVERSE/SIDE EFFECTS Hyperammonemia, hyperglycemia, electrolyte imbalances, circulatory overload. See also Amino Acid Solution.

INCOMPATIBILITIES Y-Site: ampicillin, cephadrine, tetracycline.

NURSING IMPLICATIONS

Administration

- Usually mixed with 70% dextrose.
- Initial infusion rate generally does not exceed 20–30 ml/h. Increases by increments of 10 ml/h each 24 h are recommended up to maximum of 60–100 ml/h.

Assessment & Drug Effects

- Monitor I&O. Observe patient for signs of circulatory overload (see chap 3).
- Hyperglycemia is a frequent complication in low-birth-weight infants or infants with sepsis and in uremic patients. Urine and blood glucose must be closely monitored. Exogenous insulin may be required.
- Electrolytes, calcium, phosphorus, and magnesium should be checked daily.
- Serum concentrations of potassium, phosphorus, and magnesium may decrease dramatically during therapy. Supplements may be required. Observe for signs and symptoms of hypokalemia and hypomagnesemia (see chap 3).
- Hyperammonemia commonly occurs in infants. Observe for and report promptly vomiting, lethargy, irritability.

AMINO ACID SOLUTION

(a-mee′noe)
Trade names: Aminosyn, Crystalline amino acid solution, FreAmine III, Novamine, ProcalAmine, Travasol, Trophamine
Classification: CALORIC AND ELECTROLYTIC AGENT
Pregnancy: Category C

Common side effects in *italic*; life-threatening effects underlined; generic names in **bold**; classifications in SMALL CAPS

289

A

ACTIONS/PHARMACODYNAMICS Mixture of approximately 15 essential and nonessential amino acids (but no peptides). Supplied in a variety of concentrations both alone and with electrolytes. Solutions containing 3.5% amino acids may be administered by peripheral vein. The more concentrated formulations are intended for infusion into a large (central) vein, such as the jugular or subclavian in *total parenteral nutrition (TPN):* the technique of providing total nutritional support by IV infusion of amino acids, a nonprotein source of calories (e.g., dextrose, fructose, alcohol, or fat), electrolytes, vitamins, and trace elements.

USES Adjunct in TPN to prevent nitrogen loss or to correct negative nitrogen balance when there is interference with ingestion, digestion, or absorption of proteins, particularly over long periods. Also used for short-term, protein-sparing therapy to improve nitrogen balance, e.g., surgical patients, and patients with severe trauma or sepsis. Other specially designed amino acid preparations are commercially available for patients with renal or hepatic disease or who do not tolerate conventional solutions.

ROUTE & DOSAGE

Parenteral Nutrition

Adult	IV	1–1.5 g/kg/d
Child	IV	2–3 g/kg/d

CONTRAINDICATIONS & PRECAUTIONS Contraindicated in: hypersensitivity to any component; severe uncorrected electrolyte and acid-base imbalances; decreased circulating blood volume; <u>anuria</u>, oliguria, severe kidney or liver disease, hyperammonemia, bleeding abnormalities; inborn errors of amino acid metabolism. Safe use during pregnancy (category C) and children not established. **Cautious use in:** impaired renal or hepatic function; cardiac insufficiency, hypertension; diabetes mellitus.

ADVERSE/SIDE EFFECTS Dose-related. **CNS:** headache, dizziness, mental confusion. **CV:** flushing of skin and sensations of warmth (rapid infusion); pulmonary edema, hypertension, tachycardia, CHF. **GI:** nausea, vomiting, abdominal pain, fatty liver. **Hypersensitivity:** skin rash, papular eruptions. **Infusion catheter site:** infection, phlebitis, venous thrombosis, tissue sloughing. **Metabolic:** acidosis, alkalosis, hypophosphatemia, hypocalcemia, osteoporosis, *electrolyte imbalance,* glycosuria, *hyperglycemia,* rebound hypoglycemia, hypervolemia. **Following use of hyperosmolar preparations:** osmotic diuresis, dehydration, <u>coma</u>. **Other:** increase in BUN, diaphoresis, fever.

INCOMPATIBILITIES Solution/additive: amphotericin B, ampicillin, carbenicillin, gentamicin, metronidazole, ticarcillin, tetracycline. Y-Site: ampicillin, amphotericin B, cephradine, tetracycline.

NURSING IMPLICATIONS

Administration

- Mixed solutions should be used immediately. If not used within 1 h, refrigerate and use preferably in less than 24 h, unless otherwise directed by manufacturer.
- A volumetric infusion pump is recommended with an in-line microfilter. Do not administer solution unless it is absolutely clear.
- Scrupulous observation of aseptic technique is essential when one is inserting and changing IV catheter, when changing bottles, tubing, or filters, and when giving care to catheter site.
- All IV apparatus should be replaced every 24 h. Follow agency policy.
- If infusion schedule falls behind, do not attempt to compensate by speeding up infusion rate, as this may subject patient to glucose (dextrose) overload.

Assessment & Drug Effects

- The following values are generally determined at start of TPN therapy and at regular intervals thereafter: CBC with differential and platelet count, serum electrolytes, blood glucose, urine glucose and ketones, PT, renal and hepatic function tests, trace elements (e.g., copper, zinc, manganese, iodine, cobalt, iron), plasma lipid levels.
- Check vital signs at least every 4 h; monitor I&O.
- Observe infusion catheter entry site for signs of infection, drainage, edema (extravasation).
- Sepsis is a constant threat and the most frequent serious complication of therapy. Fever or other possible signs of infection should be reported promptly. Solution and tubing are generally replaced and cultured. If source of fever still remains obscure, infusion catheter should be aseptically withdrawn and tip cultured.
- Urine should be tested for glucose, acetone, and specific gravity every 6 h until infusion rate is stabilized, then 2 times daily. Blood glucose is usually obtained daily, then twice weekly.
- Use Clinistix, Keto-Diastix, or TesTape to test for urine glucose. These specific tests for glucose are not affected by reducing substances that may be present in hyperalimentation solutions.

Common side effects in *italic*; life-threatening effects <u>underlined</u>; generic names in **bold**; classifications in SMALL CAPS

- Sudden fluctuations in urine glucose may indicate infection and should be reported.
- If TPN therapy must be interrupted for whatever reason, D5W or D10W for injection is usually given by peripheral vein to avoid rebound hypoglycemia. Weigh patient daily under standard conditions. Once patient is stabilized, weights may be done 2 or 3 times weekly.
- Be alert for signs of circulatory overload (see Signs & Symptoms, chap 3).
- Observe pediatric patients and patients with impaired hepatic function for symptoms of **hyperammonemia:** lethargy, decreased appetite, vomiting, asterixis (flapping tremor), weak pulse, irritability, decreased responsiveness, seizures.
- A BUN to creatinine ratio in excess of 1:10 may mean that patient is receiving too much protein per unit of glucose.

AMINOCAPROIC ACID

See BLOOD FORMERS & COAGULATORS, HEMOSTATIC prototype, p 131.

AMINOGLUETETHIMIDE

(a-mee-noe-gloo-teth´i-mide)
Trade name: Cytadren
Classifications: ANTINEOPLASTIC; HORMONE ANTAGONIST
Pregnancy: Category D

ACTIONS/PHARMACODYNAMICS Blocks adrenal corticosteroid biosynthesis (i.e., mineralocorticoids, glucocorticoids, and other steroids) by inhibiting enzymatic conversion of cholesterol to precursors of cortisol and aldosterone. Also blocks aromatase, thereby preventing conversion of androgens to estrogens in peripheral tissues. Because estrogens are supplied principally by the adrenals in postmenopausal and oophorectomized women, aminoglutethimide-induced lowering of plasma estrogen levels (by adrenal suppression) is reportedly as effective as that produced by surgical adrenalectomy. Goiter and mild hypothyroidism can develop with prolonged use because drug may block iodination of tyrosine. Has weak anticonvulsant properties.

USES Temporary treatment of selected patients with Cushing's syndrome associated with adrenal carcinoma, ectopic ACTH-producing tumors, or adrenal hyperplasia. **Unlabeled use:** to produce medical adrenalectomy in postmenopausal women with positive estrogen receptor test, metastatic breast cancer, or who fail or relapse with tamoxifen (Nolvadex), and for patients with prostatic carcinoma. Former use as an anticonvulsant supplement has been abandoned because of its adrenal suppressant activity.

ROUTE & DOSAGE

Cushing's Disease

Adult	PO	250 mg q6h; may be increased 250 mg/d q1–2wk if needed (max 2 g/d)

Breast Cancer

Adult	PO	250 mg b.i.d. and hydrocortisone 60 mg h.s., 20 mg in AM, and 20 mg at 2 PM daily for 2 wk; then 250 mg q.i.d. and hydrocortisone 20 mg h.s., 10 mg in AM, and 10 mg at 2 PM thereafter

PHARMACOKINETICS Onset: 3–5 d. **Distribution:** crosses placenta. **Metabolism:** hepatic metabolism. **Elimination:** half-life: 13 h (7 h with long-term use); excreted by kidneys; recovery of adrenal responsiveness to stress occurs 36–72 h after discontinuation.

CONTRAINDICATIONS & PRECAUTIONS Contraindicated in: hypothyroidism; infection. Safe use in pregnancy (category D), nursing mothers, and in children not established. **Cautious use in:** elderly.

ADVERSE/SIDE EFFECTS CNS: lethargy, drowsiness, *dizziness,* uncontrolled eye movements (dose related); clumsiness, *headache.* **CV:** *hypotension, tachycardia.* **Endocrine:** masculinization. **GI:** nausea, vomiting, anorexia. **Hematologic (rare):** neutropenia, leukopenia, thrombocytopenia, pancytopenia, agranulocytosis, decreased Hgb and Hct, anemia, Coombs' negative hemolytic anemia. **Skin:** *measles-like (morbilliform) rash,* pruritus. **Other:** hepatotoxicity.

DRUG INTERACTIONS Dexamethasone decreases pharmacologic effects of aminoglutethimide; decreases anticoagulant response to **warfarin.**

NURSING IMPLICATIONS

Administration
- Treatment with aminoglutethimide normally is administered in the hospital until a stable dosage regimen is achieved.
- If glucocorticoid replacement is needed, 20–30 mg

Common side effects in *italic*; life-threatening effects underlined; generic names in **bold**; classifications in SMALL CAPS

291

A

of hydrocortisone PO each morning may be ordered.
- Store at 15–30C (59–86F) in tightly closed containers unless otherwise directed.

Assessment & Drug Effects
- Baseline and periodic determinations should be made: 8 AM fasting plasma cortisol levels (normal: 5–30 µg/dl; excessively low levels indicate adrenal insufficiency); CBC; serum alkaline phosphatase (clue for early bone recurrence); AST (SGOT); bilirubin; thyroid function tests; urinary aldosterone (normal: 2–26 µg/24 h); serum electrolytes; CO_2.
- Baseline and regularly scheduled BP readings in the recumbent and upright positions indicate the effect of reduced aldosterone levels on BP. Orthostatic and persistent hypotension (subjectively experienced as dizziness, light-headedness, weakness) result from reduced aldosterone production.
- Dose reduction or temporary discontinuation may be indicated if any of the following occur: extreme drowsiness, severe skin rash, extremely low cortisol levels.
- The elderly are particularly sensitive to the CNS effects of aminoglutethimide (e.g., lethargy, ataxia, orthostatic dizziness, light-headedness). Note implications for ambulation.
- Patients with Cushing's syndrome may show reduced effect with continuing therapy. These patients are generally not treated beyond 3 mo with aminoglutethimide.
- *Adrenal insufficiency* (hypoadrenalism) symptoms include anorexia, nausea, vomiting, weight loss, weakness, hypotension, dizziness, hypoglycemia, oliguria, low serum sodium, elevated potassium and BUN, arthralgia, myalgia, hyperpigmentation.
- Development of adrenal insufficiency is an indication for discontinuation of the drug.
- Report symptoms of hypothyroidism (see Signs & Symptoms, chap 3) should they appear.

Patient & Family Education
- Make position changes gradually, pausing between each change. Do not stand still for prolonged periods. Support hose may be helpful. Consult physician.
- Drowsiness, nausea, and anorexia often disappear spontaneously within 1–2 wk of continuing therapy. Caution patient not to stop taking drug but to inform physician if symptoms persist or become pronounced.
- Report skin rash that persists beyond 5–8 d. Physician may discontinue drug.

- Tolerance to lethargy and ataxia usually develops after 4 wk of therapy. If symptoms are severe, however, drug discontinuation may be necessary. Keep physician informed.
- Contact physician immediately in times of stress such as surgery, dental work, acute illness, acute emotional situations. Steroid supplements may be indicated or physician may temporarily stop aminoglutethimide.
- Notify physician immediately if pregnancy is suspected.
- Because of the possibility of drowsiness and dizziness, warn patient to avoid driving and other potentially hazardous activities until the reaction to drug is known.
- Advise patient to carry card or jewelry (e.g., Medic Alert) indicating medical diagnosis, medication(s), physician's name, address, and telephone number.

Prototype: theophylline, p 136

AMINOPHYLLINE (THEOPHYLLINE ETHYLENEDIAMIDE)

(am-in-off´i-lin)
Trade names: Phyllocontin, Somophyllin, Somophyllin-DF, Truphylline
Classifications: BRONCHODILATOR; (RESPIRATORY SMOOTH MUSCLE RELAXANT)
Pregnancy: Category C

ACTIONS/PHARMACODYNAMICS Aminophylline is an ethylenediamide salt of theophylline with effects similar to those of other xanthines, e.g., caffeine and theobromine. Action is dependent on theophylline content (approximately 80%) and is measured as theophylline in the serum.

USES To prevent and relieve symptoms of acute bronchial asthma and treatment of bronchospasm associated with chronic bronchitis and emphysema. **Unlabeled use:** as a respiratory stimulant in Cheyne-Stokes respiration; for treatment of apnea and bradycardia in prematures; as cardiac stimulant and diuretic in treatment of CHF. Use as antispasmodic for acute biliary attack has largely been replaced by more effective drugs.

PHARMACOKINETICS Absorption: most products are 100% absorbed from GI tract. **Peak:** IV 30 min; uncoated tablet 1 h; sustained release 4–6 h. **Duration:** 4–8 h; varies with age, smoking, and liver function. **Distribution:** crosses placenta. **Metabolism:** extensively metabolized in liver. **Elimination:** parent drug and metabolites excreted by kidneys; excreted in breast milk.

ROUTE & DOSAGE

Bronchospasm (all doses based on ideal body weight)

Adult	Loading dose	6 mg/kg IV over 30 min
	Maintenance dose	IV by continuous infusion; PO divided q6h
Nonsmoker	PO/IV	0.5 mg/kg/h
Smoker	PO/IV	0.75 mg/kg/h
With CHF or cirrhosis	PO/IV	0.25 mg/kg/h
Child	Loading dose	6 mg/kg IV over 30 min
	Maintenance dose	IV by continuous infusion; PO divided q6h
		>9 y: 0.75 mg/kg/h
		1–9 y: 1 mg/kg/h
Infant	PO/IV	6–11 mo: 0.87 g/kg/h
		2–6 mo: 0.5 mg/kg/h
Neonate	PO/IV	0.16 mg/kg/h

CONTRAINDICATIONS & PRECAUTIONS Contraindicated in: hypersensitivity to xanthine derivatives or to ethylenediamine component; cardiac arrhythmias. Safe use during pregnancy (category C) and in nursing mothers not established. **Cautious use in:** severe hypertension, cardiac disease, arrhythmias; impaired hepatic function; diabetes mellitus; hyperthyroidism; glaucoma; prostatic hypertrophy; fibrocystic breast disease; history of peptic ulcer; neonates and young children, patients over 55 y; COPD, acute influenza or patients receiving influenza immunization.

ADVERSE/SIDE EFFECTS CNS: *nervousness,* restlessness, depression, insomnia, irritability, headache, dizziness, muscle hyperactivity, convulsions. **CV:** <u>cardiac arrhythmias,</u> tachycardia, with rapid IV: hyperventilation, chest pain, severe hypotension, <u>cardiac arrest.</u> **GI:** *nausea, vomiting, anorexia,* hematemesis, diarrhea, epigastric pain.

DRUG INTERACTIONS Increases **lithium** excretion, lowering lithium levels; **cimetidine,** high-dose **allopurinol** (600 mg/d), **ciprofloxacin, erythromycin, troleandomycin** can significantly increase **theophylline** levels.

INCOMPATIBILITIES Solution/Additive: amikacin, bleomycin, CEPHALOSPORINS, **chlorpromazine, clindamycin, codeine phosphate, dimenhydrinate, dobutamine, dopamine, doxapram, doxorubicin, epinephrine, hydralazine, hydroxyzine, insulin, isoproterenol, levorphanol, meperidine, methadone, methylprednisolone, morphine, nafcillin, norepinephrine, oxytetracycline, papaverine, penicillin G, pentazocine, procaine, prochlorperazine, promazine, promethazine, tetracycline, verapamil, vitamin B complex with C. Y-Site: amiodarone, codeine phosphate, clindamycin,** PHENOTHIAZINES **(chlorpromazine, prochlorperazine,** etc), **epinephrine, dobutamine, dopamine, levorphanol, morphine, meperidine, methadone, norepinephrine, verapamil.**

NURSING IMPLICATIONS

Administration

- Oral drug is absorbed faster if taken with a full glass of water on an empty stomach (1/2–1 h before or 2 h after meals).
- Absorption may be delayed but is not reduced by presence of food in stomach.
- GI symptoms may be minimized by taking immediately after a meal or with food.
- Extended (controlled) release preparations should not be chewed or crushed before swallowing; however, if tablet is scored, it can be broken in half, then swallowed.
- The contents of extended release capsules may be mixed with soft, moist food and swallowed without chewing.
- Rectal preparations are generally ordered when the patient must fast or cannot tolerate the drug orally. Drug absorption is enhanced if rectum is empty.
- Administered IV, aminophylline solution should be at room temperature.
- Rapid infusion of IV aminophylline may cause cardiac arrest. Monitor infusion rate carefully.
- IV aminophylline, 25 mg/ml, may be given by direct IV undiluted at a rate of 25 mg/min.
- IV aminophylline, 25 mg/ml, may be further diluted in 100–200 ml of D5W or NS and infused at a rate not to exceed 25 mg/min.

Common side effects in *italic*; life-threatening effects <u>underlined</u>; generic names in **bold**; classifications in SMALL CAPS

293

- IM route is generally avoided because injection causes prolonged intense pain. Note that IV and IM preparations are not interchangeable.
- Aminophylline should not be mixed in a syringe with other drugs.
- Do not use aminophylline solutions if discolored or if crystals are present.
- Store at 15–30C (59–86F) in tightly closed containers unless otherwise directed. Follow manufacturer's directions regarding storage of suppositories. Some are stored at room temperature; others must be refrigerated.

Assessment & Drug Effects

- Toxic effects are generally related to theophylline serum levels over 20 µg/ml (therapeutic range 10–20 µg/ml).
- High incidence of toxicity is associated with rectal suppository use because of erratic rate of absorption.
- Patients receiving parenteral aminophylline should be closely observed for signs of hypotension, arrhythmias, and convulsions until serum theophylline stabilizes within the therapeutic range.
- Monitor vital signs; measure and record I&O. Improvements in quality and rate of pulse and respiration, as well as diuresis, are expected clinical effects. A sudden, sharp, unexplained rise in heart rate is a useful clinical indicator of toxicity.
- The elderly, acutely ill, and patients with severe respiratory problems, liver dysfunction, or pulmonary edema are at greater risk of toxicity because of reduced drug clearance.
- Children appear to be more susceptible than adults to the CNS stimulating effects of xanthines (nervousness, restlessness, insomnia, hyperactive reflexes, twitching, convulsions). Dosage reduction may be indicated.

Patient & Family Education

- Smoking (tobacco or marijuana) tends to increase aminophylline elimination (prolongs half-life) and therefore dosage requirements may be higher and dosage intervals shorter than in nonsmokers.
- Advise patient to report excessive nervousness or insomnia. Dosage reduction may be indicated.
- Dizziness is a relatively common side effect, particularly in the elderly. Advise patient to take necessary safety precautions.
- Many popular OTC remedies for treatment of asthma or cough contain ephedrine in combination with various salts of theophylline. Caution patient to take only those medications approved by physician.

Prototype: isoniazid, p 83

AMINOSALICYLATE SODIUM (*PARA*-AMINO-SALICYLATE SODIUM)

(a-mee-noe-sal-i´si-late)
Trade names: Parasal Sodium, P.A.S. Sodium, Teebacin

AMINOSALICYLIC ACID (*PARA*-AMINOSALICYLIC ACID)

(a-mee-noe-sal-i-sil´ik)
Trade name: P.A.S.
Classifications: ANTIINFECTIVE; ANTITUBERCULOSIS AGENT

ACTIONS/PHARMACODYNAMICS Structurally similar to *para*-aminobenzoic acid (PABA); mechanism of action resembles that of sulfonamides. Aminosalicylic acid and salts are highly specific bacteriostatic agents that suppress growth and multiplication of *Mycobacterium tuberculosis* by preventing folic acid synthesis. Despite close chemical relationship to salicylic acid (aspirin), pharmacodynamics are not similar, and apparently it does not produce syndrome of salicylism. Aminosalicylates reportedly have potent hypolipemic action and reduce serum cholesterol and triglycerides by lowering LDL and VLDL. Mechanism of this effect has not been established. Incidence of GI disturbances and crystalluria is reportedly greater with aminosalicylic acid than with its salts. Aminosalicylate sodium contains 73% aminosalicylic acid equivalent and 54.5 mg sodium per 500 mg tablet.

USES In combination with streptomycin or isoniazid or both in treatment of pulmonary and extrapulmonary tuberculosis to delay emergence of strains resistant to these drugs. **Unlabeled use:** has been used for its lipid-lowering effect.

PHARMACOKINETICS Absorption: readily and almost completely absorbed from GI tract; aminosalicylate sodium is more rapidly and completely absorbed than the acid. **Peak effect:** 1.5–2 h. **Duration:** 4 h. **Distribution:** well distributed to most tissue and body fluids except CSF unless meninges are inflamed. **Metabolism:** metabolized in liver. **Elimination:** half-life: 1 h; >80% excreted in urine in 7–10 h.

Common side effects in *italic*; life-threatening effects underlined; generic names in **bold**; classifications in SMALL CAPS

ROUTE & DOSAGE

Tuberculosis
Aminosalicylic Acid

Adult   PO   10–12 g/d in 2–3 divided doses

Child   PO   150–300 mg/kg/d in 3–4 divided doses

Aminosalicylate Sodium

Adult   12–15 g/d in 2–4 divided doses

Child   240–360 mg/kg/d in 2–4 divided doses

CONTRAINDICATIONS & PRECAUTIONS Contraindicated in: hypersensitivity to aminosalicylates, salicylates, or to compounds containing *para*-aminophenyl groups (e.g., sulfonamides, certain hair dyes), G6PD deficiency, use of the sodium salt in patients on sodium restriction or CHF. Safe use during pregnancy not established. **Cautious use in:** impaired renal and hepatic function; blood dyscrasias; goiter; gastric ulcer.

ADVERSE/SIDE EFFECTS CNS: psychotic reactions. **GI:** *anorexia, nausea, vomiting, abdominal distress, diarrhea,* peptic ulceration. **Hematologic:** leukopenia, agranulocytosis, eosinophilia, lymphocytosis, thrombocytopenia, hemolytic anemia, (G6PD deficiency). **Hypersensitivity:** fever, chills, generalized malaise, joint pain, rash, fixed-drug eruptions, pruritus; vasculitis; Loeffler's syndrome. **Metabolic:** acute hepatitis, prothrombinemia. **Renal:** renal irritation, crystalluria. **Other:** malabsorption. With long-term administration, goiter.

DIAGNOSTIC TEST INTERFERENCES Aminosalicylates (PAS) may interfere with urine *urobilinogen* determinations (using *Ehrlich's reagent*), and may cause false-positive *urinary protein* and *VMA* determinations (with *diazoreagent*); false-positive *urine glucose* may result with *cupric sulfate tests,* e.g., *Benedict's solution,* but reportedly not with glucose oxidase reagents, e.g., Tes-Tape, Clinistix. Reduces *serum cholesterol,* and possibly *serum potassium, serum PBI,* and 24-hour *I-131 thyroidal uptake* (effect may last almost 14 days).

DRUG INTERACTIONS Increases hypoprothrombinemic effects of ORAL ANTICOAGULANTS; increased risk of crystalluria with **ammonium chloride, ascorbic acid;** decreased intestinal absorption of **cyanocobalamin, folic acid;** may decrease absorption of **digoxin;** ANTIHISTAMINES may inhibit PAS absorption; may increase or decrease **phenytoin** levels; **probenecid, sulfinpyrazone** decrease PAS elimination; SALICYLATES may enhance PAS toxicity.

NURSING IMPLICATIONS

Administration

- Administer with or immediately following meals to reduce irritative gastric effects. Physician may order an antacid to be given concomitantly. Generally, GI side effects disappear after a few days of therapy.
- Aminosalicylic acid is mildly sour to the taste, and it sometimes leaves a bitter aftertaste that may be relieved by rinsing mouth with clear water or by chewing sugar-free gum or candy.
- Crystalluria may be minimized by keeping urine neutral or alkaline with adjunctive drugs, such as antacids or with diet.
- Aminosalicylic acid is an unstable drug that deteriorates rapidly on contact with heat, air, and moisture. Store in tight, light-resistant containers in a cool, dry place, preferably at 15–30C (59–86F), unless otherwise directed.

Assessment & Drug Effects

- I&O should be monitored and fluids encouraged. High concentrations are excreted in urine, and this can cause crystalluria and hematuria.
- Abrupt onset of fever, particularly during the early weeks of therapy, and clinical picture resembling that of *infectious mononucleosis* (malaise, fatigue, generalized lymphadenopathy, splenomegaly, sore throat), as well as minor complaints of pruritus, joint pains, and headache, are strongly suggestive of hypersensitivity; these symptoms should be reported promptly.

Patient & Family Education

- Inform patient that urine may turn red on contact with hypochlorite bleach used in commercial toilet bowl cleaners.
- Hypersensitivity reactions may occur after a few days, but most commonly in the fourth or fifth week. Advise patient to report them promptly.
- Instruct patient to notify physician if sore throat or mouth, malaise, unusual fatigue, bleeding or bruising occur (symptoms of blood dyscrasia).
- Generally, chemotherapy is continued about 2 y. Patient and responsible family members must understand signs and symptoms of drug toxicity, importance of maintaining an established drug regimen, and need for remaining under close medical supervision to detect covert adverse drug effects. Point out that resistant strains develop more rapidly when drug regimen is interrupted or is sporadic.

Common side effects in *italic*; life-threatening effects underlined; generic names in **bold**; classifications in SMALL CAPS

295

A

- Caution patient not to take aspirin or other OTC drugs without physician's approval.
- A brownish or purplish discoloration of the drug signifies decomposition; should this occur, discard drug.

Prototype: procainamide, p 140

AMIODARONE HYDROCHLORIDE
(a-mee´oh-da-rone)
Trade name: Cordarone
Classifications: CARDIOVASCULAR AGENT; ANTIARRHYTHMIC
Pregnancy: Category C

ACTIONS/PHARMACODYNAMICS Structurally related to thyroxine. Class III antiarrhythmic; also has antianginal and antiadrenergic properties. Totally unrelated to other antiarrhythmics. Acts directly on all cardiac tissues. Prolongs duration of action potential and refractory period without significantly affecting resting membrane potential. By direct action on smooth muscle, decreases peripheral resistance and increases coronary blood flow. Blocks effects of sympathetic stimulation. During early treatment period (first 3 mo) thyroid hormone metabolism is altered as evidenced by serum T_4 and T_3 concentration changes. Usually normal levels are restored (unknown reason) after this period even with continued therapy.

USES Prophylaxis and treatment of life-threatening ventricular arrhythmias and supraventricular arrhythmias, particularly with atrial fibrillation. **Unlabeled use:** treatment of nonexertional angina.

ROUTE & DOSAGE

Arrhythmias

Adult	PO	*Loading dose:* 800–1600 mg/d in 1–2 doses for 1–3 wk.
		Maintenance dose: 400–600 mg/d in 1–2 doses

PHARMACOKINETICS Absorption: approximately 50% absorbed (22–86%). **Onset:** 2–3 d to 1–3 wk. **Peak:** 3–7 h. **Distribution:** concentrates in adipose tissue, lungs, kidneys, spleen; crosses placenta. **Metabolism:** extensively hepatically metabolized; undergoes some enterohepatic cycling. **Elimination:** half-life:

biphasic—initial 2.5–10 d, terminal 40–55 d; excreted chiefly in bile and feces; also excreted in breast milk.

CONTRAINDICATIONS & PRECAUTIONS Contraindicated in: severe sinus bradycardia, advanced AV block; severe liver disease. Safe use during pregnancy (category C), in nursing women, and in children not established. **Cautious use in:** Hashimoto's thyroiditis, goiter, or history of other thyroid dysfunction; CHF; electrolyte imbalance; preexisting lung disease; open heart surgery; history of hypersensitivity to iodine.

ADVERSE/SIDE EFFECTS CNS: peripheral neuropathy (*muscle weakness,* wasting numbness, tingling), *fatigue,* abnormal gait, dyskinesias, *dizziness,* parathesia, headache. **CV:** bradycardia, hypotension, sinus arrest, <u>cardiogenic shock</u>, CHF, arrhythmias. **Eye:** *corneal microdeposits,* blurred vision. **GI:** *anorexia, nausea, vomiting, constipation.* **Respiratory (pulmonary toxicity):** alveolitis, pneumonitis (fever, dry cough, dyspnea), interstitial pulmonary fibrosis. **Skin:** slate-blue pigmentation, *photosensitivity,* rash. **Other (with chronic use):** hyperthyroidism or hypothyroidism, hepatoxicity.

DIAGNOSTIC TEST INTERFERENCES *Thyroid function* test abnormalities (in the absence of thyroid function impairment).

DRUG INTERACTIONS Significantly increases **digoxin** levels; enhances pharmacologic effects and toxicities of **procainamide, quinidine, flecanide;** anticoagulant effects of ORAL ANTICOAGULANTS enhanced; **verapamil, diltiazem,** BETA-ADRENERGIC BLOCKING AGENTS may potentiate sinus bradycardia, sinus arrest, or AV block; may increase **phenytoin** levels 2–3 fold; **cholestyramine** may decrease amiodarone levels.

NURSING IMPLICATIONS

Administration
- GI symptoms occur commonly during high-dose therapy, especially with loading doses. Symptoms usually respond to dose reduction or to administration in divided dose and with food, including milk.
- Store at 15–30C (59–86F) protected from light, unless otherwise directed.

Assessment & Drug Effects
- Sustained monitoring is essential because drug has an unusually long half-life (see Pharmacokinetics).

Common side effects in *italic*; life-threatening effects <u>underlined</u>; generic names in **bold**; classifications in SMALL CAPS

- Baseline and periodic assessments should be made of liver, lung, thyroid, ocular, neurologic, and GI function.
- Report adverse reactions promptly. Bear in mind that long elimination half-life means that drug effects will persist long after dosage adjustments are made or drug is discontinued.
- Be alert to signs of *pulmonary toxicity:* progressive dyspnea, fatigue, cough, pleuritic pain, fever.
- Auscultate chest periodically or when patient complains of respiratory symptoms. Check for diminished breath sounds, rales, pleuritic friction rub; observe breathing pattern. Drug-induced pulmonary function problems must be distinguished from CHF or pneumonia. Keep physician informed.
- Monitor heart rate and rhythm and BP until drug response has stabilized. Report promptly symptomatic bradycardia (see Signs & Symptoms, chap 3).
- Significant elevations of liver enzymes AST (SGOT) and ALT (SGPT) transaminases occur frequently without producing symptoms. If elevations persist or if they are 2–3 times above normal baseline readings, dosage should be reduced or drug promptly withdrawn, to prevent hepatotoxicity and liver damage.
- CNS symptoms generally develop within a week after amiodarone therapy begins. Proximal muscle weakness, a common side effect, intensified by tremors presents a great hazard to the ambulating patient. Assess severity of symptoms. Supervision of ambulation may be indicated.
- During early treatment period, especially, watch for and report symptoms of drug-induced hypothyroidism or hyperthyroidism (see Signs & Symptoms, chap 3).
- Noncardiac side effects of amiodarone (especially lipofuscinosis, photophobia, insomnia) are major factors in noncompliance. Reinforce importance of adhering to established drug regimen.
- Patients already receiving antiarrhythmic therapy when amiodarone is started must be closely observed for adverse effects, particularly conduction disturbances and exacerbation of arrhythmias. Dosage of previous agent should be reduced by 30–50% several days after amiodarone therapy is started (anticipating onset of amiodarone antiarrhythmic effect).

Patient & Family Education

- Once stabilized, pulse should be checked daily (or as prescribed) by patient or primary caregiver. Instruct patient to report a pulse <60.
- Skin and corneal pigmentation (lipofuscinosis),

seen in most patients who receive the drug for > 2 mo, is reportedly reversible but may take 1–7 mo to fade completely because of amiodarone's long half-life. Generally, corneal deposits do not interfere with vision.
- Blue-gray skin pigmentation (associated with use >1 y) disappears slowly after amiodarone is discontinued. Occasionally, reversal is not complete.
- Photophobia may be eased by dark glasses, but some patients may be unable to go outdoors at all in the daytime even with such protection.
- Alert patient to the possibility of a photosensitivity reaction (erythema, pruritus). For maximum protection, patient should wear protective clothing and a barrier-type sunscreen that physically blocks penetration of skin by ultraviolet light (e.g., titanium oxide or zinc formulations) and should avoid exposure to sun and sunlamps.

Prototype: imipramine, p 184

AMITRIPTYLINE HYDROCHLORIDE

(a-mee-trip´ti-leen)
Trade names: Amitril, Apo-Amitriptyline, Elavil, Emitrip, Endep, Enovil, Levate, Meravil, Novotriptyn, SK-Amitriptyline
Classifications: CNS AGENT; PSYCHOTHERAPEUTIC; TRICYCLIC ANTIDEPRESSANT
Pregnancy: Category C

ACTIONS/PHARMACODYNAMICS Similar to pharmacodynamics of imipramine but with relatively greater anticholinergic and sedative actions. Among the most active of the tricyclic antidepressants (TCAs) in inhibition of serotonin uptake from synaptic gap; also inhibits norepinephrine reuptake to a moderate degree. Restoration of the levels of these neurotransmitters is a proposed mechanism of antidepressant action. Has H_2-receptor blocking activity (inhibits gastric acid secretion) and prominent anticholinergic and sedative actions.

USES Endogenous depression. **Unlabeled use:** prophylaxis for cluster, migraine, and chronic tension headaches; intractable pain, peptic ulcer disease, to increase muscle strength in myotonic dystrophy, to

---

Common side effects in *italic*; life-threatening effects underlined; generic names in **bold**; classifications in SMALL CAPS

297

treat pathologic weeping and laughing secondary to forebrain disease, for eating disorders associated with depression (anorexia or bulimia), and as sedative for nondepressed patients.

ROUTE & DOSAGE

Antidepressant

Adult	PO	75–100 mg/d; may gradually increase to 150–300 mg/d (use lower doses in outpatients)
	IM	20–30 mg q.i.d. until patient can take PO
Adolescent	PO	10 mg t.i.d. and 20 mg h.s.

PHARMACOKINETICS Absorption: rapidly absorbed from GI and injection sites. **Peak levels:** 2–12 h. **Distribution:** crosses placenta. **Metabolism:** metabolized in liver to active metabolite. **Elimination:** half-life 10–50 h; primarily excreted in urine; enters breast milk.

CONTRAINDICATIONS & PRECAUTIONS

Contraindicated in: acute recovery period after MI; history of seizure disorders; pregnancy (category C), nursing mothers, children under 12 y. **Cautious use in:** prostatic hypertrophy, history of urinary retention or obstruction; angle-closure glaucoma; diabetes mellitus; hyperthyroidism; patient with cardiovascular, hepatic, or renal dysfunction; patient with suicidal tendency, electroshock therapy; elective surgery; schizophrenia; respiratory disorders; elderly, adolescents.

ADVERSE/SIDE EFFECTS CNS: *drowsiness, sedation, dizziness,* nervousness, restlessness, fatigue, headache, insomnia, abnormal movements (extrapyramidal symptoms), seizures. **CV:** *orthostatic hypotension,* tachycardia, palpitation, ECG changes. **Eye:** blurred vision, mydriasis. **GI:** *dry mouth,* increased appetite especially for sweets , *constipation,* weight gain, sour or metallic taste, nausea, vomiting. **Other:** *urinary retention,* bone marrow depression.

DRUG INTERACTIONS ANTIHYPERTENSIVES may decrease some antihypertensive response; CNS DEPRESSANTS, **alcohol,** HYPNOTICS, BARBITURATES, SEDATIVES potentiate CNS depression; ANTICOAGULANTS, ORAL, may increase hypoprothombinemic effect; **ethchlorvynol,** transient delirium; **levodopa,** SYMPATHOMIMETICS (e.g., **epinephrine, norepinephrine**), possibility of sympathetic hyperactivity with hypertension and hyperpyrexia; MAO INHIBITORS, possibility of severe reactions, toxic psychosis, cardiovascular instability; **methylphenidate** increases plasma TCA levels; THYROID DRUGS may increase possibility of arrhythmias; **cimetidine** may increase plasma TCA levels.

NURSING IMPLICATIONS

Administration

- Oral drug may be taken with or immediately after food to reduce possibility of GI irritation. Tablet may be crushed if patient is unwilling to take it whole; administer with food or fluid.
- Dose increases by 25–50 mg are preferably made in late afternoon or at bedtime because sedative action precedes antidepressant effect.
- A single dose at bedtime is useful to promote sleep or for patients who complain of dizziness or when daytime sedation interferes with work productivity. Drug effect on depression is not affected by time of day dose is taken.
- Maintenance regimen is usually continued for at least 3 mo to prevent relapse. Typical length of therapy for depression is 6 mo–1 y.
- Abrupt discontinuation of therapy can precipitate withdrawal symptoms (headache, nausea, malaise, musculoskeletal pain, panic attack, weakness). This reaction can be avoided by tapering dosage over 2-wk.
- Store drug at 15–30C (59–86F) unless otherwise directed by manufacturer. Protect from light.

Assessment & Drug Effects

- Baseline and periodic leukocyte and differential counts, BP, cardiac, renal, and hepatic function tests, and eye examinations (including glaucoma testing) are recommended particularly for the elderly, adolescents, and for patients receiving high doses or prolonged therapy.
- Monitor BP and pulse rate in patients with preexisting cardiovascular disease. Withhold drug if there is a rise or fall in systolic BP (by 10–20 mm Hg), or a sudden increase or a significant change in pulse rate or rhythm. Notify physician.
- Monitor I&O, including bowel elimination pattern.
- During initial therapy be alert to manifestations of pronounced anticholinergic activity (see chap. 3), especially in the elderly. Institute measures to prevent falling.
- If a patient uses excessive amounts of alcohol it should be borne in mind that the potentiation of amitriptyline effects may increase the dangers of overdosage or suicide attempt.
- When used for migraine prophylaxis, therapeutic effect may occur in 1–6 wk. Drug is usually dis-

continued after patient has been headache-free for 1–2 mo. If headache recurs, physician may prescribe another course of treatment.

Patient & Family Education

- Monitor weight. Amitriptyline may increase the appetite and cause weight gain; some patients develop a craving for sweets.
- Tolerance or adaptation to distressing anticholinergic actions (see Chapter 3) usually develops after patient goes on maintenance regimen. Keep physician informed.
- Advise patient that dry mouth can be relieved by taking frequent sips of water and by increasing total fluid intake.
- Instruct patient to change from recumbency to upright position slowly and in stages. Support stockings may help. Consult physician.
- Avoid potentially hazardous activities, such as driving, until response to the drug is known.
- Desired therapeutic effects for depression may not be evident until after 3–4 wk of therapy, because of long serum half-life.
- Advise patient not to use OTC drugs while he or she is on TCA therapy. Many preparations contain sympathomimetic amines.
- Inform patient that amitriptyline may make urine blue-green.

AMMONIA SPIRIT, AROMATIC

(ah-mo´nia)
Classifications: CNS AGENT; RESPIRATORY AND CEREBRAL STIMULANT
Pregnancy: Category C

ACTIONS/PHARMACODYNAMICS Aromatic solution of ammonia, alcohol, and a mixture of oils (lemon, lavender, nutmeg). Stimulates respiratory and vasomotor centers in medulla reflexly by peripheral irritation of sensory receptors in nasal membrane, mucosa of esophagus, and fundus of stomach. Also acts as an antacid and carminative.

USES Mild stimulant ("smelling salts") to prevent or treat fainting.

ROUTE & DOSAGE

Fainting

Adult	Inhalation	Inhale vapors as required
	PO	2–4 ml in at least 30 ml water

NURSING IMPLICATIONS

Administration

- For inhalation, available in single-dose glass vials covered with woven fabric. Wrap in gauze or cloth and crush between fingers.
- Preserve in tight, light-resistant containers in a cool place not exceeding 30C (86F), unless otherwise directed.

Assessment & Drug Effects

- Medical referral is indicated if patient has had other recent episodes of fainting or if person is 40 y of age or over.

AMMONIUM CHLORIDE

(ah-mo´nium)
Classification: ELECTROLYTIC BALANCE AGENT
Pregnancy: Category B

ACTIONS/PHARMACODYNAMICS Acidifying property is due to conversion of ammonium ion (NH_4^+) to urea in liver with liberation of H^+ and Cl^-. Chloride anions displace bicarbonate, producing acidosis that causes temporary (1–3 d) increased excretion of Na^+ and hence diuresis. Potassium excretion also increases, but to a lesser extent. Tolerance to diuretic effect occurs within 2–3 d by compensatory mechanisms, including renal excretion of H^+ and K^+ cations and formation of ammonia by renal cells, with recovery of corresponding amounts of Na^+. Also has mild expectorant action. It has been proposed that gastric irritation after PO administration may cause reflex stimulation of bronchial mucous glands.

USES Systemic acidifier in patients with metabolic alkalosis; to correct chloride depletion after diuretic therapy; as adjunct to lower urinary pH in treatment of UTI; and as an aid in excretion of certain alkalinizing drugs, e.g., amphetamines. Limited use as a primary diuretic. Has been used to increase solubility of calcium and phosphate ions in urinary phosphatic calculi, and in treatment of bromism and lead poisoning, and for diuretic effect in premenstrual tension and Meniere's syndrome. Common ingredient in OTC cough mixtures for its expectorant action.

PHARMACOKINETICS Absorption: completely absorbed in 3–6 h. **Metabolism:** metabolized in liver to HCl and urea. **Elimination:** primarily excreted in urine.

Common side effects in *italic*; life-threatening effects <u>underlined</u>; generic names in **bold**; classifications in SMALL CAPS

299

ROUTE & DOSAGE

Urine Acidifier, Diuretic

Adult	PO	4–12 g/d divided q4–6h
Child	PO	75 mg/kg/d in 4 divided doses

Metabolic Acidosis

Adult	IM/IV	Dose calculated on basis of CO_2 combining power or serum Cl deficit; 50% of calculated deficit is administered slowly
Child	IM/IV	Same as for adult

CONTRAINDICATIONS & PRECAUTIONS Contraindicated in: severe renal or hepatic insufficiency; primary respiratory acidosis. Safe use during pregnancy (category B) not established. **Cautious use in:** cardiac edema, pulmonary insufficiency.

ADVERSE/SIDE EFFECTS Most are secondary to ammonia toxicity. **CNS:** headache, depression, drowsiness, twitching, excitability. **CV:** bradycardia and other arrhythmias. **GI:** gastric irritation, nausea, vomiting, anorexia. **Metabolic/Electrolytes:** metabolic acidosis, hyperammonia. **Other:** skin rash, glycosuria, hyperventilation, EEG abnormalities; pain and irritation at IV site.

DIAGNOSTIC TEST INTERFERENCES Ammonium chloride may increase *blood ammonia* and *SGOT (AST),* decrease *serum magnesium* (by increasing urinary magnesium excretion), and decrease urine *urobilinogen.*

DRUG INTERACTIONS Aminosalicylic acid may cause crystalluria; increases urinary excretion of AMPHETAMINES, **flecainide, mexiletine, methadone, ephedrine, pseudoephedrine;** decreased urinary excretion of SULFONYLUREAS, SALICYLATES.

INCOMPATIBILITIES Solution/additive: codeine phosphate, levorphanol, methadone, nitrofurantoin, warfarin.

NURSING IMPLICATIONS

Administration

- GI side effects may be minimized by giving drug immediately after meals or by use of enteric-coated tablets. Tablets should be swallowed whole.
- Note that ammonium chloride for injection is available in two strengths: 2.14% (0.4 mEq/ml) in 500 ml

containers may be given without further dilution. The 26.75% (5 mEq/ml) concentrate in 20 ml vials must be diluted before administration. The concentrate may be prepared by diluting each 20 ml of ammonium chloride with 500 ml of 0.9% NaCl injection.

- Parenteral preparations of ammonium chloride should be administered slowly by IV infusion to avoid serious side effects (ammonia toxicity) and local irritation and pain.
- Administer diluted solution at a rate not to exceed 5 ml/min. Rate is much slower for infants (check with physician).
- Store in airtight container. Avoid freezing. Concentrated solutions of ammonium chloride tend to crystallize at low temperatures. Crystals can be dissolved by placing intact container in a warm water bath and warming to room temperature.

Assessment & Drug Effects

- Baseline and periodic determinations of CO_2 combining power, serum electrolytes, and urinary and arterial pH should be made during therapy to avoid serious acidosis. For some patients, dosage may be monitored by repeated serum chloride and CO_2 content (bicarbonate) determinations and urinary pH.
- Monitor rate and depth of respirations. Shortness of breath on exertion and increased ventilation at rest are signs of acidosis and should be reported promptly.
- Monitor I&O ratio and pattern. Because of compensatory mechanisms the diuretic effect of ammonium chloride lasts only 1 or 2 d.
- In the elderly, vigorous diuresis may precipitate renal insufficiency, urinary retention in men with prostatic hypertrophy, incontinence in both sexes, and acute Na^+ and K^+ depletion. Report signs of weakness and confusion and changes in voiding pattern and comfort.
- Check urine specific gravity of elderly patients on diuretic therapy. Elevation accompanying even mild diuresis is suggestive of renal insufficiency.

Patient & Family Education

- Unless contraindicated, diet of patients on diuretic therapy should include foods high in potassium, e.g., bananas, oranges, dried fruits, cantaloupe, honeydew melon, milk (all types), tomatoes, potatoes, winter squash.
- Hyperglycemia and glycosuria are potential side effects. Note implications for the diabetic patient and instruct him or her accordingly.

Common side effects in *italic*; life-threatening effects underlined; generic names in **bold**; classifications in SMALL CAPS

Prototype: phenobarbital, p 167

AMOBARBITAL
(am-oh-bar'bi-tal)
Trade names: Amytal, Isobec, Novamobarb

AMOBARBITAL SODIUM
Trade name: Amytal Sodium
Classifications: CNS AGENT; BARBITURATE
ANTICONVULSANT; SEDATIVE-HYPNOTIC
Pregnancy: Category D
Controlled substance: Schedule II

ACTIONS/PHARMACODYNAMICS Intermediate-acting barbiturate similar to phenobarbital. CNS depressant action appears to be related to ability to interfere with ascending impulse transmission from reticular activating system (concerned with body and behavioral alertness) to cerebral cortex. Does not impair pain perception.

USES Sedative, to relieve anxiety, and as short-term hypnotic to treat insomnia. Also used parenterally to control status epilepticus or acute convulsive episodes, agitated behavior, and for narcoanalysis and narcotherapy.

ROUTE & DOSAGE

Sedative

Adult	PO	30–50 mg b.i.d. or t.i.d.
Child	PO	2 mg/kg or 70 mg/m²/d in 4 divided doses

Preoperative Sedation

Adult	PO/IM	200 mg 1 h before surgery

Labor

Adult	PO	200–400 mg repeated at 1–3 h intervals (max 1 g)

Hypnotic

Adult	PO/IM	65–200 mg (max 500 mg)
Child	IM	2–3 mg/kg

Anticonvulsant, Agitated Behavior, Hypnotic

Adult	IV	65–500 mg, not to exceed 1 g
Child	IV	Same as for adult

PHARMACOKINETICS Onset: 1 h PO; 5 min IV. **Duration:** 6–8 h PO; 3–6 h IV. **Distribution:** crosses placenta; appears in breast milk. **Metabolism:** metabolized primarily in liver. **Elimination:** half-life: 20–25 h; 40–50% of dose excreted in urine.

CONTRAINDICATIONS & PRECAUTIONS Contraindicated in: hypersensitivity to barbiturates; history of addiction; family or patient history of porphyria; severe respiratory, hepatic, or renal disease. Safe use during pregnancy (category D), in nursing women, and in children <6 y not established. **Cautious use in:** hypotension, hypertension, cardiac disease; acute or chronic pain; elderly patients.

ADVERSE/SIDE EFFECTS CNS: *drowsiness,* dizziness, hang-over, unsteadiness, lethargy, paradoxical excitement. **Hematologic (rare):** agranulocytosis, thrombocytopenia. **Hypersensitivity:** rash, angioedema, urticaria, serum sickness. **Other:** pain at IM injection site, Stevens-Johnson syndrome, hypotension, respiratory depression.

DRUG INTERACTIONS Antagonizes effects of **phenmetrazine;** CNS DEPRESSANTS, **alcohol,** SEDATIVES compound CNS depression; MAO INHIBITORS cause excessive CNS depression; **methoxyflurane** presents risk of nephrotoxicity.

INCOMPATIBILITIES Solution/additive: codeine phosphate, dimenhydrinate, phenytoin, hydrocortisone, hydroxyzine, insulin, levophanol, meperidine, methadone, morphine, norepinephrine, pentazocine, procaine, streptomycin, tetracycline, vancomycin, penicillin G, PHENOTHIAZINES, **cimetidine, pancuronium.**

NURSING IMPLICATIONS

Administration

- Rate of absorption is increased if oral drug is taken on an empty stomach.
- For insomnia (hypnotic), dose is generally administered 30–60 min before bedtime. Hypnotic use should be limited to 2 wk. Amobarbital effectiveness appears to decrease by second week of continued use.
- Drug should be injected within 30 min after vial is opened.
- Parenteral solution is reconstituted with sterile water for injection. Add diluent slowly and rotate vial. Do not shake vial. If solution does not clear within 5 min or contains a precipitate, do not use.

Common side effects in *italic*; life-threatening effects underlined;
generic names in **bold**; classifications in SMALL CAPS

Consult manufacturer's package insert for reconstitution direction to prepare specific concentrations.

- IM injection should be deep in a large muscle mass, e.g., upper outer quadrant of gluteus maximus. Superficial injections are painful and can cause sterile abscess or sloughing. No more than 5 ml should be injected IM into any one site.
- IV administration rate should not exceed 100 mg/min for adults or 60 mg/m²/min for children.
- Reactions occur most frequently with rapid IV administration.
- Store at 15–30C (59–86F) unless otherwise directed. Avoid freezing.

Assessment & Drug Effects

- Vital signs should be monitored during IV infusion and for several hours after drug administration. Caution patient not to get out of bed without assistance. Side rails are indicated.
- Personnel and equipment for management of respiratory depression and hypotension should be immediately available when drug is administered IV.
- Observe IV injection site during and after administration. Extravasation or inadvertent intraarterial injection can cause thrombophlebitis and tissue necrosis.
- Barbiturates may produce paradoxical restlessness, excitement, confusion, and depression in the elderly and in some children. Note implications for safety. Dosage adjustments may be required.

Patient & Family Education

- Caution patient not to take alcoholic beverages or other CNS depressants.
- Paradoxical excitement may also occur with onset of pain. Instruct patient to report this occurrence.
- Advise patient not to drive or engage in potentially hazardous activities until reaction to drug is known.
- Prolonged use may lead to tolerance and dependence. Advise patient to take drug only as ordered.

Prototype: imipramine, p 184

AMOXAPINE

(a-mox´a-peen)
Trade name: Asendin
Classifications: CNS AGENT; PSYCHOTHERAPEUTIC; TRICYCLIC ANTIDEPRESSANT
Pregnancy: Category C

ACTIONS/PHARMACODYNAMICS Tricyclic antidepressant (TCA) and secondary amine with mixed antidepressant and neuroleptic properties. Action mechanism not clear. Appears to reduce reuptake of norepinephrine (particularly) and serotonin and also blocks response to dopamine by dopaminergic receptors. Antidepressant activity is equivalent to that of imipramine, but additionally it is reportedly effective in relieving accompanying agitation and anxiety. Unlike other TCAs, not associated with severe cardiotoxicity, has mild sedative action, and causes slight orthostatic hypotension. Anticholinergic activity is also minimal; therefore it usually does not cause significant confusional episodes in the elderly, constipation, or exacerbation of glaucoma. Similar to imipramine in actions, uses, limitations, and interactions.

USES Neurotic and endogenous depression accompanied by anxiety or agitation.

ROUTE & DOSAGE

Antidepressant

Adult PO Start at 50 mg b.i.d. or t.i.d.; may increase on third day to 100 mg t.i.d.; *maintenance doses* ≤300 mg/d may be given as a single dose at bedtime.

PHARMACOKINETICS Absorption: rapidly absorbed. **Peak:** 1–2 h. **Distribution:** probably crosses placenta; distributed into breast milk. **Metabolism:** metabolized active metabolite. **Elimination:** half-life: 8 h parent drug, 30 h metabolite; 60% excreted in urine in 6 d; 7–18% excreted in feces.

CONTRAINDICATIONS & PRECAUTIONS Contraindicated in: hypersensitivity to other tricyclic compounds; acute recovery period after MI; children <16 y of age; pregnancy (Category C), nursing mothers. **Cautious use in:** history of convulsive disorders, schizophrenia, manic depression, electroshock therapy; alcohol abuse; history of urinary retention, benign prostatic hypertrophy; angle-closure glaucoma or increased intraocular pressure; cardiovascular disorders; impaired renal or hepatic function; elective surgery.

ADVERSE/SIDE EFFECTS CNS: *drowsiness,* dizziness, headache, fatigue, *sedation,* lethargy; (infrequent): extrapyramidal effects (acute dystonic reactions, panic attacks, parkinsonism, tardive dyskinesia), seizures (overdosage). **CV:** orthostatic hypotension; arrhythmias. **GI:** constipation, diarrhea,

Common side effects in *italic*; life-threatening effects underlined; generic names in **bold**; classifications in SMALL CAPS

flatulence, *dry mouth,* peculiar taste, nausea, heartburn. **Other:** blurred vision, nephrotoxicity (overdosage), agranulocytosis, dry eyes.

DRUG INTERACTIONS May decrease response to ANTIHYPERTENSIVES; CNS DEPRESSANTS, **alcohol,** HYPNOTICS, BARBITURATES, SEDATIVES potentiate CNS depression; may increase hypoprothombinemic effect of ORAL ANTICOAGULANTS; **ethchlorvynol,** transient delirium; with **levodopa,** SYMPATHOMIMETICS (e.g., **epinephrine, norepinephrine**), possibility of sympathetic hyperactivity with hypertension and hyperpyrexia; with MAO INHIBITORS, possibility of severe reactions: toxic psychosis, cardiovascular instability; **methylphenidiate** increases plasma TCA levels; THYROID DRUGS may increase possibility of arrhythmias; **cimetidine** may increase plasma TCA levels.

NURSING IMPLICATIONS

Administration

- May be taken with or after food to reduce GI irritation. Tablet may be crushed and taken with food or fluid of choice.
- Maintenance dose is generally taken as a single dose at bedtime to minimize daytime sedation and other annoying drug side effects.
- Store at 15–30C (59–86F) in tightly closed container unless otherwise directed.

Assessment & Drug Effects

- Initial antidepressant effect (mild euphoria, increased energy) may occur within 4–7 d; however, in most patients minimal clinical response does not occur until after 2 or 3 wk of drug therapy.
- Suicide risk may remain even when there is significant improvement. Supervise patient closely during therapy.
- Monitor I&O ratio and bowel elimination pattern. Report continuing constipation.
- Patient may experience sedation during early therapy, mostly when dosage increases are made. Note implications for ambulation, particularly in the elderly.
- Extrapyramidal reactions including parkinsonism, symptoms related to the reproductive system, and neuroleptic malignant syndrome reportedly occur more frequently with amoxapine than with other TCAs.
- Report immediately the onset of signs suggestive of tardive dyskinesia (see Signs & Symptoms, chap 3). Careful observations and prompt reporting may prevent irreversibility.
- Immediately report **signs of neuroleptic malignant syndrome:** fever, sweating, rigidity (catatonia), unstable BP, rapid, irregular pulse; changes in level of consciousness, coma. Although rare, it can be life-threatening if drug is not stopped immediately. Death can result from acute respiratory, renal, or cardiovascular failure.
- Tolerance to amoxapine antidepressant effects develops in some patients after 1–3 mo of drug therapy. Close medical follow-up is essential.

Patient & Family Education

- Excessive alcohol may potentiate drug effects, thus increasing the dangers of overdosage or suicide.
- Drinking at least 2000 ml fluid daily and eating foods with high fiber content (if allowed) will provide needed roughage.
- Amoxapine may increase the appetite and cause weight gain. Some patients develop a craving for sweets.
- Alertness and skill in performing hazardous tasks, such as driving, may be impaired, particularly during early therapy.
- Xerostomia may be relieved by frequent sips of water, increasing total fluid intake, if allowed, and by use of sugarless gum or sourballs.
- Withdrawal symptoms (headache, nausea, musculoskeletal pain, weakness) can be avoided by tapering dosage over 2 wk.
- Impress on patient the necessity of maintaining established dosage regimen. Tell patient not to skip, reduce, or double doses or change dose intervals.
- OTC drug use should be approved by the physician.
- Smoking reportedly increases metabolism of tricyclic compounds. Higher doses may be required in some smokers.

Prototype: ampicillin, p 69

AMOXICILLIN
(a-mox-i-sill´in)

Trade names: Amoxil, Larotid, Moxilean, Novamoxin, Polymox, Sumox, Trimox, Utimox, Wymox

Classifications: ANTIINFECTIVE; BETA-LACTAM ANTIBIOTIC; AMINOPENICILLIN

Pregnancy: Category B

ACTIONS/PHARMACODYNAMICS Broadspectrum, acid-stable, semisynthetic aminopenicillin

Common side effects in *italic*; life-threatening effects underlined; generic names in **bold**; classifications in SMALL CAPS

303

and analogue of ampicillin. Acts by inhibiting muco-protein synthesis in cell wall of rapidly multiplying bacteria. Like ampicillin, it is bactericidal, has essentially the same antibacterial spectrum, and is inactivated by penicillinase. Reportedly rash and diarrhea occur less frequently than with ampicillin, and at equal doses amoxicillin produces higher serum levels because it is more completely absorbed. Less effective in treatment of shigellosis than ampicillin.

USES Infections of ear, nose, and throat, GU tract, skin and soft tissue caused by susceptible bacteria. Also used in uncomplicated gonorrhea. Available in combination with potassium clavulanate, which extends antibacterial spectrum of amoxicillin to include beta-lactamase-producing strains.

ROUTE & DOSAGE

Mild to Moderate Infections

Adult	PO	250–500 mg q8h
Child	PO	20–40 mg/kd/d divided q8h

Gonorrhea

Adult	PO	3 g as single dose with 1 g probenecid

PHARMACOKINETICS Absorption: rapid and nearly complete absorption. **Peak:** 1–2 h. **Distribution:** diffuses into most tissues and body fluids, except synovial fluid and CSF (unless meninges are inflamed); crosses placenta; distributed into breast milk in small amounts. **Metabolism:** metabolized in liver. **Elimination:** half-life: 1–1.3 h; 60% of dose excreted in urine in 6–8 h.

CONTRAINDICATIONS & PRECAUTIONS Contraindicated in: hypersensitivity to penicillins; infectious mononucleosis. Safe use during pregnancy (category B) not established. **Cautious use in:** history of or suspected atopy or allergy (hives, eczema, hay fever, asthma); severely impaired renal function; history of cephalosporin allergy.

ADVERSE/SIDE EFFECTS As with other penicillins. **GI:** diarrhea, nausea, vomiting, pseudomembranous colitis (rare). **Hematologic:** hemolytic anemia, thrombocytopenia, purpura, eosinophilia, leukopenia, agranulocytosis. **Hypersensitivity:** rash, anaphylaxis. **Skin:** pruritus, urticaria, or other skin eruptions. **Other:** superinfections, conjunctival ecchymosis.

DRUG INTERACTIONS TETRACYCLINES may inhibit activity of amoxicillin; **probenecid** prolongs the activity of amoxicillin.

NURSING IMPLICATIONS

Administration

- Chewable tablet should be chewed or crushed before being swallowed with a liquid.
- May be given without regard to meals.
- For children, reconstituted pediatric drops may be placed directly on child's tongue for swallowing or added to formula, milk, fruit juice, water, ginger ale, or other soft drink. Have child drink all the prepared dose promptly.
- Store in tightly covered containers at 15–30C (59–86F) unless otherwise directed.

Assessment & Drug Effects

- Before therapy determine previous hypersensitivity reactions to penicillins, cephalosporins, and other allergens.
- Culture and sensitivity tests are done prior to initiation of therapy. Drug may be started pending results.
- Periodic assessments of renal, hepatic, and hematologic functions should be made during prolonged therapy.
- Diarrhea warrants appropriate diagnostic measures to rule out pseudomembranous colitis.
- Generalized, erythematous, maculopapular rash (ampicillin rash) is not due to hypersensitivity. It is usually mild, but can be severe. Report onset of rash to physician; hypersensitivity should be ruled out.
- An urticarial rash that occurs within a few days after start of amoxicillin is suggestive of a hypersensitivity reaction. If it occurs, look for other **signs of hypersensitivity** (fever, wheezing, generalized itching, dyspnea), and report to physician immediately.

Patient & Family Education

- Oral suspension and pediatric drops are reconstituted when they are dispensed from pharmacy. Date and time of reconstitution and discard date should appear on container. Stable for 7 d at room temperature, i.e., around 25C (77F) or 14 d if refrigerated, depending on manufacturer. Shake well before pouring.
- Instruct patient to take medication around the clock, not to miss a dose, and to continue therapy until all medication is taken, unless otherwise directed by physician.
- For most infections, treatment is continued for a minimum of 48–72 h beyond the time that patient is asymptomatic or cultures are negative.
- Patients with hemolytic streptococcal infections should receive at least 10 d of treatment to prevent occurrence of acute rheumatic fever.

Common side effects in *italic*; life-threatening effects underlined; generic names in **bold**; classifications in SMALL CAPS

■ Advise patient to report to physician the onset of diarrhea and other possible symptoms of superinfection (see Signs & Symptoms, chap 3).

Prototype: ampicillin, p 69

AMOXICILLIN AND CLAVULANATE POTASSIUM

(a-mox-i-sill´in)

Trade names: Augmentin, Clavulin
Classification: ANTIINFECTIVE; AMINOPENICILLIN
Pregnancy: Category B

ACTIONS/PHARMACODYNAMICS Semisynthetic broad-spectrum antibiotic. Fixed combination of amoxicillin, an aminopenicillin, and the potassium salt to clavulanic acid, a competitive beta-lactamase inhibitor. Used alone, clavulanic acid antibacterial activity is weak. In combination it inhibits enzyme (beta-lactamase) degradation of amoxicillin and by synergism extends both spectrum of activity and bactericidal effect of amoxicillin against many strains of beta-lactamase-producing bacteria resistant to amoxicillin alone. Active against gram-positive bacteria including *Staphylococcus aureus, Streptococcus pneumoniae, Clostridium, Peptococcus, Bacteroides fragilis* group, and many gram-negative organisms including *Branhamella catarrhalis* (formerly *Neisseria catarrhalis*), *Haemophilus influenzae, Proteus mirabilis; Salmonella, Shigella,* and *Klebsiella* sp. Generally inactive against *Pseudomonas.*

USES Infections caused by susceptible beta-lactamase-producing organisms: lower respiratory tract infections, otitis media, sinusitis, skin and skin structure infections, and UTI.

ROUTE & DOSAGE

Mild to Moderate Infections

Adult	PO	250 or 500 mg tablet (each with 125 mg clavulanic acid) q8h
Child	PO	20–40 mg/kg/d (based on amoxicillin component) divided q8h

PHARMACOKINETICS **Absorption:** rapid and nearly complete absorption. **Peak:** 1–2 h. **Distribution:** diffuses into most tissues and body fluids, except synovial fluid and CSF (unless meninges are inflamed); crosses placenta; distributed into breast milk in very small amounts. **Metabolism:** metabolized in liver. **Elimination:** half-life: amoxicillin 1–1.3 h, clavulanate 0.78–1.2 h; 50–73% of the amoxicillin and 25–45% of the clavulanate dose excreted in urine in 2 h.

CONTRAINDICATIONS & PRECAUTIONS Contraindicated in: combination shares toxic potentials of ampicillin. Hypersensitivity to penicillins; infectious mononucleosis. **Cautious use in:** lactation, pregnancy (category B).

ADVERSE/SIDE EFFECTS GI: *diarrhea,* nausea, vomiting. **Skin:** rash, urticaria. **Other:** candidal vaginitis, moderate increases in serum ALT, AST; slight thrombocytosis, bone marrow depression, glomerulonephritis.

DIAGNOSTIC TEST INTERFERENCES May interfere with *urinary glucose* determinations using *cupric sulfate, Benedict's solution, Clinitest;* does not affect glucose oxidase methods, e.g., Clinistix, TesTape. Positive direct *antiglobulin (Coombs')* test results may be reported, a reaction that could interfere with *hematologic studies* or with *transfusion cross-matching* procedures.

DRUG INTERACTIONS TETRACYCLINES may inhibit activity of amoxicillin; **probenecid** prolongs the activity of amoxicillin.

NURSING IMPLICATIONS

Administration

■ Both 250 and 500 mg tablets contain the exact amount of clavulanic acid (125 mg and potassium salt); therefore, two 250 mg tablets are not equivalent to one 500 mg tablet.
■ May be given without regard to meals.
■ Oral probenecid administered before or with amoxicillin–clavulanate potassium competitively inhibits tubular secretion of amoxicillin, thereby increasing its concentration and prolonging its effects.
■ Reconstitute oral suspension by adding amount of water specified to provide suspension containing 125 mg amoxicillin per 31.25 mg clavulanic acid, or 250 mg amoxicillin per 62.5 mg clavulanic acid per 5 ml. Tap bottle before adding water to loosen

Common side effects in *italic*; life-threatening effects underlined; generic names in **bold**; classifications in SMALL CAPS

305

A

powder, then add water in 2 portions, agitating suspension well before each addition. Discard reconstituted suspension after 10 d.

▪ Suspension should be agitated well just before administration of each dose.

▪ Patient compliance may be aided by using the chewable formulation with its lemon-lime flavor.

▪ A suggested schedule for the dialysis period: a 500 mg tablet (500 mg amoxicillin/125 mg clavulanate potassium) halfway through period and an additional 500 mg tablet at its conclusion.

▪ Store tablets in tight containers at <24C (71F). Reconstituted oral suspension should be refrigerated at 2–8C (36–46F).

Assessment & Drug Effects

▪ Before therapy is initiated, determine previous hypersensitivity to penicillins, cephalosporins, and other drugs.

▪ Before establishing a therapeutic regimen, culture and susceptibility tests are run. Drug may be started pending results.

▪ Generalized, erythematous, maculopapular rash (ampicillin rash) is not due to hypersensitivity. It is usually mild but can be severe. Report onset of rash to physician.

▪ A urticarial rash that occurs within a few days after start of amoxicillin is suggestive of a hypersensitivity reaction. Assess for other signs of hypersensitivity (see chap 3).

Patient & Family Education

▪ Advise female patient to report onset of symptoms of candidal vaginitis. Therapy may have to be discontinued. **Candidal vaginitis symptoms:** moderate amount of white, cheesy, nonodorous vaginal discharge, vaginal inflammation and itching; vulvar excoriation, inflammation, burning, itching. Miconazol (topical) or oral nystatin are effective treatment agents.

▪ Caution patient with diabetes mellitus to use Clinistix or TesTape for monitoring urinary glucose to avoid false readings.

AMPHETAMINE SULFATE

See CENTRAL NERVOUS SYSTEM AGENTS, AMPHETAMINE RESPIRATORY AND CEREBRAL STIMULANT prototype, p 194.

AMPHOTERICIN B

See ANTIINFECTIVES, ANTIFUNGAL ANTIBIOTIC prototype, p 56.

AMPICILLIN

See ANTIINFECTIVES, AMINOPENICILLIN ANTIBIOTIC prototype, p 69.

Prototype: ampicillin, p 69

AMPICILLIN SODIUM AND SULBACTAM SODIUM

(am-pi-sill´in/sul-bak´tam)
Trade name: Unasyn
Classifications: ANTIINFECTIVE; BETA-LACTAM ANTIBIOTIC; AMINOPENICILLIN
Pregnancy: Category B

ACTIONS/PHARMACODYNAMICS Antibiotic agent with broad spectrum of activity resulting from beta-lactamase inhibition; fixed combination of ampicillin sodium with sulbactam sodium in 2:1 ratio. Sulbactam inhibits beta-lactamases most frequently responsible for transferred drug resistance. Because of this action, a wide range of beta-lactamases found in organisms resistant to penicillins and cephalosporins are irreversibily inhibited. The combination of sulbactam with ampicillin restores susceptibility to the antibiotic activity of ampicillin in resistant organisms and extends into antimicrobial spectrum to include many bacteria normally resistant to it (including anaerobes).

USES Treatment of infections due to susceptible organisms in skin and skin structures (e.g., *Klebsiella pneumoniae, Staphylococcus aureus)* and intraabdominal infections (e.g., *Escherichia coli* and for gynecologic infections (e.g., *Bacteroides* sp including *B. fragilis*). Also used for infections caused by ampicillin-susceptible organisms.

Common side effects in *italic*; life-threatening effects underlined; generic names in **bold**; classifications in SMALL CAPS

ROUTE & DOSAGE

Systemic Infections

Adult	IM/IV	1.5 (1 g ampicillin, 0.5 g sulbactam) to 3 g (2 g ampicillin, 1 g sulbactam) q6h (max 4 g sulbactam/d)

PHARMACOKINETICS Peak: immediate after IV. **Duration:** 6–8 h. **Distribution:** most body tissues; high CNS concentrations only with inflamed meninges; crosses placenta; appears in breast milk. **Metabolism:** minimal hepatic metabolism. **Elimination:** half-life: 1 h; excreted in urine.

CONTRAINDICATIONS & PRECAUTIONS Contraindicated in: hypersensitivity to penicillins; mononucleosis. Safe use during pregnancy (category B), by nursing mothers, or children <12 y not established. **Cautious use in:** hypersensitivity to cephalosporins.

ADVERSE/SIDE EFFECTS GI: *diarrhea, nausea,* vomiting, abdominal distension, candidiasis. **Hematologic:** neutropenia, thrombocytopenia; increased lymphocytes, monocytes, basophils, eosinophils, BUN, creatinine, AST, ALT, alkaline phosphatase, LDH. **Hypersensitivity:** rash, itching, anaphylactoid reaction. **Renal:** dysuria. **Other:** fatigue, malaise, headache, chills, seizures, edema. **Local:** pain at injection sites; thrombophlebitis.

DRUG INTERACTIONS Allopurinol increases incidence of rash; effectiveness of the AMINOGLYCOSIDES may be impaired in patients with severe end-stage renal disease; **chloramphenicol, erythromycin, tetracycline** may reduce bactericidal effects of ampicillin—this interaction is primarily significant when low doses are used; ampicillin may interfere with the contraceptive action of ORAL CONTRACEPTIVES—female patients should be advised to consider nonhormonal contraception while on antibiotics.

INCOMPATIBILITIES Solution/Additive: incompatible in any dextrose-containing solution, including parenteral nutrition solutions. **Y-Site: clindamycin, erythromycin,** AMINOGLYCOSIDES, **lidocaine, verapamil.**

NURSING IMPLICATIONS

Administration

- **IV solution:** reconstitute each 1.5 g with 4 ml of sterile water for injection to yield solutions of 375 mg/ml (250 mg ampicillin/125 mg sulbactam); then with suitable diluent, immediately add sufficient volume to yield solutions of 3–45 mg/ml (2–30 mg ampicillin/1–11 mg sulbactam/ml).
- Administer properly diluted IV solution slowly over at least 10–15 min. Convulsions may be induced by too rapid administration.
- Use only freshly prepared solution; administer within 1 h after preparation.
- **IM solution:** Reconstitute with sterile water for injection. Consult manufacturer's directions. IM injections should be made deeply into a large muscle such as the gluteus maximus. Rotate injection sites.
- Store powder for injection at 15–30C (59–86F) before reconstitution. Storage times and temperatures vary for different concentrations of reconstituted solutions. Consult manufacturer's directions.

Assessment & Drug Effects

- Culture and sensitivity studies should be done before therapy is begun. Therapy may be started before results of susceptibility testing are known.
- Before therapy is begun, inquiry should be made regarding past hypersensitivity reactions to penicillin, cephalosporins, and other allergens.
- Report promptly unexplained bleeding (e.g., epistaxis, purpura, ecchymoses). These may be hypersensitivity phenomena and are usually reversible when drug is withdrawn.
- Monitor patient carefully during the first 30 min after initiation of IV therapy for signs of hypersensitivity and anaphylactoid reaction (see chap 3).
- Serious anaphylactoid reactions require immediate use of epinephrine, oxygen, IV steroids, and airway management.
- Observe for and report symptoms of superinfections (see Signs & Symptoms, chap 3). Ampicillin-sulbactam should be withdrawn.
- Monitor renal function: I&O ratio and pattern. Report dysuria, urine retention, and hematuria (adverse effects of ampicillin).

Patient & Family Education

- Instruct patient to immediately report chills, wheezing, pruritus, respiratory distress, or palpitations.

Common side effects in *italic*; life-threatening effects underlined; generic names in **bold**; classifications in SMALL CAPS

307

A

AMRINONE LACTATE

(am´ri-none)

Trade name: Inocor

Classifications: CARDIAC INOTROPIC AGENT;
ENZYME INHIBITOR; VASODILATOR

Pregnancy: Category C

ACTIONS/PHARMACODYNAMICS Bipyridine derivative, the first of a new chemical class of cardiac inotropic agents with vasodilator activity. Action mechanism involved in stimulation of myocardial contractility is thought to be related to inhibition of phosphodiesterase activity with resultant increase in cellular levels of cAMP. Mode of action appears to differ from that of the digitalis glycosides and beta-adrenergic stimulants. In patients with depressed myocardial function, it enhances myocardial contractility, increases cardiac output and stroke volume, and reduces right and left ventricular filling pressure, pulmonary capillary wedge pressure (PCWP), and systemic vascular resistance. Vasodilating action, produced by direct relaxant effect on vascular smooth muscle, reduces strain on failing heart. Improves hemodynamics at rest and during exercise, and increases exercise capacity without adverse effects on heart rate, rhythm, or BP.

USES Short-term management of CHF in patients not adequately controlled by traditional therapy, such as digitalis, diuretics, and vasodilators, and may be used in conjunction with these agents.

ROUTE & DOSAGE

Congestive Heart Failure

Adult IV 0.75 mg/kg bolus given slowly over 2–3 min; then start infusion at 5–10 µg/kg/min; may repeat bolus in 30 min; should not exceed 10 mg/kg/d

PHARMACOKINETICS Onset: 2–5 min. **Peak:** 10 min. **Duration:** about 2 h. **Distribution:** unknown if it crosses placenta or into breast milk. **Metabolism:** metabolized in liver. **Elimination:** half-life: 3.6–7.5 h; excreted primarily in urine.

CONTRAINDICATIONS & PRECAUTIONS Contraindicated in: hypersensitivity to amrinone or to bisulfites; severe aortic or pulmonic valvular disease in lieu of appropriate surgery, acute MI; uncorrected hypokalemia or dehydration. Safe use during pregnancy (category C), in nursing women, and in children not established. **Cautious use in:** compromised renal or hepatic function, hypertrophic subaortic stenosis. Concomitant cardiac glycoside therapy recommended in patients with atrial flutter or fibrillation.

ADVERSE/SIDE EFFECTS CV: hypotension, arrhythmias. **Endocrine:** nephrogenic diabetes insipidus. **GI:** nausea, vomiting, anorexia, abdominal cramps, hepatotoxicity. **Hematologic:** asymptomatic thrombocytopenia. **Hypersensitivity:** pericarditis, pleuritis; myositis with interstitial shadows on chest x-ray and elevated sedimentation rate; vasculitis with nodular pulmonary densities, hypoxemia, ascites, jaundice.

DRUG INTERACTIONS Possibility of excessive hypotension with **disopyramide.**

INCOMPATIBILITIES Solution/Additive: sodium bicarbonate, dextrose-containing solutions. **Y-Site:** furosemide.

NURSING IMPLICATIONS

Administration

- Intravenous amrinone therapy is indicated only for patients who can be closely monitored.
- Natural color of IV amrinone is clear yellow. Discard discolored solutions and those that contain a precipitate.
- Do not dilute IV amrinone with dextrose solutions because a chemical interaction occurs slowly over 24 h. However, manufacturer states that amrinone may be injected into a running dextrose infusion through Y-connector or directly into tubing.
- Amrinone is reportedly compatible with 0.45 and 0.9% NaCl injection. All diluted solutions should be used within 24 h.
- IV amrinone may be administered undiluted by direct IV in a single dose over 2–3 min.
- IV amrinone may be diluted by adding 1 ml of NS or 0.45% saline to each 5 mg (1 ml) of medication. The diluted solution may be infused at a rate of 5 µg/kg/min.
- Store at 15–30C (59–86F) unless otherwise directed. Protect ampuls from light.

Assessment & Drug Effects

- During IV administration, monitor BP, heart rate, and respirations and keep physician informed. Rate of administration and duration of therapy are prescribed according to clinical response and adverse effects.

Common side effects in *italic*; life-threatening effects underlined; generic names in **bold**; classifications in SMALL CAPS

- Consult physician for guidelines. In general, rate of infusion should be slowed or stopped with excessive drop in BP or arrhythmias.
- Monitor infusion site to prevent extravasation.
- Monitor I&O ratio and pattern and daily weights. Improvement in cardiac output enhances diuresis with consequent danger of hypokalemia and arrhythmias, particularly in digitalized patients. Hypokalemia should be corrected before and during amrinone therapy.
- Principal hemodynamic parameters indicating clinical improvement include: increased cardiac output, decreased PCWP. Central venous pressure may be used to assess hypotension and blood volume (hydration state).
- The following laboratory values should also be closely monitored throughout therapy to detect adverse effects of amrinone: platelet counts, liver enzymes, fluid and electrolyte balances, renal function studies.
- Another measurement used to evaluate patient response is relief of symptoms of CHF.
- Thrombocytopenia may occur during prolonged therapy or with high dosages. Platelet counts should be taken before treatment begins and frequently during therapy. Close monitoring of platelet counts, appropriate dosage reduction or drug discontinuation should prevent symptoms of thrombocytopenia and allow reversibility. If platelet count falls below 150,000/mm^3, report immediately to physician.
- Amrinone IV preparation contains sodium metabisulfite, a reducing agent to which certain susceptible individuals are allergic. Drug should be discontinued immediately if patient manifests clinical symptoms suggestive of hypersensitivity reactions.
- Patient must be closely observed when drug is withdrawn after prolonged therapy because clinical deterioration may occur within hours.

Prototype: nitroglycerin, p 149

AMYL NITRITE
(am´il)
Classifications: CARDIOVASCULAR AGENT; NITRATE VASODILATOR; ANTIDOTE
Pregnancy: Category C

ACTIONS/PHARMACODYNAMICS Short-acting vasodilator and smooth muscle relaxant with actions, contraindications, and adverse reactions similar to those of nitroglycerin. Action in treatment of cyanide poisoning based on ability of amyl nitrite to convert hemoglobin to methemoglobin, which forms a nontoxic complex with cyanide ion.

USES To relieve pain of renal and gallbladder colic. Also used as an adjunct antidote in the immediate treatment of cyanide poisoning. (Because of adverse effects, unpleasant odor, and expense, infrequently used to treat angina pectoris.) **Unlabeled uses:** change intensity of heart murmurs.

ROUTE & DOSAGE

Acute Angina

Adult	Inhalation	0.18–0.3 ml prn

Cyanide Poisoning

Adult	Inhalation	0.3 ml Pearl crushed every minute and inhaled for 15–30 s until sodium nitrite infusion is ready
Child	Inhalation	Same as for adult

PHARMACOKINETICS Absorption: rapidly absorbed from mucous membranes. **Onset:** 10–30 s. **Duration:** 3–5 min.

CONTRAINDICATIONS & PRECAUTIONS Contraindicated in: hypersensitivity to nitrites or nitrates; cerebral hemorrhage, head trauma; hypotension; glaucoma; severe anemia; hyperthyroidism; recent MI; acute alcoholism. Safe use during pregnancy (category C) and in nursing women not established.

ADVERSE/SIDE EFFECTS *Headache,* transient flushing, orthostatic hypotension, dizziness, weakness, syncope, palpitation, respiratory depression, nausea, vomiting, agitation, cardiovascular collapse, tachycardia, methemoglobinemia (large doses).

NURSING IMPLICATIONS

Administration

- Available in 0.18 ml and 0.3 ml Perls (thin, friable glass ampuls enveloped with woven fabric cover). To prepare for administration, wrap ampul in gauze or cloth and crush between fingers.
- Syncope, due to a sudden drop in systolic BP, sometimes follows amyl nitrite inhalation, particularly in the elderly. Patient should be sitting while and immediately after drug is administered.
- Amyl nitrite is volatile and highly flammable. When mixed with air or oxygen, it forms a mixture that can explode if ignited.

Common side effects in *italic*; life-threatening effects underlined; generic names in **bold**; classifications in SMALL CAPS

309

A

▪ Store at 8–15C (46–59F), unless otherwise directed. Protect from light.

Assessment & Drug Effects

▪ After administration of drug, note length of time required for pain to subside; monitor vital signs until they are stable. Rapid pulse, which usually lasts for a brief period, is an expected baroreceptor response to the fall in BP produced by the nitrite ion.

▪ When amyl nitrite is used to change the intensity of heart murmur, those resulting from stenotic valves become louder; those associated with aortic or mitral regurgitation become softer.

▪ Tolerance may develop with repeated use over prolonged periods.

Patient & Family Education

▪ Inform patient that drug has a strongly fruity odor.

▪ Patients taking amyl nitrite for angina pectoris should be advised to consult physician or go to the hospital emergency room immediately if no relief is experienced after 3 doses 5 min apart.

Prototype: atropine, p 116

ANISOTROPINE METHYLBROMIDE

(a-nis´o-tro-pine)
Trade name: Valpin 50
Classifications: AUTONOMIC NERVOUS SYSTEM AGENT; ANTICHOLINERGIC (PARASYMPATHOLYTIC); ANTIMUSCARINIC; ANTISPASMODIC
Pregnancy: Category C

ACTIONS/PHARMACODYNAMICS Synthetic quaternary ammonium antimuscarinic drug with pharmacologic effects similar to those of atropine. Inhibits muscarinic actions of acetylcholine or autonomic neuroeffector sites innervated by postganglionic cholinergic nerves.

USES Indicated as an adjunct in the treatment of peptic ulcer disease.

ROUTE & DOSAGE

Adjunct for Peptic Ulcer Disease

Adult PO 50 mg t.i.d.; higher doses may be necessary

PHARMACOKINETICS Absorption: <10% absorbed from GI tract. **Elimination:** excreted in urine, unabsorbed drug excreted in feces.

CONTRAINDICATIONS & PRECAUTIONS Contraindicated in: severe ulcerative colitis, obstructive disease of the GI tract, achalasia, paralytic ileus, intestinal atony, especially in geriatric patients; hypersensitivity to anisotropine methylbromide; angle-closure glaucoma; obstructive uropathy; tachycardia, acute hemorrhage, and myasthenia gravis. **Cautious use in:** patients in hot or humid environments, patients who are febrile or exposed to elevated temperatures; geriatric patients, infants, children; hyperthyroidism; hepatic or renal failure; hypertension, tachyarrhythmias, CHF, coronary artery disease; COPD; autonomic neuropathy; esophageal reflux, hiatal hernia, GI infections, and diarrhea; pregnancy (category C).

ADVERSE/SIDE EFFECTS CNS: headache, nervousness, drowsiness, weakness, dizziness, depression, insomnia, mental confusion or excitement especially in geriatric patients. **CV:** *palpitations, tachycardia,* hypotension, circulatory collapse. **Eye:** blurred vision, mydriasis. **GI:** *xerostomia,* loss of taste, *constipation,* nausea, vomiting. **GU:** anhidrosis, urinary hesitancy and retention. **Hypersensitivity:** anaphylaxis, urticaria, rash. **Overdosage:** curariform neuromuscular block and ganglionic blockage manifested by respiratory paralysis.

DRUG INTERACTIONS Amantadine, ANTIHISTAMINES, TRICYCLIC ANTIDEPRESSANTS, **quinidine, disopyramide, procainamide** compound anticholinergic effects; decreases **levodopa** effects; **methotrimeprazine** may precipitate extrapyramidal effects; decreases antipsychotic effects (decreased absorption) of PHENOTHIAZINES.

NURSING IMPLICATIONS

Administration

▪ Administer cautiously with febrile patients.
▪ Administer before meals and at bedtime.
▪ Dosage should be according to patient's response and tolerance.
▪ Store at room temperature (15–30C).

Assessment & Drug Effects

▪ Monitor I&O, vital signs, and cardiac rate and rhythm.
▪ Evaluate for absence of GI problems (i.e., pain, bleeding, nausea, vomiting, constipation).

Common side effects in *italic*; life-threatening effects underlined; generic names in **bold**; classifications in SMALL CAPS

- Monitor adverse effects of drug, which are generally dose related.
- Report palpitations and tachycardia, which may indicate need for dosage adjustment.

Patient & Family Education

- Advise patient to take medication 30–60 min before meals and at bedtime.
- Instruct patient to increase fluid intake to a minimum of 600–1000 ml/d (if not contraindicated) to prevent constipation.
- Instruct patient to avoid driving and other hazardous activities until reaction to drug is known.
- Inform patient that drug-induced heat intolerance may develop in hot and humid environments.
- Advise patient to use hard candy or gum to relieve dry mouth.

Prototype: streptokinase, p 134

ANISTREPLASE (APSAC)

(a-ni´strep-lase)
Trade name: Eminase
Classifications: BLOOD FORMERS AND COAGULATORS; THROMBOLYTIC ENZYME
Pregnancy: Category C

ACTIONS/PHARMACODYNAMICS A derivative of plasminogen streptokinase activator complex (APSAC). Activation of anistreplase occurs with deacylation of the drug. The production of plasmin from plasminogen by deacylated anistreplase can take place in the bloodstream or within the thrombus. The latter process is more efficient, but both may contribute to thrombolysis.

USES Management of acute MI in adults by lysis of thrombi obstructing coronary arteries and reduction of infarct size. Initiation of treatment occurs immediately after the onset of acute MI.

ROUTE & DOSAGE

Acute MI
Adult   IV   30 U IV push over 2–5 min

PHARMACOKINETICS Onset: immediate. **Peak:** 45 min after end of injection. **Duration:** 4–6 h.

Metabolism: metabolized in plasma. **Elimination:** half-life: 105–120 min.

CONTRAINDICATIONS & PRECAUTIONS Contraindicated in: active internal bleeding, history of CVA, recent (within 2 mo) intracranial or intraspinal surgery or trauma, intracranial neoplasms, uncontrolled hypertension; severe allergic reactions to either anistreplase or streptokinase. **Cautious use in:** pregnancy (category C), major surgery within preceding 10 d, cerebral vascular disease, recent GI or GU bleeding, recent trauma, hypertension, age >75 y, hemorrhagic ophthalmic conditions, current use of oral anticoagulants.

ADVERSE/SIDE EFFECTS CV: <u>hemorrhage</u>, *reperfusion arrhythmias, hypotension.* **Hypersensitivity:** <u>anaphylactic and anaphylactoid reactions</u> in <1% of patients.

NURSING IMPLICATIONS

Administration

- The drug should be instituted as soon as possible following the onset of clinical symptoms of acute MI.
- Dilute each dose with 5 ml sterile water for injection. Slowly add diluent, rolling vial to mix; do not shake.
- Diluted solution may be clear to pale yellow. Do not administer if particulate matter is present.
- Do not further dilute reconstituted solution and discard if it is not used within 30 min.
- Inject over 2–5 min directly into vein or IV line through the most proximal port.
- During administration only essential handling or moving of the patient should be done.

Assessment & Drug Effects

- Prior to administration, coagulation tests need to be done including APTT, bleeding time, PT, TT.
- Blood for Hct, Hgb, and platelet counts should be drawn before administration for baseline values in case of bleeding.
- Monitor vital signs q15min for first 6 h, including BP, pulse, respirations, and temperature. Watch for bradycardia and allergic reaction.
- Monitor neurological checks q30min for 6 h.
- Spontaneous bleeding occurs twice as often with anistreplase as with heparin. Protect patient from invasive procedures: IM injections are contraindicated. Also prevent manipulation during thrombolytic therapy to prevent bruising.
- Monitor for excess external or internal bleeding q15min for the first hour of therapy, every 30 min for second to eighth hour, then every 8 h.

Common side effects in *italic*; life-threatening effects <u>underlined</u>; generic names in **bold**; classifications in SMALL CAPS

■ Report signs of bleeding: gum bleeding, epistaxis, hematoma, spontaneous ecchymoses, oozing at catheter site, increased pain from internal bleeding. The anistreplase infusion should be interrupted, then resumed when bleeding stops.

■ If a blood gas determination is needed, select the radial rather than the femoral artery because a pressure dressing can more easily be applied to it to control oozing. It may be necessary to apply pressure to puncture sites for as long as 30 min.

■ Patient is at risk for postthrombolytic bleeding for 2–4 d after intracoronary anistreplase treatment. Continue monitoring vital signs until laboratory reports confirm anticoagulant control.

■ Following administration, coagulation tests, coronary angiography, and myocardial scanning should be done to determine effectiveness of treatment.

■ Hct should be drawn to detect possible blood loss following administration.

Patient & Family Education
■ Incidents of bleeding need to be reported to the nurse or doctor. Report blood in urine and bloody or tarry stools.

■ Bedrest is essential during therapy to prevent bleeding.

ANTHRALIN

See SKIN & MUCOUS MEMBRANE AGENTS, ANTIPSORIATIC prototype, p. 259.

ANTIHEMOPHILIC FACTOR, HUMAN (FACTOR VIII)

(an-tee-hee-moe-fill′ik)
Trade names: H.T. Factorate, H.T. Factorate Generation II, Hemofil CT, Humate, Koate-HS, Koate HT, Monoclate, Profilate
Classifications: BLOOD FORMER & COAGULATOR; HEMOSTATIC
Pregnancy: Category C

ACTIONS/PHRAMACODYNAMICS Stable lyophilized concentrate of human antihemophilic factor (AHF) obtained from large pools of fresh normal human plasma. Commercial factor VIII preparations are now subjected to heat treatment to reduce potential for transmitting HIV and viral hepatitis. Verification studies are ongoing. Potential for transmitting AIDS is yet to be proven with use of heat-treated AHF preparations. Factor VIII is essential in the body for conversion of prothrombin to thrombin by the intrinsic pathway and for maintaining effective hemostasis. Administration of AHF corrects or prevents bleeding episodes by replacing the missing clotting factor and obviates the need of administering large volumes of plasma, thus avoiding risk of hypervolemia and hyperproteinemia. Contains relatively small amounts of fibrinogen and other plasma proteins.

USES Hemophilia A (genetic deficiency of Factor VIII) and in patients with acquired circulating factor VIII inhibitors.

ROUTE & DOSAGE

Acute Bleeding Episode

Adult	IV	8–30 U/kg q8–12h
Child	IV	Same as for adult

Prophylaxis

Adult	IV	>50 kg: 500 U/d in AM
Child	IV	>50 kg: 500 U/d in AM
Adult	IV	<50 kg: 250 U/d in AM
Child	IV	<50 kg: 250 U/d in AM

PHARMACOKINETICS Distribution: does not readily cross placenta. **Metabolism:** rapidly cleared from body. **Elimination:** half-life: 12 h (4–24 h).

CONTRAINDICATIONS & PRECAUTIONS Contraindicated in: von Willebrand's disease since it is not effective for controlling bleeding. Safe use during pregnancy (category C) not established. **Cautious use in:** hepatic disease, large or frequently repeated doses to patients with blood types A, B, and AB.

ADVERSE/SIDE EFFECTS Generally related to rate of administration. **CNS:** headache, paresthesias, somnolence, lethargy, clouding or loss of consciousness. **CV:** hypotension, tachycardia. **Hypersensitivity:** anaphylactic or febrile reaction; hemolysis. **Other:** dizziness, nausea, vomiting, transient chest discomfort and cough, bronchospasm; disturbed vision; jaundice, viral hepatisis; AIDS; thrombosis.

NURSING IMPLICATIONS

Administration

- Reconstitute according to manufacturer's directions and with diluent supplied. Before reconstitution the dried concentrate and diluent should be warmed to room temperature 20–30C (68–86F). Temperature should not exceed 37C (98.6F).
- After the addition of diluent to vial, rotate or agitate gently until concentrate is completely dissolved. Administer within 3 h to avoid microbial contamination. Do not refrigerate or keep at less than room temperature after reconstitution, as precipitation may occur.
- Expiration date should be checked carefully.
- If syringe is necessary, use a plastic one (AHF solutions tend to stick to surface of ground glass).
- Physician will prescribe IV flow rate. Preparations containing 34 or more AHF U/ml should be administered at a carefully controlled rate, not exceeding 2 ml/min. Preparations containing less than 34 AHF U/ml are administered at rate of 10–20 ml over 3 min, as prescribed.
- Cryoprecipitated factor VIII must be kept frozen until ready to use. Then it should be thawed to room temperature by placing it in a warm water bath at no higher than 37C (98.6F). Higher temperatures may destroy factor VIII activity. Bag should be gently agitated to assure dissolution. Once thawed, it should be used within 3 h. It is administered through a filter.
- Cryoprecipitated factor VIII is especially appropriate for patients with von Willebrand's disease because, in addition to factor VIII, it also supplies about 250 mg fibrinogen (factor I), which these patients lack.
- Store dried concentrate preparations in refrigerator at 2–8C (35–46F) unless otherwise directed. Avoid freezing.

Assessment & Drug Effects

- Observe for vasomotor and hypersensitivity reactions. Take vital signs before and during therapy. If there is a significant increase in pulse rate, IV flow rate should be reduced or administration stopped.
- Some patients manifest an acute, transient allergic reaction (erythema, urticaria, backache, fever) during or after administration of certain preparations. The reaction generally subsides within 20 min. Notify physician.
- Factor VIII activity is determined before therapy and daily during therapy. Normal value is 100% (range 50–200%).
- Tests for factor VIII inhibitor also should be done

before initiation of therapy. Patients with inhibitor levels greater than 5–10 Bethesda U/ml may not respond to AHF or may require larger doses.

- Hct and direct Coombs' test should be monitored in patients with blood types A, B, or AB who are receiving large or frequently repeated doses to detect signs of **intravascular hemolysis:** fever, chills, tachycardia, rapid breathing, backache, hematuria, increased serum bilirubin, LDH, and reticulocytes. (AHF preparations contain small amounts of group A and B isohemagglutinins.) Reaction is life threatening and must be recognized and treated promptly.
- **Laboratory values generally characteristic of hemophilia:** factor VIII activity assay: 0–3% of normal; PTT: prolonged; platelet count and function, bleeding time, and PT normal.

Patient & Family Education

- Instruct patient to immediately report any subjective symptoms of a hypersensitivity reaction (see chap 3).

APOMORPHINE HYDROCHLORIDE

(a-poe-mor′feen)
Classification: EMETIC
Pregnancy: Category C
Controlled substance: Schedule II

ACTIONS/PHARMACODYNAMICS Centrally acting emetic prepared by treating morphine with dilute hydrochloric acid; results in marked reduction of analgesic activity but enhanced emetic action. Produces CNS excitation and depression; induces vomiting by direct stimulant action on chemoreceptor trigger zone (CTZ) and possibly by excitation of vestibular centers. Depresses medullary center that controls respiration and vasomotor tone and stimulates salivation. Elevates plasma levels of human growth hormone and reduces serum prolactin levels by stimulating dopamine receptors. Used in subemetic doses as dopaminergic agonist to reduce tremor and rigidity in parkinsonism as well as levodopa-induced tremor, choreiform movements, and dyskinesia, and in alcoholism to reduce anxiety and craving for alcohol. Has sedative and hypnotic action in small nonemetic doses.

USES To produce emesis, particularly in acute oral drug overdosage or after oral ingestion of certain poi-

Common side effects in *italic*; life-threatening effects <u>underlined</u>; generic names in **bold**; classifications in SMALL CAPS

313

A

sons. **Unlabeled use:** for parkinsonism and in conditioned aversion techniques for alcoholism.

ROUTE & DOSAGE

Emesis

Adult	SC	2–10 mg as a single dose (average 5–6 mg)
Child	SC	0.07–0.1 mg/kg as a single dose

PHARMACOKINETICS Onset: 10–15 min in adults; 1–2 min in children. **Duration:** sedative effects may last 2 h. **Metabolism:** metabolized in liver. **Elimination:** excreted in urine.

CONTRAINDICATIONS & PRECAUTIONS Contraindicated in: hypersensitivity to morphine and related opiates; after ingestion of caustics or corrosives (e.g., lye, acids) or volatile oils. Use for petroleum distillates or liquid hydrocarbons (gasoline, kerosene and the like) depends on amount ingested and relative toxicity of substance. Other contraindications: strychnine poisoning, unconsciousness, during seizures; absent gag reflex, severely inebriated patients, shock; narcosis due to alcohol, barbiturates, opiates, and other CNS or respiratory depressants. Safe use during pregnancy (category C) and in nursing mothers not established. **Cautious use in:** children, elderly and debilitated patients; impaired cardiac function; epilepsy; predisposition to nausea and vomiting; acute overdosage of digitalis glycosides (may potentiate heart block) or convulsant drugs (may precipitate convulsions).

ADVERSE/SIDE EFFECTS Increased salivation, nausea, perspiration, weakness, drowsiness, orthostatic hypotension, syncope; CNS stimulation (restlessness, tremors, tachycardia). **With large doses:** violent and persistent vomiting, retching; <u>CNS depression</u> (dyspnea, <u>depressed respirations, coma,</u> bradycardia, <u>acute circulatory failure</u>).

NURSING IMPLICATIONS

Administration

- For the adult patient, administration of 200–300 ml of water or preferably evaporated milk immediately before injection induces more efficient emesis. Smaller amounts of liquid are recommended for the small child.
- Emesis may be enhanced by gently bouncing the child. Emetic effect is reportedly potentiated by motion and reduced by recumbency.
- Position patient on side to prevent aspiration of vomitus.

- If apomorphine fails to induce vomiting, dose is not repeated because it is not likely to work and would increase the risk of CNS or respiratory depression.
- If patient has ingested an absorbable poison, activated charcoal may be given immediately after apomorphine-induced vomiting is completed. If delay in giving the emetic is anticipated, activated charcoal is administered before the injection to reduce absorption of poisons in stomach.
- Apomorphine deteriorates with age and on exposure to light and air. Solutions that are green or brown or otherwise discolored or that contain a precipitate should not be used. Note expiration date of prepared solutions of apomorphine.
- Stable for 48 h when protected from light and air and stored in refrigerator at 2–8C (36–46F). Solution should be labeled and dated.
- Store tablets in tight, light-resistant container, preferably at 15–30C (59–86F), unless otherwise directed.

Assessment & Drug Effects

- Vomiting occurs in about 5 min and may be preceded by salivation and nausea. Save all emesis unless otherwise directed by physician. When vomiting ceases, patient usually falls into a profound sleep. Sedative effects persist for about 2 h. Side rails are indicated. Caution patient not to get out of bed without assistance.
- Monitor vital signs closely for at least 2 h after drug administration. As apomorphine may not evacuate all of the toxic substance ingested, patient should be observed closely for signs of poisoning after vomiting is complete.
- Have on hand equipment for gastric lavage, suction, seizure precautions, and respiratory assistance; naloxone (opiate antagonist) to combat respiratory depression and sedation, and atropine (for treatment of cardiac depression).

Prototype: pilocarpine, p 209

APRACLONIDINE

(a-pra-clo´ni-deen)
Trade name: Iopidine
Classifications: EYE PREPARATION; MIOTIC (ANTIGLAUCOMA AGENT)
Pregnancy: Category C

ACTIONS/PHARMACODYNAMICS A relatively selective alpha-2-adrenergic agonist. When instilled into the eye, apraclonidine ophthalmic solution reduces intraocular pressure (IOP). The precise mechanism of action has not been established; however, aqueous fluorophotometry studies in humans suggest that the predominant action may be related to a reduction in the formation of aqueous humor.

USES Indicated to control or prevent intraoperative and postsurgical elevations in IOP that occur in patients after argon laser trabeculoplasty or argon laser iridotomy. **Unlabeled use:** limited use in open-angle glaucoma.

ROUTE & DOSAGE

Intraoperative and Postsurgical Increase in IOP

Adult	Ophthalmic	1 drop of 1% solution in affected eye 1 h before surgery and 1 drop in same eye immediately after surgery

Open-angle Glaucoma

Adult	Ophthalmic	1 drop of 1% solution in affected eye q12h

PHARMACOKINETICS Absorption: minimal systemic absorption. **Onset:** <1 h. **Peak:** 3–5 h. **Duration:** 12 h.

CONTRAINDICATIONS & PRECAUTIONS Contraindicated in: hypersensitivity to apraclonidine, clonidine, pregnancy (category C), lactation, children. **Cautious use in:** severe cardiac disease, hypertension, history of vasovagal attacks.

ADVERSE/SIDE EFFECTS Eye: *conjunctival blanching, mydriasis, raising of upper eyelid,* burning, discomfort, foreign body sensation, tired eyes, dryness, itching, low IOP, blurred or dimmed vision, conjunctival microhemorrhage/erythema, conjunctival hyperemia, eyelid swelling, and tearing. **CV:** bradycardia, chest heaviness or burning, palpitation, reduced systolic and diastolic pressures, and orthostatic hypotension. **GI:** *dry mouth or nose,* abdominal pain, diarrhea, gastric discomfort, nausea, dyspepsia, and vomiting. **CNS:** *lethargy,* irritability, headache, decreased libido.

DRUG INTERACTIONS Additive effects with OCULAR BETA-BLOCKERS or **pilocarpine.**

NURSING IMPLICATIONS

Administration

- Immediately after instillation of drops, apply gentle digital pressure to periphery of nasolacrimal drainage system for 1–2 min.
- Excess solution around eyes or hands should be removed immediately with a tissue.
- Store at 15–30C (59–86F) away from direct light.

Assessment & Drug Effects

- Monitor BP for hypotension and heart rate for bradycardia.
- Monitor for vasovagal attack (marked bradycardia from vagal stimulation) during surgical procedure.

Patient & Family Education

- Instruct patient in proper technique for eye-drop instillation.
- Advise patient to notify physician of any unusual or allergic reaction to apraclonidine, clonidine, or the preservative benzalkonium chloride found in medications.
- Caution about possibility of orthostatic hypotension.

Prototype: secobarbital, p 175

APROBARBITAL
(a-pro-bar´bi-tol)
Trade name: Alurate
Classifications: CNS AGENT; BARBITURATE ANXIOLYTIC, SEDATIVE-HYPNOTIC
Pregnancy: Category D

ACTIONS/PHARMACODYNAMICS Intermediate-acting barbiturate. Barbiturates can produce all levels of CNS mood alteration from excitation to mild sedation, hypnosis, and deep coma. In sufficiently high therapeutic doses, barbiturates induce anesthesia. Overdosage can produce death. These agents depress the sensory cortex, decrease motor activity, alter cerebellar function and produce drowsiness, sedation, and hypnosis. Barbiturates appear to act at the level of the thalamus where they inhibit ascending conduction in the reticular formation, thereby interfering with impulse transmission to the cortex. Barbiturates have little analgesic action at subanesthetic doses and may increase the reaction to painful

Common side effects in *italic*; life-threatening effects <u>underlined</u>; generic names in **bold**; classifications in SMALL CAPS

315

stimuli. All barbiturates exhibit anticonvulsant activity in anesthetic doses. However, only phenobarbital, mephobarbital, and metharbital are effective as oral anticonvulsants in subhypnotic doses. Barbiturates are respiratory depressants; the degree of respiratory depression is dose dependent. With hypnotic doses, respiratory depression is similar to that which occurs during physiologic sleep.

USES Indicated for routine sedation and as a hypnotic in the short-term treatment of insomnia for up to 2 wk. Barbiturates seem to lose their efficacy for sleep induction and maintenance after this period of time.

ROUTE & DOSAGE

Sedative
Adult   PO   40 mg t.i.d.

Hypnotic
Adult   PO   40–160 mg

PHARMACOKINETICS Absorption: well absorbed from GI tract. **Onset:** 45–60 min. **Duration:** 3 h. **Distribution:** crosses placenta; distributed into breast milk. **Metabolism:** metabolized in the liver. **Elimination:** half-life: 14–40 h; excreted in urine.

CONTRAINDICATIONS & PRECAUTIONS Contraindicated in: barbiturate hypersensitivity; history of manifest or latent porphyria; impaired liver function; impaired renal function; severe respiratory distress, respiratory disease where dyspnea, obstruction, or cor pulmonale is present; previous addiction to the sedative-hypnotic group; acute or chronic pain; pregnancy and lactation; children. **Cautious use in:** elderly or debilitated patients, presence of fever, hyperthyroidism, diabetes mellitus, severe anemia, debility, severely impaired liver function, pulmonary or cardiac disease, status asthmaticus, shock, uremia, borderline hypoadrenal function.

ADVERSE/SIDE EFFECTS CNS: *Somnolence,* agitation, confusion, hyperkinesia, ataxia, vertigo, CNS depression, nightmares, lethargy, *residual sedation (hangover effect),* paradoxical excitement, nervousness, psychiatric disturbance, hallucinations, insomnia, anxiety, dizziness, thinking abnormalities, delirium and stupor with excessive amounts. **Respiratory:** hypoventilation, apnea, respiratory depression, laryngospasm, bronchospasm, circulatory collapse. **CV:** bradycardia, hypotension, syncope. **GI:** nausea, vomiting, constipation, diarrhea, epigastric pain.

Hematologic: blood dyscrasia, i.e., agranulocytosis, thrombocytopenia. **Skin:** rashes, urticaria, easy bruising, petechiae. **Other:** sore throat, nosebleed, myalgia, neuralgia, arthritic pain.

DIAGNOSTIC TEST INTERFERENCES BARBITURATES may cause a false-positive *phentolamine test* and decrease *serum bilirubin concentrations.*

DRUG INTERACTIONS CNS DEPRESSANTS, **alcohol,** SEDATIVES compound CNS depression; MAO INHIBITORS cause excessive CNS depression; ANTICONVULSANTS, **rifampin, phenmetrazine** may decrease effects of aprobarbital.

NURSING IMPLICATIONS

Administration

- In patients with impaired renal or hepatic function, lower doses should be used initially.
- Patients on dialysis may require an increase in dosage.
- Prolonged administration is not recommended because drug has not been shown to be effective for a period of more than 2 wk.
- Store away from heat and direct light in air-tight container at 15–30C (59–86F).

Assessment & Drug Effects

- Monitor for severe drowsiness, severe confusion, severe weakness, shortness of breath, slow or troubled breathing, slurred speech, staggering, and bradycardia.
- Monitor hematologic studies for blood dyscrasia.
- Monitor liver function studies with continuous or prolonged use.
- Monitor elderly patients for paradoxical response (i.e., irritability, marked excitement, depression, and confusion).
- Monitor phenytoin and barbiturate blood levels frequently if these drugs are given concurrently, as the effect of barbiturates on metabolism is unpredictable.

Patient & Family Education

The patient (family) should be advised—
- Not to increase the dose of the drug without consulting a physician.
- Not to drive, operate machinery, or perform other tasks until response to drug is known.
- To avoid use of alcohol or other CNS depressants.
- To notify physician if any of the following occur: fever, sore throat, mouth sores, easy bruising or bleeding, nosebleed, or petechiae.

Common side effects in *italic*; life-threatening effects underlined; generic names in **bold**; classifications in SMALL CAPS

- To make regular visits to physician to check progress during prolonged use.
- Not to discontinue use of medication abruptly, as physician may want to gradually decrease dosage to avoid possibility of withdrawal symptoms
- To check with physician for suspected psychological or physical dependence.
- To get emergency help at once for suspected overdose.
- To increase vitamin D–fortified foods (e.g., milk products), as drug increases vitamin D metabolism, leading to subtherapeutic levels and possible onset of osteomalacia or rickets.

ASCORBIC ACID (VITAMIN C)

Trade names: Arco-Cee, Ascorbicap, Cebid, Cecon, Cenolate, C-Long, Cemill, C-Span, Cetane, Cevalin, Cevi-Bid, Ce-Vi-Sol, Cevita, Dull-C, Flavorcee, Redoxon, Schiff Effervescent Vitamin C, Vita-C, Vitamin C

ASCORBATE, SODIUM

(a-skor´bate)
Trade names: Cenolate, Cevita
Classification: VITAMIN
Pregnancy: Category C

ACTIONS/PHARMACODYNAMICS Water-soluble vitamin essential for synthesis and maintenance of collagen and intercellular ground substance of body tissue cells, blood vessels, cartilage, bones, teeth, skin, and tendons. Increases protection mechanism of the immune system, thus supporting wound healing. Inhibits formation of carcinogenic nitrosoamines and nitrosoureas; however, role in reducing established malignancies is controversial. Necessary for wound healing and resistance to infection. Powerful antioxidant and reducing agent essential for many cellular enzymatic activities and electron transport processes. Functions in carbohydrate metabolism, the conversion of folic acid (folacin) to folinic acid (leucovorin), metabolism of phenylalanine and tyrosine, reduction of plasma transferrin to liver ferritin, the formation of serotonin, and in maintenance of vascular tone and integrity. Unlike most mammals, humans are unable to synthesize ascorbic acid in the body; therefore it must be consumed daily.

USES Prophylaxis and treatment of scurvy and as a dietary supplement. **Unlabeled use:** to acidify urine; to prevent and treat cancer; to treat idiopathic methemoglobinemia; as adjuvant during deferoxamine therapy for iron toxicity; in megadoses will possibly reduce severity and duration of common cold. Widely used as an antioxidant in formulations of parenteral tetracycline and other drugs.

ROUTE & DOSAGE

Therapeutic

Adult	PO/IM/IV/SC	150–500 mg in 1–2 doses
Child	PO/IM/IV/SC	100–300 mg/d in divided doses

Prophylactic

Adult	PO/IM/IV/SC	45–60 mg/d
Child	PO/IM/IV/SC	20–50 mg/d

Urinary Acidifier

Adult	PO/IM/IV/SC	4–12 g/d in divided doses

PHARMACOKINETICS Absorption: readily absorbed PO; however, absorption may be limited with large doses. **Distribution:** widely distributed to body tissues; crosses placenta; distributed into breast milk. **Metabolism:** metabolized in liver. **Elimination:** rapidly excreted from body in urine when plasma level exceeds renal threshold of 1.4 mg/dl.

CONTRAINDICATIONS & PRECAUTIONS Contraindicated in: use of sodium ascorbate in patients on sodium restriction; use of calcium ascorbate in patients receiving digitalis. Safe use during pregnancy (category C) and in nursing mothers not established. **Cautious use in:** excessive doses in patients with G6PD deficiency; hemochromatosis, thalassemia, sideroblastic anemia, sickle cell anemia; patients prone to gout or renal calculi.

ADVERSE/SIDE EFFECTS Acute hemolytic anemia (patients with deficiency of G6PD); sickle cell crisis. **With high doses:** *nausea, vomiting, heartburn, diarrhea, abdominal cramps, headache;* insomnia, increase in urination, urethritis, dysuria, crystalluria, hyperuricemia, dental erosion with prolonged use of chewable tablets. **Parenteral:** mild soreness at injection site; dizziness and temporary faintness with rapid IV administration, deep venous thrombosis.

DIAGNOSTIC TEST INTERFERENCES High doses of absorbic acid can produce false-negative results for **urine glucose** with **glucose oxidase**

Common side effects in *italic*; life-threatening effects underlined; generic names in **bold**; classifications in SMALL CAPS

317

methods (e.g., Clinitest, Tes-Tape, Diastix); false-positive results with **copper reduction methods** (e.g., Benedict's solution, Clinitest); and false increases in **serum uric acid** determinations (by **enzymatic methods**). Interferes with **urinary steroid** (17-OHCS) determinations (by **modified Reddy, Jenkins, Thorn procedure**), decreases in **serum bilirubin,** and may cause increases in **serum cholesterol, creatinine,** and **uric acid** (methodologic inferences). May produce false-negative tests for **occult blood** in stools if taken with 48–72 h of test.

DRUG INTERACTIONS Large doses may attenuate hypoprothombinemic effects of ORAL ANTICOAGULANTS; SALICYLATES may inhibit ascorbic acid uptake by leukocytes and tissues, and ascorbic acid may decrease elimination of salicylates; chronic high doses of ascorbic acid may diminish the effects of **disulfiram.**

INCOMPATIBILITIES Solution/Additive: aminophylline, bleomycin, cephapirin, erythromycin, nafcillin, sodium bicarbonate, warfarin. Y-Site: cefazolin, doxapram, sodium bicarbonate.

NURSING IMPLICATIONS

Administration

- Open ampuls with caution. After prolonged storage, decomposition may occur with release of carbon dioxide and resulting increase in pressure within ampul.
- Ascorbic acid injection may gradually darken on exposure to light. Slight coloration reportedly does not affect its therapeutic action.
- Parenteral vitamin C is incompatible with many drugs. Consult pharmacist for compatibility information.
- IV ascorbic acid may be given undiluted at a rate of 100 mg or a fraction thereof over 1 min.
- IV ascorbic acid may be diluted in IV solutions and given as a continuous infusion.
- Oral solutions may be mixed with food.
- Effervescent tablet form should be dissolved in a glass of water immediately before ingestion.
- Store in airtight, light-resistant, nonmetallic containers, away from heat and sunlight, preferably at 15–30C (59–86F), unless otherwise specified by manufacturer.

Patient & Family Education

- High doses of vitamin C are not recommended during pregnancy. It has been suggested that the fetus may adapt to high levels of the vitamin by developing the capacity to inactivate it, leading to rebound scurvy in the offspring when vitamin C intake is reduced to normal.
- The nonprescription use of megadoses (more than 10 times the RDA) is not warranted and can be toxic for some individuals.
- Large doses of vitamin C should be prescribed in divided amounts because the body uses only what is needed at a particular time and excretes the rest in urine.
- Megadoses can increase pH of the small intestine leading to interference with absorption of vitamin B_{12}. Rebound scurvy has been reported when treatment with high doses is abruptly stopped.
- Reportedly, patients taking oral contraceptives also require vitamin C supplements.
- Smokers appear to have increased requirements for ascorbic acid because the vitamin is oxidized and excreted more rapidly than in nonsmokers. Advise patient with vitamin C deficiency to modify or stop smoking. Replacement dosages will be higher for the smoker.
- Review the importance of foods as primary sources of vitamin C.
- Vitamin C is rapidly oxidized when exposed to air (deterioration is accelerated by light and heat). Slight darkening of tablets may occur without loss of potency.
- Vitamin C increases the absorption of iron when taken at the same time as iron-rich foods.

ASPARAGINASE

(a-spar´a-gi-nase)
Trade names: Colaspase, Elspar, Kidrolase, L-Asparaginase
Classification: ANTINEOPLASTIC ENZYME
Pregnancy: Category C

ACTIONS/PHARMACODYNAMICS A highly toxic drug with a low therapeutic index. This high molecular weight enzyme isolated from *Escherichia coli* is active in solution at pH 6.5–8.0 and functions chiefly during postmitotic G_1 phase of cell division. Catalyzes hydrolysis (breakdown) of asparagine to aspartic acid and ammonia, thus depleting extracellular supply of an amino acid essential to synthesis of DNA and other nucleoproteins. Reduced availability of asparagine causes death of tumor cells, since unlike normal cells, tumor cells are unable to synthesize their own supply. Because some normal cells have high rates of protein synthesis, they also depend on an extracellular source of asparagine; thus drug-induced deficiency interferes with synthesis of important proteins by cells in, e.g., liver (prothrombin and other clotting factors, albumin), parathyroid hormone, pancreas (insulin), lymphocytes (antibodies), RNA, and kidney. Bone marrow depression or cytotoxic effects on cells of GI tract, oral mucosa, hair follicles rarely occurs. Resistance to cytotoxic action develops rapidly; therefore asparaginase is not effective in treatment of solid tumors and is not recommended for maintenance therapy. Has antiviral action but not used for this purpose because it is cytotoxic. No cross-resistance to other antineoplastic agents has been demonstrated.

USES Primarily in combination regimens with other antineoplastic agents to treat acute lymphocytic leukemia (ALL). **Unlabeled use:** other leukemias, lymphosarcoma, and (intraarterially) in treatment of hypoglycemia due to pancreatic islet cell tumor.

ROUTE & DOSAGE

Induction Agent

Adult	IV	200 IU/kg/d for 28 d; inject over at least 30 min into running IV
Child	IV	Same as for adult

PHARMACOKINETICS Distribution: distributed primarily into intravascular space (80%) and lymph; low levels in CSF, pleural and peritoneal fluids. **Metabolism:** unknown. **Elimination:** half-life: 8–30 h; small amounts found in urine.

CONTRAINDICATIONS & PRECAUTIONS Contraindicated in: history of or existing pancreatitis; chickenpox (existing or recent illness or exposure), herpetic infection. Safe use during pregnancy (category C) and in nursing mothers not established. **Cautious use in:** liver impairment; diabetes mellitus; infections; history of urate calculi or gout; antineoplastic or radiation therapy.

ADVERSE/SIDE EFFECTS CNS: depression, fatique, lethargy, drowsiness, confusion, agitation, hallucinations, dizziness, Parkinson-like syndrome with tremor and progressive increase in muscle tone. **GI:** *severe vomiting, nausea,* anorexia, abdominal cramps, diarrhea, acute pancreatitis. **GU:** uric acid nephropathy, azotemia, proteinuria, renal failure. **Hematologic:** transient bone marrow depression, *reduced clotting factors* (especially V, VII, VIII, IX), *decreased circulating platelets and fibrinogen,* leukopenia. **Hepatotoxicity:** liver function abnormali-

ties. **Hypersensitivity:** *skin rashes, urticaria,* respiratory distress, anaphylaxis. **Other:** chills, fever, fatal hyperthermia, perspiration, weight loss, hyperglycemia, glycosuria, polyuria, hypoalbuminemia, hypocalcemia, hyperuricemia; flank pain, infections.

DIAGNOSTIC TEST INTERFERENCES Asparaginase may interfere with **thyroid function** tests: decreased total **serum thyroxine** and increased **thyroxine-binding globulin index;** pretreatment values return within 4 wk after drug is discontinued.

DRUG INTERACTIONS decreased hypoglycemic effects of SULFONYLUREAS, **insulin;** increased potential for toxicity if asparaginase is given concurrently or immediately before CORTICOSTEROIDS, **vincristine; methotrexate's** antitumor effect blocked if asparaginase is given concurrently or immediately before it.

NURSING IMPLICATIONS

Administration

- Because of the possibility of unpredictable allergic reactions, an intradermal skin test is performed before the initial dose and when the drug is readministered after an interval of a week or more.
- Observe test site for at least 1 h for evidence of positive reaction (wheal, erythema). A negative skin test, however, does not preclude possibility of an allergic reaction.
- Unlike many other desensitization schedules, asparaginase desensitization does not eliminate risk of subsequent allergic reactions with retreatments.
- Administered under constant supervision by clinician experienced in cancer chemotherapy.
- Reconstituted with sterile water for injection for IV administration or with 0.9% NaCl for injection for IV and IM administration. Each 10,000 IU vial is diluted with 5 ml of diluent to yield 2000 IU/ml. Shake vial well to promote dissolution of powder. Avoid vigorous shaking. Ordinary shaking does not inactivate the enzyme or cause foaming of content.
- For IV infusion the reconstituted solution should be further diluted with 0.9% NaCl injection or 5% dextrose injection by administration into tubing of an already free flowing infusion of one of these solutions; administer over a period of not less than 30 min.
- Gelatinous fiberlike particles can develop in asparaginase solutions on standing. Use of a 5μm filter will remove particles without affecting potency.
- Limit the IM injection volume to 2 ml in one site.
- Unless otherwise directed by manufacturer, store sealed vial of lyophilized powder below 8C (46F).

Common side effects in *italic*; life-threatening effects underlined; generic names in **bold**; classifications in SMALL CAPS

319

A

Store reconstituted solutions and solutions diluted for IV infusion at 2–8C (36–46F) for up to 8 h; then discard. Use only clear solutions.

Assessment & Drug Effects

- **Have immediately available:** personnel, drugs (epinephrine, antihistamine, diphenhydramine, IV corticosteroid), oxygen, and equipment for treating allergic reaction (which may range from urticaria to anaphylactic shock) whenever drug is administered, including skin testing.
- During administration, monitor vital signs and be alert to evidence of hypersensitivity or anaphylactoid reaction (see Signs & Symptoms, chap 3). Anaphylaxis usually occurs within 30–60 min after dose has been given. It is more apt to happen with intermittent administrations, particularly when interval between doses is 7 d or more and when IM route is used.
- When asparaginase is given with or immediately before a course of prednisone and vincristine, toxicity potential is increased. When administered after these drugs, reportedly toxicity appears to be less pronounced.
- Monitor I&O and maintain adequate fluid intake.
- Because asparaginase may interfere with the synthesis of insulin, tests for glycosuria should be done regularly. Report polyuria, polydipsia, or positive urine test to the physician.
- Serum amylase, calcium blood glucose, coagulation factor determinations, ammonia and uric acid levels, hepatic and renal function tests, peripheral blood counts, and bone marrow function are monitored regularly during treatment. Liver function tests are done at least twice weekly during therapy.
- Circulating lymphoblasts decrease markedly in the first several days of treatment, and leukocyte counts may fall below normal. Protection from infection during this period is crucial. Protective isolation may be indicated. Signs of infection (chill, fever, aches, sore throat) should be reported promptly.
- Report sudden severe abdominal pain with nausea and vomiting, particularly if these symptoms occur after medication is discontinued (possible indicators of pancreatitis).
- Elevations of BUN and serum ammonia are expected findings because of enzymatic action. In most patients, blood ammonia levels are as high as 700–900 µg/dl (normal 80–110 µg/dl). Watch for signs of **hyperammonemia:** anorexia, vomiting, lethargy, weak pulse, depressed temperature, irritability, asterixis, seizures, coma. Generally, the treatment consists of low-protein diet with ample amounts of simple carbohydrates.
- Because of potential serious hepatic dysfunction the enzymatic detoxification of other drugs may be reduced. Therefore anticipate the possibility of prolonged or exaggerated effects of concurrently given drugs or their toxicity; report incidence promptly.
- CNS function (general behavior, emotional status, level of consciousness, thought content, motor function) should be evaluated before and during therapy.
- Neurotoxic reaction usually appears within the first few days of therapy. It is manifested by tiredness and changing levels of consciousness (ranging from confusion to coma) and occurs in approximately 25% of patients.

Patient & Family Education

- Patient should be informed before initiation of treatment of the positive and negative effects of drug therapy. A therapeutic response will most likely be accompanied by some toxicity in all patients; toxicity is reportedly greater in adults than in children.
- Instruct patient to notify physician of continued loss of weight or onset of foot and ankle swelling.
- Nausea, vomiting, or anorexia can interrupt scheduled doses at first, but these symptoms lessen with continued treatment. Instruct patient to try to continue all prescribed medications if at all possible; if not possible, physician should be notified without delay.
- Advise patient to report the onset of unusual bleeding, bruising, petechiae, melena, skin rash or itching, yellowed skin and sclera, joint pain, puffy face, or dyspnea.
- Drowsiness, decreased alertness, and shakiness are symptoms that can accompany treatment with this drug. Driving or operating equipment that requires alertness and skill can be hazardous. Urge caution and inform patient that these effects can continue several weeks after last dose of the drug.
- Reinforce necessity to keep scheduled appointments for evaluation of therapy.

ASPIRIN

See CENTRAL NERVOUS SYSTEM AGENTS, SALICYLATE ANALGESIC, ANTIPYRETIC prototype, p 161.

Common side effects in *italic*; life-threatening effects underlined; generic names in **bold**; classifications in SMALL CAPS

Prototype: diphenhydramine, p 47

ASTEMIZOLE
(ah stem´me zole)
Trade name: Hismanal
Classifications: ANTIHISTAMINE (H$_1$-RECEPTOR ANTAGONIST)
Pregnancy: Category C

ACTIONS/PHARMACODYNAMICS A long-acting selective histamine H$_1$-receptor antagonist. Binds preferentially to peripheral rather than central H$_1$ receptors. Does not block histamine release, antibody production, or antigen-antibody interactions. Has little or no anticholinergic and sedative effects as compared to diphenhydramine.

USES Indicated for relief of symptoms associated with seasonal allergic rhinitis and chronic idiopathic urticaria.

ROUTE & DOSAGE

Allergic Rhinitis

Adult   PO   10 mg once daily; to reduce time to steady-state concentrations may give 30 mg on day 1, 20 mg on day 2, then 10 mg/d thereafter.

PHARMACOKINETICS Absorption: readily absorbed from GI tract; absorption decreased by food. **Peak:** 1–4 h. **Duration:** up to 24 h. **Distribution:** crosses placenta; distributed into breast milk. **Metabolism:** extensively metabolized in liver (including first pass metabolism) to an active metabolite. **Elimination:** half-life: 20–24 h, metabolities 12–20 d; 54–73% excreted in feces; 25–50% excreted in urine.

CONTRAINDICATIONS & PRECAUTIONS Contraindicated in: hypersensitivity to antihistamines of similar structure, narrow-angle glaucoma, stenosing peptic ulcer, symptomatic prostatic hypertrophy, asthmatic attack, bladder neck obstruction, pyloroduodenal obstruction, children less than age 12, lactation, pregnancy (category C). **Cautious use in:** history of asthma, increased intraocular pressure, renal or hepatic impairment, elderly patients, young children.

ADVERSE/SIDE EFFECTS CNS: headache, appetite increase, weight gain, nervousness, dizziness, depression. **GI:** nausea, diarrhea, abdominal pain. **ENT:** pharyngitis, conjunctivitis, epistaxis. **Respiratory:** bronchospasm. **CV:** angioedema, palpitation. **Skin:** photosensitivity, pruritus, rash, edema. **Other:** arthralgia, myalgia.

NURSING IMPLICATIONS

Administration
- Take at least 2 h after a meal. Have no food for 1 h after taking the drug.
- Store in tightly closed containers at 15–30C (59–86F) unless otherwise directed by manufacturer.

Assessment & Drug Effects
- If taken for allergic manifestations, obtain careful history including change from usual pattern of recently ingested foods and drugs and social or emotional stress.

Patient & Family Education
Patients should be advised—
- To avoid use of alcohol or other CNS depressants.
- To observe caution while driving or performing other tasks requiring alertness.
- To inform physician of a history of glaucoma, peptic ulcer, urinary retention, or pregnancy before antihistamine therapy is begun.
- To carry medical information card or jewelry indicating type of allergy, medication, physician's name, address, and telephone number.
- That antihistamines have no therapeutic effect on the common cold.

Prototype: propranolol, p 109

ATENOLOL
(a-ten´oh-lole)
Trade name: Tenormin
Classifications: AUTONOMIC NERVOUS SYSTEM AGENT; BETA-ADRENERGIC ANTAGONIST (SYMPATHOLYTIC, BLOCKING AGENT); CARDIOVASCULAR AGENT; ANTIHYPERTENSIVE; ANTIANGINAL
Pregnancy: Category C

Common side effects in *italic*; life-threatening effects <u>underlined</u>; generic names in **bold**; classifications in SMALL CAPS

ACTIONS/PHARMACODYNAMICS In therapeutic doses, atenolol selectively blocks $beta_1$-adrenergic receptors located chiefly in cardiac muscle. With large doses preferential effect is lost and inhibition of $beta_2$-adrenergic receptors (especially in bronchial and vascular musculature) may lead to increased airway resistance, especially in patients with asthma or COPD. Compared to propranolol, it essentially lacks membrane-stabilizing and intrinsic sympathomimetic activities, is less lipophilic, and has longer antihypertensive effect, thus permitting once-a-day dosing. Being less lipophilic than propranolol, it does not readily cross blood-brain barrier and therefore is not associated with severe mental depression. Mechanisms for antihypertensive action include central effect leading to decreased sympathetic outflow to periphery, reduction in renin activity with consequent suppression of the renin-angiotensin-aldosterone system, and competitive inhibition of catecholamine binding at beta-adrenergic receptor sites. Reduces rate and force of cardiac contractions (negative inotropic action); cardiac output is reduced, as well as systolic and diastolic BP. Atenolol increases peripheral vascular resistance both at rest and with exercise. Unlike nonselective beta blockers, e.g., propranolol, atenolol does not appear to potentiate insulin-induced hypoglycemia and is less likely to produce hypertension during hypoglycemia or to impair peripheral circulation. It may inhibit hypoglycemia-induced tachycardia, but sweating is usually not affected or may even be increased.

USES Management of hypertension (step 1 drug) as a single agent or concomitantly with other antihypertensive agents, especially a diuretic, and in treatment of stable angina pectoris, MI. **Unlabeled use:** antiarrhythmic, mitral valve prolapse, adjunct in treatment of pheochromocytoma and of thyrotoxicosis; and for vascular headache prophylaxis.

ROUTE & DOSAGE

Hypertension, Angina

Adult	PO	25–50 mg/d; may increase to 100 mg/d

MI

Adult	PO	10 min after second IV dose, start 50 mg/d
	IV	5 mg q5min × 2 doses; then switch to PO

PHARMACOKINETICS Absorption: 50% of PO dose absorbed. **Peak:** 2–4 h PO; 5 min IV. **Duration:** 24 h. **Distribution:** does not readily cross blood-brain barrier. **Metabolism:** no hepatic metabolism. **Elimination:** half-life: 6–7 h; 40–50% excreted in urine; 50–60% excreted in feces.

CONTRAINDICATIONS & PRECAUTIONS Contraindicated in: sinus bradycardia, greater than first-degree heart block, overt cardiac failure, cardiogenic shock. Safe use during pregnancy (category C), in nursing women, and in children not established. **Cautious use in:** hypertensive patients with CHF controlled by digitalis and diuretics, asthma and COPD; diabetes mellitus; impaired renal function; hyperthyroidism.

ADVERSE/SIDE EFFECTS Usually well tolerated. **CNS:** dizziness, vertigo, light-headedness, syncopy, fatigue or weakness, lethargy, drowsiness, insomnia, mental changes, depression. **CV:** *bradycardia, hypotension, CHF,* cold extremities, leg pains, dysrhythmias. **GI:** nausea, vomiting, diarrhea. **Respiratory:** pulmonary edema, dyspnea, bronchospasm. **Other:** may mask symptoms of hypoglycemia; decreased sexual ability.

DRUG INTERACTIONS Atropine and other ANTICHOLINERGICS may increase atenolol absorption from GI tract; NSAIDs may decrease hypotensive effects; may mask symptoms of a hypoglycemic reaction induced by **insulin,** SULFONYLUREAS; may increase **lidocaine** levels and toxicity; pharmacologic and toxic effects of both atenolol and **verapamil** are increased. **Prazosin, terazocin** may increase severe hypotensive response to first dose of atenolol.

NURSING IMPLICATIONS

Administration

- If necessary, tablet may be crushed before administration and taken with fluid of patient's choice.
- IV atenolol may be given undiluted by direct IV at a rate of one dose per 5 min.
- IV atenolol may be diluted in up to 50 ml of D5W, 0.45% NS, or NS and given as an infusion over 15–30 min.
- Store in tightly closed, light-resistant container at 15–30C (59–86F) unless otherwise directed.

Assessment & Drug Effects

- Check apical pulse before administration of drug, especially in patients receiving digitalis (both drugs slow AV conduction). If below 60 bpm, withhold dose and consult physician.

Common side effects in *italic*; life-threatening effects <u>underlined</u>; generic names in **bold**; classifications in SMALL CAPS

- Monitor apical pulse, BP, respirations, and peripheral circulation throughout dosage adjustment period. Consult physician for acceptable parameters.

Patient & Family Education
- Advise patients to adhere rigidly to dose regimen. Sudden discontinuation of drug can exacerbate angina and precipitate tachycardia or MI in patients with coronary artery disease, and thyroid storm in patients with hyperthyroidism.
- Caution patients to make position changes slowly and in stages, particularly from recumbent to upright posture.

Prototype: tubocurarine, p 124

ATRACURIUM BESYLATE
(a-tra-kyoor´ee-um)
Trade name: Tracrium
Classifications: SKELETAL MUSCLE RELAXANT, NONDEPOLARIZING; NEUROMUSCULAR BLOCKER
Pregnancy: Category C

ACTIONS/PHARMACODYNAMICS Synthetic nondepolarizing skeletal muscle relaxant with intermediate duration of action. Pharmacologically similar to tubocurarine but produces shorter duration of neuromuscular blockade, exhibits minimal direct effects on cardiovascular system, and has less histamine-releasing action. Has minimal cumulative tendency with subsequent doses if recovery from the drug begins before dose is repeated. Unlike other skeletal muscle relaxants, does not require pseudocholinesterase or hepatic or renal routes for its elimination. Inhibits neuromuscular transmission by binding competitively with acetylcholine to muscle end plate receptors. Lacks analgesic action and has no apparent effect on pain threshold, consciousness, or cerebration. Given in general anesthesia only after unconsciousness has been induced by other drugs.

USES Adjunct for general anesthesia to produce skeletal muscle relaxation during surgery; to facilitate endotracheal intubation. Especially useful for patients with severe renal or hepatic disease, limited cardiac reserve, and in patients with low or atypical pseudocholinesterase levels.

ROUTE & DOSAGE

Skeletal Muscle Relaxation

Adult	IV	0.4–0.5 mg/kg initial dose; then 0.08–0.1 mg/kg 20–45 min after the first dose if necessary; reduce doses if used with general anesthetics
Child	IV	(≥2 y): Same as for adult

Mechanical Ventilation

Adult	IV	5–9 µg/kg/min by continuous infusion

PHARMACOKINETICS Onset: 2 min. **Peak:** 3–5 min. **Duration:** 60–70 min. **Distribution:** well distributed to tissues and extracellular fluids; crosses placenta; distribution into breast milk unknown. **Metabolism:** rapid nonenzymatic degradation in bloodstream. **Elimination:** half-life: 20 min; 70–90% excreted in urine in 5–7 h.

CONTRAINDICATIONS & PRECAUTIONS Contraindicated in: myasthenia gravis; safe use during pregnancy (category C), lactation, in children <2 y not established. **Cautious use in:** when appreciable histamine release would be hazardous (as in asthma or anaphylactoid reactions), significant cardiovascular disease), neuromuscular disease (e.g., Eaton-Lambert syndrome), carcinomatosis, electrolyte or acid-base imbalances, dehydration, impaired pulmonary function.

ADVERSE/SIDE EFFECTS CV: bradycardia, tachycardia. **Respiratory:** bronchospasm, cyanosis, _respiratory depression_. **Other:** periorbital and conjunctival edema; increased salivation, _anaphylaxis_.

DRUG INTERACTIONS GENERAL ANESTHETICS increase magnitude and duration of neuromuscular blocking action; AMINOGLYCOSIDES, **bacitracin, polymyxin B, clindamycin, lidocaine, parenteral magnesium, quinidine, quinine, trimethaphan, verapamil** increase neuromuscular blockade; DIURETICS may increase or decrease neuromuscular blockade; **lithium** prolongs duration of neuromuscular blockade; NARCOTIC ANALGESICS present possibility of additive respiratory depression; **succinylcholine** increases onset and depth of neuromuscular blockade; **phenytoin** may cause resistance to or reversal of neuromuscular blockade.

NURSING IMPLICATIONS

Administration
- Initial IV bolus dose may be given undiluted over 30–60 seconds.

Common side effects in _italic_; life-threatening effects underlined; generic names in **bold**; classifications in SMALL CAPS

323

A

- Maintenance dose is further diluted with NS or D5W and is given as a continuous infusion.
- Incompatible with alkaline solutions (e.g., barbiturates). Do not mix in same syringe or administer through same needle as used for alkaline solutions. Reportedly compatible with 5% dextrose and 0.9% NaCl.
- To preserve potency, store at 2–8C (36–46F) unless otherwise directed. Avoid freezing.

Assessment & Drug Effects

- Baseline determinations of serum electrolytes, acid-base balance, and renal function are generally done as part of preanesthetic assessment.
- Personnel and equipment required for endotracheal intubation, administration of oxygen under positive pressure, artificial respiration, and assisted or controlled ventilation should be immediately available.
- Use of peripheral nerve stimulator by qualified individual is recommended to evaluate degree of neuromuscular blockade and muscle paralysis and thus avoid risk of overdosage. Nerve stimulator is also used to identify residual paralysis during recovery period. It is especially indicated when cautious use of atracurium is specified.
- Monitor BP, pulse, and respirations and evaluate patient's recovery from neuromuscular blocking (curare-like) effect as evidenced by ability to breathe naturally or to take deep breaths and cough, keep eyes open, lift head keeping mouth closed, adequacy of hand-grip strength. Notify physician if recovery is delayed.
- Patient may find oral communication difficult until head and neck muscles recover from blockade effects.
- Recovery from neuromuscular blockade usually begins 35–45 min after drug administration and is almost complete in about 1 h. Note that recovery time may be delayed in patients with cardiovascular disease, edematous states, and in the elderly.

ATROPINE SULFATE

See AUTONOMIC NERVOUS SYSTEM AGENTS, ANTICHOLINERGIC (PARASYMPATHOLYTIC), ANTIMUSCARINIC, ANTISPASMODIC prototype, p 116.

Prototype: aurothioglucose, p 223

AURANOFIN

(au-rane´eh-fin)

Trade name: Ridaura
Classifications: GOLD COMPOUND; ANTIRHEUMATIC; ANTIINFLAMMATORY
Pregnancy: Category C

ACTIONS/PHARMACODYNAMICS Contains 29% gold (compared with aurothioglucose, which contains approximately 50%). Strongly lipophilic and almost neutral in solution, properties that may facilitate transport of agent across cell membranes. Action (complex and not fully understood) appears to be immunomodulatory: serum immunoglobulin concentrations and rheumatoid factor titers are decreased; and antiinflammatory: gold is taken up by macrophages with resulting inhibition of phagocytosis and lysosomal enzyme release. Suppresses or prevents, but does not cure, synovitis and arthritis or reverse structural damage to bone or cartilage. It does not induce rheumatoid arthritis remission.

USES Management of active stage of classic or definite rheumatoid arthritis in adults who do not respond to or tolerate other antiarthritis agents (e.g., NSAIDs, other gold compounds). **Unlabeled use:** juvenile rheumatoid arthritis, active SLE, psoriatic arthritis.

ROUTE & DOSAGE

Rheumatoid Arthritis

Adult	PO	6 mg/d in 1–2 divided doses; may increase to 6–9 mg/d in 3 divided doses after 6 mo if tolerated and needed (max 9 mg/d)

PHARMACOKINETICS Absorption: 20% absorbed from small intestine. **Peak:** 2 h. **Distribution:** highest concentrations in kidneys, spleen, lungs, adrenals, and liver; not known if crosses placenta; small amounts distributed into breast milk. **Elimination:** half-life: 11–23 d; 60% of absorbed gold eliminated in urine, remainder in feces.

CONTRAINDICATIONS & PRECAUTIONS Contraindicated in: history of gold-induced necrotizing en-

Common side effects in *italic*; life-threatening effects underlined; generic names in **bold**; classifications in SMALL CAPS

terocolitis, renal disease, exfoliative dermatitis or bone marrow aplasia; patient who has recently received radiation therapy, history of severe toxicity from previous exposure to gold or other heavy metals. Safe use during pregnancy (category C), lactation, or by children not established. Cautious use in inflammatory bowel disease, rash, liver disease, history of bone marrow depression; elderly patients; diabetes mellitus, CHF.

ADVERSE/SIDE EFFECTS GI: *diarrhea, abdominal cramping* and pain; *nausea,* vomiting, anorexia, dysphagia; *stomatitis,* glossitis, metallic taste; flatulence, constipation, GI bleeding, melena. **Hematologic:** thrombocytopenia, leukopenia, eosinophilia, agranulocytosis, aplastic anemia. **Renal:** proteinuria, hematuria, renal failure. **Skin:** *rash, pruritus,* dermatitis, urticaria. **Other:** increased AST, ALT, alkaline phosphatase.

DIAGNOSTIC TEST INTERFERENCES Auranofin may enhance response to a *tuberculin skin test.*

NURSING IMPLICATIONS

Administration
- Administer capsule with food or fluid of patient's choice.
- Store at 15–30C (59–86F); protect from light and moisture. Expiration date: 4 y after date of manufacture.

Assessment & Drug Effects
- Auranofin has many adverse side effects, but they appear to be less toxic and better tolerated than those of other gold compounds. They occur frequently in the first 6 mo of treatment but can occur at any time.
- The following symptoms should be reported promptly: unexplained bleeding or bruising, metallic taste, sore mouth; pruritus, rash; diarrhea and melena; yellow skin and sclera; unexplained cough or dyspnea.
- Therapeutic effects from auranofin treatment develop slowly and are not usually apparent for 3–4 mo.
- Drug-induced thrombocytopenia (mechanism not clear) is usually spontaneously reversible several weeks after drug is withdrawn; however, platelet

transfusions or corticosteroids or both may be required if condition is severe.
- *Laboratory signs of possible impending gold toxicity:* decreased Hgb; leukocytes <4000/mm^3; granulocytes <1500/mm^3; platelets <150,000/mm^3; proteinurea >500 mg/dl
- If drug is discontinued, adverse effects may persist for many months requiring continued medical surveillance and supportive therapy: difficulty in breathing, diarrhea and abdominal pain, fatigue, weakness, unexplained bleeding and bruising, metallic taste.
- *Overdose symptoms (limited data):* severe neurotoxicity (encephalopathy and peripheral neuropathy), multifocal myoclonus, bilateral foot drop, facial dyskinesias, fecal and urinary incontinence.

Patient & Family Education
- Instruct patient to report adverse effects of therapy.
- Do not change dosage (dose or dose interval) by omission, increase, or decrease without first consulting physician.
- Drug-induced diarrhea may respond well to treatment with an antidiarrheal drug and high-fiber diet.
- Abdominal cramping and pain should be reported; discontinuance of therapy may be necessary.
- Exposure to sunlight (especially between 10 AM and 4 PM) or to artificial ultraviolet light should be kept to a minimum to prevent photosensitivity reaction.
- Among earliest subjective symptoms of impending gold toxicity are metallic taste and pruritus with or without rash. Report promptly to physician.
- Urge patient to maintain contact with physician at appointed times (usually monthly) for assessment of disease status and monitoring of the following: urinary protein, CBC with differential and platelet count; hepatic function.
- For symptomatic treatment of mild stomatitis, the manufacturer suggests rinsing mouth with a hypotonic NaCl solution. Avoid commercial mouth rinses; clean teeth with soft tooth brush and gentle brushing to avoid gingival trauma. Floss at least once daily.

AUROTHIOGLUCOSE

See GOLD COMPOUND prototype, p 223.

Common side effects in *italic*; life-threatening effects underlined; generic names in **bold**; classifications in SMALL CAPS

325

A

Prototype: diphenhydramine, p 47

AZATADINE MALEATE

(a-za´ta-deen)
Trade name: Optimine, Trinalin
Classifications: ANTIHISTAMINE (H$_1$-RECEPTOR ANTAGONIST)
Pregnancy: Category B

ACTIONS/PHARMACODYNAMICS Long-acting antihistamine pharmacologically similar to cyproheptadine. Acts by competitively antagonizing the stimulating effects of histamine at H$_1$-receptor sites on smooth muscle of blood vessels and respiratory and GI tract. This action blocks or reduces intensity of allergic responses associated with histamine release, such as vasodilation, capillary permeability and tissue edema, and itching. In common with other antihistamines, has antiserotonin, anticholinergic, and sedative actions. Has no antiemetic effect.

USES Symptomatic relief of hay fever (seasonal allergic rhinitis), perennial (or nonseasonal) allergic rhinitis, and chronic urticaria.

ROUTE & DOSAGE

Allergic Rhinitis
Adult   PO   1–2 mg b.i.d.

PHARMACOKINETICS Absorption: readily absorbed from GI tract. **Peak:** 4 h. **Distribution:** probably crosses blood-brain barrier; crosses placenta; distribution into breast milk unknown. **Metabolism:** partially metabolized in liver. **Elimination:** half-life: 9–12 h; 50% excreted in urine in 5 d.

CONTRAINDICATIONS & PRECAUTIONS Contraindicated in: hypersensitivity to azatadine or to other H$_1$-receptor antagonists; MAO inhibitor therapy. Safe use during pregnancy (category B), in nursing women, and in children <12 y not established. **Cautious use in:** increased intraocular pressure, narrow-angle glaucoma; pyloroduodenal obstruction, stenosing peptic ulcer; prostatic hypertrophy, bladder neck obstruction; hyperthyroidism; hypertension, cardiovascular disease; convulsive disorders; history of asthma or COPD.

ADVERSE/SIDE EFFECTS CNS: *drowsiness,* sedation, dizziness, disturbed coordination, fatigue, confusion, paresthesias, neuritis, euphoria, excitation, nervousness, restlessness, insomnia, tremor, irritability, convulsions. **CV:** hypotension, palpitation, tachycardia, extrasystoles. **ENT:** nasal stuffiness; dryness of nose and throat; tinnitus. **Eye:** blurred vision. **GI:** *dry mouth,* epigastric distress, nausea, vomiting, anorexia, diarrhea, or constipation. **GU:** urinary frequency, urinary retention, early menses. **Hematologic:** hemolytic anemia, thrombocytopenia, agranulocytosis. **Respiratory:** thickening of bronchial secretions. **Other:** excessive perspiration, chills, headache.

DIAGNOSTIC TEST INTERFERENCES As a general rule, H$_1$-receptor antagonists are discontinued about 4 d before *skin testing* procedures are to be performed since they may produce false-negative results.

DRUG INTERACTIONS Alcohol, CNS DEPRESSANTS add to sedation, drowsiness; MAO INHIBITORS may prolong anticholinergic effects of azatadine; TRICYCLIC ANTIDEPRESSANTS augment anticholinergic effects.

NURSING IMPLICATIONS

Administration
- GI side effects may be minimized by administering drug with food or milk.
- Store in tightly closed container at 2–30C (36–86F), unless otherwise directed.

Assessment & Drug Effects
- Most likely to cause sedation, dizziness, hypotension, and confusion in the elderly. Advise patient to report these effects. Reduction in dosage may be indicated.
- There may be additive CNS depression with alcohol and other CNS depressants (e.g., sedatives, tranquilizers, sleep medications).

Patient & Family Education
- Commonly causes drowsiness, sedation, and dizziness; caution patient not to drive a car or engage in other potentially hazardous activities until reaction to drug is known.

Common side effects in *italic*; life-threatening effects underlined; generic names in **bold**; classifications in SMALL CAPS

- Instruct patient to avoid concurrent use of alcohol because of potential for additive CNS depression.
- Advise patient to avoid prolonged exposure to sunlight or to artificial ultraviolet light. Photosensitivity is a possible adverse effect.
- Dry mouth (xerostomia) may be relieved by the following measures: (1) frequent rinses with tepid water, preferred to commercial mouth washes, overuse of which can change oral flora; also, many contain alcohol, which enhances drying; (2) increase fluid intake (if allowed) or at least maintain normal intake; (3) brush with soft toothbrush after every meal; (4) floss teeth daily with waxed floss (before brushing); (5) sugarless gum or sugarless sourballs; (6) use of artificial saliva, e.g., Xero-Lube, Moi-Stir.

Prototype: cyclosporine, p 248

AZATHIOPRINE

(ay-za-thye´oh-preen)
Trade name: Imuran
Classification: IMMUNOSUPPRESSANT
Pregnancy: Category D

ACTIONS/PHARMACODYNAMICS Metabolized to 6-mercaptopurine in body, which accounts for most of its actions. Precise mechanism of immunosuppressant and antiinflammatory actions not determined. Antagonizes purine metabolism and appears to inhibit DNA, RNA, and normal protein synthesis in rapidly growing cells. Suppresses T cell effects before transplant rejection, i.e., during induction phase of antibody response.

USES Adjunctive agent to prevent rejection of kidney allografts, usually with other immunosuppressants. Also used in selective adult patients with severe, active rheumatoid arthritis; unresponsive to conventional therapy. **Unlabeled use:** SLE, ulcerative colitis, pemphigus, nephrotic syndrome, and other inflammatory and immunologic diseases.

PHARMACOKINETICS Absorption: readily absorbed from GI tract. **Distribution:** crosses placenta. **Metabolism:** extensively metabolized in liver to active metabolite mercaptopurine. **Elimination:** half-life: 3 h; eliminated in urine.

ROUTE & DOSAGE

Renal Transplantation

Adult	PO	3–5 mg/kg/d initially; may be able to reduce to 1–3 mg/kg/d
	IV	3–5 mg/kg/d initially; may be able to reduce to 1–3 mg/kg/d

Rheumatoid Arthritis

Adult	PO	1 mg/kg/d initially; may be increased by 0.5 mg/kg/d at 4–6 wk intervals if needed up to 2.5 mg/kg/d

---

CONTRAINDICATIONS & PRECAUTIONS Contraindicated in: hypersensitivity to azathioprine or mercaptopurine; clinically active infection, immunization of patient or close family members with live virus vaccines; anuria; pancreatitis; patients receiving alkylating agents (increased risk of neoplasms), concurrent radiation therapy. Safe use during pregnancy (category D) and lactation not established. **Cautious use in:** impaired kidney and liver function; patients receiving cadaver kidney; myasthenia gravis.

ADVERSE/SIDE EFFECTS GI: nausea, vomiting, anorexia, stomatitis, esophagitis, diarrhea, steatorrhea, pancreatitis. **Hematologic:** bone marrow depression, thrombocytopenia, leukopenia, anemia, agranulocytosis, pancytopenia. **Hepatic:** hepatitis with elevations in bilirubin, alkaline phosphatase, AST, ALT, biliary stasis, toxic hepatitis. **Hypersensitivity:** skin eruptions, rash, arthralgia. **Other:** *secondary infection (immunosuppression);* dysarthria, alopecia, muscle wasting, drug fever, retinopathy. Carcinogenic and teratogenic potential reported.

DIAGNOSTIC TEST INTERFERENCES Azathioprine may decrease plasma and urinary ***uric acid*** in patients with gout.

DRUG INTERACTIONS Allopurinol increases effects and toxicity of azathioprine by reducing metabolism of the active metabolite—allopurinol doses should be decreased by one third or one fourth; **tubocurarine** and other NONDEPOLARIZING SKELETAL MUSCLE RELAXANTS may reverse or inhibit neuromuscular blocking effects.

NURSING IMPLICATIONS

Administration
- Gastric disturbances may be minimized by administering oral drug in divided doses (prescribed), or

---

Common side effects in *italic*; life-threatening effects underlined; generic names in **bold**; classifications in SMALL CAPS

327

with food or immediately after meals, or by dosage reduction.

- Azathioprine sodium for IV injection is reconstituted by adding 10 ml sterile water for injection into vial. Swirl vial until drug is dissolved. For IV infusion, reconstituted solution may be further diluted with 50 ml NaCl injection or 5% dextrose in NaCl injection.
- IV azathioprine properly diluted may be administered by infusion over 30–60 min. Note: the final volume of the IV solution depends on time for infusion, which may range from 5 min to 8 h. Check with physician.
- Azathioprine therapy is usually started 1–5 d before kidney transplantation and restarted within 24 h after transplantation.
- Reconstituted IV solution may be stored at room temperature; but use within 24 h after reconstitution (contains no preservatives).
- Preserve in tightly closed, light-resistant containers at 15–30C (59–86F) unless otherwise directed.

Assessment & Drug Effects

- Monitor vital signs. Report signs of infection.
- CBC, including Hgb and platelet counts, should be performed before and at least weekly during first month of therapy, twice monthly during second and third months, and monthly, or more frequently therafter if indicated (e.g., by dosage or therapy changes).
- Kidney function is monitored to prevent drug accumulation (urine protein, urine electrolytes, creatinine clearance, serum creatinine, BUN).
- Surveillance of I&O ratio is crucial. Up to a twofold increase in toxicity is possible in anephric or anuric patients. Note color, character, and specific gravity of urine. Report an abrupt decrease in urinary output or any change in I&O ratio.
- Azathioprine has a high toxic potential. Because it may have delayed action, dosage should be reduced or drug withdrawn at the first indication of an abnormally large or persistent decrease in leukocyte or platelet count to avoid irreversible bone marrow depression.
- Thrombocytopenia occurs less commonly than leukopenia; however, be alert to signs of abnormal bleeding (easy bruising, bleeding gums, petechiae, purpura, melena, epistaxis, dark urine [hematuria], hemoptysis, hematemesis). If thrombocytopenia occurs, invasive procedures should be withheld, if possible.
- Liver function tests (alkaline phosphatase, AST, ALT, serum bilirubin) should be repeated at least every 3 mo or more frequently if indicated. If hepatic toxicity (see Signs & Symptoms, chap 3) develops, therapy may have to be withdrawn.
- Protective isolation may be indicated for the hospitalized patient to reduce risk of infections.

Patient & Family Education

- Therapeutic effectiveness in patients with rheumatoid arthritis usually occurs in 6–8 wk of therapy (improvement in morning stiffness and grip strength). If no improvement has occurred after 12 wk trial period, drug is generally discontinued.
- Intercurrent infection is a constant hazard of immunosuppressive therapy. Warn patient to avoid contact with persons who have colds or other infections and to report signs of impending infection, which are also possible symptoms of agranulocytosis. Personal hygiene should be scrupulous.
- Pregnancy should be ruled out before azathioprine therapy begins. Women of childbearing age should be warned about potential hazards and advised to practice birth control during therapy and for 4 mo after drug is discontinued.
- Vaccinations or other immunity-conferring agents are contraindicated because they may precipitate unusually severe reactions due to the immunosuppressive effects of azathioprine.

Prototype: ampicillin, p 69

AZLOCILLIN
(az-loe-sill′in)
Trade name: Azlin
Classifications: ANTIINFECTIVE; BETA-LACTAM ANTIBIOTIC; PENICILLIN
Pregnancy: Category B

ACTIONS/PHARMACODYNAMICS Semisynthetic, extended spectrum, bactericidal penicillin. Antibacterial spectrum similar to that of mezlocillin (Mezlin); but is more active against *Pseudomonas aeruginosa* and less active against *Klebsiella*. Believed to act by interfering with bacterial cell wall synthesis. Effective against *Streptococcus faecalis* and most other gram-positive cocci (but not penicillinase-producing strains of staphylococci), certain gram-negative bacilli, particularly *Pseudomonas aeruginosa,* and other species of *Pseudomonas, Escherichia coli, Haemophilus influenzae, Proteus mirabilis, Bacteroides fragilis,* and other anaerobes. Susceptible to inactivation by beta-lactamases produced by Enterobacteriaceae.

USES Primarily for treatment of serious infections caused by *Pseudomonas aeruginosa* in lower respiratory tract, urinary tract, skin and skin structures, bone and joints, and for bacterial septicemia. Most often used concurrently with an aminoglycoside antibiotic, e.g., amikacin, gentamicin, tobramycin, for synergistic effects against *Pseudomonas* strains. Also used with cephalosporins, e.g., cefotaxime, to treat life-threatening infections.

ROUTE & DOSAGE

Moderate to Severe Infections
Adult   IV   3–4 g q4–6h, up to 24 g/d

Pulmonary Exacerbation of Cystic Fibrosis
Child   IV   75 mg/kg q4h, up to 24 g/d

PHARMACOKINETICS Distribution: distributed in bile, urine, bronchial secretions, bone, and other tissues; poor CSF penetration unless meninges are inflamed; crosses placenta; distributed into breast milk in low concentrations. **Metabolism:** <10% metabolized in liver. **Elimination:** half-life: 55–70 min; 50–70% eliminated in urine; 20–25% excreted in bile.

CONTRAINDICATIONS & PRECAUTIONS Contraindicated in: hypersensitivity to any of the penicillins; common bile duct obstruction. Safe use during pregnancy (category B) and in neonates not established. **Cautious use in:** impaired renal or hepatic function; history of hypersensitivity to cephalosporins; nursing mothers; history of bleeding disorders; GI disease; patients on restricted sodium intake, hypokalemia and other electrolyte imbalances, dehydration.

ADVERSE/SIDE EFFECTS CNS: neuromuscular hyperirritability, convulsions. **GI:** *nausea,* steatorrhea, vomiting, *diarrhea,* epigastric pain. **Hematologic:** bone marrow depression, leukopenia, neutropenia, thrombocytopenia; prolonged prothrombin and bleeding times, hypokalemia, hypernatremia. **Hypersensitivity:** rash, pruritus, urticaria, hypersensitivity pancreatitis, arthralgia, myalgia, drug fever, chills, chest discomfort, anaphylactic reactions. **Other:** superinfections, transient chest discomfort with rapid IV injection: pain and thrombophlebitis at IV site, increased serum creatinine, BUN, glomerulonephritis.

DIAGNOSTIC TEST INTERFERENCES Transient lowering of **serum uric acid** levels. False-positive **urinary protein** reactions (pseudoproteinuria) with many methods; bromphenol blue (multi-stix) method reportedly reliable. **Platelet abnormalities** may persist for as long as 2 wk following drug discontinuation.

DRUG INTERACTIONS ORAL ANTICOAGULANTS, **heparin** increase risk of bleeding with large doses of azlocillin; **chloramphenicol** possibly antagonistic; **probenecid** decreases azlocillin elimination.

INCOMPATIBILITIES Solution/additive: AMINO-GLYCOSIDES. **Y-site:** AMINOGLYCOSIDES.

NURSING IMPLICATIONS

Administration

- **For direct IV injection:** Each gram of azlocillin should be reconstituted with at least 10 ml of sterile water, 5% dextrose, or 0.9% NaCl injection. Shake vigorously until dissolved. To minimize venous irritations, drug concentration should not exceed 10%. Resulting solution may be administered by direct IV injection or into IV tubing over 5 min or more. Rapid IV injection can cause transient chest pains.
- **For intermittent IV infusion:** Initial dilution (see above) should be diluted further with suitable diluent (sterile water, 0.9% NaCl, 5% dextrose in 0.225% NaCl, 5% dextrose in 0.45% NaCl for injection, lactated Ringer's injection) to desired volume (50–100 ml) and administered over 30 min period.
- Reconstituted solutions should be clear, colorless to pale yellow, and free of particulate matter. Solutions are stable at room temperature for 24 h (potency loss less than 10%) in suitable diluents (see above). Concentrations up to 100 mg/ml are stable for 24 h when refrigerated below 8C (46.4F).
- Prior to reconstitution, store vial containing azlocillin below 30C (86F) unless otherwise directed by manufacturer.
- When other antibiotics are prescribed concomitantly, administer each drug separately because mutual inactivation may occur when drugs are mixed together.

Assessment & Drug Effects

- Culture and susceptibility tests should be performed before initiation of drug therapy.
- A careful drug history should be obtained before initiation of therapy to determine patient's previous exposure and sensitivity to penicillin, cephalosporin, and other allergens.
- During initial drug administration, carefully moni-

Common side effects in *italic*; life-threatening effects underlined; generic names in **bold**; classifications in SMALL CAPS

329

tor for hypersensitivity or anaphylactic reactions (see Signs & Symptoms, chap 3). Report their appearance immediately.

- Baseline and periodic evaluation of renal, hepatic, and hematopoietic functions and serum electrolytes, especially potassium and sodium, is advisable during prolonged therapy.
- Monitor I&O ratio and pattern, particularly in patients with impaired renal function or who are receiving another antibiotic concurrently. Serum drug and creatinine levels and creatinine clearance are recommended to determine appropriate dosages.
- Although such incidents are rare, azlocillin can cause abnormalities in coagulation tests (thrombocytopenia), particularly in patients with renal impairment. Check values of clotting time, platelet aggregation, PT, and PTT. Instruct patient to report any unexplained bleeding or bruising (hematomas, petechiae, ecchymoses).
- Be alert to signs of superinfection (see chap 3) and report their onset immediately.

Prototype: imipenem-cilastatin, p 67

AZTREONAM

(az-tree´oh-nam)

Trade name: Azactam
Classifications: ANTIINFECTIVE; BETA-LACTAM ANTIBIOTIC
Pregnancy: Category B

ACTIONS/PHARMACODYNAMICS Synthetic monobactam antibiotic (a new class of beta lactams) with bacterial action. Differs structurally from other beta-lactam antibiotics (penicillins and cephalosporins) in having a monocyclic rather than a bicyclic nucleus. Acts by inhibiting synthesis of bacterial cell wall, which results from its high affinity for penicillin-binding protein (PBP_3), found primarily in aerobic, gram-negative bacteria. Highly resistant to beta-lactamases and does not readily induce their formation. Spectrum of activity limited to aerobic, gram-negative bacteria. Activity almost equal to that of aminoglycosides but reportedly does not cause nephrotoxicity or ototoxicity. Active against *Haemophilus influenzae, Pseudomonas aeruginosa, Neisseria gonorrhoeae,* and against Enterobacteriaceae including most strains of *E. coli, Enterobacter, Klebsiella, Proteus, Providencia, Shigella, Salmonella,* and *Serratia.* There appears to be little cross-allergenicity with penicillins and cephalosporins.

USES Gram-negative infections of urinary tract, lower respiratory tract, skin and skin structures; and for intraabdominal and gynecologic infections, septicemia, and as adjunctive therapy for surgical infections. Often used in combination with other antibiotics active against gram-positive and anaerobic bacteria in mixed infections.

ROUTE & DOSAGE

Urinary Tract Infection
Adult   IM/IV   0.5–1 g q8–12h

Moderate to Severe Infections
Adult   IM/IV   1–2 g q6–8h (max 8 g/24h)

PHARMACOKINETICS Peak: 1 h IM. **Distribution:** widely distributed including synovial and blister fluid, bile, bronchial secretions, prostate, bone, and CSF; crosses placenta; distributed into breast milk in small amounts. **Metabolism:** not extensively metabolized. **Elimination:** half-life: 1.6–2.1 h; 60–70% excreted in urine within 24 h.

CONTRAINDICATIONS & PRECAUTIONS Contraindicated in: safe use during pregnancy (category B), in nursing women, infants, and children not established. **Cautious use in:** history of hypersensitivity reaction to penicillin, cephalosporins, or to other drugs; impaired renal or hepatic function.

ADVERSE/SIDE EFFECTS CNS: headache, dizziness, confusion, paresthesias, insomnia, seizures. **CV:** hypotension, transient ECG changes, dyspnea. **ENT:** tinnitus, nasal congestion, sneezing. **Eye:** diplopia. **GI:** nausea, *diarrhea,* vomiting, mouth ulcers, halitosis, altered taste, abdominal cramps. **Hematologic:** pancytopenia, neutropenia, thrombocytopenia, anemia, leukocytosis, thrombocytosis, prolonged bleeding time. **Hepatic:** hepatitis, jaundice, elevations of liver function tests. **Hypersensitivity:** urticaria, eosinophilia, <u>anaphylaxis.</u> **Local reactions:** phlebitis, thrombophlebitis (following IV), pain at injection sites. **Skin:** rash, purpura, erythema multiforme, exfoliative dermatitis, diaphoresis; petechiae, pruritus. **Other:** superinfections (gram-positive cocci), vaginal candidiasis, vaginitis, fever.

DIAGNOSTIC TEST INTERFERENCES Aztreonam may cause transient elevations of ***liver function tests,*** increases in ***PT*** and ***PTT,*** minor changes in ***Hgb,*** and positive ***Coombs' test.***

DRUG INTERACTIONS Imipenem-cilastatin, cefoxitin may be antagonistic; **probenecid** slows renal elimination of aztreonam.

INCOMPATIBILITIES Solution/additive: **ampicillin, metronidazole, nafcillin.**

NURSING IMPLICATIONS

Administration

- For IM injection, reconstitute 15 ml vial with at least 3 ml of diluent per gram of aztreonam. Suitable diluents include sterile water for injection; bacteriostatic water for injection (with benzyl alcohol and propyl parabens); NaCl 0.9% for injection.
- IM injections should be made deeply into large muscle mass such as the upper outer quadrant of the gluteus maximus or lateral thigh. Rotate injections sites.
- IV aztreonam may be given direct IV with a single dose diluted in 6–10 ml of sterile water for injection. Immediately shake it until it is dissolved. Give over 3–5 min.
- Reconstituted solutions are colorless to light straw yellow and turn slightly pink on standing. Reportedly this does not affect potency.
- Refer to manufacturer's package insert for complete details of solution preparation for IV administration, stability information, and drug compatibility data.

Assessment & Drug Effects

- Culture and susceptibility tests should be performed before initiation of therapy.
- Before treatment is initiated, a detailed history should be obtained of drug allergies so that necessary precautions may be observed.
- Renal function should be monitored, particularly in the elderly and in those with history of renal impairment. Estimates of creatinine clearance should be made initially and at regular intervals during therapy and used as a guide to dosage.
- Be watchful for signs of opportunistic infections (diarrhea, rectal or vaginal itching or discharge, fever, cough), and promptly report this onset to physician. Overgrowth of nonsusceptible organisms, particularly staphylococci, streptococci, and fungi, is a threat, especially in patients receiving prolonged or repeated therapy.
- Inspect IV injection sites daily for signs of inflammation. Reportedly pain and phlebitis occur in over 2% of patients.

Prototype: ampicillin, p 69

BACAMPICILLIN HYDROCHLORIDE

(ba-kam-pɪ-sill in)
Trade name: Spectrobid
Classifications: ANTIINFECTIVE; ANTIBIOTIC; AMINOPENICILLIN
Pregnancy: Category B

ACTIONS/PHARMACODYNAMICS Acid-stable, penicillinase-sensitive aminopenicillin that is rapidly hydrolyzed to ampicillin in body. Has broad spectrum of antimicrobial activity and exerts antibacterial action by inhibiting bacterial cell wall biosynthesis. More rapidly and completely absorbed from GI tract than ampicillin is, and serum concentrations attained are higher.

USES Infections caused by susceptible microorganisms of upper and lower respiratory tract, urinary tract, skin and skin structures; acute uncomplicated gonorrhea.

ROUTE & DOSAGE

Moderate to Severe Infections

Adult	PO	400–800 mg q12h
Child	PO	12.5 25 mg/kg q12h

Gonorrhea

Adult	PO	1.6 g with 1 g probenecid x 1

PHARMACOKINETICS Absorption: rapidly and almost completely absorbed; hydrolyzed to ampicillin. **Distribution:** most body tissues; crosses placenta; appears in breast milk. **Metabolism:** metabolized in liver. **Elimination:** half-life: 0.7–1.1 h; 75% eliminated as ampicillin in urine within 8 h.

CONTRAINDICATIONS & PRECAUTIONS Contraindicated in: hypersensitivity to penicillins; pregnancy (category B); infectious mononucleosis or other viral diseases; children <25 kg. **Cautious use in:** history of allergy to cephalosporins; nursing mothers.

ADVERSE/SIDE EFFECTS GI: *nausea,* vomiting, anorexia, *diarrhea.* **Hematologic:** leukopenia, agranulocytosis, thrombocytopenia, eosinophilia, anemia.

Hypersensitivity: erythematous rash; anaphylaxis (rare). **Other:** superinfections, fixed drug eruption.

DIAGNOSTIC TEST INTERFERENCES High urine bacampicillin concentrations can result in false positive *urine glucose determinations with copper sulfate tests* (Benedict's, Clinitest, Fehling's); glucose oxidase methods (Clinistix, TesTape) are not affected. *Serum ALT* (SGPT) and *AST* (SGOT) may increase.

DRUG INTERACTIONS Allopurinol increases incidence of rash; since ampicillin may interfere with ORAL CONTRACEPTIVE action, female patients should be advised to consider nonhormonal contraception while on antibiotics. **Drug-food interactions:** food may decrease absorption of bacampicillin; give 1 h before or 2 h after meals.

NURSING IMPLICATIONS

Administration

- Food does not retard or reduce absorption of bacampicillin in tablet form.
- Oral suspension is affected by food and therefore should be taken on an empty stomach. Administer preferably with a full glass (240 ml) of water either 1 h before or 2 h after meals.
- The oral suspension is intended for use in children and infants weighing <25 kg, or in children who are unable to swallow tablets.
- When dispensed, oral suspension should include a calibrated liquid measuring device.
- Store in tight container at 15–30C (59–86F) unless otherwise directed.

Assessment & Drug Effects

- Careful inquiry should be made before initiation of therapy concerning previous hypersensitivity reactions to penicillins, cephalosporins, and other allergens.
- Culture and susceptibility tests should be performed before therapy is begun.
- Baseline and periodic checks of renal, hepatic, and hematopoietic status are advised during prolonged therapy, particularly in patients with history of impaired function of these systems, and in prematures and neonates.

Patient & Family Education

- Instruct patient to report symptoms of an allergic hypersensitivity reaction immediately (see chap 3).

- Advise patient to report signs of superinfection (see chap 3).
- Emphasize need to take medication for the full course of therapy as prescribed.
- Stubborn infections may require several months of clinical or bacteriologic follow-up, or both, after therapy has stopped. Urge patient to keep follow-up appointments.

BACITRACIN

(bass-i-tray´sin)
Trade names: Baciguent, Baciguent Ophthalmic, Bacitin, Bacitracin Ophthalmic
Classifications: ANTIINFECTIVE; ANTIBIOTIC
Pregnancy: Category C

ACTIONS/PHARMACODYNAMICS Polypeptide antibiotic derived from cultures of *Bacillus subtilis*. Precise mechanism of action not known. Appears to interfere with function of bacterial cell membrane by inhibiting cell wall synthesis. Spectrum of antibacterial activity similar to that of penicillin. Bactericidal or bacteriostatic depending on concentration and susceptibility of organism. Active against many gram-positive organisms including streptococci, staphylococci, pneumococci, corynebacteria, *Clostridia, Neisseria, Haemophilus influenzae,* and *Treponema pallidum*. Also active against gonococci and meningococci; ineffective against most other gram-negative organisms. Has neuromuscular blocking action.

USES Parenteral therapy restricted to infants with staphylococcal pneumonia and empyema due to susceptible organisms where adequate laboratory facilities and constant supervision are available. Used topically in treatment of superficial infections of skin and eye. **Unlabeled use:** orally for treatment of antibiotic-associated colitis. Has been used investigationally by various routes (intrathecal, intrapleural, intrasynovial) for serious infections.

PHARMACOKINETICS Absorption: poorly absorbed from intact or denuded skin or mucous membranes. **Peak:** 1–2 h IM. **Duration:** 6–8 h. **Distribution:** widely distributed including peritoneal and ascitic fluids. **Elimination:** slow renal excretion (10–40% in 24 h).

ROUTE & DOSAGE

Systemic Infections

Child	IM	<2.5 kg: up to 900 U/kg/24h divided q8–12h
		>2.5 kg: up to 1000 U/kg/24h divided q8–12h

Skin Infections

Adult	Topical	Apply thin layer of ointment b.i.d. or t.i.d. or use a solution of 250–1000 U/ml as a wet dressing
		ophthalmic ointment: applied to conjunctival sac 1 or more times/d

CONTRAINDICATIONS & PRECAUTIONS Contraindicated in: toxic reaction or renal dysfunction associated with bacitracin; impaired renal function; atopic individuals; pregnancy (category C). **Cautious use in:** myasthenia gravis or other neuromuscular disease. Patients allergic to neomycin may be sensitive to bacitracin.

ADVERSE/SIDE EFFECTS Eye: delayed corneal healing. **GI:** anorexia, nausea, vomiting, diarrhea, rectal itching and burning. **Hematologic** (systemic use): bone marrow depression, blood dyscrasias; eosinophilia. **Hypersensitivity** (associated with both systemic and topical use): erythema, anaphylaxis. **Nephrotoxicity** (dose related): increased BUN, uremia, renal tubular and glomerular necrosis. **Other:** pain and inflammation at injection site, fever, superinfection, neuromuscular blockade with respiratory depression; tinnitus.

DRUG INTERACTIONS With AMINOGLYCOSIDES, possibility of additive nephrotoxic and neuromuscular blocking effects; with **tubocurarine** and other NONDEPOLARIZING SKELETAL MUSCLE RELAXANTS, possibility of additive neuromuscular blocking effects.

NURSING IMPLICATIONS

Administration

- Bacitracin should not be reconstituted with diluents containing parabens because solution may precipitate or become cloudy.
- Parenteral solution (for IM use only) should be dissolved in 0.9% NaCl injection containing 2% procaine hydrochloride (prescribed). Alternate injection sites since injections are painful.
- Administration of parenteral bacitracin for longer than 12 d is not advised.
- Intramuscular bacitracin solution is stable for 1 wk

if refrigerated; inactivation occurs at room temperature. Dry bacitracin should be stored in refrigerator at 2–8C (36–46F). Topical ointments should be stored in tightly closed containers at 15–30C (59–86F) unless otherwise directed.

Assessment & Drug Effects

- Culture and susceptibility tests should be performed before therapy begins and periodically during therapy.
- Before systemic therapy is begun, determinations should be made of BUN and nonprotein nitrogen (NPN), and urine should be examined for albumin, casts, and cellular elements. Renal function should be monitored daily throughout therapy.
- Be alert to signs of local allergic manifestations (itching, burning, redness) with topical skin applications. Local reactions have preceded life-threatening anaphylactic episodes.
- Monitor I&O during parenteral therapy. Adequate urinary output should be maintained to reduce possibility of renal toxicity. If fluid intake is inadequate or urinary output decreases, report to physician.
- Inspect urine for turbidity and hematuria, and be on the alert for other signs and symptoms of urinary tract dysfunction. Note and report any changes in urination pattern, e.g., oliguria, urinary frequency, nocturia.
- Prolonged use may result in overgrowth of nonsusceptible organisms, especially *Candida albicans.*

Patient & Family Education

- Instruct patient taking ophthalmic preparation to stop drug and notify physician if signs of hypersensitivity appear: itching, burning, swelling of eyelids.
- Instruct patient to report local allergic manifestations with topical applications, e.g., itching, burning, redness.

Prototype: cyclobenzaprine, p 122

BACLOFEN
(bak´loe-fen)
Trade names: Lioresal, Lioresal DS
Classifications: AUTONOMIC NERVOUS SYSTEM AGENT; CENTRAL ACTING SKELETAL MUSCLE RELAXANT
Pregnancy: Category C

Common side effects in *italic*; life-threatening effects underlined; generic names in **bold**; classifications in SMALL CAPS

333

ACTIONS/PHARMACODYNAMICS Centrally acting skeletal muscle relaxant, derivative of gamma-aminobutyric acid (GABA), an inhibitory neurotransmitter. Precise mechanism of action not determined. Depresses monosynaptic and polysynaptic afferent reflex activity at spinal cord level thereby reducing skeletal muscle spasm caused by upper motor neuron lesions. Drug may also have some activity at supraspinal sites because it can produce CNS depression in high doses. Relaxes external sphincter of the hyperreflexic urinary bladder and appears to have an anticholinergic-like effect on involuntary bladder contractions.

USES To provide symptomatic relief of painful spasms in multiple sclerosis and in the management of detrusor sphincter dyssynergia in spinal cord injury or disease. **Unlabeled use:** treatment of trigeminal neuralgia, and tardive dystonia associated with antipsychotic medications.

ROUTE & DOSAGE

Muscle Spasm

Adult	PO	5 mg t.i.d.; may increase by 5 mg/dose q3d prn (max 80 mg/d)

PHARMACOKINETICS Absorption: readily absorbed from GI tract. **Peak:** 2–3 h. **Duration:** 8 h. **Distribution:** minimal amounts cross blood-brain barrier; crosses placenta; distribution into breast milk unknown. **Metabolism:** 15% of dose metabolized in liver. **Elimination:** half-life: 3–4 h; 70–85% excreted in urine within 72 h; some elimination in feces.

CONTRAINDICATIONS & PRECAUTIONS Contraindicated in: safe use during pregnancy (category C), in nursing mothers, and in children <12 yr not established. **Cautious use in:** impaired renal and hepatic function; epilepsy; diabetes mellitus; stroke; psychiatric or brain disorders; elderly patients.

ADVERSE/SIDE EFFECTS CNS: *transient drowsiness,* vertigo, dizziness, weakness, fatigue, headache, confusion, insomnia; ataxia, loss of seizure control in epileptic patients. **CV:** hypotension. **ENT:** tinnitus, nasal congestion. **Eye:** blurred vision, mydriasis, nystagmus, diplopia, strabismus, miosis. **GI:** nausea, constipation, vomiting. **GU:** urinary frequency. **Hepatic:** mild increases in AST (SGOT), and alkaline phosphatase, jaundice. **Hypersensitivity:** (uncommon): pruritus, skin eruptions, fever. **Other:** ankle edema, weight gain, hyperglycemia, excessive perspiration.

DIAGNOSTIC TEST INTERFERENCES Possibility of increases in **blood glucose,** serum **alkaline phosphatase,** and **AST** levels.

DRUG INTERACTIONS Alcohol, CNS DEPRESSANTS, MAO INHIBITORS, ANTIHISTAMINES compound CNS depression; baclofen may increase blood glucose levels, making it necessary to increase dosage of SULFONYLUREAS, **insulin.**

NURSING IMPLICATIONS

Administration

- If patient complains of GI distress, drug may be administered with food or milk.
- Store at 15–30C (59–86F) in tightly closed container unless otherwise directed.

Assessment & Drug Effects

- Supervise ambulation. Initially the loss of spasticity induced by baclofen may affect patient's ability to stand or walk.
- Baseline and periodic checks should be made of BP, weight, blood sugar, hepatic function tests, and urine.
- Advise patient to report adverse reactions to physician. Most can be reduced by decreasing dosage. Incidence of CNS symptoms (drowsiness, dizziness, ataxia) are reportedly high in patients >40 y of age.
- Many of the adverse neuropsychiatric or genitourinary symptoms resemble those of the underlying disease. Carefully assess them and report them to the physician.
- The elderly are especially sensitive to this drug. Observe carefully for side effects: mental confusion, depression, hallucinations.
- Patients with epilepsy should be closely monitored by EEG, clinical observation, and interview at regular intervals for possible loss of seizure control.
- Observe for and record response to drug. Therapeutic effectiveness may be noted in a few hours to weeks.

Patient & Family Education

- Warn patient that CNS depressant effects will be additive to other CNS depressants, including alcohol.
- Inform diabetics that baclofen may raise blood glucose levels. Urge patient to report promptly changes in urine or blood tests to the physician. Dose adjustment of insulin and hypoglycemic agents may be indicated.
- Warn patient to avoid driving and other potentially

Common side effects in *italic*; life-threatening effects underlined; generic names in **bold**; classifications in SMALL CAPS

hazardous activities until the reaction to baclofen is determined.

- Caution patient not to self-dose with OTC drugs without physician's approval.
- Inform patient that drug withdrawal should be accomplished gradually over a period of 2 wk or more. Abrupt withdrawal following prolonged administration may cause anxiety, agitated behavior, auditory and visual hallucinations, severe tachycardia, acute exacerbation of spasticity, and seizures.

Prototype: hydrocortisone, p 255

BECLOMETHASONE DIPROPRIONATE
(be-kloe-meth´a-sone)

Trade names: Beclovent, Beconase Nasal Inhaler, Vancenase Nasal Inhaler, Vanceril

Classifications: SYNTHETIC HORMONE; ADRENAL CORTICOSTEROID; GLUCOCORTICOID; ANTIINFLAMMATORY AGENT

Pregnancy: Category C

ACTIONS/PHARMACODYNAMICS Synthetic corticosteroid, structurally related to hydrocortisone, with potent glucocorticoid (antiinflammatory) and weak mineralocorticoid activity. Precise mechanism of action not known but may be related to its ability to stabilize leukocyte lysosomal membranes, reduce cellular histamine stores, and prevent release of arachidonic acid from cell membranes, thereby inhibiting production of substances that adversely affect airway function. Rapid drug metabolism plus use of metered sprays permit smaller doses, and thus there are fewer adverse reactions than with systemic corticosteroids. Unlike hydrocortisone, therapeutic doses do not suppress the hypothalamic-pituitary-adrenocortical (HPA) function or produce other systemic effects.

USES Oral inhalation to treat chronic steroid-dependent bronchial asthma adjunctively with other therapy (sympathomimetics, xanthines); nasal inhalation to treat seasonal and perennial rhinitis and to prevent postsurgical recurrence of polyposis. Beclomethasone is prophylactic and fails to provide immediate benefit in acute asthma.

PHARMACOKINETICS Absorption: readily absorbed from respiratory and GI tracts following in-

halation. **Peak:** peak effect after 1–2 wk of continuous use. **Distribution:** possibly crosses placenta; distributed into breast milk. **Metabolism:** metabolized in lung, GI tissues, and liver to inactive metabolites. **Elimination:** half-life: 3–15 h (if swallowed); 90% eliminated in feces.

ROUTE & DOSAGE

Asthma

Adult	Oral inhaler	2 inhalations t.i.d. or q.i.d. up to 20 inhalations per day; may try to reduce systemic steroids after 1 wk of concomitant therapy
Child	Oral inhaler	1–2 inhalations t.i.d. or q.i.d. up to 10 inhalations per day

Allergic Rhinitis

Adult	Nasal inhaler	1 spray in each nostril b.i.d. to q.i.d.

CONTRAINDICATIONS & PRECAUTIONS Contraindicated in: hypersensitivity to beclomethasone or to any ingredient in the formulation (e.g., oleic acid, fluorocarbons). Use of oral inhaler therapy in asthma adequately controlled by bronchodilators or nonsteroidal medication; nonasthmatic bronchitis, primary treatment of status asthmaticus, acute attack of asthma. Safe use during pregnancy (category C), in nursing mothers and in children <6 y (oral inhaler) or <12 y (nasal inhaler) not established. **Cautious use in:** patients receiving systemic corticosteroids; use with extreme caution if at all in respiratory tuberculosis, untreated fungal, bacterial, or viral infections, and ocular herpes simplex; nasal inhalation therapy for nasal septal ulcers, nasal trauma, or surgery.

ADVERSE/SIDE EFFECTS Oral inhalation: *candidal infection of oropharynx* and occasionally larynx, hoarseness, dry mouth, sore throat, sore mouth. **Nasal (inhaler):** *transient nasal irritation, burning, sneezing,* epistaxis, bloody mucus, nasopharyngeal itching, dryness, crusting, and ulceration; headache, nausea, vomiting. **Other:** with excessive doses, symptoms of hypercorticism.

NURSING IMPLICATIONS

Administration

- Note that oral inhalation and nasal inhalation products are not to be used interchangeably.

Common side effects in *italic*; life-threatening effects underlined; generic names in **bold**; classifications in SMALL CAPS

335

B

- Instructions for oral inhaler use are included with package. Review information with patient to assure complete understanding.
- If patient is also receiving a bronchodilator by inhalation (e.g., isoproterenol, metaproterenol, epinephrine), bronchodilator should be used several minutes before beclomethasone oral inhaler to enhance penetration of the steroid into the bronchial tree and to reduce the potential toxicity of fluorocarbon propellants in the two aerosols.
- *Oral inhaler:* emphasize the following: (1) Shake inhaler well before using. (2) After exhaling fully, place mouthpiece well into mouth with lips closed firmly around it. (3) Inhale slowly through mouth while activating the inhaler. (4) Hold breath 5–10 s, if possible, then exhale slowly. (5) Wait 1 min between puffs.
- Rinsing mouth and gargling with warm water after each oral inhalation removes residual medication from oropharyngeal area. Mouth care may also delay or prevent onset of oral dryness, hoarseness, and candidiasis.
- *Nasal inhaler:* Directions for use of nasal inhaler provided by manufacturer should be carefully reviewed with patient. Emphasize the following points: (1) Gently blow nose to clear nostrils. (2) Shake inhaler well before using. (3) If 2 sprays in each nostril are prescribed, direct one spray toward upper, and the other toward lower part of nostril. (4) Wash cap and plastic nosepiece daily with warm water; dry thoroughly.
- Store at 2–30C (36–86F) unless otherwise directed.

Assessment & Drug Effects

- Improvement in pulmonary function may require as long as 1–4 wk when beclomethasone is given to patient not receiving systemic steroids.
- Oral membranes should be inspected frequently for indications of *Candida* infection (white patches, red, sore membranes) and patient should be questioned about new symptoms, e.g., cough, sore mouth or throat. If symptoms of *Candida* are present, antifungal therapy (e.g., Nystatin) will be instituted.
- Patients should be closely monitored during and for several months or longer after withdrawal of systemic corticosteroids. Death from acute adrenal suppression has been reported. Steroid withdrawal must be accomplished slowly to avoid precipitating symptoms of **adrenal insufficiency** (joint discomfort, muscle pain, depression, lassitude, fatigue, weakness, dizziness, light-headedness [hypotension]), nausea, and vomiting. Symptoms may occur in spite of maintenance and even improvement of respiratory function.
- Monitor BP and weight during withdrawal-transfer period. Hypotension and weight loss (objective signs of adrenal insufficiency) indicate need for temporary boost in systemic steroid and slower withdrawal schedule.
- When symptoms for which beclomethasone was prescribed are relieved, dosage should be reduced gradually to lowest effective level. Keep physician informed.

Patient & Family Education

- Beclomethasone does not provide immediate symptomatic relief and is not prescribed for this purpose.
- Emphasize importance of taking drug precisely as directed. Therapeutic effectiveness of beclomethasone via oral or nasal inhaler depends on administering it at regular intervals, as prescribed.
- Warn patient not to use higher than prescribed dosage. If symptoms worsen, or signs of irritation appear, or symptomatic improvement does not occur within 2 or 3 wk, notify physician.
- Long-term effects of beclomethasone are not known. Therefore periodic evaluations are essential.
- Clean inhaler daily. Separate parts as directed in package insert, rinse them with warm water, and dry them thoroughly.
- During transfer from systemic steroid therapy to aerosol administration, allergic conditions previously suppressed (rhinitis, conjunctivitis, eczema) may be unmasked. Instruct patient to report them to physician promptly.
- Relief of seasonal or perennial rhinitis usually occurs over a period of a few days to 2 wk. Nasal polyps may require several weeks of treatment before effectiveness can be determined. Beclomethasone should not be continued beyond 3 wk in the absence of significant improvement.
- Keep inhalers (oral and nasal) away from open flame or heat above 49C (120F) (may explode—contents are under pressure). Do not puncture container and do not discard into fire or incinerator.

Common side effects in *italic*; life-threatening effects underlined; generic names in **bold**; classifications in SMALL CAPS

Prototype: atropine, p 116

BELLADONNA EXTRACT

BELLADONNA TINCTURE

(bell-a-don´a)

Classifications: AUTONOMIC NERVOUS SYSTEM AGENT; ANTICHOLINERGIC (PARASYMPATHOLYTIC); ANTIMUSCARINIC, ANTISPASMODIC

Pregnancy: Category C

ACTIONS/PHARMACODYNAMICS

Prepared from leaf of *Atropa belladonna* (deadly nightshade). Reversibly blocks action of acetylcholine at parasympathetic neuroeffector sites, thereby inhibiting smooth muscle contractions and suppressing secretions of secretory glands. Belladonna extract contains 12.5 mg of belladonna alkaloids per gram, and the tincture contains 0.3 mg/ml.

USES

Adjunct in treatment of peptic ulcer disease, irritable bowel syndrome, and neurogenic bowel disturbances. Also has been used for dysmenorrhea, nocturnal enuresis, spasms of urinary tract, nausea and vomiting of pregnancy, vertigo, and for symptomatic relief of parkinsonism.

ROUTE & DOSAGE

Antispasmodic

Adult	PO	15–30 mg of extract t.i.d. or q.i.d.
		0.6–1 ml of tincture t.i.d. or q.i.d.
Child	PO	0.1 ml/kg/d of tincture in 3–4 divided doses (max 3.5 ml/d)

PHARMACOKINETICS

Absorption: readily absorbed from GI tract. **Onset:** 1–2 h. **Distribution:** well distributed in body; crosses blood-brain barrier. **Elimination:** excreted unchanged in urine.

CONTRAINDICATIONS & PRECAUTIONS

Contraindicated in: hypersensitivity to anticholinergic drugs; obstructive uropathy, atony of urinary bladder; esophageal reflux, obstructive disease of GI tract, intestinal atony, paralytic ileus, severe ulcerative colitis, toxic megacolon; myasthenia gravis; narrow-angle glaucoma; unstable cardiovascular status in acute hemorrhages. Safe use during pregnancy (category C), in nursing women, and of belladonna extract tablets in children not established. **Cautious use in:** autonomic neuropathy; heart disease, hypertension; patients >40 y (higher incidence of glaucoma).

ADVERSE/SIDE EFFECTS

Dose related. **CNS:** excitement (young children and the elderly), confusion, drowsiness, delirium, headache. **CV:** rapid heart beat, tachycardia, palpitation. **Eye:** blurred vision, mydriasis, photophobia, increased intraocular pressure. **GI:** *dry mouth, constipation,* nausea, vomiting. **GU:** urinary retention, urgency. **Other:** decreased sweating, flushing, drug-induced fever, heat stroke.

DRUG INTERACTIONS

Amantadine, ANTIHISTAMINES, TRICYCLIC ANTIDEPRESSANTS, **quinidine, disopyramide, procainamide** have additive anticholinergic effects; **levodopa** effects decreased; **methotrimeprazine** may precipitate extrapyramidal effects; antipsychotic effects of PHENOTHIAZINES decreased (decreased absorption).

NURSING IMPLICATIONS

Administration

- Usually administered 30–60 min before meals and at bedtime.
- If patient is receiving antacid therapy, the antacid is given after meals. Space administration of antacid and belladonna preparations at least 1 h apart.
- Store at 15–30C (59–86F) in tightly covered, light-resistant containers, unless otherwise directed.

Assessment & Drug Effects

- Assess patient for therapeutic drug effects.
- Since drug may cause drowsiness and confusion, carefully monitor ambulation of elderly or debilitated patient.
- Monitor I&O and assess for urinary retention.

Patient & Family Education

- Instruct patient to be aware of I&O. Increase in fluid intake and bulk in diet may be allowed to prevent or relieve constipation. If it persists, notify physician.
- Caution patient to avoid hot baths, saunas, and strenuous work or exercise during hot and humid weather.
- Advise patient to refrain from driving and other potentially hazardous activities until reaction to drug is determined.
- If mouth dryness is a problem, instruct patient to practice meticulous oral hygiene. Sugarless gum or lemon drops and frequent sips of water may help.

Common side effects in *italic*; life-threatening effects <u>underlined</u>; generic names in **bold**; classifications in SMALL CAPS

337

B

Prototype: hydrochlorothiazide, p 203

BENDROFLUMETHIAZIDE

(ben-droe-floo-meth-eye´a-zide)

Trade name: Naturetin

Classifications: WATER BALANCE AGENT; THIAZIDE DIURETIC

ACTIONS/PHARMACODYNAMICS Thiazide (benzothiadazine) diuretic chemically related to the sulfonamides. Similar to hydrochlorothiazide in pharmacologic actions, uses, contraindications, precautions, adverse effects, and interactions. Reportedly does not alter serum electrolyte concentrations appreciably at recommended doses.

USES Management of edema associated with CHF, mild hypertension. **Unlabeled use:** lithium-associated diabetes insipidus.

ROUTE & DOSAGE

Hypertension

Adult	PO	2.5–20 mg/d in 1–2 divided doses
Child	PO	0.05–0.4 mg/kg/d in 1–2 divided doses

PHARMACOKINETICS Absorption: readily absorbed from GI tract. **Onset:** 1–2 h. **Peak:** 6–12 h. **Duration:** 18–24 h. **Elimination:** excreted unchanged in urine within 24 h.

CONTRAINDICATIONS & PRECAUTIONS Contraindicated in: anuria, hypersensitivity to thiazides, sulfonamides; pregnancy, lactation. **Cautious use in:** renal and hepatic disease; gout; diabetes mellitus.

ADVERSE/SIDE EFFECTS Xerostomia, sialadenitis, anorexia, unusual fatigue, paresthesias, photosensitivity, vasculitis, orthostatic hypotension, agranulocytosis, electrolyte imbalance, hypokalemia, hyperglycemia, impaired glucose tolerance, hyperuricemia, exacerbation of gout, SLE.

DRUG INTERACTIONS Cholestyramine, colestipol decrease absorption of the diuretic; **diazoxide** has additive effects; with **digoxin,** the hypokalemia may increase risk of digitalis toxicity; increases **lithium** levels and toxicity; may increase blood glucose levels, necessitating adjustment of hypoglycemic therapy, i.e., SULFONYLUREAS, **insulin.**

NURSING IMPLICATIONS

Administration

- Administer drug early in AM after patient has eaten to reduce gastric irritation and to prevent possibility of interrupted sleep because of diuresis. If 2 doses are ordered, administer second dose no later than 3 PM.
- Store tablets in tightly closed container at 15–30C (59–86F) unless otherwise specified.

Assessment & Drug Effects

- Antihypertensive effects are generally noted in 3–4 d; maximal effects may require 3–4 wk.
- Monitor BP, I&O ratio and pattern, and weight, particularly during first phase of antihypertensive therapy. Report a sudden fall in BP, which may initiate severe postural hypotension and potentially dangerous perfusion problems of the extremities, especially in older patients.
- Orthostatic hypotension and hypokalemia can be distressing side effects in the elderly.
- Monitor for hypokalemia (see Signs & Symptoms, chap 3). Report promptly.
- Hyperuricemia can be asymptomatic because thiazides interfere with uric acid excretion, although rarely precipitate acute gout. Report onset of joint pain and limitation of motion.
- The prediabetic or diabetes mellitus patient should be watched carefully for loss of control of diabetes or early signs of hyperglycemia (see Signs & Symptoms, chap 3). These symptoms are slow to develop and difficult to recognize. Notify physician, and question need to adjust insulin dosage.

Patient & Family Education

- Hypokalemia is rarely severe with thiazides. However, to prevent onset, urge patient to eat potassium-rich foods such as fruit juices, potatoes, cereals, skim milk, and bananas.
- Counsel patient to avoid OTC drugs unless they are approved by physician. Many preparations contain both potassium and sodium and if misused, or if patient overdoses, could induce electrolyte imbalance side effects.

BENTIROMIDE

(ben-teer´oh-mide)

Trade name: Chymex

Classification: DIAGNOSTIC AGENT

Pregnancy: Category B

Common side effects in *italic*; life-threatening effects underlined; generic names in **bold**; classifications in SMALL CAPS

ACTIONS/PHARMACODYNAMICS Synthetic peptide containing PABA (para-aminobenzoic acid). Each 500 mg of bentiromide contains 170 mg of PABA. Use in evaluating exocrine pancreatic function is based on pancreatic chymotrypsin metabolism of bentiromide in small intestine and its ultimate absorption and elimination as PABA. Percentage of PABA metabolites recovered in urine reflects the enzymatic activity of chymotrypsin and thus provides an indirect measure of pancreatic function. Compared with other pancreatic tests, the bentiromide test is practical and noninvasive. It is reportedly reliable in patients with severe or moderately severe insufficiency but appears to be less sensitive in patients with only slight impairment.

USES Screening test in diagnosis of pancreatic exocrine insufficiency and to monitor adequacy of pancreatic enzyme replacement therapy in patients with insufficiency. To increase test specificity, a modification utilizes a tracer dose of PABA labeled with radioactive carbon (^{14}C) concomitantly with bentiromide.

ROUTE & DOSAGE

Diagnostic Test

Adult	PO	500 mg as single dose
Child	PO	14 mg/kg as single dose

PHARMACOKINETICS Absorption: rapidly hydrolyzed to PABA in small intestine; PABA is readily absorbed from GI tract with first pass metabolism through liver. **Peak:** 2–3 h. **Distribution:** distribution to brain, placenta, and breast milk is not known. **Metabolism:** metabolized in liver. **Elimination:** 40–45% of PABA metabolites are excreted in urine within 6 h.

CONTRAINDICATIONS & PRECAUTIONS Contraindicated in: history of hypersensitivity to bentiromide or PABA or to ingredients in formulation, e.g., propylene glycol. Safe use during pregnancy (category B), in nursing mothers, and in children <6 y not established.

ADVERSE/SIDE EFFECTS Low incidence and usually transient. **CNS:** *headache,* drowsiness, lightheadedness. **GI:** *diarrhea,* flatulence, nausea, vomiting, abdominal pain, heartburn. **Other:** elevations in liver function tests, weakness.

DIAGNOSTIC TEST INTERFERENCES *False-positive bentiromide test results* can occur in patients who are vomiting, or who have malabsorption syndrome, gastric retention, or severe hepatic or renal insufficiency. *False-negative bentiromide test results* can occur with foods containing arylamines, e.g., apples, cranberries, plums, prunes, and drugs that are metabolized to primary arylamines, and subsequently excreted in urine. These foods and drugs should be discontinued 3 d prior to bentiromide administration: **acetaminophen, benzocaine, chloramphenicol, lidocaine, procaine, procainamide,** SULFONAMIDE DIURETICS (e.g., **bumetanide** [Bumex], **furosemide** [Lasix]); THIAZIDE DIURETICS; PABA-CONTAINING DRUGS, e.g., selected MULTIPLE VITAMINS, SUNSCREENS. PANCREATIC ENZYME SUPPLEMENTS, e.g., **pancreatin, pancrelipase** can also cause false-negative bentiromide test results. In adults these enzymes should be discontinued at least 5 d before administration of bentiromide and 1 d before in children with cystic fibrosis.

DRUG INTERACTIONS May increase **methotrexate** levels (increasing its toxicity); PANCREATIC ENZYMES (Pancrease, Cotazyme, etc) can cause false-negative test results; may antagonize antibacterial effects of SULFONAMIDES.

NURSING IMPLICATIONS

Administration
- Bentiromide is taken as a single dose, followed by 250 ml of water.
- To promote diuresis, another 250 ml of water is taken 2 h later, and an additional 500 ml of water during the following 4 h.
- Store bentiromide at 15–30C (59–86F) unless otherwise directed.

Patient & Family Education
- Bentiromide test (for exocrine pancreatic function) demands minute attention to detail for accuracy.
- Careful instructions should be given to patient and responsible family member(s) regarding foods and drugs that should be omitted prior to the test.
- Foods containing *arylamines* (e.g., apples, cranberries, plums, prunes) may interfere with bentiromide test results. These foods should be avoided for at least 3 d before drug is administered.

BENZALKONIUM CHLORIDE
(benz-al-koe´nee-um)

Trade names: Benza, Benzalchlor-50, Germicin, Sabol, Zephiran
Classifications: SKIN & MUCOUS MEMBRANE AGENT; TOPICAL ANTIINFECTIVE; ANTIBIOTIC
Pregnancy: Category C

Common side effects in *italic*; life-threatening effects underlined; generic names in **bold**; classifications in SMALL CAPS

339

B

ACTIONS/PHARMACODYNAMICS Quaternary ammonium cationic surfactant with low surface tension and detergent, keratolytic, wetting, and emulsifying actions. Bactericidal or bacteriostatic action (depending on concentration), probably due to inactivation of bacterial enzyme. Effective against bacteria, some fungi (including yeasts) and certain protozoa, e.g., *Trichomonas vaginalis*. Generally not effective against spore-forming organisms.

USES Antisepsis of intact skin, mucous membranes, superficial injuries, and infected wounds; also for irrigations of the eye and body cavities and for vaginal douching. A component of several contact lens wetting and cushioning solutions, and a preservative for ophthalmic solutions.

ROUTE & DOSAGE

Minor Wounds or Preoperative Disinfection

Adult   Topical   1:750 tincture or spray

Preoperative Disinfection of Denuded Skin and Mucous Membranes

Adult   Topical   1:10,000–1:2000 solution

Wet Dressings

Adult   Topical   1:5000 solution

Urinary Bladder Irrigation

Adult   Topical   1:20,000–1:5000 solution

Urinary Bladder Instillation

Adult   Topical   1:40,000–1:20,000 solution

Irrigation of Deep Infected Wounds

Adult   Topical   1:20,000–1:3000 solution

Vaginal Irrigation

Adult   Topical   1:5000–1:2000 solution

Sterile Storage of Instruments, Thermometers, Ampules

Adult   Topical   1:750 solution

CONTRAINDICATIONS & PRECAUTIONS Contraindicated in: casts, occlusive dressings, anal or vaginal packs. Pregnancy: category C. **Cautious use in:** irrigation of body cavities.

ADVERSE/SIDE EFFECTS Few or no toxic effects in recommended dilutions. Erythema, local burning, hypersensitivity reactions.

NURSING IMPLICATIONS

Administration

- Detergent action is antagonized by pus and other organic matter, and by soap substitutes (e.g., pHisoHex, pHisoderm). If these agents have been used, rinse skin thoroughly with water, dry, and then apply benzalkonium.
- For preoperative skin preparation, follow use of soap with thorough rinsing, first with water, then with 70% alcohol, before applying benzalkonium. Avoid pooling or prolonged contact of solution with skin.
- Use sterile water for injection as diluent for aqueous solutions to be instilled in wounds or body cavities. For other uses, fresh sterile distilled water is used. Tap water (especially hard water) should not be used because it may contain metallic ions and organic matter that reduce antibacterial potency of benzalkonium chloride.
- The tincture and spray preparations contain flammable solvents and should not be used near an open flame or cautery. Keep away from eyes and mucous membranes.
- If solution stronger than 1:5000 enters the eyes, irrigate immediately and repeatedly with water; see a physician promptly.
- Solutions used on denuded skin or inflamed or irritated tissues should be more dilute than those used on normal tissue.
- Store at room temperature in airtight container, protected from light.

Prototype: procaine, p 166

BENZOCAINE

(ben´zoe-caine)

Trade names: Americaine, Americaine Anesthetic Lubricant, Americaine-Otic, Anbesol, Benzocol, Biocozene, Chigger-Tox, Dermoplast, Ethyl Aminobenzoate, Foille, Hurricaine, Orabase with Benzocaine, Oracin, Orajel, Rhulicaine, Semets, Soft 'n Soothe, Solarcaine, T-caine, Unguentine

Classifications: CNS AGENT; LOCAL ANESTHETIC (ESTER TYPE); ANTIPRURITIC

Pregnancy: Category C

ACTIONS/PHARMACODYNAMICS Ethyl ester of PABA. Produces surface anesthesia by inhibiting conduction of nerve impulses from sensory nerve endings. Probable action in certain OTC appetite suppressants is dulling taste for foods. Almost identical to procaine in chemical structure but has lower solubility; therefore it is slowly absorbed and has prolonged duration of anesthetic action.

USES Temporary relief of pain and discomfort in pruritic skin problems, minor burns and sunburn, minor wounds, and insect bites. Otic preparations are used to relieve pain and itching in acute congestive and serous otitis media, swimmer's ear, and otitis externa. Preparations are also available for toothache, minor sore throat pain, canker sores, hemorrhoids, rectal fissures, pruritus ani or vulvae, as male genital desensitizer to slow onset of ejaculation, and for use as anesthetic-lubricant for passage of catheters and endoscopic tubes.

ROUTE & DOSAGE

Anesthetic

Adult	Topical	Lowest effective dose
Child	Topical	Lower strengths

PHARMACOKINETICS Absorption: poorly absorbed through intact skin; readily absorbed from mucous membranes. **Peak:** 1 min. **Duration:** 15–30 min. **Metabolism:** metabolized by plasma cholinesterases and to a lesser extent by hepatic cholinesterases. **Elimination:** metabolites excreted in urine.

CONTRAINDICATIONS & PRECAUTIONS Contraindicated in: hypersensitivity to benzocaine or other PABA derivatives (e.g., sunscreen preparations), or to any of the components in the formulation; use of ear preparation in patients with perforated eardrum or ear discharge; applications to large areas; use in children <2 y. Safe use during pregnancy (category C) not established. **Cautious use in:** history of drug sensitivity; denuded skin or severely traumatized mucosa; children <6 y.

ADVERSE/SIDE EFFECTS Low toxicity. Sensitization in susceptible individuals; allergic reactions, anaphylaxis. Methemoglobinemia reported in infants.

DRUG INTERACTIONS Benzocaine may antagonize antibacterial activity of SULFONAMIDES.

NURSING IMPLICATIONS

Administration

- Avoid contact of all preparations with eyes and be careful not to inhale mist when spray form is used. Do not use spray near open flame or in an area and do not expose to high temperatures. Hold can at least 12 inches (30 cm) away from affected area when spraying.
- Chemical burns should be washed and neutralized before benzocaine is applied.
- Before administration of hemorrhoidal preparation, rectal area should be thoroughly cleaned and dried. Usually administered morning and evening and after each bowel movement.
- Store at 15–30C (59–86F) in tight, light-resistant containers unless otherwise specified.

Patient & Family Education

- Bear in mind that when used on oral mucosa, benzocaine may interfere with second (pharyngeal) stage of swallowing. If possible, liquids and foods should not be taken for about 1 h following administration to prevent possible aspiration and mouth injury (biting tongue or buccal mucosa).
- Use specific benzocaine preparation only for problem for which prescribed or recommended by manufacturer.
- Most local anesthetics are potentially sensitizing to susceptible individuals when applied repeatedly or over extensive areas. Instruct patient to discontinue medication if the condition being treated persists, worsens, or if signs of sensitivity, irritation, or infection occur.

BENZOIN TINCTURE, COMPOUND

(ben´zoin)
Trade names: Aerozoin, Benzoin Spray
Classification: PROTECTANT, TOPICAL

ACTIONS/PHARMACODYNAMICS Mixture of benzoin, aloes, prepared storax, and tolu balsam in 90% alcohol. Reported to have local antiseptic, astringent, and protective properties.

USES To protect skin under occlusive plasters and bandages; also has been used as an antiseptic and astringent in treatment of cracked nipples and skin fissures. A common ingredient in OTC products for treatment of diaper rash and prickly heat.

Common side effects in *italic*; life-threatening effects underlined; generic names in **bold**; classifications in SMALL CAPS

341

B

ROUTE & DOSAGE

Antiseptic

Adult   Topical   Apply 1–2 times/d

CONTRAINDICATIONS & PRECAUTIONS Contraindicated in: acutely inflamed skin.

ADVERSE/SIDE EFFECTS Hypersensitivity reactions, contact dermatitis.

NURSING IMPLICATIONS

Administration

- Skin should be clean and thoroughly dry before benzoin is applied since it forms an occlusive coating and may foster retention of moisture and bacterial growth.
- Care must be taken to allow tincture of benzoin to dry thoroughly following its application to skin because it is tacky when moist and can strip skin if it sticks to bedclothing.
- Tincture of benzoin compound is frequently mixed with other topical medications, such as zinc oxide, or with aluminum and magnesium hydroxides for treatment of bedsores. Consult physician before applying such mixtures.
- For steam inhalation add 1 tsp of tincture of benzoin compound to 480 ml (1 pint) of hot water. (Benzoin spray is not intended for inhalation.) Review procedure carefully with patient to prevent burning.
- Store in a cool place.

Assessment & Drug Effects

- Inspect skin for signs of a hypersensitivity response.
- Decubitus ulcer cannot be prevented by the application of tincture of benzoin or any other topical medication.

BENZONATATE

See ANTITUSSIVE prototype, p 99.

Prototype: isotretinoin, p 253

BENZOYL PEROXIDE

(ben´zoe-ill per-ox´ide)

Trade names: Acne-Aid, Ben-Aqua, Benoxyl, Benzac, Benzagel, Clearasil Lotion, Clear By Design, Cuticura Acne, Del Aqua, Desquam-X, Dry and Clear, Fostex, Loroxide, Oxy-5, Oxy-10, PanOxyl, Persa-Gel, pHisoAc BP, Vanoxide, Xerac BP, Zeroxin

Classifications: SKIN AGENT; ANTIACNE AGENT

Pregnancy: Category C

ACTIONS/PHARMACODYNAMICS Slow release of oxygen exerts bactericidal action on *Propionibacterium (Corynebacterium) acnes* by oxidizing bacterial proteins. These anaerobic rods are found in sebaceous follicles and comedones and are responsible for formation of irritating free fatty acids in sebum. In addition to being an oxidizing agent, it also has antiseborrheic (drying) and keratolytic (peeling) actions that help to keep pilosebaceous orifices open and draining properly. Reportedly not as effective as retinoic acid in comedolytic activity.

USES Adjunctive treatment of mild to moderate acne vulgaris and acne rosacea. **Unlabeled use:** treatment of decubital or stasis ulcers.

ROUTE & DOSAGE

Acne

Adult   Topical   Apply 1–2 times/d; fair-skinned individuals should start with lower strength once/d h.s.

PHARMACOKINETICS Absorption: 50% may be absorbed through skin. **Metabolism:** metabolized to benzoic acid. **Elimination:** excreted in urine.

CONTRAINDICATIONS & PRECAUTIONS Contraindicated in: hypersensitivity to benzoyl peroxide and to benzoic acid derivatives; inflamed, denuded, thin skin. Safe use during pregnancy (category C), in nursing mothers, and in children <12 y not established. **Cautious use in:** highly sensitive skin.

ADVERSE/SIDE EFFECTS Local skin irritation, feeling of warmth, stinging; excessive scaling, erythema, edema (especially with gel preparation), allergic contact dermatitis.

Common side effects in *italic*; life-threatening effects underlined; generic names in **bold**; classifications in SMALL CAPS

NURSING IMPLICATIONS

Administration

- Avoid contact of medication with eyes, eyelids, lips, inside of nose, and sensitive skin areas of neck.
- It is usually advisable to initiate acne therapy with a single application of a small amount of medication until patient's reaction to drug is known.
- Store at 15–30C (59–86F) unless otherwise directed.

Patient & Family Education

- Mild peeling and dryness are anticipated therapeutic actions. If these effects are not observed within 3 or 4 d, application should be increased to twice daily. If peeling or drying is bothersome, dosage should be reduced.
- Medication may cause transitory redness and feeling of warmth or slight smarting. If symptoms are excessive, patient should remove medication with mild soap and water and dry skin well. Application may be attempted cautiously the following day using less medication at reduced frequency. If reaction occurs, check with physician.
- Skin irritation may be further aggravated by harsh soap, vigorous scrubbing of skin, and by other acne medications.
- Benzoyl peroxide may be worn under makeup if desired.
- If improvement does not occur within 2 wk, patient should consult a physician.

Prototype: amphetamine, p 194

BENZPHETAMINE HYDROCHLORIDE

(benz-fet´a-meen)
Trade name: Didrex
Classifications: CNS AGENT; RESPIRATORY AND CEREBRAL STIMULANT; ANOREXIANT
Pregnancy: Category X
Controlled substance: Schedule III

ACTIONS/PHARMACODYNAMICS   Indirect acting sympathomimetic amine with amphetamine-like actions but with fewer side effects than amphetamine. Anorexiant effect thought to be secondary to stimulation of hypothalamus to release stored catecholamines in the CNS.

USES Short-term adjunct in management of exogenous obesity.

ROUTE & DOSAGE

Obesity

Adult	PO	25–50 mg 1–3 times/d

PHARMACOKINETICS **Absorption:** readily absorbed from GI tract. **Duration:** 4 h. **Elimination:** renal elimination.

CONTRAINDICATIONS & PRECAUTIONS Contraindicated in: known hypersensitivity to sympathomimetic amines; angle-closure glaucoma; advanced arteriosclerosis, angina pectoris, severe cardiovascular disease, moderate to severe hypertension; hyperthyroidism, agitated states; history of drug abuse; children <12 y. Safe use during pregnancy (category X) not established. **Cautious use in:** diabetes mellitus; the elderly; psychosis.

ADVERSE/SIDE EFFECTS CNS: euphoria, irritability, hyperactivity, nervousness, *restlessness, insomnia,* tremor, headache, light-headedness, dizziness, depression following stimulant effects. **CV:** *palpitation,* tachycardia, elevated BP, irregular heart beat. **GI:** xerostomia, unpleasant taste, nausea, vomiting, diarrhea or constipation, abdominal cramps. **Other:** urticaria and other allergic skin reactions, sweating, changes in libido. **Chronic intoxication:** marked insomnia, irritability, hyperactivity, personality changes, psychosis, severe dermatoses.

DRUG INTERACTIONS Acetazolamide, sodium bicarbonate decrease amphetamine elimination; **ammonium chloride, ascorbic acid** increase amphetamine elimination; BARBITURATES may antagonize the effects of both drugs; **furazolidone** may increase BP effects of amphetamines, and interaction may persist for several weeks after discontinuation of furazolidone; **guanethidine, guanadryl** antagonize antihypertensive effects; because MAO INHIBITORS, **selegiline** can cause hypertensive crisis (fatalities reported), do not administer amphetamines during or within 14 d of these drugs; PHENOTHIAZINES may inhibit mood-elevating effects of amphetamines; TRICYCLIC ANTIDEPRESSANTS enhance amphetamine effects because they increase norepinephrine release; BETA-AGONISTS increase amphetamines' adverse cardiovascular effects.

NURSING IMPLICATIONS

Administration

- A single daily dose is taken, preferably midmorning or midafternoon, according to patient's eating habits.

Common side effects in *italic*; life-threatening effects <u>underlined</u>; generic names in **bold**; classifications in SMALL CAPS

B

- To avoid insomnia, the daily dose should be scheduled no later than 6 h before patient retires.
- Preserved in tight, light-resistant containers at 15–30C (59–86F) unless otherwise directed.

Assessment & Drug Effects

- Assess for *signs of excessive CNS stimulation:* insomnia, restlessness, tremor, palpitations. These may indicate need for dosage adjustment.
- Monitor vital signs; report elevated BP, tachycardia, and irregular heart rhythm.

Patient & Family Education

- Anorexiant effects are temporary, seldom lasting more than a few weeks; tolerance may occur. Therefore long-term use is not indicated.
- Dosage of antidiabetic drug may require adjustment in diabetic patients because their food intake may change.
- Because dizziness and light-headedness are possible side effects, caution patient against driving a car or performing any other potentially hazardous activities until reaction to drug is determined.
- Abrupt termination of therapy following prolonged high dosages can result in GI distress, stomach cramps, trembling, unusual tiredness, weakness, and mental depression.
- The possibility of psychic dependence should be noted.

> **Prototype: prochlorperazine, p 215**

BENZQUINAMIDE HYDROCHLORIDE

(benz-kwin´a-mide)
Trade name: Emete-Con
Classifications: GI AGENT; ANTIEMETIC
Pregnancy: Category C

ACTIONS/PHARMACODYNAMICS
Antiemetic activity similar to that of phenothiazines and antihistamine antiemetics but chemically unrelated to both. Mechanism of antiemetic action unknown but is believed to be by depression of chemoreceptor trigger zone (CTZ). Also exhibits antihistaminic, antiserotonin, anticholinergic, and sedative properties.

USES
Prevention and treatment of nausea and vomiting associated with anesthesia and surgery. **Unlabeled use:** management of nausea and vomiting secondary to antineoplastic therapy; as an antipsychotic agent; and as a cardiovascular stimulant.

ROUTE & DOSAGE

Antiemetic

Adult	IM	50 mg (0.5–1 mg/kg); may repeat q3–4h if necessary
	IV	25 mg (0.2–0.4 mg/kg) administered slowly at no more than 1 ml/min

PHARMACOKINETICS Absorption: readily absorbed from IM injection site. **Onset:** 15 min. **Peak:** 30 min IM. **Duration:** 3–4 h. **Distribution:** distributed throughout body tissues, with highest concentrations in liver and kidneys; distribution to placenta and breast milk unknown. **Metabolism:** metabolized in liver. **Elimination:** half-life: 40 min; 95% of dose excreted in urine and feces within 72 h.

CONTRAINDICATIONS & PRECAUTIONS Contraindicated in: IV administration to patients with cardiovascular disease, moderate to severe hypertension, or to those who have received preanesthetic or concomitant cardiovascular drugs. Safe use during pregnancy (category C), in nursing women, and in children <12 y not established. **Cautious use in:** elderly and debilitated patients.

ADVERSE/SIDE EFFECTS CNS: *drowsiness,* insomnia, headache, dizziness, excitement, restlessness, nervousness; extrapyramidal symptoms (in large doses). **CV:** (particularly following IV): flushing, sudden increase in BP and respiration; hypotension, dizziness, tachycardia, atrial fibrillation, premature atrial and ventricular contractions. **GI:** dry mouth, salivation, anorexia, nausea, vomiting, abdominal cramps. **Other:** blurred vision, sweating, shivering, chills, hiccups.

INCOMPATIBILITIES Solution/additive: **chlordiazepoxide, diazepam, pentobarbital, phenobarbital, secobarbital, thiopental.**

NURSING IMPLICATIONS

Administration

- For IV administration, reconstitute with 2.2 ml sterile water for injection; for IM administration, reconstitute with bacteriostatic water for injection (with benzyl alcohol or parabens). Do not reconstitute with NaCl because precipitation may result.
- IV benzquinamide may be given direct IV over 30–60 seconds.
- IM injection should be made well into mass of a large muscle. Aspirate carefully to avoid inadvertent intravascular injection.

Common side effects in *italic*; life-threatening effects underlined; generic names in **bold**; classifications in SMALL CAPS

- Deltoid area may be used only if well developed.
- When given for prophylaxis of nausea and vomiting, should be administered IM at least 15 min prior to expected emergence from anesthesia.
- Reconstituted solutions maintain potency for 14 d at room temperature. Do not refrigerate.
- Preserve in light-resistant containers.

Assessment & Drug Effects
- Monitor patient for cardiovascular effects such as hypertension or hypotension and arrhythmias, particularly when drug is administered IV.
- Drowsiness is a common side effect. Be aware of implications for the postoperative patient and particularly the elderly.

Prototype: hydrochlorothiazide, p 203

BENZTHIAZIDE
(bens-thye´a-zide)
Trade names: Aquatag, Exna, Hydrex, Marazide, Proaqua
Classifications: WATER BALANCE AGENT; THIAZIDE DIURETIC; ANTIHYPERTENSIVE
Pregnancy: Category D

ACTIONS/PHARMACODYNAMICS Thiazide diuretic chemically related to sulfonamides. Similar to hydrochlorothiazide. Inhibits renal tubular reabsorption of sodium and chloride, resulting in excretion of sodium and water, accompanied by some loss of bicarbonate and potassium.

USES Edema and adjunctively (step 1) with other agents in stepped care approach for treatment of mild hypertension.

ROUTE & DOSAGE

Edema

Adult	PO	25–200 mg/d or q.o.d.
Child	PO	1–4 mg/kg/d in 3 divided doses

Hypertension

Adult	PO	25–100 mg/d after breakfast, up to 200 mg/d in 2–4 divided doses

PHARMACOKINETICS Absorption: readily absorbed from GI tract. **Onset:** 2 h. **Peak:** 4–6 h. **Duration:** 12–18 h. **Distribution:** crosses placenta; distributed into breast milk. **Elimination:** excreted in urine within 24 h.

CONTRAINDICATIONS & PRECAUTIONS Contraindicated in: hypersensitivity to thiazides or sulfonamides; anuria; pregnancy (category D), lactation. **Cautious use in:** history of renal, hepatic, or pancreatic disease; history of gout; diabetes mellitus; hypercalcemia, hypokalemia.

ADVERSE/SIDE EFFECTS CNS: headache, confusion, unusual fatigue, paresthesia. **CV:** irregular heartbeat, vasculitis, orthostatic hypotension, volume depletion. **GI:** dry mouth, nausea, vomiting, anorexia, constipation, cramps. **Hematologic:** thrombocytopenia, agranulocytosis, hyperglycemia, hypokalemia; hyperuricemia. **Hypersensitivity:** dermatitis, photosensitivity, urticaria. **Other:** jaundice, increased thirst.

DIAGNOSTIC TEST INTERFERENCES *Serum PBI* levels may be decreased. Thiazides should be discontinued before *parathyroid function* tests because they tend to reduce calcium excretion.

DRUG INTERACTIONS Cholestyramine, colestipol decrease absorption of the diuretic; **diazoxide** has additive effects; with **digoxin,** hypokalemia may increase risk of digitalis toxicity; increases **lithium** levels and toxicity; may increase blood glucose levels, necessitating adjustment of dosage of SULFONYLUREAS, **insulin.**

NURSING IMPLICATIONS

Administration
- May be taken with food or milk to minimize gastric irritation unless otherwise directed by physician.
- When benzthiazide is used to promote diuresis, a single daily dose is administered, preferably early in the morning to prevent interrupted sleep because of diuresis.
- Store tablets in tightly closed container at 15–30C (59–86F) unless otherwise directed.

Assessment & Drug Effects
- Antihypertensive dosage regimens are highly individualized. Effects may be noted in 3 or 4 d; maximal effects usually require 3–4 wk.
- The elderly are more sensitive to the average adult dose. Monitor serum potassium levels and observe patient carefully for signs of hypokalemia (see Signs & Symptoms, chap 3).
- Baseline and periodic determinations should be

Common side effects in *italic*; life-threatening effects underlined; generic names in **bold**; classifications in SMALL CAPS

345

made of blood counts, serum electrolytes, uric acid, blood sugar, NPN, BUN, and serum creatinine.

- Monitor I&O ratio and pattern.
- The prediabetic or diabetes mellitus patient should be watched for loss of control of diabetes or early signs of hyperglycemia (see chap 3). These signs are slow to develop and difficult to recognize. Notify physician of their appearance, since an adjustment of insulin dosage may be needed.

Patient & Family Education

- To prevent onset of hypokalemia (rarely severe in most patients even on long-term therapy with thiazides), urge patient to eat potassium-rich foods such as fruit juices and bananas.
- Instruct patient to weigh daily and report sudden weight gain.
- To prevent dehydration, caution patient to notify doctor if severe nausea, vomiting, or diarrhea occurs.
- Counsel patient to avoid use of OTC drugs unless approved by the physician. Many preparations contain potassium and sodium.
- Warn patient about the possibility of photosensitivity reaction (like an exaggerated sunburn). Notify physician if it occurs. Thiazide-related photosensitivity is considered a photoallergy. It occurs 1 1/2–2 wk after initial sun exposure.

Prototype: levodopa, p 114

BENZTROPINE MESYLATE
(benz´troe-peen)

Trade names: Apo-Benzotropine, Bensylate, Cogentin, PMS Benzotropine
Classifications: AUTONOMIC NERVOUS SYSTEM AGENT; ANTICHOLINERGIC (PARASYMPATHOLYTIC); ANTIPARKINSONISM AGENT
Pregnancy: Category C

ACTIONS/PHARMACODYNAMICS Synthetic centrally acting anticholinergic (antimuscarinic) agent, chemically similar to atropine and diphenhydramine. Also exhibits antihistaminic and local anesthetic activity. Acts by diminishing excess cholinergic effect associated with dopamine deficiency. (Normal motor activity relies upon a balance between cholinergic and dopaminergic activity in corpus striatum.) Suppresses tremor and rigidity; does not alleviate tardive dyskinesia.

USES Symptomatic treatment of all forms of parkinsonism (arteriosclerotic, idiopathic, postencephalitic) and to relieve extrapyramidal symptoms associated with neuroleptic drugs, e.g., haloperidol (Haldol), phenothiazines, thiothixene (Navane). Commonly used as supplement with trihexyphenidyl, carbidopa, or levodopa therapy.

ROUTE & DOSAGE

Parkinsonism

Adult	PO	0.5–1 mg/d; gradually increased as needed up to 6 mg/d

Extrapyramidal Reactions

Adult	PO	1–2 mg b.i.d.
	IM/IV	1–2 mg as needed

PHARMACOKINETICS Onset: 15 min IM/IV; 1 h PO. **Duration:** 6–10 h.

CONTRAINDICATIONS & PRECAUTIONS Contraindicated in: narrow angle glaucoma; myasthenia gravis; obstructive diseases of GU and GI tracts; tendency to tachycardia; tardive dyskinesia, children <3 y. Safe use during pregnancy (category C) and in nursing women not established. **Cautious use in:** older children, elderly or debilitated patients, patients with poor mental outlook, mental disorders; enlarged prostate; hypertension; history of renal or hepatic disease.

ADVERSE/SIDE EFFECTS CNS: *sedation,* drowsiness, dizziness, paresthesias; agitation, irritability, restlessness, nervousness, insomnia, hallucinations, delirium, mental confusion, toxic psychosis, muscular weakness, ataxia, inability to move certain muscle groups. **CV:** palpitation, tachycardia, flushing. **Eye:** blurred vision, mydriasis, photophobia. **GI:** nausea, vomiting, *constipation, dry mouth,* distension, paralytic ileus. **GU:** dysuria. **Other:** anhidrosis, muscle cramps, skin rash.

DRUG INTERACTIONS Alcohol, CNS DEPRESSANTS have additive sedation and depressant effects; **amantidine,** TRICYCLIC ANTIDEPRESSANTS, MAO INHIBITORS, PHENOTHIAZINES, **procainamide, quinidine** have additive anticholinergic effects and cause confusion, hallucinations, paralytic ileus.

NURSING IMPLICATIONS

Administration

- Administration of oral drug immediately after meals

or with food may help to prevent gastric irritation. Tablet can be crushed prior to administration and sprinkled on or mixed with food.

- Patients with arteriosclerotic or idiopathic parkinsonism generally experience greatest relief by taking benztropine at bedtime.
- IV benztropine mesylate may be given undiluted by direct IV at a rate of 1 mg or a fraction thereof over 1 min.
- Drug therapy should be initiated and withdrawn gradually. Effects of benztropine are cumulative.
- Preserve in tightly covered, light-resistant container at 15–30C (59–86F) unless otherwise directed.

Assessment & Drug Effects

- Clinical improvement may not be evident until 2 or 3 d after oral drug is started.
- The elderly and patients with mental illness should be closely observed for intensification of mental symptoms, particularly during early therapy or whenever dosage increases are made.
- Acute extrapyramidal symptoms associated with initiation of antipsychotic therapy are generally transient. Report even minor symptoms to physician. Most adverse/side effects respond to dosage reduction or temporary withdrawal of drug.
- Monitor I&O ratio and pattern. Advise patient to report difficulty in urination or infrequent voiding. Dosage reduction may be indicated.
- Appearance of intermittent constipation, abdominal pain, diminution of bowel sounds on auscultation, and distension may herald onset of paralytic ileus. Patients receiving combination drugs with anticholinergic action should be closely monitored for these symptoms.
- Muscle weakness or inability to move certain muscle groups are adverse side effects and require dosage reduction.
- Most of the atropinelike side effects of benztropine are controlled by adjustment of dosage. However, severe reactions, such as signs and symptoms of CNS depression or stimulation (see chap 3), usually require interruption of drug therapy.

Patient & Family Education

- Caution patient about possibility of drowsiness and blurred vision and advise against operating vehicles or machinery or other activities requiring alertness until reaction to the drug is known. Supervision of ambulation and side rails may be indicated.
- Alcohol and other CNS depressants may cause additive drowsiness and therefore should be avoided.

Also advise patient not to take OTC cold, cough, or hay fever remedies unless approved by physician.

- Mouth dryness may be relieved by frequent rinsing of mouth with tepid water or by sugarless gum or hard candy.
- Anhidrosis (diminished sweating), especially in hot weather, may require dose adjustments because of possibility of heat stroke. This condition is most apt to occur in the elderly patient. Caution patient to avoid doing manual labor or strenuous exercise in a hot environment.

BETA CAROTENE
(bay-ta kare´oh-teen)
Trade name: Solatene
Classification: VITAMIN A PRECURSOR
Pregnancy: Category C

ACTIONS/PHARMACODYNAMICS Fat-soluble precursor of vitamin A found in green and yellow vegetables. Provides photoprotection by unclear mechanism, but it may be a quelling effect on free radicals and singlet excited oxygen (antioxidant activity), through which photosensitizers appear to act. Bioavailability is dependent on bile in intestinal tract for its absorption, fat as a carrier, and adequate protein intake. In relation to vitamin activity, 6 μg dietary beta carotene is considered to be equivalent to 1 μg vitamin A (retinol).

USES To protect against and to reduce severity of photosensitivity reactions in patients with erythropoietic protoporphyria.

ROUTE & DOSAGE

Photosensitivity Reactions

Adult	PO	30–300 mg/d
Child	PO	<14 y: 30–150 mg/d

PHARMACOKINETICS Absorption: readily absorbed from GI tract as vitamin A. **Distribution:** widely distributed, especially to skin and fat tissue; small amounts of vitamin A are stored in liver. **Metabolism:** metabolized in small intestine to vitamin A in presence of fat and bile acids; further metabolized to retinol in body. **Elimination:** metabolites are excreted in urine and feces.

Common side effects in *italic*; life-threatening effects underlined; generic names in **bold**; classifications in SMALL CAPS

347

CONTRAINDICATIONS & PRECAUTIONS Contraindicated in: pregnancy (category C); chronic diarrhea, steatorrhea. **Cautious use in:** impaired renal and hepatic function, nursing mothers.

ADVERSE/SIDE EFFECTS Diarrhea (sporadic); arthralgia; hypercarotenemia, carotenodermia (yellow or orange skin pigmentation).

NURSING IMPLICATIONS

Administration

- Administer preferably with meals.
- Capsules may be opened and contents mixed with fruit juice to aid in administration. Dry contents (powder) should not be swallowed dry but always swallowed with food or liquid.
- Store in tightly-covered, light-resistant container.

Assessment & Drug Effects

- Photoprotection, i.e., therapeutic effect of this drug, requires from 2–6 wk to develop and is correlated with development of carotenodermia (yellowness of skin due to carotenemia).
- Carotenodermia is differentiated from jaundice by the absence of yellow sclera and pruritus.

Patient & Family Education

- When palms, soles, and possibly face skin are yellowish, gradual exposure to sun or artificial (xenon arc) lights may begin.
- Drug-induced photoprotection is not complete nor is it a "sunscreen."
- Reportedly, about 86% of patients treated with this drug quadrupled the time they can be out in the sun; 8% have doubled acceptable exposure time.
- Intolerance to light returns in 1–2 wk after drug is discontinued.
- Warn patient against self-dosing with supplemental vitamin A because the usual dose of beta carotene provides the normal daily requirement.
- Yellow (especially carrots and yellow corn) and green vegetables contain beta carotene. Warn patient not to substitute these vegetables for the prescribed medication.

Prototype: hydrocortisone, p 255

BETAMETHASONE
(bay-ta-meth´a-sone)
Trade names: Betaderm Scalp Lotion, Betnelan, Celestone

BETAMETHASONE ACETATE AND BETAMETHASONE SODIUM PHOSPHATE
Trade name: Celestone Soluspan

BETAMETHASONE BENZOATE
Trade names: Beben, Benisone, Uticort

BETAMETHASONE DIPROPRIONATE
Trade names: Alphatrex, Diprogen, Diprolene, Diprosalic, Diprosone

BETAMETHASONE SODIUM PHOSPHATE (pH 8.5)
Trade names: Betameth, Betnesol, Celestone Phosphate, Celestone S, Cel-U-Jec, Selestoject

BETAMETHASONE VALERATE
Trade names: Betacort, Betaderm, Betatrex, Beta-Val, Betnovate, Celestodeem, Ectosone Lotion, Ectosone Scalp Lotion, Metaderm, Novobetamet, Valisone, Valisone Scalp Lotion, Valnac
Classifications: HORMONE; ADRENAL CORTICO-STEROID; GLUCOCORTICOID; ANTIINFLAMMATORY
Pregnancy: Category C

ACTIONS/PHARMACODYNAMICS Synthetic, long-acting glucocorticoid with minor mineralocorticoid properties but strong immunosuppressive, antiinflammatory, and metabolic actions. For contraindications & precautions and adverse/side effects, see hydrocortisone.

USES Topical use provides relief of inflammatory manifestations of corticosteroid-responsive dermatoses. With exception of use as replacement therapy in adrenocortical insufficiency and salt-losing forms of adrenogenital syndromes, betamethasone has the same indications for use, limitations, and adverse/side effects as hydrocortisone. **Unlabeled use:** prevention of neonatal respiratory distress syndrome (hyaline membrane disease).

ROUTE & DOSAGE

Antiinflammatory Agent

Adult	PO	0.6–7.2 mg/d
	IM/IV	0.5–9 mg/d as sodium phosphate
	Topical	Thin film applied to affected area 1–3 times/d

Respiratory Distress Syndrome

Adult	IM/IV	2 ml of sodium phosphate IM to mother once daily 2–3 d before delivery

PHARMACOKINETICS Unknown.

DRUG INTERACTIONS Barbiturates, phenytoin, rifampin may reduce pharmacologic effect of betamethasone by increasing its metabolism.

NURSING IMPLICATIONS

Administration

- Administer oral betamethasone with food or milk to lessen stomach irritation.
- IV betamethasone sodium phosphate may be given by direct IV undiluted at a rate of 1 dose/min. Medication may be further diluted in dextrose or saline solution and infused at a prescribed rate.
- Celestone Soluspan is used for intraarticular, IM, and intralesional injection. The preparation is not intended for IV use. Do not mix with diluents containing preservatives, e.g., parabens, phenol. If prescribed, 1% or 2% lidocaine hydrochloride may be used. (Withdraw betamethasone mixture first, then lidocaine; shake syringe briefly.)
- Consult physician regarding cleansing skin before treatments with topical drug. Some clinicians recommend washing before each application; others prefer that area not be disturbed.
- Absorption following use of aerosol preparation (Valisone) equals that of oral and parenteral administration. Avoid inhaling drug; do not spray mucous membranes or external ear canal. Protect eyes.
- The topically treated skin area should not be covered unless prescribed by physician.
- Betamethasone valerate ointment 0.1% has been used for painful nonviral ulcerations of the mouth. It is applied to the affected area 4 times daily, and

patient is instructed not to eat or drink for 30 min after application.

Assessment & Drug Effects

- Response following intraarticular, intralesional, or intrasynovial administration occurs within a few hours and persists for 1–4 wk. Following IM administration response occurs in 2–3 h and persists for 3–7 d.
- Carefully and routinely note condition of skin to which topical betamethasone has been applied. Report evidence of irritation, dryness, hypopigmentation, skin atrophy, limited response, or intercurrent infection.

Patient & Family Education

- Betamethasone appears to cause weight gain. Advise patient to monitor weight at least weekly.
- Steroids should be discontinued slowly after systemic use of ≥1 wk. Abrupt withdrawal, especially following high doses or prolonged use, can cause dizziness, nausea, vomiting, fever, muscle and joint pain, weakness.
- Advise patient to avoid exposure of topically treated areas to sunlight. Severe burns have been reported.

Prototype: propranolol, p 109

BETAXOLOL HYDROCHLORIDE
(be-tax´oh-lol)

Trade names: Betoptic, Betoptic-S
Classifications: EYE PREPARATION; MIOTIC (ANTIGLAUCOMA AGENT); AUTONOMIC NERVOUS SYSTEM AGENT; BETA-ADRENERGIC BLOCKER
Pregnancy: Category C

ACTIONS/PHARMACODYNAMICS $Beta_1$-adrenergic blocking agent (cardioselective). Following topical application to the eye, it reduces both normal and abnormal intraocular pressure (IOP) in patients with and without glaucoma. Action unclear, but reduction of IOP appears to be due to decrease in aqueous production. Betaxolol does not affect visual acuity or tear secretion and has minimal anesthetic effect. Has little or no effect on pupil size; therefore it is usually given in conjunction with a topical miotic (e.g., pilocarpine) to patient with angle-closure glaucoma. Has a low potential for systemic cardiovascu-

Common side effects in *italic*; life-threatening effects underlined; generic names in **bold**; classifications in SMALL CAPS

349

lar and pulmonary effects. The IOP-lowering effect is well maintained for at least 4 y on a continuous medication regimen, but tolerance to this action has been reported.

USES Intraocular hypertension and chronic open angle glaucoma. May be used as a single agent or in combination with other antiglaucoma drugs.

ROUTE & DOSAGE

Glaucoma

Adult	Topical	(ophthalmic) 1 drop of 0.5% solution or 0.25% suspension in affected eye twice daily; may try to reduce or eliminate other drugs at a rate of 1 drug per week after one full day of betaxolol therapy

PHARMACOKINETICS Absorption: some systemic absorption from topical administration. **Onset:** 0.5–1 h. **Peak:** 2 h. **Duration:** ≥12 h. **Distribution:** unknown after systemic absorption. **Metabolism:** metabolized in liver to at least 5 metabolites. **Elimination:** believed to be renally eliminated.

CONTRAINDICATIONS & PRECAUTIONS Contraindicated in: sinus bradycardia, AV block greater than first degree, cardiogenic shock, glaucoma, angle closure (unless with a miotic). Safe use during pregnancy (category C) and in children <18 y has not been established. **Cautious use in:** concomitant use of a systemic beta-adrenergic blocking agent; history of heart failure; diabetes mellitus; in patient with evidence of airflow obstruction or reactive airway disease; lactation.

ADVERSE/SIDE EFFECTS Topical (eye): *mild ocular stinging* and discomfort; *tearing.* **Systemic** (infrequent): slight decrease in mean systolic and diastolic BP, increased airway resistance, bradycardia, hypotension, heart failure, clinical depression.

DRUG INTERACTIONS Reserpine and other CATECHOLAMINE-DEPLETING AGENTS may cause additive hypotensive effects or bradycardia when betaxolol absorbed systemically.

NURSING IMPLICATIONS

Administration

- Avoid touching eye surface with dropper. Drop medication into conjunctival sac of affected eye.

- Store at 15–30C (59–86F) unless manufacturer recommends otherwise. Avoid freezing; keep Drop-Tainer bottle tightly closed.

Assessment & Drug Effects

- At initiation of therapy with betaxolol, IOP should be measured at different times during the day to be assured that adequate hypotensive effect is being maintained.
- IOP may not stabilize for a few weeks in some patients.

Patient & Family Education

- If other eye medications are being prescribed, determine if patient completely understands when to administer all drugs with respect to sequence.
- Be sure that patient understands how to administer medication safely.
- If dose is missed, patient should apply it as soon as possible unless it is near time (within 2 h) of next dose, in which case, patient should apply next dose at scheduled time.
- Special instructions for *patient with diabetes mellitus:* symptoms of acute hypoglycemia (tachycardia, tremor, but not sweating) may be masked by betaxolol; therefore, accuracy in blood glucose determinations by the diabetic is especially important.
- Special instructions for *patient with hyperthyroidism:* abrupt withdrawal of betaxolol may precipitate thyroid storm.
- Although systemic effects are rare, inform patient of symptoms and signs that should be reported promptly: edema of ankles, dyspnea, bradycardia, wheezing, clinical depression (lethargy, insomnia, anorexia, bouts of crying).
- Urge patient to keep in contact with physician for scheduled assessment of IOP response to medication.

BETHANECHOL CHLORIDE

See AUTONOMIC NERVOUS SYSTEM AGENTS, DIRECT-ACTING CHOLINERGIC prototype, p 120.

Prototype: levodopa, p 114

BIPERIDEN HYDROCHLORIDE
(bye-per'i-den)

Trade name: Akineton Hydrochloride

BIPERIDEN LACTATE

Trade name: Akineton Lactate

Classifications: AUTONOMIC NERVOUS SYSTEM
AGENT; ANTICHOLINERGIC (PARASYMPATHOLYTIC);
ANTIPARKINSONISM AGENT

Pregnancy: Category C

ACTIONS/PHARMACODYNAMICS Synthetic tertiary amine, antimuscarinic. In common with other antiparkinsonism drugs has atropinelike (anticholinergic) actions. Antiparkinsonism activity is thought to be by reducing central excitatory action of acetylcholine on cholinergic receptors in the extrapyramidal system. This action helps to establish some balance between cholinergic (excitatory) and dopaminergic (inhibitory) activity in the basal ganglia. Also has weak peripheral atropinelike blocking action on muscarinic receptors.

USES Adjunct in all forms of parkinsonism, particularly postencephalitic and idiopathic parkinsonism (appears to be less effective in arteriosclerotic type). Also used to control drug-induced parkinsonism (extrapyramidal symptoms) associated with reserpine and phenothiazine therapy.

ROUTE & DOSAGE

Parkinsonism

Adult	PO	2 mg 1–4 times/d
	IM/IV	2 mg injected slowly; may repeat q30min up to 8 mg/24h
Child	IM/IV	0.04 mg/kg or 1.2 mg/m²; may repeat q30min up to 8 mg/24h

PHARMACOKINETICS Unknown.

CONTRAINDICATIONS & PRECAUTIONS Contraindicated in: narrow-angle glaucoma; GI or GU obstruction, megacolon; tardive dyskinesia. Safe use during pregnancy (category C), in nursing women, and in children not established. **Cautious use in:** elderly or debilitated patients; prostatic hypertrophy; glaucoma; cardiac arrhythmias; epilepsy.

ADVERSE/SIDE EFFECTS (Dose-related): **CNS:** drowsiness, dizziness, muscle weakness, lack of coordination, disorientation, euphoria, agitation, confusion. **CV:** mild, transient postural hypotension (following IM), tachycardia. **Eye:** *blurred vision,* photophobia. **GI:** *dry mouth,* nausea, vomiting, constipation.

DRUG INTERACTIONS Alcohol and other CNS DEPRESSANTS increase sedation; **haloperidol,** PHENOTHIAZINES, OPIATES, TRICYCLIC ANTIDEPRESSANTS, **quinidine** increase risk of anticholinergic side effects.

NURSING IMPLICATIONS

Administration

- GI disturbances may be relieved by administering PO doses with or after meals.
- IV biperiden lactate may be given by direct IV undiluted at a rate of 2 mg or a fraction thereof over 1 min.
- Patient should be recumbent when receiving parenteral biperiden. Postural hypotension, disturbances of coordination, and temporary euphoria can occur following IV administration.
- Preserve in tightly closed, light-resistant containers at 15–30C (59–86F) unless otherwise directed.

Assessment & Drug Effects

- Monitor BP and pulse after IV administration. Advise patient to make position changes slowly and in stages, particularly from recumbent to upright position.
- It is reported that certain susceptible patients may manifest mental confusion, drowsiness, dizziness, agitation, hematuria, and decrease in urinary flow. Report these symptoms immediately.
- Slight dryness of mouth and blurred vision are common dose-related side effects and may be relieved or eliminated by dosage reduction.
- Monitor I&O ratio and pattern. If constipation is a problem, increase in dietary fiber and fluid intake may help.
- Biperiden usually reduces sweating, drooling, excessive oiliness of skin, and muscle rigidity. In patients with severe parkinsonism, tremors may increase as spasticity is relieved.

Patient & Family Education

- Caution patient to avoid driving and other poten-

Common side effects in *italic*; life-threatening effects underlined; generic names in **bold**; classifications in SMALL CAPS

351

tially hazardous activities until reaction to drug is determined.

- Patients on prolonged therapy can develop tolerance; an increase in dosage may be required.

BISACODYL

See GASTROINTESTINAL AGENT, STIMULANT LAXATIVE prototype, p 221.

Prototype: diphenoxylate with atropine, p 213

BISMUTH SUBSALICYLATE

Trade name: Pepto-Bismol
Classifications: GI AGENT; ANTIDIARRHEAL; SALICYLATE

ACTIONS/PHARMACODYNAMICS Hydrolyzed in GI tract to salicylate, which is believed to inhibit synthesis of prostaglandins responsible for GI hypermotility and inflammation. Effectiveness as an antidiarrheal also appears to be due to direct antimicrobial action and to an antisecretory effect on intestinal secretions exposed to toxins particularly of *Escherichia coli* and *Vibrio cholerae*. It is thought to relieve indigestion by forming insoluble complexes with gastric compounds, thus terminating their noxious effects, and by its protective coating action.

USES Prophylaxis and treatment of traveler's diarrhea (turista) and for temporary relief of indigestion. **Unlabeled use:** *Helicobacter pylori* associated with peptic ulcer disease.

ROUTE & DOSAGE

Diarrhea

Adult	PO	30 ml or 2 tab q30–60min prn up to 8 doses/d
Child	PO	10–12 y: 15 ml or 1 tab q30–60min prn up to 8 doses/d
		3–6 y: 5 ml or 1/2 tab q30–60min prn up to 8 doses/d

Traveler's Diarrhea

Adult	PO	2–4 tab or 15–30 ml q.i.d. for 3 wk

PHARMACOKINETICS Absorption: undergoes chemical dissociation in GI tract to bismuth subcarbonate and sodium salicylate; bismuth is minimally absorbed, but the salicylate is readily absorbed.

CONTRAINDICATIONS & PRECAUTIONS Contraindicated in: hypersensitivity to aspirin or other salicylates; use for more than 2 d in presence of high fever or in children <3 y unless prescribed by physician. **Cautious use in:** patient taking salicylates.

ADVERSE/SIDE EFFECTS Temporary *darkening of stool* and tongue. With high doses: fecal impaction, bismuth toxicity: encephalopathy (disorientation, muscle twitching), incontinence, metallic taste, bluish gum line; salicylism: tinnitus, hearing loss, bleeding tendencies.

DIAGNOSTIC TEST INTERFERENCES Because bismuth subsalicylate is radiopaque, it may interfere with radiographic studies of GI tract.

DRUG INTERACTIONS Bismuth may decrease the absorption of TETRACYCLINES, QUINOLONES (**ciprofloxacin, norfloxacin, ofloxacin**).

NURSING IMPLICATIONS

Patient & Family Education

- Chew chewable tablet or allow it to dissolve in mouth.
- Drug contains salicylate and therefore must be used with caution with aspirin and other salicylates. (Many OTC medications for colds, fever, and pain contain salicylates.)
- Consult physician if diarrhea is accompanied by fever or continues for more than 2 d.
- Prophylactic use should be limited to 3 wk or less. (Normal bismuth level should be less than 5 μg/L.)
- Temporary grayish black discoloration of tongue and stool may occur. (Note that this side effect may mask GI bleeding.)
- Store at room temperature and protect drug from light unless otherwise directed.

Prototype, isoproterenol, p 105

BITOLTEROL MESYLATE

(bye-tole´ter-ole)
Trade name: Tornalate
Classifications: AUTONOMIC NERVOUS SYSTEM AGENT; BETA-ADRENERGIC AGONIST (SYMPATHOMIMETIC); BRONCHODILATOR
Pregnancy: Category C

ACTIONS/PHARMACODYNAMICS Selective beta-adrenergic agonist. Hydrolyzed by an esterase

Common side effects in *italic*; life-threatening effects underlined; generic names in **bold**; classifications in SMALL CAPS

formed in greatest concentrations in lung tissues to an active catecholamine. Produces prolonged bronchodilation as a beta-adrenergic agent. Stimulates adenyl cyclase enzyme that catalyzes conversion of ATP to cAMP. The resulting increase in cAMP levels causes relaxation of bronchial smooth muscle and inhibits the release of mediators of immediate hypersensitivity (e.g., histamine) from lung tissue cells. Decreases airway resistance and increases vital capacity; bronchodilation is greater and longer in duration than that produced by isoproterenol. Cardiovascular effects appear to be similar to or less than those produced by isoproterenol. May cause CNS stimulation and other adverse nervous system effects. Tolerance to bronchodilatory effect has not been reported.

USES Prophylaxis and treatment of bronchial asthma and reversible bronchospasm in monotherapy, or concomitantly with theophylline or corticosteroids or both.

ROUTE & DOSAGE

Bronchospasm

Adult	Inhalation	2 inhalations spaced 1–3 min apart q6–8h; max of 12 inhalations/d

PHARMACOKINETICS Absorption: absorption from lungs not fully described. **Onset:** 3–5 min. **Peak:** 0.5–2 h. **Duration:** up to 8 h. **Distribution:** not known if crosses placenta or is distributed into breast milk. **Elimination:** half-life: 3 h.

CONTRAINDICATIONS & PRECAUTIONS Contraindicated in: safe use during pregnancy (category C), in nursing mothers, or in children <12 y not established. **Cautious use in:** cardiovascular disease, hypertension, hyperthyroidism, diabetes mellitus, convulsive disorders, unusual sensitivity to catecholamines; elderly patients, psychoneurosis; patient with longstanding bronchial asthma, and emphysema with degenerative heart disease.

ADVERSE/SIDE EFFECTS CNS (mild, transient): *tremors,* nervousness, headache, dizziness, lightheadedness, insomnia; hyperkinesia. **CV:** palpitations, chest discomfort; tachycardia, flushing, PVCs. **Respiratory:** *throat irritation,* cough, paradoxical bronchoconstriction, dyspnea, chest tightness. **Other:** nausea, dyspepsia; increased ALT concentration.

DRUG INTERACTIONS Effects of BETA-ADRENERGIC BLOCKERS (e.g., **propranolol**) and bitolterol may be antagonized.

NURSING IMPLICATIONS

Administration

- Patient should be given a copy of patient instructions for administration of drug by aerosol metered dose inhaler. Supervise patient a few times to be certain drug delivery is accomplished.
- Manufacturer recommends that the bottle containing the drug be removed from the inhaler and that the plastic mouthpiece be cleansed in warm tap water and thoroughly dried once daily.
- Avoid contacting eyes with bitolterol. If it should happen, flush out with copious amounts of water.
- If an adrenocorticoid inhalation is also being used, the two drugs should be administered 15 min apart unless otherwise directed by physician. This is to diminish the risk of fluorocarbon (propellant) toxicity.
- Store at 15–30C (59–86F); protect from freezing.

Assessment & Drug Effects

- Tremors, a common adverse effect and one due to skeletal muscle stimulation, tends to diminish with continued use of bitolterol. Some find the effect intolerable.
- Immediate hypersensitivity reactions (see Signs & Symptoms, chap 3) can occur with this drug. Epinephrine 1:1000 should be readily available until reaction to drug is known.
- Overdosage leads to exaggerated drug effects listed in Adverse/Side Effects.

Patient & Family Education

- Caution patient not to change dose or dose intervals, i.e., not to omit, increase, or decrease number of inhalations. Patient should notify physician immediately if condition worsens or if patient fails to respond to the usual dose.
- Warn patient not to use any other inhaler medication (OTC or left-over medication) unless the physician approves.
- Contents of the inhaler are under pressure; therefore, caution patient not to puncture the canister, use or store it near heat or an open flame, and not to place it in a fire or incinerator for disposal.

BLEOMYCIN SULFATE

(blee-oh-mye´sin)
Trade name: Blenoxane
Classifications: ANTINEOPLASTIC; ANTIBIOTIC
Pregnancy: Category D

Common side effects in *italic*; life-threatening effects underlined; generic names in **bold**; classifications in SMALL CAPS

353

ACTIONS/PHARMACODYNAMICS Mixture of cytotoxic glycopeptide antibiotics from a strain of *Streptomyces verticillus*. A toxic drug with low therapeutic index; intensely cytotoxic. By unclear mechanism, blocks DNA, RNA, and protein synthesis. A cell cycle–phase nonspecific. Weak antibiotic activity is overshadowed by potent cytotoxic effects. Has strong affinity for skin and lung tumor cells, in contrast to its low affinity for cells in hematopoietic tissue (perhaps due to the high levels of bleomycin-degrading enzymes found in bone marrow). Widely used in combination with other chemotherapeutic agents because it lacks significant myelosuppressive activity.

USES As single agent or in combination with other chemotherapeutic agents, as adjunct to surgery and radiation therapy. Squamous cell carcinomas of head, neck, penis, cervix, and vulva; also lymphomas (including reticular cell sarcoma, lymphosarcoma, Hodgkin's), and testicular carcinoma. **Unlabeled use:** intrapleural administration to prevent pleural fluid accumulation; mycosis fungoides and *Verucca vulgaris* (common warts).

ROUTE & DOSAGE

Squamous Cell Carcinoma, Testicular Carcinoma

Adult	SC, IM, IV	10–20 U/m² or 0.25–0.5 U/kg 1–2 times/wk up to a total dose of 300–400 U

Lymphomas

Adult	SC, IM, IV	10–20 U/m² 1–2 times/wk after a 1–2 U test dose x 2 doses

Hodgkin's Disease, Maintenance

Adult	SC, IM, IV	1 U IM or IV/d or 5 U/wk

PHARMACOKINETICS Distribution: concentrates mainly in skin, lungs, kidneys, lymphocytes, and peritoneum. **Metabolism:** unknown. **Elimination:** half-life: 2 h; 60–70% recovered in urine as parent compound.

CONTRAINDICATIONS & PRECAUTIONS Contraindicated in: history of hypersensitivity or idiosyncrasy to bleomycin, pregnancy (category D), women of childbearing age. **Cautious use in:** compromised hepatic, renal, or pulmonary function; previous cytotoxic drug or radiation therapy.

ADVERSE/SIDE EFFECTS CNS: headache, mental confusion. **GI:** stomatitis, ulcerations of tongue and lips, anorexia, nausea, vomiting, diarrhea, weight loss. **Hematologic (rare):** thrombocytopenia, leukopenia, mild anemia. **Respiratory:** <u>pulmonary toxicity</u> (dose- and age-related): interstitial pneumonitis, pneumonia, or fibrosis. **Skin:** diffuse alopecia (reversible), *hyperpigmentation*, *pruritic erythema*, vesiculation, acne, thickening of skin and nail beds, *patchy hyperkeratosis*, striae, peeling, bleeding. **Other:** *mild febrile reaction*, <u>anaphylactoid reaction</u>, pain at tumor site, phlebitis; renal, hepatic, and CNS toxicity; necrosis at injection site.

DRUG INTERACTIONS Other ANTINEOPLASTIC AGENTS increase bone marrow toxicity; decreases effects of **digoxin, phenytoin.**

INCOMPATIBILITIES Solution/additive: aminophylline, ascorbic acid, carbenicillin, CEPHALOSPORINS, **diazepam, hydrocortisone, methotrexate, mitomycin, nafcillin, penicillin G, terbutaline.**

NURSING IMPLICATIONS

Administration

- Used only under constant supervision by medical personnel experienced in cancer chemotherapy.
- For IV administration, dilute each 15 U with at least 5 ml of sterile water for injection, D5W, or NaCl for injection. May be further diluted in 50–100 ml of chosen diluent.
- Administer properly diluted IV solution at a rate of 15 U/10 min through Y-tube of free-flowing IV.
- Inject IM bleomycin deeply into upper outer quadrant of buttock; change sites with each injection.
- Although this drug causes nausea and vomiting, it is important that the established administration schedule for injections be maintained. Antiemetic drugs may be prescribed.
- Aspirin and diphenhydramine may be prescribed as premedication to reduce onset of drug fever and risk of anaphylaxis; however, these drugs are ineffective as treatment for drug-induced hyperpyrexia.
- Reconstituted solutions are stable at room temperature for 2 wk or for 4 wk if refrigerated. Discard unused solutions.
- Store unopened ampuls at 15–30C (59–86F) unless otherwise specified by manufacturer.

Assessment & Drug Effects

- Anaphylactoid reaction (see Signs & Symptoms, chap 3) can be fatal. It may occur immediately or

Common side effects in *italic*; life-threatening effects <u>underlined</u>; generic names in **bold**; classifications in SMALL CAPS

several hours after first or second dose, especially in lymphoma patients (10%). Usually a test dose of 2 U or less of bleomycin is given to these patients for the first 2 doses. Patient is closely monitored (vital signs, auscultation of chest, careful observations) for at least 24 h. If there is no acute reaction (hypotension, hyperpyrexia, chills, confusion, wheezing, cardiopulmonary collapse), regular dosage schedule is resumed.

- Favorable response, if any is to occur, is expected within 2 wk for treatment of Hodgkin's or testicular tumor, and within 3 wk for squamous cell cancers.
- Monitor vital signs. Febrile reaction (mild chills and fever) is relatively common in patients receiving bleomycin therapy. It usually occurs within the first few hours after administration of a large single dose and lasts about 4–12 h. Reaction tends to become less frequent with continued drug administration but can recur at any time.
- Although bone marrow toxicity is rare, unexplained bleeding or bruising should be promptly reported to the physician.
- Monitor patient for evidence of deterioration of renal function, i.e., changed I&O ratio and pattern, weight gain (edema), decreasing creatinine clearance.
- Pulmonary toxicity occurs in about 10% of all patients and most frequently in patients >70 y or when the total of all doses approaches 400 U. It may also occur in young people, however, and with lower doses.
- Monitor for nonproductive cough, chest pain, dyspnea; by auscultation for fine rales.
- Be alert to evidence of radiation recall, i.e., erythema that develops in a previously irradiated field. Most frequently occurs when chemotherapy is started during or shortly after radiation therapy, but it also may be observed several years after the treatment.
- Stomatitis can be a dose-limiting factor because oral ulcerations may interfere with adequate nutrient intake, leading to severe debilitation. Consult physician if an oral local anesthetic is indicated. It may help patient to eat if applied about 10 min before meals.
- Check weight at regular intervals under standard conditions. Weight loss and anorexia may persist a long time after therapy has been discontinued.

Patient & Family Education

- Counsel patient to avoid using OTC drugs during antineoplastic treatment period unless such drugs are approved by physician.

- Skin toxicity usually develops in second or third week of treatment and after 150–200 U of bleomycin have been administered. Report symptoms (hypoesthesias, urticaria, tender swollen hands) promptly; therapy may be discontinued.
- Hyperpigmentation may occur in areas subject to friction and pressure, skin folds, nail cuticles, scars, and intramuscular sites.
- Raynaud's phenomenon has been reported in a few patients receiving bleomycin for testicular carcinoma. Advise patient to observe and report early signs: hands and feet constantly cold especially when exposed; intermittent blanching and cyanosis in finger and toe tips; swelling of fingers and toes. Signs can occur during or after therapy has been discontinued.

Prototype: procainamide, p 140

BRETYLIUM TOSYLATE

(bre-til´ee-um)
Trade name: Bretylate, Bretylol
Classifications: CARDIOVASCULAR AGENT; ANTIARRHYTHMIC; AUTONOMIC NERVOUS SYSTEM AGENT; ADRENERGIC ANTAGONIST (SYMPATHOLYTIC, BLOCKING AGENT)
Pregnancy: Category C

ACTIONS/PHARMACODYNAMICS Quaternary ammonium compound; mechanism of action is complex and not fully understood. Suppresses ventricular fibrillation by direct action on the myocardium and ventricular tachycardia by adrenergic blockade. Shortly after administration, norepinephrine is released from adrenergic postganglionic nerve terminals, resulting in a moderate increase in BP, heart rate, and ventricular irritability. Subsequently (1–2 h) drug-induced release and reuptake of norepinephrine are blocked, leading to a state resembling surgical sympathectomy. *Electrophysiologic events:* initially bretylium causes hyperpolarization during diastole, increases conduction velocity, and shortens action potential (AP) and effective refractory period. After adrenergic blockade is established, phase 3 (repolarization) is prolonged (class III antiarrhythmic characteristic). Phase 4 (spontaneous depolarization of conducting system cells) is unaffected. These effects suppress arrhythmias with a reentry mechanism and decrease dispersion of ectopic foci. PR, QT, and

Common side effects in *italic*; life-threatening effects <u>underlined</u>; generic names in **bold**; classifications in SMALL CAPS

355

B

QRS intervals are unchanged. Orthostatic hypotension occurs commonly as a result of peripheral adrenergic blockade; some degree of hypotension may occur even while patient is supine. Tolerance to this effect develops after several days in most patients as adrenergic receptors become more responsive to circulating catecholamines (as opposed to synaptic catecholamine). Appears to lack CNS or cholinergic blockade effects, and effect on GI motility is less than with other adrenergic blockers. Has weak local anesthetic properties. Because onset of desired action is delayed, bretylium is not a first-line antiarrhythmic agent.

USES Short-term prophylaxis and treatment of ventricular fibrillation; life-threatening arrhythmias such as ventricular fibrillation not responsive to conventional therapy, e.g., lidocaine, procainamide, direct current (cardioversion).

ROUTE & DOSAGE

Ventricular Fibrillation

Adult	IV	5 mg/kg rapid IV injection; may increase to 10 mg/kg and repeat q15–30min up to 30 mg/kg/d; may also give by continuous infusion at 1–2 mg/min
	IM	5–10 mg/kg; may repeat in 1–2 h if arrhythmia persists, then 5–10 mg/kg q6–8h for maintenance
Child	IV	5 mg/kg followed by 10 mg/kg if arrhythmia persists

PHARMACOKINETICS Onset: minutes after IV; up to 6 h IM. **Peak:** 6–9 h. **Duration:** 6–24 h. **Distribution:** does not cross blood-brain barrier; not known if crosses placenta or distributed into breast milk. **Metabolism:** not metabolized. **Elimination:** half-life: 4–17 h; 70–80% excreted in urine in 24 h.

CONTRAINDICATIONS & PRECAUTIONS No contraindications for use in life-threatening refractory ventricular arrhythmias. Safe use during pregnancy (category C), in nursing mothers, and in children not established. **Cautious use in:** digitalis-induced arrhythmias, patients with fixed cardiac output, e.g., severe aortic stenosis or severe pulmonary hypertension (profound hypotension can result without compensatory increase in cardiac output); sinus bradycardia, patients on digitalis maintenance, angina pectoris; impaired renal function.

ADVERSE/SIDE EFFECTS CV: both supine and postural *hypotension* with dizziness, vertigo, light-headedness, faintness, syncope, transitory hypertension, bradycardia, increased frequency of PVCs, exacerbation of digitalis-induced arrhythmias, precipitation of angina, sensation of substernal pressure. **GI:** *nausea, vomiting* (particularly with rapid IV), parotid pain, loose stools, diarrhea, anorexia. **Other:** nasal stuffiness, mild conjunctivitis, hiccups, IM injection site reactions, respiratory depression, hyperthermia, muscle weakness.

DIAGNOSTIC TEST INTERFERENCES *Urinary VMA, epinephrine,* and *norepinephrine* levels may be decreased during bretylium therapy.

DRUG INTERACTIONS Lidocaine, procainamide, quinidine, propranolol may antagonize antiarrhythmic effects and compound hypotension; ANTIHYPERTENSIVE AGENTS will add to hypotensive effects; DIGITALIS GLYCOSIDES may worsen arrhythmias through digitalis toxicity.

INCOMPATIBILITIES Solution/additive: **dobutamine, nitroglycerin, phenytoin.** Y-site: **phenytoin.**

NURSING IMPLICATIONS

Administration

- Use of bretylium should be limited to patients in facilities adequately equipped and staffed for constant monitoring of ECG and BP and for cardiopulmonary resuscitation and cardioversion if necessary.
- In ventricular fibrillation, IV bretylium may be given by direct IV undiluted at a rate of 1 dose/15 seconds.
- IV bretylium may be diluted in 50 ml or more of NS or D5W and infused at a rate of 1–2 mg/min.
- Administer no more than 5 ml in any one IM site. Avoid injecting into or near a major nerve. Keep a record of injection sites. Injection into same site can cause muscle atrophy, necrosis, and fibrosis.
- Store at 15–30C (59–86F) unless otherwise directed.

Assessment & Drug Effects

- Anticipate vomiting. IV administration is associated with a high incidence of nausea and vomiting. These side effects can be minimized by slow administration of drug (≥10 min).
- Establish baseline readings and monitor BP and ECG when drug is administered. Observe for initial transient rise in BP, increased heart rate, PVCs and other arrhythmias, or worsening of existing arrhythmias, which may occur within a few minutes to 1 h after drug administration. Keep physician in-

Common side effects in *italic*; life-threatening effects underlined; generic names in **bold**; classifications in SMALL CAPS

formed. Usually patients eventually adjust to these effects and stabilize.

- Initial effect of hypertension is usually followed within 1 h by a fall in supine BP and by orthostatic hypotension.
- The supine position is recommended until patient develops tolerance to the hypotensive effect of bretylium (generally in several days). Hypotension can occur in the supine position, particularly in patients with severely compromised cardiac function. It may not readily respond to therapy (e.g., vasopressors, fluids); early reporting is essential.
- To prevent orthostatic hypotension, raise or lower head of bed slowly and advise patient to make position changes slowly. If patient is allowed to be out of bed, caution to dangle legs for a few minutes before standing and not to stand still for prolonged periods. Advise men to sit on toilet to urinate.
- Monitor I&O, particularly in patients with impaired renal function. Usually these patients are given lower dosages or longer dosage intervals.

Prototype: ergotamine, p 112

BROMOCRIPTINE MESYLATE
(broe-moe-krip´teen)
Trade name: Parlodel
Classifications: AUTONOMIC NERVOUS SYSTEM AGENT; ERGOT ALKALOID; ANTIPARKINSONISM AGENT
Pregnancy: Category C

ACTIONS/PHARMACODYNAMICS Semisynthetic ergot alkaloid derivative, but devoid of oxytocic activity generally attributed to drugs of this class. Reduces elevated serum prolactin levels in men and women by activating postsynaptic dopaminergic receptors in hypothalamus to stimulate release of prolactin-inhibiting factor and possibly luteinizing hormone release factor. Ovulation and ovarian function in amenorrheic women are restored (by direct action on ovary), thus correcting female infertility secondary to elevated prolactin levels. (Correction of male infertility has not been documented.) Growth hormone secretion is increased transiently in patient with normal concentrations but paradoxically is suppressed in some patients with acromegaly. Pretreatment levels are restored 2–4 wk after bromocriptine is discontinued. Activates dopaminergic receptors in neostriatum of CNS, which may explain action in parkinsonism. Also reduces BP in the hypertensive

and normotensive individual and may cause peripheral vasoconstriction (large doses) and increased sodium excretion.

USES Short-term management of amenorrhea/galactorrhea or female infertility associated with hyperprolactemia (when there is no indication of pituitary tumor) and to prevent postpartum lactation. Also used as adjunctive to levodopa or levodopa/carbidopa therapy to relieve symptoms of Parkinson's disease and to lower plasma growth hormone in patients with acromegaly. **Unlabeled use:** to relieve premenstrual symptoms, to treat hypogonadism and galactorrhea in hyperprolactinemic men; for management of hepatic encephalopathy, Cushing's syndrome, drug-induced neuroleptic malignant syndrome, and cocaine withdrawal.

ROUTE & DOSAGE

Amenorrhea or Galactorrhea, Female Infertility

Adult	PO	1.25–2.5 mg/d up to 2.5 mg 2–3 times/d

Suppression of Postpartum Lactation

Adult	PO	2.5 mg b.i.d. starting at least 4 h after delivery for 14–21 d

Parkinson's Disease

Adult	PO	1.25–2.5 mg/d up to 100 mg/d in divided doses

Acromegaly

Adult	PO	1.25–2.5 mg/d for 3 d; then increase by 1.25–2.5 mg q3–7d until desired effect achieved; usually 30–60 mg/d in divided doses

PHARMACOKINETICS Absorption: approximately 28% absorbed from GI tract. **Peak:** 1–2 h. **Duration:** 4–8 h. **Metabolism:** metabolized in liver. **Elimination:** half-life: 50 h; 85% excreted in feces in 5 d; 3–6% eliminated in urine.

CONTRAINDICATIONS & PRECAUTIONS Contraindicated in: hypersensitivity to ergot alkaloids; uncontrolled hypertension; severe ischemic heart disease or peripheral vascular disease; pituitary tumor; normal prolactin levels, nursing women. Safe use during pregnancy (category C) and in children <15 y not established. **Cautious use in:** hepatic and renal dysfunction; history of psychiatric disorder; history of MI with residual arrhythmia.

ADVERSE/SIDE EFFECTS Mostly dose related. **CNS:** headache, dizziness, vertigo, light-headedness,

Common side effects in *italic*; life-threatening effects <u>underlined</u>; generic names in **bold**; classifications in SMALL CAPS

357

fainting, sedation, nightmares, insomnia, dyskinesia, ataxia; mania, nervousness, anxiety, depression. **CV:** *orthostatic hypotension,* shock, postpartum hypertension, cerebrovascular accident, palpitation, extrasystoles, Raynaud's phenomenon, red, tender, hot, edematous extremities (erythromelalgia), exacerbation of angina, arrhythmias, acute MI. **Eye:** blurred vision, burning sensation in eyes, blepharospasm, diplopia. **GI:** *nausea,* vomiting, abdominal cramps, epigastric pain, constipation (long-term use) or diarrhea; metallic taste, dry mouth, dysphagia, anorexia, peptic ulcers, GI tract hemorrhage. **Skin:** urticaria, rash, mottling, livedo reticularis. **Other:** fatigue, nasal congestion, asthenia, pulmonary infiltration, pleural effusion and thickening with long-term therapy (6–36 mo).

DRUG INTERACTIONS Possibility of decreased tolerance to **alcohol;** ANTIHYPERTENSIVE AGENTS add to hypotensive effects; ORAL CONTRACEPTIVES, **estrogen, progestins** may interfere with effect of bromocriptine by causing amenorrhea and galactorrhea; PHENOTHIAZINES, TRICYCLIC ANTIDEPRESSANTS, **methyldopa, reserpine** can cause an increase in prolactin, which may interfere with bromocriptine activity.

NURSING IMPLICATIONS

Administration
- Administer with meals, milk, or other food to reduce incidence of GI side effects.
- Hypotension with dizziness and fainting may occur, particularly following first dose in sensitive patients. For this reason, initial dose is usually prescribed for evening administration.
- *Suppression of puerperal lactation:* Because hypotension occurs most commonly in the postpartum patient, it is recommended that therapy not be started any sooner than 4 h after delivery and then only if vital signs have stabilized.
- Store in tightly closed, light-resistant containers, preferably at 15–30C (59–86F) unless otherwise directed.

Assessment & Drug Effects
- Establish data regarding baseline vital signs. Therapy should not be initiated until vital signs are stable.
- BP should be monitored closely during the first few days of therapy and periodically throughout therapy for all patients. Compare readings with baseline data.
- Side effects are common, but they are usually mild

to moderate in degree and respond to dosage reduction or discontinuation of drug.
- Periodic evaluations should be made of hepatic, hematologic, cardiovascular, and renal function in patients on prolonged therapy.
- Note that dosages for Parkinson's disease may be almost 10 times larger than those for galactorrhea and amenorrhea. Therefore, psychotic symptoms and other adverse reactions occur most frequently in Parkinson's patients.
- Improvement in Parkinson's disease may be noted in 30–90 min following administration of bromocriptine, with maximum effect in 2 h.
- Recurrence rates of amenorrhea and galactorrhea are high (70–80%) following withdrawal of bromocriptine. Amenorrhea usually returns within 4–24 wk; galactorrhea within 2–12 wk; serum prolactin increases to pretreatment levels within 1–6 wk.

Patient & Family Education
- Instruct patient to make position changes slowly and in stages, especially from recumbent to upright posture, and to dangle legs over bed for a few minutes before ambulating. Caution patient to lie down immediately if light-headedness or dizziness occurs.
- Inform patient that a mild diuresis may occur because of vasodilating action of bromocriptine on renal arteries.
- Since bromocriptine is associated with dose-related lightheadedness, dizziness, and syncope, caution patient to avoid driving and other potentially hazardous activities until reaction to drug has been determined.
- Bromocriptine can cause digital vasospasm, particularly in patients with acromegaly and patients receiving high dosages. Advise patient to avoid exposure to cold and to report the onset of pallor of fingers or toes.
- Advise patient that bromocriptine may increase sensitivity to the effects of alcohol.
- Patients receiving bromocriptine to suppress postpartum lactation may have temporary rebound breast enlargement and pain following drug withdrawal.
- Patients being treated for amenorrhea or galactorrhea should be informed that restoration of regular menses usually occurs in 6–8 wk (range: a few days to 24 wk). (If patient has been amenorrheic more than 4 y, restoration of menses may require considerable time.) Galactorrhea suppression is usually seen after 7–12 wk of therapy but may not occur for more than 24 wk. Because long-term drug effects are not known, it is recommended that dura-

Common side effects in *italic*; life-threatening effects underlined; generic names in **bold**; classifications in SMALL CAPS

tion of therapy for amenorrhea and galactorrhea not exceed 6 mo.

- Since restoration of fertility may result during therapy, patients being treated for amenorrhea and galactorrhea should be advised to use barrier type contraceptive measures until normal ovulating cycle is restored. Oral contraceptives are contraindicated because they may cause amenorrhea and galactorrhea.
- Inform physician immediately if pregnancy occurs during therapy. Bromocriptine should be discontinued without delay. These patients should be carefully observed throughout pregnancy.

Prototype: diphenhydramine, p 47

BROMPHENIRAMINE MALEATE

(brome-fen-ir´a-meen)
Trade names: Bromphen, Codimal-A, Conjec-B, Cophene-B, Dehist, Diamine T.D., Dimetane, Dimetane Extentabs, Histaject, Nasahist B, Sinusol-B, Veltane
Classifications: ANTIHISTAMINE (H$_1$-RECEPTOR ANTAGONIST)
Pregnancy: Category C

ACTIONS/PHARMACODYNAMICS Antihistamine similar to diphenhydramine; shares properties of other antihistamines. Competes with histamine for H$_1$-receptor sites on effector cells, thus blocking histamine-mediated responses. Has less sedative effect than diphenhydramine.

USES Symptomatic treatment of allergic manifestations. Also used in various cough mixtures and antihistamine-decongestant cold formulations.

PHARMACOKINETICS Peak: 3–9 h. **Duration:** up to 48 h. **Distribution:** crosses placenta. **Elimination:** half-life: 12–34 h; 40% excreted in urine within 72 h; 2% in feces.

CONTRAINDICATIONS & PRECAUTIONS Contraindicated in: hypersensitivity to antihistamines; newborns, nursing mothers; acute asthma. Pregnancy: category C. **Cautious use in:** the elderly; prostatic hypertrophy; narrow-angle glaucoma; cardiovascular or renal disease; hyperthyroidism.

ROUTE & DOSAGE

Allergy

Adult	PO	4–8 mg t.i.d. or q.i.d. *or* 8–12 mg of sustained release b.i.d. or t.i.d.
	IM/IV	5–20 mg q6–12h (max 40 mg/24 h)
Child	PO	>6 y: 2–4 mg t.i.d. or q.i.d. *or* 8–12 mg of sustained release b.i.d. (max 12 mg/24 h)
		<6 y: 0.5 mg/kg in 3–4 divided doses
	IM/IV	>6 y: 0.5 mg/kg/24 h in 3–4 divided doses

ADVERSE/SIDE EFFECTS *Sedation,* drowsiness, dry mouth, throat, and nose, ringing or buzzing in ears, hypotension, dizziness, headache, disturbed coordination, urticaria, rash, increased sweating, stomach upset, constipation, photosensitivity, hypersensitivity reaction, agranulocytosis, thrombocytopenia.

DIAGNOSTIC TEST INTERFERENCES May cause false-negative *allergy skin tests.*

DRUG INTERACTIONS Alcohol and other CNS DEPRESSANTS add to sedation.

INCOMPATIBILITIES Solution/additive: Radiocontrast media (diatrizoate, iothalomalate).

NURSING IMPLICATIONS

Administration

- If gastric distress occurs, advise patient to take medication with meals or a snack.
- IV brompheniramine maleate may be given undiluted or diluted with 10 ml 0.9% NaCl injection unless otherwise specified by manufacturer. Administer one dose direct IV over 1 min.
- Initially diluted IV solution may be further diluted with NS for injection or D5W and infused at the ordered rate.
- Read labels carefully. Note that the 100 mg/ml concentration is not recommended for IV use. It is intended for IM administration and is given either without further dilution or diluted 1:10 with sterile saline for injection.
- Store in tightly covered container at 15–30C (59–86F) unless otherwise directed. Elixir and parenteral form should be protected from light. Avoid freezing.

Assessment & Drug Effects

- Acute hypersensitivity reaction with sudden severe agranulocytosis reportedly can occur within min-

---

Common side effects in *italic*; life-threatening effects underlined; generic names in **bold**; classifications in SMALL CAPS

utes to hours after drug ingestion. The reaction is manifested by high fever, chills, and possible development of gangrenous ulcerations of mouth and throat, pneumonia, and prostration. Patient should seek medical attention immediately.

■ Drowsiness, sweating, transient hypotension, and syncope may follow IV administration. Patient should be recumbent while receiving injection, and reaction to drug should be evaluated. Keep physician informed.

■ Elderly patients tend to be particularly susceptible to sedative effect, dizziness, and hypotension. Most symptoms respond to reduction in dosage.

■ Bear in mind that brompheniramine has an atropinelike effect (thickens bronchial secretions) that may make expectoration difficult.

■ Blood counts should be performed in patients receiving long-term therapy to reduce possibility of blood dyscrasias.

Patient & Family Education

■ Thickened bronchial secretions and dry mouth, nose, and throat may be relieved by increasing fluid intake (check with physician). Advise patient that relief of dry mouth may be provided by sugarless gum or lemon drops, frequent rinses with warm water, diligent mouth care.

■ Caution patient to avoid driving a car or other potentially hazardous activities until reaction to drug is known.

■ Advise patient not to take alcoholic beverages and other CNS depressants, e.g., tranquilizers, sedatives, pain or sleeping medicines, without consulting physician.

■ May cause false-negative allergy skin tests. The drug should be discontinued about 4 d before such tests are done.

Prototype: meclizine, p 50

BUCLIZINE HYDROCHLORIDE
(byoo-cli´zeen)

Trade name: Bucladin-S Softab
Classifications: ANTIHISTAMINE; ANTIVERTIGO; ANTIEMETIC
Pregnancy: Category C

ACTIONS/PHARMACODYNAMICS Buclizine is a piperazine derivative structurally and pharmaco-

logically related to meclizine and cyclizine used as an antiemetic. Mechanism of action not precisely known but may be related to its central anticholinergic actions. It diminishes vestibular stimulation and depresses labyrinthine function. An action on the medullary chemoreceptive trigger zone (CTZ) may also be involved in the antiemetic effect. Exhibits antihistaminic, anticholinergic, antivertigo, CNS depressant, and local anesthetic effects.

USES Prevention and treatment of motion sickness and the symptomatic treatment of vertigo.

ROUTE & DOSAGE

Motion Sickness

Adult	PO	50 mg 30 min before travel; may repeat in 4–6 h if needed

Vertigo

Adult	PO	50 mg 1–3 times/d

PHARMACOKINETICS Absorption: readily absorbed from GI tract. **Onset:** 1 h. **Duration:** 4–6 h.

CONTRAINDICATIONS & PRECAUTIONS Contraindicated in: hypersensitivity to buclizine hydrochloride, pediatric patients, elderly, lactation, pregnancy (category C). **Cautious use in:** patients receiving other CNS depressants or depressant drugs, angle-closure glaucoma, prostatic hypertrophy, bladder neck obstruction, pyloroduodenal obstruction.

ADVERSE/SIDE EFFECTS *Drowsiness,* dry mouth, headache, nausea, jitteriness.

DIAGNOSTIC TEST INTERFERENCES May interfere with *allergy skin tests.*

DRUG INTERACTIONS Alcohol and other CNS DEPRESSANTS compound CNS depression.

NURSING IMPLICATIONS

Administration
■ Administer with food, water, or milk to minimize gastric irritation.
■ Tablet may be swallowed whole, chewed, or allowed to dissolve in mouth without water.
■ Store away from heat, light, or moist areas at 15–30C in a tightly closed container.

Assessment & Drug Effects
■ Inquire about history of aspirin allergy. Withhold buclizine if aspirin hypersensitivity reported.

- May suppress dizziness, nausea, and vomiting associated with drug toxicity and serious disease conditions.
- May mask ototoxic effects of large doses of salicylates.

Patient & Family Education
- Advise patient to take at least 30 min before traveling for motion sickness.
- Do not take more medication than recommended.
- Observe caution while driving or performing other tasks requiring alertness until reaction to drug is known.
- Avoid alcohol and other CNS depressants.
- This drug may interfere with skin tests using allergens; inform physician of use.

Prototype: furosemide, p 198

BUMETANIDE
(byoo-met´a-nide)
Trade name: Bumex
Classifications: WATER BALANCE AGENT; LOOP DIURETIC
Pregnancy: Category C

ACTIONS/PHARMACODYNAMICS Sulfonamide derivative structurally related to furosemide and with similar pharmacologic effects. Diuretic activity is 40 times greater, however, and duration of action is shorter than that of furosemide. Inhibits sodium and chloride reabsorption by direct action on proximal ascending limb of the loop of Henle. Also appears to inhibit phosphate and bicarbonate reabsorption. Produces only mild hypotensive effects at usual diuretic doses. Causes both potassium and magnesium wastage.

USES Edema associated with CHF; hepatic or renal disease, including nephrotic syndrome. Has been used in management of postoperative and premenstrual edema, edema accompanying disseminated carcinoma, and mild hypertension. May be used concomitantly with a potassium-sparing diuretic.

PHARMACOKINETICS Absorption: readily absorbed from GI tract. **Onset:** 30–60 min PO; 40 min IV. **Peak:** 0.5–2 h. **Duration:** 4–6 h. **Distribution:** distributed into breast milk. **Metabolism:** partially metabolized in liver. **Elimination:** half-life: 60–90 min; 80% excreted in urine in 48 h, 10–20% excreted in feces.

ROUTE & DOSAGE

Edema

Adult	PO	0.5–2 mg once/d; may repeat at 4–5 h intervals if needed (max 10 mg/d)
	IM/IV	0.5–1 mg over 1–2 min; repeated q2–3h prn (max 10 mg/d)

CONTRAINDICATIONS & PRECAUTIONS Contraindicated in: hypersensitivity to bumetanide or to other sulfonamides; anuria, markedly elevated BUN; hepatic coma; severe electrolyte deficiency. Safe use during pregnancy (category C), in nursing mothers, and in children <18 y not established. **Cautious use in:** hepatic cirrhosis, ascites; history of gout; history of hypersensitivity to furosemide.

ADVERSE/SIDE EFFECTS CNS: dizziness, headache, weakness, fatigue. **CV:** hypotension, ECG changes, chest pain, *hypovolemia*. **GI:** nausea, vomiting, abdominal or stomach pain, GI distress, diarrhea, dry mouth. **Electrolytes:** *hypokalemia,* hyponatremia, hyperuricemia, hyperglycemia; *hypomagnesemia;* decreased calcium, chloride, ammonium, bicarbonate, phosphorus. **Hepatic:** increased or decreased serum cholesterol, increased LDH, AST, ALT, alkaline phosphatase. **Musculoskeletal:** muscle cramps, muscle pain, stiffness or tenderness; arthritic pain. **Ototoxicity:** ear discomfort, ringing or buzzing in ears, impaired hearing. **Other:** sweating, hyperventilation, glycosuria.

DRUG INTERACTIONS AMINOGLYCOSIDES, **cisplatin** increase risk of ototoxicity; bumetanide increases risk of hypokalemia-induced **digoxin** toxicity; NONSTEROIDAL ANTIINFLAMMATORY DRUGS may attenuate diuretic and hypotensive response; **probenecid** may antagonize diuretic activity; bumetanide may decrease renal elimination of **lithium.**

INCOMPATIBILITIES Solution/additive: dobutamine.

NURSING IMPLICATIONS

Administration
- May be taken with food or milk to reduce risk of gastrointestinal irritation.
- Usually administered in the morning as a single

Common side effects in *italic*; life-threatening effects underlined; generic names in **bold**; classifications in SMALL CAPS

361

dose, either daily or by intermittent schedule. For some patients, diuresis is reportedly more effective when administered in two divided doses, morning and evening.

- IV bumetanide may be given direct IV undiluted at a rate of a single dose over 1–2 min.
- For IV infusion, parenteral bumetanide is compatible with 5% dextrose, 0.9% NaCl, and lactated Ringer's. Infusion should be used within 24 h after preparation.
- Drug will discolor on exposure to light. Inspect parenteral bumetanide before administration. Discard if it contains particles or is discolored.
- Store in tight, light-resistant container at 15–30C (59–86F) unless otherwise directed.

Assessment & Drug Effects

- Monitor I&O, BUN, and serum creatinine. Report promptly the onset of oliguria or other changes in I&O ratio and pattern and significant increases in BUN or serum creatinine.
- Monitor weight, BP, and pulse rate. Assess for hypovolemia by assessing BP and pulse rate while patient is lying, sitting, and standing.
- High doses or frequent administration, particularly in the elderly, can cause profound diuresis, hypovolemia, and resulting circulatory collapse with development of thrombi and emboli. Careful monitoring is essential.
- Both hypomagnesemia and hypokalemia (see Signs & Symptoms, chap 3) pose a constant threat to all patients and particularly those receiving digitalis or who have CHF, hepatic cirrhosis, ascites, diarrhea, or potassium-depleting nephropathy. Careful monitoring and hospitalization during initial therapy and dosage adjustment periods are advised in these patients.
- Patients with hepatic disease should be carefully observed. Alterations in fluid and electrolyte balance can precipitate encephalopathy (inappropriate behavior, altered mood, impaired judgment, confusion, drowsiness, coma).
- Be alert to complaints about hearing difficulty or ear discomfort. Patients at risk of ototoxic effects (see Signs & Symptoms, chap 3) include those receiving the drug IV, especially at high doses, those with severely impaired renal function, and those receiving other potentially ototoxic or nephrotoxic drugs. Hearing tests at periodic intervals are indicated for these patients.
- Serum electrolytes, blood studies, liver and kidney function tests, uric acid (particularly patients with history of gout), and blood sugar (particularly diabetics) values should be determined initially and at regular intervals. These determinations are especially important in patients receiving prolonged treatment, high doses, or who are on sodium restriction.

Patient & Family Education

- Advise patient to report symptoms of electrolyte imbalance promptly to physician: weakness, dizziness, fatigue, faintness, confusion, muscle cramps, headache, paresthesias.
- Inform patient that serum magnesium, potassium, and sodium should be monitored during therapy.
- It is important for patient to maintain an adequate daily intake of potassium while taking bumetanide.
- Advise patient to promptly report signs and symptoms of ototoxicity.
- Advise diabetics that drug may cause loss of glycemic control and that they should inform physician of their diabetes, since adjustment in insulin dose may be required.

Prototype: procaine, p 166

BUPIVACAINE HYDROCHLORIDE
(byoo-piv´a-kane)
Trade names: Marcaine, Sensorcaine
Classifications: CNS AGENT; LOCAL ANESTHETIC (AMIDE-TYPE)
Pregnancy: Category C

ACTIONS/PHARMACODYNAMICS Anesthetic of the amide type. Decreases sodium flux into nerve cell, inhibiting initial depolarization, and prevents propagation and conduction of the nerve impulse. Progression of anesthesia, related to diameter, myelination, and conduction velocity of affected fibers manifests clinically as sequential loss of nerve function: pain, temperature, touch, proprioception, and skeletal muscle tone. CV system effects are minimal; toxic blood concentrations depress cardiac condition and excitability and myocardial contractility and cause vasodilation. Bupivacaine may stimulate or depress the CNS or do both. Primary depressant effect is in medulla and higher centers.

USES Infiltration anesthesia; peripheral, sympathetic nerve, and epidural (including caudal) block anesthesia; 0.75% bupivacaine solution in dextrose is used for spinal anesthesia.

ROUTE & DOSAGE

Infiltration Anesthesia

Adult   IM   *Local infiltration, sympathetic block:* 0.25% solution

Lumbar epidural: 0.25%, 0.5%, 0.75% solutions

Caudal block, peripheral nerve block: 0.25%, 0.5% solutions

Retrobulbar block: 0.75% solution

Child   IM   Same as for adult

PHARMACOKINETICS Onset: 4–17 min for epidural, caudal, peripheral, or sympathetic block; within 1 min for spinal block. **Duration:** 3–5 h for epidural, caudal, peripheral, or sympathetic block; 1.25–2.5 h for spinal block. **Distribution:** crosses placenta. **Metabolism:** metabolized in liver. **Elimination:** half-life: 1.5–5.5 h in adults, 8.1 h in neonates; 6% excreted unchanged in urine.

CONTRAINDICATIONS & PRECAUTIONS Contraindicated in: known sensitivity to bupivacaine or to other amide-type anesthetics or to parabens or metabisulfites; acidosis; heart block; severe hemorrhage; hypotension and shock; hypertension, cerebrospinal diseases; obstetrical paracervical anesthesia or spinal anesthesia in septicemia; topical or IV regional anesthesia; intercurrent use with chloroprocaine; history of malignant hyperthermia. Safe use during pregnancy (category C) other than during labor and lactation or in children <12 y not established. **Cautious use in:** the elderly or debilitated patient; hepatic or renal disease; known drug allergies and sensitivities, dysrhythmias, children >12 y, obstetrical delivery.

ADVERSE/SIDE EFFECTS CNS: nervousness, unusual anxiety, excitement, dizziness, drowsiness, tremors, convulsions, unconsciousness, <u>respiratory arrest</u>. Associated with epidural anesthesia: total spinal block, urinary retention, fecal incontinence, loss of perineal sensation and sexual function; persistent analgesia, paresthesia, slowing of labor, increased incidence of forceps delivery, cranial nerve palsies (with inadvertent intrathecal injection). **CV:** hypotension, ventricular arrhythmias, myocardial depression, decreased cardiac output, <u>bradycardia (fatal bradycardia during delivery)</u>, maternal hypotension, <u>cardiac arrest</u>. **Eye:** pupillary constriction; blurred or double vision. **GI:** nausea, vomiting. **Hypersensitivity:** cutaneous lesions, urticaria, sneezing, diaphoresis, syncope, hyperthermia, angioneurotic edema (in-

cluding laryngeal edema), <u>anaphylaxis, anaphylactoid reactions</u>. **Ototoxicity:** tinnitus. **Other:** inflammation or sepsis at injection site, chills, pupillary constriction.

DRUG INTERACTIONS CNS DEPRESSANTS augment CNS depression; with **isoproterenol, ergonovine** there is persistent hypertension and a risk of CVA if bupivacaine used with **epinephrine:** MAO INHIBITORS, TRICYCLIC ANTIDEPRESSANTS, PHENOTHIAZINES cause severe or prolonged hypotension or hypertension if bupivacaine used with epinephrine.

NURSING IMPLICATIONS

Administration

- Preparations containing preservatives should not be used for epidural or spinal anesthesia.
- Resuscitation equipment, oxygen, resuscitative drugs, vasopressors, should be immediately available when bupivacaine is used.
- Local anesthetics react with certain heavy metals (e.g., zinc, mercury, copper) and may release their ions from solutions. Since such ions can cause severe local irritation, avoid use of disinfecting agents containing heavy metals for skin or mucous membrane disinfection or for ampul surface disinfection.
- Bupivacaine solutions may be autoclaved at 15 psi at 121C (249.8F) for 15 min; solutions containing epinephrine should not be autoclaved. Use 91% isopropyl alcohol or 70% ethyl alcohol without denaturants to disinfect ampul surfaces.
- Bupivacaine with dextrose may be autoclaved once (repeated autoclaving or prolonged storage discolors solution because of caramelizing of dextrose).
- Do not use multiple dose vial for lumbar or caudal epidural block; it is not known whether intrathecal administration of the preservatives in this vial is safe.
- The addition of a vasoconstrictor (epinephrine) to decrease rate of absorption also reduces risk of systemic toxic reaction, prolongs anesthetic effect, and permits administration of a larger maximum single dose of anesthetic.
- It is not known whether amidetype anesthetics will trigger familial malignant hyperthermia.
- Store ampuls at 15–30C (59–85F); protect from freezing. Solutions with epinephrine should be protected from light.

Assessment & Drug Effects

- Observe for clinical response to an inadvertent intravascular injection, which can produce within

Common side effects in *italic*; life-threatening effects <u>underlined</u>; generic names in **bold**; classifications in SMALL CAPS

363

B

45 seconds a transient "epinephrine response" (increased heart rate or systolic BP or both, circumoral pallor, palpitations, nervousness) in the unsedated patient and an increase by 20 bpm or more in heart rate for at least 15 seconds in sedated patient.

- Risk of toxicity and degree of motor block increase with repeated doses (e.g., 2 doses of 0.5% solution can produce complete motor block).
- Vasoconstrictor-containing solution should be administered cautiously, if at all, to areas with end arteries (e.g., digits, penis) or to areas that have a compromised blood supply; ischemia and gangrene can result. Inspect areas for evidence of reduced perfusion because of vasospasm: pale, cold, sensitive skin.
- Systemic reactions (toxicity) are more apt to occur in children or the elderly and may develop rapidly or be delayed for as long as 30 min after administration.
- CNS stimulation (unusual anxiety, excitement, restlessness) usually occurs first, followed by CNS depression (drowsiness, unconsciousness, respiratory arrest). However, because stimulation is apt to be transient or absent, drowsiness may be the first sign of toxicity in some patients (especially children, elderly).
- Maternal hypotension may accompany regional anesthesia. Place mother on left side with legs elevated; monitor BP and fetal heart rate continuously.
- Monitor fetal heart rate during paracervical anesthesia. The risk of fetal bradycardia is high in prematurity, postmaturity, preeclampsia, uteroplacental insufficiency, and fetal distress.
- Patients receiving retrobulbar and dental blocks should have continuous monitoring of cardiac and respiratory status.
- During preparation for retrobulbar or dental anesthesia, inadvertent intraarterial injection of bupivacaine with subsequent retrograde flow into cerebral circulation may cause confusion, respiratory depression or arrest, convulsions, and CV stimulation or depression.

Patient & Family Education

- Tell patient who is given spinal anesthesia that sensation to lower extremities may not return for 2 1/2–3 1/2 h.

Prototype: morphine, p 156

BUPRENORPHINE HYDROCHLORIDE

(byoo-pre-nor´feen)
Trade name: Buprenex
Classifications: CNS AGENT; ANALGESIC; NARCOTIC (OPIATE) AGONIST-ANTAGONIST
Pregnancy: Category C
Controlled substance: Schedule V

ACTIONS/PHARMACODYNAMICS Opiate agonist-antagonist with agonist activity approximately 30 times that of morphine and antagonist activity equal to or up to 3 times greater than that of naloxone. Dose-related analgesia results from a high affinity of buprenorphine for mu- and possibly kappa-opiate receptors in the CNS. Respiratory depression occurs infrequently and is of limited clinical significance to most patients. General absence of dose-related respiratory depression at higher than usual doses may be due to drug's opiate antagonist activity. Psychologic and limited physical dependence develops infrequently. Tolerance to drug rarely develops.

USES Principally for moderate to severe postoperative pain. Also for pain associated with cancer and trigeminal neuralgia, accidental trauma, ureteral calculi, MI. **Unlabeled use:** to reverse fentanyl-induced anesthesia, to reduce opiate consumption in physical dependence on opiates (e.g., heroin).

ROUTE & DOSAGE

Postoperative Pain

Adult	IM/IV	0.3 mg q6h up to 0.6 mg q4h *or* 25–50 µg/h by IV infusion, *or* 60–180 µg over 48 h by epidural injection

---

PHARMACOKINETICS Onset: 10–30 min. **Peak:** 1 h. **Duration:** 6–10 h. **Metabolism:** metabolized extensively in liver. **Elimination:** half-life: 2.2 h; 70% eliminated in feces and 20% in urine in 7 d.

CONTRAINDICATIONS & PRECAUTIONS Contraindicated in: known hypersensitivity to buprenorphine. Safe use in children <13 y and during pregnancy (category C) and lactation not established. **Cautious use in:** patient with history of opiate use, compromised respiratory function, concomitant use of other respiratory depressants; hypothyroidism,

---

Common side effects in *italic*; life-threatening effects underlined; generic names in **bold**; classifications in SMALL CAPS

myxedema, Addison's disease; severe renal or hepatic impairment; geriatric or debilitated patients; acute alcoholism, delirium tremens; prostatic hypertrophy, urethral stricture; comatose patient; patients with CNS depression, head injury or intracranial lesion; biliary tract dysfunction.

ADVERSE/SIDE EFFECTS CNS: *sedation, drowsiness,* dizziness, vertigo, headache, amnesia, euphoria, paresthesia, depersonalization. **CV:** hypotension. **Eye:** miosis, amblyopia, mydriasis. **GI:** *nausea,* vomiting, dry mouth, constipation, abdominal cramps, flatulence, anorexia, diarrhea. **Hematologic:** decreased RBC, Hgb, Hct, sedimentation rate, total serum protein concentrations. **Respiratory:** respiratory depression, hyperventilation, dyspnea, cyanosis. **Skin:** pruritus, injection site reactions; rash, urticaria. **Other:** diaphoresis, decreased libido, flushing and sensation of warmth, tremors, chills and sensation of cold; hiccups, pallor.

DRUG INTERACTIONS Alcohol, OPIATES, other CNS DEPRESSANTS, BENZODIAZEPINES augment CNS depression; **diazepam** may cause respiratory or cardiovascular collapse.

NURSING IMPLICATIONS

Administration

- Inspect buprenorphine solution visually for particulate matter and discoloration before administration.
- IV buprenorphine HCl may be given undiluted by direct IV at a rate of 0.3 mg over 2 min.
- IV administration precautions include patient in recumbent position during infusion and for short period afterward and immediately available emergency equipment and drugs.
- Check with physician before discontinuing this drug. Gradual dose reduction may be necessary to avoid withdrawal symptoms.
- Store at 15–30C (59–86F); avoid freezing.

Assessment & Drug Effects

- Monitor respiratory status during therapy. Buprenorphine-induced respiratory depression is about equal to that produced by 10 mg morphine, but onset is slower, and if it occurs, it lasts longer.
- It may be difficult to identify respiratory depression because compensatory increases in depth of respiration prevent changes in arterial blood gas values. Also reduced pain intensity can reduce rate of respirations.
- Respiratory depression in the healthy adult plateaus or may even decrease in severity with

doses more than 1.2 mg because of antagonist activity of the drug.
- Additive analgesic effect with a concurrent NSAID or other nonnarcotic analgesic permits lower dosing of buprenorphine.
- Treatment of chronic pain is thought to be more effective if scheduled rather than on an as-needed basis. This regimen is more likely to prevent peaks and troughs of pain and to provide sustained freedom from pain.
- Monitor I&O ratio and pattern during buprenorphine therapy; urinary retention is a potential adverse effect.
- Drowsiness occurs in about 66% of patients on this drug. Dizziness and vertigo are experienced by about 10% of patients.

Patient & Family Education

- Supervise ambulation. Also warn patient that the drug may impair ability to perform hazardous activities requiring mental alertness or physical coordination (e.g., driving a car).
- Instruct patient on measures to relieve dry mouth.
- Inform patient of additive effect of other CNS depressants including alcohol.
- Warn patient not to take diazepam without medical supervision.

BUPROPION HYDROCHLORIDE
(byoo-pro´pi-on)
Trade name: Wellbutrin
Classification: ANTIDEPRESSANT
Pregnancy: Category B

ACTIONS/PHARMACODYNAMICS The neurochemical mechanism of bupropion is unknown. It does not inhibit monamine oxidase. Compared to tricyclic antidepressants it is a weak blocker of neural uptake of serotonin and norepinephrine.

USES Indicated for mental depression. Since it has been associated with increased risk of seizures, it is not the agent of first choice. **Unlabeled use:** cyclic mood disorders, schizoaffective disorders.

PHARMACOKINETICS Absorption: readily absorbed from GI tract. **Onset:** 3–4 wk. **Peak:** 1–3 h. **Metabolism:** metabolized in liver (including first pass metabolism) to active metabolites. **Elimination:** half-life: 8–24 h; 80% excreted in urine as inactive metabolites.

ROUTE & DOSAGE

Depression

Adult	PO	75–100 mg t.i.d.; doses >450 mg/d are associated with an increased risk of adverse reactions (including seizures); max 150 mg/dose; start with 75 mg t.i.d. or 100 mg b.i.d. and increase dose q3d to 300 mg/d

CONTRAINDICATIONS & PRECAUTIONS Contraindicated in: hypersensitivity to drug, history of seizure disorder, current or prior diagnosis of bulimia or anorexia nervosa, concurrent administration of MAO inhibitor, head trauma, CNS tumor; recent MI and nursing mothers. **Cautious use in:** renal or hepatic function impairment, drug abuse or dependence, and pregnancy (category B).

ADVERSE/SIDE EFFECTS CNS: <u>seizures.</u> The risk of seizure appears to be strongly associated with dose (especially >450 mg/d) and may be increased by predisposing factors (e.g., head trauma, CNS tumor) or a history of prior seizure; *agitation, insomnia, dry mouth, blurred vision, headache, dizziness, tremor.* **GI:** *nausea, vomiting, constipation.* **CV:** tachycardia. **Other:** weight loss, weight gain, rash.

DRUG INTERACTIONS Bupropion may increase metabolism of **carbamazepine, cimetidine, phenytoin, phenobarbital,** decreasing their effect; may increase incidence of adverse effects of **levodopa,** MAO INHIBITORS.

NURSING IMPLICATIONS

Administration
- May be administered with meals to decrease the incidence of nausea and vomiting.
- Increases in dosage should not exceed 100 mg/d over a 3 d period. Greater increments increase the seizure potential.
- Store away from heat and direct light as well as moist areas.

Assessment & Drug Effects
- Use extreme caution when administering drug to patient with history of seizures, cranial trauma, or other factors predisposing to seizures.
- During sudden and large increments in dose, seizure potential is increased.

- A substantial proportion of patients experience some degree of increased restlessness, agitation, anxiety, and insomnia. Symptoms may require treatment or discontinuation of drug.
- Monitor for delusions, hallucinations, psychotic episodes, confusion, and paranoia.
- May cause ECG changes such as premature beats and nonspecific ST-T changes with long-term use.
- Hepatic and renal function tests should be monitored while patient is on this drug.
- The full antidepressant effect of drug may not be realized for 4 or more weeks.

Patient & Family Education
- Drug should be taken at same times each day.
- Weight gain of ≥2 kg (5 lb.) may occur.
- Alcohol increases the risk of seizures. Therefore, its consumption should be minimized or preferably avoided.
- Ability to perform tasks requiring judgment or motor and cognitive skills may be impaired. Patient should refrain from driving or other hazardous activities until reaction to drug is known.
- Patient should check with physician before discontinuing this medication. Gradual dosage reduction may be necessary to prevent adverse effects.
- Advise patient not to take any OTC drugs without informing physician.

Prototype: lorazepam, p 177

BUSPIRONE HYDROCHLORIDE
(byoo-spye´rone)
Trade name: BuSpar
Classifications: CNS AGENT; ANXIOLYTIC
Pregnancy: Category B

ACTIONS/PHARMACODYNAMICS First generation agent in a new class of anxiolytics. Has chemical and pharmacologic properties unrelated to those of the benzodiazepines or other psychotherapeutic agents. Action is unclear but appears to be focused mainly on the brain dopamine system. Buspirone has agonist effects on presynaptic dopamine receptors and also a high affinity for serotonin receptors. Does not directly bind to the benzodiazepine–gamma aminobutyric acid (GABA)–chloride complex but may do so indirectly. Has slight alpha-adrenergic blocking action. Lacks the anticonvulsant, sedative,

Common side effects in *italic*; life-threatening effects <u>underlined</u>; generic names in **bold**; classifications in SMALL CAPS

muscle relaxant properties of the benzodiazepines, and its abuse potential appears to be minimal. Identifiable abstinence syndrome with withdrawal after long-term use has not been reported. Unlike other anxiolytics, it seems to cause less clinically significant impairment of cognitive and motor performance and produces minimal if any interaction with other brain depressants, including alcohol. Inhibits conditioned avoidance response and apomorphine-induced sterotypy without inducing catalepsy. Classed as a midbrain modulator because of its varied effects on midbrain receptors.

USES Management of anxiety disorders and for short-term treatment of generalized anxiety. **Unlabeled use:** adjuvant for nicotine withdrawal.

ROUTE & DOSAGE

Anxiety

Adult   PO   10–15 mg/d in divided doses; may increase by 5 mg/d q2–3d as needed (max 60 mg/d).

PHARMACOKINETICS Absorption: readily absorbed from GI tract but undergoes first pass metabolism. **Onset:** 5 7 d. **Peak:** 1 h. **Metabolism:** metabolized in liver. **Elimination:** half-life: 2–4 h; 30–63% excreted in urine as metabolites within 24 h.

CONTRAINDICATIONS & PRECAUTIONS Contraindicated in: safe use during pregnancy (category B), lactation, or in children <18 y not established. **Cautious use in:** renal or hepatic impairment.

ADVERSE/SIDE EFFECTS CNS: numbness, paresthesia, tremors, *dizziness, headache,* nervousness, *drowsiness,* lightheadedness, dream disturbances, decreased concentration, excitement, mood changes, depersonalization, akathesia, claustrophobia, cold intolerance. **CV:** tachycardia, palpitation, cardiac disorders. **ENT:** tinnitus, sore throat, nasal congestion. **Eye:** blurred vision, itching and redness of eyes. **GI:** *nausea,* vomiting, dry mouth, abdominal/gastric distress, diarrhea, constipation. **GU:** urinary frequency, hesitancy. **Musculoskeletal:** aches, pains, muscle cramps, spasms, stiffness, arthralgias. **Respiratory:** hyperventilation, shortness of breath. **Skin:** rash, edema, pruritus, flushing, easy bruising, hair loss, dry skin. **Other:** headache, fatigue, weakness, sweatiness, clamminess; roaring sensation in head, weight gain.

DIAGNOSTIC TEST INTERFERENCES Buspirone may increase serum concentrations of *hepatic aminotransferases* (ALT, AST).

DRUG INTERACTIONS MAO INHIBITORS, hypertension; **trazadone,** possible increase in liver transaminases; increased **haloperidol** serum levels.

NURSING IMPLICATIONS

Administration

- Administer with food to decrease first-pass metabolism. Rate of absorption may be delayed, but administration with food increases bioavailability of drug.
- Store at 15–30C (59–86F) in tightly closed container unless otherwise directed.

Assessment & Drug Effects

- May displace digoxin from its serum binding. This could increase the potential for toxic serum levels of digoxin. If the two drugs must be given concomitantly, monitor cardiovascular parameters (BP, pulse) until dosage has been stabilized.
- Benzodiazepines or sedative-hypnotic drugs are withdrawn gradually before buspirone therapy is started. Observe patient for rebound symptoms, which may occur over varying time periods during first phase of treatment.
- Involuntary movements may manifest in a small number of patients during early therapy. Symptoms include dystonia, motor restlessness, and involuntary repetitious movement of facial or cervical muscle and should be reported.
- Observe for swollen ankles, decreased urinary output, changes in voiding pattern. These symptoms as well as symptoms of hepatic impairment (jaundice, itching, nausea, vomiting) should be reported promptly.

Patient & Family Education

- Buspirone should be taken exactly as prescribed: specifically patient should not omit, skip, increase or decrease doses without advice of the physician.
- Concomitant self-medication with OTC drugs without advice of the physician should be discouraged.
- Desired therapeutic response may begin within 7–10 d; however, optimal results are not achieved for 3–4 wk. Inform patient of this expected lag in effects and reinforce the importance of continuing treatment.
- Compliance during the initial therapy period requires reinforcement because adverse/side effects usually appear early in therapy. Assure patient that these effects subside during continued therapy with or without dosage adjustment.
- Buspirone's CNS effects are not always predictable. Caution patient about driving or working with dan-

Common side effects in *italic*; life-threatening effects underlined; generic names in **bold**; classifications in SMALL CAPS

367

B

gerous equipment until reaction to the drug is known.
- Drug will be discontinued during pregnancy.
- Any changes that persist such as decreased acuity of smell, roaring noises in head, blurred vision, nightmares, weakness, should be reported.
- Patient should discuss limits of alcohol intake with physician. Cautious use is generally advised.
- Incidence of withdrawal or rebound symptoms when buspirone therapy is completed is low; when drug use is to be discontinued, be certain patient understands the planned schedule for changes in doses and intervals.

Prototype: cyclophosphamide, p 91

BUSULFAN

(byoo-sul´fan)
Trade name: Myleran
Classification: ANTINEOPLASTIC; ALKYLATING AGENT
Pregnancy: Category D

ACTIONS/PHARMACODYNAMICS Potent cytotoxic alkylating agent that may be a carcinogen in itself. Cell cycle nonspecific. Acts predominantly on slowly proliferating stem cells by inducing cross linkage in DNA, thus blocking replication and causing cell death. Reduces total granulocyte mass but has little effect on lymphocytes and platelets except in large doses. May cause widespread epithelial cellular dysplasia severe enough to make it difficult to interpret exfoliative cytologic examinations from lung, breast, bladder, and uterine cervix. May be mutagenic and carcinogenic. Acquired resistance may develop and is thought to be due to intracellular inactivation of busulfan before it reaches nuclear DNA.

USES Palliative treatment of chronic myelogenous (myeloid, granulocytic, myelocytic) leukemia for patients no longer responsive to radiation therapy or to previously tried antineoplastics. Does not appreciably extend survival time. **Unlabeled use:** polycythemia vera, severe thrombocytosis, and as adjunct in treatment of myelofibrosis.

PHARMACOKINETICS Absorption: readily absorbed from GI tract. **Peak:** 4 h. **Duration:** 4 h. **Metabolism:** metabolized in liver. **Elimination:** half-life: unknown; 10–50% excreted in urine within 48 h.

ROUTE & DOSAGE

Chronic Myelogenous Leukemia

Adult	PO	4–8 mg/d until maximal clinical and hematologic improvement; may use 1–4 mg/d if remission is shorter than 3 mo
Child	PO	0.06–0.12 mg/kg/d or 1.8–4.6 mg/m^2

CONTRAINDICATIONS & PRECAUTIONS Contraindicated in: therapy-resistant chronic lymphocytic leukemia; "blastic" crisis of chronic myelogenous leukemia; bone marrow depression, immunizations (patient and household members), chickenpox (including recent exposure), herpetic infections. Safe use during pregnancy (category D) and in nursing mothers not established. **Cautious use in:** men and women in childbearing years; history of gout or urate renal stones; prior irradiation or chemotherapy.

ADVERSE/SIDE EFFECTS Major toxic effects are related to bone marrow failure. **GI:** nausea, vomiting, diarrhea, glossitis, stomatitis, anorexia, GI bleeding. **GU:** flank pain, renal calculi, uric acid nephropathy, acute renal failure, gynecomastia, testicular atrophy, azoospermia, impotence, sterility in males, ovarian suppression, menstrual changes, amenorrhea (potentially irreversible), menopausal symptoms. **Hematologic:** agranulocytosis (rare), pancytopenia, thrombocytopenia, leukopenia, *anemia*. **Respiratory:** irreversible pulmonary fibrosis ("busulfan lung"). **Skin:** alopecia, hyperpigmentation. **Other:** endocardial fibrosis, dizziness, cholestatic jaundice, cataracts, myasthenia gravis, Addison-like syndrome; swelling of feet and lower legs, arthralgia, cellular dysplasia, superinfections, hemorrhagic complications.

DIAGNOSTIC TEST INTERFERENCES Busulfan may decrease **urinary 17-OHCS excretion,** and may increase **blood and urine uric acid** levels. Drug-induced cellular dysplasia may interfere with interpretation of **cytologic studies.**

DRUG INTERACTIONS Probenecid, sulfinpyrazone may increase uric acid levels.

NURSING IMPLICATIONS

Administration
- Medication should be taken at same time each day.
- Taking drug on an empty stomach may minimize nausea and vomiting.
- Store drug in tightly capped, light-resistant con-

Common side effects in *italic*; life-threatening effects underlined; generic names in **bold**; classifications in SMALL CAPS

tainer at 15–30C (59 and 86F), unless otherwise specified.

Assessment & Drug Effects

- Establish data base with flow chart, recording initial vital signs and weight.
- Hgb, Hct, total and differential WBC counts, platelet counts, liver and kidney function tests, serum uric acid are obtained initially and at least weekly during therapy with busulfan.
- During remission, patient is examined at monthly intervals at least. When total leukocyte count increases to approximately 50,000/mm³, induction dosage is resumed.
- With recommended dosage of busulfan, the normal leukocyte count is usually achieved in about 2 mo
- May be abrupt onset of hematotoxicity. Recovery from busulfan-induced pancytopenia may take 1 mo–2 y. It can be irreversible in some patients.
- Usually the WBC count does not start to decrease for about 10–15 d after therapy begins; it may actually increase during this period. Since the count continues to fall for more than 1 mo after busulfan is withdrawn, usually therapy will be discontinued when the total leukocyte count reaches approximately 15,000/mm³; i.e., before the count reaches normal range.
- Be alert to symptoms suggestive of superinfection (see Signs & Symptoms, chap 3), particularly when patient develops leukopenia.
- Remissions are characterized by increased appetite and sense of well-being within a few days after therapy begins.
- Weigh patient at least weekly. A slow but steady change in weight should be communicated to physician.
- Monitor I&O ratio and pattern. Urge patient to increase fluid intake to 10–12 (240 ml [8 oz]) glasses daily (if allowed) to assure adequate urinary output.
- Inspect skin and oral membranes daily and carefully examine urine and stools for abnormal bleeding due to thrombocytopenia. Ecchymotic or petechial bleeding, epistaxis, bleeding gums, cloudy or pink urine, and dark or black stools should be reported promptly.
- Auscultate lungs on a regular basis and monitor temperature. Advise patient to report immediately the onset of cough, low-grade fever, dyspnea, possible symptoms of pulmonary fibrosis (busulfan lung).
- Ovarian suppression and amenorrhea with menopausal symptoms commonly occur in premenopausal women. Effects are not apparent for 4–6 mo. Amenorrhea may be irreversible.

Patient & Family Education

- Busulfan should be taken as directed, at the same time each day.
- If possible, intrusive procedures should be avoided or at least limited during period of decreased platelet count. Caution patient to avoid trauma, floss teeth gently, use a soft toothbrush, and shave with a safety razor. Occult blood tests of urine, stool, and emesis may be indicated.
- Because of hyperpigmentation, signs of jaundice may be overlooked. Patient should report yellow sclera, dark urine, light-colored stools, abdominal discomfort, or pruritus.
- Instruct patient to report easy bruising or bleeding, sore mouth or throat, unusual fatigue (agranulocytosis), blurred vision (cataract), flank or joint pain, swelling of lower legs and feet (hyperuricemia).
- Contraceptive measures should be used during busulfan therapy and for at least 3 mo after drug is withdrawn.
- Discuss possibility of alopecia. Advise patient to brush hair gently and not more than is necessary.
- Busulfan is a highly toxic drug, and some patients eventually develop resistance to it. Keep follow-up appointments.

Prototype: phenobarbital, p 167

BUTABARBITAL SODIUM
(byoo-ta-bar´bi-tal)

Trade names: Barbased, Butalan, Butatran, Buticaps, Butisol Sodium, Day-Barb, Neo-Barb, Sarisol No. 2, Secbutobarbitone Sodium

Classifications: CNS AGENT; BARBITURATE ANXIOLYTIC, SEDATIVE-HYPNOTIC

Pregnancy: Category D

Controlled substance: Schedule III

ACTIONS/PHARMACODYNAMICS Intermediate-acting barbiturate, similar to phenobarbital. Appears to act at thalamus level, where it interferes with transmission of impulses to the cerebral cortex.

USES Hypnotic in short-term treatment of simple insomnia, as sedative for relief of anxiety, and to provide sedation preoperatively.

PHARMACOKINETICS Absorption: readily absorbed from GI tract. **Onset:** 40–60 min. **Peak:** 3–4 h.

Common side effects in *italic*; life-threatening effects <u>underlined</u>; generic names in **bold**; classifications in SMALL CAPS

369

Duration: 6–8 h. **Distribution:** crosses placenta; distributed into breast milk. **Metabolism:** metabolized in liver. **Elimination:** half-life: average 100 h; excreted in urine primarily as metabolites.

ROUTE & DOSAGE

Daytime Sedation

Adult	PO	15–30 mg t.i.d. or q.i.d.
Child	PO	7.5–30 mg t.i.d.

Preoperative Sedation

Adult	PO	50–100 mg 60–90 min before surgery
Child	PO	2–6 mg/kg in 3 equally divided doses (max 100 mg)

Hypnotic

Adult	PO	50–100 mg h.s.

CONTRAINDICATIONS & PRECAUTIONS Contraindicated in: porphyria; uncontrolled pain; severe respiratory disease; history of addiction. Pregnancy: category D. **Cautious use in:** renal or hepatic impairment.

ADVERSE/SIDE EFFECTS Drowsiness, *residual sedation* ("hangover"), headache, nausea, vomiting, constipation, diarrhea, urticaria, skin rash, muscle or joint pain.

DRUG INTERACTIONS Alcohol and other CNS DEPRESSANTS add to CNS and respiratory depression; butabarbital increases the metabolism of ORAL ANTICOAGULANTS, BETA BLOCKERS, CORTICOSTEROIDS, **doxycycline, griseofulvin, quinidine,** THEOPHYLLINES, ORAL CONTRACEPTIVES, decreasing their effectiveness.

NURSING IMPLICATIONS

Administration

- Prolonged administration is not recommended because tolerance to butabarbital occurs in about 14 d.
- Physical and psychological dependence may develop with prolonged use. Following long-term use, drug should be withdrawn slowly to avoid precipitating withdrawal symptoms.
- Store in tightly covered containers, preferably at 15–30C (59–86F), unless otherwise directed by manufacturer.

Assessment & Drug Effects

- Elderly and debilitated patients sometimes manifest morbid excitement, confusion, or depression. Some children also react with paradoxical excitement. Side rails may be advisable. Report these reactions to physician.

Patient & Family Education

- May cause drowsiness; caution patient not to drive and to avoid other potentially hazardous activities until reaction to drug is known.
- Advise patient not to drink alcoholic beverages while taking this drug. Other CNS depressants may produce additive drowsiness and should not be taken without approval of physician.

Prototype: amphotericin B, p 56

BUTOCONAZOLE NITRATE
(byoo-toe-koe´na-zole)
Trade name: Femstat
Classification: ANTIINFECTIVE; ANTIFUNGAL ANTIBIOTIC
Pregnancy: Category C

ACTIONS/PHARMACODYNAMICS Imidazole derivative with antifungal activity. Alters fungal cell membrane permeability, permitting loss of phosphorous compounds, potassium, and other essential intracellular constituents with consequent loss of ability to replicate. Action takes place primarily on medicated infected surface tissues. Has fungicidal activity against *Candida, Trichophyton, Microsporum,* and *Epidermophyton* as well as some gram-positive bacteria.

USES Local treatment of vulvovaginal candidiasis.

ROUTE & DOSAGE

Vulvovaginal Candidiasis

Adult	Topical	1 applicatorful intravaginally h.s. for 3 d; may be extended another 3 d if needed
Pregnant women	Topical	1 applicatorful intravaginally h.s. for 6 d

PHARMACOKINETICS Absorption: small amount absorbed systemically from intravaginal administration. **Distribution:** crosses placenta in animals. **Metabolism:** metabolized in liver. **Elimination:** half-life:

Common side effects in *italic*; life-threatening effects underlined; generic names in **bold**; classifications in SMALL CAPS

21–24 h; excreted in equal amounts in urine and feces within 4–7 d.

CONTRAINDICATIONS & PRECAUTIONS Contraindicated in: first trimester of pregnancy (category C). Safe use in nursing mothers and in children not established. Cautious use in: second and third trimester of pregnancy.

ADVERSE/SIDE EFFECTS Vulvar or vaginal burning, vulvar itching, discharge, soreness, swelling; itching of fingers; urinary frequency and burning; headache.

NURSING IMPLICATIONS

Administration

- The usual course of treatment is 3 d. Vulvovaginal candidiasis may be more difficult to control during pregnancy; consequently a 6 d regimen is commonly prescribed.
- Treatment should be continued even during menstruation.
- Store medication at 15–30C (59–86F); avoid extreme temperature and freezing.

Assessment & Drug Effects

- Candidiasis in nonpregnant women is usually controlled in 3 d.

Patient & Family Education

- Butoconazole can be used with oral contraceptives and antibiotic therapy.
- Caution patient to take medication exactly as prescribed; she should not increase or decrease dosage or discontinue or extend the treatment period. If symptoms (vaginal burning, discharge, or itching) persist, she should contact the physician. Drug should be discontinued if irritation occurs.
- Patient's sexual partner should wear a condom during intercourse.

Prototype: morphine, p 156

BUTORPHANOL TARTRATE

(byoo-tor´fa-nole)
Trade name: Stadol
Classifications: CNS AGENT; ANALGESIC; NARCOTIC (OPIATE) AGONIST-ANTAGONIST
Pregnancy: Category C

ACTIONS/PHARMACODYNAMICS Synthetic, centrally acting analgesic with mixed narcotic agonist and antagonist actions. Acts as agonist on one type of opioid receptor and as a competitive antagonist at others. Pharmacologic properties closely resemble those of pentazocine. Site of analgesic action believed to be subcortical, possibly in the limbic system. On a weight basis, analgesic potency appears to be about 5 times that of morphine, 40 times that of merperidine, and 15–30 times that of pentazocine. Narcotic antagonist potential is approximately 30 times that of pentazocine and 1/40 that of naloxone. Two milligrams of butorphanol produce about the same degree of respiratory depression as 10 mg morphine. Respiratory depression does not increase appreciably with higher doses, as it does with morphine, but duration of action increases. Like pentazocine, analgesic doses may increase pulmonary arterial pressure and cardiac work load. Appears to have low potential for dependence. Tends to inhibit release of antidiuretic hormone (ADH) from hypothalamus.

USES Relief of moderate to severe pain, preoperative or preanesthetic sedation and analgesia, obstetrical analgesia during labor, cancer pain, renal colic, burns. Unlabeled use: musculoskeletal and postepesiotomy pain.

ROUTE & DOSAGE

Pain Relief

Adult	IM	1–4 mg q3–4h as needed (max 4 mg/dose)
	IV	0.5–2 mg q3–4h as needed

PHARMACOKINETICS Onset: 10–30 min IM; 1 min IV. Peak: 0.5–1 h IM; 4–5 min IV. Duration: 3–4 h IM; 2–4 h IV. Distribution: crosses placenta; distributed into breast milk. Metabolism: metabolized in liver in inactive metabolites. Elimination: half-life: 3–4 h; excreted primarily in urine.

CONTRAINDICATIONS & PRECAUTIONS Contraindicated in: narcotic-dependent patients. Safe use during pregnancy prior to labor (category C), in nursing women, and in children <18 y not established. Cautious use in: history of drug abuse or dependence, emotionally unstable individuals; head injury, increased intracranial pressure; acute MI, ventricular dysfunction, coronary insufficiency, hypertension; patients undergoing biliary tract surgery; respiratory depression, bronchial asthma, obstructive respiratory disease; and renal or hepatic dysfunction.

Common side effects in *italic*; life-threatening effects <u>underlined</u>; generic names in **bold**; classifications in SMALL CAPS

371

ADVERSE/SIDE EFFECTS CNS: drowsiness, *sedation,* headache, vertigo, dizziness, floating feeling, weakness, lethargy, confusion, light-headedness, insomnia, nervousness, <u>respiratory depression</u>. **CV:** increase or decrease in BP, palpitation, bradycardia. **GI:** nausea. **Skin:** clammy skin, tingling sensation, flushing and warmth, cyanosis of extremities, diaphoresis, sensitivity to cold, skin rash, urticaria, pruritus. **Other:** transient increase in urinary output, difficulty in urinating; biliary spasm, tinnitus.

DRUG INTERACTIONS Alcohol and other CNS DEPRESSANTS augment CNS and respiratory depression.

INCOMPATIBILITIES Solution/additive: dimenhydrinate, pentobarbital. Y-site: pentobarbital.

NURSING IMPLICATIONS

Administration

- IV butorphanol tartrate may be given undiluted at a rate of 2 mg over 3–5 min.
- Store at 15–30C (59–86F) unless otherwise directed. Protect from light.

Assessment & Drug Effects

- Monitor for respiratory depression. Do not administer drug if respiratory rate is <12 breaths/min.
- Monitor vital signs. Report marked changes in BP or bradycardia.
- If butorphanol is used during labor or delivery, observe neonate for signs of respiratory depression.
- When prescirbed for emotionally unstable patients, butorphanol should be used only for relief of pain and never in anticipation of pain.
- Butorphanol has habit-forming potential.
- Because butorphanol has agonist as well as antagonist actions, it can induce acute withdrawal symptoms in opiate-dependent patients.
- Abrupt withdrawal following chronic administration may produce vomiting, loss of appetite, restlessness, abdominal cramps, increase in BP and temperature, mydriasis, faintness. Withdrawal symptoms peak 48 h after discontinuation of drug.

Patient & Family Education

- Drug-induced nausea may be controlled by lying down.
- Warn patient not to take alcohol or other CNS depressant without consulting physician because of possible additive effects.
- Butorphanol causes sedation and dizziness; therefore, observe safety precautions.

CAFFEINE

See CNS AGENTS, XANTHINE RESPIRATORY & CEREBRAL STIMULANT prototype, p 197.

CALCIFEDIOL (25-HYDROXYVITAMIN D$_3$)

(kal-si-fe-dye´ole)
Trade name: Calderol
Classifications: HORMONE; VITAMIN D ANALOG
Pregnancy: Category C

ACTIONS/PHARMACODYNAMICS Vitamin D analog and major transport form of cholecalciferol (D$_3$); fat soluble. Because it is activated in the body and has regulatory effects, it is considered a hormone. Primary action leads to regulation of serum calcium, which is affected also by the activity of other vitamin D analogs (e.g., ergocalciferol), parathyroid hormone, and calcitonin. Pharmacologic effects of calcifediol are related to its intrinsic vitamin D activity as well as to the properties of active metabolites (e.g., calcitriol), which result from renal metabolism.

USES Management of metabolic bone disease and hypocalcemia associated with chronic renal failure in patients undergoing renal dialysis. **Unlabeled uses:** osteopenia caused by prolonged glucocorticoid therapy and osteomalacia secondary to hepatic disease.

ROUTE & DOSAGE

Metabolic Bone Disease in Patients with Chronic Renal Failure

Adult	PO	Initially 300–350 µg/wk administered on a daily or alternate day schedule; may increase at 4 wk intervals if necessary; patients with normal calcium may only need 20 µg q.o.d. (usual range 50–100 µg/d *or* 100–200 µg q.o.d.)

PHARMACOKINETICS Absorption: readily absorbed from small intestines. **Peak:** 4 h. **Duration:** 15–20 d. **Distribution:** stored chiefly in liver and fat deposits. **Metabolism:** activated in kidneys. **Elimination:** half-life: 12–22 d; excreted primarily in bile and feces.

Common side effects in *italic*; life-threatening effects <u>underlined</u>; generic names in **bold**; classifications in SMALL CAPS

CONTRAINDICATIONS & PRECAUTIONS Contraindicated in: hypersensitivity to vitamin D, vitamin D toxicity, hypercalcemia. Safe use of doses in excess of RDA during pregnancy (category C), in nursing women, and in children not established. **Cautious use in:** patients receiving digitalis glycosides.

ADVERSE/SIDE EFFECTS Vitamin D intoxication and hypercalcemia. **CNS:** drowsiness, lethargy, headache, weakness, vertigo. **Eye:** blurred vision, photophobia, conjunctivitis. **GI:** anorexia, nausea, vomiting, dry mouth, thirst, constipation, diarrhea, abdominal cramps, metallic taste. **Other:** muscle or bone pain, polyuria, hypercalciuria, hyperphosphatemia; idiosyncratic reaction (headache, nausea, vomiting, diarrhea, fever).

DRUG INTERACTIONS THIAZIDE DIURETICS may cause hypercalcemia; calcifediol-induced hypercalcemia may decrease the effectiveness of **verapamil** and other CALCIUM CHANNEL BLOCKERS; calcifediol-induced hypercalcemia may precipitate digitalis arrhythmias in patients taking DIGITALIS GLYCOSIDES.

NURSING IMPLICATIONS

Administration

- Can be taken without regard to food.
- Patients undergoing dialysis may require aluminum carbonate or hydroxide gels to bind intestinal phosphate and thus lower serum phosphate levels.
- Since calcitriol is a metabolite of vitamin D_3, all sources of vitamin D are usually withheld during therapy or at least must be considered when calculating dosage.
- Store at 15–30C (59–86F) in tightly covered, light-resistant container unless otherwise directed.

Assessment & Drug Effects

- Baseline and periodic determinations should be made of serum calcium, phosphorus, magnesium, and alkaline phosphatase, and urinary calcium and phosphorus levels should be measured q24h.
- Effectiveness of therapy depends on an adequate daily intake of calcium. Since dietary calcium and phosphate are difficult to control, the physician may prescribe a calcium supplement as needed.
- Serum calcium levels particularly should be monitored at least once weekly, or whenever dosage adjustments are made, and at periodic intervals thereafter.
- Monitor for manifestations of hypercalcemia (see Signs & Symptoms, chap 3). If hypercalcemia oc-

curs, calcifediol should be discontinued until serum calcium returns to normal (9–10.6 mg/dl).
- A fall in serum alkaline phosphatase usually signals the onset of hypercalcemia.

Patient & Family Education

- Instruct patient to withhold drug and report immediately signs and symptoms of hypercalcemia (see chap 3).
- Advise patient to consult physician before taking an OTC medication. Calcium, phosphate, or magnesium-containing laxatives and antacids, mineral oil, and vitamin D preparations may increase side effects of calcifediol and therefore should be avoided.

CALCITONIN (HUMAN)
(kal-si-toe′nin)
Trade name: Cibacalcin

CALCITONIN (SALMON)
Trade names: Calcimar, Miacalcin
Classification: HORMONE; BONE METABOLISM REGULATOR
Pregnancy: Category C

ACTIONS/PHARMACODYNAMICS Calcitonin human and calcitonin salmon are synthetic polypeptides. Pharmacologic actions are the same, but calcitonin salmon is considerably more potent and has a longer duration of action. Antibody formation occurs commonly with calcitonin salmon and only rarely with calcitonin human. Calcitonin opposes the effects of parathyroid hormone on bone and kidneys, reduces serum calcium by binding to specific receptor site on osteoclast cell membrane, and alters transmembrane passage of calcium and phosphorus. Inhibition of osteoclastic bone resorption decreases both mineral release and collagen breakdown. Promotes renal excretion of calcium and phosphorus and causes transient sodium and water loss. Decreased volume and acidity of gastric juice and decreased volume of pancreatic trypsin and amylase are also transient effects. In Paget's disease, slows rate of bone turnover, with resultant decreases in serum alkaline phosphatase and urinary hydroxyproline, biochemical changes that seem to correspond to more normal bone formation. In some patients, long-term use initiates drug resistance through formation of neutralizing antibodies.

Common side effects in *italic*; life-threatening effects underlined; generic names in **bold**; classifications in SMALL CAPS

373

USES Treatment of symptomatic Paget's disease of bone (osteitis deformans). **Orphan drug approval (calcitonin human):** short-term adjunctive treatment of severe hypercalcemic emergencies, and in treatment of postmenopausal osteoporosis. **Unlabeled use:** diagnosis and management of medullary carcinoma of thyroid; treatment of osteogenesis imperfecta.

ROUTE & DOSAGE

Paget's Disease

Adult	SC	Human 0.5 mg/d or 2–3 times/wk or 0.25 mg/d up to 0.5 mg b.i.d.
	SC/IM	Salmon 100 IU/d; may decrease to 50–100 IU/d or q.o.d.

Hypercalcemia

Adult	SC/IM	Salmon 4 IU/kg q12h; may increase to 8 U/kg q6h if needed

Postmenopausal Osteoporosis

Adult	SC/IM	Salmon 100 IU/d

PHARMACOKINETICS (SALMON CALCITONIN).
Onset: 15 min. **Peak:** 4 h. **Duration:** 8–24 h. **Distribution:** does not cross placenta; distribution into breast milk unknown. **Metabolism:** metabolized in kidneys. **Elimination:** half-life: 1.25 h (1 h for human calcitonin); excreted in urine.

CONTRAINDICATIONS & PRECAUTIONS **Con-traindicated in:** hypersensitivity to fish proteins or to synthetic calcitonins; history of allergy. Safe use in children, pregnancy (category C), nursing mothers not established. **Cautious use in:** renal impairment; osteoporosis; pernicious anemia; Zollinger-Ellison syndrome.

ADVERSE/SIDE EFFECTS **GI:** *transient nausea,* vomiting, anorexia, unusual taste sensation, abdominal pain, diarrhea. **Skin:** inflammatory reactions at injection site, flushing of face or hands, pruritus of ear lobes, edema of feet, skin rashes. **Other:** headache, eye pain, nocturia, diuresis, feverish sensation, hypersensitivity reactions, <u>anaphylaxis</u>, abnormal urine sediment. Reported for calcitonin human only: urinary frequency, chills, chest pressure, weakness, paresthesias, tender palms and soles, dizziness, nasal congestion, shortness of breath, mild hypercalcemia (asymptomatic).

NURSING IMPLICATIONS

Administration

- Note that calcitonin human is administered only by SC injection; dosages are smaller than those of calcitonin salmon and are expressed in milligrams. Calcitonin salmon may be administered by SC or IM injection.
- When the volume of calcitonin salmon to be injected is more than 2 ml, the IM route is employed. Rotate injection sites.
- The transient flushing that commonly occurs following injection of calcitonin, particularly during early therapy, may be minimized by administrating the drug at bedtime. Consult physician.
- Store calcitonin (human) at 25C (77F) or less, protected from light, unless otherwise specified by manufacturer.
- Store calcitonin (salmon) in refrigerator, preferably at 2–8C (36–46F) unless otherwise directed.

Assessment & Drug Effects

- An allergy skin test is usually done prior to initiation of therapy. The appearance of more than mild erythema or wheal 15 min after intracutaneous injection indicates that the drug should not be given.
- Have on hand epinephrine 1:1000, antihistamines, oxygen in the event of a reaction. Also have readily available parenteral calcium, particularly during early therapy. Hypocalcemic tetany is a theoretical possibility.
- Periodic laboratory examination of urine specimens for sediment is recommended with long-term therapy.
- Monitor for hypocalcemia (see Signs & Symptoms, chap 3). Theoretically, calcitonin can lead to hypocalcemic tetany. Latent tetany may be demonstrated by Chvostek's or Trousseau's signs and by serum calcium values: 7–8 mg/dl (latent tetany); below 7 mg/dl (manifest tetany).

Patient & Family Education

- SC route is preferred for self-administration.
- Teach patient to recognize and seek advice about local inflammatory reaction at site of injection.
- Teach patient the importance of maintaining drug regimen even though symptoms have been ameliorated, to prevent early relapses.
- Advise patient to consult physician before using OTC preparations. Some supervitamins, hematinics, and antacids contain calcium and vitamin D (vitamin may antagonize calcitonin effects).

Common side effects in *italic*; life-threatening effects <u>underlined</u>; generic names in **bold**; classifications in SMALL CAPS

CALCITRIOL

(kal-si-trye´ole)
Trade name: Calcifex, Rocaltrol
Classifications: HORMONE; VITAMIN D ANALOG
Pregnancy: Category C

ACTIONS/PHARMACODYNAMICS Synthetic form of an active metabolite of ergocalciferol (vitamin D_2). In the liver, cholecalciferol (vitamin D_3) and ergocalciferol (vitamin D_2) are enzymatically metabolized to calcifediol, an activated form of vitamin D_3. Calcifediol is biodegraded in the kidney to calcitriol, the most potent form of vitamin D_3. Patients with nonfunctioning kidneys are unable to synthesize sufficient calcitriol and therefore must receive it pharmacologically. By promoting intestinal absorption and renal retention of calcium, calcitriol elevates serum calcium levels, decreases elevated blood levels of phosphatase and parathyroid hormone, and decreases subperiosteal bone resorption and mineralization defects in some patients.

USES Management of hypocalcemia in patients undergoing chronic renal dialysis and in patients with hypoparathyroidism or pseudohypoparathyroidism. **Unlabeled use:** in selected patients with vitamin D–dependent rickets, familial hypophosphatemia (vitamin D–resistant rickets), and in management of hypocalcemia in premature infants.

ROUTE & DOSAGE

Hypocalcemia

Adult	PO	0.25 µg/d; may be increased by 0.25 µg/d q4–8wk for dialysis patients or q2–4wk for hypoparathyroid patients if necessary
	IV	0.5 µg 3 times/wk at the end of dialysis; may need up to 3 µg 3 times/wk
Child	PO	On hemodialysis: 0.25–2 µg/d
		Renal failure without dialysis: 0.014–0.041 µg/kg/d

PHARMACOKINETICS Absorption: readily absorbed from GI tract. **Onset:** 2–6 h. **Peak:** 10–12 h. **Duration:** 3–5 d. **Metabolism:** metabolized in liver. **Elimination:** half-life: 3–6 h; excreted mainly in feces.

CONTRAINDICATIONS & PRECAUTIONS Contraindicated in: hypercalcemia or vitamin D toxicity. Safe use during pregnancy (category C), in nursing women, and in children not established. **Cautious use in:** hyperphosphatemia, patients receiving digitalis glycosides.

ADVERSE/SIDE EFFECTS Vitamin D intoxication and hypercalcemia. **CNS:** drowsiness, headache, weakness. **Eye:** blurred vision, conjunctivitis, photophobia. **GI:** anorexia, nausea, vomiting, dry mouth, thirst, constipation, abdominal cramps, metallic taste. **Other:** palpitation, increased urination, runny nose, muscle or bone pain, hypercalciuria, hyperphosphatemia.

DRUG INTERACTIONS THIAZIDE DIURETICS may cause hypercalcemia; calcifediol-induced hypercalcemia may decrease the effectiveness of **verapamil** and other CALCIUM CHANNEL BLOCKERS; calcifediol-induced hypercalcemia may precipitate digitalis arrhythmias in patients receiving DIGITALIS GLYCOSIDES.

NURSING IMPLICATIONS

Administration

- Calcitriol is given direct IV over 30–60 seconds.
- Oral dose can be taken either with food or milk or on an empty stomach. Discuss with physician.
- When given for hypoparathyroidism, the dose is given in the morning.
- Effectiveness of therapy depends on an adequate daily intake of calcium and phosphate. The physician may prescribe a calcium supplement on an as-needed basis.
- Patients undergoing dialysis may require aluminum carbonate or hydroxide gels to bind intestinal phosphate and thus lower serum phosphate levels.
- Capsules should be protected from heat, light, and moisture. Store in tightly closed container, preferably at 15–30C (59–86F) unless otherwise directed.

Assessment & Drug Effects

- Baseline and periodic determinations should be made of serum calcium, phosphorus, magnesium, alkaline phosphatase, creatinine; urinary calcium and phosphorus levels should be measured q24h.
- Monitor for hypercalcemia (see Signs & Symptoms, chap 3). During dosage adjustment period, serum calcium levels particularly should be monitored twice weekly to avoid hypercalcemia.
- Excessive intake of calcium and phosphate can cause hypercalcemia, hypercalciuria, and hyperphosphatemia.

- If hypercalcemia develops, calcitriol and calcium supplements should be discontinued until serum calcium returns to normal. Reduction of dietary calcium intake should also be considered.

Patient & Family Education

- Review symptoms of hypercalcemia (see chap 3) and advise patient to withhold drug and contact physician if they occur.
- Since calcitriol is the most potent form of vitamin D$_3$, all sources of vitamin D should be withheld during therapy to avoid possibility of hypercalcemia.
- Advise patient to consult physician before taking an OTC medication. (Many products contain calcium, vitamin D, phosphates, or magnesium, which can increase adverse effects of calcitriol.)
- Patients with normal renal function should maintain an adequate fluid intake.

Prototype: calcium gluconate, p 204

CALCIUM CARBONATE

Trade names: Amitone, Apo-Cal, BioCal, Calcite-500, Calsan, Cal-Sup, Caltrate, Chooz, Dicarbosil, Equilet, Mallamint, Mega-Cal, Nu-Cal, Os-Cal, Oystercal, Titralac, Tums
Classifications: ELECTROLYTIC BALANCE AGENT; REPLACEMENT SOLUTION; ANTACID
Pregnancy: Category C

ACTIONS/PHARMACODYNAMICS Rapid-acting antacid with high neutralizing capacity and relatively prolonged duration of action. Decreases gastric acidity (raises gastric pH), thereby inhibiting proteolytic action of pepsin on gastric mucosa. (Pepsin is inactivated above pH 4.) Also increases lower esophageal sphincter tone. Although classified as a nonsystemic antacid, a slight to moderate alkalosis usually develops with prolonged therapy. Acid rebound, which may follow even low doses, is thought to be caused by release of gastrin triggered by action of calcium in small intestines. Liberation of carbon dioxide in stomach causes belching in some patients.

USES Relief of transient symptoms of hyperacidity as in acid indigestion, heartburn, peptic esophagitis, and hiatal hernia. Also used as calcium supplement when calcium intake may be inadequate and in treatment of mild calcium deficiency states. **Unlabeled use:** for treatment of hyperphosphatemia in patients with chronic renal failure and to lower BP in selected patients with hypertension.

ROUTE & DOSAGE

All doses are in terms of *elemental calcium;* 1 g calcium carbonate = 400 mg (20 mEq) elemental calcium

Supplement for Osteoporosis
Adult   PO   1–2 g b.i.d. or t.i.d.

Antacid
Adult   PO   0.5–2 g 4–6 times/d

PHARMACOKINETICS Absorption: approximately 1/3 of dose absorbed from small intestine. **Distribution:** crosses placenta. **Elimination:** primarily excreted in feces; small amounts excreted in urine, pancreatic juice, saliva, and breast milk.

CONTRAINDICATIONS & PRECAUTIONS Contraindicated in: hypercalcemia and hypercalciuria (e.g., hyperparathyroidism, vitamin D overdosage, decalcifying tumors, bone metastases), calcium loss due to immobilization, severe renal disease, renal calculi, GI hemorrhage or obstruction, dehydration, hypochloremic alkalosis, ventricular fibrillation, cardiac disease, pregnancy (category C). **Cautious use in:** decreased bowel motility (e.g., patients receiving anticholinergics, antidiarrheals, antispasmodics), elderly patients.

ADVERSE/SIDE EFFECTS *Constipation* or laxative effect, acid rebound, nausea, eructation, *flatulence*. With prolonged use of high doses: hypercalcemia with alkalosis and conjunctival and episcleral suffusion; metastatic calcinosis, hypercalciuria, hypomagnesemia, hypophosphatemia (when phosphate intake is low), mood and mental changes, polyuria, renal calculi, renal dysfunction, vomiting, GI hemorrhage, fecal concretions, appendicolithiasis, milk-alkali syndrome.

DRUG INTERACTIONS May enhance inotropic and toxic effects of **digoxin; magnesium** may compete for GI absorption; decreases absorption of TETRACYCLINES, QUINOLONES **(ciprofloxacin);** antagonizes the effects of **verapamil** and possibly other CALCIUM CHANNEL BLOCKERS.

Common side effects in *italic*; life-threatening effects <u>underlined</u>; generic names in **bold**; classifications in SMALL CAPS

NURSING IMPLICATIONS

Administration

- When used as antacid, it is taken 1 h after meals and at bedtime. When used as calcium supplement, it is taken 1–1 1/2 h after meals, unless otherwise directed by physician.
- Chewable tablet should be chewed well before swallowing or allowed to dissolve completely in mouth, followed with water. Powder form may be mixed with water.
- Store at 15–30C (59–86F) in tightly closed container unless otherwise directed.

Assessment & Drug Effects

- Note number and consistency of stools. If constipation is a problem, physician may prescribe alternate or combination therapy with a magnesium antacid or advise patient to take a laxative or stool softener as necessary.
- Weekly serum and urine calcium determinations are recommended in patients receiving prolonged therapy and in patients with renal dysfunction.
- Record amelioration of symptoms of hypocalcemia (see Signs & Symptoms, chap 3).
- Observe for signs and symptoms of hypercalcemia in patients receiving frequent or high doses, or who have impaired renal function (see Signs & Symptoms, chap 3).

Patient & Family Education

- Because of acid rebound, which generally occurs after repeated use for 1 or 2 wk, one can quickly become a chronic user of calcium carbonate. Explain to patient the potential dangers of self-medication. Caution not to take antacids longer than 2 wk without medical supervision.
- Avoid taking calcium carbonate with cereals or other foods high in oxylates. Oxalates combine with calcium carbonate to form insoluble, nonabsorbable compounds.
- Chronic use of calcium carbonate taken together with foods high in vitamin D (such as milk) or sodium bicarbonate can cause *milk-alkali syndrome:* hypercalcemia, distaste for food, headache, confusion, nausea, vomiting, abdominal pain, metabolic alkalosis, hypercalciuria, polyuria, soft tissue calcification (calcinosis), hyperphosphatemia and renal insufficiency. Predisposing factors include renal dysfunction, dehydration, electrolyte imbalance, and hypertension.

Prototype: calcium gluconate, p 204

CALCIUM CHLORIDE

Classifications: ELECTROLYTIC BALANCE AGENT; REPLACEMENT SOLUTION
Pregnancy: Category C

ACTIONS/PHARMACODYNAMICS Actions similar to those of calcium gluconate. Ionizes more readily and thus is more potent than calcium gluconate and more irritating to tissues. Provides excess chloride ions that promote acidosis and temporary (1–2 d) diuresis secondary to excretion of sodium.

USES Treatment of cardiac resuscitation when epinephrine fails to improve myocardial contractions; for treatment of acute hypocalcemia (as in tetany due to parathyroid deficiency, vitamin D deficiency, alkalosis, insect bites or stings, and during exchange transfusions), for treatment of hypermagnesemia, and for cardiac disturbances of hyperkalemia.

ROUTE & DOSAGE

All doses are in terms of *elemental calcium;* 1 g calcium chloride = 272 mg (13.6 mEq) elemental calcium

Hypocalcemia

Adult	IV	0.5–1 g (7–14 mEq) at 1–3 d intervals as determined by patient response and serum calcium levels
Child	IV	25 mg/kg (1–7 mEq) administered slowly
Neonate	IV	<1 mEq/d

Hypocalcemic Tetany

Adult	IV	4.5–16 mEq prn
Child	IV	0.5–0.7 mEq/kg t.i.d. or q.i.d.
Neonate	IV	2.4 mEq/kg/d in divided doses

CPR

Adult	IV	2.7–3.7 mEq x 1

PHARMACOKINETICS Distribution: crosses placenta. **Elimination:** primarily excreted in feces; small amounts excreted in urine, pancreatic juice, saliva, and breast milk.

Common side effects in *italic*; life-threatening effects <u>underlined</u>; generic names in **bold**; classifications in SMALL CAPS

377

CONTRAINDICATIONS & PRECAUTIONS Contraindicated in: ventricular fibrillation, hypercalcemia, digitalis toxicity, injection into myocardium or other tissue. Safe use during pregnancy (category C), in nursing women, and in children not established. **Cautious use in:** digitalized patients; sarcoidosis, renal insufficiency, history of renal stone formation; cor pulmonale, respiratory acidosis, respiratory failure.

ADVERSE/SIDE EFFECTS Tingling sensation, chalky taste. With rapid IV, sensations of heat waves (peripheral vasodilation), fainting, hypotension, bradycardia, cardiac arrhythmias, <u>cardiac arrest</u>, pain and burning at IV site, severe venous thrombosis, necrosis and sloughing (with extravasation).

DRUG INTERACTIONS May enhance inotropic and toxic effects of **digoxin;** antagonizes the effects of **verapamil** and possibly other CALCIUM CHANNEL BLOCKERS.

NURSING IMPLICATIONS

Administration

- Solution should be warmed to body temperature before administration.
- May be given undiluted or diluted (preferred) with an equal volume of NS for injection. Give at a rate of 0.5–1 ml/min or slower if irritation develops.
- IV injection should be made through small-bore needle into a large vein to minimize venous irritation and undesirable reactions.
- Severe thromboses of peripheral veins have been reported in patients receiving calcium chloride by IV push for treatment of hypovolemic shock.
- Extravasation must be avoided during IV injection, since cellulitis, necrosis, and sloughing can result. Local necrosis can occur with leakage from vein. If given IV to children, scalp veins should be avoided.
- Calcium chloride should never be given subcutaneously or IM or by gavage, as it is a tissue irritant.
- The presence of alkalosis reduces ionization and thus absorption of calcium chloride. The presence of acidosis has the opposite effect.
- Calcium chloride is incompatible with bicarbonates, carbonates, phosphates, sulfates, and tartrates. Consult pharmacist for compatible admixtures.
- Store at 15–30C (59–86F) unless otherwise directed.

Assessment & Drug Effects

- Monitor ECG, BP, and flow rate and observe patient closely during administration.

- IV injection may be accompanied by cutaneous burning sensation and peripheral vasodilation, with moderate fall in BP. Following injection, advise ambulatory patient to remain in bed for 15–30 min or more depending on response.
- Digitalized patients must be closely observed since an increase in serum calcium increases risk of digitalis toxicity.
- Frequent determinations of serum pH, calcium, and other electrolytes should be performed as guides to dosage adjustments.

Prototype: calcium gluconate, p 204

CALCIUM GLUCEPTATE

(gloo-sep´tate)
Classifications: ELECTROLYTIC BALANCE AGENT; REPLACEMENT SOLUTION
Pregnancy: Category C

ACTIONS/PHARMACODYNAMICS Contains approximately 8% calcium per gram. Similar to calcium gluconate in actions, uses, and contraindications and precautions but reportedly is less irritating. Preferred for use when IM administration is required as in neonatal tetany. Contains 82 mg (4.1 mEq) of calcium per gram.

USES To correct hypocalcemia and following each 100 ml of exchange transfusion in newborns.

ROUTE & DOSAGE

All doses are in terms of *elemental calcium;* 1 g calcium gluceptate = 82 mg (4.1 mEq) elemental calcium

Hypocalcemia

Adult	IV	1.1–4.4 g/d
	IM	0.5–1.1 g/d

Exchange Transfusions with Citrated Blood

Neonate	IV	0.5 ml after each 100 ml of blood exchanged

PHARMACOKINETICS Duration: 2–3 h IV; 1–4 h IM. **Distribution:** crosses placenta. **Elimination:** primarily excreted in feces; small amounts excreted in urine, pancreatic juice, saliva, and breast milk.

DRUG INTERACTIONS May enhance inotropic and toxic effects of **digoxin**; antagonizes the effects of **verapamil** and possibly other CALCIUM CHANNEL BLOCKERS.

NURSING IMPLICATIONS

Administration

- May be given undiluted by direct IV at a rate not to exceed 1 ml/min or slower if irritation develops.
- Patient may complain of a transient tingling sensation and metallic taste following IV administration.
- IM injection may produce mild local reactions. Generally, this route is used only in adults when IV administration is not feasible.
- Recommended IM site for adults is the upper outer quadrant of the buttock and in infants (if prescribed) the midlateral thigh.

See calcium gluconate for additonal nursing implications, contraindications & precautions, and adverse/side effects.

CALCIUM GLUCONATE

See ELECTROLYTIC BALANCE AGENT, REPLACEMENT SOLUTION prototype, p 204.

Prototype: calcium gluconate, p 204

CALCIUM LACTATE
(lak´tate)
Classifications: ELECTROLYTIC BALANCE AGENT; REPLACEMENT SOLUTION

ACTIONS/PHARMACODYNAMICS Oral calcium preparation reportedly well tolerated. Similar to calcium gluconate in actions, contraindications, and adverse reactions. Contains 13% elemental calcium (130 mg/g).

USES Mild hypocalcemia and maintenance calcium therapy.

PHARMACOKINETICS Absorption: approximately 1/3 of dose absorbed from small intestine. **Distribution:** crosses placenta. **Elimination:** primarily excreted in feces; small amounts excreted in urine, pancreatic juice, saliva, and breast milk.

ROUTE & DOSAGE

All doses are in terms of *elemental calcium;* 1 g calcium lactate = 130 mg (6.5 mEq) elemental calcium

Supplement for Mild Hypocalcemia		
Adult	PO	325 mg–1.3 g t.i.d. with meals
Child	PO	500 mg/kg/d in divided doses

DRUG INTERACTIONS May enhance inotropic and toxic effects of **digoxin; magnesium** may compete for GI absorption; decreases absorption of TETRACYCLINES, QUINOLONES **(ciprofloxacin);** antagonizes the effects of **verapamil** and possibly other CALCIUM CHANNEL BLOCKERS.

NURSING IMPLICATIONS

Administration

- Tablets or powder can be dissolved in hot water; then add cool water to patient's taste.
- May be administered with lactose (amount pre scribed) to increase solubility.
- Store in airtight containers.

Assessment & Drug Effects

- Monitor for hypercalcemia (see Signs & Symptoms, chap 3).
- Blood calcium levels should be checked periodically. Hypercalcemia can occur during prolonged administration particularly if patient is also taking vitamin D.
- Bear in mind that an increase in serum calcium in digitalized patients increases risk of digitalis toxicity.

Patient & Family Education

- Advise patient to confer with physician regarding need for vitamin D supplementation.
- Advise patient that calcium absorption can be inhibited by zinc-rich foods such as nuts, sprouts, legumes, and soy products.

Prototype: psyllium hydrophilic muciloid, p 219

CALCIUM POLYCARBOPHIL
(pol-ee-kar´boe-fil)
Trade names: FiberCon, Mitrolan
Classifications: GI AGENT; BULK LAXATIVE; ANTIDIARRHEAL
Pregnancy: Category C

Common side effects in *italic*; life-threatening effects underlined; generic names in **bold**; classifications in SMALL CAPS

379

ACTIONS/PHARMACODYNAMICS Hydrophilic, bulk-producing laxative that restores normal moisture level and bulk content of intestinal tract. In constipation, retains free water in intestinal lumen, thereby indirectly opposing dehydrating forces of the bowel; in diarrhea, when intestinal mucosa is incapable of absorbing fluid, drug absorbs fecal fluid to form a gel. In both conditions, peristalsis is encouraged and a well-formed stool is produced.

USES Constipation or diarrhea associated with diverticulitis or irritable bowel syndrome; acute nonspecific diarrhea.

ROUTE & DOSAGE

Constipation or Diarrhea

Adult	PO	1 g q.i.d. as needed (max 6 g/24 h)
Child	PO	6–12 y: 500 mg 1–3 times/d (max 3 g/24 h)
		< 6 y: 500 mg 1–2 times/d (max 1.5 g/24 h)

CONTRAINDICATIONS & PRECAUTIONS Contraindicated in: GI obstruction; children <6 y. **Cautious use in:** pregnancy (category C); nursing mothers.

ADVERSE/SIDE EFFECTS *Flatulence,* abdominal fullness, <u>intestinal obstruction</u>; laxative dependence (long-term use).

NURSING IMPLICATIONS

Administration

- Tablets should be chewed before swallowing them. Administer with at least 180–240 ml (6–8 oz) water or other fluid of patient's choice when used as a laxative and with at least 60–90 ml (2–3 oz) of fluid when used as an antidiarrheal. Chewed tablets should not be swallowed dry.
- If diarrhea is severe, dose can be repeated every half hour up to maximum daily dose.
- Store at 15–30C (59–86F).

Assessment & Drug Effects

- Evaluate effectiveness of medication. If it is ineffective as an antidiarrheal, report to physician.
- Rectal bleeding, very dark stools, or abdominal pain should be reported promptly.

Patient & Family Education

- Drug generally produces a bowel movement within 12–72 h.

- This is an OTC product. Discuss with patient the importance of taking the drug exactly as ordered. Patient should be cautioned not to increase the dose if response is inadequate. Consult physician. Advise patients not to use another laxative while they are taking calcium polycarbophil.

Prototype: isoniazid, p 83

CAPREOMYCIN SULFATE
(kap-ree-oh-mye´sin)
Trade name: Capastat Sulfate
Classifications: ANTIINFECTIVE; ANTITUBERCULOSIS AGENT
Pregnancy: Category C

ACTIONS/PHARMACODYNAMICS Polypeptide antibiotic derived from *Streptomyces capreolus.* Action mechanism not clear. Bacteriostatic against human strains of *Mycobacterium tuberculosis* and other strains of *Mycobacterium.* Cross-resistance between capreomycin and both kanamycin and neomycin has been reported. Bacterial resistance can develop rapidly when used alone. Produces neuromuscular blockade in large doses.

USES Only in conjunction with other appropriate antitubercular drugs in treatment of pulmonary tuberculosis when bactericidal agents, e.g., isoniazid and rifampin, cannot be tolerated or when causative organism has become resistant.

ROUTE & DOSAGE

Tuberculosis

Adult	IM	1 g/d (not to exceed 20 mg/kg/d) for 60–120 d; then 1 g 2–3 times/wk

PHARMACOKINETICS Peak: 1–2 h. **Distribution:** does not cross blood-brain barrier; crosses placenta; distribution into breast milk unknown. **Elimination:** half-life: 4–6 h; 52% excreted in urine unchanged in 12 h; small amount excreted in bile.

CONTRAINDICATIONS & PRECAUTIONS Contraindicated in: safe use during pregnancy (category C), in nursing women, infants, and children not established. **Cautious use in:** renal insufficiency (extreme caution); acoustic nerve impairment; history of allergies (especially to drugs); preexisting liver disease; myasthenia gravis; parkinsonism.

ADVERSE/SIDE EFFECTS CNS: neuromuscular blockage (large doses); skeletal muscle weakness, <u>respiratory</u> <u>depression</u> <u>or</u> <u>arrest</u>. **Hematologic:** leukocytosis, leukopenia, *eosinophilia*. **Hypersensitivity:** urticaria, maculopapular rash, photosensitivity. **Renal:** <u>nephrotoxicity</u> (long-term therapy), <u>tubular necrosis</u>. **Ear:** ototoxicity: eighth nerve (auditory and vestibular) damage. **Other:** hypokalemia, and other electrolyte imbalances; impaired hepatic function (decreased BSP excretion); IM site reactions: pain, induration, excessive bleeding, sterile abscesses.

DIAGNOSTIC TEST INTERFERENCES *BSP* and *PSP* excretion tests may be decreased.

DRUG INTERACTIONS Increased risk of nephrotoxicity and ototoxicity with AMINOGLYCOSIDES, **amphotericin B, colistin, polymyxin B, cisplatin, vancomycin.**

NURSING IMPLICATIONS

Administration
- Observe injection sites for signs of excessive bleeding and inflammation.
- Reconstituted by adding 2 ml of 0.9% isotonic NaCl injection or sterile water for injection to each 1 g vial. Allow 2–3 min for drug to dissolve completely.
- IM injections should be made deep into large muscle mass. Superficial injections are more painful and are associated with sterile abscess. Rotate injection sites.
- Solution may become pale straw color and darken with time, but this does not indicate loss of potency.
- After reconstitution, solution may be stored 48 h at room temperature and up to 14 d under refrigeration unless otherwise directed.
- Store at 15–30C (59–86F) unless otherwise directed.

Assessment & Drug Effects
- The following determinations are used as guidelines for therapy and should be performed before drug is started and at regular intervals during therapy: (1) appropriate bacterial susceptibility tests; (2) audiometric measurements (twice weekly or weekly) and tests of vestibular function (periodically); (3) CBC; SMA-12 screening weekly; (4) weekly renal function studies (BUN, NPN, creatinine clearance, sediment); (5) liver function tests

(periodically); (6) serum potassium levels (monthly).
- Capreomycin is cumulative in patients with impaired renal function. Dosage should be reduced in these patients and renal function tests closely followed.
- Monitor I&O. Report immediately any change in output or I&O ratio, any unusual appearance of urine, or elevation of BUN above 30 mg/dl. (**Normal BUN:** 10–20 mg/dl.)

Patient & Family Education
- Instruct patient to report any change in hearing or disturbance of balance. These effects are sometimes reversible if drug is withdrawn promptly when first symptoms appear.
- Patient and responsible family members should be completely informed about adverse reactions. They should be urged to report immediately the appearance of any unusual symptom, regardless of how vague it may seem.

CAPTOPRIL

See CARDIOVASCULAR AGENTS, ANGIOTENSIN CONVERTING ENZYME INHIBITOR prototype, p 138.

Prototype: pilocarpine, p 209

CARBACHOL INTRAOCULAR
(kar´ba-kole)
Trade name: Miostat

CARBACHOL TOPICAL

Trade name: Isopto Carbachol
Classifications: EYE PREPARATION; MIOTIC; AUTONOMIC NERVOUS SYSTEM AGENT; DIRECT-ACTING CHOLINERGIC (PARASYMPATHOMIMETIC)
Pregnancy: Category C

ACTIONS/PHARMACODYNAMICS Potent muscarinic agonist and synthetic choline ester with pharmacologic properties similar to those of acetylcholine. Inactivation of carbachol by cholinesterase is slow; therefore its actions are more prolonged than

Common side effects in *italic*; life-threatening effects <u>underlined</u>; generic names in **bold**; classifications in SMALL CAPS

381

those of acetylcholine, also more potent and longer-acting than those of pilocarpine. Acts directly on neuroeffectors of circular pupillary constrictor and ciliary muscles, producing miosis and spasms of accommodation, thus facilitating drainage from anterior chamber with consequent lowering of IOP. Usually prepared with wetting agent such as benzalkonium chloride to enhance corneal penetration.

USES Intraocularly to produce pupillary miosis during ocular surgery. Used topically to reduce IOP in open-angle or narrow-angle glaucoma, particularly when patient has become intolerant of or resistant to pilocarpine.

ROUTE & DOSAGE

Miosis

| Adult | Topical | 1–2 drops of 0.75–3% solution in lower conjunctival sac q4–8h |
| | Intraocular | 0.5 ml of 0.01% solution injected into anterior chamber of eye |

PHARMACOKINETICS Absorption: poor penetration of intact cornea. **Onset:** 10–20 min topical; 2–5 min intraocular. **Duration:** 4–8 h topical; 24 h intraocular. **Metabolism:** inactivated by cholinesterases.

CONTRAINDICATIONS & PRECAUTIONS Contraindicated in: corneal abrasions, acute iritis. Safe use during pregnancy (category C), in nursing women, and in children not established. **Cautious use in:** acute cardiac failure; bronchial asthma; peptic ulcer, GI spasms, obstructive ileus; hyperthyroidism; urinary tract obstruction; Parkinson's disease; following topical anesthetics or tonometry; history of retinal detachment.

ADVERSE/SIDE EFFECTS Headache, brow and eye pain, conjunctival hyperemia, ciliary spasm with temporary reduction in visual acuity, iritis. **Systemic absorption:** sweating, flushing, ciliary spasm, abdominal cramps, increased peristalsis, diarrhea, nausea, vomiting, salivation, urge to urinate, transient fall in blood pressure with reflex tachycardia, asthma.

NURSING IMPLICATIONS

Administration

- Eye drops are sterile and therefore should be handled so as to avoid contamination.
- Systemic absorption may be minimized by applying pressure against inner canthus of eye (lacrimal duct) during and 1–2 min after instillation.

- Intraocular carbachol (e.g., Miostat) is intended for single-dose intraocular use only (administered by physician). Unused portions should be discarded.
- Store preferably at 15–30C (59–86F) unless otherwise directed by manufacturer.

Assessment & Drug Effects

- Frequency and strength of drops are determined by patient's response and tolerance. Resistance may develop suddenly in some patients.
- Monitor for signs of systemic absorption (see adverse/side effects). Report them to physician.

Patient & Family Education

- Instruct patient in proper technique of eye drop instillation.
- Instruct patient to blot excess medication with a clean tissue but not to rub or squeeze lids together.
- The patient with glaucoma should remain under medical supervision for periodic tonometer measurements. The patient must understand that even in the absence of symptoms, progressive ocular damage can occur unless appropriate treatment is received.
- Drug may temporarily impair visual acuity, particularly adaptation to dark, and therefore safety precautions should be taken.

Prototype: phenytoin, p 172

CARBAMAZEPINE

(kar-ba-maz´e-peen)
Trade names: Apo-Carbamazepine, Mazepine, PMS-Carbamazepine, Tegretol
Classifications: CNS AGENT; ANTICONVULSANT
Pregnancy: Category C

ACTIONS/PHARMACODYNAMICS Structurally related to tricyclic antidepressants (TCAs) but lacks antidepressant properties. Anticonvulsant actions appear qualitatively similar to those of phenytoin (Dilantin). Like phenytoin, provides relief in trigeminal neuralgia by reducing synaptic transmission within trigeminal nucleus. Also has sedative, anticholinergic, antidepressant, and muscle relaxant (by inhibition of neuromuscular transmission) and slight analgesic actions.

Common side effects in *italic*; life-threatening effects <u>underlined</u>; generic names in **bold**; classifications in SMALL CAPS

USES Alone or concomitantly with other anticonvulsants in treatment of grand mal and psychomotor or temporal lobe epilepsy and mixed seizures in patients who have not responded satisfactorily to other agents. Also used for symptomatic treatment of trigeminal (tic douloureux) and glossopharyngeal neuralgias and for pain and paroxysmal symptoms associated with multiple sclerosis and other neurologic disorders. **Unlabeled use:** certain psychiatric disorders including prophylaxis and treatment of manic-depressive illness, treatment of schizoaffective illness, resistant schizophrenia, dyscontrol syndrome; for management of alcohol withdrawal, rage outbursts, and for antidiuretic effect in diabetes insipidus.

ROUTE & DOSAGE

Epilepsy

Adult	PO	200 mg b.i.d., gradually increased to 800–1200 mg/d in 3–4 divided doses
Child	PO	6–12 y: 100 mg b.i.d., gradually increased to 400–800 mg/d in 3–4 divided doses (max 1 g/d)

Trigeminal Neuralgia

Adult	PO	100 mg b.i.d., gradually increased by 100 mg increments q12h until relief; usual dose 200–800 mg/d in 3–4 divided doses (max 1.2 g/d)

PHARMACOKINETICS Absorption: slowly absorbed from GI tract. **Peak:** 2–8 h. **Distribution:** widely distributed; high concentrations in CSF; crosses placenta; distributed into breast milk. **Metabolism:** metabolized in liver; can induce liver microsomal enzymes. **Elimination:** half-life: 14–16 h (decreases with long-term use); excreted in urine and feces.

CONTRAINDICATIONS & PRECAUTIONS Contraindicated in: hypersensitivity to carbamazepine and to TCAs; history of myelosuppression or hematologic reaction to other drugs; increased IOP; SLE; cardiac, hepatic, or renal disease; coronary artery disease; hypertension. Safe use during pregnancy (category C), in nursing women, and in children <6 y not established. **Cautious use in:** the elderly; history of cardiac disease.

ADVERSE/SIDE EFFECTS CNS: dizziness, vertigo, drowsiness, disturbances of coordination, ataxia, confusion, headache, fatigue, listlessness, speech difficulty, development of minor motor seizures, hyperreflexia, akathisia, involuntary movements, tremors, visual hallucinations, activation of latent psychosis, aggression; agitation, respiratory depression. **CV:** edema, CHF, aggravation of coronary artery disease, hypertension, hypotension, syncope, arrhythmias, heart block. **ENT:** abnormal hearing acuity. **Eye:** scotomas, retinopathy, lens opacities, conjunctivitis, blurred vision, transient diplopia, oculomotor disturbances, oscillopsia, nystagmus, mydriasis. **GI:** nausea, vomiting, anorexia, abdominal pain, diarrhea, constipation, dry mouth and pharynx, glossitis, stomatitis. **GU:** urinary frequency or retention, oliguria, impotence, albuminuria, glycosuria, elevated BUN. **Hematologic:** aplastic anemia, reticulocytosis, *leukopenia,* leukocytosis, agranulocytosis, eosinophilia, thrombocytopenia. **Hepatic:** abnormal liver function tests, hepatitis, cholestatic and hepatocellular jaundice. **Skin:** skin rashes, urticaria, petechiae, extreme multiforme, Stevens-Johnson syndrome, photosensitivity reactions, altered skin pigmentation, exfoliative dermatitis, alopecia; pneumonitis, wheezing, aggravation of SLE. **Other:** myalgia, arthralgia, leg cramps, carbamazepine-induced SLE, pancreatitis, hypothyroidism, SIADH.

DIAGNOSTIC TEST INTERFERENCES False negative *pregnancy test* results with tests involving human chorionic gonadotropin.

DRUG INTERACTIONS Serum concentrations of other ANTICONVULSANTS may decrease because of increased metabolism; **verapamil, erythromycin** may increase carbamazepine levels; decreases hypoprothrombinemic effects of ORAL ANTICOAGULANTS; increases metabolism of estrogens, thus decreasing effectiveness of ORAL CONTRACEPTIVES.

NURSING IMPLICATIONS

Administration

- Absorption of drug is enhanced by administration with meals.
- Store at 15–30C (59–86F) unless otherwise directed.

Assessment & Drug Effects

- Before initiation of carbamazepine therapy the following procedures for eliciting baseline data are recommended: (1) detailed health history; (2) physical examination, including ophthalmoscopy and ECG; (3) laboratory studies: CBCs including platelets, reticulocytes, serum electrolytes and serum iron, liver function tests, BUN, and complete urinalysis.
- At least 3 mo into therapy it is recommended that physician attempt dosage reduction or termination

---

Common side effects in *italic*; life-threatening effects underlined; generic names in **bold**; classifications in SMALL CAPS

383

of drug therapy, if possible, in patients with trigeminal neuralgia. Some patients develop tolerance to the effects of carbamazepine.

- The following reactions commonly occur during early therapy: drowsiness, dizziness, light-headedness, ataxia, gastric upset. If these symptoms do not subside within a few days, dosage adjustments may be indicated.
- In general, therapy should be discontinued if any of the following signs of myelosuppression occur: RBC <4 million/mm³, Hct <32%, Hgb <11 g/dl, WBC <4000/mm³, platelet count <100,000/mm³, reticulocyte count <20,000/mm³, serum iron > 150 μg/dl.
- Toxicity can develop when serum concentrations are even slightly above the therapeutic range.
- The pain of tic douloureux is so excruciating that it has driven some patients to suicide. Common triggering stimuli include drafts, shaving, washing face, talking, chewing, hot or cold fluids or foods, jarring the bed, sudden noises. Carbamazepine relieves pain for 24–72 h in these patients.
- Monitor I&O ratio and vital signs during period of dosage adjustment. Report oliguria, signs of fluid retention, changes in I&O ratio, and changes in BP or pulse patterns.
- Cardiac syncope may resemble epileptic seizures. Therefore it is recommended that patients who experience an apparent increase in frequency of seizures or a change in their character should be checked by continuous ECG monitoring for 24 h.
- Doses higher than 600 mg/d may precipitate arrhythmias in patients with heart disease.
- Confusion and agitation may be aggravated in the elderly; therefore side rails and supervision of ambulation may be indicated.

Patient & Family Education

- Home patients and responsible family members should be instructed to withhold drug and notify physician immediately if early signs of toxicity or a possible hematologic problem appear, e.g., anorexia, fever, sore throat or mouth, malaise, unusual fatigue, tendency to bruise or bleed, petechiae, ecchymoses, bleeding gums, nose bleeds.
- Because dizziness, drowsiness, and ataxia are common side effects, warn patient to avoid hazardous tasks requiring mental alertness and physical coordination until reaction to drug is known.
- Impress on the patient and family the importance of remaining under close medical supervision throughout therapy.
- Photosensitivity reactions have been reported; therefore caution patient to avoid excessive sunlight. Suggest application of a sunscreen (if allowed) with SPF of 12 or above.
- Patients taking oral contraceptives should be informed that carbamazepine may cause breakthrough bleeding and may also affect the reliability of oral contraceptives.
- In patients with epilepsy, abrupt withdrawal of any anticonvulsant drug may precipitate seizures or even status epilepticus.

CARBAMIDE PEROXIDE

(kar´ba-mide per-ox´ide)

Trade names: Auro Ear Drops, Cankaid, Debrox, Gly-Oxide, Murine Ear Drops, Orajel Brace-aid Rinse, Proxigel, Urea Peroxide

Classifications: SKIN & MUCOUS MEMBRANE AGENT; ANTIINFECTIVE

ACTIONS/PHARMACODYNAMICS Urea compound combined with hydrogen peroxide 1:1 with foaming action and weak antibacterial properties due to release of nascent oxygen when carbamide exposed to moisture. Effervescence of liberated oxygen mechanically facilitates cleansing by loosening tissue debris or impacted or excessive ear wax. Commercial formulations contain anhydrous glycerin, which helps to penetrate and soften wax.

USES Preparations intended for topical oral application are used for minor irritation, infection, and inflammation of mouth and gums, such as aphthous ulcers (canker sores), gingivitis, stomatitis, Vincent's infection, and denture irritations. Also used as adjunct in oral hygiene. Otic formulations are used as aid in removal of excessive or hardened cerumen and to help prevent cerumenosis.

ROUTE & DOSAGE

Mouth Lesions

Adult	Topical	Apply several drops to affected area q.i.d.; expectorate after 1–3 min; not to be used for >7 d

Ear Wax

Adult	Topical	Instill 5–10 drops in affected ear b.i.d. for 3–4 d

CONTRAINDICATIONS & PRECAUTIONS Contraindicated in: otic preparations following otic surgery; perforated ear drum; ear redness, tenderness, or pain; dizziness; ear drainage; children <12 y. Topical mouth formulations in children <3 y.

ADVERSE/SIDE EFFECTS Redness, irritation, superinfections.

NURSING IMPLICATIONS

Administration

- Protect medication from heat and direct sunlight.
- Store medication in tightly covered container in a cool place. Protect from light.

Patient & Family Education
Topical Oral Preparation

- Used preferably after meals and at bedtime. Advise patient to rinse mouth of food debris before doing treatment.
- Forewarn patient that medication will foam on contact with saliva.
- Advise patient to discontinue treatment and notify physician if redness, irritation, swelling, or pain increases or persists.
- Instruct patient to examine mouth periodically for signs of superinfection.

Otic Preparation

- Medication should be discontinued and physician notified promptly if dizziness, ear drainage, pain, tenderness, or redness develop.
- The most common causes of wax buildup are lack of humidity (causing wax to dry and harden), excessive hair growth in ears, attempts to remove wax with cotton swab, which only jams the wax farther into ears.

Prototype: penicillin G potassium, p 71

CARBENICILLIN DISODIUM
(kar-ben-i-sill′in)
Trade names: Geopen, Pyopen
Classifications: ANTIINFECTIVE; PENICILLIN ANTIBIOTIC
Pregnancy: Category B

ACTIONS/PHARMACODYNAMICS Extended spectrum, penicillinase-sensitive, semisynthetic penicillin derived from penicillin G (benzylpenicillin). Similar to penicillin G in actions and adverse effects

but differs in having a broader range of antibacterial activity. Bactericidal against a variety of gram-negative and gram-positive microorganisms. Particularly effective against gram-negative infections including *Pseudomonas aeruginosa, Proteus,* susceptible strains of *Escherichia coli, Enterobacter (Aerobacter), Haemophilus influenzae,* and *Neisseria gonorrhoeae.* Effective also in severe infections caused by gram-positive organisms, e.g., *Streptococcus pneumoniae,* and enterocci (*Streptococcus faecalis*). Inhibits aggregation of newly formed and circulating platelets with resultant prolongation of bleeding and prothrombin times, particularly in high doses and in patients with impaired renal function.

USES Septicemia, meningitis, infections of respiratory tract, soft tissue infections, pelvic and urinary tract infections. May be used concurrently with gentamicin or tobramycin pending results of culture and susceptibility test, or with probenecid to attain higher and more prolonged serum levels.

ROUTE & DOSAGE

Urinary Tract Infections

Adult	IV/IM	200 mg/kg/d in 4 divided doses or 1–2 g q6h
Child	IV/IM	50–200 mg/kg/d in 4 divided doses

Systemic Infections

Adult	IV/IM	15–40 g/d in 6 divided doses (max 40 g/d)
Child	IV/IM	250–500 mg/kg/d in 6 divided doses (max 40 g/d)

PHARMACOKINETICS Peak: 1–2 h IM. **Distribution:** low concentrations in CSF unless meninges are inflamed; crosses placenta; distributed into breast milk. **Elimination:** half-life: 67 min; 80–99% excreted unchanged in urine within 24 h.

CONTRAINDICATIONS & PRECAUTIONS Contraindicated in: hypersensitivity to penicillins. Safe use during pregnancy (category B) not established. **Cautious use in:** history of or suspected atopy or allergies; renal or hepatic disease; coagulation disorders; electrolyte imbalance, patients on sodium restriction; history of cephalosporin allergy.

ADVERSE/SIDE EFFECTS As for penicillin G: **GI:** nausea, vomiting, unpleasant taste, *diarrhea.* **Hematologic:** unusual bleeding or bruising (abnormal clotting and prothrombin times), hypernatremia and <u>fluid overload</u>, hypokalemia, hypokalemic alkalosis,

Common side effects in *italic*; life-threatening effects <u>underlined</u>; generic names in **bold**; classifications in SMALL CAPS

385

hemolytic anemia, positive Coombs' test neutropenia, leukopenia, thrombocytopenia, elevations of AST and ALT, particularly in children; elevated CPK (from muscle injury following IM use). **Hypersensitivity:** pruritus, urticaria, skin rash, fever, chills, eosinophilia, anaphylactic reaction. **Renal:** hematuria, interstitial nephritis. **Other:** pain and induration (IM site), thrombophlebitis (IV site), superinfections.

DIAGNOSTIC TEST INTERFERENCES Elevated *serum sodium* levels can occur with large carbenicillin doses because of its high sodium content.

DRUG INTERACTIONS Synergistic action when AMINOGLYCOSIDES administered concurrently; high carbenicillin doses increase risk of bleeding with ORAL ANTICOAGULANTS, **heparin;** TETRACYCLINES may reduce bactericidal activity of carbenicillin—combination generally avoided.

INCOMPATIBILITIES Solution/additive: AMINOGLYCOSIDES, **amphotericin B, bleomycin, chloramphenicol, cytarabine, doxapram, lincomycin,** TETRACYCLINES, **vitamin B complex with C. Y-site:** AMINOGLYCOSIDES, **promethazine.**

NURSING IMPLICATIONS

Administration

- Culture and susceptibility tests are performed initially and at regular intervals throughout therapy to monitor drug effectiveness. Therapy may begin pending test results.
- Careful inquiry should be made concerning hypersensitivity reactions to penicillin, cephalosporins, and other allergens.
- IM injections should not exceed 2 g per individual injection site. Administer IM well into body of large muscle. Gluteus maximus and midlateral thigh are preferred sites for adults; midlateral thigh is the preferred site for children (follow agency policy). Rotate injection sites.
- Pain and other local reactions associated with IM injections may be minimized by reconstituting drug with 0.5% lidocaine hydrochloride without epinephrine (prescribed by physician) or with bacteriostatic water for injection containing 0.9% benzyl alcohol. The latter must not be used in neonates.
- Follow manufacturer's directions explicitly regarding diluent and amount to use for initial reconstitution and for further dilution to avoid tissue irritation and phlebitis.
- After reconstitution, IM solutions retain their stability for 24 h at room temperature, and for 72 h if refrigerated. Indicate time and date of reconstitution on container.
- Carbenicillin may be given by intermittent or continuous infusion. When administered intermittently, it is generally infused over 30 min–2 h for adults and over 15 min for neonates.
- Store at 15–30C (59–86F) unless otherwise directed.

Assessment & Drug Effects

- Monitor I&O. Report any change in I&O ratio, pattern, and unusual appearance of urine. Consult physician regarding advisable fluid intake.
- Patients with impaired renal function are particularly susceptible to nephrotoxicity, neurotoxicity, and hemorrhagic manifestations and therefore must be closely monitored.
- Bleeding tendency is most likely to occur 12–24 h after initiation of therapy, in patients receiving high dose therapy, and in those with impaired renal function. If bleeding occurs, drug should be stopped. Report promptly to physician.
- Serum sodium and potassium determinations, renal, hepatic, and cardiac status, hematopoietic function, and bleeding time assessments should be made prior to and at regular intervals during prolonged therapy and in patients receiving high doses or who have impaired renal or hepatic function.
- Observe patients for symptoms of hypernatremia, CHF, and hypokalemia (see chap 3).
- Report immediately signs and symptoms of hypersensitivity reaction. Have on hand: epinephrine, IV corticosteroids, oxygen, suction, endotracheal tube, tracheostomy equipment.
- Bear in mind that superinfections (see Signs & Symptoms, chap 3) are particularly likely to occur in patients receiving extended spectrum penicillins.

Prototype: penicillin G potassium, p 71

CARBENICILLIN INDANYL SODIUM
(kar-ben-i-sill´in)
Trade names: Geocillin, Geopen Oral
Classifications: ANTIINFECTIVE; PENICILLIN ANTIBIOTIC
Pregnancy: Category B

ACTIONS/PHARMACODYNAMICS Broad spectrum, semisynthetic penicillin and acid stable ester of carbenicillin prepared for oral use. Rapidly hydrolyzed to carbenicillin in body. Like carbenicillin disodium, it is bactericidal and penicillinase sensitive and has similar antimicrobial activity but achieves lower blood concentrations than parent compound.

USES Mainly in the treatment of prostatitis and acute and chronic infections of upper and lower urinary tract caused by susceptible strains of *Escherichia coli, Enterobacter, Enterococcus, Proteus,* and *Pseudomonas* species.

ROUTE & DOSAGE

Urinary Tract Infections

Adult   PO   382–764 mg q6h for 10 d; continue for 2–4 wk for prostatitis

PHARMACOKINETICS Absorption: incompletely absorbed from GI tract. **Peak:** 0.5–1 h. **Distribution:** very low systemic concentrations; crosses placenta; distributed into breast milk. **Elimination:** half-life: 67 min; 80–99% excreted unchanged in urine within 24 h.

CONTRAINDICATIONS & PRECAUTIONS Contraindicated in: hypersensitivity to penicillins. Safe use in children and during pregnancy (category B) not established. **Cautious use in:** history of or suspected atopy or allergies; history of allergy to cephalosporins; impaired renal and hepatic function; patients on sodium restriction.

ADVERSE/SIDE EFFECTS Dose related. GI: *nausea,* vomiting, heartburn; *diarrhea,* abdominal cramps, flatulence, unpleasant aftertaste, dry mouth. **Hematologic:** neutropenia, leukopenia, thrombocytopenia, hemolytic anemia, increased AST. **Hypersensitivity:** rash, fever, urticaria, eosinophilia, pruritus, anaphylaxis. **Other:** superinfections, especially of vagina.

NURSING IMPLICATIONS

Administration

- Best taken with a full glass (240 ml) of water on an empty stomach (either 1 h before or 2 h after meals) to attain maximum therapeutic drug levels in urine. Consult physician.
- Protect tablets from moisture. Unless otherwise specified, store at 15–30C (59–86F).

Assessment & Drug Effects

- Culture and susceptibility test should be performed prior to and at regular intervals throughout therapy. Therapy may be initiated pending test results.

- Before treatment is initiated, a careful inquiry should be made concerning patient's previous exposure and sensitivity to penicillin and cephalosporins and other allergic reactions of any kind.
- Drug-induced nausea, unpleasant aftertaste and smell, dry mouth, and furry tongue may be so objectionable as to necessitate drug withdrawal. Report to physician if symptoms persist.
- During prolonged therapy, evaluations of renal, hepatic, and hematopoietic systems are advised at regular intervals. Patients with creatinine clearance of less than 10 ml/min (**normal:** 105–130 ml/min) will not attain therapeutic urine levels.
- Check with physician regarding optimum daily fluid intake. Report any change in quality or quantity of urine or in I&O ratio.
- Observe patient for signs of electrolyte imbalance. Each 1 g of drug contains approximately 1 mEq of sodium.

Patient & Family Education

- Instruct patient to take with a full glass of water on an empty stomach.
- Instruct patient to take medication around the clock, not to miss any doses, and to continue taking medication until it is all gone unless otherwise directed by physician.

Prototype: levodopa, p 114

CARBIDOPA-LEVODOPA

(kar-bi-doe′pa)
Trade name: Sinemet

CARBIDOPA

Trade name: Lodosyn
Classifications: AUTONOMIC NERVOUS SYSTEM AGENT; ANTICHOLINERGIC (PARASYMPATHOLYTIC); ANTIPARKINSONISM AGENT
Pregnancy: Category C

ACTIONS/PHARMACODYNAMICS Carbidopa, a derivative of methyldopa, is a peripheral dopa-decarboxylase inhibitor. When levodopa is given alone, large doses must be administered to compensate for peripheral decarboxylation in order to provide ade-

Common side effects in *italic*; life-threatening effects underlined; generic names in **bold**; classifications in SMALL CAPS

387

C

quate amounts of dopamine at appropriate sites in the corpus striatum. Carbidopa prevents peripheral metabolism (decarboxylation) of levodopa and thereby makes more levodopa available for transport to the brain. Carbidopa does not cross blood-brain barrier and therefore does not affect metabolism of levodopa within the brain. Addition of carbidopa reduces amount of levodopa required by about 75%, because levodopa plasma levels and plasma half-life are increased. Carbidopa also prevents the inhibitory effect of pyridoxine (vitamin B_6) on levodopa. Additionally, incidence of nausea and vomiting associated with levodopa is decreased. However, adverse CNS effects (e.g., dyskinesias) may occur at lower dosages and sooner with carbidopa-levodopa than with levodopa alone, and the combination does not appear to benefit patients with markedly irregular "on-off" response to levodopa.

USES Symptomatic treatment of idiopathic Parkinson's disease (paralysis agitans), postencephalitic parkinsonism, and parkinsonism following carbon dioxide and manganese intoxication. Carbidopa is available alone from manufacturer, on request by physician, for use with levodopa when separate titration of each agent is indicated and for investigational purposes.

ROUTE & DOSAGE

Parkinson's Disease in Patients not Currently Receiving Levodopa

Adult	PO	1 tablet containing 10 mg carbidopa/100 mg levodopa or 25 mg carbidopa/100 mg levodopa t.i.d., increased by 1 tablet q.d. or q.o.d. up to 6 tablets/d

Patients Receiving Levodopa

Adult	PO	1 tablet of the 25/250 mixture t.i.d. or q.i.d., adjusted by 1/2–1 tablet as needed up to 8 tablets/d (start at 20–25% of initial dose of levodopa)

PHARMACOKINETICS Absorption: 40–70% of carbidopa absorbed after PO dose; carbidopa may enhance absorption of levodopa. **Distribution:** widely distributed in most body tissues except CNS; crosses placenta; excreted in breast milk. **Elimination:** half-life: 2 h; excreted in urine.

CONTRAINDICATIONS & PRECAUTIONS Contraindicated in: hypersensitivity to carbidopa or levodopa; narrow-angle glaucoma; history of or sus-

pected melanoma. Safe use in women of childbearing potential, during pregnancy (category C), in nursing mothers, and in children <18 y not established. **Cautious use in:** cardiovascular, hepatic, pulmonary, or renal disorders; urinary retention; history of peptic ulcer; psychiatric states; endocrine disease; chronic wide-angle glaucoma; seizure disorders.

ADVERSE/SIDE EFFECTS No reactions reported for carbidopa alone. Adverse reactions are those of enhanced levodopa effects: **CNS:** *involuntary movements (dyskinetic, dystonic, choreiform)*, ataxia, muscle twitching, increase in hand tremor, numbness, headache, dizziness, euphoria, fatigue, confusion, insomnia, nightmares, mental disturbances, anxiety, depression with suicidal tendencies, delirium, seizures. **CV:** orthostatic hypotension, irregular heart beat, palpitation, arrhythmias, phlebitis, edema. **Eye:** blepharospasm, mydriasis, miosis, blurred vision, diplopia, oculogyric crisis. **GI:** nausea, anorexia, dry mouth, bruxism, vomiting, excess salivation. **GU:** dark urine, priapism, urinary frequency, retention, incontinence. **Hematologic:** hemolytic and nonhemolytic anemia, thrombocytopenia, agranulocytosis. **Skin:** body odor, skin rash, dark sweat, loss of hair. **Other:** hoarseness, unusual breathing patterns, neuroleptic malignant syndrome, abnormal liver function tests, abnormal PBI, BUN.

DIAGNOSTIC TEST INTERFERENCES *Urine glucose:* false-negative tests may result with use of *glucose oxidase methods* (e.g., *Clinistix, Tes-Tape*) and false-positive results with *copper reduction methods* (e.g., *Benedict's, Clinitest*), especially in patients receiving large doses. It is reported that Clinistix and Tes-Tape may be used if reading is taken at margin of wet and dry tape. There is also the possibility of false-positive tests for *urinary ketones* by *dipstick tests,* e.g., *Acetest* (equivocal), *Ketostix, Labstix;* false elevation of *serum* and *urinary uric acid* levels by colorimetric methods (not with uricase); and interference with *urine PKU test* results.

DRUG INTERACTIONS MAO INHIBITERS may precipitate hypertensive crisis; TRICYCLIC ANTIDEPRESSANTS potentiate postural hypotension; PHENOTHIAZINES, **haloperidol** may antagonize effects of levodopa; ANTICHOLINERGIC AGENTS may enhance levodopa effects but can exacerbate involuntary movements; **methyldopa, guanethidine** increase hypotensive and CNS effects; **phenytoin, papaverine** may interfere with levodopa effects.

Common side effects in *italic*; life-threatening effects underlined; generic names in **bold**; classifications in SMALL CAPS

NURSING IMPLICATIONS

Administration

- Administer with meals or food, unless otherwise directed by physician.
- Food-drug relationship: Ingestion of levodopa with meals high in protein appears to interfere with plasma-to-CNS transport of the drug.
- When patient has been taking levodopa alone, carbidopa-levodopa is usually initiated with a morning dose after patient has been without levodopa for at least 8 h.
- Store in tight, light-resistant containers at 15–30C (59–86F) unless otherwise directed.

Assessment & Drug Effects

- Rate of dosage increase is determined primarily by patient's tolerance and response to levodopa. Make accurate observations and report promptly adverse reactions and therapeutic effects.
- Monitor vital signs, particularly during period of dosage adjustment. Report alterations in BP, pulse, and respiratory rate and rhythm.
- All patients should be closely monitored for behavior changes. Patients in depression should be closely observed for suicidal tendencies.
- Patients with chronic wide-angle glaucoma should be monitored during therapy for changes in intraocular pressure.
- Monitor patients with diabetes carefully for alterations in diabetes control. Frequent monitoring of blood sugar is advised.
- All patients on extended therapy should be checked periodically for symptoms of diabetes and acromegaly and for functioning of hematopoietic, hepatic, and renal systems.
- About 50% of patients on full therapeutic doses for 1 y or longer develop abnormal involuntary movement such as facial grimacing, exaggerated chewing, protrusion of tongue, rhythmic opening and closing of mouth, bobbing of head, jerky arm and leg movements, and exaggerated respiration. Report immediately to physician.
- Chronic management may be accompanied by the **"on-off" phenomenon:** sudden, unpredictable loss of drug effectiveness ("off" effect), which lasts 1 min–1 h. This is followed by an equally abrupt return of function ("on" effect). Sometimes symptoms can be controlled by increasing number of doses per day.
- Some patients manifest increase in bradykinesia ("leg freezing" or slow body movement). The patient is unable to start walking and frequently falls.

Reduction of dosage may be indicated in these patients.

- Patients who require more frequent drug administration are most likely to manifest gradual return of parkinsonian symptoms toward the end of a dose period.

Patient & Family Education

- Patients who have been taking levodopa must be carefully instructed regarding continuation or discontinuation of levodopa as prescribed by physician. Both adverse reactions and therapeutic effects occur more rapidly with carbidopa-levodopa combination than with levodopa alone.
- Orthostatic hypotension is usually asymptomatic, but some patients experience weakness, dizziness, and faintness. Advise patient to make positional changes slowly and in stages, particularly from recumbent to upright position, to dangle legs a few minutes before standing, and to walk in place before ambulating. Tolerance to this effect usually develops within a few months of therapy. Support stockings may help. Consult physician.
- Muscle twitching and spasmodic winking are early signs of overdosage; report them promptly.
- Elevation of mood and sense of well-being may precede objective improvement. Stress the importance of resuming activities gradually and observing safety precautions to avoid injury.
- Urge patient to maintain prescribed drug regimen. Abrupt withdrawal can lead to parkinsonian crisis with return of marked muscle rigidity, akinesia, tremor, hyperpyrexia, mental changes.
- Caution patient to avoid driving or other hazardous activities until reaction to drug is determined.
- Levodopa may cause urine to darken on standing and may also cause sweat to be dark-colored. This effect is not clinically significant.
- Advise patient to wear medical identification. All health care providers should be informed that patient is taking carbidopa-levodopa.

Prototype: dinoprostone, p 251

CARBOPROST TROMETHAMINE
(kar´boe-prost)
Trade names: Hemabate, Prostin/15 M
Classifications: OXYTOCIC; PROSTAGLANDIN; ABORTIFACIENT
Pregnancy: Category C

Common side effects in *italic*; life-threatening effects <u>underlined</u>; generic names in **bold**; classifications in SMALL CAPS

389

ACTIONS/PHARMACODYNAMICS Synthetic analog of naturally occurring prostaglandin F_2 alpha with longer duration of biologic activity. Stimulates myometrial contractions of gravid uterus; contractions are qualitatively similar to those occurring at term labor. Mean time to abortion 16 h; mean dose required 2.6 ml. Length of time to abortion and total dose of carboprost required decrease with greater parity but increase with greater gestational age. Can be employed as abortifacient even if membranes are ruptured. Also stimulates smooth muscles in GI tract and bronchi, the cause of several troublesome adverse effects.

USES To induce abortion between 13th and 20th week of pregnancy, as calculated from first day of last menstrual period. Also for refractory postpartum bleeding. **Unlabeled uses:** to reduce blood loss secondary to uterine atony; to induce labor in intrauterine fetal death and hydatidiform mole.

ROUTE & DOSAGE

Adult	IM	Initial: 250 µg (1 ml) repeated at 1 1/2 – 3 1/2-h intervals if indicated by uterine response; dosage may be increased to 500 µg (2 ml) if uterine contractility is inadequate after several doses of 250 µg (1 ml); not to exceed total dose of 12 mg or continuous administration for more than 2 d

CONTRAINDICATIONS & PRECAUTIONS Contraindicated in: acute pelvic inflammatory disease, active cardiac, pulmonary, renal, or hepatic disease. Pregnancy (category C). **Cautious use in:** history of asthma; adrenal disease; anemia, hypotension, hypertension; diabetes mellitus; epilepsy, history of uterine surgery; cervical stenosis, fibroids.

ADVERSE/SIDE EFFECTS Generally transient and reversible with discontinuation of drug. Nausea, diarrhea, vomiting, fever, flushing, chills, cough, headache, pain (muscles, joints, lower abdomen, eyes), hiccups, breast tenderness.

NURSING IMPLICATIONS

Administration

- Should be administered only by trained personnel in hospital settings with intensive care and operating room facilities.
- Because nausea and diarrhea occur in about 60% of patients, an antiemetic and an antidiarrheal agent

may be prescribed before and during carboprost administration.
- Administer deeply into muscle. Aspirate carefully before injecting drug to avoid inadvertent entry into blood vessel which can result in bronchospasm, tetanic contractions, and shock. Do not use same site for subsequent doses.
- Store drug in refrigerator at 2–4C (36–39F) unless otherwise specified.

Assessment & Drug Effects

- Complete medical history and baseline physical examination should be performed before drug is administered. Patient should be completely informed of the potential risks associated with carboprost-induced abortions.
- Patient should not be left unattended during induced labor. Monitor uterine contractions and observe and report excessive vaginal bleeding and cramping pain. Save all clots and tissue for physician inspection and laboratory analysis.
- Check vital signs at regular intervals. Carboprost-induced febrile reaction occurs in more than 10% of patients and must be differentiated from endometritis, which occurs around third day after abortion.

Patient & Family Education

- Report promptly onset of bleeding, foul-smelling lochia, abdominal pain, or fever.
- In some women, ovulation may be reinstated as early as 2 wk postabortion. Patient should be informed so that appropriate contraception may be started if desired.

Prototype: cyclobenzaprine, p 122

CARISOPRODOL

(kar-eye-soe-proe′dole)
Trade name: Rela, Soma, Soprodol
Classifications: AUTONOMIC NERVOUS SYSTEM AGENT; CENTRAL ACTING SKELETAL MUSCLE RELAXANT
Pregnancy: Category C

ACTIONS/PHARMACODYNAMICS Propanediol derivative carbamate with central depressant action pharmacologically related to meprobamate. CNS depressant precise action mechanism is not clear. Skeletal muscle relaxant effect, unlike that of neuromuscular blocking agents, appears to be due to sedative action. Voluntary motor function is not lost, but there may be slight reduction in muscle tone leading to relief of pain and discomfort of muscle spasm.

USES Skeletal muscle spasm, stiffness, and pain in a variety of musculoskeletal disorders and to relieve spasticity and rigidity in cerebral palsy.

ROUTE & DOSAGE

Adult	PO	350 mg t.i.d.
Child	PO	>5 y: 25 mg/kg/d in 4 divided doses

PHARMACOKINETICS Onset: 30 min. **Duration:** 4–6 h. **Distribution:** crosses placenta. **Metabolism:** metabolized in liver. **Elimination:** half-life: 8 h; excreted by kidneys; excreted in breast milk (2–4 times the plasma concentrations).

CONTRAINDICATIONS & PRECAUTIONS Contraindicated in: hypersensitivity to carisoprodol and related compounds (e.g., meprobamate, tybamate); acute intermittent porphyria; children <12 y. Safe use during pregnancy (category C) and in nursing women not established. **Cautious use in:** impaired liver or kidney function, addiction-prone individuals.

ADVERSE/SIDE EFFECTS Low incidence of toxicity. **CNS:** *drowsiness, dizziness,* vertigo, ataxia, tremor, headache, irritability, depressive reactions, syncope, insomnia. **CV:** tachycardia, postural hypotension, facial flushing. **GI:** nausea, vomiting, hiccups. **Hypersensitivity:** skin rash, erythema multiforme, pruritus, eosinophilia, asthma, fever, <u>anaphylactic shock</u>.

DRUG INTERACTIONS Alcohol, CNS DEPRESSANTS potentiate CNS effects.

NURSING IMPLICATIONS

Administration

- May be taken with food to reduce GI symptoms. Last dose should be taken at bedtime.
- Store in tightly closed container at 15–30C (59–86F) unless otherwise directed.

Assessment & Drug Effects

- Allergic or idiosyncratic reactions generally occur within the period from the first to the fourth dose

in patients taking the drug for the first time. Symptoms usually subside after several hours; they are treated by supportive and symptomatic measures.
- There are some indications that psychologic dependence may occur with long-term use.

Patient & Family Education

- Drowsiness is a common side effect and may require reduction in dosage. Driving and other potentially hazardous activities should be avoided until response to the drug has been evaluated.
- May cause dizziness and faintness. Symptoms may be controlled by making position changes slowly and in stages. Patient should report to physician if symptoms persist.
- Caution patient not to take alcohol or other CNS depressants (effects may be additive) unless otherwise directed by physician.
- Advise patient to discontinue drug and notify physician if skin rash, diplopia, dizziness, or other unusual signs or symptoms appear.

Prototype: cyclophosphamide, p 91

CARMUSTINE
(kar-mus´teen)
Trade names: BCNU, BiCNU
Classifications: ANTINEOPLASTIC; ALKYLATING AGENT
Pregnancy: Category D

ACTIONS/PHARMACODYNAMICS Highly lipid-soluble nitrosourea derivative with cell-cycle-nonspecific activity against rapidly proliferating cell populations. Produces cross-linkage of DNA strands, thereby blocking DNA, RNA, and protein synthesis. Drug metabolites thought to be responsible for antineoplastic and toxic activities. Major toxic effect is bone marrow suppression.

USES As single agent or in combination with other antineoplastics in treatment of Hodgkin's disease and other lymphomas, melanoma, primary and metastatic tumors of brain, and GI tract malignancies. **Unlabeled uses:** treatment of carcinomas of breast, lungs; Ewing's sarcoma, Burkitt's tumor, malignant melanoma, and topically for mycosis fungoides.

Common side effects in *italic*; life-threatening effects <u>underlined</u>; generic names in **bold**; classifications in SMALL CAPS

391

ROUTE & DOSAGE

Previously Untreated Patients—Carcinoma

Adult	IV	150–200 mg/m² q6wk in one dose or given over 2 d. Doses adjusted based on hematologic parameters

Mycosis Fungoides

Adult	Topical	0.05–0.4% solution or ointment 1–2 times/d for 6–8 wk (10 mg/d)

PHARMACOKINETICS **Distribution:** readily crosses blood-brain barrier; CSF concentrations 15–70% of plasma concentrations. **Metabolism:** rapidly metabolized; metabolic fate not completely known. **Elimination:** 60–70% excreted in urine in 96 h; 6% excreted through lungs, 1% in feces; excreted in breast milk.

CONTRAINDICATIONS & PRECAUTIONS **Contraindicated in:** history of pulmonary function impairment; recent illness with or exposure to chickenpox or herpes zoster; infection, decreased circulating platelets, leukocytes, or erythrocytes. Safe use during pregnancy (category D) and in nursing women not established. **Cautious use in:** hepatic and renal insufficiency; patient with previous cytotoxic medication, or radiation therapy.

ADVERSE/SIDE EFFECTS **CNS:** dizziness, ataxia. **Eye (with high doses):** infarctions, retinal hemorrhage, suffusion of conjunctiva. **GI:** stomatitis, *nausea, vomiting*. **Hematologic:** delayed myelosuppression (dose-related); thrombocytopenia. **Hepatic (high doses):** increases in transaminases, alkaline phosphatase, bilirubin, jaundice, encephalopathy. **Renal:** decrease in kidney size, progressive azotemia, renal failure. **Respiratory:** pulmonary infiltration or fibrosis. **Other:** skin flushing and burning pain at injection site, hyperpigmentation of skin (from contact).

DRUG INTERACTIONS **Cimetidine** may potentiate neutropenia and thrombocytopenia.

NURSING IMPLICATIONS

Administration

- Used only when a physician experienced in cancer chemotherapy can provide constant supervision.
- Wear disposable gloves when preparing carmustine. Contact of drug with skin can cause burning, dermatitis, and hyperpigmentation.
- To prepare for IV administration, add supplied diluent to the 100 mg vial. Further dilute with 27 ml of sterile water for injection to yield a concentration of 3.3 mg/ml. Each dose is then added to 100–500 ml of D5W or NS and infused over at least 1 h.
- If possible avoid starting infusion into dorsum of hand, wrist, or the antecubital veins; extravasation in these areas can damage underlying tendons and nerves leading to loss of mobility of entire limb.
- Slow infusion over 1–2 h (by IV drip) and adequate dilution will reduce pain of administration. Frequently check rate of flow and blood return; palpate injection site for extravasation. If there is any question about patency, line should be restarted.
- Nausea and vomiting (dose related) may occur within 2 h after drug administration and persist for up to 6 h. Prior administration of an antiemetic may help to decrease or prevent these side effects.
- Reconstituted solutions of carmustine are clear and colorless and may be stored at 2–8C (36–46F) for 24 h protected from light.
- Store unopened vials at 2–8C (36–46F), protected from light, unless otherwise directed by manufacturer.
- Signs of decomposition of carmustine in unopened vial: liquefaction and appearance of oil film at bottom of vial. Discard drug in this condition.

Assessment & Drug Effects

- Platelet nadir usually occurs within 4–5 wk, and leukocyte nadir within 5–6 wk after therapy is terminated. Thrombocytopenia may be more severe than leukopenia; anemia is less severe. Blood studies are continued following infusion, at weekly intervals, for at least 6 wk.
- Check temperature daily. Avoid use of rectal thermometer to prevent injury to mucosa. An elevation of 0.6F or more above usual temperature warrants reporting.
- Baseline and periodic tests of hepatic, pulmonary, and renal function are recommended throughout therapy. Most patients receiving carmustine inevitably show some signs of toxicity.
- Symptoms of lung toxicity (cough, shortness of breath, fever) should be reported to the physician immediately.
- Be alert to signs of hepatic toxicity (jaundice, dark urine, pruritus, light colored stools) and renal insufficiency (dysuria, oliguria, hematuria, swelling of lower legs and feet).

Patient & Family Education

- Carmustine can cause burning discomfort even in the absence of extravasation. Report burning sensation immediately. Infusion will be discontinued

- and restarted in another site. Ice application over the area may decrease the discomfort.
- Intense flushing of skin may occur during IV infusion. This usually disappears in 2–4 h.
- Patient will be highly susceptible to infection and to hemorrhagic disorders. Be alert to hazardous periods that occur 4–6 wk after a dose of carmustine. If possible, invasive procedures (e.g., IM injections, enemas, rectal temperatures) should be avoided during this period.
- Report promptly the onset of sore throat, weakness, fever, chills, infection of any kind, or abnormal bleeding (ecchymosis, petechiae, epistaxis, bleeding gums, hematemesis, melena).

Prototype: propranolol, p 109

CARTEOLOL HYDROCHLORIDE
(car´tee-oh-lole)
Trade name: Cartrol
Classifications: AUTONOMIC NERVOUS SYSTEM AGENT; BETA-ADRENERGIC ANTAGONIST (BLOCKING AGENT, SYMPATHOLYTIC); ANTIHYPERTENSIVE
Pregnancy: Category C

ACTIONS/PHARMACODYNAMICS Carteolol is a beta-adrenergic blocking agent that competes for available beta receptor sites. It inhibits both B_1 receptors (chiefly in cardiac muscle) and B_2 receptors (chiefly in the bronchial and vascular musculature). It decreases standing and supine hypertension.

USES Alone as a step 1 agent for hypertension or in combination with other drugs, particularly a thiazide diuretic. Not indicated for hypertensive crisis. **Unlabeled use:** to reduce the frequency of anginal attacks.

ROUTE & DOSAGE

Hypertension
Adult PO 2.5 mg once/d; may increase to 5–10 mg if needed (max 10 mg/d)

PHARMACOKINETICS Absorption: readily absorbed from GI tract; 85% reaches systemic circulation. **Peak:** 1–3 h. **Duration:** 24–48 h. **Distribution:** crosses placenta; distributed into breast milk. **Metabolism:** metabolized in liver to active metabolite. **Elimination:** half-life: 4–6 h; excreted primarily in urine.

CONTRAINDICATIONS & PRECAUTIONS Contraindicated in: sinus bradycardia, greater than first-degree heart block, cardiogenic shock, CHF secondary to tachycardia treatable with beta-blockers, overt cardiac failure, hypersensitivity to beta-blocking agents, persistent severe bradycardia, bronchial asthma or bronchospasm, and severe COPD. **Cautious use in:** CHF patients treated with digitalis and diuretics, peripheral vascular disease; diabetes, hypoglycemia, thyrotoxicosis; pregnancy (category C) and nursing mothers.

ADVERSE/SIDE EFFECTS CV: increased angina, hypotension, CHF, bradycardia. **CNS:** *headache, dizziness,* drowsiness, insomnia, anxiety, tremor, paresthesia, weakness. **Endocrine:** hyperglycemia, hypoglycemia. **GI:** abdominal pain, diarrhea, nausea. **Other:** rash, muscle cramps.

DRUG INTERACTIONS DIURETICS and other HYPOTENSIVE AGENTS increase hypotensive effect; carteolol and **albuterol, metoproterenol, terbutaline, pirbuterol** are mutually antagonistic; NSAID's may blunt hypotensive effect; decreases hypoglycemic effect of **glyburide**; may increase bradycardia and sinus arrest with **amiodarone.**

NURSING IMPLICATIONS

Administration
- Doses above 10 mg/d are not advised and may actually decrease response.
- For patients with renal impairment, dose is lowered according to creatinine clearance.
- Since rate of absorption is not appreciably slowed by food, it may be given without regard to meals.
- Administer capsule or tablet whole. Do not crush or break and instruct patient not to chew before swallowing.
- Store away from heat, light, or moisture.

Assessment & Drug Effects
- Before administration, assess heart rate. If pulse is less than 50 bpm, withhold drug and notify physician
- Do not administer to patients with asthma or severe COPD.
- Monitor BP and pulse frequently during period of adjustment and periodically throughout therapy.
- If hypotension (systolic BP ≤ 90 mm Hg) occurs, discontinue the drug and carefully assess the hemodynamic status of the patient.
- Monitor daily weight and assess for evidence of fluid overload since drug may precipitate CHF (see Signs & Symptoms, chap 3).

Common side effects in *italic*; life-threatening effects <u>underlined</u>; generic names in **bold**; classifications in SMALL CAPS

393

- Mental depression may be increased by use of this drug.
- If the patient has history of bronchitis or emphysema, assess for respiratory difficulty.
- Drug may prevent the appearance of early signs and symptoms of acute hypoglycemia (see chap 3).
- Monitor diabetic for signs and symptoms of loss of diabetic control.
- Drug may reduce tolerance to cold temperatures in elderly patients or in those who have circulatory problems.

Patient & Family Education
- Advise patient to report the first sign or symptom of impending CHF (see Signs & Symptoms, chap 3) or unexplained respiratory symptoms.
- Advise patient not to discontinue medication abruptly, since sudden withdrawal may precipitate or exacerbate angina.
- Advise patient not to use any OTC products such as nasal decongestants and cold preparations without consultation.
- Instruct patient to report slow pulse rate, confusion or depression, dizziness or lightheadedness, skin rash, fever, sore throat, or unusual bleeding or bruising.
- Advise patient to be cautious while driving or performing other hazardous activities until response to drug is known.
- Stress the importance of compliance no matter how well the patient feels.
- Instruct patient to take BP at least twice a week and to report siginficant changes.
- Instruct patient to take pulse before and after taking the medication. If it is much slower than normal rate (or less than 50 bpm), check with the physician.

Prototype: bisacodyl, p 221

CASCARA SAGRADA
(kas-kar´a)

Trade names: Cascara Sagrada Aromatic Fluidextract, Cascara Sagrada Fluidextract
Classifications: GI AGENT; STIMULANT LAXATIVE
Pregnancy: Category C

ACTIONS/PHARMACODYNAMICS   Anthraquinone derivative obtained from bark of buckhorn tree (*Rhamnus purshiana*). Acts principally in large intestine by stimulating propulsive movements of colon through direct chemical irritation. Casanthrol, which is present in a variety of OTC mixtures, is a derivative of cascara sagrada.

USES Temporary relief of constipation and to prevent straining at stool in various disease conditions. Sometimes used with milk of magnesia.

ROUTE & DOSAGE

Laxative

Adult	PO	Tablet: 325–1000 mg/d; fluidextract: 0.5–1.5 ml/d; aromatic fluidextract: 2–6 ml/d
Child	PO	2–12 y: $^1/_2$ of adult dose; <2 y: $^1/_4$ of adult dose

PHARMOCOKINETICS Absorption: minimal absorption from GI tract. **Onset:** 6–12 h. **Metabolism:** metabolized in liver. **Elimination:** eliminated in feces and urine; excreted in breast milk.

CONTRAINDICATIONS & PRECAUTIONS Contraindicated in: abdominal pain, fecal impaction; GI bleeding, ulcerations; appendicitis, gastroenteritis, intestinal obstruction, nursing mothers, CHF.

ADVERSE/SIDE EFFECTS Large doses: anorexia, nausea, gripping, abnormally loose stools, hypokalemia, impaired glucose tolerance, calcium deficiency, discoloration of urine. **Chronic use:** constipation rebound, melanosis of colon.

DIAGNOSTIC TEST INTERFERENCES Possibility of interference with *PSP excretion test* because of urine discoloration.

NURSING IMPLICATIONS

Administration
- For best results administer with a full glass of water on an empty stomach. Results may be delayed somewhat by food.
- Stored preferably between 15 and 30C (59 and 86F), in tightly covered, light-resistant containers, unless otherwise directed by manufacturer.

Patient & Family Education
- A single dose taken before retiring usually results in evacuation of soft stool 6–12 h later.
- Frequent or prolonged use of irritant cathartics disrupts normal reflex activity of colon and rectum and can lead to drug dependence for evacuation.
See bisacodyl for other patient teaching points.

Common side effects in *italic*; life-threatening effects underlined; generic names in **bold**; classifications in SMALL CAPS

Prototype: bisacodyl, p 221

CASTOR OIL

Trade names: Alphamul, Emulsoil, Fleet Castor Oil Stimulant Laxative, Kellogg's Castor Oil, Neoloid, Oleum Ricini, Purge, Unisoil
Classification: GI AGENT; STIMULANT LAXATIVE
Pregnancy: Category X

ACTIONS/PHARMACODYNAMICS Obtained from the seeds of *Ricinus communis*. Hydrolyzed in small intestine to glycerol and ricinoleic acid, a local irritant. Stimulates motor activity in small intestine and inhibits antiperistalsis in colon, thus preventing normal fluid absorption from intestinal contents. Rapid evacuation of copious liquid or semiliquid stools follows, with little or no colic.

USES To prepare abdomen for radiographic examination of colon and kidneys and to evacuate irritants and poisons from intestinal tract. Rarely used to relieve constipation. Also applied locally to skin as emollient and protectant and to conjunctivae (sterile) to alleviate irritation caused by the presence of a foreign body.

ROUTE & DOSAGE

Colonic Evacuation

Adult	PO	15–60 ml administered as single dose 16 h before procedure.
Child	PO	2–12 y: 5–15 ml
		<2 y: 1–5 ml

PHARMACOKINETICS Absorption: poorly absorbed. **Onset:** 2–3 h. **Distribution:** appears in breast milk.

CONTRAINDICATIONS & PRECAUTIONS Contraindicated in: hypersensitivity to castor bean; dehydration, fecal impaction, abdominal pain, nausea, vomiting, appendicitis; GI bleeding, ulcerations, perforation, obstruction; use in conjunction with fat-soluble vermifuges; pregnancy (category X), nursing women, menstruation.

ADVERSE/SIDE EFFECTS Severe purgation, nausea, vomiting, abdominal cramps, flatus, rebound constipation, irritation of colon, pelvic congestion (rare); dehydration, electrolyte imbalance, elevation of blood glucose levels (extended use).

NURSING IMPLICATIONS

Administration
- More active if taken on empty stomach. Because castor oil is a fat, it may retard gastric emptying time.
- In general it is best not to schedule a laxative within 2 h of taking other medications.
- Action begins in 2–3 h, depending on dose. Time the administration so as not to interfere with patient's sleep.
- Castor oil has objectionable odor, taste, and consistency. It may be made somewhat more palatable by chilling it and administering it with cold fruit juice or a carbonated beverage chaser.
- Emulsified forms are reported to be less disagreeable to taste. Shake emulsion well before pouring. Mix with 1/2–1 glass (120–240 ml) of liquid (water, soft drink, fruit juice, milk).
- Store in tightly covered containers at 15–30C (59–86F) unless otherwise directed. Avoid exposure to excessive light. Protect from freezing.

Assessment & Drug Effects
- Assess effectiveness of medication, especially when it is used in preparation for roentgenographic examination.

Patient & Family Education
- Castor oil causes complete emptying of intestinal contents, and therefore normal evacuation may be delayed for 2 d or more.
- Long-term use may result in laxative dependence.

Prototype: cefonicid, p 60

CEFACLOR

(sef´a-klor)
Trade name: Ceclor
Classifications: ANTIINFECTIVE; ANTIBIOTIC; SECOND GENERATION CEPHALOSPORIN
Pregnancy: Category B

ACTIONS/PHARMACODYNAMICS Semisynthetic, second generation oral cephalosporin antibiotic similar to cefonicid. Possibly more active than

Common side effects in *italic*; life-threatening effects <u>underlined</u>; generic names in **bold**; classifications in SMALL CAPS

395

other oral cephalosporins against gram-negative bacilli, especially beta-lactamase-producing *Haemophilus influenzae,* including ampicillin-resistant strains. Also active against *Escherichia coli, Proteus mirabilis, Klebsiella* sp and certain gram-positive strains, e.g., *Streptococcus pneumoniae, S. pyogenes,* and *Staphylococcus aureus.* Preferentially binds to one or more of the penicillin-binding proteins (PBPs) located on cell walls of susceptible organisms. This inhibits third and final stage of bacterial cell wall synthesis, thus killing the bacterium. Partial cross-allergenicity between penicillins and cephalosporins has been reported. Cefaclor has not been associated with hemostatic defects or pseudomembranous enterocolitis.

USES Treatment of otitis media and infections of upper and lower respiratory tract, urinary tract, and skin and skin structures caused by ampicillin-resistant *H. influenzae;* acute uncomplicated UTI.

ROUTE & DOSAGE

Mild to Moderate Infections

Adult	PO	250–500 mg q8h
Child	PO	20–40 mg/kg/d divided q8h (max 1 g/d)

PHARMACOKINETICS Absorption: well absorbed; acid stable. **Peak:** 30–60 min. **Elimination:** half-life 0.5–1 h; 60% of dose eliminated renally in 8 h; crosses placenta; excreted in breast milk.

CONTRAINDICATIONS & PRECAUTIONS Contraindicated in: hypersensitivity to cephalosporins and related antibiotics. Safe use during pregnancy (category B), in nursing mothers, and infants < 1 mo not established. **Cautious use in:** history of sensitivity to penicillins or other drug allergies; markedly impaired renal function.

ADVERSE/SIDE EFFECTS GI: *diarrhea;* nausea, vomiting, anorexia, pseudomembranous colitis. **Hematologic:** transient leukopenia, transient leukocytosis, slight elevations of AST, ALT, alkaline phosphatase, BUN, serum creatinine; positive direct Coombs' test. **Hypersensitivity:** serum sickness–like reaction: urticaria, pruritus, morbilliform eruptions, eosinophilia, joint pain or swelling, fever. **Other:** superinfections.

DIAGNOSTIC TEST INTERFERENCES Cefaclor may produce positive direct Coombs' test, which can complicate ***cross-matching procedures*** and ***hematologic studies.*** False-positive ***urine glucose*** determinations may result with use of copper sulfate reduction methods, e.g., Clinitest or Benedict's reagent, but not with glucose oxidase (enzymatic) tests such as Clinistix, Diastix, Tes-Tape.

DRUG INTERACTIONS Probenecid decreases renal excretion of cefaclor.

NURSING IMPLICATIONS

Administration
- Administered with food if nausea and vomiting appear to be associated with gastric irritation. Although food in the intestinal tract delays absorption and reduces blood level totals, amount absorbed is unchanged.
- After stock oral suspension is prepared, it should be kept refrigerated. Expiration date should appear on label. Discard unused portion after 14 d. Shake well before pouring.
- Store pulvules at 15–30C (59–86F) in tightly closed container unless otherwise directed.

Assessment & Drug Effects
- Culture and susceptibility tests recommended prior to and periodically during therapy.
- Before therapy is initiated, a careful inquiry should be made concerning previous hypersensitivity to cephalosporins, penicillins, and other drug allergies.
- Diarrhea, the most frequent adverse effect, may be due to a pharmacologic effect or to associated change in intestinal flora. If it persists, interruption of therapy may be necessary.
- Monitor for manifestations of drug hypersensitivity (see Signs & Symptoms, chap 3). Discontinue drug and promptly report them if they appear.
- Monitor for manifestations of superinfection (see Signs & Symptoms, chap 3). Promptly report their appearance.

Patient & Family Education
- Urge patient to report promptly signs and symptoms of superinfection (see chap 3).
- Yogurt or buttermilk (if allowed) may serve as a prophylactic against intestinal superinfections by helping to maintain normal intestinal flora.
- Instruct patient to take medication for the full course of therapy as directed by physician.

Common side effects in *italic;* life-threatening effects underlined; generic names in **bold;** classifications in SMALL CAPS

Prototype: cephalothin, p 58

CEFADROXIL

(set-a-drox´ill)
Trade names: Duricef, Ultracef
Classifications: ANTIINFECTIVE; ANTIBIOTIC;
FIRST GENERATION CEPHALOSPORIN
Pregnancy: Category B

ACTIONS/PHARMACODYNAMICS
Semi-synthetic, first generation cephalosporin antibiotic with antibacterial spectrum similar to that of cephalothin. Bactericidal action (similar to that of penicillins): drug penetrates bacterial cell wall, resists beta-lactamases and inactivates enzymes essential to cell wall synthesis. At equivalent doses, reportedly attains greater concentrations in serum and urine than other oral cephalosporins. Active against organisms that liberate cephalosporinase and penicillinase (beta-lactamases). According to clinical and laboratory evidence, partial cross-allergenicity exists between penicillins and cephalosporins.

USES Primarily in treatment of urinary tract infections caused by *Escherichia coli*, *Proteus mirabilis*, and *Klebsiella* sp; infections of skin and skin structures caused by staphylococci and streptococci; and for treatment of group A beta-hemolytic streptococcal pharyngitis and tonsillitis.

ROUTE & DOSAGE

Uncomplicated Urinary Tract Infection

Adult	PO	1–2 g/d in 1–2 divided doses
Child	PO	30 mg/kg/d in 2 divided doses

Skin and Skin Structure Infections, Streptococcal Pharyngitis, or Tonsillitis

Adult	PO	1 g/d in 1–2 divided doses
Child	PO	30 mg/kg/d in 2 divided doses

Renal Impairment (Creatinine Clearance <25 ml/min)

Adult	PO	1 g q24h
Child	PO	15 mg/kg q24h

PHARMACOKINETICS Absorption: acid stable; rapidly absorbed from GI tract. **Peak:** 1 h. **Elimination:** half-life 1–12 h; 90% excreted unchanged in urine within 8 h; bacterial inhibitory levels persist 20–22 h; crosses placenta; excreted in breast milk.

CONTRAINDICATIONS & PRECAUTIONS Contraindicated in: hypersensitivity to cephalosporins and related antibiotics. Safe use during pregnancy (category B), in nursing mothers, and in children not established. **Cautious use in:** sensitivity to penicillins or other drug allergies; impaired renal function, history of colitis.

ADVERSE/SIDE EFFECTS GI: nausea, *diarrhea*, vomiting, heartburn, gastritis, bloating, abdominal cramps. **Hypersensitivity:** rash, swollen eyelids (angioedema), pruritus, chills. **Other:** dysuria, dizziness, headache, fatigue, positive direct Coombs' test; increased AST, ALT, alkaline phosphatase; transient neutropenia, superinfections.

DIAGNOSTIC TEST INTERFERENCES False-positive *urine glucose* determinations using copper sulfate reduction reagents, such as Clinitest or Benedict's reagent, but not with glucose oxidase tests, e.g., Clinistix, Diastix, Tes-Tape. Cefadroxil-induced positive direct Coombs' test may interfere with *cross-matching procedures* and *hematologic studies.*

DRUG INTERACTIONS Probenecid decreases renal excretion of cefadroxil.

NURSING IMPLICATIONS

Administration

- Nausea may be reduced by administration of drug with food or milk. If nausea persists, termination of therapy may be necessary.
- Directions for mixing the oral suspension are on the label. Reconstituted solution contains 125 mg or 250 mg cefadroxil per 5 ml suspension. Shake well before use; discard after 14 d.
- Store in tight container at 15–30C (59–86F) unless otherwise directed. Oral suspensions are stable for 14 d under refrigeration at 2–8C (36–46F). Avoid freezing. Note expiration date on label.

Assessment & Drug Effects

- Culture and susceptibility testing are recommended prior to and periodically during therapy.
- Before therapy is initiated, a careful inquiry should be made concerning previous hypersensitivity to cephalosporins, penicillins, and other drug allergies.
- Baseline and periodic renal function studies should be performed in patients with renal function impairment, and I&O ratio and pattern should be monitored.

Common side effects in *italic*; life-threatening effects underlined; generic names in **bold**; classifications in SMALL CAPS

397

- Monitor for manifestations of drug hypersensitivity (see Signs & Symptoms, chap 3). Discontinue drug and promptly report them if they appear.
- Monitor for manifestations of superinfection (see Signs & Symptoms, chap 3). Promptly report their appearance.

Patient & Family Education

- If patient is allergic to penicillin, the possibility of an allergic reaction is high. Report promptly the onset of rash, urticaria, pruritus, fever.
- Instruct patient to take medication for the full course of therapy as directed by the physician.
- Report promptly signs and symptoms of superinfections (see chap 3).

Prototype: cefonicid, p 60

CEFAMANDOLE NAFATE

(sef-a-man´dole)
Trade name: Mandol
Classifications: ANTIINFECTIVE; ANTIBIOTIC; SECOND GENERATION CEPHALOSPORIN
Pregnancy: Category B

ACTIONS/PHARMACODYNAMICS Semisynthetic, second generation cephalosporin antibiotic similar to other drugs of this class. Preferentially binds to one or more of the penicillin-binding proteins (PBP) located on cell walls of susceptible organisms. This inhibits third and final stage of bacterial wall synthesis, thus killing the bacterium. Usually active against organisms susceptible to first generation cephalosporins. In addition it is active against the anaerobes *Clostridium* sp, *Peptococcus* sp, *Fusobacterium* sp; and against some strains of *Providencia* sp, *Enterobacter, Serratia, Proteus, E. coli,* and *Klebsiella* resistant to first generation cephalosporins. Inactive against enterococci, methicillin-resistant staphylococci, *Listeria monocytogenes* and *Pseudomonas.* Partial cross-allergenicity between penicillins and cephalosporins has been reported. Chemical structure contains a methyltetrazolethiol side chain that is associated with coagulation abnormalities.

USES Serious infections of respiratory, genitourinary, and biliary tracts, skin and soft tissue, bones and joints, and in septicemia and peritonitis (caused by *E. coli* and other coliform microbes); also perioperative prophylaxis to reduce infections in patient undergoing potentially contaminated procedure.

ROUTE & DOSAGE

Moderate to Severe Infections

Adult	IV/IM	500 mg–1 g q4–8h, up to 2 g q4h
Child	IV/IM	50–100 mg/kg/d in 3–6 divided doses, up to 150 mg/kg/d (not to exceed adult doses)

Surgical Prophylaxis

Adult	IV/IM	1–2 g 30–60 min before surgery, then q6h for 24 h
Child	IV/IM	50–100 mg/kg 30–60 min before surgery, then q6h for 24 h

PHARMACOKINETICS Peak levels: 0.5–2 h after IM; 10 min after IV. **Distribution:** poor CNS penetration even with inflamed meninges; extensive enterohepatic circulation; high concentrations in bile. **Metabolism:** rapidly hydrolyzed in plasma to active metabolite. **Elimination:** half-life: 30–120 min; 68–85% excreted unchanged in urine in 6–8 h.

CONTRAINDICATIONS & PRECAUTIONS Contraindicated in: hypersensitivity to cephalosporins and related antibiotics. Safe use during pregnancy (category B), in nursing mothers, and in children between 1 and 6 mo not established. **Cautious use in:** history of sensitivity to penicillins or other drug allergies; renal function impairment; history of GI disease, particularly colitis.

ADVERSE/SIDE EFFECTS GI: abdominal cramps, *diarrhea,* pseudomembranous colitis. **Hematologic:** (rare): neutropenia, thrombocytopenia, hypoprothrombinemia (vitamin K deficiency), positive Coombs' test, transient elevations in AST, ALT, alkaline phosphatase, BUN. **Hypersensitivity:** rash, urticaria, drug fever, eosinophilia. **Other:** pain, redness and induration, sterile abscess at injection site, superinfections.

DIAGNOSTIC TEST INTERFERENCES False-positive *urine glucose* determinations using copper sulfate reduction methods, e.g., Clinitest or Benedict's reagent, but not with glucose oxidase (enzymatic) tests such as Clinistix, Diastix, Tes-Tape. Cefamandole-induced positive direct Coombs' test may interfere with *cross-matching procedures* and *hematologic studies.*

Common side effects in *italic*; life-threatening effects underlined; generic names in **bold**; classifications in SMALL CAPS

DRUG INTERACTIONS **Probenecid** decreases renal elimination of cefamandole; **alcohol** causes disulfiram reaction.

INCOMPATIBILITIES **Solution/additive:** Ringer's lactate, calcium gluconate, calcium gluceptate, cimetidine, AMINOGLYCOSIDES, **metronidazole**, **magnesium.** **Y-Site:** AMINOGLYCOSIDES.

NURSING IMPLICATIONS

Administration
- *For IM administration:* to each gram of cefamandole add 3 ml of sterile water for injection or bacteriostatic water for injection, 0.9% NaCl injection or 0.9% bacteriostatic NaCl injection. Resulting solution will contain 285 mg cefamandole per milliliter.
- Administer IM deep into a large muscle mass such as gluteus maximus or lateral thigh.
- After reconstitution, cefamandole may liberate CO_2. Do not store medication in syringes, as pressure build-up from CO_2 may force plunger out of barrel.
- *For direct IV administration:* each gram of cefamandole should be reconstituted with 10 ml sterile water for injection, 5% dextrose injection, or 0.9% NaCl injection. Appropriate dose is administered slowly over 3–5 min.
- Cefamandole may be further diluted in 100–1000 ml of D5W or NS and given by IV intermittent or continuous infusion. The rate of infusion is determined by the amount of solution.
- Prolonged exposure to light causes cefamandole powder to discolor. Once reconstituted, cefamandole is no longer light sensitive. Solutions appear light yellow to amber. Do not use if otherwise colored or if a precipitate is present.
- Because cefamandole is formulated with sodium carbonate, it is incompatible with fluids containing magnesium or calcium ions. Consult package insert for compatible IV infusion fluids and stability and storage times.
- Store cefamandole powder at 15–30C (59–86F). Protect from light. Reconstituted drug remains stable at 15–30C (59–86F) for 24 h and when refrigerated at 5C (41F), for 96 h.

Assessment & Drug Effects
- Culture and susceptibility testing recommended prior to and periodically during therapy. Cefamandole therapy may be instituted pending test results.
- Before therapy is initiated, determine previous hypersensitivity to cephalosporins, penicillins, and other drugs.

- Baseline and periodic studies of renal function and PT determinations should be performed.
- Monitor I&O ratio and pattern, particularly in patients with impaired renal function, patients > 50 y, or patients who are receiving high doses.
- Antibiotic associated pseudomembranous enterocolitis (life-threatening) is a superinfection caused by *Clostridia difficile* (spore- and toxin-forming bacteria) and may occur in 4–9 d or as long as 6 wk after cefamandole is discontinued (see Signs & Symptoms, chap 3). Most likely to occur in the chronically ill or debilitated elderly patient especially if undergoing abdominal surgery or if in an ICU.
- At onset of diarrhea, patient should check for fever and report fever and diarrhea to physician.
- Monitor for manifestations of hypersensitivity (see Signs & Symptoms, chap 3). If they appear, discontinue drug and report them promptly.

Patient & Family Education
- Advise patient to avoid use of alcohol during and for 48–72 h after taking cefamandole. A drug-induced disulfiram-like reaction (see Signs & Symptoms, chap 3) may follow alcohol intake.
- Drug therapy for beta-hemolytic streptococcal infections should continue for at least 10 d to guard against risk of rheumatic fever and glomerulonephritis.
- Superinfections may occur, particularly during prolonged use of cephalosporins. Report promptly signs and symptoms of superinfection (see chap 3).
- Patient should report loose stools or diarrhea.
- Yogurt or buttermilk, 120 ml (4 oz) of either (if allowed), may serve as a prophylactic against intestinal superinfection by helping to maintain normal intestinal flora.

Prototype: cephalothin, p 58

CEFAZOLIN SODIUM
(sef-a´zoe-lin)
Trade names: Ancef, Kefzol
Classifications: ANTIINFECTIVE; ANTIBIOTIC; FIRST GENERATION CEPHALOSPORIN
Pregnancy: Category B

ACTIONS/PHARMACODYNAMICS Semisynthetic, first generation derivative of cephalosporin C; antibiotic activity similar to that of cephalothin. Activity against gram-negative organisms is limited.

Common side effects in *italic*; life-threatening effects underlined; generic names in **bold**; classifications in SMALL CAPS

399

C

Reported to be less irritating to tissue and less nephrotoxic than cephalothin, and to produce higher and more sustained serum levels at equivalent dosages. Bactericidal action: preferentially binds to one or more of the penicillin-binding proteins (PBP) located on cell walls of susceptible organisms. This inhibits third and final stage of bacterial cell wall synthesis, thus killing the bacterium. Appears to be less resistant to bacterial beta-lactamases (cephalosporinases and penicillinases) than other cephalosporins.

USES Severe infections of urinary and biliary tracts, skin, soft tissue, and bone, and for bacteremia and endocarditis caused by susceptible organisms; also perioperative prophylaxis in patients undergoing procedures associated with high risk of infection, e.g., open heart surgery.

ROUTE & DOSAGE

Moderate to Severe Infections

Adult	IV/IM	250 mg–2 g q8h, up to 2 g q4h (max 12 g/d)
Child	IV/IM	25–50 mg/kg/d in 3–4 divided doses, up to 100 mg/kg/d (not to exceed adult doses)

Surgical Prophylaxis

Adult	IV/IM	1–2 g 30–60 min before surgery, then q8h for 24 h
Child	IV/IM	25–50 mg/kg 30–60 min before surgery, then q8h for 24 h

PHARMACOKINETICS Peak: 1–2 h after IM; 5 min after IV. **Distribution:** poor CNS penetration even with inflamed meninges; high concentrations in bile and in diseased bone; crosses placenta. **Elimination:** half-life: 90–130 min; 70% excreted unchanged in urine in 6 h; small amount excreted in breast milk.

CONTRAINDICATIONS & PRECAUTIONS Contraindicated in: hypersensitivity to any cephalosporin and related antibiotics. Safe use during pregnancy (category B), in nursing mothers, and in infants < 1 mo not established. **Cautious use in:** history of penicillin sensitivity, impaired renal function, patients on sodium restriction.

ADVERSE/SIDE EFFECTS GI: *diarrhea,* anorexia, abdominal cramps. **Hematologic:** neutropenia, leukopenia, thrombocytopenia, positive direct and indirect Coombs' test, transient rise in BUN, AST, ALT, alkaline phosphatase. **Hypersensitivity:** <u>anaphylaxis</u>, maculopapular rash, urticaria, fever, eosinophilia. **Other:**

superinfections, seizure (high doses in patients with renal insufficiency), hemostatic defects.

DIAGNOSTIC TEST INTERFERENCES Because of cefazolin effect on the direct Coombs' test, transfusion ***cross-matching procedures*** and ***hematologic studies*** may be complicated. False-positive ***urine glucose*** determinations are possible with use of copper sulfate tests (e.g., Clinitest or Benedict's reagent) but not with glucose oxidase tests such as Tes-Tape, Diastix, or Clinistix.

DRUG INTERACTIONS Probenecid decreases renal elimination of cefazolin.

INCOMPATIBILITIES Solution/additive: AMINOGLYCOSIDES, **bleomycin, ascorbic acid, cimetidine, lidocaine, vitamin B complex with C, amobarbital, calcium chloride, calcium gluceptate, calcium gluconate, colistin, erythromycin,** TETRACYCLINES, **pentobarbital, polymyxin B. Y-Site:** AMINOGLYCOSIDES.

NURSING IMPLICATIONS

Administration

- IM injections should be made deep into large muscle mass. Pain on injection is usually minimal. Rotate injection sites.
- Preparation of IM solution: reconstituted with sterile water for injection, bacteriostatic water for injection, or 0.9% sodium chloride injection. Reconstituted solutions are stable for 24 hr at room temperature and for 96 hr refrigerated.
- For IV administration, dilute each 1 g with 10 ml of sterile water for injection. May be further diluted with 50–100 ml of NS or D5W. Infuse 1 g over 5 min or longer as determined by the amount of solution.
- The risk of IV site reactions may be reduced by proper dilution of IV solution, use of small bore IV needle in a large vein, and by rotating injection sites.
- Store vials preferably between 15 and 30C (59 and 86F), unless otherwise directed by manufacturer.

Assessment & Drug Effects

- Before therapy is initiated determine history of hypersensitivity to cephalosporins, penicillins, and other drugs.
- Culture and susceptibility testing is recommended prior to and during therapy. Therapy may be initiated pending results.
- Monitor intake and output ratio and pattern. Be alert to changes in BUN, serum creatinine.

Common side effects in *italic;* life-threatening effects <u>underlined;</u> generic names in **bold**; classifications in SMALL CAPS

- If patient has had a reaction to penicillin, be alert to signs of hypersensitivity with use of cefazolin. Cross-allergenicity between cephalosporins and penicillin has been reported. Prompt attention should be given to onset of signs of hypersensitivity (see chap 3).
- Promptly report the onset of diarrhea, which may or may not be dose related. It is seen especially in patients with history of drug-related GI disturbances. Pseudomembranous colitis, a potentially life-threatening condition, starts with diarrhea.

Patient & Family Education
- Report promptly signs and symptoms of superinfection (see chap 3).
- Report signs of hemostatic defects: ecchymoses, petechiae, nose bleed.

Prototype: cefotaxime, p 62

CEFIXIME
(ce-fi´xim)
Trade name: Suprax
Classifications: ANTIINFECTIVE; ANTIBIOTIC; THIRD GENERATION CEPHALOSPORIN
Pregnancy: Category B

ACTIONS/PHARMACODYNAMICS
A third generation cephalosporin that is highly stable in the presence of beta-lactamases (penicillinases and cephalosporinases) and therefore has excellent activity against a wide range of gram-negative bacteria. It is bactericidal against susceptible bacteria. Cephalosporins inhibit mucopeptide synthesis in the bacterial cell wall.

USES
Effective against *Streptococcus pyogenes, Streptococcus pneumoniae,* and gram-negative bacilli, including *Haemophilus influenzae, Branhamella catarrhalis,* and *Neisseria gonorrhoeae.* Little activity against staphylococci, and no activity against *Pseudomonas aeruginosa;* also uncomplicated UTI, otitis media, pharyngitis, tonsillitis, and bronchitis.

ROUTE & DOSAGE

Infection

Adult	PO	400 mg/d in 1–2 divided doses
Child	PO	8 mg/kg/d in 1–2 divided doses

PHARMACOKINETICS
Absorption: 40–50% absorbed from GI tract. **Peak:** 2–6 h. **Distribution:** distributed into breast milk. **Elimination:** half-life: 3–4 h; 50% excreted in urine, 50% in bile.

CONTRAINDICATIONS & PRECAUTIONS
Contraindicated in: patients with known allergy to the cephalosporin group of antibiotics. **Cautious use in:** allergy to penicillin, history of colitis, renal insufficiency.

ADVERSE/SIDE EFFECTS
GI: *diarrhea,* loose stools, nausea, vomiting, dyspepsia, flatulence. **CNS:** drug fever, headache, dizziness. **Other:** rash, pruritus, vaginitis, genital pruritus, thrombocytopenia, leukopenia.

NURSING IMPLICATIONS

Administration
- Oral drug may be administered without regard to meals.
- Because of lack of bioequivalence, tablets should not be substituted for liquid in treatment of otitis media.
- After reconstitution, suspension may be kept for 14 d at room temperature or refrigerated. Store away from heat and light. Keep tightly closed and shake well before using.

Assessment & Drug Effects
- Culture and susceptibility tests should be performed prior to initiation of therapy and periodically during therapy. Therapy may be implemented pending test results.
- Before therapy is initiated a careful inquiry should be made to determine previous hypersensitivity reactions to cephalosporins, penicillins, and history of other allergies, particularly to drugs.
- If seizures associated with the drug therapy occur, the drug should be discontinued.
- Superinfections (see Signs & Symptoms, chap 3) caused by overgrowth of nonsusceptible organisms may occur, particularly during prolonged use.
- Monitor I&O ratio and pattern. Nephrotoxicity occurs more frequently in patients > 50 y, with impaired renal function, in the debilitated, and in patients receiving high doses or other nephrotoxic drugs.
- Carefully monitor anyone with a history of allergies, especially to drugs. Report manifestations of hypersensitivity (see Signs & Symptoms, chap 3).
- Promptly report loose stools or diarrhea, which may indicate pseudomembranous colitis (see Signs

---

Common side effects in *italic*; life-threatening effects <u>underlined</u>; generic names in **bold**; classifications in SMALL CAPS

& Symptoms, chap 3). Discontinuation of drug may be necessary.

Patient & Family Education
- Instruct patient to report loose stools or diarrhea during drug therapy and for several weeks after. Elderly patients are especially susceptible to pseudomembranous colitis.
- Instruct patient to take antibiotic for the full course of treatment.
- Instruct patient not to miss any doses and to take the doses at evenly spaced times, day and night.

Prototype: cefotaxime, p 62

CEFMETAZOLE
(sef-met´a-zol)
Trade name: Zefazone
Classifications: ANTIINFECTIVE; ANTIBIOTIC; THIRD GENERATION CEPHALOSPORIN
Pregnancy: Category B

ACTIONS/PHARMACODYNAMICS Cefmetazole is a synthetic cephalosporin antibiotic. Its bactericidal action results from inhibition of cell wall synthesis. It is active against a wide range of aerobic and anaerobic gram-positive and gram-negative bacteria.

USES UTI infections caused by *Escherichia coli*, lower respiratory tract infections, namely pneumonia and bronchitis caused by *Streptococcus pneumoniae*, *Staphylococcus aureus*, *E. coli*, *Haemophilus influenzae*. In addition, it is effective against *Staphylococcus epidermidis*, *Streptococcus pyogenes*, *Streptococcus agalactiae*, *Proteus vulgaris*, and *Bacteroides fragilis*; preoperative prophylaxis of cesarean section, hysterectomy, cholecystectomy, and colorectal surgery.

ROUTE & DOSAGE

Systemic Infections
Adult   IV   2 g q6–12h

Surgical Prophylaxis
Adult   IV   1–2 g 30–90 min before surgery; then q8h for 2 more doses

PHARMACOKINETICS Elimination: half-life: 1.2 h; excreted unchanged in urine.

CONTRAINDICATIONS & PRECAUTIONS Contraindicated in: patients with known allergy to cefmetazole or to any other cephalosporin antibiotic. **Cautious use in:** allergy to penicillin, history of colitis, renal insufficiency.

ADVERSE/SIDE EFFECTS GI: *diarrhea,* loose stools, nausea, vomiting, dyspepsia, flatulence. **CNS:** drug fever, headache, dizziness. **Other:** rash, pruritus, vaginitis, genital pruritus.

DRUG INTERACTIONS Probenecid decreases renal elimination of cefmetazole.

INCOMPATIBILITIES Solution/additive: AMINOGLYCOSIDES. **Y-Site:** AMINOGLYCOSIDES.

NURSING IMPLICATIONS

Administration
- Reconstitute with sterile water for injection, bacteriostatic water for injection, or 0.9% NaCl injection. Dilute 1 g with 3.7 ml to yield 250 mg/ml or with 10 ml to yield 100 mg/ml. Dilute 2 g with 7 ml to yield 250 mg/ml or with 15 ml to yield 125 mg/ml.
- May be further diluted to concentrations ranging from 1–20 mg/ml by adding it to 0.9% NaCl, 5% dextrose, or lactate Ringer's injection.
- Drug can be given direct IV over 3–5 min or infused over 10–60 min.
- Observe IV sites for evidence of inflammatory reaction. Risk of phlebitis may be reduced by use of a small needle in a large vein.
- Potency is retained for 24 h after reconstitution at room temperature, 7 d under refrigeration, and for 6 wk if frozen. Store away from heat, light, and moisture; do not refreeze.

Assessment & Drug Effects
- Culture and susceptibility tests should be performed before initiation of therapy and periodically during therapy. Therapy may be implemented pending test results.
- Before therapy is initiated a careful inquiry should be made to determine previous hypersensitivity to cephalosporins, penicillins, and history of other allergies, particularly to drugs.
- Assess for signs and symptoms of superinfections (see chap 3) caused by overgrowth of nonsusceptible organisms, particularly with prolonged use.
- Monitor PT in patients with renal or hepatic disease or those receiving a long course of antibiotic therapy.
- Promptly report loose stools or diarrhea because of risk of pseudomembranous colitis (see Signs & Symptoms, chap 3). Elderly are especially susceptible. Drug may be discontinued.

Common side effects in *italic*; life-threatening effects underlined; generic names in **bold**; classifications in SMALL CAPS

Patient & Family Education

- Patient should report onset of loose stools or diarrhea even for several weeks after drug is discontinued.
- Advise patient that ingestion of alcohol within 24 hours of drug may cause a disulfiram like reaction (see signs & symptoms, chap 3).

CEFONICID SODIUM

See ANTIINFECTIVES, ANTIBIOTIC, SECOND GENERATION CEPHALOSPORIN prototype, p 60.

Prototype: cefotaxime, p 62

CEFOPERAZONE SODIUM

(sef-oh-per′a-zone)
Trade name: Cefobid
Classifications: ANTIINFECTIVE; ANTIBIOTIC; THIRD GENERATION CEPHALOSPORIN
Pregnancy: Category B

ACTIONS/PHARMACODYNAMICS Semisynthetic third generation cephalosporin antibiotic. Preferentially binds to one or more of the penicillin-binding proteins (PBP) located on cell walls of susceptible organisms. This inhibits third and final stage of bacterial cell wall synthesis, thus killing the bacterium. Spectrum of activity is similar to that of cefotaxime. Generally active against a wide variety of gram-negative bacteria, including some strains of *Pseudomonas aeruginosa.* Also active against some organisms resistant to first and second generation cephalosporins and currently available aminoglycoside antibiotics and penicillins: e.g., *Escherichia coli, Klebsiella pneumoniae,* and *Serratia marcescens.* Other susceptible organisms include *Proteus mirabilis, Salmonella, Shigella, Haemophilus influenzae, Neisseria gonorrhoeae,* groups A and B streptococci, *Staphylococcus aureus,* and some strains of *Pseudomonas* sp. Cefoperazone inhibits some strains of *Clostridium,* but *C. difficile* is resistant to the drug, as is *Listeria monocytogenes.* Partial cross-allergenicity between penicillins and cephalosporins has been reported (unpredictable). Chemical structure contains a side chain, which is associated with coagulation abnormalities.

USES Infections of skin and skin structures, urinary tract, respiratory tract; and peritonitis and other intraabdominal infections, pelvic inflammatory disease, endometritis and other infections of the female genital tract, and bacterial septicemia. **Unlabeled use:** children <12 y.

ROUTE & DOSAGE

Moderate to Severe Infections

Adult	IV/IM	1–2 g q12h; 16 g/d in 2–4 divided doses
Child	IV/IM	<12 y: 25–100 mg/kg q12h

PHARMACOKINETICS Peak levels: 1–2 h after IM; 15–20 min after IV. **Distribution:** low CNS penetration except with inflamed meninges; highest concentrations in bile; crosses placenta. **Elimination:** half-life: 2 h, 70–75% excreted unchanged in bile in 6–12 h, small amount excreted in breast milk.

CONTRAINDICATIONS & PRECAUTIONS Contraindicated in: hypersensitivity to cephalosporins and related beta-lactam antibiotics. Safe use during pregnancy (category B) and in children <12 y not established. **Cautious use in:** history of hypersensitivity to penicillins, history of allergy, particularly to drugs; hepatic disease, history of colitis or other GI disease, history of bleeding disorders; nursing mothers.

ADVERSE/SIDE EFFECTS GI: abdominal cramps, bloating, loose stools or *diarrhea.* **Hematologic:** reversible neutropenia (with prolonged use); reduction in neutrophils, Hgb, Hct; abnormal PT and PTT; hypoprothrombinemia. **Hepatic:** hepatitis (rare), elevated liver function tests: AST, ALT, alkaline phosphatase. **Hypersensitivity:** skin rash, urticaria, pruritus, fever, eosinophilia. **Renal:** transient increases in serum creatinine and BUN, oliguria. **Other:** phlebitis (IV site), transient pain (IM site), superinfections.

DIAGNOSTIC TEST INTERFERENCES Cefoperazone can cause positive direct ***Coombs' test,*** which may result in interferences with ***hematologic studies*** and ***cross-matching*** procedures. False-positive results for ***urine glucose*** using copper sulfate tests (Benedict's, Clinitest), but not with glucose enzymatic tests, e.g., Clinistix, Tes-Tape, Diastix. Also causes prolonged prothrombin twice during therapy.

DRUG INTERACTIONS Probenecid decreases renal elimination of cefoperazone; **alcohol** produces disulfiram reaction.

Common side effects in *italic*; life-threatening effects <u>underlined</u>; generic names in **bold**; classifications in SMALL CAPS

403

INCOMPATIBILITIES Solution/additive: AMINO-GLYCOSIDES, **doxapram.** Y-Site: AMINOGLYCOSIDES, **labetalol, meperidine, perphenazine.**

NURSING IMPLICATIONS

Administration

- Dilute each 1 g with 5 ml sterile water. Shake vigorously to dissolve. May be further diluted in 50–100 ml of D5W or NS for intermittent infusion or 500–1000 ml for continuous infusion. See manufacturer's directions for reconstitution and dilution and for compatible diluents.
- Rapid, direct (bolus) IV injections not recommended. Cefoperazone may be administered by intermittent IV over a 15–30 min period or by continuous IV infusion, as prescribed.
- To prepare IM injections, appropriate diluents include sterile water for injection, bacteriostatic water for injection, and 0.5% lidocaine. See package insert for reconstitution procedure.
- Protect sterile powder and piggyback units from light and store at or below 25C (77F). Reconstituted solutions may be stored in original containers for 24 h at 15–25C (59–77F); for 5 d under refrigeration at 5C (41F) or less, or for at least 3 wk in freezer.

Assessment & Drug Effects

- Culture and susceptibility studies should be performed before initiation of therapy and during therapy, as indicated. Therapy may begin pending test results.
- Before therapy begins, determine hypersensitivity to cephalosporins, penicillins, and other drug allergies.
- PTT and PT should be performed before and during therapy.
- Observe for and question patient about signs of hemostatic defects: wound bleeding (e.g., surgical patient), nose bleeds, bleeding gums, bloody sputum, hematuria. Hypoprothrombinemia and vitamin K deficiency are possible complications of therapy and can result in significant blood loss in some patients. Reversible with vitamin K and plasma if necessary.
- Drug-induced vitamin K deficiency develops in conditions that reduce vitamin K–producing bacteria in GI tract. Patients at risk are those with poor nutritional states, malabsorption problems, patients on hyperalimentation regimens, and alcoholism. Vitamin K supplements may be prescribed for these patients, if indicated.
- Report the onset of loose stools or diarrhea. Most patients respond to replacement of fluids, electrolytes, and proteins. Discontinuation of drug may be required for some patients.
- Cefoperazone serum levels (at steady state: 150 µg/ml) should be monitored in patients with hepatic disease or biliary obstruction who are receiving over 4 g/d, patients with both hepatic and renal disease receiving over 1–2 g/d, and patients with renal impairment on high dose therapy.

Patient & Family Education

- Warn patient that ingestion of alcohol within 72 h after drug administration will cause a disulfiram-like reaction (see Signs & Symptoms, chap 3). Effects generally appear within 15–30 min after alcohol is taken and disappear spontaneously 1–2 h later.
- Instruct patient to report promptly signs and symptoms of superinfection (see chap 3).

Prototype: cefonicid, p 60

CEFORANIDE

(se-for´a-nide)
Trade name: Precef
Classifications: ANTIINFECTIVE; ANTIBIOTIC; SECOND GENERATION CEPHALOSPORIN
Pregnancy: Category B

ACTIONS/PHARMACODYNAMICS Semisynthetic, second generation cephalosporin antibiotic with drug structure characterized by a beta-lactam ring (like the penicillin structure); generally resistant to hydrolysis by beta-lactamases. Bactericidal action: preferentially binds to one or more of the penicillin-binding proteins (PBP) located on cell wall of susceptible organisms. This inhibits third and final stage of bacterial cell walls synthesis, thus killing the bacterium. Ceforanide is usually active against the organisms susceptible to first generation cephalosporins. In addition, it is bactericidal against *Providencia* sp, *Clostridium* sp, *Peptococcus* sp, and against strains of *Citrobacter, Enterobacter, Serratia, Neisseria, Proteus, Escherichia coli,* and *Klebsiella* that are resistant to first generation cephalosporins; generally inactive against enterococci, methicillin-resistant staphylococci, *Acinetobacter, Listeria monocytogenes,* and *Pseudomonas*. Partial cross-allergenicity between other beta-lactam antibiotics and cephalosporins has been reported.

Common side effects in *italic*; life-threatening effects <u>underlined</u>; generic names in **bold**; classifications in SMALL CAPS

USES To treat infections caused by susceptible organisms in the lower respiratory tract, urinary tract, skin and skin structures, bones and joints, endocarditis, and septicemia and for perioperative prophylaxis in patient undergoing prosthetic arthroplasty or cardiovascular surgery. **Unlabeled use:** prophylaxis during biliary tract or gastric bypass surgery.

ROUTE & DOSAGE

Moderate to Severe Infections

Adult	IV/IM	500 mg–1 g q12h
Child	IV/IM	20–40 mg/kg/d in 2 divided doses

Surgical Prophylaxis

Adult	IV/IM	500 mg–1 g 60 min before surgery, then q12h for 24 h
Child	IV/IM	20–40 mg/kg 60 min before surgery, then q12h for 24 h

PHARMACOKINETICS Peak: 1 h after IM; 30 min after IV. **Distribution:** poor CNS penetration even with inflamed meninges; crosses placenta. **Metabolism:** not metabolized. **Elimination:** half-life: 2.3–3.3 h; 78–95% excreted unchanged in urine; small amount excreted in breast milk.

CONTRAINDICATIONS & PRECAUTIONS Contraindicated in: hypersensitivity to cephalosporins and related antibiotics; severely impaired renal or hepatic function. Safe use during pregnancy (category B) and in children not established. **Cautious use in:** nursing mothers.

ADVERSE/SIDE EFFECTS GI: nausea, vomiting, *diarrhea,* abdominal cramps. **Hematologic:** *transient thrombocytosis* (20% of patients); eosinophilia, neutropenia, decreased hematocrit. **Other:** superinfections; infection site reactions; hypersensitivity reactions.

DIAGNOSTIC TEST INTERFERENCES Ceforanide causes false-positive direct Coombs' test (may interfere with *cross-matching procedures* and *hematologic studies*).

DRUG INTERACTIONS Probenecid decreases renal elimination of ceforanide.

INCOMPATIBILITIES Solution/Additive: AMINOGLYCOSIDES. **Y-Site:** AMINOGLYCOSIDES.

NURSING IMPLICATIONS

Administration

- IM injections should be made deeply into large muscle mass. Pain and discomfort at IM site occurs commonly. Rotate injection sites
- *Reconstitution: IM:* 500 mg vial with 1.7 ml diluent to make 250 mg/ml solution (see manufacturer's directions).
- *IV:* Dilute contents of 500 mg vial in 5 ml of sterile water or NS for injection; administer slowly by direct IV administration over 3–5 min or further dilute in 50–100 ml D5W or NS and infuse over 30 min.
- Reconstituted solution may become discolored (usually light yellow to amber) if exposed to high temperatures; however, potency is not affected. Solution may be cloudy immediately after reconstitution; let stand and it will clear.
- A supplemental dose (1 g) is generally given immediately following hemodialysis.
- After reconstitution, solution is stable for 48 h at 25C (77F); 14 d when refrigerated at 4C (39F), or 90 d when frozen at −15C (5F). Do not refreeze.

Assessment & Drug Effects

- Before therapy begins determine history of hypersensitivity to cephalosporins, penicillins, or other beta-lactam antibiotics.
- Report onset of diarrhea (may be dose related). If severe, pseudomembranous colitis (see Signs & Symptoms, chap 3) must be ruled out. Elderly patients are especially susceptible.
- Ceforanide serum concentrations should be monitored when drug is used for patient with renal impairment.
- Monitor for manifestations of hypersensitivity (see Signs & Symptoms, chap 3).

Patient & Family Education

- Report promptly signs and symptoms of superinfection (see chap 3). Discontinue drug and promptly report this to physician.

CEFOTAXIME SODIUM

See ANTIINFECTIVES, ANTIBIOTIC, THIRD GENERATION CEPHALOSPORIN prototype, p 62.

Common side effects in *italic*; life-threatening effects <u>underlined</u>; generic names in **bold**; classifications in SMALL CAPS

Prototype: cefotaxime, p 62

CEFOTETAN DISODIUM

(sef´oh-tee-tan)
Trade name: Cefotan
Classifications: ANTIINFECTIVE; ANTIBIOTIC; THIRD GENERATION CEPHALOSPORIN
Pregnancy: Category B

ACTIONS/PHARMACODYNAMICS

Semisynthetic beta-lactam antibiotic, classified as a third generation cephalosporin. Preferentially binds to one or more of the penicillin-binding proteins (PBP) located on cell walls of susceptible organisms. This inhibits third and final stage of bacterial cell wall synthesis, thus killing the bacterium. Generally less active against susceptible staphylococci than first generation cephalosporins are but has broad spectrum of activity against gram-negative bacteria when compared to first and second generation cephalosporins. Spectrum of activity is like that of cefotaxime including *Escherichia coli, Klebsiella* sp, *Enterobacter* sp, *Proteus* sp, *Streptococcus pneumoniae, Staphylococcus aureus,* penicillinase- and nonpenicillinase-producing *Haemophilus influenzae, Salmonella, Shigella, Neisseria gonorrhoeae,* and many anaerobes. Generally inactive against *Pseudomonas aeruginosa.* Chemical structure contains a side chain that is associated with coagulation abnormalities. Partial cross-allergenicity between cephalosporins and other beta-lactam antibiotics has been reported (unpredictable).

USES

Infections caused by susceptible organisms in urinary tract, lower respiratory tract, skin and skin structures, bones and joints, gynecologic tract; also intraabdominal infections, bacteremia, and perioperative prophylaxis.

ROUTE & DOSAGE

Moderate to Severe Infections
Adult IV/IM 1–2 g q12h

Surgical Prophylaxis
Adult IV/IM 1–2 g 30–60 min before surgery

PHARMACOKINETICS

Peak: 1.5–3 h after IM. **Distribution:** poor CNS penetration; widely distributed to body tissues and fluids, including bile, sputum, prostatic and peritoneal fluids; crosses placenta. **Elimination:** half-life: 180–270 min; 51–81% excreted unchanged in urine; 20% excreted in bile; small amount excreted in breast milk.

CONTRAINDICATIONS & PRECAUTIONS

Contraindicated in: hypersensitivity to cephalosporins and related beta-lactam antibiotics. Safe use in pregnancy (category B) and children not established. **Cautious use in:** nursing mothers.

ADVERSE/SIDE EFFECTS

GI: nausea, vomiting, *diarrhea,* abdominal pain. **Hematologic:** eosinophilia, thrombocytopenia, prolongation of bleeding time or prothrombin time. **Hypersensitivity:** rash, pruritus, fever, chills. **Other:** injection site pain, inflammation, disulfiram-like reaction.

DIAGNOSTIC TEST INTERFERENCES

May cause falsely elevated **serum** or **urine creatinine** values (Jaffe reaction). False-positive reactions for **urine glucose** have not been reported using copper sulfate reduction methods, e.g., Benedict's, Clinitest; however, since it has occurred with other cephalosporins, it may be advisable to use glucose oxidase tests (Clinistix, Tes Tape, Diastix). Positive direct antiglobulin (Coombs') test results may interfere with **hematologic studies** and **cross-matching** procedures.

DRUG INTERACTIONS

Probenecid decreases renal elimination of cefotetan; **alcohol** produces disulfiram reaction.

INCOMPATIBILITIES

Solution/additive: AMINOGLYCOSIDES, **doxapram,** TETRACYCLINES, heparin. **Y-Site:** AMINOGLYCOSIDES.

NURSING IMPLICATIONS

Administration

- For direct IV administration, dilute each 1 g with 10 ml of sterile water for injection. May be given by direct IV over 3–5 min.
- For intermittent IV infusion, dilute each 1 g with 50–100 ml of D5W or NS and administer a single dose over 30 min.
- For IV infusion, solution may be given for longer period of time through tubing system through which other IV solutions are being given. Butterfly or scalp vein–type needles are preferred. During infusion, temporarily discontinue administration of other solutions at same site.
- For IM reconstitution (follow manufacturer's directions for selection of diluent), add 2 ml diluent to 1 g size vial; withdraw approximately 2.4 ml to yield 375 mg drug/ml.

- For IM administration, inject well into body of large muscle such as upper outer quadrant of buttock (gluteus maximus).
- Protect sterile powder from light; store at 22C (71.6F) or less; remains stable 24 mo after date of manufacture. May darken with age, but potency is unaffected. Reconstituted solutions: stable for 24 h at 25C (77F); 96 h when refrigerated at 5C (41F); or at least 1 wk when frozen at −20C (−4F). Piggyback reconstituted solutions: stable for 24 h at 25C (77F) or for 96 h at 5C (41F). Reconstituted solutions transferred to plastic syringes: stable for 24 h at room temperature, or 96 h when refrigerated. Thaw frozen solutions at room temperature. Do not refreeze.

Assessment & Drug Effects

- Culture and susceptibility studies should be performed before initiation of therapy and during therapy, as indicated. Therapy may begin pending test results.
- Before therapy begins, determine history of hypersensitivity to cephalosporins and penicillins, and other drug allergies.
- Monitor renal function, especially if cefotetan dose is high or if therapy is prolonged in order to recognize symptoms of nephrotoxicity and ototoxicity (see chap 3).
- Report onset of loose stools or diarrhea. If diarrhea is severe, suspect pseudomembranous colitis (see chap 3) caused by *Clostridium difficile*. Check temperature. Report fever and severe diarrhea to physician; drug should be discontinued.

Patient & Family Education

- Report promptly signs and symptoms of superinfection (see chap 3).
- Report loose stools or diarrhea.

Prototype: cefonicid, p 60

CEFOXITIN SODIUM

(se-fox´i-tin)

Trade name: Mefoxin

Classifications: ANTIINFECTIVE; ANTIBIOTIC; SECOND GENERATION CEPHALOSPORIN

Pregnancy: Category B

ACTIONS/PHARMACODYNAMICS Semisynthetic, broad-spectrum beta-lactam antibiotic derivative of cephamycin C (produced by *Streptomyces lactamdurans*). Classified as second generation cephalosporin; structurally and pharmacologically related to cephalosporins and penicillins. Antimicrobial spectrum of activity resembles that of cefonicid. Considerably less active than most cephalosporins against staphylococci. Preferentially binds to one or more of the penicillin-binding proteins (PBP) located on cell walls of susceptible organisms. This inhibits third and final stage of bacterial cell wall synthesis, thus killing the bacterium. Partial cross-allergenicity between other beta-lactam antibiotics and cephalosporins has been reported. Because of potential for incompatibility, manufacturer states that cefoxitin should not be administered with aminoglycoside antibiotics.

USES Infections caused by susceptible organisms in the lower respiratory tract, urinary tract, skin and skin structures, bones and joints; also intraabdominal endocarditis, gynecological infections, septicemia, uncomplicated gonorrhea, and perioperative prophylaxis in prosthetic arthroplasty or cardiovascular surgery. May be cephalosporin of choice for mixed aerobic-anaerobic infections (e.g., *Bacteroides fragilis*).

ROUTE & DOSAGE

Moderate to Severe Infections

Adult	IV/IM	1–2 g q6–8 h; up to 12 g/d
Child	IV/IM	80–160 mg/kg/d in 4–6 divided doses (max 12 g/d)

Surgical Prophylaxis

Adult	IV/IM	2 g 30–60 min before surgery; then 2 g q6h for 24 h
Child	IV/IM	30–40 mg/kg 30–60 min before surgery; then 2 g q6h for 24 h

Uncomplicated Gonorrhea

Adult	IV/IM	2 g given concurrently with 1 g probenecid PO

PHARMACOKINETICS Peak: 20–30 min after IM; 5 min after IV. **Distribution:** poor CNS penetration even with inflamed meninges; widely distributed in body tissues including pleural, synovial, and ascitic fluid and bile; crosses placenta. **Elimination:** half-life: 45–60 min, 85% excreted unchanged in urine in 6 h, small amount excreted in breast milk.

CONTRAINDICATIONS & PRECAUTIONS Contraindicated in: hypersensitivity to cephalosporins and related antibiotics. Safe use during pregnancy (cate-

Common side effects in *italic*; life-threatening effects <u>underlined</u>; generic names in **bold**; classifications in SMALL CAPS

407

gory B), in nursing mothers, and in children <3 mo not established. **Cautious use in:** history of sensitivity to penicillin or other allergies, particularly to drugs, impaired renal function.

ADVERSE/SIDE EFFECTS GI: *diarrhea,* pseudomembranous colitis. **Hematologic (rare):** transient leukopenia, neutropenia, pancytopenia, hemolytic anemia, positive direct Coombs' test, elevated serum creatinine, BUN, AST, ALT, LDH (lactic dehydrogenase), alkaline phosphatase. **Hypersensitivity:** rash, exfoliative dermatitis, pruritus, urticaria, drug fever, eosinophilia. **Other:** superinfections, local reactions: pain, tenderness, and induration (IM site), thrombophlebitis (IV site); nephrotoxicity, interstitial nephritis.

DIAGNOSTIC TEST INTERFERENCES Cefoxitin causes false-positive (black-brown or green-brown color) *urine glucose* reaction with copper reduction reagents such as Benedict's or Clinitest, but not with enzymatic glucose oxidase reagents (Clinistix, Tes-Tape). With high doses, falsely elevated *serum and urine creatinine* (with Jaffee reaction) reported. False-positive direct Coombs' test (may interfere with *cross-matching procedures* and *hematologic studies*) has also been reported.

DRUG INTERACTIONS Probenecid decreases renal elimination of cefoxitin.

INCOMPATIBILITIES Solution/Additive: AMINOGLYCOSIDES. **Y-Site:** AMINOGLYCOSIDES.

NURSING IMPLICATIONS

Administration

- Recommended diluents for IM solution include sterile water for injection or 0.5 or 1% lidocaine hydrochloride (without epinephrine), used to reduce discomfort of IM injection. Consult physician before using lidocaine.
- After reconstitution for IM use, shake vial and allow solution to stand until it becomes clear. Solutions retain potency for 24 h at room temperature, for 7 d if refrigerated, and for at least 26 wk if frozen.
- Administer IM injections deep into large muscle mass such as upper outer quadrant of gluteus maximus. Aspirate before injecting drug. Rotate injection sites.
- For direct IV administration, dilute each 1 g with 10 ml sterile water, D5W, or NS. May be given by direct IV over 3–5 min.
- For IV infusion, dilute one dose (1–2 g) in 50–1000

ml of compatible solution and give at a rate determined by the volume of solution.

- Drug therapy for beta-hemolytic streptococcal infections should continue for at least 10 d to guard against risk of rheumatic fever.
- Reconstituted solution may become discolored (usually light yellow to amber) if exposed to high temperatures; however, potency is not affected. Solution may be cloudy immediately after reconstitution; let stand and it will clear.
- After reconstitution, solution is stable for 24 h at room temperature 25C (77F); 7 d when refrigerated at 4C (39F), or 30 wk when frozen at −20C (−4F).

Assessment & Drug Effects

- Before therapy is initiated, determine previous hypersensitivity to cephalosporins, penicillins, and other drug allergies.
- Culture and susceptibility testing is advised prior to and periodically during therapy.
- Inspect injection sites regularly. Report evidence of inflammation and patient's complaint of pain.
- Monitor I&O ratio and pattern. Nephrotoxicity occurs most frequently in patients >50 y, in patients with impaired renal function, the debilitated, and in patients receiving high doses or other nephrotoxic drugs.
- Be alert to signs and symptoms of superinfections (see chap 3). This condition is most apt to occur in elderly patients, especially when drug has been used for prolonged period.
- Report onset of diarrhea (may be dose related). If severe, pseudomembranous colitis (see Signs & Symptoms, chap 3) must be ruled out. Elderly patients are especially susceptible.

Prototype: cefotaxime, p 62

CEFTAZIDIME

(sef´tay-zi-deem)
Trade names: Fortaz, Tazicef, Tazidime
Classifications: ANTIINFECTIVE; ANTIBIOTIC; THIRD GENERATION CEPHALOSPORIN
Pregnancy: Category B

ACTIONS/PHARMACODYNAMICS Semisynthetic, third generation broad-spectrum cephalosporin similar to cefotaxime but more active against *Pseudomonas aeruginosa* and less active against

Common side effects in *italic*; life-threatening effects underlined; generic names in **bold**; classifications in SMALL CAPS

staphylococci and *Bacteroides fragilis*. Preferentially binds to one or more of the penicillin-binding proteins (PBP) located on cell walls of susceptible microbes; this inhibits third and final stage of bacterial cell wall synthesis, leading to cell death. Most strains of gonococci, meningococci and *Haemophilus influenzae* are highly susceptible to ceftazidime; *Listeria monocytogenes* organisms are resistant. Emergence of resistance during treatment has been reported. May be used concomitantly with other antibiotics (e.g., aminoglycosides, vancomycin, clindamycin).

USES To treat infections of lower respiratory tract, skin and skin structures, urinary tract, bones and joints; also used to treat bacteremia, gynecological, intraabdominal and CNS infections (including meningitis). **Unlabeled uses:** surgical prophylaxis.

ROUTE & DOSAGE

Moderate to Severe Infections

Adult	IV/IM	1–2 g q8–12h; up to 2 g q6h
Child	IV/IM	<4 wk: 30 mg/kg q12h
		1 mo–12 y: 30–50 mg/kg/d in 3 divided doses (max 6 g/d)

PHARMACOKINETICS Peak: 1 h after IM or IV. **Distribution:** CNS penetration with inflamed meninges; also penetrates bone, gallbladder, bile, endometrium, heart, skin, and ascitic and pleural fluids; crosses placenta. **Metabolism:** not metabolized. **Elimination:** half-life: 25–60 min; 80–90% excreted unchanged in urine in 24 h; small amount excreted in breast milk.

CONTRAINDICATIONS & PRECAUTIONS Contraindicated in: hypersensitivity to cephalosporins and related beta-lactam antibiotics. Safe use in pregnancy (category B) and children not established. **Cautious use in:** nursing mothers.

ADVERSE/SIDE EFFECTS GI: nausea, vomiting, *diarrhea,* abdominal pain, metallic taste, drug-associated pseudomembranous colitis. **GU:** vaginitis, candidiasis. **Hematologic:** eosinophilia, thrombocytosis. **Hypersensitivity:** (1–3%): pruritus, rash, urticaria, fever. **Other:** phlebitis, pain or inflammation at injection site, superinfections, transient elevation of hepatic enzymes.

DIAGNOSTIC TEST INTERFERENCES False-positive reactions for **urine glucose** have been reported using copper sulfate (e.g., Benedict's solution, Clinitest). Glucose oxidase tests (Clinistix, TesTape)

are unaffected. May cause positive direct antiglobulin (Coombs') test results which can interfere with *hematologic studies* and *transfusion cross-matching procedures.*

DRUG INTERACTIONS Probenecid decreases renal elimination of ceftazidine.

INCOMPATIBILITIES Solution/Additive: AMINOGLYCOSIDES. **Y-Site:** AMINOGLYCOSIDES.

NURSING IMPLICATIONS

Administration
- **Reconstitution:** Refer to manufacturer's directions regarding diluent and method. IM: add 3 ml diluent to 1 g-size vial to yield 280 mg/ml.
- **IM:** inject into large muscle mass (e.g., upper outer quadrant of gluteus maximus or lateral part of thigh).
- For IV administration, add 10 ml of sterile water for injection to 1 g to yield 280 mg/ml. May be given direct IV over 3–5 min or may be further diluted with 50–100 ml of D5W or NS and infused over 30 min.
- Give through tubing or administration set while patient is also receiving one of the compatible IV fluids. Intermittent administration with Y-type set: during infusion of ceftazidime solution, discontinue other solutions.
- Protect sterile powder from light; store at 15–30C (59–86F). Store commercially available frozen ceftazidime at temperature no greater than −20C (−4F). Reconstituted solution is stable 7 d when refrigerated at 4–5C (39–41F); for 18–24 h when stored at 15–30C (59–86F).

Assessment & Drug Effects
- Culture and susceptibility studies should be performed before initiation of therapy and during therapy as indicated. Therapy may begin pending test results.
- Before therapy begins, determine history of hypersensitivity to cephalosporins and penicillins, and other drug allergies.
- If administered concomitantly with another antibiotic, monitor renal function and report if dysfunction symptoms appear (e.g., changes in I&O ratio and pattern, dysuria).
- Be alert to onset of rash, itching, and dyspnea. Check patient's temperature. If it is elevated, suspect onset of hypersensitivity reaction (see Signs & Symptoms, chap 3).
- Superinfections have occurred and are usually

Common side effects in *italic*; life-threatening effects underlined; generic names in **bold**; classifications in SMALL CAPS

409

caused by *Enterobacter, Pseudomonas* or *Candida* (see Signs & Symptoms, chap 3).

- If diarrhea occurs and is severe, suspect pseudomembranous colitis (caused by *Clostridium difficile*). Check temperature: Report fever and severe diarrhea to physician; drug should be discontinued.

Patient & Family Education

- Instruct patient to report loose stools or diarrhea promptly.
- Advise patient to report signs and symptoms of superinfection promptly.

Prototype: cefotaxime, p 62

CEFTIZOXIME SODIUM

(sef-ti-zox´eem)

Trade name: Cefizox

Classifications: ANTIINFECTIVE; ANTIBIOTIC; THIRD GENERATION CEPHALOSPORIN

Pregnancy: Category B

ACTIONS/PHARMACODYNAMICS Semisynthetic third generation cephalosporin antibiotic. Bactericidal action: preferentially binds to one or more of the penicillin-binding proteins (PBP) located on cell walls of susceptible organisms. This inhibits third and final stage of bacterial cell wall synthesis, thus killing the bacterium. Spectrum of activity similar to that of cefotaxime. Generally resistant to inactivation by beta-lactamases that act principally as cephalosporinases and penicillinases. *Clostridium difficile,* enterococci including *Streptococcus faecalis,* and most strains of *Listeria monocytogenes* are resistant to ceftizoxime. Incompatible with the aminoglycoside antibiotics. Evidence of partial cross-allergenicity among cephalosporins and other beta-lactamase antibiotics has been reported.

USES Infections caused by susceptible organisms in lower respiratory tract, skin and skin structures, urinary tract, bones and joints; also used to treat intraabdominal infections, pelvic inflammatory disease, uncomplicated gonorrhea, meningitis *(Haemophilus influenzae, Streptococcus pneumoniae),* and for surgical prophylaxis. **Unlabeled use:** meningitis caused by *Neisseria meningitidis* and *Escherichia coli.*

PHARMACOKINETICS Peak: 1 h after IM or IV. **Distribution:** crosses placenta. **Metabolism:** not metabo-

lized. **Elimination:** half-life: 25–60 min; 80–90% excreted unchanged in urine in 24 h; small amount excreted in breast milk.

ROUTE & DOSAGE

Moderate to Severe Infections

Adult	IV/IM	1–2 g q8–12h, up to 2 g q4h
Child	IV/IM	≥ 6 mo: 50 mg/kg q6–8h, up to 200 mg/kg/d

CONTRAINDICATIONS & PRECAUTIONS Contraindicated in: hypersensitivity to cephalosporins and other beta-lactam antibiotics. Safe use during pregnancy (category B) and for infants and children not established.

ADVERSE/SIDE EFFECTS GI: nausea, vomiting, diarrhea, pseudomembranous colitis. **Hematologic:** transient eosinophilia, thrombocytosis. **Hypersensitivity:** rash, pruritus, fever. **Other:** transient elevations of BUN, creatinine; phlebitis. *Vaginitis (local):* burning, cellulitis. *Injection sites:* pain, induration, paresthesia.

DIAGNOSTIC TEST INTERFERENCES Ceftizoxime causes false-positive direct Coombs' test (may interfere with *cross-matching procedures* and *hematologic studies*).

DRUG INTERACTIONS Probenecid decreases renal elimination of ceftizoxime.

INCOMPATIBILITIES Solution/Additive: AMINOGLYCOSIDES. **Y-Site:** AMINOGLYCOSIDES.

NURSING IMPLICATIONS

Administration

- For IV administration, dilute each 1 g with 10 ml sterile water. May be given by direct IV over 3–5 min or further diluted in 50–100 ml of D5W or NS and infused over 30 min.
- Store sterile powder at 15–30C (59–86F); protect from light. Consult manufacturer's directions concerning storage of reconstituted solutions.

Assessment & Drug Effects

- Before therapy is instituted, determine history of hypersensitivity reactions to cephalosporins, penicillin, or other drugs. Report to physician history of allergy, particularly to drugs.
- Culture and sensitivity tests should be performed before initiation of therapy and periodically during

Common side effects in *italic*; life-threatening effects underlined; generic names in **bold**; classifications in SMALL CAPS

therapy if indicated. Therapy may be instituted pending test results.

- Be alert to symptoms of hypersensitivity reaction (see chap 3). Serious reactions may require emergency measures.
- It is not known whether this cephalosporin causes false-positive results with urine glucose determination using cupric sulfate solution (Benedict's reagent, or Clinitest).

Patient & Family Education

- Instruct patient to report loose stools or diarrhea promptly.
- Advise patient to report symptoms of hypersensitivity (see chap 3) promptly.

Prototype: cefotaxime, p 62

CEFTRIAXONE SODIUM

(sef-try-ax´one)
Trade name: Rocephin
Classifications: ANTIINFECTIVE; ANTIBIOTIC; THIRD GENERATION CEPHALOSPORIN
Pregnancy: Category B

ACTIONS/PHARMACODYNAMICS
Semisynthetic third generation cephalosporin antibiotic. Bactericidal action: preferentially binds to one or more of the penicillin-binding proteins (PBP) located on cell walls of susceptible organisms. This inhibits third and final stage of bacterial cell wall synthesis, thus killing the bacterium. Spectrum of activity similar to that of cefotaxime including most Enterobacteriaceae, most gram-positive aerobic cocci, *Neisseria meningitidis,* and most strains of penicillinase-producing and nonpenicillinase-producing *Neisseria gonorrhoeae.* Has some activity against *Treponema pallidum* but none against most strains of clostridia. Should not be admixed with other antiinfectives because of potential for incompatibility.

USES
Infections caused by susceptible organisms in lower respiratory tract, skin and skin structures, urinary tract, bones and joints; also intraabdominal infections, pelvic inflammatory disease, uncomplicated gonorrhea, meningitis, and surgical prophylaxis.

PHARMACOKINETICS
Peak: 1.5–4 h after IM; immediately after IV infusion. **Distribution:** widely distributed in body tissues and fluids; good CNS penetration, especially with inflamed meninges; crosses placenta. **Metabolism:** not metabolized. **Elimination:** half-life: 5–10 h; 33–65% excreted unchanged in urine; also excreted in bile; small amount excreted in breast milk.

ROUTE & DOSAGE

Moderate to Severe Infections

Adult	IV/IM	1–2 g q12–24h (max 4 g/d)
Child	IV/IM	50–75 mg/kg/d in 2 divided doses (max 2 g/d)

Meningitis

Adult	IV/IM	2 g q12h
Child	IV/IM	75 mg/kg loading dose, then 100 mg/kg/d in 2 divided doses (max 4 g/d)

Surgical Prophylaxis

Adult	IV/IM	1 g 30–120 min before surgery

Uncomplicated Gonorrhea

Adult	IM	250 mg as single dose

CONTRAINDICATIONS & PRECAUTIONS Contraindicated in: hypersensitivity to cephalosporins and related antibiotics. Safe use during pregnancy (category B) not established. **Cautious use in:** nursing mothers.

ADVERSE/SIDE EFFECTS GI: *diarrhea,* abdominal cramps, <u>pseudomembranous colitis</u>. **Gynecologic:** genital pruritus; moniliasis. **Hematologic:** eosinophilia, thrombocytosis, leukopenia. **Hypersensitivity:** pruritus, fever, chills. **Other:** pain, induration at IM injection site; phlebitis (IV site).

DIAGNOSTIC TEST INTERFERENCES Causes prolonged PT during therapy.

DRUG INTERACTIONS Probenecid decreases renal elimination of ceftriaxone; **alcohol** produces disulfiram reaction.

INCOMPATIBILITIES Solution/Additive: AMINOGLYCOSIDES, **clindamycin. Y-Site:** AMINOGLYCOSIDES.

NURSING IMPLICATIONS

Administration

- For IV administration, dilute each 250 mg with 2.4 ml of sterile water, D5W, or NS to yield 100 mg/ml.

Common side effects in *italic*; life-threatening effects <u>underlined</u>; generic names in **bold**; classifications in SMALL CAPS

411

Further dilute with 50–100 ml D5W or NS and infuse over 30 min.

- Reconstituted solutions should be light yellow to amber.
- Because of its long elimination half-life, ceftriaxone can be given in a single daily dose instead of multiple doses.
- Treatment is continued at least 2 d after symptoms and infections disappear; 4–14 d is usual. For infections caused by *Streptococcus pyogenes,* therapy is continued at least 10 d.
- Protect sterile powder from light. Store at 15–25C (59–77F). Reconstituted solutions: diluent, concentration of solutions are determinants of stability. See manufacturer's instructions.

Assessment & Drug Effects

- Culture and sensitivity tests should be performed before initiation of therapy and periodically during therapy. Dosage may be started pending test results.
- Before therapy is initiated, determine history of hypersensitivity reactions to cephalosporins and penicillins and history of other allergies, particularly to drugs.
- Inspect injection sites for induration and inflammation. Rotate sites. Note IV injection sites for signs of phlebitis (redness, swelling, pain).
- No dosage adjustment is necessary if patient has hepatic or renal impairment; however, if impairment is severe, blood levels are carefully monitored.
- Monitor for manifestations of hypersensitivity (see Signs & Symptoms, chap 3). Report their appearance promptly and discontinue drug.
- Ceftriaxone appears to alter vitamin K–producing gut bacteria; therefore, hypoprothrombinemic bleeding may occur. Watch for and report signs: petechiae, ecchymotic areas, epistaxis, or any unexplained bleeding.
- The incidence of antibiotic-produced pseudomembranous colitis (see Signs & Symptoms, chap 3) is higher than with most cephalosporins. Most vulnerable patients: chronically ill or debilitated elderly patients undergoing abdominal surgery and those who may be in intensive care. If diarrhea occurs, check for fever. Report both promptly.

Patient & Family Education

- Report any signs of bleeding.
- Report loose stools or diarrhea promptly.

Prototype: cefonicid, p 60

CEFUROXIME SODIUM

(se-fyoor-ox´eem)
Trade name: Zinacef

CEFUROXIME AXETIL

Trade name: Ceftin
Classifications: ANTIINFECTIVE; ANTIBIOTIC; SECOND GENERATION CEPHALOSPORIN
Pregnancy: Category B

ACTIONS/PHARMACODYNAMICS Semisynthetic second generation cephalosporin antibiotic with structure similar to that of the penicillins. Resistance against beta-lactamase-producing strains exceeds that of first generation cephalosporins. Antimicrobial spectrum of activity resembles that of cefonicid. Preferentially binds to one or more of the penicillin-binding proteins (PBP) located on cell walls of susceptible organisms. This inhibits third and final stage of bacterial cell wall synthesis, thus killing the bacterium. Partial cross-allergenicity between other beta-lactam antibiotics and cephalosporins has been reported. Cefuroxime may be incompatible with aminoglycoside antibiotics.

USES Infections caused by susceptible organisms in the lower respiratory tract, urinary tract, skin, and skin structures; also used for treatment of meningitis, gonorrhea, and otitis media and for perioperative prophylaxis (e.g., open-heart surgery).

PHARMACOKINETICS Absorption: axetil salt well absorbed from GI tract; hydrolyzed to active drug in GI mucosa. **Peak effect:** PO 2 h; IM 30 min. **Distribution:** widely distributed in body tissues and fluids; adequate CNS penetration with inflamed meninges; crosses placenta. **Elimination:** half-life: 1–2 h; 66–100% excreted in urine in 24 h; excreted in breast milk.

CONTRAINDICATIONS & PRECAUTIONS Contraindicated in: hypersensitivity to cephalosporins and related antibiotics. Safe use during pregnancy (category B) and in children <3 mo not established.

Cautious use in: history of allergy, particularly to drugs; penicillin sensitivity; renal insufficiency; history of colitis or other GI disease; nursing women.

<u>ROUTE & DOSAGE</u>

Moderate to Severe Infections

Adult	PO	250–500 mg q12h
	IV/IM	750 mg–1.5 g q6–8h
Child	PO	125–250 mg q12h
	IV/IM	50–100 mg/kg/d divided q6–8h

Bacterial Meningitis

Adult	IV/IM	3 g q8h
Child	IV/IM	200–240 mg/kg/d divided q6–8h; reduced to 100 mg/kg/d upon improvement

Surgical Prophylaxis

Adult	IV/IM	1.5 g 30–60 min before surgery, then 750 mg q8h for 24 h
Child	IV/IM	Same as for adult

ADVERSE/SIDE EFFECTS GI: *diarrhea,* nausea, colitis. **Hematologic:** decreased Hgb and Hct, transient eosinophilia, neutropenia, leukopenia. **Hepatic:** transient increases in AST, ALT, alkaline phosphatase, LDH, and bilirubin. **Hypersensitivity:** rash, pruritus, urticaria, positive Coombs' test. **Renal:** increased serum creatinine and BUN, decreased creatinine clearance. **Other:** local reactions: thrombophlebitis (IV site); pain, burning, cellulitis (IM site); superinfections.

DIAGNOSTIC TEST INTERFERENCES Cefuroxime causes false-positive (black-brown or green-brown color) *urine glucose* reaction with copper reduction reagents, e.g., Benedict's or Clinitest, but not with enzymatic glucose oxidase reagents, e.g., Clinistix, Tes-Tape. False-positive direct Coombs' test (may interfere with *cross-matching procedures* and *hematologic studies*) has been reported.

DRUG INTERACTIONS Probenecid decreases renal elimination of cefuroxime, thus prolonging its action.

INCOMPATIBILITIES Solution/Additive: AMINOGLYCOSIDES, **doxapram, sodium bicarbonate.** Y-**Site:** AMINOGLYCOSIDES, **sodium bicarbonate.**

NURSING IMPLICATIONS

Administration

- Shake IM suspension gently before administration. IM injections should be made deeply into large muscle mass. Rotate injection sites.
- Most patients complain of pain after IM administration, which lasts about 5 min. Reportedly, IM injections are less painful if IM concentrations recommended by manufacturer are used and if injections are made into gluteus maximus rather than lateral aspect of thigh.
- For IV administration, dilute each 750 mg with 9 ml sterile water, D5W, or NS. May be given by direct IV or further diluted in 50–100 ml of compatible solution. May also be added to 1000 ml of IV solution for continuous infusion.
- For direct intermittent IV, solution is injected slowly into a vein over 3–5 min, or injection may be made slowly through tubing system of a freely running compatible IV solution.
- For intermittent infusion, administer over 30 min. Rate of continuous infusion should be ordered by physician.
- Cefuroxime powder and solutions of the drug may range in color from light yellow to amber without adversely affecting product potency.
- When reconstituted as directed with sterile water for injection, solutions retain potency 24 h at room temperature and 48 h under refrigeration (5C); then they should be discarded.
- Store powder at 15–30C (59–86F) protected from light unless otherwise directed.

Assessment & Drug Effects

- Culture and susceptibility tests should be performed before initiation of therapy and periodically during therapy, if indicated. Therapy may be instituted pending test results.
- Before therapy is initiated, determine history of hypersensitivity reactions to cephalosporins, penicillins, and history of allergies, particularly to drugs.
- Inspect IM and IV injection sites frequently for signs of phlebitis.
- Report onset of loose stools or diarrhea. Although pseudomembranous colitis (see Signs & Symptoms, chap 3) rarely occurs, this potentially life-threatening complication should be ruled out as the cause of diarrhea during and after antibiotic therapy.
- Monitor for manifestations of hypersensitivity (see Signs & Symptoms, chap 3). Discontinue drug and report their appearance promptly.
- Monitor I&O ratio and pattern, especially in

severely ill patients receiving high doses. Report any significant changes.

Patient & Family Education

- Advise patient to report loose stools or diarrhea promptly.
- Advise patient to report signs and symptoms of hypersensitivity (see chap 3).

CELLULOSE SODIUM PHOSPHATE (CSP)

Trade name: Calcibind
Classifications: RESIN EXCHANGE AGENT, CATION; ANTILITHIC
Pregnancy: Category C

ACTIONS/PHARMACODYNAMICS Synthetic sodium salt of the phosphate ester of cellulose; cation exchange resin. When taken with meals, releases sodium in exchange for bivalent cations (e.g., dietary and secreted calcium and magnesium) in intestines to form a nonabsorbable complex. Binding of these bivalent ions renders them unavailable for complexing with oxalate (e.g., calcium oxalate or calcium phosphate in urine); thus formation of renal calculi is inhibited. Does not generally cause significant alterations in serum phosphate or calcium in most patients. Serum magnesium is predictably reduced, however, and therefore supplemention is necessary. Does not appear to affect serum concentrations of trace elements copper, zinc, or iron. Contains about 25–50 mEq of exchangeable sodium per 15 g of CSP (1 mEq of sodium contains approximately 23 mg).

USES Adjunct to dietary restriction to reduce renal calculi formation in absorptive hypercalciuria type I with recurrent calcium oxalate and calcium phosphate nephrolithiasis. **Unlabeled uses:** adjunct in treatment of hypercalcemia (e.g., associated with parathyroid carcinoma or sarcoidosis) and in management of calcinosis cutis.

ROUTE & DOSAGE

Urinary Calcium Exceeding 300 mg/d

Adult	PO	Initial: 5 g t.i.d. with each meal; decrease to 5 g with the main meal and 2.5 g with the other 2 meals when urinary calcium is <150 mg/d

PHARMACOKINETICS Absorption: not absorbed from GI tract. **Metabolism:** partially hydrolyzed in intestines, causing release of phosphorous ions, which are absorbed by the intestines. **Elimination:** nonabsorbable complex of calcium and cellulose phosphate excreted in feces along with unchanged resin.

CONTRAINDICATIONS & PRECAUTIONS Contraindicated in: bone disease, hypocalcemia, hypomagnesemia, hyperoxaluria; primary and secondary hyperparathyroidism, including renal hypercalciuria; high fasting urinary calcium or hypophosphatemia; conditions associated with high skeletal mobilization of calcium. Safe use during pregnancy (category C), in nursing mothers, and in children <16 y not established. **Cautious use in:** sodium restriction, CHF, ascites, nephrotic syndrome.

ADVERSE/SIDE EFFECTS GI: *loose stools, diarrhea, GI discomfort, dyspepsia, anorexia, nausea, vomiting.* **With long-term use:** <u>hypomagnesemia</u>, hypomagnesuria, hyperoxaluria, acute arthritis, arthralgia, hyperparathyroid bone disease, symptoms related to electrolyte imbalances, or depletion of trace elements copper, zinc, and iron.

DRUG INTERACTIONS CALCIUM SUPPLEMENTS counteract calcium-lowering effects of CSP; CSP also binds **magnesium,** decreasing its absorption—separate administration by at least 1 h; THIAZIDE DIURETICS may have additive effects; **ascorbic acid** is metabolized to oxalate and can counteract oxalate-lowering effects of CSP.

NURSING IMPLICATIONS

Administration

- Powder can be mixed with full glass (240 ml) of water, soft drink, or fruit juice and taken with meals. CSP is not palatable.
- Oral magnesium supplement (e.g., magnesium gluconate) should be administered to prevent hypomagnesemia. It can be given at any time as long as it is at least 1 h before or after CSP to avoid binding of magnesium.
- Doses of oral magnesium supplement depend on dose of CSP. Patients receiving 15 g/d of CSP should take 1.5 g magnesium gluconate before breakfast and again at bedtime (separately from CSP). Patients taking 10 g/d of CSP should take 1 g magnesium gluconate twice a day.
- Store in tightly closed container at 15–30C (59–86F), protected from moisture, unless otherwise directed.

Common side effects in *italic*; life-threatening effects <u>underlined</u>; generic names in **bold**; classifications in SMALL CAPS

Assessment & Drug Effects

- Monitor I&O ratio and pattern. Fluid intake should be encouraged to maintain a urinary output of at least 2 L/d (approximately 240 ml/h while awake).
- Serum parathyroid hormone (PTH) levels should be evaluated at least once between first 2 wk–5 mo of therapy, and then every 3–6 mo during therapy. Serum and urinary calcium and oxalate, serum magnesium, copper, iron, and zinc, and CBC should be monitored every 3–6 mo throughout therapy.
- Observe urinary calcium levels. A reduction of less than 30 mg/5 g in urinary calcium in patients on moderate calcium and sodium restriction indicates treatment failure. Drug is usually discontinued.
- Discontinuation of therapy is also indicated in patients on moderate oxalate restriction with urinary oxalate levels in excess of 55 mg/d. A rise in serum PTH above normal also points to the need to adjust dosage or stop the drug.
- To increase therapeutic effectiveness of CSP, dietary restriction of sodium, calcium, oxalate, and ascorbic acid is essential. Collaborate with physician and dietitian.
- With long-term use, monitor for manifestations of hypomagnesemia (see Signs & Symptoms, chap 3).

Patient & Family Education

- Be sure that patient understands drug will not work unless it is taken with meals or at least within 30 min of a meal.
- Instruct patients on long-term therapy to report signs and symptoms of hypomagnesemia (see chap 3).

Prototype: cephalothin, p 58

CEPHALEXIN

(sef-a-lex´in)
Trade names: Cefanex, Keflex, Keftab
Classifications: ANTIINFECTIVE; ANTIBIOTIC; FIRST GENERATION CEPHALOSPORIN
Pregnancy: Category B

ACTIONS/PHARMACODYNAMICS Semisynthetic derivative of cephalosporin C. Broad-spectrum, first generation cephalosporin antibiotic with antiinfective activity similar to that of cephalothin but reportedly less potent. Preferentially binds to one or more of the penicillin-binding proteins (PBP) located on cell walls of susceptible organisms. This inhibits third and final stage of bacterial cell wall synthesis, thus killing the bacterium. Ineffective against many gram-negative or anaerobic organisms. Cross-allergenicity between cephalosporins and penicillins has been reported.

USES To treat infections caused by susceptible pathogens in respiratory and urinary tracts, middle ear, skin, soft tissue, and bone.

ROUTE & DOSAGE

Mild to Moderate Infection

Adult	PO	250–500 mg q6h
Child	PO	25–50 mg/kg/d in 4 divided doses

Skin and Skin Structure Infections

Adult	PO	500 mg q12h

Otitis Media

Child	PO	75–100 mg/kg/d in 4 divided doses

PHARMACOKINETICS Absorption: rapidly absorbed from GI tract; stable in stomach acid. **Peak:** 1 h. **Distribution:** widely distributed in body fluids with highest concentration in kidney; crosses placenta. **Elimination:** half-life: 38–70 min; 80–100% eliminated unchanged in urine in 8 h; excreted in breast milk.

CONTRAINDICATIONS & PRECAUTIONS Contraindicated in: hypersensitivity to cephalosporins and related antibiotics. Safe use during pregnancy (category B), by nursing mothers, and infants <1 mo not established. **Cautious use in:** history of hypersensitivity to penicillin or other drug allergy; severely impaired renal function.

ADVERSE/SIDE EFFECTS CNS: dizziness, headache, fatigue. **GI:** *diarrhea* (generally mild), nausea, vomiting, anorexia, abdominal pain. **Hematologic:** slightly elevated ALT, AST, alkaline phosphatase; eosinophilia, positive direct Coombs' test. **Hypersensitivity:** angioedema, rash, urticaria, anaphylaxis. **Other:** superinfections, hemostatic defects.

DIAGNOSTIC TEST INTERFERENCES False-positive **urine glucose** determinations using copper

Common side effects in *italic*; life-threatening effects underlined; generic names in **bold**; classifications in SMALL CAPS

415

sulfate reagents, e.g., Clinitest, Benedict's reagent, but not with glucose oxidase (enzymatic) tests, e.g., Tes-Tape, Diastix, Clinistix. Positive direct Coombs' test may complicate transfusion *cross-matching procedures* and *hematologic studies.*

DRUG INTERACTIONS **Probenecid** decreases renal elimination of cephalexin.

NURSING IMPLICATIONS

Administration
- Cephalexin is not destroyed by gastric acid, but peak blood levels are slightly lower and delayed when cephalexin is administered with food. Total amount absorbed, however, is unchanged.
- Cephalexin oral suspension should be refrigerated; discard unused portions 14 d after preparation. Label should indicate expiration date. Keep tightly covered. Shake suspension well before pouring.
- Store capsules and tablets at 15–30C (59–86F) unless otherwise specified.

Assessment & Drug Effects
- Periodic evaluations of renal and hepatic function should be made in patients receiving prolonged therapy.
- Monitor for manifestations of hyposensitivity (see Signs & Symptoms, chap 3). Discontinue drug and report their appearance promptly.

Patient & Family Education
- Take medication for the full course of therapy as directed by physician.
- Drug therapy for beta-hemolytic streptococcal infections should continue for at least 10 d to guard against risk of rheumatic fever and glomerulonephritis.
- Keep physician informed if adverse reactions appear.
- Be alert to signs and symptoms of superinfections (see chap 3). These symptoms should be reported promptly and appropriate therapy instituted.

CEPHALOTHIN SODIUM

See ANTIINFECTIVES, ANTIBIOTIC, FIRST GENERATION CEPHALOSPORIN prototype, p 58

> **Prototype: cephalothin, p 58**

CEPHAPIRIN SODIUM

(sef-a-pye´rin)
Trade name: Cefadyl
Classifications: ANTIINFECTIVE; ANTIBIOTIC; FIRST GENERATION CEPHALOSPORIN
Pregnancy: Category B

ACTIONS/PHARMACODYNAMICS Semisynthetic, first generation, broad-spectrum cephalosporin antibiotic similar to cephalothin. Reported to cause less tissue irritation and to be less nephrotoxic than cephalothin. Preferentially binds to one or more of the penicillin-binding proteins (PBP) located on cell walls of susceptible organisms. This inhibits third and final stage of bacterial cell wall synthesis, thus killing the bacterium. Cross-allergenicity between cephalosporins and penicillins has been reported.

USES Serious infections of respiratory and urinary tracts, skin and soft tissue, and for osteomyelitis, septicemia, and endocarditis caused by susceptible pathogens, e.g., group A beta-hemolytic streptococci, penicillinase- and non-penicillinase-producing *Staphylococcus aureus, Streptococcus pneumoniae, viridans streptococci, Haemophilus influenzae, Escherichia coli, Proteus mirabilis,* and *Klebsiella* sp; also to prevent postoperative infection when infection at operative site is a risk.

ROUTE & DOSAGE

Mild to Moderate Infection

Adult	IM/IV	500 mg–1 g q4–6h up to 12 g/d
Child	IM/IV	40–80 mg/kg/d in 4 divided doses

Perioperative Prophylaxis

Adult	IM/IV	1–2 g 30–60 min before surgery; 1–2 g during surgery; then 1–2 g q6h for 24 h

Renal Impairment

Adult	IM/IV	Serum creatinine < 5 mg/dl: 7.5–15 mg/kg q12h

PHARMACOKINETICS **Peak:** 30 min after IM; 5 min after IV. **Distribution:** widely distributed in body fluids with highest concentration in kidney; crosses placenta. **Metabolism:** partially metabolized in liver and kidneys. **Elimination:** half-life: 36–54 min; 60–85% eliminated unchanged in urine in 6 h; excreted in breast milk.

CONTRAINDICATIONS & PRECAUTIONS Contraindicated in: hypersensitivity to cephalosporins and related antibiotics. Safe use during pregnancy (category B), in nursing mothers, and in children <3 mo not established. **Cautious use in:** history of sensitivity to penicillins and other allergies, particularly to drugs; sodium restriction, impaired renal function.

ADVERSE/SIDE EFFECTS GI: nausea, vomiting, *diarrhea,* abdominal cramps. **Hematologic** (rare): neutropenia, leukopenia, anemia, positive direct Coombs' test. **Hypersensitivity:** rash, urticaria, drug fever, eosinophilia, serum sickness–like reactions, anaphylaxis. **Other:** needle site reactions (infrequent); elevations in AST, ALT, alkaline phosphatase, bilirubin, BUN.

DIAGNOSTIC TEST INTERFERENCES False-positive *urine glucose* determinations, using copper sulfate reduction methods, e.g., Clinitest or Benedict's reagent, but not with glucose oxidase (enzymatic) tests, e.g., Clinistix, Diastix, Tes-Tape. Positive Coombs' test may complicate *cross-matching procedures* and *hematologic studies.*

DRUG INTERACTIONS Probenecid decreases renal elimination of cephapirin.

INCOMPATIBILITIES Solution/Additive: AMINO-GLYCOSIDES, **aminophylline, ascorbic acid, epinephrine, norepinephrine, mannitol, phenytoin,** TETRACYCLINES, **thiopental. Y-Site:** AMINO-GLYCOSIDES, TETRACYCLINES, **thiopental, phenytoin.**

NURSING IMPLICATIONS

Administration

- IM injections should be made deep into large muscle mass. Rotate injection sites.
- For IM use, the 500 mg and 1 g vials are reconstituted with 1 or 2 ml sterile water for injection or bacteriostatic water for injection, respectively. Resulting solutions will contain 500 mg of cephapirin per 1.2 ml.
- For direct IV injection the 1 g or 2 g vial is reconstituted with 10 ml or more 0.9% NaCl injection, bacteriostatic water for injection, or dextrose injection. May be given by direct IV over 5 min or may be further diluted with 50–100 ml of D5W or NS and infused over 30 min.

- After reconstitution, depending on diluent and amount used, solutions retain potency for 12–48 h at room temperature or for 10 d if refrigerated at 4C. See package insert for specific information.
- Solutions may become slightly yellow, but this does not affect potency.

Assessment & Drug Effects

- Culture and susceptibility testing should be performed before treatment is begun. Therapy may be initiated before results are obtained.
- Before therapy begins, determine history of previous hypersensitivity to cephalosporins, penicillins, and other allergies, particularly to drugs.
- Periodic monitoring of renal function is important. Advise patient to report changes in I&O ratio and pattern or evidence of blood or pus in urine.
- Monitor for manifestations of hypersensitivity (see Signs & Symptoms, chap 3). Discontinue drug and report their appearance promptly.

Patient & Family Education

- Advise patient to report promptly signs and symptoms of superinfections (see chap 3).
- Advise patient to report signs and symptoms of hypersensitivity (see chap 3).

Prototype: cephalothin, p 58

CEPHRADINE

(sef´ra-deen)
Trade names: Anspor, Velosef
Classifications: ANTIINFECTIVE; ANTIBIOTIC; FIRST GENERATION CEPHALOSPORIN
Pregnancy: Category B

ACTIONS/PHARMACODYNAMICS Semisynthetic acid-stable, first generation, broad-spectrum cephalosporin similar to cephalothin. Preferentially binds to one or more of the penicillin-binding proteins (PBP) located on cell walls of susceptible organisms. This inhibits third and final stage of bacterial cell wall synthesis, thus killing the bacterium. Cross-allergenicity between cephalosporins and penicillins has been reported.

USES Serious infections of respiratory and urinary tracts, skin and soft tissues, and for otitis media caused by susceptible pathogens; for perioperative prophylaxis, in cesarean section (intraoperative and postoperative); in septicemia (due to *Streptococcus pneumoniae, Staphylococcus aureus, Proteus mirabilis*, and *Escherichia coli*). Also used to treat urinary tract infections due to *Klebsiella* sp and enterococci (*Streptococcus faecalis*).

ROUTE & DOSAGE

Mild to Moderate Infection

Adult	PO	250–500 mg q6h or 500 mg–1 g q12h up to 4 g/d
	IM/IV	2–4 g/d in 4 divided doses (max 8 g/d)
Child doses	PO	25–50 mg/kg/d in 2–4 divided up to 4 g/d
	IM/IV	50–100 mg/kg/d in 4 divided doses up to 8 g/d

Perioperative Prophylaxis

Adult	PO	1 g 30–60 min before surgery; 1 g during surgery; then 1 g q4–6h for 24 h

PHARMACOKINETICS Absorption: well absorbed from GI tract. **Peak:** 1 h after PO; 1–2 h after IM; 5 min after IV. **Distribution:** widely distributed in body fluids, with highest concentration in kidney; crosses placenta. **Elimination:** half-life: 1–2 h; 80–90% eliminated unchanged in urine in 6 h; excreted in breast milk.

CONTRAINDICATIONS & PRECAUTIONS Contraindicated in: hypersensitivity to cephalosporins and related antibiotics. Safe use during pregnancy (category B), in nursing mothers, and children <9 mo not established. **Cautious use in:** history of penicillin or other allergies, particularly to drugs; impaired renal function, sodium restriction (parenteral cephradine).

ADVERSE/SIDE EFFECTS GI: *diarrhea* or loose stools, abdominal pain, heartburn. **Hematologic:** neutropenia, leukopenia, positive direct Coombs' test, elevations of ALT, AST, alkaline phosphatase, serum bilirubin, lactic dehydrogenase (following parenteral use), BUN. **Hypersensitivity:** urticaria, rash, pruritus, joint pains, eosinophilia. **Other:** dizziness, tightness in chest, pain, induration and tissue sloughing (IM injection site); thrombophlebitis (IV site); paresthesias, superinfections.

DIAGNOSTIC TEST INTERFERENCES Cephradine causes false-positive (black-brown or green-brown color) *urine glucose* reaction with copper reduction reagents, e.g., as Benedict's or Clinitest, but not with enzymatic glucose oxidase reagents, e.g.,

Clinistix, Tes-Tape. False-positive direct Coombs' test (may interfere with ***cross-matching procedures*** and ***hematologic studies***) has also been reported.

DRUG INTERACTIONS Probenecid decreases renal elimination of cephradine.

INCOMPATIBILITIES Solution/Additive: AMINOGLYCOSIDES, TPN SOLUTIONS, OTHER ANTIBIOTICS. **Y-Site:** AMINOGLYCOSIDES, TPN SOLUTIONS, OTHER ANTIBIOTICS.

NURSING IMPLICATIONS

Administration

- Oral cephradine may be given without regard to meals (acid stable); however, the presence of food may delay absorption.
- To minimize pain and induration of IM site, inject deep into large muscle mass such as gluteus maximus or lateral aspect of thigh.
- For IV administration, dilute each 500 mg with 5 ml sterile water for injection. May be further diluted (preferred) in 10–20 ml of D5W or NS.
- Give properly diluted solution by direct IV over 3–5 min. May be further diluted in 50–100 ml and infused over 30–60 min.
- After reconstitution, IM or IV solutions should be used within 2 h at room temperature. With refrigeration (5C), potency is retained 24 h. Reconstituted solutions may vary in color from light straw to yellow; this does not affect potency.
- The risk of thrombophlebitis may be reduced by proper dilution of IV fluid, use of small IV needles and large veins, and by alternating injection sites.
- Following reconstitution, oral suspension may be stored at room temperature up to 7 d or in refrigerator for up to 14 d. Shake well before pouring.
- All forms of cephradine are stored at 15–30C (59–86F) unless otherwise directed. Protect from concentrated light or direct sunlight.

Assessment & Drug Effects

- Before therapy is initiated, determine history of previous hypersensitivity to cephalosporins, penicillins, and other drug allergies.
- Culture and sensitivity tests and renal function studies should be performed before and periodically during drug therapy.
- Recommended dosage schedule in patients with reduced renal function is lowered based on creatinine clearance determinations and severity of infection.
- Inspect IV insertion site frequently for thrombophlebitis (see Signs & Symptoms, chap 3).

Common side effects in *italic*; life-threatening effects underlined; generic names in **bold**; classifications in SMALL CAPS

■ Pseudomembranous enterocolitis, a potentially life-threatening superinfection caused by *Clostridia difficile,* may occur during or after cephalosporin therapy. If diarrhea occurs, check for fever. Report diarrhea and fever promptly.

■ Monitor for signs of superinfection (see chap 3). Report their appearance promptly.

Patient & Family Education

■ Instruct patient to take medication for the full course of therapy as directed by physician. Therapy is usually continued for at least 48–72 h after patient becomes asymptomatic.

■ Superinfections caused by overgrowth of nonsusceptible organisms may occur. Instruct patient to report early signs and symptoms (see chap 3) promptly.

■ Instruct patient to report loose stools or diarrhea promptly.

CHARCOAL, ACTIVATED (LIQUID ANTIDOTE)

Trade names: Charcocaps, CharcolantiDote
Classifications: ANTIDOTE; ADSORBENT
Pregnancy: Category C

ACTIONS/PHARMACODYNAMICS Residue from destructive distillation of organic materials treated to reduce particle size, which increases surface area and adsorptive power (referred to as activation). Activated charcoal (carbon) is a chemically inert, odorless, tasteless, fine black powder with wide spectrum of adsorptive activity. Acts by binding (adsorbing) toxic substances, thereby inhibiting their GI absorption, enterohepatic circulation, and thus bioavailability. Recent studies indicate that administration by "gastric dialysis" (repetitive doses) effectively increases clearance of drugs already absorbed into the systemic circulation. Action appears to result from increased rate of drug diffusion from plasma into GI tract where it is adsorbed by activated charcoal.

USES General purpose emergency antidote in the treatment of poisonings by most drugs and chemicals, e.g., acetaminophen, aspirin, atropine, barbiturates, digitalis glycosides, phenytoin, propoxyphene, strychnine, tricyclic antidepressants, among many others. Gastric dialysis (repetitive doses) in uremia to adsorb various waste products from GI tract; severe acute poisoning. Has been used to adsorb intestinal gases in treatment of dyspepsia, flatulence, and distension (value in these conditions not established). Sometimes used topically as a deodorant for foul-smelling wounds and ulcers.

ROUTE & DOSAGE

Acute Poisonings

Adult	PO	30–100 g in at least 180–240 ml (6–8 oz) of water or 1 g/kg
Child	PO	Same as for adult

Gastric Dialysis

Adult	PO	20–40 g q6h for 1 or 2 d

GI Disturbances

Adult	PO	520–975 mg p.c. up to 5 g/d

PHARMACOKINETICS Absorption: not absorbed. **Elimination:** excreted in feces.

CONTRAINDICATIONS & PRECAUTIONS Contraindicated in: reportedly not effective for poisonings by cyanide, mineral acids, caustic alkalis, organic solvents, iron, ethanol, methanol. Safe use as antiflatulent in children <3 y not established.

ADVERSE/SIDE EFFECTS *Vomiting (rapid ingestion of high doses), constipation, diarrhea.*

DRUG INTERACTIONS May decrease absorption of all other oral medications—administer at least 2 h apart.

NURSING IMPLICATIONS

Administration

■ Before using charcoal as an antidote, call a poison control center, an emergency room, or a physician immediately for advice.

■ Activated charcoal tablets or capsules are less adsorptive and thus less effective than powder or liquid form; therefore they are not recommended in treatment of acute poisoning.

■ Drug is most effective when administered as soon as possible after acute poisoning (preferably within 30 min).

■ In an emergency, dose may be approximated by stirring sufficient activated charcoal into tap water to make a slurry the consistency of soup (about 20–30 g in at least 240 ml of water).

■ It is common practice to administer a single dose of activated charcoal simultaneously with a laxative, such as magnesium citrate, magnesium sulfate, or

Common side effects in *italic*; life-threatening effects <u>underlined</u>; generic names in **bold**; classifications in SMALL CAPS

419

C

sodium sulfate, to hasten drug elimination and to prevent constipation and possible impaction.

- Activated charcoal can be swallowed or given through a nasogastric tube. If administered too rapidly, patient may vomit.

- If necessary, palatability may be improved by adding a small amount of concentrated fruit juice or chocolate powder to the slurry. Reportedly, these agents do not appreciably alter adsorptive activity.

- To prevent adsorption of gases from the air, store in tightly covered container at 15–30C (59–86F) unless otherwise directed.

Assessment & Drug Effects

- Record appearance, color, consistency, frequency, and relative amount of stools. Inform patient that activated charcoal will color feces black.

CHENODIOL (CHENODEOXYCHOLIC ACID)

(kee-noe-dye´ole)
Trade name: Chenix
Classification: GALLSTONE SOLUBILIZING AGENT
Pregnancy: Category X

ACTIONS/PHARMACODYNAMICS Naturally occurring human bile acid synthesized by liver. After PO administration of chenodiol, biliary cholesterol saturation decreases, perhaps because of drug-induced suppression of hepatic synthesis of cholesterol and cholic acid and decreased biliary cholesterol secretion. By reducing cholesterol saturation in bile, chenodiol promotes dissolution of uncalcified cholesterol gallstones. Chenodiol has no effect on bile pigment stones. Inhibition of fluid absorption in colon by chenodiol and perhaps increase in fluid secretion may be the cause of loose stools or diarrhea. Increases in low-density lipoproteins (LDL) may pose a potential risk to patients with atherosclerosis. Prophylactic use of low doses in preventing stone recurrence is ineffective.

USES To dissolve small or floatable radiolucent cholesterol gallstones in carefully selected patients with radiographically well-visualized gallbladders and who are high surgical risks because of systemic disease or age.

PHARMACOKINETICS Absorption: rapidly absorbed from small intestine. **Distribution:** distributed mainly into bile; crosses placenta. **Metabolism:** par-

tially metabolized in intestines by anaerobic bacteria to lithocolic acid. **Elimination:** half-life (biphasic): 3.1 min and 16.4 min; 80% excreted in bile and feces; excreted in breast milk.

ROUTE & DOSAGE

Cholesterol Gallstones

Adult	PO	250 mg b.i.d., AM and PM, for first 2 wk therapy; increase by 250 mg at weekly intervals to 13–16 mg/kg/d in 2 divided doses for up to 24 mo

CONTRAINDICATIONS & PRECAUTIONS Contraindicated in: hepatocellular dysfunction, bile duct abnormalities, nonvisualized gallbladder after two consecutive single doses of PO cholecystographic agent; patients with radiopaque or radiolucent bile pigment stones, gallstone complications, compelling reasons for gallbladder surgery (e.g., unremitting acute cholecystitis, biliary obstruction, biliary GI fistula). Safe use during pregnancy (category X), in fertile women, nursing mothers, and children, and for longer than 6 mo not established. **Cautious use in:** atherosclerosis.

ADVERSE/SIDE EFFECTS GI: *mild diarrhea* (dose related), severe diarrhea (overdosage), fecal urgency, nausea, vomiting, dyspepsia, epigastric distress, anorexia, heartburn, flatulence, abdominal cramps. **Hepatic:** *transient elevations of serum transaminases,* particularly ALT or AST, *elevated serum total cholesterol, elevated LDL,* slight reduction of serum triglycerides, hepatitis. **Other:** leukopenia.

DRUG INTERACTIONS Cholestyramine, colistipol, ANION EXCHANGE RESINS, ALUMINUM–CONTAINING ANTACIDS decrease absorption of chenodiol; ESTROGENS, ORAL CONTRACEPTIVES may counteract chenodiol effects by increasing biliary cholesterol secretion.

NURSING IMPLICATIONS

Administration

- Chenodiol should be taken with meals or milk. Food generally decreases rate but not extent of absorption.

- Store at 15–30C (59–86F) in tightly closed container unless otherwise directed.

Assessment & Drug Effects

- If partial stone dissolution does not occur by 9–12 mo, it is unlikely that further treatment will be ef-

Common side effects in *italic*; life-threatening effects underlined; generic names in **bold**; classifications in SMALL CAPS

fective. Therapy should be discontinued if no response has occurred by 16–18 mo following therapy initiation.

- Diarrhea is usually mild, transient, and dose related. It occurs in about 30–40% of patients, more frequently at beginning of therapy, but may occur at any time during therapy. Treatment generally consists of temporary dosage reduction (by about 1/2) until diarrhea is controlled; dosage is then gradually increased to original level. Antidiarrheal agents may also be prescribed.

Patient & Family Education

- Advise patient that the crampy abdominal pain that sometimes accompanies bouts of diarrhea is to be distinguished from the pain of biliary colic. The pain of biliary colic occurs in right upper quadrant or epigastric region, is frequently associated with nausea and vomiting, and should be reported to physician immediately.
- To reduce risk of stone recurrence, attain and maintain ideal body weight, include high-fiber foods in diet, and reduce cholesterol and carbohydrate intake.

Prototype: secobarbital, p 175

CHLORAL HYDRATE

(klor´al hye´drate)

Trade names: Aquachloral Supprettes, Noctec, Novochlorhydrate

Classifications: CNS AGENT; ANXIOLYTIC, SEDATIVE-HYPNOTIC

Pregnancy: Category C

Controlled Substance: Schedule IV

ACTIONS/PHARMACODYNAMICS Produces "physiologic sleep" by mild cerebral depression with little effect on respirations or BP and little or no hangover. Principal action thought to be due in part to trichloroethanol, its reduction product. Does not affect sleep physiology (e.g., REM sleep) in low doses. It is the oldest chloral derivative and is still regarded as a relatively safe, effective, and inexpensive sedative-hypnotic. Has little or no analgesic action. May cause enzyme induction and displace certain drugs from protein-binding sites.

USES Short-term management of insomnia, for general sedation (especially in the young and the elderly), for sedation before and after surgery, to reduce anxiety associated with drug withdrawal, and alone or with paraldehyde to prevent or suppress alcohol withdrawal symptoms.

ROUTE & DOSAGE

Sedative

Adult	PO/PR	250 mg t.i.d. p.c.
Child	PO/PR	8.3 mg/kg t.i.d. p.c. (max 1 g)

Hypnotic

Adult	PO/PR	500 mg–1 g 15–30 min before h.s. or 30 min before surgery
Child	PO/PR	50 mg/kg 15–30 min before h.s. or 30 min before surgery (max 1 g)

EEG Premedication

Child	PO/PR	20–25 mg/kg

PHARMACOKINETICS Absorption: readily absorbed from oral or rectal administration. **Onset:** 30–60 min. **Peak:** 1–3 h. **Duration:** 4–8 h. **Distribution:** well distributed to all tissues; 70–80% protein bound; crosses placenta. **Metabolism:** metabolized in liver to the active metabolite trichloroethanol. **Elimination:** half-life: 8–11 h; excreted primarily by kidneys, with a small amount excreted in feces via bile.

CONTRAINDICATIONS & PRECAUTIONS Contraindicated in: known hypersensitivity to drug; severe hepatic, renal, or cardiac disease; rectal dosage form in patients with proctitis; oral use in patients with esophagitis, gastritis, gastric or duodenal ulcers. Safe use during pregnancy (category C) and in nursing women not established. **Cautious use in:** history of intermittent porphyria, asthma, history of or proneness to drug dependence, depression, suicidal tendencies.

ADVERSE/SIDE EFFECTS Generally well tolerated. **CNS:** dizziness, motor incoordination, headache, hangover (infrequent). **CV (overdosage):** arrhythmias, cardiac arrest. **GI:** *nausea, vomiting, diarrhea.* **Hypersensitivity:** purpura, urticaria, erythematous rash, eczema, erythema multiforme, angioedema, eosinophilia. **Other:** breath odor, leukopenia, ketonuria, conjunctivitis. **Chronic use:** fixed drug eruptions, severe gastritis, renal, and hepatic damage, sudden death.

DIAGNOSTIC TEST INTERFERENCES False-positive results for ***urine glucose*** with Benedict's solutions, and possibly with Clinitest but not with glucose oxidase methods (e.g., Clinistix, Diastix,

---

Common side effects in *italic*; life-threatening effects underlined; generic names in **bold**; classifications in SMALL CAPS

421

Tes-Tape). Possible interference with fluorometric test for **urine catecholamines** (if chloral hydrate is administered within 48 h of test) and **urinary 17-OHCS** determinations (by modification of Reddy, Jenkins, Thorn procedure).

DRUG INTERACTIONS Alcohol, BARBITURATES, **paraldehyde,** other CNS DEPRESSANTS potentiate CNS depression; tachycardia may also occur with **alcohol;** increases anticoagulant effect of ORAL ANTICOAGULANTS; **furosemide** IV can produce flushing, diaphoresis, BP changes.

NURSING IMPLICATIONS

Administration

- Corrosive to skin and mucous membranes unless well diluted. Has an aromatic, pungent odor and bitter, pungent taste; these may be minimized by use of the capsule form or by dilution of liquid preparations in chilled fluids.
- Watch to see that drug is not cheeked and hoarded.
- Solutions are preserved in tightly covered, light-resistant containers. All forms preferably stored at 15–30C (59–86F) unless otherwise directed.

Assessment & Drug Effects

- Chloral hydrate is not intended for relief of pain. When used in the presence of pain, it may cause excitement and delirium.
- Remove matches, cigarettes, etc., if patient is a smoker. Side rails may be advisable for the elderly patient.
- Prolonged use can lead to tolerance, physical dependence, and addiction. Sudden withdrawal from dependent patients may produce delirium, mania, or convulsions.
- Allergic skin reactions may occur within several hours or as long as 10 d after drug administration.
- Evaluate patient's response to chloral hydrate and continued need for the drug.

Patient & Family Education

- Because hypnotic doses may cause dizziness, caution patient not to ambulate without assistance.
- Caution patient to avoid concomitant use of alcoholic beverages.
- Driving and other potentially hazardous activities should be avoided while patient is under the influence of chloral hydrate.

Prototype: mechlorethamine, p 96

CHLORAMBUCIL
(klor-am´byoo-sil)
Trade name: Leukeran
Classifications: ANTINEOPLASTIC; ALKYLATING AGENT; NITROGEN MUSTARD
Pregnancy: Category D

ACTIONS/PHARMACODYNAMICS Potent aromatic derivative of the alkylating agent nitrogen mustard and slowest acting and least toxic of the nitrogen mustards. A cell-cycle nonspecific (kills both resting and dividing cells), it causes cytotoxic cross linkage in DNA, thus preventing synthesis of DNA, RNA, and proteins. Myelosuppression in therapeutic doses is moderate and rapidly reversible. Lymphocytic effect is marked. Has mutagenic and embryotoxic properties.

USES As single agent or in combination with other antineoplastics in treatment of chronic lymphocytic leukemia, malignant lymphomas including lymphosarcoma, Hodgkin's disease, and giant follicular lymphoma, and in treatment of carcinoma of the ovary, breast, and testes. **Unlabeled uses:** nonneoplastic conditions: vasculitis complicating rheumatoid arthritis, autoimmune hemolytic anemias associated with cold agglutinins, lupus glomerulonephritis, idiopathic nephrotic syndrome, polycythemia vera, and macroglobulinemia.

ROUTE & DOSAGE

Malignant Diseases (Lymphomas, Hodgkin's Disease, etc)

Adult	PO	0.1–0.2 mg/kg/d (usual dose 4–10 mg/d)
Child	PO	0.1–0.2 mg/kg/d in single or divided doses

PHARMACOKINETICS Absorption: rapidly and completely absorbed from GI tract. **Peak:** 1 h. **Distribution:** extensively bound to plasma and tissue proteins; crosses placenta. **Metabolism:** extensively metabolized in liver. **Elimination:** half-life: 1.5–2.5 h; 60% eliminated in urine as metabolites within 24 h.

CONTRAINDICATIONS & PRECAUTIONS Contraindicated in: hypersensitivity to chlorambucil or to other alkylating agents; administration within 4 wk of a full course of radiation or chemotherapy; full dosage if bone marrow is infiltrated with lymphomatous tissue or is hypoplastic; smallpox and other vaccines. Safe use during pregnancy (category D) and in nursing women not established. **Cautious use in:** excessive or prolonged dosage, pneumococcus vaccination, history of seizures or head trauma.

ADVERSE/SIDE EFFECTS Hematologic: bone marrow depression: *leukopenia,* thrombocytopenia, anemia. **Metabolic:** sterility, hyperuricemia. **GI:** low incidence of gastric discomfort. **Other:** drug fever, skin rashes, papilledema, alopecia, peripheral neuropathy, sterile cystitis, pulmonary complications, hepatotoxicity, seizures (high doses).

DRUG INTERACTIONS May have to adjust dose of **allopurinol, colchicine** because of chlorambucil-associated hyperuricemia.

NURSING IMPLICATIONS

Administration

- Nausea and vomiting may be controlled by giving entire daily dose at one time, 1 h before breakfast or 2 h after evening meal, or at bedtime. Consult physician.
- During maintenance therapy, physician may occasionally interrupt drug schedule to determine if patient is in remission.
- With confirmation of bone marrow depression (low platelet and neutrophil counts or peripheral lymphocytosis), it is recommended that dosage not exceed 0.1 mg/kg.
- Store at 15–30C (59–86F) in tightly closed, light-resistant container.

Assessment & Drug Effects

- CBC, hemoglobin, total and differential leukocyte counts, and serum uric acid should be checked initially and at least once weekly during treatment.
- Body weight, size of spleen, and temperature charted before initiation of therapy and at the time of blood counts provide a useful profile for determining degree of bone marrow suppression.
- Leukopenia usually develops after the third week of treatment; it may continue for up to 10 d after last dose, then rapidly return to normal. About 25% of patients receiving a total dose of approximately 450 mg and 50% of those receiving this dosage for ≥ 8 wk may develop severe neutropenia.
- If possible, avoid or reduce to minimum injections and other invasive procedures (e.g., rectal temperatures, enemas) when platelet count is low because of danger of bleeding.

Patient & Family Education

- During treatment it is dangerous to go longer than 2 wk without a clinical examination and blood studies. Keeping appointments with the physician is imperative.
- Advise patient to notify physician if the following symptoms occur: unusual bleeding or bruising, sores on lips or in mouth; flank, stomach or joint pain; fever, chills, or other signs of infection, sore throat, cough, dyspnea.
- Skin reactions are rare, but all appear to show a consistent pattern: pustular eruption on mouth, chin, cheeks; urticarial erythema on trunk that spreads to legs. The rash occurs early in treatment period and lasts about 10 d after last dose. Urge the patient to report immediately the onset of cutaneous reaction.
- If physician agrees, urge patient to drink at least 10–12 glasses (240 ml [8 oz] each) of fluid per day and to report to physician if urine output decreases below normal amounts.
- Advise patient to report to physician immediately if she becomes pregnant. She should be informed of the potential hazard to the fetus.
- Discuss possibility of gonadal suppression with patient (amenorrhea or azoospermia may be irreversible), which occurs especially with high doses.

CHLORAMPHENICOL

(klor-am-fen´i-kole)
Trade names: Chlorofair, Chloromycetin, Chloroptic, Chloroptic S.O.P., Fenicol, Isopto Fenicol, Novochlorocap, Ophthochlor, Pentamycetin

CHLORAMPHENICOL PALMITATE

Trade name: Chloromycetin Palmitate

CHLORAMPHENICOL SODIUM SUCCINATE

Trade name: Chloromycetin Sodium Succinate
Classifications: ANTIINFECTIVE; ANTIBIOTIC
Pregnancy: Category C

ACTIONS/PHARMACODYNAMICS Synthetic broad-spectrum antibiotic formerly derived from

Common side effects in *italic*; life-threatening effects underlined; generic names in **bold**; classifications in SMALL CAPS

423

Streptomyces venezuelae. Principally bacteriostatic but may be bactericidal in certain species (e.g., *Haemophilus influenzae*) or when given in higher concentrations. Effective against a wide variety of gram-negative and gram-positive bacteria and most anaerobic microorganisms. Believed to act by binding to the 50S ribosome of bacteria and by interfering with protein synthesis.

USES Severe infections when other antibiotics are ineffective or are contraindicated. Particularly effective against *Salmonella typhi* and other *Salmonella* sp, *Streptococcus pneumoniae, Neisseria,* meningeal infections caused by *H. influenzae,* and infections involving *Bacteroides fragilis* and other anaerobic organisms, *Rickettsia rickettsii* (cause of Rocky Mountain spotted fever) and other rickettsiae, the lymphogranuloma-psittacosis group *(Chlamydia),* and *Mycoplasma.* Also used in cystic fibrosis antiinfective regimens and topically for infections of skin, eyes, and external auditory canal.

ROUTE & DOSAGE

Serious Infections

Adult	PO/IV	50 mg/kg/d in 4 divided doses
	Topical	1–2 drops of ophthalmic solution q3–6h or small strip of ophthalmic ointment in lower conjunctival sac q3–6h or 2–3 drops of otic solution in ear t.i.d.
Child	PO/IV	50 mg/kg/d in 4 divided doses
Infant	PO/IV	25 mg/kg/d divided q6h

Meningitis

| Adult | IV | 75–100 mg/kg/d divided q6h |
| Child | IV | Same as for adult |

PHARMACOKINETICS Absorption: rapidly absorbed from GI tract. **Peak:** PO: 1–3 h; IV: 1 h. **Distribution:** widely distributed to most body tissues including saliva and ascitic, pleural and synovial fluid; concentrates in liver and kidneys; penetrates CNS; crosses placenta. **Metabolism:** primarily inactivated in liver. **Elimination:** half-life: 1.5–4.1 h; much longer in neonates; metabolite and free drug excreted in urine; excreted in breast milk.

CONTRAINDICATIONS & PRECAUTIONS Contraindicated in: history of hypersensitivity or toxic reaction to chloramphenicol; treatment of minor infections, prophylactic use; typhoid carrier state, history or family history of drug-induced bone marrow depression, concomitant therapy with drugs that produce bone marrow depression. Safe use during pregnancy (category C) and in nursing mothers not established. **Cautious use in:** impaired hepatic or renal function; premature and full-term infants, children; intermittent porphyria; patients with G6PD deficiency; patient or family history of drug-induced bone marrow depression.

ADVERSE/SIDE EFFECTS CNS: Neurotoxicity: headache, mental depression, confusion, delirium, digital paresthesias, peripheral neuritis. **Eye:** visual disturbances, optic neuritis, optic nerve atrophy, contact conjunctivitis. **GI:** nausea, vomiting, diarrhea, perianal irritation, enterocolitis, glossitis, stomatitis, unpleasant taste, xerostomia. **Hematologic:** bone marrow depression (dose-related and reversible): reticulocytosis, leukopenia, granulocytopenia, thrombocytopenia, increased plasma iron, reduced Hgb, hypoplastic anemia. Non-dose-related and irreversible; pancytopenia, agranulocytosis, aplastic anemia, paroxysmal nocturnal hemoglobinuria, leukemia. **Hypersensitivity:** angioedema, urticaria, contact dermatitis, maculopapular and vesicular rashes, dyspnea, fever, anaphylaxis. **Other:** jaundice, hypoprothrombinemia, fixed-drug eruptions, superinfections, gray syndrome.

DIAGNOSTIC TEST INTERFERENCES Possibility of false-positive results for **urine glucose** by copper reduction methods (e.g., Benedict's solution, Clinitest). Chloramphenicol may interfere with **17-OHCS** (urinary steroid) determinations (modification of Reddy, Jenkins, Thorn procedure not affected), with **urobilinogen excretion,** and with responses to **tetanus toxoid** and possibly other active immunizing agents.

DRUG INTERACTIONS The metabolism of **chlorpropamide, dicumarol, phenytoin, tolbutamide** may be decreased, prolonging their activity. **Phenobarbital** decreases chloramphenicol levels. The response to iron preparations, folic acid, and vitamin B_{12} may be delayed.

INCOMPATIBILITIES Solutions/Additives: chlorpromazine, polymyxin-B, prochlorperazine, promethazine, TETRACYCLINES, vancomycin, glycopyrrolate, metoclopramide.

NURSING IMPLICATIONS

Administration

- Oral drug is taken preferably with a full glass of water on an empty stomach, at least 1 h before or

Common side effects in *italic*; life-threatening effects underlined; generic names in **bold**; classifications in SMALL CAPS

2 h after a meal, to achieve optimum blood levels.

- Chloramphenicol sodium succinate is intended for IV administration only. Dilute each 1 g with 10 ml of sterile water or D5W. Give direct IV slowly over a period of at least 1 min.
- IV solution may be further diluted in 50–100 ml of 5% dextrose and infused over 30–60 min.
- Solution for injection may form crystals or a second layer when stored at low temperatures. Solution can be clarified by shaking vial. Do not use cloudy solutions.
- *Instillation of eye drops:* after instillation apply light pressure to lacrimal duct for 1–2 min to prevent drainage into nasopharynx and systemic absorption. This is an extremely important step to decrease absorption. Several cases of aplastic anemia have been associated with use of ophthalmic preparations.
- Store topical ophthalmic, otic, and skin preparations, PO forms, and unopened ampuls preferably between 15–30C (59–86F) and protected from light unless otherwise directed by manufacturer.

Assessment & Drug Effects

- Bacterial culture and susceptibility tests are performed prior to first dose and periodically thereafter.
- Baseline CBC, platelets, serum iron, and reticulocyte cell counts are recommended before initiation of therapy, at 48 h intervals during therapy, and periodically during follow-up period. Chloramphenicol should be discontinued upon appearance of leukopenia, reticulocytopenia, thrombocytopenia, or anemia.
- Nondose-related irreversible bone marrow depression may appear weeks or months after drug therapy is terminated. The potential for this side effect is greatest in patients with impaired hepatic or renal function, infants, children, and premenopausal women.
- Close observation of the patient is also crucial, because blood studies are not always reliable predictors of irreversible bone marrow depression.
- Chloramphenicol blood levels should be closely monitored weekly. More frequent determinations are made in patients with hepatic dysfunction and in patients receiving therapy for longer than 2 wk. Desired concentrations: peak 10–20 μg/ml; through 5–10 μg/ml.
- Check temperature at least q4h. Usually chloramphenicol is discontinued if temperature remains normal for 48 h.
- Report any appreciable change in I&O ratio or pattern.

- More frequent determinations of serum glucose are recommended in patients receiving oral antidiabetic agents.
- Gray syndrome has occurred 2–9 d after initiation of high dose chloramphenicol therapy in premature infants and neonates and in children ≤ 2 y. It appears to be associated with initiation of therapy within the first 48 h of life and in children with preexisting liver dysfunction. Report early signs: abdominal distension, failure to feed, pallor, changes in vital signs. Early detection and prompt termination of therapy can interrupt a potentially fatal course.

Patient & Family Education

- Inform patient that bitter taste may occur 15–20 s after IV injection and that it usually lasts only 2–3 min.
- Report immediately sore throat, fever, fatigue, petechiae, nose bleeds, bleeding gums, or other unusual bleeding or bruising, or any other suspicious sign of symptom. Drug therapy should be discontinued if abnormal bleeding occurs.
- Watch for signs and symptoms of superinfection (see chap 3).
- Advise patient to follow dosage and duration of therapy as prescribed by physician.
- Prolonged or frequent intermittent use of topical preparations should be avoided because systemic absorption and toxicity can occur.
- Withhold medication and check with physician immediately if signs of hypersensitivity reaction (see chap 3), irritation, superinfection, or other adverse reactions appear.
- Applications to skin are generally preceded by a soap and water cleansing and thorough drying of part before reapplication of medication. Consult physician.

Prototype: lorazepam, p 177

CHLORDIAZEPOXIDE HYDROCHLORIDE
(klor-dye-az-e-pox´ide)
Trade names: A-poxide, Libritabs, Librium, Lipoxide, Medilium, Murcil, Novopoxide, Reponans, Sereen, SK-Lygen, Solium
Classifications: CNS AGENT; PSYCHOTHERAPEUTIC; BENZODIAZEPINE ANXIOLYTIC, SEDATIVE-HYPNOTIC
Pregnancy: Category D
Controlled substance: Schedule IV

Common side effects in *italic*; life-threatening effects underlined; generic names in **bold**; classifications in SMALL CAPS

425

ACTIONS/PHARMACODYNAMICS Benzodiazepine derivative. Acts on the limbic, thalamic, and hypothalamic areas of the CNS. Produces mild sedative, anticonvulsant, anxiolytic, and skeletal muscle relaxant effects. Has long-acting hypnotic properties. Causes mild suppression of REM sleep and of deeper phases, particularly stage 4, while increasing total sleep time.

USES Relief of various anxiety and tension states, preoperative apprehension and anxiety, and for management of alcohol withdrawal. **Unlabeled use:** essential, familial, and senile action tremors.

ROUTE & DOSAGE

Mild Anxiety, Preoperative Anxiety

Adult	PO	5–10 mg t.i.d. or q.i.d.
	IM/IV	50–100 mg 1 h before surgery
Child	PO	5 mg b.i.d. to q.i.d.; may be increased to 10 mg t.i.d.

Severe Anxiety and Tension

Adult	PO	20–25 mg t.i.d. or q.i.d.
	IM/IV	50–100 mg; then 25–50 mg t.i.d. or q.i.d.

Alcohol Withdrawal Syndrome

Adult	PO	50–100 mg prn up to 300 mg/d
	IM/IV	50–100 mg; may repeat in 2–3 h if necessary

PHARMACOKINETICS Absorption: well absorbed from GI tract; slow erratic absorption from IM. **Peak:** 1–4 h PO; 15–30 min IM; 3–30 min IV. **Distribution:** widely distributed throughout body; crosses placenta. **Metabolism:** metabolized in liver to long-acting active metabolite. **Elimination:** half-life: 5–30 h; slowly excreted in urine (may last several days); excreted in breast milk.

CONTRAINDICATIONS & PRECAUTIONS Contraindicated in: hypersensitivity to chlordiazepoxide and other benzodiazepines; narrow angle glaucoma, prostatic hypertrophy, shock, comatose states, primary depressive disorder or psychoses, pregnancy (category D), nursing mothers, lactation, oral use in children <6 y, parenteral use in children <12 y, acute alcohol intoxication. **Cautious use in:** anxiety states associated with impending depression, history of impaired hepatic or renal function; addiction-prone individuals, blood dyscrasias; in the elderly, debilitated patients, children; hyperkinesis, COPD.

ADVERSE/SIDE EFFECTS CNS: *drowsiness,* dizziness, *lethargy,* changes in EEG pattern; vivid dreams, nightmares, headache, extrapyramidal symptoms, vertigo, syncope, tinnitus, confusion, hallucinations, parodoxic rage, depression, delirium, ataxia. **CV:** orthostatic hypotension, tachycardia, changes in ECG patterns seen with rapid IV administration. **GI:** nausea, dry mouth, vomiting, constipation, increased appetite. **GU:** urinary frequency. **Other:** edema, pain in injection site, photosensitivity, skin rash, blood dyscrasias, jaundice, acute intermittent porphyria, hiccups, elevation of LDH, <u>respiratory depression</u>.

DIAGNOSTIC TEST INTERFERENCES Chlordiazepoxide increases **serum bilirubin, AST** and **ALT;** decreases **radioactive iodine uptake;** and may falsely increase readings for urinary **17-OHCS** (modified Glenn-Nelson technique).

DRUG INTERACTIONS Alcohol, CNS DEPRESSANTS, ANTICONVULSANTS potentiate CNS depression; **cimetidine** increases **chlordiazepoxide** plasma levels, thus increasing toxicity; may decrease antiparkinson effects of **levodopa;** may increase **phenytoin** levels; smoking decreases sedative and antianxiety effects.

NURSING IMPLICATIONS

Administration

- Patients who complain of gastric distress may obtain relief by taking the drug with or immediately after meals or with milk. If an antacid is prescribed, it should be taken at least 1 h before or after chlordiazepoxide to prevent delay in drug absorption.
- Supervise drug ingestion to prevent "cheeking" pills, a maneuver that leads to hoarding or omission of drug.
- Prepare parenteral solution immediately before use; discard unused portion. Drug is unstable in light and when in solution.
- Use special diluent provided by manufacturer to make the IM solution. Add diluent carefully to avoid bubble formation; gently agitate until solution is clear. Resulting solution: 50 mg/ml. Discard diluent if it is not clear.
- For IV injection, 5 ml of sterile water for injection or NaCl 0.9% is added to each 100 mg ampule of dry powder and agitated gently until dissolved. Do not use IM diluent for the IV solution because it may contain air bubbles.
- Do not mix any other drug with chlordiazepoxide solution.
- IV chlordiazepoxide is administered by direct IV,

Common side effects in *italic*; life-threatening effects <u>underlined</u>; generic names in **bold**; classifications in SMALL CAPS

properly diluted, at a rate of 100 mg or a fraction thereof over 1 min.

▪ Store in tight, light-resistant containers at 15–30C (59–86F) unless otherwise specified by manufacturer. The special diluent supplied by manufacturer for IM preparation should be kept refrigerated, preferably at 2–8C (36–46F) until ready for use.

Assessment & Drug Effects

▪ In early part of therapy, check BP and pulse before giving benzodiazepine. If blood pressure falls 20 mm Hg or more or if pulse rate is above 120 bpm, delay medication and consult physician.

▪ Orthostatic hypotension and tachycardia occur more frequently with parenteral administration. Patient should stay recumbent 2–3 h after IM or IV injection; observe closely and monitor vital signs.

▪ Until drug dosage is stabilized, monitor I&O. Report changes in I&O ratio and dysuria to physician. Cumulative (overdosage) effects can result with renal dysfunction. The elderly are especially vulnerable.

▪ Observe intake of patient who is seriously agitated or depressed; willful reduction of fluids can be hazardous.

▪ **Paradoxic reactions:** excitement, stimulation, disturbed sleep patterns, acute rage; may occur during first few weeks of therapy in psychiatric patients and in hyperactive and aggressive children receiving chlordiazepoxide. Withhold drug and report to physician.

▪ Observe patient's sleep pattern and quality. If dreams or nightmares interfere with rest, notify physician. A change in the dosing schedule, dose, or an alternate drug may be prescribed.

▪ If drug has been prescribed for anxiety-induced insomnia and is used every day, its effect begins in 2 or 3 nights; however, usefulness for this problem lasts only a few weeks.

▪ Periodic blood cell counts and liver function tests are recommended during prolonged therapy.

▪ Sore throat or mouth, upper respiratory infection, fever, and malaise should alert one to the possibility of agranulocytosis. Total and differential WBC counts should be ordered immediately, and protective isolation instituted.

▪ Adverse reactions are dose related but even at lower ranges may occur in elderly and debilitated patients. Supervision of ambulation is indicated, and possibly side rails.

▪ Some studies suggest that smoking increases clearance rate of chlordiazepoxide. The heavy smoker may require higher dosage of the drug for therapeutic effectiveness than the nonsmoker.

▪ Habituation and physical dependence can occur.

▪ Observe for signs of developing physical or psychologic dependency such as requests for change in drug regimen (dose and dose interval), diminishing favorable response (e.g., disturbed sleep pattern, increase in psychomotor activity), manipulative behavior, withdrawal symptoms. Investigate the symptoms of ataxia, vertigo, slurred speech; the patient may be taking more than the prescribed dose.

▪ Abrupt discontinuation of drug in patients receiving high doses for long periods (≥4 mo) has precipitated withdrawal symptoms, but not for at least 5–7 d because of slow elimination. Symptoms may include restlessness, headache, unreal or distant feelings, parethesias, abdominal and muscle cramps, abnormal perceptions of motion, tremors, insomnia, vomiting, anorexia, profuse sweating, psychomotor activity including convulsions and delirium. In most cases, after usual doses there is no withdrawal syndrome.

Patient & Family Education

▪ Advise patient to take drug specifically as prescribed: not to skip, increase, or decrease doses, change intervals, or terminate therapy without physician's advice and not to lend or offer any of drug to another person.

▪ Advise patient that OTC drugs should not be taken unless prescribed.

▪ Long-term use of this drug may cause xerostomia. Inform patient that good oral hygiene can alleviate the discomfort.

▪ Sedation may occur during early therapy. Advise patient that activities requiring mental alertness and precision should be avoided until reaction to the drug has been evaluated.

▪ Caution against drinking alcoholic beverages. When combined with chlordiazepoxide, effects of both are potentiated.

▪ If patient becomes pregnant during therapy or intends to become pregnant, advise her to communicate with physician about continuing therapy.

▪ Caution patient to avoid excessive sunlight. Photosensitivity has been reported. A sun screen lotion (SPF 12 or above) should be used (if allowed).

Common side effects in *italic*; life-threatening effects <u>underlined</u>; generic names in **bold**; classifications in SMALL CAPS

427

CHLORHEXIDINE GLUCONATE

(klor-hex´i-deen)
Trade names: Hibiclens, Hibistat, Peridex
Classifications: SKIN & MUCOUS MEMBRANE
AGENT; ANTIINFECTIVE
Pregnancy: Category B

ACTIONS/PHARMACODYNAMICS Gluconic
salt of chlorhexidine in near neutral solution with the
unique property of persisting residual antimicrobial
activity. Active against a wide variety of microorganisms including gram-positive bacteria and gram-negative bacteria such as *Pseudomonas aeruginosa*.
Adsorption onto cell walls of bacteria changes permeability, permitting leakage of essential intracellular components, thereby preventing reproduction.
Chlorhexidine is not significantly affected by presence of blood or other organic material and is not absorbed systemically through intact skin. Has shown a
50–97% reduction in counts of both aerobic and
anaerobic bacteria in plaque after 3 mo of controlled
use. No significant change in bacterial resistance, no
superinfections, or other adverse changes occur in
oral microbial ecosystem with chlorhexidine use.

USES Skin cleanser for surgical scrub and preoperative showering and bathing. Also used to cleanse
skin wounds, as a germicidal hand rinse, and as antibacterial dental rinse.

ROUTE & DOSAGE

Gingivitis

Adult	Topical	Rinse mouth with 15 ml (1/2 oz) of the 0.12% solution for 30 s twice daily (in the morning and evening) after toothbrushing; oral mouth rinse should be expectorated after rinsing since it is not intended for ingestion
Child	Topical	Same as for adult

Skin Disinfectant

Adult	Topical	Swab or scrub area with a 4% solution for 2–3 min
Child	Topical	Same as for adult

PHARMACOKINETICS Absorption: not absorbed
through intact skin and mucous membranes. **Onset:**
immediate. **Duration:** 4–5 h.

**CONTRAINDICATIONS & PRECAUTIONS Con-
traindicated in:** hypersensitivity to chlorhexidine gluconate. Safe use during pregnancy (category B), in
nursing mothers, or in children < 18 y not established. **Cautious use in:** front-tooth restorations, peri-
odontitis.

ADVERSE/SIDE EFFECTS PO: *staining of oral
surfaces* (including dentures, tooth fillings), change
in taste perception; increase in supragingival calculus
formation; stomatitis, especially in children 10–18 y;
irritation of tongue tip; superficial desquamation of
oral mucosa (especially in children). **Skin:** skin irritation, dermatitis, photosensitivity. **Other:** deafness
(when instilled into middle ear).

NURSING IMPLICATIONS

Administration

- Avoid contacting eyes and ears with chlorhexidine;
  should it happen, rinse out promptly and thoroughly with water.
- *Treatment of denture stomatitis:* Soak dentures in
  chlorhexidine oral rinse (Peridex) for 1–2 min 2
  times a day. Rinse mouth (swish solution in mouth
  for 30 s) before replacing dentures.
- Use should be discontinued if skin irritation, dermatitis, or photosensitivity develop.
- Store chlorhexidine at 15–30C (59–86F); avoid exposure to heat above 40C (104F); do not freeze.

Prototype: procaine, p 166

CHLOROPROCAINE HYDROCHLORIDE

(klor-oh-proe´kane)
Trade names: Nesacaine, Nesacaine-CE
Classifications: CNS AGENT; LOCAL ANESTHETIC
(ESTER-TYPE)
Pregnancy: Category C

ACTIONS/PHARMACODYNAMICS Short-act-
ing ester-type local anesthetic similar to procaine.
Decreases sodium flux into nerve cells, thus preventing initial depolarization, propagation, and conduction of the nerve impulse. Not used for spinal,
topical, or IV regional anesthesia.

USES Infiltration anesthesia and for peripheral, sympathetic, and epidural (including caudal) block anesthesia.

Common side effects in *italic*; life-threatening effects <u>underlined</u>;
generic names in **bold**; classifications in SMALL CAPS

ROUTE & DOSAGE

Infiltration and Nerve Block

Adult 1–2% solution: max 800 mg without epinephrine, 1 g with epinephrine

Caudal and Epidural Block (Without Preservatives)

Adult 2–3% solution: max 800 mg without epinephrine, 1 g with epinephrine

PHARMACOKINETICS Onset: 6–12 min. **Duration:** 30–60 min without epinephrine; 60–90 min with epinephrine. **Metabolism:** hydrolyzed by plasma pseudocholinesterases. **Elimination:** excreted by kidneys.

CONTRAINDICATIONS & PRECAUTIONS con-traindicated in: known sensitivity to ester-type anesthetics, bisulfites, parabens (preservative) or PABA; intercurrent use of bupivacaine. Safe use during pregnancy (category C), by nursing mothers or children <12 y not established. **Cautious use in:** cardiac function impairment; history of drug hypersensitivity; debilitated, elderly, or acutely ill patients; dysrhythmias.

ADVERSE/SIDE EFFECTS CNS: anxiety, nervousness, tremors, sedation, circumoral paresthesia, convulsions followed by drowsiness, respiratory arrest. **CV:** myocardial depression, hypotension, arrhythmias, bradycardia, cardiac arrest. **Eye:** blurred or double vision. **Ear:** tinnitus. **GI:** nausea, vomiting. **Hypersensitivity:** cutaneous lesions of delayed onset; urticaria, sneezing, anaphylactoid reactions. **Other:** with caudal or epidural anesthesia: urinary retention, fecal or urinary incontinence, slowing of labor and increased incidence of forceps delivery, headache, backache, edema, status asthmaticus.

NURSING IMPLICATIONS

Administration

- A test dose (3 ml of 3% solution or 5 ml of 2% solution) is given before epidural use to check for intravascular or subarachnoid injection. *Signs of intravascular injection:* "epinephrine response" (tachycardia, circumoral pallor, palpitations, nervousness). *Signs of subarachnoid injection:* motor paralysis and extensive sensory anesthesia.
- If patient is moved with potential displacement of epidural catheter, test dose is repeated. At least 5 min should elapse between each test dose. Total dose for anesthesia is administered in fractional doses.
- Nesacaine formulation incorporates parabens

(preservative) and sodium bisulfite; Nesacaine-CE is preservative-free but incorporates sodium bisulfite. Both parabens and bisulfites may initiate an allergic reaction in some individuals. Determine patient's sensitivity before administration of drug.

- Chloroprocaine is incompatible with alkali hydroxides and their carbonates: soaps, iodine, iodides, silver salts. Avoid use of any of these agents for skin or mucous membrane disinfection before chloroprocaine administration.
- Low temperatures may cause crystallization of drug; exposure to room temperature should promote dissolution. If crystals remain, discard vial.
- Do not administer solution that is colored. Discard partially used solutions that are preservative-free.
- Vials can be autoclaved for terminal sterilization. Sterilization with ethylene oxide is not recommended because of its potential absorption through vial closure.
- Store vials at 15–30C (59–86F); protect from freezing and from direct light.

Assessment & Drug Effects

- Monitor vital signs throughout period of drug use.
- Resuscitation equipment, oxygen, resuscitative drugs, and vasopressors should be immediately available when chloroprocaine is in use.

CHLOROQUINE HYDROCHLORIDE

See ANTIINFECTIVE, ANTIMALARIAL prototype p 79.

Prototype: hydrochlorothiazide, p 203

CHLOROTHIAZIDE

(klor-oh-thye´a-zide)
Trade names: Diachlor, Diuril, SK-Chlorothiazide

CHLOROTHIAZIDE SODIUM

Trade name: Sodium Diuril
Classifications: WATER BALANCE AGENT; THIAZIDE DIURETIC; ANTIHYPERTENSIVE
Pregnancy: Category B

ACTIONS/PHARMACODYNAMICS Thiazide diuretic chemically related to sulfonamides. Primary ac-

Common side effects in *italic*; life-threatening effects underlined; generic names in **bold**; classifications in SMALL CAPS

429

C

tion is production of diuresis by direct action on the distal convoluted tubules. Inhibits reabsorption of sodium, potassium, and chloride ions. Promotes renal excretion of sodium (and water), bicarbonate, and potassium; decreases renal calcium excretion and supports uric acid retention. Antihypertensive mechanism is unclear but correlates with contraction of extracellular and intravascular fluid volumes and direct vasodilatory effect on vascular wall. This initially reduces cardiac output with subsequent decrease in peripheral resistance through autoregulatory mechanisms. Thiazide-induced hypokalemia may promote hyperglycemia by suppressing release of endogenous insulin. Has paradoxic antidiuretic effect in diabetes insipidus, and increases total serum cholesterol and triglyceride levels. Cross-allergy reported among chemically related drugs, e.g., furosemide (Lasix), sulfonylureas, acetazolamide (Diamox), and other sulfonamides.

USES Adjunctively to manage edema associated with CHF, hepatic cirrhosis, renal dysfunction, corticosteroid, or estrogen therapy. Used alone as step 1 agent in stepped-care approach, or in combination with other agents for treatment of hypertension. **Unlabeled use:** to reduce polyuria of central and nephrogenic diabetes insipidus, to prevent calcium-containing renal stones, and to treat renal tubular acidosis.

ROUTE & DOSAGE

Hypertension, Edema

Adult	PO	250 mg–1 g/d in 1–2 divided doses
	IV	250 mg–1 g/d in 1–2 divided doses

Edema

Child	PO	<6 mo: 10–30 mg/kg/d in 1–2 divided doses
		≥6 mo: 20–22 mg/kg/d in 1–2 divided doses

PHARMACOKINETICS Absorption: incompletely absorbed PO. **Onset:** 2 h PO; 15 min IV. **Peak:** 3–6 h PO; 30 min IV. **Duration:** 6–12 h PO; 2 h IV. **Distribution:** distributed throughout extracellular tissue; concentrates in kidney; crosses placenta. **Metabolism:** does not appear to be metabolized. **Elimination:** half-life: 45–120 min; excreted in urine and breast milk.

CONTRAINDICATIONS & PRECAUTIONS Contraindicated in: hypersensitivity to thiazides or sulfonamides; anuria; hypokalemia; IV use in infants and children; during pregnancy (category B) and in nursing mothers. **Cautious use in:** history of sulfa allergy; impaired renal or hepatic function or gout; hypercalcemia, diabetes mellitus, elderly or debilitated patients, pancreatitis, sympathectomy, jaundiced children.

ADVERSE/SIDE EFFECTS CNS: unusual fatigue, dizziness, mental changes, vertigo, headache, paresthesias. **CV:** irregular heart beat, weak pulse, orthostatic hypotension. **GI:** vomiting, heartburn, acute pancreatitis, diarrhea. **Hematologic:** leukopenia, agranulocytosis, thrombocytopenia, aplastic anemia, electrolyte imbalance, asymptomatic hyperuricemia, hyperglycemia, glycosuria, rise in blood ammonia level, SIADH secretion. **Hypersensitivity:** urticaria, photosensitivity, skin rash, fever, respiratory distress, anaphylactic reaction. **Other:** *hypokalemia*, hypercalcemia, elevated cholesterol and triglyceride levels.

DIAGNOSTIC TEST INTERFERENCES Chlorothiazide (thiazides) may cause: marked increases in *serum amylase* values, decrease in *PBI* determinations; increase in excretion of *PSP*; increase in *BSP retention;* false-negative *phentolamine* and *tyramine* tests; interference with *urine steroid* determinations, and possibly the *histamine test* for pheochromocytoma. Thiazides should be discontinued at least 3 d before *bentiromide test* (thiazides can invalidate test) and before *parathyroid function tests* because they tend to decrease calcium excretion.

DRUG INTERACTIONS Amphotericin B, CORTICOSTEROIDS increase hypokalemic effects of chlorothiazide; the hypoglycemic effects of SULFONYLUREAS and **insulin** may be antagonized; **cholestyramine, colestipol** decrease thiazide absorption; intensifies hypoglycemic and hypotensive effects of **diazoxide;** increased potassium and magnesium loss may cause **digoxin** toxicity; decreases **lithium** excretion, increasing its toxicity; increases risk of NSAID-induced renal failure and may attenuate diuresis.

INCOMPATIBILITIES Y-Site: chlorpromazine, amikacin, codeine phosphate, hydralazine, insulin, levorphanol, methadone, morphine, norepinephrine, polymyxin B, procaine, prochlorperazine, promazine, promethazine, strep-

tomycin, TETRACYCLINES, **trifluromazine, vancomycin,** MULTIVITAMINS.

NURSING IMPLICATIONS

Administration

- Oral drug may be administered with or after food to prevent gastric irritation. Extent of absorption appears to be increased by taking it with food.
- Schedule daily doses to avoid nocturia and interrupted sleep.
- **IV solution:** Reconstitute with no less than 18 ml sterile water for injection (500 mg/20 ml vial). Solution may be further diluted for IV administration with dextrose or NaCl injection. May be given by direct IV at a rate of 0.5 gram over 5 min.
- Chlorothiazide is not compatible with whole blood or its derivatives. See manufacturer's directions regarding dilutions, stability, storage, and compatible IV fluids.
- Do not administer chlorothiazide solution SC or IM. Thiazide preparations are extremely irritating to the tissues, and great care must be taken to avoid extravasation. Palpate IV catheter/needle entry site occasionally to confirm needle position. If infiltration occurs, stop medication, remove needle, and apply ice if area is small.
- Store tablets, PO solutions, and parenteral dosage forms at 15–30C (59–86F) unless otherwise directed by manufacturer. Unused reconstituted IV solutions may be stored at room temperature up to 24 h. Use only clear solutions.

Assessment & Drug Effects

- Baseline and periodic determinations are indicated for blood count, serum electrolytes, CO_2, BUN, creatinine, uric acid, and blood sugar.
- Thiazide therapy can cause hyperglycemia (see Signs & Symptoms, chap 3) and glycosuria in diabetic and diabetic-prone individuals. Dosage adjustment of hypoglycemic drugs may be required.
- Asymptomatic hyperuricemia can be produced because of interference with uric acid excretion. Patient with history of gout may be continued on a thiazide with adjusted doses of uricosuric agent.
- Establish baseline weight before initiation of therapy. Weigh patient at the same time each AM under standard conditions. Usually a gain of more than 1 kg (2 lb) within 2 or 3 d and a gradual weight gain over the week's period is reportable. Tell patient to check for signs of edema (hands, ankles, pretibial areas).
- BP should be closely monitored during early drug therapy. Physician may want initial measurements for patients with hypertension taken with patient standing, sitting, and to evaluate drug effects.
- Skin and mucous membranes should be inspected daily for evidence of petechiae in patients receiving large doses and those on prolonged therapy.
- In an attempt to relieve dry mouth, patient may significantly increase fluid intake. Consult physician about permissible intake volume.
- Patients on digitalis therapy should be observed closely for signs and symptoms of hypokalemia (see chap 3). Even moderate reduction in serum potassium can precipitate digitalis intoxication in these patients.

Patient & Family Education

- Explain to patient that he or she will be urinating greater amounts and more frequently than usual and that there will be an unusual sense of tiredness. With continued therapy, diuretic action decreases; hypotensive effects usually are maintained, and sense of tiredness diminishes.
- Antihypertensive action of a thiazide diuretic requires several days before effects are observed; usually optimum therapeutic effect is not established for 3–4 wk.
- Monitor I&O ratio. Excessive diuresis or oliguria may cause electrolyte imbalance and necessitate prompt dosage adjustment. To prevent dehydration, urge patient to report GI illness accompanied by protracted vomiting or prolonged period of diarrhea.
- If orthostatic hypotension is a troublesome symptom (and it may be, especially in the elderly), inform patient of measures that may help him or her tolerate the effect and to prevent falling.
- Because of the possibility of dehydration, caution patient against drinking large quantities of coffee or other caffeine drinks. Caffeine is a CNS stimulant with diuretic effects.
- Advise patient to watch for and report signs and symptoms of hypokalemia, hypercalcemia, or hyperglycemia (see chap 3).
- Hypokalemia may be prevented if the daily diet contains potassium-rich foods. Urge patient to eat a banana and drink at least 6 oz orange juice every day. Collaborate with dietitian and physician.
- Warn patient about the possibility of photosensitivity reaction and to notify physician if it occurs. Thiazide-related photosensitivity is considered a photoallergy (radiation changes drug structure and makes it allergenic for some individuals). It occurs 1 1/2–2 wk after initial sun exposure.

C

Prototype: estradiol, p 236

CHLOROTRIANISENE
(klor-oh-trye-an´i-seen)
Trade name: TACE
Classifications: HORMONE; SYNTHETIC ESTROGEN
Pregnancy: Category X

ACTIONS/PHARMACODYNAMICS Nonesteroidal synthetic estrogen derived from diethylstilbestrol. Properties similar to those of other estrogens. Has weak estrogenic properties until metabolized.

USES Inoperable progressing prostatic cancer; short-term treatment of symptoms of estrogen deficiency, e.g., atrophic vaginitis, female hypogonadism, kraurosis vulvae, vasomotor symptoms of menopause. Use for prevention of postpartum breast engorgement no longer recommended because large doses required increase risk of thrombophlebitis.

ROUTE & DOSAGE

Menopausal Symptoms
Adult   PO   12–25 mg/d x 30 d

Prostatic Cancer
Adult   PO   12–25 mg/d

Female Hypogonadism
Adult   PO   12–25 mg/d x 21 d followed by IM progesterone or PO progestin for 5 d

PHARMACOKINETICS Onset: approximately day 14 of therapy. **Distribution:** stored in fat tissues, from where it is slowly released. **Metabolism:** converted in liver to active estrogen.

CONTRAINDICATIONS & PRECAUTIONS Contraindicated in: thrombophlebitis or thromboembolic disorders, breast cancer, undiagnosed abnormal vaginal bleeding, pregnancy (category X). Safe use during lactation not established. **Cautious use in:** history of jaundice, metabolic bone diseases, hypertension, impaired renal function, asthma, history of gallbladder disease, diabetes mellitus.

ADVERSE/SIDE EFFECTS CNS: headache, dizziness, sudden loss of coordination, slurred speech, mental depression, irritability. **CV:** thromboembolism, thrombophlebitis, edema. **GI:** abdominal cramps, anorexia, *nausea,* vomiting, diarrhea. **Gynecologic:** spotting, breakthrough bleeding, prolonged bleeding, amenorrhea, decrease in libido; testicular atrophy, gynecomastia (males); lumps in breast, breast tenderness, pigmentation of nipples and areola. **Other:** jaundice, loss of hair, shortness of breath, aggravation of migraine, photosensitivity, visual disturbances, intolerance to contact lenses.

NURSING IMPLICATIONS

Administration
- Instruct patient to swallow the capsule whole. It may be taken with or immediately after food to reduce nausea.
- Because of its long-acting effects, chlorotrianisene is less suitable for cyclic therapy than the shorter acting estrogens.
- When chlorotrianisene is administered for postpartum breast engorgement, first dose should be given within the first 8 h after delivery.
- Capsules should be stored in tightly closed container in a dry place, preferably at 15–30C (59–86F). Protect from extremes of temperature and humidity above 50%.

Assessment & Drug Effects
- Monitor for signs and symptoms of thrombophlebitis (see chap 3) in the lower extremities.
- Monitor BP, especially in hypertensive patients, as drug may cause fluid retention.

Patient & Family Education
- May cause loss of diabetes control. Monitor blood and urine glucose closely.
- If pregnancy occurs during therapy, stop medication and report promptly to physician.
- Inform patient of the importance of keeping follow-up appointments.
- Instruct patient to report signs and symptoms of thrombophlebitis (see chap 3).

Prototype: diphenhydramine, p 47

CHLORPHENIRAMINE MALEATE

(klor-fen-cer´a-meen)

Trade names: Aller-Chlor, Chlo-Amine, Chlorate, Chlor-Pro, Chlorspan, Chlortab, Chlor-Trimeton, Pfeiffer Allergy, Phenetron, Telachlor, Teldrin, Trymegan

Classifications: ANTIHISTAMINE (H₁-RECEPTOR ANTAGONIST)

Pregnancy: Category B

ACTIONS/PHARMACODYNAMICS Antihistamine that generally produces less drowsiness than other antihistamines, but side effects involving CNS stimulation may be more common. Competes with histamine for H₁-receptor sites on effector cells, thus prevents histamine action that promotes capillary permeability and edema formation and constrictive action on respiratory, gastrointestinal, and vascular smooth muscles. Has antiemetic, antitussive, anticholinergic, and local anesthetic actions.

USES Symptomatic relief of various uncomplicated allergic conditions; to prevent transfusion and drug reactions in susceptible patients, and as adjunct to epinephrine and other standard measures in anaphylactic reactions.

ROUTE & DOSAGE

Symptomatic Allergy Relief

Adult	PO	2–4 mg t.i.d. or q.i.d.; 8–12 mg b.i.d. or t.i.d.; max 24 mg/d
Child	PO	6–12 y: 2 mg q4–6h (max 12 mg/d)
		2–6 y: 1 mg q4–6h

Allergic Reactions to Blood

Adult	SC/IV/IM	10–20 mg (max 40 mg/d)

PHARMACOKINETICS Absorption: well absorbed from GI tract; about 45% of dose reaches systemic circulation intact. **Onset:** within 6 h. **Peak:** 2–6 h. **Distribution:** highest concentrations in lung, heart, kidney, brain, small intestine, and spleen. **Elimination:** half-life: 12–43 h.

CONTRAINDICATIONS & PRECAUTIONS

Contraindicated in: Hypersensitivity to antihistamines of similar structure; lower respiratory tract symptoms, narrow-angle glaucoma, obstructive prostatic hypertrophy or other bladder neck obstruction, GI obstruction or stenosis, pregnancy (category B), nursing mothers, premature and newborn infants, during or within 14 days of MAO inhibitor therapy. **Cautious use in:** convulsive disorders, increased intraocular pressure, hyperthyroidism, cardiovascular disease, hypertension, diabetes mellitus, history of bronchial asthma, elderly patients, patients with G6PD deficiency.

ADVERSE/SIDE EFFECTS Low incidence of side effects. **CNS:** *drowsiness,* sedation, headache, dizziness, vertigo, tinnitus, fatigue, disturbed coordination, tingling, heaviness, weakness of hands, tremors, euphoria, nervousness, restlessness, insomnia. **CV:** palpitation, tachycardia, mild hypotension or hypertension. **ENT:** *dryness of mouth,* nose, and throat, tinnitus, vertigo, acute labyrinthitis, thickened bronchial secretions, wheezing, sensation of chest tightness. **Eye:** blurred vision, diplopia. **GI:** epigastric distress, anorexia, nausea, vomiting, constipation or diarrhea. **GU:** urinary frequency or retention, dysuria.

DIAGNOSTIC TEST INTERFERENCES Antihistamines should be discontinued 4 d before **skin testing** procedures for allergy because they may obscure otherwise positive reactions.

DRUG INTERACTIONS Alcohol (ethanol) and other CNS DEPRESSANTS produce additive sedation and CNS depression.

NURSING IMPLICATIONS

Administration

- Sustained release tablets should be swallowed whole and not crushed or chewed.
- In patients receiving antihistamines for allergic manifestations, a careful history should be taken to discover the allergen involved, if possible.
- The 100 mg/ml preparation is intended for IM or SC use only. It should not be administered IV because it contains preservatives. The 10 mg/ml injection can be given IV, IM, or SC. It contains no preservatives.
- IV chlorpheniramine may be given by direct IV undiluted. Administer 10 mg or fraction thereof over at least 1 min.
- Solutions for injection should not be given intradermally.
- If patient manifests any reaction after parenteral administration, drug should be discontinued. (Excep-

Common side effects in *italic*; life-threatening effects underlined; generic names in **bold**; classifications in SMALL CAPS

433

tion: patient may experience transitory stinging sensation that rarely lasts longer than a few minutes.)

- Store preferably between 15 and 30C (59 and 86F) unless otherwise directed by manufacturer. Syrup and injection forms should be protected from light to prevent discoloration.

Assessment & Drug Effects

- Monitor for CNS depression and sedation, especially when chlorpheniramine is given in combination with other CNS depressants.
- Monitor BP in hypertensive patients since chlorpheniramine may elevate BP.

Patient & Family Education

- Driving a car and other potentially hazardous activities should be avoided until drug response has been determined.
- Antihistamines have additive effects with alcohol. Therefore advise cautious use.
- Patients on prolonged therapy should have periodic blood cell counts.
- Store antihistamines out of reach of children. Fatalities have been reported.
- Patients with allergies should be advised to carry at all times medical identification jewelry or card indicating specific allergy, name, and physician's name, address, and telephone number.

CHLORPROMAZINE

See CNS AGENTS, PSYCHOTHERAPEUTIC, PHENOTHIAZINE ANTIPSYCHOTIC (TRANQUILIZER) prototype, p 191.

Prototype: tolbutamide, p 234

CHLORPROPAMIDE
(klor-proe´pa-mide)

Trade names: Apo-Chlorpropamide, Chloronase, Diabinese, Glucamide, Novopropamide

Classifications: HORMONE; SULFONYLUREA ANTIDIABETIC

Pregnancy: Category C

ACTIONS/PHARMACODYNAMICS Longest-acting first generation sulfonylurea compound, structurally and pharmacologically related to tolbutamide. Although a sulfonamide derivative, it has no antiinfective activity. Lowers blood glucose by stimulating beta cells in pancreas to release endogenous insulin. May potentiate available antidiuretic hormone (ADH) secretion, a property not shared by other sulfonylureas. Has longer duration of action and about 6 times the potency of tolbutamide, as well as a higher incidence of side effects. Reported to be associated with fewer primary and secondary failures. There is no evidence that cardiovascular mortality is associated with the use of sulfonylureas.

USES Mild to moderately severe, stable non-insulin-dependent diabetes mellitus (type II, NIDDM) in patients who cannot be controlled by diet alone and who do not have complications of diabetes. **Unlabeled use:** neurogenic diabetes insipidus.

ROUTE & DOSAGE

Antidiabetic

Adult	PO	Initial: 100–250 mg/d with breakfast; adjust by 50–125 mg/d q3–5d until glycemic control is achieved, up to 750 mg/d

Antidiuretic

Adult	PO	100–250 mg/d; may adjust q2–3d up to 500 mg/d

PHARMACOKINETICS Absorption: readily absorbed from GI tract. **Onset:** 1 h. **Peak:** 3–6 h. **Distribution:** highly protein bound; distributed into breast milk. **Metabolism:** metabolized in liver. **Elimination:** half-life: 36 h; 80–90% excreted in urine in 96 h.

CONTRAINDICATIONS & PRECAUTIONS Contraindicated in: known hypersensitivity to sulfonylureas and to sulfonamides; as sole therapy for type I (IDDM) diabetes; diabetes complicated by severe infection; acidosis; severe renal, hepatic, or thyroid insufficiency. Safe use during pregnancy (category C), in nursing mothers, and in children not established. **Cautious use in:** elderly patients, Addison's disease, CHF, and hepatic porphyria.

ADVERSE/SIDE EFFECTS CNS: drowsiness, muscle cramps, weakness, paresthesias. **GI:** GI distress, anorexia, nausea, diarrhea, constipation, cholestatic jaundice. **Hematologic:** leukopenia, thrombocytopenia, anemia (rare); <u>agranulocytosis</u>. **Hypersensitivity:** rash, pruritus. **Other:** <u>hypoglycemia</u>, antidiuretic effect (SIADH): dilutional hyponatremia, water intoxication, hyposthenuria, flushing, photosensitivity.

DRUG INTERACTIONS Adverse effects of ORAL ANTICOAGULANTS, **phenytoin,** SALICYLATES, NSAIDS may be increased along with those of chlorpropamide; THIAZIDE DIURETICS may increase blood sugar; **alcohol** produces disulfiram reaction; **probenecid,** MAO INHIBITORS may increase hypoglycemic effects.

NURSING IMPLICATIONS

Administration

- Chlorpropamide is generally prescribed as a single morning dose with breakfast. Alternatively, it may be prescribed to be divided into 2 or 3 doses and taken with meals to minimize GI side effects and to achieve maximum diabetes control.
- Store below 40C (104F), preferably at 15–30C (59–86F) in a tightly closed container, unless otherwise directed.

Assessment & Drug Effects

- Monitor blood and urine glucose to determine effectiveness of glycemic control.
- Glycosylated hemoglobin levels should be determined every 2–3 mo.
- Monitor for signs and symptoms of hypoglycemia (see chap 3).
- Baseline and periodic hematologic and hepatic studies are advisable, particularly in patients receiving high doses. A CBC should be performed if symptoms of anemia appear; advise patient to report dizziness, shortness of breath, malaise, fatigue.
- In the treatment of diabetes insipidus the expected therapeutic effect of chlorpropamide is the promotion of a significant decrease in urinary output. Monitor I&O ratio and check with physician regarding allowable parameters.

Patient & Family Education

- With long-acting hypoglycemic agents such as chlorpropamide, mild CNS symptoms of hypoglycemia predominate, whereas other symptoms may go unnoticed or simply may be tolerated.
- Because chlorpropamide has a long half-life, hypoglycemia can be severe, although onset is not as fast or as dramatic as with use of insulin.
- The more severe toxic effects, jaundice and agranulocytosis, are often preceded by skin eruptions, malaise, fever, or photosensitivity. Immediately report these symptoms to the physician. A change to another hypoglycemic agent may be indicated.
- Caution patient not to self-dose with OTC drugs unless approved or prescribed by the physician.
- Instruct the controlled diabetic patient to monitor weight and to be aware of I&O ratio and pattern. Infrequently chlorpropamide produces an antidiuretic effect, with resulting severe hyponatremia, edema, and water intoxication. If fluid intake far exceeds output and edema develops (weight gain), the patient should report to the physician.

Prototype: chlorpromazine, p 191

CHLORPROTHIXENE
(klor-proe-thix´een)
Trade names: Taractan, Tarasan
Classifications: CNS AGENT; PSYCHOTHERAPEUTIC; PHENOTHIAZINE ANTIPSYCHOTIC (TRANQUILIZER)
Pregnancy: Category C

ACTIONS/PHARMACODYNAMICS Structurally and pharmacologically similar to the phenothiazines. Believed to act by blocking dopamine receptor sites in brain. Produces strong antiemetic effect by inhibiting medullary chemoreceptor trigger zone (CTZ). Also has prominent sedative effect but less hypotensive, anticholinergic, and antihistaminic activity than chlorpromazine, and incidence of extrapyramidal symptoms is less.

USES Management of manifestations of psychotic disorders.

ROUTE & DOSAGE

Antipsychotic

Adult	PO	25–50 mg t.i.d. or q.i.d. (max 600 mg/d)
	IM	25–50 mg; may repeat t.i.d. or q.i.d. if needed
Child	PO	10–25 mg t.i.d. or q.i.d.

PHARMACOKINETICS Absorption: partially absorbed from GI tract. **Onset:** 10–30 min IM. **Metabolism:** metabolized in liver. **Elimination:** half-life: 30 h; excreted primarily in urine with some elimination in feces.

Common side effects in *italic*; life-threatening effects <u>underlined</u>; generic names in **bold**; classifications in SMALL CAPS

435

CONTRAINDICATIONS & PRECAUTIONS Contraindicated in: hypersensitivity to phenothiazine derivatives; bone marrow depression, circulatory collapse, coronary artery disease, cerebrovascular disorders, CHF, alcoholism, comatose states. Safe use during pregnancy (category C) or in nursing mothers or safe PO use in children <6 y or parenteral use in those <12 y not established. **Cautious use in:** persons exposed to extreme heat or organophosphate insecticides, persons with suicide tendency; history of drug abuse, peptic ulcer, cardiovascular or respiratory disease, breast cancer, persons receiving electroshock treatment.

ADVERSE/SIDE EFFECTS CNS: *sedation,* drowsiness, lethargy, dizziness, ataxia, convulsions, tardive dyskinesia, pseudoparkinsonism and other extrapyramidal symptoms. **CV:** orthostatic hypotension, Q and T wave distortions, tachycardia. **Eye:** blurred vision, ocular disturbances. **GI:** *dry mouth,* constipation. **GU:** difficult urination, urinary retention, galactorrhea, gynecomastia, increased libido, impotence, amenorrhea. **Hematologic:** transient leukopenia, agranulocytosis, thrombocytopenic purpura. **Skin:** inability to sweat, contact dermatitis, photosensitivity, urticaria. **Other:** uricosuria, increased appetite, excessive weight gain, thirst, nasal stuffiness, jaundice.

DIAGNOSTIC TEST INTERFERENCES *Immunologic urine pregnancy tests* may produce false-positive or false-negative results depending on test used. *Urine bilinogen test* results may be false-positive.

DRUG INTERACTIONS Alcohol, other CNS DEPRESSANTS increase sedation and CNS depression.

NURSING IMPLICATIONS

Administration

- May be taken with food or a full glass of water or milk to reduce risk of gastric irritation.
- Oral concentrate may be given alone or diluted in water, milk, fruit juice, coffee, or carbonated beverage just before administration. Warn patient not to spill oral liquid on skin or clothing because drug can cause contact dermatitis.
- Administer IM in upper outer quadrant of buttock or midlateral thigh. Rotate injection sites.
- Since postural hypotension may occur in some patients, IM injection should be given with patient recumbent. Patient should remain lying down for at least 1/2 h. Observe patient until weakness or dizziness, if present, passes. Caution patient to make position changes slowly, and in stages, particularly from recumbent to upright position.
- Monitor patient closely when changeover from parenteral to oral dose is made. Oral dose is alternated with parenteral dose on same day, then oral dose only.
- When therapy is to be discontinued, doses should be reduced gradually over a several-day period. Abrupt withdrawal may produce nausea, vomiting, gastritis, dizziness, and tremulousness.
- Store in light-resistant, tightly covered container at 15–30C (59–86F) unless otherwise specified.

Assessment & Drug Effects

- Before treatment is initiated, establish baseline BP readings (standing and recumbent) and pulse and respiratory patterns.
- Geriatric and debilitated patients should be closely supervised particularly during ambulation. Lethargy and drowsiness are easily controlled by dosage adjustment.
- Monitor I&O ratio and bowel elimination pattern. Patient should know what laxative to use if necessary. Consult physician about prescribing a high-fiber diet.
- Patients on high dose or prolonged therapy should have the following follow-up checks at periodic intervals: blood cell counts and differential, liver function tests, urine tests for bile and bilirubin, ophthalmologic examinations.
- Hepatotoxicity (see Signs & Symptoms, chap 3) generally occurs after 4–10 wk of continuous therapy. Agranulocytosis (see Signs & Symptoms, chap 3) is most likely to occur after 2–4 wk of treatment.
- Therapy may be accompanied by inability to sweat, which can increase body temperature. Patient exposed to extremes in environmental temperature or to high fever due to illness may develop heat stroke. Inform physician and prepare to institute measures (evaporative cooling, and antipyretics) to rapidly lower body temperature.

Patient & Family Education

- Be certain patient understands dosing regimen and the importance of not changing or omitting doses.
- Patients for whom prolonged therapy is contemplated should be informed about the risk of developing tardive dyskinesia (see Signs & Symptoms, chap 3). Early symptoms, such as wormlike movements of the tongue and bizarre, rhythmic movements of mouth and face, should be reported immediately.
- Alcohol and other CNS depressants should be avoided during treatment with chlorprothixene.

Common side effects in *italic*; life-threatening effects underlined; generic names in **bold**; classifications in SMALL CAPS

- Caution patient to avoid excessive exposure to sunlight. Use sunscreen lotion (SPF above 12) when outdoors, even if it is a cloudy day.
- Warn patient to avoid driving and other potentially hazardous activities until his or her reaction to drug is known.
- Urge patient to keep follow-up appointments. Periodic evaluations should be made to determine possibility of dosage reduction or termination of drug therapy.
- May discolor urine pink to red, or red brown.

Prototype: tetracycline, p 74

CHLORTETRACYCLINE HYDROCHLORIDE
(klor-te-tra-sye´kleen)
Trade names: Aureomycin Ointment 3%, Aureomycin Ophthalmic 1%
Classifications: ANTIINFECTIVE; TETRACYCLINE ANTIBIOTIC
Pregnancy: Category D

ACTIONS/PHARMACODYNAMICS Broad-spectrum antibiotic derived from *Streptomyces aureofaciens*. Effective against most *Chlamydia, Mycoplasma, Rickettsia* spirochetes, and a variety of gram-negative and gram-positive pathogens. Primarily bacteriostatic in action; inhibits protein synthesis. See antibiotic, tetracycline, prototype for specific modes of action and range of antimicrobial activity.

USES Ophthalmic ointment is used as adjunct with oral therapy in the treatment of *Chlamydia* trachoma and inclusion conjunctivitis and for superficial ocular infections caused by susceptible organisms. Skin ointment is used for treatment of superficial pyogenic skin infections and for prophylaxis of minor skin abrasions.

ROUTE & DOSAGE

Eye Infection

Adult	Topical	Apply thin strip of ophthalmic ointment to lower conjunctival sac of infected eye q2h or more often as needed

Skin Infection

Adult	Topical	Apply skin ointment 1 or more times/d

CONTRAINDICATIONS & PRECAUTIONS Contraindicated in: hypersensitivity to tetracyclines. Safe use during pregnancy (category D), in nursing women, and in children <8 y not established.

ADVERSE/SIDE EFFECTS Hypersensitivity: itching, burning, urticaria, dermatitis, angioneurotic edema. **Other:** superinfection; possible interference with color vision (ophthalmic preparation), skin dryness.

NURSING IMPLICATIONS

Administration
- The ophthalmic ointment and skin ointment are not interchangeable.
- Chlortetracycline preparations (ophthalmic and skin) are stored in tightly closed, light-resistant containers at 15–30C (59–86F) unless otherwise directed.

Assessment & Drug Effects
- Culture and susceptibility tests should be initiated before start of therapy to determine sensitivity of infecting organisms to chlortetracycline.
- Monitor for signs and symptoms of hypersensitivity or superinfection (see chap 3). Report their appearance promptly.

Patient & Family Education
- Discontinue medication and notify physician if an adverse reaction occurs or if infection shows no improvement or appears to be worsening.
- Advise patient to apply medication as directed by physician and not to exceed prescribed duration of therapy. Prolonged or frequent intermittent use of an antibiotic should be avoided because of danger of hypersensitization and superinfection.

Prototype: hydrochlorothiazide, p 203

CHLORTHALIDONE
(klor-thal´i-done)
Trade names: Hygroton, Hylidone, Novothalidone, Thalitone, Uridon
Classifications: WATER BALANCE AGENT; THIAZIDE DIURETIC; ANTIHYPERTENSIVE
Pregnancy: Category B

ACTIONS/PHARMACODYNAMICS Sulfonamide derivative. Differs chemically from thiazides

Common side effects in *italic*; life-threatening effects underlined; generic names in **bold**; classifications in SMALL CAPS

437

but shares similar actions, uses, contraindications, adverse reactions, and drug interactions. Increases excretion of sodium and chloride by inhibiting their reabsorption in the cortical diluting segment of the ascending loop of Henle. Reportedly causes elevations in total cholesterol, LDL cholesterol, and triglycerides, in some patients.

USES Edema associated with CHF, renal decompensation, hepatic cirrhosis, corticosteroid and estrogen therapy; as sole agent or with other antihypertensives to treat hypertension.

ROUTE & DOSAGE

Hypertension

Adult	PO	12.5–25 mg/d; may be increased to 100 mg/d if needed
Child	PO	2 mg/kg 3 times/wk

Edema

Adult	PO	50–100 mg/d; may be increased to 200 mg/d if needed

PHARMACOKINETICS Absorption: readily absorbed from GI tract. **Onset:** 2 h. **Peak:** 3–6 h. **Duration:** 24–72 h. **Distribution:** crosses placenta; appears in breast milk. **Elimination:** half-life: 54 h; 30–60% excreted in urine in 24 h.

CONTRAINDICATIONS & PRECAUTIONS Contraindicated in: hypersensitivity to sulfonamide derivatives; anuria, hypokalemia. Safe use during pregnancy (category B), in nursing mothers, and children not established. **Cautious use in:** history of renal and hepatic disease, gout, SLE, diabetes mellitus.

ADVERSE/SIDE EFFECTS CNS: dizziness, vertigo, paresthesias, headache, xanthopsia (yellow vision). **CV:** orthostatic hypotension. **GI:** anorexia, nausea, vomiting, diarrhea, constipation, cramping, jaundice, pancreatitis. **Hematologic:** *hypokalemia,* hyponatremia, hypochloremia, hypercalcemia, leukopenia, agranulocytosis, thrombocytopenia, aplastic anemia. **Skin/Hypersensitivity:** rash, urticaria, photosensitivity, vasculitis. **Other:** glycosuria, hyperglycemia, impotence, exacerbation of gout.

DRUG INTERACTIONS Increased risk of **digoxin** toxicity because of hypokalemia; CORTICOSTEROIDS, **amphotericin B** increase hypokalemia; decreases **lithium** elimination; may antagonize the hypoglycemic effects of SULFONYLUREAS; NSAIDs may attenuate diuretic effects; **cholestyramine** decreases thiazide absorption.

NURSING IMPLICATIONS

Administration
- When chlorthalidone is used as a diuretic, an intermittent dose schedule may reduce incidence of adverse reactions.
- Administered as single dose in AM to reduce potential for interrupted sleep because of diuresis.
- Store tablets in tightly closed container at 15–30C (59–86F) unless otherwise advised.

Assessment & Drug Effects
- When chlorthalidone is used for hypertension, establish baseline BP measurements and check at regular intervals during period of dosage adjustment.
- Elderly patients are more sensitive to adverse effects of drug-induced diuresis because of age-related changes in the cardiovascular and renal systems. Be alert to signs of hypokalemia (see chap 3).
- The following laboratory values should be obtained initially and periodically throughout therapy: serum electrolytes (particularly K, Mg, Ca), serum uric acid, creatinine, BUN, and uric acid and blood sugar (especially in patients with diabetes).

Patient & Family Education
- Advise patient to maintain adequate potassium intake, to monitor weight, and to make a daily estimate of I&O ratio.

Prototype: cyclobenzaprine, p 122

CHLORZOXAZONE
(klor-zox´a-zone)
Trade name: Paraflex, Parafon Forte
Classifications: AUTONOMIC NERVOUS SYSTEM AGENT; CENTRAL ACTING SKELETAL MUSCLE RELAXANT
Pregnancy: Category C

ACTIONS/PHARMACODYNAMICS Centrally acting skeletal muscle relaxant. Acts indirectly by depressing nerve transmission through polysynaptic pathways in spinal cord, subcortical centers, and brainstem and possibly by sedative effect. Not effective for spastic or dyskinetic CNS disorders, e.g., cerebral palsy.

Common side effects in *italic*; life-threatening effects underlined; generic names in **bold**; classifications in SMALL CAPS

USES Symptomatic treatment of muscle spasm and pain associated with various musculoskeletal conditions.

ROUTE & DOSAGE

Skeletal Muscle Relaxant

Adult	PO	250–500 mg t.i.d. or q.i.d. (max 3 g/d)
Child	PO	20 mg/kg/d in 3–4 divided doses

PHARMACOKINETICS Absorption: readily absorbed from GI tract. **Onset:** 1 h. **Peak:** 1–4 h. **Duration:** 3–4 h. **Distribution:** not known if crosses placenta or distributed into breast milk. **Metabolism:** metabolized in liver. **Elimination:** half-life: 66 min; excreted in urine.

CONTRAINDICATIONS & PRECAUTIONS Contraindicated in: impaired liver function. Safe use during pregnancy (category C) not established. **Cautious use in:** patients with known allergies or history of drug allergies; history of liver disease; elderly patients.

ADVERSE/SIDE EFFECTS CNS: *drowsiness, dizziness,* lightheadedness, headache, malaise, overstimulation. **GI:** anorexia, heartburn, nausea, vomiting, constipation, diarrhea, abdominal pain. **Hypersensitivity:** erythema, rash, pruritus, urticaria, petechiae, ecchymoses. **Other:** hepatotoxicity. jaundice, liver damage.

DRUG INTERACTIONS Alcohol, CNS DEPRESSANTS add to CNS depression.

NURSING IMPLICATIONS

Administration

- May be taken with food or meals to prevent gastric distress. If necessary, tablet may be crushed and mixed with food or liquid, e.g., milk, fruit juice.
- Store in tight container at 15–30C (59–86F) unless otherwise directed.

Assessment & Drug Effects

- Some patients may require supervision of ambulation during early drug therapy.
- Periodic liver function tests are advised in patients receiving long-term therapy even if sporadic.
- Since chlorzoxazone metabolite may discolor urine, dark urine cannot be a reliable sign of a hepatotoxic reaction.

Patient & Family Education

- Since sedation, drowsiness, and dizziness may occur, advise patient not to undertake activities requiring mental alertness, judgment, and physical coordination until reaction to drug is known.
- Drug may discolor urine orange to purplish red, but this is of no clinical significance.
- Drug should be discontinued if signs of hypersensitivity (see chap 3) or of liver dysfunction appear (abdominal discomfort, yellow sclerae or skin, pruritus, malaise, nausea, vomiting).
- Advise patient to check with physician before taking an OTC depressant (e.g., antihistamine, sedative, alcohol) since effects may be additive.

CHOLESTYRAMINE RESIN

See CARDIOVASCULAR AGENT, ANTILIPEMIC, BILE ACID SEQUESTRANT prototype, p 142.

Prototype: aspirin, p 161

CHOLINE MAGNESIUM TRISALICYLATE

(cho´leen mag-ne´si-um tri-sal´i-ci-late)
Trade name: Trilisate
Classifications: CNS AGENT; SALICYLATE ANALGESIC, ANTIPYRETIC; NSAID
Pregnancy: Category C

ACTIONS/PHARMACODYNAMICS Trilisate is a nonsteroidal, antiinflammatory preparation combining choline salicylate and magnesium salicylate. It also has analgesic and antipyretic action. Mode of action is by inhibiting prostaglandin synthesis. Platelet aggregation is not affected.

USES Osteoarthritis, rheumatoid arthritis, and other arthrides. Preferable to aspirin for patients with GI bleeding.

ROUTE & DOSAGE

Arthritis

Adult	PO	1.5–2.5 g/d in 1–3 divided doses (max 4.5 g/d)

Mild to Moderate Pain, Fever

Adult	PO	2–3 g/d in 2 divided doses
Child	PO	50 mg/kg/d in 2 divided doses

Common side effects in *italic*; life-threatening effects underlined; generic names in **bold**; classifications in SMALL CAPS

PHARMACOKINETICS Absorption: readily absorbed from small intestine. **Onset:** 30 min. **Peak:** 1–3 h. **Metabolism:** metabolized in liver. **Elimination:** half-life: 2–3 h; excreted in urine.

CONTRAINDICATIONS & PRECAUTIONS Contraindicated in: hypersensitivity to nonacetylated salicylates. **Cautious use in:** chronic renal and hepatic failure, peptic ulcer; patients on coumadin or heparin; pregnancy (category C); children and teenagers with chickenpox, influenza, or flu symptoms because of the potential for Reye's syndrome.

ADVERSE/SIDE EFFECTS CNS: headache, vertigo, confusion, drowsiness. **GI:** vomiting, diarrhea. **Ear:** tinnitus.

DRUG INTERACTIONS Aminosalicylic acid increases risk of salicylate toxicity; **ammonium chloride** and other **acidifying agents** decrease its renal elimination, increasing risk of salicylate toxicity; ANTICOAGULANTS increase risk of bleeding; CARBONIC ANHYDRASE INHIBITORS enhance salicylate toxicity; CORTICOSTEROIDS compound ulcerogenic effects; increases **methotrexate** toxicity; low doses of salicylates may antagonize uricosuric effects of **probenecid, sulfinpyrazone.**

NURSING IMPLICATIONS

Administration
- May be given with food to reduce gastric upset. Do not give with antacids.
- Use cautiously in chronic renal failure, peptic ulcer disease, and with known allergies to salicylates.
- Drug should not be given to children or teenagers with chickenpox, influenza, or flu symptoms because of association with Reye's syndrome.
- Store at 59–86F (15–30C).

Assessment & Drug Effects
- As with other NSAIDs, the antipyretic and antiinflammatory effects may mask usual signs and symptoms of infection or other diseases.
- Assess for GI discomfort; nausea, gastric irritation, indigestion, diarrhea, and constipation are frequent complaints.
- If used concurrently with warfarin, monitor for signs and symptoms of bleeding and closely monitor PT.

Patient & Family Education
- Avoid taking aspirin or acetaminophen concurrently with drug.

- Inform patient of possible CNS effects (e.g., vertigo, drowsiness) and caution to avoid dangerous activities until reaction to drug is determined.
- Instruct patient to report tinnitus to physician.
- Instruct patient to report persistent gastric irritation and epigastric pain.
- Instruct patients with type II diabetes who are taking an oral hypoglycemic agent (OHA) that hypoglycemic effects may be enhanced.
- Do not give to children or teenagers with chickenpox, influenza, or flu symptoms because of association with Reye's Syndrome.

Prototype: aspirin, p 161

CHOLINE SALICYLATE

(koe´leen)
Trade name: Arthropan
Classifications: CNS AGENT; SALICYLATE ANALGESIC, ANTIPYRETIC; NSAID
Pregnancy: Category C

ACTIONS/PHARMACODYNAMICS Choline salt of salicylic acid available commercially as a liquid salicylate preparation. Reported to be less potent than aspirin as an analgesic, antiinflammatory, and antipyretic, and produces less gastric irritation and bleeding. Clinical significance of the claim that it is absorbed more rapidly than aspirin is unclear. Unlike aspirin, believed to have no appreciable effect on platelet function.

USES Analgesic and antiinflammatory in rheumatoid arthritis, rheumatic fever, osteoarthritis, and other conditions for which oral salicylates are usually recommended. May be indicated for patients who have difficulty swallowing tablets or capsules or as an alternative preparation for patients who show gastric intolerance to aspirin or who should avoid sodium-containing salicylates.

PHARMACOKINETICS Absorption: readily absorbed from GI tract. **Peak:** 10–30 min. **Distribution:** widely distributed in most body tissues; crosses placenta; distributed in breast milk. **Elimination:** half-life: 2–3 h; excreted in urine.

CONTRAINDICATIONS & PRECAUTIONS Contraindicated in: salicylate hypersensitivity. **Cautious use in:** history of peptic ulcer disease.

Common side effects in *italic*; life-threatening effects underlined; generic names in **bold**; classifications in SMALL CAPS

ROUTE & DOSAGE

Analgesic, Antipyretic

Adult	PO	435–870 mg (2.5–5 ml) q4h
Child	PO	2–11 y: 2 g (11.5 ml)/m² in 4–6 divided doses

Arthritis

Adult	PO	4.8–7.2 g (28–41 ml)/d in 4–6 divided doses
Child	PO	107–134 mg (0.6–0.8 ml)/kg/d in 4–6 divided doses

ADVERSE/SIDE EFFECTS *Nausea,* vomiting. **High doses:** tinnitus, deafness, dizziness, sweating, mental confusion, hyperventilation; hepatotoxicity.

DIAGNOSTIC TEST INTERFERENCES As for aspirin with the exception of *5-HIAA* which is not affected by choline salicylate.

DRUG INTERACTIONS Aminosalicylate increases risk of salicylate toxicity; increases risk of bleeding with ORAL ANTICOAGULANTS; SULFONYLUREAS pose increased risk of hypoglycemia with large doses of salicylates; CARBONIC ANHYDRASE INHIBITORS cause metabolic acidosis that may increase salicylate toxicity; CORTICOSTEROIDS add to ulcerogenic effects; may increase **methotrexate** levels; small doses of salicylates may blunt uricosuric effects of **probenecid, sulfinpyrazone.**

NURSING IMPLICATIONS

Administration

- Although the preparation is mint flavored, the taste is objectionable to some patients. May be mixed with or followed by fruit juice, a carbonated beverage, or water. Do not administer with an antacid.
- If patient requires an antacid, administer choline salicylate before meals and the antacid 2 hr after meals.
- Store in tightly capped container at temperature between 15 and 30C (59 and 86F). Protect from freezing.

Assessment & Drug Effects

- Monitor effectiveness of drug in relieving pain in arthritic joints.
- Assess for signs of bleeding, especially in patients on anticoagulant therapy.

Patient & Family Education

- Available OTC. Caution patient not to exceed recommended dosage and to keep medicine out of the reach of children.

- Avoid concurrent use of other drugs containing aspirin or salicylates unless otherwise advised by physician.

CHORIONIC GONADOTROPIN

(go-nad´oh-troe-pin)

Trade names: Antuitrin, A.P.L., Chorex, Chorigon, Choron 10, Corgonject-5, Follutein, Glukor, Gonic, HCG, Pregnyl, Profasi HP

Classification: HORMONE

Pregnancy: Category C

ACTIONS/PHARMACODYNAMICS Human chorionic gonadotropin (HCG) is a polypeptide hormone produced by the placenta and extracted from urine during first trimester of pregnancy. Actions nearly identical to those of pituitary luteinizing hormone (LH). Promotes production of gonadal steroid hormones by stimulating interstitial cells of the testes (Leydig cells) to produce androgen, and the corpus luteum of the ovary to produce progesterone. Androgen stimulation in the male produces secondary sex characteristics and may cause testicular descent if there is no anatomic impediment. Administration of HCG to women of childbearing age with normal functioning ovaries causes maturation of the ovarian follicle and triggers ovulation. When given during normal pregnancy, it maintains corpus luteum after LH decreases, supports continuing secretion of estrogen and progesterone, and prevents ovulation. HCG has no known effect on fat metabolism, appetite, sense of hunger, or body fat distribution.

USES Prepubertal cryptorchidism not due to anatomic obstruction and male hypogonadism secondary to pituitary deficiency. Also used in conjunction with menotropins to induce ovulation and pregnancy in infertile women in whom the cause of anovulation is secondary (ovulation usually occurs within 18 h). To stimulate spermatogenesis in males with hypogonadism. **Unlabeled use:** corpus luteum dysfunction.

PHARMACOKINETICS Onset: 2 h. **Peak:** 6 h. **Distribution:** testes in males, ovaries in females. **Elimination:** half-life: 23 h; 10–12% excreted in urine within 24 h.

ROUTE & DOSAGE

Prepubertal Cryptorchidism

Child	IM	4000 units 3 times/wk for 3 wk, *or* 5000 U q.o.d. for 4 doses, *or* 500–1000 U 3 times/wk for 4–6 wk

Hypogonadotropic Hypogonadism

Adult	IM	500–1000 U 3 times/wk for 3 wk; then 2 times/wk for 3 wk *or* 4000 U 3 times/wk for 6–9 mo followed by 2000 U 3 times/wk for 3 mo

Stimulation of Spermatogenesis

Adult	IM	5000 U 3 times/wk until normal testosterone levels are achieved (4–6 mo), then 2000 U 2 times/wk with menotropins for 4 mo

Induction of Ovulation

Adult	IM	500–1000 U 1 d following last dose of menotropins

CONTRAINDICATIONS & PRECAUTIONS Contraindicated in: known hypersensitivity to HCG, hypogonadism of testicular origin, hypertrophy or tumor of pituitary, prostatic carcinoma or other androgen-dependent neoplasms, precocious puberty. Safe use during pregnancy (category C) not established. **Cautious use in:** epilepsy, migraine, asthma, cardiac or renal disease.

ADVERSE/SIDE EFFECTS Headache, irritability, restlessness, depression, fatigue, gynecomastia, edema, precocious puberty, pain at injection site, increased urinary steroid excretion, ectopic pregnancy (incidence low). When used with menotropins (human menopausal gonadotropin): ovarian hyperstimulation (ascites with or without pain, pleural effusion, ruptured ovarian cysts with resultant hemoperitoneum, multiple births), arterial thromboembolism.

DIAGNOSTIC TEST INTERFERENCES *Pregnancy tests:* possibility of false results.

NURSING IMPLICATIONS

Administration

- Following reconstitution (diluent furnished by manufacturer), solution is stable for 30–90 d, depending on manufacturer, when refrigerated; thereafter potency decreases.

- Store powder for infection at 15–30C (59–86F) unless otherwise directed.

Patient & Family Education

- Given to the anovulatory patient after failure to respond to therapy with clomiphene citrate.
- Treatment for prepubertal cryptorchidism is usually started between 4 and 9 y. HCG can help predict whether orchidopexy will be needed in the future.
- When used for treatment of infertility, timing of coitus is important. Daily intercourse is encouraged from day before HCG is given until ovulation occurs.
- Instruct patient to report promptly onset of abdominal pain and distension (ovarian hyperstimulation syndrome).
- Induction of androgen secretion by HCG may induce precocious puberty in patient treated for cryptorchidism. Instruct parent to report to physician if the following appear: axillary, facial, pubic hair, penile growth, acne, deepening of voice.
- Observe for signs of fluid retention. A weight chart should be maintained for a bi-weekly record. Report to physician if weight gain is associated with edema.
- Vaginal bleeding during treatment of corpus luteum deficiency should be reported; drug will be discontinued.

CHYMOPAPAIN

(kye´moe-pa-pane)
Trade names: Chymodiactin, Discase
Classification: ENZYME
Pregnancy: Category C

ACTIONS/PHARMACODYNAMICS Proteolytic enzyme isolated from crude latex of papaya (Carica papaya). When injected into the herniated nucleus pulposus, causes solubilization of protein core of the chondromucoprotein. Net effect is reduction in intradiscal osmotic pressure, with resulting decrease in fluid absorption and accumulation and, ultimately, intradiscal pressure.

USES Chemonucleolytic agent as an alternative to surgery in patients with documented herniated lumbar intervertebral discs who have not responded to adequate trial(s) of conservative therapy.

PHARMACOKINETICS Distribution: detectable in plasma within 30 min. **Metabolism:** inactivated in plasma. **Elimination:** small portions detected in urine.

Common side effects in *italic*; life-threatening effects underlined; generic names in **bold**; classifications in SMALL CAPS

ROUTE & DOSAGE

Herniated Lumbar Disc

Adult Intradiscal 2000–4000 U/disc (max cumulative dose not to exceed 8000 U); at least 15 min should elapse between discography and administration. Not recommended to inject >2 discs

CONTRAINDICATIONS & PRECAUTIONS Contraindicated in: hypersensitivity to papaya, chymopapain, and other papaya derivatives (as in certain meat tenderizers, beers, and contact lens cleaners); previous injections of chymopapain or surgical treatment for the spinal disorder; use for other than lumbar spine severe spondylolisthesis, progressing paralysis, or neurologic dysfunction; spinal cord or cauda equina lesion, intrathecal administration. Safe use during pregnancy (category C) and in children not established.

ADVERSE/SIDE EFFECTS GI: nausea. **Hypersensitivity:** erythema, piloerection, rash, pruritus, urticaria, vasomotor rhinitis, angioedema, conjunctivitis. Anaphylaxis: bronchospasm, laryngeal edema, arrhythmias, cardiac arrest, coma, death. **Neuromuscular:** *back pain, stiffness, soreness,* back spasms, sacral burning sensation, paresthesias, lessened sensitivity to pain, leg weakness, cramping in both calves, pain in opposite leg; acute transverse myelitis or myelopathy with paraplegia and paraparesis; cerebral hemorrhage. **Other:** headache, dizziness, urinary retention.

DRUG INTERACTIONS RADIOCONTRAST MEDIA increase risk of adverse effects; do not use until 3–4 d after chymopapain administration.

NURSING IMPLICATIONS

Administration
- Only used in hospital settings by physicians with specialized training in the use of chymopapain.
- To reconstitute, clean top of vial stopper with alcohol. Allow alcohol to evaporate before inserting needle into vial (alcohol inactivates chymopapain).
- Following reconstitution with sterile water for injection, chymopapain solutions are enzymatically stable for 1 h. Since solutions contain no preservative, they should be used within 1 h. Discard unused portions.
- Do not use bacteriostatic water for injection for reconstitution since it may inactivate chymopapain.

- Store powder for injection in refrigerator at 2–8C (36–46F) until ready to be reconstituted unless otherwise directed.

Assessment & Drug Effects
- Candidates for therapy should be carefully questioned about allergies, especially to papaya or its derivatives, and about history of any previous chymopapain injection.
- Papain is widely used in a variety of applications. Therefore a large part of the U.S. population has probably developed sensitivity to papain.
- In the period immediately following drug administration, patient must be monitored closely for at least 2 h for anaphylactic reaction. Patients should be informed that delayed reactions have occurred as late as 15 d after injection.
- Anaphylaxis appears to occur 10 times more frequently in female patients, particularly those with erythrocyte sedimentation rates greater than 20 mm/h (**Normal:** 0–20 mm/h).
- Monitor vital signs. Anticipate the possibility of anaphylaxis. Also be alert to arrhythmias and signs of shock.

Patient & Family Education
- To allay anxiety, inform patient of the possibility of neuromuscular symptoms after drug administration. Back pain, stiffness, and soreness occur in 50% and back spasm in 30% of patients and may last for several days. Rarely, residual stiffness and soreness may persist for several months. Notify physician of any abnormalities.

CICLOPIROX OLAMINE
(sye-kloe-peer´ox)
Trade name: Loprox
Classifications: ANTIINFECTIVE; ANTIFUNGAL ANTIBIOTIC
Pregnancy: Category B

ACTIONS/PHARMACODYNAMICS Synthetic broad spectrum antifungal agent with activity against pathogenic fungi including dermatophytes, yeasts, and *Malassezia furfur,* some species of *Mycoplasma* and *Trichomonas vaginalis,* and certain strains of gram-positive and gram-negative bacteria. Inhibits transport of amino acids within fungal cell, thereby interfering with synthesis of protein, RNA, and DNA.

Common side effects in *italic*; life-threatening effects <u>underlined</u>; generic names in **bold**; classifications in SMALL CAPS

443

USES Topically for treatment of tinea cruris and tinea corporis (ringworm) due to *Trichophyton rubrum, Trichophyton mentagrophytes, Epidermophyton floccosum,* and *Microsporum canis,* and for tinea (pityriasis) versicolor due to *Malassezia furfur;* also cutaneous candidiasis (moniliasis) caused by *Candida albicans.*

ROUTE & DOSAGE

Tinea

Adult	Topical	Massage cream into affected area and surrounding skin twice daily, morning and evening

PHARMACOKINETICS Absorption: 1.3% absorbed through intact skin. **Distribution:** distributed to epidermis, corium (dermis), including hair and hair follicles and sebaceous glands; not known if crosses placenta or is distributed into breast milk. **Elimination:** half-life: 1.7 h; excreted primarily by kidneys.

CONTRAINDICATIONS & PRECAUTIONS Contraindicated in: hypersensitivity to ciclopirox olamine or to any excipients in the formulation. Safe use during pregnancy (category B), in nursing women, and in children <10 y not established.

ADVERSE/SIDE EFFECTS Irritation, pruritus, burning, worsening of clinical condition.

NURSING IMPLICATIONS

Administration

- Wash hands thoroughly before and after treatments.
- Consult with physician about specific procedure for cleansing the skin before medication is applied. Regardless of method used, dry skin thoroughly before drug application.
- Store at 15–30C (59–86F) unless otherwise directed.

Assessment & Drug Effects

- In general, tinea versicolor responds to drug treatment in about 2 wk. Tinea pedis ("athlete's foot"), tinea corporis (ringworm), tinea cruris ("jock itch"), and candidiasis (moniliasis) require about 4 wk of therapy.
- Recurrences are especially likely to occur in patients with diabetes or other predisposing illnesses.

Patient & Family Education

- Instruct patient to use medication for the prescribed time even though symptoms improve.
- Report skin irritation or other possible signs of sensitization. A reaction suggestive of sensitization warrants drug discontinuation.
- Caution patient not to use occlusive dressings or wrappings.
- Warn patient to avoid contact of drug in or near the eyes.
- Wear light clothing and footwear that will allow ventilation. Loose-fitting cotton underwear or socks are ideal.

CIMETIDINE

See GASTROINTESTINAL AGENT, ANTISECRETORY (H$_2$-RECEPTOR ANTAGONIST) prototype, p 216.

Prototype: trimethoprim, p 90

CINOXACIN

(sin-ox′a-sin)
Trade name: Cinobac
Classifications: URINARY TRACT ANTIINFECTIVE; QUINOLONE
Pregnancy: Category B

ACTIONS/PHARMACODYNAMICS Synthetic bactericidal agent with properties similar to those of nalidixic acid but with fewer side effects. Acts intracellularly to inhibit bacterial DNA replication and protein synthesis. Effective against a wide variety of gram-negative pathogens, particularly most strains of *Escherichia coli, Klebsiella* and *Enterobacter* species, *Proteus mirabilis,* and *Proteus vulgaris.* Not active against staphylococci, enterococci, or *Pseudomonas.*

USES Initial and recurrent UTIs in adults caused by susceptible microorganisms.

ROUTE & DOSAGE

UTI

Adult	PO	1 g/d in 2–4 divided doses

PHARMACOKINETICS Absorption: readily absorbed from GI tract. **Peak:** 2–3 h. **Duration:** 12 h. **Distribution:** concentrates in renal and prostatic tissues; crosses placenta   listribution into breast milk

Common side effects in *italic*; life-threatening effects underlined; generic names in **bold**; classifications in SMALL CAPS

unknown. **Elimination:** half-life: 1.5 h; 97% excreted in urine within 24 h.

CONTRAINDICATIONS & PRECAUTIONS Contraindicated in: hypersensitivity to cinoxacin or to other quinolones; anuria. Safe use during pregnancy (category B), in nursing mothers, and in prepubertal children not established. **Cautious use in:** impaired renal or hepatic function.

ADVERSE/SIDE EFFECTS CNS: *headache, dizziness,* insomnia, tingling sensations, agitation, anxiety. **Ear:** tinnitus. **Eye:** photophobia, blurred vision. **GI:** *nausea,* vomiting, anorexia, constipation, rectal itching, metallic taste, sore gums, abdominal cramps, diarrhea. **Hypersensitivity:** urticaria, pruritus, rash, edema. **Other:** swelling of extremities, arthropathy; elevations of AST, ALT, alkaline phosphatase, BUN, and serum creatinine.

DRUG INTERACTIONS Probenecid decreases renal elimination of cinoxacin.

NURSING IMPLICATIONS

Administration

- May be taken with food. Although presence of food in stomach may reduce peak serum concentrations, total amount absorbed is not affected.
- Therapeutic effectiveness is enhanced by taking the drug at evenly spaced intervals throughout 24 h so that urinary drug concentration is maintained.

Assessment & Drug Effects

- Susceptibility tests should be performed before start of therapy and during therapy if response is not satisfactory.
- Since dizziness is a possible side effect, supervision of ambulation, especially with the elderly and debilitated, may be warranted.

Patient & Family Education

- Advise patient to take drug for the full course of therapy as prescribed.
- Instruct patient to report to physician if symptoms do not improve within a few days or if they become worse.
- Caution patient to avoid driving and other potentially hazardous tasks until reaction to drug is known.
- Photophobia may be relieved by wearing dark glasses.

CIPROFLOXACIN HYDROCHLORIDE

See ANTIINFECTIVE, QUINOLONE, prototype, p 87.

Prototype: cyclophosphamide, p 91

CISPLATIN (*CIS*-DDP, *CIS*-PLATINUM II)
(sis´pla-tin)
Trade name: Platinol
Classifications: ANTINEOPLASTIC; ALKYLATING AGENT
Pregnancy: Category D

ACTIONS/PHARMACODYNAMICS A heavy metal complex with platinum as central atom surrounded by 2 chloride atoms and 2 ammonia molecules in the *cis* position. Biochemical properties similar to those of bifunctional alkylating agents. Produces interstrand and intrastrand crosslinkage in DNA of rapidly dividing cells, thus preventing DNA, RNA, and protein synthesis. Cell-cycle nonspecific, i.e., effective throughout the entire cell life cycle. Carcinogenicity has not been fully studied, but other compounds with similar action mechanisms and mutogenicity have been reported to be carcinogenic.

USES Established combination therapy (cisplatin, vinblastine, bleomycin) in patient with metastatic testicular tumors and with doxorubicin for metastatic ovarian tumors following appropriate surgical or radiation therapy. **Unlabeled uses:** carcinoma of endometrium, bladder, head, and neck.

ROUTE & DOSAGE

Testicular neoplasms

Adult	IV	20 mg/m²/d for 5 d q3–4wk for 3 courses

Ovarian neoplasms

Adult		*Combination therapy:* 50 mg/m² once q3–4wk
		Single agent: 100 mg/m² once q3–4wk

PHARMACOKINETICS Peak: immediately after end of infusion. **Distribution:** widely distributed in body fluids and tissues; concentrated in kidneys, liver, and prostate; accumulated in tissues. **Metabolism:** not completely known. **Elimination:** half-life:

Common side effects in *italic*; life-threatening effects <u>underlined</u>; generic names in **bold**; classifications in SMALL CAPS

445

73–290 h; 15–50% of dose excreted in urine within 24–48 h.

CONTRAINDICATIONS & PRECAUTIONS

Contraindicated in: history of hypersensitivity to cisplatin or other platinum-containing compounds; impaired renal function; myelosuppression; impaired hearing; history of gout and urate renal stones. Safe use during pregnancy (category D), in nursing women, and in children not established. **Cautious use in:** previous cytoxic drug or radiation therapy; with other ototoxic and nephrotoxic drugs.

ADVERSE/SIDE EFFECTS

CNS: seizures, headache; peripheral neuropathies (may be irreversible): paresthesia, unsteady gait, clumsiness of hands and feet, exacerbation of neuropathy with exercise, loss of taste. **ENT:** <u>ototoxicity</u> (may be irreversible): tinnitus, hearing loss, deafness, vertigo. **Eye:** blurred vision, changes in ability to see colors (optic neuritis, papilledema). **GI:** *marked nausea, vomiting*, anorexia, stomatitis, xerostomia, diarrhea, constipation. **Hematologic:** myelosuppression (25–30% patients): leukopenia, thrombocytopenia; hemolytic anemia, hemolysis. **Hypersensitivity:** <u>anaphylactic-like reactions</u>. **Renal** (dose-related; cumulative): nephrotoxicity. **Other:** cardiac abnormalities, hypocalcemia, *hypomagnesemia*, hyperuricemia, elevated AST, SIADH.

DRUG INTERACTIONS

AMINOGLYCOSIDES, **amphotericin B, vancomycin,** other NEPHROTOXIC DRUGS increase nephrotoxicity and acute renal failure—try to separate by at least 1–2 wk; AMINOGLYCOSIDES, **furosemide** increase risk of ototoxicity.

INCOMPATIBILITIES

Solution/Additive: 5% dextrose, sodium bicarbonate, metoclopramide.

NURSING IMPLICATIONS

Administration

- Administered only under supervision of a qualified physician experienced in the use of antineoplastics.
- About 8–12 h before the initial dose a Foley catheter is inserted and hydration is started with 1–2 L IV infusion fluid to reduce risk of nephrotoxicity and ototoxicity. Drug is then diluted in 2 L 5% dextrose in 1/2 or 1/3 normal saline containing 37.5 g mannitol (an osmotic diuretic) and infused over 6–8 h. Hydration and forced diuresis are continued for at least 24 h after drug administration to ensure adequate urinary output.

- Usually a parenteral antiemetic agent is administered 1/2 h before cisplatin therapy is instituted and given on a scheduled basis throughout day and night as long as necessary.
- Use disposable gloves when preparing cisplatin solutions. If drug accidentally contacts skin or mucosa, wash immediately and thoroughly with soap and water.
- Reconstituted drug with sterile water for injection (1 mg/ml dilution) should be clear and colorless. Keep reconstituted solutions at room temperature; refrigeration will cause a precipitate to form. Since it lacks bacterial preservatives, it should be used within 20 h.
- Unless otherwise specified by manufacturer, store unopened vials in refrigerator at 2–8C (36–46F).

Assessment & Drug Effects

- A pretreatment ECG and cardiac monitoring during induction therapy are indicated because of possible myocarditis or focal irritability.
- Monitor urine output and specific gravity for 4 consecutive hours before treatment and for 24 h after therapy. Report if output is less than 100 ml/h or if specific gravity is more than 1.030. A urine output of less than 75 ml/h necessitates medical intervention to avert a renal emergency.
- Audiometric testing should be performed before the first dose and before each subsequent dose. Ototoxicity (reported in 31% of patients) may occur after a single dose of 50 mg/m². Children who receive repeated doses are especially susceptible.
- Anaphylactoid reactions (particularly in patient previously exposed to cisplatin) may occur within minutes of drug administration.
- The following tests should be done *before* initiating every course of therapy and repeated each week during treatment period: serum uric acid, serum creatinine, BUN, urinary creatinine clearance.
- Patient should be closely monitored for dose-related adverse reactions. Drug action is cumulative; therefore severity of most adverse effects increases with repeated doses.
- A single course of therapy is given no more frequently than once every 3 or 4 wk. A repeat course should not be given until (1) serum creatinine is below 1.5 mg/dl; (2) BUN is below 25 mg/dl; (3) platelets ≥ 100,000/mm³; (4) WBC ≥ 4000/mm³; (5) audiometric test is within normal limits.
- Nephrotoxicity (reported in 28–36% of patients receiving a single dose of 50 mg/m²) usually occurs within 2 wk after drug administration and becomes more severe and prolonged with repeated courses of cisplatin.

Common side effects in *italic*; life-threatening effects <u>underlined</u>; generic names in **bold**; classifications in SMALL CAPS

C

- Suspect ototoxicity if patient manifests tinnitus or difficulty hearing in the high frequency range.
- Intractable nausea and vomiting severe enough to warrant discontinuation of drug usually begin 1–4 h after treatment and may last 24 h or persist for up to 1 wk after treatment is ended.
- Monitor and report abnormal electrolyte levels: sodium > 145 or < 135 mEq/L, and potassium > 5 or < 3.5 mEq/L.
- CBC and platelet counts are done weekly for 2 wk after each course of treatment. The nadirs in platelet and leukocyte counts occur between day 18 and 23 (range: 7.5–45) with most patients recovering in 13–62 d. A decrease in hemoglobin (more than 2 g/dl) occurs at approximately the same time and with the same frequency.
- Check BP, mental status, pupils, and fundi every hour during therapy. Hydration and mannitol may increase the danger of elevated intracranial pressure (ICP).
- Neurologic examinations at regular intervals should include tests of muscle strength, Romberg, vibratory and position sense, tests of sensation.
- Monitor and report abnormal bowel elimination pattern. Constipation and the possibility of fecal impaction may be caused by neurotoxicity; diarrhea is a possible response to GI irritation.
- Inspect oral membranes daily for xerostomia (white patches and ulcerations) and tongue for signs of fungal overgrowth (black, furry appearance).
- Infection precautions should be instituted promptly if a temperature increase of 0.6F over the previous reading is noted.
- The patient should be weighed under standard conditions (same time, clothing, scale) every day. A gradual ascending weight profile occurring over a period of several days should be reported.

Patient & Family Education

- Continue maintenance of adequate hydration (at least 3000 ml/24 h oral fluid if physician agrees) and report promptly the symptoms of nephrotoxicity: reduced urinary output, flank pain, anorexia, nausea, vomiting, dry mucosae, itching skin, urine odor on breath, fluid retention, and weight gain.
- Keep vestibular stimulation to the minimum to avoid dizziness or falling: avoid unnecessary turning in bed, and change position gradually and slowly.
- Tingling, numbness, and tremors of extremities, loss of position sense and taste, and constipation are early signs of neurotoxicity. Report their occurrence promptly to prevent irreversibility. Pain with

heel walking and difficulty in getting out of bed or chair are late indicators of nerve damage.
- If patient's oral discomfort interferes with eating, report to physician.
- Report promptly evidence of unexplained bleeding and easy bruising.
- Report unusual fatigue, fever, sore mouth and throat, abnormal body discharges.

Prototype: diphenhydramine, p 47

CLEMASTINE FUMARATE

(klem´as-teen)
Trade names: Tavist, Tavist-1
Classifications: ANTIHISTAMINE (H₁-RECEPTOR ANTAGONIST)
Pregnancy: Category C

ACTIONS/PHARMACODYNAMICS An antihistamine (H_1-receptor antagonist) with prominent antipruritic activity and low incidence of unpleasant side effects. Anticholinergic effects are weak, and central sedative effects are generally mild.

USES Symptomatic relief of allergic rhinitis (sneezing, rhinorrhea, pruritus) and mild uncomplicated allergic skin manifestations such as urticaria and angioedema.

ROUTE & DOSAGE

Allergic Rhinitis

Adult	PO	1.34 mg b.i.d.; may increase up to 8.04 mg/d
Child	PO	0.67 mg b.i.d.; may increase up to 4.02 mg/d

Allergic Urticaria

Adult	PO	2.68 mg b.i.d. or t.i.d.; may increase up to 8.04 mg/d
Child	PO	1.34 mg b.i.d.; may increase up to 4.02 mg/d

PHARMACOKINETICS Absorption: readily absorbed from GI tract. **Peak:** 5–7 h. **Duration:** 10–12 h. **Distribution:** distributed into breast milk. **Metabolism:** metabolized in liver. **Elimination:** excreted chiefly in urine.

Common side effects in *italic*; life-threatening effects underlined; generic names in **bold**; classifications in SMALL CAPS

447

CONTRAINDICATIONS & PRECAUTIONS Contraindicated in: hypersensitivity to clemastine or to other antihistamines of similar chemical structure; lower respiratory tract symptoms, including acute asthma; concomitant MAO inhibitor therapy. Safe use during pregnancy (category C) and in nursing mothers not established. **Cautious use in:** history of bronchial asthma, increased intraocular pressure, GI or GU obstruction, hyperthyroidism, cardiovascular disease, hypertension, elderly patients.

ADVERSE/SIDE EFFECTS CNS: Sedation, *transient drowsiness,* dry nose and throat, headache, dizziness, weakness, fatigue, disturbed coordination; confusion, restlessness, nervousness, hysteria, convulsions, tremors, irritability, euphoria, insomnia, paresthesias, neuritis. **CV:** hypotension, palpitation, tachycardia, extrasystoles. **ENT:** vertigo, tinnitus, acute labyrinthitis. **Eye:** blurred vision, diplopia. **GI:** *dry mouth,* epigastric distress, anorexia, nausea, vomiting, diarrhea, constipation. **GU:** difficult urination, urinary retention, early menses. **Hematologic:** hemolytic anemia, thrombocytopenia, agranulocytosis. **Hypersensitivity:** urticaria, rash, photosensitivity, anaphylaxis. **Respiratory:** dry nose and throat, thickening of bronchial secretions, tightness of chest, wheezing, nasal stuffiness. **Other:** excess perspiration, chills.

DRUG INTERACTIONS Alcohol and other CNS DEPRESSANTS increase sedation; MAO INHIBITORS may prolong and intensify anticholinergic effects.

NURSING IMPLICATIONS

Administration
- May be administered with food, water, or milk to reduce possibility of gastric irritation.
- Elderly patients usually require less than average adult dose.
- Store at 15–30C (59–86F) unless otherwise directed.

Assessment & Drug Effects
- Monitor for drowsiness, poor coordination, or dizziness, especially in the elderly or debilitated. Supervision of ambulation may be warranted.
- Assess for symptomatic relief with use of the medication.

Patient & Family Education
- Advise patient to check with physician before taking alcohol or other CNS depressants, since effects may be additive.

- Clemastine may cause lethargy and drowsiness; therefore necessary safety precautions should be taken.
- Advise elderly patients to make position changes slowly and in stages, particularly from recumbent to upright posture since they are more likely to experience dizziness and hypotension than younger patients.
- Caution patient not to drive and to avoid other potentially hazardous activities until response to the drug has been established.
- Should be discontinued about 4 d before skin testing procedures since it may prevent otherwise positive reactions.
- Advise frequent sips of water or sugarless hard candy to relieve dry mouth.

CLINDAMYCIN HYDROCHLORIDE

See ANTIINFECTIVE, ANTIBIOTIC, CLINDAMYCIN prototype, p 64.

Prototype: amphotericin B, p 56

CLIOQUINOL (IODOCHLORHYDROXYQUIN)
(klee-oh-kwee´nole)
Trade names: Torofor, Vioform
Classifications: ANTIINFECTIVE; ANTIBIOTIC; ANTIFUNGAL
Pregnancy: Category C

ACTIONS/PHARMACODYNAMICS Halogenated hydroxyquinoline with broad spectrum of antifungal and antibacterial activity. Available OTC.

USES Topically for treatment of inflamed cutaneous conditions such as eczema, athlete's foot, and other fungal conditions.

ROUTE & DOSAGE

Inflamed Cutaneous Conditions

Adult	Topical	Apply thin layer to affected area b.i.d. or t.i.d. for 1 wk only

PHARMACOKINETICS Absorption: minimally absorbed through intact skin. **Elimination:** some is

Common side effects in *italic*; life-threatening effects <u>underlined</u>; generic names in **bold**; classifications in SMALL CAPS

rapidly excreted in urine; the rest may persist in body 1 mo or more.

CONTRAINDICATIONS & PRECAUTIONS Contraindicated in: hypersensitivity to chloroxine, iodine, or iodine-containing preparations; tuberculosis; vaccinia, varicella, or other viral skin conditions; severe renal disease; hepatic damage; thyroid disorder. Safe use during pregnancy (category C) and in nursing mothers not established.

ADVERSE/SIDE EFFECTS Infrequent: local burning, irritation, redness, swelling, itching, rash, staining of hair and skin. Systemic reactions (if used on large skin areas): iodism, hypersensitivity reaction, slight enlargement of thyroid gland, hair loss, agranulocytosis, subacute myeloptic neuropathy.

DIAGNOSTIC TEST INTERFERENCES Possibility of elevated *PBI*, decreased *iodine 131 thyroidal uptake*, and elevation of butanol-extractable iodine *(BEI)*. False-positive ferric chloride test for phenylketonuria *(PKU)* may result if clioquinol is present on diaper or in urine.

NURSING IMPLICATIONS

Administration

- Area to be treated is generally washed with soap and water and dried thoroughly before each application. Consult physician.
- Do not apply an occlusive dressing without a physician's order.
- Preserve in tightly covered, light-resistant containers at 15–30C (59–86F) unless otherwise directed.

Assessment & Drug Effects

- Monitor for signs of skin irritation. Notify physician if they appear. Drug may be discontinued.
- Monitor for signs of systemic absorption such as thyroid enlargement and hair loss. Notify physician if they occur. Drug may be discontinued.

Patient & Family Education

- Avoid contact of drug in or around eyes. Drug may stain fabric, skin, or hair yellow on contact.
- Clioquinol should be discontinued if skin irritation, rash, or other signs of sensitivity or systemic absorption develop. Report to physician.
- Treatment is usually continued 4 wk for athlete's foot or ringworm and 2 wk for jock itch.

- Notify physician if there is no improvement within 1–2 wk. Apply the drug as directed and only for the period of time prescribed.

Prototype: hydrocortisone, p 255

CLOBETASOL PROPIONATE
(cloe-bay´ta-sol)
Trade names: Dermovate, Temovate
Classifications: SKIN AND MUCOUS MEMBRANE AGENT; ANTIINFLAMMATORY; HORMONE; ADRENAL CORTICOSTEROID; GLUCOCORTICOID
Pregnancy: Category C

ACTIONS/PHARMACODYNAMICS Topical synthetic corticosteroid and analog of prednisolone with a high level of glucocorticoid activity and slight degree of mineralocorticoid activity. Mechanism of action is related to suppression of mitotic activity, vasoconstriction, the immune response, membrane permeability, and release of inflammatory mediators. After percutaneous absorption, clobetasol enters the same pharmacokinetic pathways as systemically administered corticosteroids and, like other corticosteroids, has antiinflammatory and antipruritic properties. May cause reversible hypothalmic–pituitary–adrenocortical (HPA) axis suppression, especially in children. One of the most potent topical corticosteroids available.

USES Short-term relief of inflammation and pruritic manifestations of moderate to severe corticosteroid-responsive dermatoses.

ROUTE & DOSAGE

Inflamed Cutaneous Conditions

Adult	Topical	Apply thin layer to affected area b.i.d. for no more than 14 d (max 50 g/wk), *or* b.i.d. 3 d/wk, *or* 1–2 times/wk for up to 6 mo

PHARMACOKINETICS Absorption: minimally absorbed through intact skin unless occlusive dressing is used. **Metabolism:** some liver metabolism. **Elimination:** excreted in urine and bile.

CONTRAINDICATIONS & PRECAUTIONS Contraindicated in: hypersensitivity to clobetasol, other

Common side effects in *italic*; life-threatening effects underlined; generic names in **bold**; classifications in SMALL CAPS

449

corticosteroids; rosacea, perioral dermatitis, acne. Safe use during pregnancy (category C) and in children <12 y not established. **Cautious use in:** hepatic impairment, application to large areas of skin, or to face, groin or axilla; viral skin diseases (e.g., varicella, vaccinia, herpes simplex), fungal or bacterial infections of skin; nursing mothers.

ADVERSE/SIDE EFFECTS Local: stinging and burning sensations, hypertrichosis, hypopigmentation especially in blacks; pruritus; *skin atrophy,* striae, miliaria; cracking, erythema, folliculitis, numbness of fingers, fissuring of skin, *telangiectasia, acneiform eruptions.* **Systemic:** <u>reversible HPA-axis suppression</u>; Cushing's syndrome, hyperglycemia, glucosuria.

NURSING IMPLICATIONS

Administration

- Gently wash area to be treated, then apply medication in a thin layer with gentle rubbing. If application is to hairy area, part hair and apply medication directly to lesions.
- Avoid applying clobetasol near eyes or around mouth.
- Store at controlled room temperature (15–30C [59–86F]) in tightly capped tubes. Do not refrigerate.

Assessment & Drug Effects

- When drug is applied to highly absorptive areas, such as the face, groin, or axilla, frequently observe for signs of skin atrophy (shiny, thin, wrinkled skin) and report to physician.
- Observe for and report any adverse effects, especially when drug is used for prolonged periods or with elderly patients with atrophic skin.

Patient & Family Education

- Discuss with patient limitations on use of medication: amount of drug available in container, how long it should last, and method of application.
- Caution patient not to cover or wrap the treated area. An occlusive dressing or wrap can increase systemic absorption as much as tenfold and therefore is contraindicated.
- If medication does not provide relief within 3–5 d or if irritation develops or worsens in involved areas, notify the physician.

Prototype: hydrocortisone, p 255

CLOCORTOLONE PIVALATE
(kloe-kor´toe-lone)
Trade name: Cloderm
Classifications: SKIN AND MUCOUS MEMBRANE AGENT, ANTIINFLAMMATORY, ADRENAL CORTICOSTEROID, GLUCOCORTICOID
Pregnancy: Category C

ACTIONS/PHARMACODYNAMICS In common with other topical corticosteroids has antiinflammatory, antipruritic, and vasoconstrictor properties.

USES Relief of inflammatory and pruritic manifestations of corticosteroid-responsive dermatoses.

ROUTE & DOSAGE

Inflamed Cutaneous Conditions

| Adult | Topical | Apply thin layer to affected area 1–4 times/d |

PHARMACOKINETICS Absorption: minimally absorbed through intact skin unless occlusive dressing is used. **Metabolism:** some liver metabolism. **Elimination:** excreted in urine.

CONTRAINDICATIONS & PRECAUTIONS Contraindicated in: hypersensitivity to corticosteroids. Safe use during pregnancy (category C), in nursing women, and in children not established. **Cautious use in:** herpetic lesions.

ADVERSE/SIDE EFFECTS Generally well tolerated. Burning, itching, irritation, folliculitis, dryness, acneiform eruptions, hypertrichosis, hypopigmentation, perioral dermatitis, allergic contact dermatitis, skin maceration and *atrophy,* striae, and miliaria, especially with occlusive dressings or wrappings.

NURSING IMPLICATIONS

Administration

- Discuss with physician specific procedure for cleansing skin before each application and proper use of occlusive dressings.
- Antipruritic and antiinflammatory effectiveness of drug is enhanced by occlusive dressings since percutaneous absorption is substantially increased.
- Occlusive dressings should not be used on weep-

Common side effects in *italic*; life-threatening effects <u>underlined</u>; generic names in **bold**; classifications in SMALL CAPS

ing or exudative lesions. Patients with this type of lesion should be advised not to wear tight-fitting clothing or wrappings that could act as an occlusive dressing.

- If infection develops, occlusive dressing should be discontinued and appropriate antimicrobial treatment initiated.
- Store at 15–30C (59–86F) unless otherwise directed.

Assessment & Drug Effects

- Patients receiving prolonged therapy or applications to large areas or in whom occlusive dressings are being used should be closely observed for signs of systemic absorption.
- Tests of urinary free cortisol and ACTH stimulation tests are advised at regular intervals to evaluate hypothalmic–pituitary–adrenocortical (HPA) axis suppression.
- Elderly patients with atrophic skin are more susceptible to systemic toxicity because they tend to absorb proportionately larger amounts than young adults. (Children also absorb high amounts because of larger skin surface area–to–body weight ratio.)

Patient & Family Education

- Advise patient to notify physician if local irritation, signs of infection, hypersensitivity, or systemic reaction develop.
- Caution patient to use medication as directed and only for the disorder prescribed.
- Avoid contact of drug in or near the eyes.

Prototype: dapsone, p 77

CLOFAZIMINE
(kloe-faʹzi-meen)
Trade name: Lamprene
Classifications: ANTIINFECTIVE, ANTILEPROSY AGENT
Pregnancy: Category C

ACTIONS/PHARMACODYNAMICS Exerts a slow bactericidal effect on *Mycobacterium leprae* (Hansen's bacillus) and has antiinflammatory activity. Binds preferentially to DNA of all mycobacteria and inhibits their growth. Its antiinflammatory action (precise mechanism unknown) controls erythema nodosum leprosum reactions. Bacterial killing is not

detectable in biopsy tissue from leprosy patient until 50 d after start of therapy. Clofazimine is not effective against all forms of leprosy. Does not show cross-resistance with rifampin or dapsone. Has no clinically useful activity against microorganisms other than mycobacteria.

USES Chiefly in multiinfective therapy of multibacillary leprosy (with dapsone, rifampin, ethionamide) to prevent development of drug resistance. Also in lepromatous leprosy, including dapsone-resistant lepromatous leprosy and leprosy complicated by erythema nodosum leprosum (lepra) reaction. **Unlabeled use:** *Mycobacterium avium-intracellulare* complex infections in patients with AIDS.

ROUTE & DOSAGE

Dapsone-resistant Leprosy

Adult	PO	100 mg/d in combination with 1 or more antileprosy drugs for 3 y, then 100 mg/d as monotherapy

Erythema Nodosum Leprosum

Adult	PO	100–300 mg/d for up to 3 mo; taper dose to 100 mg/d as soon as possible

Mycobacterium avium-intracellulare

Adult	PO	100 mg 1–3 times/d

PHARMACOKINETICS Absorption: slowly absorbed from GI tract; approximately 50% absorbed. **Peak:** 4–12 h. **Distribution:** distributed predominantly to fatty tissues and reticuloendothelial system; crosses placenta; distributed into breast milk. **Elimination:** half-life: 70 d; primarily eliminated in feces through bile.

CONTRAINDICATIONS & PRECAUTIONS Contraindicated in: safe use during pregnancy (category C) and by nursing mothers not established. **Cautious use in:** patient with GI problems, children.

ADVERSE/SIDE EFFECTS CNS: drowsiness, fatigue, headache, giddiness, dizziness, neuralgia, taste disorder. **Eye:** *conjunctival and corneal discoloration,* dryness, burning, itching, irritation. **GI:** *abdominal/epigastric pain* (dose-related), *nausea, vomiting, diarrhea,* bowel obstruction, hepatitis, jaundice, enlarged liver. **Skin:** *pink-brown skin discoloration, ichthyosis, dryness,* rash, pruritus, phototoxicity. **Other:** hypokalemia; elevated albumin, serum bilirubin, and AST; eosinophilia; erythema nodosum leprosum (lepra) reaction.

Common side effects in *italic*; life-threatening effects underlined; generic names in **bold**; classifications in SMALL CAPS

DRUG INTERACTIONS Isoniazid may decrease clofazimine concentrations in skin. **Food-drug interactions:** food will increase absorption.

NURSING IMPLICATIONS

Administration

- Drug should be taken with meals or milk to reduce gastric irritation.
- Doses of more than 100 mg/d are given for as short a period of time as possible and should be administered under close medical supervision.
- Store capsules at 15–30C (59–86F); protect from moisture.

Assessment & Drug Effects

- Clofazimine is well tolerated in dosages no greater than 100 mg/d. Most adverse effects are dose related and reversible with discontinuation of drug.
- Abnormal crystalline deposits may result and cause serious side effects (e.g., pain in bones and joints, GI bleeding, diminished vision). Reactions are usually reversible but may require months or years to diminish.
- Severe abdominal symptoms (including splenic infarction, bowel obstruction, and GI bleeding) have occurred (although rarely), requiring explorative laparotomies. Deaths have been reported.
- Drug-induced reddish-brown discoloration of skin, cornea, conjunctiva, and body fluids (including tears, sweat, sputum, urine, and feces) occur in 75–90% of patients within a few weeks of treatment. Skin discoloration may take months or years to disappear after drug is discontinued.
- The onset of tender, erythematous nodules with lymphadenopathy, joint swelling, epistaxis, iritis suggests a type 2 leprosy reactional state. Dosage may be increased to 200 mg/d. After reactive episode is controlled, dosage is tapered to 100 mg/d as soon as possible. Patient should remain under medical surveillance during the episode.

Patient & Family Education

- Caution patient to adhere strictly to established drug regimen. No drug dosage should be omitted, increased, or decreased without advice of physician.
- Advise patient to report promptly bone and joint pain; GI bleeding, colicky abdominal pain, nausea, vomiting, diarrhea; diminished vision.
- Skin dryness and ichthyosis (thickening and scaling of skin) may respond well to hydration and lubrication measures. Advise patient to minimize use of

soap, avoid applying it directly to dry skin, and to thoroughly rinse it off.
- When dizziness, drowsiness, or visual impairment side effects are experienced, patient should not drive or work with hazardous equipment. These symptoms are generally dose related. Discuss with physician.

Prototype: lovastatin, p 143

CLOFIBRATE

(kloe-fry´brate)
Trade names: Atromid-S, Claripex, Novofibrate
Classifications: CARDIOVASCULAR DRUG; ANTILIPEMIC; LIPID-LOWERING AGENT
Pregnancy: Category C

ACTIONS/PHARMACODYNAMICS Structurally related to gemfibrozil. Reduces very low density lipoproteins (VLDL) to a greater extent than it reduces low density lipoproteins (LDL). Mechanism of action is unclear; it appears to inhibit cholesterol biosynthesis prior to mevalonate formation and transfer of triglycerides from liver to serum. Interferes with binding of free fatty acids to albumin and increases fecal excretion of neutral sterols. Its ability to cause regression of xanthomatous lesions is thought to be due to mobilization of cholesterol from tissue. Reduces platelet adhesiveness and increases release of ADH from posterior pituitary. Studies suggest that incidence of hepatic cancer may increase in patients on high doses of clofibrate. Effects of drug-induced lowering of serum cholesterol and other lipids on morbidity and mortality due to atherosclerosis or coronary heart disease have not been determined. The risk of cholelithiasis and cholecystitis requiring surgery is reportedly double that for nonusers.

USES Adjunct for treatment of severe primary (type III) hyperlipidemia. **Unlabeled use:** management of diabetes insipidus.

ROUTE & DOSAGE

Hyperlipidemia

Adult	PO	2 g/d in 2–4 divided doses

Diabetes Insipidus

Adult	PO	1.5–2 g/d in 2–4 divided doses

Common side effects in *italic*; life-threatening effects underlined; generic names in **bold**; classifications in SMALL CAPS

PHARMACOKINETICS Absorption: readily absorbed from GI tract. **Peak:** 4–6 h. **Distribution:** distributed to extracellular space; crosses placenta; distribution into breast milk unknown. **Metabolism:** hydrolyzed in plasma to clofibric acid, which is further metabolized in liver. **Elimination:** half-life 10–35 h; excreted in urine.

CONTRAINDICATIONS & PRECAUTIONS Contraindicated in: impaired renal or hepatic function, primary biliary cirrhosis. Safe use during pregnancy (category C), in nursing mothers, and in children <14 y not established. **Cautious use in:** history of jaundice or hepatic disease; gallstones; peptic ulcer; hypothyroidism; cardiovascular disease.

ADVERSE/SIDE EFFECTS CNS: drowsiness, dizziness, headache. **CV:** increase or decrease in angina, CHF, arrhythmias. **GI:** *nausea,* vomiting, loose stools, diarrhea, flatulence, abdominal distress, gastritis, stomatitis, cholelithiasis. **GU:** renal insufficiency. **Gynecologic:** impotence, decreased libido. **Hematologic:** neutropenia, leukopenia, anemia, eosinophilia, <u>agranulocytosis</u>, potentiation of anticoagulant effect. **Musculoskeletal:** flulike symptoms. **Skin:** swelling and phlebitis at xanthoma sites, skin rash, allergy, urticaria, pruritus. **Other:** tremor, diaphoresis, SLE syndrome, rheumatoid arthritis, thrombocytopenic purpura, gynecomastia, malignancy, blurred vision.

DIAGNOSTIC TEST INTERFERENCES Clofibrate therapy may lead to increased *BSP* retention, *thymol* turbidity; increased *serum creatine phosphokinase (CPK); proteinuria,* parodoxical increase in *LDL* or *cholesterol* levels (if there is a large decrease in VLDL level). Lower fasting *blood glucose* and *serum insulin* levels in patients with diabetes mellitus.

DRUG INTERACTIONS ORAL ANTICOAGULANTS increase hypoprothrombinemia and increase risk of bleeding; **probenecid** increases effects of clofibrate; SULFONYLUREAS increase hypoglycemic effects.

NURSING IMPLICATIONS

Administration

- If gastric distress is a problem, administer drug with meals.
- Preserve in closed, light-resistant containers at 15–30C (59–86F) unless otherwise directed.

Assessment & Drug Effects

- Serum LDL and VLDL levels should be determined initially and evaluated every 2 wk during first few months of therapy, and then at monthly intervals. If tests show a steady rise or are otherwise abnormal, clofibrate should be withdrawn.
- Frequent serum transaminase and other liver tests are advocated, as well as periodic CBC, renal function tests, and determinations of plasma and urine steroid levels, serum electrolyte levels, and blood sugar.
- Therapeutic response generally occurs during the first or second month of therapy. Rebound may occur in second or third month, followed by a further decrease, and may also occur with sudden withdrawal of drug.
- Clofibrate therapy for increased serum cholesterol and triglycerides is generally withdrawn after 3 mo if the response is not adequate.

Patient & Family Education

- Flulike symptoms (malaise, muscle soreness, aching, weakness) should be reported promptly to the physician. Other reportable conditions include leukopenia, pulmonary edema, and renal insufficiency (see Signs & Symptoms, chap 3) and gastric pain, nausea, and vomiting.
- Women of childbearing years should be on birth control regimen. If pregnancy is desired, clofibrate therapy should be discontinued at least 2 mo before conception.
- Advise patient to adhere to drug regimen as established and not to stop taking the drug without consulting the physician.
- Caution patient about self-dosing with OTC drugs without the approval of the physician.

CLOMIPHENE CITRATE

(kloe'mi-feen)
Trade names: Clomid, Milophene, Serophene
Classifications: OVULATION STIMULANT;
ANTIESTROGENIC
Pregnancy: Category X

ACTIONS/PHARMACODYNAMICS Oral nonsteroidal estrogen agonist or antagonist. Induces ovulation in selected anovulatory women. Lacks androgenic, antiandrogenic, or progestational effects and does not appear to effect pituitary-adrenal or pituitary-thyroid functions. May act by binding to hypothalamic estrogen receptors, decreasing their num-

Common side effects in *italic*; life-threatening effects <u>underlined</u>; generic names in **bold**; classifications in SMALL CAPS

453

bers, and by inhibiting receptor replenishment. Resulting false hypoestrogenic state stimulates pituitary release of luteinizing hormone (LH), follicle stimulating hormone (FSH), and gonadotropins, leading to ovarian stimulation (maturation of ovarian follicle, ovulation, and development and function of the corpus luteum). Ineffective in presence of panhypopituitarism, endometrial carcinoma, ovarian failure, thyroid or adrenal disease, azoospermia in the partner. Normal ovulatory function does not usually resume after treatment or after pregnancy.

USES Infertility in appropriately selected women desiring pregnancy whose partners are fertile and potent. **Unlabeled use:** male infertility, menstrual abnormalities, gynecomastia, fibrocystic breast disease, regulation of cycles in patients using rhythm method of contraception, endometrial hyperplasia, persistent lactation.

ROUTE & DOSAGE

Infertility

Adult	PO	First course: 50 mg/d for 5 d; start on 5th day of cycle following start of spontaneous or induced bleeding (with progestin) or at any time in the patient who has had no recent uterine bleeding
		Second course if ovulation: repeat first course until conception or for 3 cycles
		Second course if no ovulation: 100 mg/d for 5 d as above (max 100 mg/d)

PHARMACOKINETICS Absorption: readily absorbed from GI tract. **Metabolism:** metabolized in liver. **Elimination:** half-life: 5 d; excreted primarily in feces in 5 d; the remainder is excreted slowly from enterohepatic pool or is stored in body fat for later release.

CONTRAINDICATIONS & PRECAUTIONS Contraindicated in: pregnancy (category X); neoplastic lesions, ovarian cyst; hepatic disease or dysfunction; abnormal bleeding; visual abnormalities; mental depression; thrombophlebitis. **Cautious use in:** polycystic ovarian enlargement, pelvic discomfort, sensitivity to pituitary gonadotropins.

ADVERSE/SIDE EFFECTS Dose related. **GI:** nausea, vomiting, increased appetite with weight gain, constipation, bloating. **GU:** urinary frequency, polyuria. **Eye (reversible and of short duration):** transient blurring, diplopia, scotomas, photophobia, floaters, prolonged after-images. **Reproductive:** spontaneous abortion, multiple ovulations, ovarian failure.

Ovarian hyperstimulation syndrome; enlarged ovaries with multiple follicular cysts. **Other:** *vasomotor flushes,* breast discomfort, abdominal pain, heavy menses, exacerbation of endometriosis; mental depression, headache, fatigue, insomnia, dizziness, vertigo.

DIAGNOSTIC TEST INTERFERENCES Clomiphene may increase BSP retention; *plasma transcortin, thyroxine* and *sex hormone binding globulin* levels. Also increases *follicle-stimulating* and *luteinizing hormone* secretion in most patients.

NURSING IMPLICATIONS

Administration

- Pretreatment with estrogen is indicated for the patient who has been hypoestrogenic for a long time. Estrogen therapy is stopped immediately before clomiphene therapy begins.
- Each course of therapy should start on or about the 5th cycle day once ovulation has been established.
- Store at 15–30C (59–86F) in tightly capped, light-resistant container.

Assessment & Drug Effects

- If abnormal bleeding occurs, full diagnostic measures are crucial. Report it immediately.
- If patient needs to wear dark glasses even inside or if she has blurred or decreased vision or scotomas (signs of ocular toxicity), she should promptly report for a complete ophthalmologic evaluation. Drug will be stopped until symptoms subside.
- If clomiphene is continued more than 1 y, patient should have an ophthalmologic examination at regular intervals.
- Pelvic pain indicates the need for immediate pelvic examination for diagnostic purposes.

Patient & Family Education

- Advise patient to take the medicine at same time every day to maintain drug levels and prevent forgetting a dose.
- Missed dose: instruct patient to take drug as soon as possible. If not remembered until time for next dose, double the dose, then resume regular dosing schedule. If more than one dose is missed, patient should check with physician.
- Incidence of multiple births during clomiphene use is reportedly increased to 6 times normal and appears to increase with dose increases. Multiple births other than twins are rare.

Common side effects in *italic*; life-threatening effects underlined; generic names in **bold**; classifications in SMALL CAPS

- Patient who is going to respond usually ovulates 4–10 d after last day of treatment.
- The likelihood of conception diminishes with each succeeding course of therapy. If pregnancy is not achieved after 3 ovulatory responses, further treatment with clomiphene is not recommended.
- Usually, the couple is told to attempt conception 2 d before ovulation and to have intercourse every other day starting within 48 h after ovulation.
- Symptoms that should be reported: hot flushes resembling those associated with menopause; nausea, vomiting, headache. Appropriate drug therapy may be prescribed. Symptoms disappear after clomiphene is discontinued.
- Yellowing of eyes, light-colored stools, yellow, itchy skin, and fever symptomatic of jaundice should be reported promptly.
- Instruct patient to stop taking clomiphene if she suspects pregnancy and to contact physician for a confirmatory examination.
- Because of the possibility of light-headedness, dizziness, and visual disturbances, caution the patient against performing hazardous tasks requiring skill and coordination in an environment with variable lighting.
- Warn patient to report promptly excessive weight gain, signs of edema, bloating, decreased urinary output.

Prototype: diazepam, p 170

CLONAZEPAM

(kloe-na´zi-pam)
Trade names: Klonopin, Rivotril
Classifications: CENTRAL NERVOUS SYSTEM AGENT; ANTICONVULSANT; BENZODIAZEPINE
Pregnancy: Category C
Controlled substance: Schedule IV

ACTIONS/PHARMACODYNAMICS Benzodiazepine derivative with strong anticonvulsant activity and several other pharmacologic properties characteristic of the drug class. Suppresses spike and wave discharge in absence seizures (petit mal) and decreases amplitude, frequency, duration, and spread of discharge in minor motor seizures.

USES Alone or with other drugs in absence, myoclonic, and akinetic seizures, Lennox-Gastaut syndrome, absence seizures refractory to succinimides or valproic acid, and for infantile spasms and restless legs. **Unlabeled uses:** complex partial seizure pattern and generalized tonic-clonic convulsions.

ROUTE & DOSAGE

Seizures

Adult	PO	1.5 mg/d in 3 divided doses, increased by 0.5–1 mg q3d until seizures are controlled or until intolerable side effects (max recommended dose 20 mg/d)
Child	PO	<10 y: 0.01–0.03 mg/kg/d (not to exceed 0.05 mg/kg/d) in 3 divided doses; may increase by 0.25–0.5 mg q3d until seizures are controlled or until intolerable side effects (max recommended dose 0.2 mg/kg/d)

PHARMACOKINETICS Absorption: readily absorbed from GI tract. **Onset:** 60 min. **Peak:** 1–2 h. **Duration:** up to 12 h in adults; 6–8 h in children. **Distribution:** crosses placenta; distributed into breast milk. **Metabolism:** metabolized in liver. **Elimination:** half-life: 18–40 h; excreted in urine primarily as metabolites.

CONTRAINDICATIONS & PRECAUTIONS Contraindicated in: hypersensitivity to benzodiazepines; liver disease; acute narrow-angle glaucoma; breast feeding. Safe use in pregnancy (category C) not established. **Cautious use in:** renal disease; COPD; drug-controlled open-angle glaucoma; addiction-prone individuals; children (because of unknown consequences of long-term use on growth and development); patient with mixed seizure disorders.

ADVERSE/SIDE EFFECTS CNS: *drowsiness, sedation, ataxia,* insomnia, aphonia, choreiform movements, <u>coma</u>, dysarthria, "glassy-eyed" appearance, headache, hemiparesis, hypotonia, slurred speech, tremor, vertigo. **CV:** palpitations, bradycardia. **Eye:** diplopia, nystagmus, abnormal eye movements. **GI:** dry mouth, sore gums, anorexia, coated tongue, increased salivation, increased appetite, nausea, constipation, diarrhea. **GU:** increased libido, dysuria, enuresis, nocturia, urinary retention. **Hematologic:** anemia, leukopenia, thrombocytopenia, eosinophilia. **Psychiatric:** confusion, depression, hallucinations, aggressive behavior problems, hysteria, suicide attempt. **Respiratory:** chest congestion, <u>respiratory depression</u>, rhinorrhea, dyspnea, hypersecretion in upper respiratory passages. **Skin:** hirsutism, hair loss, skin rash, ankle and facial edema.

Common side effects in *italic*; life-threatening effects <u>underlined</u>; generic names in **bold**; classifications in SMALL CAPS

DIAGNOSTIC TEST INTERFERENCES Clonazepam causes transient elevations of *serum transaminase* and *alkaline phosphatase.*

DRUG INTERACTIONS Alcohol and other CNS DEPRESSANTS increase sedation and CNS depression; may increase **phenytoin** levels.

NURSING IMPLICATIONS

Administration

- If a new anticonvulsant is to be substituted, it is usually added to the drug regimen as the former medication is gradually withdrawn. Slow tapering of dose over several days' time is imperative. Abrupt withdrawal in patient on high doses or long-term therapy can precipitate status epilepticus. Other withdrawal symptoms include convulsion, tremor, abdominal and muscle cramps, vomiting, sweating.
- Store in tightly closed container protected from light at 15–30C (59–86F) unless otherwise specified.

Assessment & Drug Effects

- Monitor I&O ratio and other indicators of renal function. Excess accumulation of metabolites because of impaired excretion leads to toxicity.
- If multiple anticonvulsants are being given, watch patient carefully for signs of overdosage or drug interaction, i.e., increased depressant adverse effects.
- Liver function tests, platelet counts, blood counts, and clinical evaluation of drug efficacy should be a part of the follow-up care of the patient on clonazepam.
- Both psychological and physical dependence may occur in the patient on long-term, high-dose therapy. Watch patient to see that he or she does not cheek the tablet. Limit availability of large amounts of drug in the addiction-prone individual.
- *Overdose:* somnolence, confusion, irritability, sweating, muscle and abdominal cramps, diminished reflexes, coma.

Patient & Family Education

- Anticonvulsant activity is often lost after 3 mo of therapy; dosage adjustment may reestablish efficacy. Patient should be aware of necessity to report loss of seizure control promptly.
- Counsel patient to take drug as prescribed and not to alter dosing regimen or stop medication without consulting physician.
- Caution patient not to self-medicate with OTC drugs before consulting the physician.

- Advise patient not to drive a car or engage in other activities requiring mental alertness and physical coordination until reaction to the drug is known. Drowsiness occurs in approximately 50% of patients.
- Patient should carry identification (e.g., Medic Alert) bearing information about medication in use and the diagnosis.

Prototype: methyldopa, p 148

CLONIDINE HYDROCHLORIDE
(kloe´ni-deen)

Trade names: Catapres, Catapres-TTS
Classifications: CARDIOVASCULAR AGENT; CENTRAL ACTING ANTIHYPERTENSIVE
Pregnancy: Category C

ACTIONS/PHARMACODYNAMICS Centrally acting antiadrenergic imidazoline derivative chemically related to tolazoline. Stimulates α_2-adrenergic receptors in CNS to inhibit sympathetic vasomotor centers. Central actions reduce plasma concentrations of norepinephrine and decrease systolic and diastolic BP and heart rate. Orthostatic effects tend to be mild and occur infrequently. Initial dose is followed by enhanced tubular reabsorption of sodium and chloride; after 3 to 4 d, sodium retention is reversed and natriuresis occurs. Also inhibits renin release from kidneys. Reportedly minimizes or eliminates many of the common clinical signs and symptoms associated with withdrawal of heroin, methadone, or other opiates. This action is believed to be related to stimulation of inhibitory receptors in locus coeruleus, a major noradrenergic nucleus in brain.

USES Step 2 drug in stepped care approach to treatment of hypertension, either alone or with diuretic or other antihypertensive agents. **Unlabeled uses:** prophylaxis for migraine, treatment of dysmenorrhea, menopausal flushing, diarrhea, paroxysmal localized hyperhidroses; alcohol, smoking, opiate, and benzodiazepine withdrawal, in the clonidine suppression test for diagnosis of pheochromocytoma and for treatment of Gilles de la Tourette syndrome.

PHARMACOKINETICS Absorption: readily absorbed from GI tract. **Onset:** 30–60 min PO; 1–3 d transdermal. **Peak:** 2–4 h PO; 2–3 d transdermal.

Duration: 8 h PO; 7 d transdermal. **Distribution:** widely distributed; crosses blood-brain barrier; not known if crosses placenta or distributed into breast milk. **Metabolism:** metabolized in liver. **Elimination:** half-life: 6–20 h; 80% excreted in urine, 20% in feces.

ROUTE & DOSAGE

Hypertension

Adult	PO	0.1 mg b.i.d. or t.i.d.; may increase by 0.1–0.2 mg/d until desired response is achieved (max 2.4 mg/d)
	Transdermal	0.1 mg patch once q7d; may increase by 0.1 mg q1–2wk

CONTRAINDICATIONS & PRECAUTIONS Contraindicated in: safe use during pregnancy (category C), in nursing women, and in children not established. Use of clonidine patch in polyarteritis nodosa, scleroderma, SLE. **Cautious use in:** severe coronary insufficiency, recent MI, sinus node dysfunction, cerebrovascular disease; chronic renal failure; Raynaud's disease, thromboangiitis obliterans; history of mental depression.

ADVERSE/SIDE EFFECTS CNS: *drowsiness, sedation,* dizziness, headache, fatigue, weakness, sluggishness, dyspnea, vivid dreams, nightmares, insomnia, behavior changes, agitation, hallucination, nervousness, restlessness, anxiety, mental depression. **CV:** postural hypotension (mild), peripheral edema, ECG changes, bradycardia, tachycardia, irregular heartbeat, palpitation, flushes, rapid increase in BP with abrupt withdrawal. **Eye:** dry eyes. **GI/Metabolic:** *dry mouth, constipation,* abdominal pain, pseudo-obstruction of large bowel, altered taste, parotitis, nausea, vomiting, hepatitis, hyperbilirubinemia, weight gain (sodium retention). **GU:** impotence, loss of libido. **Skin:** rash, pruritus, thinning of hair, exacerbation of psoriasis; with transdermal patch: hyperpigmentation, recurrent herpes simplex, skin irritation, contact dermatitis, mild erythema.

DIAGNOSTIC TEST INTERFERENCES Possibility of decreased urinary excretion of *aldosterone, catecholamines,* and *VMA* (however, sudden withdrawal of clonidine may cause increases in these values); transient increases in blood glucose; weakly positive direct antiglobulin (Coombs') tests.

DRUG INTERACTIONS Alcohol and other CNS DEPRESSANTS add to CNS depression; TRICYCLIC ANTIDEPRESSANTS may reduce antihypertensive effects.

NURSING IMPLICATIONS

Administration

▪ Last PO dose is commonly administered immediately before patient retires to ensure overnight BP control and to minimize daytime drowsiness.

▪ Dosage is increased gradually over a period of weeks so as not to lower BP abruptly (especially important in the elderly). Follow-up visits should be scheduled every 2–4 wk until BP stabilizes, then every 2–4 mo.

▪ Apply transdermal patch to dry skin, free of hair and rash. Avoid irritated, abraded, or scarred skin.

▪ Recommended areas for applying transdermal patch: upper outer arm, anterior chest. Less drug is absorbed from thighs. Rotate application sites and keep a record.

▪ During change from PO clonidine to transdermal system, PO clonidine should be maintained for at least 24 h after patch is applied. If patient is taking high PO doses, PO dosage may have to be tapered over several days. Directions should be written out and reviewed with patient so there is no misunderstanding.

▪ If drug is to be discontinued, it is withdrawn over a period of 2–4 d. Abrupt withdrawal resembles sympathetic stimulation and may result in restlessness and headache 2–3 h after a missed dose and a hypertensive crisis within 8–18 h.

▪ Store in tightly closed container at 15–30C (59–86F) unless otherwise directed.

Assessment & Drug Effects

▪ Discuss with physician schedule for BP determinations: when to take readings, how often to take readings; position of patient (supine, sitting, standing; after exercise).

▪ BP should be closely monitored whenever a drug is added to or withdrawn from therapeutic regimen.

▪ Tolerance sometimes develops in some patients. Physician may increase dosage or prescribe concomitant administration of a diuretic to enhance antihypertensive response.

▪ Monitor I&O during period of dosage adjustment. Report change in I&O ratio or change in voiding pattern.

▪ Determine weight daily. Patients not receiving a concomitant diuretic agent may gain weight, particularly during first 3 or 4 d of therapy, because of marked sodium and water retention.

Common side effects in *italic*; life-threatening effects underlined; generic names in **bold**; classifications in SMALL CAPS

457

- Patients with history of mental depression require close supervision, as they may be subject to further depressive episodes.

Patient & Family Education
- Although postural hypotension occurs infrequently, advise patient to make position changes slowly, and in stages, particularly from recumbent to upright position, and to dangle and move legs a few minutes before standing. Caution patient to lie down immediately if faintness or dizziness occurs.
- Inform patient of the possible sedative effect and caution against potentially hazardous activities until reaction to drug has been determined.
- Warn patient of the danger of omitting doses or of stopping the drug without consulting the physician.
- Advise patient to carry Medic Alert or other appropriate medical identification card.
- Caution patient not to take OTC medications, alcohol, or other CNS depressants without prior discussion with physician.
- Instruct patient to examine site when transdermal patch is removed and to report to physician if erythema, rash, irritation, or hyperpigmentation occurs.
- Advise patient that if transdermal patch loosens, it can be taped in place with adhesive. The patch should never be cut or trimmed.

Prototype: lorazepam, p 177

CLORAZEPATE DIPOTASSIUM
(klor-az´e-pate)
Trade names: Tranxene, Tranxene-SD
Classifications: CENTRAL NERVOUS SYSTEM AGENT; BENZODIAZEPINE; ANXIOLYTIC, SEDATIVE-HYPNOTIC; ANTICONVULSANT
Pregnancy: Category C
Controlled substance: Schedule IV

ACTIONS/PHARMACODYNAMICS Anxiolytic with actions, uses, and interactions qualitatively similar to those of lorazepam but with fewer unwanted side effects, e.g., sedation.

USES Management of anxiety disorders, short-term relief of anxiety symptoms, as adjunct in management of partial seizures, and symptomatic relief of acute alcohol withdrawal.

ROUTE & DOSAGE

Anxiety

Adult	PO	15 mg/d h.s.; may increase to 15–60 mg/d in divided doses (max 60 mg/d)

Acute Alcohol Withdrawal

Adult	PO	30 mg followed by 30–60 mg in divided doses (max 90 mg/d); taper by 15 mg/d over 4 d to 7.5–15 mg/d until patient is stable

Partial Seizures

Adult	PO	7.5 mg t.i.d.
Child	PO	9–12 y: 7.5 mg b.i.d.; may increase by no more than 7.5 mg/wk (max 60 mg/d)

PHARMACOKINETICS Absorption: decarboxylated in stomach; absorbed as active metabolite, desmethyldiazepam. **Peak:** 1 h. **Duration:** 24 h. **Distribution:** crosses placenta; distributed into breast milk. **Metabolism:** metabolized in liver to oxazepam. **Elimination:** half-life: 30–200 h; excreted primarily in urine.

CONTRAINDICATIONS & PRECAUTIONS Contraindicated in: hypersensitivity to clorazepate and other benzodiazepines; patients <9 y; acute narrow-angle glaucoma; depressive neuroses, psychotic reactions, drug abusers. Safe use during pregnancy (category C), in nursing mothers, and in children <9 y not established. **Cautious use in:** elderly, debilitated patients; hepatic disease; kidney disease.

ADVERSE/SIDE EFFECTS *Drowsiness,* ataxia, GI disturbances, xerostomia, diplopia, blurred vision, dizziness, headache, paradoxical excitement, mental confusion, insomnia, hypotension; abnormal liver and kidney function tests, decreased Hct, blood dyscrasias; allergic reactions.

DRUG INTERACTIONS Alcohol and other CNS DEPRESSANTS compound CNS depression; clorazepate increases effects of **cimetidine, disulfiram,** causing excessive sedation.

NURSING IMPLICATIONS

Administration
- Antacids delay absorption of drug. If patient has gastric distress, advise taking drug with food or

---

Common side effects in *italic*; life-threatening effects <u>underlined</u>; generic names in **bold**; classifications in SMALL CAPS

milk. If necessary to use an antacid (with approval), it should be taken no less than 1 h before or 1 h after drug ingestion.

■ Drug dose should be tapered gradually over several day's time when regimen is to be discontinued. Abrupt termination may lead to memory impairment, severe GI symptoms, muscle pain, restlessness, irritability, fatigue, insomnia.

■ Store in light-resistant container at 15–30C (59–86F) unless otherwise specified.

Assessment & Drug Effects

■ Effectiveness of clorazepate for long-term use (more than 4 mo) has not been determined. Usefulness of drug should be periodically reassessed.

■ Drowsiness, a common side effect, is more likely to occur at initiation of therapy and with dose increments on successive days.

■ Periodic blood counts and tests of liver and kidney function should be performed throughout therapy.

■ Patient with history of or actual cardiovascular disease should be monitored in early therapy for drug-induced responses. If systolic BP drops more than 20 mm Hg or if there is a sudden increase in pulse rate, withhold drug and notify physician.

Patient & Family Education

■ Counsel patient to take drug as prescribed and not to change dose or abruptly stop taking the drug without physician's approval.

■ Caution patient not to self-dose with OTC drugs (cold remedies, sleep medications, antacids) without consulting physician.

■ Caution patient to avoid driving and other potentially hazardous activities until reaction to drug is known.

■ Warn patient not to use alcohol and other CNS depressants while on clorazepate therapy.

■ Patient should be advised that if she becomes pregnant during therapy or intends to become pregnant, she should communicate with her physician about the desirability of discontinuing the drug.

■ Alert responsible family member(s) to report signs of possible drug abuse and dependency to physician: nervousness, insomnia, memory impairment, diarrhea.

Prototype: amphotericin B, p 56

CLOTRIMAZOLE

(kloe-trim´a-zole)
Trade names: Gyne-Lotrimin, Lotrimin, Mycelex, Mycelex-G
Classifications: ANTIINFECTIVE; ANTIBIOTIC; ANTIFUNGAL
Pregnancy: Category B (topical); category C (oral)

ACTIONS/PHARMACODYNAMICS Has broad spectrum fungicidal activity. Acts by altering fungal cell membrane permeability, permitting loss of phosphorous compounds, potassium, and other essential intracellular constituents with consequent loss of ability to replicate. Active against *Trichophyton rubrum, Trichophyton mentagrophytes, Epidermophyton floccosum, Microsporum canis, Malassezia furfur,* and *Candida* sp, including *Candida albicans.* Natural or acquired fungal resistance to clotrimazole is rare.

USES Dermal infections including tinea pedis, tinea cruris, tinea corporis, tinea versicolor; also vulvovaginal and oropharyngeal candidiasis. **Unlabeled use:** trichomoniasis.

ROUTE & DOSAGE

Dermal Infections

Adult	Topical	Apply small amount onto affected areas b.i.d. AM and PM

Vulvovaginal Infections

Adult	Topical	Insert 1 applicatorful or one 100 mg vaginal tablet into vagina at bedtime for 7 d, *or* one 500 mg vaginal tablet at bedtime for 1 dose

Oropharyngeal Candidiasis

Adult	PO	1 troche (lozenge) 5 times/d q3h for 14 d

PHARMACOKINETICS Absorption: minimal systemic absorption; minimally absorbed topically. **Peak:** high saliva concentrations <3h; high vaginal concentrations in 8–24 h. **Metabolism:** metabolized in liver. **Elimination:** eliminated as metabolite in bile.

CONTRAINDICATIONS & PRECAUTIONS Contraindicated in: ophthalmic uses; systemic mycoses.

Common side effects in *italic*; life-threatening effects underlined; generic names in **bold**; classifications in SMALL CAPS

459

Safe use during pregnancy (category C for oral troches, category B for topical preparations), in nursing mothers, and in children <3 y not established. **Cautious use in:** hepatic impairment.

ADVERSE/SIDE EFFECTS Skin preparations: stinging, erythema, edema, vesication, desquamation, pruritus, urticaria, skin fissures. **Vaginal preparations:** mild burning sensation, lower abdominal cramps, bloating, cystitis, urethritis, mild urinary frequency, vulval erythema and itching, pain and vaginal soreness during intercourse. **Other:** abnormal liver function tests; occasional nausea and vomiting (with oral troche).

NURSING IMPLICATIONS

Administration

- Instruct patient taking the oral lozenge to allow it to dissolve slowly in mouth over 15–30 min for maximum effectiveness.
- Vaginal preparations are effective only for candidiasis.
- Skin cream and solution preparations should be applied sparingly. Protect hands with latex gloves when applying medication.
- Avoid contact of clotrimazole preparations with the eyes.
- Occlusive dressings should not be applied unless otherwise directed by physician.
- Consult physician about skin cleansing procedure before applying medication. Regardless of procedure used, dry skin thoroughly.
- Store cream and solution formulations at 15–30C (59–86F); do not store troches or vaginal tablets above 35 (95F) unless otherwise directed.

Assessment & Drug Effects

- Evaluate effectiveness of treatment. Report any signs of skin irritation with dermal preparations.
- Anticipate signs of clinical improvement within the first week of drug use.

Patient & Family Education

- Advise patient to use clotrimazole as directed and for the length of time prescribed by physician.
- Generally, clinical improvement is apparent during first week of therapy. Advise patient to report to physician if condition worsens or if signs of irritation or sensitivity develop, or if no improvement is noted after 4 wk of therapy.
- Inform patient receiving the drug vaginally that sexual partner may experience burning and irritation of penis or urethritis and advise refraining

from sexual intercourse during therapy or that sexual partner wear a condom.

Prototype: penicillin G, p 71

CLOXACILLIN, SODIUM
(klox-a-sill´in)

Trade names: Cloxapen, Cloxilean, Tegopen
Classifications: ANTIINFECTIVE; ANTIBIOTIC, NATURAL PENICILLIN; BETA-LACTAM
Pregnancy: Category B

ACTIONS/PHARMACODYNAMICS Semisynthetic, acid-stable, penicillinase-resistant, isoxazolyl penicillin. Mechanism of bactericidal action, contraindications, precautions, and adverse reactions as for penicillin G. In common with other isoxazolyl penicillins (dicloxacillin, oxacillin), highly active against most penicillinase-producing staphylococci, less potent than penicillin G against penicillin-sensitive microorganisms, and generally ineffective against gram-negative bacteria and methicillin-resistant staphylococci.

USES Primarily in infections caused by penicillinase-producing staphylococci and penicillin-resistant staphylococci. May be used to initiate therapy in suspected staphylococcal infections pending culture and susceptibility test results. As with other penicillins, serum concentrations are enhanced by concurrent use of probenecid.

ROUTE & DOSAGE

Mild to Moderate Infections

Adult	PO	250–500 mg q6h
Child	PO	<20 kg: 12.5–25 mg/kg q6h (max 4 g/d)

PHARMACOKINETICS Absorption: 37–60% absorbed from GI tract. **Peak:** 0.5–2 h. **Duration:** 4–6 h. **Distribution:** distributed throughout body with highest concentrations in liver, kidney, spleen, bone, bile, and pleural fluid; low CSF penetration; crosses placenta; distributed into breast milk. **Metabolism:** metabolized in liver. **Elimination:** half-life: 30–60 min; excreted primarily in urine with some elimination through bile.

CONTRAINDICATIONS & PRECAUTIONS Contraindicated in: sensitivity to penicillins. Safe use during pregnancy (category B), in nursing mothers, and in neonates not established. **Cautious use in:** history of or suspected atopy or allergy (asthma, eczema, hives, hay fever), renal or hepatic function impairment, history of allergy to cephalosporins.

ADVERSE/SIDE EFFECTS GI: *nausea,* vomiting, flatulence, *diarrhea.* **Hematologic:** eosinophilia, leukopenia, agranulocytosis. **Hypersensitivity:** pruritus, urticaria, rash, wheezing, sneezing, chills, drug fever, anaphylaxis. **Other:** elevated AST, ALT; jaundice (possibly of allergic etiology); superinfections.

DRUG INTERACTIONS Probenecid decreases cloxacillin elimination.

NURSING IMPLICATIONS

Administration

- Best taken on an empty stomach (at least 1 h before or 2 h after meals) unless otherwise advised by physician. Food reduces rate and extent of drug absorption.
- After reconstitution (by pharmacist), PO solution retains potency for 14 d if refrigerated (container should be so labeled and dated). Shake well before pouring.
- Unless otherwise advised, store capsules at 15–30C (59–86F).

Assessment & Drug Effects

- Before treatment is initiated, determine previous exposure and sensitivity to penicillins and cephalosporins and other allergic reactions of any kind.
- As with other penicillins, monitor for signs and symptoms of anaphylactoid reaction (see chap 3) or other signs or symptoms of hypersensitivity reaction (see chap 3).
- Periodic assessments of renal, hepatic, and hematopoietic function are advised in patients on long-term therapy.

Patient & Family Education

- Instruct patient to take medication around the clock, not to miss a dose, and to continue taking the medication until it is all gone, unless otherwise directed by physician.
- Inform patient to report to physician the onset of hypersensitivity reaction (see Signs & Symptoms, chap 3) and superinfections.
- Advise patient to check with physician if GI side effects (nausea, vomiting, diarrhea) appear.

CLOZAPINE

(clo´za-pin)
Trade names: Clozaril, Leponex
Classifications: ANTIPSYCHOTIC; NEUROLEPTIC AGENT
Pregnancy: Category B

ACTIONS/PHARMACODYNAMICS Mechanism is not defined. Interferes with binding of dopamine to D_1 and D_2 receptors in the limbic region of brain. It binds primarily to nondopaminergic sites (e.g., alpha-adrenergic, serotonergic, and cholinergic receptors).

USES Indicated only in the management of severely ill schizophrenic patients who have failed to respond to other neuroleptic agents.

ROUTE & DOSAGE

Schizophrenia

Adult	PO	>16 y: Initiate at 25–50 mg/d and titrate to a target dose of 350–450 mg/d in 3 divided doses at 2 wk intervals; further increases can be made if necessary; max 900 mg/d

PHARMACOKINETICS Absorption: readily absorbed from GI tract. **Onset:** 2–4 wk. **Peak:** 2.5 h. **Distribution:** possibly distributed into breast milk. **Metabolism:** metabolized in liver. **Elimination:** half-life: 8–12 h; 50% excreted in urine, 30% in feces.

CONTRAINDICATIONS & PRECAUTIONS Contraindicated in: severe CNS depression, blood dyscrasia, or history of bone marrow depression. **Cautious use in:** arrhythmias, GI disorders, narrow-angle glaucoma, hepatic and renal impairment, prostatic hypertrophy, and history of seizures

ADVERSE/SIDE EFFECTS CNS: seizures, *transient fever,* sedation. **CV:** orthostatic hypotension, *tachycardia,* ECG changes. **GI:** nausea, dry mouth, constipation, hypersalivation. **Other:** agranulocytosis, urinary retention.

DRUG INTERACTIONS Alcohol and other CNS DEPRESSANTS compound depressant effects; ANTI-

---

CHOLINERGIC AGENTS potentiate anticholinergic effects; ANTIHYPERTENSIVE AGENTS may potentiate hypotension.

NURSING IMPLICATIONS

Administration

- If therapy must be discontinued, the drug is usually withdrawn gradually over 1–2 wk.
- Store the drug away from heat or light.

Assessment & Drug Effects

- Because of risk of agranulocytosis (see Signs & Symptoms, chap 3) a baseline white blood count and differential count must be made before initial treatment, every week throughout treatment, and for 4 wk after the drug is discontinued.
- Monitor for seizure activity; seizure potential increases at the higher dose level.
- If the drug is being discontinued, closely monitor for recurrence of psychotic symptoms.
- Monitor for development of tachycardia or hypotension, which may pose a serious risk for patients with compromised cardiovascular function.
- Monitor daily temperature and report fever. Transient elevation above 38C (100.4F), with peak incidence during first 3 wk of drug therapy, may occur.

Patient & Family Education

- Advise patient not to engage in any hazardous activity until response to the drug is known. Drowsiness and sedation are common side effects.
- Warn patient about the risk of agranulocytosis (see Signs & Symptoms, chap 3). Emphasize importance of complying with blood test regimen. Advise patient to report flulike symptoms, fever, sore throat, lethargy, malaise, or other signs of infection.
- Instruct patient to rise slowly to avoid orthostatic hypotension.
- Instruct patient that drug should be taken exactly as ordered.
- Instruct patient not to use OTC drugs or alcohol without permission of physician.
- Instruct patient to notify physician of pregnancy, as drug is not normally administered during pregnancy.
- Instruct patient not to breast feed while she is taking clozapine.

Prototype: procaine, p 166

COCAINE
(koe-kane´)

COCAINE HYDROCHLORIDE

Classifications: CENTRAL NERVOUS SYSTEM AGENT; ANESTHETIC, LOCAL
Pregnancy: Category C
Controlled substance: Schedule II

ACTIONS/PHARMACODYNAMICS Alkaloid obtained from leaves of *Erythroxylon coca*. Topical application blocks nerve conduction and produces surface anesthesia accompanied by local vasoconstriction. Exerts adrenergic effect by potentiating action of endogenous (and injected) epinephrine and norepinephrine, possibly by inhibiting reuptake of catecholamines into sympathetic nerve terminals. Effective nasal decongestant but rarely used for this purpose because of abuse potential. Systemic absorption produces descending CNS stimulation, with intense, short-lived euphoria accompanied by indifference to pain or hunger and with illusions of great strength, endurance, and mental capacity, all the bases for drug abuse.

USES Surface anesthesia of ear, nose, throat, rectum, and vagina. Ophthalmic use largely abandoned because of its tendency to cause corneal sloughing. Sometimes used as ingredient in Brompton's cocktail.

ROUTE & DOSAGE

Surface Anesthesia

Adult	Topical	1–10% solution (use > 4% solution with caution); max single dose 1 mg/kg

---

PHARMACOKINETICS Absorption: readily absorbed from mucous membranes; absorption limited by vasoconstriction. **Onset:** 1 min. **Peak:** 15–120 min. **Duration:** 30 min–2 h. **Distribution:** crosses placenta; distributed into breast milk. **Metabolism:** hydrolyzed in serum. **Elimination:** half-life: 1–2.5 h; excreted in urine; detectable for up to 30 h.

Common side effects in *italic*; life-threatening effects <u>underlined</u>; generic names in **bold**; classifications in SMALL CAPS

CONTRAINDICATIONS & PRECAUTIONS Contraindicated in: hypersensitivity to local anesthetics; sepsis in region of proposed application. Safe use during pregnancy (category C), and in nursing mothers not established. **Cautious use in:** history of drug sensitivities, history of drug abuse.

ADVERSE/SIDE EFFECTS CNS: *CNS stimulation* and CNS depression (respiratory and circulatory failure). **CV:** tachycardia, ventricular fibrillation, MI, angina pectoris. **ENT:** runny nose, perforated nasal septum. **Eye:** clouding, pitting, and ulceration of cornea. **GI:** nausea, vomiting, anorexia, abdominal pain. **Other:** formication ("cocaine bugs"), hypersensitivity reactions; pneumonia, lung damage (chronic cocaine smoking).

DRUG INTERACTIONS Epinephrine entails risk of severe hypertension and arrhythmias; MAO INHIBITORS potentiate pharmacologic effects of cocaine.

NURSING IMPLICATIONS

Administration

- To discourage illegal use, cocaine solutions for topical application are often tinted with an antiseptic dye such as methylene blue. This dye also inhibits mold growth in the solution.
- Preserve in tightly closed, light-resistant containers.

Assessment & Drug Effects

- When used for anesthesia of throat, cocaine causes temporary paralysis of cilia of respiratory tract cells, reducing protection against aspiration. It also may interfere with pharyngeal stage of swallowing. Give nothing by mouth until sensation returns.
- Monitor cardiovascular status, especially in patients with known cardiac disease. Report promptly cardiac arrhythmias.

Patient & Family Education

- Instruct patients with a known history of cardiac disease to promptly report angina or other distress.

Prototype: morphine, p 156

CODEINE
(koe´deen)
Trade name: Methylmorphine

CODEINE PHOSPHATE
Trade name: Paveral

CODEINE SULFATE

Classifications: CNS AGENT; NARCOTIC (OPIATE) AGONIST ANALGESIC; ANTITUSSIVE
Pregnancy: Category C
Controlled substance: Schedule II

ACTIONS/PHARMACODYNAMICS Opium derivative made by methylation of morphine. Similar to morphine in actions, uses, contraindications, precautions, and adverse reactions. Not as potent as morphine and has shorter duration of action, thus producing less severe adverse reactions. However, in equianalgesic doses parenteral codeine produces degree of respiratory depression similar to that of morphine. In contrast to morphine, orally administered codeine is about 60% as potent as the parenteral form. Histamine-releasing action appears to be more potent than that of morphine and may result in hypotension, flushing, and rarely bronchoconstriction. Analgesic potency is about one-sixth that of morphine; antitussive activity is also a little less than that of morphine. The analgesic effect of oral codeine 65 mg is approximately equivalent to that of aspirin 650 mg. Reportedly not as effective for uterine or dental pain as are prostaglandin inhibitors such as aspirin.

USES Symptomatic relief of mild to moderately severe pain when control cannot be obtained by nonnarcotic analgesics and to suppress hyperactive or nonproductive cough.

PHARMACOKINETICS Absorption: readily absorbed from GI tract. **Onset:** 15–30 min. **Peak:** 1–1.5 h. **Duration:** 4–6 h. **Distribution:** crosses placenta; distributed into breast milk. **Metabolism:** metabolized in liver. **Elimination:** half-life: 2.5–4 h; excreted in urine.

CONTRAINDICATIONS & PRECAUTIONS Contraindicated in: hypersensitivity to codeine or other morphine derivatives; acute asthma, COPD; increased intracranial pressure, head injury, acute alco-

---

Common side effects in *italic*; life-threatening effects underlined; generic names in **bold**; classifications in SMALL CAPS

463

holism, hepatic or renal dysfunction, hypothyroidism. Safe use during pregnancy (category C), in nursing mothers, and in neonates not established. **Cautious use in:** prostatic hypertrophy, debilitated patients, very young and very old patients; history of drug abuse.

ROUTE & DOSAGE

Analgesic

Adult	PO/IM/SC	15–60 mg q.i.d.
Child	PO/IM/SC	3 mg/kg/d in 6 divided doses

Antitussive

Adult	PO	10–20 mg q4–6h prn (max 120 mg/24h)
Child	PO	6–12 y: 5–10 mg q4–6h (max 60 mg/24 h)
		2–6 y: 2.5–5 mg q4–6h (max 30 mg/24 h)

ADVERSE/SIDE EFFECTS CNS: *dizziness,* lightheadedness, *drowsiness,* sedation, lethargy, euphoria, agitation; restlessness, exhilaration, convulsions, narcosis, <u>respiratory depression</u>. **CV:** palpitation, hypotension, orthostatic hypotension, bradycardia, tachycardia, <u>circulatory collapse</u>. **GI:** *nausea,* vomiting, *constipation.* **GU:** urinary retention. **Hypersensitivity:** diffuse erythema, rash, urticaria, *pruritus,* excessive perspiration, facial flushing, shortness of breath, <u>anaphylactoid reaction</u>. **Other:** miosis, fixed-drug eruption.

DRUG INTERACTIONS Alcohol and other CNS DEPRESSANTS augment CNS depressant effects.

NURSING IMPLICATIONS

Administration

- Administer PO codeine with milk or other food to reduce possibility of GI distress.
- Patient's individual need for medication should be evaluated before each administration.
- Preserve in tight, light-resistant containers at 15–30C (59–86F) unless otherwise directed.

Assessment & Drug Effects

- Record relief of pain and duration of analgesia.
- Treatment of cough is directed toward decreasing frequency and intensity of cough without abolishing protective cough reflex, which serves the important function of removing bronchial secretions.
- Although codeine has less abuse liability than morphine, dependence is a major unwanted effect.

- Since drug may cause dizziness and lightheadedness, supervision of ambulation and other safety precautions may be warranted.
- Nausea is a common side effect. Report nausea accompanied by vomiting. Change to another analgesic may be warranted.

Patient & Family Education

- Because orthostatic hypotension is a possible side effect, instruct patient to make position changes slowly and in stages particularly from recumbent to upright posture. Also advise patient to lie down immediately if light-headedness or dizziness occurs.
- Nausea appears to be aggravated by ambulation. Advise patient to lie down when feeling nauseated and to notify physician if this symptom persists.
- Inform patient that codeine may impair ability to perform tasks requiring mental alertness and therefore to avoid driving and other potentially hazardous activities until reaction to drug is known.
- Advise patient not to take alcohol or other CNS depressants unless approved by physician.
- Inform patient that hyperactive cough may be lessened by avoiding irritants such as smoking, dust, fumes, and other air pollutants. Humidification of ambient air may provide some relief.

COLCHICINE

See ANTIGOUT AGENT prototype, p 46.

Prototype: cholestyramine, p 142

COLESTIPOL HYDROCHLORIDE
(koe-les´ti-pole)
Trade name: Colestid
Classifications: CARDIOVASCULAR DRUG; ANTILIPEMIC; BILE ACID SEQUESTRANT
Pregnancy: Category C

ACTIONS/PHARMACODYNAMICS Insoluble chloride salt of a basic anion exchange resin, with high molecular weight. Binds with bile acids in intestinal tract to form an insoluble complex that is excreted in the feces, thus reducing circulating cholesterol and increasing serum LDL removal rate. Serum triglycerides are not affected or are minimally increased. Route and dosage, contraindications, adverse reactions, interactions are similar to those of cholestyramine.

USES Pruritus associated with partial biliary obstruction; also as adjunct to diet therapy of patient with primary hypercholesterolemia (type IIa hyperlipoproteinemia) or with coronary artery disease unresponsive to diet or other measures alone. **Unlabeled uses:** digitoxin overdose and hyperoxaluria and to control postoperative diarrhea caused by excess bile acids in colon.

ROUTE & DOSAGE

Hypercholesterolemia
Adult   PO   15–30 g/d in 2–4 doses a.c. and h.s.

Digitalis Toxicity
Adult   PO   10 g followed by 5 g q6–8h as needed

PHARMACOKINETICS Absorption: not absorbed from GI tract. **Elimination:** excreted in feces as insoluble complex.

CONTRAINDICATIONS & PRECAUTIONS Contraindicated in: complete biliary obstruction, hypersensitivity to bile acid sequestrants. Safe use during pregnancy (category C), in nursing mothers, and in children not established. **Cautious use in:** hemorrhoids; bleeding disorders; malabsorption states; the elderly.

ADVERSE/SIDE EFFECTS GI: *constipation,* abdominal pain or distension, belching, flatulence, nausea, vomiting, diarrhea. **Other:** dermatitis, urticaria, joint and muscle pain, arthritis, shortness of breath, transient increases in liver enzyme tests, serum phosphorus and chloride; decreases in serum sodium and potassium.

DRUG INTERACTIONS Because it decreases the absorption from the GI tract of ORAL ANTICOAGULANTS, **digoxin**, TETRACYCLINES, PENICILLINS, **phenobarbital**, THYROID HORMONES, THIAZIDE DIURETICS, IRON SALTS, FAT-SOLUBLE VITAMINS (A,D,E,K), administer cholestyramine 4 h before or 2 h after these drugs.

NURSING IMPLICATIONS

Administration
- To prevent accidental inhalation or esophageal distress with dry form, always mix with liquids, juices, soups, cereals, or pulpy fruits. Add powder to at

least 90 ml fluid. When carbonated drink is used, slowly stir in a large glass because excess foaming may occur. Rinse glass with small amount extra fluid to be sure all the drug is taken.
- Drugs given concomitantly should be scheduled at least 1 h before or 4 h after ingestion of colestipol to reduce interference with their absorption (see drug interactions).
- Store at 15–30C (59–86F) in tightly closed container unless otherwise instructed.

Assessment & Drug Effects
- Watch for changes in bowel elimination pattern. Constipation should not be allowed to persist without medical attention.
- Monitor serum sodium and potassium levels. Monitor for and report signs and symptoms of hyponatremia and hypokalemia (see chap 3).

Patient & Family Education
- Be sure patient understands importance of established regimens for colestipol and other drugs that patient is taking. Patient should not change the times for taking each drug, nor omit or increase doses. Any change in established regimens should be approved by the physician.
- Patients receiving prolonged therapy should report unusual bleeding (vitamin K deficiency). Colestipol prevents absorption of fat-soluble vitamins (A, D, E, K).
- Urge patient not to use OTC drugs unless physician has given approval.
- Check with physician regarding permitted amount of alcohol intake.

Prototype: trimethoprim, p 90

COLISTIMETHATE SODIUM
(koe-lis-ti-meth'ate)
Trade name: Coly-mycin M
Classification: URINARY TRACT ANTIINFECTIVE

ACTIONS/PHARMACODYNAMICS Polymyxin antibiotic and parenteral form of colistin. Similar to polymyxin B in structure and actions but about one-third to one-fifth as potent. Antibacterial activity and overall toxicity are less, but nephrotoxic potential is almost identical with that of polymyxin B. Believed to act by affecting phospholipid component in bacterial cytoplasmic membranes with resulting damage

Common side effects in *italic*; life-threatening effects underlined; generic names in **bold**; classifications in SMALL CAPS

465

and leakage of essential intracellular components. Bactericidal against most gram-negative organisms including *Pseudomonas aeruginosa*, *Escherichia coli*, *Enterobacter aerogenes*, *Haemophilus* sp, *Klebsiella pneumoniae*, *Brucella*, *Salmonella*, *Shigella*, *Bordetella*, *Pasteurella*, and *Vibrio*. Not effective against *Proteus* or *Neisseria* species. Complete cross-resistance and cross-sensitivity to polymyxin B reported but not to broad-spectrum antibiotics.

USES Particularly for severe, acute and chronic UTIs caused by susceptible strains of gram-negative organisms resistant to other antibiotics. Has been used with carbenicillin for *Pseudomonas* sepsis in children with acute leukopenia.

ROUTE & DOSAGE

Urinary Tract Infections

Adult	IM/IV	2.5–5 mg/kg/d divided in 2–4 doses; max 5 mg/kg/d
Child	IM/IV	Same as for adult

PHARMACOKINETICS Peak: 1–2 h IM. **Duration:** 8–12 h. **Distribution:** widely distributed in most tissues except CNS; crosses placenta; distributed into breast milk. **Metabolism:** metabolized in liver. **Elimination:** half-life: 2–3 h; 66–75% excreted in urine within 24h.

CONTRAINDICATIONS & PRECAUTIONS Contraindicated in: hypersensitivity to polypeptide antibiotics; concomitant use of drugs that potentiate neuromuscular blocking effect (aminoglycoside antibiotics, other polymyxins, anticholinesterases, curariform muscle relaxants, ether, sodium citrate); nephrotoxic and ototoxic drugs. Safe use during pregnancy not established. **Cautious use in:** impaired renal function; myasthenia gravis; elderly patients, infants.

ADVERSE/SIDE EFFECTS Respiratory arrest after IM injection. **CNS:** circumoral, lingual, and peripheral paresthesias; visual and speech disturbances, neuromuscular blockade (generalized muscle weakness, dyspnea, respiratory depression or paralysis), seizures, psychosis. **Ear:** ototoxicity. **Hypersensitivity:** drug fever, pruritus, urticaria, dermatoses. **Renal:** nephrotoxicity. **Other:** GI disturbances, pain at IM site.

DRUG INTERACTIONS Tubocurarine, pancuronium, atracurium, AMINOGLYCOSIDES may compound and prolong respiratory depression; AMINOGLYCOSIDES, **amphotericin B, vancomycin** augment nephrotoxicity.

INCOMPATIBILITIES Solution/Additive: carbenicillin, cephalothin, erythromycin, hydrocortisone, kanamycin.

NURSING IMPLICATIONS

Administration

- IM injection should be made deep into upper outer quadrant of buttock. Patients commonly experience pain at injection site. Rotate sites.
- Infusion solution should be freshly prepared and used within 24 h.
- Reconstitute each 150 mg vial with 2 ml of sterile water for injection to yield a concentration of 75 mg/ml. Swirl vial gently during reconstitution to avoid bubble formation. Further dilute with 20 ml sterile water for injection.
- A single initial dose properly diluted is given by direct IV at a rate of 75 mg over 5 min.
- Subsequent doses are usually further diluted in an additional 50 ml or more of compatible solution and infused over a period of hours.
- IV infusion rate is prescribed by physician. (Rate of 5–6 mg/h is recommended for patients with normal renal function.)
- Reconstituted solution may be stored in refrigerator at 2–8C (36–46F) or at controlled room temperature of 15–30C (59–86F). Use within 7 d. Store unopened vials at controlled room temperature.

Assessment & Drug Effects

- Culture and susceptibility tests should be performed initially and periodically during therapy to determine responsiveness of causative organisms.
- Respiratory arrest has been reported after IM administration. Report restlessness or dyspnea promptly.
- Baseline renal function tests should be performed prior to therapy; frequent monitoring of renal function and urine drug levels is advisable during therapy. Impaired renal function increases the possibility of nephrotoxicity, apnea, and neuromuscular blockade.
- Monitor I&O. Decrease in urine output or change in I&O ratio and rising BUN, serum creatinine, and serum drug levels (without dosage increase) are indications of renal toxicity. If they occur, withhold drug and report to physician.
- Elderly patients and infants are particularly prone to renal toxicity because they tend to have inadequate renal reserves. Close monitoring is essential.
- Be alert to neurologic symptoms: changes in speech and hearing, visual changes, drowsiness,

dizziness, ataxia, and transient paresthesias, and keep physician informed.
- Postoperative patients who have received curariform muscle relaxants, ether, or sodium citrate should be closely monitored for signs of neuromuscular blockade (delayed recovery, muscle weakness, depressed respiration).

Patient & Family Education
- Because of the possibility of transient neurologic disturbances, caution ambulatory patient to avoid operating a vehicle or other potentially hazardous activities while on drug therapy.

Prototype: trimethoprim, p 90

COLISTIN SULFATE
(koe-lis´tin)
Trade names: Coly-Mycin S, Polymyxin E
Classifications: ANTIINFECTIVE; ANTIBIOTIC

ACTIONS/PHARMACODYNAMICS Polymyxin antibiotic derived from *Bacillus polymyxa* var. *colistinus*. Antibacterial potency appears to be equal to that of polymyxin B. Bactericidal against most gram-negative enteric pathogens, especially *Escherichia coli, Shigella, Pseudomonas aeruginosa, Klebsiella pneumoniae,* and *Aerobacter aerogenes.* Not effective against *Proteus, Neisseria,* or gram-positive microorganisms.

USES Diarrhea in infants and children caused by susceptible organisms.

ROUTE & DOSAGE

Diarrhea

Child	PO	5–15 mg/kg/d divided q8h

PHARMACOKINETICS Absorption: only slightly absorbed from GI tract. **Elimination:** half-life: 2–3 h; excreted in urine.

CONTRAINDICATIONS & PRECAUTIONS Contraindicated in: hypersensitivity to colistin derivatives. **Cautious use in:** renal impairment. See also colistimethate.

ADVERSE/SIDE EFFECTS Infrequent within recommended dosage range: nausea, vomiting, hyper-

sensitivity reactions, superinfections. Same potential for nephrotoxicity and neurotoxicity as colistimethate.

NURSING IMPLICATIONS

Administration
- Oral suspension is prepared by reconstituting powder with 37 ml distilled water. Slowly add one half of diluent to bottle, replace cap, and shake well. Add remaining diluent and repeat shaking. Indicate expiration date on label.
- After reconstitution, oral solution is stable for 2 wk when kept below 15C (59F). Store in tightly covered container; protect from light. Unopened bottles may be stored at controlled room temperature 15–30C (59–86F) unless otherwise directed.

Assessment & Drug Effects
- Renal function should be assessed prior to initiation of therapy, and frequent measurements should be made during therapy in patients with impaired renal function.
- Monitor I&O. Urine output alone is not a reliable index of renal toxicity. Hematuria and proteinuria and increases in BUN and serum creatinine can occur without oliguria.

Patient & Family Education
- Report signs and symptoms of a hypersensitivity reaction (see chap 3) promptly.
- Report signs and symptoms of superinfection (see chap 3) promptly.

COLLAGENASE
(kol´la-je-nase)
Trade names: Biozyme-C, Santyl
Classifications: DEBRIDING AGENT; ENZYME
Pregnancy: Category C

ACTIONS/PHARMACODYNAMICS Enzymatic debriding agent derived from fermentation of *Clostridium histolyticum.* Possesses specific ability to hydrolyze (digest) peptide bonds of denatured and undenatured collagen as well as cellular and bacterial debris. Proteolytic action results in liquefaction of necrotic tissue without affecting collagen in newly formed granulation tissue or other healthy tissue, facilitation of tissue granulation, and subsequent

Common side effects in *italic*; life-threatening effects underlined; generic names in **bold**; classifications in SMALL CAPS

467

wound epithelialization. Although it lacks direct anti-infective properties, it discourages bacterial growth by removing debris that might invite bacterial proliferation.

USES To debride necrotic tissue of severe burns or dermal ulcers including decubiti and stasis ulcers.

ROUTE & DOSAGE

Debridement of Necrotic Tissue

Adult Topical Apply once/d or q.o.d. as directed

CONTRAINDICATIONS & PRECAUTIONS Contraindicated in: local or systemic hypersensitivity to collagenase. Pregnancy category C. **Cautious use in:** debilitated patients.

ADVERSE/SIDE EFFECTS Local: pain, burning, redness, *irritation.* **Other:** hypersensitivity reactions reported following long-term use in combination with cortisone; bacteremia.

DRUG INTERACTIONS Benzalkonium chloride, hexachloraphene, nitrofurazone, tincture of iodine, silver sulfadiazine, silver nitrate, Burow's solution, ALUMINUM-CONTAINING SOLUTIONS inactivate collagenase.

NURSING IMPLICATIONS

Administration

- Before each collagenase application, necrotic debris should be removed by gently cleansing lesion with cotton or gauze saturated with hydrogen peroxide or Dakin's solution, followed by sterile normal saline. Check with physician about specific procedure.
- If lesion has had prior treatment with incompatible topical agent, site should be carefully cleansed by repeated washings with normal saline before applying collagenase.
- Irritation or redness of surrounding skin can be prevented by confining ointment to lesion being treated and by applying a protectant such as zinc oxide paste to skin.
- Store ointment at temperatures not exceeding 37C (98.6F) unless otherwise directed.

Assessment & Drug Effects

- Complete wound debridement generally occurs in about 7 to 14 d. Collagenase should be discontinued when necrotic tissue has been debrided and healthy granulation tissue is present.

- There is some risk of bacteremia associated with the use of debriding enzymes, particularly in debilitated patients. Monitor vital signs.

Patient & Family Education

- Avoid contact of drug in or near eyes. If contact occurs, irrigate immediately with copious amounts of water.

Prototype: prednisone, p 225

CORTICOTROPIN
(kor-ti-koe-troe´pin)
Trade names: ACTH, Acthar

CORTICOTROPIN REPOSITORY

Trade names: ACTH Gel, Acthron, Cortigel, Cortrophin-Gel, Cotropic Gel, H.P. Acthar Gel

CORTICOTROPIN ZINC HYDROXIDE

Trade name: Cortrophin-Zinc
Classifications: HORMONE; ADRENAL CORTICOSTEROID
Pregnancy: Category C

ACTIONS/PHARMACODYNAMICS Adrenocorticotropic hormone (ACTH) extracted from pituitary of domestic animals (usually pigs). Stimulates functioning adrenal cortex to produce and secrete corticosterone, cortisol (hydrocortisone), several weak androgens, and limited amounts of aldosterone. Therapeutic effects appear more rapidly than do those of prednisone. Suppresses further release of corticotropin by negative feedback mechanism. Chronic administration of exogenous corticosteroids decreases ACTH store and causes structural changes in pituitary. Lack of ACTH stimulation can lead to adrenal cortex atrophy.

USES Diagnostic test of adrenocortical function and adjunctively to treat adrenal insufficiency secondary to inadequate corticotropin secretion. Effective in treatment of adrenocorticoid-responsive diseases, such as multiple sclerosis, but adrenocorticoid therapy is preferred.

PHARMACOKINETICS Absorption: readily absorbed from IM site. **Onset:** 6 h. **Duration:** 2–4 h IV/IM;

12–24 h repository. **Distribution:** concentrated in many tissues; not known if crosses placenta or distributed into breast milk. **Metabolism:** metabolized in liver. **Elimination:** half-life: <20 min; excreted in urine.

ROUTE & DOSAGE

Diagnostic Test

Adult	IV	10–25 U in 500 ml D5W infused over 8 h

Therapeutic

Adult	IM/SC	40–80 U/d; dose and frequency individualized
		Repository: 40–80 U q24–72h
	IM	Zinc Hydroxide: 40 U q12–24h

Acute Multiple Sclerosis

Adult	IM/SC	80–120 U/d for 2–3 wk
		Repository: 80–120 U/d for 2–3 wk

CONTRAINDICATIONS & PRECAUTIONS Contraindicated in: ocular herpes simplex; recent surgery; CHF; scleroderma; osteoporosis; systemic fungoid infections; hypertension; sensitivity to porcine proteins; conditions accompanied by primary adrenocortical insufficiency or hyperfunction. Use during pregnancy (category C) or in lactating women requires evaluation of expected benefits against possible hazards to mother and child. **Cautious use in:** patients with latent tuberculosis or those reacting to tuberculin; hypothyroiditis, impaired hepatic function.

ADVERSE/SIDE EFFECTS CNS: euphoria, insomnia, headache, convulsions, papilledema, mood swings, depression. **Eye:** cataract, glaucoma. **GI:** nausea, vomiting, abdominal distension, peptic ulcer with perforation and hemorrhage. **Gynecologic:** hirsutism, amenorrhea. **Metabolic:** sodium and water retention; potassium and calcium loss, negative nitrogen balance, hyperglycemia. **Skin:** acne, impaired wound healing, fragile skin, petechiae, ecchymosis. **Other:** osteoporosis, loss of muscle mass, hypersensitivity, cushingoid state, activation of latent diabetes mellitus or tuberculosis, vertebral compression fracture.

DRUG INTERACTIONS Aspirin, NSAIDS increase potential for hypoprothrombinemia; because of enzyme induction, BARBITURATES, **phenytoin, rifampin** decrease effects of corticotropin; ESTROGENS may increase corticotropin binding and effects; **amphotericin B,** DIURETICS increase potassium loss.

INCOMPATIBILITIES Solution/Additive: aminophylline, sodium bicarbonate.

NURSING IMPLICATIONS

Administration

- Dosage is individualized. Changes in dosage regimen are gradual and only after full drug effects have become apparent.
- Corticotropin zinc hydroxide and corticotropin repository forms are not suitable for IV use.
- Shake corticotropin zinc hydroxide bottle well before injecting drug deep into gluteal muscle.
- For IV administration, dilute powder with 2 ml sterile water or NS for injection; desired dose is withdrawn from vial and further diluted with 500 ml of D5W and infused over 8 h.
- Administration of the hormone at high dosage levels is tapered rather than withdrawn suddenly. A 2–5 d period of adrenocortical hypofunction follows discontinuation of corticotropin.
- *Storage: Corticotropin for Injection (reconstituted solution):* stable for 24 h or 7 d, depending on product, when stored at 2–8C (36–46F). Corticotropin repository: store at 2–15C (36–59F). Corticotropin zinc hydroxide: store at 15–30C (59–86F).

Assessment & Drug Effects

- Before giving corticotropin to patient with suspected sensitivity to porcine proteins, hypersensitivity skin testing should be performed.
- Observe patient closely for 15 min for hypersensitivity reactions during IV administration or immediately after SC or IM injections (urticaria, pruritus, dizziness, nausea, vomiting, anaphylactic shock). Epinephrine 1:1000 should be readily available for emergency treatment.
- Adrenal response to corticotropin is measured against a baseline plasma cortisol level 1 h before the 8 h test. Another plasma level is determined after at least 1 h of the infusion.
- *Test results:* Patient with normal adrenal reserve: an increase in plasma cortisol levels of 15–40 µg/dl by the eighth hour of the 8 h corticotropin infusion (plasma cortisol levels more than 45 µg/dl by 8 h, urinary 17-OHCS increase to 12–25 mg/g creatinine; 17-KS increase by 1.5–2.5 times control level). Patient with complete primary adrenal suppression: no change from baseline plasma cortisol or urinary 17-OHCS or 17-KS excretion levels. Patient with hypopituitarism: plasma cortisol levels and

Common side effects in *italic*; life-threatening effects <u>underlined</u>; generic names in **bold**; classifications in SMALL CAPS

469

C

urinary 17-OHCS increase in subnormal increments after the 8 h test daily for 5 d.

- Corticotropin may suppress signs and symptoms of chronic disease.
- New infections can appear during treatment. Because of decreased resistance and inability to localize the infection, it may be severe. Report immediately.
- Prolonged use of corticotropin increases risk of hypersensitivity reaction (see Signs & Symptoms, chap 3).
- Growth and development of a child receiving this drug should be carefully monitored.

Patient & Family Education

- Corticotropin administration increases requirements for insulin and oral antidiabetic agents. Make patient with diabetes mellitus aware of the need to monitor blood glucose closely until response to the drug is stabilized.
- Advise patient to monitor weight and report a steady gain, especially if accompanied by edema. Patient should also promptly report headache, muscle weakness, abdominal pain.
- Caution patient against self-medicating with OTC drugs without consulting physician.
- Eye examinations should be done before initiation of expected long-term therapy and periodically during treatment. Instruct patient to report to physician if blurred vision occurs.
- Dietary salt restriction and potassium supplementation may be necessary to minimize edema caused by overstimulation of the adrenal cortex by corticotropin.
- Patient should not be immunized with live vaccines while receiving corticotropin.

Prototype: prednisone, p 225

CORTISONE ACETATE
(kor´ti-sone)

Trade names: Cortistan, Cortone
Classifications: HORMONE; SYNTHETIC ADRENAL CORTICOSTEROID; GLUCOCORTICOID; MINERALOCORTICOID; ANTIINFLAMMATORY
Pregnancy: Category D

ACTIONS/PHARMACODYNAMICS Short-acting synthetic steroid with prominent glucocorticoid activity and mineralocorticoid effects approximately equal to those of prednisone (cortisol). Because therapeutic activity of cortisone results from its conversion in body to cortisol, its effects simulate those of hydrocortisone. Has antiinflammatory and immunosuppressive actions. Metabolic effects include promotion of protein, carbohydrate, and fat metabolism and interference with linear growth in children. Mineralocorticoid actions include promotion of sodium retention and potassium excretion. May foster development of osteoporosis.

USES Replacement therapy for primary or secondary adrenocortical insufficiency and inflammatory and allergic disorders.

ROUTE & DOSAGE

Replacement or Inflammatory Disorders

Adult	PO/IM	20–300 mg/d in 1 or more divided doses; try to reduce periodically by 10–25 mg/d to lowest effective dose
Child	PO/IM	0.7–10 mg/kg/d or 20–300 mg/m² in 4 divided doses

PHARMACOKINETICS Absorption: readily absorbed from GI tract. **Onset:** rapid PO; 24–48 h IM. **Peak:** 2 h PO; 24–48 h IM. **Duration:** 1.25–1.5 d. **Distribution:** concentrated in many tissues; crosses placenta; distributed into breast milk. **Metabolism:** metabolized in liver. **Elimination:** half-life: 0.5 h; HPA suppression: 8–12 h; excreted in urine.

CONTRAINDICATIONS & PRECAUTIONS Contraindicated in: hypersensitivity to glucocorticoids; psychoses; viral or bacterial diseases of skin; Cushing's syndrome, immunologic procedures. Safe use in pregnancy (category D), by nursing mothers, and children not established. **Cautious use in:** diabetes mellitus; hypertension, CHF; active or arrested tuberculosis; active or latent peptic ulcer.

ADVERSE/SIDE EFFECTS CNS: euphoria, insomnia, vertigo, nystagmus. **CV:** CHF, hypertension, *edema*. **Endocrine:** hyperglycemia. **Eye:** *cataracts,* glaucoma, blurred vision. **GI:** *nausea,* peptic ulcer, pancreatitis. **Hematologic:** thrombocytopenia. **Musculoskeletal:** *compression fracture,* osteoporosis, muscle weakness. **Skin:** impaired wound healing, petechiae, ecchymosis, acne.

Common side effects in *italic*; life-threatening effects underlined; generic names in **bold**; classifications in SMALL CAPS

DRUG INTERACTIONS BARBITURATES, **pheny-toin, rifampin,** because of enzyme induction, decrease effects of cortisone.

NURSING IMPLICATIONS

Administration

- Administer cortisone (usually in AM) with food or fluid of patient's choice to reduce gastric irritation.
- Sodium chloride and a mineralocorticoid are usually given with cortisone as part of replacement therapy.
- Parenteral cortisone is a suspension (25 mg/ml) and therefore should not be used IV. Shake bottle well before withdrawing dose.
- Admixtures with other parenteral medications are not recommended because of state of suspension and altered absorption rate.
- Alternate-day therapy with an oral intermediate acting glucocorticoid may decrease growth retardation effect in children.
- Store at 15–30C (59–86F) in tightly closed container unless otherwise directed by manufacturer. Protect from heat and freezing.

Assessment & Drug Effects

- Monitor for signs and symptoms of Cushing's syndrome (see chap 3), especially in patients on long-term therapy.
- Cortisone may mask some signs of infection, and new infections may appear.
- Be alert to *clinical indications of infection:* malaise, anorexia, depression, and evidence of delayed healing. (Classic signs of inflammation are suppressed by cortisone.)
- Ecchymotic areas, unexplained bleeding, and easy bruising are reportable signs.

Patient & Family Education

- Advise patient to take drug exactly as prescribed and caution against altering dose intervals or stopping therapy abruptly.
- Patient should monitor weight and report a steady gain especially if it is accompanied by signs of fluid retention (e.g., edema of ankles or hands).
- Changes in visual acuity, including blurring, should be reported promptly.
- Inform physician or dentist that cortisone is being taken. Patient should carry identification card or jewelry that states drug being taken and physician's name.

Prototype: prednisone, p 225

COSYNTROPIN

(koe-sin-troe´pin)
Trade names: Cortrosyn, Synacthen Depot
Classification: DIAGNOSTIC AGENT
Pregnancy: Category C

ACTIONS/PHARMACODYNAMICS Synthetic polypeptide resembling corticotropin (ACTH) in the first 24 of the 39 amino acids in naturally occurring ACTH. Has less immunologic activity and is associated with less risk of sensitivity than corticotropin. In patient with normal adrenocortical function, stimulates adrenal cortex to secrete corticosterone, cortisol (hydrocortisone), several weak androgenic substances, and limited amounts of aldosterone (steroidogenic activity). Extraadrenal actions, not used therapeutically, include melanotropic and adipokinetic effects and increased secretion of growth hormone.

USES Diagnostic tool to differentiate primary adrenal from secondary (pituitary) adrenocortical insufficiency. **Unlabeled use:** in patients with normal adrenocortical function for the long-term treatment of chronic inflammatory or degenerative disorders responsive to glucocorticoids.

ROUTE & DOSAGE

Rapid Screening Test

Adult	IM/IV	0.25 mg injected over 2 min
Child	IM	<2 y: 0.125 mg injected over 2 min
	IV	<2 y: 0.125 mg IV at 0.04 mg/h over 6 h

PHARMACOKINETICS Absorption: plasma cortisol levels double in 15–30 min. **Peak:** 1 h. **Duration:** 2–4 h. **Distribution:** unknown; does not cross placenta. **Metabolism:** unknown.

CONTRAINDICATIONS & PRECAUTIONS Contraindicated in: history of allergic disorders. Safe use during pregnancy (category C) and in nursing women not established.

Common side effects in *italic*; life-threatening effects underlined;
generic names in **bold**; classifications in SMALL CAPS

471

ADVERSE/SIDE EFFECTS Hypersensitivity reactions (rare); pruritus; mild fever, chronic pancreatitis.

DIAGNOSTIC TEST INTERFERENCES Cortisone, hydrocortisone, estrogen, spironolactone, elevated bilirubin, and presence of free Hgb in plasma may interfere with *plasma cortisol* determinations.

NURSING IMPLICATIONS

Administration

- Reconstitute cosyntropin powder by adding 1.1 ml 0.9% NaCl injection (diluent provided by manufacturer) to vial labeled 0.25 mg to provide solution containing 0.25 mg cosyntropin/ml.
- Reconstituted drug may be given by direct IV over 2 min or further diluted in D5W or NS and infused over 4–8 h.
- Reconstituted solutions remain stable 24 h at room temperature or 21 d at 2–8C.
- Cosyntropin should not be added to blood or to plasma infusions.

Assessment & Drug Effects

- Although plasma cortisol levels are better indicators of adrenal function, the response can also be measured by 24 h urinary 17-KS or 17-OHCS excretion before and at end of IV infusion.
- *Normal 17-KS levels:* men: 10–25 mg/24 h; women <50 y: 5–15 mg/24 hr; >50 y: 4–8 mg/24h.
- *Normal 17-OHCS levels:* men: 5–12 mg/24 h; women: 3–10 mg/24 h; children 8–12 y: <4.5 mg/24 h; younger children: 1.5 mg/24 h. May be slightly higher in obese or muscular individuals.
- Urine collection for study of 17-KS excretion may have to be postponed if female patient is menstruating.
- If patient is on prednisone, dexamethasone, or betamethasone, therapy can continue through the test period because these drugs do not interfere with analysis of serum cortisol.

CROMOLYN SODIUM

(kroe´moe-lin)

Trade names: Disodium Cromoglycate, DSCG, Intal, Nasalcrom, Opticrom, Rynacrom
Classifications: ANTIASTHMATIC; MAST CELL STABILIZER
Pregnancy: Category B

ACTIONS/PHARMACODYNAMICS Synthetic asthma-prophylactic agent with unique action. Inhibits release of bronchoconstrictors—histamine and SRS-A (slow-reacting substance of anaphylaxis)—from sensitized pulmonary mast cells, thereby suppressing an allergic response. Believed to act by interfering with calcium transport across mast cell membrane and probably by phosphorylation of mast cell protein. Has no intrinsic bronchodilator, antihistaminic, or vasoconstrictor properties, thus only of value when taken prophylactically. Particularly effective for IgE-mediated or "extrinsic asthma" precipitated by exposure to specific allergen, e.g., pollens, dust, animal dander. Has also benefited many patients with nonatopic or "intrinsic asthma" triggered by nonallergic factors such as infections, irritants, emotions, or exercise.

USES Primarily for prophylaxis of mild to moderate seasonal and perennial bronchial asthma and allergic rhinitis. Also used for prevention of exercise-related bronchospasm, prevention of acute bronchospasm induced by known pollutants or antigens, and for prevention and treatment of allergic rhinitis. **Ophthalmic use:** allergic ocular disorders. **Unlabeled uses:** orally for systemic mastocytosis and for prophylaxis of GI and systemic reactions to food allergy. **Orphan drug:** Proposed use: mastocytosis; vernal keratoconjunctivitis.

ROUTE & DOSAGE

Allergies

Adult	Inhalation	Metered dose inhaler or capsule: 1 spray or 1 capsule inhaled q.i.d.
		Nasal solution: 1 spray in each nostril 3–6 times/d at regular intervals
	Ophthalmic	1–2 drops in each eye 4–6 times/d at regular intervals
Child	Inhalation	>6 y: Metered dose inhaler or capsule: Same as for adult
		>6 y: Nasal solution: Same as for adult
	Ophthalmic	>6 y: Same as for adult

PHARMACOKINETICS Absorption: approximately 8% of dose absorbed from lungs. **Onset:** 1 wk with regular use. **Peak:** 15 min. **Duration:** 4–6 h; may last as long as 2–3 wk. **Elimination:** half-life: 80 min; excreted in bile and urine in equal amounts.

Common side effects in *italic*; life-threatening effects underlined; generic names in **bold**; classifications in SMALL CAPS

CONTRAINDICATIONS & PRECAUTIONS Contraindicated in: use of aerosol (because of fluorocarbon propellants) in patients with coronary artery disease or history of arrhythmias; dyspnea, acute asthma, status asthmaticus, patients unable to coordinate actions or follow instructions. Safe use in children <6 y not determined; use of capsule not recommended for children. Safe use during (category B) and in nursing women not established. **Cautious use in:** renal or hepatic dysfunction.

ADVERSE/SIDE EFFECTS Generally well tolerated. **CNS:** headache, dizziness, peripheral neuritis. **ENT:** *sneezing, nasal stinging and burning,* dryness and *irritation of throat and trachea; cough;* nasal congestion. **Eye:** itchy, puffy eyes, lacrimation, *transient burning, stinging.* **GI:** swelling of parotid glands, dry mouth, slightly bitter after-taste, *nausea,* vomiting, esophagitis. **Hypersensitivity:** erythema, urticaria, rash, contact dermatitis, peripheral eosinophilia, angioedema, bronchospasm, anaphylaxis (rare).

NURSING IMPLICATIONS

Administration

- Patients should receive detailed instructions for loading and administering the spinhaler or nasalmatic device. See manufacturer's instructions. Therapeutic effect is dependent on proper inhalation technique.
- Advise patient to clear as much mucus as possible before inhalation treatments.
- Instruct patient to exhale as completely as possible before placing inhaler mouthpiece between lips, tilt head backward and inhale rapidly and deeply with steady, even breaths. Remove inhaler from mouth, hold breath for a few seconds, then exhale into the air. Repeat until entire dose is taken.
- Caution patient not to exhale into inhaler because moisture from breath will interfere with its proper operation. Also inform patient that capsule is intended for inhalation only and is ineffective if swallowed.
- Protect cromolyn from moisture and heat. Store in tightly closed, light-resistant container at 15–30C (59–86F) unless otherwise directed.

Assessment & Drug Effects

- A drug history is advisable before treatment is initiated. Cromolyn capsules contain a lactose vehicle to which patients with lactose deficiency may react.
- Exacerbation of asthmatic symptoms including breathlessness and cough may occur in patients re-

ceiving cromolyn during corticosteroid withdrawal. The same is true of patients on maintenance steroid therapy when cromolyn is withdrawn.
- Cromolyn does not eliminate the continued need for therapy with bronchodilators, expectorants, antibiotics, or corticosteroids, but the amount and frequency of use of these medications may be appreciably reduced.
- Eosinophil count is a reliable indicator of developing allergy and therefore should be monitored.
- For patients with asthma, therapeutic effects may be noted within a few days but generally not until after 1–2 wk of therapy.

Patient & Family Education

- Inform patient that throat irritation, cough, and hoarseness can be minimized by gargling with water, drinking a few swallows of water, or by sucking on a lozenge after each treatment.
- Provide patient with specific instructions regarding what to do in the event of an acute asthmatic attack. Cromolyn is of no value in acute asthma.
- Advise patient to report any unusual signs or symptoms. Hypersensitivity reactions (see Signs & Symptoms, chap 3) can be severe and life-threatening. Drug should be discontinued if an allergic reaction occurs.
- Treatment with cromolyn 15 min before doing protracted exercises reportedly blunts the effects of vigorous exercise as well as cold air.
- ***Ophthalmic use:*** Patient should be advised not to wear soft contact lenses during therapy with ophthalmic drug. They may be worn within a few hours after therapy is discontinued.
- Instruct patient in the proper technique for instillation of ophthalmic drops.

Prototype: lindane, p 263

CROTAMITON

(kroe-tam´i-tonn)
Trade name: Eurax
Classifications: SKIN AND MUCOUS MEMBRANE AGENT; SCABICIDE; ANTIPRURITIC
Pregnancy: Category C

ACTIONS/PHARMACODYNAMICS Scabicidal and antipruritic agent. Available in an emollient-lo-

Common side effects in *italic*; life-threatening effects underlined; generic names in **bold**; classifications in SMALL CAPS

473

tion base or in a vanishing cream. By unknown mechanisms, drug eradicates *Sarcoptes scabiei* and effectively relieves itching. Carcinogenesis, mutagenesis, and impairment to fertility: data not available.

USES Treatment of scabies and for symptomatic treatment of pruritus.

ROUTE & DOSAGE

Scabies

Adult	Topical	Apply a thin layer of cream from neck to toes; apply a second layer 24 h later; bathe 48 h after last application to remove drug

CONTRAINDICATIONS & PRECAUTIONS Contraindicated in: application to acutely inflamed skin, raw or weeping surfaces, eyes, or mouth; history of previous sensitivity to crotamiton. Safe use during pregnancy (category C) or in children not established.

ADVERSE/SIDE EFFECTS Skin irritation (particularly with prolonged use), rash, erythema, sensation of warmth, allergic sensitization.

NURSING IMPLICATIONS

Administration
- Shake container well before use of solution.
- The skin must be thoroughly dry before applying medication.
- If drug accidentally contacts eyes, thoroughly flush out medication with water.
- *Pruritus treatment:* Massage medication gently into affected areas until it is completely absorbed. Repeat as needed (usually effective for 6–10 h).
- Store in tightly closed containers at 15–30C (59–86F). Do not freeze.

Patient & Family Education
- Review package insert with patient before treatment begins.
- Instruct the patient to discontinue medication and report to physician if irritation or sensitization develops.

CYANOCOBALAMIN

(sye-an-oh-koe-bal´a-min)
Trade names: Anacobin, Bedoz, Berubigen, Betalin 12, Cobex, Crystamine, Crysti-12, Cyanabin, Cyanoject, Kaybovite, Redisol, Rubesol, Rubion, Rubramin PC, Sytobex
Classification: VITAMIN B_{12}
Pregnancy: Category A; C (parenteral)

ACTIONS/PHARMACODYNAMICS Vitamin B_{12} is a cobalt-containing B complex vitamin produced by *Streptomyces griseus*. Essential for normal growth, cell reproduction, maturation of RBCs, nucleoprotein synthesis, maintenance of nervous system (myelin synthesis), and believed to be involved in protein and carbohydrate metabolism. Also acts as coenzyme in various biologic reactions. Stimulates reticulocytes and together with folic acid is involved in formation of oxyribonucleotides from ribonucleotides. Vitamin B_{12} deficiency results in megaloblastic anemia, dysfunction of spinal cord with paralysis, GI lesions.

USES Vitamin B_{12} deficiency due to malabsorption syndrome as in pernicious (Addison's) anemia, sprue; GI pathology, dysfunction, or surgery; fish tapeworm infestation, and gluten enteropathy. Also used in B_{12} deficiency caused by increased physiologic requirements or inadequate dietary intake, and in vitamin B_{12} absorption (Schilling) test. **Unlabeled use:** to prevent and treat toxicity associated with sodium nitroprusside.

PHARMACOKINETICS Absorption: intestinal absorption requires presence of intrinsic factor in terminal ileum. **Distribution:** widely distributed; principally stored in liver, kidneys, and adrenals; crosses placenta. **Metabolism:** converted in tissues to active co-enzymes; enterohepatically cycled. **Elimination:** 50–95% of doses ≥100 µg are excreted in urine in 48 h; excreted in breast milk.

CONTRAINDICATIONS & PRECAUTIONS Contraindicated in: history of sensitivity to vitamin B_{12}, other cobalamins, or cobalt; early Leber's disease (hereditary optic nerve atrophy), indiscriminate use in folic acid deficiency. Safe use during pregnancy (category C), in nursing women, and in children not established. **Cautious use in:** heart disease, anemia, pulmonary disease.

ROUTE & DOSAGE

Vitamin B₁₂ Deficiency

Adult	IM/Deep SC	30 µg/d for 5–10 d; then 100–200 µg/mo
Child	IM/Deep SC	100 µg doses to a total of 1–5 mg over 2 wk; then 60 µg/mo

Pernicious Anemia

Adult	IM/Deep SC	100–1000 µg/d for 2–3 wk; then 100–1000 µg q2–4wk

Diagnosis of Megaloblastic Anemia

Adult	IM/Deep SC	1 µg/d for 10 d while maintaining a low folate and vitamin B₁₂ diet

Schilling Test

Adult	IM/Deep SC	1000 µg × 1 dose

Nutritional Supplement

Adult	PO	1–25 µg/d
Child	PO	<1 y: 0.3 µg/d ≥1 y: 1 µg/d

ADVERSE/SIDE EFFECTS CV: feeling of swelling of body, peripheral vascular thrombosis, pulmonary edema, CHF. **GI:** mild transient diarrhea. **Skin:** itching, rash, flushing. **Other:** hypokalemia, sudden death; severe optic nerve atrophy (patients with Leber's disease), anaphylactic shock; unmasking of poly cythemia vera (with correction of vitamin B₁₂ deficiency); precipitation of gout.

DIAGNOSTIC TEST INTERFERENCES Most antibiotics, methotrexate, and pyrimethamine may produce invalid diagnostic *blood assays for vitamin B₁₂.* Possibility of false-positive test for *intrinsic factor antibodies.*

DRUG INTERACTIONS Alcohol, **aminosalicylic acid, neomycin, colchicine** may decrease absorption of oral cyanocobalamin; **chloramphenicol** may interfere with therapeutic response to cyanocobalamin.

NURSING IMPLICATIONS

Administration

- PO preparations may be mixed with fruit juices. However, administer promptly since ascorbic acid affects the stability of vitamin B₁₂.

- Administration of oral vitamin B₁₂ with meals increases its absorption, presumably by stimulating production of intrinsic factor.
- Parenteral therapy is the preferred treatment for patients with pernicious anemia, since oral administration may be unreliable. However, oral therapy may be used when the condition is mild and is without neurologic signs or in rare patients who are sensitive to the parenteral form or who refuse it.
- Preserved in light-resistant containers at room temperature preferably at 15–30C (59–86F) unless otherwise directed by manufacturer.

Assessment & Drug Effects

- Before initiation of therapy, reticulocyte and erythrocyte counts, Hgb, Hct, vitamin B₁₂ and serum folate levels should be determined; these studies should be repeated between 5 and 7 d after start of therapy and at regular intervals during therapy.
- A careful history of sensitivities should be obtained. Sensitization to cyanocobalamin can take as long as 8 y to develop.
- Potassium levels should be monitored during the first 48 h, particularly in patients with Addisonian pernicious anemia or megaloblastic anemia. Conversion to normal erythropoiesis increases erythrocyte potassium requirement and can result in severe hypokalemia and sudden death.
- Monitor vital signs in patients with cardiac disease and in those receiving parenteral cyanocobalamin, and be alert to symptoms of pulmonary edema, which generally occur early in therapy.
- Therapeutic response to drug therapy is usually dramatic, occurring within 48 h. Effectiveness is measured by laboratory values and improvement in manifestations of vitamin B₁₂ deficiency.
- Characteristically, reticulocyte concentration rises in 3–4 d, peaks in 5–8 d, and then gradually declines as erythrocyte count and hemoglobin rise to normal levels (in 4–6 wk).
- Usually, demonstrable neurologic damage is considered irreversible if there is no improvement after 1–1 1/2 y of adequate therapy.
- Bowel regularity is essential for consistent absorption of oral preparations.
- Smokers appear to have increased requirements for vitamin B₁₂.
- A complete diet and drug history and an inquiry into alcohol drinking patterns should be obtained on all patients receiving cyanocobalamin to identify and correct poor habits.

Common side effects in *italic*; life-threatening effects underlined; generic names in **bold**; classifications in SMALL CAPS

475

Patient & Family Education

- Advise patient to notify physician of any intercurrent disease or infection. Increased dosage may be required.
- It is imperative that the patient with pernicious anemia understand that parenteral drug therapy must be continued throughout life to prevent irreversible neurologic damage.
- Dietary deficiency of vitamin B_{12} has been observed in strict vegetarians (vegans) and their breast-fed infants and in the elderly. Advise vegetarians of the relationship between vitamin B_{12} deficiency and their diet.
- Rich food sources: nutrient-added breakfast cereals, vitamin B_{12}–fortified soy milk, organ meats, clams, oysters; egg yolk, crab, salmon, sardines, muscle meat, milk, and dairy products.

Prototype: ampicillin, p 69

CYCLACILLIN
(sye-kla-sill´in)
Trade name: Cyclapen-W
Classifications: ANTIINFECTIVE; ANTIBIOTIC; AMINOPENICILLIN; BETA-LACTAM
Pregnancy: Category B

ACTIONS/PHARMACODYNAMICS Acid stable, semisynthetic aminopenicillin derivative with broad antibacterial spectrum almost identical to that of ampicillin. Like ampicillin, it is also penicillinase sensitive and is bactericidal. Acts by inhibiting biosynthesis of cell wall mucopeptide in actively multiplying organisms. Reported to have no appreciable advantage over ampicillin except that it is more completely absorbed and may have lower incidence of diarrhea and skin rash.

USES UTIs caused by *Escherichia coli* and *Proteus mirabilis;* otitis media and respiratory tract infections caused by *Streptococcus pneumoniae, Haemophilus influenzae,* and group A beta-hemolytic streptococci; skin and soft tissue infections caused by group A beta-hemolytic streptococci and non-penicillinase-producing staphylococci.

PHARMACOKINETICS Absorption: well absorbed from GI tract. **Peak effect:** 30–60 min. **Duration:** 6–8 h. **Distribution:** distribution to placenta and breast milk unknown. **Elimination:** half-life: 30–40 min; excreted in urine.

ROUTE & DOSAGE

Systemic Infections

Adult	PO	250–500 mg q8h
Child	PO	<20 kg: 125 mg q8h
		>20 kg: 250 mg q8h up to 100 mg/kg/d (max 2 g/d)

CONTRAINDICATIONS & PRECAUTIONS Contraindicated in: history of penicillin allergy. Safe use during pregnancy (category B), in nursing mothers, and in children <2 mo not established. **Cautious use in:** history of or suspected atopy or allergy (hay fever, asthma, hives, eczema); history of cephalosporin allergy; impaired renal function.

ADVERSE/SIDE EFFECTS GI: *diarrhea,* nausea, vomiting, abdominal pain. **Hematologic:** anemia, thrombocytopenia with or without purpura, leukopenia, neutropenia, eosinophilia. **Hypersensitivity:** rash, urticaria, pruritus, anaphylaxis. **Other:** dizziness, headache, superinfections, interstitial nephritis.

DIAGNOSTIC TEST INTERFERENCES As with other semisynthetic penicillins, cyclacillin may cause elevations of *AST.*

DRUG INTERACTIONS Allopurinol increases incidence of rash; effectiveness of AMINOGLYCOSIDES may be impaired in patients with severe end stage renal disease; **chloramphenicol, erythromycin, tetracycline** may reduce bactericidal effects of cyclacillin—this interaction is primarily significant when low doses are used; cyclacillin may interfere with contraceptive action of ORAL CONTRACEPTIVES—female patients should be advised to consider nonhormonal contraception while on any antibiotic.

NURSING IMPLICATIONS

Administration

- Absorption is faster and more complete if cyclacillin is taken on an empty stomach (either 1 h before or 2 h after meals).
- Shake suspension form well before pouring it.
- For patients with impaired renal function, dosage intervals may be adjusted on basis of creatinine clearance values.
- After reconstitution, suspension retains potency for 7 d at room temperature and for 14 d under refrigeration. Expiration date should appear on label. A calibrated measuring device should be dispensed with suspension.

Common side effects in *italic*; life-threatening effects underlined; generic names in **bold**; classifications in SMALL CAPS

- Store tablets in a tight container preferably at 25C (77F) unless otherwise directed.

Assessment & Drug Effects

- Culture and susceptibility tests should be performed before and during therapy. Therapy may be initiated pending test results.
- Before therapy is initiated, determine previous hypersensitivity to penicillins, cephalosporins, or other drugs.
- Be alert for signs & symptoms of a hypersensitivity or anaphylactoid reaction (see chap 3). Report their appearance promptly.
- Monitor for signs and symptoms of superinfection (see chap 3). Report their appearance promptly.

Patient & Family Education

- Instruct patient to take medication at equally spaced intervals and to continue medication for the full course of therapy as prescribed by physician.
- Advise patient to keep physician informed of progress and adverse reactions and also to report symptoms of superinfection (see chap 3).

Prototype: hydralazine, p 152

CYCLANDELATE

(sye-klan´de-late)
Trade names: Cyclan, Cyclospasmol
Classifications: CARDIOVASCULAR DRUG;
NONNITRATE VASODILATOR
Pregnancy: Category C

ACTIONS/PHARMACODYNAMICS Produces vasodilation by papaverinelike relaxation of peripheral vascular smooth muscle. Has no significant adrenergic stimulating or blocking actions.

USES Adjunctive therapy in arteriosclerosis obliterans, intermittent claudication, thrombophlebitis (to control associated vasospasm and muscular ischemia), nocturnal leg cramps, Raynaud's phenomenon.

PHARMACOKINETICS Absorption: readily absorbed from GI tract. **Peak:** 1–1.5 h. **Duration:** 3–4 h. **Metabolism:** unknown.

CONTRAINDICATIONS & PRECAUTIONS Contraindicated in: safe use during pregnancy (category

C), in women of childbearing age, or in nursing mothers not established. **Cautious use in:** severe obliterative coronary artery or cerebrovascular disease, recent MI, bleeding tendencies, active bleeding, glaucoma.

ROUTE & DOSAGE

Vasospasm

Adult	PO	200–400 mg q.i.d. a.c. and h.s.; may reduce by 200 mg increments once response achieved; usual range 400–800 mg/d in 2–4 divided doses

ADVERSE/SIDE EFFECTS Relatively nontoxic. *Dizziness, facial flushing, sweating, tingling sensation in face, fingers, toes; tachycardia, weakness, headache;* GI disturbances: heartburn, eructation, stomach pain, possible prolongation of bleeding time (high doses).

NURSING IMPLICATIONS

Administration

- GI distress may be relieved by taking medication with meals, milk, or an antacid (if prescribed).
- Store in tightly-closed container at 15–30C (59–86F) unless otherwise directed.

Assessment & Drug Effects

- Some patients experience mild flushing, headaches, weakness, and tachycardia during the first week of therapy, requiring dosage reduction.
- Therapeutic effect on peripheral circulation may be manifested by slight rise in skin temperature, increased pulse volume, the ability to walk longer distances without discomfort, and lessened pain.
- Since drug may cause dizziness, supervision of ambulation and other safety precautions may be warranted.

Patient & Family Education

- Inform patient that improvement usually occurs gradually and that prolonged therapy may be necessary.
- Caution patient to make position changes slowly and in stages, particularly from recumbent to upright posture, to dangle legs over bed for a few minutes before ambulating; to lie down if feels faint or dizzy, and to avoid driving or other potentially hazardous activities. Patient should notify physician if symptoms persist.
- Since nicotine constricts blood vessels, patient should be advised to stop smoking.

Common side effects in *italic*; life-threatening effects underlined; generic names in **bold**; classifications in SMALL CAPS

477

Prototype: meclizine, p 50

CYCLIZINE HYDROCHLORIDE

(sye´kli-zeen)

Trade name: Marezine Hydrochloride

CYCLIZINE LACTATE

Trade names: Marezine Lactate, Marzine
Classifications: ANTIHISTAMINE (H₁-RECEPTOR ANTAGONIST); ANTIVERTIGO AGENT; ANTIEMETIC
Pregnancy: Category B

ACTIONS/PHARMACODYNAMICS Piperazine antihistamine (H₁-receptor blocking agent) structurally and pharmacologically related to other cyclizine compounds (e.g., buclizine, hydroxyzine, meclizine). In common with these agents, it exhibits CNS depression and anticholinergic, antispasmodic, local anesthetic, and antihistaminic activity. Has prominent depressant action on labyrinthine excitability and on conduction in vestibular-cerebellar pathways, thus producing marked antimotion and antiemetic effects. Mechanism of action not known.

USES Chiefly for prevention and treatment of motion sickness and postoperative nausea and vomiting.

ROUTE & DOSAGE

Motion Sickness

Adult	PO	50 mg 30 min before travel; then q4–6h prn (max 200 mg/d)
	IM	50 mg q4–6h prn
Child	PO	6–12y: 25 mg q4–6h prn (max 75 mg/d)
	IM	6–12 y: 1 mg/kg t.i.d. prn (max 75 mg/d)

Postoperative Vomiting

Adult	IM	50 mg 15–30 min before end of operation; may repeat q4–6h (t.i.d.) prn during first few days after surgery

PHARMACOKINETICS Onset: rapid. **Duration:** 4–6 h. **Metabolism:** unknown.

CONTRAINDICATIONS & PRECAUTIONS Contraindicated in: pregnancy (category B), nursing mothers, children <6 y. **Cautious use in:** narrow-angle glaucoma; prostatic hypertrophy; obstructive disease of GU or GI tracts; postoperative patients.

ADVERSE/SIDE EFFECTS Usually dose-related. **CNS:** *drowsiness,* excitement, euphoria, auditory and visual hallucinations, hyperexcitability alternating with drowsiness, convulsions, underlined respiratory paralysis. **CV:** hypotension, palpitation, tachycardia. **EENT:** *dry mouth,* nose, and throat; blurred vision, diplopia, tinnitus. **GI:** anorexia, nausea, vomiting, diarrhea, or constipation. **Hypersensitivity:** urticaria, rash, cholestatic jaundice. **Other:** pain at IM injection site.

DIAGNOSTIC TEST INTERFERENCES Because cyclizine is an antihistamine, inform patient that *skin testing* procedures should not be scheduled for about 4 d after drug is discontinued or false-negative reactions may result.

DRUG INTERACTIONS Alcohol, BARBITURATES, CNS DEPRESSANTS (e.g., HYPNOTICS, SEDATIVES, and ANXIOLYTICS) may compound effects of cyclizine.

NURSING IMPLICATIONS

Administration

- Aspirate needle carefully before injecting IM. Anaphylactic reactions following inadvertent IV injection have been reported.
- For prophylaxis of postoperative nausea and vomiting, drug usually prescribed with preoperative medication or is administered 20–30 min before expected termination of surgery.
- Store tablets in tight, light-resistant container at 15–30C (59–86F) unless otherwise directed. Store parenteral form in a cold place at 5–10C (41–50F). When parenteral solution is stored at room temperature for prolonged periods, it may become slightly yellow, but this does not indicate loss of potency.

Assessment & Drug Effects

- Because cyclizine can cause hypotension, the postoperative patient receiving the drug will require close monitoring of vital signs.
- Monitor for and report signs of CNS stimulation (e.g., hyperexcitability, euphoria). Dose reduction or discontinuation of drug may be indicated.

Patient & Family Education

- Advise patient to take cyclizine with food or a glass of milk or water to minimize GI irritation.
- Forewarn patient about side effects of drowsiness and dizziness and advise not to drive a car or engage in other potentially hazardous activities until reaction to the drug is known.
- Caution patient that alcohol, barbiturates, narcotic

Common side effects in *italic*; life-threatening effects underlined; generic names in **bold**; classifications in SMALL CAPS

analgesic, and other CNS depressants may compound sedative action.

CYCLOBENZAPRINE HYDROCHLORIDE

See AUTONOMIC NERVOUS SYSTEM AGENT, SKELETAL MUSCLE RELAXANT, CENTRAL ACTING, prototype, p 122.

CYCLOPENTOLATE HYDROCHLORIDE

See EYE PREPARATION, CYCLOPLEGIC, prototype, p 208.

CYCLOPHOSPHAMIDE

See ANTINEOPLASTIC, ALKYLATING AGENT prototype, p 91.

Prototype: isoniazid, p 83

CYCLOSERINE

(sye-kloe-ser´een)
Trade name: Seromycin
Classifications: ANTIINFECTIVE;
ANTITUBERCULOSIS AGENT
Pregnancy: Category C

ACTIONS/PHARMACODYNAMICS Broad-spectrum antiinfective derived from strains of *Streptomyces orchidaceus* or *S. garyphalus;* also produced synthetically. Structural analog of the amino acid D-alanine. Inhibits cell wall synthesis in susceptible strains of gram-positive and gram-negative bacteria and in *Mycobacterium tuberculosis* by competitively interfering with the incorporation of D-alanine into the bacterial cell wall. Bacteriostatic or bactericidal depending on concentration and susceptibility of organism.

USES In conjunction with other tuberculostatic drugs in treatment of active pulmonary and extrapulmonary tuberculosis when primary agents isoniazid, rifampin, ethambutol, streptomycin have failed. Also used in treatment of acute UTI caused by *Enterobacter* sp and *Escherichia coli* that are unresponsive to conventional treatment. **Unlabeled use:** treatment of tuberculosis meningitis and nocardiosis.

ROUTE & DOSAGE

Tuberculosis

Adult	PO	250 mg q12h for 2 wk; may increase to 500 mg q12h (max 1g/d)

Urinary Tract Infection

Adult	PO	250 mg q12h for 2 wk

PHARMACOKINETICS Absorption: 70–90% absorbed from GI tract. **Peak:** 3–4 h. **Distribution:** distributed to lung, ascitic, pleural and synovial fluids, and CSF; crosses placenta; distributed into breast milk. **Metabolism:** not metabolized. **Elimination:** half-life: 10 h; 60–70% excreted in urine within 72 h; small amount in feces.

CONTRAINDICATIONS & PRECAUTIONS Contraindicated in: epilepsy; depression, severe anxiety, history of psychoses; severe renal insufficiency; chronic alcoholism. Safe use during pregnancy (category C), in nursing women, and in children not established.

ADVERSE/SIDE EFFECTS CNS: *drowsiness,* anxiety, *headache,* tremors, myoclonic jerking, convulsions, vertigo, visual disturbances, speech difficulties (dysarthria), lethargy, depression, disorientation with loss of memory, confusion, nervousness, psychoses, tic episodes, character changes, hyperirritability, aggression, hyperreflexia, peripheral neuropathy, paresthesias, paresis, dyskinesias. **CV:** arrhythmias, CHF. **Eye:** eye pain (optic neuritis), photophobia. **Hematologic:** vitamin B_{12} and folic acid deficiency, megaloblastic or sideroblastic anemia. **Hypersensitivity:** dermatitis, photosensitivity.

DRUG INTERACTIONS Alcohol increases risk of seizures; **ethionamide, isoniazid** potentiate neurotoxic effects; may inhibit **phenytoin** metabolism, increasing its toxicity.

NURSING IMPLICATIONS

Administration

- Pyridoxine 200–300 mg/d may be ordered concurrently to prevent neurotoxic effects of cycloserine.

Common side effects in *italic*; life-threatening effects underlined; generic names in **bold**; classifications in SMALL CAPS

479

- Store in tightly closed container at 15–30C (59–86F) unless otherwise directed.

Assessment & Drug Effects

- Culture and susceptibility tests should be performed before initiation of therapy and periodically thereafter to detect possible bacterial resistance.
- Monitoring of blood-drug levels and hematologic, renal, and hepatic function at regular intervals is advised.
- Maintenance of blood-drug level below 30 μg/ml considerably reduces incidence of neurotoxicity. Possibility of neurotoxicity increases when dose is 500 mg or more or when renal clearance is inadequate. Blood-drug levels should be determined at least weekly in these patients.
- Observe patient carefully for signs of hypersensitivity and neurologic effects. Neurotoxicity generally appears within first 2 wk of therapy and disappears after drug is discontinued.
- Drug should be discontinued or dosage reduced if symptoms of CNS toxicity or hypersensitivity reaction (see chap 3) develop.

Patient & Family Education

- Advise patient to take cycloserine after meals to prevent GI irritation.
- Advise patient or responsible family member to notify physician immediately of the onset of skin rash and early signs of CNS toxicity (see chap 3).
- Advise patient to avoid potentially hazardous tasks such as driving until reaction to cycloserine has been determined.
- Instruct patient to take drug precisely as prescribed and to keep follow-up appointments. Continuous therapy may extend into months or years.

CYCLOSPORINE

See IMMUNOSUPPRESSANT prototype, p 248.

Prototype: diphenhydramine, p 47

CYPROHEPTADINE HYDROCHLORIDE

(si-proe-hep′ta-deen)
Trade names: Periactin, Vimicon
Classifications: ANTIHISTAMINE; ANTIPRURITIC
Pregnancy: Category B

ACTIONS/PHARMACODYNAMICS Potent piperidine antihistamine with pharmacologic actions similar to those of azatadine. Acts by competing with histamine for H_1-receptor sites on effector cells, thus preventing histamine-mediated responses. Also competes with serotonin for receptor sites, thereby blocking response to serotonin. Produces mild central depression and moderate anticholinergic effects; lacks antiemetic action. Has significant antipruritic, local anesthetic, and antiserotonin activity. Also stimulates appetite, perhaps by activation of hypothalamic appetite-regulating center.

USES Symptomatic relief of various allergic conditions, including hay fever, vasomotor rhinitis, allergic conjunctivitis, urticaria caused by cold sensitivity, and pruritus of allergic dermatoses. Effective in treatment of anaphylactoid reactions as adjunct to epinephrine and other standard measures after acute symptoms have been controlled. **Unlabeled uses:** Cushing's disease, carcinoid syndrome, vascular headaches, and as appetite stimulant.

ROUTE & DOSAGE

Allergies

Adult	PO	4 mg t.i.d. or q.i.d.; (4–20 mg/d) max 0.5 mg/kg/d
Child	PO	0.25 mg/kg/d in 3–4 divided doses (max 12 mg/d for 2–6 y, 16 mg/d for 6–12 y)

PHARMACOKINETICS Absorption: readily absorbed from GI tract. **Duration:** 6–9 h. **Distribution:** distribution into breast milk not known. **Metabolism:** metabolized in liver. **Elimination:** excreted in urine.

CONTRAINDICATIONS & PRECAUTIONS Contraindicated in: hypersensitivity to cyproheptadine or other H_1-receptor antagonist antihistamines; acute asthma attack. Safe use during pregnancy (category B), in nursing mothers, and in children <2 y not established. **Cautious use in:** elderly and debilitated patients; patients predisposed to urinary retention; glaucoma; asthma; hyperthyroidism; cardiovascular disease, hypertension; GI or GU tract obstruction.

ADVERSE/SIDE EFFECTS CNS: *drowsiness,* dizziness, faintness, headache, tremulousness, fatigue, disturbed coordination. **ENT:** dry nose and throat. **GI:** *dry mouth,* nausea, vomiting, epigastric distress, appetite stimulation, weight gain, transient decrease in fasting blood sugar level, increased serum amylase level, cholestatic jaundice. **GU:** urinary frequency, retention, and difficult urination. **Other:** thickened bronchial secretions, skin rash.

DIAGNOSTIC TEST INTERFERENCES As a general rule, antihistamines are discontinued about 4 d before skin testing procedures are to be performed because they may produce false-negative results.

NURSING IMPLICATIONS

Administration

- GI side effects may be minimized by administering drug with food or milk.
- Store in tightly covered container at 15–30C (59–86F) unless otherwise directed.

Assessment & Drug Effects

- In some patients, the sedative effect disappears spontaneously after 3–4 d of drug administration.
- Since drug may cause dizziness, supervision of ambulation and other safety precautions may be warranted.

Patient & Family Education

- Warn the patient to avoid activities requiring mental alertness and physical coordination, such as driving a car, until reaction to the drug is known.
- Causes sedation, dizziness, and hypotension in the elderly. Advise patient to report these symptoms. Children are more apt to manifest CNS stimulation, e.g., confusion, agitation, tremors, hallucinations. Reduction in dosage may be indicated.
- Cyproheptadine may increase and prolong the effects of alcohol, barbiturates, narcotic analgesics, anxiolytics, and other CNS depressants.
- Patient should monitor weight and keep physician informed of any significant weight gain.
- Maintaining sufficient fluid intake may help to relieve dry mouth and also may reduce risk of cholestatic jaundice.

Prototype: fluorouracil, p 94

CYTARABINE
(sye-tare´a-been)
Trade names: ARA-C, Cytosar-U, Cytosine Arabinoside
Classifications: ANTINEOPLASTIC; ANTIMETABOLITE; IMMUNOSUPPRESSANT
Pregnancy: Category D

ACTIONS/PHARMACODYNAMICS Pyrimidine analog with cell phase specificity affecting rapidly dividing cells in S phase (DNA synthesis). In certain conditions prevents development of cell from G_1 to S phase. Interferes with DNA synthesis by blocking conversion of cytidine to deoxycytidine and may be incorporated into RNA molecule. Has strong myelosuppressant activity. Immunosuppressant properties are exhibited by obliterated cell-mediated immune responses, such as delayed hypersensitivity skin reactions.

USES To induce and maintain remission in acute myelocytic leukemia, acute lymphocytic leukemia, and meningeal leukemia and for treatment of lymphomas. Used in combination with other antineoplastics in established chemotherapeutic protocols.

ROUTE & DOSAGE

Leukemias		
Adult	IV	200 mg/m² by continuous infusion over 24 h
	SC	1 mg/kg 1–2 times/wk
	Intrathecal	5–75 mg once q4d or once/d for 4 d
Child	IV	Same as for adult
	SC	Same as for adult
	Intrathecal	Same as for adult

PHARMACOKINETICS Peak: 20–60 min SC. **Distribution:** crosses blood-brain barrier in moderate amounts; crosses placenta. **Metabolism:** metabolized primarily in liver. **Elimination:** half-life: 1–3 h; 80% excreted in urine in 24 h.

CONTRAINDICATIONS & PRECAUTIONS Contraindicated in: history of drug-induced myelosuppression; immunization procedures. Safe use during pregnancy (category D) particularly during first trimester, nursing mothers, and infants not established. **Cautious use in:** impaired renal or hepatic function, gout, drug-induced myelosuppression.

ADVERSE/SIDE EFFECTS CNS: headache, neurotoxicity; peripheral neuropathy, brachial plexus neuropathy, personality change, neuritis, vertigo, lethargy, somnolence, confusion. **Eye:** conjunctivitis, keratitis, photophobia. **GI:** *nausea, vomiting,* diarrhea, stomatitis, oral or anal inflammation or ulceration, esophagitis, anorexia, hemorrhage. **Hematologic:** *leukopenia, thrombocytopenia,* anemia, megaloblast

---

Common side effects in *italic*; life-threatening effects underlined; generic names in **bold**; classifications in SMALL CAPS

481

tosis, myelosuppression (reversible); transient hyper-uricemia. **Hepatic:** hepatotoxicity, jaundice. **Renal:** renal dysfunction, urinary retention. **Skin:** rash, erythema, freckling, cellulitis, skin ulcerations, pruritus, urticaria, bulla formation, desquamation. **Other:** weight loss, sore throat, fever, thrombophlebitis and pain at injection site; pericarditis, bleeding (any site), pneumonia. Potentially carcinogenic and mutagenic.

DRUG INTERACTIONS GI toxicity may decrease **digoxin** absorption; decreases AMINOGLYCOSIDES activity against *Klebsiella pneumoniae*.

INCOMPATIBILITIES Solution/Additive: cephalothin, fluorouracil, gentamicin, heparin, insulin, nafcillin, oxacillin, penicillin G.

NURSING IMPLICATIONS

Administration

- The 100 mg and 500 mg vials are reconstituted with 5 ml and 10 ml, respectively, of bacteriostatic water for injection. (Diluents containing benzyl alcohol must not be used for neonates. A fatal toxic syndrome could result.)
- Reconstitued drug may be given by direct IV at a rate of 100 mg or a fracion thereof over 3 min.
- For IV infusion the reconstituted solution may be further diluted with 5% dextrose or 0.9% NaCl injection and infused over 1–24 h.
- Nausea and vomiting of several hours' duration complicate rapid direct IV injection. Effects are less severe with IV infusion. Administration of cytarabine 1 h before meals or giving an antiemetic before the drug may reduce these side effects. Noncontinuous dosage schedules may permit the patient to tolerate larger amounts of drug.
- For intrathecal injection, reconstitute with an isotonic, buffered diluent without preservatives. Follow manufacturer's recommendations. Solution should be administered as soon as possible after preparation.
- Store cytarabine in refrigerator until reconstituted. Reconstituted solutions may be stored at 15–30C (59–86F) for 48 h. Solutions with a slight haze should be discarded.

Assessment & Drug Effects

- Inspect patient's mouth before the administration of each dose. Toxicity necessitating dosage alterations almost always occurs. Report adverse reactions immediately.
- Hematocrit and platelet counts and total and differential leukocyte counts should be evaluated daily during initial therapy. Serum uric acid and hepatic function tests should be performed at regular intervals throughout treatment period.

- Hyperuricemia due to rapid destruction of neoplastic cells may accompany cytarabine therapy. A regimen that includes a uricosuric agent such as allopurinol, urine alkalinization, and adequate hydration may be started. To reduce potential for urate stone formation, fluids are forced in excess of 2 L, if tolerated. Consult physician.
- Monitor I&O ratio and pattern.
- During granulocytic periods, development of usual signs of inflammation may be inhibited. Monitor body temperature. Be alert to the most subtle signs of infection, especially low-grade fever, and report promptly.
- When platelet count falls below 50,000/mm^3 and polymorphonuclear leukocytes to below 1000/mm^3, therapy may be suspended. WBC nadir is usually reached in 5–7 d after therapy has been stopped. Therapy is restarted with appearance of bone marrow recovery and when preceding cell counts are reached.
- Provide good oral hygiene to diminish side effects and chance of superinfection. Stomatitis and cheilosis usually appear 5–10 d into the therapy.

Patient & Family Education

- Advise patient to report promptly protracted vomiting or signs of nephrotoxicity (see chap 3).
- Flulike syndrome occurs usually within 6–12 wk after drug administration and may recur with successive therapy. Instruct patient to report chills, fever, achy joints and muscles.
- Advise patient to report any signs and symptoms of superinfection (see chap 3).

Prototype: cyclophosphamide, p 91

DACARBAZINE

(da-kar´ba-zeen)

Trade names: DTIC, DTIC-Dome, Imidazole carboxamide

Classifications: ANTINEOPLASTIC; ALKYLATING AGENT

Pregnancy: Category C

ACTIONS/PHARMACODYNAMICS Cytotoxic agent with alkylating properties. Cell-cycle nonspecific. Interferes with purine metabolism and with

Common side effects in *italic*; life-threatening effects underlined; generic names in **bold**; classifications in SMALL CAPS

RNA and protein synthesis in rapidly proliferating cells. Has minimal immunosuppressive activity; reportedly carcinogenic, mutagenic, and teratogenic.

USES As single agent or in combination with other antineoplastics in treatment of metastatic malignant melanoma, refractory Hodgkin's disease, various sarcomas, and neuroblastoma. **Unlabeled use:** soft tissue metastatic sarcoma and malignant glucagonoma.

ROUTE & DOSAGE

Neoplasms

Adult	IV	2–4.5 mg/kg/d for 10 d repeated at 4 wk intervals, *or* 250 mg/m²/d for 5 d repeated at 3 wk intervals

PHARMACOKINETICS Distribution: localizes primarily in liver. **Metabolism:** extensively metabolized in liver. **Elimination:** half-life: 5 h; 35–50% excreted in urine in 6 h.

CONTRAINDICATIONS & PRECAUTIONS Contraindicated in: safe use during pregnancy (category C) not established.

ADVERSE/SIDE EFFECTS CNS: confusion, headache, seizures, blurred vision. **GI:** *anorexia, nausea, vomiting.* **Hematologic:** severe leukopenia and thrombocytopenia, mild anemia. **Hypersensitivity:** erythematosus, urticarial rashes; hepatotoxicity, photosensitivity. **Other:** alopecia, facial paresthesia and flushing, flu-like syndrome, myalgia, malaise, anaphylaxis, *pain along injected vein.*

INCOMPATIBILITIES Solution/Additive: heparin.

NURSING IMPLICATIONS

Administration

■ Should be administered to hospitalized patients because close observation and frequent laboratory studies are required during and after therapy.

■ All handlers of dacarbazine should wear gloves. If solution gets into the eyes, wash them with soap and water immediately, then irrigate with water or isotonic saline.

■ Reconstitute drug with sterile water for injection to make a solution containing 10 mg/ml dacarbazine (pH 3.0–4.0) by adding 9.9 ml to 100 mg or 19.8 ml to 200 mg. The reconstituted solution may be further diluted.

■ Resulting solution is administered through a free-flowing IV with 5% dextrose injection or NaCl in-

jection. Administered by direct IV over 1 min or by IV infusion over 30 min.

■ *IV extravasation:* Monitor injection site frequently (instruct patient to do so, if able): Give prompt attention to patient's complaint of swelling, stinging, and burning sensation around injection site. Extravasation can occur painlessly and without visual signs.

■ *Danger areas for extravasation:* dorsum of hand or ankle (especially if peripheral arteriosclerosis is present), joint spaces and previously irradiated areas. If possible avoid using antecubital vein or veins on dorsum of hand or wrist where extravasation could lead to loss of mobility of entire limb. Avoid veins in extremity with compromised venous or lymphatic drainage and veins near joint spaces.

■ If extravasation is suspected, infusion should be stopped immediately and restarted in another in vein. Report to the physician. Prompt institution of local treatment is imperative.

■ Store reconstituted solution up to 72 h at 4C (39F) or at room temperature for up to 8 h. Store diluted reconstituted solution for 24 h at 4C (39F) or at room temperature for up to 8 h. Protect from light.

Assessment & Drug Effects

■ Check patient's mouth for ulcerative stomatitis prior to the administration of each dose.

■ Skin damage by dacarbazine can lead to deep necrosis requiring surgical debridement, skin grafting, and even amputation. At risk are the elderly, very young, comatose, and debilitated patients. Other risk factors include establishing an IV line in a vein previously punctured several times and nonplastic catheters.

■ Hematopoietic toxicity usually appears about 4 wk after first dose. Generally a leukocyte count of <3000/mm³ and a platelet count of <100,000/mm³ require suspension or cessation of therapy. Leukopenia and thrombocytopenia can be severe enough to cause death.

■ Restriction of oral fluids and food for 4–6 h prior to treatment may prevent vomiting. Palliation and prevention of vomiting may be provided also by administration of an antiemetic.

■ During platelet nadir avoid if possible all tests and treatments (e.g., IM) requiring needle punctures. Observe carefully and report evidence of unexplained bleeding.

■ Protect patient from excess expenditure of energy and from infection, especially during leukocyte nadir. Monitor temperature and report any elevation immediately.

■ Severe nausea and vomiting (>90% of patients) be-

Common side effects in *italic*; life-threatening effects <u>underlined</u>; generic names in **bold**; classifications in SMALL CAPS

483

gins within 1 h after drug administration and may last for as long as 12 h.

- Most patients develop tolerance to vomiting and diarrhea after the first 1 or 2 d. If vomiting persists, discontinuation of therapy may be necessary.
- Monitor I&O ratio and pattern and daily temperature. Renal impairment extends the half-life and increases danger of toxicity. Report symptoms of renal dysfunction and even a slight elevation of temperature.

Patient & Family Education

- Flulike syndrome may occur during or even a week after treatment is terminated and last 7–21 d. Symptoms frequently recur with successive treatments. Advise patient to report them to physician.
- Caution patient to avoid prolonged exposure to sunlight or to ultraviolet light during treatment period and for at least 2 wk after last dose. Protect exposed skin with sun screen lotion (≥SPF 15) and avoid exposure in midday.
- Warn patient to report promptly the onset of blurred vision or paresthesia.

Prototype: mechlorethamine, p 96

DACTINOMYCIN

(dak-ti-noe-mye´sin)
Trade names: Actinomycin, Cosmegen, Lyovac
Classifications: ANTINEOPLASTIC, ANTIINFECTIVE; ANTIBIOTIC; IMMUNOSUPPRESSANT
Pregnancy: Category C

ACTIONS/PHARMACODYNAMICS Potent cytotoxic antibiotic derived from mixture of actinomycins produced by *Streptomyces parvullus.* Toxic properties preclude its use as antibiotic. Complexes with DNA, thereby inhibiting DNA, RNA, and protein synthesis. Causes delayed myelosuppression; is strongly tissue corrosive and has a low therapeutic index. Potentiates effects of x-ray therapy; the converse also appears likely. Recent reports indicate increased potential for secondary primary tumors following treatment with x-ray and dactinomycin.

USES As single agent or in combination with other antineoplastics or radiation to treat Wilms' tumor, rhabdomyosarcoma, carcinoma of testes and uterus, Ewing's sarcoma, and sarcoma botryoides. **Unlabeled**

use: malignant melanoma, trophoblastic tumors, Kaposi's sarcoma, osteogenic sarcoma, among others.

ROUTE & DOSAGE

Neoplasms

Adult	IV	500 µg/d for a maximum of 5 d; may repeat at 2–4 wk intervals if tolerated
Child	IV	15 µg/kg/d (max 500 µg) for 5 d *or* 2.5 mg/m² over 7 d; may repeat at 2–4 wk intervals if tolerated

Isolation Perfusion

Adult	IV	50 µg/kg for lower extremity or pelvis; 35 µg/kg for upper extremity

PHARMACOKINETICS Distribution: concentrated in liver, spleen, kidneys, and bone marrow; does not cross blood-brain barrier; crosses placenta; distribution into breast milk not known. **Elimination:** half-life: 36 h; 50% excreted unchanged in bile and 10% in urine; only 30% excreted in urine over 9 d.

CONTRAINDICATIONS & PRECAUTIONS Contraindicated in: chickenpox, herpes zoster, and other viral infections; pregnancy (category C), lactation, infants <6 mo. **Cautious use in:** previous therapy with antineoplastics or radiation within 3–6 wk, bone marrow depression; infections; history of gout; impairment of kidney or liver function; obesity.

ADVERSE/SIDE EFFECTS GI: cheilitis, ulcerative stomatitis, esophagitis, dysphagia, hepatotoxicity, hepatomegaly, proctitis, anorexia, *nausea, vomiting,* abdominal pain, diarrhea, GI ulceration. **Hematologic:** anemia (including aplastic anemia), agranulocytosis, leukopenia, thrombocytopenia, pancytopenia, reticulopenia. **Skin:** acne, desquamation, hyperpigmentation and reactivation of erythema especially over previously irradiated areas, *alopecia* (reversible). **Other:** malaise, fatigue, lethargy, fever, myalgia, anaphylaxis, gonadal suppression, hypocalcemia, hyperuricemia, thrombophlebitis; *necrosis, sloughing and contractures at site of extravasation.*

DRUG INTERACTIONS Elevated uric acid level produced by dactinomycin may necessitate dose adjustment of ANTIGOUT AGENTS; effects of both dactinomycin and other MYELOSUPPRESSANTS are potentiated; effects of both **radiation** and dactinomycin are potentiated, and dactinomycin may reactivate erythema from previous radiation therapy; **vitamin K** effects (antihemorrhagic) decreased, leading to prolonged clotting time and potential hemorrhage.

NURSING IMPLICATIONS

Administration

- Manufacturer advises use of gloves and eye shield to protect the person making the solution. If skin is contaminated, rinse with running water for 10 min, then rinse with buffered phosphate solution. If solution gets into the eyes, wash with water immediately; then irrigate with water or isotonic saline for 10 min.
- Reconstitute by adding 1.1 mg sterile water for injection (without preservative); the resulting solution will contain approximately 0.5 mg/ml.
- Once reconstituted, dactinomycin may be added directly to infusion solutions of 5% dextrose injection or NaCl injection, or into tubing or side arm of a running IV infusion, and administered over a 10–15 min period. Discard unused portion.
- Following IV injection, some clinicians recommend injecting 5–10 ml IV solution into the side arm or flushing the vein with running IV infusion for 2–5 min to remove any remaining drug from tubing.
- Observe injection site frequently; if extravasation occurs, stop infusion immediately. Infusion should be restarted in another vein. Report to physician. Prompt institution of local treatment to prevent thrombophlebitis and necrosis is imperative.
- The obese or edematous patient is given a lower dose of dactinomycin calculated at 400–600 $\mu g/m^2$ to relate dosage to lean body mass. Monitor for symptoms of toxicity from overdosage.
- Store drug at 15–30C (59–86F) unless otherwise advised. Protect from heat and light.

Assessment & Drug Effects

- Severe, sometimes fatal, toxic effects occur with high frequency. Effects usually appear 2–4 d after a course of therapy is stopped and may reach maximal severity 1–2 wk following discontinuation of therapy.
- Nausea and vomiting usually occur a few hours after drug administration and are generally controlled by an antiemetic drug. Vomiting may be severe enough to require intermittent therapy. Observe patient daily for signs of drug toxicity.
- Frequent determinations of renal, hepatic, and bone marrow function are advised. WBC counts should be performed daily and platelet counts every 3 d to detect hematopoietic depression.
- Monitor temperature and inspect oral membranes daily for stomatitis.
- The combination of stomatitis, diarrhea, and severe hematopoietic depression usually requires prompt interruption of therapy until drug toxicity subsides.

- Report onset of unexplained bleeding, jaundice, and wheezing. Also, be alert to signs of agranulocytosis (see chap 3). Report to physician. Antibiotic therapy, protective isolation, and discontinuation of the antineoplastic are indicated.
- Dactinomycin is usually given no later than the first 5–7 d of radiation therapy because of risk of severe drug-induced skin reactions (erythema, desquamation, pigmentation).
- Radiation therapy is generally continued despite the occurrence of drug-induced skin reactions and the side effects of radiation (gastric distress and severe mucositis near site of radiation).
- Observe and report symptoms of hyperuricemia (see chap 3). Urge patient to increase fluid intake up to 3000 ml/d if allowed.

Patient & Family Education

- Discuss possibility of gonadal suppression (amenorrhea or azoospermia) with patient before therapy is instituted. This may be an irreversible side effect.
- Patient should be advised of the potential for nausea and vomiting and of what preventative measures will be taken to minimize these side effects.
- Patient should be informed that reversible alopecia is an anticipated side effect. Appropriate supportive guidance should be provided.

Prototype: testosterone, p 229

DANAZOL

(da´na-zole)

Trade names: Cyclomen, Danocrine

Classifications: SYNTHETIC HORMONE; ANDROGEN/ANABOLIC STEROID

Pregnancy: Category C

ACTIONS/PHARMACODYNAMICS Synthetic androgen steroid; derivative of testosterone with dose-related mild androgenic effects but no estrogenic or progestational activity. Suppresses pituitary output of FSH and LH, resulting in anovulation and associated amenorrhea. Interrupts progress and pain of endometriosis by causing atrophy and involution of both normal and ectopic endometrial tissue. Has no effect on large endometriomas or on anatomic deformities associated with pain of dysmenorrhea.

USES Palliative treatment of endometriosis when alternative hormonal therapy is ineffective, contraindi-

Common side effects in *italic*; life-threatening effects underlined; generic names in **bold**; classifications in SMALL CAPS

485

D

cated, or intolerable. Also used to treat fibrocystic breast disease and hereditary angioedema. **Unlabeled uses:** to treat precocious puberty, gynecomastia, menorrhagia, premenstrual syndrome (PMS), chronic immune thrombocytopenic purpura (ITP), autoimmune hemolytic anemia, hemophilia A and B.

ROUTE & DOSAGE

Endometriosis

Adult	PO	400 mg b.i.d. for 3–6 mo; start during menstruation or if pregnancy test is negative; therapy may be extended to 9 mo if necessary; regimen cannot be repeated

Fibrocystic Breast Disease

Adult	PO	100–400 mg in 2 divided doses; start during menstruation or if pregnancy test is negative

Hereditary Angioedema

Adult	PO	200 mg b.i.d. or t.i.d.; may decrease by 50% at intervals of 1–3 mo or longer; start during menstruation or if pregnancy test is negative

PHARMACOKINETICS Elimination: half-life: 4.5 h; other pharmacokinetic information is not known.

CONTRAINDICATIONS & PRECAUTIONS Contraindicated in: pregnancy (category C), nursing mothers, children, undiagnosed abnormal genital bleeding; impaired renal, cardiac, or hepatic function. **Cautious use in:** migraine headache, epilepsy.

ADVERSE/SIDE EFFECTS Androgenic (virilization): acne, mild hirsutism, deepening of voice, oily skin and hair, hair loss, edema, weight gain, pitch breaks, voice weakness, decrease in breast size. **CNS:** dizziness, sleep disorders, fatigue, tremor, irritability. **Eye:** conjunctival edema. **GI:** gastroenteritis. **GU:** decreased libido. **Hypersensitivity:** skin rashes, nasal congestion. **Hypoestrogenic:** *hot flushes;* sweating; emotional lability; nervousness; vaginitis with itching, drying, burning, or bleeding; amenorrhea, irregular menstrual patterns. **Musculoskeletal:** carpal tunnel syndrome, joint lock-up, joint swelling. **Other:** elevated BP, possibility of cholestatic jaundice, hepatitis, <u>hepatic damage</u>, thrombocytopenia, increased LDL; decreased HDL; impairment in glucose tolerance.

NURSING IMPLICATIONS

Administration

- For patients with endometriosis or irregular periods or fibrocystic breast disease, therapy should start during menstruation, or a pregnancy test should be performed before treatment is initiated.
- Store capsules at 15–30C (59–86F) in tightly closed container.

Assessment & Drug Effects

- Routine breast examinations should be carried out during therapy. Carcinoma of the breast should be ruled out prior to start of therapy for fibrocystic breast disease. Advise patient to report to physician if any nodule enlarges or becomes tender or hard during therapy.
- In fibrocystic breast disease, inform patient that pain and discomfort is usually relieved in 2 or 3 mo; the nodularity in 4–6 mo. Menses may be regular or irregular in pattern during therapy.
- Because danazol may cause fluid retention, patients with cardiac or renal dysfunction, epilepsy, or migraine should be observed closely during therapy, as these problems could worsen. Monitor weight.
- Drug-induced edema may compress the median nerve, producing symptoms of carpal tunnel syndrome. If patient complains of wrist pain that worsens at night, paresthesias in radial palmar aspect of the hand and fingers, consult physician.
- Baseline and periodic liver function tests should be performed in all patients. Patients with diabetes (or history of) should have blood glucose tests.
- Semen of adolescents, especially, should be checked q3–4 mo for volume, viscosity, motility, and sperm count.

Patient & Family Education

- Drug-induced amenorrhea is reversible. Ovulation and cyclic bleeding usually return within 60–90 d after therapeutic regimen is discontinued. Advise patient that potential for conception may also be restored at that time.
- A nonhormonal contraceptive should be used during danazol treatment (because ovulation may not be suppressed) until 6–8 wk of therapy. If pregnancy occurs while patient is receiving the drug, danazol should be discontinued, and the question of continuing the pregnancy considered.
- Advise patient to report voice changes promptly. Drug should be stopped to avoid permanent damage to voice. Virilizing side effects may persist even after drug therapy is terminated.

Common side effects in *italic*; life-threatening effects <u>underlined</u>; generic names in **bold**; classifications in SMALL CAPS

Prototype: cyclobenzaprine, p 122

DANTROLENE SODIUM
(dan´troe-leen)
Trade name: Dantrium
Classifications: AUTONOMIC NERVOUS SYSTEM AGENT; SKELETAL MUSCLE RELAXANT, CENTRAL
Pregnancy: Category C

ACTIONS/PHARMACODYNAMICS Hydantoin derivative, structurally related to phenytoin, with peripheral skeletal muscle relaxant action. Directly relaxes the spastic muscle by interfering with calcium ion (contraction activator) release from sarcoplasmic reticulum. Clinical doses produce about a 50% decrease in contractility of skeletal muscles but no effect on smooth or cardiac muscles. Relief of spasticity may be accompanied by muscle weakness sufficient to affect overall functional capacity of the patient. Reduces spastic or reflex contractions more than voluntary activity.

USES Orally for the symptomatic treatment of skeletal muscle spasms secondary to spinal cord injury, stroke, cerebral palsy, multiple sclerosis. Used intravenously for the management of malignant hyperthermia. Oral dantrolene has been used prophylactically (2 or 3 d before anesthesia) for patients with a history of malignant hyperthermia or with a family history of the disorder. **Unlabeled use:** neuroleptic malignant syndrome, exercise-induced muscle pain, and flexor spasms.

PHARMACOKINETICS Absorption: about 35% slowly and incompletely absorbed from GI tract. **Peak:** 5 h. **Distribution:** crosses placenta. **Metabolism:** metabolized in liver. **Elimination:** half-life: 8.7 h; excreted in urine chiefly as metabolites.

CONTRAINDICATIONS & PRECAUTIONS Contraindicated in: active hepatic disease; when spasticity is necessary to sustain upright posture and balance in locomotion or to maintain increased body function; spasticity due to rheumatic disorders. Safe use during pregnancy (category C), in nursing mothers, and in children <5 y not established. **Cautious use in:** impaired cardiac or pulmonary function, patients >35 y, especially women.

ROUTE & DOSAGE

Relief of Spasticity

Adult	PO	25 mg once/d; increase to 25 mg b.i.d. to q.i.d.; may increase q4–7d up to 100 mg b.i.d. to q.i.d.
Child	PO	0.5 mg/kg b.i.d.; increase to 0.5 mg/kg t.i.d. or q.i.d.; may increase by 0.5 mg/kg up to 3 mg/kg b.i.d. to q.i.d. (max 100 mg q.i.d.)

Malignant Hyperthermia

Adult	IV	1 mg/kg rapid IV push repeated prn up to a total of 10 mg/kg
	PO	May be necessary to continue orally with 1–2 mg/kg q.i.d. for 1–3 d to prevent recurrence
Child	IV	Same as for adult
	PO	Same as for adult

ADVERSE/SIDE EFFECTS CNS: drowsiness, *muscle weakness,* dizziness, light-headedness, unusual fatigue, speech disturbances, headache, confusion, nervousness, mental depression, insomnia, euphoria, seizures. **CV:** tachycardia, erratic BP. **Eye:** blurred vision, diplopia, photophobia. **GI:** *diarrhea,* constipation, nausea, vomiting, anorexia, swallowing difficulty, alterations of taste, gastric irritation, abdominal cramps, GI bleeding. **GU:** crystalluria with pain or burning with urination, urinary frequency, urinary retention, nocturia, enuresis, difficult erection. **Hepatic** (prolonged use of high doses): hepatitis, jaundice, hepatomegaly, <u>hepatic necrosis</u>. **Hypersensitivity:** pruritus, urticaria, eczematoid skin eruption, photosensitivity, eosinophilic pleural effusion.

DRUG INTERACTIONS Alcohol and other CNS DEPRESSANTS compound CNS depression; ESTROGENS increase risk of hepatotoxicity in women >35 y; **verapamil** and other CALCIUM CHANNEL BLOCKERS increase risk of ventricular fibrillation and cardiovascular collapse with IV dantrolene.

NURSING IMPLICATIONS

Administration

- If necessary, an oral suspension for a single dose may be made by emptying contents of capsule(s) into fruit juice or other liquid. Pharmacist can prepare a multiple dose suspension on request. Suspension should be shaken well before it is poured. Since it will not contain a preservative, avoid contamination, keep refrigerated, and use within several days.

- For IV administration, dilute each 20 mg with 60 ml sterile water without preservatives. Shake until clear; then give by rapid direct IV injection.
- IV extravasation should be avoided. Solution has a high pH and therefore is extremely irritating to tissue. Observe and palpate entry site frequently during therapy.
- Store capsules in tightly closed light-resistant container. Contents of vial (for IV use) must be protected from direct light and used within 6 h after reconstitution, since it does not contain a preservative. Both PO and parenteral forms are stored at 15–30C (59–86F) unless otherwise directed.

Assessment & Drug Effects

- Prior to initiation of therapy, an assessment should be made of patient's neuromuscular function as a baseline for comparison.
- During IV infusion, monitor vital signs. ECG, CVP, and serum potassium should also be monitored.
- Supervise ambulation until patient's reaction to drug is known. Relief of spasticity may be accompanied by some loss of voluntary strength, which may impede patient's ability to maintain balance and an upright posture.
- The most common side effects are drowsiness, dizziness, fatigue, muscular weakness, general malaise, headache, diarrhea. Symptoms are generally transient, lasting up to 14 d after initiation of therapy. Keep physician informed.
- Patients with impaired cardiac or pulmonary function should be closely monitored for cardiovascular or respiratory symptoms such as tachycardia, BP changes, feeling of suffocation.
- Because of the possibility of hepatotoxicity (see Signs & Symptoms, chap 3), it is recommended that drug be discontinued if improvement is not evident within 45 d.
- Improvement may not be apparent until 1 wk or more of drug therapy.
- Baseline and regularly scheduled hepatic function tests (alkaline phosphatase, AST, ALT, total bilirubin), blood cell counts, and renal function tests should be performed.
- Risk of hepatotoxicity is greater in females >35 y, patients taking other medications, and in patients taking high dantrolene doses (400 mg or more daily) for prolonged periods.
- Monitor bowel function. Persistent diarrhea may necessitate drug withdrawal. Severe constipation with abdominal distension and signs of intestinal obstruction have been reported.

Patient & Family Education

- Instruct patient to report promptly the onset of jaundice: yellow skin, or sclerae; dark urine, clay-colored stools, itching, abdominal discomfort. Hepatotoxicity more frequently occurs between 3rd and 12th mo of therapy.
- Patients with malignant hyperthermia should be advised to wear medical identification (e.g., Medic Alert), indicating diagnosis, physician, telephone number, and drug.
- Advise patient to report symptoms of allergy and of *allergic pleural effusion:* shortness of breath, pleuritic pain, dry cough.
- Forewarn patient of the possibility of dizziness and drowsiness and advise to avoid driving and other potentially hazardous activities until reaction to drug is known.
- Since hepatotoxicity occurs more commonly when other drugs are taken concurrently, advise patient not to take OTC medications, alcoholic beverages, or other CNS depressants unless otherwise advised by physician.

DAPSONE

See ANTIINFECTIVE, ANTILEPROSY (SULFONE) AGENT prototype, p 77.

Prototype: mechlorethamine, p 96

DAUNORUBICIN HYDROCHLORIDE
(daw-noe-roo´bi-sin)
Trade names: Cerubidine, DNR
Classifications: ANTINEOPLASTIC; ANTIINFECTIVE; ANTIBIOTIC; IMMUNOSUPPRESSANT
Pregnancy: Category D

ACTIONS/PHARMACODYNAMICS Cytotoxic and antimitotic glycoside antibiotic; cell-cycle specific for S-phase of cell division. Toxic properties preclude its use as an antibiotic. Action mechanism unclear but may be due to rapid intercalating of DNA molecule resulting in inhibition of DNA, RNA, and protein synthesis. A potent bone marrow suppressant, with immunosuppressive properties. Induces cardiac toxicity and may be mutagenic and carcinogenic (development of secondary carcinomas).

Common side effects in *italic*; life-threatening effects <u>underlined</u>; generic names in **bold**; classifications in SMALL CAPS

USES To induce remission in acute nonlymphocytic leukemia (myelogenous, monocytic, erythroid) in adults. **Unlabeled use:** solid tumors of childhood and non-Hodgkin's lymphoma.

ROUTE & DOSAGE

Neoplasms

Adult	IV	Single agent: 30–60 mg/m²/d for 3–5 d q3–4wk (maximum total cumulative dose 500–600 mg/m²)
		Combination therapy: 30–45 mg/m²/d on days 1, 2, 3 of first course and days 1 and 2 of subsequent courses
Child	IV	Combination therapy: ≥2 y: 25–45 mg/m²
		<2 y: calculated on body weight (mg/kg) rather than body surface area

PHARMACOKINETICS Distribution: highest concentrations in spleen, kidneys, liver, lungs, and heart; does not cross blood-brain barrier; crosses placenta; distribution into breast milk not known. **Metabolism:** metabolized in liver to active metabolite. **Elimination:** half-life: 18.5–26.7 h; 25% excreted in urine, 40% in bile.

CONTRAINDICATIONS & PRECAUTIONS Contraindicated in: severe myelosuppression; immunizations (patient, family), and preexisting cardiac disease unless risk-benefit is evaluated; lactation; uncontrolled systemic infection. Safe use during pregnancy (category D) and in nursing women not established. **Cautious use in:** history of gout, urate calculi, hepatic or renal function impairment; elderly patients with inadequate bone reserve due to age or previous cytotoxic drug therapy, tumor cell infiltration of bone marrow, patient who has received potentially cardiotoxic drugs or related antineoplastics.

ADVERSE/SIDE EFFECTS CV: pericarditis, myocarditis, arrhythmias, peripheral edema, CHF. **GI:** *acute nausea and vomiting* (mild), anorexia, *stomatitis,* mucositis, diarrhea (occasionally). **Hematopoietic:** bone marrow depression, thrombocytopenia, leukopenia, anemia. **Skin:** generalized *alopecia* (reversible), transverse pigmentation of nails, contact dermatitis, urticaria. **Other:** hyperuricemia, fever, gonadal suppression, severe cellulitis or tissue necrosis at site of drug extravasation.

INCOMPATIBILITIES Solution/Additive: dexamethasone, heparin.

NURSING IMPLICATIONS

Administration

- Use of gloves during preparation of the solution for infusion is recommended to prevent skin contact with the drug. If this occurs, decontaminate with copious amounts of water with soap.
- Reconstitute 20 mg vial with 4 ml sterile water for injection. Concentrations of the solution will be 5 mg/ml. Withdraw dose into syringe containing 10–15 ml normal saline and inject over approximately 3 min into the tubing or side arm of a rapidly flowing IV infusion of 5% glucose or normal saline solution.
- Daunorubicin should never be administered IM or SC, and it should never be mixed with other drugs.
- If serum bilirubin is 1.2–3.0 mg/dl, the recommended dose is 3/4 normal dose; if serum bilirubin is >3 mg/dl, 1/2 normal dose is recommended; *normal serum bilirubin:* 0.7 mg/dl.
- When serum creatinine is > 3 mg/dl, the dose is reduced to 1/2 normal value; *normal serum creatinine:* 0.7–1.5 mg/dl.
- Reconstituted solution is stable 24 h at room temperature and 48 h under refrigeration at 2–8C (36–46F) protected from light.

Assessment & Drug Effects

- Extravasation can cause severe tissue necrosis and therefore must be avoided.
- Hct, platelet count, total and differential leukocyte count, serum uric acid, chest x ray, and cardiac, hepatic, and renal function tests should be performed prior to and periodically during therapy.
- Prior to each course of therapy, tests are performed to recognize patients at greatest risk for development of acute CHF.
- Monitor BP, temperature, pulse, and respiratory function during treatment.
- Acute CHF can occur suddenly, especially when total dosage exceeds 550 mg/m², or in patients with compromised heart function because of previous radiation therapy to heart area.
- Report immediately breathlessness, orthopnea, change in pulse and BP parameters. Early clinical diagnosis of drug-induced CHF is essential for successful treatment.
- A profound suppression of bone marrow is required to induce a complete remission. Nadirs for thrombocytes and leukocytes are usually reached in 10–14 d.
- Myelosuppression imposes risk of superimposed infection. Promptly report elevation of temperature, chills, symptoms of upper respiratory tract in-

Common side effects in *italic*; life-threatening effects underlined; generic names in **bold**; classifications in SMALL CAPS

489

D

fection, tachycardia, symptoms of overgrowth with opportunistic organisms—superinfection (see chap 3).

- Protect patient from contact with persons with infections. The most hazardous period is during nadirs of thrombocytes and leukocytes.
- Drug-induced hyperuricemia (see Signs & Symptoms, chap 3) may occur because of rapid lysis of leukemic cells. Monitor serum uric acid levels; *normal serum uric acid:* 3–7 mg/dl.
- Nausea and vomiting are usually mild and may be controlled by antiemetic therapy.
- Inspect oral membranes daily. Mucositis may occur 3–7 d after drug is administered.

Patient & Family Education

- Discuss probability of onset of alopecia but inform patient that recovery is usual in 6–10 wk.
- Discuss possibility of gonadal suppression (amenorrhea or azoospermia) before treatment begins. Patient should understand that usually it is an irreversible side effect.
- Advise against conception during treatment because of teratogenic properties of the drug. Advise patient to report to the physician should she become pregnant.
- Forewarn patient that daunorubicin may turn urine red (a transient effect) on the day of infusion.

DEFEROXAMINE MESYLATE

(de-fer-ox´a-meen)
Trade name: Desferal
Classifications: CHELATING AGENT; ANTIDOTE
Pregnancy: Category C

ACTIONS/PHARMACODYNAMICS Chelating agent isolated from *Streptomyces pilosus* with specific affinity for ferric ion and low affinity for calcium. Binds ferric ions to form ferrioxamine complex, a stable water-soluble chelate readily excreted by kidneys. Main effect is removal of iron from ferritin, hemosiderin, and transferrin. Does not affect hemoglobin or cytochromes or increase excretion of electrolytes and other trace elements. Has histamine-releasing properties when administered rapidly by IV route. Theoretically, 100 mg of deferoxamine can chelate 8.5 mg of ferric iron. Deferoxamine also chelates aluminum.

USES Adjunct in treatment of acute iron intoxication. Has been used in management of hemochromatosis

and hemosiderosis secondary to increased iron storage as from multiple transfusions used in treatment of congenital anemias, e.g., thalassemia (Cooley's or Mediterranean anemia), sickle cell anemia, and other chronic anemias. **Unlabeled use:** to promote aluminum excretion in aluminum-associated dialysis encephalopathy and aluminum accumulation in bones of patients in renal failure.

ROUTE & DOSAGE

Acute Iron Intoxication

Adult	IM/IV	1 g followed by 500 mg at 4 h intervals for 2 doses; subsequent doses of 500 mg q4–12h may be given if necessary (max 6 g/24 h); infuse at ≤ 15 mg/kg/h
Child	IM/IV	20 mg/kg followed by 10 mg/kg at 4 h intervals for 2 doses; subsequent doses of 10 mg/kg q4–12h may be given if necessary (max 6 g/24 h); infuse at ≤ 15 mg/kg/h

Chronic Iron Overload

Adult	IM	500 mg–1 g/d
	IV	2 g with each unit of blood transfused; infuse at ≤ 15 mg/kg/h
Child	IM	Same as for adult
	IV	Same as for adult

PHARMACOKINETICS Distribution: widely distributed in body tissues. **Metabolism:** forms nontoxic complex with iron. **Elimination:** excreted primarily in urine; some excreted in feces.

CONTRAINDICATIONS & PRECAUTIONS Contraindicated in: severe renal disease, anuria, pyelonephritis; pregnancy (category C), and children <3 y of age. **Cautious use in:** history of pyelonephritis.

ADVERSE/SIDE EFFECTS CV: hypotension, tachycardia. **ENT:** decreased hearing. **Eye:** blurred vision, decreased visual acuity and visual fields, color vision abnormalities, night blindness, retinal pigmentary degeneration, cataracts. **GI:** abdominal discomfort, diarrhea. **GU:** dysuria, exacerbation of pyelonephritis. **Hypersensitivity:** generalized itching, cutaneous wheal formation, rash, fever, anaphylactoid reaction. **Local:** *pain and induration at injection site.*

NURSING IMPLICATIONS

Administration

- Reconstitute by adding 2 ml sterile water for injection to 500 mg vial. Make certain that drug is completely dissolved before withdrawing it from vial. For IM or SC administration, the reconstituted solution can be given without further dilution. Rotate injection sites.

- IV route is used only for patients in shock. For IV administration, reconstitute as for IM or SC use. After drug is completely dissolved, withdraw prescribed amount from vial and add to 0.9% NaCl, D5W, or lactated Ringer's solution.
- Physician will prescribe specific infusion flow rate (should not exceed 15 mg/kg/h) and volume of solution. Monitor vital signs.
- Solutions reconstituted with sterile water may be stored at room temperature for not longer than 1 wk. Protect from light.

Assessment & Drug Effects

- Baseline tests of kidney function should be performed prior to drug administration.
- Monitor injection site. If pain and induration occur, infusion should be moved to another site.
- Side effects occur more often with too rapid IV infusion. Notify physician of side effects.
- Monitor I&O ratio and pattern. Report any change. Observe stools for blood (iron intoxication frequently causes necrosis of GI tract).
- Periodic ophthalmoscopic (slit lamp) examinations and audiometry are advisable for patients on prolonged or high dose therapy for chronic iron overload.

Patient & Family Education

- Deferoxamine chelate imparts a characteristic reddish color to urine (presumptive evidence of elevated serum iron and indication for further therapy). Keep physician informed.
- Instruct patient to report blurred vision or any other visual abnormality.

Prototype: Pilocarpine, p 209

DEMECARIUM BROMIDE

(dem-e-kare´ee-um)

Trade name: Humorsol
Classifications: EYE PREPARATION; MIOTIC (ANTIGLAUCOMA); AUTONOMIC NERVOUS SYSTEM AGENT; CHOLINERGIC; CHOLINESTERASE INHIBITOR
Pregnancy: Category C

ACTIONS/PHARMACODYNAMICS Potent, indirect-acting quaternary ammonium compound with prolonged effect. Action attributed to reversible cholinesterase inhibition, which permits accumulation and sustained action of endogenous acetylcholine at cholinergic synapses. Local application to conjunctiva produces intense miosis by contraction of iris sphincter and increased accommodation by contraction of ciliary muscle. The resultant widening of the trabecular network decreases intraocular pressure (IOP) by facilitating aqueous humor outflow. Also enhances resorption of aqueous humor by increasing permeability and dilation of conjunctival vessels.

USES Open-angle glaucoma and selected cases of glaucoma due to synechial formation. Also used following iridectomy and in management of accommodative esotropia (convergent strabismus) when less potent miotics have failed. Carbonic anhydrase inhibitor may be used concomitantly to enhance action.

ROUTE & DOSAGE

Glaucoma

Adult	Topical	1–2 drops of 0.125–0.25% solution 2 times/wk up to b.i.d.
Child	Topical	1 drop of 0.125–0.25% solution 2 times/wk up to b.i.d.

Convergent Stabismus

Child	Topical	1 drop of 0.125% solution in each eye daily for 2–3 wk; then decrease to 1 drop q.o.d. for 2–3 wk; then 1 drop 2 times/wk

PHARMACOKINETICS Absorption: absorbed through conjuctiva and intact skin. **Onset:** miosis 15–60 min; IOP 12 h. **Peak:** miosis 2–4 h; IOP 24 h. **Duration:** miosis 3–10 d, up to 4 wk; IOP 9 d.

CONTRAINDICATIONS & PRECAUTIONS Contraindicated in: narrow-angle glaucoma, history of retinal detachment, ocular hypertension accompanied by inflammation, active uveitis, glaucoma associated with iridocyclitis; bronchial asthma; spastic GI conditions, peptic ulcer; marked vagotonia, pronounced bradycardia or hypotension, recent MI, parkinsonism, epilepsy. Safe use in pregnancy not established. **Cautious use in:** myasthenia gravis, corneal abrasion, individuals exposed to organophosphate insecticides or pesticides.

Common side effects in *italic*; life-threatening effects underlined; generic names in **bold**; classifications in SMALL CAPS

491

ADVERSE/SIDE EFFECTS Local effects: *stinging, burning,* lacrimation, ciliary spasm with eye and brow pain, photophobia, frontal headache, *myopia with visual blurring,* twitching of eyelids, conjunctival and ciliary hyperemia, iris cysts (particularly in children following prolonged use), activation of latent iritis or uveitis, retinal detachment (occasionally), conjunctival thickening and obstruction of nasolacrimal canals (prolonged use), lens opacity, contact dermatitis. **Systemic effects:** parasympathetic stimulation: nausea, vomiting, abdominal pain, diarrhea, urinary frequency or incontinence, excessive salivation, nasal congestion, rhinorrhea, profuse sweating, flushing, muscular weakness, paresthesias, bronchospasm, hypotension, shock, bradycardia, depression of serum cholinesterase and erythrocytes.

DRUG INTERACTIONS Neostigmine, physostigmine augment systemic effects; **succinylcholine** may cause prolonged apnea and cardiovascular collapse.

NURSING IMPLICATIONS

Administration

- Physician may prescribe schedule so that drug is instilled at bedtime to minimize disturbing visual effects.
- The first instillation will be made by physician. Since a transient paradoxic increase in IOP may occur initially, tonometric readings should be made at least hourly for 3 or 4 h after first instillation.
- *Procedure for instilling eye drop:* To minimize overflow of solution into nasal and pharyngeal spaces, and possibly systemic absorption, patient should be in supine position. After drop is instilled into lower conjunctiva (see Fig 2-2, p 12), gentle digital pressure is applied to inner canthus against nose (lacrimal sac). Maintain pressure for 1 or 2 min after drop is instilled. Instruct patient to avoid squeezing lids together. Blot excess medication with a clean tissue. Wash hands before and immediately after administration. Maintain sterility of dropper.
- Avoid prolonged contact of drug with skin. If solution contacts skin, wash promptly with large volumes of water.
- If possible, demecarium bromide should be discontinued 2–6 wk prior to surgery.
- Preserve in tight, light-resistant containers, preferably at 15–30C (59–86F) unless otherwise directed.

Assessment & Drug Effects

- Demecarium bromide is a dangerous drug capable of producing cumulative systemic effects. It is essential to adhere precisely to prescribed drug concentration, dosage schedule, and technique of administration. Closely observe patient during initial period.
- Monitor for eye pain. Pain in affected eye is more intense with accommodative effort to near objects and with exposure to light. These effects appear more frequently in younger patients than in older patients.
- Monitor for systemic effects due to parasympathetic stimulation (see adverse/side effects).

Patient & Family Education

- Supervise ambulation. Inform patient that difficulty in accommodating to degree of light, blurred distant vision, miosis with dimmed vision, and eyelid twitching may persist for a week or more.
- Advise patient to avoid driving, particularly at night, and other potentially hazardous activities until side effects have disappeared.
- Advise patient to report promptly to the physician the onset of excessive salivation, diaphoresis, urinary incontinence, diarrhea, muscle weakness, respiratory problems, cardiac irregularities, or symptoms of shock (signs of systemic absorption). Drug should be discontinued.
- Caution patient of possible added systemic effects from skin contact or inhalation of organophosphate-type insecticides or pesticides while receiving demecarium.

Prototype: tetracycline, p 74

DEMECLOCYCLINE HYDROCHLORIDE
(dem-e-kloe-sye´kleen)
Trade names: Declomycin, Ledermycin
Classifications: ANTIINFECTIVE; ANTIBIOTIC; TETRACYCLINE
Pregnancy: Category D

ACTIONS/PHARMACODYNAMICS Broad-spectrum, tetracycline antibiotic isolated from mutant strain of *Streptomyces aureofaciens.* Similar to tetracycline but is absorbed more readily, excreted much more slowly, and has longer duration of effective blood levels; therefore intervals between doses can be longer. Primarily bacteriostatic in action (inhibits protein synthesis in susceptible organisms). Photosensitivity reactions occur more frequently and are more severe than those produced by other tetracyclines. Allergic reactions also appear to be more common, and it causes the most marked tooth discoloration if given during tooth development period. Demeclocycline is the only tetracycline capable of producing dose-related reversible nephrogenic diabetes insipidus syndrome. Promotes water diuresis by inhibiting ADH-induced water reabsorption in renal distal convoluted tubules and collecting tubules.

USES Similar to those of tetracycline. **Unlabeled use:** treatment of chronic SIADH (syndrome of inappropriate [excessive] antidiuretic hormone) secretion.

ROUTE & DOSAGE

Antiinfective

Adult	PO	150 mg q6h or 300 mg q12h (max 2.4 g/d)
Child	PO	>8 y: 6.6–13.2 mg/kg/d in 4 divided doses

Gonorrhea

Adult	PO	600 mg followed by 300 mg q12h for 4 d

SIADH

Adult	PO	600–1200 mg/d in 3–4 divided doses

PHARMACOKINETICS Absorption: 60–80% absorbed from GI tract. **Peak:** 3–4 h. **Distribution:** concentrated in liver; crosses placenta; distributed into breast milk. **Metabolism:** metabolized in liver; enterohepatic circulation. **Elimination:** half-life: 10–17 h; 40–50% excreted in urine and 31% in feces in 48 h.

CONTRAINDICATIONS & PRECAUTIONS Contraindicated in: hypersensitivity to any of the tetracyclines; cirrhosis, common bile duct obstruction; period of tooth development (last half of pregnancy; category D), nursing women, children <8 y (causes permanent yellow discoloration of teeth, enamel hypoplasia, and retarded bone growth). **Cautious use in:** impaired renal or hepatic function; nephrogenic diabetes insipidus; use of capsule or tablet formulations in patients with esophageal compression or obstruction.

ADVERSE/SIDE EFFECTS GI: *nausea,* vomiting, *diarrhea,* esophageal irritation or ulceration, enterocolitis, abdominal cramps, anorexia. **Hematologic:** thrombocytopenia, neutropenia, eosinophilia, hemolytic anemia. **Hypersensitivity:** *photosensitivity,* urticaria, angioneurotic edema, exacerbation of SLE,

pericarditis, anaphylaxis. **Renal:** nephrotoxicity, acute renal failure (in patients with Laennec's cirrhosis), diabetes insipidus. **Skin:** pruritus, erythematous eruptions, exfoliative dermatitis, pigmentation of nails; loosening or softening of nails.

DIAGNOSTIC TEST INTERFERENCES Like other tetracyclines, demeclocycline may cause false increases in **urine catecholamines** (fluorometric methods); false decreases in **urine urobilinogen;** and false-negative **urine glucose** with glucose oxidase methods (e.g., Clinistix, TesTape).

DRUG INTERACTIONS Antacids, iron preparation, calcium, magnesium, zinc, kaolin-pectin, sodium bicarbonate can significantly decrease demeclocycline absorption; effects of **desmopressin** and demeclocycline antagonized; increases **digoxin** absorption, increasing risk of digoxin toxicity; **methoxyflurane** increases risk of renal failure. **Food-drug interactions:** dairy products significantly decrease demeclocycline absorption; food may decrease drug absorption also.

NURSING IMPLICATIONS

Administration

- Check expiration date before administering drug. Renal damage and death have resulted from use of outdated tetracyclines.
- Absorption may be impaired by foods rich in iron such as red meat or dark green vegetables, milk, milk products, or other calcium-containing foods. Of all tetracyclines, demeclocycline has the greatest affinity for calcium ions. Administer not less than 1 h before or 2 h after meals.
- If gastric distress is a problem, physician may prescribe taking drug with a light meal even though absorption may be reduced. The meal should not contain dairy products.
- Instruct patient to take demeclocycline for prescribed length of time and to discard medication when no longer needed or if outdated.
- Preserve in tight, light-resistant containers, preferably at 15–30C (59–86F) unless otherwise directed. Tetracyclines form toxic products when outdated or when exposed to light, heat, or humidity.

Assessment & Drug Effects

- Culture and susceptibility testing is recommended prior to initiation of therapy and at periodic intervals during prolonged therapy.
- If drug therapy is prolonged, periodic evaluations of serum drug levels, electrolytes, and renal, hep-

Common side effects in *italic;* life-threatening effects underlined; generic names in **bold**; classifications in SMALL CAPS

493

atic, and hematopoietic systems are recommended.
- Monitor I&O ratio and pattern and record weights in patients with impaired kidney or liver function, or on prolonged or high dose therapy. Some patients develop diabetes insipidus–like syndrome (SIADH).

Patient & Family Education
- Should be taken on an empty stomach to enhance absorption. Because esophageal irritation and ulceration have been reported, advise patient to (1) take each dose with a full glass (240 ml) of water; (2) remain standing for at least 90 s after taking medication; and (3) avoid taking drug within 1 h of lying down or bedtime.
- For most infections, therapy is usually continued 24–48 h after fever and other symptoms have subsided. Therapy should continue for at least 10 d for streptococcal infections.
- Stress importance of reporting symptoms of superinfections (see chap 3).
- Demeclocycline-induced phototoxic reaction can be unusually severe. It is similar to a bad sunburn and may be accompanied by loosening and pigmentation of nails. Demeclocycline should be discontinued promptly at the first indication of a reaction. Paresthesias of nose, hands, and feet may be an early sign. Use of sun screens reportedly provides only limited protection.
- Caution patient to avoid exposure to sunlight or ultraviolet light during treatment and for several weeks after treatment.

Prototype: reserpine, p 154

DESERPIDINE
(de-ser´pi-deen)
Trade name: Harmonyl
Classifications: CARDIOVASCULAR AGENT; ANTIHYPERTENSIVE; RAUWOLFIA ALKALOID; ANTIPSYCHOTIC
Pregnancy: Category D

ACTIONS/PHARMACODYNAMICS Indole alkaloid obtained from *Rauwolfia serpentina*. Mechanism of action has not been established. Depletes catecholamine and serotonin stores in many organs, including the brain and adrenal medulla, and reduces uptake of catecholamines by adrenergic neurons. Depletion of catecholamine stores occurs slowly, resulting in gradual decrease in peripheral vascular resistance and BP similar to effects of reserpine. Venous dilation and peripheral pooling of blood reduces venous return to the heart and decreases cardiac output.

USES Mild to moderate hypertension and the symptomatic treatment of agitated psychotic states such as schizophrenic disorders.

ROUTE & DOSAGE

Hypertension

Adult	PO	0.75–1 mg/d; may try to decrease to 0.25 mg/d

Antipsychotic

Adult	PO	0.1–1 mg/d in 1–2 divided doses

PHARMACOKINETICS Absorption: readily absorbed from GI tract. **Onset:** 2–3 wk. **Peak:** 2 h. **Duration:** >24 h. **Distribution:** crosses blood-brain barrier and placenta; distributed into breast milk. **Metabolism:** metabolized in liver. **Elimination:** up to 60% excreted in feces; approximately 10% excreted unchanged in urine.

CONTRAINDICATIONS & PRECAUTIONS Contraindicated in: mental depression, active peptic ulcer disease, ulcerative colitis, history of hypersensitivity to rauwolfia alkaloids, ECT. Safe use during pregnancy (category D) not established. **Cautious use in:** epilepsy, impaired renal function, bronchial asthma, CVA, cardiac arrhythmias, obesity, gallstones, breast cancer, patients receiving diuretics, other hypotensive agents, cardiac glycosides, MAO inhibitors, or CNS depressants.

ADVERSE/SIDE EFFECTS CV: *bradycardia, hypotension,* chest pain, dysrhythmias. **CNS:** *drowsiness, depression,* nervousness, paradoxical anxiety, nightmares, extrapyramidal tract symptoms, *fatigue, lethargy.* **GI:** abdominal cramps, diarrhea, nausea, vomiting, anorexia, peptic ulcers, dry mouth. **Skin:** rash, pruritus, ecchymosis. **EENT:** epistaxis, deafness, ptosis, blurred vision, lacrimation, miosis, glaucoma, uveitis, optic atrophy, nasal congestion. **Hematologic:** thrombocytopenia purpura, anemia, prolonged bleeding time. **Other:** dysuria, dyspnea, impotence, decreased libido, gynecomastia, galactorrhea, edema.

DRUG INTERACTIONS Alcohol and other CNS DEPRESSANTS compound depression; **digoxin** may

Common side effects in *italic*; life-threatening effects underlined; generic names in **bold**; classifications in SMALL CAPS

increase risk of arrhythmias; MAO INHIBITORS may cause excitation or hypertension; may decrease effects of **levodopa.**

NURSING IMPLICATIONS

Administration

- Administer with meals or milk to reduce GI irritation.
- If the pill cannot be swallowed whole, it may be crushed and given in applesauce.
- Withdraw medication 2 wk before ECT is employed.

Assessment & Drug Effects

- Monitor BP for severe hypotension and heart rate for bradycardia and arrhythmias, especially in patients on digitalis or quinidine. Evaluate signs and symptoms of CHF (see chap 3).
- Assess bleeding time and check for ecchymosis or other signs of thrombocytopenia.
- Assess I&O, especially in patient with renal impairment. Evaluate daily weight and assess for edema.
- Monitor for signs and symptoms of dehydration (see chap 3).
- Monitor patient with history of peptic ulcer, ulcerative colitis, or gallstones, since drug increases GI motility and secretions.
- Monitor for signs and symptoms of depression such as changes in sleep patterns and loss of appetite.

Patient & Family Education

- Advise patient to take drug same time each day, not to skip or double doses, and not to stop therapy without advice of physician.
- Advise patient not to take other medications, especially OTC drugs, unless discussed with physician.
- Advise caution with alcohol or other CNS depressants.
- Advise caution when driving or doing other hazardous activities because of possible drowsiness or dizziness.
- Instruct patient to report dizziness, confusion, depression, fever, or sore throat.
- Inform patient that impotence and gynecomastia may occur but are reversible.
- Inform patient that therapeutic effect may take 2–4 wk.

Prototype: imipramine, p 184

DESIPRAMINE HYDROCHLORIDE
(dess-ip´ra-meen)
Trade names: Norpramin, Pertofrane
Classification: CNS AGENT; PSYCHOTHERAPEUTIC; TRICYCLIC ANTIDEPRESSANT
Pregnancy: Category C

ACTIONS/PHARMACODYNAMICS Dibenzoxazepine tricyclic antidepressant (TCA) and secondary amine. Desipramine is the active metabolite of imipramine and has similar pharmacologic actions. Unlike imipramine, onset of action is more rapid, and it has lower potential for producing sedative and anticholinergic effects and orthostatic hypotension. In common with other TCAs, antidepressant activity appears to be related to inhibition of reuptake of norepinephrine (most prominent action) and serotonin in the CNS. Restoration of the levels of these neurotransmitters is a proposed mechanism of antidepressant action.

USES Endogenous depression and various depression syndromes. **Unlabeled uses:** attention deficit disorder in children >6 y and adolescents; to prevent depression in cocaine withdrawal.

ROUTE & DOSAGE

Antidepressant

Adult	PO	75–100 mg/d at bedtime or in divided doses; may gradually increase to 150–300 mg/d (use lower doses in elderly patients)
Adolescent	PO	25–50 mg/d (max 100 mg/d) in divided doses

PHARMACOKINETICS Absorption: rapidly absorbed from GI tract and injection sites. **Peak:** 4–6 h. **Distribution:** crosses placenta. **Metabolism:** metabolized in liver. **Elimination:** half-life: 7–60 h; primarily excreted in urine.

CONTRAINDICATIONS & PRECAUTIONS Contraindicated in: hypersensitivity to tricyclic compounds; recent MI. Safe use during pregnancy (category C), in nursing mothers, and in children <12 y not established. **Cautious use in:** urinary retention, prostatic hypertrophy; narrow-angle glaucoma; epilepsy; alcoholism; adolescents, the elderly; thyroid; cardio-

Common side effects in *italic*; life-threatening effects underlined; generic names in **bold**; classifications in SMALL CAPS

495

vascular, renal, and hepatic disease; suicidal tendency; ECT; elective surgery.

ADVERSE/SIDE EFFECTS CNS: *drowsiness,* dizziness, weakness, fatigue, headache, insomnia, confusional states, depressive reaction, paresthesias, ataxia, extrapyramidal effects. **CV:** *postural hypotension,* hypotension, hypertension, palpitation, tachycardia, ECG changes, flushing, heart block. **ENT:** tinnitus, parotid swelling. **Eye:** blurred vision, disturbances in accommodation, mydriasis, increased IOP. **GI:** *dry mouth, constipation,* bad taste, diarrhea, stomatitis, nausea. **GU:** *urinary retention,* frequency, delayed micturition, nocturia. **Hematologic:** eosinophilia, bone marrow depression (leukopenia, agranulocytosis, thrombocytopenia). **Hypersensitivity:** rash, urticaria, photosensitivity. **Reproduction:** impaired sexual function, galactorrhea. **Other:** sweating, craving for sweets, weight gain or loss, SIADH secretion, hyperpyrexia, eosinophilic pneumonia.

DRUG INTERACTIONS May somewhat decrease response to ANTIHYPERTENSIVES; CNS DEPRESSANTS, **alcohol,** HYPNOTICS, BARBITURATES, SEDATIVES potentiate CNS depression; may increase hypoprothombinemic effect of ORAL ANTICOAGULANTS; **ethchlorvynol** may cause transient delirium; **levodopa,** SYMPATHOMIMETICS (e.g., **epinephrine, norepinephrine**) pose possibility of sympathetic hyperactivity with hypertension and hyperpyrexia; MAO INHIBITORS pose possibility of severe reactions, toxic psychosis, cardiovascular instability; **methylphenidate** increases plasma TCA levels; THYROID AGENTS may increase possibility of arrhythmias; **cimetidine** may increase plasma TCA levels.

NURSING IMPLICATIONS

Administration

- May be taken with or immediately after food to reduce possibility of gastric irritation.
- Maintenance dose is generally prescribed as a single dose at bedtime to minimize daytime sedation and other annoying drug side effects.
- Store drug in tightly closed container at 15–30C (59–86F) unless otherwise specified.

Assessment & Drug Effects

- Full therapeutic effect usually not realized until at least 2 wk of therapy.
- Careful observation for desired effects is important during early therapy. Drug metabolism may vary as much as 36-fold among users of desipramine, leading to wide differences in dose requirements.

- Monitor BP and pulse rate during early phase of therapy, particularly in the elderly, debilitated, and cardiovascular patients. If BP rises or falls more than 20 mm Hg or if there is a sudden increase in pulse rate or change in rhythm, withhold drug and inform physician.
- Drowsiness, dizziness, and orthostatic hypotension in patient on long-term, high dosage therapy are signs of impending toxicity. Prolonged QT or QRS intervals indicate possible toxicity. Report to physician.
- Observe patient with history of glaucoma. Symptoms that may signal acute attack (severe headache, eye pain, dilated pupils, halos of light, nausea, vomiting) should be reported promptly.
- Monitor bowel elimination pattern and I&O ratio. Severe constipation and urinary retention are potential problems of TCA therapy.
- If a patient uses excessive amounts of alcohol it should be borne in mind that the potentiation of drug effects may increase the danger of overdosage or suicide attempt.
- Suicide is an inherent risk with any depressed patient. Supervise drug ingestion and observe patient closely.
- Norpramin tablets may contain tartrazine, which can cause allergic-type reactions including bronchial asthma in susceptible individuals. Such individuals are frequently also sensitive to aspirin.

Patient & Family Education

- Instruct patient to make all position changes slowly and in stages, particularly from recumbent to standing position.
- Caution patient to avoid potentially hazardous activities such as driving until reaction to drug is known.
- Patient instructions: take medication exactly as ordered; do not change dose or dose intervals.
- Abrupt discontinuation of desipramine can precipitate withdrawal symptoms in patients who have received high dosages for prolonged periods: headache, nausea, musculoskeletal pain, weakness.
- OTC drugs should not be taken unless the physician has approved their use.
- Smoking may increase the metabolism of desipramine, thereby diminishing its therapeutic action. Advise patient to stop or at least limit smoking.

Common side effects in *italic*; life-threatening effects underlined; generic names in **bold**; classifications in SMALL CAPS

Prototype: digoxin, p 146

DESLANOSIDE
(des-lan′oh-side)
Trade names: Cedilanid-D, Cedilanid Injection, Desacetyl-lanatoside C
Classification: CARDIOVASCULAR DRUG; ANTIARRHYTHMIC; CARDIAC GLYCOSIDE
Pregnancy: Category C

ACTIONS/PHARMACODYNAMICS Rapid-acting parenteral digitalis glycoside obtained by alkaline hydrolysis of lanatoside C, a glycoside of *Digitalis lanata*. Shares essentially the same actions, contraindications, and adverse reactions of digoxin but is administered parenterally only.

USES Rapid digitalizing effect in emergency treatment of CHF, cardiac arrhythmias, such as atrial fibrillation or flutter, paroxysmal atrial tachycardia, and cardiogenic shock.

ROUTE & DOSAGE

Digitalizing Dose

Adult IV/IM 1.6 mg in 1–2 divided doses or 0.8 mg followed by 0.2–0.4 mg at 2–4 h intervals until adequate response or toxic effects occur (max 1.6–2 mg)

PHARMACOKINETICS Onset: within 10 min. **Duration:** 2–4 h. **Elimination:** half-life: 33–36 h; approximately 20% excreted in urine daily.

CONTRAINDICATIONS & PRECAUTIONS Contraindicated in: hypersensitivity to digitalis preparations; patients with digitalis toxicity; loading dose to patients who have received a digitalis preparation within previous 2–3 wk; ventricular tachycardia or fibrillation. Severe pulmonary disease, idiopathic hypertrophic subaortic stenosis, hypokalemia or hypercalcemia. Safe use during pregnancy (category C) not established. **Cautious use in:** elderly patients, acute MI, electrical conversion of arrhythmias, incomplete AV block, constrictive pericarditis, hypothyroidism, impaired renal function, nursing mothers.

ADVERSE/SIDE EFFECTS Anorexia, nausea, vomiting, diarrhea, headache, weakness, fatigue, apathy, visual disturbances, arrhythmias, heart block.

NURSING IMPLICATIONS

Administration
- IV deslanoside may be given by direct IV undiluted or diluted in 10 ml NS. Administer at a rate of 0.2 mg/min through a Y-tube of IV infusion tubing.
- Maintenance therapy with an oral digitalis glycoside is preferred and may be instituted within 12–24 h after digitalization with deslanoside.
- Deslanoside should be protected from light. Store at 15–30C (59–86F) unless otherwise directed.

Assessment & Drug Effects
- Effectiveness of drug is manifested in 5–15 min and lasts up to 3 d.
- Monitor for hypercalcemia (see Signs & Symptoms, chap 3). This drug is contraindicated until normal calcium balance is restored.
- Monitor for hypokalemia (see Signs & Symptoms, chap 3), since digitalis toxicity risk will be increased.
- Patient must be closely observed during deslanoside therapy with monitoring of ECG, serum electrolytes, and renal function.

Prototype: vasopressin, p 239

DESMOPRESSIN ACETATE
(des-moe-press′in)
Trade names: DDAVP, Stimate
Classifications: SYNTHETIC PITUITARY HORMONE (ANTIDIURETIC); VASOPRESSOR; OXYTOCIC
Pregnancy: Category B

ACTIONS/PHARMACODYNAMICS Synthetic analog of the natural human posterior pituitary (antidiuretic) hormone, arginine vasopressin. Has more specific and longer duration of action than antidiuretic hormone and lower incidence of allergic reactions. Also, oxytocic and vasopressor actions are not apparent at therapeutic dosages. Unlike vasopressin, it does not stimulate release of adrenocorticotropic hormone nor does it increase plasma cortisol, growth hormone, prolactin, or luteinizing hormone levels. Reduces urine volume and osmolality in patients with central diabetes insipidus by increasing reabsorption of water by kidney collecting tubules. Produces a dose-related increase in factor VIII (antihemophilic factor) and von Willebrand's factor. Not effective in treatment of nephrogenic diabetes insipidus. Toler-

Common side effects in *italic*; life-threatening effects underlined; generic names in **bold**; classifications in SMALL CAPS

497

ance to drug effect rarely develops during prolonged therapy.

USES To control and prevent symptoms and complications of central (neurohypophyseal) diabetes insipidus, and to relieve temporary polyuria and polydipsia associated with trauma or surgery in the pituitary region. **Unlabeled use:** to increase factor VIII activity in selected patients with mild to moderate hemophilia A and in type I von Willebrand's disease, or uremia, and to control enuresis in children.

ROUTE & DOSAGE

(0.1 ml = 10 µg)

Diabetes Insipidus

Adult	Intranasal	0.1–0.4 ml in 1–3 divided doses
	IV/SC	2–4 µg in 2 divided doses
Child	Intranasal	3 mo–12 y: 0.05–0.3 ml in 1–2 divided doses
	IV/SC	0.3 µg/kg infused over 15–30 min

Enuresis

Adult	Intranasal	5–40 µg h.s.
Child	Intransasl	3–12 y: Same as for adult

von Willebrand's Disease

Adult	IV/SC	0.3 µg/kg 30 min preop; may repeat in 48 h if needed
Child	IV/SC	Same as for adult

PHARMACOKINETICS Absorption: 10–20% absorbed through nasal mucosa. **Onset:** 15–60 min. **Peak:** 1–5 h. **Duration:** 5–21 h. **Distribution:** small amount crosses blood-brain barrier; distributed into breast milk. **Elimination:** half-life: 76 min.

CONTRAINDICATIONS & PRECAUTIONS Contraindicated in: nephrogenic diabetes insipidus, type II B von Willebrand's disease. Safe use during pregnancy (category B) and in nursing mothers not established. **Cautious use in:** coronary artery insufficiency, hypertensive cardiovascular disease.

ADVERSE/SIDE EFFECTS Dose-related. **CNS:** transient headache, drowsiness, listlessness. **ENT:** nasal congestion, rhinitis, nasal irritation. **GI:** nausea, heartburn, mild abdominal cramps. **Other:** vulval pain, shortness of breath, slight rise in BP, facial flushing, pain and swelling at injection site.

DRUG INTERACTIONS Demeclocycline, lithium, other VASOPRESSORS may decrease antidiuretic response; **carbamazepine, chlorpropamide, clofibrate** may prolong antidiuretic response.

NURSING IMPLICATIONS

Administration

- Follow manufacturer's instructions for proper technique with nasal spray.
- Initial dose usually administered in the evening, and antidiuretic effect observed. Dose is increased each evening until uninterrupted sleep is obtained. If daily urine volume is more than 2 L after nocturia is controlled, morning dose is started and adjusted daily until urine volume does not exceed 1.5–2 L/24 h.
- When given IV for diabetes insipidus, may be given undiluted by direct IV over 30 seconds.
- When desmopressin is given IV for von Willebrand's disease (type I), 0.3 µg/kg is diluted in 10 ml of NS (children ≤ 10 kg) or 50 ml of NS (children > 10 kg and adults) and infused over 15–30 min.
- Store parenteral solution and nasal spray in refrigerator preferably at 4C (39.2F) unless otherwise directed. Avoid freezing. Discard solutions that are discolored or contain particulate matter.

Assessment & Drug Effects

- Monitor I&O ratio and pattern (intervals). Fluid intake must be carefully controlled, particularly in the elderly and in the very young to avoid water retention and sodium depletion.
- Weigh patient daily and observe for edema. Severe water retention may require reduction in dosage and use of a diuretic.
- Monitor BP during dosage-regulating period and whenever drug is administered parenterally.
- Therapeutic effectiveness is judged by control of polyuria and nocturia and relief of polydipsia.
- Monitor urine osmolality and plasma osmolality. An increase in urine osmolality and a decrease in plasma osmolality indicate effectiveness of treatment in diabetes insipidus.

Patient & Family Education

- Report upper respiratory tract infection or nasal congestion.
- Demonstrate administration technique to patient. Follow manufacturer's instructions to insure delivery of drug high into nasal cavity and not down throat. A flexible calibrated plastic tube is provided.

Common side effects in *italic*; life-threatening effects <u>underlined</u>; generic names in **bold**; classifications in SMALL CAPS

Prototype: hydrocortisone, p 255

DESONIDE

(dess′oh-nide)
Trade names: DesOwen, Tridesilon
Classifications: SKIN & MUCOUS MEMBRANE;
ANTIINFLAMMATORY; SYNTHETIC ADRENAL
CORTICOSTEROID HORMONE; GLUCOCORTICOID
Pregnancy: Category C

ACTIONS/PHARMACODYNAMICS Synthetic nonfluorinated corticosteroid with antiinflammatory, antipruritic, and vasoconstrictive activity. Action is thought to result in part from complexing of drug with cytoplasmic steroid receptors. Decreases inflammation, reduces capillary wall permeability and edema formation, antagonizes histamine activity and release of kinin, and reduces fibroblast proliferation. Percutaneous penetration is minimal on intact skin.

USES To relieve inflammatory and pruritic symptoms of a variety of skin disorders responsive to corticosteroids.

ROUTE & DOSAGE

Inflammation
Adult   Topical   Apply thin layer b.i.d. to q.i.d.

PHARMACOKINETICS Absorption: minimum absorption through intact skin; increased absorption from axilla, eyelid, face, scalp, scrotum, or with occlusive dressing.

CONTRAINDICATIONS & PRECAUTIONS Contraindicated in: safe use during pregnancy (category C) and by nursing mothers not established. **Cautious use in:** children.

ADVERSE/SIDE EFFECTS Skin: burning sensation, pruritus, acneiform eruptions, hypopigmentation, hypertrichosis, folliculitis, perioral dermatitis, allergic contact dermatitis. With occlusive dressing: maceration of skin, atrophy, striae, secondary infection, miliaria.

NURSING IMPLICATIONS

Administration
- Avoid putting medication in or near eyes.
- Before application, cleanse skin area, dry thoroughly, then gently rub in a thin layer of the drug.
- Do not use an occlusive dressing unless specifically directed to do so by physician. Occlusion will greatly enhance drug absorption.
- Store drug at 15–30C (59–86F); protect from light and heat unless otherwise directed.

Assessment & Drug Effects
- Inspect skin for infection, striae, atrophy (often associated with occlusive dressings). If present, patient should stop the drug and notify the physician.
- Children may demonstrate greater susceptibility to drug-induced linear growth retardation and delayed weight gain.

Patient & Family Education
- If signs of systemic absorption, skin irritation or ulceration, hypersensitivity (see Signs & Symptoms, chap 3), or infection occurs, patient should notify the physician.
- Caution patient to apply medication exactly as prescribed, not to change intervals or amount, and not to use the preparation for any other skin disorder.
- Bandage or wrap treated area only if prescribed.
- Advise parent not to use tightfitting diapers or plastic pants on a child receiving drug in the diaper area; these garments can act as occlusive dressings.

Prototype: hydrocortisone, p 255

DESOXIMETASONE

(des-ox-i-met′a-sone)
Trade name: Topicort, Topicort-LP
Classifications: SKIN & MUCOUS MEMBRANE;
ANTIINFLAMMATORY; SYNTHETIC ADRENAL
CORTICOSTEROID HORMONE; GLUCOCORTICOID
Pregnancy: Category C

ACTIONS/PHARMACODYNAMICS Synthetic fluorinated corticosteroid with antiinflammatory, antipruritic, and vasoconstrictive activity. Thought to result in part from complexing of drug with cytoplasmic steroid receptors. Decreases inflammation, reduces capillary wall permeability and edema formation, antagonizes histamine activity and release of kinin, and reduces fibroblast proliferation. Percutaneous penetration is minimal on intact skin.

USES To relieve inflammatory and pruritic symptoms of a variety of skin disorders responsive to corticosteroids.

ROUTE & DOSAGE

Inflammation

Adult	Topical	Apply thin layer b.i.d.

PHARMACOKINETICS Absorption: minimum absorption through intact skin; increased absorption from axilla, eyelid, face, scalp, scrotum, or with occlusive dressing.

CONTRAINDICATIONS & PRECAUTIONS Contraindicated in: safe use during pregnancy (category C) and by nursing mothers not established. **Cautious use in:** children.

ADVERSE/SIDE EFFECTS Skin: pruritus, acneiform eruptions, burning sensation, irritation, erythema, dryness, hypopigmentation, hypertrichosis, folliculitis, allergic contact dermatitis, vesiculitis. **Systemic:** hypothalamic-pituitary-adrenocortical (HPA) axis suppression, Cushing's syndrome, hyperglycemia, glycosuria. In children: intracranial hypertension, interference with growth and development (chronic therapy).

NURSING IMPLICATIONS

Administration

- Not for ophthalmic use. Take care not to put medication near eyes. Do not apply to vulvovaginal or perianal areas.
- Before application of topical medication, cleanse skin area, dry thoroughly, then gently rub in a thin layer of the drug.
- Do not use an occlusive dressing unless specifically directed to do so by physician. Occlusion will greatly enhance drug absorption.
- Store drug at 15–30C (59–86F); protect from light and heat unless otherwise directed by manufacturer.

Assessment & Drug Effects

- Inspect skin for infection, striae, atrophy (often associated with occlusive dressings). If any of these are present, stop the drug and notify the physician.
- Children may demonstrate greater susceptibility to drug-induced linear growth retardation and delayed weight gain.

Patient & Family Education

- Should not be used over extensive areas, in large amounts, or for prolonged periods.
- If signs of systemic absorption, skin irritation or ulceration, hypersensitivity, or infection occur, patient should notify physician.
- Caution patient to apply medication exactly as prescribed as scheduled and not to change intervals or use the preparation for any other skin disorder.
- Bandage or wrap treated area only if prescribed.
- Advise parent not to use tightfitting diapers or plastic pants on a child receiving drug in the diaper area; these garments can act as occlusive dressings.

Prototype: prednisone, p 225

DEXAMETHASONE

(dex-a-meth´a-sone)
Trade names: Aeroseb-Dex, Decaderm, Decadron, Decaspray, Deronil, Dexameth, Dexamethasone Intensol, Dexasone, Dexone, Hexadrol, Maxidex, Mymethasone

DEXAMETHASONE ACETATE

Trade names: Dalalone D.P., Dalalone-LA, Decadron-LA, Decaject-LA, Dexacen LA-8, Dexasone-LA, Dexo-LA, Dexon LA, Dexone LA, Solurex-LA

DEXAMETHASONE SODIUM PHOSPHATE

Trade names: Ak-Dex, Alba Dex, Dalalone, Decadrol, Decadron Phosphate, Decaject, Dex-4, Dexacen-4, Dexasone, Dexon, Dexone, Hexadrol Phosphate, Maxidex ophthalmic, Savacort-D, Solurex
Classifications: HORMONE; SYNTHETIC ADRENAL CORTICOSTEROID; GLUCOCORTICOID; IMMUNOSUPPRESSANT; DIAGNOSTIC AGENT; ANTIEMETIC
Pregnancy: Category C

ACTIONS/PHARMACODYNAMICS Long-acting synthetic adrenocorticoid with intense antiinflammatory (glucocorticoid) activity and minimal mineralocorticoid activity. **Antiinflammatory action:** prevents accumulation of inflammatory cells at sites of infection; inhibits phagocytosis, lysosomal enzyme release, and synthesis of selected chemical mediators of inflammation; reduces capillary dilation and permeability. *Immunosuppression:* not clearly understood, but may be due to prevention or suppression of delayed hypersensitivity immune reaction. Also reduces number of circulating T lymphocytes, monocytes, eosinophils, decreases binding of immunoglobulin to cell surface receptors, and suppresses synthesis or release of interleukins. Because of minimal mineralocorticoid activity, dexamethasone is inadequate as the sole agent in treatment of adrenal insufficiency.

USES Adrenal insufficiency concomitantly with a mineralocorticoid; inflammatory conditions, allergic states, collagen diseases, hematologic disorders, cerebral edema, and addisonian shock. Also palliative treatment of neoplastic disease, as adjunctive short-term therapy in acute rheumatic disorders and GI diseases, and as a diagnostic test for Cushing's syndrome and for differential diagnosis of adrenal hyperplasia and adrenal adenoma. **Unlabeled uses:** as an antiemetic in cancer chemotherapy; as a diagnostic test for endogenous depression; and to prevent hyaline membrane disease in prematures.

PHARMACOKINETICS Absorption: readily absorbed from GI tract. **Onset:** rapid onset. **Peak:** 1–2 h PO; 8 h IM. **Duration:** 2.75 d PO; 6 d IM; 1–3 wk intralesional, intraarticular. **Distribution:** crosses placenta; distributed into breast milk. **Elimination:** half-life: 3–4.5 h; hypothalamus-pituitary axis suppression: 36–54 h.

CONTRAINDICATIONS & PRECAUTIONS Contraindicated in: systemic fungal infection, acute infections, active or resting tuberculosis, vaccinia, varicella, administration of live virus vaccines (to patient, family members), latent or active amebiasis. *Ophthalmic use:* primary open-angle glaucoma, eye infections, superficial ocular herpes simplex, keratitis and tuberculosis of eye. Safe use during pregnancy (category C), in nursing mothers, and in children not established. **Cautious use in:** stromal herpes simplex, keratitis, GI ulceration, renal disease, diabetes mellitus, hypothyroidism, myasthenia gravis, CHF, cirrhosis, psychic disorders, seizures.

ADVERSE/SIDE EFFECTS *Aerosol therapy: nasal irritation,* dryness, epistaxis, rebound congestion, bronchial asthma, anosmia, perforation of nasal septum. *Systemic absorption:* **CNS:** euphoria, insomnia, convulsions, increased ICP, vertigo, headache, psychic disturbances. **CV:** CHF, hypertension, *edema.* **Endocrine:** menstrual irregularities, *hyperglycemia;* cushingoid state; growth suppression in children; hir-

sutism. **Eye:** *posterior subcapsular cataract,* increased IOP, glaucoma, exophthalmos. **GI:** peptic ulcer with possible perforation, abdominal distension, nausea, increased appetite, heartburn, dyspepsia, pancreatitis, bowel perforation, *oral candidiasis.* **Musculoskeletal:** muscle weakness, loss of muscle mass, vertebral compression fracture, pathologic fracture of long bones, tendon rupture. **Skin:** acne, *impaired wound healing,* petechiae, ecchymoses, diaphoresis, allergic dermatitis, hypo- or hyperpigmentation, SC and cutaneous atrophy, burning and tingling in perineal area (following IV injection).

ROUTE & DOSAGE

Allergies, Inflammation, Neoplasias

Adult	PO	0.25–4 mg b.i.d. to q.i.d.
	IM	8–16 mg q1–3 wk or 0.8–1.6 mg intralesional q1–3wk
Child	PO	0.2 mg/kg/d in divided doses

Cerebral Edema

Adult	IV	10 mg followed by 4 mg q4h; reduce dose after 2–4 d; then taper over 5–7 d
Child	PO	0.2 mg/kg/d in divided doses

Shock

Adult	IV	1–6 mg/kg as a single dose or 40 mg repeated q2–6h if needed

Dexamethasone Suppression Test

Adult	PO	0.5 mg q6h for 48 h

Inflammation

Adult	Ophthalmic	1–2 drops in conjunctival sac up to 4–6 times/d; may instill hourly for severe disease
	Topical	Apply sparingly t.i.d. or q.i.d.
	Oral Inhalation	Up to 3 inhalations t.i.d. or q.i.d. (max 12 inhalations/d)
	Intranasal	2 sprays in each nostril b.i.d. or t.i.d. (max 12 sprays/d)
Child	Oral Inhalation	Up to 2 inhalations q.i.d. (max 8 inhalations/d)
	Intranasal	1 or 2 sprays in each nostril b.i.d. (max 8 sprays/d)

DIAGNOSTIC TEST INTERFERENCES *Dexamethasone suppression test for endogenous depression:* false-positive results may be caused by **alcohol, glutethimide, meprobamate;** false-negative results may be caused by high doses of BENZODI-AZEPINES (e.g., **chlordiazepoxide** and **cyprohepta-dine**), long-term GLUCOCORTICOID treatment, **indomethacin. Ephedrine,** ESTROGENS or HEPATIC ENZYME–INDUCING AGENTS **(phenytoin)** may also cause false-positive results in *test for Cushing's syndrome.*

DRUG INTERACTIONS BARBITURATES, **phenytoin, rifampin** increase steroid metabolism— dosage of dexamethasone may need to be increased; **amphotericin B,** DIURETICS compound potassium loss; **ambenonium, neostigmine, pyridostigmine** may cause severe muscle weakness in patients with myasthenia gravis; may inhibit antibody response to VACCINES, TOXOIDS.

INCOMPATIBILITIES Solution/Additive: daunoru-bicin, doxorubicin, doxapram, glycopyrrolate, metaraminol, vancomycin.

NURSING IMPLICATIONS

Administration
- Because dexamethasone prolongs HPA axis sup-pression, alternate day therapy (ADT) is not rec-ommended.
- Once-daily doses should be administered in the AM with food or liquid of patient's choice.
- Administer IM injection deep into a large muscle mass (e.g., gluteus maximus). Avoid SC injection: atrophy and sterile abscesses may occur.
- The repository form, dexamethasone acetate (for IM or local injection only), is a white suspension that settles on standing; mild shaking will resus-pend the drug.
- IV dexamethasone may be given undiluted by di-rect IV over 30 seconds or less. Drug may be added to an infusion of D5W or NS and administered over a prescribed period.
- Because adrenal suppression can occur with pro-longed use, dosage should be tapered over a pe-riod of time before it is discontinued.
- When large doses of dexamethasone are necessary, the patient may be given an antacid between meals to reduce risk of peptic ulcer.
- Eye ointment is instilled by same procedure as eye drops. After administration, lids should be kept closed at least 1 min to allow ointment to melt.
- Hold aerosol container upright approximately 15 cm (6 in) from area being treated. Shake well be-fore spraying. If spray is to be applied about the face, the eyes should be protected, and spray should not be inhaled.

- Do not store or expose aerosol to temperature above 48.9C (120F); do not puncture or discard into a fire or an incinerator.
- Store at 15–30C (59–86F) unless otherwise directed.

Assessment & Drug Effects
- Cushing's syndrome (see Signs & Symptoms, chap 3) and other systemic effects can occur from over-administration of dexamethasone by any route.
- Hiccups occurring for several hours following each drug dose constitute an annoying complication of high-dose oral dexamethasone (treatment regimen of the cancer patient). Conventional measures do not seem to bring relief. Swallowing an antacid may help; frequently the drug dose must be ta-pered or discontinued.
- The neonate born to a mother who has been re-ceiving a corticosteroid during pregnancy should be monitored for symptoms of hypoadrenocorti-cism.
- The acetate and sodium phosphate formulations may contain bisulfites or parabens or both. These inactive ingredients are allergenic to some individ-uals. Monitor for signs and symptoms of a hyper-sensitivity reaction (see chap 3).
- Observe eyelids and eye surfaces being treated with solution or ointment. If irritation develops, stop the treatment and consult physician.

Patient & Family Education
- Make certain patient is aware of the importance of taking dexamethasone exactly as prescribed. Specifically, he or she should not omit, increase, decrease, or skip doses without advice of the physician. Patient should also understand what to do when a dose of dexamethasone is missed.
- Lack of response to the medication may signal hy-poadrenocorticism and be evidenced by malaise, orthostatic hypotension, muscular weakness and pain, nausea, vomiting, anorexia, hypoglycemic re-actions (see Signs & Symptoms, chap 3), mental de-pression. Patient should be instructed to report these symptoms.
- *Symptoms of early hyperadrenocorticism* may be sub-tle: increased appetite and weight gain, increased facial hair (women), full-looking face (moon fa-cies), abdominal distension, easy bruising, extreme weakness, amenorrhea. Alert patient (and family) to potential changes in appearance; physician should be contacted if they appear.
- Electrolytes and BP should be evaluated during therapy at regular intervals. Urge patient to keep appointments for check-ups.
- If patient is also receiving a potassium-depleting di-

uretic, dexamethasone-induced potassium loss may be enhanced. Encourage patient to add potassium-rich foods to diet and to report signs of hypokalemia (see chap 3).

- The dexamethasone dose regimen may need to be altered if patient is subjected to stress; e.g., surgery, infections, emotional stress, illness, acute bronchial attacks, trauma. Consult physician if change in living or working environment is anticipated.
- Caution patient not to change the prescribed regimen without physician's approval.
- Inform patient that discontinuation of dexamethasone should be accomplished gradually and under the guidance of the physician.
- Urge patient to report exacerbation of symptoms, inadequate response, and onset of side effects promptly.
- Emphasize the implications of immunosuppression with regard to prevention of exposure to infection, trauma, and to sudden changes in environmental factors.
- Instruct patient to report steady weight gain, especially if accompanied by edema of legs and ankles.
- Warn patient receiving ophthalmic preparation to consult physician promptly and to interrupt treatment if changes in visual acuity or diminished visual fields occur. Frequent measurement of IOP, slit-lamp microscopy, and examination of optic nerve head should accompany long-term therapy.
- For aerosol preparations the order should be specific as to number of sprays for each nostril, for each administration.
- Instruct patient to rinse mouth with warm water after each inhalation treatment to prevent excessive drying of oral and pharyngeal membranes (prevent cough, hoarseness, sore throat) and to prevent development of superinfections (see Signs & Symptoms, chap 3).

Prototype: diphenhydramine, p 47

DEXCHLORPHENIRAMINE MALEATE
(dex-klor-fen-eer′a meen)
Trade names: Dexchlor, Poladex T.D., Polaramine, Polargen
Classification: ANTIHISTAMINE; (H_1-RECEPTOR ANTAGONIST)
Pregnancy: Category B

ACTIONS/PHARMACODYNAMICS H_1-receptor antagonist and alkylamine antihistamine derived

from chlorpheniramine, with which it shares actions, uses, contraindications, precautions, and adverse reactions. In common with other antihistamines, has anticholinergic properties and produces mild-to-moderate drowsiness and sedation.

USES Perennial and seasonal allergic rhinitis, other manifestations of allergy, and vasomotor rhinitis. Also as adjunct to epinephrine in treatment of anaphylactic reactions.

ROUTE & DOSAGE

Allergic Rhinitis

Adult	PO	2 mg q4–6h *or* 4–6 mg of repeat-action tablets h.s. *or* q8–10h during the day
Child	PO	6–11 y: 1 mg q4–6h (not to exceed 6 mg/24 h) *or* 4 mg of repeat-action tablets h.s.
	PO	2–5 y: 0.5 mg q4–6h (not to exceed 3 mg/24 h)

PHARMACOKINETICS Absorption: readily absorbed from GI tract. **Onset:** 15–30 min. **Peak:** 3 h. **Distribution:** small amounts distributed into breast milk. **Metabolism:** metabolized in liver. **Elimination:** excreted in urine within 24 h.

CONTRAINDICATIONS & PRECAUTIONS Contraindicated in: hypersensitivity to antihistamines of similar class; acute asthmatic attack, lower respiratory tract symptoms, newborns, premature infants. Safe use during pregnancy (category B) and in nursing mothers not established. **Cautious use in:** increased intraocular pressure; prostatic hypertrophy; hyperthyroidism; renal and cardiovascular disease, elderly patients.

ADVERSE/SIDE EFFECTS CNS: *drowsiness,* dizziness, weakness, headache, excitation, neuritis, disturbed coordination, insomnia, euphoria, paresthesias. **ENT:** vertigo, tinnitus, acute labyrinthitis. **CV:** palpitation, tachycardia, hypotension, extrasystoles. **GI:** nausea, vomiting, anorexia, *dry mouth,* constipation, diarrhea. **GU:** difficulty in urinating, *urinary retention,* urinary frequency, early menses. **Hematologic:** thrombocytopenia, agranulocytosis, hemolytic or hypoplastic anemia. **Other:** blurred vision, skin eruptions, photosensitivity.

DIAGNOSTIC TEST INTERFERENCES In common with other antihistamines, dexchlorpheniramine may interfere with *Skin tests for allergy;* discontinue dexchlorpheniramine at least 72 h before tests.

DRUG INTERACTIONS Alcohol and other CNS DEPRESSANTS, MAO INHIBITORS compound CNS depression.

NURSING IMPLICATIONS

Administration
- Advise patient to take medication with food, water, or milk to lessen GI distress.
- Regular tablet may be crushed and taken with fluid or mixed with food.
- Store at 15–30C (59–86F) unless otherwise directed.

Assessment & Drug Effects
- Supervise ambulation and take safety precautions.
- Monitor I&O and assess for difficulty voiding (e.g., frequency or retention).

Patient & Family Education
- Instruct patient to swallow timed-release tablet whole. It should not be broken, crushed, or chewed.
- Because of the possibility of drowsiness, dizziness, and blurred vision, caution patient to avoid driving and other potentially hazardous activities until reaction to drug is known.
- Advise patient to ask physician about the use of alcohol, tranquilizers, sedatives, or other CNS depressants because the effects of dexchlorpheniramine will be additive.
- Dexchlorpheniramine should be discontinued about 4 d before skin tests for allergies, since it can affect test results, making them inaccurate.

Prototype: bethanechol, p 120

DEXPANTHENOL
(dex-pan´the-nole)
Trade names: Dexol, Ilopan, Panthoderm
Classifications: AUTONOMIC NERVOUS SYSTEM AGENT; CHOLINERGIC, DIRECT ACTING; VITAMIN B COMPLEX
Pregnancy: Category C

ACTIONS/PHARMACODYNAMICS Alcohol analog of the coenzyme vitamin pantothenic acid, to which it is readily converted. A member of the B-complex group and precursor of coenzyme A, which is essential to normal epithelial function and biosynthesis of fatty acids, amino acids, and acetylcholine. Increases GI peristalsis and intestinal tone by stimulating acetylation of choline to acetylcholine. Topical application reportedly relieves itching and may aid healing of skin lesions by stimulating epithelialization and granulation. Also has antibacterial activity.

USES Prevention or treatment of postoperative abdominal distension, intestinal atony, and paralytic ileus. Topically to relieve itching and to promote healing in minor skin lesions.

ROUTE & DOSAGE

Postoperative Abdominal Distension, Intestinal Atony, Paralytic Ileus

Adult	IM	250–500 mg; repeat in 2 h; then repeat q4–12h prn
	IV	500 mg by slow IV infusion
Child	IM	11–12.5 mg/kg; repeat in 2 h; then repeat q4–12h prn

Itching

Adult	Topical	Apply to affected area 1–2 times/d

PHARMACOKINETICS Absorption: readily absorbed from IM site. **Distribution:** highest concentration in liver, adrenals, heart, and kidneys; small amount distributed into breast milk. **Metabolism:** rapidly converted to pantothenic acid, the active moiety. **Elimination:** 70% excreted in urine, 30% in feces.

CONTRAINDICATIONS & PRECAUTIONS Contraindicated in: hemophilia; ileus due to mechanical obstruction. Safe use during pregnancy (category C), in nursing women, and in children not established. **Cautious use in:** hypokalemia.

ADVERSE/SIDE EFFECTS Generally well tolerated. Rare: allergic manifestations, hyperperistalsis, *diarrhea*, prolonge.d bleeding time.

DRUG INTERACTIONS Prolongs muscle relaxation effects of **succinylcholine.**

NURSING IMPLICATIONS

Administration
- Do not administer within 1 h of succinylcholine administration.
- IV dexpanthenol is not intended for direct IV administration.
- IV dexpanthenol is diluted in at least 500 ml of D5W or lactated Ringer's solution and infused slowly over 3–6 h.

- Store at 15–30C (59–86F); protect from freezing and excessive heat.

Assessment & Drug Effects
- Observe for and report bleeding tendency. Dexpanthenol may prolong bleeding time in some patients.
- Report immediately any evidence of a hypersensitivity reaction (see Signs & Symptoms, chap 3); drug should be discontinued.
- Therapeutic results may not be obtained in patients with hypokalemia.

Patient & Family Education
- Instruct patient to report abdominal cramping or diarrhea.

Prototype: albumin, p 126

DEXTRAN 40
(dex´tran)

Trade names: Gentran 40, Hyskon, 10% LMD, Rheomacrodex
Classifications. BLOOD DERIVATIVE, PLASMA VOLUME EXPANDER; REPLACEMENT SOLUTION
Pregnancy: Category C

ACTIONS/PHARMACODYNAMICS Low molecular weight polysaccharide formed by the action of *Leuconostoc mesenteroides* on sucrose. Average molecular weight is approximately 40,000 (range 10,000–90,000). As a hypertonic colloidal solution, produces immediate and short-lived expansion of plasma volume by increasing colloidal osmotic pressure and drawing fluid from interstitial to intravascular spaces. Cardiovascular response to volume expansion includes increased BP, pulse pressure, CVP, cardiac output, venous return to heart, and urinary output. In addition to plasma volume expansion, it improves microcirculation, possibly by decreasing blood viscosity (lower Hct) and by retarding RBC sludging that may accompany shock. Reduces possibility of deep venous thrombosis and pulmonary embolism, primarily by inhibiting venous stasis and platelet adhesiveness. Lower incidence of allergic reactions than with higher molecular weight products.

USES Adjunctively to expand plasma volume and provide fluid replacement in treatment of shock or impending shock caused by hemorrhage, burns, surgery, or other trauma. Also used in prophylaxis and therapy of venous thrombosis and pulmonary embolism. Used as priming fluid or as additive to other primers during extracorporeal circulation.

ROUTE & DOSAGE

Shock

Adult	IV	500 ml administered rapidly (over 15–30 min); additional doses may be given more slowly up to 20 ml/kg in the first 24 h; doses up to 10 ml/kg/d may be given for an additional 4 d if needed
Child	IV	Same as for adult

Prophylaxis for Thromboembolic Complications

Adult	IV	500–1000 ml (10 ml/kg) on the day of operation followed by 500 ml/d for 2–3 d; may continue with 500 ml q2–3d for up to 2 wk if necessary

Priming for Extracorporeal Circulation

Adult	IV	10–20 ml/kg added to perfusion circuit

PHARMACOKINETICS Onset: volume expansion within minutes of infusion. **Duration:** 12 h. **Metabolism:** degraded to glucose and metabolized to CO_2 and water over a period of a few weeks. **Elimination:** 75% excreted in urine within 24 h; small amount excreted in feces.

CONTRAINDICATIONS & PRECAUTIONS Contraindicated in: hypersensitivity to dextrans, renal failure, hypervolemic conditions, severe CHF, thrombocytopenia, significant anemia, hypofibrinogenemia or other marked hemostatic defects including those caused by drugs, e.g., heparin, warfarin. Safe use during pregnancy (category C) not established. **Cautious use in:** active hemorrhage; severe dehydration; chronic liver disease; impaired renal function; patients susceptible to pulmonary edema or CHF.

ADVERSE/SIDE EFFECTS Hypersensitivity: mild to generalized urticaria, pruritus, angioedema, nasal congestion, *dyspnea*, wheezing, tightness in chest, nausea, vomiting, arthralgia, anaphylactic shock. **Other:** renal tubular vacuolization (osmotic nephrosis), stasis, and blocking; oliguria, renal failure; increased AST and ALT. **Hematologic:** decreased factor VIII levels, interference with platelet function, prolonged bleeding and coagulation times; decreased Hct and plasma protein levels, arrhythmias.

DIAGNOSTIC TEST INTERFERENCES When blood samples are drawn for study, notify laboratory

Common side effects in *italic*; life-threatening effects <u>underlined</u>; generic names in **bold**; classifications in SMALL CAPS

505

that patient has received dextran. **Blood glucose:** false increases (utilizing ortho-toluidine methods or sulfuric or acetic acid hydrolysis). **Urinary protein:** false increases (utilizing Lowry method). **Bilirubin assays:** false increases when alcohol is used. **Total protein assays:** false increases using biuret reagent. **Rh testing, blood typing** and **cross-matching** procedures: dextran may interfere with results (by inducing rouleaux formation) when proteolytic enzyme techniques are used (saline agglutination and indirect antiglobulin methods reportedly not affected).

NURSING IMPLICATIONS

Administration

- Use only if seal is intact, vacuum is detectable, and solution is absolutely clear.
- When stored for long periods, dextran flakes may form. To dissolve flakes, place unopened bottle in warm water bath until solution clears.
- If blood is to be administered, a cross-match specimen should be drawn before dextran infusion.
- Specific flow rate should be prescribed by physician. Usually administered at a rate of 500 ml over 15–30 min.
- Dextran should be stored at a constant temperature, preferably 25C (77F). Once opened, unused portion should be discarded because dextran contains no preservative.

Assessment & Drug Effects

- Patient's state of hydration should be evaluated before dextran therapy begins. Administration of dextran to severely dehydrated patients can result in renal failure.
- Baseline Hct should be taken prior to and after initiation of dextran (dextran usually lowers Hct). Notify physician if Hct is depressed below 30% by volume.
- Hypersensitivity reaction is most likely to occur during the first few minutes of administration. Monitor vital signs and observe patient closely for at least the first 30 min of infusion. Therapy should be terminated at the first sign of a hypersensitivity reaction (see chap 3).
- Monitoring CVP is advised as an estimate of blood volume status and as a guide for determining dosage. **Normal CVP:** 5–10 cm H_2O.
- Observe patient for clinical signs of circulatory overload (see chap 3).
- In patients for whom sodium restriction is indicated, it should be noted that 500 ml of dextran 40 in 0.9% normal saline contains 77 mEq of both sodium and chloride.

- Monitor I&O ratio and check urine specific gravity at regular intervals. Low urine specific gravity may signify failure of renal dextran clearance and is an indication for discontinuing therapy.
- State of hydration should be monitored throughout therapy by I&O ratio and by determinations of urine and serum osmolarity.
- In poorly hydrated patients dextran may attract water from extravascular spaces and cause dehydration. Monitor for signs of dehydration (see chap 3).
- Report oliguria, anuria, or lack of improvement in urinary output (dextran usually causes an increase in urinary output). Dextran should be discontinued at the first indication of renal dysfunction.
- Low urine specific gravity may signify failure of renal dextran clearance and is an indication for discontinuing therapy.
- Transient prolongation of bleeding time and interference with normal blood coagulation may occur with high doses.

Prototype: albumin, p 126

DEXTRAN 70
(dex´tran)
Trade name: Macrodex

DEXTRAN 75
Trade name: Gentran 75
Classifications: BLOOD DERIVATIVE; PLASMA VOLUME EXPANDER; REPLACEMENT SOLUTION

ACTIONS/PHARMACODYNAMICS High molecular weight polysaccharides. Dextran 70 has an average molecular weight of 70,000; that of dextran 75 is 75,000 (molecular weight range for both: 20,000–200,000). Colloidal properties approximate those of serum albumin. Differs from dextran 40 in molecular weight and in having less effect on rouleaux formation and sludging of red blood cells and a higher incidence of severe allergic reactions.

USES Primarily for emergency treatment of hypovolemic shock or impending shock caused by hemorrhage, burns, surgery, or other trauma. Intended for emergency treatment only when whole blood or blood products are not available or when haste precludes cross-matching of blood. **Unlabeled use:**

Common side effects in *italic*; life-threatening effects underlined; generic names in **bold**; classifications in SMALL CAPS

nephrosis, toxemia of pregnancy, and prophylaxis of deep-vein thrombosis.

ROUTE & DOSAGE

Shock

Adult	IV	500 ml administered rapidly (over 15–30 min); additional doses may be given more slowly up to 20 ml/kg in the first 24 h; doses up to 10 ml/kg/d may be given for an additional 4 d if needed

PHARMACOKINETICS Onset: volume expansion within minutes of infusion. **Duration:** 12 h. **Metabolism:** degraded to glucose and metabolized to carbon dioxide and water over a period of a few weeks. **Elimination:** 75% excreted in urine within 24 h; small amount excreted in feces.

CONTRAINDICATIONS & PRECAUTIONS Contraindicated in: known hypersensitivity to dextrans; severe bleeding disorders; severe CHF; renal failure.

ADVERSE/SIDE EFFECTS *Allergic reactions,* severe anaphylactoid reaction, GI disturbances, lowered plasma protein levels (high doses).

NURSING IMPLICATIONS

Administration
- Use only if seal is intact, vacuum is detectable, and solution is absolutely clear.
- Specific flow rate should be prescribed by physician. (For emergency treatment of shock, rate of administration for first 500 ml may be 20–40 ml/min. In normovolemic patients, flow rate should not exceed 4 ml/min.)
- Store at a constant temperature, preferably 25C (77F).

Assessment & Drug Effects
- Bleeding time may be temporarily prolonged in patients receiving more than 1000 ml of dextran 70 or 75.
- Patient should be observed closely for signs of anaphylaxis (see chap 3), especially during first 30 min of infusion. Severe reactions occasionally have resulted in fatalities.
- Monitor I&O ratio and pattern. Monitor vital signs frequently as warranted by condition of patient.

DEXTRANOMER

(dex-tran´oh-mer)

Trade name: Debrisan

Classification: WOUND CLEANSING AGENT

ACTIONS/PHARMACODYNAMICS Consists of small, spherical, dry, hydrophilic beads of a dextran polymer that when applied to secreting wound surface absorbs tissue exudate. Dextranomer has no debriding action. Also effective in removing bacteria and protein, particularly fibrin and fibrinogen degradation products. Shortens healing time by retarding eschar or scab formation and by reducing inflammation and edema. Each gram of dextranomer absorbs about 4 ml of exudate. Dextranomer beads are made up of cross-linked dextran arranged in a 3-dimensional network large enough to allow low molecular weight substances (e.g., exudates) to be absorbed readily into beads; high molecular weight substances (such as plasma proteins, fibrinogen) remain in bead interspaces. Not effective for cleansing nonsecreting wounds. Systemic absorption does not occur; drug appears to have low sensitizing potential.

USES To cleanse exudating wounds such as venous stasis ulcers; decubitus ulcers; infected burns; and infected, traumatic, and surgical wounds.

ROUTE & DOSAGE

Exudative Wounds

Adult	Topical	Apply to affected area 1–2 times/d; may need more frequent changes for profusely draining wounds

CONTRAINDICATIONS & PRECAUTIONS Contraindicated in: deep fistulas, sinus tracts, deep body cavities where complete removal is not assured, dry wounds.

ADVERSE/SIDE EFFECTS Reportedly well-tolerated. Erythema, pain, irritation, bleeding, blistering, usually associated with dressing changes.

NURSING IMPLICATIONS

Administration
- Content of container should be reserved for use in a single patient to avoid possibility of cross contamination.
- Before application, debride and wash wound as di-

Common side effects in *italic*; life-threatening effects underlined; generic names in **bold**; classifications in SMALL CAPS

507

rected by physician. Leave wound surface moist. Pour dextranomer into wound to depth of at least 6 mm (1/4 inch). Cover with sterile gauze pad and tape in place loose enough to allow for expansion of beads. Do not use occlusive dressings because maceration of tissue surrounding wound may result.

- Do not apply beads or paste to deep fistulas, sinuses, or any body cavity where complete removal is not possible.
- For wounds in hard-to-reach body areas, a freshly-prepared paste may be made by mixing 3 parts Debrisan beads with 1 part sterile glycerin in a receptacle. Apply to wound with sterile spatala. Debrisan is available in a convenient premixed sterile paste.
- For reapplication, beads should be removed before becoming fully saturated and dried out, to prevent difficult removal from wound surface. When saturated, beads appear grayish-yellow.
- Beads can be removed by irrigating with sterile water, saline, or other cleansing solution. Removal should be as complete as possible. Soaking or whirlpool may be required to remove stubborn patches of beads.
- Store in tightly closed container in a dry place at a constant room temperature, preferably 25C (77F), unless otherwise directed.

Assessment & Drug Effects

- Reduction of wound edema, which occurs during first few days of therapy, may make wound appear larger.
- Dextranomer should be discontinued when wound is no longer draining and healthy granulation tissue is established.

Prototype: amphetamine, p 194

DEXTROAMPHETAMINE SULFATE

(dex-troe-am-fet´a-meen)

Trade names: Dexampex, Dexedrine, Ferndex, Oxydess II, Spancap No. 1

Classifications: CNS AGENT; RESPIRATORY & CEREBRAL STIMULANT; AMPHETAMINE; ANOREXIANT

Controlled substance: Schedule II

ACTIONS/PHARMACODYNAMICS Dextrorotatory isomer of amphetamine, with which it shares actions, uses, contraindications, precautions, and adverse reactions. On a weight basis, has less pronounced action on cardiovascular and peripheral nervous systems and is a more potent appetite suppressant. CNS stimulating effect approximately twice that of racemic amphetamine. Anorexigenic effect is thought to result from CNS stimulation and possibly from loss of acuity of smell and taste. In hyperkinetic children, amphetamines reduce motor restlessness by an unknown mechanism.

USES Adjunct in short-term treatment of exogenous obesity, narcolepsy, and attention deficit disorder with hyperactivity in children (also called minimal brain dysfunction or hyperkinetic syndrome). **Unlabeled uses:** adjunct in epilepsy to control ataxia and drowsiness induced by barbiturates; to combat sedative effects of trimethadione in absence seizures.

ROUTE & DOSAGE

Narcolepsy

Adult	PO	5–20 mg 1–3 times/d at 4–6 h intervals
Child	PO	>12 y: 10 mg/d; may increase by 10 mg at weekly intervals
		6–12 y: 5 mg/d; may increase by 5 mg at weekly intervals

Attention Deficit Disorder

Child	PO	≥ 6 y: 5 mg 1–2 times/d; may increase by 5 mg at weekly intervals (max 40 mg/d)
	PO	3–5 y: 2.5 mg 1–2 times/d; may increase by 2.5 mg at weekly intervals

Obesity

Adult	PO	5–10 mg 1–3 times/d or 10–15 mg of sustained release once/d 30–60 min a.c.

PHARMACOKINETICS **Absorption:** rapid. **Peak:** 1–5 h. **Duration:** up to 10 h. **Distribution:** all tissues especially the CNS. **Metabolism:** metabolized in liver. **Elimination:** half-life: 10–30 h; renal elimination; excreted in breast milk.

CONTRAINDICATIONS & PRECAUTIONS Contraindicated in: hypersensitivity to sympathomimetic amines, glaucoma, agitated states, psychoses (especially in children), advanced arteriosclerosis, symptomatic heart disease, moderate to severe hypertension, hyperthyroidism, history of drug abuse, during or within 14 d of MAO inhibitor therapy, as anorexiant in children <12 y, for attention deficit disorder in children <3 y.

Common side effects in *italic*; life-threatening effects underlined; generic names in **bold**; classifications in SMALL CAPS

ADVERSE/SIDE EFFECTS CNS: nervousness, *restlessness,* hyperactivity, *insomnia,* euphoria, dizziness, headache; **with prolonged use:** severe depression, psychotic reactions. **CV:** palpitation, tachycardia, elevated BP. **GI:** dry mouth, unpleasant taste, anorexia, weight loss, diarrhea, constipation, abdominal pain. **Other:** impotence, changes in libido, unusual fatigue, increased intraocular pressure, marked dystonia of head, neck, and extremities; sweating.

DIAGNOSTIC TEST INTERFERENCES Dextroamphetamine may cause significant elevations in *plasma corticosteroids* (evening levels are highest) and increases in **urinary epinephrine** excretion (during first 3 h after drug administration).

DRUG INTERACTIONS Acetazolamide, sodium bicarbonate decrease dextroamphetamine elimination; **ammonium chloride, ascorbic acid** increase dextroamphetamine elimination; effects of both BAR-BITURATES and dextroamphetamine may be antagonized; **furazolidone** may increase BP effects of amphetamines—interaction may persist for several weeks after discontinuing furazolidone; antagonizes antihypertensive effects of **guanethidine, guanadryl;** MAO INHIBITORS, **selegiline** can cause hypertensive crisis (fatalities reported)—do not administer amphetamines during or within 14 d of these drugs; PHENOTHIAZINES may inhibit mood elevating effects of amphetamines; TRICYCLIC ANTIDEPRESSANTS enhance dextroamphetamine effects because of increased norepinephrine release; BETA ADRENERGIC AGONISTS increase cardiovascular adverse effects.

NURSING IMPLICATIONS

Administration

- Administered 30–60 min before meals for treatment of obesity. Long-acting form is administered in the morning.
- To avoid insomnia, administer last dose no later than 6 h before patient retires (10–14 h before bedtime for sustained-release form).
- Store in tightly closed containers at 15–30C (59–86F) unless otherwise directed.

Assessment & Drug Effects

- Growth rate should be closely monitored in children.
- Periodic interruption of therapy or reduction in dosage is recommended to assess effectiveness of therapy in behavior disorders.
- Tolerance to anorexiant effects may develop after a few weeks; however, tolerance does not appear to develop when dextroamphetamine used in treatment of narcolepsy.

Patient & Family Education

- Instruct patient to swallow sustained-release capsule whole with a liquid and not to chew or crush it.
- Inform patient that drug may impair ability to drive or perform other potentially hazardous activities.
- Discontinuation of drug following long-term use should be accomplished gradually to avoid extreme fatigue, mental depression, and prolonged sleep pattern that follows abrupt withdrawal.

D

Prototype: benzonatate, p 99

DEXTROMETHORPHAN HYDROBROMIDE

(dex-troe-meth-or´fan)
Trade names: Benylin DM, Cremacoat 1, Delsym, DM Cough, Hold, Koffex, Mediquell, Neo-DM, Ornex DM, Pedia Care, Pertussin 8 Hour Cough Formula, Robidex, Robitussin DM, Romilar CF, Romilar Children's Cough, Sedatuss, Sucrets Cough Control
Classification: ANTITUSSIVE
Pregnancy: Category C

ACTIONS/PHARMACODYNAMICS Nonnarcotic derivative of levorphanol. Chemically related to morphine but without central hypnotic or analgesic effect or capacity to cause tolerance or addiction. Controls cough spasms by depressing cough center in medulla. Does not depress respiration or inhibit ciliary action. Antitussive activity comparable to that of codeine but is less likely than codeine to cause constipation, drowsiness, or GI disturbances.

USES Temporary relief of cough spasms in nonproductive coughs due to colds, pertussis, and influenza.

PHARMACOKINETICS Absorption: readily absorbed from GI tract. **Onset:** 15–30 min. **Duration:** 3–6 h. **Metabolism:** metabolized in liver. **Elimination:** excreted in urine.

CONTRAINDICATIONS & PRECAUTIONS Contraindicated in: children <2 y, asthma, productive

Common side effects in *italic*; life-threatening effects <u>underlined</u>;
generic names in **bold**; classifications in SMALL CAPS

509

cough, persistent or chronic cough; hepatic function impairment; pregnancy, category C. **Cautious use in:** chronic pulmonary disease; enlarged prostate; patients on MAO inhibitors.

ROUTE & DOSAGE

Cough

Adult	PO	10–20 mg q4h *or* 30 mg q6–8h (max 120 mg/d); *or* 60 mg of sustained-action liquid b.i.d
Child	PO	6–12 y: 5–10 mg q4h *or* 15 mg q6–8h (max 60 mg/d) *or* 30 mg sustained-action liquid b.i.d.
		2–6 y: 2.5–5 mg q4h *or* 7.5 mg q6–8h (max 30 mg/d) *or* 15 mg sustained-action liquid b.i.d.

ADVERSE/SIDE EFFECTS Rare: *dizziness, drowsiness,* CNS depression with very large doses; excitability, especially in children; GI upset, constipation, abdominal discomfort.

DRUG INTERACTIONS High risk of excitation, hypotension, and hyperpyrexia with MAO INHIBITORS.

NURSING IMPLICATIONS

Administration

▪ Although soothing local effect of the syrup may be enhanced if administered undiluted, depression of cough center depends on systemic absorption of drug.

Patient & Family Education

▪ Unnecessary cough may be lessened by avoiding irritants such as smoking, dust, fumes, and other air pollutants. Humidification of ambient air may provide some relief.
▪ Treatment is directed toward decreasing the frequency and intensity of cough without completely eliminating protective cough reflex.
▪ Dextromethorphan can be purchased over the counter. Advise patient that any cough persisting longer than 1 wk or 10 d should be medically diagnosed.

Prototype: lovastatin, p 143

DEXTROTHYROXINE SODIUM
(dex-troe-thye-rox´een)
Trade name: Choloxin
Classification: CARDIOVASCULAR DRUG; ANTILIPEMIC; LIPID-LOWERING AGENT
Pregnancy: Category C

ACTIONS/PHARMACODYNAMICS Sodium salt and dextrorotatory isomer of thyroxine. Reduces serum cholesterol and LDL levels in hyperlipidemia; triglycerides and beta lipoproteins may also be lowered from previously elevated levels, but effect is variable. By an unclear mechanism, liver is stimulated to increase catabolism and excretion of cholesterol and its degradation products via the biliary route into feces. Greatest decrease in serum cholesterol occurs in patients with highest baseline concentrations, with maximum therapeutic effects in 1 or 2 mo. Cholesterol synthesis is increased, but metabolic end products do not accumulate in the blood. It has not been determined whether drug-induced lowering of serum cholesterol or other lipids has beneficial, detrimental, or no effects on morbidity or mortality due to atherosclerosis or coronary heart disease.

USES Adjunct to other medications in the treatment of primary hypercholesterolemia (type IIa hyperlipidemia), particularly euthyroid patients with significant risk but no evidence of coronary artery disease.

ROUTE & DOSAGE

Euthyroid Hyperlipidemia

Adult	PO	1–2 mg/d, increased by 1 or 2 mg every month if needed (max 8 mg/d)
Child	PO	0.05 mg/kg/d, increased by not more than 0.05 mg/kg every month if needed (max 4 mg/d)

PHARMACOKINETICS Absorption: about 25% absorbed from GI tract. **Distribution:** crosses placenta; distribution into breast milk not known. **Metabolism:** metabolized in liver. **Elimination:** half-life: 18 h; excreted in urine and feces.

CONTRAINDICATIONS & PRECAUTIONS Contraindicated in: euthyroids: known organic heart disease including angina pectoris, arrhythmias, decompensated or borderline compensated cardiac states; history of MI or CHF; rheumatic heart disease; hypertension; advanced liver or kidney disease; history of iodism; pregnancy (category C), nursing mothers; 2 wk prior to elective surgery. **Cautious use in:** hypothyroid patients with concomitant coronary artery disease; women of childbearing age with familial hypercholesterolemia; diabetes mellitus; liver and kidney impairment; children, the elderly.

ADVERSE/SIDE EFFECTS Mainly due to increased metabolism. **CNS:** insomnia, nervousness, dizziness, psychic changes, paresthesias. **CV:** angina pectoris, palpitation, cardiac arrhythmia, ECG evidence of ischemic myocardial changes, increase in heart size; <u>MI</u> (relationship not conclusive), worsening of peripheral vascular disease. **ENT:** tinnitus, hoarseness. **Eye:** visual disturbances, exophthalmos, retinopathy, lid lag. **GI:** nausea, constipation, diarrhea, bitter taste, weight loss. **Iodism:** acneiform rash, pruritus, coryza, conjunctivitis, stomatitis, brassy taste, laryngitis, bronchitis.

DRUG INTERACTIONS Cholestyramine, colestipol decrease absorption of dextrothyroxine; compounds thyroid effects of other THYROID PREPARATIONS; increases risk of hypoprothrombinemia associated with **warfarin; digoxin** may enhance myocardial stimulation; may increase blood glucose, requiring adjustment of **insulin** and SULFONYLUREAS.

NURSING IMPLICATIONS

Administration

- Store medication in light and moisture proof container at 15–30C (59–86F) unless otherwise specified.

Assessment & Drug Effects

- Serum lipids should be determined initially and evaluated at monthly intervals during therapy. Patient should be on a normal diet for several days prior to the test.
- Initial decrease in cholesterol levels may not occur until 2 wk–1 mo after initiation of therapy. Maximum decrease usually occurs during second or third month of therapy.
- Patients with cardiac disease should be observed closely, particularly during early therapy, and checked at frequent intervals throughout the treatment period.
- Hypothyroid patients with organic heart disease have a high incidence of adverse/side effects.
- Report immediately new signs and symptoms of

cardiac disease or increased decompensation in the borderline compensated patient. Dose adjustment may be indicated.

- Patients with diabetes should be closely monitored. Dosage adjustment of insulin or oral antidiabetic agent may be required. Advise patient to report diminishing control of diabetes.

Patient & Family Education

- Goal of therapy is to prevent further atherosclerosis. Encourage patient to adhere to diet regimen, an important adjunct to therapeutic plan.
- Since hypercholesterolemia is frequently genetically determined, family members of patient, especially children 5 y and older, should be screened for abnormal lipid values.
- Serum lipids generally return to pretreatment levels within 6 wk–3 mo after drug is withdrawn.
- Teratogenic studies have been inconclusive; thus strict birth control measures are advised for women of childbearing potential.
- Instruct patient to report chest pain, palpitations, sweating, diarrhea, headache, or skin rash.
- Advise patient to report promptly the onset of iodism (see adverse/side effects). If iodism is developing, the drug will be withdrawn.
- Instruct patient not to self-dose with OTC medications unless physician's approval is obtained.
- Advise patient not to change dosage regimen in any way without consulting the physician.
- Patient should inform physician or dentist in an emergency situation that he or she is taking dextrothyroxine before any surgery is performed.

DIAZEPAM

See CNS AGENTS, ANTICONVULSANT, BENZODIAZEPINE, prototype, p 170.

Prototype: hydralazine, p 152

DIAZOXIDE

(dye-az-ox´ide)
Trade names: Hyperstat I.V., Proglycem
Classifications: CARDIOVASCULAR DRUG;
ANTIHYPERTENSIVE; VASODILATOR; SULFONYLUREA
Pregnancy: Category C

Common side effects in *italic*; life-threatening effects <u>underlined</u>; generic names in **bold**; classifications in SMALL CAPS

511

ACTIONS/PHARMACODYNAMICS Rapid-acting thiazide (benzothiadiazine) nondiuretic hypotensive and hyperglycemic agent. In contrast to thiazide diuretics, causes sodium and water retention and decreases urinary output, probably because it increases proximal tubular reabsorption of sodium and decreases glomerular filtration rate. Produces hyperglycemia by inhibiting pancreatic insulin secretion and by stimulating endogenous catecholamine release. Reduces peripheral vascular resistance and BP by direct vasodilatory effect on peripheral arteriolar smooth muscles, perhaps by direct competition for calcium receptor sites. Hypotensive effect may be accompanied by marked reflex increase in heart rate, cardiac output, and stroke volume; thus cerebral and coronary blood flow are usually maintained. Renal blood flow initially decreases then increases. Oral drug has more prominent hyperglycemic action and less marked antihypertensive effect than parenteral drug. Diazoxide may inhibit ureteral and GI motility and is a powerful uterine relaxant.

USES Intravenously for emergency lowering of BP in hospitalized patients with malignant hypertension, particularly when associated with renal impairment. Not effective in pheochromocytoma. Commonly used with a diuretic such as furosemide (Lasix) to counteract diazoxide-induced sodium and water retention. Orally in treatment of various diagnosed hypoglycemic states due to hyperinsulinism when other medical treatment or surgical management has been unsuccessful or is not feasible.

ROUTE & DOSAGE

Severe Hypertension

Adult	IV	1–3 mg/kg up to 150 mg repeated at 5–15 min intervals if necessary
Child	IV	Same as for adult

Hypoglycemia

Adult	PO	3–8 mg/kg/d divided q8–12h
Child	PO	Neonates/Infants: 8–15 mg/kg/d divided q8–12h

PHARMACOKINETICS Onset: 30–60 s IV; 1 h PO. **Peak:** 5 min IV. **Duration:** 2–12 or more h IV; 8 h PO. **Distribution:** crosses blood-brain barrier and placenta. **Metabolism:** partially metabolized in the liver. **Elimination:** half-life: 21–45 h; excreted in urine.

CONTRAINDICATIONS & PRECAUTIONS Contraindicated in: hypersensitivity to diazoxide or to other thiazides; cerebral bleeding, eclampsia; aortic coarctation; AV shunt, significant coronary artery disease. Safe use during pregnancy (category C) and in nursing mothers not established. Use of oral diazoxide for functional hypoglycemia or in presence of increased bilirubin in newborns. **Cautious use in:** diabetes mellitus; impaired cerebral or cardiac circulation; impaired renal function; patients taking corticosteroids or estrogen-progestogen combinations; hyperuricemia, history of gout, uremia.

ADVERSE/SIDE EFFECTS CNS: tinnitus, momentary hearing loss, headache, weakness, malaise, dizziness, polyneuritis, sleepiness, insomnia, euphoria, anxiety, extrapyramidal signs. **CV:** palpitations, atrial and ventricular arrhythmias, flushing, shock; *orthostatic hypotension,* CHF, transient hypertension. **Eye:** blurred vision, transient cataracts, subconjunctival hemorrhage, ring scotoma, diplopia, lacrimation, papilledema. **GI:** *nausea, vomiting,* abdominal discomfort, diarrhea, constipation, ileus, anorexia, transient loss of taste, parotid swelling, dry mouth. **Hematologic:** transient neutropenia, eosinophilia, decreased Hgb/Hct, decreased IgG. **Hypersensitivity:** rash, fever, leukopenia. **Renal:** decreased urinary output, nephrotic syndrome (reversible), hematuria, increased nocturia, proteinuria, azotemia. **Skin:** pruritus, flushing, monilial dermatitis, herpes, hirsutism; loss of scalp hair, sweating, sensation of warmth, burning, or itching. **Other:** impaired hepatic function, chest and back pain, muscle cramps; acute pancreatitis, pancreatic necrosis, advance in bone age (children); *sodium and water retention, edema,* hyperuricemia, glycosuria, inhibition of labor, enlargement of breast lump, galactorrhea; decreased immunoglobinemia.

DIAGNOSTIC TEST INTERFERENCES Diazoxide can cause false-negative response to **glucagon.**

DRUG INTERACTIONS SULFONYLUREAS antagonize effects; THIAZIDE DIURETICS may intensify hyperglycemia and antihypertensive effects; **phenytoin** increases risk of hyperglycemia, and diazoxide may increase phenytoin metabolism, causing loss of seizure control.

NURSING IMPLICATIONS

Administration

- IV diazoxide is given undiluted by rapid direct IV injection.
- Patient should be recumbent while receiving IV diazoxide and should remain in bed for at least 30 min following administration.

Common side effects in *italic*; life-threatening effects underlined; generic names in **bold**; classifications in SMALL CAPS

- Since diazoxide causes sodium and water retention, a diuretic is generally prescribed to avoid CHF and drug resistance and to maximize hypotensive effect.
- When a diuretic, e.g., furosemide (Lasix), is prescribed, it is generally given 30–60 min prior to IV diazoxide. Patient should remain recumbent 8–10 h because of possible additive hypotensive effect.
- Alternate oral antihypertensive therapy should be started as soon as possible after emergency is controlled. It is rarely necessary to give IV diazoxide therapy for more than 4 or 5 d.
- Darkened solutions may have lost potency and should not be administered.
- Store capsules, oral suspension, and injection at 2–30C (35.6–86F) unless otherwise directed. Protect from light, heat, and freezing.

Assessment & Drug Effects

- Check IV injection sites daily. Solution is strongly alkaline. Extravasation of medication into SC or IV tissues can cause severe inflammatory reaction. Diazoxide is administered only by peripheral vein.
- Diazoxide is discontinued if not effective in 2 or 3 wk.
- Blood glucose, serum electrolytes, and CBC should be determined at start of IV therapy and regularly thereafter in patients receiving multiple doses.
- Monitor BP q5min for the first 15–30 min or until stabilized, then hourly for balance of drug effect.
- If BP continues to fall 30 min or more after IV drug administration, suspect cause other than drug effect. Notify physician immediately.
- Monitor pulse: tachycardia has occurred immediately following IV; palpitation and bradycardia have also been reported.
- Report promptly any change in I&O ratio.
- Observe patient closely for signs and symptoms of CHF (see chap 3).
- Serum electrolyte levels should be evaluated at regular intervals, particularly in patient with impaired renal function. (Hypokalemia potentiates hyperglycemic effect of diazoxide.)
- In contrast to IV diazoxide, oral administration usually does not produce marked effects on BP. However, periodic measurements of BP and vital signs should be made.
- Prolonged surveillance of symptoms for up to 7 d may be essential because of long half-life of diazoxide (for both oral and parenteral forms).

Patient & Family Education

- Diazoxide may cause hyperglycemia and glycosuria in diabetic and diabetic-prone individuals.

Blood and urine glucose should be closely monitored; report any abnormalities to physician.
- Instruct patient to report palpitations, chest pain, dizziness, fainting, or severe headache.
- Lanugo type hirsutism occurs frequently and is most common in children and women. Reassure patient that it is reversible with discontinuation of drug.

Prototype: procaine, p 166

DIBUCAINE
(dye´byoo-kane)
Trade name: Nupercainal
Classification: CNS AGENT; ANESTHETIC, LOCAL (AMIDE-TYPE)
Pregnancy: Category C

ACTIONS/PHARMACODYNAMICS Long-acting anesthetic of the amide type and reportedly one of the most potent and most toxic. Appears to inhibit initiation and conduction of nerve impulses by reducing permeability of nerve cell membrane to sodium ions. Duration of action is about 3 times longer than that of procaine, and it is approximately 15 times more toxic.

USES Fast, temporary relief of pain and itching due to hemorrhoids and other anorectal disorders, nonpoisonous insect bites, sunburn, minor burns, cuts, and scratches.

ROUTE & DOSAGE

Itching Due to Insect Bites or Hemorrhoids

Adult	Topical	Apply skin cream or ointment to affected area as needed (max 1 oz [28 g]/24 h); insert rectal ointment morning and evening and after each bowel movement
Child	Topical	Apply skin cream or ointment to affected area as needed (max 1/4 oz [7 g]/24 h)

PHARMACOKINETICS Absorption: poorly absorbed from intact skin; readily absorbed from mucous membranes or abraded skin. **Onset:** 15 min. **Duration:** 2–4 h.

CONTRAINDICATIONS & PRECAUTIONS Contraindicated in: hypersensitivity to amide-type anesthetics. Pregnancy: category C.

Common side effects in *italic*; life-threatening effects underlined; generic names in **bold**; classifications in SMALL CAPS

513

ADVERSE/SIDE EFFECTS Irritation, contact dermatitis; rectal bleeding (suppository).

NURSING IMPLICATIONS

Administration

- The cream preparation is water soluble and therefore should be applied after bathing or swimming.
- Dibucaine preparations are stored at 15–30C (59–86F) in tight, light-resistant containers.

Patient & Family Education

- Instruct patient to use OTC preparations as directed. Review package instructions with patient.
- Caution patient to discontinue medication if irritation or rectal bleeding (following use of rectal preparations) develops and to consult physician.
- Remind patient that hemorrhoids can be caused or worsened by constipation, excessive straining at stool, and excessive standing, sitting, and coughing.
- Physician may prescribe sitz baths 3 or 4 times daily to reduce the swelling and pain of hemorrhoids.
- Medication is intended only for temporary relief of mild to moderate itching or pain.
- Seek medical advice for continuing discomfort, pain or bleeding, or sensation of rectal pressure.

Prototype: acetazolamide, p 206

DICHLORPHENAMIDE
(dye-klor-fen´a-mide)

Trade names: Daranide, Oratrol
Classifications: EYE PREPARATION; CARBONIC ANHYDRASE INHIBITOR; ANTIGLAUCOMA
Pregnancy: Category C

ACTIONS/PHARMACODYNAMICS Nonbacteriostatic sulfonamide derivative similar to acetazolamide except that chloride excretion is increased, and thus potential for significant metabolic acidosis is less. Lowers IOP by decreasing production of aqueous humor. Produces diuresis but is not used as a diuretic because effect is lost with chronic use. Contraindications, precautions, and adverse reactions are the same as for acetazolamide.

USES Adjunctive treatment of open-angle glaucoma and preoperatively in narrow-angle glaucoma when delay of surgery is desired to lower IOP. Commonly used in conjunction with a miotic; an osmotic agent may also be used to enhance reduction of IOP in acute angle-closure glaucoma.

ROUTE & DOSAGE

Glaucoma

Adult	PO	100–200 mg followed by 100 mg q12h until desired response is obtained
		Maintenance: 25–50 mg 1–3 times/d

PHARMACOKINETICS Absorption: well absorbed from GI tract. **Onset:** 0.5–1 h. **Peak:** 2–4 h. **Duration:** 6–12 h.

CONTRAINDICATIONS & PRECAUTIONS Contraindicated in: hypersensitivity to sulfonamides and sulfonamide derivative diuretics; depressed sodium and potassium levels, severe pulmonary obstruction, marked kidney or liver dysfunction, hyperchloremic acidosis, adrenocortical insufficiency, long-term use in noncongestive angle-closure glaucoma. Safe use during pregnancy (category C) and in nursing mothers not established. **Cautious use in:** respiratory acidosis, reduced respiratory capacity, diabetes mellitus.

ADVERSE/SIDE EFFECTS CNS: paresthesia, sedation, drowsiness, fatigue, dizziness, ataxia. **GI:** anorexia, nausea, vomiting, metallic taste, diarrhea, abdominal discomfort. **Hematologic:** leukopenia, agranulocytosis, thrombocytopenia, hemolytic anemia. **Renal:** urinary frequency, crystalluria, renal calculi. **Skin:** urticaria, pruritus, rash. **Other:** weight loss, fever, glycosuria, asymptomatic hyperuricemia.

DRUG INTERACTIONS Renal excretion of AMPHETAMINES, **ephedrine, flecainide, quinidine, procainamide,** TRICYCLIC ANTIDEPRESSANTS may be decreased, thereby enhancing or prolonging their effects; increases renal excretion of **lithium;** excretion of **phenobarbital** may be increased; **amphotericin B,** CORTICOSTEROIDS may increase potassium loss; dichlorphenamide-induced hypokalemia may predispose patients taking DIGITALIS GLYCOSIDES to digitalis toxicity; patients on high doses of SALICYLATES are at higher risk for salicylate toxicity.

NURSING IMPLICATIONS

Administration

- May be taken with meals to reduce gastric irritation.

Assessment & Drug Effects

- Since drug may cause dizziness and ataxia, supervision of ambulation and other safety precautions may be warranted.

- Monitor for hematologic reactions common to sulfonamides. Obtain baseline CBC and platelet counts before initiating therapy and at regular intervals during therapy.

Patient & Family Education

- High fluid intake is generally recommended to reduce risk of renal calculi. Consult physician.
- Advise patient to report to physician the onset of sore throat, fever, unusual bleeding or bruising, tremors, flank or loin pain, skin rash.
- Caution patient to avoid driving and other potentially hazardous activities until reaction to drug is known.
- Brand interchange is not recommended. Bioavailability problems have been reported.

Prototype: ibuprofen, p 160

DICLOFENAC SODIUM
(di-klo´fen-ak)

Trade name: Voltaren
Classifications: CNS AGENT; NSAID; ANALGESIC, NONNARCOTIC; ANTIPYRETIC
Pregnancy: Category B

ACTIONS/PHARMACODYNAMICS Nonsteroidal antiinflammatory drug (NSAID) with analgesic and antipyretic activity. Although its exact mechanism of action has not been fully elucidated, it appears to be a potent inhibitor of cyclooxygenase, thereby decreasing the synthesis of prostaglandins, prostacyclin, and thromboxane. At therapeutic doses, has little effect on platelet aggregation.

USES Analgesic and antipyretic effects in symptomatic treatment of rheumatoid arthritis, osteoarthritis, and ankylosing spondylitis. Also acute gout; juvenile rheumatoid arthritis; various rheumatic conditions including bursitis, myalgia, sciatica, and tendinitis; acute soft tissue injuries including sprains and strains; dysmenorrhea; headache, migraine, and dental, minor surgical, and postpartum pain; and renal or biliary colic.

PHARMACOKINETICS Absorption: readily absorbed from GI tract; 50–60% reaches systemic circulation. **Peak:** 2–3 h. **Distribution:** widely distributed including synovial fluid and into breast milk. **Metabolism:** extensively metabolized in liver. **Elimination:** half-life: 1.2–2 h; 50–70% excreted in urine, 30–35% in feces.

ROUTE & DOSAGE

Rheumatoid Arthritis

Adult	PO	150–200 mg/d in 3–4 divided doses
Child	PO	25 mg b.i.d. or t.i.d.

Osteoarthritis

Adult	PO	100–150 mg/d in 3–4 divided doses

Ankylosing Spondylitis

Adult	PO	25 mg q.i.d. and 25 mg h.s.

CONTRAINDICATIONS & PRECAUTIONS Contraindicated in: hypersensitivity to diclofenac, patients in whom asthma, urticaria, angioedema, bronchospasm, severe rhinitis, shock, or other sensitivity reaction is precipitated by aspirin or other NSAIDs, pregnancy, lactation. **Cautious use in:** geriatric patients and children; patients receiving anticoagulant therapy; history of GI disease; GU tract problems such as dysuria, cystitis, hematuria, nephritis, nephrotic syndrome, patients who must restrict their sodium intake; impaired hepatic function; SLE; heart failure; hypertension.

ADVERSE/SIDE EFFECTS CNS: dizziness, headache, drowsiness. **ENT:** tinnitus. **Skin:** rash, pruritus. **GI:** *dyspepsia,* nausea, vomiting, abdominal pain, cramps, constipation, diarrhea, indigestion, abdominal distension, flatulence, peptic ulcer. **CV:** fluid retention, hypertension, CHF. **Hepatic:** liver enzymes, transaminases increased. **Respiratory:** asthma. **Other:** liver test abnormalities, back, leg, or joint pain, hyperglycemia, prolonged bleeding time; inhibits platelet aggregation.

DIAGNOSTIC TEST INTERFERENCES Liver function test values may be increased. Liver function test abnormalities may return to normal despite continued use; however, if significant abnormalities occur, clinical signs and symptoms consistent with liver disease develop, or systemic manifestations such as eosinophilia or rash occur, the medication should be discontinued. Serum uric acid concentrations may be decreased because of increased renal clearance.

DRUG INTERACTIONS Increases **cyclosporine**-induced nephrotoxicity; increases **methotrexate** levels (increases toxicity); may decrease BP-lowering effects of DIURETICS; may increase levels and toxicity of **lithium;** may increase **digoxin** levels.

Common side effects in *italic*; life-threatening effects <u>underlined</u>; generic names in **bold**; classifications in SMALL CAPS

515

NURSING IMPLICATIONS

Administration

- Administer on an empty stomach, 1 h before or after a meal, as absorption is delayed markedly by food.
- Schedule administration 30 min before physical therapy or planned exercise to keep discomfort at a minimum.
- Gastric irritation may be minimized by administering it with a full glass of water.
- Do not crush tablets or dissolve in water. They should be swallowed whole.
- When prescribed for dysmenorrhea, administer 1 or 2 d before menses when prostaglandin levels are higher.
- To reduce risk of bleeding, discontinue therapy about 1 wk before surgery.
- Use with caution in those who must restrict sodium intake.
- Store at 15–30C (59–86F) away from heat and direct light.

Assessment & Drug Effects

- Monitor liver function and serum uric acid concentrations.
- Observe and report signs of bleeding (e.g., petechiae, ecchymoses, bleeding gums, bloody or black stools, cloudy or bloody urine). Monitor Hct and PT.
- Monitor BP for hypertension and blood sugar for hyperglycemia.
- Monitor for increased serum sodium and potassium in patients receiving potassium-sparing diuretics.
- Monitor weight and report gains greater than 1 kg (2 lb)/24 h.
- Monitor for signs and symptoms of GI irritation and ulceration.

Patient & Family Education

- Instruct patient not to lie down for 15–30 min after taking the medicine to decrease esophageal irritation.
- Advise patient to discontinue use with onset of ringing or buzzing in the ears, impaired hearing, dizziness, GI discomfort, or bleeding.
- Advise patient not to take aspirin or other OTC analgesics without permission of the physician.
- Instruct patient to avoid alcohol or other CNS depressants.
- Advise caution while driving, operating machines, or other hazardous activities until reaction to drug is known.
- Advise patient to stay out of direct sunlight, wear protective clothing, apply a sunblock product with SPF of at least 15.

Prototype: penicillin G potassium, p 71

DICLOXACILLIN SODIUM

(dye-klox-a-sill´in)
Trade names: Dycill, Dynapen, Pathocil
Classifications: ANTIINFECTIVE; BETA-LACTAM ANTIBIOTIC; SEMISYNTHETIC PENICILLIN
Pregnancy: Category B

ACTIONS/PHARMACODYNAMICS Semisynthetic, acid-stable, penicillinase-resistant isoxazolyl penicillin. Mechanism of action similar to that of penicillin G; however, platelet dysfunction not reported for dicloxacillin. Action is bactericidal. Inhibits biosynthesis of bacterial cell wall during stage of active multiplication. Reportedly the most active of the isoxazolyl penicillins (cloxacillin, oxacillin) against penicillinase-producing staphylococci. Less potent than penicillin G against penicillin-sensitive microorganisms and generally ineffective against methicillin-resistant staphylococci and gram-negative bacteria. Contains 0.6 mEq (13.8 mg) sodium (250 mg capsule).

USES Primarily in systemic infections caused by penicillinase-producing staphylococci and penicillin-resistant staphylococci.

ROUTE & DOSAGE

Mild to Moderate Infections

Adult	PO	125–500 mg q6h
Child	PO	<40 kg: 12.5–25 mg/kg q6h (max 4 g/d)

PHARMACOKINETICS Absorption: 35–76% absorbed from GI tract. **Peak:** 0.5–2 h. **Duration:** 4–6 h. **Distribution:** distributed throughout body with highest concentrations in liver and kidney; low CSF penetration; crosses placenta; distributed into breast milk. **Metabolism:** metabolized in liver. **Elimination:** half-life: 30–60 min; excreted primarily in urine with some elimination through bile.

CONTRAINDICATIONS & PRECAUTIONS Contraindicated in: hypersensitivity to penicillins. Safe use during pregnancy (category B) and in neonates not

---

Common side effects in *italic*; life-threatening effects <u>underlined</u>; generic names in **bold**; classifications in SMALL CAPS

established. **Cautious use in:** history of or suspected atopy or allergy (asthma, eczema, hives, hay fever); history of hypersensitivity to cephalosporins.

ADVERSE/SIDE EFFECTS GI: nausea, vomiting, flatulence, *diarrhea,* abdominal pain. **Hypersensitivity:** pruritus, urticaria, rash, wheezing, sneezing, anaphylaxis; eosinophilia. **Other:** transient elevations of ALT, superinfections.

DRUG INTERACTIONS Probenecid decreases dicloxacillin elimination.

NURSING IMPLICATIONS

Administration

- Best taken on an empty stomach at least 1 h before or 2 h after meals. Food reduces drug absorption.
- Following reconstitution (by pharmacist), oral suspensions are stable for 7 d at room temperature or 14 d under refrigeration at 2–8C (35.6–46.4F). Container should be so labeled and dated. Shake well before pouring.
- Capsules are stored at 15–30C (59–86F) in tight containers unless otherwise directed.

Assessment & Drug Effects

- Before initiation of therapy a careful inquiry should be made concerning patient's previous exposure and sensitivity to penicillins and cephalosporins, and other allergic reactions of any kind.
- Bacteriologic studies should be done prior to initiation of therapy to determine susceptibility of causative organism. Therapy may begin pending test results.
- Blood cultures, WBC, and differential counts are recommended before therapy begins and at least weekly for patients on prolonged therapy. Periodic ALT and AST determinations, urinalysis, BUN, and creatinine are also advised for these patients.

Patient & Family Education

- Instruct patient to take medication around the clock, not to miss a dose, and to continue taking the medication until it is all gone, unless otherwise directed by physician.
- Advise patient to check with physician if GI side effects appear.
- Instruct patient to watch for and report the signs of hypersensitivity reactions and superinfections (see chap 3).

Prototype: warfarin, p 127

DICUMAROL

(dye-koo'ma-role)
Trade name: Bishydroxycoumarin
Classifications: BLOOD FORMERS & COAGULATORS; ORAL ANTICOAGULANT
Pregnancy: Category D

ACTIONS/PHARMACODYNAMICS Long-acting coumarin derivative. Interferes with blood clotting by depressing hepatic synthesis of vitamin K–dependent coagulation factors: II, VII, IX, X. Similar to other drugs of this series in actions, uses, contraindications, precautions, and adverse effects.

ROUTE & DOSAGE

Anticoagulant

Adult	PO	200–300 mg on day 1, then 25–200 mg/d based on PTs

PHARMACOKINETICS Absorption: slowly and incompletely absorbed from GI tract. **Peak:** 1–4 d. **Duration:** 2–10 d. **Distribution:** crosses placenta; distributed into breast milk. **Metabolism:** metabolized in liver. **Elimination:** half-life: 1–2 d; 70–85% excreted in urine, 15–30% in feces.

CONTRAINDICATIONS & PRECAUTIONS Contraindicated in: hemorrhagic tendencies: hemophilia, thrombocytopenia, leukemia; open wounds or ulcers; renal or hepatic impairment, vitamin C or K deficiency; severe hypertension; subacute bacterial endocarditis; visceral carcinoma. Safe use during pregnancy (category D), in nursing women, and in children not established. **Cautious use in:** active tuberculosis, major surgery, indwelling catheters.

ADVERSE/SIDE EFFECTS GI: diarrhea, flatulence, nausea, vomiting, anorexia, abdominal cramping. **GU:** hematuria, priapism. **Hematologic:** leukopenia, agranulocytosis. **Skin:** unusual hair loss, urticaria, dermatitis. **Other:** hypersensitivity, fever, hemorrhage.

DRUG INTERACTIONS See warfarin, p 127.

NURSING IMPLICATIONS

Administration

- Frequent dosage adjustment may be necessary during first 1 or 2 wk of therapy because drug absorp-

---

Common side effects in *italic*; life-threatening effects <u>underlined</u>; generic names in **bold**; classifications in SMALL CAPS

517

tion is so variable. Administration with food enhances drug absorption.

- Store in tightly closed container at 15–30C (59–86F) unless otherwise directed.

Assessment & Drug Effects

- During period of dosage adjustment, prothrombin activity should be checked daily and dose order obtained.
- Blood for PT should be drawn at least 5 h after an IV bolus dose of heparin or 24 h following a full therapeutic SC dose. Continuous IV infusion or low doses of heparin SC usually do not cause a significant increase in PT; therefore blood can be drawn at any time.
- When patient is controlled on maintenance dose, PTs may be checked semiweekly, weekly for 3–4 wk, then at 1–4 wk intervals, depending on stability of patient's response.

Patient & Family Education

- Instruct patient to inform physician if any other medication is being taken, including OTC drugs.
- Caution patient not to add or discontinue any medication without approval of physician or pharmacist.
- Instruct patient to report immediately any unexplained bleeding, easy bruising, or prolonged bleeding time.
- Advise patient to tell all doctors and dentists who may administer care that he or she is on anticoagulant therapy.
- Stress importance of avoiding unusual changes in vitamin intake, diet or life-style without consulting physician. Also advise patient to notify physician of any changes in health status. Illness may increase anticoagulant requirement.

Prototype: atropine, p 116

DICYCLOMINE HYDROCHLORIDE

(dye-sye´kloe-meen)

Trade names: Antispas, A-spas, Bentyl, Bentylol, Byclomine, Cyclocen, Dibent, Dicen, Di-Cyclonex, Dilomine, Di-Spaz, Formulex, Neoquess, Nospaz, Or-Tyl, Spasmoject, Viscerol
Classifications: AUTONOMIC NERVOUS SYSTEM AGENT; ANTICHOLINERGIC (PARASYMPATHOLYTIC); ANTISPASMODIC
Pregnancy: Category B

ACTIONS/PHARMACODYNAMICS Synthetic tertiary amine with antispasmodic properties. Relieves smooth muscle spasm in GI and biliary tracts, uterus, and ureters by nonspecific direct relaxant action. Atropinelike (antimuscarinic) side effects on salivary and sweat glands, gastric secretions, eyes, and cardiovascular system are generally slight with average dosage. Exhibits local (membrane) anesthetic properties.

USES Adjunctively in treatment of functional bowel disorders/irritable bowel syndrome. **Unlabeled uses:** acute enterocolitis, peptic ulcer, and infant colic.

ROUTE & DOSAGE

Irritable Bowel Disorders

Adult	PO	20–40 mg q.i.d.
	IM	20 mg q.i.d.
Child	PO	10 mg t.i.d. or q.i.d. (max 40 mg/d)
Infants	PO	5 mg t.i.d. or q.i.d.

PHARMACOKINETICS Absorption: readily absorbed from GI tract. **Onset:** 1–2 h. **Duration:** 4 h. **Metabolism:** metabolized in liver. **Elimination:** half-life: 9–10 h; 80% excreted in urine, 10% in feces.

CONTRAINDICATIONS & PRECAUTIONS Contraindicated in: hypersensitivity to anticholinergic drugs; obstructive diseases of GU and GI tracts, paralytic ileus, intestinal atony, biliary tract disease; unstable cardiovascular status; severe ulcerative colitis, toxic megacolon; myasthenia gravis; infants <6 mo. Safe use during pregnancy (category B), in nursing mothers, and in children not established. **Cautious use in:** glaucoma; prostatic hypertrophy; autonomic neuropathy; ulcerative colitis; hyperthyroidism; coronary heart disease, CHF, arrhythmias, hypertension; hepatic or renal disease; hiatal hernia associated with esophageal reflux; infants ≤6 mo.

ADVERSE/SIDE EFFECTS Dose related. **CNS:** lightheadedness, drowsiness, headache, insomnia, brief euphoria, fever, restlessness, irritability, coma, seizures. **CV:** fluctuations in heart rate, palpitation, tachycardia. **GI:** *dry mouth,* nausea, *constipation,* paralytic ileus, vomiting, diminished sense of taste, bloated feeling. **GU:** urinary hesitancy, *urinary retention,* impotence. **Other:** blurred vision, decreased sweating, suppression of lactation, urticaria, allergic reactions; curarelike effect (cyanosis, apnea, respiratory arrest).

Common side effects in *italic*; life-threatening effects <u>underlined</u>; generic names in **bold**; classifications in SMALL CAPS

D

NURSING IMPLICATIONS

Administration

- Administered 30 min before meals and at bedtime.
- Store below 30C (86F) unless otherwise directed.

Assessment & Drug Effects

- Treatment of infant colic with dicyclomine is not without some risk, especially in infants <2 mo of age. Doubling the usual dose of 5 mg can produce serious toxic effects.
- Infants ≤6 wk have developed respiratory symptoms as well as seizures, fluctuations in heart rate, weakness, and coma within minutes after taking syrup formulation. Symptoms generally last 20–30 min and are believed to be due to local irritation.
- Monitor I&O.
- If drug produces drowsiness and lightheadedness, supervision of ambulation and other safety precautions are warranted.

Patient & Family Education

- Dicyclomine may increase risk of heatstroke by decreasing sweating, especially in the elderly.
- Since dicyclomine may produce drowsiness and blurred vision, avoid activities requiring mental alertness until reaction to drug is known.
- Report changes in urine volume, voiding pattern.

Prototype: estradiol, p 236

DIENESTROL

(dye-en-ess´trole)

Trade names: DV, Estraguard, Ortho Dienestrol

Classifications: SYNTHETIC HORMONE; ESTROGEN

Pregnancy: Category X

ACTIONS/PHARMACODYNAMICS Synthetic nonsteroidal estrogen structurally related to diethylstilbestrol. See estradiol for actions and contraindications.

USES Atrophic vaginitis and kraurosis vulvae associated with menopause.

ADVERSE/SIDE EFFECTS Increased risk of endometrial cancer and gallbladder disease; thromboembolism. **GU:** vaginal candidiasis, breakthrough bleeding. **GI:** nausea, vomiting, abdominal cramps, bloating. **Skin:** erythema multiforme, loss of scalp hair, hirsutism. **CNS:** mental depression, headache, migraine, dizziness.

ROUTE & DOSAGE

Atrophic Vaginitis

Adult	Intravaginal	1–2 applicatorsful/d for 1–2 wk; then decrease dose by half for another 1–2 wk
		Maintenance: 1 applicatorful 1–3 times/wk

NURSING IMPLICATIONS

Administration

- Administration at bedtime increases absorption and thus effectiveness.
- Insert cream applicator (or suppository inserter) approximately 2 in. (5 cm), directing it slightly back toward sacrum. Patient should remain in recumbent position about 30 min to prevent losing the medication.
- If patient is to administer medication to herself, instruct her to wash her hands well before and after procedure; also advise her not to use tampons while on vaginal therapy.
- Protect cream from light. Store at 8–15C (46–59F) in a tight container unless otherwise directed.

Patient & Family Education

- Review package insert with patient.

DIETHYLPROPION HYDROCHLORIDE

See CENTRAL NERVOUS SYSTEM AGENTS, RESPIRATORY & CEREBRAL STIMULANT, ANOREXIANT prototype, p 196.

Prototype: estradiol, p 236

DIETHYLSTILBESTROL (DES)

(dye-eth-il-stil-bess´trole)

Trade name: Stilbestrol

DIETHYLSTILBESTROL DIPHOSPHATE

Trade names: Honval, Stilphostrol

Classifications: SYNTHETIC HORMONE; ESTROGEN, ANTINEOPLASTIC

Pregnancy: Category X

Common side effects in *italic*; life-threatening effects <u>underlined</u>; generic names in **bold**; classifications in SMALL CAPS

519

ACTIONS/PHARMACODYNAMICS Potent non-steroidal synthetic estrogen compound with strong teratogenic potential: may cause vaginal or cervical cancer in offspring if mother is treated with diethylstilbestrol (DES) during pregnancy. Competes for androgen or estrogen receptors on tumor cells, thereby changing the hormonal environment essential for their survival. Also interferes with release of FSH and LH with resultant inhibition of lactation, ovulation, and androgen secretion. Long-term therapy with 5 mg/d for prostatic carcinoma reportedly associated with increased risk of cardiovascular deaths. DES 1 mg is approximately equivalent to 1.6 mg diethylstilbestrol diphosphate.

USES Estrogen deficiency states, including female hypogonadism or castration, primary ovarian failure, menopausal symptoms, atrophic vaginitis, kraurosis vulvae, and for palliative treatment of advanced metastatic carcinoma of the breast in selected men and postmenopausal women and advanced inoperable carcinoma of prostate. **Unlabeled use:** emergency postcoital contraceptive ("morning after pill").

ROUTE & DOSAGE

Carcinoma Palliation

Adult   PO   Breast: 15 mg/d

Prostate: 1–3 mg/d; may increase in advanced cases

Postcoital Contraception

Adult   PO   25 mg b.i.d. for 5 d; must start within 72 h after coitus

Prostate Carcinoma

Adult   PO   50 mg t.i.d.; may increase to 200 mg or more t.i.d. depending on tolerance of patient

IV   0.5 g followed by 1 g/d for 5 or more days; then may reduce to 0.25–0.5 g 1–2 times/wk

PHARMACOKINETICS Absorption: readily absorbed from GI tract. **Metabolism:** metabolized in liver. **Elimination:** excreted in urine and feces.

CONTRAINDICATIONS & PRECAUTIONS Contraindicated in: use for birth control (except emergency postcoital contraception); malignancies or precarcinomatous lesions (vagina, vulva, or breasts); pregnancy (category X); blood clotting disorders; hepatic dysfunction; undiagnosed vaginal bleeding; long-term use during menopause. **Cautious use in:** hypertension; migraine; diabetes mellitus; asthma.

ADVERSE/SIDE EFFECTS CV: <u>thromboembolic disorders</u>, hypertension, edema, <u>MI</u>. **CNS:** headache, dizziness, chronic depression. **Eye:** intolerance to contact lenses, worsening of myopia. **GI:** *nausea,* vomiting, diarrhea, anorexia, constipation, cramps, bloating, cholestatic jaundice. **Metabolic:** reduced carbohydrate tolerance, hypercalcemia, folic acid deficiency. **Reproduction:** gynecomastia, mastodynia, breast secretions, breakthrough bleeding, changes in menstrual flow, dysmenorrhea, amenorrhea, vaginal candidiasis, changes in libido. **Skin:** melasma (discoloration), erythema multiforme or nodosum, loss of scalp hair, hirsutism. **Other:** weight changes, leg cramps.

DRUG INTERACTIONS Rifampin may increase DES metabolism; may antagonize anticoagulant effects of **warfarin.**

NURSING IMPLICATIONS

Administration
- Enteric-coated tablets should be swallowed whole.
- Cyclic therapy generally consists of 3 wk on DES (once daily), followed by 1 wk without the drug. Some clinicians add progestin therapy for 7–13 d of the cycle on the theory that this will reduce risk of endometrial hyperplasia.
- Dosage reduction or discontinuation of therapy is generally attempted at 3–6-mo intervals.
- *Diethylstilbestrol diphosphate IV solution:* dissolve dose in 300 ml 0.9% NaCl for injection or 5% dextrose for injection. Infusion: administer slowly (1–2 ml/min) during first 10–15 min and then flow rate is adjusted to permit remainder of solution to be given over a period of 1 h.
- Patient should be lying down during infusion to reduce incidence of dizziness.
- When used as an emergency postcoital contraceptive, drug is started preferably within 24 h and not later than 72 h after sexual intercourse. Conception is prevented, but pregnancy is not terminated. Full course of the regimen must be taken if pregnancy is to be prevented.
- After reconstitution, solution may be stored at room temperature if protected from direct light. Under these conditions, solution is stable for about 5 d. Do not use if a precipitate or cloudiness is present.
- Store tablets and ampuls at 15–30C (59–86F) in a tightly closed container. Protect from light and freezing.

Assessment & Drug Effects
- Nausea and vomiting are common in the menopausal group of patients receiving ≥1 mg/d

and relatively uncommon in men and nonpregnant women even when doses are 3–5 mg/d.

- Severe nausea and vomiting with contraceptive doses can lead to noncompliance. An antiemetic may be required.
- Risk of blood clot formation is high. Monitor for signs & symptoms of deep vein thrombosis or thrombophlebitis (see chap 3).

Patient & Family Education

- Patients with intact uterus should be closely monitored for endometrial cancer. Advise patient to report the onset of vaginal bleeding or any other unusual sign or symptom.
- Reassure the postmenopausal patient that withdrawal bleeding is not a sign of fertility because ovulation is not possible.
- Women should have breasts and pelvic organs examined before treatment begins and at intervals throughout therapy. Teach the patient self-examination of breasts. Urge her to keep check-up appointments.
- A pregnancy test is advised before the patient is started on therapy with DES. Patient should be informed of the teratogenic potential of this drug.
- In the event of contraceptive failure the risk of teratogenic effects is substantially increased. DES administration increases risk of vaginal carcinoma.
- Reassure the male patient that drug-induced loss of libido and development of feminine characteristics will disappear with termination of therapy.
- Urge patient to maintain established regimen, i.e., the dose should not be increased, decreased, or omitted, without physician's advice.

Prototype: hydrocortisone, p 255

DIFLORASONE DIACETATE

(dye-flor´a-sone)

Trade names: Florone, Florone E, Maxiflor, Psorcon

Classifications: SKIN AGENT; ANTIINFLAMMATORY; SYNTHETIC ADRENAL CORTICOSTEROID HORMONE; GLUCOCORTICOID

Pregnancy: Category C

ACTIONS/PHARMACODYNAMICS Topical synthetic fluorinated high potency corticosteroid with antiinflammatory, antipruritic, and vasoconstric-tive activity. Thought to result in part from complexing of drug with cytoplasmic steroid receptors. Decreases inflammation, reduces capillary wall permeability and edema formation, antagonizes histamine activity and release of kinin, and reduces fibroblast proliferation. Percutaneous penetration is minimal on intact skin.

USES To relieve inflammatory and pruritic symptoms of a variety of skin disorders responsive to corticosteroids.

ROUTE & DOSAGE

Inflammation

Adult	Topical	Apply thin layer of ointment 1–3 times/d or cream 2–4 times/d

PHARMACOKINETICS Absorption: minimum absorption through intact skin; increased absorption from axilla, eyelid, face, scalp, scrotum, or with occlusive dressing.

CONTRAINDICATIONS & PRECAUTIONS Contraindicated in: safe use during pregnancy (category C) and by nursing mothers not established. **Cautious use in:** children, viral diseases of skin, fungal and bacterial infections.

ADVERSE/SIDE EFFECTS Skin: acneiform eruptions, burning sensation, pruritus, hypertrichosis, hypopigmentation, folliculitis.

NURSING IMPLICATIONS

Administration

- Before application of topical medication, gently cleanse skin area, then lightly rub in a thin layer of the drug. When treating hairy area, part the hair and apply drug directly to the site.
- Do not apply occlusive dressing unless specifically prescribed.
- Store drug in cool place and protect from light and heat.

Assessment & Drug Effects

- Monitor for and report signs of hypersensitivity (see chap 3) or other signs of skin irritation.

Patient & Family Education

- Caution patient to apply medication as scheduled and not to change intervals or amount.
- If there are signs of systemic absorption (e.g., skin irritation or ulceration, hypersensitivity, infection),

Common side effects in *italic*; life-threatening effects underlined; generic names in **bold**; classifications in SMALL CAPS

521

patient should notify physician.

- Systemic absorption is usually associated with long-term therapy, extensive body surface treatment, or with use of an occlusive dressing. Caution patient not to bandage, wrap, or otherwise tightly cover affected area unless it is prescribed.
- Inspect skin for infection, striae, atrophy. If present, patient should stop the drug and notify the physician.

D

Prototype: Ibuprofen, p 160

DIFLUNISAL
(dye-floo´ni-sal)
Trade name: Dolobid
Classifications: CNS AGENT; ANALGESIC; NSAID
Pregnancy: Category C

ACTIONS/PHARMACODYNAMICS Long-acting nonsteroidal antiinflammatory drug (NSAID) with peripheral analgesic properties classified as a nonacetylated salicylate. Derived from salicylic acid but is not hydrolyzed to salicylate in the body. Precise mode of action not known but appears to be related principally to inhibition of prostaglandin synthesis. In common with other NSAIDs, inhibits cyclooxygenase, an enzyme that catalyzes the formation of prostaglandin from arachidonic acid (precursor). More potent than aspirin and acetaminophen in equianalgesic doses and has longer duration of effect. However, onset of analgesic action may be delayed unless loading dose is used. Unlike aspirin, inhibition of platelet function and effect on bleeding time are dose related and reversible, lasting only about 24 h after drug is discontinued. Reportedly has lower incidence of gastric erosion, significant fecal blood loss, tinnitus, and hearing problems than aspirin has. Exerts mild antipyretic effect; therefore not used clinically for this purpose. Has some uricosuric activity at usual dosages.

USES Acute and long-term relief of mild to moderate pain and symptomatic treatment of osteoarthritis and rheumatoid arthritis.

PHARMACOKINETICS Absorption: readily absorbed from GI tract. **Onset:** 1 h. **Peak:** 2–3 h. **Duration:** 12 h. **Distribution:** probably crosses placenta; distributed into breast milk. **Metabolism:** metabolized in liver. **Elimination:** half-life: 8–12 h; excreted in urine.

ROUTE & DOSAGE

Analgesia

Adult	PO	1000 mg followed by 500 mg q8–12h

Arthritis

Adult	PO	500–1000 mg/d in 2 divided doses (max 1500 mg/d)

CONTRAINDICATIONS & PRECAUTIONS Contraindicated in: patients in whom aspirin or other NSAIDs precipitate an acute asthmatic attack (bronchospasm), urticaria, angioedema, severe rhinitis, or shock; active peptic ulcer, GI bleeding. Safe use during pregnancy (category C), in nursing mothers, and in children <12 y not established. Use during third trimester of pregnancy specifically contraindicated because NSAIDs are known to cause premature closure on ductus arteriosus in fetus. **Cautious use in:** history of upper GI disease; impaired renal or hepatic function; compromised cardiac function, and other conditions associated with fluid retention; patients receiving diuretics; geriatric patients; hypertension; patients who may be adversely affected by prolonged bleeding time.

ADVERSE/SIDE EFFECTS CNS: headache, drowsiness, insomnia, dizziness, vertigo, lightheadedness, fatigue, weakness, nervousness, hallucinations, confusion, disorientation, stupor. **CV:** palpitation, syncope, tachycardia, *peripheral edema.* **ENT:** tinnitus, hearing loss. **Eye:** blurred vision, reduced visual acuity, changes in color vision, scotomas, corneal deposits, retinal disturbances. **GI:** *nausea,* GI pain, flatulence, GI bleeding, stomatitis, peptic ulcer, anorexia, eructation, cholestatic jaundice, severe hepatic dysfunction. **GU:** dysuria, hematuria, proteinuria, interstitial nephritis, renal failure. **Hematologic:** prolonged PT, anemia, leukopenia, thrombocytopenia, decreased serum uric acid, transient elevations of liver function tests. **Hypersensitivity syndrome:** fever, chills, rash, eosinophilia, changes in renal and hepatic function, <u>anaphylactic reactions with bronchospasm.</u> **Skin:** rash, toxic epidermal necrolysis, exfoliative dermatitis, urticaria. **Other:** weight gain, chest pain, hyperventilation, dyspnea, muscle cramps, photosensitivity.

DIAGNOSTIC TEST INTERFERENCES Diflunisal can lower *serum uric acid* concentrations by as much as 1.4 mg/dl and increased renal clearance of uric acid.

DRUG INTERACTIONS ANTACIDS decrease diflunisal absorption; **aspirin** and other NSAIDs increase risk of GI bleeding; increases risk of **warfarin**-induced hypoprothombinemia; increases **methotrexate** levels and toxicity.

NURSING IMPLICATIONS

Administration

- Diflunisal can be taken with water, milk, or food to reduce GI irritation. Food causes slight reduction in absorption rate but does not affect total amount absorbed.
- Store at 15–30C (59–86F) in tightly closed containers unless otherwise directed.

Assessment & Drug Effects

- Full antiinflammatory effect for arthritis may not occur until 8 d to several weeks into therapy in some patients.
- Diflunisal should be discontinued if patient presents signs of hepatic toxicity (see chap 3).
- Although the antipyretic effect is mild, chronic or high doses may mask fever in some patients.

Patient & Family Education

- Instruct patient to swallow tablet whole. It should not be crushed or chewed.
- Caution patient to take drug as prescribed. Doubling the dosage can produce greater than doubling of drug accumulation, particularly in patients receiving repetitive doses.
- Advise patient to report the onset of eye problems immediately to physician.
- Patients with impaired renal function should be closely monitored. Instruct patient to be aware of I&O ratio and pattern and to check for and report peripheral edema and unusual weight gain.
- Advise all patients and particularly those with history of GI problems to report promptly to physician the onset of melena, hematemesis, or severe stomach pain.
- Caution patient about potentially hazardous activities until reaction to drug is known.

DIGOXIN

See CARDIOVASCULAR DRUGS, CARDIAC GLYCOSIDE prototype, p 146.

DIGOXIN IMMUNE FAB (OVINE)

Trade name: Digibind
Classification: ANTIDOTE
Pregnancy: Category C

ACTIONS/PHARMACODYNAMICS Purified fragments of antibodies specific for digoxin (but also effective for digitoxin) produced in sheep immunized with digoxin-albumin conjugate. Use of fragments of antidigoxin antibodies (Fab) instead of whole antibody molecules permits more extensive and faster distribution to serum and toxic cellular sites. Acts by selectively complexing with circulating digoxin or digitoxin, thereby preventing drug from binding at receptor sites; the complex is then eliminated in urine. Each 40 mg vial binds approximately 0.6 mg of digoxin or digitoxin.

USES Treatment of potentially life-threatening digoxin or digitoxin intoxication in carefully selected patients.

ROUTE & DOSAGE

Serious Digoxin Toxicity Secondary to Overdose

IV Dosages vary according to amount of digoxin to be neutralized; dosages are based on total body load or steady state serum digoxin concentrations (see package insert); some patients may require a second dose after several hours

PHARMACOKINETICS Onset: <1 min after IV administration. **Elimination:** half-life: 14–20 h; excreted in urine over 5–7 d.

CONTRAINDICATIONS & PRECAUTIONS Contraindicated in: hypersensitivity to sheep products; renal or cardiac failure. Safe use during pregnancy (category C) or in nursing women not established. **Cautious use in:** prior treatment with sheep antibodies or ovine Fab fragments; history of allergies; impaired renal function.

ADVERSE/SIDE EFFECTS Adverse reactions associated with use of digoxin immune Fab are related primarily to the effects of digitalis withdrawal on the heart (see Nursing Implications). Allergic reactions have been reported rarely. Hypokalemia.

DIAGNOSTIC TEST INTERFERENCES Digoxin immune Fab may interfere with *serum digoxin* determinations by immunoassay tests.

D

Common side effects in *italic*; life-threatening effects <u>underlined</u>; generic names in **bold**; classifications in SMALL CAPS

523

DRUG INTERACTIONS Not established.

NURSING IMPLICATIONS

Administration

- Reconstitute by dissolving 40 mg (1 vial) in 4 ml of sterile water for injection; mix gently (solution will contain 10 mg/ml). For administration by IV infusion, reconstituted solution may be diluted further with sterile isotonic saline injection.
- After reconstitution, digoxin immune Fab is administered by IV infusion over 30 min, preferably through a 0.22 µm membrane filter, or as bolus injection if cardiac arrest is imminent.
- For infants, reconstitute as directed and administer with a tuberculin syringe. For small doses (e.g., 2 mg or less), dilute the reconstituted 40 mg vial with 36 ml of sterile isotonic saline injection to make a concentration of 1 mg/ml. Children must be closely monitored for fluid overload.
- Reconstituted solutions should be used promptly or refrigerated at 2–8C (36–46F) for up to 4 h.

Assessment & Drug Effects

- Skin testing for allergy is performed prior to administration of immune Fab, particularly in patients with history of allergy or who have had previous therapy with immune Fab.
- As a precaution, emergency equipment and drugs should be immediately available before skin testing is done or first dose is given and should be kept readily accessible until patient is out of danger.
- The following measurements should be determined before administration of digoxin immune Fab and repeated at frequent intervals during therapy: temperature; BP; ECG; serum potassium; serum digoxin or digitoxin concentration (this measurement will not be accurate for at least 5–7 d after therapy begins because of test interference by immune Fab).
- Make note also of presenting symptoms of digoxin (digitoxin) toxicity. Effective treatment should be reflected in improvement in cardiac rhythm abnormalities, mental orientation and other neurologic symptoms, and GI and visual disturbances.
- Reversal of signs and symptoms of digitalis toxicity occurs in 15–60 min in adults and usually within minutes in children.
- Cardiac status may deteriorate as inotropic action of digitalis is withdrawn by action of immune Fab. Closely monitor for CHF, arrhythmias, increase in heart rate, and hypokalemia.
- Digoxin intoxication causes hyperkalemia. Following treatment with immune Fab, potassium rapidly shifts back into cells with resulting hypokalemia. Close monitoring of serum potassium is particularly critical during first several hours following administration of immune Fab.
- Follow-up serum digoxin levels and ECG readings are recommended for at least 2–3 wk.

Prototype: ergotamine, p 112

DIHYDROERGOTAMINE MESYLATE
(dye-hye-droe-er-got´a-meen)
Trade name: D.H.E. 45
Classifications: AUTONOMIC NERVOUS SYSTEM AGENT; ALPHA-ADRENERGIC ANTAGONIST; ERGOT ALKALOID
Pregnancy: Category X

ACTIONS/PHARMACODYNAMICS Alpha-adrenergic blocking agent and dihydrogenated ergot alkaloid with direct constricting effect on smooth muscle of peripheral and cranial blood vessels. Maintains elevated levels of circulating norepinephrine (vasoconstrictor action) by inhibiting its reuptake. Vasoconstrictor action is more prominent on capacitance vessels (veins, venules) than on resistance vessels (arteries, arterioles). Reduces rate of serotonin-induced platelet aggregation. Has somewhat weaker vasoconstrictor action than ergotamine but greater adrenergic blocking activity. Toxicity potential is about one-tenth that of parent drug. Lacks uterine stimulating action in therapeutic dose.

USES To prevent or abort vascular headache (e.g., migraine or histaminic cephalalgia) when rapid control is desired or other routes are not feasible. With low dose heparin therapy to prevent postoperative deep-vein thrombosis and pulmonary embolism. **Other use:** to treat postural hypotension.

ROUTE & DOSAGE

Migraine Headache
Adult	IM/IV	1 mg; may be repeated at 1 h intervals to a total of 3 mg IM or 2 mg IV (max 6 mg/wk)

PHARMACOKINETICS Onset: 15–30 min IM; <5 min IV. **Duration:** 3–4 h. **Distribution:** probably distributed into breast milk. **Metabolism:** metabolized in liver. **Elimination:** half-life: 21–32 h; excreted primarily in urine; some excreted in feces.

Common side effects in *italic*; life-threatening effects underlined; generic names in **bold**; classifications in SMALL CAPS

CONTRAINDICATIONS & PRECAUTIONS Contraindicated in: history of hypersensitivity to ergot preparations; peripheral vascular disease, coronary heart disease, hypertension; peptic ulcer; impaired hepatic or renal function; sepsis. Safe use during pregnancy (category X), in nursing women, and in children not established.

ADVERSE/SIDE EFFECTS CV: vasospasm: coldness, numbness and tingling in fingers and toes, muscle pains and weakness of legs, precordial distress and pain, transient tachycardia or bradycardia, hypertension (large doses). **GI:** *nausea, vomiting.* **Other:** dizziness, dysphoria, *localized edema and itching;* ergotism (excessive doses).

DRUG INTERACTIONS BETA-BLOCKERS, **erythromycin** increase peripheral vasoconstriction with risk of ischemia.

NURSING IMPLICATIONS

Administration
- Drug should be given at first warning of migraine headache. Optimum results are obtained by titrating the doses required to give relief for several headaches to determine the minimal effective dose. This dose is used for subsequent attacks.
- Onset of action after IM injection is delayed about 20 min; therefore, when more rapid relief is required, the IV route is prescribed.
- IV dihydroergotamine may be given by direct IV undiluted at a rate of 1 mg/60 seconds.
- Protect ampuls from heat and light; do not freeze. Discard ampul if solution appears discolored.
- Store at 15–30C (59–86F) unless otherwise directed.

Patient & Family Education
- Advise patient to lie down in a quiet, darkened room for several hours after drug administration for best results.
- Report the onset of nausea vomiting, change in heart beat, numbness, tingling, pain or weakness of extremities.

DIHYDROTACHYSTEROL
(dye-hye-droe-tak-iss´ter-ole)
Trade names: DHT, DHT Intensol, Hytakerol
Classifications: VITAMIN D; REGULATOR, SERUM CALCIUM
Pregnancy: Category A

ACTIONS/PHARMACODYNAMICS Oil-soluble reduction product of ergocalciferol (vitamin D_2) with pharmacologic actions similar to those of both ergocalciferol and parathyroid hormone. In comparison with ergocalciferol, dihydrotachysterol has weak antirachitic activity, promotes less intestinal absorption of calcium but almost equal phosphate diuresis. In equivalent high doses has shorter duration of action and thus less potential hazards of hypercalcemia than ergocalciferol and is more effective in mobilization of calcium from bone. (1 mg = 120,000 U of ergocalciferol.) Acts like parathyroid hormone in ability to raise serum calcium concentrations rapidly; also reported to increase intestinal absorption of sodium, potassium, and magnesium.

USES Hypocalcemia associated with hypoparathyroidism, both postoperative and idiopathic, and in pseudohypoparathyroidism. Also for prophylaxis of hypocalcemic tetany following thyroid surgery. **Unlabeled uses:** vitamin D–resistant rickets (familial hypophosphatemia), osteoporosis, and renal osteodystrophy.

ROUTE & DOSAGE

Hypoparathyroidism, Pseudohypoparathyroidism

Adult	PO	0.75–2.5 mg/d for several days; then 0.2–1 mg/d (may need 1.5 mg/d)
Child	PO	1–5 mg/d for 4 d; then 0.5–1.5 mg/d

Thyroidectomy-induced Hypocalcemia

Adult	PO	0.25 mg/d

Renal Osteodystrophy

Adult	PO	0.1–0.6 mg/d
Child	PO	0.1–0.5 mg/d

PHARMACOKINETICS Absorption: readily absorbed from small intestines. **Peak:** 2 wk. **Duration:** 2 wk. **Distribution:** distributed in breast milk. **Metabolism:** metabolized in liver to active metabolite. **Elimination:** excreted primarily in bile and feces.

CONTRAINDICATIONS & PRECAUTIONS Contraindicated in: sensitivity to vitamin D; hypercalcemia and hypocalcemia associated with renal insufficiency and hyperphosphatemia; renal stones, hypervitaminosis D. Safe use during pregnancy (category A), in nursing mothers, and in children in amounts exceeding RDA not established.

Common side effects in *italic*; life-threatening effects underlined; generic names in **bold**; classifications in SMALL CAPS

525

ADVERSE/SIDE EFFECTS Hypercalcemia. **CNS:** drowsiness, headache, weakness, vertigo, ataxia, atonia, mental depression. **GI:** anorexia, nausea, vomiting, metallic taste, dry mouth, thirst, diarrhea, constipation, abdominal pain. **GU:** nocturia, polyuria, renal calculi. **Other:** tinnitus.

DRUG INTERACTIONS Not established.

NURSING IMPLICATIONS

Administration

- Withhold drug if signs and symptoms of hypercalcemia appear (see chap 3) and report to physician.
- Store in tightly closed, light-resistant containers at 15–30C (59–86F) unless otherwise directed.

Assessment & Drug Effects

- Determine serum and urinary calcium levels at least weekly during first month of therapy until they are stabilized, then monthly thereafter.
- Adequate calcium intake is necessary for clinical response to therapy. Usually supplemented with 10–15 g of oral calcium lactate or gluconate daily.
- Patients with hyperphosphatemia will require dietary restriction of phosphate or administration of calcium carbonate supplements with meals, or both, to bind intestinal phosphates and improve calcium balance.
- Hypoparathyroid patients receiving thiazide diuretics are prone to develop hypercalcemia and therefore require close monitoring.

Patient & Family Education

- Inform patients of the signs and symptoms of hypercalcemia (see chap 3).

Prototype: aluminum hydroxide, p 212

DIHYDROXYALUMINUM SODIUM CARBONATE
(dye-hye-drox-ia-lu-min-um)
Trade name: Rolaids
Classification: GI AGENT; ANTACID & ADSORBENT
Pregnancy: Category C

ACTIONS/PHARMACODYNAMICS Combines antacid properties of sodium bicarbonate (as sodium carbonate) and aluminum hydroxide and therefore has both systemic and nonsystemic effects. Has rapid onset of action because of sodium carbonate; pro-

longed action is attributed to aluminum hydroxide. Each tablet contains 53 mg (2.30 mEq) of sodium. Acid neutralizing capacity (ANC): 7.5.

ROUTE & DOSAGE

Antacid

Adult   PO   Chew 1–2 tab prn

CONTRAINDICATIONS & PRECAUTIONS Contraindicated in: aluminum sensitivity, severe renal disease, patients on sodium-restricted diets, dehydration. **Cautious use in:** elderly patients; history of CHF, decreased GI motility; pregnancy (category C).

ADVERSE/SIDE EFFECTS Constipation, intestinal concretions, anorexia.

DRUG INTERACTIONS Decreases absorption of ANTIINFECTIVES: TETRACYCLINES, QUINOLONES **(ciprofloxacin, norfloxacin).**

NURSING IMPLICATIONS

Patient & Family Education

- Instruct patient to chew tablet thoroughly before swallowing and to take it with water or milk.
- Constipation occurs commonly and may be managed by alternating with a magnesium-containing antacid.
- Rolaids are not suitable for long-term or frequent use.
- In common with other antacids, this drug can cause premature disintegration and absorption of enteric-coated tablets and may interfere with absorption of other oral medications. In general, it is advisable not to take other oral drugs within 1 or 2 h of an antacid.

Prototype: verapamil, p 144

DILTIAZEM
(dil-tye´a-zem)
Trade name: Cardizem, Cardizem SR
Classifications: CARDIOVASCULAR AGENT; CALCIUM CHANNEL BLOCKING AGENT; ANTIARRHYTHMIC; VASODILATOR; ANTIHYPERTENSIVE
Pregnancy: Category C

D

ACTIONS/PHARMACODYNAMICS Slow channel blocker with pharmacologic actions similar to those of verapamil. Inhibits calcium ion influx through slow channels into cell of myocardial and arterial smooth muscle (both coronary and peripheral blood vessels). As a result, intracellular calcium remains at subthreshold levels insufficient to stimulate cell excitation and contraction. Dilates coronary arteries and arterioles and inhibits coronary artery spasm; thus myocardial oxygen delivery is increased (antianginal effect). Slows SA and AV node conduction (antiarrhythmic effect) without affecting normal arterial action potential or intraventricular conduction. By vasodilation of peripheral arterioles drug decreases total peripheral vascular resistance and reduces arterial BP at rest (antihypertensive effect). May cause slight decrease in heart rate. Does not alter total serum calcium levels.

USES Vasospastic angina (Printzmetal's variant or at rest angina), chronic stable (classic effort-associated) angina, essential hypertension. **Unlabeled use:** prevention of reinfarction in non-Q-wave, MI.

ROUTE & DOSAGE

Angina

Adult	PO	30 mg q.i.d.; may increase q1–2d as required; usual dose range 180–360 mg/d in divided doses

Hypertension

Adult	PO	60–120 mg sustained release b.i.d. (usual range: 240–360 mg/d)

PHARMACOKINETICS Absorption: approximately 80% absorbed from GI tract, with 40% reaching systemic circulation. **Peak:** 2–3 h; 6–11 h sustained release. **Distribution:** distributed into breast milk. **Metabolism:** metabolized in liver. **Elimination:** half-life: 3.5–9 h; excreted primarily in urine with some elimination in feces.

CONTRAINDICATIONS & PRECAUTIONS Contraindicated in: known hypersensitivity to drug; sick sinus syndrome (unless pacemaker is in place and functioning); second- or third-degree AV block; severe hypotension (systolic <90 mm Hg or diastolic <60 mm Hg); patients undergoing intracranial surgery; bleeding aneurysms. Safe use during pregnancy (category C), in nursing mothers, and in children not established. **Cautious use in:** CHF (especially if patient is also receiving beta blocker), conduction abnormalities; renal or hepatic impairment; the elderly; nursing mothers.

ADVERSE/SIDE EFFECTS CNS: *headache, fatigue, dizziness, asthenia, drowsiness, nervousness, insomnia, confusion, tremor, gait abnormality.* **CV:** edema, arrhythmias, angina, second- or third-degree AV block, bradycardia, CHF, asymptomatic systole, flushing, hypotension, syncope, palpitations. **ENT:** nasal congestion, tinnitus, epistaxis. **Eye:** irritation, amblyopia. **GI:** nausea, constipation, anorexia, vomiting, diarrhea, impaired taste, weight increase. **Renal:** nocturia, hematuria, acute renal failure. **Skin:** rash, petechiae, pruritus; urticaria. **Other:** elevation of hepatic enzymes, hyperglycemia, osteoarticular pain, sexual difficulties; dyspnea; hair loss.

DRUG INTERACTIONS BETA-BLOCKERS, **digoxin** may have additive effects on AV node conduction prolongation; may increase **digoxin** levels; **cimetidine** may increase diltiazem levels, thus increasing effects; may increase **cyclosporine** levels.

NURSING IMPLICATIONS

Administration

- Administer before meals and at bedtime.
- Withhold drug if systolic BP is < 90 mm Hg or diastolic is < 60 mm Hg.
- Store at 15–30C (59–86F) in tightly closed container unless otherwise directed.

Assessment & Drug Effects

- BP and ECG should be evaluated before initiation of therapy and monitored particularly during dosage adjustment period. Baseline and periodic tests of liver and renal function are also recommended.
- Monitor for headache. An analgesic may be required.
- Drug may induce hyperglycemia. Monitor diabetes closely.

Patient & Family Education

- Because of the possibility of light-headedness, dizziness (hypotension), advise patient to make position changes slowly and in stages. Supervision of ambulation may be indicated.
- Caution patient to avoid driving and other potentially hazardous activities until reaction to drug is known.
- Stress importance of keeping follow-up appointments and of keeping physician informed.

D

Prototype: diphenhydramine, p 47

DIMENHYDRINATE
(dye-men-hye´dri-nate)

Trade names: Apo-Dimenhydrinate, Calm-X, Dimenhydrinate Injection, Dimentabs, Dinate, Dommanate, Dramanate, Dramamine, Dramilin, Dramocen, Dramoject, Dymenate, Gravol, Hydrate, Marmine, Motion-Aid, Nauseatol, Novodimenate, PMS Dimenhydrinate, Reidamine, Travamine, Travel Aid, Travel Eze, Wehamine

Classifications: ANTIHISTAMINE (H$_1$ RECEPTOR ANTAGONIST); ANTIEMETIC; ANTIVERTIGO AGENT
Pregnancy: Category B

ACTIONS/PHARMACODYNAMICS H$_1$-receptor antagonist and chlorotheophylline salt of diphenhydramine, with which it shares similar properties. Precise mode of antinauseant action not known, but thought to involve ability to inhibit cholinergic stimulation in vestibular and associated neural pathways.

USES Chiefly in prevention and treatment of motion sickness. Also has been used in management of vertigo, nausea, and vomiting associated with radiation sickness, labyrinthitis, Meniere's syndrome, stapedectomy, anesthesia, and various medications.

ROUTE & DOSAGE

Motion Sickness

Adult	PO	50–100 mg q4–6h (max 400 mg/24h)
	IM/IV	50 mg as needed
Child	PO	6–12 y: 25–50 mg q6–8h (max 150 mg/24h)
		2–6 y: up to 25 mg q6–8h (max 75 mg/24h)
	IM/IV	6–12 y: 1.25 mg/kg q.i.d. up to 300 mg/d
		2–6 y: 1.25 mg/kg q.i.d. up to 300 mg/d

PHARMACOKINETICS Absorption: readily absorbed from GI tract. **Onset:** 15–30 min PO; immediate IV; 20–30 min IM. **Duration:** 3–6 h. **Distribution:** distributed into breast milk. **Elimination:** excreted in urine.

CONTRAINDICATIONS & PRECAUTIONS Contraindicated in: narrow-angle glaucoma, prostatic hypertrophy. Safe use during pregnancy (category B), in nursing women, and in children <2 y not established. **Cautious use in:** convulsive disorders.

ADVERSE/SIDE EFFECTS. CNS: *drowsiness,* headache, incoordination, dizziness, blurred vision, nervousness, restlessness, *insomnia (especially children)*. **CV:** hypotension, palpitation. **Other:** dry mouth, nose, throat. Less frequently: anorexia, constipation or diarrhea, urinary frequency, dysuria.

DIAGNOSTIC TEST INTERFERENCE *Skin testing* procedures should not be performed within 72 h after use of an antihistamine.

DRUG INTERACTIONS Alcohol and other CNS DEPRESSANTS enhance CNS depression, drowsiness; TRICYCLIC ANTIDEPRESSANTS compound anticholinergic effects.

INCOMPATIBILITIES Solution/Additive: aminophylline, amobarbital, butorphanol, chlorpromazine, glycopyrrolate, hydroxyzine, midazolam, pentobarbital, prochlorperazine, promazine, promethazine, thiopental.

NURSING IMPLICATIONS

Administration
- *IV injection:* IV dimenhydrinate may be given by direct IV. Dilute each 50 mg in 10 ml of NS. Administer 50 mg or fraction thereof over 2 min.
- To prevent radiation sickness, drug is usually administered 30–60 min before treatment, then repeated 1 1/2 h after treatment, and again in 3 h.
- Store preferably at 15–30C (59–86F), unless otherwise directed by manufacturer. Examine parenteral preparation for particulate matter and discoloration. Do not use unless absolutely clear.

Assessment & Drug Effects
- High incidence of drowsiness. Side rails and supervision of ambulation may be indicated.
- Tolerance to CNS depressant effects usually occurs after a few days of drug therapy. Some decrease in antiemetic action may result with prolonged use.
- Antihistamines can obscure signs of dizziness, nausea, and vomiting, associated with drug toxicity and serious disease conditions.

Patient & Family Education

- Caution ambulatory patient not to drive or operate dangerous machinery until reaction to drug is known.
- To prevent motion sickness, dimenhydrinate should be taken 30 min before departure and should be repeated before meals and upon retiring.

DIMERCAPROL

(dye-mer-kap´role)
Trade names: BAL in Oil, British Anti-Lewisite
Classifications: CHELATING AGENT; ANTIDOTE
Pregnancy: Category D

ACTIONS/PHARMACODYNAMICS Dithiol compound originally developed as antidote for Lewisite, an arsenic-containing chemical warfare agent. Combines with ions of various heavy metals to form relatively stable, nontoxic, soluble complexes called chelates (mercaptides), which can be excreted; inhibition of sulfhydryl enzymes by toxic metals is thus prevented. May also reactivate affected enzymes but is most effective when administered prior to enzyme damage.

USES Acute poisoning by arsenic, gold, and mercury; as adjunct to edetate calcium disodium (EDTA) in treatment of lead encephalopathy. **Unlabeled use (topical):** chromium dermatitis; ocular and dermatologic manifestations of arsenic poisoning, as adjunct to penicillamine to increase rate of copper excretion in Wilson's disease, and for poisoning with antimony, bismuth, chromium, copper, nickel, tungsten, zinc.

ROUTE & DOSAGE

Arsenic or Gold Poisoning

Adult	IM	2.5–3 mg/kg q4h for first 2 d; then q.i.d. on third day; then b.i.d. for 10 d
Child	IM	Same as for adult

Mercury Poisoning

Adult	IM	5 mg/kg initially; followed by 2.5 mg/kg 1–2 times/d for 10 d
Child	IM	Same as for adult

Acute Lead Encephalopathy

Adult	IM	4 mg/kg initially; then 3–4 mg/kg q4h with EDTA for 2–7 d depending on response
Child	IM	Same as for adult

PHARMACOKINETICS Peak: 30–60 min. **Distribution:** distributed mainly in intracellular spaces, including brain; highest concentrations in liver and kidneys. **Elimination:** half-life: short; completely excreted in urine and bile within 4 h.

CONTRAINDICATIONS & PRECAUTIONS Contraindicated in: hepatic insufficiency (with exception of postarsenical jaundice); severe renal insufficiency; poisoning due to cadmium, iron, selenium, or uranium. Safe use during pregnancy (category D) and in nursing women not established. **Cautious use in:** hypertension, patients with G6PD deficiency.

ADVERSE/SIDE EFFECTS CNS: headache, anxiety, muscle pain or weakness, restlessness, paresthesias, tremors, *convulsions*, shock. **CV:** *elevated BP*, tachycardia. **ENT:** rhinorrhea; burning sensation, feeling of pain and constriction in throat. **GI:** nausea, *vomiting*; burning sensation in lips and mouth, halitosis, salivation; abdominal pain, metabolic acidosis. **GU:** burning sensation in penis, <u>renal damage</u>. **Other:** pains in chest or hands, pain and sterile abscess at injection site, sweating, reduction in polymorphonuclear leukocytes, dental pain.

DIAGNOSTIC TEST INTERFERENCES ^{131}I *thyroidal uptake* values may be decreased if test is done during or immediately following dimercaprol therapy.

DRUG INTERACTIONS Iron, cadmium, selenium, uranium form toxic complexes with dimercaprol.

NURSING IMPLICATIONS

Administration

- Because irreversible tissue damage may occur quickly, particularly in mercury poisoning, dimercaprol therapy must be initiated as soon as possible (within 1–2 h) after ingestion of the poison.
- Administered by deep IM injection only. Local pain, gluteal abscess, and skin sensitization reported. Rotate injection sites and observe daily.
- Contact of drug with skin may produce erythema, edema, dermatitis. Handle with caution.
- Presence of sediment in ampul reportedly does not indicate drug deterioration.

Assessment & Drug Effects

- Monitor vital signs. Elevations of systolic and diastolic BPs accompanied by tachycardia frequently occur within a few minutes following injection and

Common side effects in *italic*; life-threatening effects <u>underlined</u>; generic names in **bold**; classifications in SMALL CAPS

529

may remain elevated up to 2 h.

- Fever occurs in approximately 30% of children receiving treatment and may persist throughout therapy.
- I&O should be monitored. Drug is potentially nephrotoxic. Report oliguria or change in I&O ratio.
- Urine should be kept alkaline to reduce possibility of renal damage during elimination of dimercaprol chelate.
- Daily urine examinations should be made for albumin, blood, casts, and pH. Blood and urinary levels of the metal serve as guides for dosage adjustments.
- Minor adverse reactions usually reach maximum 15–20 min after drug administration and generally subside in 30–90 min. Ephedrine or an antihistamine is sometimes administered to prevent symptoms.

DIMETHYL SULFOXIDE

(dye-meth´il sul-fox´ide)
Trade names: DMSO, Rimso-50
Classifications: SKIN & MUCOUS MEMBRANE AGENT; ANTIINFLAMMATORY, LOCAL
Pregnancy: Category C

ACTIONS/PHARMACODYNAMICS Mechanism of action not known. Reported actions and effects include antiinflammatory effects, membrane penetration, collagen dissolution, peripheral nerve blockade (local analgesia), vasodilation, muscle relaxation, diuresis, weak bacteriostatic and antifungal actions, initiation of histamine release at administration site, cholinesterase inhibition. Enhances percutaneous absorption of many drugs by increasing permeability of skin.

USES Symptomatic treatment of interstitial cystitis. **Unlabeled uses:** topical treatment of a variety of musculoskeletal disorders, arthritis, scleroderma, tendinitis, breast and prostate malignancies, retinitis pigmentosa, herpes virus infections, head and spinal cord injuries, shock, and as a carrier to enhance penetration and absorption of other drugs. Also used to protect living cells and tissues during cold storage (cryoprotection). Widely used as an industrial solvent and in veterinary medicine for treatment of musculoskeletal injuries.

ROUTE & DOSAGE

Interstitial Cystitis

Adult Intravesicular Instillation: 50 ml of 50% solution instilled slowly into urinary bladder and retained for 15 min; may repeat q2wk until maximum relief obtained; then increase intervals between treatments

PHARMACOKINETICS Absorption: readily absorbed systemically. **Peak:** 4–8 h. **Distribution:** widely distributed in tissues and body fluids; penetrates blood-brain barrier; distributed into breast milk. **Metabolism:** metabolized to dimethyl sulfide (garlic breath) and dimethyl sulfone. **Elimination:** dimethyl sulfide excreted through lungs and skin; dimethyl sulfone may remain in serum > 2 wk and is excreted in urine and feces.

CONTRAINDICATIONS & PRECAUTIONS Contraindicated in: safe use during pregnancy (category C), in nursing mothers, and in children not established. **Cautious use in:** hepatic or renal dysfunction.

ADVERSE/SIDE EFFECTS Eye: transient disturbances in color vision, photophobia (lens opacities have occurred in laboratory animals). **GI:** nausea, diarrhea. **Hypersensitivity:** local or generalized rash, erythema, pruritus, urticaria, swelling of face, dyspnea (anaphylactoid reaction). **Other:** nasal congestion, headache, sedation, drowsiness. **Following intravesicular instillation:** *garliclike odor on breath and skin; garliclike taste;* discomfort during administration; transient cystitis. **Following topical application:** vesicle formation.

DRUG INTERACTIONS Decreases effectiveness of **sulindac,** possibly causing severe peripheral neuropathy.

NURSING IMPLICATIONS

Administration

- Manufacturer suggests application of analgesic lubricant such as lidocaine jelly to urethra to facilitate insertion of catheter.
- Patient retains instillation for 15 min and then expels it by spontaneous voiding.
- Discomfort associated with instillation usually becomes less prominent with repeated administration. Physician may prescribe an oral analgesic or suppository containing belladonna and an opiate prior to instillation to reduce bladder spasm.
- Store at 15–30C (59–86F) unless otherwise directed by manufacturer. Protect from strong light and avoid contact with plastics.

Common side effects in *italic*; life-threatening effects underlined; generic names in **bold**; classifications in SMALL CAPS

Assessment & Drug Effects

- CBCs and liver and renal function tests are recommended, initially and at 6 mo intervals.
- Complete eye evaluation including slit-lamp examination is recommended prior to and at regular intervals during therapy.

Patient & Family Education

- Garliclike taste may be experienced within minutes after drug instillation and may last for several hours. Garliclike odor on breath and skin may last as long as 72 h.
- Caution patient not to use OTC topical medications without consulting physician.

DINOPROSTONE

See PROSTAGLANDIN prototype, p 251.

DIPHENHYDRAMINE HYDROCHLORIDE

See ANTIHISTAMINE (H$_1$-RECEPTOR ANTAGONIST) prototype, p 47.

Prototype: prochlorperazine, p 215

DIPHENIDOL

(di-phen´i-dol)
Trade name: Vontrol
Classifications: GI AGENT; ANTIEMETIC; ANTIVERTIGO
Pregnancy: Category C

ACTIONS/PHARMACODYNAMICS Mechanism of action not precisely known but may exert a specific effect on the vestibular apparatus to control vertigo and inhibit the chemoreceptor trigger zone (CTZ) to control nausea and vomiting. Has a weak peripheral anticholinergic effect.

USES Peripheral (labyrinthine) vertigo and associated nausea and vomiting, in Meniere's syndrome and middle and inner ear surgery (labyrinthitis). Also control of nausea and vomiting in postoperative states, malignant neoplasms, and labyrinthine disturbances.

ROUTE & DOSAGE

Nausea, Vomiting, Vertigo

Adult	PO	25–50 mg q4h prn (max 300 mg/d)
Child	PO	> 11 kg or > 6 mo: 0.88 mg/kg; may repeat in 1 h if needed, then q4h prn (max 5.5 mg/kg/d)

PHARMACOKINETICS Absorption: readily absorbed form GI tract. **Peak:** 1.5–3 h. **Metabolism:** metabolized in liver. **Elimination:** half-life: 4 h; excreted primarily in urine, small amount of feces.

CONTRAINDICATIONS & PRECAUTIONS Contraindicated in: hypersensitivity to diphenidol, anuria, pregnancy (category C), lactation, children <25 kg (50 lb). **Cautious use in:** glaucoma, obstructive lesions of the GI and GU tracts such as stenosing peptic ulcer, prostatic hypertrophy, pyloric and duodenal obstruction, organic cardiospasm.

ADVERSE/SIDE EFFECTS CNS: Auditory and visual hallucinations, disorientation, confusion, drowsiness, overstimulation, depression, blurred vision. **GI:** dry mouth, nausea, indigestion.

DRUG INTERACTIONS None noted.

NURSING IMPLICATIONS

Administration

- Tablets may be swallowed whole, chewed, or allowed to dissolve in mouth.
- Administer with food, water, or milk to minimize gastric irritation.
- Do not administer to children weighing less than 25 kg (50 lb).
- Should be administered only to patients under close medical supervision.
- Store at 15–30C (59–86F) in a tight, light resistant container unless otherwise specified.

Assessment & Drug Effects

- Inquire about history of anuria, hypotension, or renal function impairment before starting therapy.
- Monitor I&O and assess weight daily.
- Assess BP for signs of hypotension.
- Observe for blurred vision, confusion, or hallucinations.
- Observe for signs of toxicity of other drugs (e.g., digitalis) or masking of symptoms of disease (e.g., brain tumor, intestinal obstruction).
- Because of anticholinergic effect of drug, patients with glaucoma and obstructive lesions of the GI or GU tract should be closely monitored for worsening of the condition.

Common side effects in *italic*; life-threatening effects underlined; generic names in **bold**; classifications in SMALL CAPS

531

Patient & Family Education

- Instruct patient not to take more medication than prescribed.
- Instruct patient to take as soon as possible if dose is missed but not to take if almost time for next dose nor to double dose.
- Instruct patient to avoid use of alcohol or other CNS depressants.
- Advise against driving or performing other hazardous activities until response to drug is known.
- Instruct patient to report severe or persistent nausea and vomiting.

D

DIPHENOXYLATE HYDROCHLORIDE WITH ATROPINE SULFATE

See GASTROINTESTINAL AGENTS, ANTIDIARRHEAL prototype, p 213.

Prototype: Pilocarpine, p 209

DIPIVEFRIN HYDROCHLORIDE

(dye-pi´ve-frin)

Trade name: Propine
Classifications: EYE PREPARATION; MYDRIATIC; AUTONOMIC NERVOUS SYSTEM AGENT; ADRENERGIC AGONIST (SYMPATHOMIMETIC)
Pregnancy: Category B

ACTIONS/PHARMACODYNAMICS Formed by diesterification of epinephrine in pivalic acid, which enhances lipophilic and penetrating properties. Classified as a prodrug of epinephrine. (Prodrugs are compounds that are therapeutically inactive until biotransformed to parent compound.) Converted to epinephrine by esterases in the eye. IOP-lowering effect and mydriatic action are substantially greater than produced by epinephrine. Unlike epinephrine, produces only minimal systemic sympathomimetic effects. Appears to lower IOP by reducing production of aqueous humor and by enhancing its outflow. Does not produce miosis or accommodative spasms, blurred vision, or night blindness associated with miotic agents.

USES Alone or in combination with other antiglaucomatous agents to control IOP in chronic open-angle glaucoma. **Unlabeled use:** to reduce IOP in ocular hypertension, low tension and secondary glaucomas.

ROUTE & DOSAGE

Glaucoma

Adult	Topical	1 drop in eye q12h

PHARMACOKINETICS Absorption: rapidly absorbed into aqueous humor, where it is hydrolyzed to epinephrine by esterases in the cornea, conjunctiva, and aqueous humor. **Onset:** 30 min. **Peak:** 1 h. **Duration:** ≥12 h (up to 2 wk in some patients). **Distribution:** systemic distribution not determined. **Elimination:** half-life: 0.9–3.1 h.

CONTRAINDICATIONS & PRECAUTIONS Contraindicated in: hypersensitivity to epinephrine; angle-closure glaucoma. Safe use during pregnancy (category B), in nursing mothers, and in children not established. **Cautious use in:** asthma, atopic nonasthmatic individuals; aphakia (absence of crystalline lens); hypertension; cardiac disorders.

ADVERSE/SIDE EFFECTS Eye: *mydriasis, blurred vision, ocular pain, headache, burning or stinging, conjunctival injection and irritation, photophobia;* adrenochrome deposits on conjunctiva and cornea, macular edema (aphakic patients); bulbar conjunctival follicles. **Hypersensitivity:** blepharoconjunctivitis, chemosis of conjunctiva, eczematoid dermatitis, pruritus, blepharitis.

NURSING IMPLICATIONS

Administration

- Apply light finger pressure to lacrimal duct during and for 1 or 2 min following instillation. Blot excess medication with clean tissue.
- Withhold medication and consult physician if signs of sensitivity develop or if irritation increases or persists.
- Store at 15–30C (59–86F) unless otherwise directed.

Assessment & Drug Effects

- Patient may experience a temporary stinging and burning sensation with initial instillation.
- Monitor for signs of hypersensitivity (see adverse/side effects). If these appear, withhold drug and report to physician.
- Carefully monitor patient with a history of hypertension.

DIPYRIDAMOLE

(dye-peer-id´a-mole)

Trade names: Apo-Dipyridamole, Persantine, Pyridamole, IV Persantine

Classifications: CARDIOVASCULAR DRUG; NONNITRATE VASODILATOR

Pregnancy: Category C

ACTIONS/PHARMACODYNAMICS Nonnitrate coronary vasodilator with many properties similar to those of papaverine. Increases coronary blood flow by selectively dilating coronary arteries, thereby increasing myocardial oxygen supply. Exhibits mild inotropic action. Has little effect on BP and blood flow in peripheral arteries. Inhibits ADP-induced platelet aggregation. Does not affect prothrombin activity.

USES To prevent postoperative thromboembolic complications associated with prosthetic heart valves and as adjunct for thallium stress testing. **Unlabeled use:** to reduce rate of reinfarction following MI; to prevent TIAs (transient ischemic attacks) and coronary by-pass graft occlusion.

ROUTE & DOSAGE

Prevention of Thromboembolism in Cardiac Valve Replacement

Adult   PO   75–100 mg q.i.d.

Thromboembolic Disorders

Adult   PO   150–400 mg/d in divided doses

Thallium Stress Test

Adult   IV   0.142 mg/kg/min for 4 min

PHARMACOKINETICS Absorption: readily absorbed from GI tract. **Peak:** 45–150 min. **Distribution:** small amount crosses placenta. **Metabolism:** metabolized in liver. **Elimination:** half-life: 10–12 h; mainly excreted in feces.

CONTRAINDICATIONS & PRECAUTIONS Contraindicated in: safe use in pregnancy (category C) and nursing mothers not established. **Cautious use in:** hypotension, anticoagulant therapy.

ADVERSE/SIDE EFFECTS Usually dose related, minimal, and transient. **CNS:** headache, dizziness, faintness, syncope, weakness. **CV:** peripheral vasodilation, flushing. **GI:** nausea, vomiting, diarrhea, abdominal distress. **Other:** skin rash, pruritus.

NURSING IMPLICATIONS

Administration

- Preferable to take on an empty stomach at least 1 h before or 2 h after meals, with a full glass of water. Physician may prescribe it to be taken with food if gastric distress persists.
- Product interchange is not advisable. Bioavailability differences among dipyridamole preparations have been reported.
- Before IV administration, dilute to at least a 1:2 ratio with 0.5N NaCl injection, 1N NaCl injection, or 5% dextrose injection for a total volume of 20 to 50 ml.
- The recommended IV dose is 0.142 mg/kg/min infused over 4 min.
- Store in tightly closed container at 15–30C (59–86F) unless otherwise directed. Protect IV dipyridamole from direct light.

Assessment & Drug Effects

- Clinical response may not be evident before second or third month of continuous therapy.
- Expected therapeutic effects: reduced frequency or elimination of anginal episodes, improved exercise tolerance, reduced requirement for nitrates.

Patient & Family Education

- Counsel patient to notify physician of any side effects.
- If postural (orthostatic) hypotension is a problem, advise patient to make all position changes slowly and in stages, especially from recumbent to upright posture.

DISOPYRAMIDE PHOSPHATE

(dye-soe-peer´a-mide)

Trade names: DSP, Napamide, Norpace, Norpace CR, Rythmodan, Rythmodan-LA

Classifications: CARDIOVASCULAR AGENT; ANTIARRHYTHMIC

Pregnancy: Category C

ACTIONS/PHARMACODYNAMICS Class IA antiarrhythmic agent with pharmacologic actions similar to those of quinidine and procainamide, although

---

Common side effects in *italic*; life-threatening effects <u>underlined</u>; generic names in **bold**; classifications in SMALL CAPS

D

chemically unrelated. Acts as myocardial depressant by reducing rate of spontaneous diastolic depolarization in pacemaker cells, thereby suppressing ectopic focal activity. In usual doses, retards upstroke velocity, lengthens action potential of normal cardiac cells, and reduces differences in duration of action potential between normal and infarcted tissue. Disopyramide shortens sinus node recovery time and increases atrial and ventricular effective refractory period but has minimal effect on refractoriness and conduction time of AV node or on conduction time of His-Purkinje system or QRS duration. Has prominent atropinelike (anticholinergic) effects particularly on GI and urogenital systems.

USES To suppress and prevent recurrence of premature ventricular contractions (unifocal, multifocal, paired) and ventricular tachycardia not severe enough to require cardioversion. **Unlabeled uses:** in combination with other antiarrhythmic drugs to treat or prevent serious refractory arrhythmias. To convert atrial fibrillation, atrial flutter, and paroxysmal atrial tachycardia to normal sinus rhythm.

ROUTE & DOSAGE

Arrhythmias

Adult	PO	>50 kg: 100–200 mg q6h or 300 mg controlled release capsule q12h
		<50 kg: 100 mg q6h or 200 mg controlled release q12h
Child	PO	12–18 y: 6–15 mg/kg/d in divided doses q6h
		4–12 y: 10–15 mg/kg/d in divided doses q6h
		1–4 y: 10–20 mg/kg/d in divided doses q6h
		<1y: 10–30 mg/kg/d in divided doses q6h

PHARMACOKINETICS Absorption: readily absorbed from GI tract; 60–83% reaches systemic circulation. **Onset:** 30 min–3.5 h. **Peak:** 1–2 h. **Duration:** 1.5–8.5 h. **Distribution:** distributed in extracellular fluid; crosses placenta; distributed into breast milk. **Metabolism:** metabolized in liver. **Elimination:** half-life: 4–10 h; 80% excreted in urine, 10% in feces.

CONTRAINDICATIONS & PRECAUTIONS Contraindicated in: cardiogenic shock, preexisting 2nd or 3rd degree AV block (if no pacemaker is present); uncompensated or inadequately compensated CHF, hypotension (unless secondary to cardiac arrhyth-

mia), hypokalemia. Safe use during pregnancy (category C), in nursing women, and in children not established. **Cautious use in:** sick sinus syndrome (bradycardia-tachycardia); Wolff-Parkinson-White (WPW) syndrome or bundle branch block, myocarditis or other cardiomyopathy, underlying cardiac conduction abnormalities; hepatic or renal impairment; urinary tract disease (especially prostatic hypertrophy); myasthenia gravis; narrow-angle glaucoma, family history of glaucoma.

ADVERSE/SIDE EFFECTS CNS: dizziness, headache, fatigue, muscle weakness, convulsions, paresthesias, peripheral neuropathy, nervousness, depression, acute psychosis. **CV:** *hypotension,* chest pain, edema, dyspnea, syncope, bradycardia, tachycardia; worsening of CHF or cardiac arrhythmia; <u>cardiogenic shock</u>, <u>heart block</u>; edema with weight gain. **Eye:** *blurred vision,* dry eyes, increased IOP, precipitation of acute angle-closure glaucoma. **GI:** *dry mouth, constipation,* epigastric or abdominal pain, cholestatic jaundice. **GU:** *hesitancy and retention,* urinary frequency, urgency, renal insufficiency, impotence. **Hypersensitivity:** pruritus, urticaria, rash, photosensitivity, <u>laryngospasm</u>. **Other:** dry nose and throat, *hypokalemia,* <u>agranulocytosis,</u> thrombocytopenia, drying of bronchial secretions, initiation of uterine contractions (pregnant patient); muscle aches, precipitation of myasthenia gravis.

DRUG INTERACTIONS ANTICHOLINERGIC DRUGS (e.g., TRICYCLIC ANTIDEPRESSANTS, ANTIHISTAMINES) compound anticholinergic effects; other ANTIARRHYTHMICS compound toxicities; **phenytoin, rifampin** may increase disopyramide metabolism and decrease levels; may increase **warfarin**-induced hypoprothrombinemia.

NURSING IMPLICATIONS

Administration

- For patients who have been receiving either quinidine or procainamide, manufacturer suggests starting disopyramide 6–12 h after last quinidine dose and 3–6 h after last procainamide dose.
- Loading doses are not recommended for patients with cardiomyopathy, cardiac decompensation, or renal or hepatic impairment.
- Controlled release capsules are not appropriate for use in loading doses when rapid control is required or in patients with creatinine clearance of ≤ 40 ml/min.
- When patient is to be transferred from conventional capsule to controlled release capsule, start

Common side effects in *italic*; life-threatening effects <u>underlined</u>; generic names in **bold**; classifications in SMALL CAPS

the latter 6 h after last dose of conventional capsule.

- Store at 15–30C (59–86F) unless otherwise directed.

Assessment & Drug Effects

- Check apical pulse before administering drug. Withhold drug and notify physician if pulse rate is slower than 60 bpm, faster than 120 bpm, or if there is any unusual change in rate, rhythm, or quality.
- ECG should be closely monitored. The following signs are indications for drug withdrawal: prolongation of QT interval and worsening of arrhythmia interval, QRS widening (> 25%).
- Baseline and periodic determinations should be made of hepatic and renal function, blood glucose, and serum potassium. Hypokalemia or other imbalances are corrected before initiation of therapy.
- Closely monitor BP in all patients during periods of dosage adjustment and in those receiving high dosages.
- Monitor I&O, particularly in the elderly and patients with impaired renal function or prostatic hypertrophy. Persistent urinary hesitancy or retention may necessitate lower dosage or discontinuation of drug.
- Patients with atrial flutter or fibrillation are usually digitalized prior to initiation of therapy to ensure that improvement in AV conduction does not lead to a dangerously rapid ventricular rate.
- Toxic effects are enhanced by hyperkalemia. Report signs and symptoms (see chap 3).
- Patients with a family history of glaucoma should have IOP measured before treatment begins.
- Blood glucose levels should be monitored in patients with CHF, hepatic or renal disease, patients taking beta adrenergic blocking agents, and the elderly.
- Monitor for signs and symptoms of CHF (see chap 3).
- Disopyramide should be discontinued promptly if signs and symptoms of agranulocytosis, or peripheral neuritis, or jaundice (see chap 3) appear.

Patient & Family Education

- Instruct patient to weigh daily under standard conditions and to check ankles and tibiae daily for edema. Report to physician a weekly weight gain of ≥ 1–2 kg (2–4 lb).
- Instruct patient to report signs and symptoms of hypoglycemia (see chap 3).
- Because of the possibility of hypotension, advise patient to make position changes slowly, particularly from recumbent posture, to dangle legs for a few minutes before ambulating, and not to stand still for prolonged periods. Instruct patient to lie down or sit down if he or she feels light-headed.
- To maintain regularity of heartbeat, drug must be taken precisely as prescribed. Emphasize importance of not skipping or stopping medication or changing dose without consulting physician.
- Urge patient to keep appointments for periodic clinical evaluation.
- Advise patient not to take OTC medications unless approved by physician.
- May cause photosensitivity; therefore exposure to sunlight or ultraviolet light should be avoided.
- Since drug may cause dizziness and blurring of vision, caution patient to avoid driving and other potentially hazardous activities until reaction to drug effects is known.
- Warn patient not to drink alcoholic beverages while taking disopyramide.

DISULFIRAM
(dye-sul´fi-ram)
Trade names: Antabuse, Cronetal, Ro-sulfiram
Classifications: ENZYME INHIBITOR; ANTIALCOHOL AGENT
Pregnancy: Category X

ACTIONS/PHARMACODYNAMICS Acts as a deterrent to alcohol ingestion by inhibiting the enzyme acetaldehyde dehydrogenase, which normally metabolizes alcohol in the body. As a result, when a small amount of alcohol is ingested, acetaldehyde concentration of blood rises 5–10 times above normal. This causes a complex of highly unpleasant symptoms known as the disulfiram reaction, which serves as a deterrent to further drinking. Disulfiram possesses antithyroid and sedative actions usually unimportant unless alcohol is ingested. Does not produce tolerance and is not a cure for alcoholism.

USES Adjunct in treatment of the patient with chronic alcoholism who sincerely wants to maintain sobriety.

ROUTE & DOSAGE

Alcoholism

Adult	PO	500 mg/d for 1–2 wk; then 125–500 mg/d (max 500 mg/d)

Common side effects in *italic*; life-threatening effects underlined; generic names in **bold**; classifications in SMALL CAPS

535

PHARMACOKINETICS Absorption: readily absorbed from GI tract. **Onset:** up to 12 h. **Duration:** up to 2 wk. **Distribution:** initially deposited in fat. **Metabolism:** metabolized slowly in liver. **Elimination:** 5–20% excreted in feces; 20% remains in body for 1–2 wk; some may be excreted in breath as carbon disulfide.

CONTRAINDICATIONS & PRECAUTIONS Contraindicated in: severe myocardial disease; psychoses; pregnancy (category X); or patients who have recently received alcohol, metronidazole, paraldehyde; multiple drug dependence. **Cautious use in:** diabetes mellitus; epilepsy; hypothyroidism; coronary artery disease, cerebral damage; chronic and acute nephritis; hepatic cirrhosis or insufficiency; abnormal EEG.

ADVERSE/SIDE EFFECTS Disulfiram reaction (with alcohol ingestion): flushing of face, chest, arms, pulsating headache, nausea, violent vomiting, thirst, sweating, marked uneasiness, confusion, weakness, vertigo, blurred vision, pruritic skin rash, hyperventilation, abnormal gait, slurred speech, disorientation, confusion, personality changes, bizarre behavior, psychoses, tachycardia, palpitation, chest pain. Severe reactions: hypotension to shock level, arrhythmias, acute congestive failure, marked respiratory depression, unconsciousness, convulsions, sudden death. **CNS:** drowsiness, fatigue, restlessness, headache, tremor, psychoses (usually with high doses); polyneuritis, peripheral neuropathy, optic neuritis. **GI:** Mild GI disturbances, garliclike or metallic taste, hepatotoxicity, hypersensitivity hepatitis. **GU:** impotence. **Hypersensitivity:** allergic or acneiform dermatitis; urticaria; fixed-drug eruption.

DIAGNOSTIC TEST INTERFERENCES Disulfiram can reduce *uptake of I-131;* or decreases *PBI* test results (rare).

DRUG INTERACTIONS Alcohol (including in liquid OTC drugs, **IV nitroglycerin, IV cotrimoxazole**), **metronidazole, paraldehyde** will produce disulfiram reaction; **isoniazid** can produce neurological symptoms; may increase blood levels and toxicity of **warfarin, paraldehyde,** BARBITURATES, **phenytoin.**

NURSING IMPLICATIONS

Administration

- Daily dose should be taken in the morning when the resolve not to drink may be strongest.
- To minimize sedative effect the drug may be prescribed to be taken at bedtime. Decrease in dose may also reduce sedative effect.
- Therapy is not initiated until patient has abstained from alcohol and alcohol-containing preparations for at least 12 h and preferably 48 h.
- Maintenance therapy with disulfiram may be required for months or even years. Compliance should be determined periodically.
- Protect tablets from light. Store at 15–30C (59–86F) unless otherwise directed.

Assessment & Drug Effects

- Complete physical examination, and careful drug history are advised prior to therapy. Baseline and follow-up transaminase studies every 10–14 d are suggested to detect hepatic dysfunction. In addition, CBC and sequential multiple analysis (SMA-12) tests should be performed every 6 mo.
- Disulfiram reaction occurs within 5–10 min following ingestion of alcohol and may last 30 min to several hours. When symptoms subside, patient may sleep for several hours, after which patient is well again. Some patients have disagreeable breath because of a disulfiram metabolite.
- Intensity of reaction varies with each individual, but it is generally proportional to the amount of alcohol ingested.
- Psychotic responses (usually associated with high dosages) may unmask underlying psychosis in some patients stressed by alcohol withdrawal.
- Treat patient with severe disulfiram reaction as though he or she were in shock. Monitor potassium levels, especially if patient has diabetes mellitus.

Patient & Family Education

- Patient should be completely aware of and should consent to therapy with disulfiram. Patient and family should be fully informed of possible dangers if alcohol is ingested during disulfiram treatment.
- Instruct patient to report promptly to physician the onset of nausea with right upper quadrant pain or discomfort, itching, jaundiced sclerae or skin, dark urine, clay-colored stools. Disulfiram should be withheld pending liver function studies.
- Ingestion of even small amounts of alcohol or use of external applications that contain alcohol may be sufficient to produce a reaction. Teach patient to read labels and to avoid use of anything containing alcohol.
- Patient should be informed that prolonged administration of disulfiram does not produce tolerance; the longer one remains on therapy, the more sensitive one becomes to alcohol.
- Warn patient that alcohol sensitivity may last as

long as 2 wk after disulfiram has been discontinued.

- During first 2 wk of therapy, patient may experience side effects of disulfiram itself (See Adverse/Side Effects). These symptoms usually disappear with continued therapy or with dose reduction.
- Advise patient to carry an identification card stating that patient is on disulfiram therapy and describing the symptoms of disulfiram reaction. The names of the physician or institution to contact in an emergency should also be provided.
- During early therapy when drowsiness may be a problem, the patient should avoid driving or performing other tasks requiring alertness.

Prototype: isoproterenol, p 105

DOBUTAMINE HYDROCHLORIDE
(doe-byoo′ta-meen)
Trade name: Dobutrex
Classifications: AUTONOMIC NERVOUS SYSTEM AGENT; BETA-ADRENERGIC AGONIST; CATECHOLAMINE
Pregnancy: Category C

ACTIONS/PHARMACODYNAMICS Synthetic, direct-acting sympathomimetic amine with electrophysiologic effects on heart similar to those of isoproterenol and dopamine. Produces inotropic effect by acting on beta receptors and primarily on myocardial adrenergic alpha receptors. Increases cardiac output and decreases pulmonary wedge pressure and total systemic vascular resistance with comparatively little or no effect on BP. Also increases conduction through AV node. Has lower potential for precipitating arrhythmias than dopamine. In CHF, increase in cardiac output enhances renal perfusion and increases renal output and renal sodium excretion. Studies have shown that clinical benefits of dobutamine in these patients may continue for weeks to months after drug has been discontinued. Exact mechanism underlying this sustained effect is not known.

USES Inotropic support in short-term treatment of adults with cardiac decompensation due to depressed myocardial contractility (cardiogenic shock) resulting from either organic heart disease or from cardiac surgery. **Unlabeled use:** to augment cardiovascular function in children undergoing cardiac catheterization.

ROUTE & DOSAGE

Cardiac Decompensation

Adult	IV	2.5–10 µg/kg/min (up to 40 µg/kg/min); has been given for up to 72 h without decrease in effectiveness
Child	IV	Same as for adult

PHARMACOKINETICS Onset: 2–10 min. **Peak:** 10–20 min. **Metabolism:** metabolized in liver and other tissues by COMT. **Elimination:** half-life: 2 min; excreted in urine.

CONTRAINDICATIONS & PRECAUTIONS Contraindicated in: history of hypersensitivity to other sympathomimetic amines, ventricular tachycardia, idiopathic hypertrophic subaortic stenosis. Safe use during pregnancy (category C), in nursing mothers and children, or following acute MI not established. **Cautious use in:** preexisting hypertension, atrial fibrillation.

ADVERSE/SIDE EFFECTS Generally dose related. **CNS:** headache, tremors, paresthesias, mild leg cramps, nervousness, fatigue (with overdosage). **CV:** *increased heart rate and BP,* premature ventricular beats, palpitation, *anginal pain.* **GI:** nausea, vomiting. **Other:** nonspecific chest pain, shortness of breath.

DRUG INTERACTIONS GENERAL ANESTHETICS (especially **cyclopropane** and **halothane**) may sensitize myocardium to effects of CATECHOLAMINES such as dobutamine and lead to serious arrhythmias— used with extreme caution; BETA-ADRENERGIC BLOCKING AGENTS, e.g., **metoprolol, propranolol**, may make dobutamine ineffective in increasing cardiac output, but total peripheral resistance may increase— concomitant use generally avoided; MAO INHIBITORS, tricylic antidepressants potentiate pressor effects— used with extreme caution.

INCOMPATIBILITIES Solution/Additive: sodium bicarbonate, aminophylline, bretylium, bumetanide, calcium chloride, calcium gluconate, diazepam, doxapram, digoxin, epinephrine, furosemide, heparin, insulin, magnesium sulfate, phenytoin, potassium chloride, potassium phosphate. Y-site: acyclovir, aminophylline, sodium bicarbonate.

Common side effects in *italic*; life-threatening effects underlined; generic names in **bold**; classifications in SMALL CAPS

537

NURSING IMPLICATIONS

Administration

- Hypovolemia should be corrected by administration of appropriate volume expanders prior to initiation of therapy.
- Since dobutamine enhances AV conduction, patients with atrial fibrillation are generally given a digitalis preparation prior to initiation of therapy to reduce risk of ventricular tachycardia.
- Dobutamine may be reconstituted by adding 10 ml sterile water for injection or 5% dextrose injection to 250 mg vial. If not completely dissolved, additional 10 ml of diluent may be added.
- For IV infusion, reconstituted solution must be further diluted before administration to at least 50 ml with 5% dextrose, 0.9% NaCl, or sodium lactate injection. IV solutions should be used within 24 h.
- Rate of infusion should be controlled by an infusion pump (preferred) or a microdrip IV infusion set.
- Solutions containing dobutamine may exhibit color changes because of slight oxidation of drug. This does not affect potency.
- Dobutamine is incompatible with sodium bicarbonate and other alkaline solutions.
- Reconstituted solution may be refrigerated at 2–15C (36–59F) for 48 h or for 6 h at room temperature.

Assessment & Drug Effects

- At any given dosage level, drug takes 10–20 min to produce peak effects.
- ECG and BP should be monitored continuously during administration of dobutamine.
- IV infusion rate and duration of therapy are determined by heart rate, blood pressure, ectopic activity, urine output, and whenever possible, by measurements of cardiac output and central venous or pulmonary wedge pressures.
- Patients are usually managed with a Swan-Ganz catheter so that pulmonary artery wedge pressure (PAWP) and cardiac output can be monitored during drug administration.
- Marked increases in blood pressure (systolic pressure is the most likely to be affected) and heart rate, or the appearance of arrhythmias or other adverse cardiac effects are usually reversed promptly by reduction in dosage.
- Patients with preexisting hypertension must be closely observed for exaggerated pressor response.
- Tolerance has been observed with continuous or prolonged dobutamine infusions. However, adverse reactions are no different than those seen with shorter infusions.

- Monitor intake and output ratio and pattern. Urine output and sodium excretion generally increase because of improved cardiac output and renal perfusion.

Patient & Family Education

- Instruct patient to promptly report anginal pain.

DOCUSATE CALCIUM (DIOCTYL CALCIUM SULFOSUCCINATE)

See GASTROINTESTINAL AGENT, STOOL SOFTENER prototype, p 222.

Prototype: epinephrine, p 102

DOPAMINE HYDROCHLORIDE

(doe´pa-meen)
Trade names: Dopastat, Intropin, Revimine
Classifications: AUTONOMIC NERVOUS SYSTEM AGENT; ALPHA- AND BETA-ADRENERGIC AGONIST (SYMPATHOMIMETIC)
Pregnancy: Category C

ACTIONS/PHARMACODYNAMICS   Naturally occurring neurotransmitter and immediate precursor of norepinephrine. Major cardiovascular effects produced by direct action on alpha- and beta-adrenergic receptors and on specific dopaminergic receptors in mesenteric and renal vascular beds. Positive inotropic effect on myocardium increases cardiac output with increase in systolic and pulse pressure and little or no effect on diastolic pressure. Improves circulation to renal vascular bed by decreasing renal vascular resistance with resulting increase in glomerular filtration rate and urinary output. Blood flow to peripheral vascular bed may decrease while mesenteric flow increases. Less prone to cause substantial decrease in systemic vascular resistance, tachyarrhythmias, or increased myocardial oxygen consumption than are other catecholamines. More effective when therapy is started shortly after signs and symptoms of shock appear and before urine flow has decreased to < 0.3 ml/min.

USES   To correct hemodynamic imbalance in shock syndrome due to MI (cardiogenic shock), trauma, endotoxic septicemia (septic shock), open heart surgery, and CHF. **Unlabeled uses:** acute renal failure; cirrhosis; hepatorenal syndrome; barbituate intoxication.

ROUTE & DOSAGE

Shock

Adult	IV	2–5 µg/kg/min increased gradually up to 20–50 µg/kg/min if necessary
Child	IV	Same as for adult

PHARMACOKINETICS Onset: <5 min. **Duration:** <10 min. **Distribution:** Widely distributed; does not cross blood-brain barrier. **Metabolism:** Inactive in the liver, kidney, and plasma by monoamine oxidase and COMT. **Elimination:** Half-life: 2 min; excreted in urine.

CONTRAINDICATIONS & PRECAUTIONS Contraindicated in: pheochromocytoma; tachyarrhythmias or ventricular fibrillation. Safe use during pregnancy (category C), in nursing women, and in children not established. **Cautious use in:** patients with history of occlusive vascular disease (e.g., Buerger's or Raynaud's disease); cold injury; diabetic endarteritis, arterial embolism.

ADVERSE/SIDE EFFECTS CV: *hypotension,* ectopic beats, *tachycardia,* anginal pain, palpitation, vasoconstriction (indicated by disproportionate rise in diastolic pressure); cold extremities; less frequent: aberrant conduction, bradycardia, widening of QRS complex, elevated blood pressure. **GI:** nausea, vomiting **Other:** headache necrosis, tissue sloughing with extravasation, gangrene, azotemia, piloerection, dyspnea, dilated pupils (high doses).

DIAGNOSTIC TEST INTERFERENCES Dopamine may modify test response when histamine is used as a control for *intradermal skin tests*.

DRUG INTERACTIONS MAO INHIBITORS, ERGOT ALKALOIDS, **furazolidine** increase alpha-adrenergic effects (headache, hyperpyrexia, hypertension); **guanethidine, phenytoin** may decrease dopamine action; BETA-BLOCKERS antagonize cardiac effects; ALPHA-BLOCKERS antagonize peripheral vasoconstriction; **halothane, cyclopropane** increase risk of hypertension and ventricular arrhythmias.

INCOMPATIBILITIES Solution/Additive: sodium bicarbonate, **aminophylline, amphotericin B, ampicillin, cephalothin, penicillin G. Y-Site:** acyclovir, **aminophylline, amphotericin B,** sodium bicarbonate.

NURSING IMPLICATIONS

Administration

- Before initiation of dopamine therapy, hypovolemia should be corrected, if possible, with either whole blood or plasma
- Dilution should be made just prior to administration, although reportedly the solution may remain stable for 24 h after dilution.
- IV infusion rate and guidelines for adjusting rate of flow in relation to changes in blood pressure will be prescribed by physician. Microdrip or other reliable metering device should be used for accuracy of flow rate.
- Infusion rate must be continuously monitored for free flow, and care must be taken to avoid extravasation, which can result in tissue sloughing and gangrene. For this reason, infusion is made preferably into a large vein of the antecubital fossa. Phentolamine mesylate (Regitine) should be readily available when dopamine is being administered.
- Dopamine is a potent drug. Patient must be under constant observation.
- Protect dopamine from light. Discolored solutions should not be used. Reconstituted solution is stable for 48 h when stored at 2–15C (36–59F) or 6 h at room temperature 15–30C (59–86F).

Assessment & Drug Effects

- Monitor blood pressure, pulse, peripheral pulses, and urinary output at intervals prescribed by physician. Precise measurements are essential for accurate titration of dosage.
- Close observation is critical when patient is receiving dopamine. The following indicators are used for decreasing or temporarily suspending dose (report promptly to physician): reduced urine flow rate in absence of hypotension; ascending tachycardia; dysrhythmias; disproportionate rise in diastolic pressure (marked decrease in pulse pressure); signs of peripheral ischemia: pallor, cyanosis, mottling, coldness, complaints of tenderness, pain, numbness, or burning sensation. Presence of peripheral pulses is not always indicative of adequate circulation.
- Signs and symptoms of overdosage generally respond to dosage reduction or temporary discontinuation of drug, since dopamine has short duration of action. However, if these measures fail, a short-acting alpha-adrenergic blocking agent (e.g., phentolamine) may be given to antagonize peripheral vasoconstriction.
- ***Antidote for extravasation:*** Stop infusion promptly and remove needle. Immediately infiltrate the is-

Common side effects in *italic*; life-threatening effects underlined; generic names in **bold**; classifications in SMALL CAPS

539

chemic are, using syringe and fine needle. Recommended dose is 5–10 mg phentolamine mesylate in 10–15 ml of normal saline, using syringe and fine needle.

■ In addition to improvement in vital signs and urine flow, other indices of adequate dosage and perfusion of vital organs include loss of pallor, increase in toe temperature, adequacy of nail bed capillary filling, and reversal of confusion or comatose state.

D

Prototype: caffeine, p 197

DOXAPRAM HYDROCHLORIDE

(dox´a-pram)
Trade name: Dopram
Classifications: CNS AGENT; RESPIRATORY AND CEREBRAL STIMULANT
Pregnancy: Category B

ACTIONS/PHARMACODYNAMICS Short-acting analeptic capable of stimulating all levels of the cerebrospinal axis. Has minor effect on cortex. Respiratory stimulation by direct medullary action or possibly by indirect activation of peripheral chemoreceptors increases tidal volume and slightly increases respiratory rate. Decreases P_{CO_2} and increases P_{O_2} by increasing alveolar ventilation; may elevate BP and pulse rate by stimulation of brainstem vasomotor areas. Also increases salivation and release of gastric acids and epinephrine.

USES Short-term adjunctive therapy to alleviate postanesthesia and drug-induced respiratory depression and to hasten arousal and return of pharyngeal and laryngeal reflexes. Also as a temporary measure (approximately 2 h) in hospitalized patients with COPD associated with acute respiratory insufficiency as an aid to prevent elevation of $PaCO_2$ during administration of oxygen. (Not used in conjunction with mechanical ventilation.) **Unlabeled use:** neonatal apnea refractory to xanthine therapy.

PHARMACOKINETICS Onset: 20–40 s. **Peak:** 1–2 min. **Duration:** 5–12 min. **Metabolism:** rapidly metabolized. **Elimination:** excreted in urine as metabolites.

CONTRAINDICATIONS & PRECAUTIONS Contraindicated in: epilepsy and other convulsive disorders; incompetence of ventilatory mechanism due to muscle paresis, pulmonary fibrosis, flail chest, pneu-

ROUTE & DOSAGE

Postanesthesia

Adult   IV   0.5–1 mg/kg single injection not to exceed 1.5 mg/kg or 2 mg/kg total dose when repeated at 5 min intervals, or 1–3 mg/min infusion (max 4 mg/kg or 300 mg, not to exceed 3 g/d)

Drug-induced CNS Depression

Adult   IV   1–2 mg/kg; repeat in 5 min; then q1–2h until patient awakens; if relapse occurs, resume q1–2h injections (max total dose 3 g); if no response after priming dose, may give 1–3 mg/min for up to 2 h until patient awakens

Chronic Obstructive Pulmonary Disease

Adult   IV   1–2 mg/min for a max of 2 h (max rate 3 mg/min)

mothorax, airway obstruction, extreme dyspnea, or acute bronchial asthma; severe hypertension, coronary artery disease, uncompensated heart failure, CVA. Safe use during pregnancy (category B), in nursing mothers, and in children <12 y not established. **Cautious use in:** history of bronchial asthma, COPD; cardiac disease, severe tachycardia, arrhythmias, hypertension; hyperthyroidism; pheochromocytoma; head injury, cerebral edema, increased intracranial pressure; peptic ulcer, patients undergoing gastric surgery; acute agitation.

ADVERSE/SIDE EFFECTS CNS: dizziness, sneezing, apprehension, confusion, *involuntary movements,* hyperactivity, paresthesias; feeling of warmth and burning, especially of genitalia and perineum; flushing, sweating, hyperpyrexia, headache, pilomotor erection, pruritus, muscle tremor, rigidity, convulsions, *increased deep-tendon reflexes,* bilateral Babinski sign, *carpopedal spasm,* pupillary dilation, mild delayed narcosis. **CV:** *mild to moderate increase in BP, sinus tachycardia,* bradycardia, extrasystoles, lowered T waves, PVCs, chest pains, tightness in chest. **GI:** nausea, vomiting, diarrhea, salivation, sour taste. **GU:** urinary retention, frequency, incontinence. **Respiratory:** dyspnea, tachypnea, cough, <u>laryngospasm, bronchospasm</u>, hiccups, rebound hypoventilation, hypocapnia with tetany. **Other:** local skin irritation, thrombophlebitis with extravasation; decreased Hgb, Hct, and RBC count; elevated BUN; albuminuria.

DRUG INTERACTIONS MAO INHIBITORS, SYMPATHOMIMETIC AGENTS add to pressor effects.

Common side effects in *italic*; life-threatening effects <u>underlined</u>; generic names in **bold**; classifications in SMALL CAPS

INCOMPATIBILITIES Solution/Additive: amino-phylline, ascorbic acid, CEPHALOSPORINS, **carbenicillin, dexamethasone, diazepam, digoxin, dobutamine, folic acid, furosemide, hydrocortisone, ketamine, methylprednisolone, minocycline, thiopental, ticarcillin.**

NURSING IMPLICATIONS

Administration

- Contains benzyl alcohol; therefore, do not use in newborns.
- Adequacy of airway and oxygenation must be assured before initiation of doxapram therapy.
- Drug is available prediluted. For undiluted ampules, follow manufacturer's recommendations for dilution.
- IV flow rate is prescribed by physician. Infusion rate may start at 1 mg/min until satisfactory respiratory response is observed. It should then be maintained at 1–2 mg/min and be adjusted to maintain desired respiratory response. An infusion pump is advisable for regulatory flow rate.
- Store at 15–30C (59–86F) unless otherwise directed.

Assessment & Drug Effects

- Extravasation or use of same IV site for prolonged periods can cause thrombophlebitis (see Signs & Symptoms, chap 3) or tissue irritation.
- Careful monitoring and accurate observations of BP, pulse, deep tendon reflexes, airway, and arterial blood gases are essential guides for determining minimum effective dosage and preventing overdosage. Baseline determinations should be made for comparison.
- In patients with COPD, arterial Po_2 and Pco_2 and O_2 saturation should be drawn prior to initiation of doxapram infusion and oxygen administration and then at least every 30 min during infusion. Infusion should not be administered for longer than 2 h.
- Doxapram should be discontinued if arterial blood gases show evidence of deterioration and when mechanical ventilation is initiated.
- Observe patient continuously during therapy and maintain vigilance until patient is fully alert (usually about 1 h) and protective pharyngeal and laryngeal reflexes are completely restored.
- Notify physician immediately of any side effects. Be alert for early signs of toxicity: tachycardia, muscle tremor, spasticity, hyperactive reflexes.
- A mild to moderate increase in BP commonly occurs.
- If sudden hypotension or dyspnea develops, doxapram should be discontinued.

Prototype: imipramine, p 184

DOXEPIN HYDROCHLORIDE
(dox'e-pin)
Trade names: Adapin, Sinequan
Classifications: CNS AGENT;
PSYCHOTHERAPEUTIC; TRICYCLIC ANTIDEPRESSANT
Pregnancy: Category C

ACTIONS/PHARMACODYNAMICS Dibenzoxepin tricyclic antidepressant (TCA). Actions, limitations, and interactions are similar to those of imipramine. Reportedly one of the most sedating of the TCAs.

USES Psychoneurotic anxiety or depressive reactions, mixed symptoms of anxiety and depression; anxiety or depression associated with alcoholism, organic disease, psychotic depressive disorders. **Unlabeled uses:** peptic ulcer disease, neuralgia, pruritus.

ROUTE & DOSAGE

Antidepressant

Adult	PO	30–150 mg/d h.s. or in divided doses; may gradually increase to 300 mg/d (use lower doses in elderly patients)

PHARMACOKINETICS Absorption: rapidly absorbed from GI and injection sites. **Peak:** 2 h. **Distribution:** crosses placenta; distributed into breast milk. **Metabolism:** metabolized in liver. **Elimination:** half-life: 6–8 h; primarily excreted in urine.

CONTRAINDICATIONS & PRECAUTIONS Contraindicated in: prior sensitivity to any TCA; during acute recovery phase following MI; glaucoma; prostatic hypertrophy; tendency to urinary retention; concurrent use of MAO inhibitors. Safe use during pregnancy (category C), in nursing women, and in children <12 y not established. **Cautious use in:** patients receiving ECT, patients with suicidal tendency; renal, cardiovascular or hepatic dysfunction.

ADVERSE/SIDE EFFECTS Anticholinergic: **CNS:** *drowsiness,* dizziness, weakness, fatigue, headache, hypomania, confusion, tremors, paresthesias. **CV:** *orthostatic hypotension,* palpitation, hypertension, tachycardia, ECG changes. **Eye:** mydriasis, blurred vision, photophobia. **GI:** *dry mouth,* sour or metallic

Common side effects in *italic*; life-threatening effects underlined; generic names in **bold**; classifications in SMALL CAPS

541

taste, epigastric distress, constipation. **GU:** urinary retention, delayed micturition, urinary frequency. **Other:** increased perspiration, tinnitus, weight gain, photosensitivity reaction, skin rash, <u>agranulocytosis</u>.

DRUG INTERACTIONS May decrease some antihypertensive response to ANTIHYPERTENSIVES; CNS DEPRESSANTS, **alcohol,** HYPNOTICS, BARBITURATES, SEDATIVES potentiate CNS depression; may increase hypoprothombinemic effect of ORAL ANTICOAGULANTS; **ethchlorvynol** may cause transient delirium; **levodopa,** SYMPATHOMIMETICS (e.g., **epinephrine, norepinephrine**) introduce possibility of sympathetic hyperactivity with hypertension and hyperpyrexia; MAO INHIBITORS introduce possibility of severe reactions, toxic psychosis, cardiovascular instability; **methylphenidate** increases plasma TCA levels; thyroid agents may increase possibility of arhythmias; **cimetidine** may increase plasma TCA levels.

NURSING IMPLICATIONS

Administration

- Oral concentrate must be diluted with approximately 120 ml water, milk, or fruit juice just before administration.
- Capsule may be emptied and contents swallowed with fluid or mixed with food.
- If daytime sedation is pronounced, inform physician. Entire daily dose (up to 150 mg) may be prescribed for bedtime administration.
- Store at 15–30C (59–86F) in tightly closed light-resistant container.

Assessment & Drug Effects

- If a patient uses excessive amounts of alcohol, potentiation of doxepin effects may increase the danger of overdosage or suicide attempt.
- Doxepin has moderate to strong anticholinergic effects. Be alert to changes in I&O ratio and check patient for constipation and abdominal distension.

Patient & Family Education

- Teach the necessity to maintain established dosage regimen and to avoid change of intervals, doubling, reducing, or skipping doses.
- The actions of both alcohol and doxepin are potentiated when used together during therapy and for up to 2 wk after doxepin is discontinued. Consult physician about safe amount of alcohol, if any, that can be taken.
- Caution patient to avoid driving and other potentially hazardous activities until reaction to drug is

known. Doxepin has a pronounced sedative effect; symptom tends to disappear with continued therapy.

DOXORUBICIN HYDROCHLORIDE

(dox-oh-roo′bi-sin)
Trade names: Adriamycin, ADR
Classifications: ANTINEOPLASTIC ANTIBIOTIC; IMMUNOSUPPRESSANT
Pregnancy: Category D

ACTIONS/PHARMACODYNAMICS Cytotoxic anthracycline antibiotic isolated from *Streptomyces peucetius,* with wide spectrum of antitumor activity and strong immunosuppressive properties. Intercalates with preformed DNA residues, blocking effective DNA and RNA transcription. Highly destructive to rapidly proliferating cells and slowly developing carcinomas; selectively toxic to cardiac tissue. A potent radiosensitizer capable of enhancing radiation reactions. No clinical cross-resistance to standard antineoplastics; therefore, it may be especially effective in patients with less advanced disease. Cytotoxicity precludes its use as antiinfective agent. Tests on experimental models have shown mutagenic and carcinogenic properties.

USES To produce regression in neoplastic conditions, including acute lymphoblastic and myeloblastic leukemias, Wilms' tumor, neuroblastoma, soft tissue and bone sarcomas, breast and ovary carcinomas, lymphomas, bronchogenic carcinoma. Generally used in combined modalities with surgery, radiation, and immunotherapy. Also effective pretreatment to sensitize superficial tumors to local radiation therapy. **Unlabeled use:** multiple myeloma.

ROUTE & DOSAGE

Neoplasm

Adult	IV	60–75 mg/m² as single dose at 21 d intervals *or* 30 mg/m² on each of 3 consecutive days repeated every 4 wk (max total cumulative dose 500–550 mg/m²)

PHARMACOKINETICS Distribution: widely distributed; does not cross blood-brain barrier; crosses placenta; distribution into breast milk not known. **Metabolism:** metabolized in liver to active metabolite. **Elimination:** half-life: 16.7–31.7 h; excreted primarily in bile.

Common side effects in *italic*; life-threatening effects <u>underlined</u>; generic names in **bold**; classifications in SMALL CAPS

CONTRAINDICATIONS & PRECAUTIONS Contraindicated in: myelosuppression, impaired cardiac function, obstructive jaundice, previous treatment with complete cumulative doses of doxorubicin or daunorubicin. Safe use during pregnancy (category D) not established. Cautious use in: impaired hepatic or renal function; patients who have received cyclophosphamide or pelvic irradiation or radiotherapy to areas surrounding heart; history of atopic dermatitis.

ADVERSE/SIDE EFFECTS CV: serious, irreversible myocardial toxicity with delayed CHF, ventricular arrhythmias, acute left ventricular failure, hypertension, hypotension. GI: *stomatitis*, esophagitis with ulcerations; nausea, vomiting, anorexia, inanition, diarrhea. Hematopoietic: *severe myelosuppression (60–85% of patients)*; leukopenia (principally granulocytes), thrombocytopenia, anemia. Hypersensitivity: red flare around injection site, erythema, skin rash, pruritus, angioedema, urticaria, eosinophilia, fever, chills, anaphylactoid reaction. Skin: hyperpigmentation of nail beds, tongue, and buccal mucosa (especially in blacks); *complete alopecia* (reversible), hyperpigmentation of dermal creases (especially in children), rash, *recall phenomenon (skin reaction due to prior radiotherapy)*. Other: conjunctivitis (rare), lacrimation, drowsiness, fever, facial flush with too rapid IV infusion rate, microscopic hematuria, hyperuricemia. *With extravasation: severe cellulitis, vesication, tissue necrosis,* lymphangitis, phlebosclerosis.

DRUG INTERACTIONS BARBITURATES may decrease pharmacologic effects of doxorubicin by increasing its hepatic metabolism—increase in doxorubicin dosage may be needed; **streptozocin** (Zanosar) may prolong doxorubicin half-life—dosage reduction of doxorubicin may be indicated.

INCOMPATIBILITIES Solution/Additive: **aminophylline, cephalothin, dexamethasone, diazepam, fluorouracil, furosemide, hydrocortisone, heparin, vinblastine. Y-site: furosemide, heparin.**

NURSING IMPLICATIONS

Administration

- Caution should be observed in preparing doxorubicin solution. Wear gloves. If powder or solution contacts skin or mucosa, wash copiously with soap and water.
- Dilute the powder with 0.9% NaCl to yield a final

concentration of 2 mg/ml. Bacteriostatic diluents are not recommended.

- Administered slowly into side arm of freely running IV infusion of NaCl injection or 5% dextrose injection. Tubing should be attached to a butterfly needle inserted into a large vein.
- Do not mix this drug with other drugs.
- Infusion rate usually permits administration of the dose in a 3–5 min period. Rate will be specifically ordered. Facial flushing and local red streaking along the vein may occur if drug is administered too rapidly. Urticaria around injection site is usually self-limiting.
- If possible, avoid using antecubital vein or veins on dorsum of hand or wrist where extravasation could damage underlying tendons and nerves. Also avoid veins in extremity with compromised venous or lymphatic drainage.
- Personnel who handle or are exposed to doxorubicin during the first trimester of pregnancy are at high risk of losing the fetus.
- Reconstituted solution is stable for 24 h at room temperature and for 48 h under refrigeration (4–10C) (39–50F). Protect from sunlight; discard unused solution.

Assessment & Drug Effects

- Give prompt attention to complaint of stinging or burning sensation at the injection site. Infusion should be stopped promptly and IV needle removed. Notify physician promptly.
- Monitor area of extravasation closely for 3–4 wk. If ulceration begins (usually 1–4 wk after extravasation), a plastic surgeon should be consulted.
- Begin a flow chart to establish baseline data. Include temperature, pulse, respiration, BP, body weight, laboratory values, and I&O ratio and pattern.
- Evaluation of hepatic, renal, hematopoietic, and cardiac function (ECG) should be performed prior to initiation of therapy, at regular intervals thereafter, and at end of therapy.
- CHF may occur several weeks to months after cessation of therapy.
- Doxorubicin cardiomyopathy is associated with persistent reduction in voltage of QRS wave, prolonged systolic (time) interval, and reduced ejection fraction.
- Be alert to and report early signs of cardiotoxicity (see chap 3). Monitor pulse and BP frequently. Acute life-threatening arrhythmias may occur within a few hours of drug administration.
- Objective signs of hepatic dysfunction (jaundice, dark urine, pruritus) or kidney dysfunction (altered

Common side effects in *italic*; life-threatening effects underlined; generic names in **bold**; classifications in SMALL CAPS

543

I&O ratio and pattern, local discomfort with voiding) should be reported promptly.
- Stomatitis, generally maximal in second week of therapy, frequently begins with a burning sensation accompanied by erythema of oral mucosa that may progress to ulceration and dysphagia in 2 or 3 d. Fastidious oral hygiene is required, especially before and after meals.
- Immunosuppressive properties of doxorubicin require careful screening of visitors and attending personnel to shield the patient from infection, especially during leukopenic periods.
- The nadir of leukopenia (an expected 1000/mm^3) typically occurs 10–14 d after single dose, with recovery occurring within 21 d.
- Superinfections may result from antibiotic therapy during leukopenic period. Report signs of superinfection (see chap 3) promptly.
- Bloody diarrhea may result from an antiblastic effect on rapidly growing intestinal mucosal cells. Avoid rectal medications and use of rectal thermometer to prevent trauma.

Patient & Family Education
- Complete alopecia (reversible) is an expected side effect.
- Inform patient that alopecia may also involve eyelashes and eyebrows, beard and mustache, pubic and axillary hair. Regrowth of hair usually begins 2–3 mo after drug is discontinued.
- Advise patient that drug turns urine red for 1–2 d after administration.
- Increased lacrimation for 5–10 d after a single dose is a possibility. Caution patient to keep hands away from eyes to prevent conjunctivitis.

Prototype: tetracycline, p 74

DOXYCYCLINE HYCLATE
(dox-i-sye′kleen)
Trade names: AK-Ramycin, AK-Ratabs, Doryx, Doxy, Doxy-Caps, Doxychel, Doxy-Lemmon, SK-Doxycycline, Vibramycin, Vibra-Tabs, Vivox
Classifications: ANTIINFECTIVE; ANTIBIOTIC; TETRACYCLINE
Pregnancy: Category D

ACTIONS/PHARMACODYNAMICS Semisynthetic broad-spectrum tetracycline antibiotic derived from oxytetracycline. More completely absorbed, effective blood levels maintained for longer periods and excreted more slowly than most other tetracyclines, thus requiring smaller and less frequent dosing. Reportedly low incidence of phototoxic reactions and has less affinity for calcium ions than other tetracyclines. Primarily bacteriostatic in action (inhibits protein synthesis in susceptible organisms). Recommended doses of doxycycline do not ordinarily lead to excessive drug accumulation; therefore it is useful in patients with renal impairment.

USES Similar to those of tetracycline, e.g., chlamydial and mycoplasmal infections; gonorrhea, syphilis in penicillin-allergic patients; rickettsial diseases; acute exacerbations of chronic bronchitis. **Unlabeled use:** treatment of acute PID, leptospirosis, prophylaxis for rape victims, suppression and chemoprophylaxis of chloroquine-resistant *Plasmodium falciparum* malaria, short-term prophylaxis and treatment of travelers' diarrhea caused by enterotoxigenic strains of *Escherichia coli*.

ROUTE & DOSAGE

Antiinfective

Adult	PO/IV	100 mg q12h on day 1; then 100 mg/d as single dose up to 100 mg q12h
Child	PO/IV	> 8 y: 4.4 mg/kg in 1–2 doses on day 1; then 2.2–4.4 mg/kg/d in 1–2 divided doses

Gonorrhea

Adult	PO	200 mg immediately, followed by 100 mg h.s.; then 100 mg b.i.d. for 3 d

Primary and Secondary Syphilis

Adult	PO	300 mg/d in divided doses for at least 10 d

Travelers' Diarrhea

Adult	PO	100 mg/d during risk period (up to 2 wk) beginning day 1 of travel

---

PHARMACOKINETICS Absorption: completely absorbed from GI tract. **Peak:** 1.5–4 h. **Distribution:** penetrates eye, prostate, and CSF; crosses placenta; distributed into breast milk. **Metabolism:** not metabolized. **Elimination:** half-life: 14–24 h; 20–30% excreted in urine and 20–40% in feces in 48 h.

CONTRAINDICATIONS & PRECAUTIONS Contraindicated in: sensitivity to any of the tetracyclines; use during period of tooth development: last half of

Common side effects in *italic*; life-threatening effects underlined; generic names in **bold**; classifications in SMALL CAPS

pregnancy, nursing women, infants, and children <8 y (causes permanent yellow discoloration of teeth, enamel hypoplasia, and retardation of bone growth). **Cautious use in:** alcoholism.

ADVERSE/SIDE EFFECTS CNS: Intracranial hypertension. **Eye:** interference with color vision. **GI:** anorexia, *nausea,* vomiting, diarrhea, enterocolitis; esophageal irritation (oral capsule and tablet). **Hematologic:** neutropenia, eosinophilia, thrombocytopenia, hemolytic anemia. **Skin:** rashes, photosensitivity reaction. **Other:** thrombophlebitis (IV use), superinfections, increase in BUN (dose-related), hypersensitivity reactions.

DIAGNOSTIC TEST INTERFERENCES Like other tetracyclines, doxycycline may cause false increases in *urinary catecholamines* (fluorometric methods); false decreases in *urinary urobilinogen;* false-negative *urine glucose* with glucose oxidase methods (e.g., Clinistix, Tes-Tape); parenteral doxycycline (containing ascorbic acid) may cause false-positive determinations using Benedict's reagent or Clinitest.

DRUG INTERACTIONS ANTACIDS, **iron** preparation, **calcium, magnesium, zinc, kaolin-pectin, sodium bicarbonate** can significantly decrease absorption; effects of both doxycycline and **desmopressin** antagonized; increases **digoxin** absorption, thus increasing risk of digoxin toxicity; **methoxyflurane** increases risk of renal failure.

NURSING IMPLICATIONS

Administration

- Check expiration date. Degradation products of tetracycline are nephrotoxic.
- Unlike most tetracyclines, oral doxycycline may be taken with food or milk to minimize nausea without significantly affecting bioavailability of drug.
- Consult physician about ordering the oral suspension for patients who are bedridden or have difficulty swallowing.
- *Preparation and storage of IV solutions:* Reconstitute by adding 10 ml sterile water for injection, or other diluent recommended by manufacturer, to each 100 mg of drug. Before administration the reconstituted solution must then be diluted further with 100–1000 ml (per 100 mg of drug) of compatible infusion solution to produce concentrations ranging from 0.1 to 1 mg/ml.
- Administer properly diluted doxycycline at a rate of 100 mg over 1–4 h. Infusion should be completed within 12 h of dilution.

- IV infusion rate will be prescribed by physician. Duration of infusion varies with dose but is usually 1–4 h. Recommended minimum infusion time for 100 mg of 0.5 mg/ml solution is 1 h.
- When diluted with lactated Ringer's or dextrose 5% in lactated Ringer's injection, infusion must be completed within 6 h to ensure adequate stability.
- During infusion, all solutions must be protected from direct sunlight.
- Reconstituted solutions are stable for 72 h if refrigerated. After this time infusion must be completed within 12 h.
- Doxycycline, oral and parenteral forms (prior to reconstitution), should be stored in tightly covered, light-resistant containers at 15–30C (59–86F) unless otherwise directed.

Assessment & Drug Effects

- Doxycycline (capsule and tablet forms) is associated with a comparatively high incidence of esophagitis, especially in patients > 40 y. Sudden onset of painful or difficult swallowing should be reported promptly to physician.
- Monitor IV insertion site for signs of thrombophlebitis (see chap 3). If these develop, discontinue IV and begin it in another site.
- Be alert for and report evidence of superinfections (see Signs & Symptoms, chap 3).

Patient & Family Education

- Instructions for patients taking capsule or tablet forms (to prevent esophageal ulceration): Take drug with a full glass (240 ml) of water to assure passage into stomach. Remain standing for about 90 s after taking medication. Avoid taking capsule or tablet within 1 h of lying down or retiring.
- To reduce risk of phototoxic reaction, caution patient to avoid exposure to direct sunlight and ultraviolet light while taking doxycycline and for 4 or 5 d after therapy is terminated. Phototoxic reaction appears like an exaggerated sunburn. Sunscreens provide little protection.
- Advise patient to take medication for full course of therapy, as prescribed.

DRONABINOL

(droe-nab´i-nol)
Trade names: Marinol, THC
Classifications: CNS AGENT; ANTIEMETIC; CANNABINOID
Pregnancy: Category B
Controlled substance: Schedule II

Common side effects in *italic*; life-threatening effects underlined; generic names in **bold**; classifications in SMALL CAPS

545

ACTIONS/PHARMACODYNAMICS Synthetic derivative of tetrahydrocannabinol (THC), the principal psychoactive constituent of marijuana *(Cannabis sativa)*. Action (mechanism unclear): inhibits vomiting control mechanism in the medulla oblongata, producing potent antiemetic effect; nontherapeutic actions are exactly like those of marijuana. Has complex CNS effect that necessitates close supervision of the patient during drug use. Decreases REM sleep; effect on BP is unpredictable; oral temperature may be decreased, and heart rate may be increased. Risk of drug abuse is high since dronabinol produces both physical and psychologic dependence.

USES To treat chemotherapy-induced nausea and vomiting in cancer patients who fail to respond to conventional antiemetic therapy. **Unlabeled use:** glaucoma.

ROUTE & DOSAGE

Chemotherapy-induced Nausea

Adult	PO	5 mg/m^2 1–3 h before administration of chemotherapy; then q2–4h after chemotherapy for a total of 4–6 doses; dose may be increased by 2.5 mg/m^2 up to a max of 15 mg/m^2 if necessary

PHARMACOKINETICS Absorption: rapidly absorbed from GI tract, with bioavailability of 10–20%. **Peak:** 2–3 h. **Distribution:** fat soluble; distributed to many organs; distributed into breast milk. **Metabolism:** metabolized in liver; extensive first pass metabolism. **Elimination:** half-life: 25–36 h; excreted principally in bile; 50% excreted in feces within 72 h; 10–15% excreted in urine.

CONTRAINDICATIONS & PRECAUTIONS Contraindicated in: nausea and vomiting caused by other than chemotherapeutic agents; hypersensitivity to dronabinol or sesame oil; used during pregnancy (category B) only if clearly necessary. **Cautious use in:** first exposure, especially in elderly or cardiac patient; hypertension, cardiovascular disorders; epilepsy; psychiatric illness, patient receiving other psychoactive drugs; severe hepatic dysfunction.

ADVERSE/SIDE EFFECTS CNS: *drowsiness,* psychologic high, dizziness, anxiety, confusion, euphoria, sensory or perceptual difficulties, impaired coordination, depression (7%), irritability, headache, hallucinations (rare), ataxia (4%), memory lapse, paresthesias, paranoia, depersonalization, disorientation, tinnitus, nightmares, speech difficulty, facial flush, diaphoresis. **CV:** tachycardia, orthostatic hypotension, hypertension, syncope. **GI:** dry mouth, diarrhea, fecal incontinence. **Other:** muscular pains.

DRUG INTERACTIONS Alcohol and other CNS DEPRESSANTS may exaggerate psychoactive effects of dronabinol; TRICYCLIC ANTIDEPRESSANTS, **atropine** may cause tachycardia.

NURSING IMPLICATIONS

Administration

- Doses are not repeated following a reaction until patient's mental state has returned to normal and the circumstances have been evaluated.
- Store dronabinol at 8–15C (46–59F).

Assessment & Drug Effects

- Patients with hypertension or heart disease should have monitoring of BP and cardiac status.
- Response to dronabinol is varied, and previous uneventful use does not guarantee that adverse reactions will not occur. Effects of drug may persist an unpredictably long time (days). Extended use at therapeutic dosage may cause accumulation of toxic amounts of dronabinol and its metabolites.
- If dose is increased, watch for disturbing psychiatric symptoms such as altered mental state, loss of coordination, evidence of a psychologic high (easy laughing, elation and heightened awareness), or depression.
- Overdosage may occur at both therapeutic and at higher nontherapeutic doses. At therapeutic doses, overdosage produces disturbing psychiatric symptoms. Physical examination: pupils unchanged, conjunctivae injected. Observe patient in a quiet, controlled setting, provide supportive measures, withhold drug until patient has returned to baseline (usually within 24 h).
- Withdrawal symptoms have been observed within 12 h after abrupt withdrawal of the drug: irritability, insomnia, restlessness. Peak intensity of symptoms occurs at about 24 h: hot flashes, diaphoresis, rhinorrhea, watery diarrhea, hiccups, anorexia. Usually syndrome is over in 96 h.

Patient & Family Education

- Caution patient to avoid driving or other potentially hazardous activities that require alertness and judgment because of high incidence of dizziness and drowsiness.
- Alert and prepare patient and family for possible (reversible) drug-induced mood changes or behavior changes that may occur during dronabinol use.

Common side effects in *italic*; life-threatening effects <u>underlined</u>; generic names in **bold**; classifications in SMALL CAPS

- Caution against ingestion of **alcohol** during period of systemic dronabinol effect. Effect on blood ethanol levels are complex and unpredictable.

Prototype: haloperidol, p 189

DROPERIDOL
(droe-per´i-dole)
Trade name: Inapsine
Classifications: CNS AGENT; ANTIPSYCHOTIC (TRANQUILIZER); BUTYROPHENONE; ANTIEMETIC
Pregnancy: Category C

ACTIONS/PHARMACODYNAMICS Butyrophenone derivative structurally and pharmacologically related to haloperidol. Antagonizes emetic effects of morphinelike analgesics and other drugs that act on CTZ. Mild alpha-adrenergic blocking activity and direct vasodilator effect may cause hypotension. Acts primarily at subcortical level to produce sedation. Sedative property reduces anxiety and motor activity without necessarily inducing sleep; patient remains responsive. Potentiates other CNS depressants. Reduces pressor effects of epinephrine and decreases epinephrine-induced arrhythmias but does not prevent cardiac arrythmias. May decrease pulmonary arterial pressure. Has greater tendency to produce extrapyramidal symptoms than haloperidol has.

USES To produce tranquilizing effect and to reduce nausea and vomiting during surgical and diagnostic procedures. Also for premedication, during induction, and as adjunct in maintenance of general or regional anesthesia. Principally used in fixed combination with the potent narcotic analgesic fentanyl (Innovar) to produce neuroleptanalgesia (quiescence, reduced motor activity, and indifference to pain and environmental stimuli) to permit carrying out a variety of diagnostic and minor surgical procedures. **Unlabeled use:** IV antiemetic in cancer chemotherapy.

PHARMACOKINETICS Onset: 3–10 min. **Peak:** 30 min. **Duration:** 2–4 h; may persist up to 12 h. **Distribution:** crosses placenta. **Metabolism:** metabolized in liver. **Elimination:** excreted in urine and feces.

ROUTE & DOSAGE

Premedication

Adult	IM/IV	2.5–10 mg 30–60 min preoperatively
Child	IM/IV	0.088–0.165 mg/kg 30–60 min preoperatively

Maintenance of General Anesthesia

Adult	IM/IV	Induction: 0.22–0.275 mg/kg Maintenance: 1.25–2.5 mg
Child	IM/IV	0.088–0.165 mg/kg

CONTRAINDICATIONS & PRECAUTIONS Contraindicated in: known intolerance to droperidol. Safe use during pregnancy (category C) and in children <2 y not established. **Cautious use in:** elderly, debilitated, and other poor-risk patients; Parkinson's disease; hypotension; liver, kidney, cardiac disease; cardiac bradyarrhythmias.

ADVERSE/SIDE EFFECTS CNS: *postoperative drowsiness, extrapyramidal symptoms:* dystonia, akathisia, oculogyric crisis; dizziness, restlessness, anxiety, hallucinations, mental depression. **CV:** *hypotension, tachycardia.* **Other:** chills, shivering, <u>laryngospasm</u>, <u>bronchospasm</u>.

INCOMPATIBILITIES Solution/Additive: **fluorouracil, furosemide, heparin, leucovorin, methotrexate, pentobarbital. Y-site: fluorouracil, furosemide, heparin, leucovorin, methotrexate, nafcillin.**

NURSING IMPLICATIONS

Administration
- When patient is under the effect of another CNS depressant, the required dose of droperidol may be less than usual. Postoperative narcotics or other CNS depressants are prescribed in reduced doses since they have additive or potentiating effects.
- IV droperidol may be given undiluted by direct IV at a rate of 10 mg or fraction thereof over 30–60 seconds.
- Drug incompatibilities: do not mix with parenteral barbiturates, since a precipitate may occur.
- Protect from light. Store at 15–30C (59–86F), unless otherwise directed by manufacturer.

Assessment & Drug Effects
- Monitor vital signs closely. Hypotension and tachycardia are common side effects.
- Because of possibility of severe orthostatic hypotension, always exercise care in moving and po-

Common side effects in *italic*; life-threatening effects <u>underlined</u>; generic names in **bold**; classifications in SMALL CAPS

547

sitioning the medicated patient. Avoid abrupt changes in position.

- Patient who receives a narcotic analgesic concurrently should be observed carefully for signs of impending respiratory depression.
- Elevated BP has been reported following administration of droperidol with parenteral analgesics.
- During the postoperative period, EEG patterns are slow to return to normal.
- Extrapyramidal symptoms may occur within 24–48 h postoperatively. Observe patient carefully for early signs of acute dystonia: facial grimacing, restlessness, tremors, torticollis, oculogyric crisis. Report promptly.
- Droperidol may aggravate symptoms of acute depression.

Prototype: procaine, p 166

DYCLONINE HYDROCHLORIDE
(dye-kloe-neen)
Trade name: Dyclone
Classifications: CNS AGENT; ANESTHETIC, LOCAL (MUCOSAL); ANTIPRURITIC
Pregnancy: Category C

ACTIONS/PHARMACODYNAMICS Organic ketone, synthetic local topical anesthetic agent. Unrelated to amide derivatives. Produces local anesthesia by blocking impulses at peripheral nerve endings in skin and mucous membranes.

USES Topical anesthesia of mucous membranes preparatory for endoscopic examinations and gynecologic and proctologic procedures. Also to suppress gag reflex, to relieve pain of minor burns or trauma, and to alleviate itching of pruritus ani or vulvae. **Unlabeled use:** to provide relief from discomfort of fever blisters.

PHARMACOKINETICS Absorption: absorbed through skin and mucous membranes. **Onset:** 2–10 min. **Duration:** up to 1 h.

CONTRAINDICATIONS & PRECAUTIONS Contraindicated in: cystoscopic procedures following IV pyelography (because contrast media containing iodine may precipitate and interfere with visualization); applications to extensive areas or to bleeding surfaces. Safe use during pregnancy (category C) not es-

tablished. **Cautious use in:** debilitated or elderly patients, children, patients with drug sensitivities or family history of allergies; severe trauma or sepsis in region of application.

ROUTE & DOSAGE

Topical Anesthesia

Adult	Topical	Apply 0.5–1% solution by swabbing, gargling, spray, instillation, wet compress, or rinse

Before Urologic Endoscopy

Adult	Topical	Instill 30–60 ml of 0.5–1% solution into urethra and retain 5–10 min before procedure

ADVERSE/SIDE EFFECTS Skin: urticaria, edema, contact dermatitis (local): burning, tenderness, swelling, irritation, urethritis. **Systemic absorption:** nervousness, dizziness, drowsiness, excitement or depression, tremors, *seizures,* blurred vision, hypotension, bradycardia, cardiac or respiratory arrest.

DIAGNOSTIC TEST INTERFERENCES Dyclonine may interfere with visualization in cystoscopic procedures by causing precipitation of iodine in *contrast media.*

NURSING IMPLICATIONS

Administration

- To relieve pain of esophageal lesions, 5–15 ml of 0.5% dyclonine solution may be swallowed (prescribed).
- Avoid contact with eyes or eyelids. Applications to large areas should be avoided.
- Store at 15–30C (59–86F) in tight, light-resistant container unless otherwise directed.

Assessment & Drug Effects

- When applied orally, dyclonine may interfere with second stage of swallowing. Do not give patient anything by mouth within 60 min (until return of gag reflex) following drug administration.
- If necessary, gag reflex may be tested by gently stroking soft palate with a cotton swab (while holding tongue down with a depressor). If patient does not gag or swallow, give nothing by mouth. Suctioning of secretions may be necessary to prevent aspiration.
- A sip of clear water should be the first thing swallowed when gag reflex returns.

Patient & Family Education

- If patient is to self-administer medication orally, he or she should be instructed on suppression of gag reflex and appropriate safety precautions.

Prototype: theophylline, p 136

DYPHYLLINE

(dye´fi-lin)

Trade names: Asminyl, Dilin, Dilor, Dyflex, Dylline, Lufyllin, Neothylline, Oxystat, Protophylline

Classifications: BRONCHODILATOR; RESPIRATORY SMOOTH MUSCLE RELAXANT; CNS AGENT; RESPIRATORY STIMULANT; XANTHINE

Pregnancy: Category C

ACTIONS/PHARMACODYNAMICS Xanthine and derivative of theophylline with which it shares similar pharmacologic effects: bronchodilation, myocardial stimulation, vasodilation, diuresis, and smooth muscle relaxation. Unlike other xanthines, dyphylline is not metabolized to theophylline in body; therefore serum theophylline levels are not useful. (Specific assay for dyphylline must be used.) Claimed to cause less gastric distress than theophylline because of its neutral pH. Appears to be more uniformly and predictably absorbed than theophylline, but levels and activity are lower, and it has a short half-life; thus higher and more frequent dosing may be required to attain comparable sustained effects.

USES Acute bronchial asthma and reversible bronchospasm associated with chronic bronchitis and emphysema.

ROUTE & DOSAGE

Asthma

Adult	PO	200–800 mg q6h up to 15 mg/kg q.i.d.
	IM	250–500 mg q6h up to 15 mg/kg q.i.d.
Child	PO/IM	≥ 6 y: 4.4–6.6 mg/kg/d in divided doses

PHARMACOKINETICS Absorption: readily absorbed from GI tract. **Peak:** 1 h. **Metabolism:** metabolized in liver (but not to theophylline). **Elimination:** half-life: 2 h; excreted in urine.

CONTRAINDICATIONS & PRECAUTIONS Contraindicated in: hypersensitivity to xanthine compounds; apnea in newborns. Safe use during pregnancy (category C) and in nursing mothers not established. **Cautious use in:** severe cardiac disease, hypertension, acute myocardial injury, renal or hepatic dysfunction, glaucoma, hyperthyroidism, peptic ulcer, in the elderly and in children; concomitant administration of other xanthine formulations or other CNS-stimulating drugs.

ADVERSE/SIDE EFFECTS CNS: headache, irritability, restlessness, dizziness, insomnia, light-headedness, muscle twitching, <u>convulsions</u>. **CV:** palpitation, *tachycardia,* extrasystoles, flushing, hypotension. **GI:** *nausea,* vomiting, diarrhea, anorexia, epigastric distress. **Respiratory:** tachypnea. **Other:** albuminuria, fever, dehydration.

DRUG INTERACTIONS BETA-BLOCKERS may antagonize bronchodilating effects of dyphylline; **halothane** increases risk of cardiac arrhythmias; **probenecid** may decrease dyphylline elimination.

NURSING IMPLICATIONS

Administration

- Absorption is enhanced by taking oral preparation with a full glass of water on an empty stomach, e.g., 1 h before or 2 h after meals. However, administration after meals may help to relieve gastric discomfort.
- Care should be exercised in the amount of elixir given to children because it has a high alcohol content (18–20%).
- For IM administration, aspirate carefully before injecting and inject slowly.
- Do not use parenteral form if a precipitate is present.
- Store at 15–30C (59–86F) unless otherwise directed. Protect dyphylline injection from light.

Assessment & Drug Effects

- Baseline and periodic pulmonary function tests may be done to assess therapeutic effectiveness of dyphylline.
- Minimal effective therapeutic dyphylline blood level is reported to be 12 μg/ml.
- Toxic diphylline plasma levels, although rare with normal dosage, are a risk in patients with a diminished capacity for diphylline clearance, e.g., those with CHF or hepatic impairment or who are >55 y or <1 y of age.

Common side effects in *italic*; life-threatening effects <u>underlined</u>; generic names in **bold**; classifications in SMALL CAPS

549

Patient & Family Education

- Instruct patient to consistently take medication with or without food at the same time each day.
- Instruct patient to notify physician of adverse effects: nausea, vomiting, insomnia, jitteriness, headache, rash, severe GI pain, restlessness, convulsions, or irregular heart beat.
- Instruct patient not to accept brand interchange except under physician guidance.
- Caution patient to avoid alcohol and also large amounts of coffee and other xanthine-containing beverages, e.g., tea, cocoa, colas, during therapy.
- Many OTC drugs for coughs, colds, and allergies contain ephedrine or other sympathomimetics and xanthines (e.g., caffeine, theophylline, aminophylline). Advise patient to consult physician before taking OTC preparations.

Prototype: pilocarpine hydrochloride, p 209

ECHOTHIOPHATE IODIDE

(ek-oh-thye´oh-fate)
Trade name: Phospholine Iodide
Classifications: EYE PREPARATION; MIOTIC (ANTIGLAUCOMA AGENT)
Pregnancy: Category C

ACTIONS/PHARMACODYNAMICS Potent, long-acting cholinesterase inhibitor and organophosphate. Produces cholinesterase inhibition (relatively irreversible), which persists for days or weeks until new enzyme is synthesized. Inhibition prevents hydrolysis of ACh, leaving it free to stimulate iris sphincter and ciliary muscle to produce miosis and spasm of accommodation.

USES Chronic open-angle glaucoma, conditions obstructing aqueous outflow, e.g., synechia formation, following iridectomy or cataract surgery, and for diagnosis and treatment of accommodative esotropia. Use is usually reserved for patients not satisfactorily controlled by less potent miotics.

PHARMACOKINETICS Absorption: readily absorbed through conjunctival sac. **Onset:** 10 min miosis; 4–8 h IOP. **Peak:** 30 min miosis; 24 h IOP. **Duration:** 1–4 wk.

ROUTE & DOSAGE

Glaucoma

Adult	Topical	1 drop of 0.03–0.25% solution in conjunctival sac 1–2 times/d

Accommodative Esotropia

Adult	Topical	*Diagnosis:* 1 drop of 0.125% solution in both eyes once/d at bedtime for 2–3 wk
		Treatment: 1 drop of 0.125% solution q.o.d. or 1 drop of 0.06% solution daily (max 1 drop 0.125% solution daily)

CONTRAINDICATIONS & PRECAUTIONS Contraindicated in: acute angle-closure glaucoma, history of or active uveitis. Safe use during pregnancy (category C) not established. **Cautious use in:** history of retinal detachment, corneal abrasion; disorders that may respond adversely to vagotonic action, e.g., bronchial asthma, spastic diseases of GI tract, bradycardia, epilepsy, Parkinson's disease; patients routinely exposed to organophosphate insecticides.

ADVERSE/SIDE EFFECTS CNS: headache, muscle weakness, hyperactivity (children with Down's syndrome). **CV:** cardiac irregularities, flushing, bradycardia. **Eye:** browache, lacrimation, stinging, *dimness or blurring of vision,* photosensitivity, *ciliary or accommodative spasm,* lid muscle twitching, *iris cysts* (especially in children), conjunctival redness and thickening. **GI:** *diarrhea, abdominal cramps,* salivation, *nausea, vomiting.* **GU:** frequent urination or incontinence. **Other:** profuse sweating, respiratory difficulties, nasal congestion.

DRUG INTERACTIONS Ambenonium, edrophonium, neostigmine, pyridostigmine compound systemic cholinergic effects; **succinylcholine** may cause prolonged apnea, cardiovascular collapse

NURSING IMPLICATION

Administration

- When possible, instillation of daily dose or one of the daily doses should be made at bedtime to minimize patient distress from blurred vision.
- *Administration technique:* Gentle finger pressure should be applied against nasolacrimal sac while drug is being instilled; maintain pressure for 1 or 2 min following instillation.
- Reconstituted solutions remain stable for 1 mo at room temperature. Expiration date should appear

on label. The time solutions remain stable under refrigeration varies with manufacturer.

- Before reconstitution, store at 15–30C (59–86F) in a tight container, unless otherwise directed.

Assessment & Drug Effects

- Slit-lamp examinations and tonometric measurements are performed before and during therapy.
- All patients should remain under close supervision while receiving echothiophate.
- Echothiophate therapy is generally discontinued 2–6 wk before surgery. If necessary, alternate miotic therapy is substituted.
- Tolerance may develop after prolonged use, but the response is usually restored by a prescribed rest period from the drug.

Patient & Family Education

- Browache, headache, dimness or blurring of vision may occur at onset of therapy, but these symptoms usually disappear within 5–10 d. If symptoms persist, notify physician.
- It is generally advisable for patient to remove soft contact lenses before instilling eye drops. Consult physician about this teaching point.
- Inform patient that vision may be especially poor in dim light and at night and therefore to avoid night driving.
- Since toxicity is cumulative, symptoms may not appear for several weeks after start of therapy. Advise patient to notify physician promptly of any unusual signs or symptoms or any new or worsening visual problem.
- Duration of echothiophate therapy for convergent strabismus ranges from 1–5 y. If eyes deviate following drug withdrawal, surgery is usually considered.
- Patient should be informed that alcoholic beverages may increase severity of systemic drug effects.
- It may be advisable for some patients to carry a medical identification card indicating use of echothiophate.
- Caution patient to report salivation, diarrhea, profuse sweating, urinary incontinence, or muscle weakness. These systemic effects indicate the need to terminate medication.
- Warn patients of possible additive systemic effects from exposure to organophosphorus-type insecticides and pesticides, e.g., parathion, malathion. If exposure to these substances is unavoidable, advise the patient to wear a respiratory mask and to wash and change clothing frequently.

Prototype: amphotericin B, p 56

ECONAZOLE NITRATE

(e-kone´ a-zole)

Trade names: Ecostatin, Spectazole

Classifications: ANTIINFECTIVE; ANTIBIOTIC; ANTIFUNGAL

Pregnancy: Category C

E

ACTIONS/PHARMACODYNAMICS Synthetic imidazole derivative with broad antifungal spectrum of activity similar to that of miconazole. Exerts fungistatic action but may be fungicidal for certain microorganisms or at high concentrations. Mechanism of action not known but appears to be related to altered cellular membrane permeability and to interference with RNA, protein, and lipid biosynthesis. Active against dermatophytes (including *Trichophyton mentagrophytes, T. rubrum, T. tonsurans, Epidermophyton floccosum, Microsporum audouini, M. canis*), yeasts, e.g., *Candida albicans, Pityrosporum obiculare* (tinea versicolor), and many other genera of fungi. Also appears to be active against some gram-positive bacteria (e.g., *Staphylococcus aureus, Streptococcus pyogenes,* and *Corynebacterium diphtheriae*).

USES Topically for treatment of tinea pedis (athlete's foot or ringworm of foot), tinea cruris ("jock itch" or ringworm of groin), tinea corporis (ringworm of body), tinea versicolor, and cutaneous candidiasis (moniliasis). **Unlabeled uses:** has been used for topical treatment of erythrasma and with corticosteroids for fungal or bacterial dermatoses associated with inflammation.

ROUTE & DOSAGE

Tinea Cruris, Tinea Corporis, Tinea Pedis, Cutaneous Candidiasis

Adult	Topical	Apply sufficient amount to affected areas twice daily, morning and evening

Tinea Versicolor

Adult	Topical	Apply sufficient amount to affected areas once daily

PHARMACOKINETICS Absorption: minimal percutaneous absorption through intact skin; increased absorption from denuded skin. **Peak:** 0.5–5 h.

Common side effects in *italic*; life-threatening effects underlined; generic names in **bold**; classifications in SMALL CAPS

551

Elimination: < 1% of applied dose is eliminated in urine and feces.

CONTRAINDICATIONS & PRECAUTIONS Contraindicated in: safe use during pregnancy (category C) and in nursing women not established.

ADVERSE/SIDE EFFECTS Burning, stinging sensation, pruritus, erythema.

NURSING IMPLICATIONS

Administration
- Cleanse skin with soap and water and dry thoroughly before applying medication (unless otherwise directed by physician). Wash hands thoroughly before and after treatments.
- Do not use occlusive dressings unless prescribed by physician.
- Store at temperature less than 30C (86F) unless otherwise directed.

Patient & Family Education
- Instruct patient to use medication for the prescribed time even if symptoms improve and to report to physician skin reactions suggestive of irritation or sensitization.
- Clinical improvement should occur within the first 1 or 2 wk of therapy. Advise patient to notify physician if full course of therapy does not result in improvement. Diagnosis should be reevaluated.
- Caution patient not to apply the topical cream in or near the eyes or intravaginally.

EDETATE CALCIUM DISODIUM
(ed´e-tate)
Trade names: Calcium Disodium Versenate, Calcium EDTA
Classification: CHELATING AGENT
Pregnancy: Category C

ACTIONS/PHARMACODYNAMICS Chelating agent that combines with divalent and trivalent metals to form stable, nonionizing soluble complexes that can be readily excreted by kidneys. Action is dependent on ability of heavy metal to displace the less strongly bound calcium in the drug molecule.

USES Principally as adjunct in treatment of acute and chronic lead poisoning (plumbism). Generally used in combination with dimercaprol (BAL) in treatment of lead encephalopathy or when blood lead level exceeds 100 µg/dl. Also used to diagnose suspected lead poisoning. **Unlabeled uses:** treatment of poisoning from other heavy metals such as chromium, manganese, nickel, zinc, and possibly vanadium; removal of radioactive and nuclear fission products such as plutonium, yttrium, uranium. Not effective in poisoning from arsenic, gold, or mercury.

ROUTE & DOSAGE

Diagnosis of Lead Poisoning

Adult	IM/IV	500 mg/m^2 (max 1 g) over 1 h IV or IM; then collect urine for 24 h; if µg lead:mg EDTA ratio in urine is > 1, the test is positive
Child	IM/IV	50 mg/kg (max 1 g) IM; then collect urine for 6–8 h; if µg lead:mg EDTA ratio in urine is > 0.5, the test is positive

Treatment of Lead Poisoning

Adult	IM/IV	1–1.5 g/m^2 in 250–500 ml D5W or NS over 1 h IV q12h for up to 5 d; if patient is symptomatic, infuse over 2 h; may give the second dose 6 h after the first dose; then q12h
Child	IM/IV	35 mg/kg b.i.d. (not to exceed 50 mg/kg/d in mild cases) for 3–5 d

PHARMACOKINETICS Absorption: well absorbed IM. **Onset:** 1 h. **Peak:** peak chelation 24–48 h. **Distribution:** distributed to extracellular fluid; does not enter CSF. **Metabolism:** not metabolized. **Elimination:** half-life: 20–60 min IV, 90 min IM; chelated lead excreted in urine; 50% excreted in 1 h.

CONTRAINDICATIONS & PRECAUTIONS Contraindicated in: severe renal disease, anuria; IV use in patients with lead encephalopathy not generally recommended (because of possible increase in intracranial pressure); during pregnancy (category C). **Cautious use in:** renal dysfunction; active tubercular lesions; history of gout.

ADVERSE/SIDE EFFECTS CNS: numbness, tingling sensations (paresthesias), headache, weakness, muscle cramps, malaise, fatigue. **CV:** hypotension, thrombophlebitis. **GI:** anorexia, nausea, vomiting, diarrhea, abdominal cramps, cheilosis. **Hematologic:** transient bone marrow depression, depletion of blood metals. **Renal:** <u>nephrotoxicity</u>. **Other:** *Febrile reaction:* excessive thirst, fever, chills, severe myalgia, arthralgia, GI distress, and accompanied by **histamine-**

Common side effects in *italic*; life-threatening effects <u>underlined</u>; generic names in **bold**; classifications in SMALL CAPS

like reactions: flushing, throbbing headache, sweating, sneezing, nasal congestion, lacrimation, postural hypotension, tachycardia.

DIAGNOSTIC TEST INTERFERENCES Edetate calcium disodium may decrease **serum cholesterol, plasma lipid** levels (if elevated), and **serum potassium** values. **Glycosuria** may occur with toxic doses.

DRUG INTERACTIONS None established.

INCOMPATIBILITIES Solution/Additive: **amphotericin B, hydralazine.**

NURSING IMPLICATIONS

Administration

- The IM route is preferred for symptomatic children and is recommended for patients with incipient or overt lead-induced encephalopathy.
- *Warning:* rapid IV infusion may be lethal by suddenly increasing intracranial pressure in patients who already have cerebral edema.
- Procaine hydrochloride should be added to minimize pain at IM injection site (usually 1 ml of procaine 1% to each 1 ml of concentrated drug). Consult physician.
- When dimercaprol (BAL) and Calcium EDTA are given concurrently, each should be injected into separate IM sites.
- For IV administration, dilute the 5 ml ampule with 250–500 ml of NS or D5W.
- Calcium disodium edetate can produce potentially fatal effects when higher than recommended doses are used or when it is continued after toxic effects appear.
- Calcium EDTA interferes with duration of action of zinc insulin preparations (forms chelate with zinc); therefore do not administer them concurrently.

Assessment & Drug Effects

- Adequacy of urinary output must be determined before therapy is initiated. This may be done by administering IV fluids before giving first dose.
- Fluid intake is generally increased to enhance urinary excretion of chelates. Excess fluid intake, however, should be avoided in patients with lead encephalopathy because of the danger of further increasing intracranial pressure. Consult physician regarding allowable intake.
- Monitor I&O. Since drug is excreted almost exclusively via kidneys, toxicity may develop if output is inadequate. Therapy should be stopped if urine

flow is markedly diminished or absent. Report any change in output or I&O ratio to physician.
- Routine urinalyses including tests for coproporphyrins should be performed prior to therapy and daily during entire course of therapy. Presence of large renal epithelial cells or increasing hematuria and proteinuria are indications to terminate drug immediately.
- Serum creatinine, calcium, and phosphorus determinations should be done before and during each course of therapy.
- Baseline and frequent determinations of BUN and ECG should be monitored during therapy.
- Patients on prolonged therapy should have periodic determinations of blood trace element metals (e.g., copper, zinc, magnesium).
- Be alert for occurrence of febrile reaction that may appear 4–8 h after drug infusion (see Adverse/Side Effects).

EDETATE DISODIUM

(ed´e-tate)
Trade names: Disotate, Disodium EDTA, Endrate
Classifications: CHELATING AGENT; REGULATOR, SERUM CALCIUM
Pregnancy: Category C

ACTIONS/PHARMACODYNAMICS Structurally distinct from edetate calcium disodium. Forms chelates with many bivalent and trivalent metals, e.g., magnesium, zinc, and other trace metals, but has particular affinity for calcium. Forms a stable, nonionizing soluble complex that can be readily excreted via kidneys. Does not chelate potassium but promotes its urinary excretion and may reduce serum potassium levels. Not recommended for treatment of lead toxicity because it may cause severe hypocalcemia. Exerts negative inotropic effect on heart and may antagonize the inotropic and chronotropic effects of digitalis glycosides.

USES In selected patients for emergency treatment of hypercalcemia and to control ventricular arrhythmias and heart block associated with digitalis toxicity when other drugs, e.g., phenytoin and potassium are contraindicated or ineffective. **Unlabeled use:** in ophthalmology to remove corneal calcium deposits (topically or by iontophoresis).

Common side effects in *italic*; life-threatening effects <u>underlined</u>; generic names in **bold**; classifications in SMALL CAPS

553

E

ROUTE & DOSAGE

Hypercalcemia

Adult	IV	50 mg/kg/d (up to 3 g/d) diluted in 500 ml of D5W or NS and infused over 3–4 h
Child	IV	40 mg/kg/d (up to 70 mg/kg/d) diluted to at least 30 mg/ml in D5W or NS and infused over 3–4 h

Digitalis-induced Ventricular Arrhythmia

Adult	IV	15 mg/kg/h up to 60 mg/kg/d by IV infusion in D5W
Child	IV	Same as for adult

PHARMACOKINETICS Metabolism: not metabolized. **Elimination:** approximately 95% of dose excreted renally as calcium chelate.

CONTRAINDICATIONS & PRECAUTIONS Contraindicated in: significant renal disease, anuria, hypocalcemia, history of seizure disorders or intracranial lesions, active or healed calcified tubercular lesions, generalized arteriosclerosis associated with advancing age, coronary or peripheral vascular disease. Safe use during pregnancy (category C) not established. **Cautious use in:** limited cardiac reserve, incipient CHF, potassium deficiency states.

ADVERSE/SIDE EFFECTS CNS: transient numbness, circumoral paresthesias, muscle cramps, muscle weakness, back pain, lassitude, malaise, headache, fatigue, convulsions. **CV:** hypotension, hypertension, arrhythmias, thrombophlebitis. **GI:** *nausea, vomiting, anorexia, diarrhea, abdominal cramps.* **Renal:** (with excessive dosage): <u>nephrotoxicity</u>: urgency, dysuria, nocturia, oliguria, polyuria, proteinuria, tubular necrosis. **Skin:** exfoliative dermatitis and other skin and mucous membrane lesions resembling those of pyridoxine (vitamin B_6) deficiency. **Other:** fever, chills, anemia, glycosuria, hyperuricemia, <u>severe hypocalcemia</u> (rapid IV or high dosages), tetany, hypomagnesemia (prolonged therapy), calcium embolization, damage to reticuloendothelial system with hemorrhagic tendencies (excessive dosage). *Local reactions: pain,* erythema, dermatitis at infusion site.

DIAGNOSTIC TEST INTERFERENCES Colorimetric method of determining ***serum calcium*** levels will not be accurate; oxalate method may yield artificially low serum calcium values. Greater accuracy may be possible by performing test immediately before dose due is administered or by acidifying the sample (atomic absorption spectrometry reportedly not affected). ***Serum alkaline phosphatase*** may

be decreased (thought to be induced by low ***serum magnesium*** levels).

DRUG INTERACTIONS Edetate disodium may lower blood glucose levels and thus reduce **insulin** requirements in (IDDM) diabetic patients; reaction is thought to be due to chelation of the zinc in insulin preparations.

NURSING IMPLICATIONS

Administration

- The commercially available injection must be diluted before administration. Drug is extremely irritating to tissue and therefore should be well diluted before infusion.
- Dilute a single dose in 500 ml of D5W or NS and infuse over 3 or more hours.
- Monitor IV infusion rate as prescribed by physician. Rapid IV infusion (or high serum drug levels) can produce hypocalcemic tetany, cardiac arrhythmias, seizures, and cardiac arrest.
- Extravasation must be prevented.

Assessment & Drug Effects

- Serum calcium levels should be determined after each administration. Observe for and report immediately early signs and symptoms of hypocalcemia (see chap 3).
- Cardiac function should be monitored, particularly in patients with arrhythmias and those with history of seizure disorders or intracranial lesions.
- Determine BP and HR before patient ambulates. Be alert to the possibility of postural hypotension.
- Monitor and report any significant change in I&O ratio to physician.
- Urinalyses should be done daily throughout therapy, and renal function studies (BUN, serum creatinine) should be performed prior to initiation of therapy, every 48 h during therapy, and 48 h after therapy is discontinued. Nephrotoxicity is usually reversible if drug is stopped promptly at the first appearance of symptoms.
- Insulin-dependent diabetic (IDDM) patients may require reduction of insulin dosage while receiving edetate disodium therapy (See Drug Interactions).

Patient & Family Education

- Advise patient to remain in bed for about 20 to 30 min after infusion because of the possibility of postural hypotension. Instruct patient to make position changes slowly, to dangle legs and move ankles and toes for a few minutes before getting out of

Common side effects in *italic*; life-threatening effects <u>underlined</u>; generic names in **bold**; classifications in SMALL CAPS

bed, and to avoid standing still. Supervise ambulation.

Prototype: Neostigmine, p 118

EDROPHONIUM CHLORIDE
(ed-roe-foe´nee-um)

Trade name: Tensilon
Classifications: AUTONOMIC NERVOUS SYSTEM AGENT; CHOLINERGIC (PARASYMPATHOMIMETIC) CHOLINESTERASE INHIBITOR; ANTIDOTE; DIAGNOSTIC AGENT
Pregnancy: Category C

ACTIONS/PHARMACODYNAMICS Rapidly reversible indirect-acting cholinesterase inhibitor (quaternary ammonium compound) similar to neostigmine. Acts as antidote to curariform drugs by displacing them from muscle cell receptor sites, thus permitting resumption of normal transmission of neuromuscular impulses. However, like neostigmine, it prolongs skeletal muscle relaxant action of succinylcholine chloride and decamethonium bromide. Use in myasthenia gravis is based on its ability to inhibit breakdown of ACh (acetylcholine) at postsynaptic membrane. The result is increased availability of the neurotransmitter for stimulation of ACh receptors.

USES Differential diagnosis and as adjunct in evaluation of treatment requirements of myasthenia gravis, for differentiating myasthenic from cholinergic crisis, and to reverse neuromuscular blockade produced by overdosage of nondepolarizing skeletal muscle relaxants, e.g., tubocurarine, gallamine. Not recommended for maintenance therapy in myasthenia gravis because of its short duration of action. **Unlabeled uses:** to terminate paroxysmal atrial tachycardia, as an aid in diagnosing supraventricular tachyarrhythmias, and to evaluate function of demand pacemakers.

PHARMACOKINETICS Onset: 30–60 s IV; 2–10 min IM. **Duration:** 5–10 min IV; 5–30 min IM.

CONTRAINDICATIONS & PRECAUTIONS Contraindicated in: hypersensitivity to anticholinesterase agents; intestinal and urinary obstruction. Safe use during pregnancy (category C) and in nursing mothers not established. **Cautious use in:** bronchial asthma; cardiac arrhythmias; patients receiving digitalis.

ROUTE & DOSAGE

Edrophonium Test for Myasthenia Gravis

Adult	IV	Prepare 10 mg in a syringe; inject 2 mg over 15–30 s; if no reaction after 45 s, inject the remaining 8 mg; may repeat test after 30 min
	IM	Inject 10 mg IM; if cholinergic reaction occurs, retest after 30 min with 2 mg to rule out false-negative reaction
Child	IV	≤ 34 kg: 1 mg IV; if no response after 45 s, dose may be titrated up to 5 mg
	IM	2 mg
	IV	> 34 kg: 2 mg IV; if no response after 45 s, dose may be titrated up to 10 mg
	IM	5 mg
	IM	Infants: 0.5–1 mg

Evaluation of Myasthenia Treatment

Adult	IV	1–2 mg administered 1 h after last PO dose of anticholinesterase medication

Curare Antagonist

Adult	IV	10 mg administered over 30–45 s; may repeat q5–10min as needed up to 40 mg

ADVERSE/SIDE EFFECTS Severe side effects uncommon with usual doses. **CNS:** weakness, muscle cramps, dysphoria, fasciculations, incoordination, dysarthria, dysphagia, convulsions, respiratory paralysis. **CV:** bradycardia, irregular pulse, hypotension, pulmonary edema. **Eye:** miosis, blurred vision, diplopia, lacrimation. **GI:** diarrhea, abdominal cramps, nausea, vomiting, excessive salivation. **Respiratory:** increased bronchial secretions, bronchospasm, laryngospasm, pulmonary edema. **Other:** excessive sweating, urinary frequency, incontinence.

DRUG INTERACTIONS Procainamide, quinidine may antagonize the effects of edrophonium; DIGITALIS GLYCOSIDES increase the sensitivity of the heart to edrophonium; **succinylcholine, decamethonium** may prolong neuromuscular blockade.

NURSING IMPLICATIONS

Administration

- Edrophonium usually is administered by a physician. Monitor vital signs. Observe for signs of respiratory distress. Patients > 50 y are particularly likely to develop bradycardia, hypotension, and cardiac arrest.
- Some clinicians recommend giving a 1–2 mg test dose of edrophonium to elderly patients, to those

Common side effects in *italic*; life-threatening effects underlined; generic names in **bold**; classifications in SMALL CAPS

555

with history of heart disease or who take digitalis, and possibly to all patients.

- Antidote (atropine sulfate) and facilities for endotracheal intubation, tracheostomy, suction, assisted respiration, and cardiac monitoring should be immediately available for treatment of cholinergic reaction.

Assessment & Drug Effects

- **Edrophonium test for myasthenia gravis:** All cholinesterase inhibitors (anticholinesterases) should be discontinued for at least 8 h before test. Estimates of muscle strength should be made before and after administration of edrophonium. Positive response to edrophonium test consists of brief improvement in muscle strength unaccompanied by lingual or skeletal muscle fasciculations. In nonmyasthenic patients, edrophonium produces a cholinergic reaction (muscarinic side effects): skeletal muscle fasciculations, muscle weakness.
- **Evaluation of myasthenic treatment:** *Myasthenic response:* immediate subjective improvement with increased muscle strength (improvement of ptosis, respiration, ability to speak, swallow, and talk), absence of fasciculations; generally indicates that patient requires larger dose of anticholinesterase agent or longer-acting drug. *Cholinergic response* (muscarinic side effects): lacrimation, diaphoresis, salivation, abdominal cramps, diarrhea, nausea, vomiting; accompanied by decrease in muscle strength. Muscle weakness may appear in the following order: muscles of neck, chewing, swallowing, shoulder girdle, upper extremities, pelvic girdle, extraocular muscles, legs; fasciculations may be present or absent. Usually indicates overtreatment with cholinesterase inhibitor. *Adequate response:* no change in muscle strength; fasciculations may be present or absent; minimal cholinergic side effects (observed in patients at or near optimal dosage level).
- **Test to differentiate myasthenic crisis from cholinergic crisis:** *Myasthenic crisis:* edrophonium will cause improvement of respiration, indicating need for longer-acting anticholinesterase drug. *Cholinergic crisis* (caused by excessive cholinesterase inhibition or by overdosage of cholinergic drug): edrophonium will produce increase in oropharyngeal secretions and further weakness of muscles of respiration; usually indicates need for discontinuing anticholinesterase drug.

EMETINE HYDROCHLORIDE

See ANTIINFECTIVES, AMEBICIDE prototype, p 51.

Prototype: captopril, p 138

ENALAPRIL MALEATE
(e-nal´a-pril)
Trade name: Vasotec

ENALAPRILAT
Trade name: Vasotec I.V.
Classifications: CARDIOVASCULAR AGENT; ANGIOTENSION-CONVERTING ENZYME (ACE) INHIBITOR; ANTIHYPERTENSIVE
Pregnancy: Category C

ACTIONS/PHARMACODYNAMICS Vasotec is an angiotension-converting enzyme (ACE) inhibitor that catalyzes the conversion of angiotension I to angiotension II, a vasoconstrictor substance. Therefore inhibition of ACE decreases angiotension II levels, which decreases vasopressor activity and aldosterone secretion. Both actions achieve an antihypertensive effect by suppression of the renin-angiotension-aldosterone system. ACE inhibitors also reduce peripheral arterial resistance (afterload), pulmonary capillary wedge pressure (PCWP), a measure of preload, and pulmonary vascular resistance and improve cardiac output as well as exercise tolerance.

USES Management of mild to moderate hypertension as monotherapy or with a diuretic. Malignant, refractory, accelerated, and renovascular hypertension (except in bilateral renal artery stenosis or renal artery stenosis in a solitary kidney). Also used with diuretics and digitalis in treatment of CHF not responding to other measures. **Unlabeled use:** hypertension or renal crisis in scleroderma.

PHARMACOKINETICS Absorption: 70% absorbed from GI tract. **Onset:** 1 h PO; 15 min IV. **Peak:** 4–8 h PO; 4 h IV. **Duration:** 12–24 h PO; 6 h IV. **Distribution:** limited amount crosses blood-brain barrier; crosses placenta. **Metabolism:** oral dose undergoes first-pass metabolism in liver to active form, enalaprilat. **Elimination:** half-life: 2 h; 60% excreted in urine, 33% in feces within 24 h.

ROUTE & DOSAGE

Hypertension

Adult   PO   5 mg/d; may increase to 10–40 mg/d in 1–2 divided doses

         IV   1.25 q6h; may give up to 5 mg q6h in hypertensive emergencies

Congestive Heart Failure

Adult   PO   2.5 mg 1–2 times/d; may increase up to 5–20 mg/d in 1–2 divided doses (max 40 mg/d)

CONTRAINDICATIONS & PRECAUTIONS Contraindicated in: hypersensitivity to enalapril or captopril. Safe use during pregnancy (category C), in nursing mothers, or in children not established. **Cautious use in:** renal impairment, renal-artery stenosis; patients with hypovolemia, receiving diuretics, undergoing dialysis; patients in whom excessive hypotension would present a hazard (e.g., cerebrovascular insufficiency); CHF; hepatic impairment; diabetes mellitus.

ADVERSE/SIDE EFFECTS CNS: *headache, dizziness,* fatigue, nervousness, paresthesias, asthenia, insomnia, somnolence. **CV:** *hypotension including postural hypotension;* syncope, palpitations, chest pain. **GI:** diarrhea, nausea, abdominal pain, loss of taste, dyspepsia. **Hematologic:** decreased Hgb and Hct; neutropenia, <u>agranulocytosis</u>, eosinophilia. **Renal:** (patient with CHF): <u>acute renal failure</u>, deterioration in renal function. **Skin:** pruritus with and without *rash,* angioedema, erythema. **Other:** hypoglycemia in patient with diabetes mellitus; hyperkalemia; cough, difficult breathing; muscle cramps; impotence.

DRUG INTERACTIONS Indomethacin and other NSAIDS may decrease antihypertensive activity; POTASSIUM SUPPLEMENTS, POTASSIUM-SPARING DIURETICS may cause hyperkalemia; may increase **lithium** levels and toxicity.

NURSING IMPLICATIONS

Administration

- Symptomatic hypotension occasionally may occur following the initial dose of enalapril. If possible, diuretics should be discontinued for 2–3 d prior to initial PO dose to reduce incidence of hypotension. If the diuretic cannot be discontinued, an initial dose of 2.5 mg is given PO. Keep patient under medical supervision for at least 2 h and until BP has stabilized for at least an additional hour.

- To control hypertension, 1.25 mg/ml of enalaprilat is administered slowly IV over at least 5 min through a port of a free flowing infusion of D5W or NS. It may be used as provided or diluted with up to 50 ml of a compatible diluent (i.e., D5W, NS) as indicated. Patients may receive the drug for up to 7 d.

- For conversion from IV to oral therapy the recommended initial dose is 5 mg once a day with a creatinine clearance of (Cl_{cr}) >30 ml/min, and 2.5 mg once daily with a Cl_{cr} <30 ml/min.

- Oral enalapril may be administered with food or drink of patient's choice.

- Store tablets at <30C (86F); protect from heat and light. Expiration date: 30 mo following date of manufacture if stored at <30C.

Assessment & Drug Effects

- The peak effects after the first IV dose may not occur for up to 4 h. The peak effects of subsequent doses may exceed those of the first.

- First dose phenomenon (i.e., a sudden exaggerated hypotensive response) may occur within 1–3 h of first IV dose, especially in the patient with very high blood pressure or one on a diuretic and controlled salt intake regimen. An IV infusion of normal saline for volume expansion may be ordered to counteract the hypotensive response. (This initial response is not an indicator to stop therapy.)

- Bedrest and BP monitoring are advised for the first 3 h after the initial IV dose.

- The hypotensive effect of ACE inhibitors is the same in both standing and supine positions.

- Monitor BP for first several days of therapy. If antihypertensive effect is diminished before 24 h, the total dose may be given as 2 divided doses.

- Hypotension during initiation of enalapril treatment for the patient with CHF may be prevented by liberalizing sodium intake or withholding diuretics and other vasodilators several days before starting ACE inhibition. In the patient with severe hypertension, adrenergic drugs may be stopped for a few days. Monitor these patients carefully for at least 1 wk after first dose of enalapril.

- Transient hypotension with lightheadedness is not an indication to discontinue enalapril treatment but should be reported to physician. Until BP has stabilized, patient should be cautious about ambulation and should not engage in hazardous activities including driving a car.

- Keep in mind that the elderly are particularly sensitive to drug-induced hypotension.

- Patients who have diabetes, impaired renal function, or CHF may receive drugs that increase serum potassium; these patients especially are at risk of

E

developing hyperkalemia during enalapril treatment. Monitor serum potassium and be alert to symptoms of hyperkalemia ($K^+ > 5.7$ mEq/L).

- Hearing loss that develops or worsens during enalapril treatment has been reported.
- Renal function should be monitored closely during first few weeks of therapy. Advise patient to be aware of I&O ratio and pattern and to report significant changes (e.g., hematuria, dysuria) to physician.
- Periodic monitoring of WBC counts in patients with collagen vascular disease and renal disease is advisable.

Patient & Family Education

- Antihypertensive effect may not be experienced until several weeks after enalapril therapy starts.
- Usually patient describes a feeling of well-being with enalapril therapy, and therefore the risk of manipulating the regimen is high. Caution patient not to omit, decrease, or increase dose or to alter the dosing interval without advice of the physician.
- If drug has to be discontinued because of syncope or severe hypotension, patient should be informed that the hypotensive effect may persist a week or longer after termination of therapy because of long duration of drug action.
- Advise against a self-selected low-sodium diet (e.g., low-sodium foods or low-sodium milk) without approval from physician.
- Because of the potential for hyperkalemia, patient should avoid use of a salt substitute (principal ingredient: potassium salt) and potassium supplements.
- A persistent nonproductive cough, especially at night, may be a disturbing side effect. This problem sometimes accompanied by nasal congestion should not be tolerated. Advise patient to report symptoms to physician. Enalapril may be discontinued.
- Angioedema is a rare side effect and, if accompanied by laryngeal edema, may be fatal. Advise patient to report to physician promptly if swelling of face, eyelids, tongue, lips, or extremities occurs.
- If chest pain is relieved by enalapril, patient should understand that pain-free overexertion still may be hazardous. Urge patient to respect guidelines for exercise outlined by physician or physical therapist.
- Caution patient not to use OTC medications without advice of physician.

Prototype: epinephrine, p 102

EPHEDRINE HYDROCHLORIDE
(e-fed´rin)
Trade name: Efedron

EPHEDRINE SULFATE

Trade names: Ectasule, Ephedsol, Vatronol
Classifications: AUTONOMIC NERVOUS SYSTEM AGENT; ALPHA- AND BETA-ADRENERGIC AGONIST (SYMPATHOMIMETIC); BRONCHODILATOR; DECONGESTANT
Pregnancy: Category C

ACTIONS/PHARMACODYNAMICS Both indirect and direct acting sympathomimetic amine. Pharmacologically similar to epinephrine but less potent, with slower onset and more prolonged action; effective by oral route. Elevates blood sugar less than epinephrine does and has more pronounced central stimulatory actions. Thought to act indirectly by releasing tissue stores of norepinephrine and directly by stimulation of α and β_1 and β_2 adrenergic receptors. Cardiovascular actions (positive inotropic and pressor effects) persist 7–10 times as long as those of epinephrine; although bronchodilation is less prominent, it is more sustained. Like epinephrine, it contracts dilated arterioles of nasal mucosa, thus reducing engorgement and edema and facilitating ventilation and drainage. Local application to eye produces mydriasis without loss of light reflexes or accommodation or change in intraocular pressure (IOP). Use in enuresis is based on ability to contract urinary bladder sphincter and on central effects, which decrease depth of sleep. Potentiates action of acetylcholine at neuromuscular junctions; thus it may increase skeletal muscle tone in myasthenia gravis.

USES Temporary relief of congestion of hay fever, allergic rhinitis, and sinusitis; and in treatment and prophylaxis of mild cases of acute asthma and in patients with chronic asthma requiring continuing treatment. Also has been used for its CNS stimulant actions in treatment of narcolepsy, to improve respiration in narcotic and barbiturate poisoning, to combat hypotensive states, especially those associated with spinal anesthesia; in management of enuresis or impaired bladder control; as adjunct in treatment of myasthenia gravis; as mydriatic; to relieve dysmenorrhea; and for temporary support of ventric-

---

Common side effects in *italic*; life-threatening effects <u>underlined</u>;
generic names in **bold**; classifications in SMALL CAPS

ular rate in Adams-Stokes syndrome; for peripheral edema secondary to type I diabetic neuropathy.

ROUTE & DOSAGE

Bronchodilator, Nasal Decongestant

Adult	PO	25–50 mg q3–4h prn (max 150 mg/24 h)
	IM/IV/SC	12.5–25 mg
Child	PO	> 2 y: 2–3 mg/kg/d in 4–6 divided doses
	PO	6–12 y: 6.25–12.5 mg q4h (max 75 mg/24 h)

Hypotension

Adult	PO	25 mg 1–4 times/d (max 150 mg/24 h)
	IM/SC/IV	10–50 mg IM/SC or 10–25 mg slow IV; may repeat in 5–10 min if necessary (max 150 mg/24 h)
Child	PO/IM/SC/IV	3 mg/kg/d in 4–6 divided doses (max 75 mg/24 h)

Myasthenia Gravis

Adult	PO	25 mg t.i.d. or q.i.d.

Enuresis

Adult	PO	25 mg h.s.

Nasal Decongestant

Adult	Intranasal	2–4 drops or a small amount of jelly in each nostril no more than q.i.d. for 3–4 consecutive days

PHARMACOKINETICS Absorption: readily absorbed from GI tract. **Peak:** 15 min–1 h. **Duration:** bronchodilation 2–4 h; cardiac & pressor effects up to 4 h PO and 1 h IV. **Distribution:** widely distributed; crosses blood-brain barrier and placenta; distributed into breast milk. **Metabolism:** small amounts metabolized in liver. **Elimination:** half-life: 3–6 h; excreted in urine.

CONTRAINDICATIONS & PRECAUTIONS Contraindicated in: history of hypersensitivity to ephedrine or other sympathomimetics; narrow-angle glaucoma. Safe use during pregnancy (category C) and in nursing women not established. **Cautious use in:** Use with extreme caution if at all in hypertension, arteriosclerosis, angina pectoris, coronary insufficiency, chronic heart disease; diabetes mellitus; hyperthyroidism; prostatic hypertrophy.

ADVERSE/SIDE EFFECTS Systemic (usually with large doses): CNS: headache, insomnia, *nervousness,* anxiety, tremulousness, giddiness. **CV:** palpitation, tachycardia, precordial pain, cardiac arrhythmias. **GU:** difficult or painful urination, acute urinary retention (especially older men with prostatism). **GI:** nausea, vomiting, anorexia. **Other:** sweating, thirst, fixed-drug eruption. **Topical use:** *burning, stinging,* dryness of nasal mucosa, sneezing, rebound congestion. **Overdosage:** euphoria, confusion, delirium, convulsions, pyrexia, CNS depression (somnolence, coma), hypertension, rebound hypotension, respiratory depression, paranoid psychosis, visual and auditory hallucinations.

DIAGNOSTIC TEST INTERFERENCES Ephedrine is generally withdrawn at least 12 h before ***sensitivity tests*** are made to prevent false-positive reactions.

DRUG INTERACTIONS MAO INHIBITORS, TRICYCLIC ANTIDEPRESSANTS, **furazolidine, guanethidine** may increase alpha-adrenergic effects (headache, hyperpyrexia, hypertension); **sodium bicarbonate** decreases renal elimination of ephedrine, increasing its CNS effects; **epinephrine, norepinephrine** compound sympathomimetic effects; effects of ALPHA AND BETA BLOCKERS and ephedrine antagonized.

INCOMPATIBILITIES Solution/Additive: hydrocortisone, pentobarbital, phenobarbital, secobarbital, thiopental.

NURSING IMPLICATIONS

Administration

- Insomnia is common, particularly with continued therapy. Timing of administration and size of dosage are important considerations. If possible, administer last dose a few hours before bedtime.
- Have patient clear nose before instilling drops. Instruct patient to blow gently with both nostrils open. Generally, nose drops are instilled with head in lateral, head-low position (see Fig 2-4) to avoid entry of drug into throat. Check with physician.
- IV ephedrine may be given undiluted by direct IV at a rate of 10 mg or fraction thereof over 30–60 seconds.
- Preserve in tightly closed, light-resistant containers at 15–30C (59–86F) unless otherwise directed by manufacturer. Do not administer liquid medication unless absolutely clear.

Common side effects in *italic*; life-threatening effects underlined; generic names in **bold**; classifications in SMALL CAPS

559

Assessment & Drug Effects

- Patients receiving ephedrine IV must be under constant supervision. Take baseline BP and other vital signs. Check BP repeatedly during first 5 min, then q3–5min until stabilized.
- When ephedrine is given IV, initially it constricts renal blood vessels, consequently reducing urine formation. As BP rises toward normal levels, renal function is restored. However, if BP increases to hypertensive levels, renal blood flow and urine output again decrease.
- Monitor I&O ratio and pattern, especially in older male patients. Encourage patient to void before taking medication (see Adverse/Side Effects).
- Frequent dosing in patients with hypertension can result in rebound hypotension. Monitoring of central venous pressure or left ventricular filling pressure is advisable in these patients.
- Systemic effects of nose drops can occur because of excessive dosage from rapid absorption of drug solution through nasal mucosa. This is most likely to occur in the elderly.
- In general, topical treatment should not be continued for more than 3–5 consecutive days. Diminished response with rebound congestion may occur if drug is administered in rapidly repeated doses or over prolonged period. Prescribed withdrawal of drug over several days frequently enables the patient to attain former responsiveness.

Patient & Family Education

- Ephedrine is a commonly abused drug. Patients should be advised of side effects and dangers and should be cautioned to take medication only as prescribed.
- Warn patient not to take OTC medications for coughs, colds, allergies, or asthma unless approved by physician. Ephedrine is a common ingredient in these preparations.

EPINEPHRINE

See AUTONOMIC NERVOUS SYSTEM AGENTS, ALPHA- AND BETA-ADRENERGIC AGONIST (SYMPATHO-MIMETIC) prototype, p 102.

EPOETIN ALFA (HUMAN RECOMBINANT ERYTHROPOIETIN)

See BLOOD FORMERS & COAGULATORS, HEMATOPOIETIC GROWTH FACTOR prototype, p 130.

ERGOCALCIFEROL

(er-goe-kal-sif′e-role)

Trade names: Activated Ergosterol, Calciferol, Deltalin, Drisdol, D-Vi-Sol, Ostoforte, Radiostol, Radiostol Forte, Viosterol, Vitamin D_2

Classification: VITAMIN D

Pregnancy: Category C

ACTIONS/PHARMACODYNAMICS The name vitamin D encompasses two related fat-soluble substances (sterols) that occur in nature or are synthetically prepared. One is cholecalciferol (vitamin D_3) formed by activation of provitamin 7-dehydrocholesterol in skin following exposure to ultraviolet irradiation; it is also found in fish liver oils and in livers of fish-eating animals. Cholecalciferol is commercially available only in combination products. (Cod liver oil contains about 2 μg cholecalciferol per milliliter plus 780 U of vitamin A per milliliter.) The other, ergocalciferol (vitamin D_2), is formed by ultraviolet irradiation of ergosterol, a provitamin found in yeasts and fungi. Each has essentially equal antirachitic and hypercalcemic potency. Vitamin D acts like a hormone in that it is distributed through the circulation and plays a major regulatory role. Maintains normal blood calcium and phosphate ion levels by enhancing their intestinal absorption and by promoting mobilization of calcium from bone and renal tubular resorption of phosphate. Essential for normal bone development; stimulates production and prolongs life span of osteoclasts and promotes mineral resorption by bones. Functions in magnesium metabolism and in maintenance of normal parathyroid activity and neuromuscular function. Vitamin D deficiency causes rickets in children and osteomalacia in adults. Activity of cholecalciferol and ergocalciferol may be expressed as USP U or IU (international units) of vitamin D, which are equivalent (40 USP U or IU = biologic activity of 1 μg of ergocalciferol or cholecalciferol).

USES Familial hypophosphatemia (vitamin D–resistant rickets), osteomalacia (adult rickets), anticonvulsant-induced rickets and osteomalacia, osteoporosis, renal osteodystrophy, hypocalcemia associated with hypoparathyroidism; prophylaxis and treatment of nutritional rickets. Also hypophosphatemia in Fanconi's syndrome. **Unlabeled uses:** with varying clinical results in lupus vulgaris, psoriasis, and rheumatoid arthritis.

ROUTE & DOSAGE

40 U = 1 μg

Nutritional Rickets, Osteomalacia

Adult	PO/IM	25–125 μg/d for 6–12 wk; may need up to 7.5 mg/d in patients with malabsorption
Child	PO/IM	50–125 μg/d; may need up to 250–625 μg/d in patients with malabsorption

Vitamin D–dependent Rickets

Adult	PO/IM	250 μg–1.5 mg/d; may need up to 12.5 mg/d (prolonged therapy with > 2.5 mg/d increases risk of toxicity)
Child	PO/IM	75–125 μg/d; may need up to 1.5 mg/d

Hypoparathyroidism, Pseudohypoparathyroidism

Adult	PO/IM	625 μg–5 mg/d; may need up to 10 mg/d (prolonged therapy with > 2.5 mg/d increases risk of toxicity)
Child	PO/IM	1.25–5 mg/d; (prolonged therapy with > 2.5 mg/d increases risk of toxicity)

PHARMACOKINETICS Absorption: readily absorbed from GI tract. **Peak activity:** after 4 wk. **Duration:** 2 mo or more. **Distribution:** most of drug first appears in lymph, then concentrates in liver; stored chiefly in liver and to a lesser extent in skin, brain, spleen, and bones. **Metabolism:** metabolized in liver and kidney to active metabolites. **Elimination:** half-life: 12–24 h; about 50% of oral dose excreted in bile; may be stored in tissues for months.

CONTRAINDICATIONS & PRECAUTIONS Contraindicated in: hypersensitivity to vitamin D, hypervitaminosis D, hypercalcemia, hyperphosphatemia, renal osteodystrophy with hyperphosphatemia, malabsorption syndrome, decreased renal function. Safe use of amounts in excess of 400 IU (10 μg) daily in pregnancy (category C) not established. **Cautious use in:** coronary disease; nursing women; arteriosclerosis (especially in the elderly); history of renal stones.

ADVERSE/SIDE EFFECTS Vitamin D toxicity (hypervitaminosis D): produces symptoms of hypercalcemia. Initial: *fatigue, weakness, headache, drowsiness, metallic taste, dry mouth, anorexia, nausea, vomiting, diarrhea, constipation, abdominal cramps, vertigo, tinnitus, ataxia, muscle and joint pain, hypotonia (infants),* exanthema. Later: anemia, calcification of soft tissues (kidneys, blood vessels, myocardium, lungs, skin); nephrotoxicity: polyuria, hyposthenuria, polydipsia, nocturia, casts, albuminuria, hematuria; hypertension, conjunctivitis (calcific), photophobia, rhinorrhea, pruritus; overt psychosis (rare), mild acidosis, convulsions, cardiac arrhythmias, osteoporosis (adults), weight loss, renal failure. **Chronic hypervitaminosis D in children:** <u>mental and physical retardation</u>, suppression of linear growth.

DIAGNOSTIC TEST INTERFERENCES Vitamin D may cause false increase in *serum cholesterol* measurements (Zlatkis-Zak reaction).

DRUG INTERACTIONS Cholestyramine, colistipol, mineral oil may decrease absorption of vitamin D.

NURSING IMPLICATIONS

Administration

- IM injection should be made deeply, preferably into gluteus maximus and injected slowly. Aspirate carefully. Rotate injection sites.
- Physician may prescribe ergocalciferol IM for patients with malabsorption syndrome or impaired hepatic or biliary function since bile is necessary for absorption of the oral form.
- Once symptoms of vitamin D deficiency are relieved, dosage should be reduced to prevent hypercalcemia.
- Preserve in tightly covered, light-resistant containers at 15–30C (59–86F), unless otherwise directed. Decomposes on exposure to light and air.

Assessment & Drug Effects

- Patients receiving therapeutic doses of vitamin D must remain under close medical supervision.

Common side effects in *italic*; life-threatening effects <u>underlined</u>; generic names in **bold**; classifications in SMALL CAPS

561

- When high therapeutic doses are used, progress is followed by frequent determinations (q2wk or more often) of serum calcium, phosphorus, magnesium, alkaline phosphatase, BUN, and determinations of urine calcium (quantitative), casts, albumin, and RBC. Blood calcium concentration is generally kept between 9–10 mg/dl.
- In patients with osteomalacia a decrease in serum alkaline phosphatase may signal the onset of hypercalcemia.
- *Treatment of vitamin D toxicity* consists of prompt discontinuation of the vitamin, a low-calcium diet, generous fluid intake and acidification of urine (to prevent calculus formation and enhance urinary excretion of calcium), and general symptomatic and supportive treatment.

Patient & Family Education

- Most foods contain little or no vitamin D. High concentrations are found in liver oil from cod, turbot, and halibut. Other good sources include salmon, sardines, herring, egg yolk, fortified milk, butter, and margarine. Patients receiving therapeutic doses of vitamin D should be informed regarding allowable intake of these foods. Collaborate with dietitian.
- Magnesium-containing antacids and laxatives should be avoided in patients with chronic renal failure receiving vitamin D preparations since they are more prone to develop magnesium intoxication than other patients.
- Advise patient not to use OTC medications unless approved by physician.

Prototype: ergotamine, p 112

ERGOLOID MESYLATE

(er´goe-loid mess´i-late)

Trade names: Deapril-ST, Gerimal, Hydergine, Hydroloid-G, Niloric

Classifications: AUTONOMIC NERVOUS SYSTEM AGENT; ALPHA-ADRENERGIC ANTAGONIST (BLOCKING AGENT, SYMPATHOLYTIC); ERGOT ALKALOID

Pregnancy: Category C

ACTIONS/PHARMACODYNAMICS Combination of three hydrogenated derivatives of ergot alkaloids. Produces peripheral vasodilation primarily by central action and may cause slight reduction in BP and heart rate. Lacks vasoconstrictor and oxytocic properties of the natural ergot alkaloids. Reportedly relieves symptoms of cerebral arteriosclerosis, possibly by increasing cerebral metabolism with consequent increase in blood flow. Conclusive evidence of therapeutic effectiveness for senile dementia is lacking. However, short-term clinical studies have demonstrated modest improvement in some patients.

USES Senile dementia of Alzheimer type.

ROUTE & DOSAGE

Senile Dementia of Alzheimer Type

Adult   PO/SL   1 mg t.i.d.; doses up to 4.5–12 mg/d have been used

PHARMACOKINETICS Absorption: incompletely absorbed from GI tract; approximately 50% reaches systemic circulation. **Peak:** 1.5–3 h. **Metabolism:** undergoes rapid first-pass metabolism in liver. **Elimination:** half-life: 2–12 h; primarily excreted in feces.

CONTRAINDICATIONS & PRECAUTIONS Contraindicated in: acute or chronic psychosis. Safe use during pregnancy (category C), in nursing women, and in children not determined. **Cautious use in:** acute intermittent porphyria.

ADVERSE/SIDE EFFECTS Mostly dose related. **CV:** orthostatic hypotension, dizziness or lightheadedness, flushing, sinus bradycardia. **EENT:** blurred vision, nasal stuffiness, increased nasopharyngeal secretions. **GI:** sublingual irritation, anorexia, stomach cramps, transient nausea and vomiting, heartburn. **Other:** skin rash, drowsiness, headache, precipitation of acute intermittent porphyria.

NURSING IMPLICATIONS

Administration

- Instruct patient to allow SL tablet to dissolve under tongue and not to drink, eat, or smoke while tablet is in place. SL tablets should not be crushed.
- Store at 15–30C (59–86F) in tightly closed container unless otherwise directed.

Assessment & Drug Effects

- Establish baseline values of BP and pulse; check at regular intervals throughout therapy.
- Sinus bradycardia (40 bpm) has been reported in patients receiving 1.5 mg doses. Report to physi-

Common side effects in *italic*; life-threatening effects underlined; generic names in **bold**; classifications in SMALL CAPS

cian. Pulse rate usually returns to normal within 2 d after drug is discontinued.

- Drug should be permanently withdrawn if marked bradycardia or hypotension occurs.
- Continuous clinical evaluations must be made to determine effect of therapy. The following items suggested by manufacturer might be used as guidelines for observations: mental alertness, emotional lability, ability to do self-care, improvement in depression, anxieties, fears, cooperativeness, sociability, appetite, fatigue, dizziness.
- Up to 6 mo of treatment may be necessary. Optimal dose and duration of therapy are not known. Improvement may not be apparent until after 3–4 wk of therapy.

Patient & Family Education

- Advise patient to make position changes slowly, particularly from recumbent to upright posture, and to move ankles and feet for a few minutes before ambulating.

Prototype: ergotamine tartrate, p 112

ERGONOVINE MALEATE

(er-goe-noe´veen)
Trade name: Ergotrate Maleate
Classifications: AUTONOMIC NERVOUS SYSTEM AGENTS; ALPHA-ADRENERGIC ANTAGONIST (BLOCKING AGENT, SYMPATHOLYTIC); ERGOT ALKALOID; OXYTOCIC

ACTIONS/PHARMACODYNAMICS Ergot alkaloid with slow but powerful oxytocic effect; less toxic and less prone to cause gangrene than other ergot derivatives. Exerts moderate cerebral vascular constriction but is inferior to ergotamine as a migraine specific. Produces prolonged nonphasic uterine contractions. Like other oxytocics, may evoke severe hypertensive episodes in hypertensive or toxemic patients or when regional anesthesia (caudal or spinal) containing vasoconstrictors has been used.

USES To prevent or reduce postpartum and postabortal hemorrhage due to uterine atony. **Unlabeled use:** aid in diagnosis of variant angina pectoris.

PHARMACOKINETICS Absorption: readily absorbed from GI tract. **Onset:** 5–15 min PO; 2–5 min

ROUTE & DOSAGE

Postpartum Hemorrhage

Adult	PO	0.2–0.4 mg q6–12h until danger of atony passes (2–7 d)
	IM/IV	0.2 mg q2–4h up to a max of 5 doses

IM; immediately IV. **Duration:** 3 or more h PO; 3 h IM; 45 min IV. **Distribution:** distributed into breast milk. **Metabolism:** slowly metabolized in liver. **Elimination:** half-life: 0.5–2 h; excreted in feces; small amount excreted in urine.

CONTRAINDICATIONS & PRECAUTIONS Contraindicated in: hypersensitivity to ergot preparations, to induce labor, use prior to delivery of placenta, threatened spontaneous abortion, prolonged use, uterine sepsis, hypertension, toxemia.

ADVERSE/SIDE EFFECTS *Nausea, vomiting* (especially with IV doses), severe hypertensive episodes, bradycardia, allergic phenomena including shock, ergotism.

DRUG INTERACTIONS PARENTERAL SYMPATHOMIMETICS, OTHER ERGOT ALKALOIDS add to pressor effects with possible hypertension.

NURSING IMPLICATIONS

Administration

- Before labor is induced, consult with physician about route to be used for administration of ergonovine during delivery. Have drug prepared so that there is no delay.
- PO tablets may also be administered on tongue (perlingually) or by rectum (suspended in water as retention enema).
- IV ergonovine, given in second stage of labor as head is born, induces contractions in 1 min. IM injection as infant is being born produces, in 2–5 min, uterine contractions that separate placenta and prevent blood loss.
- *IV injection:* IV ergonovine maleate may be given by direct IV undiluted at a rate of 0.2 mg or a fraction thereof over 1 min.
- If solution for injection is discolored or contains particles, do not use.
- Store drug in cool place, below 8C (46F). However, delivery room stocks may be kept at room temperature for up to 60 d.

Assessment & Drug Effects

- Assess and record character of uterine contractions.
- IM injection initially produces firm, titanic contrac-

Common side effects in *italic*; life-threatening effects underlined; generic names in **bold**; classifications in SMALL CAPS

563

tion of postpartum uterus; a succession of minor relaxations and contractions then occur with relaxation increasing over the next 1.5 h. Vigorous rhythmic contractions continue for 3 h or more after injection.

- Desired oxytocic action of ergonovine may be antagonized by hypocalcemia. Assess serum calcium level.
- Severe cramping following oral doses is evidence of effectiveness; however, it may also indicate need to reduce dose.
- Monitor BP, pulse, and uterine response following injection until postpartum condition is stabilized (about 1 or 2 h).
- Report sudden increase in BP, pulse changes, and frequent periods of uterine relaxation. (Uterus may fail to respond in hypocalcemic patients.)
- High incidence of nausea and danger of hypertension and CVA have limited the use of IV route for emergency treatment.

Patient & Family Education
- Advise patient to anticipate moderate to severe cramping with oral dose.
- Instruct patient to report any of the following: headache, dizziness, tinnitus. (These may indicate ergotism.)

ERGOTAMINE TARTRATE

See AUTONOMIC NERVOUS SYSTEM AGENTS, ADRENERGIC ANTAGONIST (SYMPATHOLYTIC), ERGOT ALKALOID prototype, p 112.

Prototype: nitroglycerin, p 149

ERYTHRITYL TETRANITRATE

(e-ryth´-rityl te´tra-ni´trate)
Trade name: Cardilate
Classifications: CARDIOVASCULAR AGENT; NITRATE VASODILATOR
Pregnancy: Category C

ACTIONS/PHARMACODYNAMICS Organic nitrate with pharmacologic actions similar to those of nitroglycerin. Mechanism of action not specifically understood. Relaxes vascular smooth muscle with resulting vasodilation. Dilation of peripheral blood vessels tends to cause peripheral pooling of blood, decreased venous return to heart, decreased left ventricular end-diastolic pressure, with consequent reduction in myocardial oxygen consumption. Cross tolerance with other nitrates is possible. Not used for acute relief of angina attacks.

USES Prophylactic management of long-term angina pectoris and situations likely to provoke angina attacks. **Unlabeled use:** diffuse esophageal spasm without gastroesophageal reflux.

ROUTE & DOSAGE

Prophylaxis for Situational Angina Attacks

Adult	PO	5–10 mg
	SL	5–10 mg

Long-term Prophylaxis for Angina

Adult	PO	10 mg a.c. and h.s. t.i.d. or q.i.d. (max 100 mg/d)

Diffuse Esophageal Spasm

Adult	PO	10–15 mg q.i.d.

PHARMACOKINETICS Absorption: readily absorbed from GI tract with significant first pass metabolism. **Onset:** 5 min SL; 15–30 min PO. **Peak:** 15 min SL; 60 min PO. **Duration:** 3 h SL; 6 h PO. **Metabolism:** metabolized in liver. **Elimination:** excreted in urine.

CONTRAINDICATIONS & PRECAUTIONS Contraindicated in: history of hypersensitivity to nitrates or nitrites, severe anemia, acute MI; extended-release preparations in patients with functional or organic GI hypermotility or malabsorption syndrome; pregnancy (category C). **Cautious use in:** increased intracranial pressure (e.g., head trauma, cerebral hemorrhage), diuretic-induced fluid depletion, and hypotension.

ADVERSE/SIDE EFFECTS CNS: *headache,* dizziness, weakness, restlessness, blurred vision, syncope. **CV:** *tachycardia, hypotension,* cardiovascular collapse, transient pulselessness. **GI:** nausea, vomiting, dry mouth, incontinent of urine and feces. **Skin:** *flushing,* pallor, perspiration, rash, dermatitis. **Other:** hypersensitivity reaction, methemoglobinemia.

DIAGNOSTIC TEST INTERFERENCES May interfere with the Zlatkis-Zak color reaction for serum cholesterol causing a false report of decreased serum value.

Common side effects in *italic*; life-threatening effects underlined; generic names in **bold**; classifications in SMALL CAPS

DRUG INTERACTIONS Alcohol, BETA-BLOCKERS, PHENOTHIAZINES may potentiate hypotensive effects.

NURSING IMPLICATIONS

Administration

- Oral drug is most effective if taken on an empty stomach.
- Chewable tablets must not be swallowed whole.
- Store in tightly closed container in a cool, dry place at 15–30C.

Assessment & Drug Effects

- Take apical pulse for 1 min, assessing for possible tachycardia.
- Assess BP frequently as drug may cause orthostatic hypotension.
- Monitor vital signs more closely if client is on other cardiac drugs (e.g., antihypertensive, antianginal). Assess for hypotensive effects of other drugs that the patient may be taking.
- Assess character of anginal pain as drug is not used for active relief of angina attack.
- Assess for GI problems, flushing, perspiration, and rashes.
- Determine effectiveness of dose by assessing frequency and duration of anginal attacks.

Patient & Family Education

- Advise patient that drug should be taken 30 min before meals and if necessary at midmorning, midafternoon, and at bedtime with a maximum dose of 100 mg/d.
- Advise patient that drug is not to be used to relieve an acute episode of anginal pain.
- Advise patient to anticipate situations that may provoke anginal attack and take SL tablet 5–10 min prior to stressful situation.
- Instruct patient to change positions slowly until tolerance to hypotensive effects of drug is known.
- Instruct patient to lie down at the first indication of lightheadedness or faintness and to take deep breaths and move arms and legs to relieve symptoms.
- Advise patient not to drink alcohol because it may increase possibility of lightheadedness and faintness.
- Instruct patient to report onset of skin rash or persistent headaches and report increased incidences of other side effects to physician.
- Headaches are common during initiation of therapy. Advise patient that tolerance to this side effect usually develops.

ERYTHROMYCIN

See ANTIINFECTIVES, ANTIBIOTIC, ERYTHROMYCIN prototype, p 65.

Prototype: erythromycin, p 65

ERYTHROMYCIN ESTOLATE

Trade names: Ilosone, Nororythro
Classifications: ANTIINFECTIVE; ANTIBIOTIC; ERYTHROMYCIN
Pregnancy: Category B

ACTIONS/PHARMACODYNAMICS Acid ester salt of erythromycin. Reported to be acid stable and thus less susceptible to action of gastric juices or food in stomach and to give higher, more predictable, and more prolonged antibiotic blood levels than other oral erythromycins. Greater potential for producing hepatotoxicity than by erythromycin (base).

USES See erythromycin.

ROUTE & DOSAGE

Infections		
Adult	PO	250 mg q6h up to 4 g/d according to severity of infection
Child	PO	30–50 mg/kg/d in 4 divided doses up to 100 mg/kg/d for severe infections

PHARMACOKINETICS Absorption: readily absorbed from GI tract. **Peak:** 2 h. **Distribution:** concentrates in liver; crosses placenta; distributed into breast milk. **Metabolism:** metabolized in liver. **Elimination:** half-life: 3–5 h; excreted primarily in bile and feces.

CONTRAINDICATIONS & PRECAUTIONS Contraindicated in: hypersensitivity to erythromycins; history of erythromycin-associated hepatitis; hepatic dysfunction; treatment of skin disorders such as acne or furunculosis, prophylaxis of rheumatic fever. Safe use during pregnancy (category B) not established.

ADVERSE/SIDE EFFECTS Cholestatic hepatitis syndrome. **GI:** *nausea,* vomiting, heartburn, *abdominal cramps,* right upper quadrant pain or tenderness, jaundice. **Hypersensitivity:** fever, disturbance in color

Common side effects in *italic*; life-threatening effects <u>underlined</u>; generic names in **bold**; classifications in SMALL CAPS

565

vision, headache, myalgia, abnormal liver function tests, eosinophilia, leukocytosis; slight increase in prothrombin time. **Other:** superinfections.

DRUG INTERACTIONS May increase **carbamazepine, cyclosporine, theophylline** levels and toxicity; **warfarin** may increase prothrombin time (PT); **ergotamine** may induce ischemia and peripheral vasospasm.

NURSING IMPLICATIONS

Administration
- Serum levels are comparable whether drug is taken with or after food or when the patient is in the fasting state. It therefore may be taken without regard to meals.
- Chewable tablets should be chewed or crushed, not swallowed whole.
- After reconstitution, suspensions are stable for 14 d at room temperature; however, to preserve palatability, keep refrigerated. Protect from light.

Assessment & Drug Effects
- Culture and susceptibility testing should be performed before initiation of treatment.
- Cholestatic hepatitis syndrome is most likely to occur in adults who have received erythromycin estolate for more than 10 d or who have had repeated courses of therapy. The condition is generally reversible within 3–5 d after cessation of therapy.
- Hepatic function tests and blood cell counts should be conducted initially and periodically if therapy is prolonged 10 d or more.

Patient & Family Education
- Advise patients to report immediately the onset of adverse reactions and to be on the alert for signs and symptoms associated with jaundice (see chap 3).

Prototype: erythromycin, p 65

ERYTHROMYCIN ETHYLSUCCINATE

Trade names: Apo-Erythro-ES, E.E.S., EES-200, EES-400, E-Mycin E, EryPed Pediamycin, Erytkocin, Wyamycin E
Classifications: ANTIINFECTIVE; ANTIBIOTIC; ERYTHROMYCIN
Pregnancy: Category B

ACTIONS/PHARMACODYNAMICS Acid-stable ester salt of erythromycin.

USES See erythromycin.

ROUTE & DOSAGE

400 mg erythromycin ethylsuccinate is approximately equal to 250 mg erythromycin base

Infection

Adult	PO	400 mg q6h up to 4 g/d according to severity of infection
Child	PO	30–50 mg/kg/d in 4 divided doses up to 100 mg/kg/d for severe infections

PHARMACOKINETICS Absorption: readily absorbed from GI tract. **Peak:** 2 h. **Distribution:** concentrates in liver; crosses placenta; distributed into breast milk. **Metabolism:** metabolized in liver. **Elimination:** half-life: 2–5 h; excreted primarily in bile and feces.

CONTRAINDICATIONS & PRECAUTIONS Contraindicated in: hypersensitivity to erythromycins; history of erythromycin-associated hepatitis; preexisting liver disease. Safe use during pregnancy (category B) not established.

ADVERSE/SIDE EFFECTS GI: diarrhea, *nausea,* vomiting, stomatitis, *abdominal cramps,* anorexia. **Other:** skin eruptions, hepatotoxicity and ototoxicity potential, superinfections.

DRUG INTERACTIONS May increase **carbamazepine, cyclosporine, theophylline** levels and toxicity; **warfarin** may increase prothrombin time (PT); **ergotamine** may induce ischemia and peripheral vasospasm.

NURSING IMPLICATIONS

Administration
- PO formulations may be administered without regard to meals in patients ≥ 2 y.
- Chewable tablets should be chewed and not swallowed whole.
- PO suspensions are stable for 14 d at room temperature unless otherwise stated by manufacturer. Note expiration date.
- Store tablets in tight containers at 15–30C (59–86F) unless otherwise directed.

Assessment & Drug Effects
- Culture and susceptibility testing should be performed before initiation of treatment.

Common side effects in *italic*; life-threatening effects <u>underlined</u>; generic names in **bold**; classifications in SMALL CAPS

- Cholestatic hepatitis syndrome is most likely to occur in adults who have received erythromycin estolate for more than 10 d or who have had repeated courses of therapy. The condition is generally reversible within 3–5 d after cessation of therapy.
- Hepatic function tests and blood cell counts should be conducted periodically if therapy is prolonged 10 d or more.
- Ototoxicity is most likely to occur in patients receiving high dosage or who have impaired renal function. Report immediately the onset of tinnitus, vertigo, or hearing impairment.

Patient & Family Education

- Advise to report immediately the onset of adverse reactions and to be on the alert for signs and symptoms associated with jaundice (see chap 3).

Prototype: erythromycin, p 65

ERYTHROMYCIN GLUCEPTATE

Trade name: Ilotycin Gluceptate
Classifications: ANTIINFECTIVE; ANTIBIOTIC; ERYTHROMYCIN
Pregnancy: Category B

ACTIONS/PHARMACODYNAMICS Soluble salt of erythromycin.

USES When oral administration is not possible or the severity of infection requires immediate high serum levels. See erythromycin.

ROUTE & DOSAGE

Infections

Adult	IV	250 mg–1 g q6h up to 4 g/d according to severity of infection
Child	IV	15–20 mg/kg/d in 4 divided doses up to 100 mg/kg/d for severe infections

PHARMACOKINETICS Peak: 1 h. **Distribution:** concentrates in liver; crosses placenta; distributed into breast milk. **Metabolism:** metabolized in liver. **Elimination:** half-life: 3–5 h; excreted primarily in bile and feces; 12–15% excreted in urine.

CONTRAINDICATIONS & PRECAUTIONS Contraindicated in: hypersensitivity to erythromycins. Safe use during pregnancy (category B) not established. **Cautious use in:** impaired hepatic function.

ADVERSE/SIDE EFFECTS *Pain and venous irritation after IV injection;* allergic reactions, <u>anaphylaxis (rare)</u>; superinfections; variations in liver function tests following prolonged or repeated therapy. **GI:** *nausea, vomiting, diarrhea, abdominal cramps.*

DRUG INTERACTIONS May increase **carbamazepine, cyclosporine, theophylline** levels and toxicity; **warfarin** may increase prothrombin time (PT); **ergotamine** may induce ischemia and peripheral vasospasm.

INCOMPATIBILITIES Solution/Additive: amikacin, aminophylline, heparin, TETRACYCLINES, **pentobarbital, secobarbital. Y-Site: aminophylline, heparin,** TETRACYCLINES.

NURSING IMPLICATIONS

Administration

- Initial solution is prepared by adding 10 ml sterile water for injection without preservatives to each 500 mg or fraction thereof (see manufacturer's directions for dilution). Shake vial until drug is completely dissolved.
- Before administration, initial solution is further diluted with 80–250 ml of NS, lactated Ringer's or Normosol-R and buffer to neutrality (see manufacturer's directions). Stability of solution is dependent on pH and is optimal at pH 6–8.
- Continuous infusion is administered slowly within 24 h after dilution to a volume of 500 ml.
- Physician will prescribe specific IV infusion rate. Rate should be slow to avoid pain along course of vein.
- PO therapy should replace IV administration as soon as possible.
- Initially reconstituted solution is stable up to 7 d if refrigerated at 2–8C (36–46F).
- Store sterile powder at 15–30C (59–86F) unless otherwise directed.

Assessment & Drug Effects

- Culture and susceptibility testing should be performed prior to initiation of therapy.
- Hearing impairment may occur with large doses of this drug. It may occur as early as the second day and as late as the third week of therapy.
- IV infusion of large doses reported to increase risk of thrombophlebitis. Assess for Signs & Symptoms (see chap 3).

E

Common side effects in *italic*; life-threatening effects <u>underlined</u>; generic names in **bold**; classifications in SMALL CAPS

567

- Periodic hepatic function tests are advised in patients receiving daily high doses or prolonged or repeated therapy.

Patient & Family Education
- Instruct patient to report immediately tinnitus, dizziness or hearing impairment.

Prototype: erythromycin, p 65

ERYTHROMYCIN LACTOBIONATE

Trade name: Erythrocin Lactobionate-I.V.
Classifications: ANTIINFECTIVE; ANTIBIOTIC; ERYTHROMYCIN
Pregnancy: Category B

ACTIONS/PHARMACODYNAMICS Lactobionate salt of erythromycin.

USES When oral administration is not possible or severity of infection requires immediate high serum levels. See erythromycin.

ROUTE & DOSAGE

Infections

Adult	IV	250 mg–1 g q6h up to 4 g/d according to severity of infection
Child	IV	15–20 mg/kg/d in 4 divided doses up to 100 mg/kg/d for severe infections

PHARMACOKINETICS Peak: 1 h. **Distribution:** concentrates in liver; crosses placenta; distributed into breast milk. **Metabolism:** metabolized in liver. **Elimination:** half-life: 3–5 h; excreted primarily in bile and feces; 12–15% excreted in urine.

CONTRAINDICATIONS & PRECAUTIONS Contraindicated in: hypersensitivity to erythromycins. Safe use during pregnancy (category B) not established. **Cautious use in:** impaired hepatic function.

ADVERSE/SIDE EFFECTS Anorexia, *abdominal discomfort,* diarrhea, *nausea,* vomiting, allergic reactions, *thrombophlebitis at injection site;* ototoxicity associated with IV infusions of 4 g/d or more (reversible), PVCs, torsades de pointes; superinfections.

DRUG INTERACTIONS May increase **carbamazepine, cyclosporine, theophylline** levels and toxicity; **warfarin** may increase prothrombin time (PT); **ergotamine** may induce ischemia and peripheral vasospasm.

INCOMPATIBILITIES Solution/Additive: **ampicillin, ascorbic acid, cephalothin, colistimethate, heparin, metaraminol, metoclopramide, tetracycline, vitamin B complex with C.**

NURSING IMPLICATIONS

Administration
- Initial solution is prepared by adding 10 ml sterile water for injection without preservatives to each 500 mg or fraction thereof. Shake vial until drug is completely dissolved.
- Before administration, initial solution is further diluted with 80–250 ml of NS, lactated Ringer's, or Normosol-R and buffer to neutrality (see manufacturer's directions). Stability of solution is dependent on pH and is optimal at pH 6–8.
- Continuous infusion is administered slowly within 24 h after dilution to a volume of 500 ml.
- Physician will prescribe specific IV infusion rate. Rate should be slow to avoid pain along course of vein.
- Continuous infusion is preferable, but intermittent infusion in 20 to 60 min periods at intervals of ≥q6h is also effective.
- IV therapy should be replaced by oral dosage form as soon as possible.
- Store sterile powder at 15–30C (59–86F) unless otherwise directed.
- Initially reconstituted solution is stable up to 7 d if refrigerated at 2–8C (36–46F).

Assessment & Drug Effects
- Culture and susceptibility tests should be performed prior to initiation of therapy.
- IV infusions of large doses reportedly are associated with thrombophlebitis. Assess for signs and symptoms (see chap 3).
- Hearing impairment may occur with large doses of the drug and may occur as early as the second day and as late as the third week of therapy.
- Periodic hepatic function tests are advised in patients receiving daily high doses or prolonged or repeated therapy.

Patient & Family Education
- Instruct patient to report immediately tinnitus, dizziness or hearing impairment.

Prototype: erythromycin, p 65

ERYTHROMYCIN STEARATE

Trade names: Apo-Erythro-S, Eramycin, Erypar, Ethril, Erythrocin Stearate, SK-Erythromycin, Wyamycin S
Classifications: ANTIINFECTIVE; ANTIBIOTIC; ERYTHROMYCIN
Pregnancy: Category B

ACTIONS/PHARMACODYNAMICS Reportedly one of the most completely and reliably absorbed forms of erythromycin.

USES See erythromycin.

ROUTE & DOSAGE

Infections

Adult	PO	250 mg q6h up to 4 g/d according to severity of infection
Child	PO	30–50 mg/kg/d in 4 divided doses up to 100 mg/kg/d for severe infections

PHARMACOKINETICS Absorption: readily absorbed from GI tract. **Peak:** 2 h. **Distribution:** concentrates in liver; crosses placenta; distributed into breast milk. **Metabolism:** metabolized in liver. **Elimination:** half-life: 5.5 h; excreted primarily in bile and feces.

CONTRAINDICATIONS & PRECAUTIONS Contraindicated in: hypersensitivity to erythromycins; history of erythromycin stearate–induced hepatitis. Safe use during pregnancy (category B) not established. **Cautious use in:** impaired hepatic function.

ADVERSE/SIDE EFFECTS *Abdominal cramps,* diarrhea, *nausea,* vomiting, urticaria, skin eruptions, superinfections.

DRUG INTERACTIONS May increase **carbamazepine, cyclosporine, theophylline** levels and toxicity; **warfarin** may increase prothrombin time (PT); **ergotamine** may induce ischemia and peripheral vasospasm.

NURSING IMPLICATIONS

Administration
- Optimum blood levels are obtained when drug is taken on empty stomach.
- Protect tablets from light.

Assessment & Drug Effects
- Culture and susceptibility testing should be performed before initiation of therapy.

Patient & Family Education
- Instruct patient not to chew or crush film-coated tablet.
- May be taken with food.
- Advise patient to take at evenly spaced intervals during the day and preferably around the clock.
- In treatment of group A beta-hemolytic streptococcal infections, therapeutic dosage should be administered for at least 10 d.
- Advise patient to notify physician of nausea, vomiting, diarrhea or stomach cramps, severe abdominal pain, yellow discoloration of skin or eyes, darkened urine, pale stools, or unusual tiredness.

Prototype: propranolol, p 109

ESMOLOL HYDROCHLORIDE
(ess´moe-lol)

Trade name: Brevibloc
Classifications: AUTONOMIC NERVOUS SYSTEM AGENT; BETA-ADRENERGIC ANTAGONIST (BLOCKING AGENT, SYMPATHOLYTIC); ANTIARRHYTHMIC
Pregnancy: Category C

ACTIONS/PHARMACODYNAMICS Ultrashort-acting $beta_1$-adrenergic blocking agent with cardioselective properties but devoid of intrinsic sympathetic activity (ISA) or membrane-stabilizing (quinidinelike) activity. Its unique properties, i.e., rapid onset of action and ultrashort elimination half-life, allow precise titration of levels of beta-blockade. Thus onset of undesirable side effects can be quickly reversed or terminated. Its hemodynamic effects are mild, with potency as a beta blocker about 1/100th that of propranolol. By competitive binding at beta-adrenergic receptors, inhibits the agonist effect of catecholamines. Since it binds predominantly to $beta_1$-receptors in cardiac tissue, sympathetically mediated increases in cardiac rate and BP are blocked. Esmolol rapidly reduces systolic hypertension and attenuates heart rate acceleration that accompanies anesthesia induction and intubation. Compatible with commonly used anesthetics.

USES Supraventricular tachyarrhythmias (SVT) in perioperative and postoperative periods or in other

---

Common side effects in *italic*; life-threatening effects <u>underlined</u>; generic names in **bold**; classifications in SMALL CAPS

569

critical situations. Also short-term treatment of non-compensating sinus tachycardia and in the control of heart rate for patients with MI. **Unlabeled uses:** moderate postoperative hypertension; treatment of intense transient adrenergic response to surgical stress in cardiac as well as noncardiac surgery.

ROUTE & DOSAGE

Supraventricular Tachyarrhythmias

Adult   IV   500 µg/kg loading dose followed by 50 µg/kg/min; may increase dose q5–10min prn (max 200 µg/kg/min)

PHARMACOKINETICS **Onset:** <5 min. **Peak:** 10–20 min. **Duration:** 10–30 min. **Metabolism:** rapidly hydrolyzed by RBC esterases. **Elimination:** half-life: 9 min; eliminated in urine.

CONTRAINDICATIONS & PRECAUTIONS **Contraindicated in:** cardiac failure, heart block greater than first degree, sinus bradycardia, cardiogenic shock. Safe use during pregnancy (category C), in nursing mothers, and in children not established. **Cautious use in:** history of allergy or bronchial asthma, bronchospasm, emphysema; CHF; diabetes mellitus; renal function impairment.

ADVERSE/SIDE EFFECTS **CNS:** headache, speech disorder, *dizziness,* diaphoresis, somnolence, confusion, paresthesia, asthenia, lightheadedness, grand mal seizures. **CV:** *hypotension* (dose related), cold hands and feet, bradyarrhythmias, flushing, myocardial depression. **GI:** nausea, vomiting, dysgeusia. **Respiratory:** dyspnea, chest pain, rhonchi, <u>bronchospasm</u>. **Skin:** *infusion site inflammation* (redness, swelling, induration), skin discoloration and burning; diaphoresis. **Other:** fever, urinary retention, muscle stiffness, midscapular pain, pallor, flushing.

DRUG INTERACTIONS May increase **digoxin** IV levels 10–20%; **morphine** IV may increase esmolol levels by 45%; **succinylcholine** may prolong neuromuscular blockade.

INCOMPATIBILITIES **Y-Site: furosemide.**

NURSING IMPLICATIONS

Administration

- Esmolol must be diluted before administration (available as a solution: 250 mg/ml in 10 ml ampuls).
- Preparation of infusion: dilute each 5 g with 20 ml of D5W, NS, or other appropriate diluent (see manufacturer's directions). Resulting solution yields 10 mg/ml. Caution: a stronger solution (e.g., 20 mg/ml) may cause venous irritation and thrombophlebitis.
- Do not admix with other drugs before dilution in a suitable IV fluid.
- Esmolol infusion may be administered via a central vein; use of butterfly needles is not recommended. Rate of infusion is determined by body weight (see route and dosage table).
- After heart rate control has been achieved with esmolol, transition to another antiarrhythmic agent (e.g., propranolol, digoxin, or calcium channel blocking agent) is accomplished as follows: 1/2 h after first dose of alternate agent, esmolol infusion rate is reduced by 50%. After second dose of the alternate agent, monitor response and if control is maintained for the first hour, discontinue esmolol infusion.
- Effects of abrupt withdrawal of esmolol have not been reported; however, sudden discontinuation of infusion in patient with coronary artery disease should be done with caution.
- Esmolol is intended for short-term use. A continuous infusion over a 24 h period seems to be well tolerated; limited data indicate that an infusion up to 48 h is also well tolerated.
- The diluted infusion solution is stable for at least 24 h at room temperature.
- Store ampuls at 15–30C (59–86F) unless otherwise directed.

Assessment & Drug Effects

- Monitor BP, pulse, ECG, during esmolol infusion.
- Hypotension may have its onset during the initial titration phase; thereafter the risk increases with increasing doses.
- Usually the hypotension experienced during esmolol infusion is resolved within 30 min after infusion is reduced or discontinued.
- IV site reactions (burning, erythema) or diaphoresis may develop during infusion. Both reactions are temporary, but injection site should be changed if local reaction occurs. Blood chemistry abnormalities have not been reported.
- ***Overdose symptoms:*** discontinue administration if the following symptoms appear: bradycardia, severe dizziness or drowsiness, dyspnea, bluish-colored fingernails or palms of hands, seizures.

ESTRADIOL

See HORMONES, ESTROGEN prototype, p 236.

Prototype: estradiol, p 236

ESTRADIOL CYPIONATE

Trade names: Depo-Estradiol, Cypionate, Depogen, Dura-Estrin, E-Ionate PA, Estra-D, Estro-Cyp, Estroject-LA, Hormogen Depot
Classifications: HORMONE; ESTROGEN

ACTIONS/PHARMACODYNAMICS Average duration of effects 3–8 wk.

USES See estradiol.

ROUTE & DOSAGE

Menopause
Adult   IM   1–5 mg q3–4wk

Female Hypogonadism
Adult   IM   1.5–2 mg every month

NURSING IMPLICATIONS

See numerous nursing implications under estradiol.
- Discuss package insert with patient to assure understanding of estrogen therapy.
- Store drug at controlled room temperature; protect from light.

Prototype: estradiol, p 236

ESTRADIOL VALERATE

Trade names: Delestrogen, Dioval, Duragen, Estraval-PA, Femogex, Valergen
Classifications: HORMONE; ESTROGEN

ACTIONS/PHARMACODYNAMICS Provides 2–3 wk of estrogen effects from single IM injection.

USES See estradiol.

ROUTE & DOSAGE

Menopause, Female Castration, Atrophic Vaginitis
Adult   IM   10–20 mg q4wk

Prostatic Carcinoma
Adult   IM   ≥ 30 mg q1–2wk

Prevention of Postpartum Breast Engorgement
Adult   IM   10–25 mg at end of first stage of labor

NURSING IMPLICATIONS

- See numerous nursing implications under estradiol, the prototype for estrogens.
- Discuss package insert with patient to assure understanding of estrogen therapy.
- Store drug at controlled room temperature; protect from light.

Prototype: mechlorethamine, p 96

ESTRAMUSTINE PHOSPHATE SODIUM

(ess-tra-muss´teen)
Trade name: Emcyt
Classification: ANTINEOPLASTIC; NITROGEN MUSTARD

ACTIONS/PHARMACODYNAMICS Conjugate of estradiol and the carbamate of nitrogen mustard. Extent of antitumor activity contributed by each, as well as precise mechanisms of action, unknown. Appears to act as a relatively weak alkylating agent and estrogen. Major effectiveness reported to be in patients who have been refractory to estrogen therapy alone.

USES Palliative treatment of metabolic or progressive carcinoma of prostate.

ROUTE & DOSAGE

Neoplasm
Adult   PO   14 mg/kg/d in 3–4 divided doses

PHARMACOKINETICS Absorption: readily absorbed from GI tract. **Peak:** 2–3 h. **Metabolism:** dephosphorylated in intestines to estramustine, estradiol, estrone, and nitrogen mustard; further metabolized in liver. **Elimination:** half-life: 20 h; excreted in feces via bile.

Common side effects in *italic*; life-threatening effects underlined; generic names in **bold**; classifications in SMALL CAPS

571

E

CONTRAINDICATIONS & PRECAUTIONS Con-
traindicated in: hypersensitivity to either estradiol or nitrogen mustard; active thrombophlebitis or thromboembolic disorders. **Cautious use in:** history of thrombophlebitis, thromboses, or thromboembolic disorders; cerebrovascular or coronary artery disease; gallstones or peptic ulcer; impaired liver function; metabolic bone diseases associated with hypercalcemia; diabetes mellitus; hypertension, conditions that might be aggravated by fluid retention (e.g., epilepsy, migraine, renal dysfunction); elderly patients.

ADVERSE/SIDE EFFECTS CNS: lethargy, emotional lability, insomnia, headache, anxiety, epilepsy. **CV:** hypertension, CVA, <u>MI,</u> *thrombophlebitis,* CHF, *peripheral edema.* **GI:** *nausea,* diarrhea, anorexia, flatulence, vomiting, thirst, GI bleeding. **Hematologic:** leukopenia, thrombocytopenia, hypercalcemia, *abnormalities in liver function tests.* **Respiratory:** hoarseness, burning sensation in throat, dyspnea, upper respiratory discharge, <u>pulmonary emboli.</u> **Skin:** rash, pruritus, urticaria, dry skin, easy bruising, flushing, peeling skin and fingertips, thinning hair. **Other:** tearing of eyes, gynecomastia, breast tenderness, impotence, renal dysfunction, leg cramps, decrease in glucose tolerance, bone marrow toxicity (uncommon).

FOOD-DRUG INTERACTIONS Milk, dairy products, calcium supplements, may decrease estramustine absorption.

NURSING IMPLICATIONS

Administration
- Drug can be taken with meals to reduce incidence of GI side effects. Some patients require drug withdrawal because of intolerable GI effects.
- Store in refrigerator at 2–8C (38–46F) in tight, light-resistant containers, unless otherwise directed by manufacturer.

Assessment & Drug Effects
- Check BP at regular intervals throughout therapy. Report significant elevations to physician.
- Keep track of weight and examine patient daily for peripheral edema. Be mindful that drug can cause CHF.
- Monitor I&O ratio and pattern to prevent dehydration and electrolyte imbalance, especially with vomiting or diarrhea.
- Patients with diabetes should be closely observed because of possibility of estramustine-induced reduction in glucose tolerance. Baseline and periodic glucose tolerance tests are advised.

- Baseline and periodic hepatic enzymes and bilirubin tests should be performed, then repeated after drug has been discontinued for 2 mo.
- Patient should receive therapy for 30–90 d before evaluations are made to determine adequacy of response and possible benefits of continuing treatment.
- Some patients have received therapy more than 3 y. Therapy is usually continued as long as patient demonstrates a favorable response.

Patient & Family Education
- To reduce drug-induced nausea, instruct patient to eat small feedings at frequent intervals; eat slowly; avoid fried, greasy, spicy, and overly sweet foods; and attempt cold food if food odors are offensive.
- Instruct patient to keep physically quiet when nauseated and keep upper torso elevated (for about 2 h after eating).
- Advise patient to drink liquids 1 h before or 1 h after rather than with meals; clear liquids may be more palatable.
- Patient should be advised to use a barrier contraceptive. (Drug has mutagenic and teratogenic properties.) Some patients formerly impotent have regained potency while taking estramustine.
- Advise patient who experiences thinning of hair to avoid vigorous treatment of scalp and to wash and comb hair gently.

Prototype: estradiol, p 236

ESTROGENS, CONJUGATED
(ess´tro-jenz)
Trade names: C.E.S., Estrocon, Premarin, Progens
Classifications: HORMONE; ESTROGEN
Pregnancy: Category X

ACTIONS/PHARMACODYNAMICS Short-acting estrogen mixture of conjugated estrogens including sodium estrone sulfate and sodium equilin sulfate. Binds to intracellular receptors that stimulate DNA and RNA to synthesize proteins responsible for effects of estrogen.

USES Atrophic vaginitis, kraurosis vulvae, and abnormal bleeding (hormonal imbalance); also female hypogonadism, primary ovarian failure, vasomotor symptoms associated with menopause; to retard pro-

gression of osteoporosis and as palliative therapy of breast and prostatic carcinomas. **Unlabeled use:** post-coital contraceptive.

ROUTE & DOSAGE

Menopause, Osteoporosis, Atrophic Vaginitis, Kraurosis Vulvae

Adult	PO	0.3–1.25 mg/d for 21 d each month; adjust to lowest level that gives symptom control (≤0.625 mg/d)
	IM/IV	25 mg; repeated in 6–12 h if needed
	Topical	2–4 g of cream/d

Female Hypogonadism

Adult	PO	2.5–7.5 mg/d in 1–3 divided doses for 20 d; followed by a 10 d rest period

Postcoital Contraception

Adult	PO	30 mg/d in divided doses for 5 consecutive days beginning within 72 h of coitus

Breast Cancer

Adult	PO	10 mg t.i.d. for at least 3 mo

Prostatic Cancer (Palliation)

Adult	PO	1.25–2.5 mg t.i.d.

CONTRAINDICATIONS & PRECAUTIONS Con-
traindicated in: breast cancer, known or suspected pregnancy (category X). **Cautious use in:** hypertension; gallbladder disease; diabetes mellitus; heart failure; hepatic or renal dysfunction, history of thromboembolic disease.

ADVERSE/SIDE EFFECTS CNS: headache, dizziness, depression, *libido changes*. **CV:** thromboembolic disorders, hypertension. **GI:** *nausea*, vomiting, diarrhea, bloating, cholestatic jaundice. **GU:** mastodynia, spotting, changes in menstrual flow, dysmenorrhea, amenorrhea. **Metabolic:** reduced carbohydrate tolerance, fluid retention. **Other:** leg cramps.

DRUG INTERACTIONS Carbamazepine, phen-
ytoin, rifampin decrease estrogen levels because they increase its metabolism; may enhance steroid effects of CORTICOSTEROIDS; may decrease anticoagulant effects of ORAL ANTICOAGULANTS.

NURSING IMPLICATIONS

See numerous additional implications under estradiol.

Administration

- Tablet can be taken with food or liquid of patient's choice.
- Given cyclically except when used for treatment of postpartum breast engorgement and for palliation of cancer. Cyclic regimen: dose for 3 wk followed by 1 wk off.
- Conjugated estrogens solution is compatible with D5W and NS and is incompatible with any solution with an acid pH (<7.0). Rapid IV injection may cause skin flushing.
- IV estrogen is given slowly by direct IV injection at a rate of 5 mg/min.
- Before reconstitution for IV or IM, refrigerate ampul at 2–8C (36–46F). To reconstitute, add diluent to ampul and agitate gently; use within a few hours.
- If reconstituted solution is stored in refrigerator and protected from light, it will remain stable for 60 d. Discard precipitated or discolored solution.
- ***Morning after pill:*** When used as an emergency postcoital contraceptive as for rape or for incest, drug is started within 24 h and not later than 72 h after sexual exposure. A pregnancy test is performed before dosing.
- Store vaginal cream at 15–30C (59–86F); protect from light and from freezing.

Patient & Family Education

- Severe nausea and vomiting (because of high dosage) reenforces noncompliance with morning after pill. An antiemetic may be required. Full course of the regimen must be taken if pregnancy is to be prevented. Emotional support from family or caregiver is of primary importance.
- Be certain patient is aware of importance of taking drug exactly as prescribed: specifically, doses should not be omitted, increased, or decreased without advice of physician.
- Intravaginal estrogen cream is readily absorbed and reaches blood levels approaching those of parenteral or orally administered estrogen. Systemic hyperestrogenic effects (uterine bleeding, edema, mastalgia, reactivation of endometriosis) may result from overdosage of intravaginal cream or from overexposure of denuded or abraded skin surfaces of hands to estrogen.
- A calibrated dosage applicator should be dispensed with the vaginal cream. Inform the patient.
- ***Intravaginal administration:*** If patient is to administer medication to herself, instruct her to wash her hands well before and after the application, and to avoid contact of denuded areas with the cream.

Also tell her not to use tampons while on vaginal cream therapy.
- Caution patient to report adverse symptoms of estrogen therapy to the physician promptly.
- Risk of blood clot formation is high with morning after pill. Discuss signs of thrombophlebitis (see chap 3).
- Review package insert with patient to assure understanding of estrogen therapy.

Prototype: estradiol, p 236

ESTROGENS, ESTERIFIED

Trade names: Estratab, Menest, Menrium
Classifications: HORMONE; ESTROGEN
Pregnancy: Category X

ACTIONS/PHARMACODYNAMICS Combination of same estrogens as found in conjugated estrogens (but in different proportions): sodium estrone sulfate and sodium equilin sulfate. Binds to intracellular receptors that stimulate DNA and RNA to synthesize proteins responsible for effects of estrogen.

USES Atrophic vaginitis, kraurosis vulvae and abnormal bleeding (hormonal imbalance); also used to treat female hypogonadism, and castration, primary ovarian failure, vasomotor symptoms associated with menopause; and as palliative therapy of breast and prostatic carcinomas.

ROUTE & DOSAGE

Menopause

Adult	PO	0.3–1.25 mg/d for 21 d each month; adjust to lowest level that gives symptom control (≤ 0.625 mg/d)

Female Hypogonadism, Primary Ovarian Failure, Female Castration

Adult	PO	2.5–7.5 mg/d in 1–3 divided doses for 20 d followed by a 10 d rest period; during last 5 d of estrogen, give a PO progestin

Breast Cancer

Adult	PO	10 mg t.i.d. for 2–3 mo

Prostatic Cancer (Palliation)

Adult	PO	1.25–2.5 mg t.i.d. for several weeks

CONTRAINDICATIONS & PRECAUTIONS Contraindicated in: breast cancer; known or suspected pregnancy (category X). **Cautious use in:** hypertension; gallbladder disease; diabetes mellitus; heart failure; hepatic or renal dysfunction; history of thromboembolic disease.

ADVERSE/SIDE EFFECTS CNS: headache, dizziness, depression, *libido changes*. **CV:** <u>thromboembolic disorders</u>, hypertension. **GI:** *nausea,* vomiting, diarrhea, bloating, cholestatic jaundice. **GU:** mastodynia, spotting, changes in menstrual flow, dysmenorrhea, amenorrhea. **Metabolic:** reduced carbohydrate tolerance, fluid retention. **Other:** leg cramps.

DRUG INTERACTIONS Carbamazepine, phenytoin, rifampin decrease estrogen levels because they increase its metabolism; may enhance steroid effects of CORTICOSTEROIDS; may decrease anticoagulant effects of ORAL ANTICOAGULANTS.

NURSING IMPLICATIONS
See numerous nursing implications under estradiol.

Administration
- Tablet can be taken with food or fluid of patient's choice.
- Given cyclically, except when used for palliation of cancer.
- Store tablets at 15–30C (59–86F) in a tightly closed container.

Patient & Family Education
- Be certain patient is aware of importance of taking drug exactly as prescribed: specifically, doses should not be omitted, increased, or decreased without advice of physician. Patient should also be made aware of what to do when a dose is missed.
- Review package insert with patient to assure understanding of estrogen therapy.

Common side effects in *italic*; life-threatening effects <u>underlined</u>; generic names in **bold**; classifications in SMALL CAPS

Prototype: estradiol, p 236

ESTRONE
(ess´trone)
Trade name: Femogen

ESTRONE AQUEOUS SUSPENSION
Trade names: Estronol, Kestrone-5, Theelin
Aqueous

ESTROGENIC SUBSTANCE AQUEOUS SUSPENSION
Trade names: Estaqua, Estrofol, Estroject-2,
Foygen Aqueous, Gravigen Aqueous, Gynogen
Classifications: HORMONE; ESTROGEN
Pregnancy: Category X

ACTIONS/PHARMACODYNAMICS First sex hormone isolated in pure form; present in urine of pregnant mares along with other estrogens. Binds to intracellular receptors that stimulate DNA and RNA to synthesize proteins responsible for effects of estrogen.

USES Atrophic vaginitis, kraurosis vulvae, and abnormal bleeding (hormonal imbalance); also female hypogonadism, primary ovarian failure, vasomotor symptoms associated with menopause, and as palliative therapy of prostatic carcinoma.

ROUTE & DOSAGE

Menopause
Adult   IM   0.1–0.5 mg 2–3 times/wk

Female Hypogonadism, Primary Ovarian Failure
Adult   IM   0.1–1 mg/wk in single or divided doses

Inoperable Prostatic Cancer (Palliation)
Adult   IM   2–4 mg/d 2–3 times/wk

CONTRAINDICATIONS & PRECAUTIONS Contraindicated in: breast cancer; known or suspected pregnancy (category X). **Cautious use in:** hypertension; gallbladder disease; diabetes mellitus; heart failure; hepatic or renal dysfunction; history of thromboembolic disease.

ADVERSE/SIDE EFFECTS CNS: headache, dizziness, depression, *libido changes*. **CV:** thromboem-bolic disorders, hypertension. **GI:** *nausea*, vomiting, diarrhea, bloating, cholestatic jaundice. **GU:** mastodynia, spotting, changes in menstrual flow, dysmenorrhea, amenorrhea. **Metabolic:** reduced carbohydrate tolerance, fluid retention. **Other:** leg cramps.

DRUG INTERACTIONS Carbamazepine, phenytoin, rifampin decrease estrogen levels because they increase its metabolism; may enhance steroid effects of CORTICOSTEROIDS; may decrease anticoagulant effects of ORAL ANTICOAGULANTS.

NURSING IMPLICATIONS
See numerous nursing implications under estradiol.

Administration
■ Shake vial and syringe well to suspend medication before withdrawing and injecting medication.
■ Store at 15–30C (59–86F) unless otherwise directed by manufacturer. Protect from light and from freezing.

Assessment & Drug Effects
■ Patients with conditions that may be influenced by fluid retention (migraine, cardiac or renal dysfunction, asthma, epilepsy, hypertension) should be monitored carefully. Check BP on a regular basis.
■ Spotting or breakthrough bleeding occurring when a barbiturate and estrone are taken concurrently indicates reduced availability of the estrogen.

Patient & Family Education
■ Review package insert with patient to assure understanding of estrogen therapy.
■ Advise patient to determine weight under standard conditions 1 or 2 times/wk and to report sudden weight gain or other signs of fluid retention.
■ Teach patient how to elicit **Homan's sign:** pain in calf and popliteal region with forced dorsiflexion of foot (early sign of thrombosis).
■ Instruct patient to report a positive Homan's sign and the following symptoms of thromboembolic disorders immediately: tenderness, swelling, and redness in extremity; sudden, severe headache or chest pain, slurring of speech; change in vision; tenderness, pain, sudden shortness of breath. If physician is not available, patient should go to the nearest hospital emergency room.
■ Symptoms of vaginal candidiasis (thick, white, curdlike secretions and inflamed, congested introitus) should be reported to permit appropriate treatment.
■ Advise patient to report severe abdominal pain and tenderness or abdominal mass, possible symptoms of hepatic adenoma or hepatic hemorrhage.

- If user suspects she is pregnant, she should stop taking the estrogen immediately and inform the physician. She should be apprised of the potential risk of masculinization of female fetus.
- Estrogen stimulation in women sterilized because of endometriosis may cause serious bleeding in remaining foci of endometrial tissues. Report unexplained and sudden pain.

Prototype: estradiol, p 236

ESTROPIPATE

(es-troe-pi´pate)

Trade names: Ogen, Piperazine Estrone Sulfate

Classifications: HORMONE; ESTROGEN

Pregnancy: Category X

ACTIONS/PHARMACODYNAMICS Water-soluble preparation of pure crystalline estrone (responsible for therapeutic actions conjugated as the sulfate and stabilized with piperazine). Binds to intracellular receptors that stimulate DNA and RNA to synthesize proteins responsible for effects of estrogen.

USES Atrophic vaginitis, kraurosis vulvae, and abnormal bleeding (hormonal imbalance); also female hypogonadism, primary ovarian failure, vasomotor symptoms associated with menopause, and as palliative therapy of prostatic carcinoma.

ROUTE & DOSAGE

Menopause, Atrophic Vaginitis, Kraurosis Vulvae

Adult	PO	0.75–6 mg/d for 21 d each month; adjust to lowest level that gives symptom control
	Intravaginal	2–4 g of cream once/d in a cyclic regimen

Female Hypogonadism, Primary Ovarian Failure, Female Castration

Adult	PO	1.5–9 mg/d in 1–3 divided doses for 21 d, followed by a 8–10 d drug-free period

CONTRAINDICATIONS & PRECAUTIONS Contraindicated in: estrogen hypersensitivity, breast cancer, known or suspected pregnancy (category X). **Cautious use in:** hypertension; gallbladder disease; diabetes mellitus; heart failure; hepatic or renal dysfunction; history of thromboembolic disease.

ADVERSE/SIDE EFFECTS CNS: headache, dizziness, depression, *libido changes*. **CV:** thromboembolic disorders, hypertension. **GI:** *nausea,* vomiting, diarrhea, bloating, cholestatic jaundice. **GU:** mastodynia, spotting, changes in menstrual flow, dysmenorrhea, amenorrhea. **Metabolic:** reduced carbohydrate tolerance, fluid retention. **Other:** leg cramps.

DRUG INTERACTIONS Carbamazepine, phenytoin, rifampin decrease estrogen levels because they increase its metabolism; may enhance steroid effects of CORTICOSTEROIDS; may decrease anticoagulant effects of ORAL ANTICOAGULANTS.

NURSING IMPLICATIONS

See numerous nursing implications under estradiol.

Administration

- Tablet may be taken with food or fluid of patient's choice.
- Vaginal cream is dispensed with a calibrated dosage applicator. Squeeze tube of cream to force sufficient amount into applicator so that number on plunger indicating prescribed dose is level with top of barrel.
- Store in tightly closed containers at 15–30C (59–86F) unless otherwise directed.

Patient & Family Education

- Between uses, pull plunger out of barrel and wash applicator in warm soapy water. Do not place plunger in hot or boiling water.
- Warn patient not to use tampons while on vaginal cream therapy.
- If patient is to administer medication to herself, instruct her to wash her hands well before and after the procedure.
- Estrogen in cream is readily absorbed from the vaginal mucosa and reaches blood levels approaching those of parenteral or orally administered estrogen. Systemic hyperestrogenic effects (reportable) (uterine bleeding, edema, mastalgia, reactivation of endometriosis) may result from overdosage of intravaginal drug or from overexposure of denuded or abraded skin surfaces of hands to estrogen.
- Sudden discontinuation of vaginal cream after high dosage or prolonged use may evoke withdrawal bleeding.
- Review patient package insert (PPI) with patient.

Common side effects in *italic*; life-threatening effects underlined; generic names in **bold**; classifications in SMALL CAPS

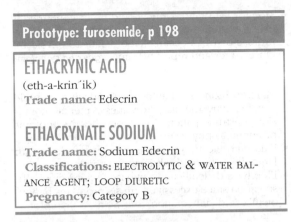

Prototype: furosemide, p 198

ETHACRYNIC ACID
(eth-a-krin′ik)
Trade name: Edecrin

ETHACRYNATE SODIUM

Trade name: Sodium Edecrin
Classifications: ELECTROLYTIC & WATER BALANCE AGENT; LOOP DIURETIC
Pregnancy: Category B

ACTIONS/PHARMACODYNAMICS Unsaturated ketone derivative of phenoxyacetic acid with rapid and potent diuretic action. Action mechanism is unclear but may involve blocking of sulfhydryl-catalyzed enzyme systems. Inhibits sodium and chloride reabsorption in proximal tubule and most segments of loop of Henle, promotes potassium and hydrogen ion excretion, and decreases urinary ammonium ion concentration and pH. Appears to have little effect on bicarbonate excretion, but chloruretic effect may foster bicarbonate retention. Promotes calcium elimination in hypercalcemia and nephrogenic diabetes insipidus. Paradoxic decrease in urine volume may follow drug-induced sodium loss. Fluid-electrolyte loss may exceed that caused by thiazides, but the effect on carbohydrate metabolism and blood glucose is less. Tends to promote urate excretion at high doses and retention at low doses. Does not inhibit carbonic anhydrase; action is independent of systemic acid-base balance. Appears to have little or no direct effect on renal blood flow or glomerular filtration rate. Aldosterone secretion may be increased, thus contributing to hypokalemia. Hypotensive effect may be due to hypovolemia secondary to diuresis and in part to decreased vascular resistance.

USES Severe edema associated with CHF, hepatic cirrhosis, ascites of malignancy, renal disease, nephrotic syndrome, lymphedema. **Unlabeled uses:** treatment of nephrogenic diabetes insipidus, hypercalcemia, mild to moderate hypertension, and as adjunct in therapy of hypertensive crisis complicated by pulmonary edema.

PHARMACOKINETICS Absorption: rapidly absorbed from GI tract. **Onset:** 30 min PO; 5 min IV. **Peak:** 2 h PO; 15–30 min IV. **Duration:** 6–8 h PO; 2 h IV. **Distribution:** does not cross CSF. **Metabolism:** me-

ROUTE & DOSAGE

Edema

Adult	PO	50–100 mg 1–2 times/d; may increase by 25–50 mg prn up to 400 mg/d
	IV	0.5–1 mg/kg or 50 mg up to 100 mg; may repeat if necessary
Child	PO	25 mg daily, may increase by 25 mg/d as needed

tabolized to cysteine conjugate. **Elimination:** half-life: 30–70 min; 30–65% excreted in urine; 35–40% excreted in bile.

CONTRAINDICATIONS & PRECAUTIONS Contraindicated in: history of hypersensitivity to ethacrynic acid; increasing azotemia, anuria; hepatic coma; severe diarrhea, dehydration, electrolyte imbalance, hypotension; pregnancy (category B), nursing mothers, infants, parenteral use in pediatric patients. **Cautious use in:** hepatic cirrhosis; elderly cardiac patients; diabetes mellitus; history of gout; pulmonary edema associated with acute MI; hyperaldosteronism; nephrotic syndrome; history of pancreatitis.

ADVERSE/SIDE EFFECTS CNS: headache, fatigue, weakness, apprehension, confusion, local irritation of IV site. **CV:** *postural hypotension* (dizziness, lightheadedness), thrombophlebitis, emboli. **Electrolyte imbalance:** hyponatremia, *hypokalemia,* hypochloremic alkalosis, hypomagnesemia, hypocalcemia, hypercalciuria, hyperuricemia, hypovolemia. **ENT:** vertigo, tinnitus, sense of fullness in ears, temporary or permanent deafness. **GI:** anorexia, diarrhea, nausea, vomiting, dysphagia, abdominal discomfort or pain, GI bleeding (IV use), acute pancreatitis (increased serum amylase), abnormal liver function tests, jaundice, hepatic damage. **Hematologic:** <u>thrombocytopenia, agranulocytosis, severe neutropenia,</u> Henloch's purpura (in patients with rheumatic fever), hypoproteinemia. **Skin:** skin rash, pruritus. **Other:** tetany, acute gout; elevated BUN, creatinine, and urate levels; uricosuria, hematuria, glycosuria, hyperglycemia, acute hypoglycemia with seizures (rare), gynecomastia, fever, chills, malaise, blurred vision.

DRUG INTERACTIONS THIAZIDE DIURETICS increase potassium loss; increased risk of **digoxin** toxicity from hypokalemia; CORTICOSTEROIDS, **amphotericin B** increase risk of hypokalemia; decreased **lithium** clearance, so increased risk of lithium toxicity; SULFONYLUREA effect may be blunted, causing hyperglycemia; ANTIHYPERTENSIVE AGENTS increase risk of orthostatic hypotension; AMINOGLYCOSIDES may in-

Common side effects in *italic*; life-threatening effects <u>underlined</u>; generic names in **bold**; classifications in SMALL CAPS

577

E

crease risk of ototoxicity; **warfarin** potentiates hypoprothrombinemia.

INCOMPATIBILITIES Solution/Additive: hydralazine, procainamide, tolazoline, triflupromazine.

NURSING IMPLICATIONS

Administration

- Administer PO drug after a meal or food to prevent gastric irritation.
- Schedule doses to avoid nocturia and thus sleep interference. Avoid administration within at least 4 h of bedtime, if possible. This recommendation may not apply to the patient who accumulates fluid and develops respiratory symptoms during sleep.
- Reconstitute for IV administration by adding 50 ml of 5% dextrose injection or 0.9% of NaCl injection to vial. Solution should be used within 24 h. Discard cloudy solutions.
- Parenteral drug is intended for IV use only. It is given slowly into tubing of a running infusion of compatible IV fluid or by direct IV injection over several minutes.
- If a second IV dose is required, a new site should be selected to prevent thrombophlebitis.
- Store oral tablet and parenteral dosage form at 15–30C (59–86F) unless otherwise directed.

Assessment & Drug Effects

- Patient should be observed closely when receiving the drug by IV infusion. Rapid, copious diuresis following IV administration can produce hypotension and peripheral vascular collapse.
- Extravasation of IV drug causes local pain and tissue irritation from dehydration and blood volume depletion.
- Baseline and periodic determinations should be made of blood count, serum electrolytes, CO_2, BUN, creatinine, blood sugar, uric acid, and liver function.
- Monitor BP during initial therapy. Because orthostatic hypotension can occur, supervision of ambulation is indicated.
- For patients with impaired cardiac function, monitor BP and pulse throughout therapy. Diuretic-induced hypovolemia may reduce cardiac output, and electrolyte loss promotes cardiotoxicity in those receiving digitalis (cardiac) glycosides.
- Establish baseline weight prior to start of therapy; weigh patient under standard conditions. Keep physician informed of weight loss or gain in excess of 1 kg (2 lb)/d.

- Monitor I&O ratio. Drug should be discontinued if excessive diuresis, oliguria, hematuria, or sudden profuse diarrhea occurs. Report signs to physician.
- Observe for and report warning *signs and symptoms of electrolyte imbalance:* anorexia, nausea, vomiting, thirst, dry mouth, polyuria, oliguria, weakness, fatigue, dizziness, faintness, headache, muscle cramps, paresthesias, drowsiness, mental confusion. Instruct patient to report these symptoms promptly to physician.
- Fluid and electrolyte depletion is most likely with large doses or rigid salt-intake restriction.
- Elderly and debilitated patients require close observation since excessive diuresis promotes hypovolemia and dehydration (see Signs & Symptoms, chap 3).
- Report immediately possible signs of thromboembolic complications (see Signs & Symptoms, chap 3).
- In patients receiving any other potentially ototoxic drug concurrently with ethacrynic acid, renal status, audiograms, and vestibular function tests are advised before initiation of therapy and regularly throughout therapy.
- Impaired glucose tolerance with hyperglycemia and glycosuria has occurred in patients receiving doses in excess of 200 mg/d. Diabetic and diabetic-prone individuals, patients with potassium depletion, or decompensated hepatic cirrhosis are especially susceptible.

Patient & Family Education

- Explain diuretic effect (increased volume and frequency of voiding) to the patient. Diuretic effect tends to diminish with continuous therapy.
- Teach patient signs and symptoms of hypokalemia and hyponatremia (see chap 3), and advise patient to report any of these promptly.
- Caution patient to make position changes slowly, particularly from recumbent to upright posture.
- GI side effects occur most frequently after 1–3 mo of PO therapy or in patients on high dosage. The onset of loose stools or other GI symptoms at any time during therapy should be reported to permit dosage adjustment or discontinuation of drug if indicated.
- Report immediately any evidence of impaired hearing. Hearing loss may be preceded by vertigo, tinnitus, or fullness in ears; it may be transient, lasting 1–24 h, or it may be permanent.

Common side effects in *italic*; life-threatening effects underlined; generic names in **bold**; classifications in SMALL CAPS

Prototype: isoniazid, p 83

ETHAMBUTOL HYDROCHLORIDE
(e-tham´byoo-tole)
Trade names: Etibi, Myambutol
Classifications: ANTIINFECTIVE;
ANTITUBERCULOSIS AGENT
Pregnancy: Category B

ACTIONS/PHARMACODYNAMICS Synthetic antituberculosis agent with bacteriostatic action. Mode of action not completely understood, but it appears to inhibit RNA synthesis and thus arrests multiplication of tubercle bacilli. Not recommended for use as sole agent. The emergence of resistant strains is delayed by administering ethambutol in combination with other antituberculosis drugs.

USES In conjunction with at least one other antituberculosis agent in treatment of pulmonary tuberculosis. **Unlabeled use:** atypical mycobacterial infections.

ROUTE & DOSAGE

Tuberculosis

Adult	PO	15 mg/kg q24h; for retreatment start with 25 mg/kg/d for 60 d; then decrease to 15 mg/kg/d
Child	PO	6–12 y: 10–15 mg/kg/d

PHARMACOKINETICS Absorption: 70–80% absorbed from GI tract. **Peak:** 2–4 h. **Distribution:** distributes to most body tissues; highest concentrations in erythrocytes, kidney, lungs, saliva; crosses placenta; distributed into breast milk. **Metabolism:** metabolized in liver. **Elimination:** half-life: 3–4 h; 50% excreted in urine within 24 h; 20–22% excreted in feces.

CONTRAINDICATIONS & PRECAUTIONS Contraindicated in: optic neuritis; children <13 y. Safe use during pregnancy (category B) not established. **Cautious use in:** patients with renal impairment; gout; ocular defects, e.g., cataract, recurrent ocular inflammatory conditions, diabetic retinopathy.

ADVERSE/SIDE EFFECTS CNS: headache, dizziness, confusion, hallucinations, paresthesias, peripheral neuritis (rare), joint pains and weakness of lower extremities. **Eye:** ocular toxicity: *retrobulbar optic neuritis;* possibility of anterior optic neuritis with decrease in visual acuity, temporary loss of vision, constriction of visual fields, red-green color blindness, central and peripheral scotomas, eye pain, photophobia; retinal hemorrhage and edema. **GI:** anorexia, nausea, vomiting, abdominal pain. **Hypersensitivity:** pruritus, dermatitis, anaphylaxis. **Other:** hyperuricemia, fever, malaise, leukopenia (rare), bloody sputum, transient impairment of liver function (possibly hepatotoxicity); nephrotoxicity, acute gouty arthritis, ECG abnormalities, excessive sweating.

NURSING IMPLICATIONS

Administration
- Ethambutol may be taken with food if GI irritation occurs. Absorption is not significantly affected by food in stomach.
- Protect ethambutol from light, moisture, and excessive heat. Store in tightly closed container at 15–30C (59–86F) unless otherwise directed.

Assessment & Drug Effects
- Culture and susceptibility tests should be performed before initiation of therapy and repeated periodically throughout therapy.
- Ocular toxicity generally appears within 1–7 mo after start of therapy. Symptoms usually disappear within several weeks to months after drug is discontinued, depending on degree of ocular damage.
- Ophthalmoscopic examination including tests of visual fields (finger perimetry), tests for visual acuity using a Snellen eye chart, and tests for color discrimination should be performed prior to start of therapy and at monthly intervals during therapy. Eyes should be tested separately as well as together.
- Monitor I&O ratio in patients with renal impairment. Report oliguria or any significant changes in ratio or in laboratory reports of renal function. Systemic accumulation with toxicity can result from delayed drug excretion.
- Hepatic and renal function tests, blood cell counts, and serum uric acid determinations should be performed at regular intervals throughout therapy.

Patient & Family Education
- Emphasize importance of adhering to drug regimen and of keeping follow-up appointments.
- In general, therapy may continue for 1–2 y or longer, although shorter treatment regimens have been used with success.
- If patient becomes pregnant during therapy, advise her to notify physician immediately. Drug should be withdrawn.
- Advise patient to report promptly to physician the onset of blurred vision, changes in color percep-

Common side effects in *italic*; life-threatening effects underlined; generic names in **bold**; classifications in SMALL CAPS

579

tion, constriction of visual fields, or any other visual symptoms. Patient should be questioned periodically about eyes.

- If detected early, visual defects generally disappear over several weeks to months. In rare instances, recovery may be delayed for a year or more or defect may be irreversible.

Prototype: hydralazine, p 152

ETHAVERINE HYDROCHLORIDE

(e´tha-ve-rine)

Trade names: Ethaquin, Ethatab, Ethavex-100, Isovex

Classifications: CARDIOVASCULAR AGENT; NONNITRATE VASODILATOR

Pregnancy: Category C

ACTIONS/PHARMACODYNAMICS Ethaverine is an alkaloid prepared synthetically or from opium. It has no narcotic properties. It directly relaxes all smooth muscles, especially when they have been spasmodically contracted. Vasodilation may be related to its ability to inhibit cyclic phosphodiesterase, thus increasing levels of intracellular cyclic AMP. When spasm is present, action is especially pronounced on coronary, cerebral, pulmonary, and peripheral arteries. Like quinidine, acts directly on myocardium, depresses conduction and irritability, and prolongs refractory period. Stimulates respiration by action on the carotid and aortic body chemoreceptors. Relaxes smooth muscles of bronchi, GI tract, ureters, and biliary system. Objective proof of therapeutic value is reportedly lacking.

USES Primarily for peripheral and cerebral vascular insufficiency associated with arterial spasm; also a smooth muscle spasmolytic in spastic conditions of the GI and GU tracts.

ROUTE & DOSAGE

Peripheral and Cerebral Vascular Insufficiency

Adult	PO	100 mg t.i.d.; may increase up to 200 mg t.i.d.

PHARMACOKINETICS Absorption: readily absorbed from GI tract. **Peak:** 1–2 h. **Duration:** 6 h regular tablets. **Metabolism:** metabolized in liver. **Elimination:** excreted in urine chiefly as metabolites.

CONTRAINDICATIONS & PRECAUTIONS Contraindicated in: complete atrioventricular dissociation (AV heart block) and severe hepatic disease. **Cautious use in:** patients with glaucoma, pregnancy (category C), nursing mothers, and myocardial depression.

ADVERSE/SIDE EFFECTS CNS: vertigo, *headache, drowsiness*. **CV:** *hypotension,* arrhythmias. **GI:** nausea, anorexia, abdominal distress, dry throat. **Other:** malaise, *flushing,* sweating, lassitude, <u>respiratory depression</u>.

DRUG INTERACTIONS May decrease **levodopa** effectiveness; **morphine** may antagonize smooth muscle relaxation effect of ethaverine.

NURSING IMPLICATIONS

Administration

- Monitor heart rate (apical pulse for 1 full minute) and BP; if significant changes occur (e.g., hypotension, arrhythmias), withhold drug and notify physician.
- Preserve in a tightly covered, light-resistant container.

Assessment & Drug Effects

- Routinely monitor apical pulse for changes in rate and rhythm. Drug may cause cardiac arrhythmias.
- Monitor BP for hypotension, and respiration rate for respiratory depression. Promptly report marked changed to physician.
- Liver function and blood tests should be performed periodically. Hepatotoxicity (thought to be a hypersensitivity reaction) is reversible with prompt drug withdrawal.

Patient & Family Education

- Since nicotine constricts blood vessels, encourage patients with peripheral vascular problems not to smoke.
- Since drug may cause dizziness and drowsiness, advise patients to avoid driving and potentially hazardous tasks until reaction to drug is known.
- Warn patient that alcohol may increase drowsiness and dizziness.
- Instruct patient to notify physician if jaundice or skin rash appear. Hepatic function tests may be indicated.
- Inform patient that drug may cause flushing, headache, and diaphoresis; physician should be notified if symptoms are pronounced.
- Advise patient to notify physician if GI distress develops and persists.

E

Common side effects in *italic*; life-threatening effects <u>underlined</u>; generic names in **bold**; classifications in SMALL CAPS

Prototype: secobarbital, p 175

ETHCHLORVYNOL

(eth-klor-vi'nole)
Trade name: Placidyl
Classifications: CNS AGENT; BARBITURATE
ANXIOLYTIC, SEDATIVE-HYPNOTIC
Pregnancy: Category C
Controlled substance: Schedule IV

ACTIONS/PHARMACODYNAMICS CNS depressant effects similar to those of chloral hydrate and barbiturates. Mechanism of action not known. Hypnotic doses produce cerebral depression and quiet, deep sleep; sedative doses reduce anxiety and apprehension. Also exhibits anticonvulsant and muscle relaxant activity. Has no analgesic properties. Effect on REM sleep not known. Not commonly used as a sedative because of its short duration of action.

USES Short-term therapy of simple insomnia for periods up to 1 wk.

ROUTE & DOSAGE

Sedative

Adult	PO	200 mg b.i.d. or t.i.d.

Hypnotic

Adult	PO	500 mg–1 g h.s.; may give an additional 200 mg if patient awakens early

PHARMACOKINETICS Absorption: readily absorbed from GI tract. **Onset:** 15–30 min. **Peak:** 1–2 h. **Duration:** 5 h. **Distribution:** localizes in adipose tissue, liver, kidney, spleen, brain, CSF, bile; crosses placenta; distribution into breast milk unknown. **Metabolism:** metabolized in liver with enterohepatic cycling and possibly in kidney. **Elimination:** half-life: 20–100 h; 10% excreted in urine within 24 h.

CONTRAINDICATIONS & PRECAUTIONS Contraindicated in: porphyria; patients with uncontrolled pain; first and second trimesters of pregnancy (category C). Safe use in nursing mothers and in children not established. **Cautious use in:** third trimester of pregnancy; patients with mental depression or suicidal tendencies, addiction-prone individuals; impaired hepatic or renal function; elderly or debilitated patients; patients who respond unpredictably to alcohol or barbiturates.

ADVERSE/SIDE EFFECTS CNS: dizziness, facial numbness, headache, mild hangover, tremors, incoordination, slurred speech, ataxia, prolonged hypnosis, profound muscular weakness, excitement, hysteria, syncope; overdosage: stupor, coma, respiratory failure. **CV:** overdosage: bradycardia, *hypotension*. **Eye:** blurred vision, nystagmus, toxic amblyopia, permanent visual defects, peripheral neuropathy. **GI:** nausea, vomiting, aftertaste. **Hypersensitivity:** urticaria, thrombocytopenia, cholestatic jaundice.

DIAGNOSTIC TEST INTERFERENCES *Phentolamine test:* false-positive test results (ethchlorvynol should be withdrawn at least 24 h before the test).

DRUG INTERACTIONS Alcohol and other CNS DEPRESSANTS amplify CNS depression; decrease anticoagulation effect of ORAL ANTICOAGULANTS.

NURSING IMPLICATIONS

Administration

- Ethchlorvynol produces transient giddiness and ataxia in some patients who apparently absorb the drug rapidly. Symptoms may be minimized by administering the drug with milk or other food.
- Preserve in tight, light-resistant containers (darkens on exposure to light; slight darkening does not affect potency). Store at 15–30C (59–86F) unless otherwise directed.

Assessment & Drug Effects

- Report the appearance of mental confusion, hallucinations, or drowsiness in patients receiving daytime sedation; decrease in dosage or drug discontinuation is indicated.
- The elderly may not tolerate average adult doses. Observe intensity and duration of drug action.
- Severe withdrawal symptoms may occur if drug is discontinued abruptly in patients taking regular doses (unusual anxiety, tremors, ataxia, irritability, slurred speech, memory loss, hallucinations, delirium, convulsions).

Patient & Family Education

- Caution patient to avoid driving a motor vehicle or engaging in other activities requiring mental alertness and physical coordination for at least 5 h after taking drug.
- Psychological and physical dependence are possible; therefore prolonged administration is not recommended. Urge patient to adhere to established drug regimen.

E

Common side effects in *italic*; life-threatening effects underlined; generic names in **bold**; classifications in SMALL CAPS

Prototype: meprobamate, p 179

ETHINAMATE

(e-thin´a-mate)
Trade name: Valmid
Classifications: CNS AGENT; CARBAMATE ANXIOLYTIC, SEDATIVE-HYPNOTIC
Pregnancy: Category C
Controlled substance: Schedule IV

ACTIONS/PHARMACODYNAMICS Carbamate derivative that is a short-acting hypnotic and a non-selective CNS depressant. Its site and mechanism of action are not known. Hypnotic doses suppress REM sleep.

USES Short-term therapy of simple insomnia for periods of up to 1 wk. Drug-free intervals greater than or equal to 1 week should elapse before retreatment is considered. It has generally been replaced by other sedative-hypnotic agents.

ROUTE & DOSAGE

Hypnotic
Adult PO 0.5–1 g 20 min before bedtime

PHARMACOKINETICS Absorption: readily absorbed from GI tract. **Onset:** 20 min. **Peak:** 1 h. **Duration:** 3–5 h. **Metabolism:** metabolized in liver. **Elimination:** half-life: 2.5 h; excreted in urine.

CONTRAINDICATIONS & PRECAUTIONS Contraindicated in: hypersensitivity to ethinamate, first and second trimesters of pregnancy (category C), and uncontrolled pain. Safe use in nursing mothers and children <15 y not established. **Cautious use in:** elderly or debilitated patients, third trimester of pregnancy (category C).

ADVERSE/SIDE EFFECTS Mild GI upset, rash, paradoxical excitement in children.

DRUG INTERACTIONS CNS DEPRESSANTS, **alcohol,** SEDATIVES compound CNS depression; MAO INHIBITORS cause excessive CNS depression; ANTICONVULSANTS, **rifampin, phenmetrazine** may decrease effects of ethinamate.

NURSING IMPLICATIONS

Administration
- May be administered with food to minimize gastric distress.

- Since elderly may be more sensitive to the effects of ethinamate and develop adverse side effects more readily, lower doses are generally prescribed and dose increases are made gradually.
- Prolonged administration is not recommended, since ethinamate has not been shown to be effective for a period of more than 7 d.

Assessment & Drug Effects
- The elderly may not tolerate average adult doses. Observe intensity and duration of adverse effects.
- Psychological and physical dependence is possible; therefore prolonged administration is not recommended.
- Discontinuation of the drug following long-term use may cause severe withdrawal symptoms; therefore the drug must be gradually withdrawn.

Patient & Family Education
- Patient should avoid alcohol and other CNS depressants because of potential addictive effects.
- Caution patient against operating machinery or driving a motor vehicle within 5 h after ingesting ethinamate, since it may cause daytime drowsiness.
- Advise patient to check with doctor before he or she discontinues drug after prolonged use. Gradual withdrawal may be necessary to avoid withdrawal symptoms.

Prototype: estradiol, p 236

ETHINYL ESTRADIOL

(eth´in-il ess-tra-dye´ole)
Trade names: Estinyl, Feminone
Classifications: HORMONE; ESTROGEN
Pregnancy: Category X

ACTIONS/PHARMACODYNAMICS Oral estrogen with actions similar to those of estradiol. Given cyclically for short-term use. Binds to intracellular receptors that stimulate DNA and RNA to synthesize proteins responsible for effects of estrogen.

USES Moderate to severe vasomotor symptoms associated with menopause; also postmenopausal osteoporosis, female gonadism, and as palliation for inoperable, metastatic cancer of female breast (at least 5 y postmenopause) and of the prostate. **Unlabeled use:** postcoital contraceptive.

Common side effects in *italic*; life-threatening effects underlined; generic names in **bold**; classifications in SMALL CAPS

ROUTE & DOSAGE

Menopause, Postmenopausal Osteoporosis

Adult   PO   0.02–0.05 mg/d for 21 d each month; adjust to lowest level that gives symptom control

Female Hypogonadism

Adult   PO   0.05 mg 1–3 times/d for 2 wk, followed by 2 wk of progestin; continue this regimen for 3–6 mo

Breast Cancer

Adult   PO   1 mg t.i.d. for 2–3 mo

Prostatic Cancer (Palliation)

Adult   PO   0.15–2 mg/d

Postcoital Contraceptive

Adult   PO   5 mg/d for 5 consecutive days beginning within 72 h of coitus

CONTRAINDICATIONS & PRECAUTIONS Contraindicated in: breast cancer, known or suspected pregnancy (category X). **Cautious use in:** hypertension; gallbladder disease; diabetes mellitus; heart failure; hepatic or renal dysfunction, history of thromboembolic disease.

ADVERSE/SIDE EFFECTS CNS: headache, dizziness, depression, *libido changes.* **CV:** <u>thromboembolic disorders</u>, hypertension. **GI:** *nausea,* vomiting, diarrhea, anorexia, weight changes, bloating, cholestatic jaundice. **Metabolic:** reduced carbohydrate tolerance, fluid retention. **Reproductive:** mastodynia, breakthrough bleeding, changes in menstrual flow, dysmenorrhea, amenorrhea, vaginal candidiasis; in men: impotence, gynecomastia, testicular atrophy. **Other:** leg cramps, edema.

DRUG INTERACTIONS Carbamazepine, phenytoin, rifampin decrease estrogen levels because they increase its metabolism; may enhance steroid effects of CORTICOSTEROIDS; may decrease anticoagulant effects of ORAL ANTICOAGULANTS.

NURSING IMPLICATIONS

Administration

- Tablet may be taken with food or fluid of patient's choice.
- Given cyclically, except when used for palliation of carcinoma. Usual cyclic regimen during menopause: once daily for 3 wk, followed by 1 wk without the drug; then repeat.
- *Morning after pill:* When used as an emergency postcoital contraceptive, as for rape or for incest, drug is started within 24 h and not later than 72 h after sexual exposure. A pregnancy test is performed before dosing.
- Store at 15–30C (59–86F) in tight, light-resistant container.

Assessment & Drug Effects

- Severe nausea and vomiting (because of high dosage) can cause noncompliance. An antiemetic may be required. Full course of the regimen must be taken if pregnancy is to be prevented. Emotional support from family or caregiver is of primary importance.
- Patients with conditions that may be influenced by fluid retention (migraine, cardiac or renal dysfunction, asthma, epilepsy, hypertension) should be monitored carefully. Check BP on a regular basis.
- Pyridoxine (vitamin B_6) levels are lowered by estrogens. A supplement may be ordered for the patient on long-term therapy, especially if undernourished.

Patient & Family Education

- Be certain patient understands dose schedule and regimen. She should understand what to do if a dose is missed.
- Teach patient how to elicit *Homan's sign:* pain in calf and popliteal region with forced dorsiflexion of foot (early sign of thrombosis).
- Risk of blood clot formation is high. Instruct patient to report immediately a positive Homan's sign and the following *symptoms of thromboembolic disorders:* tenderness, swelling, and redness in extremity; sudden, severe headache or chest pain, slurring of speech; change in vision; tenderness, pain, sudden shortness of breath. If physician is not available, patient should go to the nearest hospital emergency room.
- Estrogen stimulation in women sterilized because of endometriosis may cause serious bleeding in remaining foci of endometrial tissues. Report unexplained and sudden pain.
- Advise patient to report severe abdominal pain and tenderness, or abdominal mass, possible symptoms of hepatic adenoma or hepatic hemorrhage.
- Advise patient to determine weight under standard conditions 1 or 2 times/wk and to report sudden weight gain or other signs of fluid retention.
- A low-salt diet and diuretic may be prescribed to reduce cyclic fluid retention.
- History of jaundice in pregnancy increases the possibility of estrogen-induced jaundice. Instruct pa-

———— Common side effects in *italic*; life-threatening effects <u>underlined</u>; ————
generic names in **bold**; classifications in SMALL CAPS

583

tient to report yellow skin and sclera, pruritus, dark urine, and light-colored stools. Estrogen therapy is usually interrupted pending clinical investigation.

- High vitamin C intake, e.g., 1 g/d, may increase ethinyl estradiol levels. Abrupt withdrawal of vitamin C may lead to breakthrough bleeding.
- Symptoms of vaginal candidiasis (thick, white, curd-like secretions and inflamed congested introitus) should be reported to permit appropriate treatment.
- Reassure male patients that estrogen-induced feminization and impotence are reversible with termination of therapy.
- If user suspects she is pregnant, she should stop taking the estrogen immediately and inform the physician. She should be apprised of the potential risk of masculinization of female fetus.
- Estrogenic depression of caffeine metabolism may cause caffeinism. Urge patient to decrease caffeine intake from sources such as tea, coffee, and cola.

Prototype: isoniazid, p 83

ETHIONAMIDE

(e-thye-on-am´ide)
Trade name: Trecator-SC
Classifications: ANTIINFECTIVE;
ANTITUBERCULOSIS AGENT; ANTILEPROSY
(SULFONE) AGENT
Pregnancy: Category D

ACTIONS/PHARMACODYNAMICS Thiomide derivative of isonicotinic acid chemically related to isoniazid. Bacteriostatic or bactericidal depending on concentration used and susceptibility of organism. Mechanism of action not known, but believed to act by inhibiting bacterial peptide synthesis. Effective against human and bovine strains of *Mycobacterium tuberculosis* and against of *Mycobacterium kansasii* and some strains of *Mycobacterium avium-intracellulare* complex. Also active against *Mycobacterium leprae*. Emergence of resistant strains may be delayed or prevented when administered concurrently with other antituberculosis drugs. Cross resistance not reported. Requirements for pyridoxine may increase; ethionamide may act as a pyridoxine antagonist or possibly increase renal excretion of pyridoxine.

USES Any form of active tuberculosis when treatment with primary antituberculosis drugs (e.g., isoniazid, streptomycin, ethambutol, rifampin) has failed.

Must be given with at least one other effective antituberculosis agent. **Unlabeled use:** atypical mycobacterial infections and tuberculous meningitis.

ROUTE & DOSAGE

Tuberculosis

Adult	PO	0.5–1 g/d divided q8–12h
Child	PO	12–15 mg/kg/d in 3–4 equally divided doses (max 1 g/d)

PHARMACOKINETICS Absorption: 80% absorbed from GI tract. **Peak:** 3 h. **Duration:** 9 h. **Distribution:** widely distributed including CSF; crosses placenta; distribution into breast milk unknown. **Metabolism:** metabolized in liver. **Elimination:** half-life: 3 h; excreted in urine.

CONTRAINDICATIONS & PRECAUTIONS Contraindicated in: hypersensitivity to ethionamide and chemically related drugs, e.g., isoniazid, niacin (nicotinamide); severe hepatic damage. Safe use during pregnancy (category D), by nursing mothers or by children, and in women of childbearing potential not established. **Cautious use in:** diabetes mellitus, hepatic dysfunction.

ADVERSE/SIDE EFFECTS CNS: headache, restlessness, psychic disturbances including mental depression, hallucinations; drowsiness, dizziness, ataxia, weakness, peripheral neuritis, paresthesias, tremors, convulsions. **ENT:** olfactory disturbances. **Eye:** optic neuritis (blurred or loss of vision, eye pain, diplopia). **GI:** dose related and frequent; symptoms may be due to CNS stimulation rather than to GI irritation: anorexia, *epigastric distress, nausea, vomiting,* metallic taste, *diarrhea,* stomatitis, sialorrhea. **Hematologic:** thrombocytopenia. **Hepatic:** elevated ALT, AST; hepatitis (with jaundice). **Hypersensitivity:** (rare): skin rash, exfoliative dermatitis, photosensitivity, thrombocytopenia, purpura. **Other:** severe postural hypotension, menorrhagia, gynecomastia, impotence, acne; goiter (hypothyroidism): weight gain, cold, dry, puffy skin; hair loss, pellagralike syndrome, superinfections, joint pains, acute rheumatic symptoms, hypoglycemia.

DRUG INTERACTIONS Cycloserine, isoniazid may increase neurotoxic effects.

NURSING IMPLICATIONS

Administration

- GI side effects may be minimized by taking drug with or after meals. Some patients tolerate ethion-

Common side effects in *italic*; life-threatening effects <u>underlined</u>; generic names in **bold**; classifications in SMALL CAPS

amide best when it is taken as a single dose after the evening meal or as a single dose at bedtime. (GI symptoms appear to increase with divided doses, although serum concentrations may be higher.)

- About 50% of patients cannot tolerate a single dose larger than 500 mg because of GI side effects. Dosage may be reduced as much as one third to one half for these patients. An antiemetic is sometimes prescribed, but if symptoms persist, drug should be discontinued.
- Physician may prescribe pyridoxine (vitamin B_6) concurrently to prevent or relieve peripheral neuritis and other neurotoxic effects.
- Store in a cool, dry place at 8–15C (46–59F) in a tightly-closed container unless otherwise directed.

Assessment & Drug Effects

- Culture and susceptibility tests should be made before start of therapy.
- Report onset of skin rash. Progression to exfoliative dermatitis can occur if drug is not promptly discontinued.
- Liver function tests (AST and ALT), CBC, and renal function tests including urinalysis should be done prior to and every 2–4 wk during therapy.
- This drug may make it difficult to manage blood glucose levels in the diabetic. Alert the patient to monitor blood glucose closely until response to the drug is established. These patients appear to be especially prone to hepatotoxicity (see Signs & Symptoms, chap 3).

Patient & Family Education

- Because ethionamide may increase potential for hepatic dysfunction, physician may suggest moderation or elimination of alcohol ingestion.
- Hepatotoxicity is generally reversible if drug is promptly withdrawn. Instruct patient to report onset of signs or symptoms (see chap 3).
- If patient complains of optic symptoms (diplopia, blurred vision), ophthalmoscopic examination is advised promptly and then periodically thereafter during therapy.
- Caution patient who is experiencing postural hypotension to make position changes slowly and in stages, particularly from recumbent to upright posture and to move feet and ankles a few minutes before stepping on the floor. Instruct patient to lie down or sit down immediately if he or she is feeling faint or dizzy and not to stand still for prolonged periods or take very hot baths or showers.
- Emphasize importance of adhering to established drug regimen. Patient should not omit, increase, or

decrease dose or change dose intervals unless advised to do so by physician.

Prototype: atropine, p 116

ETHOPROPAZINE HYDROCHLORIDE

(eth-oh-pro′pa-zeen)
Trade names: Parsidol, Parsitan
Classifications: AUTONOMIC NERVOUS SYSTEM AGENT; ANTICHOLINERGIC; ANTIMUSCARINIC; ANTIPARKINSONISM
Pregnancy: Category C

ACTIONS/PHARMACODYNAMICS Phenothiazine derivative with prominent atropine-like blocking action. In addition to centrally-acting anticholinergic (parasympatholytic) effects, also exhibits some antihistaminic, local anesthetic, ganglionic blocking and adrenergic blocking actions. Differs from other phenothiazines in that it is used to control extrapyramidal reactions caused by drugs of this class, and it has no antiemetic activity. Mode of action not known but believed to be related to ability to block both muscarinic and nicotinic actions of acetylcholine.

USES Adjunctive therapy in all forms of parkinsonism (arteriosclerotic, idiopathic, postencephalitic), and to control drug-induced extrapyramidal reactions. Also being used for symptomatic treatment of hepatolenticular degeneration and for congenital athetosis.

ROUTE & DOSAGE

Parkinsonism

Adult	PO	50 mg 1–2 times/d; may increase to 100–400 mg/d in divided doses if necessary; some patients may require 500–600 mg/d

PHARMACOKINETICS Onset: 0.5–1 h. **Duration:** 4 h.

CONTRAINDICATIONS & PRECAUTIONS Contraindicated in: glaucoma, prostatic hypertrophy or bladder neck obstruction, pyloric or duodenal obstruction. Safe use during pregnancy (category C), in nursing women, and in children not established. **Cautious use in:** tardive dyskinesia, hepatic, renal, or

Common side effects in *italic*; life-threatening effects underlined; generic names in **bold**; classifications in SMALL CAPS

585

cardiac disease, myasthenia gravis, elderly patients, achalasia, chronic pulmonary disease.

ADVERSE/SIDE EFFECTS Generally dose related. **CNS:** *drowsiness, cerebral reaction (fogginess, inability to think, lassitude, forgetfulness, confusion),* dizziness, headache, paresthesias, ataxia, toxic psychosis, accentuation of parkinsonism. **CV:** hypotension, tachycardia. **Eye:** blurred vision, diplopia, mydriasis. **GI:** nausea, vomiting, epigastric distress, *dry mouth,* constipation. **GU:** *urinary retention.* **Other:** muscle cramps; sensation of heaviness of extremities; rash; theoretically possible for all phenothiazines: jaundice, ECG abnormalities, hematologic reactions (agranulocytosis, pancytopenia, purpura), endocrine disturbances, jaundice, pigmentation of cornea, lens, retina, skin, visual hallucinations.

NURSING IMPLICATIONS

Administration

- Transfer to or from ethopromazine should be done gradually to avoid aggravation of symptoms.
- Store at 15–30C (59–86F) in tightly closed container unless otherwise specified. Protect from light.

Assessment & Drug Effects

- There is a high incidence of side effects in therapeutic dosage range. Close medical supervision is necessary, especially of the elderly since they are more prone to develop adverse effects.
- Elderly patients should be examined periodically for glaucoma.
- Mentally ill patients require close observation for worsening of mental symptoms, particularly when drug therapy is initiated and whenever dosage adjustments are made.
- Caution patient to keep cool during hot weather and to avoid strenuous exercise. Ethopromazine can interfere with normal body temperature regulation by diminishing sweat secretion.
- Observe for and report therapeutic drug effects: reduction in severity of rigidity, tremor, spasms, drooling, forward-leaning walking gait, and abnormal fixation of eyeballs.

Patient & Family Education

- Caution patient to avoid driving and other potentially hazardous activities until reaction to drug is known. Drowsiness usually disappears after a few days of therapy.
- Since transient hypotension is a potential side effect, advise patient to make position changes slowly, particularly from recumbent to upright position, and to lie down or sit down if lightheadedness or dizziness occurs.
- Dry mouth may be a distressing side effect for some patients. It may be relieved by frequent sips of water, sugarless chewing gum, or sour balls. If severe enough to interfere with eating, talking, or swallowing, report to physician.
- Urge patient to keep follow-up appointments.

ETHOSUXIMIDE

See CENTRAL NERVOUS SYSTEM AGENTS, SUCCINIMIDE ANTICONVULSANT prototype, p 174.

Prototype: procaine hydrochloride, p 166

ETIDOCAINE HYDROCHLORIDE

(e-ti´doe-kane)
Trade name: Duranest
Classifications: CNS AGENT; LOCAL ANESTHETIC (AMIDE-TYPE)
Pregnancy: Category B

ACTIONS/PHARMACODYNAMICS Amide-type anesthetic similar to bupivacaine in action and uses. Inhibits sodium fluxes into nerve cell required for initial depolarization, propagation, and conduction of nerve impulse.

USES Infiltration anesthesia, peripheral nerve blocks (intercostal, ulnar, inferior alveolar, brachial plexus) and central neural block (lumbar or caudal epidural blocks).

ROUTE & DOSAGE

Percutaneous Infiltration

Adult	IM	0.5% solution; max 300 mg, 400 mg if given with epinephrine

Peripheral Nerve Block, Caudal

Adult	IM	0.5% or 1% solution; max 300 mg (400 mg if given with epinephrine)

Central Neural Block

Adult	IM	0.5% or 1.5% solution; max 300 mg (400 mg if given with epinephrine)

PHARMACOKINETICS Absorption: readily absorbed from parenteral injection sites. **Onset:** 2–8 min.

Common side effects in *italic*; life-threatening effects underlined; generic names in **bold**; classifications in SMALL CAPS

Duration: 4.5–13 h. **Distribution:** crosses blood-brain barrier and placenta. **Metabolism:** metabolized in liver. **Elimination:** half-life: 1–2 h; excreted in urine.

CONTRAINDICATIONS & PRECAUTIONS Contraindicated in: known sensitivity to amide-type anesthetics, parabens, bisulfites; acidosis, heart block, severe hemorrhage, severe hypotension, hypertension; cerebrospinal deformities or disease; spinal block, epidural anesthesia in vaginal delivery; injection into inflamed or infected area. Safe use during pregnancy (category B) (except during labor), in nursing mothers, or in children <14 y not established. **Cautious use in:** known drug sensitivities; impaired cardiac function; renal or hepatic disease; severe shock; elderly, debilitated or severely ill patients.

ADVERSE/SIDE EFFECTS CNS: nervousness, headache, anxiety, excitement, <u>convulsions followed by drowsiness, unconsciousness, respiratory arrest</u>. **CV:** myocardial depression, arrhythmias, <u>cardiac arrest, fetal bradycardia during delivery</u>, maternal hypotension. **Ear/eye:** blurred vision, tinnitus. **GI:** nausea, vomiting. **Other:** skin rash, <u>anaphylaxis, anaphylactoid reactions</u>, injection site inflammation and pain, edema, pupillary constriction, backache.

NURSING IMPLICATIONS

Administration
- Discard partially used vial of etidocaine, since it has no preservative.
- Store vials at 15–30C (59–86F); protect from freezing. Solutions with epinephrine should be protected from direct light.

Assessment & Drug Effects
- When used for peridural analgesia, drug produces a profound degree of motor blockade and abdominal relaxation.
- Small doses injected into head and neck areas may produce adverse effects similar to the systemic toxicity seen with unintentional intravascular injection of larger doses: confusion, convulsions, respiratory depression or arrest, CV stimulation or depression. Monitor patient's CV and respiratory status continuously during administration.
- Early warnings of *CNS toxicity:* restlessness, anxiety, tinnitus, dizziness, blurred vision, tremors, drowsiness. At first sign, oxygen is administered.
- Etidocaine may trigger familial malignant hyperthermia. Early unexplained signs of tachycardia, tachypnea, labile BP, metabolic acidosis, and skeletal muscle rigidity may precede temperature eleva-

tion. Prognosis depends on early recognition, prompt discontinuation of drug, institution of supportive measures, and dantrolene.
- Local anesthetics react with certain heavy metals (e.g., zinc, mercury, copper) and can cause severe local irritation; avoid use of disinfecting agents containing heavy metals for skin or mucous membrane disinfection or for vial surface disinfection.

Patient & Family Education
- Use for dental anesthesia: caution patient not to chew solid foods or test the anesthetized region by biting or probing before anesthesia wears off to prevent traumatizing tongue, lip, and buccal mucosa.
- When appropriate, inform patient that he or she may experience temporary loss of sensation and motor activity, usually in the lower part of the body, after proper administration of epidural anesthesia.

ETIDRONATE DISODIUM
(e-ti-droe´nate)
Trade names: Didronel, Didronel I.V., EHDP
Classification: REGULATOR, BONE METABOLISM
Pregnancy: Category B

ACTIONS/PHARMACODYNAMICS Diphosphate preparation with primary action on bone. Mechanism of action not fully understood. Slows rate of bone turnover (bone resorption and new bone formation) in pagetic bone lesions and in normal remodeling process. Lowers serum alkaline phosphatase and urinary hydroxyproline levels and reduces elevated cardiac output associated with Paget's disease by decreasing vascularity of bone. Induces reversible hyperphosphatemia without adverse effects.

USES Symptomatic Paget's disease and heterotopic ossification due to spinal cord injury or after total hip replacement. **Unlabeled uses:** to prevent parathyroid hormone–induced bone resorption, management of malignancy-associated hypercalcemia, treatment of osteoporosis.

PHARMACOKINETICS Absorption: variably absorbed from GI tract. **Distribution:** 50% of absorbed drug is distributed to bone. **Metabolism:** not metabolized. **Elimination:** half-life: 6 h; 50% of absorbed dose is excreted in urine.

Common side effects in *italic*; life-threatening effects <u>underlined</u>; generic names in **bold**; classifications in SMALL CAPS

587

ROUTE & DOSAGE

Paget's Disease

Adult   PO   5–10 mg/kg/d for up to 6 mo *or* 11–20 mg/kg/d for up to 3 mo; may repeat after 3–6 mo off the drug if necessary

Heterotopic Ossification Due to Spinal Cord Injury

Adult   PO   20 mg/kg/d for 2 wk; then 10 mg/kg/d for an additional 10 wk

Heterotopic Ossification Due to Total Hip Arthroplasty

Adult   PO   20 mg/kg/d starting 1 mo before the procedure and continuing for 3 mo after

Malignancy-associated Hypercalcemia

Adult   IV   7.5 mg/kg/d for 3–7 d diluted in at least 250 ml NS and infused over at least 2 h; may repeat after 7 d off if necessary

CONTRAINDICATIONS & PRECAUTIONS Contraindicated in: enterocolitis; children; pathologic fractures. Safe use during pregnancy (category B) (PO), (category C) (parenteral), in nursing women, and in children not established. **Cautious use in:** renal impairment; patients on restricted calcium and vitamin D intake.

ADVERSE/SIDE EFFECTS GI: nausea, diarrhea, *loose bowel movements,* metallic or altered taste. **Other:** increased or recurrent bone pain in pagetic sites, onset of bone pain in previously asymptomatic sites, increased risk of fractures in patient with Paget's disease, hypocalcemia, hyperphosphatemia, renal insufficiency (high IV doses), elevated serum phosphatase, suppressed mineralization of uninvolved skeleton (focal osteomalacia), angioedema, urticaria, rash.

DRUG INTERACTIONS CALCIUM SUPPLEMENTS, ANTACIDS, IRON AND OTHER MINERAL SUPPLEMENTS may decrease absorption of etidronate—give etidronate 2 h before other drugs. **Drug-Food interactions:** food, especially milk and dairy products, will decrease absorption of etidronate—give 2 h before meals.

NURSING IMPLICATIONS

Administration

- Administer as single dose on empty stomach 2 h before meals with full glass of water or juice to reduce gastric irritation.
- GI side effects may be relieved by dividing total daily dose.

- IV etidronate is prepared by diluting a single dose in 25 ml of NS.
- After dilution, it is important to administer the IV slowly over a period of at least 2 h.
- Store at 15–30C (59–86F) in tightly closed container unless otherwise directed.

Assessment & Drug Effects

- GI side effects may interfere with adequate nutritional status and should be treated promptly. Persistent nausea or diarrhea should be reported.
- Monitor I&O ratio, serum creatinine, or BUN of patient with impaired renal function.
- Hypocalcemia is a theoretical possibility and is most likely to occur after parenteral administration beyond 3 d. Signs and symptoms (see chap 3) should be reported at onset.
- Latent tetany (hypocalcemia) may be detected by Chvostek's and Trousseau's signs and a serum calcium value of 7–8 mg/dl.
- Laboratory test values may suggest clinical progress (e.g., decreased urinary excretion of hydroxyproline reflects decreased bone resorption; decreased serum alkaline phosphatase level indicates decreased bone formation). **Normal urinary hydroxyproline:** 15–50 mg/24 h. **Normal serum alkaline phosphatase:** 1.4–4.1 Bodansky units.
- Serum phosphate levels generally return to normal 2–4 wk after medication is discontinued.

Patient & Family Education

- Instruct patient to avoid eating 2 h before or after taking PO etidronate. Drug absorption is decreased by food, especially milk, milk products, and other foods high in calcium, mineral supplements, and antacids.
- Maintenance of optimum nutritional status, especially adequate intake of calcium and vitamin D, is an important adjunct to effective therapy. Advise patient to include milk, dairy products, and leafy vegetables in diet.
- The risk of pathological fractures increases when daily dose of 20 mg/kg is taken longer than 3 mo. Instruct patient to report promptly the sudden onset of unexplained pain.
- Response of Paget's disease to etidronate therapy may be slow (1–3 mo) and may continue for months after treatment is discontinued.
- Retreatment should not be instituted prematurely or before symptoms return. Instruct patient to report promptly if bone pain, restricted mobility, heat over involved bone site occur.
- Urge patient to keep appointments for periodic evaluation of clinical tests.

E

Common side effects in *italic*; life-threatening effects underlined; generic names in **bold**; classifications in SMALL CAPS

Prototype: thiopental, p 164

ETOMIDATE
(e-tom´i-date)
Trade name: Amidate
Classifications: CNS AGENT; GENERAL ANESTHETIC
Pregnancy: Category C

ACTIONS/PHARMACODYNAMICS Short-acting nonbarbiturate intravenous anesthetic induction agent with hypnotic but no analgesic action. Lowers cerebral blood flow and causes slight decrease in intracranial pressure and moderate decrease in intraocular pressure. Also, it does not liberate histamine. These characteristics and associated low incidence of cardiovascular and respiratory effects assign an advantage to the agent for anesthetic induction in high-risk patients (e.g., patients with asthma, drug allergy, cardiovascular disease, or those undergoing neurosurgery). Prolonged administration may suppress cortisol secretion, an effect that may be apparent within several hours or not for days.

USES Induction of general anesthesia, to supplement subpotent anesthetic agents (e.g., nitrous oxide), and for anesthesia maintenance during brief operative procedures.

ROUTE & DOSAGE

Anesthesia Induction
Adult   IV   0.2–0.6 mg/kg over 30–60 s

PHARMACOKINETICS Onset: 1 min. **Duration:** 3–5 min. **Metabolism:** metabolized in liver. **Elimination:** half-life: 75 min; 75% excreted in urine, 23% excreted in feces.

CONTRAINDICATIONS & PRECAUTIONS Contraindicated in: during labor and delivery; as sedation for patient requiring a respirator; in pregnancy unless clearly needed and when potential benefit outweighs unknown risk to fetus. Safe use during pregnancy (category C), in nursing women, and in children <10 y not established. **Cautious use in:** immunosuppression.

ADVERSE/SIDE EFFECTS CNS: *transient skeletal muscle movements, especially myoclonus; adverting and tonic movements; uncontrolled eye movements.*

CV: *transient venous pain,* hypertension, hypotension, tachycardia, bradycardia, and other arrhythmias. **GI:** postoperative nausea and vomiting. **Respiratory:** hypoventilation or hyperventilation, transient apnea, laryngospasm, hiccups, snoring. **Other:** adrenocortical suppression, Addisonian crisis (with prolonged use), hyperkalemia or hyponatremia or both, oliguria; fever, then hypothermia; profound weakness.

NURSING IMPLICATIONS

Administration
- Transient muscular movements can be reduced, and the recovery period shortened, by giving fentanyl IV 1–2 min before anesthesia induction.
- Store drug at 2–8C (36–46F). Avoid exposure to extreme heat; do not freeze.

Assessment & Drug Effects
- Etomidate is not intended for prolonged infusion. When drug is administered over a several hour period, the potential for an antisteroidogenic effect is magnified. Plasma cortisol levels will be monitored to detect a sudden fall leading to hypotension. *Normal free plasma cortisol range:* 5–20 µg/100 ml.
- During recovery period, monitor BP, pulse, and respirations q10–15min until stable, then q4h. Continue checking vital signs q4h for 12–24 h.
- Severe drug-induced hypotension is rapidly reversed by a corticosteroid but not by catecholamines.
- Monitor I&O ratio and pattern and serum K during recovery period; be prepared to intervene if symptoms of Addisonian crisis occur.

ETOPOSIDE
(e-toe-po´side)
Trade names: VePesid, VP-16, VP-16-213
Classification: ANTINEOPLASTIC
Pregnancy: Category D

ACTIONS/PHARMACODYNAMICS Semisynthetic derivative of podophyllotoxin, a chemical produced by podophyllin of the mandrake or May apple plant. Produces cytotoxic action by unclear mechanism. Primary action is by arresting G_2 (resting or premitotic) phase of cell cycle; also acts on S (DNA synthesis) phase. High doses cause lysis of cells entering mitotic phase, and lower doses inhibit cells from entering prophase.

Common side effects in *italic*; life-threatening effects underlined; generic names in **bold**; classifications in SMALL CAPS

589

USES Treatment of refractory testicular neoplasms, in patients who have already received appropriate surgical, chemotherapeutic, and radiation therapy; for treatment of choriosarcoma in women and small cell carcinoma of the lung. **Unlabeled uses:** Hodgkin's and non-Hodgkin's lymphomas, acute myelogenous (nonlymphocytic) leukemia.

ROUTE & DOSAGE

Testicular Carcinoma

Adult	IV	50–100 mg/m²/d for 5 consecutive days q3–4wk for 3–4 courses *or* 100 mg/m² on days 1, 3, and 5 q3–4wk for 3–4 courses
	PO	Twice the IV dose rounded to the nearest 50 mg

Small Cell Lung Carcinoma

Adult	IV	35 mg/m²/d for 4 consecutive days to 50 mg/m²/d for 5 consecutive days q3–4wk
	PO	Twice the IV dose rounded to the nearest 50 mg

PHARMACOKINETICS Absorption: approximately 50% absorbed from GI tract. **Peak:** 1–1.5 h. **Distribution:** variable penetration into CSF. **Metabolism:** probably metabolized in liver. **Elimination:** half-life: 5–10 h; 44–60% excreted in urine, 2–16% excreted in feces over 3 d.

CONTRAINDICATIONS & PRECAUTIONS Contraindicated in: severe bone marrow depression; severe hepatic or renal impairment; existing or recent viral infection, bacterial infection; intraperitoneal, intrapleural, or intrathecal administration. Safe use during pregnancy (category D), in nursing mothers, and in children not established. **Cautious use in:** impaired renal or hepatic function; gout.

ADVERSE/SIDE EFFECTS CNS: peripheral neuropathy, paresthesias, CNS toxicity: somnolence, unusual tiredness, weakness, depression, headache, ataxia (rare), transient vertigo (rare), transient confusion. **CV:** transient hypotension, palpitation, tachycardia, transient hypertension, MI, pulmonary edema (causal relationship not established). **GI:** *nausea, vomiting,* dyspepsia, anorexia, diarrhea, constipation, stomatitis, aftertaste. **Hematologic:** *leukopenia (principally granulocytopenia), thrombocytopenia,* severe myelosuppression, hyperuricemia, *anemia, pancytopenia, neutropenia.* **Hypersensitivity:** sweating, chills, fever, coryza, tachycardia; throat, back and general body pain; abdominal cramps, high fre-

quency deafness, flushing, substernal chest pain, dyspnea, bronchospasm, pulmonary edema, anaphylactoid reaction. **Respiratory:** pleural effusion, bronchospasm. **Skin:** *reversible alopecia* (can progress to total baldness); nail pigmentation, radiation recall dermatitis, rash, severe pruritus (rare), Stevens-Johnson syndrome. **Other:** necrosis, thrombophlebitis (with extravasation), *pain at IV site;* sepsis (immunosuppression), intermittent muscle cramps, fever, gonadal suppression; transient cortical blindness, nephrotoxicity, hepatotoxicity, and hematotoxicity with overdosage; possibility of carcinogenesis.

NURSING IMPLICATIONS

Administration

- Should be administered under the supervision of a qualified physician experienced in the use of antineoplastic therapy.
- Wear disposable surgical gloves when preparing or disposing of etoposide. Materials used in its preparation should be properly disposed of to prevent contamination of the environment. Follow agency policy.
- Each 100 mg must be diluted with 250–500 ml of D5W or NS to produce final concentrations of 0.2–0.4 mg/ml.
- Administer by slow IV infusion over 30–60 min to reduce risk of hypotension and bronchospasm. These symptoms can occur with rapid injection or slow infusion of higher than recommended dosages.
- Before administration, inspect solution for particulate matter and discoloration. Solution should be clear and yellow. If crystals are present, discard.
- Diluted solutions with concentration of 0.2 mg/ml are stable for 96 h, and the 0.4 mg/ml solutions are stable for 48 h under normal room fluorescent light in glass or plastic (PVC) containers
- Store unopened vials at 15–30C (59–86F) unless otherwise directed.
- Refrigerate capsules at 2–8C (36–46F) unless otherwise directed. Do not freeze.

Assessment & Drug Effects

- Check IV site during and after infusion. Extravasation can cause thrombophlebitis and necrosis.
- Be prepared to treat an anaphylactoid reaction (see Signs & Symptoms, chap 3); can develop in 1–2 min; can culminate in shock and death. If the reaction occurs, infusion should be stopped immediately.
- Most patients will manifest some evidence of toxic-

ity; therefore constant vigilance is essential. Adverse effects are generally reversible with reduction of dosage or discontinuation of drug.

- Monitor vital signs during and after infusion. If hypotension occurs, infusion should be stopped immediately.
- Patients who develop severe toxic reactions to etoposide should be closely monitored for 3–4 wk because the drug is extensively bound to plasma proteins.
- The following laboratory tests are advised before therapy is begun, at regular intervals during therapy, and before each subsequent treatment course: CBC, WBC counts; hepatic and renal function tests: AST, ALT, serum bilirubin, LDH, BUN, serum creatinine.
- Bone marrow depression, notably leukopenia and thrombocytopenia, is used as an index for dosage regulation. WBC counts reach their lowest point (nadir) over 7–14 d, and platelet nadirs occur over 9–16 d after drug administration. An absolute neutrophil count below 500/mm³ or a platelet count below 50,000/mm³ signifies need to withhold therapy.
- Be alert to evidence of patient complaints that might suggest development of leukopenia (see Signs & Symptoms, chap 3), infection (immunosuppression), and bleeding.
- During period of platelet nadir particularly, protect patient from any trauma that might precipitate bleeding. If possible, invasive procedures should be withheld.
- GI side effects are generally mild and do not appear to be dose related. Some patients may require an antiemetic dosing.

Patient & Family Education
- Before treatment begins, patient and responsible family members should be informed of the possible adverse effects of etoposide, such as blood dyscrasias, alopecia, carcinogenesis.
- Because transient hypotension after therapy is a possible side effect, caution patient to make position changes slowly, particularly from recumbent to upright position.
- Women of childbearing potential should be advised to avoid pregnancy because of possible harm to fetus.
- Inspect patient's mouth daily for ulcerations and bleeding. Stomatitis is especially likely to occur in patients who have had prior radiation therapy of head and neck. Patients with stomatitis should avoid obvious irritants such as hot or spicy foods, smoking, alcohol.

Prototype: isotretinoin, p 253

ETRETINATE
(e-tret´i-nate)
Trade name: Tegison
Classifications: SKIN AGENT; ANTIPSORIATIC; RETINOID
Pregnancy: Category X

ACTIONS/PHARMACODYNAMICS A second generation retinoid related to retinoic acid and retinol (vitamin A). Mechanism of action unknown. Reduces redness, scaling, and thickness of psoriasis lesions by normalizing epidermal differentiation; also decreases stratum corneum thickness and inflammation in epidermis and dermis. Etretinate is effective in severe recalcitrant psoriasis, both pustular and erythrodermic types; is teratogenic and has serious side effects.

USES Treatment of severe recalcitrant psoriasis in patients unresponsive to or intolerant of standard therapies.

ROUTE & DOSAGE

Psoriasis

Adult	PO	0.75–1 mg/kg/d in divided doses, not to exceed 1.5 mg/kg/d; may be able to decrease to 0.5–0.75 mg/kg/d after 8–10 wk of therapy

PHARMACOKINETICS Absorption: readily absorbed from GI tract with significant first pass metabolism. **Peak:** 2.5–5 h. **Duration:** detectable serum levels for years after discontinuation. **Distribution:** accumulates in adipose tissue, liver, and subcutaneous fat; crosses placenta; distributed into breast milk. **Metabolism:** metabolized in liver. **Elimination:** half-life: 120 h; excreted primarily in feces; some excretion in urine.

CONTRAINDICATIONS & PRECAUTIONS Contraindicated in: intolerance to isotretinoin, tretinoin, vitamin A derivatives, or to parabens (preservative in etretinate formulation); pregnancy (category X), lactation, severe obesity. **Cautious use in:** cardiovascular disease or family history of; children (used only if all alternative therapies have been ineffective); hepatic impairment; diabetes mellitus, patients predisposed to hypertriglyceridemia.

Common side effects in *italic*; life-threatening effects <u>underlined</u>; generic names in **bold**; classifications in SMALL CAPS

591

ADVERSE/SIDE EFFECTS Nearly all resemble those of hypervitaminosis A syndrome. **CNS:** *fatigue, headache, fever,* dizziness, lethargy, amnesia, anxiety, depression, <u>pseudotumor cerebri</u>, emotional lability. **CV:** edema; <u>cardiac thrombotic or obstructive events</u>; postural hypotension, coagulation disorders, <u>MI</u> (rare). **ENT:** dry nose, *nose bleeds,* rhinorrhea, change in hearing, earache, otitis externa. **Eye:** *eye irritation,* decreased night vision, *eyelid abnormalities; double vision;* corneal erosion and abrasions; dry eyes, eye pain, blurred vision, excessive tearing, conjunctivitis, scotomas, photophobia. **GI:** abdominal pain, *appetite change,* stomatitis, *sore tongue,* thirst, *nausea,* constipation, diarrhea, flatulence, weight loss, *gingival bleeding, dry mouth.* **GU:** abnormal menses, atrophic vaginitis, dysuria, polyuria, kidney stones, urinary retention. **Hematologic:** anemia; increased or decreased serum potassium, calcium, sodium, *phosphorus, chloride, fasting blood sugars,* platelets, Hgb, Hct, *PTT, MCHC,* prothrombin time; increased BUN, creatinine. **Hepatic:** *hypertriglyceridemia,* <u>hepatitis (hepatotoxicity)</u>, *hypercholesterolemia,* lowered HDL, increased AST, ALT, bilirubin. **Musculoskeletal:** *bone and joint pain,* muscle cramps, myalgia, gout, hyperkinesia, *hyperostosis.* **Respiratory:** dyspnea, coughing, pharyngitis. **Skin:** nail disorders, *photosensitivity; skin fragility and peeling;* changes in perspiration, *hair loss,* dry skin, rash, itching, skin atrophy, fissures, ulcerations; hirsutism, herpes simplex. **Other:** *chapped lips*, cheilitis; <u>malignant neoplasms</u>.

DRUG INTERACTIONS Alcohol may increase plasma triglyceride levels; **isotretinoin,** VITAMIN A PREPARATIONS compound toxic effects; **methotrexate** may increase risk of hepatotoxicity; TETRACYCLINES may increase risk of pseudotumor cerebri. **Drug-Food interactions: milk** will increase absorption of etretinate.

NURSING IMPLICATIONS

Administration
- Etretinate therapy should be managed only by a physician who is knowledgeable in the systemic use of retinoids.
- Consistent administration of etretinate with whole milk or other high-fat food increases drug absorption and allows smaller doses. It may thus be easier to titrate lowest effective dosage range. Discuss with physician.
- Store capsules at 15–30C (59–86F); protect from light and moisture.

Assessment & Drug Effects
- Transient exacerbation of psoriasis may occur during the initial treatment period.
- Hepatic function tests are performed before beginning treatment, then at 1–2 wk intervals for 1–2 mo. Periodic tests continue thereafter at intervals of 1–3 mo during the treatment period. Drug is discontinued in presence of hepatitis.
- Blood lipid determinations are performed before treatment starts and then repeated at 1–2 wk intervals until lipid response is established (usually 4–8 wk). Because hypertriglyceridemia, hypercholesterolemia, and lowered LDL may increase patient's cardiovascular risk, regular monitoring is essential.
- Patient should have a pregnancy test 2 wk before starting therapy. Etretinate is then started on second or third day of the next normal menstrual period. Effective contraception should be used at least 1 mo before starting treatment, continued during treatment, and perhaps for as long as 4 y after treatment ends. Patient should discuss this with physician.

Patient & Family Education
- Complete clearing of the disease has been observed after 4–9 mo of therapy in most patients.
- The most common sites for drug-induced hyperostosis (abnormal growth of bone tissue) in adults are in the ankles, pelvis, and knees. Pain and limitation of motion should be reported immediately; drug will be discontinued.
- If drug is prescribed for children, pretreatment x-rays of bone age (including x-rays of knees) and yearly x-rays thereafter are advised. Caution parent to report promptly the onset of pain or limitation of motion in the child.
- Caution patient to report immediately signs and symptoms of hepatitis: jaundice (see chap 3), flu-like symptoms.
- If any visual difficulties develop, drug should be discontinued and patient should have an ophthalmic examination.
- Patient may notice increased sensitivity to contact lenses because of dry eyes (side effect). Advise patient to check with physician about eye lubricating solution such as artificial tears (available OTC).
- Because dry skin or peeling is a common side effect, caution patient to avoid skin applications that may aggravate the condition, such as alcohol-containing preparations.
- High-fat foods in diet should be controlled because this drug can cause hypertriglyceridemia and increased LDLs.
- Patient should be advised to avoid vitamin A sup-

Common side effects in *italic*; life-threatening effects <u>underlined</u>; generic names in **bold**; classifications in SMALL CAPS

- plements because of the possibility of additive toxic effects.
- Caution patient to report early symptoms of *pseudotumor cerebri:* headache, vomiting, nausea, blurred vision.
- Because of potential drug-induced photosensitivity and photophobia, caution patient to avoid excessive sun exposure and sunlamp treatments. Advise use of sunglasses and sunscreen.
- Drug-induced effects on oral mucosa and gingiva because of decreased salivary flow should be reported and treated.
- Patient should be completely aware of the teratogenic danger. If patient becomes pregnant, urge her to talk with the physician about the risk of continuing pregnancy.
- Patient should be warned not to donate blood while taking etretinate and for several years after therapy. This is to prevent a pregnant woman from being given blood containing this teratogenic agent.
- Inform patient that after treatment is discontinued, some degree of relapse may occur by the end of 2 mo. If this happens, subsequent 4–9 mo course(s) of treatment (same dosage) provides a response similar to the initial therapy response.

FACTOR IX COMPLEX

Trade names: Konyne, Konyne-HT, Profilnine, Proplex, Proplex SX
Classifications: BLOOD COAGULATOR; HEMOSTATIC (SYSTEMIC)
Pregnancy: Category C

ACTIONS/PHARMACODYNAMICS Dried, purified concentrate of vitamin K–dependent blood coagulation factors II, VII, IX, and X derived from fresh pooled plasma of healthy donors. Although tested for presence of HIV and hepatitis virus, some risk of transmitting hepatitis exists. Possibility of developing hepatitis is small in patients with severe hemophilia since they have received numerous transfusions and, therefore, have developed hepatitis antibodies. Factor IX complex contains only traces of blood groups A and B isohemagglutins; however, when large doses are administered, the amount of isohemagglutins becomes significant and can cause intravascular hemolysis. Congenital deficiency of any one of the four blood coagulation factors present in factor IX complex can result in a hemorrhagic problem. Factor VII (proconvertin or serum prothrombin

conversion accelerator), factor IX (Christmas factor or plasma thromboplastin component), and factor X or Stuart-Prower factor (resembles factor VII) are all essential for conversion of factor II prothrombin to thrombin. Note that some products are heparin free (Konyne, Profilnine) and that others contain heparin as a stabilizing agent (Proplex, Proplex SX).

USES Primarily to control bleeding in patients with factor IX deficiency, i.e., hemophilia B (Christmas disease). Also to reverse effects of coumarin anticoagulants. Proplex is used to control bleeding in patients with hemophilia A (who have factor VIII inhibitors).

ROUTE & DOSAGE

Bleeding in Patient with Hemophilia A Who Has Factor VIII Inhibitors

Adult	IV	75 U/kg ideal body weight; a second dose may be given if necessary after 8–12 h

Prophylaxis for Spontaneous Bleeding Episodes

Adult	IV	500 U/wk

Prompt Reversal of Anticoagulant Effect of Coumarins or Drug-Induced Bleeding

Adult	IV	15 U/kg

PHARMACOKINETICS Metabolism: rapidly cleared from plasma after IV administration. **Elimination:** half-life: 17–32 h.

CONTRAINDICATIONS & PRECAUTIONS Contraindicated in: liver disease or suspicious signs of disseminated intravascular coagulation (DIC) or fibrinolysis; patients with mild factor IX deficiency who could be treated effectively with fresh-frozen plasma; patients who have had little exposure to blood products (at high risk of developing viral hepatitis); patients undergoing elective surgery (risk of thromboses). Safe use during pregnancy not established.

ADVERSE/SIDE EFFECTS Generally well tolerated. **With large doses:** chills, fever (pyrogenic reaction), DIC, thromboses, MI. **With rapid infusion:** vasomotor reactions (flushing, changes in BP or pulse rate), transient fever, chills, headache, tingling, urticaria, nausea, vomiting, somnolence, lethargy. **Other:** severe hypersensitivity reactions including anaphylactic shock (rare), *viral hepatitis.*

Common side effects in *italic*; life-threatening effects underlined; generic names in **bold**; classifications in SMALL CAPS

593

NURSING IMPLICATIONS

Administration

- Dilute with at least 1 ml of sterile water for injection for each 50 U (50 U/ml). A more dilute solution using 2 ml of sterile water for injection for each 50 U (25 U/ml) may be preferred. Diluent is usually provided by manufacturer.
- Before reconstitution, warm diluent (sterile water for injection) to room temperature. After diluent is added, vial should be gently agitated to assure complete dissolution of powder.
- Rate of flow is prescribed (generally not to exceed 3 ml/min).
- After reconstitution, solution should be administered within 3 h to avoid possibility of microbial contamination. It should not be refrigerated because precipitation may occur.
- Refrigerate unopened vials at 2–8C (35–46F) until reconstituted unless otherwise directed. Do not freeze.

Assessment & Drug Effects

- Typing and crossmatching should be done to reduce risk of intravascular hemolysis in patients with type A, B, or AB blood, and for general emergency purposes.
- Coagulation assays should be performed before initiation of therapy and at regular intervals during therapy to individualize dosage.
- Be alert to signs of DIC, e.g., oliguria, mucosal bleeding, ecchymoses, abnormal coagulation tests, and hypersensitivity reactions.
- Risk of DIC increases with repeated administrations since unnecessarily high levels of factors II, IX, and X, which have a particularly long half-life, are produced. The possibility of DIC is reportedly reduced by avoiding elevations of the patient's factor IX levels to more than 50% of normal.
- Monitor vital signs and I&O.

Patient & Family Education

- Instruct patient to report bleeding gums and signs and symptoms of hypersensitivity (see chap 3).
- Patients with hemophilia A (classic hemophilia) commonly have hemarthrosis (i.e., bleeding into joints causing swelling, pain, and immobility). Bleeding into soft tissues and muscle causes hematomas that compress nerves, blood vessels, and even the airway. Prompt treatment and physical therapy can prevent irreversible joint damage and muscle atrophy.

Prototype: cimetidine, p 216

FAMOTIDINE
(fa-moe´ti-deen)
Trade name: Pepcid
Classifications: GASTROINTESTINAL AGENT; ANTISECRETORY AGENT (H_2-RECEPTOR ANTAGONIST)
Pregnancy: Category B

ACTIONS/PHARMACODYNAMICS A thiazole derivative, structurally similar to histamine and pharmacologically similar to cimetidine. A potent competitive inhibitor of histamine at histamine (H_2) receptor sites in gastric parietal cells. This action reduces parietal cell output of hydrochloric acid; thus detrimental effects of acid on gastric mucosa are diminished. Inhibits basal, nocturnal, meal-stimulated, and pentogastrin-stimulated gastric secretion; also inhibits pepsin secretion. Is 20–160 times more potent than cimetidine and 3–20 times more potent than ranitidine. Does not affect gastric emptying or exocrine pancreatic function. The thiazole ring in its structure is thought to explain the lower antiandrogenic side effects and the lesser influence on hepatic cytochrome P-450 enzyme activity when compared with cimetidine.

USES Short-term treatment of active duodenal ulcer; maintenance therapy for duodenal ulcer patients on reduced dosage after healing of an active ulcer; treatment of pathologic hypersecretory conditions (e.g., Zollinger-Ellison syndrome), benign gastric ulcer. **Unlabeled uses:** gastroesophogeal reflux, gastritis, stress ulcer prophylaxis.

ROUTE & DOSAGE

Duodenal Ulcer

Adult	PO	40 mg h.s. *or* 20 mg b.i.d.
	IV	20 mg q12h

Duodenal Ulcer, Maintenance Therapy

Adult	PO	20 mg h.s.

Pathological Hypersecretory Conditions

Adult	PO	20–160 mg q6h

PHARMACOKINETICS Absorption: incompletely absorbed from GI tract (40–50% reaches systemic circulation). **Onset:** 1 h. **Peak:** 1–3 h PO; 0.5–3 h IV.

Duration: 10–12 h. **Metabolism:** metabolized in liver. **Elimination:** half-life: 2.5–4 h; excreted in urine.

CONTRAINDICATIONS & PRECAUTIONS Con-
traindicated in: safe use during pregnancy (category B), by nursing mothers, or in children not established. **Cautious use in:** renal insufficiency.

ADVERSE/SIDE EFFECTS CNS:
dizziness, headache, paresthesias, psychic disturbance including depression, anxiety, decreased libido, insomnia, somnolence. **GI:** nausea, constipation, vomiting, anorexia, dry mouth, diarrhea, abdominal discomfort, liver abnormalities, dysgeusia. **Musculoskeletal:** musculoskeletal pain; arthralgia. **Respiratory:** <u>bronchospasm</u>. **Skin:** rash, alopecia, acne, pruritus, dry skin, flushing. **Other:** asthenia, fever, fatigue, palpitations, thrombocytopenia.

DRUG INTERACTIONS None identified.

NURSING IMPLICATIONS

Administration
- Administer oral drug with liquid or food of patient's choice; an antacid may be given with famotidine if patient is also on antacid therapy.
- **_Reconstitution:_** _IV solutions:_ dilute 20 mg (2 ml) famotidine IV solution (containing 10 mg/ml) with D5W, NS, or other compatible IV diluent (see manufacturer's directions) to a total volume of 5 or 10 ml; administer direct IV over not less than 2 min. _IV infusion:_ dilute 2 ml famotidine IV with 100 ml compatible IV solution; infuse over 15–30 min.
- Famotidine IV reconstituted solutions are stable for 48 h at room temperature (15–30C) (59–86F).
- This drug is safely administered to the elderly without dosage modification except in renal impairment.
- In the patient with severe renal insufficiency, dosage adjustment may be made on basis of creatinine clearance. High plasma concentrations of famotidine do not appear to produce drug-related toxicity.
- Store at 15–30C (59–86F). Protect from moisture and strong light; do not freeze. Store IV solution at 2–8C (36–46F).

Assessment & Drug Effects
- Monitor for improvement in GI distress.
- Monitor for signs of GI bleeding.

Patient & Family Education
- Smoking increases volume of HCl secretion, especially nocturnal secretion. Advise patient to stop smoking or at least to avoid smoking after bedtime dose.
- Instruct patient to adhere to established drug regimen (i.e., drug should not be increased, decreased, or omitted and it should be taken for the full time of treatment even if patient feels better). If a dose is missed, take it as soon as possible. If it is close to next dose, do not double dose but resume dosing according to planned schedule.
- Inform patient that pain relief may not be experienced for several days after starting therapy.
- Self-dosing with OTC medications can cancel out therapeutic effects of this drug. Avoid use of any nonprescribed drug without approval of the physician.

FAT EMULSION, INTRAVENOUS
Trade names: Intralipid, Liposyn, Nutralipid, Soyacal, Travamulsion
Classification: CALORIC AGENT
Pregnancy: Category B for Soyacal 10%; C for all others

F

ACTIONS/PHARMACODYNAMICS
Intralipid (available in 10% and 20% concentrations) is a soybean oil in water emulsion containing egg yolk phospholipids and glycerin. Liposyn 10% is a safflower oil in water emulsion containing egg phosphatides and glycerin. Caloric value per milliliter of Intralipid 10% and Liposyn 10% is 1.1, and for Intralipid 20% it is 2. Fat emulsions contain a mixture of neutral triglycerides, mostly unsaturated fatty acids, the majority of which include linoleic, oleic, and palmitic acids. Intralipid also contains linolenic acid, and Liposyn also contains stearic acid. Emulsified fat particles are approximately 0.4–0.5 μm in diameter, similar in size to chylomicrons (naturally occurring fat molecules). Fatty acids are essential for normal structure and function of cell membranes. They are also utilized by the body as a source of energy and may increase heat production, decrease respiratory quotient (ratio of $CO_2:O_2$), and increase oxygen consumption. When used as a source of calories in patients receiving amino acid–dextrose infusions, fat emulsion should supply no more than 60% of total caloric input for adults and children and 40% in newborns (remainder is supplied by amino acid–dextrose mixture). When used to prevent or correct fatty acid deficiency, 8–10% of total calories

---

Common side effects in *italic*; life-threatening effects <u>underlined</u>;
generic names in **bold**; classifications in SMALL CAPS

should be supplied by fat emulsion. Fat emulsion preparations are isotonic and may be given by central or peripheral venous routes.

USES Fatty acid deficiency. Also to supply fatty acids and calories in high-density form to patients receiving prolonged TPN therapy who cannot tolerate high dextrose concentrations or when fluid intake must be restricted as in renal failure, CHF, ascites.

ROUTE & DOSAGE

Prevention of Essential Fatty Acid Deficiency

Adult	IV	500 ml of 10% *or* 250 ml of 20% solution infused over 8–12 h twice/wk (max rate of 100 ml/h)
Child	IV	1 g/kg infused slowly over 8–12 h twice/wk (max rate of 100 ml/h)

Calorie Source in Fluid-restricted Patients

Adult	IV	up to 2.5 g/kg or 60% of nonprotein calories daily infused over at least 8–12 h (max rate of 100 ml/h)
Child	IV	up to 4 g/kg or 60% of nonprotein calories daily infused over at least 8–12 h (max rate of 100 ml/h)

CONTRAINDICATIONS & PRECAUTIONS Contraindicated in: hyperlipemia; bone marrow dyscrasias; impaired fat metabolism as in pathological hyperlipemia, lipoid nephrosis, acute pancreatitis accompanied by hyperlipemia. **Cautious use in:** severe hepatic or pulmonary disease; coagulation disorders, anemia; newborns, prematures, infants with hyperbilirubinemia; when danger of fat embolism exists; diabetes mellitus; thrombocytopenia; history of gastric ulcer.

ADVERSE/SIDE EFFECTS Acute reactions: fever, chills, flushing, sweating, pain in back and chest, dyspnea, cyanosis, pressure sensation over eyes, nausea, vomiting, headache, dizziness, sleepiness, neurologic symptoms, hypersensitivity reactions (to egg protein), *hyperlipemia,* hypercoagulability, *transient increases in liver function tests,* thrombocytopenia in neonates, irritation at infusion site. **Long-term administration:** sepsis, jaundice (cholestasis), hepatomegaly, kernicterus (infants with hyperbilirubinemia); rarely: thrombophlebitis, leukopenia, anemia; "overloading syndrome" (focal seizures, lethargy, delayed clotting, fever, leukocytosis, impaired liver function, splenomegaly, shock), gastroduodenal ulcer, hemorrhagic diathesis; fat deposits in lungs, IV fat pigment (brown pigmentation in reticuloendothelial system).

DIAGNOSTIC TEST INTERFERENCES Blood samples drawn during or shortly after fat emulsion infusion may produce abnormally high *hemoglobin MCH and MCHC* values. Fat emulsions may cause transient abnormalities in *liver function tests* and may interfere with estimations of *serum bilirubin* (especially in infants).

INCOMPATIBILITIES Solution/Additive: aminophylline, ampicillin, calcium chloride, calcium gluconate, magnesium chloride, methicillin, penicillin G, phenytoin, ranitidine, tetracycline, vitamin B complex. Y-Site: phenytoin, tetracycline.

NURSING IMPLICATIONS

Administration

- If possible, allow preparations that have been refrigerated to stand at room temperature for about 30 min before using.
- Do not use if oil appears to be separating out of the emulsion.
- Fat emulsions may be administered via a separate peripheral site or by piggyback into same vein receiving amino acid injection and dextrose mixtures. Administered by piggyback through a Y connector near infusion site so that the two solutions mix only in short piece of tubing proximal to needle.
- Fat emulsion must be hung higher than hyperalimentation solution bottle to prevent back up of fat emulsion into primary line.
- An in-line filter is not recommended because size of fat particles is larger than pore size.
- Flow rate of each solution should be controlled by separate infusion pumps.
- Do not mix fat emulsions with electrolytes, vitamins, drugs, or other nutrient solutions.
- In adults, fat emulsion is usually delivered during waking hours so as not to interrupt patient's sleep. Because newborns and prematures tend to metabolize fat slowly, it is usually administered at a constant rate over 20–24 h to reduce risk of hyperlipemia.
- Unless otherwise directed by manufacturer, the 10% solutions Intralipid 10% and Liposyn 10% may be stored at room temperature (25C [77F] or below). Intralipid 20% should be refrigerated. Do not freeze.
- Contents of partly used containers should be discarded.

Assessment & Drug Effects

- Acute reactions tend to occur within the first 2 1/2 h of therapy. Observe patient closely.

Common side effects in *italic*; life-threatening effects underlined; generic names in **bold**; classifications in SMALL CAPS

- The following baseline determinations are recommended: hemogram, platelet count, blood coagulation, liver function tests, plasma lipid profile (especially serum triglycerides and cholesterol, free fatty acids in plasma). These tests are usually repeated 1 or 2 times weekly during therapy in adults, and more frequently in children. Significant deviations should be reported promptly.
- Because newborns are prone to develop thrombocytopenia, daily platelet counts are advised during first week of therapy, then every other day during second week and 3 times weekly thereafter.
- Lipemia must clear after each daily infusion. Degree of lipemia is measured by serum triglycerides and cholesterol levels 4–6 h after infusion has ceased.

Patient & Family Education

- Instruct patient to report difficulty breathing, nausea, vomiting, or headache.

Prototype: diethylpropion, p 196

FENFLURAMINE HYDROCHLORIDE
(fen-flure´a-meen)
Trade names: Pondimin, Ponderal
Classification: CNS AGENT; RESPIRATORY & CEREBRAL STIMULANT; ANOREXIANT
Pregnancy: Category C
Controlled substance: Schedule IV

ACTIONS/PHARMACODYNAMICS Indirect-acting sympathomimetic amine related to amphetamine. Differs pharmacologically from amphetamine in that it generally produces CNS depression more often than stimulation. Exact mechanism of appetite-inhibiting action not clearly defined but may be due to stimulation of hypothalamus. Reduces CSF content of 5-hydroxyindoleacetic acid, the principal active metabolite of serotonin. Believed to have intrinsic hypoglycemic activity. Appears to increase glucose uptake by skeletal muscles, thus reducing glucose available for conversion to lipid.

USES Short-term (a few weeks) adjunct in treatment of exogenous obesity. **Unlabeled use:** selected autistic children with high serotonin blood levels.

ROUTE & DOSAGE

Exogenous Obesity

Adult	PO	20 mg t.i.d. a.c.; may be increased at weekly intervals by 20 mg/d to max of 40 mg t.i.d.

PHARMACOKINETICS Absorption: readily absorbed from GI tract. **Onset:** 1–2 h. **Duration:** 4–6 h. **Metabolism:** metabolized in liver. **Elimination:** excreted in urine.

CONTRAINDICATIONS & PRECAUTIONS Contraindicated in: hypersensitivity to sympathomimetic amines; hyperthyroidism; advanced arteriosclerosis, severe hypertension; glaucoma; symptomatic cardiovascular disease including arrhythmias; alcoholism, history of drug abuse; agitated states. Safe use during pregnancy (category C), in nursing mothers, and in children <12 y not established. **Cautious use in:** mental depression; hypertension; diabetes mellitus.

ADVERSE/SIDE EFFECTS CNS: *drowsiness,* sedation, dizziness, confusion, incoordination, headache, elevated mood, dysphoria, mental depression, anxiety, nervousness, psychotic episodes, tremors, weakness, fatigue, dysarthria, insomnia, vivid dreams, nightmares. **Overdosage:** agitation, exaggerated or depressed reflexes, hyperpyrexia, convulsions, coma. **CV:** palpitation, tachycardia, chest pain, arrhythmias, hypotension, hypertension; severe, irreversible pulmonary hypertension; fainting. **Eye:** blurred vision, mydriasis, eye irritation. **GI:** *dry mouth, diarrhea,* nausea, vomiting, unpleasant taste, abdominal pain, constipation. **Gynecologic:** increased or decreased libido, impotence, menstrual irregularities. **Skin:** skin rashes, urticaria, ecchymosis, erythema, burning sensation of skin, hair loss. **Other:** myalgia, edema, dysuria, urinary frequency, grinding teeth during sleep (bruxism), sweating, fever, chills.

DRUG INTERACTIONS GENERAL ANESTHETICS may produce cardiac arrhythmias; **alcohol** and other CNS DEPRESSANTS may compound depressant effects; do not use fenfluramine within 14 d of MAO INHIBITORS, **furazolidone** since they may cause hypertensive crisis.

NURSING IMPLICATIONS

Administration

- Administered on an empty stomach 30–60 min before meals.

F

Common side effects in *italic*; life-threatening effects <u>underlined</u>; generic names in **bold**; classifications in SMALL CAPS

597

- Dose increase should be made gradually to minimize possibility of side effects.
- Store in tightly closed container at 15–30C (59–86F) unless otherwise directed.

Assessment & Drug Effects

- Patients with diabetes maintained on insulin or other antidiabetic drugs should be observed for excessive hypoglycemic activity (see Signs & Symptoms, chap 3) when fenfluramine is added to the therapeutic regimen.
- If fenfluramine is prescribed for patients with hypertension, BP should be monitored.
- Mentally depressed patients may become more depressed during therapy or after withdrawal of fenfluramine.
- If tolerance to anorexigenic effect develops, drug should be discontinued.

Patient & Family Education

- Diarrhea may occur during first week of therapy; report it to physician; dose reduction or termination of therapy may be required.
- Warn patient that fenfluramine may impair ability to perform hazardous tasks such as driving a motor vehicle.
- To achieve and maintain weight loss, patient should be adequately instructed in dietary management.
- After excessive use, abrupt discontinuation of fenfluramine may be associated with irritability and mental depression.

Prototype: Ibuprofen, p 160

FENOPROFEN CALCIUM
(fen-oh-proe´fen)
Trade name: Nalfon
Classifications: CNS AGENT; NONNARCOTIC ANALGESIC, ANTIPYRETIC; NSAID
Pregnancy: Category B (D in 3rd trimester)

ACTIONS/PHARMACODYNAMICS Propionic acid derivative chemically and pharmacologically similar to ibuprofen. Exhibits antiinflammatory, analgesic, and antipyretic properties. Exact mode of antiinflammatory action not known but believed to be related to inhibition of prostaglandin synthesis. Serum uric acid lowering and suppression of platelet aggregation reportedly less than that of aspirin. May prolong bleeding time, but prothrombin time, whole blood clotting time, and platelet counts are usually not affected. Claimed to be comparable to aspirin in antiinflammatory activity and to be associated with lower incidence of adverse GI symptoms. Studies suggest that fenoprofen may prolong labor by reducing uterine contractility. Cross-sensitivity to other nonsteroidal antiinflammatory drugs (NSAIDs) has been reported.

USES Antiinflammatory and analgesic effects in the symptomatic treatment of acute and chronic rheumatoid arthritis and osteoarthritis; relief of mild to moderate pain. **Unlabeled uses:** juvenile rheumatoid arthritis, acute gouty arthritis, ankylosing spondylitis; fever associated with pulmonary tuberculosis, type A influenza, colds; neoplasms.

ROUTE & DOSAGE

Inflammatory Disease

Adult	PO	300–600 mg t.i.d. or q.i.d. (max 3200 mg/d)
Child	PO	900 mg/m² in divided doses; may increase over 4 wk to 1.8 g/m²

Mild to Moderate Pain

Adult	PO	200 mg q4–6h prn

PHARMACOKINETICS Absorption: 80% absorbed from GI tract. **Onset:** 2 h. **Peak:** 2 h. **Duration:** 4–6 h. **Distribution:** small amounts distributed into breast milk. **Metabolism:** metabolized in liver. **Elimination:** half-life: 3 h; excreted primarily in urine; some biliary excretion.

CONTRAINDICATIONS & PRECAUTIONS Contraindicated in: history of nephrotic syndrome associated with aspirin or other NSAIDs; patient in whom urticaria, severe rhinitis, bronchospasm, angioedema, nasal polyps are precipitated by aspirin or other NSAIDs; significant renal or hepatic dysfunction. Safe use during pregnancy (category B), by nursing mothers, and in children not established. **Cautious use in:** history of upper GI tract disorders; hemophilia or other bleeding tendencies; compromised cardiac function, hypertension; impaired hearing.

ADVERSE/SIDE EFFECTS CNS: *headache, drowsiness,* dizziness, fatigue, lassitude, tremor, confusion, insomnia, nervousness, depression. **CV:** palpitation, tachycardia, peripheral edema. **Ear/eye:** tinnitus, decreased hearing, deafness; blurred vision. **GI:** *indigestion, nausea, vomiting,* anorexia, *constipation,* diarrhea, flatulence, abdominal pain, dry mouth; infrequent: gastritis, peptic ulcer, jaundice, cholestatic hepatitis, GI bleeding. **GU:** nephrotoxicity (rare): dysuria, cystitis, hematuria, oliguria, azotemia, anuria, allergic nephritis, papillary necrosis. **Hematologic (infrequent):** thrombocytopenia, hemolytic anemia, agranulocytosis, pancytopenia. **Skin:** (may or may not be hypersensitivity reaction): pruritus, rash, purpura, increased sweating, urticaria. **Other:** dyspnea, malaise, anaphylaxis.

DRUG INTERACTIONS Fenoprofen may prolong bleeding time—should not be given with ORAL ANTI-COAGULANTS, **heparin;** action and side effects of **phenytoin,** SULFONYLUREAS, SULFONAMIDES, and fenoprofen may be potentiated.

NURSING IMPLICATIONS

Administration

- For rapid absorption, best taken on an empty stomach 30–60 min before or 2 h after meals. May be administered with meals, milk, or antacid (prescribed), however, if patient experiences GI disturbances. Peak plasma levels may be delayed by food or antacids, but total amount absorbed is not affected.
- Tablet may be crushed or capsule emptied and contents swallowed with fluid or mixed with food.
- Store capsules and tablets in tightly closed containers at 15–30C (59–86F); avoid freezing.

Assessment & Drug Effects

- Baseline and periodic evaluations of hemoglobin, renal and hepatic function, and auditory and ophthalmic examinations are recommended in patients receiving prolonged or high dose therapy.
- Monitor for signs and symptoms of GI bleeding.
- When phenobarbital is added to or withdrawn from patient's drug regimen, dosage adjustment of fenoprofen may be required.
- An ophthalmologic examination is recommended if patient has eye complaints.

Patient & Family Education

- Because fenoprofen may cause dizziness and drowsiness, advise patient to exercise caution when driving or performing other potentially hazardous activities.
- Instruct patient to report immediately the onset of unexplained fever, rash, arthralgia, oliguria, edema, weight gain. Possible symptoms of nephrotic syndrome are rapidly reversible if drug is promptly withdrawn.
- Therapeutic effectiveness of fenoprofen in patients with arthritis may be evidenced within a few days with peak effect in 2–3 wk.
- Inform patient that alcohol and aspirin may increase risk of GI ulceration and bleeding tendencies and should be avoided unless otherwise advised by physician.
- Fenoprofen may prolong bleeding time; therefore advise patient to inform dentist or surgeon that he is taking this drug.

Prototype: morphine, p 156

FENTANYL CITRATE
(fen´ta-nil)
Trade names: Duragesic, Sublimaze
Classifications: CNS AGENT; ANALGESIC; NARCOTIC (OPIATE) AGONIST; GENERAL ANESTHETIC
Pregnancy: Category B (D for prolonged use or use of high doses at term)
Controlled substance: Schedule II

ACTIONS/PHARMACODYNAMICS Synthetic, potent narcotic agonist analgesic with pharmacologic actions qualitatively similar to those of morphine and meperidine, but action is more prompt and less prolonged. Principal actions: analgesia and sedation. Drug induced alterations in respiratory rate and alveolar ventilation may persist beyond the analgesic effect. As dose increases, pulmonary exchange deficit increases; large doses may produce apnea. Emetic effect is less than with either morphine or meperidine. Exhibits little hypnotic activity and rarely causes histamine release.

USES Short-acting analgesic during operative and perioperative periods, as a narcotic analgesic supplement in general and regional anesthesia, and with droperidol or with diazepam to produce neuroleptoanalgesia. Also given with oxygen and a skeletal muscle relaxant (neuroleptoanesthesia) to selected high-risk patients (e.g., those undergoing open heart surgery) when attenuation of the response to surgical stress without use of additional anesthesia agents is important.

PHARMACOKINETICS Absorption: absorbed through the skin, leveling off between 12–24 h. **Onset:** immediate IV; 7–15 min IM; 12–24 h transdermal. **Peak:** 3–5 min IV;24–72 h transdermal. **Duration:** 30–60

F

ROUTE & DOSAGE

Premedication

Adult	IM	50–100 µg 30–60 min before surgery

Adjunct for Regional Anesthesia

Adult	IM	50–100 µg
	IV	2–20 µg/kg over 1–2 min up to 50 µg/kg

General Anesthesia

Adult	IV	up to 150 µg/kg as required

Postoperative Pain

Adult	IM	50–100 µg q1–2h prn
Child	IM	1.7–3.3 µg/kg q1–2h prn

Chronic Pain

Adult	Transdermal	Doses of transdermal fentanyl must be individualized and should be regularly reassessed; for patient not already receiving an opioid, the initial dose should be a 25 µg/h patch q3d; for patients already on opioids, see package insert for conversions

min IV; 1–2 h IM; 72 h transdermal. **Metabolism:** metabolized in liver. **Elimination:** excreted in urine.

CONTRAINDICATIONS & PRECAUTIONS Contraindicated in: patients who have received MAO inhibitors within 14 d; myasthenia gravis. Safe use during pregnancy (category C) and in children <2 y not established. **Cautious use in:** head injuries, increased intracranial pressure; elderly, debilitated, poor-risk patients; COPD, other respiratory problems; liver and kidney dysfunction; bradyarrhythmias, by nursing mothers.

ADVERSE/SIDE EFFECTS CNS: *sedation,* euphoria, dizziness, diaphoresis, delirium, convulsions with high doses. **CV:** hypotension, bradycardia, <u>circulatory depression, cardiac arrest</u>. **Eye:** miosis, blurred vision. **GI:** *nausea,* vomiting, constipation, ileus. **Respiratory:** <u>laryngospasm</u>, bronchoconstriction, <u>respiratory depression or arrest</u>. **Other:** muscle rigidity, especially muscles of respiration after rapid IV infusion, urinary retention, rash, contact dermatitis from patch.

DRUG INTERACTIONS Alcohol and other CNS DEPRESSANTS potentiate effects; MAO INHIBITORS may precipitate hypertensive crisis.

INCOMPATIBILITIES Solution/Additive: pentobarbital, thiopental.

NURSING IMPLICATIONS

Administration

- May be given undiluted or diluted in 5 ml sterile water or NS. Administered by direct IV over 1–2 min.
- Narcotics and other CNS depressants have additive or potentiating effects. If one is prescribed, initial dosage of narcotic analgesic should be reduced to 1/4 or 1/3 of that usually employed.
- Store at 15–30C (59–86F) unless otherwise directed. Protect drug from light.

Assessment & Drug Effects

- Monitor vital signs and observe patient for signs of skeletal and thoracic muscle (depressed respirations) rigidity and weakness.
- During postoperative period, watch carefully for respiratory depression and for movements of various groups of skeletal muscle in extremities, external eye, and neck. These movements may present patient management problems and should be reported promptly.
- Duration of respiratory depressant effect may be considerably longer than narcotic analgesic effect. Have immediately available: oxygen, resuscitative and intubation equipment, and an opioid antagonist such as naloxone.

Prototype: ferrous sulfate, p 132

FERROUS FUMARATE

(foo´ma-rate)

Trade names: Feco-T, Femiron, Feostat, Fersamal, Fumasorb, Fumerin, Hemocyte, Ircon-FA, Neo-Fer-50, Novofumar, Palafer, Palmiron

Classifications: BLOOD FORMER; IRON PREPARATION

Pregnancy: Category A

ACTIONS/PHARMACODYNAMICS Comparable to ferrous sulfate in actions, uses, contraindications, and adverse reactions. Contains 330 mg/g elemental iron (33%).

Common side effects in *italic*; life-threatening effects <u>underlined</u>; generic names in **bold**; classifications in SMALL CAPS

ROUTE & DOSAGE

Therapeutic

Adult	PO	200 mg t.i.d. or q.i.d.
Child	PO	3 mg/kg t.i.d.

Prophylactic

Adult	PO	200 mg once/d
Child	PO	3 mg/kg once/d

NURSING IMPLICATIONS

See ferrous sulfate for nursing implications, diagnostic test interferences, and drug interactions.

Prototype: ferrous sulfate, p 132

FERROUS GLUCONATE

(gloo´koe-nate)

Trade names: Fergon, Ferralet, Fertinic, Novoferrogluc, Simron

Classifications: BLOOD FORMER; IRON PREPARATION

Pregnancy: Category A

ACTIONS/PHARMACODYNAMICS Claimed to cause less gastric irritation and to be better tolerated than ferrous sulfate. Has same actions, uses, contraindications, and adverse reactions as ferrous sulfate. Contains 120 mg/g elemental iron (12%).

ROUTE & DOSAGE

Therapeutic

Adult	PO	325–600 mg q.i.d.; may be gradually increased to 650 mg q.i.d. as needed and tolerated
Child	PO	6–12 y: 100–300 mg t.i.d.
		<6 y: 100–300 mg/d in divided doses

Prophylactic

Adult	PO	325–600 mg once/d
Child	PO	6–12 y: 100–300 mg once/d
		<6 y: 100–300 mg/d in divided doses

NURSING IMPLICATIONS

See ferrous sulfate for nursing implications, diagnostic test interferences, and drug interactions.

FERROUS SULFATE

See BLOOD FORMERS & COAGULATORS, IRON PREPARATION prototype, p 132.

FIBRINOLYSIN AND DESOXYRIBONUCLEASE

(fye-bri-noe-lye´sin)

Trade name: Elase

Classification: DEBRIDING ENZYME

Pregnancy: Category C

ACTIONS/PHARMACODYNAMICS Combination of two bovine proteolytic enzymes: fibrinolysin extracted from bovine plasma acts primarily on fibrin in blood clots and exudates, and desoxyribonuclease derived from beef pancreas attacks DNA in devitalized tissue and disintegrating cells. Enzymatic debridement is directed primarily against denatured proteins in dead tissue; normal tissue remains relatively unaffected. Lacks antiinfective activity, but debriding action reduces necrotic material that tends to favor bacterial growth.

USES Debriding agent in a variety of inflammatory and infected lesions such as general surgical wounds, abscesses, fistulas, and sinus tracts; ulcerative lesions, second- and third-degree burns, circumcision and episiotomy, cervicitis, and vaginitis.

ROUTE & DOSAGE

Vaginitis

Adult	Topical	5 g of ointment intravaginally at bedtime for 5 d, or 10 ml of solution instilled into vagina and held in place with a cotton tampon for 24 h followed by the ointment

Infected Wounds, Empyema Cavities, Fistulas, Sinus Tracts, Subcutaneous Hematomas

Adult	Topical	Irrigate with the solution; solution should be drained and replaced q6–8h

CONTRAINDICATIONS & PRECAUTIONS Contraindicated in: hypersensitivity to bovine products or to mercury derivatives (e.g., thimerosal): not recommended for parenteral use; hematomas adjacent to or within adipose tissue.

F

Common side effects in *italic*; life-threatening effects <u>underlined</u>; generic names in **bold**; classifications in SMALL CAPS

601

ADVERSE/SIDE EFFECTS With higher than recommended dosage: local hyperemia.

NURSING IMPLICATIONS

Administration

- Reconstitute contents of vial with 10 ml sterile isotonic NaCl solution.
- Solution must be freshly prepared before use. Loss of potency is delayed somewhat by refrigeration; however, solution must be used within 24 h.
- For maximal effectiveness, (1) dense eschars should be removed surgically before therapy is initiated; (2) accumulated necrotic debris must be removed periodically to ensure contact of medication with substrate; (3) dressing should be changed at least once daily, preferably two or three times daily.
- *Application of ointment:* flush away necrotic debris and exudates with hydrogen peroxide, sterile warm water, or normal saline (as prescribed), and gently dry area. Apply thin layer of ointment and cover with vaseline gauze or other nonocclusive dressing (as prescribed).
- *Application of solution (wet-to-dry dressing method):* (1) Mix vial of powder with 10–50 ml of saline. (2) Saturate fine mesh gauze or unfolded sterile gauze sponge with the solution. (3) Carefully pack ulcerated area with the saturated gauze. (4) Allow gauze to dry in contact with wound for 6–8 h (as prescribed). (5) Wound is mechanically debrided when dried gauze is removed. (6) Repeat 3 or 4 times daily (as prescribed).
- Manufacturer states that Elase is compatible with chloramphenicol, penicillin, streptomycin, and tetracycline. It is inactivated by plasma, serum, urea, and heat.
- The dry powder is stable at room temperature (59–86F). Note expiration date printed on package.

Prototype: epoetin alfa, p 130

FILGRASTIM
(fil-gras´tim)
Trade name: Neupogen
Classification: BLOOD FORMATION;
HEMATOPOIETIC GROWTH FACTOR
Pregnancy: Category C

ACTIONS/PHARMACODYNAMICS Filgrastim is a human granulocyte colony stimulating factor (G-

CSF) produced by recombinant DNA technology. Endogenous G-CSF regulates the production of neutrophils within the bone marrow. It is not species specific and primarily affects neutrophil progenitor proliferation, differentiation and selected end-cell functional activity (including enhanced phagocytic activity, antibody-dependent killing, and the increased expression of some functions associated with cell-surface antigens).

USES To decrease the incidence of infection, as manifested by febrile neutropenia, in patients with nonmyeloid malignancies receiving myelosuppressive anticancer drugs associated with a significant incidence of severe neutropenia with fever.

ROUTE & DOSAGE

Neutropenia

Adult	IV	5 µg/kg/d by 30 min infusion; dose may be increased by 5 µg/kg/d (max 30 µg/kg/d)
	SC	5 µg/kg/d as single dose; dose may be increased by 5 µg/kg/d (max 20 µg/kg/d)
Child	IV	Same as for adult
	SC	Same as for adult

PHARMACOKINETICS Absorption: readily absorbed from SC site. **Onset:** 4 h. **Peak:** 1 h. **Elimination:** half-life: 1.4–7.2 h; probably excreted in urine.

CONTRAINDICATIONS & PRECAUTIONS Contraindicated in: hypersensitivity to *Escherichia coli*–derived proteins, simultaneous administration with chemotherapy, and myeloid cancers. **Cautious use in:** pregnancy (category C) and nursing mothers.

ADVERSE/SIDE EFFECTS CV: abnormal ST segment depression. **Hematologic:** anemia. **GI:** nausea, anorexia. **Other:** *bone pain*, hyperuricemia, *fever.*

INTERACTIONS Drug-Laboratory modifications: elevations in leukocyte alkaline phosphatase, serum alkaline phosphatase, lactate dehydrogenase, and uric acid have been reported. These elevations appear to be related to increased bone marrow activity.

NURSING IMPLICATIONS

Administration

- Do not administer filgrastim 24 h before or after cytotoxic chemotherapy.

Common side effects in *italic*; life-threatening effects underlined; generic names in **bold**; classifications in SMALL CAPS

- Filgrastim administration is normally continued until the absolute neutrophil count (ANC) is 10,000/mm^3 after chemotherapy-induced nadir.
- Prior to injection, filgrastim may be allowed to reach room temperature for a maximum of 6 h. Discard any vial left at room temperature for > 6 h.
- Administer prescribed dose SC or IV as ordered. Dose may be increased in 5 μg/kg increments for each chemotherapy cycle.
- Use only one dose per vial; do not reenter the vial.
- Refrigerate at 2–8C (36–46F). Do not freeze. Avoid shaking.

Assessment & Drug Effects
- A baseline CBC with differential and platelet count is obtained prior to administering drug.
- CBC should be done twice weekly during therapy to monitor neutrophil count and leukocytosis. WBC ≥ 100,000/mm^3 have been observed with no apparent adverse effect.
- Discontinue filgrastim if absolute neutrophil count surpasses 10,000/mm^3 after the chemotherapy induced nadir.
- With the discontinuation of filgrastim therapy, neutrophil counts return to normal.
- Regular monitoring of hematocrit and platelet count is recommended.
- If the patient develops sternal pain, the drug should be discontinued.
- Closely monitor patients with preexisting cardiac conditions. MI and arrhythmias have been associated with a small percent of patients receiving filgrastim.
- Monitor temperature q4h. Incidence of infection should be reduced after administration of filgrastim.
- Assess degree of bone pain if present. Physician should be consulted if nonnarcotic analgesics do not provide relief.
- The safety and efficacy of chronic administration of filgrastim over a period of several years has yet to be established.

Patient & Family Education
- Instruct patient to report bone pain and, if necessary, to request analgesics to control pain.
- If home use is prescribed, instruct patient in the importance of proper drug administration and disposal. A puncture-resistant container for the disposal of used syringes and needles should be available to the patient.

Prototype: atropine, p 116

FLAVOXATE HYDROCHLORIDE
(fla-vox´ate)
Trade name: Urispas
Classifications: AUTONOMIC NERVOUS SYSTEM AGENT; ANTICHOLINERGIC (PARASYMPATHOLYTIC); ANTISPASMODIC
Pregnancy: Category C

ACTIONS/PHARMACODYNAMICS Exerts spasmolytic (papaverinelike) action on smooth muscle. Reported to produce an increase in urinary bladder capacity in patients with spastic bladder, possibly by direct action on detrusor muscle. Also demonstrates local anesthetic and analgesic action.

USES Symptomatic relief of dysuria, frequency, urgency, nocturia, incontinence, and suprapubic pain associated with various urologic disorders.

ROUTE & DOSAGE

Dysuria, Nocturia, Incontinence

Adult	PO	100–200 mg t.i.d. or q.i.d.

PHARMACOKINETICS Elimination: 10–30% excreted in urine within 6 h.

CONTRAINDICATIONS & PRECAUTIONS Contraindicated in: pyloric or duodenal obstruction, obstructive intestinal lesions, ileus, achalasia, GI hemorrhage; obstructive uropathies of lower urinary tract. Safe use during pregnancy (category C) and in children <12 y not established. **Cautious use in:** suspected glaucoma.

ADVERSE/SIDE EFFECTS CNS: headache, vertigo, drowsiness, mental confusion (especially in the elderly), difficulty with concentration, nervousness. **CV:** palpitation, tachycardia. **Eye:** blurred vision, increased intraocular tension, disturbances of eye accommodation. **GI:** nausea, vomiting, dry mouth (and throat), abdominal pain, constipation (with high doses). **Skin:** dermatosis, urticaria. **Other:** dysuria, hyperpyrexia, eosinophilia, leukopenia (rare).

NURSING IMPLICATIONS

Administration
- Store at 15–30C (59–86F) unless otherwise directed.

Common side effects in *italic*; life-threatening effects <u>underlined</u>; generic names in **bold**; classifications in SMALL CAPS

603

F

Assessment & Drug Effects

- Monitor heart rate. Take apical pulse for 1 full minute. Report tachycardia.
- Periodic evaluation of blood counts is advisable during therapy.

Patient & Family Education

- Because of the possibility of drowsiness, mental confusion, and blurred vision, advise patients to avoid driving or performing tasks that require mental alertness and physical coordination until reaction to drug is known.
- Advise patient to report to physician adverse reactions, clinical improvement, or the lack of a favorable response.

Prototype: procainamide, p 140

FLECAINIDE

(fle-kay´nide)
Trade name: Tambocor
Classification: CARDIOVASCULAR AGENT;
ANTIARRHYTHMIC
Pregnancy: Category C

ACTIONS/PHARMACODYNAMICS

Local (membrane) anesthetic and antiarrhythmic with electrophysiologic properties similar to other class IC antiarrhythmic drugs. Slows conduction velocity throughout myocardial conduction system, increases ventricular refractoriness but has little effect on repolarization. Prolongs His-ventricular (HQ) and QRS intervals at therapeutic doses. Clinically, flecainide causes both hypotension and negative inotropy (in higher dose ranges) and is an effective suppressant of PVCs and a variety of atrial and ventricular arrhythmias. Generally does not alter cardiac function, but with IV administration, pulmonary capillary wedge pressure may be increased in patient with coronary disease.

USES

Life-threatening ventricular arrhythmias.
Unlabeled uses: atrial tachycardia and other arrhythmias unresponsive to standard agents (e.g., quinidine), Wolff-Parkinson-White syndrome, and recurrent ventricular tachycardias.

ROUTE & DOSAGE

Life-threatening Ventricular Arrhythmias

Adult	PO	100 mg q12h; may increase by 50 mg b.i.d. q4d to a max of 400 mg/d

PHARMACOKINETICS

Absorption: readily absorbed from GI tract. **Peak:** 2–3 h. **Distribution:** crosses placenta; distributed into breast milk. **Metabolism:** metabolized in liver. **Elimination:** half-life: 7–22 h; excreted mainly in urine.

CONTRAINDICATIONS & PRECAUTIONS

Contraindicated in: hypersensitivity to flecainide; preexisting second- or third-degree AV block, right bundle branch block when associated with a left hemiblock unless a pacemaker is present; cardiogenic shock, significant hepatic impairment. Safe use during pregnancy (category C), in nursing mothers, and in children <18 y not established. **Cautious use in:** CHF, sick sinus syndrome, renal impairment.

ADVERSE/SIDE EFFECTS

Usually dose-related. **CNS:** *dizziness,* headache, lightheadedness, unsteadiness, paresthesias. **CV:** arrhythmias, chest pain, worsening of CHF. **Eye:** *blurred vision, difficulty in focusing,* spots before eyes. **GI:** *nausea,* constipation, change in taste perception. **Hematologic:** thrombocytopenia, leukopenia. **Other:** dyspnea, fever, edema, speech disorders, polyuria, urinary retention (rare), leg cramps.

DRUG INTERACTIONS

Cimetidine may increase flecainide levels; may increase **digoxin** levels 15–25%; BETA-BLOCKERS may have additive negative inotropic effects.

NURSING IMPLICATIONS

Administration

- May be given without regard to food.
- Dosage increases more frequently than every 4 d are not recommended. Steady state plasma levels may not be achieved for 3–5 d, and flecainide has a long half-life.
- Store in tightly covered light-resistant containers at 15–30C (59–86F) unless otherwise directed.

Assessment & Drug Effects

- Preexisting hypokalemia or hyperkalemia should be corrected before treatment is initiated.
- ECG monitoring, including Holter monitor for ambulating patients, is essential because of the possibility of drug-induced arrhythmias.
- Patients with pacemakers should have pacing threshold determination before initiation of therapy, after 1 wk of therapy, and at regular intervals thereafter.
- Plasma level monitoring is recommended, especially in patients with severe CHF or renal failure

Common side effects in *italic*; life-threatening effects underlined;
generic names in **bold**; classifications in SMALL CAPS

because drug elimination may be delayed in these patients.

- Effective trough plasma levels are between 0.7–1 µg/ml. The probability of adverse reactions increases when trough levels exceed 1 µg/ml.
- Once arrhythmia is controlled, dosage reduction may be attempted with caution.

Patient & Family Education

- Impress on patient the importance of taking drug at the prescribed times.
- Instruct patient to report visual disturbances.

Prototype: fluorouracil, p 94

FLOXURIDINE

(flox-yoor´i-deen)
Trade name: FUDR
Classifications: ANTINEOPLASTIC;
ANTIMETABOLITE
Pregnancy: Category D

ACTIONS/PHARMACODYNAMICS Pyrimidine antagonist and cell-cycle specific. Catabolized to fluorouracil in vivo, thus producing same systemic effects as fluorouracil.

USES Palliative agent in management of selected patients with GI metastasis to liver. **Unlabeled use:** carcinoma of breast, ovary, cervix, urinary bladder, and prostate not responsive to other antimetabolites.

ROUTE & DOSAGE

Carcinoma

Adult	Intraarterial	0.1–0.6 mg/kg/d by continuous intraarterial infusion

PHARMACOKINETICS Distribution: distributed to tumor, intestinal mucosa, bone marrow, liver, and CSF; probably crosses placenta. **Metabolism:** rapidly metabolized in liver to fluorouracil. **Elimination:** half-life: 16 min; 15% excreted in urine, 60-80% excreted through lungs as carbon dioxide.

CONTRAINDICATIONS & PRECAUTIONS Contraindicated in: existing or recent viral infections. Pregnancy (category D). **Cautious use in:** poor nutritional status, bone marrow depression, serious infections; high-risk patients: prior high-dose pelvic irradiation, use of alkylating agents; impaired renal or hepatic function.

ADVERSE/SIDE EFFECTS CNS: vertigo, convulsions, depression, euphoria, hemiplegia. **CV:** myocardial ischemia, angina. **GI:** *nausea, vomiting, stomatitis,* diarrhea, cramps, anorexia, enteritis, gastritis, esophagopharyngitis. **Hematologic:** leukopenia, *thrombocytopenia.* **Skin:** dermatitis, alopecia (usually reversible), *erythema* or increased skin pigmentation (photosensitivity), nail change, dry skin, pruritic ulcerations, rash. **Other:** hiccups, renal insufficiency, gonadal suppression, fever, epistaxis, decreased resistance to disease.

NURSING IMPLICATIONS

Administration

- Drug is reconstituted with 5 ml sterile distilled water for injection. It is further diluted with 5% dextrose or 0.9% NaCl injection to a volume appropriate for the infusion apparatus to be used. It is administered by pump only to overcome pressure in large arteries and to ensure a uniform rate.
- Because of serious toxicity potential, patient should be hospitalized at least during the initial course of therapy.
- Reconstituted solutions are stable at 2–8C (36–46F) for no more than 2 wk.
- Store at 15–30C (59–86F) unless otherwise directed.

Assessment & Drug Effects

- Examine infusion site frequently for signs of extravasation. If this occurs, infusion should be stopped and restarted in another vessel.
- Therapeutic response is likely to be accompanied by some evidence of toxicity. Supervise patient carefully to note onset of serious side effects. Examine mouth for ulcerations before each dose is to be administered.
- Therapy should be discontinued promptly with onset of any of the following: stomatitis, esophagopharyngitis, intractable vomiting, diarrhea, leukopenia (WBC <3500/mm^3), or rapidly falling WBC count, thrombocytopenia (platelets 100,000/mm^3), GI bleeding, hemorrhage from any site.
- Baseline and periodic determinations should be made of total and differential leukocyte counts, Hct, platelet count, serum uric acid creatinine, and liver function tests.

Patient & Family Education

- Inform patient that floxuridine sometimes causes temporary thinning of hair.

Common side effects in *italic*; life-threatening effects underlined; generic names in **bold**; classifications in SMALL CAPS

605

- Inform patient of potential for nausea and vomiting and measures to alleviate them.

Prototype: amphotericin B, p 56

FLUCONAZOLE
(flu-con´a-zole)
Trade name: Diflucan
Classifications: ANTIINFECTIVE; ANTIBIOTIC; ANTIFUNGAL
Pregnancy: Category C

ACTIONS/PHARMACODYNAMICS Fungistatic but may be fungicidal depending on concentration. It interferes with cytochrome P-450 activity, which is necessary for the formation of ergosterol. Ergosterol, the principal sterol in the fungal cell membrane, becomes depleted and interferes with membrane function.

USES Cryptococcal meningitis and oropharyngeal and systemic candidiasis, both commonly found in AIDS and other immunocompromised patients. **Unlabeled use:** vaginal candidiasis.

ROUTE & DOSAGE

Oropharyngeal Candidiasis

Adult	PO/IV	200 mg day 1, then 100 mg q.d. x 2 wk
Child	PO/IV	3–6 mg/kg/d

Esophageal Candidiasis

Adult	PO/IV	200 mg day 1, then 100 mg q.d. x 3 wk
Child	PO/IV	3–6 mg/kg/d

Systemic Candidiasis

Adult	PO/IV	400 mg day 1, then 200 mg q.d. x 4 wk
Child	PO/IV	3–6 mg/kg/d

Cryptococcal Meningitis

Adult	PO/IV	400 mg day 1, then 200 mg q.d. x 10–12 wk
Child	PO/IV	3–6 mg/kg/d

PHARMACOKINETICS Absorption: 90% absorbed from GI tract. **Peak:** 1–2 h. **Distribution:** widely distributed, including CSF. **Metabolism:** 11% of dose metabolized in liver. **Elimination:** half-life: 20–50 h; excreted in urine.

CONTRAINDICATIONS & PRECAUTIONS Contraindicated in: hypersensitivity to fluconazole or other azole antifungals. **Cautious use in:** pregnancy (category C).

ADVERSE/SIDE EFFECTS CNS: headache. **GI:** nausea, vomiting, abdominal pain, diarrhea. **Other:** rash, increase in AST in patients with cryptococcal meningitis and AIDS.

DRUG INTERACTIONS Increased PT in patients on **warfarin;** increased **phenytoin, cyclosporine** levels; hypoglycemic reactions with ORAL SULFONYLUREAS; decreased fluconazole levels with **rifampin, cimetidine.**

NURSING IMPLICATIONS

Administration
- IV fluconazole should be administered at a maximum rate of approximately 200 mg/h if given as a continuous infusion.
- IV admixtures of fluconazole and other medications are not recommended.
- Administer the drug after hemodialysis is completed.

Assessment & Drug Effects
- Patients allergic to other azole antifungals may be allergic to fluconazole.
- The drug may cause elevations of the following laboratory serum values: ALT, AST, alkaline phosphatase, bilirubin.
- Since renal impairment requires dosage adjustment, monitor BUN and serum creatinine concentrations.
- Since the drug can cause hepatotoxicity, liver function tests should be monitored.
- Monitor for signs and symptoms of hepatotoxicity (see chap 3).

Patient & Family Education
- It is important that the medication be taken for the full course of therapy, which may take weeks or months.
- If a dose is missed, it should be taken as soon as possible; however, it should not be taken if it is almost time for next dose.

Common side effects in *italic*; life-threatening effects underlined; generic names in **bold**; classifications in SMALL CAPS

FLUCYTOSINE

(floo-sye'toe-seen)

Trade names: Ancobon, Ancotil, 5-FC, 5-Fluorocytosine

Classifications: ANTIINFECTIVE; ANTIBIOTIC; ANTIFUNGAL

Pregnancy: Category C

ACTIONS/PHARMACODYNAMICS

Fluorinated pyrimidine structurally related to fluorouracil. Ineffective for cancerous tumors possibly because it does not enter mammalian cells. Precise mechanism of action poorly understood, but it appears to involve interference with nucleic acid and protein synthesis. Selectively penetrates fungal cell and is converted to fluorouracil, an antimetabolite believed to be responsible for antifungal activity. Conversion to fluorouracil in body of host is considerably less than in fungi.

USES

Alone or in combination with amphotericin B for serious systemic infections caused by susceptible strains of *Cryptococcus* and *Candida* species. **Unlabeled use:** chromomycosis.

ROUTE & DOSAGE

Fungal Infection

Adult	PO	50–150 mg/kg/d divided q6h
Child	PO	> 50 kg: 50–150 mg/kg/d divided q6h
		<50 kg: 1.5–4.5 g/m²/d divided q6h

PHARMACOKINETICS

Absorption: readily absorbed from GI tract. **Peak:** 2 h. **Distribution:** widely distributed in body tissues including aqueous humor and CSF; crosses placenta. **Metabolism:** minimally metabolized. **Elimination:** half-life: 3–6 h; 75–90% excreted in urine unchanged.

CONTRAINDICATIONS & PRECAUTIONS

Contraindicated in: safe use during pregnancy (category C) and in nursing women not established. Extreme caution in impaired renal function; bone marrow depression, hematologic disorders, patients being treated with or having received radiation or bone marrow depressant drugs.

ADVERSE/SIDE EFFECTS

CNS: confusion, hallucinations, headache, sedation, vertigo. **GI:** nausea, vomiting, diarrhea, abdominal bloating, enterocolitis, bowel perforation (rare). **Hematologic:** hypoplasia of bone marrow: anemia, leukopenia, thrombocytopenia, agranulocytosis, eosinophilia. **Other:** rash; elevated levels of serum alkaline phosphatase, AST, ALT, BUN, serum creatinine; hepatomegaly, hepatitis.

DIAGNOSTIC TEST INTERFERENCES

False elevations of *serum creatinine* can occur with *Ektachem analyzer.*

DRUG INTERACTIONS

Amphotericin B produces additive or synergistic effects and can increase flucytosine toxicity by inhibiting its renal clearance.

NURSING IMPLICATIONS

Administration

- Lower dosages and longer dosage intervals are recommended in patients with serum creatinine of 1.7 mg/dl or higher.
- Incidence and severity of nausea and vomiting may be decreased by giving capsules a few at a time over 15 min.
- Preserve in light-resistant containers at 15–30C (59–86F).

Assessment & Drug Effects

- Culture and susceptibility tests should be performed before initiation of therapy and at weekly intervals during therapy. Organism resistance has been reported.
- Hematologic, renal, and hepatic function tests should be performed on all patients before and at frequent intervals during therapy. Twice weekly leukocyte and platelet counts are recommended.
- Frequent assays of blood drug level are recommended, especially in patients with impaired renal function to determine adequacy of drug excretion (therapeutic range: 25–120 µg/ml).
- Monitor I&O. Report change in I&O ratio or pattern. Because most of drug is eliminated unchanged by kidneys, compromised function can lead to drug accumulation.

Patient & Family Education

- Instruct patient to report fever, sore mouth or throat, and unusual bleeding or bruising tendency.
- Duration of therapy is generally 4–6 wk, but it may continue for several months.

F

Common side effects in *italic*; life-threatening effects underlined; generic names in **bold**; classifications in SMALL CAPS

607

FLUDROCORTISONE

See HORMONES, ADRENAL CORTICOSTEROID, MINERALOCORTICOID prototype, p 227.

Prototype: hydrocortisone, p 255

FLUNISOLIDE

(floo-niss'oh-lide)
Trade names: AeroBid, Nasalide
Classifications: SKIN & MUCOUS MEMBRANE AGENT; ANTIINFLAMMATORY; ADRENAL CORTICOSTEROID
Pregnancy: Category C

ACTIONS/PHARMACODYNAMICS Modified steroid preparation with topical antiinflammatory and vasoconstrictor activity, structurally related to hydrocortisone. Exact mechanism of action not known. Glucocorticoid activity is more potent than mineralocorticoid action. Does not suppress hypothalamus-pituitary-adrenal function (HPA) except in excessive doses. Commercial preparations contain no propellant (fluorocarbon), which has been associated with excessive dryness of nasal mucosa.

USES Symptomatic relief of seasonal and perennial rhinitis in patients who have developed tolerance or poor response to conventional therapy; steroid-dependent asthma. **Unlabeled use:** Serous otitis media in children.

ROUTE & DOSAGE

Allergic Rhinitis

Adult	Inhaled/Intranasal	2 sprays orally, or intranasally in each nostril, b.i.d.; may increase to t.i.d. if needed
Child	Inhaled/Intranasal	6–14 y: 1 spray orally, or intranasally in each nostril, t.i.d. or 2 sprays b.i.d.

PHARMACOKINETICS Absorption: approximately 50% reaches systemic circulation. **Onset:** 3–5 d. **Peak:** 10–30 min. **Metabolism:** metabolized in liver to active metabolites. **Elimination:** half-life: 1–2 h; 50% excreted in urine, 50% excreted in feces.

CONTRAINDICATIONS & PRECAUTIONS Contraindicated in: hypersensitivity to any ingredients in the formulation; children <6 y. Safe use during pregnancy (category C) and by nursing women not established. **Cautious use in:** recent nasal ulcers, nasal surgery or trauma, active or latent tuberculosis (respiratory tract); untreated fungal, bacterial, or systemic viral infection; ocular herpes, patients receiving systemic corticosteroids.

ADVERSE/SIDE EFFECTS CNS: headache, dizziness. **ENT:** *mild transient nasal burning or stinging,* nasal congestion, sneezing, epistaxis or bloody nasal discharge, nasal irritation or dryness, sore throat, hoarseness, bitter taste, loss of taste or smell. **GI:** dry mouth, nausea, vomiting, abdominal bloating. **Other:** HPA suppression with excessive dosages, increase in AST; watery eyes; nasal septal perforation (rare, causal relationships not established); localized candidal infections.

NURSING IMPLICATIONS

Administration
- Have patient clear nasal passages of secretions before he or she takes medication.
- Store at 15–30C (59–86F) in light-resistant containers unless otherwise directed. Opened containers of flunisolide should be discarded after 3 mo.

Assessment & Drug Effects
- If transfer from prolonged systemic steroid therapy to flunisolide is too rapid, symptoms of corticosteroid withdrawal (joint or muscle pain, lassitude, depression), acute adrenal insufficiency, or exacerbation of asthma may occur.

Patient & Family Education
- Instruct patient who is using a bronchodilator by oral inhalation to use it several minutes before inhaling flunisolide to increase its penetration and to reduce possibility of toxicity from aerosol propellant (fluorocarbons).
- Inform patient that maximum therapeutic effects are achieved by taking medication exactly as directed (prescribed dosage, intervals, and procedure). Review patient instructions provided by manufacturer with patient.
- Mild transient nasal burning or stinging occurs commonly (almost 45% of patients). If symptoms persist or increase in severity or if no improvement is noted within 3 wk, physician should be notified. Discontinuation of therapy may be necessary.

Prototype: hydrocortisone, p 255

FLUOCINOLONE ACETONIDE

(floo-oh-sin´oh-lone)

Trade names: Dermalar, Dermophyl, Fluoderm, Fluolar, Fluonid, Flurosyn, Synalar, Synalar-HP, Synemol

Classifications: SKIN AGENT; ANTIINFLAMMATORY; ADRENAL CORTICOSTEROID

Pregnancy: Category C

ACTIONS/PHARMACODYNAMICS Synthetic fluorinated steroid with strong antiinflammatory, antipruritic, and vasoconstrictive actions but negligible mineralocorticoid effects. More effective than hydrocortisone.

USES To relieve inflammatory manifestations of corticosteroid-responsive dermatoses.

ROUTE & DOSAGE

Inflammation

Adult   Topical   Apply thin layer b.i.d. to q.i.d.

PHARMACOKINETICS Absorption: minimum absorption through intact skin; increased absorption from axilla, eyelid, face, scalp, scrotum, or with occlusive dressing.

CONTRAINDICATIONS & PRECAUTIONS Contraindicated in: infants <2 y; ophthalmic use.

ADVERSE/SIDE EFFECTS See hydrocortisone.

NURSING IMPLICATIONS

■ Protect drug from light.
See numerous nursing implications under hydrocortisone.

Prototype: hydrocortisone, p 255

FLUOCINONIDE

(floo-oh-sin´oh-nide)

Trade names: Lidemol, Lidex, Lidex-E, Lyderm, Topsyn

Classifications: SKIN AGENT; ANTIINFLAMMATORY; ADRENAL CORTICOSTEROID

Pregnancy: Category C

ACTIONS/PHARMACODYNAMICS Synthetic fluorinated glucocorticoid used only topically for antiinflammatory effects in glucocorticoid-responsive dermatoses. See hydrocortisone for contraindications and precautions, drug interactions.

ROUTE & DOSAGE

Inflammation

Adult   Topical   Apply thin layer b.i.d. to q.i.d.

PHARMACOKINETICS Absorption: minimum absorption through intact skin; increased absorption from axilla, eyelid, face, scalp, scrotum, or with occlusive dressing.

ADVERSE/SIDE EFFECTS Burning, itching, hypertrichosis, dermatitis; see hydrocortisone.

NURSING IMPLICATIONS

See numerous nursing implications under hydrocortisone.

FLUORESCEIN SODIUM

(flure´e-seen)

Trade names: AK-Fluor, Fluorescite, Fluor-I-Strip, Fluor-I-Ful-Glo, Funduscein, Strip A.T.

Classification: DIAGNOSTIC AGENT

Pregnancy: Category C

ACTIONS/PHARMACODYNAMICS Mildly antiseptic fluorescent dye related chemically to phenolphthalein.

USES An aid in fitting hard contact lenses, applanation tonometry, detecting corneal epithelial defects, and testing potency of lacrimal system. Used IV as a diagnostic aid in retinal angiography. Also used as an antidote for aniline dye.

CONTRAINDICATIONS & PRECAUTIONS Contraindicated in: topical use with soft contact lenses not recommended. **Cautious use in:** history of hypersensitivity, allergies, bronchial asthma.

F

Common side effects in *italic*; life-threatening effects underlined; generic names in **bold**; classifications in SMALL CAPS

609

ROUTE & DOSAGE

Diagnostic Aid

Adult	Topical	Instill 1–2 drops and have patient keep eyelid closed for 60 s; or moisten strip with sterile water, touch conjunctiva or fornix with moistened tip, and have patient blink to distribute

Retinal Angiography

Adult	IV	5 ml of 10% solution or 3 ml of 25% solution injected rapidly in antecubital vein
Child	IV	7.5 mg/kg injected rapidly in antecubital vein

ADVERSE/SIDE EFFECTS *Topical use: temporary stinging, burning sensation,* conjunctival redness. *IV administration:* **CNS:** headache, paresthesias, dizziness, pyrexia, convulsions. **CV:** hypotension, transient dyspnea, acute pulmonary edema, basilar artery ischemia, syncope, <u>severe shock, cardiac arrest</u>. **GI:** nausea, vomiting. **Hypersensitivity:** urticaria, pruritus, angioneurotic edema, <u>anaphylactic reaction</u>. **Other:** thrombophlebitis at injection site, temporary discoloration of skin and urine, strong metallic taste following high dosage.

NURSING IMPLICATIONS

Administration

- Avoid touching eyelids of surrounding area with eyedropper when instilling medication.
- Fluorescein inactivates preservatives commonly used in ophthalmic preparations; therefore, solutions can be easily contaminated, particularly with *Pseudomonas*. Unit-dose containers or individually wrapped filter paper strips impregnated with fluorescein offer greater assurance of sterility.
- *To fit hard contact lenses:* fluorescein is instilled with contact lenses in place. Patient should be instructed to blink several times to distribute dye. Under blue light, areas that lack fluorescein will appear black, indicating that contact lens is touching cornea at these points.
- *To test for potency of lacrimal system:* 1 drop of 2% solution is instilled into conjunctival sac. Instruct patient to blink at least 4 times. After 6 min nasal secretions are examined under blue light. Traces of dye in secretions indicate that nasolacrimal drainage system is open.
- *As an antidote for aniline dye* (in indelible pencils): After removal of pencil point, eye is irrigated with 2% solution every 10 min until visible precipitate is no longer present. Irrigations are repeated every 30 min for 12–24 h.
- Solution container should be kept tightly closed when not in use.
- Store below 27C (80F). Protect from light and freezing.

Assessment & Drug Effects

- Facilities for treatment of anaphylactic reaction should be immediately available, e.g., epinephrine 1:1000 for IV or IM use, an antihistamine, and oxygen.
- Surface eye defects absorb more fluorescein than intact tissue. Thus corneal abrasions or ulcerations appear green under normal light or bright yellow under cobalt blue illumination. Foreign bodies are surrounded by a green ring. Similar lesions in conjunctiva will appear orange-yellow. Aqueous humor (being more alkaline) will cause bright green fluorescence (useful for detecting wound leaks).
- Fluorescein should be discontinued immediately if signs of sensitivity develop.

Patient & Family Education

- IV administration may impart a yellowish orange discoloration to skin and to urine. Skin discoloration usually fades in 6–12 h; urine clears in 24–36 h.

Prototype: hydrocortisone, p 255

FLUOROMETHOLONE

(flure-oh-meth´oh-lone)
Trade names: Fluor-Op, FML Forte, FML Liquifilm Ophthalmic
Classifications: SKIN & MUCOUS MEMBRANE AGENT; ANTIINFLAMMATORY; ADRENAL CORTICOSTEROID

ACTIONS/PHARMACODYNAMICS Fluorinated adrenal corticosteroid with actions, contraindications, and adverse/side effects similar to those of hydrocortisone.

USES Topically in management of glucocorticoid-responsive ocular inflammations.

ADVERSE/SIDE EFFECTS Eye: increased intraocular pressure, especially in the elderly patient, corneal pathology; with excessive use: diminished visual field, optic nerve damage, cataracts, glaucoma exacerbation.

——— Common side effects in *italic*; life-threatening effects <u>underlined</u>; ——— generic names in **bold**; classifications in SMALL CAPS

ROUTE & DOSAGE

Ocular Inflammation

Adult	Topical	1–2 drops of suspension in conjunctival sac qh for the first 24–48 h; then h.i.d. to q.i.d.; or a thin strip of ointment q4h for the first 24–48 h; then 1–3 times/d
Child	Topical	> 2 y: Same as for adult

NURSING IMPLICATIONS

Patient & Family Education

- Eye drops are not to be used for extended periods.
- Depress lacrimal duct after instilling eye drops.
- Caution patient to follow established dose regimen.
- If visual acuity decreases or visual field diminishes, patient should stop drug and notify physician.

See nursing implications under hydrocortisone.

FLUOROURACIL

See ANTINEOPLASTICS, ANTIMETABOLITE prototype, p 94.

FLUOXETINE

See CNS AGENTS, PSYCHOTHERAPEUTIC, BICYCLIC ANTIDEPRESSANT prototype, p 180.

Prototype: testosterone, p 229

FLUOXYMESTERONE

(floo-ox-ee-mess′te-rone)
Trade names: Android-F, Halotestin, Ora Testryl
Classifications: SYNTHETIC HORMONE; ANDROGEN/ANABOLIC STEROID
Pregnancy: Category X
Controlled substance: Schedule III

ACTIONS/PHARMACODYNAMICS Short-acting, orally effective halogenated derivative of testosterone with up to 5 times the androgenic/anabolic activity of methyltestosterone. Has hypercholesterolemic effect. Retention of sodium is minimal; thus hypertension and edema rarely complicate therapy.

Reduces nitrogen, potassium, and calcium excretion and promotes recalcification of osseous metastases and regression of soft tissue lesions.

USES In men as replacement therapy in conditions associated with testicular hormone deficiency; in women to antagonize effects of estrogen in androgen-responsive inoperable breast cancer. Also in combination with estrogens for management of severe postmenopausal vasomotor symptoms.

ROUTE & DOSAGE

Male Hypogonadism

Adult	PO	2.5–20 mg/d

Metastatic Carcinoma of Female Breast

Adult	PO	10–40 mg/d in divided doses

Postpartum Breast Engorgement

Adult	PO	2.5 mg shortly after delivery; then 5–10 mg/d in divided doses for 4–5 d

PHARMACOKINETICS Absorption: readily absorbed from GI tract. **Metabolism:** metabolized in liver. **Elimination:** half-life: 9.5 h.

CONTRAINDICATIONS & PRECAUTIONS Contraindicated in: breast cancer in men, prostatic cancer, benign obstructive prostatic hypertrophy; hypercalcemia; diabetes mellitus; severe cardiorenal disease or liver damage; nephrosis or nephrotic phase of nephritis; history of MI; athletes; infants; women with inoperable mammary cancer <1 y or >5 y after menopause; pregnancy (category X), nursing mothers.

ADVERSE/SIDE EFFECTS Virilization (women); priapism, impotence, gynecomastia (men); jaundice (reversible), hypoglycemia, hypercalcemia, <u>hepatocellular carcinoma</u>, peliosis hepatitis, nausea, vomiting, diarrhea, symptoms resembling peptic ulcer, <u>anaphylactic reactions</u> (rare), *edema, acne.*

DRUG INTERACTIONS ORAL ANTICOAGULANTS increase risk of bleeding. Possibly increases risk of **cyclosporine** toxicity. **Insulin** and ORAL HYPOGLYCEMIC AGENTS may decrease glucose level; dose will need to be adjusted.

NURSING IMPLICATIONS

Administration

- Administer drug immediately before or with meals to diminish GI distress.

Common side effects in *italic*; life-threatening effects <u>underlined</u>; generic names in **bold**; classifications in SMALL CAPS

611

Assessment & Drug Effects

- Baseline and periodic determinations of liver function and serum electrolytes are indicated. Serial determinations of serum cholesterol are advised in patients with history of MI or coronary artery disease. **Normal total cholesterol:** 150–280 mg/dl.
- Monitor I&O ratio and pattern and weight, and check for edema; report significant changes. Edema is generally controllable with salt restriction or diuretic therapy.
- Monitor for signs of hypercalcemia (see Chapter 3), which is particularly likely to occur in patients with metastatic breast carcinoma and may indicate bone metastases. Anabolic therapy will be stopped if it develops; consult physician about hydration and activity of patient.
- Be alert for voice change in female patient, an early sign of virilism. Virilism may be irreversible even after prompt discontinuation of therapy.
- When used in pediatrics, therapy is preceded by x-ray of wrist bones to establish level of bone maturation. During treatment, bone maturation may proceed more rapidly than linear growth; therefore intermittent dosage schedule and periodic x-rays are usual.
- Children <7 y are particularly sensitive to androgenic effects and therefore should be closely observed for precocious development of male sexual characteristics or masculinization. They should be questioned about the presence of priapism (inappropriate and frequent erections). These symptoms may necessitate drug withdrawal.
- Anabolic treatment may reduce blood glucose in diabetic patients. Watch for symptoms of hypoglycemia (see Chapter 3) and report to physician.
- Observe patient on concomitant anticoagulant therapy for ecchymotic areas, petechiae, or abnormal bleeding from any site. Close monitoring of prothrombin time is essential.
- When fluoxymesterone is used for palliation of mammary cancer, subjective effects of therapy may not be experienced for about 1 mo; objective symptoms may be delayed for as long as 3 mo.
- Anabolic response may be evidenced by euphoria and gain in weight and appetite, especially in emaciated and debilitated patient.
- Baseline and periodic determinations should be made of Hgb, Hct, hepatic function, and serum and urine calcium.

Patient & Family Education

- Drugs are most effective when combined with a therapeutic dietary regimen, physical therapy, and optimum health-promoting habits.
- Reinforce adherence to scheduled appointments for physical therapy and laboratory tests. Stress importance of good personal hygiene, including meticulous skin care (females and prepubertal males are especially likely to develop acne).
- Teach patient to note and report symptoms of jaundice (see Chapter 3) to physician. Dose adjustment may reverse the condition.
- Instruct female patient to report menstrual irregularities. Usually the physician will discontinue medication pending determination of cause.
- Because skeletal stimulation continues about 6 mo after treatment has been stopped, x-rays are used as determinants for discontinuing therapy well before bone maturation reaches the norm for chronologic age. Teach parents the importance of keeping child's appointments for bone maturation studies (usually every 3–6 mo) to prevent compromised adult height.
- Instruct to report priapism (symptom of overdosage) promptly; temporary interruption of regimen is indicated. Also advise to report persistent GI distress, diarrhea, or the onset of jaundice.
- Explain to female on drug for palliation of mammary cancer that virilization usually occurs. Urge early reporting of voice change (hoarseness or deepening), increased libido (associated with clitoral enlargement), hirsutism. Usually, stopping therapy will end further development of symptoms but will not reverse hirsutism or voice change.

Prototype: chlorpromazine, p 191

FLUPHENAZINE DECANOATE

(floo-fen´a-zeen)
Trade names: Prolixin Decanoate, Modecate Decanoate

FLUPHENAZINE ENANTHATE

Trade names: Moditen Enanthate, Prolixin Enanthate

FLUPHENAZINE HYDROCHLORIDE

Trade names: Moditen Hydrochloride, Permitil, Prolixin
Classifications: CNS AGENT; PSYCHOTHERAPEUTIC; ANTIPSYCHOTIC; PHENOTHIAZINE
Pregnancy: Category C

Common side effects in *italic*; life-threatening effects underlined; generic names in **bold**; classifications in SMALL CAPS

ACTIONS/PHARMACODYNAMICS Potent piperazine derivative of phenothiazine. In common with other phenothiazines, blocks postsynaptic dopamine receptors in the brain. Similar to other phenothiazines with the following exceptions: more potent per weight, higher incidence of extrapyramidal complications, and lower frequency of sedative and hypotensive effects. Has weak antiemetic and anticholinergic actions. Fluphenazine hydrochloride has more rapid action and shorter duration of action and thus may be used initially to determine the patient's response or to establish appropriate dosage. Fluphenazine decanoate and enanthate are esterified forms of fluphenazine (esterification markedly prolongs duration of effects). These preparations are indicated primarily for maintenance therapy in patients who cannot be relied on to take daily PO formulations.

USES Management of manifestations of psychotic disorders. **Unlabeled use:** as antineuralgia adjunct.

ROUTE & DOSAGE

Psychosis

Adult	PO	0.5–10 mg/d in 1–4 divided doses, up to a usual max of 20 mg/d
	IM/SC	HCl: 2.5–10 mg/d divided q6–8h up to usual max of 10 mg/d
		Decanoate: 12.5–25 mg q1–4 wk
		Enanthate: 25 mg q2wk

PHARMACOKINETICS Absorption: HCl is readily absorbed PO and IM; decanoate, enanthate have delayed IM absorption. **Onset:** 1 h HCl; 24–72 h decanoate, enanthate. **Peak:** 0.5 h PO; 1.5–2 h IM HCl. **Duration:** 6–8 h HCl; 1–6 wk decanoate; 2–4 wk enanthate. **Distribution:** crosses blood-brain barrier and placenta. **Metabolism:** metabolized in liver. **Elimination:** half-life: 15 h HCl; 3.6 d enanthate; 7–10 d decanoate.

CONTRAINDICATIONS & PRECAUTIONS Contraindicated in: known hypersensitivity to phenothiazines; subcortical brain damage, comatose or severely depressed states, blood dyscrasias, renal or hepatic disease. Safe use during pregnancy (category C) or in nursing women not established. Parenteral form not recommended for children <12 y. **Cautious use in:** with anticholinergic agents, other CNS depressants; elderly patients, previously diagnosed breast cancer; cardiovascular diseases; pheochromocytoma; history of convulsive disorders; patients exposed to extreme heat or phosphorous insecticides; peptic ulcer; respiratory impairment.

ADVERSE/SIDE EFFECTS CNS: *extrapyramidal symptoms* (resembling Parkinson's disease), tardive dyskinesia, sedation, drowsiness, dizziness, headache, mental depression, catatonic-like state, impaired thermoregulation, grand mal seizures. **CV:** tachycardia, hypertension, hypotension. **GI:** dry mouth, nausea, epigastric pain, constipation, fecal impaction, cholecystic jaundice. **GU:** urinary retention, polyuria. **Gynecologic:** inhibition of ejaculation. **Hematologic:** transient leukopenia, agranulocytosis. **Other:** SLE-like syndrome, contact dermatitis, peripheral edema, nasal congestion, blurred vision, increased intraocular pressure, *photosensitivity,* "silent pneumonia," hyperprolactinemia.

DRUG INTERACTIONS Alcohol and other CNS DEPRESSANTS may potentiate depressive effects; decreases seizure threshold—may need to adjust dosage of ANTICONVULSANTS.

NURSING IMPLICATIONS

Administration

- Extended release tablet should be swallowed whole. (Not recommended for children.)
- Dilute PO concentrate in fruit juice, water, carbonated beverage, milk, soup. Avoid caffeine-containing beverages (cola, coffee) as a diluent, also tannic acid (tea) or pectinates (apple juice).
- Persons preparing PO concentrate or liquid preparations for injection should be careful not to contact skin or clothing with drug. Warn patient to avoid spilling drug. If skin is contacted, it should be rinsed promptly with warm water.
- Antacids diminish absorption; therefore administer PO preparations at least 1 h before or 1 h after the antacid.
- Dry syringe and needle (at least 21 gauge) should be used for administering fluphenazine decanoate or enanthate. Moisture may cause solution to become cloudy.
- Fluphenazine enanthate and decanoate are given IM or SC.
- All preparations of fluphenazine should be protected from light and from freezing. Solutions may safely vary in color from almost colorless to light amber. Discard dark or otherwise discolored solutions.
- Store in tightly closed container at 15–30C (59–86F) unless otherwise specified by manufacturer.

Assessment & Drug Effects

- Report immediately the onset of mental depression and extrapyramidal symptoms. They occur fre-

Common side effects in *italic*; life-threatening effects underlined; generic names in **bold**; classifications in SMALL CAPS

613

quently, particularly with long-acting forms (decanoate and enanthate). Be alert for appearance of acute dystonia (see Signs & Symptoms, chap 3). Symptoms can be controlled by reducing fluphenazine dosage or by adding an antiparkinsonism drug such as benztropine (Cogentin).

- Extended exposure to high environmental temperature, to sun's rays, or to a high fever associated with serious illness places this patient at risk for heat stroke. Be alert to red, dry, hot skin; full, bounding pulse, dilated pupils, dyspnea, mental confusion, elevated BP, temperature over 40.6C (105F). Inform physician and institute measures to reduce body temperature rapidly.
- Renal function should be monitored in patients on long-term treatment. The drug should be discontinued if BUN is elevated (**normal BUN:** 10–20 mg/dl). Blood studies, hepatic function tests, and ophthalmologic examinations should also be performed periodically.
- Monitor BP during early therapy. Hypotension is rarely a problem; however, fluctuations in BP have occurred in some patients. If systolic drop is more than 20 mm Hg, inform physician.
- Monitor I&O ratio and bowel elimination pattern. Check for abdominal distension and pain. Monitor for xerostomia and constipation. The depressed patient may not seek help for either of these conditions, or for urinary retention.
- Patients on large doses who undergo surgery and those with cerebrovascular, cardiac, or renal insufficiency are especially prone to hypotensive effects.

Patient & Family Education

- Caution patient against driving motor vehicle or other hazardous activities until reaction to the drug is known.
- Advise patient not to alter dosage regimen or stop it abruptly. Caution patient not to give the drug to any other person.
- The physician should give approval before patient self-doses with OTC drugs.
- Because both decanoate and enanthate formulations have a long duration of action, early detection of adverse effects is critical. Patient should inform the physician promptly if the following symptoms appear: light-colored stools, changes in vision, sore throat, fever, cellulitis, rash, any interference with volitional movement.
- Encourage adequate food and fluid intake as prophylaxis for constipation and for xerostomia.
- Patient may be unable to adjust to extreme temperatures. Advise caution because of possible impaired thermoregulation.

- Warn patient to avoid exposure to sun, especially from 10 AM to 2 PM; also, to wear protective clothing and cover exposed skin surfaces with sun screen lotion (SPF above 12). Photosensitivity is a fairly common side effect for the person on long-term therapy.
- Alcohol should be avoided while patient is on fluphenazine therapy.
- Inform patient that fluphenazine may discolor urine pink to red or reddish brown.

Prototype: hydrocortisone, p 255

FLURANDRENOLIDE
(flure-an-dren´oh-lide)
Trade names: Cordran, Cordran SP, Drenison
Classifications: SKIN AGENT;
ANTIINFLAMMATORY; ADRENAL CORTICOSTEROID
Pregnancy: Category C

ACTIONS/PHARMACODYNAMICS Topical fluorinated steroid with substituted 17-hydroxyl group. Crosses skin cell membrane, complexes with nuclear DNA, and stimulates synthesis of enzymes thought to be responsible for antiinflammatory effects. Also has antipruritic and vasoconstrictive properties. Systemic absorption leads to actions, limitations, and drug interactions of hydrocortisone.

USES Relief of pruritus and inflammatory manifestations of corticosteroid-responsive dermatoses.

ROUTE & DOSAGE

Inflammation

Adult	Topical	Apply thin layer b.i.d. or t.i.d.; apply tape 1–2 times/d at 12 h intervals
Child	Topical	Apply thin layer 1–2 times/d; apply tape once/d

PHARMACOKINETICS Absorption: minimum absorption through intact skin; increased absorption and depot effect with repeated applications resulting in increased potential for systemic effects and more severe side effects.

CONTRAINDICATIONS & PRECAUTIONS Contraindicated in: fungal infections, tuberculosis of skin, herpes simplex, vaccinia, varicella, in ear if drum is perforated, impaired circulation to the part being

Common side effects in *italic*; life-threatening effects <u>underlined</u>; generic names in **bold**; classifications in SMALL CAPS

treated, ophthalmic use, application to face and intertriginous areas or to weeping or exudative surfaces; concomitant use with more potent steroids. Safe use during pregnancy (category C) and in nursing women not determined. **Cautious use in:** application to large surface areas, prolonged use, occlusive dressings, application to scrotal, vulval, perineal areas; use in children.

ADVERSE/SIDE EFFECTS Especially with occlusive dressings. **Eye:** cataracts and glaucoma (prolonged application around eyes). **Skin:** burning, itching, irritation, dryness, folliculitis, hypertrichosis, hypopigmentation, allergic contact dermatitis, acneiform eruptions, perioral dermatitis, skin maceration and atrophy, striae, purpura (on diffusedly atrophied skin), photosensitivity, miliaria (cutaneous changes associated with sweat retention). **Other:** secondary infection, adrenal suppression; in adults: Cushing's syndrome, hyperglycemia, glycosuria; in children (reversible): benign intracranial hypertension, development of Cushingoid features and edema, delayed linear growth and weight gain, low plasma cortisol, absence of response to ACTH.

NURSING IMPLICATIONS

Administration

- The ointment is usually indicated for dry, scaly skin; the cream and lotion are appropriate for moist lesions.
- Always wash patient's skin before applying flurandrenolide to prevent buildup of drug. Do not use alcohol or alcohol base solutions to cleanse affected area. Lightly rub in the thin film of medication. If area is hairy, shave or clip the hair and apply lotion or ointment directly to skin.
- Occlusive dressings are not applied unless specifically prescribed. Avoid use of occlusive dressing if skin surface is weeping or if exudative lesion is present.
- If an occlusive dressing is to be used, apply a generous layer of cream or ointment, cover with a thin, pliable plastic film, and then seal to skin with hypoallergenic tape.
- Because a tight fitting diaper or one covered with plastic pants may serve as an occlusive dressing, it should be avoided if drug is to be applied to skin in diaper area.
- Cordran tape is a flexible polyethelene film impregnated with flurandrenolide in the acrylic adhesive. It serves as an occlusive dressing and should not be applied to exudative lesions. Apply tape to clean and dry affected area. Remove carefully; it

can strip the epidermis. It may also cause purpura in treated area.
- Topical corticosteroid therapy is terminated gradually to prevent withdrawal symptoms.
- Store at 15–30C (59–86F). Protect from moisture heat, freezing, or light.

Assessment & Drug Effects

- Close surveillance and periodic evaluation for evidence of systemic absorption (i.e., Cushing's syndrome) are indicated when occlusive dressings are used, when patient is receiving long-term therapy, and when large areas of skin surface are covered with topical steroid.
- If systemic absorption is noted, an attempt will be made to withdraw the drug by decreasing frequency of applications or by substituting a less potent steroid.
- Pediatric treatment for > 2 wk with tape or with ointment or cream of potency of 0.05% should be evaluated carefully by the physician.
- Children and infants are more susceptible to topical corticosteroid–induced adrenal suppression than adults because of a larger skin surface area to body weight ratio.
- Frequently inspect treated area for signs of exudation, infection, irritation, ulceration, hypersensitivity. If present, stop application of topical corticosteroid and notify physician.
- If large surface area is covered with an occlusive dressing, check body temperature. (Thermoregulation may be impaired.) If temperature is elevated, use of topical corticosteroid should be discontinued.
- The antiinflammatory action may mask signs of infection. Monitor treated areas carefully for presence of infection and apparent extension of inflammation. Report to physician.
- Occasionally *steroid withdrawal symptoms* (rebound inflammation, fainting, dyspnea, anorexia, hypoglycemia, hypotension, fever, weakness, arthralgia) develop even though medication dosage is gradually tapered.

Patient & Family Education

- During long-term therapy it is advisable for women to use contraceptive measures. If the patient suspects pregnancy, she should promptly consult the physician.
- Advise patient to avoid exposure of affected areas to ultraviolet rays or to direct sunlight because of danger of photosensitivity.

F

Prototype: lorazepam, p 177

FLURAZEPAM HYDROCHLORIDE
(flure-az´e-pam)
Trade names: Apo-Flurazepam, Dalmane, Durapam, Novoflupam
Classifications: CNS AGENT; BENZODIAZEPINE ANXIOLYTIC, SEDATIVE-HYPNOTIC
Pregnancy: Category X
Controlled substance: Schedule IV

ACTIONS/PHARMACODYNAMICS
Benzodiazepine derivative, with hypnotic activity equal to or greater than that produced by barbiturates or chloral hydrate. Mode and site of action not known but appears to act at limbic and subcortical levels of CNS to produce sedation, skeletal muscle relaxation, and anticonvulsant effects. Reduces sleep induction time; produces slight if any suppression of REM time (dream sleep) but marked reduction of stage 4 sleep (deepest sleep stage) while at the same time increasing duration of total sleep time. Significance of sleep alterations not understood.

USES
Hypnotic in management of all kinds of insomnia, e.g., difficulty in falling asleep, frequent nocturnal awakening or early morning awakening or both. Also for treatment of poor sleeping habits.

ROUTE & DOSAGE

Sedative, Hypnotic
Adult   PO   ≥ 15 y: 15–30 mg h.s.

PHARMACOKINETICS
Absorption: readily absorbed from GI tract. **Onset:** 15–45 min. **Duration:** 7–8 h. **Distribution:** crosses blood-brain barrier and placenta; distributed into breast milk. **Metabolism:** metabolized in liver to active metabolites. **Elimination:** half-life: 47–100 h; excreted primarily in urine.

CONTRAINDICATIONS & PRECAUTIONS
Contraindicated in: prolonged administration; sleep apnea; intermittent porphyria; acute narrow-angle glaucoma; children <15 y; pregnancy, nursing mothers. **Cautious use in:** impaired renal or hepatic function; mental depression, psychoses, history of suicidal tendencies, addiction-prone individuals; elderly or debilitated patients; COPD.

ADVERSE/SIDE EFFECTS
CNS: *residual sedation, drowsiness,* lightheadedness, dizziness, ataxia, headache, nervousness, apprehension, talkativeness, irritability, depression, hallucinations, nightmares, confusion, paradoxic reactions: excitement, euphoria, hyperactivity, disorientation, coma (overdosage). **Eye:** blurred vision, burning eyes. **GI:** heartburn, nausea, vomiting, diarrhea, abdominal pain. Rarely: xerostomia, excessive salivation, bitter taste, swollen tongue. **Hematologic:** (rare): blood dyscrasias (granulocytopenia, leukopenia). **Other:** immediate allergic reaction, chest pain, muscle and joint pain, genitourinary complaints, shortness of breath, hypotension, sweating, jaundice (rare).

DIAGNOSTIC TEST INTERFERENCES
Flurazepam may increase serum levels of *total and direct bilirubin, alkaline phosphatase, AST,* and *ALT.* False-negative *urine glucose* reactions may occur with *Clinistix* and *Diastix;* no effect with TesTape.

DRUG INTERACTIONS
Alcohol, CNS DEPRESSANTS, ANTICONVULSANTS potentiate CNS depression; **cimetidine, disulfiram** may increase flurazepam levels, thus increasing its toxicity.

NURSING IMPLICATIONS

Administration
- Encourage patient to remain upright in bed (e.g., reading) for 20–30 min after taking the drug. This may help patient experience the onset of natural sleepiness.
- Store in light-resistant container with child-proof cap at 15–30C (59–86F) unless otherwise specified.

Assessment & Drug Effects
- Hypnotic effect is apparent on second or third night of consecutive use and continues 1 or 2 nights after drug is stopped (drug has a long half-life).
- Residual sedation and drowsiness are relatively common. Excessive drowsiness, ataxia, vertigo, and falling occur more frequently in elderly or debilitated patients. Supervise ambulation. Side rails may be advisable.
- Prolonged use of large doses can result in psychic and physical dependence. If patient has a history of drug abuse, monitor drug ingestion.
- With repeated use, blood counts and liver and kidney function tests are advised.
- Withdrawal symptoms have occurred 3 d after abrupt discontinuation of flurazepam after prolonged use: worsening of insomnia, dizziness, blurred vision, anorexia, GI upset, nasal congestion, paresthesias.

Common side effects in *italic;* life-threatening effects underlined; generic names in **bold**; classifications in SMALL CAPS

Patient & Family Education

- Because flurazepam has cumulative effects, warn patients to avoid potentially hazardous activities such as driving a motor vehicle or operating machinery until reaction to drug is known.
- Caution patient to avoid alcohol. Concurrent ingestion with flurazepam intensifies CNS depressant effects. Symptoms may occur even when alcohol is ingested as long as 10 h after last flurazepam dose (because it has a long half-life).
- Caution patients about the possibility of additive depressant effects if flurazepam is combined with barbiturates, tranquilizers, or other CNS depressants.
- Advise patient to seek approval from physician before self-dosing with OTC drugs.
- Dose intervals or dosage should not be changed. Instruct patient not to use it for a self-diagnosed problem.
- Patient should be advised that if she becomes pregnant during therapy or intends to become pregnant, she should ask her physician about the desirability of discontinuing the drug.
- Because insomnia is usually transient, the prolonged use of this hypnotic is inadvisable.

Prototype: ibuprofen, p 160

FLURBIPROFEN SODIUM

(flure-bi´proe-fen)
Trade names: Ansaid, Ocufen
Classifications: CNS AGENT; NONNARCOTIC ANALGESIC, ANTIPYRETIC; NSAID
Pregnancy: Category C

ACTIONS/PHARMACODYNAMICS Inhibitor of prostaglandin synthesis including in the conjunctiva and uvea; structurally and pharmacologically related to ibuprofen. Potency as an inhibitor of prostaglandin synthesis is greater than that of other NSAIDs (e.g., ibuprofen, indomethacin, aspirin). Blocks synthesis of prostaglandin by inhibition of the enzyme cyclooxygenase, which catalyzes formation of prostaglandin precursors (endoperoxides) from arachidonic acid. (Prostaglandins mediate intraocular inflammation, disruption of blood–aqueous humor barrier, vasodilation, and increases in vascular permeability, intraocular pressure (IOP), and leukocytosis.) When administered prophylactically ocular flurbiprofen reduces miosis, permitting maintenance of drug-induced mydriasis during surgical procedures. Also inhibits migration of leukocytes into inflamed tissues, depresses monocyte function, and may inhibit platelet aggregation. Has no significant effect on IOP. Potential for cross-sensitivity to aspirin and other NSAIDs exists. Risk of systemic effect appears to be minimal after topical ophthalmic use.

USES Inhibition of intraoperative miosis; arthritis and other inflammatory diseases; mild to moderate pain. **Unlabeled use:** management of postoperative ocular inflammation, prevention of postcystoid macular edema.

ROUTE & DOSAGE

Inflammatory Disease

Adult	PO	200–300 mg/d in 2–4 divided doses (max 300 mg/d)

Mild-to-moderate Pain

Adult	PO	50–100 mg q6–8h

Inhibition of Intraoperative Miosis

Adult	Topical	1 drop in eye approximately q30min beginning 2 h before surgery for a total of 4 drops per affected eye

PHARMACOKINETICS Absorption: 80% absorbed from GI tract. **Onset:** 2 h. **Peak:** 2 h. **Duration:** 6–8 h. **Distribution:** small amounts distributed into breast milk. **Metabolism:** metabolized in liver. **Elimination:** half-life: 5 h; excreted primarily in urine; some biliary excretion.

CONTRAINDICATIONS & PRECAUTIONS Contraindicated in: epithelial herpes simplex keratitis. Safe use during pregnancy (category C), by nursing mothers, or children not established. **Cautious use in:** concomitant use with other NSAIDs; patient who may be adversely affected by prolonged bleeding time; patient in whom asthma, rhinitis, or urticaria is precipitated by aspirin or other NSAIDs. For contraindications to oral use, see ibuprofen.

ADVERSE/SIDE EFFECTS Ocular: (transient): *mild ocular stinging*, burning, itching, or foreign body sensation. **Other:** slowed corneal healing; increased bleeding time. For adverse/side effects to oral preparations, see ibuprofen.

DRUG INTERACTIONS ORAL ANTICOAGULANTS, **heparin** may prolong bleeding time; actions and side effects of both flurbiprofen and **phenytoin**, SULFONYLUREAS, or SULFONAMIDES may be potentiated.

NURSING IMPLICATIONS

For nursing implications for oral preparation, see ibuprofen.

Administration of Eye Preparation

- Administer ophthalmic preparation with great care to avoid contamination of solution. Do not touch eye surface with dropper.
- Store at 15–30C (59–86F) in tight, light-resistant container.

Patient & Family Education for Eye Preparation

- Ocular irritation that persists after flurbiprofen use during surgery (tearing, dry eye sensation, dull eye pain, photophobia) should be reported to physician.
- Advise patient with bleeding tendency to report unexplained bleeding, prolongation of bleeding time, or bruises. Minor systemic absorption of flurbiprofen may temporarily increase bleeding time.

FOLIC ACID (VITAMIN B₉, PTEROYLGLUTAMIC ACID)

Trade names: Apo-Folic, Folacin, Folvite, Novofolacid

FOLATE SODIUM

Trade name: Folvite Sodium
Classification: VITAMIN B₉
Pregnancy: Category A

ACTIONS/ PHARMACODYNAMICS Member of vitamin B complex essential for nucleoprotein synthesis and maintenance of normal erythropoiesis. Stimulates production of RBCs, WBCs, and platelets in patients with megaloblastic anemias. Folic acid is not metabolically active but is reduced in the body to the coenzyme tetrahydrofolic acid, involved in the 1-carbon transfer reactions in purine and thymidylate biosynthesis. In folic acid deficiency, impaired thymidylate synthesis results in production of defective DNA that leads to megaloblast formation and arrest of bone marrow maturation.

USES Folate deficiency, macrocytic anemia, and megaloblastic anemias associated with malabsorption syndromes, alcoholism, primary liver disease, inadequate dietary intake, pregnancy, infancy, and childhood.

PHARMACOKINETICS Absorption: readily absorbed from proximal small intestine. **Peak:** 30–60 min PO. **Distribution:** distributed to all body tissues; high concentrations in CSF; crosses placenta; distributed into breast milk. **Metabolism:** metabolized in liver to active metabolites. **Elimination:** small amounts eliminated in urine in folate-deficient patients; large amounts excreted in urine with high doses.

ROUTE & DOSAGE

Therapeutic

Adult	PO/IM/SC/IV	≤ 1 mg/d
Child	PO/IM/SC/IV	≤1 mg/d

Maintenance

Adult	PO/IM/SC/IV	≤ 0.4 mg/d
Child	PO/IM/SC/IV	> 4 y: ≤ 0.4 mg/d
		< 4 y: ≤ 0.3 mg/d
		Infants: ≤ 0.1 mg/d

CONTRAINDICATIONS & PRECAUTIONS Contraindicated in: folic acid alone for pernicious anemia or other vitamin B₁₂ deficiency states; normocytic, refractory, aplastic, or undiagnosed anemia.

ADVERSE/SIDE EFFECTS Reportedly nontoxic. Rare: allergic sensitization (rash, pruritus, general malaise, bronchospasm). Slight flushing and feeling of warmth following IV administration.

DIAGNOSTIC TEST INTERFERENCES Falsely low serum *folate levels* may occur with *Lactobacillus casei assay* in patients receiving antibiotics such as tetracyclines.

DRUG INTERACTIONS Chloramphenicol may antagonize effects of folate therapy; **phenytoin** metabolism may be increased, thus decreasing its levels in folate-deficient patients.

INCOMPATIBILITIES Solution/Additive: doxapram.

NURSING IMPLICATIONS

Administration

- IV folic acid may be given by direct IV undiluted over 30–60 seconds. May also be added to a continuous infusion.
- Store at 15–30C (59–86F) in tightly closed containers protected from light, unless otherwise directed.

Assessment & Drug Effects

- A careful history of dietary intake and drug and alcohol usage should be obtained before start of therapy. Drugs reported to cause folate deficiency include oral contraceptives, alcohol, barbiturates, methotrexate, phenytoin, primidone, and trimethoprim. Folate deficiency may also result from renal dialysis

Folic acid can obscure diagnosis of pernicious anemia by alleviating hematologic manifestations of vitamin B_{12} deficiency while allowing irreparable neurologic damage to remain progressive.

- Therapeutic effects of folic acid therapy include improvement in blood picture and gradual reversal of *symptoms of folic acid deficiency:* glossitis, diarrhea, constipation, weight loss, irritability, fatigue, restless legs, diffuse muscular pain, insomnia, forgetfulness, mental depression, pallor. Keep physician informed of patient's response.

Patient & Family Education

- The recommended daily allowances (RDA) of folic acid are as follows: infants, 30 µg; children, 100–300 µg; adults, 400 µg; during pregnancy, 800 µg; during lactation, 500 µg.
- Folates are present in a wide variety of foods; rich sources include yeast, liver, whole grain, bran, fresh leafy vegetables, asparagus, dried beans and lentils, nuts, and fruits. Approximately 50–90% of folate content is destroyed by long cooking or by canning.
- Emphasize the need for the patient to remain under close medical supervision while he or she is receiving folic acid therapy. Adjustment of maintenance dose should be made if there is threat of relapse.

FURAZOLIDONE

(fur-a-zoe´li-done)
Trade name: Furoxone
Classifications: ANTIINFECTIVE; MAO INHIBITOR
Pregnancy: Category C

ACTIONS/PHARMACODYNAMICS Synthetic nitrofuran with antibacterial and antiprotozoal properties. Acts by interfering with several bacterial enzyme systems. Bactericidal against majority of GI pathogens, including species of *Enterobacter aerogenes, Escherichia coli, Giardia lamblia, Proteus, Salmonella, Shigella, Staphylococcus,* and *Vibrio cholerae.* Also has MAO inhibitor action that is cumulative and dose related (occurring after 4 or 5 d of therapy) and is thought to be due to a metabolite.

USES Bacterial or protozoal diarrhea and enteritis caused by susceptible organisms.

ROUTE & DOSAGE

Diarrhea and Enteritis

Adult	PO	100 mg q.i.d.
Child	PO	≥ 5 y: 25–50 mg q.i.d. (max 8.8 mg/kg/d)
		1–4 y: 17–25 mg q.i.d.
		1 mo–1 y: 8–17 mg q.i.d.

PHARMACOKINETICS Absorption: poorly absorbed from GI tract. **Metabolism:** metabolized in intestines. **Elimination:** excreted in urine.

CONTRAINDICATIONS & PRECAUTIONS Contraindicated in: hypersensitivity to furazolidone, concurrent use with alcohol, other MAO inhibitors, tyramine-containing foods, indirect-acting sympathomimetic amines; infants <1 mo. Safe use during pregnancy (category C) and in nursing mothers not established. **Cautious use in:** if at all, patients with glucose-6-phosphate dehydrogenase (G6PD) deficiency.

ADVERSE/SIDE EFFECTS GI: anorexia, *nausea, vomiting,* abdominal pain, diarrhea, colitis, proctitis, staphylococcic enteritis. **Hypersensitivity:** fever, arthralgia, hypotension, urticaria, angioedema, vesicular or morbilliform rash. **Other:** headache, malaise, dizziness, hypoglycemia, intravascular hemolysis in patients with G6PD deficiency (reversible), agranulocytosis (rare), partial deafness (rare).

DIAGNOSTIC TEST INTERFERENCES Furazolidone metabolite reportedly may cause false-positive reactions for *urine glucose* with copper sulfate reduction methods, e.g., *Benedict's reagent, Clinitest,* and *Fehling's solution.*

DRUG INTERACTIONS Alcohol may elicit disulfiram-type reaction up to 4 d after the drug is stopped; MAO INHIBITORS, NARCOTICS, SYMPATHOMIMETIC AMINES, **ephedrine, phenylpropanolamine** may cause a hypertensive reaction; TRICYCLIC ANTIDEPRESSANTS may cause toxic psychosis. **Food-Drug interactions:** may interact with tyramine-containing foods, resulting in flushing, tachycardia, and hypertensive crisis. See phenelzine (MAO inhibitor prototype) p 182.

F

NURSING IMPLICATIONS

Administration

- Preserve in tight, light-resistant containers (drug darkens on exposure to light). Protect from excessive heat.

Assessment & Drug Effects

- Nausea and vomiting occur commonly but may be relieved by reducing dosage. If symptoms persist, drug discontinuation may be necessary.
- Bed rest and fluid and electrolyte replacement (as indicated) are important adjuncts to drug therapy. Consult physician regarding dietary allowances.
- Keep physician informed of signs of dehydration (see chap 3) and electrolyte imbalance.
- Since drug may cause hypoglycemia (see Signs & Symptoms, chap 3), diabetic patients will require close monitoring. Use glucose oxidase methods for urine testing, e.g., Clinistix, Diastix, TesTape.
- Patients with G6PD deficiency (e.g., patients of Mediterranean or Near East origin and blacks) should be closely observed by blood and urine studies for intravascular hemolysis: hematuria (pink or red urine), hemoglobinuria, hemoglobinemia.

Patient & Family Education

- Advise patient or family member to record number of stools passed, fluid intake, and daily weight.
- Caution patient not to exceed prescribed dosage and to contact physician if diarrhea persists or worsens or if side effects develop. If satisfactory clinical response does not occur within 7 d, drug should be discontinued.
- Faintness, weakness, and lightheadedness may be symptoms of hypersensitivity reaction or hypoglycemia and should be reported.
- Foods high in tyramine (e.g., aged and fermented food and drinks) may produce hypertensive reaction. Provide patient with list of high-tyramine foods. Hypertensive crisis is most likely to occur when drug is continued beyond 5 d or when large doses are given.
- Warn patients not to drink alcohol during furazolidone therapy and for at least 4 d after drug is stopped. Ingestion of alcohol may cause disulfiram-type reaction (see Signs & Symptoms, chap 3); symptoms may last up to 24 h.
- Advise patient not to take OTC medications unless approved by physician. Nasal decongestants, cold and hay-fever remedies, appetite suppressants, and other medications containing indirect-acting amines expose patient to hazards of hypertensive reaction.

- Inform patients that drug may impart a harmless brown color to urine.
- Advise the diabetic of potential for hypoglycemia.

FUROSEMIDE

See ELECTROLYTIC & WATER BALANCE AGENT, LOOP DIURETIC, prototype, p 198.

Prototype: tubocurarine, p 124

GALLAMINE TRIETHIODIDE
(gal′a-meen)
Trade name: Flaxedil
Classifications: AUTONOMIC NERVOUS SYSTEM AGENT; NONDEPOLARIZING SKELETAL MUSCLE RELAXANT
Pregnancy: Category C

ACTIONS/PHARMACODYNAMICS Synthetic, nondepolarizing neuromuscular blocking agent (curariform drug). Similar to tubocurarine in actions, uses, contraindications, precautions, and adverse reactions. About 20% as potent as tubocurarine; reported to produce less ganglionic blockade and to have no histamine-releasing properties except in very high doses. Has parasympatholytic effect on vagus and may cause tachycardia and occasionally hypertension.

USES Preanesthetic and intraanesthetic medication to induce skeletal muscle relaxation for treatment of GI disorders and to reverse neuromuscular blockade.

ROUTE & DOSAGE

Skeletal Muscle Relaxation
Adult IV 1 mg/kg initial dose; then 0.5–1 mg/kg q30–40min prn (max single dose 100 mg)

PHARMACOKINETICS Peak: 3 min. **Duration:** 15–20 min. **Distribution:** crosses placenta. **Elimination:** excreted primarily unchanged in urine.

CONTRAINDICATIONS & PRECAUTIONS Contraindicated in: hypersensitivity to gallamine or iodides; myasthenia gravis; impaired pulmonary or renal function; shock; infants weighing less than 5 kg; hyperthyroidism; hypertension, tachycardia, cardiac insufficiency; hypoalbuminemia. **Cautious use in:** impaired liver function.

ADVERSE/SIDE EFFECTS Decreased respiratory minute volume, transient tachycardia.

NURSING IMPLICATIONS

Administration

- Gallamine may be given undiluted by direct IV. Administer a single dose over 30 to 60 seconds.
- Store at 15–30C (59–86F) unless otherwise directed and protect from light and excessive heat.

Assessment & Drug Effects

- Tachycardia occurs almost immediately after administration, reaches maximum within 3 min, and declines gradually to premedication level.
- Patients with electrolyte imbalance, dehydration, or elevated temperature may be more sensitive to the effects of gallamine.

Prototype: lovastatin, p 143

GEMFIBROZIL

(gem-fiʹbroe-zil)
Trade name: Lopid
Classifications: CARDIOVASCULAR AGENT;
ANTILIPEMIC, LIPID-LOWERING AGENT
Pregnancy: Category B

ACTIONS/PHARMACODYNAMICS Fibric acid derivative with lipid-regulating properties. Action mechanism is unclear. Blocks lipolysis of stored triglycerides in adipose tissue and inhibits hepatic uptake of fatty acids. Both of these effects decrease delivery of fatty acids to the liver and may explain an apparent decrease in hepatic very low density lipoprotein (VLDL)–triglyceride synthesis and secretion. Produces a moderate increase in high density lipoprotein (HDL)–cholesterol levels and reduces levels of total and low density lipoprotein (LDL)–cholesterol and triglycerides. May increase cholesterol excretion into bile; therefore is said to be lithogenic. Toxicity potential is low; no adverse effects due to long-term use have been reported.

USES Patients with very high serum triglyceride levels (above 750 mg/dl) (type IV and V hyperlipidemia) who have not responded favorably to inten-

sive diet restriction and who are at risk of pancreatitis and abdominal pain. Also severe familial hypercholesterolemia (type IIa or IIb) that developed in childhood and has failed to respond to dietary control or to other cholesterol-lowering drugs.

ROUTE & DOSAGE

Hypertriglyceridemia

Adult PO 600 mg b.i.d. 30 min before morning and evening meal; may increase up to 1500 mg/d.

PHARMACOKINETICS Absorption: readily absorbed from GI tract. **Peak:** 1–2 h. **Metabolism:** undergoes enterohepatic circulation. **Elimination:** half-life: 1.3–1.5 h; excreted primarily in urine; 6% excreted in feces.

CONTRAINDICATIONS & PRECAUTIONS Contraindicated in: gallbladder disease, hepatic or severe kidney dysfunction. Safe use during pregnancy (category B), in nursing mothers, and in children not established. **Cautious use in:** diabetes mellitus, hypothyroidism.

ADVERSE/SIDE EFFECTS CNS: headache, dizziness, blurred vision. **GI:** *abdominal or epigastric pain,* diarrhea, nausea, vomiting, flatulence. **Hematologic:** anemia, eosinophilia, leukopenia, mild decreases in Hct, Hgb. **Musculoskeletal:** painful extremities, back pain, muscle cramps, myalgia, arthralgia, swollen joints. **Skin:** rash, dermatitis, pruritus, urticaria. **Other:** hypokalemia, moderate hyperglycemia. Causal relationship not established: viral or bacterial infection, fatigue, malaise, syncope, vertigo, insomnia, paresthesias, tinnitus, dry mouth, constipation, anorexia, dyspepsia, *cholelithiasis,* cholecystitis, malignancy, postcholecystectomy complications, pancreatitis, cardiac arrhythmias, intermittent claudication.

DRUG INTERACTIONS May potentiate hypoprothrombinemic effects of ORAL ANTICOAGULANTS; **lovastatin** increases risk of myopathy and rhabdomyolysis.

NURSING IMPLICATIONS

Administration

- Instruct patient to take drug 30 min before breakfast and evening meal.
- Store at 15–30C (59–86F) unless otherwise directed.

Assessment & Drug Effects

- The following laboratory tests should be monitored initially and at regular intervals during first year of therapy: serum LDL and VLDL, triglycerides, total cholesterol, CBC, blood glucose, liver function tests.
- Mild decreases in WBC, Hgb, Hct may occur during early stage of treatment but generally stabilize with continued therapy.
- Frequent PT determinations are advisable until the drug effect on platelet aggregation is evident (may be inhibited).
- Gemfibrozil should be discontinued if the lipid response is not adequate after 3 mo of therapy.
- Gallbladder studies are indicated if patient presents signs and symptoms suggestive of cholelithiasis or cholecystitis (right upper quadrant and epigastric pain frequently radiating to right shoulder blade and generally associated with nausea, vomiting, and flatulence). Symptoms often occur during the night or early morning; jaundice may or may not be present.

Patient & Family Education

- Advise patient to report promptly if unexplained bleeding occurs (e.g., easy bruising, epistaxis, hematuria).
- Because gemfibrozil may cause blurred vision and vertigo, caution patient to avoid driving and other potentially hazardous activities until reaction to drug is known.
- Patients with high serum triglyceride levels are generally advised to lose excess weight and to restrict carbohydrate and alcohol intake (alcohol increases serum triglyceride levels).
- Patients with high cholesterol are generally advised to avoid foods high in cholesterol and saturated fats.
- Fat intake may be limited to 25–30% of total calories; simple carbohydrates to 35–40% of total calories. Complex carbohydrates (cereals, pasta, vegetables, rice) are promoted over simple sugars. Cholesterol intake is usually kept at fewer than 300 mg/d.

GENTAMICIN SULFATE

See ANTIINFECTIVES, ANTIBIOTIC, AMINOGLYCOSIDE prototype, p 53.

Prototype: tolbutamide, p 234

GLIPIZIDE
(glip´i-zide)
Trade name: Glucotrol
Classifications: SULFONYLUREA ANTIDIABETIC AGENT
Pregnancy: Category C

ACTIONS/PHARMACODYNAMICS Second generation sulfonylurea hypoglycemic agent structurally similar to acetohexamide (first generation). Potency is enhanced by as much as 200-fold over first generation agents. Directly stimulates functioning pancreatic beta cells to secrete insulin, leading to an acute drop in blood glucose. Indirect action leads to altered numbers and sensitivity of peripheral insulin receptors, resulting in increased insulin binding. It also causes inhibition of hepatic glucose production and reduction in serum glucagon levels. Fasting insulin levels are not increased by long-term glipizide therapy; however, a postprandial insulin response lasting through the meal challenge continues to be enhanced for at least 6 mo. Has no antidiuretic activity and has no effect on plasma lipoproteins. Since loss of diabetic control may be transient when patient is being treated by diet alone, a short course of glipizide therapy may be adequate to restore control. It has not been established that this drug will prevent long-term cardiovascular and neurologic complications of diabetes mellitus.

USES Adjunct to diet for control of hyperglycemia in patient with type II (non-insulin-dependent) diabetes mellitus after dietary control alone has failed; also used to treat transient loss of control in patient usually controlled well on diet.

ROUTE & DOSAGE

Control of Hyperglycemia

Adult PO 2.5–5 mg/d, 30 min before breakfast; May increase by 2.5–5 mg q 1–2 wk. > 15 mg/d should be given in divided doses 30 min before morning and evening meal (max 40 mg/d)

PHARMACOKINETICS Absorption: readily absorbed from GI tract. **Onset:** 15–30 min. **Peak:** 1–2 h. **Duration:** up to 24 h. **Metabolism:** metabolized extensively in liver. **Elimination:** half-life: 3–5 h; excreted mainly in urine with some excretion via bile in feces.

Common side effects in *italic*; life-threatening effects underlined; generic names in **bold**; classifications in SMALL CAPS

CONTRAINDICATIONS & PRECAUTIONS Contraindicated in: diabetic ketoacidosis. Safe use during pregnancy (category C), in nursing mothers, and in children not established. **Cautious use in:** impaired renal and hepatic function, the elderly, debilitated, malnourished patient; patient with adrenal or pituitary insufficiency.

ADVERSE/SIDE EFFECTS GI: nausea, diarrhea, constipation, gastralgia, cholestatic jaundice (rare). **Hematologic:** leukopenia, thrombocytopenia, hemolytic anemia, aplastic anemia, agranulocytosis, pancytopenia. **Metabolic:** hepatic porphyria; disulfiram-like reactions (rare). **Skin:** erythema, morbilliform or maculopapular rash, pruritus, urticaria, eczema (transient), porphyria cutanea tarda, photosensitivity reactions. **Other:** transient: drowsiness, headache, hypersensitivity (rare). **Overdosage:** hypoglycemia, *mild:* fatigue, drowsiness, hunger, GI distress (heartburn, abdominal pain, anorexia), headache, anxiety; *severe:* visual disturbances, ataxia, confusion, tachycardia, seizures, coma.

DRUG INTERACTIONS Alcohol produces disulfiram-like reaction in some patients; ORAL ANTICOAGULANTS, **chloramphenicol, clofibrate, phenylbutazone,** MAO INHIBITORS, SALICYLATES, **probenecid,** SULFONAMIDES may potentiate hypoglycemic actions; THIAZIDES may antagonize hypoglycemic effects; **cimetidine** may increase glipizide levels, causing hypoglycemia.

NURSING IMPLICATIONS

Administration

- Take 30 min before the first meal of the day to give best protection against postprandial hyperglycemia.
- Usually 5–7 d are allowed to elapse between titration steps. If response to a single dose is unsatisfactory, the dose may be divided.
- If glipizide is used during pregnancy, it is discontinued at least 1 mo before the expected delivery date to prevent prolonged, severe hypoglycemia (4–10 d) in the neonate.
- Store in tightly closed light-resistant container at 15–30C (59–86F).

Assessment & Drug Effects

- The initial dose and establishment of a maintenance regimen in the elderly or debilitated patient is approached both conservatively and gradually. Close observation for early signs of hypglycemia (easily overlooked) is paramount.

- At the beginning of the treatment program the patient should be checked for cardiovascular risk factors, and if necessary, corrective measures should be instituted.
- Severe drug-induced skin rashes and pruritus may necessitate discontinuation of drug use. Symptoms usually subside rapidly when drug is withdrawn.
- During insulin withdrawal and transfer to glipizide, urine tests for sugar and ketone bodies should be checked at least 3 times daily. Advise patient to contact the physician if tests are abnormal.
- If the patient is being transferred from one to another sulfonylurea, no transition period is necessary. However, the patient who is transferred from one with a long half-life (e.g., chlorpropamide, half-life: 30–40 h) must be observed for hypoglycemic responses (see Signs & Symptoms, chap 3) for 1–2 wk because of potential overlapping of drug effect.
- Keep in mind that if the patient is also receiving a beta adrenergic blocking agent (suppresses reflex tachycardia) or is elderly, the first signs of hypoglycemia may be hard to detect.
- ***Overdose treatment:*** Mild hypoglycemia (reaction without loss of consciousness of neurologic symptoms) is treated with PO glucose and adjustment of dosage and meal pattern. The patient should be closely monitored for at least 5–7 d to assure reestablishment of safe control. Severe hypoglycemia requires emergency hospitalization to permit treatment to maintain a blood glucose level above 100 mg/dl.

Patient & Family Education

- Emphasize to the patient that glipizide treatment accompanies (does not substitute for) continued control of diet and (if patient is obese) a weight-loss program.
- Blood glucose testing is encouraged for the patient on a sulfonylurea.
- Inform patient about the importance of exercise as a part of the total control program.
- Advise patient who wishes to become pregnant that a transfer to insulin for blood glucose control is recommended by many clinicians.
- When a drug that affects the hypoglycemic action of sulfonylureas (see Drug Interactions) is withdrawn or added to the glipizide regimen, the patient should be alerted to the added danger of loss of control. Urine and blood glucose tests and test for ketone bodies should be carefully monitored.
- Remind patient that hypoglycemia is a potential effect of the following situations: after severe or prolonged exercise, after alcohol ingestion, when

Common side effects in *italic*; life-threatening effects underlined; generic names in **bold**; classifications in SMALL CAPS

623

caloric intake is deficient, when more than one glucose-lowering drug is being used.

■ Advise patient or primary care provider to observe for signs of cholestatic jaundice (yellow sclera, dark urine, pruritus). If they occur, inform the physician promptly. The drug may have to be discontinued and replaced by another antidiabetic agent.

GLUCAGON
(gloo´ka-gon)
Classifications: HORMONE; ANTIDIABETIC AGENT
Pregnancy: Category B

ACTIONS/PHARMACODYNAMICS
Polypeptide hormone produced by alpha cells of islets of Langerhans. Actions appear to be related to increased synthesis of cyclic adenosine monophosphate (cAMP) and phosphorylase activity, which increase hepatic gluconeogenesis. Stimulates uptake of amino acids and their conversion to glucose precursors. Promotes lipolysis in liver and adipose tissue with release of free fatty acid and glycerol, which further stimulates ketogenesis and hepatic gluconeogenesis. Action in hypoglycemia relies on presence of adequate liver glycogen stores. Under normal conditions, proper blood sugar level is maintained by homeostatic balance between glucagon and insulin. Glucagon is of little value in starvation, adrenal insufficiency, or chronic hypoglycemia; type 1 (juvenile or unstable) diabetics do not respond satisfactorily. Increases heart rate (chronotropic action) and myocardial contractility (positive inotropic action) and improves AV conduction in a manner similar to that produced by catecholamines. Actions are independent of beta blockade. Also exerts a relaxant effect on smooth muscle of GI tract and reduces gastric and pancreatic secretions.

USES
Emergency treatment of severe hypoglycemic reactions in diabetic patients who are unconscious or unable to swallow food or liquids and in psychiatric patients receiving insulin shock therapy. Also radiologic studies of GI tract to relax smooth muscle and thereby allow finer detail of mucosa; to diagnose insulinoma. **Unlabeled uses:** GI disturbances associated with spasm, cardiovascular emergencies, and to overcome cardiotoxic effects of beta-blockers, quinidine, tricyclic antidepressants; as an aid in abdominal imaging.

ROUTE & DOSAGE

Hypoglycemia

Adult	IM/IV/SC	0.5–1 U; may repeat q5–20min if no response for 1–2 more doses
Child	IM/IV/SC	0.025 U/kg; may repeat q5–20min if no response for 1–2 more doses

Insulin Shock Therapy

Adult	IM/IV/SC	0.5–1 U usually 1 h after coma develops; if no response, may repeat in 25 min

Diagnostic Aid to Relax Stomach or Upper GI Tract

Adult	IM/IV/SC	0.25–2 U 10 min before the procedure

Diagnostic Aid for Examination of Colon

Adult	IM/IV/SC	2 U 10 min before the procedure

PHARMACOKINETICS
Onset: 5–20 min. **Peak:** 30 min. **Duration:** 1–1.5 h. **Metabolism:** metabolized in liver, plasma, and kidneys. **Elimination:** half-life: 3–10 min.

CONTRAINDICATIONS & PRECAUTIONS
Contraindicated in: hypersensitivity to glucagon or protein compounds. Safe use during pregnancy (category B) and in nursing women not established. **Cautious use in:** insulinoma, pheochromocytoma.

ADVERSE/SIDE EFFECTS
Nausea and vomiting; hypersensitivity reactions; Stevens-Johnson syndrome (erythema multiforme); hyperglycemia, hypokalemia.

INCOMPATIBILITIES
Solution/Additive: sodium chloride.

NURSING IMPLICATIONS

Administration
■ Dilute 1 unit (1 mg) of glucagon with 1 ml of diluent supplied by manufacturer. Administer by direct IV. Flush line with 5% dextrose instead of NaCl solution.

■ After reconstitution of dry powder, use solution immediately.

■ Glucagon will form a precipitate in saline solutions and solutions with pH of 3–9.5 (pH of glucagon is 2.5–3). Glucagon should be considered incompatible in syringe with any other drug.

■ Reconstituted solution remains potent for up to 3 mo if kept refrigerated at 2–8C (36–46F). Use only special vehicle supplied by manufacturer for dilution. Indicate date on label. Lyophilized (dry powder) form is stable at room temperature.

Assessment & Drug Effects

■ Hypoglycemic reactions (i.e., signs & symptoms, chap 3) require immediate treatment. Prolonged hypoglycemic coma can result in brain damage.

■ IV glucose must be given if patient fails to respond to glucagon.

■ Patient usually awakens from (diabetic) hypoglycemic coma 5–20 min after glucagon injection. As soon as possible after patient regains consciousness, PO carbohydrate should be given.

■ After recovery from hypoglycemic reaction, symptoms such as headache, nausea, and weakness may persist.

Patient & Family Education

■ For patients with frequent or severe hypoglycemic reactions, physician may request that a responsible family member be taught how to administer glucagon SC or IM. Stress importance of notifying physician promptly whenever a hypoglycemic reaction occurs so that reason for the reaction can be ascertained. Also review package insert with patient and family member.

■ Remind patient that hypoglycemic episodes ("insulin reaction") follow too much insulin, delay of food intake, sickness (especially vomiting), or increased physical activity. Review the early symptoms of hypoglycemia (see chap 3). Emphasize the importance of routinely carrying candy or other readily available carbohydrate to take at first warning of an oncoming hypoglycemic reaction.

GLUTAMIC ACID HYDROCHLORIDE

(gloo-tam´ik)

Trade name: Acidulin
Classification: GASTROINTESTINAL AGENT; DIGESTANT
Pregnancy: Category C

ACTIONS/PHARMACODYNAMICS Amino acid chemically combined with hydrochloric acid, which is released on contact with water.

USES May be prescribed instead of diluted hydrochloric acid for treatment of hypochlorhydria and achlorhydria because it is convenient to carry and does not injure dental enamel.

ROUTE & DOSAGE

Hypochlorhydria
Adult   PO   1–3 capsules or tablets t.i.d. a.c.

CONTRAINDICATIONS & PRECAUTIONS Contraindicated in: gastric hyperacidity, peptic ulcer. Pregnancy (category C).

ADVERSE/SIDE EFFECTS Overdose: systemic acidosis.

NURSING IMPLICATIONS

Administration

■ Administer 30 min before meals.
■ Capsules must be swallowed whole.

Assessment & Drug Effects

■ Monitor for signs and symptoms of metabolic acidosis (see chap 3).
■ If acidosis is suspected, monitor for signs and symptoms of hypokalemia.

Patient & Family Education

■ Instruct patient to take drug 30 min before meals and not to exceed ordered dose.

Prototype: secobarbital, p 175

GLUTETHIMIDE

(gloo-teth´i-mide)

Trade names: Doriden, Doriglute
Classification: CNS AGENT; ANXIOLYTIC, SEDATIVE-HYPNOTIC
Pregnancy: Category C
Controlled substance: Schedule III

ACTIONS/PHARMACODYNAMICS Piperidine derivative structurally related to methyprylon. Pharmacologic actions similar to those of barbiturates. Can induce hypnosis without producing reliable analgesic, antitussive, or anticonvulsant action. Causes less respiratory depression but greater degree of hypotension than barbiturates. Exhibits anticholinergic activity, especially mydriasis, and inhibits salivary secretions and intestinal motility. Significantly suppresses REM sleep (dreaming stage of sleep); but following drug withdrawal after chronic administration, REM rebound occurs, and patient may experi-

G

Common side effects in *italic*; life-threatening effects <u>underlined</u>; generic names in **bold**; classifications in SMALL CAPS

625

ence markedly increased dreaming, nightmares, insomnia. Addiction liability similar to that of barbiturates. Stimulates hepatic microsomal enzymes and thus may alter metabolism of other drugs.

USES Short-term treatment of insomnia and for sedative effect preoperatively and during first stage of labor. Not indicated for routine sedation or persistent insomnia.

ROUTE & DOSAGE

Insomnia

Adult   PO   250–500 mg h.s.; may repeat prn but not <4 h before arising

Preoperative Sedation

Adult   PO   500 mg the night before surgery and 500 mg–1 g 1 h before anesthesia

PHARMACOKINETICS Absorption: erratic absorption from GI tract. **Onset:** 30 min. **Duration:** 4–8 h. **Distribution:** widely distributed; localizes in adipose tissue, liver, kidney, brain, and bile; crosses placenta; distributed into breast milk in small quantities. **Metabolism:** metabolized in liver. **Elimination:** half-life: 10–12 h; metabolites excreted in urine.

CONTRAINDICATIONS & PRECAUTIONS Contraindicated in: uncontrolled pain; intermittent porphyria; severe hepatic and renal impairment; prolonged administration; children <12 y. Safe use during pregnancy (except with caution during first stage of labor) not established. **Cautious use in:** elderly or debilitated patients; prostatic hypertrophy, bladder neck obstruction; pyloroduodenal obstruction, stenosing peptic ulcer; narrow-angle glaucoma; hypotension, cardiac arrhythmias; mental depression (particularly in patients with suicidal tendencies), history of alcoholism or drug abuse.

ADVERSE/SIDE EFFECTS CNS: CNS depression in fetus; paradoxic excitement, headache, vertigo. **GI:** gastric irritation, nausea, drug "hangover," dry mouth. **Hematologic:** blood dyscrasias; **Skin:** generalized skin rash (occasionally, purpuric or urticarial), exfoliative dermatitis. **Other:** acute hypersensitivity reactions, hiccups, blurred vision, porphyria, jaundice. **Acute overdosage (CNS depression):** coma; depressed reflexes, including corneal reflex; dilated, fixed pupils; hypotension; hypothermia followed by hyperpyrexia; tachycardia; respiratory depression, cyanosis, sudden apnea; urinary bladder atony; decreased intestinal motility, adynamic ileus; facial twitching;

intermittent spasticity; flaccid paralysis; pulmonary and cerebral edema; renal tubular necrosis; severe infections. **Chronic toxicity (toxic psychosis):** slurred speech, impaired memory, inability to concentrate, mydriasis, dry mouth, nystagmus, ataxia, hyporeflexia, tremors, peripheral neuropathy, osteomalacia (rare).

DRUG INTERACTIONS Alcohol, BARBITURATES, other CNS DEPRESSANTS compound depressant effects; TRICYCLIC ANTIDEPRESSANTS add to anticholinergic effects; decreases anticoagulant effects of ORAL ANTICOAGULANTS.

NURSING IMPLICATIONS

Administration

- If administered for insomnia, glutethimide should be given 4 h or more before the usual time of arising to avoid residual daytime effects.
- Abrupt withdrawal following regular use may produce nausea, vomiting, nervousness, tremors, abdominal cramps, nightmares, insomnia, tachycardia, chills, fever, numbness of extremities, dysphagia, delirium, hallucinations, or convulsions. Withdrawal should be gradual, with stepwise dose reduction over a period of several days or weeks.

Assessment & Drug Effects

- Sedative-hypnotic effect of glutethimide is counteracted by pain. Consult physician about prescribing an analgesic for pain if required.
- Keep physician informed of patient's response to drug. Smallest effective dosage should be used for the shortest period of time compatible with patient's needs.
- Overdosage of glutethimide is difficult to treat. Patients tend to go in and out of toxicity, possibly because of delayed absorption of the drug.
- *Treatment of acute overdosage:* gastric lavage, regardless of time that has elapsed since drug ingestion. Some physicians lavage with a 1:1 mixture of castor oil and water (glutethimide is lipid-soluble). Supportive treatment is based on presenting signs and symptoms.

Patient & Family Education

- Advise patient to report onset of rash or any other unusual symptoms. Discontinuation of drug is indicated if a rash occurs.
- Caution patient to avoid driving a motor vehicle or engaging in other activities requiring mental alertness for 7–8 h after drug ingestion.
- Warn patient about possible adverse reactions

Common side effects in *italic*; life-threatening effects underlined; generic names in **bold**; classifications in SMALL CAPS

when glutethimide is combined with alcohol or other CNS depressants.

- Prolonged use of moderate to high doses of glutethimide can produce tolerance and psychologic and physical dependence.

Prototype: tolbutamide, p 234

GLYBURIDE
(glye´byoor-ide)

Trade names: DiaBeta, Euglucon, Micronase
Classifications: SULFONYLUREA; ANTIDIABETIC AGENT
Pregnancy: Category B

ACTIONS/PHARMACODYNAMICS One of the most potent of the sulfonylurea hypoglycemic agents. Second generation sulfonylurea closely related in actions, uses, and limitations to glipizide. Potency is enhanced by as much as 200-fold over first generation agents. Appears to lower blood sugar concentration in both diabetic and nondiabetic individuals by sensitizing functioning pancreatic beta cells to release insulin in the presence of elevated serum glucose levels. Blood glucose lowering effect persists during long-term glyburide treatment, but there is a gradual decline in meal-stimulated secretion of endogenous insulin toward pretreatment levels. Extrapancreatic effects are thought to augment drug effect on the beta cells, i.e., enhanced peripheral sensitization to insulin, decrease in hepatic glucose production, and increased insulin binding to cell membrane receptors. Produces mild diuresis by enhanced free water clearance, perhaps by inhibiting reabsorption of Na⁺ in the proximal renal tubule or by blocking non-vasopressor-dependent reabsorption of water in the distal renal tubules.

USES Adjunct to diet to lower blood glucose in patients with type II diabetes mellitus (NIDDM) after dietary control alone has failed.

ROUTE & DOSAGE

Control of Hyperglycemia

Adult PO 1.25–5 mg/d with breakfast; may increase by 2.5–5 mg q1–2wk; > 15 mg/d should be given in divided doses with morning and evening meal (max 20 mg/d)

PHARMACOKINETICS Absorption: readily absorbed from GI tract. **Onset:** 15–60 min. **Peak:** 1–2 h. **Duration:** up to 24 h. **Distribution:** distributed in highest concentrations in liver, kidneys, and intestines; crosses placenta. **Metabolism:** metabolized extensively in liver. **Elimination:** half-life: 10 h; excreted equally in urine and feces.

CONTRAINDICATIONS & PRECAUTIONS Contraindicated in: diabetic ketoacidosis, as sole therapy for type II diabetes mellitus. Safe use during pregnancy (category B), in nursing mothers, and in children not established. **Cautious use in:** renal or hepatic insufficiency, elderly, debilitated, or malnourished patients; adrenal or pituitary insufficiency.

ADVERSE/SIDE EFFECTS *Hypoglycemia*, epigastric fullness, heartburn, nausea, cholestatic jaundice, pruritus, erythema, urticarial or morbilliform eruptions, photosensitivity, paresthesia, joint pain, nocturia.

DRUG INTERACTIONS Alcohol causes disulfiram-like reaction in some patients; ORAL ANTICOAGULANTS, **chloramphenicol, clofibrate, phenylbutazone,** MAO INHIBITORS, SALICYLATES, **probenecid,** SULFONAMIDES may potentiate hypoglycemic actions; THIAZIDES may antagonize hypoglycemic effects; **cimetidine** may increase glyburide levels, causing hypoglycemia.

NURSING IMPLICATIONS

Administration

- Glyburide is generally administered once daily in the morning with breakfast or with first main meal.
- Store in tightly closed, light-resistant container at 15–30C (59–86F).

Assessment & Drug Effects

- The elderly patient is especially vulnerable to glyburide-induced hypoglycemia (see Signs & Symptoms, chap 3) because the antidiabetic agent is long-acting. Blood glucose levels should be monitored carefully during the dangerous early treatment period when dosage is being individualized.
- If the patient is also receiving a beta-adrenergic blocking agent (suppresses reflex tachycardia) or if the patient is elderly, the first signs of hypoglycemia may be hard to detect.
- Monitor for signs and symptoms of cardiovascular disease (e.g., angina, intermittent claudication).
- The following indices of patient's response to ther-

G

Common side effects in *italic*; life-threatening effects <u>underlined</u>; generic names in **bold**; classifications in SMALL CAPS

627

apy should be monitored at regular intervals: blood and urine glucose determinations, glycosylated hemoglobin determinations, urine ketones.

■ It is possible that the effectiveness of any hypoglycemic agent including glyburide may diminish over time because (1) dose is not adequate; (2) patient is being careless about diet or exercise program; (3) patient has become less responsive to the drug; and (4) diabetes is worsening.

■ Persistence of acetonuria with glycosuria indicates that the patient may require insulin therapy.

Patient & Family Education

■ If symptoms of hypoglycemia occur, patient should eat or drink some form of sugar, e.g., corn syrup, orange juice with 2 or 3 tsp of table sugar. Reaction should be reported to physician promptly.

■ Remind patient that loss of control of diabetes may result from stress such as fever, surgery, trauma, infection. Blood and urine glucose and ketone body detection may need to be checked more frequently during these stress periods, and transfer from the sulfonylurea to insulin may be necessary.

■ During conversion period when both insulin and glyburide are being used, instruct patient to test urine for ketone bodies and glucose at least 3 times daily and to report promptly abnormal findings to the physician.

■ Emphasize importance of keeping follow-up medical appointments and of adhering to dietary instructions, regular exercise program, scheduled urine and blood testing.

GLYCERIN

(gli´ser-in)

Trade names: Fleet Babylax, Glycerol, Glyrol, Osmoglyn, Sani Supp

GLYCERIN ANHYDROUS

Trade name: Ophthalgan

Classifications: HYPEROSMOTIC LAXATIVE; ANTIGLAUCOMA

Pregnancy: Category C

ACTIONS/PHARMACODYNAMICS Trihydric alcohol. When administered orally, glycerin raises plasma osmotic pressure by withdrawing fluid from extravascular spaces; lowers ocular tension by decreasing volume of intraocular fluid. Also may decrease CSF pressure and produce slight diuresis. Topical application to eye reduces edema by hygroscopic effect. Glycerin suppositories apparently work by causing dehydration of exposed tissue, which produces an irritant effect, and by absorbing water from tissues, thus creating more mass. Both actions stimulate peristalsis.

USES Orally to reduce elevated intraocular pressure (IOP) before or after surgery in patients with acute narrow-angle glaucoma, retinal detachment, or cataract and to reduce elevated CSF pressure. Sterile glycerin (anhydrous) is used topically to reduce superficial corneal edema resulting from trauma, surgery, or disease and to facilitate ophthalmoscopic examination. Used rectally (suppository or enema) to relieve constipation. **Unlabeled use:** to reduce mortality due to strokes in the elderly.

ROUTE & DOSAGE

Decrease IOP

Adult	PO	1–1.8 g/kg 1–1.5 h before ocular surgery; may repeat q5h

Constipation

Adult	PR	Insert 1 suppository or 5–15 ml of enema high into rectum and retain for 15 min
Child	PR	Insert 1 suppository or 2–5 ml of enema high into rectum and retain for 15 min

Reduction of Corneal Edema

Adult	Topical	1–2 drops instilled into eye q3–4h

PHARMACOKINETICS Absorption: readily absorbed from GI tract after oral administration; rectal preparations are poorly absorbed. **Onset:** 10 min PO. **Peak:** 30 min–2 h. **Duration:** 4–8 h. **Metabolism:** 80% metabolized in liver; 10–20% metabolized in kidneys to CO_2 and water or utilized in glucose or glycogen synthesis. **Elimination:** half-life: 30–40 min; 7–14% excreted unchanged in urine.

CONTRAINDICATIONS & PRECAUTIONS Contraindicated in: safe use during pregnancy (category C) and in nursing women not established. **Cautious use in:** cardiac, renal, or hepatic disease; diabetes mellitus; dehydrated or elderly patients.

ADVERSE/SIDE EFFECTS Headache, dizziness, nausea, vomiting, thirst, diarrhea, hyperglycemia, glycosuria, dehydration, <u>hyperosmolar nonketotic</u>

coma, irregular heartbeat, disorientation, convulsive seizures (rare). **Suppository form:** abdominal cramps, rectal discomfort, hyperemia of rectal mucosa.

NURSING IMPLICATIONS

Administration

- Commercially available flavored solution may be poured over crushed ice and sipped through a straw. Lemon or lime juice and 0.9% NaCl (if allowed) may be added to unflavored solution for palatability.
- Headache (from cerebral dehydration) may be prevented or relieved by having patient lie down during and after administration of PO drug.

Assessment & Drug Effects

- Consult physician regarding fluid intake in patients receiving drug for elevated IOP. Although hypotonic fluids will relieve thirst and headache caused by the dehydrating action of glycerin, these fluids may nullify its osmotic effect.
- Many dentists discourage use of glycerin and lemon for mouth care because of its drying effect on mucous membranes. Also, lemon being highly acidic can decalcify teeth if contact is sustained.
- Monitor glycemic control in diabetics. Drug may cause hyperglycemia (see Signs & Symptoms, chap 3).

Patient & Family Education

- After administration of glycerin rectal suppository or enema, patient will usually have an evacuation within 15–30 min.
- Slight hyperglycemia and glycosuria may occur with PO use. Patients with diabetes may require adjustment in insulin dosage.

Prototype: atropine, p 116

GLYCOPYRROLATE
(glye-koe-pye´roe-late)
Trade names: Robinul, Robinul Forte
Classifications: AUTONOMIC NERVOUS SYSTEM AGENT; ANTICHOLINERGIC (PARASYMPATHOLYTIC); ANTIMUSCARINIC, ANTISPASMODIC
Pregnancy: Category B

ACTIONS/PHARMACODYNAMICS Synthetic anticholinergic (antimuscarinic) quaternary ammonium compound with pharmacologic effects similar to those of atropine. Inhibits muscarinic actions of acetylcholine or autonomic neuroeffector sites innervated by postganglionic cholinergic nerves. Also antagonizes muscarinic symptoms (e.g., excessive tracheal or bronchial secretions, bronchospasm, bradycardia) induced by cholinergic drugs, such as anticholinesterases, and anesthetic agents. Inhibits motility of GI tract and genitourinary tract and decreases volume of gastric and pancreatic secretions, saliva, and perspiration. In contrast to atropine, glycopyrrolate is highly polar and therefore does not easily penetrate lipid membranes such as the blood-brain barrier. Has lower incidence of CNS-related side effects than atropine has and reportedly has longer vagal blocking and antisialogogue effects.

USES Adjunctive management of peptic ulcer and other GI disorders associated with hyperacidity, hypermotility, and spasm. Also used parenterally as preanesthetic and intraoperative medication and to reverse neuromuscular blockade.

ROUTE & DOSAGE

Peptic Ulcer

Adult	PO	1 mg t.i.d or 2 mg b.i.d. or t.i.d. in equally divided intervals (max 8 mg/d); should then decrease to 1 mg b.i.d.
	IM/IV	0.1–0.2 mg as single dose t.i.d. or q.i.d.

Reversal of Neuromuscular Blockade

Adult	IV	0.2 mg glycopyrrolate administered with 1 mg of neostigmine or 5 mg pyridostigmine

PHARMACOKINETICS Absorption: poorly and incompletely absorbed from GI tract. **Onset:** 1 min IV; 15–30 min IM/SC; 1 h PO. **Peak:** 30–45 min IM/SC; 1 h PO. **Duration:** 2–7 h IM/SC; 8–12 h PO. **Distribution:** crosses placenta. **Metabolism:** minimally metabolized in liver. **Elimination:** 85% excreted in urine.

CONTRAINDICATIONS & PRECAUTIONS Contraindicated in: glaucoma; asthma; prostatic hypertrophy, obstructive uropathy; obstructive lesions or atony of GI tract; severe ulcerative colitis; myasthenia gravis; tachycardia; during cyclopropane anesthesia; children <12 y (except parenteral use in conjunction with anesthesia). Safe use during pregnancy (category B) or in nursing mothers not established. **Cautious use in:** autonomic neuropathy, hepatic or renal disease.

Common side effects in *italic*; life-threatening effects underlined; generic names in **bold**; classifications in SMALL CAPS

629

ADVERSE/SIDE EFFECTS *Xerostomia, decreased sweating, urinary hesitancy or retention,* blurred vision, mydriasis, constipation, palpitation, tachycardia, drowsiness, weakness, dizziness. **Overdosage:** neuromuscular blockade (curare-like action) leading to muscle weakness and paralysis is possible.

DRUG INTERACTIONS Amantadine, ANTIHISTAMINES, TRICYCLIC ANTIDEPRESSANTS, **quinidine, disopyramide, procainamide** compound anticholinergic effects; decreases **levodopa** effects; **methotrimeprazine** may precipitate extrapyramidal effects; decreases antipsychotic effects (decreased absorption) of PHENOTHIAZINES.

INCOMPATIBILITIES Solution/Additive: methylprednisolone, chloramphenicol, dexamethasone, diazepam, dimenhydrinate, methohexital, pentazocine, phenobarbital, secobarbital, sodium bicarbonate, thiopental. Y-Site: diazepam, dimenhydrinate, methohexital, pentazocine, phenobarbital, secobarbital, thiopental.

NURSING IMPLICATIONS

Administration
- Do not combine glycopyrrolate in same syringe with drugs capable of raising the pH above 6.0 (see Incompatibilities). A precipitate and gas will form.
- May be given undiluted by direct IV. Administer 0.2 mg or fraction thereof over 1–2 min.
- Inspect parenteral products for cloudiness and discoloration. Discard such solutions.

Assessment & Drug Effects
- Incidence and severity of side effects are generally dose related.
- Monitor I&O ratio and pattern particularly in the elderly. Watch for urinary hesitancy and retention.
- Monitor vital signs, especially when drug is given parenterally. Report any changes in heart rate or rhythm.

Patient & Family Education
- Caution patient to avoid high environmental temperatures. (Heat prostration can occur because of decreased sweating.)
- Because glycopyrrolate may produce dizziness and blurred vision, warn patient not to engage in activities requiring mental alertness, such as operating a motor vehicle or performing other hazardous tasks.
- Instruct patient to use good oral hygiene, frequent mouth rinses with water, and a saliva substitute to lessen effects of xerostomia (dry mouth).

Prototype: aurothioglucose, p 223

GOLD SODIUM THIOMALATE
(thye-oh-mah´late)
Trade name: Myochrysine
Classifications: GOLD COMPOUND; ANTIRHEUMATIC
Pregnancy: Category C

ACTIONS/PHARMACODYNAMICS Water-soluble gold compound similar to aurothioglucose in actions and uses. Contains approximately 50% gold. Has immunomodulatory and antiinflammatory effects. Action mechanism unclear: drug appears to act by suppression of phagocytosis, altered immune responses, and possibly by inhibition of prostaglandin synthesis. See aurothioglucose.

USES Selected patients (adults and juveniles) with acute rheumatoid arthritis. **Unlabeled uses:** psoriatic arthritis; Felty's syndrome.

ROUTE & DOSAGE

Rheumatoid Arthritis

Adult	IM	10 mg wk 1, 25 mg wk 2; then 25–50 mg/wk to a cumulative dose of 1 g; if improvement occurs, continue at 25–50 mg q2wk for 2–20 wk, then q3–4wk indefinitely or until side effects occur
Child	IM	10 mg test dose; then 1 mg/kg/wk or 2.5–5 mg for wk 1 and 2; then 1 mg/kg q1–4wk (max single dose 50 mg)

PHARMACOKINETICS Absorption: slowly and irregularly absorbed from IM site. **Peak:** 3–6 h. **Distribution:** widely distributed, especially to synovial fluid, kidney, liver, and spleen; does not cross blood-brain barrier; crosses placenta. **Metabolism:** unknown. **Elimination:** half-life: 3–168 d; 60–90% of dose ultimately excreted in urine; also eliminated in feces; traces may be found in urine for ≥ 6 mo.

CONTRAINDICATIONS & PRECAUTIONS Contraindicated in: history of severe toxicity from previous exposure to gold or other heavy metals; severe debilitation; SLE, Sjögren's syndrome in rheumatoid arthritis; renal disease; hepatic dysfunction, history of infectious hepatitis or hematologic disorders; uncontrolled diabetes, or CHF. Safe use during pregnancy (category C) not established. **Cautious use in:** history of drug allergies or hypersensitivity, hypertension.

ADVERSE/SIDE EFFECTS CNS: dizziness, syncope, sweating, flushing (nitritoid-type reactions). **CV:** bradycardia. **GI:** Metallic taste, *stomatitis,* nausea, vomiting; hepatitis, jaundice. **Hematologic** (rare): leukopenia, <u>agranulocytosis, thrombocytopenia</u>, <u>hypoplastic and aplastic anemia</u>, eosinophilia. **Renal:** nephrotic syndrome, glomerulitis with hematuria, *proteinuria.* **Skin:** transient pruritus, *erythema, dermatitis (common),* exfoliative dermatitis, fixed drug eruption, alopecia, shedding of nails, gray to blue pigmentation of skin (chrysiasis). **Other:** gold deposits in ocular tissues, *photosensitivity,* peripheral neuritis, <u>anaphylaxis</u>, angioneurotic edema, pulmonary fibrosis, interstitial pneumonitis.

DRUG INTERACTIONS ANTIMALARIALS, IMMUNO-SUPPRESSANTS, **penicillamine, phenylbutazone** increase risk of blood dyscrasias.

NURSING IMPLICATIONS

Administration

- Agitate vial before withdrawing dose to assure uniform suspension.
- Drug is usually administered deep into upper outer quadrant of gluteus with patient lying down. Patient should remain recumbent for at least 30 min after injection because of the danger of "nitritoid reaction" (transient giddiness, vertigo, facial flushing, fainting). Observe for allergic reactions.
- Preserve in tight, light-resistant containers at 15–30C (59–86F). Drug should not be used if it is any darker than pale yellow.

Assessment & Drug Effects

- Prior to each injection, urine should be analyzed for protein, blood, and sediment. Drug should be discontinued promptly if proteinuria or hematuria develops.
- Patient should be interviewed and examined before each injection to detect occurrence of transient pruritus or dermatitis (both are common early indications of toxicity), stomatitis (sore tongue, palate, or throat), metallic taste, indigestion, or other signs and symptoms of possible toxicity. Treatment should be interrupted immediately if any of these reactions occurs.
- Allergic reaction may occur almost immediately after injection, 10 min after injection, or at any time during therapy. If it is observed, treatment should be discontinued. At time of injection have antidote dimercaprol (BAL) on hand.
- Baseline Hgb and RBC determinations, WBC count, differential count, platelet count, and urinalysis should be obtained before initiation of therapy and at regular intervals thereafter.
- Rapid reduction in hemoglobin level, WBC count below 4000/mm³, eosinophil count above 5%, and platelet count below 100,000/mm³ signify possible toxicity.

Patient & Family Education

- Therapeutic effects may not appear until after 2 mo of therapy. This may be a basis for noncompliance.
- Rapid improvement in joint swelling usually indicates that patient is closely approaching drug tolerance level; report to physician.
- Patients who develop gold dermatitis should be warned that exposure to sunlight may aggravate the problem.
- The appearance of purpura or ecchymoses is always an indication for doing a platelet count; instruct patient to report them to physician.
- Patients should be informed about possible adverse reactions and warned to report any symptom suggestive of toxicity as soon as it appears. Adverse reactions may occur at any time during drug therapy or even a few months after drug is discontinued; most reactions occur during second or third month of treatment (usually after the amount injected has reached about 250–500 mg).

GONADORELIN HYDROCHLORIDE

(goe-nad-oh-rell´in)
Trade name: Factrel
Classification: SYNTHETIC HORMONE;
DIAGNOSTIC AGENT
Pregnancy: Category B

ACTIONS/PHARMACODYNAMICS Synthetic luteinizing hormone–releasing hormone (LH-RH) with structure identical to the natural hormone; also referred to as gonadotropin-releasing hormone (GnRH). Stimulates anterior pituitary to release the gonadotropin LH. Range for normal baseline LH levels: 5–25 mIU/ml in postpubertal males, postpubertal and premenopausal females. Tests are performed during early follicular phase of the menstrual cycle (days 1 to 7).

USES To evaluate functional capacity and response of the gonadotropes of anterior pituitary and in suspected gonadotropic deficiency. Also used to evaluate residual gonadotropic function of the pituitary following surgical or radiologic removal of a pituitary tumor. **Unlabeled use:** treatment of delayed puberty, amenorrhea, and infertility in males.

Common side effects in *italic*; life-threatening effects <u>underlined</u>; generic names in **bold**; classifications in SMALL CAPS

631

ROUTE & DOSAGE

Evaluation of Functional Capacity of Anterior Pituitary

Adult SC/IV 100 μg administered in women during early phase of menstrual cycle (day 1 to 7) if it can be determined

PHARMACOKINETICS Duration: 3–5 h. **Distribution:** distributed into breast milk. **Metabolism:** hydrolyzed in plasma. **Elimination:** half-life: 10–40 min; metabolites excreted in urine.

CONTRAINDICATIONS & PRECAUTIONS Contraindicated in: safe use in pregnancy (category B) not established; concurrent use of other drugs having effect on pituitary-gonadotropic function.

ADVERSE/SIDE EFFECTS CNS: headache, lightheadedness. **GI:** nausea, abdominal discomfort. **Other:** flushing, local inflammation at injection site if given SC; allergic or hypersensitivity reactions (rare); rash (rare).

DRUG INTERACTIONS ANDROGENS, ESTROGENS, PROGESTINS, GLUCOCORTICOIDS may cause false test results; **digoxin** may suppress gonadotropin levels; DOPAMINE ANTAGONISTS, PHENOTHIAZINES increase prolactin and blunt response to gonadorelin; **spironolactone, levodopa** increase gonadotropin levels.

NURSING IMPLICATIONS

Administration

- *Preparation of the solution:* reconstitute 100 μg vial with 1 ml sterile diluent (supplied by manufacturer), and the 500 μg vial with 2 ml. Solution should be used immediately after preparation.
- Administer a single dose by direct IV over 15–30 seconds.
- Overdosage has not been reported. Doses as high as 3 mg twice daily for 28 d have been used without signs of toxicity.
- After reconstitution, store drug at room temperature and use within 24 h. Discard unused diluted solution and diluent. Store ampule at room temperature.
- Test procedure is according to established protocol (see manufacturer's information).

Assessment & Drug Effects

- Repetitive high doses of gonadorelin may inhibit spermatogenesis and cause luteolysis.

Interpretation of Test

- In menopausal and postmenopausal women, baseline LH levels are elevated.
- Patient clinically diagnosed or with suspected pituitary or hypothalamus dysfunction often demonstrates subnormal or absent LH response after test dose.
- The normal response indicates presence of functional pituitary gonadotropes.

Prototype: amphotericin B, p 56

GRISEOFULVIN MICROSIZE

(gri-see-oh-ful´vin)
Trade names: Fulvicin-U/F, Grifulvin V, Grisactin, Grisovin-FP

GRISEOFULVIN ULTRAMICROSIZE

Trade names: Fulvicin P/G, Grisactin Ultra, Gris-PEG
Classifications: ANTIINFECTIVE; ANTIBIOTIC; ANTIFUNGAL
Pregnancy: Category C

ACTIONS/PHARMACODYNAMICS Fungistatic antibiotic derived from species of *Penicillium*. Arrests metaphase of cell division by disrupting mitotic spindle structure in fungal cells. Deposits in keratin precursor cells and has special affinity for diseased tissue. Tightly bound to new keratin of skin, hair, and nails, which becomes highly resistant to fungal invasion. Effective against various species of *Epidermophyton, Microsporum,* and *Trichophyton* (has no effect on other fungi, including *Candida,* bacteria, and yeasts). Has some direct vasodilatory activity. Efficacy of GI absorption of ultramicrosize formulation reported to be twice that of microsize griseofulvin. Theoretically, cross-sensitivity with penicillin is a possibility.

USES Mycotic disease of skin, hair, and nails not amenable to conventional topical measures. Concomitant use of appropriate topical agent may be required, particularly for tinea pedis. **Unlabeled uses:** Raynaud's disease, angina pectoris, and gout.

PHARMACOKINETICS Absorption: absorbed primarily from duodenum; microsize is variably and unpredictably absorbed; ultramicrosize is almost completely absorbed. **Peak:** 4–8 h. **Distribution:** concentrates in skin, hair, nails, fat, and skeletal muscle; crosses placenta. **Metabolism:** metabolized in liver. **Elimination:** half-life: 9–24 h; excreted mainly in urine; some excretion in perspiration.

ROUTE & DOSAGE

Tinea Corporis, Tinea Cruris, Tinea Capitis

Adult	PO	500 mg microsize or 330–375 mg ultramicrosize daily in single or divided doses
Child	PO	11 mg/kg/d microsize or 7.3 mg/kg/d ultramicrosize in single or divided doses

Tinea Pedis, Tinea Unguium

Adult	PO	0.75–1 g microsize or 660–750 mg ultramicrosize daily in single or divided doses; microsize dose should be decreased to 500 mg/d after response is noted
Child	PO	11 mg/kg/d microsize or 7.3 mg/kg/d ultramicrosize in single or divided doses

CONTRAINDICATIONS & PRECAUTIONS Contraindicated in: porphyria; hepatic disease; SLE. Safe use during pregnancy (category C), for children ≤ 2 y, or for prophylaxis against fungal infections not established. **Cautious use in:** penicillin-sensitive patients (possibility of cross-sensitivity with penicillin exists; however, reportedly penicillin-sensitive patients have been treated without difficulty).

ADVERSE/SIDE EFFECTS Low incidence of side effects. **CNS:** *severe headache,* insomnia, peripheral neuritis, paresthesias, fatigue, mental confusion, impaired performance of routine functions, psychotic symptoms, vertigo. **ENT:** temporary loss of hearing, dizziness. **GI:** heartburn, nausea, vomiting, diarrhea, flatulence, dry mouth, thirst, decreased taste acuity, anorexia, unpleasant taste, furred tongue, oral thrush. **Hematologic:** leukopenia, neutropenia, granulocytopenia, punctate basophilia, monocytosis. **Hypersensitivity:** urticaria, photosensitivity, lichen planus, skin rashes, pruritus, fixed drug eruption, serum sickness syndromes, severe angioedema. **Renal** (nephrotoxicity): proteinuria, cylinduria. **Other:** hepatotoxicity, estrogenlike effects (in children), aggravation of SLE, overgrowth of nonsusceptible organisms, candidal intertrigo, elevated porphyrins in feces and erythrocytes, blurred vision.

DRUG INTERACTIONS Alcohol may cause flushing and tachycardia; BARBITURATES may decrease activity of griseofulvin; may decrease hypoprothrombinemic effects of ORAL ANTICOAGULANTS; may increase **estrogen** metabolism, resulting in break through bleeding, and decrease contraceptive efficacy of ORAL CONTRACEPTIVES

NURSING IMPLICATIONS

Administration

- Giving the drug with or after meals may allay GI disturbances.
- Serum levels may be enhanced by giving the microsize formulations with a high fat content meal (increases drug absorption rate). Consult physician.
- Store griseofulvin preparations at 15–30C (59–86F) in tightly covered containers unless otherwise directed.

Assessment & Drug Effects

- Before treatment is initiated, inquire about history of sensitivity to griseofulvin, penicillins, or other allergies.
- Monitor food intake. Griseofulvin may alter taste sensations, and this may cause appetite suppression and inadequate nutrient intake.
- Blood studies should be performed at least once weekly during first month of therapy or longer. Periodic tests of renal and hepatic function are also advised.
- Treatment should be continued until there is clinical improvement or until 2 or 3 consecutive weekly cultures are negative.

Patient & Family Education

- Patient may experience symptomatic relief after 48–96 h of therapy. Stress the importance of continuing treatment as prescribed to prevent relapse.
- Duration of treatment depends on time required to replace infected skin, hair, or nails, and thus varies with infection site. Average duration of treatment for tinea capitis (scalp ringworm), 4–6 wk; tinea corporis (body ringworm), 2–4 wk; tinea pedis (athlete's foot), 4–8 wk; tinea unguium (nail fungus), at least 4 mo for fingernails, depending on rate of growth, and 6 mo or more for toenails.
- Caution patient to avoid exposure to intense natural or artificial sunlight, because photosensitivity-type reactions may occur.
- Headaches often occur during early therapy but frequently disappear with continued drug administration.
- Warn patient of possible disulfiram-type reaction (see Signs & Symptoms, chap 3) on ingestion of alcohol during therapy.
- Emphasize importance of cleanliness and keeping

Common side effects in *italic*; life-threatening effects <u>underlined</u>; generic names in **bold**; classifications in SMALL CAPS

633

skin dry (moist skin favors growth of fungi). For athlete's foot, advise patient to wear well-ventilated shoes without rubber soles, to alternate shoes, and to change socks daily. Physician may prescribe a drying powder as necessary.

- Patient should be informed that pharmacologic effects of oral contraceptives may be reduced. Breakthrough bleeding and pregnancy may occur. Alternative form of birth control may be advisable during griseofulvin therapy.

GUAIFENESIN

See ANTITUSSIVES, EXPECTORANTS, & MUCO-LYTICS, EXPECTORANT prototype, p 99.

Prototype: methyldopa, p 148

GUANABENZ ACETATE

(gwan´a-benz)
Trade name: Wytensin
Classifications: CARDIOVASCULAR AGENT; CENTRAL ACTING ANTIHYPERTENSIVE; AUTONOMIC NERVOUS SYSTEM AGENT; ALPHA-ADRENERGIC AGONIST (SYMPATHOMIMETIC)
Pregnancy: Category C

ACTIONS/PHARMACODYNAMICS Centrally acting alpha$_2$-adrenergic agonist. A derivative of guanethidine, but pharmacologic actions more closely resemble those of clonidine. Lowers BP, primarily by stimulating central alpha adrenergic receptors, which leads to inhibition of sympathetic outflow from brain. Reduces both supine and standing BP, usually without producing postural hypotension, and slightly lowers pulse rate. Peripheral resistance lowers with long-term therapy, but cardiac output and left ventricular ejection fraction are unaffected. Also has no effect on exercise tolerance or on potassium levels. It does not cause sodium retention or excretion; however, it appears to enhance urinary dilution and free water diuresis. Slight reduction in serum cholesterol and total triglycerides may occur, but HDL cholesterol fraction is not affected. Tolerance to antihypertensive actions not reported. Given the fact that central adrenergic hyperactivity causes symptoms of narcotic withdrawal, guanabenz appears to

ROUTE & DOSAGE

Hypertension
Adult   PO   4 mg b.i.d.; may increase by 4–8 mg/d q1–2wk up to 32 mg b.i.d.

Opiate Withdrawal
Adult   PO   4 mg b.i.d. to q.i.d.

help control abstinence symptoms by reducing norepinephrine output.

USES Used alone in treatment of hypertension or in combination with a thiazide diuretic (stepped-care approach: step 2.) **Unlabeled uses:** opiate detoxification, analgesic for chronic pain.

PHARMACOKINETICS Absorption: 75% absorbed from GI tract. **Onset:** 60 min. **Peak:** 2–5 h. **Duration:** 6–12 h. **Distribution:** widely distributed; crosses blood-brain barrier; not known if crosses placenta or distributed into breast milk. **Metabolism:** extensively metabolized. **Elimination:** half-life: 4–14 h; 80% excreted in urine; 20% in feces.

CONTRAINDICATIONS & PRECAUTIONS Contraindicated in: safe use during pregnancy (category C), in nursing mothers, and in children not established. **Cautious use in:** severe coronary insufficiency, recent MI, cerebrovascular disease, severe hepatic or renal failure.

ADVERSE/SIDE EFFECTS CNS: *drowsiness or sedation,* dizziness, weakness, headache, anxiety, ataxia, depression, sleep disturbances. **CV:** chest pain, edema, arrhythmias, palpitation. **GI:** *dry mouth,* nausea, epigastric pain, diarrhea, vomiting, constipation, abdominal discomfort, taste disorders. **GU:** increased urination, urinary frequency, sexual dysfunction. **Hematologic:** decreases in serum cholesterol, triglycerides, norepinephrine, dopamine, beta hydroxylase, renin; increase in hepatic enzymes (rare). **Other:** gynecomastia, blurred vision, nasal congestion, dyspnea, muscle aches, aches in extremities, rash, pruritus. **Overdosage:** hypotension; somnolence, lethargy, irritability, miosis, bradycardia, unusual fatigue or weakness, nervousness.

DRUG INTERACTIONS Alcohol and other CNS DEPRESSANTS compound CNS depression; TRICYCLIC ANTIDEPRESSANTS may reduce antihypertensive effects of guanabenz.

———— Common side effects in *italic*; life-threatening effects <u>underlined</u>; ———— generic names in **bold**; classifications in SMALL CAPS

NURSING IMPLICATIONS

Administration

- One dose is usually prescribed for bedtime administration to ensure overnight control and to reduce possibility of daytime drowsiness or sedation.
- Store at 15–30C (59–86F) in tightly closed containers unless otherwise directed.

Assessment & Drug Effects

- Baseline and periodic tests should include blood chemistry (serum potassium, CBC, creatinine, uric acid, cholesterol, glucose), urinalysis for protein and sugar, and ECG.
- Dry mouth requires early attention and specific treatment because (1) it can interfere with patient's food and fluid intake; (2) deprivation of normal salivary flow is a potential dental hazard since it favors demineralization of teeth; and (3) it can be a factor in noncompliance.

Patient & Family Education

- Elderly patients tend to be more sensitive to normal adult doses of antihypertensive drugs because of deficient baroreceptor reflexes. Therefore, although orthostatic hypotension is not an expected guanabenz effect, caution patient to make all position changes slowly and in stages.
- Dry mouth, a common side effect, may be relieved by frequent rinses with water and sugar-free gum or sour balls. Advise edentulous patients to remove dentures at least 2 or 3 times a day when rinsing mouth so that all oral tissues are moistened.
- Warn patient not to omit dosage and not to stop drug therapy without consulting the physician. Abrupt discontinuation of guanabenz may cause *sympathetic overactivity:* anxiety, nervousness, palpitation, chest pain, fast or irregular heartbeat, trembling, flushing, headache, increased sweating and salivation, elevation of BP (usually above basal level).
- Advise patient to use caution when driving or performing other potentially hazardous activities until reaction to drug is determined. Also warn patient that tolerance to alcohol and other CNS depressants may be reduced by guanabenz.

See guanethidine for patients with hypertension.

Prototype: methyldopa, p 148

GUANADREL SULFATE

(gwahn'a-drel)

Trade name: Hylorel
Classifications: CARDIOVASCULAR AGENT; ANTIHYPERTENSIVE; AUTONOMIC NERVOUS SYSTEM AGENT; ADRENERGIC ANTAGONIST (BLOCKING AGENT, SYMPATHOLYTIC)
Pregnancy: Category B

ACTIONS/PHARMACODYNAMICS Adrenergic ganglionic blocking agent structurally and pharmacologically related to guanethidine. Not as potent as guanethidine, and onset of action and duration of effects are shorter. Also, less apt to cause morning orthostatic hypotension, and incidence of diarrhea is less. Acts as a false neurotransmitter without adrenergic activity because it blocks the release of norepinephrine from adrenal medulla and adrenergic nerve endings that normally follows sympathetic nerve stimulation. The net effect is catecholamine depletion with resulting relaxation of vascular smooth muscle, reduction of peripheral vascular resistance, lowering of systolic and diastolic BP, and a relative increase in parasympathetic tone. Unlike several other step-2 drugs, hypotensive effect is not related to CNS activity and therefore produces less sedation and depression. May cause sodium and water retention and consequent expansion of plasma volume, which generally requires use of a diuretic to maintain hypotensive effect. Decreases standing (orthostatic) more than supine BP and is more effective in lowering systolic than diastolic BP.

USES Stepped-care approach: step-2 treatment of hypertension, usually with a diuretic.

ROUTE & DOSAGE

Hypertension

Adult	PO	5 mg b.i.d.; may increase up to 20–75 mg/d in 2–4 divided doses

PHARMACOKINETICS Absorption: readily absorbed from GI tract. **Onset:** 0.5–2 h. **Peak:** 4–6 h. **Duration:** 4–14 h. **Distribution:** widely distributed. **Elimination:** half-life: 10–12 h; 85% excreted in urine within 24 h.

CONTRAINDICATIONS & PRECAUTIONS Contraindicated in: pheochromocytoma, CHF, patients taking MAO inhibitors. Safe use during pregnancy (cat-

Common side effects in *italic*; life-threatening effects underlined;
generic names in **bold**; classifications in SMALL CAPS

635

egory B), in nursing women, and in children not established. **Cautious use in:** cerebrovascular, coronary artery, or peripheral vascular disease, bronchial asthma, history of peptic ulcer, diarrhea, elderly patients.

ADVERSE/SIDE EFFECTS Mostly dose related. **CNS:** *fatigue, headache, drowsiness,* paresthesias, tremors, confusion, depression or other psychologic problems, sleep disorders. **CV:** *morning orthostatic hypotension* (lightheadedness, weakness), *orthostatic hypotension during the day,* palpitation, chest pain. **GI:** *diarrhea,* or increased number of stools, indigestion, constipation, dry mouth and thirst, anorexia, glossitis, nausea, vomiting, abdominal distress or pain. **GU:** nocturia, urine retention, urinary urgency or frequency, hematuria, *impaired ejaculation,* impotence. **Other:** visual disturbances; musculoskeletal aches, pains, or inflammation; excessive weight gain or loss, peripheral edema, nasal stuffiness, cough, *shortness of breath at rest or with exercise.*

DRUG INTERACTIONS Alcohol intensifies orthostatic hypotension and sedation; ALPHA- OR BETA-ADRENERGIC BLOCKERS, **reserpine** may intensify orthostatic hypotension and bradycardia; may enhance the action of **epinephrine, norepinephrine, methoxamine;** MAO INHIBITORS, PHENOTHIAZINES, TRICYCLIC ANTIDEPRESSANTS, **ephedrine, phenylpropanolamine** may antagonize hypotensive effects of guanadrel.

NURSING IMPLICATIONS

Administration

- Because serum half-life of guanadrel averages about 10 h, dosage adjustments are generally made weekly or monthly.
- Store at 15–30C (59–86F) unless otherwise directed.

Assessment & Drug Effects

- Dosage adjustments should be based on BP response in supine position and after standing 2–20 min. Record baseline measurements for future comparison purposes.
- The full effect of guanadrel on standing (orthostatic) BP should be carefully evaluated before the hospitalized patient is discharged. For ambulatory patient, BP measurements should also be taken following exercise for complete assessment.
- Patients with cerebrovascular, coronary artery, or peripheral vascular disease are particularly prone to orthostatic hypotension and therefore should be closely monitored.

- Guanadrel tends to enhance sodium and water retention, but these effects are generally controlled by concurrent diuretic therapy. Patients are usually advised to omit obviously salty foods and to avoid adding salt to served foods.

Patient & Family Education

- Inform patient about the possibility of orthostatic hypotension. Hypotensive effect of guanadrel is most prominent in the standing position or with prolonged standing, after exercise, and with vasodilation effects associated with fever, hot shower, or tub bath, hot environment, or with ingestion of alcohol.
- Caution elderly patients particularly not to get out of bed without assistance during initial dosage adjustment period.
- Warn patient to make position changes slowly and in stages, especially from recumbent to upright posture. These precautions should be observed throughout drug therapy. Some clinicians prescribe surgical support hose and advise patient to flex arms and legs before standing to augment venous return.
- Advise patient to lie down immediately at first hint of faintness, dizziness, weakness, or lightheadedness. All are possible manifestations of orthostatic hypotension.
- Teach patient to monitor weight and to check legs and ankles for edema and in particular to note if rings or shoes suddenly seem too tight. Advise patient to notify physician of peripheral edema or unexpected weight gain of ≥ 1 kg (2 lb)/day.
- To encourage patient compliance in taking guanadrel at the same time(s) each day, suggest that it be taken in relation to a daily routine activity.
- Most side effects disappear or at least diminish in intensity after about 8 wk of therapy.
- Dry mouth may be relieved by frequent rinsing with water and use of sugar-free gum or sour balls. Advise patient against overuse of commercial mouthwashes. Most contain alcohol, which tends to cause even more dryness.
- Some patients develop tolerance to hypotensive effect of guanadrel following long-term therapy and require careful and gradual dosage increases.
- Patient should be specifically cautioned not to use OTC drugs for treatment of colds, allergy, asthma, or appetite suppressants without consulting the physician or pharmacist. Many of these products contain adrenergic (sympathomimetic) amines, which may interfere with hypotensive action of guanadrel.

Common side effects in *italic*; life-threatening effects underlined; generic names in **bold**; classifications in SMALL CAPS

GUANETHIDINE SULFATE

(gwahn eth'i-deen)

Trade name: Ismelin
Classifications: CARDIOVASCULAR AGENT; ANTIHYPERTENSIVE; AUTONOMIC NERVOUS SYSTEM AGENT; ADRENERGIC ANTAGONIST (BLOCKING AGENT, SYMPATHOLYTIC)
Pregnancy: Category C

ACTIONS/PHARMACODYNAMICS Potent, long-acting, adrenergic blocking agent. Competes with norepinephrine for reuptake into adrenergic neurons; displaces stored norepinephrine, thus exposing it to degradation by MAO. Guanethidine slowly accumulates in storage granules and is released by nerve stimulation as a "false neurotransmitter" that effectively blocks adrenergic actions of norepinephrine. Produces gradual prolonged fall in BP, usually associated with bradycardia and decreased pulse pressure. Antihypertensive effect results from venous dilatation with peripheral pooling, decreased venous return, and decreased cardiac output. Drug-induced sodium retention and expansion of plasma volume, with resulting tolerance to antihypertensive effect, may occur unless concomitant diuretic therapy is administered. Renal blood flow and glomerular filtration rate may decrease during early therapy. Guanethidine also causes decreased plasma renin activity. It diminishes or eliminates cardiovascular reflexes and is therefore more effective in lowering orthostatic than supine BP. Marked increase in GI motility is thought to be partly due to unopposed parasympathetic activity, but mechanism is poorly understood. Has weak local anesthetic effect and appears to have some antidiabetic (hypoglycemic) action. Local instillation in eye causes miosis and reduces intraocular pressure in glaucomatous eyes.

USES Stepped care approach to treatment of moderate to severe hypertension either alone or in conjunction with a thiazide diuretic or hydralazine (step 4). **Unlabeled uses:** chronic open-angle glaucoma, endocrine ophthalmopathy. **Orphan drug:** reflex sympathetic dystrophy syndrome; causalgia.

PHARMACOKINETICS Absorption: completely absorbed, but undergoes significant first pass metabolism by liver; 3–50% of dose reaches systemic circulation. **Peak effect:** 1–3 wk. **Distribution:** rapidly distributed to adrenergic neuron storage sites; does

ROUTE & DOSAGE

Hypertension

Adult	PO	10 mg once/d; may be increased by 10 mg q5–7d up to 300 mg/d; may start with 25–50 mg/d in hospitalized patients; increase by 25–50 mg q1–3d
Child	PO	0.2 mg/kg/d; may increase by 0.2 mg/kg q1–3wk if needed (max 1–1.6 mg/kg/d)

not cross blood-brain barrier. **Metabolism:** metabolized in liver to inactive metabolites. **Elimination:** half-life: 5 d; excreted in urine.

CONTRAINDICATIONS & PRECAUTIONS Contraindicated in: pheochromocytoma, frank CHF (not due to hypertension). Safe use during pregnancy (category C) not established. **Cautious use in:** diabetes mellitus, impaired renal or hepatic function, sinus bradycardia, limited cardiac reserve, coronary disease with insufficiency, recent MI, cerebrovascular insufficiency, febrile illnesses, the elderly; history of peptic ulcer, colitis, or bronchial asthma.

ADVERSE/SIDE EFFECTS CV: *marked orthostatic and exertional hypotension* with dizziness, lightheadedness, fainting; bradycardia, symptomatic sick sinus syndrome (weakness, dizziness, blurred vision); angina, *edema with weight gain,* CHF, complete heart block. **EENT:** blurred vision, ptosis of eyelids, parotid tenderness, nasal congestion. **GI:** *severe diarrhea,* nausea, vomiting, constipation, dry mouth. **GU:** nocturia, urinary retention, incontinence, inhibition of ejaculation, psychological impotence. **Skin:** skin eruptions, loss of scalp hair. **Other:** dyspnea, psychic depression, weakness, fatigue, myalgia, tremor, chest paresthesias, asthma, rise in BUN, polyarteritis nodosa.

DRUG INTERACTIONS Alcohol, levodopa, DIURETICS and other HYPOTENSIVE AGENTS increase hypotensive effects; MAO INHIBITORS may antagonize hypotensive effects; **norepinephrine, pseudoephedrine,** OTHER DECONGESTANTS, TRICYCLIC ANTIDEPRESSANTS, PHENOTHIAZINES block hypotensive effects.

NURSING IMPLICATIONS

Administration

- Tablet may be crushed before administration and taken with fluid of patient's choice.
- Because guanethidine has prolonged onset and duration of action and since its effects are cumulative, dosage should be increased slowly (at intervals of

Common side effects in *italic*; life-threatening effects underlined; generic names in **bold**; classifications in SMALL CAPS

637

no less than 5–7 d for adults and 1–3 wk in children) and only if there has been no reduction in standing BP from previous levels. BP should be monitored during dosage adjustment period.

Assessment & Drug Effects

- During period of dosage adjustment, doses must be carefully titrated on the basis of orthostatic and supine BP. The hypotensive effect of guanethidine is greater with patient in orthostatic position as opposed to supine position. Take readings before initiation of therapy as baseline for comparison.
- Ideal dosage is that which reduces orthostatic BP to within normal range without faintness, dizziness, weakness, or fatigue.
- Physician generally prescribes taking BP first in supine position and then again after patient has been standing for 10 min.
- Because hospitalized patients are given higher initial doses than ambulatory patients, standing BP determinations should be made regularly during the day if possible.
- I&O should be monitored, especially in the elderly and in patients with limited cardiac reserve or impaired renal function. Report changes in I&O ratio.
- Patients with limited cardiac reserve are particularly susceptible to guanethidine-induced sodium and water retention, with resulting edema, CHF, and drug resistance.
- Observe for evidence of edema, and weigh patients daily (or as prescribed) under standard conditions. Sudden weight gain of 1 kg (2 lb) or more should be reported to physician.
- Guanethidine is reported to have antidiabetic activity. Patients on antidiabetic therapy should be observed closely for signs of hypoglycemia.

Patient & Family Education

- To reinforce patient compliance in taking drug regularly at the same time each day, suggest that it be taken to coincide with some routine activity such as brushing teeth in the morning. Stress importance of not stopping drug without advice of physician.
- Caution patient not to get out of bed without assistance. Supervise ambulation, particularly in the elderly, since they are prone to develop orthostatic hypotension.
- Patients should be informed that orthostatic hypotension is most prominent shortly after arising from sleep and when too rapid changes are made to sitting or upright positions. Warn patients to move gradually to sitting position and to make all position changes slowly and in stages. Advise patient to flex arms and legs slowly before standing to augment venous return.

- Patients should be informed that orthostatic hypotension is intensified by prolonged standing, hot baths or showers, hot weather, alcohol ingestion, and strenuous physical exercise (particularly if followed by immobility).
- Warn patients to lie down or sit down (in head-low position) immediately at the onset of dizziness, weakness, or faintness.
- Advise patient to report character and frequency of stools. Diarrhea due to accelerated GI motility may be manifested by increased frequency of bowel movements and may be explosive and embarrassing to patient.
- Advise patient to consult physician regarding allowable salt intake.
- Dosage requirements may be reduced in presence of febrile illnesses. Advise patient to report fever to physician.
- Guanethidine may sensitize the patient to some sympathomimetic agents found in OTC cold remedies and cause hypertensive crisis. Caution patient to consult physician or pharmacist before taking any OTC drug.

Prototype: methyldopa, p 148

GUANFACINE HYDROCHLORIDE
(gwahn´fa-seen)
Trade name: Tenex
Classifications: CARDIOVASCULAR AGENT; CENTRAL ACTING ANTIHYPERTENSIVE; AUTONOMIC NERVOUS SYSTEM AGENT; ALPHA-ADRENERGIC AGONIST (SYMPATHOMIMETIC)
Pregnancy: Category B

ACTIONS/PHARMACODYNAMICS Central acting antihypertensive with alpha$_2$-adrenergic agonist properties. In cerebral cortex, stimulation of alpha$_2$-adrenoceptors triggers inhibitory neurons to reduce central sympathetic outflow, i.e., impulses from vasomotor center to heart and blood vessels, with the result that peripheral vascular resistance is decreased and heart rate is slightly reduced (5 bpm). Cardiac output is not altered by this agent. Stimulates growth hormone secretion without effect on its plasma level.

USES Management of mild to moderate hypertension, usually with a thiazide-type diuretic. In stepped-care approach, guanfacine is considered a step 2 agent added to the treatment regimen if step 1 agents are inadequate. Has limited usefulness as step 1 agent. **Unlabeled use:** adjunct in heroin withdrawal.

Common side effects in *italic*; life-threatening effects underlined; generic names in **bold**; classifications in SMALL CAPS

ROUTE & DOSAGE

Hypertension

Adult PO 1 mg/d h.s.; may be gradually increased to 3 mg/d if needed

PHARMACOKINETICS Absorption: readily absorbed from GI tract. **Onset:** 2 h. **Peak:** 6 h. **Duration:** up to 24 h. **Distribution:** crosses placenta. **Metabolism:** metabolized in liver. **Elimination:** half-life: 17 h; 80% excreted in the urine in 24 h.

CONTRAINDICATIONS & PRECAUTIONS Contraindicated in: treatment of acute hypertension associated with toxemia of pregnancy; pregnancy (category B); children <12 y. **Cautious use in:** severe coronary insufficiency, recent MI, cerebrovascular disease; chronic renal or hepatic failure; nursing mothers.

ADVERSE/SIDE EFFECTS CNS: confusion, amnesia, mental depression, drowsiness, *dizziness, sedation,* headache, paresthesia, paresis, *asthenia, fatigue,* insomnia. **CV:** bradycardia, palpitation, substernal pain. **ENT:** rhinitis, tinnitus, taste change. **Eye:** vision disturbances, conjunctivitis, iritis. **GI:** *dry mouth, constipation,* abdominal pain, diarrhea, dysphagia, nausea. **GU:** *impotence,* testicular disorder, urinary incontinence. **Musculoskeletal:** leg cramps, hypokinesia. **Skin:** dermatitis, pruritus, purpura, sweating. **Other:** dyspnea.

DRUG INTERACTIONS Alcohol and other CNS DEPRESSANTS compound sedation and CNS depression.

NURSING IMPLICATIONS

Administration

- Single dose is best taken at bedtime to reduce effect of somnolence.
- Discontinuation of guanfacine treatment is gradual with planned tapering of schedule.
- Store tablets at 15–30C (59–86F) in tightly closed container, protect from light.

Assessment & Drug Effects

- Abrupt discontinuation may cause plasma and urinary catecholamine increases, leading to symptoms of tachycardia, insomnia, anxiety, nervousness. Rebound hypertension (i.e., increases in BP to levels significantly greater than those before therapy) may occur 2–7 d after abrupt drug withdrawal, but serious effects rarely develop.

- Monitor BP until it is stabilized. Report a rise in pressure that occurs toward end of dose interval; a divided dose schedule may be ordered.
- Side effects tend to be dose-dependent, increasing significantly with doses above 3 mg/d.

Patient & Family Education

- Urge patients to continue with drug even after they feel well. Advise maintenance of dosage regimen (dose and dose intervals). If 2 or more doses are missed, consult physician about how to reestablish dosage regimen.
- Dry mouth fosters changes that promote dental problems. Urge patient to employ measures to keep mouth moist; suggest, if necessary, a saliva substitute, e.g., Moi-Stir, Xero-Lube (available OTC). If dry mouth persists > 2 wk, patient should check with dentist.
- Advise caution about driving or performing other tasks requiring alertness until reaction to drug is known.
- Tolerance for alcohol and other CNS depressants may be reduced by guanfacine. Advise patients to avoid alcohol and not to self-medicate with nonprescription drugs such as sleeping medications, or cough medications without advice of physician.

HAEMOPHILUS b CONJUGATE VACCINE

(hee-mof´il-us)
Trade names: HibTITER, PedvaxIIIB, ProHIBiT
Classification: VACCINE
Pregnancy: Category C

ACTIONS/PHARMACODYNAMICS A highly purified capsular polysaccharide extracted from *Haemophilus influenzae* type b (Hib). Hib capsular polysaccharide, principal antigen in the vaccine, promotes production of Hib anticapsular antibody, which mediates complement-dependent bacteriolyses and opsinization of *H. influenzae* type b organism. Serum antibody response is age dependent; i.e., response is poor in infants, increasing significantly between 12–24 mo. Immunization against *H. influenzae* type b disease (e.g., bacterial meningitis and other systemic bacterial infections such as pneumonia, pericarditis, cellulitis) may be considered in children 2–18 mo of age. Data concerning use and efficacy of the vaccine in older children and adults are incomplete. Studies are in progress to determine

H

need, frequency, and safety of revaccination with Hib polysaccharide vaccine, especially in children 18–23 mo.

USES To provide active immunity to *H. influenzae* type b (Hib) infection in children 2 mo–5 y. **Unlabeled uses:** adults at risk of Hib infection who have Hodgkin's disease, before immunosuppressive chemotherapy.

ROUTE & DOSAGE

Immunoprophylaxis for *H. influenzae* type b infection

Child	IM	2–6 mo: HibTITER: 0.5 ml, 3 doses 2 mo apart with booster at 15 mo
		PedvaxHIB: 0.5 ml, 2 doses 2 mo apart with booster at 12 mo
		7–11 mo: HibTITER: 0.5 ml, 2 doses 2 mo apart with booster at 15 mo
		PedvaxHIB: 0.5 ml, 2 doses 2 mo apart with booster at 15 mo
		12–14 mo: HibTITER: 0.5 ml, 1 dose with booster at 15 mo
		PedvaxHIB: 0.5 ml, 1 dose with booster at 15 mo
		15 mo–5 y: All vaccines: 0.5 ml as 1 dose

PHARMACOKINETICS Onset: antibody levels detected within 2 wk. **Peak:** 3 wk. **Duration:** 1.5–3.5 y. **Distribution:** crosses placenta; distributed into breast milk.

CONTRAINDICATIONS & PRECAUTIONS Contraindicated in: hypersensitivity to any component of vaccine (e.g., thiomerosal); febrile illness (other than upper respiratory tract infection); active infection. Safe use during pregnancy and by nursing mothers not established.

ADVERSE/SIDE EFFECTS Irritation at injection site (4–9%). **Other:** acute febrile reactions (13%), irritability, anorexia, anaphylactoid reaction (infrequent).

DIAGNOSTIC TEST INTERFERENCES Hib polysaccharide vaccine may interfere with interpretation of *antigen detection tests* (e.g., latex agglutination) used in diagnosis of systemic Hib disease.

DRUG INTERACTIONS IMMUNOSUPPRESSANT DRUGS, STEROIDS may decrease antibody response.

NURSING IMPLICATIONS

Administration

- Vaccine should not be administered intradermally or by IV.
- Reconstitute lyophilized powder with supplied diluent to provide solution containing 25 μg/0.5 ml. Use sterile needle and syringe free of preservatives or antiseptics Record date of reconstitution on vaccine label.
- Avoid injecting the vaccine near blood vessels or nerves. Draw back on plunger to avoid inadvertent entry into a blood vessel. If blood is drawn into syringe, discard and prepare a new dose of vaccine.
- Hib polysaccharide vaccine and DPT (diphtheria, pertussis, tetanus) may be given at the same time but at different sites.
- *Storage:* Expiration date for lyophilized powder for injection is 24 mo from date of issue from manufacturer's cold storage. Drug should be refrigerated at 2–8C (36–46F) but may be frozen without loss of potency. The diluent should not be frozen.

Assessment & Drug Effects

- After administration of the vaccine be prepared for anaphylactoid reaction (see Signs & Symptoms, chap 3) by having epinephrine 1:1000 available.
- Routine immunization against Hib is not recommended for children 18–23 mo unless child is at high risk of exposure or infection.

Patient & Family Education

- Inform parents that vaccine may not be completely effective if given to child 18–23 mo. However, if vaccine is given before child is 2 y, because of high-risk situation, a booster dose may be necessary at 24 mo or later, but at least 2 mo after first dose.
- Local reactions to the vaccine at the injection site (erythema, tenderness, induration, swelling, pain) may appear within 6 h after administration; usually symptoms are mild and disappear in 24 h.
- Monitor temperature after injection. An acute febrile reaction with temperature above 38.3C (101F) may follow vaccination (less than 1% of recipients). Report to physician.

Prototype: lorazepam, p 177

HALAZEPAM

(hal ah´u jmm)

Trade name: Paxipam
Classifications: CNS AGENT; BENZODIAZEPINE ANXIOLYTIC, SEDATIVE-HYPNOTIC
Pregnancy: Category D
Controlled substance: Schedule IV

ACTIONS/PHARMACODYNAMICS Psychotropic drug that shares antianxiety actions of other short-term benzodiazepine derivatives. Exact mechanism of action is unknown, but clinically it produces dose-related CNS depressant effect ranging from mild improvement of psychomotor activity to hypnosis. Clinical efficacy in long-term use (i.e., > 4 mo) has not been evaluated. Animal studies suggest that drug induces activity of hepatic microsomal enzymes; therefore metabolism of other drugs given concurrently may be increased.

USES To manage anxiety disorders or for short-term relief of anxiety symptoms.

ROUTE & DOSAGE

Anxiety
Adult   PO   20–40 mg t.i.d. or q.i.d.

PHARMACOKINETICS Absorption: readily absorbed from GI tract. **Peak:** 1–3 h. **Distribution:** crosses placenta; distributed into breast milk. **Metabolism:** metabolized in liver to active form. **Elimination:** half-life: 30–200 h (active metabolite); excreted in urine.

CONTRAINDICATIONS & PRECAUTIONS Contraindicated in: hypersensitivity to halazepam or other benzodiazepines; psychosis, anxiety-free psychiatric disorders, acute narrow-angle glaucoma. **Cautious use in:** abnormal kidney or liver function. Safe use during pregnancy (category D), in nursing mothers, and in children < 18 y not established.

ADVERSE/SIDE EFFECTS CNS: *drowsiness, sedation*, headache, confusion, ataxia, paresthesia. **CV:** hypotension, tachycardia, bradycardia. **GI:** dry mouth, increased salivation, nausea, vomiting, constipation. **Other:** allergic manifestations, motion sickness, visual disturbances, GU distress, respiratory disturbances, abnormal liver values.

DRUG INTERACTIONS Cimetidine, disulfiram, ORAL CONTRACEPTIVES may increase effects of halazepam; **alcohol,** other CNS DEPRESSANTS compound CNS depression.

NURSING IMPLICATIONS

Administration
- Patients with renal or hepatic impairment may require lower doses.
- Store at 2–30C (36–86F) unless directed otherwise.

Assessment & Drug Effects
- Ataxia, confusion, or oversedation (sleeping in the daytime) may be symptoms of overdosage and can occur at relatively low dosage in the elderly or debilitated patient.
- Smoking decreases sedative effects of benzodiazepines, including halazepam. This is especially true if patient is a heavy smoker.
- Psychic or physical dependence can develop, particularly in addiction-prone patient, who should be under careful surveillance while on this drug.
- Response to halazepam should be reassessed periodically. Effectiveness in long-term use (more than 4 mo) is not known.

Patient & Family Education
- If patient becomes pregnant or plans on pregnancy, she should discuss with physician desirability of discontinuing drug because of its potential hazard to the fetus.
- Warn patient not to alter drug regimen (dose or interval) and not to stop taking drug suddenly. Barbiturate-like withdrawal symptoms may occur (dysphoria, insomnia, abdominal and muscle cramps, vomiting, sweating, tremors, convulsions). Dosage is tapered after long-term use to discontinue its use.
- Caution patient to avoid driving and other potentially hazardous activities until reaction to drug is known.
- Warn patient that ingestion of alcohol or other CNS depressants can produce additive effects.

Prototype: hydrocortisone, p 255

HALCINONIDE

(hal-sin´oh-nide)

Trade names: Halciderm, Halog
Classifications: SKIN AGENT; ANTIINFLAMMATORY; HORMONE; ADRENAL CORTICOSTEROID
Pregnancy: Category C

H

Common side effects in *italic*; life-threatening effects underlined; generic names in **bold**; classifications in SMALL CAPS

641

ACTIONS/PHARMACODYNAMICS Fluorinated steroid with substituted 17-hydroxyl group, chemically similar to flurandrenolide (Cordran). Crosses cell membranes, complexes with nuclear DNA and stimulates synthesis of enzymes thought to be responsible for antiinflammatory effects. Systemic absorption leads to actions, limitations, and drug interactions observed with use of hydrocortisone.

USES Relief of pruritic and inflammatory manifestations of corticosteroid-responsive dermatoses.

ROUTE & DOSAGE

Inflammation

Adult	Topical	Apply thin layer b.i.d. or t.i.d.
Child	Topical	Apply thin layer once/d

PHARMACOKINETICS Absorption: minimum absorption through intact skin; increased absorption from axilla, eyelid, face, scalp, scrotum, or with occlusive dressing.

NURSING IMPLICATIONS

Administration

- Check with physician regarding specific application procedure. Generally, skin is gently washed and thoroughly dried before each application.
- Selection of medication vehicle depends on condition of lesions. Ointment is usually preferred for dry scaly lesions. Moist lesions are appropriately treated with solution.
- Not to be applied in or around the eyes.
- Occlusive dressings should not be applied over areas covered with halcinonide unless specifically prescribed.
- Store at room temperature; avoid freezing.

Assessment & Drug Effects

- Medication should be discontinued if signs of infection or irritation occur.
- Systemic corticosteroid effects may be produced when occlusive dressings are used or when topical applications cover large areas of skin. In addition there is increased risk of withdrawal symptoms when either procedure is discontinued after prolonged use.

HALOPERIDOL

See CNS AGENT, PSYCHOTHERAPEUTIC, ANTIPSYCHOTIC (TRANQUILIZER), BUTYROPHENONE prototype, p 189.

Prototype: amphotericin B, p 56

HALOPROGIN

(ha-loe-proe′jin)
Trade name: Halotex
Classifications: ANTIINFECTIVE; ANTIBIOTIC; ANTIFUNGAL
Pregnancy: Category B

ACTIONS/PHARMACODYNAMICS Synthetic iodinated phenolic ether. Fungicidal or fungistatic against various species of *Trichophyton, Epidermophyton, Microsporum, Malassezia,* and *Candida.* Also active in vitro against *Staphylococcus aureus* and *Streptococcus pyogenes.*

USES Superficial fungal infections such as tinea pedis, tinea cruris, tinea corporis, and tinea manus. Also tinea versicolor caused by *Malassezia furfur.* May be used in combination antiinfective therapy for mixed infections.

ROUTE & DOSAGE

Superficial Fungal Infections

Adult	Topical	Apply liberally to affected area b.i.d. for 2–3 wk

PHARMACOKINETICS Absorption: minimum absorption through intact skin.

CONTRAINDICATIONS & PRECAUTIONS Contraindicated in: safe use during pregnancy (category C) not established.

ADVERSE/SIDE EFFECTS Local irritation, burning sensation, vesiculation, increased maceration, exacerbation of preexisting lesions, sensitization, pruritus. Low incidence of systemic toxicity.

NURSING IMPLICATIONS

Administration

- Check with physician regarding specific application procedure. Generally, skin is gently washed and thoroughly dried before each application.
- Avoid contact of medication with eyes.

Assessment & Drug Effects

- Medication should be discontinued if signs of infection or irritation occur.

Common side effects in *italic*; life-threatening effects <u>underlined</u>; generic names in **bold**; classifications in SMALL CAPS

- Therapy should be reevaluated if no improvement is noted after 2–3 wk.

Patient & Family Education

- Advise patient to discontinue medication if condition worsens or if burning irritation, or signs of sensitization occur, and consult physician.
- Patients with tinea pedis (athlete's foot) should be advised not to wear occlusive footwear because it tends to promote systemic drug absorption and enhance fungal growth.
- To avoid spread of infection to others, instruct patient to keep facecloth, towels, and other articles of personal hygiene separate.
- Advise patient to wear freshly laundered clothes daily.

HEMIN

(hee´min)

Trade name: Panhematin
Classifications: ENZYME INHIBITOR; BLOOD DERIVATIVE
Pregnancy: Category C

ACTIONS/PHARMACODYNAMICS Sterile, nonpyrogenic ferric iron complex of protoporphyrin IX; derived from processed red blood cells. Represses synthesis of porphyrin in liver or bone marrow by blocking production of delta-aminolevulinic acid (ALA) synthetase, an essential enzyme in the porphyrin-heme biosynthetic pathway. Each vial contains hemin 313 mg with sodium carbonate 215 mg, sorbitol 300 mg (no preservatives).

USES Recurrent attacks of acute intermittent porphyria (AIP) only after an appropriate period of alternate therapy has been tried (i.e., glucose 400 g/d for 1–2 d).

ROUTE & DOSAGE

Acute Intermittent Porphyria

Adult	IV	1–4 mg/kg/d administered over 10–15 min for 3–14 d; dose should not be repeated earlier than q12h (max 6 mg/kg in 24 h)

PHARMACOKINETICS Duration: can be detected in plasma up to 5 d. **Elimination:** excess amounts eliminated in bile and urine.

CONTRAINDICATIONS & PRECAUTIONS Contraindicated in: history of hypersensitivity to hemin; porphyria cutanea tarda. Safe use during pregnancy (category C), in nursing women, and in children not established.

ADVERSE/SIDE EFFECTS *Phlebitis* (when administered into small veins); anticoagulant effect: prolonged PT, thromboplastin time, thrombocytopenia, hypofibrinogenemia; decreased Hct; reversible renal shutdown (with excessive doses).

DRUG INTERACTIONS Potentiates anticoagulant effects of ANTICOAGULANTS; BARBITURATES, ESTROGENS, SULFONAMIDES may antagonize hemin effect.

NURSING IMPLICATIONS

Administration

- Hemin is administered only by physicians experienced in the management of porphyria in hospitals equipped to perform the recommended clinical and laboratory monitoring.
- Hemin should be administered via a large arm vein or central venous catheter to reduce risk of phlebitis. Terminal filtration through a sterile 0.45 μm or smaller filter is recommended to assure that no undissolved particles are injected into patient.
- Because hemin contains no preservatives, it should be reconstituted immediately before use. Reconstitute by aseptically adding 43 ml sterile water for injection to vial. Shake well for 2–3 min to dissolve all particles. Discard unused portions.
- Freeze and store lyophilized powder until time of use.

Assessment & Drug Effects

- Monitor IV site for signs and symptoms of thrombophlebitis (see chap 3).
- The following laboratory values are monitored throughout hemin therapy (decrease in these values is an indication of a favorable clinical response): ALA, UPG (uroporphyrinogen), PBG (porphobilinogen or coproporphyrin).
- To monitor clinical effect of drug therapy, be aware of the patient's symptoms and complaints associated with acute porphyria, which may include depression, insomnia, anxiety, disorientation, hallucinations, psychoses; dark urine, nausea, vomiting, abdominal pain, low back and leg pain, pareses (neuropathy), seizures.
- Monitor I&O ratio and pattern, particularly in patients receiving high doses. Promptly report the onset of oliguria or anuria.

Common side effects in *italic*; life-threatening effects underlined; generic names in **bold**; classifications in SMALL CAPS

H

Patient & Family Education

▪ Instruct patient to report signs and symptoms of excessive anticoagulant effects including bruising, hematuria, tarry black stools, and nose bleeds.

Prototype: warfarin, p 127

HEPARIN CALCIUM

(hep´a-rin)
Trade names: Calcilean, Calciparine

HEPARIN SODIUM

Trade names: Hepalean, Heparin Sodium Lock Flush Solution, Hep-Lock, Lipo-Hepin, Liquaemin Sodium
Classifications: BLOOD FORMERS & COAGULATORS; ANTICOAGULANT
Pregnancy: Category C

ACTIONS/PHARMACODYNAMICS Strongly acidic, high molecular weight mucopolysaccharide with rapid anticoagulant effect, prepared from bovine lung tissue or porcine intestinal mucosa. Exerts direct effect on blood coagulation (clotting) by enhancing the inhibitory actions of antithrombin III (heparin cofactor) on several factors essential to normal blood clotting, thereby blocking the conversion of prothrombin to thrombin and fibrinogen to fibrin. Does not lyse already existing thrombi but may prevent their extension and propagation. Inhibits formation on new clots. Prolongs whole blood clotting time, thrombin time, partial thromboplastin time, and prothrombin time, but bleeding time (test of platelet function) is usually unaffected except with high doses. Reduces plasma triglycerides (antilipemic action), exhibits antiinflammatory and diuretic effects, and may suppress aldosterone secretion. Reportedly enhances potassium retention and possibly plays a role in immunologic reactions. The calcium salt is derived from porcine intestinal mucosa; the sodium salt is prepared from either porcine intestinal mucosa or bovine lung tissue.

USES Prophylaxis and treatment of venous thrombosis and pulmonary embolism and to prevent thromboembolic complications arising from cardiac and vascular surgery, frostbite, and during acute stage of MI. Also used in treatment of disseminated intravascular coagulation (DIC), atrial fibrillation with embolization, and as anticoagulant in blood transfusions, extracorporeal circulation, and dialysis procedures. **Unlabeled uses:** prophylaxis in hip and knee surgery. Heparin Sodium Lock Flush Solution is used to maintain potency of indwelling IV catheters in intermittent IV therapy or blood sampling. It is not intended for anticoagulant therapy.

ROUTE & DOSAGE

Treatment of Thromboembolism

Adult	IV	5000 U bolus dose; then 20,000–40,000 U infused over 24 h; dose adjusted to maintain desired APTT; *or* 5000–10,000 U IV piggyback q4–6h
	SC	10,000–20,000 U followed by 8,000–20,000 U q8–12h
Child	IV	50 U/kg bolus; then 20,000 U/m²/24 h or 50–100 U/kg q4h

Open Heart Surgery

Adult	IV	150–300 U/kg

Prophylaxis of Embolism

Adult	SC	5000 U q12h

PHARMACOKINETICS Onset: 20–60 min SC. **Peak:** within minutes. **Duration:** 2–6 h IV; 8–12 h SC. **Distribution:** does not cross placenta; not distributed into breast milk. **Metabolism:** metabolized in liver and by reticuloendothelial system. **Elimination:** half-life: 90 min; excreted slowly in urine.

CONTRAINDICATIONS & PRECAUTIONS Contraindicated in: history of hypersensitivity to heparin (white clot syndrome); active bleeding, bleeding tendencies (hemophilia, purpura, thrombocytopenia); jaundice; ascorbic acid deficiency; inaccessible ulcerative lesions; visceral carcinoma; open wounds, extensive denudation of skin, suppurative thrombophlebitis; advanced kidney, liver, or biliary disease; active tuberculosis; bacterial endocarditis; continuous tube drainage of stomach or small intestines; threatened abortion; suspected intracranial hemorrhage, severe hypertension; recent surgery of eye, brain, or spinal cord; spinal tap; shock. Teratogenic potential not established. **Cautious use in:** alcoholism; history of atopy or allergy (asthma, hives, hay fever, eczema); during menstruation, pregnancy (category C) especially the last trimester, and immediate postpartum period; patients with indwelling catheters; the elderly; use of acid-citrate-dextrose (ACD)-converted blood (may contain heparin); patients in hazardous occupations; cerebral embolism.

Common side effects in *italic*; life-threatening effects underlined; generic names in **bold**; classifications in SMALL CAPS

H

ADVERSE/SIDE EFFECTS Spontaneous bleeding, injection site reactions: pain, itching, ecchymoses, tissue irritation and sloughing; cyanosis and pains in arms or legs (vasospasm); *transient thrombocytopenia,* hypofibrinogenemia, increased AST, ALT, "white clot syndrome" (see Nursing Implications). Rarely, frequent and persistent erections (priapism). **Hypersensitivity:** fever, chills, urticaria, pruritus, skin rashes, itching and burning sensations of feet, numbness and tingling of hands and feet, elevated BP, headache, reversible transient alopecia (usually around temporal area), nasal congestion, lacrimation, conjunctivitis, chest pains, arthralgia, bronchospasm, anaphylactoid reactions. **Large doses for prolonged periods:** osteoporosis (back or rib pain, decrease in height, spontaneous fractures), hypoaldosteronism, suppressed renal function, hyperkalemia; rebound hyperlipidemia (following termination of heparin therapy).

DIAGNOSTIC TEST INTERFERENCES Notify laboratory that patient is receiving heparin, when a test is to be performed. Possibility of false-positive rise in **BSP** test and in **serum thyroxine;** and increases in **resin T_3 uptake;** false-negative ^{125}I **fibrinogen uptake.** Heparin prolongs PT. Valid readings may be obtained by drawing blood samples at least 4–6 h after an IV dose (but at any time during heparin infusion) and 12–24 h after an SC heparin dose.

DRUG INTERACTIONS May prolong PT, which is used to monitor therapy with ORAL ANTICOAGULANTS; **aspirin,** NSAIDS increase risk of bleeding; **nitroglycerin** IV may decrease anticoagulant activity; **protamine** antagonizes effects of heparin.

INCOMPATIBILITIES Solution/Additive: **amikacin, codeine, chlorpromazine, cytarabine, diazepam, dobutamine, doxorubicin, droperidol, erythromycin, gentamicin, haloperidol, hyaluronidase, hydrocortisone, kanamycin, levorphanol, meperidine, methadone, methicillin, methotrimeprazine, morphine, netilmicin, pentazocine, polymyxin B, promethazine, streptomycin, tetracycline, tobramycin, triflupromazine, vancomycin. Y-Site: amikacin, decarbazine, diazepam, doxorubicin, droperidol, ergotamine, erythromycin, gentamicin, haloperidol, kanamycin, methotrimeprazine, netilmicin, phenytoin, polymyxin B, streptomycin, tobramycin, triflupromazine, vancomycin.**

NURSING IMPLICATIONS

Administration

- Before administering heparin, coagulation test values must be checked; if results are not within therapeutic range, the physician is notified, and dosage adjustment is made. Because heparin has short half-life, it must be given on time to maintain anticoagulant effect.
- Heparin is not intended for IM administration.
- Solutions of heparin or heparin lock-flush that contain benzyl alcohol preservative should not be used in neonates.
- More concentrated heparin solutions are recommended for SC injection.
- (1) Preferably, SC injections are made into the fatty layer of the abdomen or just above the iliac crest. (2) Use a 25- or 26-gauge, 1/2- or 5/8-inch needle. (3) Avoid injecting within 5 cm (2 in) of umbilicus or any scar or bruise. Insert needle into tissue roll perpendicular to skin surface. To avoid possibility of tissue injury and hematoma do not withdraw plunger to check entry into blood vessel. (4) Apply gentle pressure to puncture site 5 to 10 s following injection but do not massage. (5) Systematically rotate injection sites and keep record.
- A single dose of IV heparin (adult 5000 U, child 50 U/kg) may be given undiluted by direct IV injection over 60 seconds.
- IV heparin may be added to NS, D5W, or Ringer's for injection and infused intermittently or continuously.
- When heparin is added to an infusion solution, manufacturer recommends inverting container at least 6 times to insure adequate mixing and to prevent pooling of heparin.
- Continuous IV infusion of heparin requires close monitoring. A constant infusion pump should be used.
- Because heparin is strongly acidic, it is incompatible with many drugs; therefore avoid mixing any drug with heparin unless specifically advised by physician or pharmacist to do so.
- Abrupt withdrawal of heparin may precipitate increased coagulability; generally, full dose heparin is followed by oral anticoagulant prophylactic therapy.
- Administration of an oral anticoagulant usually overlaps that of heparin for 3–5 d while heparin is being tapered off. To obtain valid PT, a period of at least 4–6 h after last IV dose and 12–24 h after the last SC (intrafat) dose of heparin should elapse before blood is drawn.
- Heparin is stable at 15–30C (59–86F). Protect from

H

Common side effects in *italic*; life-threatening effects underlined; generic names in **bold**; classifications in SMALL CAPS

645

freezing. Inspect all preparations for discoloration and particulate matter before administration.

Assessment & Drug Effects

- Baseline blood coagulation tests, Hct, Hgb, RBC, and platelet counts should be performed before therapy is initiated, at regular intervals throughout therapy, and whenever patient shows signs of bleeding. Some physicians also periodically test urine for hematuria and stools for occult blood.
- The APTT and the activated coagulation time (ACT) are coagulation tests commonly used to monitor heparin therapy. In general, dosage is adjusted to keep APTT between 1.5–2.5 times normal control level, and the ACT at approximately 2 to 3 times the control value in seconds. (Standards vary in different laboratories.)
- During dosage adjustment period, blood is drawn for coagulation test 30 min before each scheduled SC or intermittent IV dose and approximately q4h for patients receiving continuous IV heparin. After dosage is established, tests may be done once daily.
- Monitor platelet count, Hgb, and test for occult blood in the stool regularly during heparin therapy.
- Construct a flow chart indicating dates, coagulation time determinations, Hct, platelet counts, heparin doses, and urine and stool tests for occult bleeding.
- Patients vary widely in their reaction to heparin, and no test can reliably predict bleeding. The risk of hemorrhage appears to be greatest in women, all patients ≥ 60 y, patients receiving heparin prophylactically following surgery, and patients with liver disease or renal insufficiency.
- Monitor vital signs. Report fever, drop in BP, rapid pulse, and other signs and symptoms of hemorrhage.
- Some patients develop paradoxical thrombi ("white clot syndrome") in association with low platelet count. The complication is thought to result from irreversible platelet aggregation induced by heparin. If it occurs, heparin should be discontinued.
- Observe all needle sites daily for hematoma and signs of inflammation (swelling, heat redness, pain).
- ***Antidote:*** have on hand protamine sulfate (1% solution), specific heparin antagonist. Because heparin has a short half-life, mild overdosage can frequently be controlled by merely withdrawing heparin. In some cases, however, whole blood or plasma transfusion may be necessary. Coagulation studies should be done to confirm protamine effect.

- "Heparin resistance" has occurred in conditions associated with large amounts of fibrin deposition (e.g., early stage of thrombophlebitis, peritonitis, fever, pleurisy, cancer, MI, extensive surgery).
- A baseline APTT is recommended when Heparin Lock Flush Solution is to be used on a regular basis.

Patient & Family Education

- Inform patients without frightening them to protect themselves from injury and to report pink, red, dark brown, or cloudy urine; red or dark brown vomitus; red or black stools; bleeding gums or oral mucosa; ecchymoses, hematoma, epistaxis, bloody sputum; chest pain; abdominal or lumbar pain or swelling; unusual increase in menstrual flow; pelvic pain; severe or continuous headache, faintness, or dizziness.
- Inform women that menstruation may be somewhat increased and prolonged. Usually this is not a contraindication to continued therapy if bleeding is not excessive and patient has no underlying pathology.
- Tell patient that heparin may have a diuretic effect beginning 36–48 h after initial dose and lasting 36–48 h after termination of therapy.
- If patient is to be discharged on heparin, teach the correct technique for SC administration to the person who will be giving the injections.
- In the absence of a low platelet (thrombocyte) count, patient may carry out normal activities such as shaving with a safety razor. Usually heparin does not affect bleeding time.
- Transient alopecia sometimes occurs several months after heparin therapy. Reassure patient that condition is reversible.
- Smoking and alcohol consumption may alter response to heparin and therefore are not advised. Also, caution patient not to take aspirin, antihistamines, cough preparations containing guaifenesin (glyceryl guaiacolate), or any other OTC medication without physician's approval because they may interfere with platelet function.

HEPATITIS B IMMUNE GLOBULIN

Trade names: H-BIG, Hep-B-Gammagee, HyperHep
Classification: SERUM
Pregnancy: Category C

ACTIONS/PHARMACODYNAMICS Sterile solution of immunoglobulins [not less than 80% immunoglobulin G (IgG)] prepared by a special process using pooled human plasma. Preparation contains a high antibody titer specific to hepatitis B surface antigen (anti-HBs); plasma does not show serologic evidence of hepatitis B surface antigen (HBsAg). Serum has also been tested for and found free of antibody to human immunodeficiency virus (HIV). The possibility of transmission of hepatitis infection or AIDS from HBIG is remote.

USES Prophylactically to provide passive immunity to hepatitis B infection in individuals exposed to HBV or HBsAg-positive materials (blood plasma, serum). Also as postexposure prophylaxis after bite or percutaneous exposure, ingestion, direct mucous membrane contact, sexual or intimate contact, and in neonates born to HBsAg-positive women.

ROUTE & DOSAGE

Hepatitis B Prophylaxis

Adult	IM	0.06 ml/kg as soon as possible after exposure, preferably within 24 h, but no later than 7 d; repeat 28–30 d after exposure
Child	IM	Same as for adult

Newborn Exposure

Child	IM	0.5 ml as soon as possible after birth but no later than 24 h; repeat dose 3 and 6 mo later

PHARMACOKINETICS Absorption: slowly absorbed from IM site. **Onset:** 1–6 d. **Peak:** 3–11 d. **Duration:** 2–6 mo. **Elimination:** half-life: 21 d.

CONTRAINDICATIONS & PRECAUTIONS Cautious use in: history of systemic allergic reactions to immune globulin, thrombocytopenia or bleeding disorders, HBsAg-positive individuals, patients with specific immunoglobulin A (IgA) deficiency; pregnancy (category C).

ADVERSE/SIDE EFFECTS Usually infrequent and mild. **Skin/Hypersensitivity:** urticaria, rash, angioedema, pruritus, erythema, sensitization (following large or repeated doses), anaphylaxis (rare). **Local:** muscle stiffness; pain, tenderness, swelling, erythema of injection site. **Other:** nausea, faintness, fever, dizziness, malaise, lassitude, body and joint pain, leg cramps.

DRUG INTERACTIONS May interfere with immune response to LIVE-VIRUS VACCINES (measles, mumps, rubella, poliovirus).

NURSING IMPLICATIONS

Administration

- Hepatitis B immune globulin may be administered at the same time or up to 1 mo preceding hepatitis B vaccination (hepatitis B vaccine) without impairing the active immune response from the vaccination.
- IM injections should be made preferably into deltoid muscle or anterolateral aspect of thigh. Because of risk of injury to the sciatic nerve, injections into the gluteus are not advised routinely except when large volumes must be given or large doses must be divided into multiple injections. This route is used only for adults.
- For neonates and small children the preferred IM injection site is the anterolateral aspect of the thigh.
- Inadvertent IV administration can cause a precipitous fall in BP and an anaphylactic reaction.
- Skin testing with HBIG is not advised.
- Store at 2–8C (36–46F) unless otherwise directed. Avoid freezing. Solution should be clear, slightly amber, and moderately viscous. Do not mix with other medications.

Assessment & Drug Effects

- Hypersensitivity reactions are most likely to occur in patients receiving large doses or repeated injections. Have epinephrine 1:1000 readily available.
- Presence of HBsAg in serum indicates active hepatitis B infection or that the person is a chronic carrier. Care providers should be aware that this serum is highly infective.

Patient & Family Education

- Hepatitis B virus infection usually spreads by parenteral means, as from contaminated blood, plasma, serum, needles, contamination of cuts or mucous membranes with the virus, and by oral ingestion, e.g., pipetting accident. It has also been reported that HBsAg may be present in many body fluids (e.g., saliva, tears, urine, feces, pleural effusions, semen). Although the clinical significance of this finding has not been determined, all body fluids should be considered contaminated pending full study.
- Hepatitis B virus transmission can be prevented by following appropriate CDC precautions.

H

Common side effects in *italic*; life-threatening effects underlined; generic names in **bold**; classifications in SMALL CAPS

647

HEPATITIS B VACCINE (RECOMBINANT)

Trade names: Engerix-B, Recombivax HB
Classification: VACCINE
Pregnancy: Category C

ACTIONS/PHARMACODYNAMICS Suspension of inactivated and purified hepatitis B surface antigen (HBsAg) derived from human plasma of screened asymptomatic HBsAg-positive carriers of hepatitis B virus. (Purification process also removes or inactivates representatives of all other known groups of animal viruses.) Hepatitis B vaccine recombinant is the first vaccine produced by gene splicing. No human plasma is used in its production. The recommended 3-dose regimen produces active immunity against hepatitis B infection by inducing protective antibody (anti-HBs) formation. Children respond with a higher titer of anti-HBs than adults; response tends to be less in immunodeficient patients than in healthy individuals, lower in males than in females, and lower in older than young adults. For most healthy persons, immunity (i.e., protective anti-HBs titer) appears to persist for about 5 y. Hepatitis B vaccine will not prevent infection if it is administered during the incubation period. There is no evidence to date that suggests transmission of AIDS by this vaccine.

USES To promote active immunity in individuals at high risk of potential exposure to hepatitis B virus or HBsAg-positive materials. Has been used simultaneously (into different sites) with hepatitis B immune globulin (HBIG) for postexposure prophylaxis in selected patients and in infants born to HBsAg-positive mothers.

PHARMACOKINETICS Absorption: slowly absorbed from IM site. **Onset:** 2 wk. **Peak:** 6 mo. **Duration:** at least 3 y.

CONTRAINDICATIONS & PRECAUTIONS Contraindicated in: history of allergic reaction to hepatitis B vaccine or to any ingredient in the formulation (Heptavax-B contains alum and a mercury derivative as a preservative); HBsAg carriers. Safe use during pregnancy (category C) and in nursing mothers not established. **Cautious use in:** compromised cardiopulmonary status, serious active infection or fever; thrombocytopenia or other bleeding disorders.

ROUTE & DOSAGE

Hepatitis B Prophylaxis

Adult	IM	Recombivax: 1 ml (10 µg) at 0, 1, and 6 mo
		Engerix B: 1 ml (20 µg) at 0, 1, and 6 mo or 0, 1, 2, and 12 mo
Child	IM	Recombivax: 0.5 ml (5 µg) at 0, 1, and 6 mo
		Engerix B: 0.5 ml (10 µg) at 0, 1, and 6 mo or 0, 1, 2, and 12 mo

Dialysis and Immunodeficient Patients

Adult	IM	Recombivax: 2 ml (20 µg) at 0, 1, and 6 mo
		Engerix B: 2 ml (40 µg) at 0, 1, and 6 mo or 0, 1, 2, and 12 mo

ADVERSE/SIDE EFFECTS *Mild local tenderness at injection site, local inflammatory reaction* (swelling, heat, redness, induration, pain); *fever, malaise, fatigue,* headache, dizziness, faintness, leg cramps, myalgia, arthralgia, nausea, vomiting, urticaria, diarrhea, rash, pruritus; possibility of subcutaneous nodules following SC injections; hypersensitivity. Causal relationship not established: tremors, recurrent Bell's palsy, transverse myelitis, seizures, paresthesias, Guillain-Barré syndrome, acute radiculoneuropathy, aseptic meningitis, flu-like symptoms, joint inflammation, chest pain, hives, herpes zoster infection, psoriasis, skin and mucous membrane eruptions, erythema multiforme, optic neuritis, visual disturbances, tinnitus, thrombocytopenia.

NURSING IMPLICATIONS

Administration

- Not to be administered IV or intradermally. Hepatitis B vaccine is intended for IM use; however, it has been administered SC in patients (e.g., hemophiliacs) at risk of hemorrhage from IM injection.
- Preferably IM injection should be made into the deltoid and in neonates into the anterolateral thigh, avoiding blood vessels and nerves. Carefully aspirate to prevent inadvertent intravascular injection.
- It is a general rule that whenever a vaccine is to be administered, epinephrine should be immediately available to treat anaphylaxis.
- Shake vial well before withdrawing dose to assure uniform suspension. Use dry, sterile needle and syringe.
- Store unopened and opened vials at 2–8C (36–46F) unless otherwise directed. Avoid freezing (freezing destroys potency).

H

Common side effects in *italic*; life-threatening effects underlined; generic names in **bold**; classifications in SMALL CAPS

Assessment & Drug Effects

- The ACIP recommends serologic confirmation of postvaccination immunity in patients undergoing dialysis and in immunodeficient patients.
- Monitor temperature. Some patients develop a temperature elevation of 38.3C (101F) following vaccination that may last 1 or 2 d.

Patient & Family Education

- Following the 5 y period of immunity conferred by hepatitis B vaccine, a single booster is presently suggested to maintain immunity.
- It is estimated that the incidence of hepatitis B infection in the United States is about 200,000. Vaccination is not advised for the general public but is strongly recommended for high-risk groups including health care personnel, selected patients, and patient contacts.

Prototype: albumin, p 126

HETASTARCH

(het'a-starch)
Trade names: HES, Hespan, Hydroxyethyl Starch
Classification: PLASMA VOLUME EXPANDER
Pregnancy: Category C

ACTIONS/PHARMACODYNAMICS Synthetic starch closely resembling human glycogen. Has an average molecular weight of about 450,000 (range 10,000–1 million). Colloidal osmotic properties are approximately equal to those of human serum albumin. Acts much like albumin and dextran but is claimed to be less likely to produce anaphylaxis or to interfere with cross matching or bloodtyping procedures. Causes no significant alterations in fibrinogen or clotting time but may prolong the PPT and PT. Expansion of plasma volume is immediate and slightly greater than amount of hetastarch administered. In hypovolemic patients, it increases arterial and venous pressures, heart rate, cardiac output, urine output, and colloidal osmotic pressure. Not a substitute for blood or plasma; has no oxygen-carrying capacity or antigenic properties. Commercially available as 6% hetastarch in 0.9% NaCl in 500 mg infusion bottle.

USES Early fluid replacement and plasma volume expansion when whole blood is not available or when there is no time for necessary cross matching. Used to expand plasma volume during cardiopulmonary bypass and in adjunctive treatment of shock caused by hemorrhage, burns, surgery, sepsis, or other trauma. Also used as sedimenting agent in preparation of granulocytes by leukopheresis. **Unlabeled use:** as a priming fluid in pump oxygenators for perfusion during extracorporeal circulation and as a cryoprotective agent for long-term storage of whole blood.

ROUTE & DOSAGE

Plasma Volume Expansion

Adult	IV	500–1000 ml at a max rate of 20 ml/kg/h (max 1500 ml/d)

Leukopheresis

Adult	IV	250–750 ml infused at a constant fixed ratio of 8:1 to venous whole blood

---

PHARMACOKINETICS Duration: 24–36 h. **Distribution:** remains in intravascular space. **Metabolism:** metabolized in reticuloendothelial system. **Elimination:** excreted in urine with some biliary excretion.

CONTRAINDICATIONS & PRECAUTIONS Contraindicated in: severe bleeding disorders, CHF, renal failure with oliguria and anuria, treatment of shock not accompanied by hypovolemia. Safe use during pregnancy and in children not established. **Cautious use in:** hepatic or renal insufficiency, pulmonary edema in the very young or the elderly, patients on sodium restriction.

ADVERSE/SIDE EFFECTS CV: peripheral edema, circulatory overload, heart failure. **Hematologic:** (with large volumes) prolongation of PT, PPT, clotting time, and bleeding time; decreased Hct, Hgb, platelets, calcium, and fibrinogen; dilution of plasma proteins, hyperbilirubinemia, increased sedimentation rate. **Hypersensitivity:** pruritus, anaphylactoid reactions (periorbital edema, urticaria, wheezing). **Other:** vomiting, mild fever, chills, influenza-like symptoms, headache, muscle pains, submaxillary and parotid glandular swelling.

DRUG INTERACTIONS None established.

NURSING IMPLICATIONS

Administration

- Hetastarch is administered undiluted by IV infusion.

Common side effects in *italic*; life-threatening effects underlined; generic names in **bold**; classifications in SMALL CAPS

649

- Specific flow rate is prescribed by physician. Rate may be as high as 20 ml/kg/h in acute hemorrhagic shock.
- Solutions should be clear, pale yellow to amber in color. Discard solutions that appear turbid or discolored.
- Partially used bottles should be discarded. Hetastarch solution contains no preservatives.
- Store at room temperature. Avoid extremes of heat or cold.

Assessment & Drug Effects

- Monitor for signs and symptoms of hypersensitivity reaction (see chap 3).
- Measure and record I&O. Report oliguria or significant changes in I&O ratio.
- Monitor BP and vital signs and observe patient for unusual bruising or bleeding.
- Observe for signs of circulatory overload (see chap 3).
- Check laboratory reports of Hct values. Notify physician if there is an appreciable drop in Hct or if value approaches 30% by volume. Hct should not be allowed to drop below 30%.
- *Recommended laboratory determinations for donors undergoing repeated leukopheresis procedures* (in addition to regular and frequent clinical evaluation): CBC, total WBC and platelet counts, WBC differential count, Hgb, Hct, PT, and PTT.

H

HEXACHLOROPHENE

(hex-a-klor´oh-feen)
Trade names: Germa-Medica, HCP, pHisoHex, pHisoScrub, Septi-Soft, Septisol, WescoHEX
Classification: ANTIINFECTIVE, TOPICAL

ACTIONS/PHARMACODYNAMICS

Bacteriostatic against gram-positive bacteria, especially strains of staphylococci. Less active against gram-negative organisms and has little effect on spores. Efficacy depends on adsorption of hexachlorophene onto skin surface following repeated applications over several days. The resulting drug residue is antibacterial. Soluble in alcohol, acetone; insoluble in water.

USES

Surgical scrub and bacteriostatic skin cleanser. May also be used, only as long as necessary, to control an outbreak of gram-positive infection when other procedures have been unsuccessful.

ROUTE & DOSAGE

Surgical Scrub

Adult   Topical   Squeeze 1/2–1 tsp into palm and add water; work into lather and apply to area to be cleansed; rinse thoroughly

PHARMACOKINETICS Absorption: readily absorbed from GI tract and from intact and denuded skin. **Duration:** residual drug may remain on skin for 3–4 d after repeated use. **Distribution:** crosses placenta. **Elimination:** half-life: 6–44 h.

CONTRAINDICATIONS & PRECAUTIONS Contraindicated in: sensitivity to any of its components; primary light sensitivity to halogenated phenol derivatives; premature infants; open cuts, burns, wounds; with occlusive dressing, wet pack or lotion, vaginal pack or tampon; application to any mucous membranes, to large surface areas, or for routine prophylactic total body bathing; multiple daily handwashing with hexachlorophene during pregnancy.

ADVERSE/SIDE EFFECTS CNS: (neurotoxicity): dizziness, headache, confusion, lethargy, optic atrophy, diplopia, miosis, twitching, irritability, agitation, convulsions, respiratory arrest. **Accidental ingestion:** cramping, diarrhea, abdominal distension and pain, anorexia, nausea, vomiting, hypotension, shock. **Sensitization from excessive scrubbing:** *dermatitis,* erythema, scaling. **Other:** *photosensitivity.*

DRUG INTERACTIONS None established.

NURSING IMPLICATIONS

Administration

- A single application has little more effect than nonmedicated soaps. Regular and repeated applications are required to build up antibacterial residue (maximal concentration reached in 2–4 d).
- Presence of organic matter (e.g., pus, serum) and products containing alcohol reduce activity of hexachlorophene; activity is retained in the presence of oils and other vehicles used for topical application.
- Hexachlorophene should be rinsed thoroughly with clear water, especially from sensitive areas, to prevent possibility of systemic absorption. Antibacterial residue will be retained. However, to remove residue, use alcohol or non-hexachlorophene-containing soap or detergent.
- Since hexachlorophene is incompatible with many metals, it is stored and dispensed from specially de-

Common side effects in *italic*; life-threatening effects underlined; generic names in **bold**; classifications in SMALL CAPS

signed dispensers available from the manufacturer.
- Exposure of the emulsion to strong, direct light causes brown discoloration on the surface. Shake cleanser before use if discolored (efficacy is not affected by color change). Also hexachlorophene stains porous surfaces; rinse off spills immediately.
- Store in tight, light-resistant containers at 15–30 C.

Assessment & Drug Effects
- Infants, especially premature infants or those with dermatoses, are particularly susceptible to hexachlorophene absorption leading to systemic toxicity and brain abscess.
- Hexachlorophene may produce erythema, dryness, and scaling in patients with sensitive skin, especially when combined with excessive rubbing or exposure to heat or cold.
- Discontinue immediately if signs of cerebral irritability or other adverse reactions (suggestive of absorption) occur.

HOMATROPINE HYDROBROMIDE

See EYE, EAR, NOSE & THROAT PREPARATIONS, MYDRIATIC prototype, p 210.

HYALURONIDASE

(hye-al-yoor-on´i dase)
Trade name: Wydase
Classification: ENZYME
Pregnancy: Category C

ACTIONS/PHARMACODYNAMICS Mucolytic enzyme prepared from purified bovine testicular hyaluronidase. Hydrolyzes hyaluronidase, thereby modifying connective tissue permeability, permitting diffusion and spreading of substances injected subcutaneously and the absorption of transudates and exudates. Hastens disappearance of swelling after clysis and reduces pain related to distension.

USES To increase rate of absorption of parenteral fluids given by hypodermoclysis, to enhance diffusion of toxic or irritating drug in management of IV extravasation; to diffuse anesthetics at site of injection (including dental surgical sites); and to increase absorption of SC administered contrast media in excretion urography.

ROUTE & DOSAGE

Absorption and Dispersion of Injected Drugs

Adult SC 150 U added to each liter of drug solution or injected before clysis

SC Urography

Adult SC 75 units injected over each scapula followed by injection of contrast medium at same sites

Management of Catecholamine Extravasation

Adult SC 5–10 ml infiltrated around site of extravasation

CONTRAINDICATIONS & PRECAUTIONS Contraindicated in: injection into or around inflamed, infected, or cancerous areas; CHF; hypoproteinemia. Safe use during pregnancy and in nursing mothers not established.

ADVERSE/SIDE EFFECTS Infrequent: sensitivity, allergic reactions (urticaria), spread of infectious processes, overhydration. **Overdosage:** local edema, erythema, chills, nausea, vomiting, dizziness, hypotension, tachycardia.

DRUG INTERACTIONS When hyaluronidase is used to increase diffusion of a local anesthetic, bear in mind that absorption rate will be enhanced as much as 3- to 12-fold. Therefore watch for adverse reactions and expect a shorter duration of drug action.

INCOMPATIBILITIES Solution/Additive: epinephrine, heparin.

NURSING IMPLICATIONS

Administration
- Preliminary skin test for sensitivity is advised. Approximately 0.02 ml of 150 U/ml solution (3 U) is injected intradermally by physician; positive reaction consists of wheal with pseudopods and localized itching within 5 min, persisting 20–30 min. Erythema alone is not a positive reaction.
- Hyaluronidase is not recommended for IV use.
- Addition of hyaluronidase to hypodermoclyses may promote overhydration because it speeds water absorption. Infusion flow rate should be prescribed by physician. Patient should be closely monitored.
- *For children < 3 y:* the volume of a single clysis should be limited to 200 ml. *For premature infants and neonates:* volume should not exceed 25

H

Common side effects in *italic*; life-threatening effects underlined; generic names in **bold**; classifications in SMALL CAPS

651

ml/kg/d, and rate of administration should be no greater than 2 ml/min. *For adults:* rate and volume as employed for IV infusion.

■ Store the lyophilized powder at controlled room temperature in a dry place. Lyophilized form is unstable in solution; reconstitute with NaCl injection just before use (usually in the proportion of 1 ml/150 U of hyaluronidase). Do not use solution if it is discolored or contains a precipitate.

■ Hyaluronidase injection is reportedly stable for up to 3 mo when stored at temperature not over 25C (77F); however, manufacturer recommends storage at 2–8C (36–46F). Consult pharmacist.

HYDRALAZINE HYDROCHLORIDE

See CARDIOVASCULAR AGENTS, NONNITRATE VASODILATOR prototype, p 152.

HYDROCHLOROTHIAZIDE

See ELECTROLYTIC & WATER BALANCE AGENTS, THIAZIDE DIURETIC prototype, p 203.

Prototype: morphine, p 156

HYDROCODONE BITARTRATE
(hye-droe-koe´done)
Trade names: Dihydrocodeinone Bitartrate, Vicodin (with acetaminophen)
Classifications: CNS AGENT; NARCOTIC (OPIATE) AGONIST ANALGESIC; ANTITUSSIVE
Pregnancy: Category C
Controlled substance: Schedule III

ACTIONS/PHARMACODYNAMICS Morphine derivative similar to codeine but more addicting and with slightly greater antitussive activity. Suppresses cough reflex by direct action on cough center in medulla. Available in the United States only in combination with other drugs.

USES Symptomatic relief of hyperactive or nonproductive cough and for relief of moderate to moderately severe pain. A common ingredient in a variety of proprietary mixtures.

PHARMACOKINETICS Onset: 10–20 min. **Duration:** 3–6 h. **Distribution:** crosses placenta; distributed into breast milk. **Metabolism:** metabolized in liver. **Elimination:** half-life: 3.8 h; excreted in urine.

ROUTE & DOSAGE

Mild to Moderate Pain, Cough

Adult	PO	5–10 mg q4–6h prn (max 15mg/dose)
Child	PO	2–12 y: 1.25–5 mg q4–6h (max 10 mg/dose)

CONTRAINDICATIONS & PRECAUTIONS Cautious use in: respiratory depression, asthma, emphysema; history of drug abuse or dependence; postoperative patients; debilitated patients; children < 1 y. Pregnancy (category C). Also patients with preexisting increased intercranial pressure.

ADVERSE/SIDE EFFECTS Dry mouth, *constipation, nausea,* vomiting; lightheadedness, sedation, dizziness, *drowsiness,* euphoria, dysphoria, rash, pruritus.

DRUG INTERACTIONS Alcohol and other CNS DEPRESSANTS compound sedation and CNS depression.

NURSING IMPLICATIONS

Administration
■ May be taken with food or milk to prevent GI irritation.
■ Preserve in tight, light-resistant containers.

Assessment & Drug Effects
■ Monitor for effectiveness of drug for pain relief.
■ Monitor for nausea and vomiting. They are more prominent in ambulatory patients.
■ Monitor bowel elimination.

Patient & Family Education
■ Since hydrocodone may cause dizziness and drowsiness, caution patient to avoid hazardous activities until response to drug is determined.
■ Warn patient that alcohol and other CNS depressants may cause additive depression.
■ Adequate hydration (at least 1500–1800 ml/d) may help to liquefy tenacious sputum.
■ Caution patient not to take larger doses than prescribed. Psychic and physical dependence and tolerance may develop with repeated administration.

H

HYDROCORTISONE

See SKIN & MUCOUS MEMBRANE AGENTS, ANTIINFLAMMATORY prototype, p 255.

Prototype: hydrochlorothiazide, p 203

HYDROFLUMETHIAZIDE

(hye-droe-floo-meth-eye´a-zide)
Trade names: Diucardin, Saluron
Classifications: ELECTROLYTIC & WATER BALANCE AGENT; THIAZIDE DIURETIC; ANTIHYPERTENSIVE
Pregnancy: Category B

ACTIONS/PHARMACODYNAMICS Thiazide diuretic chemically related to sulfonamides. Similar to hydrochlorothiazide in actions, uses, contraindications, precautions, adverse reactions, and interactions.

ROUTE & DOSAGE

Edema
Adult   PO   25 mg–200 mg/d in 1–2 divided doses

Hypertension
Adult   PO   50–100 mg/d in 1–2 divided doses
Child   PO   1 mg/kg/d once/d

PHARMACOKINETICS Absorption: incompletely absorbed. **Onset:** 1–2 h. **Peak:** 3–4 h. **Duration:** 18–24 h. **Distribution:** distributed throughout extracellular tissue; concentrates in kidney; crosses placenta; distributed in breast milk. **Metabolism:** does not appear to be metabolized. **Elimination:** half-life: 17 h; excreted in urine.

CONTRAINDICATIONS & PRECAUTIONS Contraindicated in: hypersensitivity to other thiazides or sulfonamide derivatives; anuria; pregnancy (category B), lactation; hypokalemia.

ADVERSE/SIDE EFFECTS Postural hypotension, photosensitivity, *hypokalemia, hyperglycemia,* hyponatremia, *asymptomatic hyperuricemia,* agranulocytosis. See also hydrochlorothiazide.

DRUG INTERACTIONS Amphotericin B, CORTICOSTEROIDS increase hypokalemic effects; may antagonize hypoglycemic effects of ORAL HYPO-GLYCEMIC AGENTS, **insulin; cholestyramine, colistipol** decrease thiazide absorption; **diazoxide** intensifies hypoglycemic and hypotensive effects; increased potassium and magnesium loss may cause **digoxin** toxicity, decreases **lithium** excretion, thus increasing lithium toxicity; increases risk of NSAID-induced renal failure—NSAIDs may attenuate diuresis.

NURSING IMPLICATIONS

Administration
- Schedule diuretic dose early in the morning to prevent interrupted sleep. If two doses are taken each day, schedule dose 2 no later than 3 PM.
- Antihypertensive effects may be noted in 3–4 d, maximal effects may require 3–4 wk.

Assessment & Drug Effects
- Baseline and periodic determinations should be made for serum electrolytes, blood counts, BUN, blood glucose, uric acid, and CO_2.
- Monitor patient for hypokalemia and hyponatremia (see Signs & Symptoms, chap 3).
- Elderly patients are especially susceptible to the hypotensive effects that may accompany excessive diuresis.
- Dietary management is important in thiazide treatment for hypertension. The physician will specifically order goals of the diet: electrolyte, weight, or fluid control. Collaborate with dietitian and arrange for patient-dietitian planning for diet.
- Asymptomatic hyperuricemia can be produced because of interference with uric acid excretion. Report onset of joint pain and limitation of motion.
- Monitor for signs of diabetes. The diabetic patient should be watched for loss of control of diabetes.

Patient & Family Education
- Warn patient about the possibility of photosensitivity reaction. Thiazide-related photosensitivity is considered a photoallergy. It occurs 1 1/2–2 wk after initial sun exposure.
- Counsel patient to avoid use of OTC drugs unless approved by the physician.
- Store tablets in tightly closed container at 15–30C (59–86F) unless otherwise directed.

HYDROGEN PEROXIDE (H_2O_2)

(hye´droe-jen per-ox´ide)
Classifications: SKIN & MUCOUS MEMBRANE AGENT; ANTIBACTERIAL

H

ACTIONS/PHARMACODYNAMICS Comparatively weak, short-acting antibacterial agent with oxidizing properties and acidic pH. Effective as wound cleanser and deodorant. Slowly releases nascent oxygen and water on contact with catalase, an enzyme found in blood and most other tissue fluids. Effervescence caused by release of oxygen mechanically loosens wound debris and pockets of bacteria. Reduction in bacteria is believed to be more a factor of mechanical action than antibacterial activity. Each milliliter of 3% hydrogen peroxide releases about 10 ml of molecular oxygen.

USES Cleansing agent for wounds and suppurating ulcers, as mouthwash or gargle as in Vincent's stomatitis. Also to remove ear wax in ceruminosis.

ROUTE & DOSAGE

Wound Cleansing

Adult Topical 1.5–3% solution for wound cleansing

Mouthwash

Adult Dilute with equal volume of water when used as a mouthwash or gargle

CONTRAINDICATIONS & PRECAUTIONS Contraindicated in: instillation into closed body cavities or into abscesses. **Cautious use in:** deep wounds, burns.

ADVERSE/SIDE EFFECTS *Irritation of skin or mucous membranes;* superinfections (black hairy tongue), decalcification of tooth enamel (overuse as mouthwash); systemic oxygen emboli, ECG changes, shock, coma with instillation into closed body cavities; subcutaneous (oxygen) gas formation with pressurized irrigation of fresh open wounds.

NURSING IMPLICATIONS

Administration

- Use caution when opening container. Release of oxygen that occurs with decomposition may cause pressure build-up within bottle.
- May be diluted with water or normal saline. Use immediately after diluting; solution loses oxygen with storage and therefore is ineffective.
- H_2O_2 should never be instilled into closed body cavities or into abscesses that do not allow the liberated free oxygen escape, nor should bandages be applied too soon following its use for wound cleansing. Wound irrigation with H_2O_2, even when diluted, has caused near-fatal systemic oxygen mi-

croemboli by passage of oxygen into the vascular system.

- Store at 15–30C (59–86F) in tightly-covered, light-resistant container unless otherwise directed. Protect from heat and light.

Assessment & Drug Effects

- When hydrogen peroxide is used for wound cleansing, observe and record appearance of wound prior to each application. Pink granulation tissue without purulent discharge may indicate need to discontinue H_2O_2.
- If redness, swelling, pain, or irritation in or around wound increases or persists or if infection occurs, discontinue use and notify physician.

Patient & Family Education

- When used as a mouthwash, H_2O_2 should be diluted to half-strength (with water or normal saline) and used only for a short time. Discontinue promptly if irritation of tongue or buccal mucosa occurs. Full-strength H_2O_2 can harm the gums.
- Overuse of H_2O_2 as mouthwash decreases oral pH, creating an acid environment that can support superinfections, enamel decalcification, and caries.

Prototype: morphine, p 156

HYDROMORPHONE HYDROCHLORIDE

(hye-droe-mor´fone)
Trade names: Dilaudid, Dilaudid-HP
Classifications: CNS AGENT; ANALGESIC; NARCOTIC (OPIATE) AGONIST
Pregnancy: Category C
Controlled substance: Schedule II

ACTIONS/PHARMACODYNAMICS Semisynthetic phenanthrene derivative structurally similar to morphine but with 8–10 times more potent analgesic effect. Has more rapid onset and shorter duration of action than morphine and is reported to have less hypnotic action and less tendency to produce nausea and vomiting. Has antitussive properties.

USES Relief of moderate to severe pain and control of persistent nonproductive cough.

PHARMACOKINETICS Onset: 15–30 min. **Peak:** 30–90 min. **Duration:** 4–5 h. **Distribution:** crosses pla-

Common side effects in *italic*; life-threatening effects underlined; generic names in **bold**; classifications in SMALL CAPS

ROUTE & DOSAGE

Moderate to Severe Pain

Adult	PO/SC/IM/IV	1–4 mg q4–6h prn
	Rectal	3 mg q4–6h

centa; distributed into breast milk. **Metabolism:** metabolized in liver. **Elimination:** excreted in urine.

CONTRAINDICATIONS & PRECAUTIONS Contraindicated in: intolerance to opiate agonists. Safe use in pregnancy (category C) or in children not established.

ADVERSE/SIDE EFFECTS GI: nausea, vomiting, constipation. **CNS:** euphoria, dizziness, sedation, *drowsiness*. **CV:** hypotension, bradycardia or tachycardia. **Respiratory:** respiratory depression. **Other:** blurred vision.

DRUG INTERACTIONS Alcohol and other CNS DEPRESSANTS compound sedation and CNS depression.

INCOMPATIBILITIES Solution/Additive: prochlorperazine, sodium bicarbonate, thiopental. Y-Site: minocycline, prochlorperazine, tetracycline.

NURSING IMPLICATIONS

Administration

- Fullest analgesic effect is achieved if drug is given before patient experiences intense pain.
- When narcotic therapy is initiated, a fixed schedule provides more effective management than a prn schedule because blood levels can be maintained and peaks of pain can be avoided.
- For direct IV injection, dilute in at least 5 ml of sterile water or 0.9% NaCl. Administer at a rate of 2 mg over 3–5 min.
- A slight discoloration may develop in ampules or multidose vials with no loss of potency.
- Preserve in tight, light-resistant containers at 15–30C (59–86F).

Assessment & Drug Effects

- Before administration of drug, note respiratory rate, rhythm, and depth and size of pupils. Respirations of 12/min or less and mitosis are signs of toxicity. Withhold drug and promptly notify physician.
- Monitor vital signs at regular intervals. Drug-induced respiratory depression may occur even with small doses and increases progressively with higher doses.

- Tartrazine in cough syrup may cause allergic reactions, including bronchial asthma. Monitor closely after administration.
- Assess effectiveness of pain relief 30 min after medication administration.
- Carefully monitor drug effects in elderly or debilitated patients and those with impaired renal and hepatic function. These patients are especially at risk for toxic effects.
- Drug depresses cough and sigh reflexes and may induce atelectasis, especially in postoperative patients and those with pulmonary disease. Assess effectiveness of cough.
- Nausea and orthostatic hypotension most often occur in ambulatory patients or when a supine patient assumes the head-up position.
- Monitor I&O ratio and pattern. Assess lower abdomen for bladder distension. Report oliguria or urinary retention.
- Monitor bowel pattern, as drug-induced constipation may require treatment.

Patient & Family Education

- Advise patient on prn schedule to request medication at the onset of pain and not to wait until pain is severe.
- Inform patient that drug may cause drowsiness, dizziness, and blurred vision. Advise caution with activities requiring alertness.
- Advise patient to avoid alcohol and other CNS depressants while receiving drug.

HYDROQUINONE

(hye´droe-kwin-one)
Trade names: Eldopaque, Eldoquin, Esoterica Regular, Melanex, Mercolized Cocrema, Pabaquinone, Porcelana, Quinnone, Solaquin
Classifications: SKIN & MUCOUS MEMBRANE AGENT; DEPIGMENTOR
Pregnancy: Category C

ACTIONS/PHARMACODYNAMICS Topical agent that causes reversible bleaching of hyperpigmented skin due to increased melanin. Interferes with formation of new melanin but does not destroy existing pigment. Believed to act by inhibiting tyrosinase in melanocytes, thereby depressing melanin synthesis and melanocytic growth, and possibly by increasing excretion of melanin from melanocytes.

USES Gradual bleaching of hyperpigmented skin conditions such as chloasma or melasma, severe

Common side effects in *italic*; life-threatening effects underlined; generic names in **bold**; classifications in SMALL CAPS

655

freckling, senile lentigines (age spots or liver spots). Also as an antioxidant in topical preparations. Some formulations include a sunscreening agent (e.g., Porcelana with Sunscreen, Mercolized Cocrema, Pabaquinone, and Solaquin).

ROUTE & DOSAGE

Bleaching of Hyperpigmented Skin

Adult	Topical	Apply thin layer and rub into hyperpigmented skin b.i.d., morning and evening

CONTRAINDICATIONS & PRECAUTIONS Contraindicated in: prickly heat, sunburn, irritated skin, depilatory usage. Safe use during pregnancy (category C), in nursing women, and in children ≤ 12 y not established.

ADVERSE/SIDE EFFECTS Dryness and fissuring of paranasal and infraorbital areas, inflammatory reaction, erythema; stinging, tingling, burning sensations; irritation, sensitization, and contact dermatitis.

DRUG INTERACTIONS None established.

NURSING IMPLICATIONS

Administration
- Skin should be tested for sensitivity before treatment is initiated. Apply small amount of drug (about 25 mm in diameter) to an unbroken patch of skin and check in 24 h. If vesicle formation, itching, or excessive inflammation occurs, drug should not be used. Minor redness is not a contraindication.
- Applications should be limited to an area no larger than that of face and neck.

Assessment & Drug Effects
- In general, complete depigmentation occurs in 1–4 mo and lasts 2–6 mo after hydroquinone is discontinued. Once desired results are obtained, amount and frequency of applications should be reduced to the least that will maintain depigmentation.
- If bleaching or skin lightening does not occur after 2 or 3 mo of therapy, it should be discontinued.

Patient & Family Education
- Advise patient to use a sunscreen agent or a hydroquinone formulation containing a sunscreen for day time applications.
- Inform patient that sensitization and contact dermatitis have been reported. Advise using only the smallest quantity of medication necessary.

- Instruct patient to wash drug off if rash or irritation develops and to consult physician.
- Advise patient to avoid contact of hydroquinone with the eyes and not to use on open lesions, sunburned, irritated or otherwise damaged skin.
- Patient should be advised to continue use of protective clothing and sunscreening agent after treatment is terminated to reduce possibility of repigmentation.

HYDROXOCOBALAMIN (VITAMIN B$_{12\alpha}$)

(hye-drox-oh-koe-bal´a-min)
Trade names: Alphamin, AlphaRedisol, CoDROXOMIN, Hybalamin, Hydrobexan, Hydroxo-12, LA-12
Classification: Vitamin B$_{12}$
Pregnancy: Category A (C if > RDA)

ACTIONS/PHARMACODYNAMICS Cobalamin derivative similar to cyanocobalamin (vitamin B$_{12}$) in actions, uses, contraindications, precautions, and adverse reactions. More slowly absorbed from injection site than cyanocobalamin and may be taken up by liver in larger quantities. Results in higher and more sustained serum cobalamin levels and significantly less urinary excretion of cobalamin than produced by similar doses of cyanocobalamin; however, some patients reportedly develop an antibody to the plasma B$_{12}$-binding protein. **Unlabeled use:** cyanide poisoning and tobacco amblyopia.

ROUTE & DOSAGE

Vitamin B$_{12}$ Deficiency

Adult	IM	30 µg/d for 5–10 d and then 100–200 µg/mo *or* 1000 µg qod until remission and then 1000 µg/mo
Child	IM	100 µg doses to a total of 1–5 mg over 2 wk and then 30–50 µg/mo

PHARMACOKINETICS Distribution: widely distributed; principally stored in liver, kidneys, and adrenals; crosses placenta. **Metabolism:** converted in tissues to active co-enzymes; enterohepatically cycled. **Elimination:** 50–95% of doses ≥ 100 µg are excreted in urine in 48 h; excreted in breast milk.

DRUG INTERACTIONS Chloramphenicol may interfere with therapeutic response to hydroxycobalamin.

H

NURSING IMPLICATIONS
- Some patients experience mild pain at injection site after administration.

See cyanocobalamin, p 475, for additional nursing implications.

Prototype: chloroquine, p 79

HYDROXYCHLOROQUINE SULFATE
(hye-drox-ee-klor´oh-kwin)
Trade name: Plaquenil Sulfate
Classifications: ANTIINFECTIVE; ANTIMALARIAL
Pregnancy: Category C

ACTIONS/PHARMACODYNAMICS Derivative closely related to chloroquine and with similar actions, uses, contraindications, precautions, adverse reactions, and interactions.

USES Suppressive prophylaxis and treatment of acute malarial attacks due to all forms of susceptible malaria. Used adjunctively with primaquine for eradication of *Plasmodium vivax* and *Plasmodium malariae*. More commonly prescribed than chloroquine for treatment of rheumatoid arthritis and lupus erythematosus (usually in conjunction with salicylate or corticosteroid therapy). **Unlabeled use:** porphyria cutanea tarda.

PHARMACOKINETICS Absorption: rapidly and almost completely absorbed. **Peak:** 1–2 h. **Distribution:** widely distributed; concentrates in lungs, liver, erythrocytes, eyes, skin, and kidneys; crosses placenta. **Metabolism:** partially metabolized in liver to active metabolite. **Elimination:** half-life: 70–120 h; eliminated in urine; excreted in breast milk.

CONTRAINDICATIONS & PRECAUTIONS Contraindicated in: known hypersensitivity to, or retinal or visual field changes associated with, quinoline compounds; psoriasis, porphyria, long-term therapy in children; pregnancy (category C). Safe use in juvenile arthritis not established. **Cautious use in:** hepatic disease; alcoholism, with hepatotoxic drugs; impaired renal function; metabolic acidosis; patients with tendency to dermatitis.

ADVERSE/SIDE EFFECTS CNS: muscle weakness, vertigo, tinnitus, nerve deafness, headache,

ROUTE & DOSAGE

Doses are expressed in terms of hydroxychloroquine base. 400 mg tablet = 310 mg base; 800 mg tablet = 620 mg base

Acute Malaria

Adult	PO	620 mg base followed by 310 mg base at 6, 18, and 24 h
Child	PO	10 mg base/kg and then 5 mg base/kg at 6, 18, and 24 h

Malaria Suppression

Adult	PO	310 mg base the same day each week starting 2 wk before exposure and continuing for 4–6 wk after leaving the area of exposure
Child	PO	5 mg base/kg the same day each week starting 2 wk before exposure and continuing for 4–6 wk after leaving the area of exposure

Lupus Erythematosus

Adult	PO	310 mg base 1–2 times/d

Rheumatoid Arthritis

Adult	PO	400–600 mg/d until response and then decrease to lowest maintenance levels possible

mood or mental changes, *retinopathy*. **GI:** anorexia, nausea, vomiting, diarrhea, abdominal cramps, weight loss. **Hematologic:** agranulocytosis, thrombocytopenia, aplastic anemia. **Skin:** bleaching or loss of hair, unusual pigmentation (blue-black) of skin or inside mouth, skin rash, itching.

DRUG INTERACTIONS Aluminum- and **magnesium**-containing ANTACIDS and LAXATIVES decrease hydroxychloroquine absorption—separate administrations by at least 4 h; hydroxychloroquine may interfere with response to **rabies vaccine.**

NURSING IMPLICATIONS
Administration
- Administration of drug with meals or milk may reduce incidence of GI distress.
- Administer antacids and laxatives at least 4 h before or after hydroxychloroquine.
- Store at 15–30C (59–86F) unless otherwise directed.

Assessment & Drug Effects
- All patients on long-term therapy should have baseline and periodic ophthalmoscopic examinations and blood cell counts.

Common side effects in *italic*; life-threatening effects underlined; generic names in **bold**; classifications in SMALL CAPS

- In patients requiring long-term therapy, therapeutic effect may not appear for several weeks, and maximal benefit may not occur for 6 mo.
- Patients receiving prolonged therapy should be informed about adverse symptoms. Drug should be discontinued if weakness, visual symptoms, hearing loss, unusual bleeding or bruising or skin eruptions occur.

Patient & Family Education
- Counsel patient to follow drug regimen as prescribed by the physician.
- Caution patients to keep drug out of reach of children.

Prototype: progesterone, p 241

HYDROXYPROGESTERONE CAPROATE
(hye-drox-ee-proe-jess´te-rone)
Trade names: Delalutin, Duralutin, Gesterol L.A., Hydroxon, Hylutin, Hyprogest 250, Hyproval PA, Pro-Depo
Classifications: HORMONE; PROGESTIN
Pregnancy: Category X

ACTIONS/PHARMACODYNAMICS Long-acting synthetic progestational hormone. Has slower onset and longer action than progesterone. Has minimal estrogenic and androgenic activity. Induces and maintains endometrium, preventing uterine bleeding; inhibits production of pituitary gonadotropin, preventing ovulation; and produces thick cervical mucus resistant to passage of sperm.

USES Amenorrhea, abnormal uterine bleeding, advanced uterine cancer, and as "medical D and C" (conversion of proliferative endometrium to secretory endometrium and desquamation). Also as a test for endogenous estrogen production.

PHARMACOKINETICS Duration: 9–17 d. **Distribution:** crosses placenta; distributed into breast milk. **Metabolism:** metabolized in liver. **Elimination:** eliminated in urine.

CONTRAINDICATIONS & PRECAUTIONS Contraindicated in: severe hepatic disease, carcinoma of breast or genital region; thromboembolic disorders, pregnancy (category X), missed abortion, abnormal vaginal bleeding. **Cautious use in:** diabetes mellitus; asthma; epilepsy; migraine; cardiac or renal dysfunction; mental depression.

ROUTE & DOSAGE

Amenorrhea

Adult	IM	375 mg started anytime during cycle; after 4 d of desquamation or if no bleeding, 21 d after injection, start cyclic therapy; repeat cyclic therapy q4wk and stop after 4 cycles

Advanced Uterine Adenocarcinoma

Adult	IM	≥ 1 g at once, and repeat 1 or more times/wk; stop at time of relapse or if no desirable results obtained after a total of 12 wk of therapy

Test for Endogenous Estrogen Production

Adult	IM	250 mg at anytime during cycle; repeat for confirmation 4 wk after first injection; stop after second injection

ADVERSE/SIDE EFFECTS CNS: cerebral thrombosis or hemorrhage, migraine, depression. **CV:** hypertension, thromboembolic disorders, e.g., pulmonary embolism. **GI:** nausea, vomiting, cholestatic jaundice, abdominal cramps. **Reproduction:** breakthrough bleeding, changes in cervical erosion and secretions, changes in menstrual flow, dysmenorrhea, vaginal candidiasis. **Other:** edema, weight changes; breast tenderness, enlargement, or secretion; allergy-like reactions (especially at high doses); female fetus masculinization; decreased glucose tolerance. **Respiratory:** coughing, dyspnea, chest constriction. **Skin:** photosensitivity, acne, melasma, hirsutism, some loss of scalp hair, rash.

DRUG INTERACTIONS Rifampin may decrease pharmacologic effects of progestins.

NURSING IMPLICATIONS

Administration
- Not intended for IV use. Drug is packaged in an oil vehicle.
- Inject into a large muscle. Drug may cause local irritation at injection site.
- Protect drug preparation from light; store at 15–30C (59–86F).

Assessment & Drug Effects
- Record onset and duration of menstrual flow when drug is used to treat amenorrhea.

Common side effects in *italic*; life-threatening effects underlined; generic names in **bold**; classifications in SMALL CAPS

Patient & Family Education

- Stress importance of reporting immediately if pregnancy is suspected, the onset of vaginal bleeding, or thromboembolic implications (pain or numbness of legs, sudden onset of chest pain or shortness of breath, sudden severe headache or dizziness, visual problems).
- Teach patient self-breast examination.
- Diabetic patients should be advised to monitor blood glucose closely.
- Caution patient to use sunscreen and protective clothing when exposed to sun to reduce risk of photosensitivity.
- Counsel patient that onset of normal menstrual cycles may not occur for 2 or 3 mo after cessation of drug.
- Patient should be given package insert to read. This is an FDA regulation. Exception: cancer patients.
- **Test for endogenous estrogen production:** If patient is not pregnant and has a responsive endometrium (i.e., produces estrogen), bleeding (progesterone withdrawal sign) occurs 7 to 14 d after injection, indicating endogenous estrogen.

Prototype: fluorouracil, p 94

HYDROXYUREA

(hye-drox´ee-yoo-ree-ah)
Trade name: Hydrea
Classifications: ANTINEOPLASTIC;
ANTIMETABOLITE
Pregnancy: Category D

ACTIONS/PHARMACODYNAMICS Synthetic analogue of urea with antimetabolite activity. Blocks incorporation of thymidine into DNA and may damage already formed DNA molecules; does not affect synthesis of RNA or protein. Cytotoxic effect limited to tissues with high rates of cell proliferation. May reduce iron utilization by erythrocytes; has no effect on erythrocyte survival time. No cross resistance with other antineoplastics has been demonstrated.

USES Palliative treatment of metastatic melanoma, chronic myelocytic leukemia; recurrent metastatic, or inoperable ovarian cancer. Also used as adjunct to x-ray therapy for treatment of advanced primary squamous cell (epidermoid) carcinoma of head (excluding lip), neck, lungs. **Unlabeled uses:** psoriasis; combination therapy with radiation of lung carcinoma.

ROUTE & DOSAGE

Palliative Therapy
Adult PO 80 mg/kg q3d or 20–30 mg/kg/d

PHARMACOKINETICS Absorption: readily absorbed from GI tract. **Peak:** 2 h. **Distribution:** crosses blood-brain barrier. **Metabolism:** metabolized in liver. **Elimination:** eliminated as respiratory CO_2 and as urea in urine.

CONTRAINDICATIONS & PRECAUTIONS Contraindicated in: Pregnancy (category D), children, myelosuppression. **Cautious use in:** recent use of other cytotoxic drugs or irradiation; renal dysfunction; elderly patients; history of gout.

ADVERSE/SIDE EFFECTS CNS: (rare): headache, dizziness, disorientation, drowsiness (large doses), hallucinations, convulsions. **GI:** (occasional): stomatitis, anorexia, nausea, vomiting, diarrhea, constipation. **Hematologic:** <u>bone marrow suppression</u> (*leukopenia,* anemia, thrombocytopenia), megaloblastic erythropoiesis. **Skin:** maculopapular rash, facial erythema, postirradiation erythema, alopecia (rare). **Other:** renal tubular dysfunction, dysuria (rare), elevated BUN, serum, creatinine levels, hyperuricemia, abnormal BSP retention, fever, chills, malaise, elevation of hepatic enzymes.

DRUG INTERACTIONS None established.

NURSING IMPLICATIONS

Administration

- If patient has difficulty swallowing capsule, open, mix with water, and give immediately.
- Store in tightly covered container at 15–30C (59–86F) unless otherwise directed.

Assessment & Drug Effects

- Status of kidney, liver, bone marrow functions should be determined before and periodically during therapy; hemoglobin, WBC, platelet counts are monitored at least once weekly.
- IF WBC drops to 2500/mm³ or platelets to 100,000/mm³, therapy will be interrupted.
- Blood levels are rechecked after 3 d; if significant recovery is manifest, therapy may be resumed.
- Monitor I&O. Advise patients with high serum uric acid levels particularly to drink at least 10–12 240 ml (8 oz) glasses of fluid daily to prevent uric acid nephropathy.
- Patients with marked renal dysfunction may rapidly develop visual and auditory hallucinations and hematologic toxicity.

H

Common side effects in *italic*; life-threatening effects <u>underlined</u>; generic names in **bold**; classifications in SMALL CAPS

659

Patient & Family Education

- Toxicity incidence with use of hydroxyurea is as high as 66% with doses of 40 mg/kg body weight.
- Advise patient to report fever, chills, sore throat, nausea, vomiting, diarrhea, loss of appetite, and unusual bruising or bleeding.
- Advise patient to use barrier contraceptive during therapy. Drug is teratogenic.

HYDROXYZINE HYDROCHLORIDE

See ANTIHISTAMIINES, ANTIPRURITIC prototype, p 49.

Prototype: atropine, p 116

HYOSCYAMINE SULFATE

(hye-oh-sye´a-meen)
Trade names: Anaspaz, Bellaspaz, Cystospaz, Levsin, Levsinex, Neoquess
Classifications: ANTICHOLINERGIC (PARASYMPATHOLYTIC);
ANTIMUSCARINIC, ANTISPASMODIC
Pregnancy: Category C

ACTIONS/PHARMACODYNAMICS Extremely potent belladonna alkaloid with anticholinergic and antispasmodic activity. Said to be twice as potent as atropine, 4 times as potent as methantheline bromide, and 20 times as potent as homatropine methylbromide. Anticholinergic effect chiefly related to the levo isomer. Action is produced by competitive inhibition of acetylcholine at the parasympathetic neuroeffector junctions.

USES GI tract disorders caused by spasm and hypermotility, as conjunct therapy with diet and antacids for peptic ulcer management, and as an aid in the control of gastric hypersecretion and intestinal hypermotility. Also symptomatic relief of biliary and renal colic, as a "drying agent" to relieve symptoms of acute rhinitis, to control preanesthesia salivation and respiratory tract secretions, to treat symptoms of parkinsonism, and to reduce pain and hypersecretion in pancreatitis.

PHARMACOKINETICS Absorption: well absorbed from all administration sites. **Onset:** 2–3 min IV; 20–30

ROUTE & DOSAGE

GI Spasms

Adult	IV/IM/SC	0.25–0.5 mg q6h
	PO/SL	0.125–0.25 mg t.i.d. or q.i.d. prn

min PO. **Peak Effect:** 15–30 min IV; 30–60 min PO. **Duration:** 4–6 h (up to 12 h with sustained release form). **Distribution:** distributed in most body tissues; crosses blood-brain barrier and placenta; distributed in breast milk. **Metabolism:** metabolized in liver. **Elimination:** half-life: 3.5–13 h; excreted in urine.

CONTRAINDICATIONS & PRECAUTIONS Contraindicated in: hypersensitivity to belladonna alkaloids. Narrow-angle glaucoma, prostatic hypertrophy, obstructive diseases of GI or GU tract, paralytic ileus or intestinal atony; myasthenia gravis. **Cautious use in:** diabetes mellitus; cardiac disease.

ADVERSE/SIDE EFFECTS CNS: headache, unusual tiredness or weakness, confusion, *drowsiness,* excitement in elderly patients. **CV:** palpitations, tachycardia. **Eye:** *blurred vision,* increased intraocular tension, cycloplegia, mydriasis. **GI:** *dry mouth, constipation,* paralytic ileus. **Other:** *urinary retention,* anhidrosis, suppression of lactation.

DRUG INTERACTIONS Amantadine, ANTIHISTAMINES, TRICYCLIC ANTIDEPRESSANTS, **quinidine, disopyramide, procainamide** add anticholinergic effects; decreases **levodopa** effects; **methotrimeprazine** may precipitate extrapyramidal effects; decreases antipsychotic effects of PHENOTHIAZINES (decreased absorption).

NURSING IMPLICATIONS

Administration

- Administer PO preparations about 1 h before meals and at bedtime (at least 2 h after last meal).
- A single IV dose may be given by direct IV undiluted over 60 seconds.
- Dose for the elderly patient should be less than the standard adult dose. Observe patient carefully for signs of paradoxic reactions.

Assessment & Drug Effects

- Monitor bowel elimination; may cause constipation.
- Monitor urinary output.
- Risk of urinary retention is lessened if patient voids prior to each dose.
- Assess for dry mouth and advise good oral hygiene.

Patient & Family Education

- Advise patient to avoid excessive exposure to high environmental temperatures, since drug-induced heat stroke can develop.
- This drug may cause drowsiness. Advise patient to observe caution and to avoid driving and other potentially hazardous activities until response to drug is known.
- If patient complains about blurred vision, suggest use of dark glasses; but if this side effect persists, advise patient to report to physician for dose adjustment or possible change of drug.

IBUPROFEN

See CENTRAL NERVOUS SYSTEM AGENT, ANALGESIC, ANTIPYRETIC, NONSTEROIDAL ANTIINFLAMMATORY DRUG prototype, p 160.

Prototype: acyclovir, p 85

IDOXURIDINE (IDU)

(eye-dox-yoor´i-deen)
Trade names: Dendrid, Herplex, Herplex Liquifilm, IDU, Stoxil
Classifications: ANTIINFECTIVE; ANTIVIRAL
Pregnancy: Category C

ACTIONS/PHARMACODYNAMICS Topical antiviral agent. Pyrimidine nucleoside structurally related to thymidine, a metabolite essential for synthesis of DNA. Antiviral activity is primarily due to a substitution process. During viral replication, idoxuridine complexes with viral DNA by substituting for thymidine. The DNA-drug complex is more susceptible to breakage than normal DNA, resulting in increased number of errors in protein formation and inhibition of viral replication. Idoxuridine (IDU) is also incorporated into host DNA; large IV doses of the drug may adversely affect rapidly dividing host cells, e.g., in GI tract, bone marrow, and epidermal cells. Inhibits growth of herpes simplex types I and II, varicella-zoster, vaccinia, cytomegalovirus, and small animal viruses containing DNA. Not effective against RNA viruses. Epithelial viral infections characterized by a dendritic figure respond well to the antiviral activity especially during initial attacks. Chronic or recurrent viral infections that involve deep stromal structures (e.g., herpetic iritis) respond less well and do not heal. Idoxuridine has no effect on accumulated scarring, vascularization, or consequent progressive loss of vision. Some resistant strains of herpes simplex have been reported. Potentially carcinogenic. Squamous cell carcinoma at site of topical treatment has been reported.

USES Herpes simplex keratitis as single agent or conjunctively with a corticosteroid. **Unlabeled use:** cutaneous herpes simplex.

ROUTE & DOSAGE

Herpes Simplex Keratitis

Adult	Topical	1 drop instilled in conjunctival sac q1h during the day and q2h at night until improvement occurs; then decrease to q2h during the day and q4h at night; use ointment q4h during the day with the last dose at bedtime (5 applications/d)

PHARMACOKINETICS Absorption: poorly absorbed from eye tissues. **Distribution:** crosses placenta. **Metabolism:** metabolized in liver.

CONTRAINDICATIONS & PRECAUTIONS Contraindicated in: hypersensitivity to idoxuridine, iodine or iodine-containing preparations, or to any components in the formulation. **Cautious use in:** pregnancy and lactation; corticosteroids.

ADVERSE/SIDE EFFECTS Eye: local irritation, pain, burning, lacrimation, pruritus, inflammation, or edema of eyes, lids, and surrounding face; follicular conjunctivitis, photophobia; local allergic reaction (rare); corneal clouding, stippling, and small punctate defects; corneal ulceration and swelling; delayed healing. **Systemic absorption:** stomatitis, anorexia, nausea, vomiting, alopecia, leukopenia, thrombocytopenia, iodism, hepatotoxicity. **Overdosage:** (local): small defects in corneal epithelium. **Other:** sensitization.

NURSING IMPLICATIONS

Administration

- To prevent the possibility of systemic absorption, apply light finger pressure to head of lacrimal duct for 1 min when eyedrop is instilled.
- Topical corticosteroids may be used with idoxuridine for herpes simplex with stromal lesions, corneal edema, or iritis. Idoxuridine therapy should continue a few days after the steroid is discontinued.

Common side effects in *italic*; life-threatening effects <u>underlined</u>; generic names in **bold**; classifications in SMALL CAPS

661

- Do not mix idoxuridine with any other drug. Antibiotics and atropine may be given concurrently if necessary.
- Follow manufacturer's directions regarding storage. Decomposed idoxuridine not only has reduced antiviral activity but also may be toxic.
- Ophthalmic solution should be refrigerated at 2–8C (36–46F) in a tight, light-resistant container unless otherwise directed. The ointment should be stored at 2–15C (36–59F).

Assessment & Drug Effects

- Epithelial infections usually improve within 7–8 d. If patient continues to improve, therapy is generally continued ≤ 21 d.
- Patients should be closely supervised by ophthalmologist.

Patient & Family Education

- Instruct patient in proper technique for eye drop instillation.
- Boric acid should not be used during therapy with idoxuridine, since irritation may occur.
- The recommended frequency and duration of therapy must not be exceeded.
- If photosensitivity is troublesome, advise patient to wear sunglasses.

Prototype: cyclophosphamide, p 91

IFOSFAMIDE

(i-fos´-fa-mide)
Trade name: Ifex
Classifications: ANTINEOPLASTIC; ALKYLATING AGENT
Pregnancy: Category D

ACTIONS/PHARMACODYNAMICS Ifosfamide is a chemotherapeutic agent chemically related to nitrogen mustards. The alkylated metabolites of ifosfamide interact with DNA. Cytotoxic action is primarily due to cross-linking of strands of DNA and RNA, as well as inhibition of protein synthesis.

USES In combination with other agents in various regimens for germ cell testicular cancer, soft tissue sarcomas, Ewing's sarcoma, and non-Hodgkin's lymphoma. Also for lung and pancreatic sarcoma.

PHARMACOKINETICS Distribution: distributed into breast milk. **Metabolism:** metabolized in liver to

ROUTE & DOSAGE

Antineoplastic

Adult   IV   1.2 g/m²/d for 5 consecutive d; administer over at least 30 min; repeat q3wk or after recovery from hematologic toxicity (platelets ≥ 100,000/mm³; WBC ≥ 4,000/mm³)

active form. **Elimination:** half-life: 7–15 h; 70–86% excreted in urine.

CONTRAINDICATIONS & PRECAUTIONS Contraindicated in: patients with severe bone marrow depression or who have demonstrated previous hypersensitivity to ifosfamide. **Cautious use in:** impaired renal function, prior radiation or prior therapy with other cytotoxic agents; pregnancy (category D) and nursing mothers.

ADVERSE/SIDE EFFECTS CNS: *somnolence, confusion, hallucinations,* coma, dizziness, seizures, cranial nerve dysfunction. **GI:** *nausea, vomiting,* anorexia, diarrhea, metabolic acidosis, hepatic dysfunction. **Hematologic:** neutropenia, thrombocytopenia. **GU:** hemorrhagic cystitis, nephrotoxicity. **Other:** *alopecia,* skin necrosis with extravasation.

DRUG INTERACTIONS HEPATIC ENZYME INDUCERS (BARBITURATES, **phenytoin, chloral hydrate**) may increase hepatic conversion of ifosfamide to active metabolite; CORTICOSTEROIDS may inhibit conversion to active metabolites.

NURSING IMPLICATIONS

Administration

- Because of the carcinogenicity of ifosfamide, caution and proper technique is necessary in preparation, use, and disposal of the agent. Follow established guidelines.
- Prepare IV solution of drug by diluting 1 g in 20 ml of sterile water or bacteriostatic water with a final concentration of 50 mg/ml. Solution prepared with sterile water should be used within 6 h. Solution prepared with bacteriostatic solution is stable for a week at 30C or 6 wk at 5C.
- Solutions for intermittent IV infusion may be prepared by further dilution of drug with 5% dextrose injection, 0.9% NaCl injection, or lactated Ringer's injection. Administer over 30 min.
- Reconstituted solutions are stable for 1 wk at 30C (86F) and 3 wk at 5C (41F).

Assessment & Drug Effects

- Obtain a urinalysis prior to each dose. If microscopic hematuria (greater than 10 RBCs per high

Common side effects in *italic*; life-threatening effects underlined; generic names in **bold**; classifications in SMALL CAPS

power field) is present, subsequent dose should be withheld until complete resolution in order to decrease the incidence of hemorrhagic cystitis.

- Hold ifosfamide if WBC is below 2000/mm^3 or platelet count is below 50,000/mm^3
- Therapy should be discontinued if any of the following CNS symptoms occur: somnolence, confusion, depressive psychosis, and hallucinations.
- To reduce the risk of hemorrhagic cystitis, hydration with 3000 ml of fluid daily is recommended prior to ifosfamide therapy and for at least 72 h following treatment to ensure ample urine output.
- Hematologic profile (particularly neutrophils, hemoglobin, platelets) should be checked before each dose is given and at regular intervals to determine degree of hematopoietic suppression.
- Ifosfamide often causes nausea and vomiting. Since it is important to continue therapy despite these effects, ask physician for antiemetic to lessen effect.
- Carefully monitor progress of healing wounds; drug may slow wound healing.

Patient & Family Education
- Instruct patient to void frequently to lessen contact of irritating chemical with bladder mucosa.
- Advise patient that susceptibility to infection may increase and to avoid people with infection. Should report any infection, fever or chills, cough or hoarseness, lower back or side pain, painful or difficult urination.
- Advise patient to check with physician immediately if there is any unusual bleeding or bruising, black tarry stools, or blood in urine or if pinpoint red spots develop on skin.
- Advise patient of possible side effects (e.g., alopecia, nausea, and vomiting) and measures that can be taken to minimize them.

IMIPENEM-CILASTATIN SODIUM

See ANTIINFECTIVES, ANTIBIOTIC, OTHER BETA-LACTAM prototype, p 67.

IMIPRAMINE

See CENTRAL NERVOUS SYSTEM AGENTS, PSYCHOTHERAPEUTIC, TRICYCLIC ANTIDEPRESSANT prototype, p 184.

IMMUNE GLOBULIN INTRAMUSCULAR (IGIM, GAMMA GLOBULIN, IMMUNE SERUM GLOBULIN [ISG])

Trade names: Gamastan, Gammar

IMMUNE GLOBULIN INTRAVENOUS (IGIV)

Trade names: Gamimune N, Gammagard, IGIV Sandoglobulin, Venoglobulin-1
Classifications: SERUM; IMMUNIZING AGENT
Pregnancy: Category C

ACTIONS/PHARMACODYNAMICS Sterile concentrated solution containing globulin (primarily IgG) prepared from large pools of normal human plasma of either venous or placental origin and processed by a special fractionating technique. Like hepatitis B immune globulin (HBIG), contains antibody specific to hepatitis B surface antigen but in lower concentrations. Therefore not considered treatment of first choice for postexposure prophylaxis against hepatitis B but usually an acceptable alternative when HBIG is not available. Also much less expensive than HBIG. Nonreactive when tested for hepatitis B.

USES IM preparation: In susceptible persons to provide passive immunity or to modify severity of certain infectious diseases, e.g., rubeola (measles), rubella (German measles), varicella-zoster (chicken pox), type A (infectious) hepatitis, and as replacement therapy in congenital agammaglobulinemia or IgG deficiency diseases. May be used as an alternative to HBIG to provide passive immunity in hepatitis B infection. Also for postexposure prophylaxis of hepatitis non-A, non-B and nonspecific hepatitis. **Immune globulin IV:** principally as maintenance therapy in patients unable to manufacture sufficient quantities of IgG antibodies, in patients requiring an immediate increase in immunoglobulin levels, and when IM injections are contraindicated as in patients with bleeding disorders or who have small muscle mass. Also in chronic autoimmune thrombocytopenia and idiopathic thrombocytopenic purpura (ITP). **Unlabeled uses:** Kawasaki syndrome, chronic lymphocytic leukemia, AIDS, premature and low-birth-weight neonates, autoimmune neutropenia or hemolytic anemia.

Common side effects in *italic*; life-threatening effects underlined; generic names in **bold**; classifications in SMALL CAPS

663

ROUTE & DOSAGE

Hepatitis A Exposure

Adult   IM   0.02 ml/kg as soon as possible after exposure; if period of exposure will be ≥ 3
mo, give 0.05–0.06 ml/kg once q4–6mo

Child   IM   Same as for adult

Hepatitis B Exposure

Adult   IM   0.02–0.06 ml/kg as soon as possible
after exposure if HBIG is unavailable.

Child   IM   Same as for adult

Rubella Exposure

Adult   IM   20 ml as single dose in susceptible pregnant women

Rubeola Exposure

Adult   IM   0.25 ml/kg within 6 d of exposure

Child   IM   Same as for adult

Varicella-zoster Exposure

Adult   IM   0.6–1.2 ml/kg promptly

Child   IM   Same as for adult

Immunoglobulin Deficiency

Adult   IV   Gammagard, Gamimune: 100
mg/kg/mo; Sandoglobulin,
Venoglobulin: 200 mg/kg/mo

        IM   1.2 ml/kg followed by 0.6 ml/kg
q2–4wk

Child   IV   Gammagard, Gamimune; same as for
adult; Sandoglobulin, Venoglobulin:
same as for adult

        IM   Same as for adult

Idiopathic Thrombocytopenia Purpura

Adult   IV   400 mg/kg/d for 5 consecutive d or
1 g/kg q.o.d. for up to 3 doses

Child   IV   Same as for adult

PHARMACOKINETICS Peak: 2 d. **Distribution:**
rapidly and evenly distributed to intravascular and
extravascular fluid compartments. **Elimination:** half-
life: 21–23 d.

CONTRAINDICATIONS & PRECAUTIONS Con-
traindicated in: history of anaphylaxis or severe reaction to human immune serum globulin (IG) or to any
ingredient in the formulation such as thimerosal
(mercury derivative) preservative in IM formulations
and maltose (stabilizing agent) in IV formulations;
persons with clinical hepatitis A; IGIV for patients
with class-specific anti-IgA deficiencies; IGIM in severe thrombocytopenia or other bleeding disorders.

Safe use during pregnancy (category C) not established.

ADVERSE/SIDE EFFECTS IGIM: *pain, tenderness,
muscle stiffness at IM site;* local inflammatory reaction, erythema, urticaria, angioedema, headache,
malaise, fever, arthralgia, nephrotic syndrome, hypersensitivity (fever, chills, anaphylactic shock). **IGIV
(mostly related to rate of administration):** *nausea, flushing, chills,* headache, chest tightness, wheezing,
skeletal pain, back pain, abdominal cramps, anaphylaxis.

DRUG INTERACTIONS May interfere with antibody response to LIVE VIRUS VACCINES (measles,
mumps, rubella); give vaccines 14 d before or 3 mo
after immune globulins.

NURSING IMPLICATIONS

Administration

- Note that IGIM is intended only for IM use and that
  IGIV is meant only for IV use. They are not interchangeable.
- *IV solution:* Venoglobulin-1 and Gammagard are
  packaged with the diluent and transfer device.
  Gamimune N may be given undiluted or diluted to
  a 5% solution. Sandoglobulin is provided with
  enough diluent to make a 3% solution.
- Specific infusion flow rate should be prescribed by
  physician. Rates vary with product being infused.
  For example, Gamimune is generally started at
  0.01–0.02 ml/kg/min for 30 min; if tolerated, rate is
  increased to 0.02–0.04 ml/kg/min. The initial flow
  rate for Sandoglobulin is 0.5–1 ml/min. If tolerated
  after 15–30 min, rate is increased to 1.5–2.5 ml/min.
- Refer to manufacturer's directions for information
  on reconstitution, dilution, and flow rates.
- For adults and older children, IM injections are
  made preferably into deltoid or anterolateral aspect
  of thigh; in neonates and small children, into anterolateral aspect of thigh.
- Gluteal injections are generally avoided because of
  risk of injury to sciatic nerve. However, when large
  volumes of immune globulin are prescribed or
  when large doses must be divided into several injections, the upper outer quadrant of the gluteus
  has been used in adults.
- Aspirate carefully after introducing needle into
  muscle to avoid inadvertent IV injection.
- Store Gamimune at 2–8C (36–46F); store
  Sandoglobulin below 20C (68F) unless otherwise
  directed. Avoid freezing. Do not use if turbidity has
  occurred or if product has been frozen. Do not mix
  with other drugs. Discard partially used vial.

Common side effects in *italic;* life-threatening effects <u>underlined;</u>
generic names in **bold**; classifications in SMALL CAPS

Assessment & Drug Effects

- **Hepatitis A (infectious hepatitis):** immune globulin is most effective when given before or as soon as possible after exposure but not more than 2 wk after (incubation period for hepatitis A is 15–50 d). Persons who are already presenting clinical manifestations of hepatitis A should not receive immune globulin.
- **Hepatitis B (serum hepatitis):** immune globulin is administered preferably within 24 h and not more than 7 d after exposure.
- **Measles (rubeola):** after immune globulin administration, passive immunity lasts about 3–4 wk. In general, patients who are ≤ 15 mo should receive active immunization with measles virus vaccine (unless it is contraindicated) 3 mo after administration of IGIM.
- **Immunodeficiency diseases:** to prevent serious infections, serum concentrations of immune globulin are commonly kept above 200 mg/dl.
- Emergency drugs and appropriate emergency facilities should be immediately available for treatment of anaphylaxis or sensitization.
- Hypersensitivity reactions (see Signs & Symptoms, chap 3) are most likely to occur in patients receiving large IM doses, repeated injections, or rapid IV infusion of immune globulin.
- When patient is receiving IGIV, monitor vital signs continuously and closely monitor infusion rate.
- IGIV may have a mild diuretic effect in some patients because of the presence of maltose in the formulation.

Patient & Family Education

- Instruct patient to report immediately such symptoms as nausea, chills, headache, and chest tightness during IV infusion. Such side effects may be an indication to slow rate of infusion.

Prototype: hydrochlorothiazide, p 203

INDAPAMIDE
(in-dap´a-mide)
Trade name: Lozol
Classifications: ELECTROLYTIC & WATER BALANCE AGENT; THIAZIDE-LIKE DIURETIC
Pregnancy: Category B

ACTIONS/PHARMACODYNAMICS Sulfonamide derivative and first member of the indoline class of antihypertensive/diuretic agents. Has both diuretic and direct vascular effects; action mechanism is similar to that of the thiazide diuretics. Principal site of action is on the proximal portion of the distal renal tubules. Enhances excretion of sodium, potassium, and water by interfering with sodium transfer across renal epithelium. Like the thiazides, indapamide increases calcium reabsorption without causing important changes in serum calcium concentration. Free water clearance during hydration is decreased. Hypotensive activity in the hypertensive patient appears to result from a decrease in plasma and extracellular fluid volume, decreased peripheral vascular resistance, direct arteriolar dilation, and calcium channel blockade. Has little effect on cardiac output, rate, or rhythm and, unlike the thiazides, does not cause significant increase in serum cholesterol but tends to increase HDL levels. Augments the action of other hypotensive agents.

USES Alone or with other antihypertensives as step 1 agent in the management of hypertension in patients who have failed to respond to diet, exercise, or weight reduction. **Unlabeled use:** edema associated with CHF.

ROUTE & DOSAGE

Hypertension, Edema

Adult PO 2.5 mg once/d; may increase to 5 mg/d if needed

PHARMACOKINETICS Absorption: readily absorbed from GI tract. **Peak:** 2–2.5 h. **Duration:** up to 36 h. **Metabolism:** metabolized in liver. **Elimination:** half-life: 14–18 h; 60% excreted in urine; 16–23% excreted in feces.

CONTRAINDICATIONS & PRECAUTIONS Contraindicated in: hypersensitivity to indapamide or other sulfonamide derivatives, anuria. Safe use during pregnancy (category B), lactation, and in children not established. **Cautious use in:** electrolyte imbalance, severe renal disease; impaired hepatic function or progressive liver disease; hypokalemia; prediabetic and type II diabetic patient, hyperparathyroidism, thyroid disorders; SLE; sympathectomized patient; history of gout.

ADVERSE/SIDE EFFECTS CNS/Neuromuscular: headache, dizziness, fatigue, weakness, loss of energy, muscle cramps or spasm, paresthesia, tension, anxiety, nervousness, agitation, vertigo, insomnia, mental depression, blurred vision, lightheadedness,

---

Common side effects in *italic*; life-threatening effects underlined; generic names in **bold**; classifications in SMALL CAPS

665

drowsiness, CNS depression, <u>depressed respirations</u>. **CV:** orthostatic hypotension, PVCs, dysrhythmias, flushing, palpitation. **GI:** dry mouth, anorexia, nausea, vomiting, diarrhea, constipation, abdominal cramps or pain. **GU:** urinary frequency, nocturia, polyuria, glycosuria, impotence or reduced libido. **Skin:** rash, hives, pruritus, vasculitis, photosensitivity. **Other:** rhinorrhea, dilutional hyponatremia, *hyperuricemia,* exacerbation of gout; *hypokalemia,* hyperglycemia, hypochloremia, hypercalcemia, increased BUN or creatinine, weight loss, exacerbation of SLE; increased cholesterol.

DIAGNOSTIC TEST INTERFERENCES Since indapamide may cause hypercalcemia (and hypophosphatemia), it is generally withheld before tests for *parathyroid function* are performed.

DRUG INTERACTIONS Effects of **diazoxide** and indapamide intensified; increased risk of **digoxin** toxicity with hypokalemia; decreased renal **lithium** clearance may increase risk of lithium toxicity.

NURSING IMPLICATIONS

Administration
- Administer in AM to prevent nocturia. Urge patient to take at least 240 ml (8 oz) of fluid (if allowed) with the medication.
- Store in tight, light-resistant container at 15–30C (59–86F) unless otherwise directed.

Assessment & Drug Effects
- The following laboratory tests should be performed before initiation of treatment and periodically thereafter: BUN, serum creatinine, uric acid, blood glucose, and serum electrolytes.
- Individuals at risk of electrolyte imbalance include those receiving a digitalis preparation, on a salt-restricted diet or a low-potassium diet, those with a history of ventricular arrhythmias, and those receiving potassium-depleting drugs (corticosteroids, corticotropin). Elderly patients are especially sensitive to both diuretic action and the effects of potassium deficit.
- Side effects of indapamide are mild and transient; however, drug-induced electrolyte imbalances may become clinically serious in the following situations: protracted vomiting and diarrhea, excessive sweating, GI drainage, and paracentesis. Restoration of electrolyte and fluid volume may be indicated.
- Report promptly signs of hyponatremia or hypokalemia (see chap 3).
- Monitor I&O. Instruct patient to report immediately to the physician symptoms of developing renal insufficiency (see chap 3).

- Routine examinations for blood glucose level changes or for glycosuria in the patient with diabetes or patients who are diabetes prone should continue throughout indapamide treatment period. The drug may alter insulin requirements and cause borderline diabetes to manifest.
- BP measurements should be taken at periodic intervals in patients with hypertension, and results reported to physician.

Patient & Family Education
- Instruct patient to record weight at least every other day and to inspect ankles and legs for edema. Advise patient to report unexplained, progressive weight gain (e.g., 1–1.5 kg [2–3 lb] in 2–3 d).
- A diuretic regimen may be sufficient therapy for reducing mild hypertension. Urge patient to keep scheduled appointments so that hypotensive response can be monitored.)
- Teach patient the signs and symptoms of electrolyte imbalance.
- Since constipation may be a side effect, advise patient to consult physician for a laxative if needed and not to self-dose with an OTC product.

Prototype: ibuprofen, p 160

INDOMETHACIN
(in-doe-meth´a-sin)
Trade names: Indameth, Indocid, Indocin, Indocin SR, Indo-Lemmon
Classifications: CNS AGENT; NONNARCOTIC ANALGESIC, ANTIPYRETIC; NSAID
Pregnancy: Category B (D in third trimester)

ACTIONS/PHARMACODYNAMICS Potent nonsteroidal arylacetic acid compound with antiinflammatory, analgesic, and antipyretic effects similar to those of aspirin. Antipyretic and antiinflammatory actions may be related to ability to inhibit prostaglandin biosynthesis. Uncouples oxidative phosphorylation in cartilaginous and hepatic mitochondria. Appears to reduce motility of polymorphonuclear leukocytes, development of cellular exudates, and vascular permeability in injured tissue. Apparently has no uricosuric action. Inhibits platelet aggregation, but effect is of shorter duration than that of aspirin (effect usually disappears within 24 h after drug is discontinued). Enhances effect of ADH and therefore promotes sodium and water retention.

USES Palliative treatment in active stages of moderate to severe rheumatoid arthritis, ankylosing rheumatoid spondylitis, acute gouty arthritis, and osteoarthritis of hip in patients intolerant to or unresponsive to adequate trials with salicylates and other therapy. Also used IV to close patent ductus arteriosus in the premature infant. **Unlabeled use:** to relieve biliary pain and dysmenorrhea; Paget's disease, athletic injuries, juvenile arthritis, idiopathic pericarditis.

ROUTE & DOSAGE

Rheumatoid Arthritis

Adult	PO	25–50 mg b.i.d or t.i.d. (max 200 mg/d) or 75 mg sustained release 1–2 times/d

Acute Gouty Arthritis

Adult	PO	50 mg t.i.d. until pain is tolerable; then rapidly taper off

Bursitis

Adult	PO	25–50 mg t.i.d. or q.i.d. (max 200 mg/d) or 75 mg sustained release 1–2 times/d

Close Patent Ductus Arteriosus

Premature Infant	IV	<48 h: 0.2 mg/kg followed by 2 doses of 0.1 mg/kg q12–24h
		2–7 d: 0.2 mg/kg followed by 2 doses of 0.2 mg/kg q12–24h
		<7 d: 0.2 mg/kg followed by 2 doses of 0.25 mg/kg q12–24h

PHARMACOKINETICS Absorption: completely absorbed from GI tract. **Onset:** 1–2 h. **Peak:** 3 h. **Duration:** 4–6 h. **Metabolism:** metabolized in liver. **Elimination:** half-life: 2.5–124 h; excreted primarily in urine.

CONTRAINDICATIONS & PRECAUTIONS Contraindicated in: allergy to indomethacin, aspirin, or other NSAID; nasal polyps associated with angioedema, history of GI lesions; pregnancy (category B; D in third trimester), nursing mothers, children (≤14 y). **Cautious use in:** history of psychiatric illness, epilepsy, parkinsonism; impaired renal or hepatic function; uncontrolled infections; coagulation defects, CHF; elderly patients, persons in hazardous occupations.

ADVERSE/SIDE EFFECTS CNS: *headache, dizziness,* vertigo, lightheadedness, syncope, fatigue, muscle weakness, ataxia, insomnia, nightmares, drowsiness, narcolepsy, confusion, coma, convulsions, peripheral neuropathy, psychic disturbances (hallucinations, depersonalization, depression), aggravation of epilepsy, parkinsonism **CV:** elevated BP, palpitation, chest pains, tachycardia, bradycardia, CHF. **Eye/ear:** blurred vision, lacrimation, eye pain, visual field changes, corneal deposits, retinal disturbances including macula, *tinnitus,* hearing disturbances, deafness (rarely). **GI:** (common): *nausea, vomiting,* diarrhea, anorexia, bloating, abdominal distension, ulcerative stomatitis, proctitis, rectal bleeding, GI ulceration, hemorrhage, perforation. **Hematologic:** hemolytic anemia, aplastic anemia (sometimes fatal), agranulocytosis, leukopenia, thrombocytopenic purpura, inhibited platelet aggregation. **Hypersensitivity:** rash, purpura, pruritus, urticaria, angioedema, angiitis, rapid fall in blood pressure, dyspnea, asthma syndrome (in aspirin-sensitive patients). **Renal:** renal function impairment, hematuria, urinary frequency, renal failure (causal relationships not established). **Other:** epistaxis, hair loss, exfoliative dermatitis, erythema nodosum, vaginal bleeding, breast changes, hyponatremia, hypokalemia, hyperkalemia, hypoglycemia or hyperglycemia, glycosuria (rare), toxic hepatitis, edema, weight gain, flushing, sweating; tissue irritation with extravasation.

DIAGNOSTIC TEST INTERFERENCES Increased *AST, ALT, bilirubin, BUN;* positive direct *Coombs' test.*

DRUG/INTERACTIONS ORAL ANTICOAGULANTS, **heparin, alcohol** may prolong bleeding time; may increase **lithium** toxicity; effects of ORAL ANTICOAGULANTS, **phenytoin,** SALICYLATES, SULFONAMIDES, SULFONYLUREAS increased because of protein-binding displacement; increased toxicity including GI bleeding with SALICYLATES, NSAIDs; may blunt effects of ANTIHYPERTENSIVES and DIURETICS.

NURSING IMPLICATIONS

Administration

- Administer immediately after meals, or with food, milk, or antacid (if prescribed) to minimize GI side effects. Food or antacid may cause somewhat delayed and reduced absorption, but advantage of safety outweighs risk of impaired absorption.
- Indomethacin rectal suppository use is contraindicated with history of proctitis or recent bleeding.
- Dilute 1 mg with only 1 ml of NS or sterile water for injection without preservatives. Resulting concentration (1 mg/ml) may be further diluted with an additional 1 ml for each 1 mg to yield 0.5 mg/ml.

Common side effects in *italic*; life-threatening effects underlined; generic names in **bold**; classifications in SMALL CAPS

667

- Diluted solution may be administered by direct IV with a single dose given over 5–10 s.
- **Note:** Do not use diluents containing benzyl alcohol, since it is associated with toxicity in neonates.
- Discard any used IV indomethacin, since it contains no preservative.
- Store oral and rectal forms in tight, light-resistant containers at 15–30C (59–86F) unless otherwise directed. Do not freeze.

IV Administration for Patent Ductus Arteriosus

- Be careful to avoid extravasation or leakage. Indomethacin IV can be irritating to tissue. Monitor I&O closely and keep physician informed. Indomethacin can cause significant impairment of renal function. It is not unusual for urine output to decrease by 50% or more. Request specific guidelines regarding acceptable parameters. Monitor BUN, serum creatinine, glomerular filtration rate, creatinine clearance, and serum electrolytes.

Assessment & Drug Effects

- Indomethacin is contraindicated in patients allergic to aspirin. Question patient carefully regarding aspirin sensitivity before initiation of therapy.
- Incidence of adverse reactions is high (especially in elderly patients) and is dose related in most patients. Physician will rely on accurate and prompt reporting of patient's response.
- Patient should be carefully observed and should be instructed to report adverse reactions to prevent serious and sometimes irreversible or fatal effects.
- In patients with underlying cardiovascular disease the potential for sodium and water retention should be anticipated. Monitor weight and observe dependent areas for signs of edema.
- Frontal headache is the most frequent CNS side effect; it should be reported. If it persists, dosage reduction or cessation of drug may be indicated. Usually more severe in the morning, within 1 h after drug ingestion. A bedtime dose, with milk, may reduce the incidence of morning headache.
- CBC, renal and hepatic function tests, ophthalmoscopic examinations, and hearing tests should be performed periodically during prolonged therapy.
- Green urine has been reported in patients who develop indomethacin-induced hepatitis.

Patient & Family Education

- Indomethacin can cause severe GI complications (reported to be among the most common side effects). Be alert to suspicious signs and symptoms and report immediately.
- Expected therapeutic effects in rheumatoid arthritis are reduced fever, increased strength, reduced stiffness, and relief of pain, swelling, and tenderness. If improvement is not noted in 2–3 wk, alternate therapy is generally prescribed.
- Therapeutic effect in acute gouty attack (relief of joint tenderness and pain) is usually apparent in 24–36 h; swelling generally disappears in 3–5 d. Keep physician informed; dosage should be reduced once pain is tolerable.
- Because of the possibility of dizziness and lightheadedness, caution the patient to avoid activities requiring mental alertness and motor coordination until reaction to drug is known.
- Advise patient not to take aspirin; it may potentiate ulcerogenic effects.

Prototype: insulin injection, p 230

INSULIN, HUMAN

Trade names: Humulin, Insulatard, Novolin, Velosulin
Classifications: SYNTHETIC HORMONE; INSULIN ANTIDIABETIC
Pregnancy: Category B

ACTIONS/PHARMACODYNAMICS Biosynthetic human insulin is derived not from human pancreas but from cultures of *Escherichia coli* genetically modified by recombinant DNA technology. Contains less than 4 ppm of immunoreactive *E. coli* polypeptides (ECPs). Semisynthetic human insulin is prepared from pork insulin by an enzymatic process that substitutes an alanine residue of pork insulin with threonine, resulting in an insulin molecule with the amino acid sequence identical to that of human insulin. Manufacturer claims that these products are devoid of the following insulin contaminants: proinsulin, glucagon, vasoactive intestinal polypeptide, pancreatic polypeptide, somatostatin. Biological potency of 1 mg human insulin: not less than 26 USP human insulin units. Human insulin may be preferred over pork, beef, or mixed-species insulins because it is theoretically less likely to elicit formation of insulin antibodies. See insulin injection for actions.

(Human) insulin injection (Humulin R, Novolin R, Velosulin Human): a rapid-acting clear, colorless aqueous solution of antidiabetic principle of the pancreas containing 100 U/ml. The biosynthetic preparation (Humulin R) contains 10–40 µg zinc/100 U/ml. The semisynthetic preparation (Novolin R) contains only trace amounts of zinc (10–20 µg/100 U/ml). Both biosynthetic and semisynthetic preparations also contain glycerin and cresol as preservatives. The only form of human insulin that can be administered intravenously.

Isophane (human) insulin suspension (NPH) (Humulin N, Insulatard NPH, Novolin N): an intermediate-acting cloudy or milky suspension of zinc insulin crystals and protamine sulfate in buffered water. Each 100 USP units contains 10–40 µg zinc and 0.15–0.25% dibasic sodium phosphate, glycerin, cresol, and phenol. Novolin 70/30 is a mixture of 70% isophane (human) insulin suspension (NPH) and 30% (human) insulin injection.

(Human) insulin zinc suspension (Lente) (Humulin L, Novolin L): an intermediate-acting cloudy or milky suspension of insulin modified by addition of zinc chloride in buffered water. Each 100 USP units contains approximately 150 µg zinc; also contains sodium acetate, sodium chloride and methylparaben.

USES Replacement therapy in the management of the newly diagnosed patient with type I (IDDM) diabetes and for patient currently receiving pork, beef, or mixed-species insulin. Also in some patients with history of insulin allergy or resistance.

ROUTE & DOSAGE

Diabetes Mellitus

Adult	IV/IM/SC	Individualized doses; see insulin injection

PHARMACOKINETICS Onset: 0.5–1 h regular; 1–2 h NPH, Lente; 4–8 h Ultralente. **Peak:** 2–3 h regular; 8–12 h NPH, Lente; 16–18 h Ultralente. **Duration:** 5–7 h regular; 18–24 h NPH, Lente; 36 h Ultralente. **Metabolism:** metabolized in liver and kidney. **Elimination:** half-life: up to 13 h; <2% excreted unchanged in urine.

ADVERSE/SIDE EFFECTS Generalized and cutaneous allergic reactions in patient who is also allergic to animal insulins.

See also insulin injection for diagnostic test interferences and drug interactions.

INCOMPATIBILITIES Regular insulin. Solution/ Additive: aminophylline, amobarbital, chlorothi- **azide, dobutamine, pentobarbital, phenobarbital, phenytoin, secobarbital, sodium bicarbonate, thiopental.**

NURSING IMPLICATIONS

See insulin injection for nursing implications related to assessment and drug effects and patient and family education.

Administration

- (Human) insulin injection (regular human insulin) is given SC, IM, and IV. Isophane (human) insulin suspension (NPH) and (human) insulin zinc suspension (Lente) are usually given SC, never IV.
- (Human) insulin injection may be given undiluted by direct IV. Each 50 U or fraction thereof may be given over 1 min.
- (Human) insulin injection by IV infusion will be administered at a rate determined by the physician. The IV preparation of insulin is usually diluted in 0.9% or 0.45% NaCl injection.
- Any changes in insulin brand, purity, strength, type, or species should be made under medical surveillance. Monitor patient closely. Adjustments in dosage may be needed with the first dose and even with subsequent doses for a period of several weeks.
- Active principle in the suspension forms (e.g., Novolin N, Novolin L) is in the milky white precipitate. To assure complete dispersion, mix thoroughly, gently rotating vial between palms and inverting it end to end several times. Do not shake; frothing will interfere with accurate measurement. If suspension or vial walls display granules or clumps after mixing, discard vial.
- Human insulins should not be mixed with any other insulin.
- Discard partially empty vial if it has not been used for several weeks.
- Refrigerate unopened vial at 2–8C (36–46F) and store vial-in-use at 15–30C (59–86F). Avoid freezing, exposure to extremes in temperature, or to direct sunlight.

INSULIN INJECTION

See HORMONE, ANTIDIABETIC, INSULIN prototype, p 230.

Common side effects in *italic*; life-threatening effects <u>underlined</u>; generic names in **bold**; classifications in SMALL CAPS

669

INSULIN INJECTION CONCENTRATED

Trade names: Iletin II, Regular (Concentrated), U-500
Classifications: SYNTHETIC HORMONE; INSULIN ANTIDIABETIC
Pregnancy: Category B

ACTIONS/PHARMACODYNAMICS Concentrated insulin from purified pork pancreas unmodified by any agent that might prolong its action. Because of its high concentration, duration of action is similar to that of an intermediate-acting insulin. See insulin injection for actions, contraindications, precautions, and adverse reactions.

USES Only for the occasional patient who develops insulin resistance and requires daily doses greater than 200 U (even as high as several thousand units).

ROUTE & DOSAGE

Diabetes Mellitus

Adult IM/SC Individualized doses; see insulin injection

PHARMACOKINETICS Onset: 0.5–1 h regular. **Peak:** 2–3 h regular. **Duration:** 5–7 h regular. **Metabolism:** metabolized in liver and kidney. **Elimination:** half-life: up to 13 h; <2% excreted unchanged in urine.

INCOMPATIBILITIES Regular insulin. Solution/Additive: aminophylline, amobarbital, chlorothiazide, dobutamine, pentobarbital, phenobarbital, phenytoin, secobarbital, sodium bicarbonate, thiopental.

NURSING IMPLICATIONS

See also insulin injection for numerous nursing implications, diagnostic test interferences, and drug interactions.

Administration

- Label of U-500 insulin is brown-and-white striped. U-500 requires a prescription.
- This preparation should not be administered IV because of the high risk of allergic or anaphylactoid reaction.
- Discard solution that is not absolutely clear and colorless.
- Use a tuberculin syringe for accuracy in measurement. Even a slight variation can mean a large overdose or underdose.
- Store in a cold place, preferably a refrigerator, unless otherwise directed. Avoid freezing.

Assessment & Drug Effects

- Patients receiving concentrated insulin are kept under close surveillance until dosage is established. Close monitoring for symptoms of hypoglycemia, hyperglycemia, allergic or anaphylactoid reactions, and of water and electrolyte imbalance is essential.
- Severe secondary hypoglycemia reactions may develop 18–24 h after administration of drug. Have on hand glucagon, IV dextrose, epinephrine.
- There seems to be no condition of absolute resistance. All insulin-resistant patients will respond if dose is large enough.
- Frequently, responsiveness to insulin effect is regained after a short period of therapy with concentrated insulin.

INSULIN, ISOPHANE (NPH)

Trade names: Humulin N, Iletin I, Iletin II (beef), Iletin II (pork), Insulatard NPH, Mixtard, Novolin 70/30, Novolin N
Classifications: HORMONE; INSULIN ANTIDIABETIC
Pregnancy: Category B

ACTIONS/PHARMACODYNAMICS Intermediate-acting, cloudy suspension of zinc insulin crystals (derived from beef or pork pancreas or both) and modified by protamine in a neutral buffer. NPH Iletin II (beef or pork), and Insulatard are "purified" or "single component" insulins that have been purified and are less likely to cause allergic reactions than nonpurified preparations. Combines some of the advantages and eliminates some of the disadvantages of both very short-acting and very long-acting preparations. Therapeutic effect is prompt enough to control postprandial hyperglycemia, which formerly called for supplemental doses of insulin injection. See insulin injection for actions, contraindications, and adverse reactions.

USES Generally considered drug of choice to control hyperglycemia in the diabetic patient. Mixtard and

Novolin 70/30 are fixed combinations of purified regular insulin 30% and NPH 70%.

ROUTE & DOSAGE

Diabetes Mellitus

Adult	IM/SC	Individualized doses; see insulin injection

PHARMACOKINETICS Onset: 1–2 h. **Peak:** 8–12 h NPH. **Duration:** 18–24 h NPH. **Metabolism:** metabolized in liver and kidney. **Elimination:** half-life: up to 13 h; < 2% excreted unchanged in urine.

NURSING IMPLICATIONS

See also insulin injection for numerous nursing implications, diagnostic test interferences, and drug interactions.

Administration

- This preparation should never be administered IV. It is not suitable for emergency use.
- Usually given 30–60 min before first meal of the day. If necessary, a second smaller dose may be prescribed 30 min before supper or at bedtime.
- To assure complete dispersion, mix thoroughly by gently rotating vial between palms and inverting it end to end several times. Do not shake; frothing will interfere with accurate measurement. If suspension or vial walls display granules or clumps after mixing or if solution is clear and remains clear after mixing, discard vial.
- Isophane insulin may be mixed with insulin injection without altering either solution.
- Isophane insulin should not be mixed with lente forms.
- Patient receiving insulin injection (regular) may be transferred directly to isophane insulin on unit-for-unit basis: initial dose of isophane should be about two-thirds to three-fourths total daily dose of regular insulin. Monitor patient closely.
- If dosage is very high, physician may prescribe divided doses; 2/3 in morning and 1/3 30 min before supper or at bedtime.
- Insulins should not be mixed unless prescribed by physician. In general, when insulin injection (regular insulin) is to be combined, it is drawn first. Important to follow the same order of sequence with the same stock bottles every day.
- Discard partially empty vial if it has not been used for several weeks.
- Store unopened vial at 2–8C (36–46F); store vial in use at 15–30C (59–86F). Avoid freezing and exposure to extremes in temperature or to direct sunlight.

Assessment & Drug Effects

- Suspect hypoglycemia if fatigue, weakness, sweating, tremor, or nervousness occur. See insulin injection for complete description.

Patient & Family Education

- If insulin was given before breakfast, a hypoglycemic episode is most likely to occur between midafternoon and dinnertime, when insulin effect is peaking. Patient should be told to eat a snack in midafternoon and to carry sugar or candy to treat a reaction. A snack at bedtime will prevent insulin reaction during the night.
- Teach the patient the signs and symptoms of hypoglycemia and hyperglycemia (see chap 3).
- The patient should always consult physician before making changes in dosage to accommodate anticipated stress or exercise.

Prototype: insulin injection, p 230

INSULIN, PROTAMINE ZINC (PZI)

Trade names: Iletin I, Iletin II (Beef), Iletin II (Pork)
Classifications: HORMONE; INSULIN ANTIDIABETIC
Pregnancy: Category B

ACTIONS/PHARMACODYNAMICS Long-acting, cloudy suspension of insulin modified by addition of zinc chloride and protamine sulfate, which has poor solubility and thus delays absorption. Derived from beef or pork pancreas or both. May be used in combination with a shorter acting form. See insulin injection for actions, contraindications, precautions, and adverse/side effects.

USES Diabetes mellitus in patients who are not adequately controlled by unmodified insulin.

ROUTE & DOSAGE

Diabetes Mellitus

Adult	IM/SC	Individualized doses; see insulin injection

PHARMACOKINETICS Onset: 4–8 h. **Peak:** 14–24 h. **Duration:** 36 h. **Metabolism:** metabolized in liver and kidney. **Elimination:** half-life: up to 13 h; < 2% excreted unchanged in urine.

Common side effects in *italic*; life-threatening effects <u>underlined</u>; generic names in **bold**; classifications in SMALL CAPS

671

ADVERSE/SIDE EFFECTS Lymphedema around injection site, hypoglycemia, hypersensitivity reactions.

NURSING IMPLICATIONS

See also insulin injection for numerous nursing implications, diagnostic test interferences, drug interactions.

Administration

- Should not be administered IV. Not suitable for emergency use.
- Usually administered 30–60 min before breakfast.
- To assure complete dispersion, mix thoroughly by gently rotating vial between palms and inverting it end to end several times. Do not shake; frothing will interfere with accurate measurement. If suspension or vial walls display granules or clumps after mixing or if solution is clear and remains clear after mixing, discard vial.
- PZI is compatible with regular insulin. Insulins must not be mixed unless prescribed by physician.
- When mixing regular insulin with PZI, prepare solution immediately before administration. Withdraw insulin injection into syringe before PZI so that vial of insulin injection will not be contaminated with excess protamine.
- Discard partially empty vial if it has not been used for several weeks.
- Store unopened vial at 2–8C (36–46F); store vial in use at 15–30C (59–86F). Avoid freezing and exposure to extremes in temperature or to direct sunlight.

Patient & Family Education

- Teach patient that prolonged insulin effect requires careful distribution of carbohydrates in a balanced diet. Patient should not redistribute food or alter dose or time of taking insulin unless advised by physician.
- If one dose of insulin has controlled diabetes for some time, the patient may test urine and blood for glucose once a day or 2 or 3 times weekly. In the event of infection, emotional stress, or change in activity, patient should increase number of tests per day.
- The usual proportion of PZI to insulin injection prescribed is 1:2 or 1:3 to provide a preparation with both rapid onset and prolonged duration of action.
- Full therapeutic effect of PZI may be delayed several days following institution of treatment. During this interval, small supplemental doses of insulin injection are often necessary.

- Between-meal snacks may be necessary; bedtime snacks are essential.
- If injection is given in the morning, hypoglycemia is most likely to occur during the night or early morning.
- Blood glucose levels fall slowly after injection of PZI; thus, marked hypoglycemia may develop without producing an apparent cluster of symptoms. Teach patient to be alert to the significance of sweating or fatigue unwarranted by patient's activities, as well as other vague symptoms such as lassitude, drowsiness, tremulousness. The physician should be notified immediately. Without prompt and adequate treatment, patient may become unconscious.
- *Treatment of PZI-induced hypoglycemia:* requires both fast acting and complex carbohydrate (e.g., corn syrup or honey with bread) followed in 1–2 h by additional "slow" carbohydrates, such as milk and crackers. Emergency treatment: 10–20 g glucose IV followed later by food.

Prototype: insulin injection, p 230

INSULIN ZINC SUSPENSION (LENTE)

Trade names: Humulin L, Lente Iletin I, Lente Iletin II (purified beef, pork), Lente Purified Pork Insulin, Novolin

Classifications: HORMONE; INSULIN ANTIDIABETIC

Pregnancy: Category B

ACTIONS/PHARMACODYNAMICS Intermediate-acting, cloudy insulin suspension, equivalent to a mixture of 30% prompt insulin zinc (Semilente) and 70% extended zinc insulin (Ultralente) suspensions. Obtained from beef or pork pancreas or both. Because insulin zinc suspension contains no modifying foreign protein (protamine or globin), allergic reactions are rare. Time action is intermediate between those of prompt and extended insulins and is so close to that of isophane (NPH) insulin that the two forms may be used interchangeably. See insulin injection for contraindications, precautions, and adverse/side effects.

USES Hyperglycemia in diabetic patients allergic to other preparations of insulin. Also for patients with evidence of thrombotic phenomena in which protamine may be a factor.

ROUTE & DOSAGE

Diabetes Mellitus

Adult IM/SC Individualized doses; see insulin injection

PHARMACOKINETICS Onset: 1–2 h. **Peak:** 8–12 h. **Duration:** 18–24 h. **Metabolism:** metabolized in liver and kidney. **Elimination:** half-life: up to 13 h; < 2 % excreted unchanged in urine.

NURSING IMPLICATIONS

See also insulin injection for numerous nursing implications, diagnostic test interferences and drug interactions.

Administration

- Usually administered 30–60 min before breakfast. Some patients require another injection 30 min before suppertime or at bedtime.
- Should not be administered IV. This preparation is not suitable for emergency treatment.
- Zinc insulin preparations (Ultralente, Lente, Semilente) can be mixed with one another if prescribed by physician, but they must not be mixed with other modified insulins. Compatible with regular insulin.
- To assure complete dispersion, mix thoroughly by gently rotating the vial between the palms and by inverting it end-to-end several times. Do not shake; frothing will interfere with accurate measurement. If the suspension or vial walls display granules or clumps of precipitate after mixing or if solution is clear and remains clear after rotating, discard vial.
- Because time of action of insulin zinc suspension (Lente) approximates that of isophane insulin suspension (NPH), the patient can usually be transferred directly to the latter on a unit-for-unit basis. Transfer from regular insulin to insulin zinc suspension: initial dose of insulin zinc should be 2/3–3/4 total daily dose of regular insulin.
- Discard partially empty vial if it has not been used for several weeks.
- Store unopened vial at 2–8C (36–46F); store vial in use at 15–30C (59–86F). Avoid freezing and exposure to extremes in temperature or to direct sunlight.

Patient & Family Education

- Symptoms of hypoglycemia (see chap 3) are most apt to occur between midafternoon and dinner time (an early symptom may be a sense of extreme fatigue). Notify the physician promptly and immediately take soluble carbohydrate (e.g., orange juice, honey, corn syrup). If the time between the midday and evening meal is prolonged, an afternoon snack may be ordered.
- The possibility of nocturnal hypoglycemia should not be overlooked, especially during dose adjustment. Teach family to monitor for signs of restlessness or profuse sweating during sleep.

Prototype: insulin injection, p 230

INSULIN ZINC SUSPENSION, EXTENDED (ULTRALENTE)

Trade names: Humulin U; Iletin I, Ultralente; Ultralente Insulin; Ultralente Purified Beef
Classifications: HORMONE; INSULIN ANTIDIABETIC
Pregnancy: Category B

ACTIONS/PHARMACODYNAMICS Long-acting cloudy suspension of insulin modified by addition of zinc chloride. Large particle size and high zinc content delay absorption and prolong action. Obtained from beef or pork pancreas or both. No modifying protein (protamine or globin) is added; therefore incidence of allergic reactions is low. Similar to protamine zinc insulin suspension (PZI) in actions and indications. Usually administered in combination with a shorter acting insulin preparation. See insulin injection for actions, uses, contraindications, and adverse/side effects.

ROUTE & DOSAGE

Diabetes Mellitus

Adult IM/SC Individualized doses; see insulin injection

PHARMACOKINETICS Onset: 4–8 h. **Peak:** 16–18 h. **Duration:** 36 h. **Metabolism:** metabolized in liver and kidney. **Elimination:** half-life: up to 13 h; < 2% excreted unchanged in urine.

NURSING IMPLICATIONS

See also insulin injection for numerous nursing implications, diagnostic test interferences, and drug interactions.

Administration

- This drug is not to be used IV, and it is not suitable for emergency situations.

Common side effects in *italic*; life-threatening effects <u>underlined</u>; generic names in **bold**; classifications in SMALL CAPS

673

- Administered 30–60 min before breakfast by deep SC injection.
- To assure complete dispersion, mix thoroughly by gently rotating vial between palms and by inverting it end to end several times. Do not shake; frothing will interfere with accurate measurement. Discard vial if suspension on vial walls displays granules or clumps of precipitate or if solution is clear and remains clear after mixing.
- May be mixed with Semilente but not with other modified insulin preparations. Compatible with regular insulin. Insulins should not be mixed unless prescribed by physician.
- Discard partially empty vial if it has not been used for several weeks.
- Store unopened vial at 2–8C (36–46F); store vial in use at 15–30C (59–86F). Avoid freezing and exposure to extremes in temperature or to direct sunlight.

Patient & Family Education

- When switching from a standard insulin to one of the purified insulins, dosage should be reduced initially and patient closely monitored. Usually dosage reduction is about 20%.
- Hypoglycemia is most apt to occur during the night or early morning. Teach family to watch sleeping patient carefully for signs of restlessness or profuse sweating and to notify physician if it occurs. Hypoglycemia is treated by administering soluble carbohydrate (orange juice, sugar, honey) plus a slowly digestible carbohydrate (bread, crackers). Supplemental feedings may be prescribed.

Prototype: insulin injection, p 230

INSULIN ZINC SUSPENSION, PROMPT (SEMILENTE)

Trade names: Semilente Iletin I, Semilente Insulin, Semilente Purified Pork Insulin
Classifications: HORMONE; INSULIN ANTIDIABETIC
Pregnancy: Category B

ACTIONS/PHARMACODYNAMICS

Rapid-acting cloudy suspension of insulin modified by addition of zinc chloride so that solid phase of suspension is amorphous and therefore more quickly absorbed. Obtained from beef or pork pancreas or both. No modifying protein (protamine or globin) is added; therefore incidence of allergic reactions is low. See insulin injection for actions, contraindications, precautions, and adverse/side effects.

USES Most commonly to supplement intermediate and long-acting insulins. Also for routine management of diabetes, especially for patients allergic to other types of insulin, and for patients with evidence of thrombotic phenomena in which protamine may be a factor.

ROUTE & DOSAGE

Diabetes Mellitus

Adult	IM/SC	Individualized doses; see insulin injection

PHARMACOKINETICS Onset: 0.5–1 h. **Peak:** 4–7 h. **Duration:** 12–16 h. **Metabolism:** metabolized in liver and kidney. **Elimination:** half-life: up to 13 h; < 2% excreted unchanged in urine.

NURSING IMPLICATIONS

See also insulin injection for numerous nursing implications, diagnostic test interferences, and drug interactions.

Administration

- Should be dispensed in original unopened multidose container with expiration date of not later than 24 mo after vial was filled.
- Should never be administered IV. Preparation is not suitable for emergency use.
- Usually administered once daily, 30 min before breakfast. Additional doses may be required for some patients 30 min before a meal or at bedtime.
- To assure complete dispersion, mix thoroughly by gently rotating vial between palms and by inverting it end to end several times. Do not shake; frothing will interfere with accurate measurement. If the suspension on vial walls displays granules or clumps of crystalline precipitate after mixing or if solution is clear and remains clear after vial is rotated, discard vial.
- The zinc insulin preparations (Ultralente, Lente, Semilente) can be mixed with one another, but they must not be mixed with other modified insulin. Insulins should not be mixed unless prescribed by physician.
- Discard partially empty vial if it has not been used for several weeks.
- Store unopened vial at 2–8C (36–46F); store vial in use at 15–30C (59–86F). Avoid freezing and expo-

sure to extremes in temperature or to direct sunlight.

Patient & Family Education
- Symptoms of hypoglycemia are most apt to appear before lunch; glycosuria is most apt to appear during the night.
- This preparation should not be substituted for another insulin preparation without direction by a physician.

INTERFERON ALFA-2A

See IMMUNOMODULATOR prototype, p 246.

Prototype: interferon alfa-2A, p 246

INTERFERON ALFA-2B
(in-ter-feer´on)
Trade name: Intron A
Classifications: IMMUNOMODULATOR;
ANTINEOPLASTIC; ANTIVIRAL
Pregnancy: Category C

ACTIONS/PHARMACODYNAMICS Alpha (leukocyte) interferon is a natural product induced virally in peripheral WBC or lymphoblastoid cells. The drug interferon alfa-2B is obtained by recombinant DNA technology from a strain of *Escherichia coli* bearing an interferon alfa-2B gene from human leukocytes. Has the same actions (antiviral, immunomodulating, antiproliferative) as interferon alfa-2A.

USES Hairy-cell leukemia in splenectomized and nonsplenectomized patients ≥ 18 y. **Unlabeled use:** multiple sclerosis.

ROUTE & DOSAGE

Hairy Cell Leukemia

Adult	IM/SC	2 million U/m² 3 times/wk

PHARMACOKINETICS Peak: 6–8 h. **Metabolism:** metabolized in kidneys. **Elimination:** half-life: 6–7 h.

CONTRAINDICATIONS & PRECAUTIONS Contraindicated in: hypersensitivity to interferon alfa-2B or to any components of the product. Safe use during pregnancy (category C), by nursing mothers, or chil-dren < 18 y not established. **Cautious use in:** severe, preexisting cardiac, renal, or hepatic disease; pulmonary disease (e.g., COPD); diabetes mellitus prone to ketoacidosis; coagulation disorders; severe myelosuppression; recent MI; previous dysrhythmias.

ADVERSE/SIDE EFFECTS CNS: depression, nervousness, anxiety, confusion, dizziness, *fatigue,* somnolence, insomnia, altered mental states, ataxia, tremor, paresthesias, headache. **CV:** hypotension (rarely symptomatic), hypertension, tachycardia (usually associated with high fever), dyspnea, *hot flushes.* **ENT:** epistaxis, nasal congestion, pharyngitis, sneezing. **Eye:** abnormal vision, oculomotor paralysis. **GI:** taste alteration, *anorexia,* weight loss, nausea, vomiting, stomatitis, diarrhea, constipation, paralytic ileus, flatulence, stomatitis. **Hematologic:** mild thrombocytopenia, transient granulocytopenia, leukemia. **Skin:** mild pruritus, mild alopecia, rash, dry skin, herpetic eruptions, nonherpetic cold sores, urticaria. **Other:** *flulike symptoms (fever, chills) associated with myalgia and arthralgia,* leg cramps, increased saliva, hyperglycemia.

NURSING IMPLICATIONS
See interferon alfa-2A for additional nursing implications related to assessment and drug effects and patient and family education.

Administration
- Interferon alfa-2B should be administered under the guidance of a qualified physician. Usually patient is hospitalized for first 4–5 d of treatment.
- *Reconstitution:* the final concentration with the amount of required diluent is determined by the condition being treated (see manufacturer's directions). Inject diluent (bacteriostatic water for injection) into interferon alfa-2B vial; gently agitate solution before withdrawing dose with a sterile syringe. Reconstituted solution remains stable for 1 mo if refrigerated.
- Reconstituted solution should be clear and colorless to light yellow. Inspect visually for particulate material and discard solution if it is present or if solution is discolored. Sterilized glass or plastic disposable syringes may be used.
- Bedtime administration may decrease awareness of side effects.
- Store vials and reconstituted solutions at 2–8C (36–46F).

Assessment & Drug Effects
- Patient should be well hydrated, especially during initial stage of treatment. Urge fluids of choice; monitor I&O.

Common side effects in *italic*; life-threatening effects underlined; generic names in **bold**; classifications in SMALL CAPS

675

■ Coagulation disorders (as evidenced by elevated PT and PTT) may develop with this agent. Inspect body surfaces for signs: ecchymoses, petechiae; report unexplained bleeding and easy bruising.

Patient & Family Education
■ If severe reactions occur, the physician will decrease the dosage by 50%.
■ Patients with hairy cell leukemia or chronic hepatitis non-A, non-B/C may be permitted to self-administer interferon alfa-2B. Use sterilized glass or disposable syringes.

Prototype: benzonatate, p 99

IODINATED GLYCEROL
(eye´oh-di-nay-ted gli´ser-ole)
Trade names: Iophen, Organidin, R-Gen
Classification: EXPECTORANT
Pregnancy: Category X

ACTIONS/PHARMACODYNAMICS Stable complex of iodine and glycerol. Concentrates in secretions of respiratory tract. Liquefies thick, tenacious respiratory tract fluid and facilitates expectoration. Contains approximately 50% organically bound iodine, little or no inorganic iodine, and no free iodine. Does not appreciably raise protein bound iodine values.

USES Adjunctive treatment in bronchial asthma, bronchitis, emphysema, and other respiratory disorders and after surgery to help prevent atelectasis.

ROUTE & DOSAGE

Expectorant

Adult	PO	60 mg q.i.d.
Child	PO	up to 30 mg q.i.d.

CONTRAINDICATIONS & PRECAUTIONS Contraindicated in: history of marked sensitivity to inorganic iodides; hypersensitivity to iodinated glycerol (or any of its ingredients) and related compounds; goiter, hypothyroidism, pregnancy (category X); nursing mothers; neonates. **Cautious use in:** history of thyroid disease.

ADVERSE/SIDE EFFECTS Rare: GI irritation, nausea, rash, hypersensitivity. Usually associated with long-term use. **Iodism:** coryza, headache, parotitis, ulcerations of mouth and throat, metallic taste, inflam-mation of salivary glands, salivation, skin eruptions, generalized furunculosis, eye irritation, swelling of eyelids. **Other:** (rare): hypothyroidism, goiter or enlarged thyroid, parkinsonism, CNS depression, fever, glomerulonephritis, vasculitis.

DIAGNOSTIC TEST INTERFERENCES Iodinated glycerol may depress *RAI uptake* values, and alter other *thyroid function tests.*

DRUG INTERACTIONS Lithium, ANTITHYROID AGENTS potentiate goitrogenic and hypothyroid action.

NURSING IMPLICATIONS

Administration
■ All preparations should be administered with liquid. Drinking a glass of water with or after the medication may help to liquefy respiratory tract secretions.
■ Store at 15–30C (59–86F) unless otherwise directed. Avoid freezing.

Assessment & Drug Effects
■ Before administering iodinated glycerol, determine if patient is allergic to iodine or seafood.
■ If iodism (see adverse effects) occurs, discontinue iodinated glycerol and institute appropriate supportive therapy.

Patient & Family Education
■ Drug should be discontinued if skin rash or other evidence of hypersensitivity or iodism occurs.
■ Advise patient to increase fluid intake if not contraindicated.

Prototype: emetine, p 51

IODOQUINOL
(eye-oh-do-kwin´ole)
Trade names: Diiodohydroxyquin, Diodoquin, Moebiquin, Sebaquin, Yodoxin
Classifications: ANTIINFECTIVE; AMEBICIDE; ANTIPROTOZOAL
Pregnancy: Category C

ACTIONS/PHARMACODYNAMICS Dihalogenated derivative of 8-hydroxyquinoline. Iodoquinol is a direct-acting (contact) amebicide effective against both trophozoites and cyst forms of *Entamoeba histolytica* in intestinal lumen. Action mechanism unclear. Not useful for extraintestinal amebiasis. Range of antiprotozoal action includes *Trichomonas vaginalis* and *Balantidium coli;* also has some antibacterial and antifungal properties. Contains approximately 64% organically bound iodine.

USES Intestinal amebiasis and for asymptomatic passers of cysts. Commonly used either concurrently or in alternating courses with another intestinal amebicide. **Unlabeled use:** balantidiasis and *Acrodermatitis enteropathica;* traveler's diarrhea; shampoo preparation (Sebaquin) used for control of seborrheic dermatitis of scalp.

ROUTE & DOSAGE

Intestinal Amebiasis

Adult	PO	630–650 mg t.i.d. for 20 d (max 2 g/d); may repeat after a 2–3 wk drug-free interval
Child	PO	30–40 mg/kg/d in 2–3 divided doses for 20 d (max 1.95 g/d); may repeat after a 2–3 wk drug-free interval

PHARMACOKINETICS Absorption: small amount absorbed from GI tract. **Elimination:** excreted in feces.

CONTRAINDICATIONS & PRECAUTIONS Contraindicated in: hypersensitivity to any 8-hydroxyquinoline or to iodine-containing preparations or foods; hepatic or renal damage; preexisting optic neuropathy. **Cautious use in:** severe thyroid disease; minor self-limiting problems; prolonged high-dosage therapy. Safe use during pregnancy (category C) and in nursing mothers not established.

ADVERSE/SIDE EFFECTS CNS: headache, dizziness or lightheadedness, vertigo, ataxia, peripheral neuropathy (especially in children); muscle pain, weakness usually below T_{12} vertebrae, dysesthesias especially of lower limbs, paresthesias, ataxia, psychological changes, greenish discoloration of tongue. **Eye:** blurred vision, optic atrophy, optic neuritis, permanent loss of vision, subacute myelo-optic neuropathy. **GI:** nausea, vomiting, anorexia, abdominal cramps, diarrhea, constipation, rectal irritation and itching. **Hypersensitivity:** urticaria, pruritus. **Skin:** discoloration of hair and nails, acne, hair loss, urticaria, rectal itching, pruritus, various forms of skin eruptions. **Other:** increased sense of warmth, thyroid hypertrophy, agranulocytosis. **Iodism:** generalized furunculosis (iodine toxiderma), skin eruptions, rhinitis, ptyalism, frontal headache, chills, fever, weakness, emaciation, agranulocytosis.

DIAGNOSTIC TEST INTERFERENCES Iodoquinol can cause elevations of **PBI** and decrease of **I-131 uptake** (effects may last for several weeks to 6 mo even after discontinuation of therapy). **Ferric chloride test for PKU** (phenylketonuria) may yield false-positive results if iodoquinol is present in urine.

NURSING IMPLICATIONS

Administration

- Administer drug after meals to reduce GI irritation. If patient has difficulty swallowing tablet, it may be crushed and mixed with applesauce or chocolate syrup.
- Shampoo preparation (Sebaquin) should not be used over large areas or for prolonged periods. Advise patient to rinse it thoroughly from hair following shampoo and to avoid bringing it in contact with eyes.
- Store at 15–30C (59–86F) unless otherwise directed.

Assessment & Drug Effects

- Monitor I&O ratio. Record characteristics of stools: color, consistency, frequency, presence of blood, mucus, or other material.
- It is advisable for patient to have ophthalmologic examinations at regular intervals during prolonged therapy.
- Eye problems and peripheral neuropathy are especially likely to occur in children on high-dose, long-term therapy. Monitor and report immediately the onset of blurred or decreased vision or eye pain. Also report symptoms of peripheral neuropathy: pain, numbness, tingling, or weakness of extremities.

Patient & Family Education

- Instruct patient to report skin rash and symptoms of agranulocytosis (see chap 3).
- Advise patient to complete full course of treatment; ideally, patient is discharged when three stool specimens repeated daily for 3 consecutive days are negative of parasites. Stool should be examined again in 1, 3, and 6 mo after termination of treatment.
- Intestinal amebiasis is spread mainly by contaminated water, raw fruits or vegetables, flies, roaches, and hand-to-mouth transfer of infected feces. Emphasize importance of handwashing after defecation and before eating.

Common side effects in *italic*; life-threatening effects underlined; generic names in **bold**; classifications in SMALL CAPS

677

IPECAC SYRUP

(ip´e-kak)
Classifications: GASTROINTESTINAL AGENT;
EMETIC
Pregnancy: Category C

ACTIONS/PHARMACODYNAMICS Derived from dried rhizomes and roots of *Cephaelis ipecacuanha*. Contains two primary alkaloids: cephaeline (produces emesis) and emetine, a toxic alkaloid that is excreted slowly from the body. Emetine can cause potentially fatal cumulative toxicity with repeated use. It appears to inhibit protein synthesis and energy production in muscle tissue with resultant skeletal and cardiac muscle toxicity. Acts locally on gastric mucosa and centrally on chemoreceptor trigger zone (CTZ) in the medulla to induce vomiting. Also has expectorant action that is thought to result from increased bronchial secretions resulting from reflex stimulation of gastric mucosa.

USES Emergency emetic to remove unabsorbed ingested poisons.

ROUTE & DOSAGE

Emergency Emesis

Adult	PO	30 ml followed by 1–2 240 ml (8 oz) glasses of water; may repeat once in 20 min if necessary
Child	PO	> 1 y: 15 ml followed by 1–2 240 ml (8 oz) glasses of water; may repeat once in 20 min if necessary
		< 1 y: 5–10 ml followed by 120–240 ml (4–8 oz) of water; may repeat once in 20 min if necessary

PHARMACOKINETICS Onset: 15–30 min. **Duration:** 25 min. **Elimination:** metabolite can be detected in urine up to 60 d after excessive doses.

CONTRAINDICATIONS & PRECAUTIONS Contraindicated in: comatose, semicomatose, inebriated, deeply sedated patients; patients in shock; patients with depressed gag reflex; seizures, active or impending; impaired cardiac function; arteriosclerosis; treatment of ingested strong alkalis, acids, or other corrosives, strychnine, petroleum distillates, volatile oils, or rapid-acting CNS depressants. Safe use in pregnancy (category C), nursing mothers, infants under 6 mo not established.

ADVERSE/SIDE EFFECTS Diarrhea, mild GI upset, slight CNS depression, lethargy. If drug is not vomited but absorbed or if ipecac overdosage: *persistent vomiting,* gastroenteritis, bloody diarrhea, sensory disturbances, stomach cramps, tremor; achy, stiff muscles, severe myopathy (muscle weakness), including <u>cardiomyopathy, cardiotoxicity,</u> cardiac arrhythmias, atrial fibrillation, tachycardia, chest pain, dyspnea, hypotension, <u>fatal myocarditis,</u> convulsions, <u>coma.</u>

NURSING IMPLICATIONS

Administration

- Not to be confused with ipecac fluid extract, which is 14 times stronger and has caused deaths when mistakenly given at the same dosage as ipecac syrup.
- Action of ipecac syrup is facilitated by following the dose with 200–300 ml of tepid water or other clear liquid for adults, 100–200 ml for children. Avoid milk or carbonated beverages (manufacturer's recommendation) since they may delay emesis. Some clinicians allow carbonated beverages for children who will not drink water.
- Activated charcoal should not be given simultaneously with ipecac syrup because charcoal adsorbs ipecac and renders it completely ineffective.
- In small children, emetic effect is reportedly enhanced by gently bouncing the child.
- Vomiting should not be induced if victim is unconscious or semiconscious or is convulsing.
- Store in tight containers at temperature not exceeding 25C (77F).

Assessment & Drug Effects

- Emetic effect occurs in 15–30 min and continues for 20–25 min. If vomiting does not occur in 20–30 min, dose may be repeated once.
- If vomiting does not occur within 15–20 min after a second dose (given only if vomiting has not occurred following first dose), contact physician immediately. Dosage should be recovered by gastric lavage and activated charcoal if necessary.
- Ipecac syrup can be cardiotoxic if not vomited and allowed to be absorbed.
- Most patients stop vomiting within 2–3 h after ipecac syrup is given; however, if vomiting persists, report immediately to physician.
- Ipecac syrup may be ineffective if patient is also taking a drug with antiemetic action.

Patient & Family Education

- If poisoning has occurred, identify poison and relative amount taken as quickly as possible. Be pre-

Common side effects in *italic*; life-threatening effects <u>underlined</u>; generic names in **bold**; classifications in SMALL CAPS

pared to tell poison center patient's age, weight, symptoms.
- Call an emergency room, poison control center, or physician before using ipecac syrup.
- Do not exceed recommended dosage.

Prototype: atropine, p 116

IPRATROPIUM BROMIDE
(i-pra-troe´pee-um)
Trade name: Atrovent
Classifications: AUTONOMIC NERVOUS SYSTEM AGENT; ANTICHOLINERGIC (PARASYMPATHOLYTIC); BRONCHODILATOR
Pregnancy: Category B

ACTIONS/PHARMACODYNAMICS Quaternary compound, chemically related to atropine, with low solubility; does not cross blood-brain barrier. Lacks systemic effects of atropinelike drugs used as bronchodilators. Produces local, site-specific effects on the larger central airways. Bronchodilation inhibits acetylcholine at its receptor sites, thereby blocking cholinergic bronchomotor tone (bronchoconstriction); also abolishes vagally mediated reflex bronchospasm triggered by such nonspecific agents as cigarette smoke, inert dusts, cold air, and a range of inflammatory mediators (e.g., histamine). As with other long-acting anticholinergic bronchodilators, ipratropium is more effective in the patient with chronic obstructive pulmonary disease (COPD) and less effective in patients with asthma than are adrenergic bronchodilators. Has minimal effect on ciliary activity, sputum volume or viscosity, and mucus secretion; decreases pulmonary resistance in patient with stable COPD.

USES Maintenance therapy in COPD including chronic bronchitis and emphysema. **Unlabeled use:** perennial nonallergic rhinitis.

ROUTE & DOSAGE

COPD

Adult	Inhalation	2 inhalations q.i.d. at no less than 4 h intervals (max 12 inhalations in 24 h)

PHARMACOKINETICS Absorption: 10% of inhaled dose reaches lower airway; approximately 0.5% of dose is systemically absorbed. **Peak effect:** 1.5–2 h. **Duration:** 4–6 h. **Elimination:** half-life: 1.5–2 h; 48% of dose excreted in feces; < 5% excreted in urine.

CONTRAINDICATIONS & PRECAUTIONS Contraindicated in: use as primary treatment for acute episodes; hypersensitivity to atropine or derivatives. Safe use in children < 12 y not established. **Cautious use in:** pregnancy (category B), nursing mothers; narrow-angle glaucoma; prostatic hypertrophy, bladder neck obstruction.

ADVERSE/SIDE EFFECTS Systemic reactions extremely rare. **CNS:** paresthesia, dizziness, headache, fatigue, insomnia, coordination difficulty, nervousness. **CV:** hypotension, tachycardia, palpitations. **Eye:** blurred vision, difficulty in accommodation, acute eye pain, worsening of narrow-angle glaucoma. **GI:** nausea, GI distress, constipation, bitter taste, dry oropharyngeal membranes. **Respiratory:** *cough*, hoarseness, exacerbation of symptoms, drying of bronchial secretions, mucosal ulcers. **Other:** rash, hives, flushing, alopecia, urinary retention.

NURSING IMPLICATIONS

Administration
- Not indicated for the initial treatment of acute episodes of bronchospasm where rapid response is required.
- Demonstrate aerosol use and check return demonstration several times before patient is discharged from supervision. Discuss package insert with patient. Treatment failure is commonly due to improper administration. Extenders for metered dose inhalers (MDI) are available for the patient who cannot master MDI technique (e.g., InspirEase, Brethancer).
- Store inhaler below 30C (86F). Avoid freezing and exposure to excess humidity or to sunlight.

Assessment & Drug Effects
- Ipratropium does not alter mucociliary clearance or the volume or viscosity of respiratory secretions.
- Monitor respiratory status; auscultate lungs before and after inhalation.
- Treatment failure (exacerbation of respiratory symptoms) should be reported to physician. Interruption of ipratropium therapy and substitution of another bronchodilator may be ordered. Usually patient can resume treatment with this agent after interrupted therapy.

Common side effects in *italic*; life-threatening effects underlined; generic names in **bold**; classifications in SMALL CAPS

679

Patient & Family Education

- This medication is not an emergency agent because of its delayed onset and the time required to reach peak bronchodilation.
- Instruct patient to allow 30–60 s between puffs for optimum results. Caution against medication–eye contact.
- Advise patient who is using other inhalations to wait 5 min between medications. Check with physician about sequence of administration.
- Advise patient to take medication only as directed, noting some leniency in number of puffs within 24 h. Parent should supervise child's administration until certain all of dose is being administered.
- Swallowed doses may be the basis for constipation.
- Patient may find it helpful to rinse mouth after medication puffs to reduce bitter taste. Dry mouth may be relieved by a saliva substitute (e.g., Moi-Stir, available OTC). If patient complains of a cough, consult physician.
- The elderly patient may develop urinary problems and should be alerted to discuss changes in normal urinary pattern with the physician.
- Advise patients to call physician if they note changes in sputum color or amount, ankle edema, or significant weight gain.
- Do not puncture, break, or burn container. Discard when outdated.

Prototype: ferrous sulfate, p 132

IRON DEXTRAN

Trade names: Feostat, Feronim, Imferon
Classifications: BLOOD FORMER; IRON PREPARATION
Pregnancy: Category B

ACTIONS/PHARMACODYNAMICS A dark brown, slightly viscous liquid complex of ferric hydroxide with dextran in 0.9% NaCl solution for injection. Reticuloendothelial cells of liver, spleen, and bone marrow dissociate iron from iron dextran complex; the released ferric ion combines with transferrin and is transported to bone marrow, where it is incorporated into hemoglobin.

USES Only in patients with clearly established iron deficiency anemia when oral administration of iron is unsatisfactory or impossible. Each milliliter of iron dextran contains 50 mg elemental iron.

ROUTE & DOSAGE

Iron Deficiency

Adult	IM/IV	Dose is individualized and is determined from a table of correlations between patient's weight and hemoglobin (see package insert); no more than 100 mg (2 ml) of iron dextran should be administered within 24 h
Child	IM/IV	<5 kg (10 lb): no more than 0.5 ml (25 mg)/d
		5–10 kg (10–20 lb): no more than 1 ml (50 mg)/d
		> 10 kg (20 lb): no more than 2 ml (100 mg)/d

PHARMACOKINETICS Absorption: 60% absorbed from IM site by 3 d; 90% absorbed by 1–3 wk. **Distribution:** crosses placenta; distributed into breast milk. **Metabolism:** metabolized in reticuloendothelial system. **Elimination:** half-life: 6 h.

CONTRAINDICATIONS & PRECAUTIONS Contraindicated in: hypersensitivity to the product; all anemias except iron-deficiency anemia. Safe use during pregnancy (category C) not established. **Cautious use in:** rheumatoid arthritis, ankylosing spondylitis; impaired hepatic function; history of allergies or asthma.

ADVERSE/SIDE EFFECTS CNS: headache, shivering, transient paresthesias, syncope, dizziness, coma. **CV:** *peripheral vascular flushing (rapid IV), hypotension,* precordial pain or pressure sensation, tachycardia, fatal cardiac arrhythmias, circulatory collapse. **GI:** nausea, vomiting, transient loss of taste perception, metallic taste, diarrhea, melena, abdominal pain, hemorrhagic gastritis, intestinal necrosis. **Hypersensitivity:** urticaria, skin rash, allergic purpura, pruritus, fever, chills, dyspnea, arthralgia, myalgia; anaphylaxis. **Other:** sterile abscess and brown skin discoloration (IM site), local phlebitis (IV site), lymphadenopathy, hemosiderosis, risk of carcinogenesis at injection site associated with IM administration, metabolic acidosis, hyperglycemia, reactivation of quiescent rheumatoid arthritis, exogenous hemosiderosis, hepatic damage, seizures, bleeding disorder with severe toxicity, *pain at IM injection site.*

DIAGNOSTIC TEST INTERFERENCES Falsely elevated ***serum bilirubin*** and falsely decreased ***serum calcium*** values may occur. Large doses of iron dextran may impart a brown color to serum drawn 4 h after iron administration. ***Bone scans*** involving Tc-99m diphosphonate have shown dense areas of activity along contour of iliac crest 1–6 d after IM injections of iron dextran.

NURSING IMPLICATIONS

Administration

- Regardless of route used, a test dose of 0.5 ml is given over a 5 min period before the first IM or IV therapeutic dose to observe patient's response to the drug. If no reaction to the IM test dose occurs after at least 1 h, the remaining portion of initial dose is administered. If no reaction occurs after the IV test dose, the therapeutic regimen is started in 2–3 d. Fatal anaphylactic reactions have occurred. Epinephrine (0.5 ml of a 1:1000 solution) should be immediately available for hypersensitivity emergency.
- Although anaphylactic reactions (see Signs & Symptoms, chap 3) usually occur within a few minutes after injection, it is recommended that 1 h or more elapse before remainder of initial dose is given following test dose.
- IM injections should be given only into the muscle mass in upper outer quadrant of buttock (never in the upper arm or other exposed area). Use a 2- or 3-inch, 19- or 20-gauge needle. The Z-track technique is recommended to prevent drug leakage and brown staining of subcutaneous tissue. Staining of skin may also be minimized by using one needle to withdraw drug from container and another needle for injection. Brown staining of skin may persist 1–2 y, since drug is absorbed slowly from SC tissue.
- If patient is receiving IM in standing position, patient should be bearing weight on the leg opposite the injection site; if in bed, patient should be in the lateral position with injection site uppermost.
- The multiple-dose vial is used *only* for IM injections. Since it contains a preservative (phenol), it is not suitable for IV use.
- Mixing any other drug in syringe or solution with iron dextran is not advised.
- The IV route is preferred and recommended for patients with insufficient muscle mass, those with impaired absorption (as in edema), when uncontrolled bleeding is a possibility, or when massive and prolonged parenteral therapy is indicated.
- If the IV injection does not exceed 100 mg, it is administered undiluted at a prescribed rate usually no more than 50 mg (1 ml) or less per minute.
- **IV infusion:** calculated iron dextran dose is diluted in 250–1000 ml of 0.9% NaCl injection. Test dose of 25 mg (0.5 ml) is administered over 5 min. If no ad-

verse reactions occur, remainder of dose is infused (e.g., over 1–6 h). After infusion is completed, flush vein with 10 ml of 0.9% NaCl injection. Increased frequency of adverse effects may be expected with large IV doses.
- Store below 30C (86F) unless otherwise directed.

Assessment & Drug Effects

- Anticipated response to parenteral iron therapy is an average weekly hemoglobin rise of about 1 g/d. As with oral therapy, peak levels are generally reached in about 4–8 wk.
- After IV administration, the patient should remain in bed for at least 30 min to prevent orthostatic hypotension. Monitor BP and pulse.
- IV administration may exacerbate acute joint pain in patients with rheumatoid arthritis or ankylosing spondylitis. For this reason the IM route is generally preferred in these patients.
- Systemic reactions may occur over 24 h after parenteral iron has been administered.
- Periodic determinations of hemoglobin, hematocrit, and reticulocyte count should be made as a guide to therapy.

Patient & Family Education

- Patients receiving iron injections should not take iron by mouth. To do so may cause iron poisoning.
- Encourage patient to eat foods high in iron and vitamin C.
- Advise patient to notify physician of any of the following: backache or muscle ache, chills, dizziness, fever, headache, nausea or vomiting, paresthesias, pain or redness at injection site, skin rash or hives, or difficulty breathing.

Prototype: phenelzine, p 182

ISOCARBOXAZID

(eye-soe-kar-box´a-zid)
Trade name: Marplan
Classifications: CNS AGENT; PSYCHOTHERAPEUTIC; ANTIDEPRESSANT; MAO INHIBITOR
Pregnancy: Category C

ACTIONS/PHARMACODYNAMICS MAO inhibitor of the hydrazine group. Similar in actions, uses, contraindications, precautions, and adverse re-

Common side effects in *italic*; life-threatening effects <u>underlined</u>; generic names in **bold**; classifications in SMALL CAPS

681

actions to phenelzine. Inhibits monoamine oxidase, the enzyme involved in the catabolism of catecholamine neurotransmitters (dopamine, epinephrine, norepinephrine) and serotonin. Drug increases concentration of these amines in the body, the proposed basis for the antidepressant effect of MAOIs.

USES Symptomatic treatment of depressed patients refractory to or intolerant of TCAs or electroconvulsive therapy.

ROUTE & DOSAGE

Refractory Depression

Adult   PO   10–30 mg/d in 1–3 divided doses (max 30 mg/d)

PHARMACOKINETICS Duration: up to 2 wk. **Metabolism:** metabolized in liver.

CONTRAINDICATIONS & PRECAUTIONS Contraindicated in: hypersensitivity to MAO inhibitors; pheochromocytoma; CHF; children (< 16 y); elderly (> 60 y) or debilitated; severe renal or hepatic impairment. Safe use during pregnancy (category C) and in nursing mothers not established. **Cautious use in:** hypertension, hyperthyroidism, parkinsonism, cardiac arrhythmias, epilepsy, suicidal risks.

ADVERSE/SIDE EFFECTS CNS: dizziness, lightheadedness, tiredness, weakness, *drowsiness,* vertigo, headache, *overactivity,* hyperreflexia, muscle twitching, tremors, mania hypomania, *insomnia,* confusion, memory impairment. **CV:** *orthostatic hypotension,* parodoxical hypertension, palpitation, tachycardia, other arrhythmias. **Eye:** *blurred vision,* nystagmus, glaucoma, toxic amblyopia (causal relationship not confirmed). **GI:** increased appetite, weight gain, *nausea,* diarrhea, *constipation, anorexia,* black tongue, *dry mouth,* abdominal pain. **GU:** dysuria, *urinary retention,* incontinence, sexual disturbances. **Other:** peripheral edema, excessive sweating, chills, skin rash, hepatitis, jaundice.

DRUG INTERACTIONS TRICYCLIC ANTIDEPRESSANTS, **fluoxetine,** AMPHETAMINES, **ephedrine, phenylpropanolamine, reserpine, guanethidine, buspirone, methyldopa, dopamine, levodopa, tryptophan** may precipitate hypertensive crisis, headache, or hyperexcitability; **alcohol** and other CNS DEPRESSANTS compound CNS depressant effects; **meperidine** can cause fatal cardiovascular collapse; ANESTHETICS exaggerate hypotensive and CNS depressant effects; **metrizamide** increases risk of seizures; compounds hypotensive effects of DIURETICS and other ANTIHYPERTENSIVE AGENTS. **Food-Drug interactions:** all **tyramine**-containing foods (aged cheeses, processed cheeses, sour cream, wine, champagne, beer, pickled herring, anchovies, caviar, shrimp, liver, dry sausage, figs, raisins, overripe bananas or avacodos, chocolate, soy sauce, bean curd, yeast extracts, yogurt, papaya products, meat tenderizers, broad beans) may precipitate hypertensive crisis.

NURSING IMPLICATIONS

Administration

- Dosage is individually adjusted on basis of careful observations of patient. Monitor BP and report any unusual symptoms.
- Physician will reduce dosage to maintenance level as soon as improvement is observed because drug has a cumulative effect.
- Store in a tight, light-resistant container at 15–30C (59–86F).

Assessment & Drug Effects

- Most adverse reactions occur because of failure to recognize cumulative effects of isocarboxazid.
- Therapeutic effects may be apparent within 1 wk or less, but in some patients there may be a time lag of 3–4 wk before improvement occurs.
- Monitor for orthostatic hypotension by evaluating BP with patient recumbent and standing.
- Check for peripheral edema daily and monitor weight several times weekly.
- Although therapeutic effect is delayed, toxic symptoms from overdosage or from ingestion of contraindicated substances (e.g., foods high in tyramine) may occur within hours.
- Clinical effects of isocarboxazid may continue for up to 2 wk after drug is discontinued.
- Monitor I & O and bowel elimination patterns.

Patient & Family Education

- Caution patient to make position changes slowly and in stages and to lie down or sit down if faintness occurs.
- Because drowsiness or dizziness may occur, advise patient to use caution when driving or performing other potentially hazardous activities.
- Advise patient to consult physician before self-medicating with OTC agents (e.g., cough, cold, hayfever, or diet medications).
- Advise patient to avoid alcohol and excessive caffeine-containing beverages and tryptophan- and tyramine-containing foods.
- Tyramine-rich foods include cheeses, yeast, meat

Common side effects in *italic*; life-threatening effects underlined; generic names in **bold**; classifications in SMALL CAPS

extracts, smoked or pickled meat, poultry, or fish, fermented sausages, and overripe fruit.

Prototype: isoproterenol, p 105

ISOETHARINE HYDROCHLORIDE

(eye-soe-eth´a-reen)

Trade names: Arm-a-Med Isoetharine, Beta-2, Bronkosol, Dey-Lute, Disorine Day-Dose Isoetharine, Dispos-a Med Isoethorine

ISOETHARINE MESYLATE

Trade names: Bronkometer
Classifications: AUTONOMIC NERVOUS SYSTEM AGENT; BETA-ADRENERGIC AGONIST (SYMPATHOMIMETIC); BRONCHODILATOR (RESPIRATORY SMOOTH MUSCLE RELAXANT)
Pregnancy: Category C

ACTIONS/PHARMACODYNAMICS Synthetic sympathomimetic stimulant with relatively rapid onset and long duration of action. Has selective affinity for $beta_2$ adrenoceptors on bronchial and selected arteriolar musculature and a lower order of affinity for $beta_1$ receptors. Produces few cardiac side effects. Relieves reversible bronchospasm and by bronchodilation facilitates expectoration of pulmonary secretions. Increases vital capacity and decreases airway resistance. May inhibit antigen-induced release of histamine.

USES Bronchial asthma and reversible bronchospasm occurring with bronchitis and emphysema.

ROUTE & DOSAGE

Bronchospasm

Adult	Inhalation	0.5–1 ml 0.5% or 0.5 ml 1% solution diluted 1:3 with normal saline, *or* 2–4 ml 0.125% solution undiluted, *or* 2–5 ml 0.2% solution undiluted, *or* 2 ml 0.25% solution undiluted per nebulizer q4h up to 5 times/d
		1–2 inhalations from a metered dose inhaler (MDI) q4h up to 5 times/d

PHARMACOKINETICS Onset: immediate. **Peak effect:** 5–15 min. **Duration:** 1–4 h. **Metabolism:** metabo-

lized in lungs, liver, GI tract, and other tissues. **Elimination:** excreted by kidneys.

CONTRAINDICATIONS & PRECAUTIONS Contraindicated in: known hypersensitivity to sympathomimetic amines and to bisulfites; concomitant use with epinephrine or other sympathomimetic amines; patients with preexisting cardiac arrhythmias associated with tachycardia. Use during pregnancy (category C) and by nursing mothers requires judgment of risk/benefit ratio. **Cautious use in:** elderly patients; hypertension, acute coronary artery disease, CHF, cardiac asthma; hyperthyroidism, diabetes mellitus; tuberculosis; history of seizures.

ADVERSE/SIDE EFFECTS *Tachycardia, palpitations,* changes in BP, <u>cardiac arrest</u>; nausea, vomiting; headache, *anxiety,* tension, restlessness, insomnia, *tremor,* weakness, dizziness, excitement; cough, bronchial irritation and edema; tachyphylaxis.

DRUG INTERACTIONS Epinephrine, other SYMPATHOMIMETIC BRONCHODILATORS possibly have additive effects; MAO INHIBITORS, TRICYCLIC ANTIDEPRESSANTS potentiate action on vascular system; effects of both BETA-ADRENERGIC BLOCKERS and isoetharine antagonized.

NURSING IMPLICATIONS

Administration

- Patient should administer drug on arising in morning and before meals to reduce fatigue from activity by improving lung ventilation.
- Instruct patient to wait 1 full min after initial 1 or 2 inhalations (Bronkometer) to be sure of necessity for another dose. Action should begin immediately and peak within 5–15 min.
- *Oxygen aerosolization:* special recommendations for administration are that oxygen flow rate be 4–6 L/min over 15–20 min. *IPPB:* inspiratory flow rate of 15 L/min at cycling pressure of 15 cm H_2O. Highly individualized.
- Isoetharine inhalation may be alternated with epinephrine administration but may not be administered simultaneously because of danger of excessively rapid heartbeat.
- Do not use discolored or precipitated solutions.
- Protect solutions from light, freezing, and heat. Store at 15–30C (59–86F).

Assessment & Drug Effects

- The preservative sodium bisulfite is in the hydrochloride formulation. If patient has a history of allergy to sulfite agents, this product should not be used. Symptoms of throat irritation, hives, itching, chest tightness, and wheezing following nebulized drug suggest an allergy.

- Elderly patients may be especially sensitive to adrenergic drug effects. Monitor cardiac status and report tachycardia and palpitations.

Patient & Family Education

- Warn patient to keep spray away from eyes by closing eyes when actuating the nebulizer.
- Caution patient to use inhalation therapy according to prescribed regimen. Overuse because of inadequate relief may decrease desired effect and cause symptoms including tachycardia, palpitations, headache, nausea, dizziness.
- Information and instructions are furnished with the aerosol form of isoetharine. Urge patient to read and ask questions if necessary. Supervise first use of nebulizer.
- Urge patient to increase daily fluid intake to aid in liquefaction of bronchial secretions.
- For unknown reasons, paradoxical airway resistance (manifested by sudden increase in dyspnea) may occur with repeated excessive use. Should this occur, instruct patient and family to discontinue isoetharine and report to physician.
- Remind patient not to discard drug applicator. Refill units are available.

Prototype: pilocarpine, p 209

ISOFLUROPHATE

(eye-soe-flure´oh-fate)
Trade name: Floropryl
Classifications: EYE PREPARATION; MIOTIC; ANTIGLAUCOMA AGENT
Pregnancy: Category C

ACTIONS/PHARMACODYNAMICS Long-acting irreversible anticholinesterase with potent miotic effect. After topical application to conjunctival sac, isoflurophate strongly contracts iris sphincter and ciliary muscles, producing pupil constriction (miosis), reduced intraocular pressure (IOP), and increased aqueous humor outflow. Decreases activity of extraocular muscles of convergence, dilates blood vessels of iris, ciliary body, and conjunctiva, and increases premeability of blood-aqueous barrier. Tolerance to isoflurophate may develop.

USES Primary open-angle glaucoma, conditions that obstruct aqueous outflow, e.g., synechial formation; after iridectomy; accommodative convergent strabismus.

ROUTE & DOSAGE

Glaucoma

Adult	Topical	0.5 cm (1/4 in) strip of ointment in conjunctival sac q8–72h

Strabismus

Adult	Topical	0.5 cm (1/4 in) strip of ointment in conjunctival sac of each eye at bedtime for 2 wk; when accommodative factor is evident, decrease frequency to q2–7d for 2 wk

PHARMACOKINETICS Absorption: poor penetration of intact cornea. **Onset:** 5–10 min. **Peak:** 15–20 min. **Duration:** 1–4 wk. **Metabolism:** inactivated by cholinesterases in tissues.

CONTRAINDICATIONS & PRECAUTIONS Contraindicated in: hypersensitivity to components of formulation; vagotonia, active uveal inflammation; glaucoma associated with iridocyclitis; angle-closure (narrow-angle) glaucoma. Safe use during pregnancy not established. **Cautious use in:** corneal abrasion, history of detached retina; exposure to organophosphate-type insecticides and pesticides; bronchial asthma; peptic ulcer; epilepsy, parkinsonism; pronounced bradycardia and hypotension, recent MI; patient with myasthenia gravis who is receiving cholinesterase-inhibitor therapy.

ADVERSE/SIDE EFFECTS Eye: *stinging, burning, lacrimation,* lid muscle twitching, conjunctival and ciliary redness, visual blurring, iris cysts, <u>retinal detachment</u>, activation of latent iritis or uveitis; browache, headache. Prolonged use: conjunctival thickening, nasolacrimal canal obstruction, lens opacity. **Systemic effects:** nausea, vomiting, abdominal cramps, salivation, diarrhea; urinary incontinence, diaphoresis, muscle weakness, cardiac arrhythmias, respiratory difficulty, <u>shock</u>.

DRUG INTERACTIONS CORTICOSTEROIDS, ANTIHISTAMINES, **meperidine,** TRICYCLIC ANTIDEPRESSANTS, ADRENERGIC AGONISTS may antagonize miotic or ocular hypotensive effects; **epinephrine** (topical), **timolol** (topical), CARBONIC ANHYDRASE INHIBITORS increase IOP lowering effects; **ambenonium, physostigmine, succinylcholine** add to systemic effects.

NURSING IMPLICATIONS

Administration

- Administer dose with patient in supine position. Instruct patient to close (not squeeze) eyes after administration. Apply ointment at bedtime to lessen problem of blurred vision.
- Keep ointment tube tightly closed between treatments to prevent absorption of moisture and consequent loss of potency.
- Avoid wetting tip or touching tip of tube of medication to eyelid, cornea, or any other wet surface. In the presence of water, isoflurophate hydrolyzes to hydrogen fluoride, a vapor that is irritating to eyes and mucous membranes.
- This drug is extremely potent; it should be handled and given only by a person familiar with its use and thoroughly indoctrinated in application technique.
- Store at 15–30C (59–86F) in tightly closed tube unless otherwise directed.

Assessment & Drug Effects

- Iris cysts occur most frequently in children. They may be asymptomatic but can enlarge to the point of obscuring vision. Eyes should be examined at regular intervals for early detection of cysts. Usually iris cysts shrink when isoflurophate is discontinued.
- During initial isoflurophate treatment for glaucoma a decrease in IOP should occur within a few hours. Patient is usually kept under supervision during this time, and examinations are performed every hour for 3–4 h to be certain that a sharp rise in pressure does not occur.
- After long-term use, blood vessels of eyes dilate, and permeability increases. The danger of hyphemia (blood in anterior eye chamber) during ocular surgery is high; therefore drug use should be discontinued immediately before surgery.
- Routine examinations should be scheduled during long-term therapy to rule out development of lens opacities.

Patient & Family Education

- Primary efforts should be placed on preventing overdosage, especially in children. Be certain patient is aware of the importance of taking isoflurophate exactly as prescribed. Warn parent not to omit, increase, decrease, or skip doses without advice of the physician. Too much drug leading to excess miosis can impair vision and have systemic effects.
- If tolerance develops, another miotic may be used for a short while; then isoflurophate treatment can be resumed.

- Miotics and the preservatives in miotic preparations could be absorbed by soft contact lenses. Check with ophthalmologist about removal of lenses before applying the miotic.
- Warn patient to consult physician promptly and to discontinue treatment if visual acuity or visual fields diminish.
- Users of isoflurophate, especially the elderly, should not drive at night because of drug-induced spasm of accommodative muscles and poor vision in dim light.

ISONIAZID

See ANTIINFECTIVE, ANTITUBERCULOSIS AGENT prototype, p 83.

Prototype: atropine, p 116

ISOPROPAMIDE IODIDE

(i-so-pro´-pa-mide)
Trade names: Darbid
Classifications: AUTONOMIC NERVOUS SYSTEM AGENT; ANTICHOLINERGIC (PARASYMPATHOLYTIC); ANTIMUSCARINIC; ANTISPASMODIC
Pregnancy: Category C

ACTIONS/PHARMACODYNAMICS Synthetic antimuscarinic, anticholinergic that inhibits vagal activity, thus producing gastric acid antisecretory activity and inhibition of GI motility.

USES Adjunct therapy in treatment of peptic ulcers and irritable bowel syndrome; in conjunction with an H_2-receptor antagonist in the treatment of Zollinger-Ellison syndrome.

ROUTE & DOSAGE

Adjunct for Peptic Ulcer Disease

Adult	PO	5 mg q12h; may increase up to 10 mg b.i.d.

PHARMACOKINETICS Absorption: incompletely absorbed from GI tract. **Duration:** 10–12 h. **Elimination:** excreted in urine; unabsorbed drug excreted in feces.

Common side effects in *italic*; life-threatening effects underlined; generic names in **bold**; classifications in SMALL CAPS

685

CONTRAINDICATIONS & PRECAUTIONS Contraindicated in: allergies to iodine, glaucoma, obstructive uropathy, GI obstructive disease, paralytic ileus, intestinal atony, severe ulcerative colitis, toxic megacolon, myasthenia gravis, unstable cardiovascular status. **Cautious use in:** heart disease, elderly, autonomic neuropathy, hyperthyroidism, hypertension, prostatic hypertrophy, reflex esophagitis, nursing mothers, and pregnancy (category C).

ADVERSE/SIDE EFFECTS CNS: headache, nervousness, drowsiness, weakness, dizziness, depression, insomnia, mental confusion or excitement, especially in geriatric patients. **CV:** *palpitations, tachycardia,* hypotension. **Eye:** blurred vision, mydriasis. **GI:** *xerostomia,* loss of taste, *constipation,* nausea, vomiting. **GU:** anhidrosis, urinary hesitancy and retention. **Skin:** anaphylaxis, urticaria, rash. **Overdosage:** curariform neuromuscular block and ganglionic blockage manifested by respiratory paralysis.

DRUG INTERACTIONS Amantadine, ANTIHISTAMINES, TRICYCLIC ANTIDEPRESSANTS, **quinidine, disopyramide, procainamide** add to anticholinergic effects; decreases **levodopa** effects; **methotrimeprazine** may precipitate extrapyramidal effects; decreases antipsychotic effects (decreased absorption) of PHENOTHIAZINES.

NURSING IMPLICATIONS

Administration
- May delay absorption of other drugs given concurrently; therefore plan drug regimen accordingly.
- Give 30 min to 1 h before a meal to minimize interference with digestion.
- May contribute to the problem of urinary retention. Have patient void before giving drug.
- Discontinue 1 wk before thyroid function studies.
- Store in a tight, light-resistant container.

Assessment & Drug Effects
- Monitor heart rate prior to administration and withhold the drug if patient develops tachycardia.
- Drug should be administered with great caution to patient with inflammatory bowel disease; drug may cause paralytic ileus and subsequent toxic megacolon.
- Monitor I&O, especially in older patients and patients who have had surgery.
- May contribute to problem of urinary retention. Palpate lower abdomen for bladder distension.
- If constipation is a problem, check for abdominal distension and auscultate for bowel sounds. Drug may cause a paralytic ileus.

- Monitor patient's vital signs carefully, especially pulse for cardiac arrhythmias. Be alert to changes in quality, rate, and rhythm of pulse.
- Geriatric and debilitated patients sometimes manifest drowsiness or CNS depression with usual doses of drug. In addition to dosage adjustment, side rails and supervision of ambulation may be indicated.

Patient & Family Education
- Advise patient not to take medication if he or she is allergic to iodine.
- Advise patient that drug may increase incidence of fever and risk of heat stroke because it decreases sweating.
- Since drug may produce drowsiness and blurred vision, advise patient not to perform activities requiring mental alertness, such as operating a motor vehicle, until reaction to drug is known.
- Advise patient that increased fluid intake and increased bulk in diet may help to overcome constipating effect of drug.

ISOPROTERENOL HYDROCHLORIDE

See AUTONOMIC NERVOUS SYSTEM AGENTS, ADRENERGIC AGONIST (SYMPATHOMIMETIC), BETA, prototype, p 105.

Prototype: mannitol, p 200

ISOSORBIDE
(eye-soe-sor´bide)
Trade name: Ismotic
Classifications: OSMOTIC DIURETIC; EYE PREPARATION; ANTIGLAUCOMA
Pregnancy: Category B

ACTIONS/PHARMACODYNAMICS Actions similar to those of other osmotic agents, e.g., mannitol, but produces greater diuresis and does not cause hyperglycemia. Reduces intraocular pressure (IOP) by increasing plasma osmotic pressure. Commercial preparation contains sodium 105 mEq and potassium 34 mEq.

USES Short-term emergency treatment of acute angle-closure glaucoma and for reducing IOP before and after surgery for glaucoma and cataract.

Common side effects in *italic*; life-threatening effects underlined; generic names in **bold**; classifications in SMALL CAPS

ROUTE & DOSAGE

Acute Angle-closure Glaucoma

Adult PO 1–3 g/kg b.i.d. to q.i.d.

PHARMACOKINETICS Absorption: readily absorbed from GI tract. **Onset:** 30 min. **Peak:** 1–1.5 h. **Duration:** up to 5–6 h. **Elimination:** eliminated unchanged in urine.

CONTRAINDICATIONS & PRECAUTIONS Contraindicated in: hypersensitivity to isosorbide; severe renal disease, anuria; severe dehydration; frank or impending pulmonary edema; hemorrhagic glaucoma. Safe use during pregnancy (category B) not established. **Cautious use in:** diseases associated with sodium retention.

ADVERSE/SIDE EFFECTS CNS: *headache,* lethargy, vertigo, dizziness, lightheadedness, syncope, *confusion, disorientation,* irritability. **GI:** *nausea, vomiting,* diarrhea, anorexia, gastric discomfort. **Other:** thirst, hiccups, rash, hypernatremia, hyperosmolality.

NURSING IMPLICATIONS

Administration
- Isosorbide may be more palatable if poured over cracked ice and sipped.
- Apply gentle pressure to lacrimal sac during and immediately following drug instillation for about 1 min to lessen possibility of systemic absorption.

Assessment & Drug Effects
- Ensure that patient's bladder is empty before surgery since drug causes diuresis.
- Fluid and electrolyte balance should be carefully maintained with repeated doses.
- Monitor I&O. Report oliguria or significant changes in I&O ratio.

Patient & Family Education
- The patient should understand that therapy for glaucoma is prolonged and that adherence to established regimen is crucial to prevent blindness.
- Advise patient to keep follow-up appointments.

Prototype: nitroglycerin, p 149

ISOSORBIDE DINITRATE

(eye-soe-sor´bide)

Trade names: Coronex, Dilatrate-SR, Iso-Bid, Isonate, Isordil, Isotrate, Novosorbide, Onset, Sorate, Sorbide, Sorbitrate, Sorbitrate SA
Classifications: CARDIOVASCULAR AGENT; NITRATE VASODILATOR
Pregnancy: Category C

ACTIONS/PHARMACODYNAMICS Organic nitrate with pharmacologic actions similar to those of nitroglycerin. Mechanism of action not specifically understood. Relaxes vascular smooth muscle with resulting vasodilation. Dilation of peripheral blood vessels tends to cause peripheral pooling of blood, decreased venous return to heart, and decreased left ventricular end-diastolic pressure, with consequent reduction in myocardial oxygen consumption. Cross tolerance with other nitrates is possible.

USES Relief of acute anginal attacks and for management of long-term angina pectoris. **Unlabeled uses:** alone or in combination with a cardiac glycoside or with other vasodilators, e.g., hydralazine, prazosin, for refractory CHF; diffuse esophageal spasm without gastroesophageal reflux and heart failure.

ROUTE & DOSAGE

Angina Prophylaxis

Adult PO Regular tablets: 2.5–30 mg q.i.d. a.c. and h.s.

Sublingual tablet: 2.5–10 mg q4–6h

Chewable tablet: 5–30 mg chewed q2–3h

Sustained-release tablets: 40 mg q6–12h

Acute Anginal Attack

Adult PO Sublingual tablet: 2.5–10 mg q2–3h prn

Chewable tablet: 5–30 mg chewed prn for relief

PHARMACOKINETICS Absorption: significant first pass metabolism with PO absorption, with 50–60% reaching systemic circulation. **Onset:** 2–5 min SL; within 1 h regular tabs; within 3 min chewable tabs; 30 min sustained-release tabs. **Duration:** 1–2 h SL; 4–6

Common side effects in *italic*; life-threatening effects <u>underlined</u>; generic names in **bold**; classifications in SMALL CAPS

687

h regular tabs; 0.5–2 h chewable tabs; 6–12 h sustained-release tabs. **Metabolism:** metabolized in liver. **Elimination:** 80–100% excreted in urine within 24 h.

CONTRAINDICATIONS & PRECAUTIONS Contraindicated in: hypersensitivity to nitrates or nitrites; severe anemia; head trauma; increased intracranial pressure. Safe use during pregnancy (category C) and in nursing mothers not established. **Cautious use in:** glaucoma, hypotension, hyperthyroidism.

ADVERSE/SIDE EFFECTS CNS: *headache,* dizziness, weakness, *lightheadedness,* restlessness. **CV:** palpitation, postural hypotension, tachycardia. **GI:** nausea, vomiting. **Skin:** *flushing,* pallor, perspiration, rash, exfoliative dermatitis. **Other:** hypersensitivity reaction, paradoxical increase in anginal pain, methemoglobinemia (overdose).

DRUG INTERACTIONS Alcohol may enhance hypotensive effects and lead to cardiovascular collapse; ANTIHYPERTENSIVE AGENTS, PHENOTHIAZINES add to hypotensive effects.

NURSING IMPLICATIONS

Administration

- Not to be confused with isosorbide, an oral osmotic diuretic.
- Regular oral forms are best taken on an empty stomach (1 h a.c. or 2 h p.c.). If patient complains of vascular headache, however, it may be taken with meals.
- Advise patient not to eat, drink, talk, or smoke while sublingual tablet is under tongue.
- Instruct patient to place sublingual tablet under tongue at first sign of an anginal attack. If pain is not relieved, repeat dose at 5–10 min intervals to a maximum of 3 doses. If pain continues, notify physician or go to nearest hospital emergency room.
- Chewable tablet must be thoroughly chewed before it is swallowed.
- Sustained-release forms should be swallowed whole and not crushed or chewed.
- Patient should be sitting when taking rapid-acting forms of isosorbide dinitrate (sublingual and chewable tablets) because of the possibility of faintness.
- Store in tightly closed container in a cool, dry place, preferably at 15–30C (59–86F) unless otherwise directed. Do not expose to extremes of temperature.

Assessment & Drug Effects

- Monitor effectiveness of drug in relieving angina.
- Headaches tend to decrease in intensity and frequency with continued therapy but may require administration of analgesic and reduction in dosage.
- Chronic administration of large doses may produce tolerance and thus decrease effectiveness of nitrate preparations.

Patient & Family Education

- Caution patient to make position changes slowly, particularly from recumbent to upright posture, and to dangle feet and ankles before ambulating.
- Instruct patient to lie down at the first indication of lightheadedness or faintness.
- Therapeutic effectiveness of isosorbide dinitrate may be evaluated by having patient keep a record of anginal attacks and the number of sublingual tablets required to provide relief.
- Advise patient not to drink alcohol because it may increase possibility of lightheadedness and faintness.

ISOTRETINOIN

See SKIN AGENT, ANTIACNE (RETINOID) prototype, p 253.

Prototype: isoproterenol, p 105

ISOXSUPRINE HYDROCHLORIDE
(eye-sox´syoo-preen)
Trade names: Vasodilan, Voxsuprine
Classifications: AUTONOMIC NERVOUS SYSTEM AGENT; BETA-ADRENERGIC AGONIST; CARDIOVASCULAR AGENT; VASODILATOR
Pregnancy: Category C

ACTIONS/PHARMACODYNAMICS Sympathomimetic with beta-adrenergic stimulant activity and with slight effect on alpha receptors. Action is not blocked by propranolol (a beta-adrenergic blocker), suggesting that isoxuprine acts directly on vascular smooth muscle. Vasodilating action on arteries within skeletal muscles is greater than on cutaneous vessels. Also causes cardiac stimulation (increases cardiac contractility, rate, and output) and may produce bronchodilation, mild inhibition of GI motility, and uterine relaxation by direct action on smooth muscles. At high doses inhibits platelet aggregation and lowers blood viscosity.

USES Adjunctive therapy in treatment of cerebral vascular insufficiency and peripheral vascular disease, such as arteriosclerosis obliterans, thromboangitis obliterans (Buerger's disease), and Ray-naud's disease. **Unlabeled uses:** dysmenorrhea and threatened abortion and premature labor, but efficacy has not been established.

ROUTE & DOSAGE

Cerebral Vascular Insufficiency, Peripheral Vascular Disease
Adult   PO   10–20 mg t.i.d. or q.i.d.

PHARMACOKINETICS Absorption: readily absorbed from GI tract. **Peak:** 1 h. **Duration:** 3 h. **Distribution:** crosses placenta. **Metabolism:** metabolized in blood. **Elimination:** half-life: 1.25 h; excreted in urine.

CONTRAINDICATIONS & PRECAUTIONS Contraindicated in: immediately postpartum; presence of arterial bleeding; parenteral use in presence of hypotension, tachycardia. Safe use in pregnancy (category C) not established. **Cautious use in:** bleeding disorders; severe cerebrovascular disease, severe obliterative coronary artery disease, recent MI.

ADVERSE/SIDE EFFECTS CV: flushing, orthostatic hypotension with lightheadedness, faintness; palpitation, tachycardia. **CNS:** dizziness, nervousness, trembling, weakness. **GI:** nausea, vomiting, abdominal distress, abdominal distension. **Other:** severe rash, chest pain.

NURSING IMPLICATIONS

Administration

- Do not give isoxsuprine immediately after delivery, since it causes uterine relaxation, or in the presence of arterial bleeding.
- Store in tight containers at 15–30C (59–86F) unless otherwise directed.

Assessment & Drug Effects

- May cause hypotension and tachycardia. Monitor BP and pulse. Supervise ambulation.
- If isoxsuprine has been used to delay premature labor, hypotension and irregular and rapid heart-

beat may be observed in both mother and baby. Hypocalcemia, hypoglycemia, and ileus have been observed in babies born of mothers taking isoxsuprine.
- Therapeutic response to isoxsuprine in treatment of peripheral vascular disorders may take several weeks. Evaluate clinical manifestations of arterial insufficiency: pain with walking (intermittent claudication), rest pain, sensations of numbness, coldness, burning; weak or absent peripheral pulses, rapid blanching when legs are elevated; rubor (cyanosis or dusky skin color) in dependent position. Keep physician informed.

Patient & Family Education

- Advise patient to report adverse reactions (skin rash, palpitation, flushing) promptly; symptoms are usually effectively controlled by dosage reduction or discontinuation of drug.
- To prevent orthostatic hypotension, instruct patient to make position changes slowly and in stages, particularly from recumbent to upright posture and to avoid standing still.
- For treatment of menstrual cramps, isoxsuprine is usually started 1–3 d before onset of menstruation and continued until pain is relieved or menstrual flow stops.
- Prescribed adjuncts to drug therapy may include support hose, elevation of head of bed with 10–15 cm (4–6 in) blocks to relieve rest pain (by enhancing blood flow to extremities); Buerger-Allen exercises; graduated exercise program to develop collateral blood supply.

Prototype: gentamicin, p 53

KANAMYCIN

(kan-a-mye´sin)
Trade names: Anamid, Kantrex, Klebcil
Classifications: ANTIINFECTIVE; ANTIBIOTIC, AMINOGLYCOSIDE
Pregnancy: Category D

ACTIONS/PHARMACODYNAMICS Broadspectrum, aminoglycoside antibiotic derived from *Streptomyces kanamyceticus*. Usually bacterial in action. Like other aminoglycosides, appears to inhibit protein synthesis in susceptible microorganisms by binding irreversibly to 30S ribosomal subunits. Active against many gram-negative microorganisms, espe-

K

Common side effects in *italic*; life-threatening effects <u>underlined</u>; generic names in **bold**; classifications in SMALL CAPS

689

cially *Acinetobacter, Escherichia coli, Enterobacter aerogenes, Klebsiella pneumoniae, Proteus* sp, and *Serratia marcescens.* Also effective against many strains of *Staphylococcus aureus,* but it is not the drug of choice. Inhibits growth of *Mycobacterium tuberculosis* in vitro. As with other aminoglycosides, exerts curarelike effect on neuromuscular junction. Oral kanamycin reportedly decreases serum cholesterol.

USES Orally to reduce ammonia-producing bacteria in intestinal tract, as adjunctive treatment of hepatic coma, and for preoperative bowel antisepsis; parenterally for short-term treatment of serious infections; intraperitoneally after fecal spill during surgery; as irrigation solution; and as aerosol treatment. Has been used with other drugs to treat tuberculosis in patients resistant to conventional therapy.

ROUTE & DOSAGE

Preoperative Intestinal Antisepsis

Adult	PO	1 g q1h for 4 doses, then q6h for 36–72 h

Hepatic Coma

Adult	PO	8–12 g/d in divided doses

Serious Infection

Adult	IM/IV	15 mg/kg/d in equally divided dosesq8–12h
Child	IM/IV	Same as for adult
Adult	Intraperitoneal	500 mg diluted in 20 ml sterile water instilled through wound catheter
Adult	Inhalation	250 mg diluted in 3 ml normal saline administered per nebulizer q6–12h
Adult	Irrigation	0.25% solution prn

PHARMACOKINETICS Absorption: poorly absorbed from GI tract; readily absorbed from peritoneal cavity, bronchial tree, and wounds. **Peak:** 1–2 h. **Distribution:** crosses placenta; distributed into breast milk. **Elimination:** half-life: 2–4 h; 80–90% excreted in urine within 24 h.

CONTRAINDICATIONS & PRECAUTIONS Contraindicated in: history of hypersensitivity to kanamycin or other aminoglycosides; history of drug-induced ototoxicity, preexisting hearing loss, vertigo, or tinnitus; long-term therapy; PO use in intestinal obstruction or ulcerative bowel lesions; intraperitoneally to patients under effects of inhalation anes-

thetics or skeletal muscle relaxants. Safe use during pregnancy (category D) and in nursing women not established. **Cautious use in:** impaired renal function; elderly patients, neonates, and infants (immature renal systems); myasthenia gravis; parkinsonian syndrome.

ADVERSE/SIDE EFFECTS Dose related: **CNS:** dizziness, circumoral and other paresthesias, optic neuritis, peripheral neuritis, headache, restlessness, tremors, lethargy, convulsions; rarely: neuromuscular paralysis, respiratory depression. **ENT:** *ototoxicity:* deafness (can be irreversible), *tinnitus, vertigo* or *dizziness,* ataxia, nystagmus. **GI:** nausea, vomiting, diarrhea, appetite changes, abdominal discomfort, stomatitis, proctitis, malabsorption syndrome (with prolonged oral administration). **Hematologic:** anemia, increased or decreased reticulocytes, granulocytopenia, agranulocytosis, thrombocytopenia, purpura. **Hypersensitivity:** eosinophilia, maculopapular rash, pruritus, urticaria, drug fever, anaphylaxis. **Renal:** nephrotoxicity; hematuria, urine casts and cells, proteinuria; elevated serum creatinine and BUN, acute tubular necrosis (rare). **Other:** superinfections; local pain; nodular formation at injection site. See gentamicin for other possible adverse/side effects.

DRUG INTERACTIONS Amphotericin B, cisplatin, methoxyflurane, vancomycin add to nephrotoxicity; GENERAL ANESTHETICS, SKELETAL MUSCLE RELAXANTS add to neuromuscular blocking effects; **capreomycin** compounds ototoxicity and nephrotoxicity; LOOP AND THIAZIDE DIURETICS may increase risk of ototoxicity.

INCOMPATIBILITIES Solution/Additive: cephalothin, cephapirin, chlorpheniramine, colistimethate, heparin, hydrocortisone, methohexital, ampicillin, carbenicillin, methicillin, penicillin, mezlocillin, piperacillin. Y-Site: heparin, methohexital.

NURSING IMPLICATIONS

Administration

- PO kanamycin can be taken on a full or empty stomach.
- Administer IM injection deep into upper outer quadrant of gluteal muscle (often painful). Observe sites daily for signs of irritation; rotate injection sites.
- *Preparation of IV infusion:* each 500 mg must be diluted with at least 100 to 200 ml 0.9% NaCl or 5%

K

dextrose injection and administered over 30–60 min. Physician will prescribe the specific flow rate (usually does not exceed 3 or 4 ml/min).

- Kanamycin should not be mixed with other drugs.
- Kanamycin is stable for 24 h at room temperature in most IV solutions. Consult manufacturer's literature for storage and compatibility information.
- Store unopened vials and capsules at 15–30C (59–86F) unless otherwise directed. Some vials may darken with time, but this does not affect potency.

Assessment & Drug Effects

- Culture and susceptibility studies should be performed before initiation of therapy and periodically thereafter.
- Baseline weight, vital signs, urinalysis, and kidney function tests should be assessed before and at regular intervals during therapy.
- Monitoring of peak and trough serum kanamycin concentrations is advised, especially in patients with impaired renal function and the elderly. Generally peak concentrations above 30 µg/ml are not recommended; trough concentrations should not exceed 5–10 µg/ml.
- Blood specimens for peak kanamycin concentrations are generally drawn 30–60 min after IM administration and 30 min after completion of a 30–60 min IV infusion. For trough levels, blood specimens are drawn just before the next IM or IV dose.
- Parenteral kanamycin is highly concentrated in the urinary system; patient should be well hydrated to prevent chemical irritation of renal tubules.
- Monitor I&O. Report decrease in urine output or change in I&O ratio.
- Check urinalysis and kidney function and notify physician immediately of signs of renal irritation: albuminuria, casts, red and white cells in urine, increasing NPN, BUN, and serum creatinine, decreasing urine specific gravity, and creatinine clearance, oliguria, and edema.
- Risk of ototoxicity is high in patients with impaired renal function, the elderly, poorly hydrated patients, and when therapy is expected to last ≥5 d.
- Patient should be monitored for hearing and balance problems. Kanamycin-induced ototoxicity is greatest in the auditory branch of the eighth cranial (acoustic) nerve. ***Symptoms of auditory branch involvement:*** tinnitus, roaring or sensation of fullness in ears, hearing impairment. High-frequency deafness, detected only by audiometry, occurs first. ***Symptoms of vestibular branch involvement:*** headache, vertigo or dizziness, nystagmus, ataxia, and nausea and vomiting with motion. Drug should be stopped if ototoxicity occurs.

- Tinnitus is not a reliable index of ototoxicity in the very old.
- In patients with impaired renal function, deafness has occurred 2–7 d or more after termination of therapy.
- Patients receiving kanamycin in the immediate postoperative period should be closely monitored for neuromuscular blockade (muscle weakness, apnea, and respiratory depression).
- Be alert to signs of superinfection (see chap 3).

Patient & Family Education

- In treatment of urinary tract infections, physician may prescribe concomitant administration of an alkalinizing agent or patient may be advised to omit foods that enhance urine acidity, e.g., prunes and prune juice, cranberries and cranberry juice.
- Advise patient to report ototoxic symptoms.

Prototype: diphenoxylate with atropine, p 213

KAOLIN AND PECTIN

(kay´oh-lin and pek´tin)
Trade names: Kaopectate, Kao-tin, Kapectolin, Kaypectol, K P, K Pek, Pecto Kay
Classifications: GI AGENT; ANTIDIARRHEAL
Pregnancy: Category C

ACTIONS/PHARMACODYNAMICS Kaolin (sometimes called porcelain clay) is native hydrated aluminum silicate, powdered and freed from impurities for pharmaceutical use. Pectin is purified carbohydrate obtained by acid extraction of the inner rind of citrus fruits or apple pomace. Kaolin is reported to have adsorbent, protectant, and demulcent properties. Pectin's mechanism of action is unknown; it is believed to act as an adsorbent and demulcent and may help consolidate stool. Efficacy of kaolin or pectin in diarrhea is not clearly established.

USES Adjunct in symptomatic treatment of mild to moderately severe acute diarrhea. Commonly used in antidiarrheal combination products.

PHARMACOKINETICS Absorption: not absorbed from GI tract.

CONTRAINDICATIONS & PRECAUTIONS Contraindicated in: suspected obstructive bowel lesion, pseudomembranous colitis, diarrhea associated with

Common side effects in *italic*; life-threatening effects underlined; generic names in **bold**; classifications in SMALL CAPS

691

ROUTE & DOSAGE

Diarrhea

Adult	PO	60–120 ml of regular suspension *or* 45–90 ml of concentrated suspension after each loose bowel movement
Child	PO	3–5 y: 15–30 ml regular suspension *or* 15 ml concentrated suspension after each loose bowel movement
		6–11 y: 30–60 ml regular suspension *or* 30 ml concentrated suspension after each loose bowel movement
		≥ 12 y: 60 ml regular suspension *or* 45 ml concentrated suspension after each loose bowel movement

bacterial toxins; presence of fever; use for more than 48 h without medical direction. Safe use during pregnancy (category C) and breast feeding not established. **Cautious use in:** infants or children ≤ 3 y, elderly patients.

ADVERSE/SIDE EFFECTS Constipation usually mild and transient; fecal impaction (rare).

DRUG INTERACTIONS Chloroquine, digoxin, penicillamine, tetracycline, ciprofloxacin, and most other drugs, since it may decrease absorption of any orally administered medication. Administer at least 2–4 h before other oral medications.

NURSING IMPLICATIONS

Administration
- Shake suspension well before pouring.
- Store in tightly closed container at 15–30C (59–86F) unless otherwise directed. Protect from freezing.

Assessment & Drug Effects
- Assess for abdominal distension, number of stools per day.
- Be aware that fecal impaction may result from taking kaolin and pectin, especially in the elderly.

Patient & Family Education
- Instruct patient not to exceed prescribed dosage.
- Advise patient to notify physician if diarrhea is not controlled within 48 h or if fever develops.
- Prolonged use of kaolin can interfere with normal absorption of nutrients.

K

KETAMINE HYDROCHLORIDE

(keet´a-meen)
Trade name: Ketalar
Classifications: CNS AGENT; GENERAL ANESTHETIC
Pregnancy: Category C

ACTIONS/PHARMACODYNAMICS Rapid-acting phencyclidine derivative. Produces profound anesthesia that may be accompanied by increase in salivary secretions, depression of pharyngeal and laryngeal reflexes, and slight stimulation of skeletal muscle tone, cardiovascular action, and increase in cerebral blood flow and intracranial pressure. Precise action mechanism unknown but is believed to be related to ability to block afferent impulses associated with affective-emotional components of pain perception. Acts primarily on cortex and limbic system, which probably accounts for emergence reactions of recovery period. (See nursing implications.) Produces "dissociative anesthesia," which describes the feeling of separation from surroundings experienced by patient. Because it does not relax skeletal muscles effectively, it is not used for intraabdominal or intrathoracic procedures unless supplemented with another inhalation anesthetic.

USES As sole anesthetic agent for diagnostic and surgical procedures of short duration that do not require skeletal muscle relaxation. Also to induce anesthesia before administration of other general anesthetics or to supplement low potency anesthetics such as nitrous oxide.

ROUTE & DOSAGE

Anesthesia

Adult	IV	1–4.5 mg/kg slowly over 60 s
	IM	6.5–13 mg/kg; half of initial dose may be repeated as needed

PHARMACOKINETICS Onset: 30 s IV; 3–8 min IM. **Duration:** 5–10 min IV; 12–25 min IM. **Distribution:** widely distributed with high concentrations in the brain, lungs, liver, and body fat; crosses placenta. **Metabolism:** metabolized in liver. **Elimination:** half-life: 2.5 h; 90% excreted in urine, 5% in feces.

CONTRAINDICATIONS & PRECAUTIONS Contraindicated in: severe hypertension, severe coronary heart disease or cardiac decompensation, increased intracranial pressure, history of cerebrovascular accident, increased intraocular pressure, psychiatric disorders; for surgery or diagnostic procedures of pharynx, larynx, and bronchial tree. Safe use during pregnancy (category C) including obstetrics not established. **Cautious use in:** thyroid replacement therapy; chronic alcoholism; convulsive disorders.

ADVERSE/SIDE EFFECTS CNS: *emergence reactions (hallucinations, delirium, confusion, excitement, irrational behavior),* dissociation, polyneuropathy, athetoid movements of mouth and tongue, muscular rigidity, fasciculations, tremors, tonic and clonic movements resembling convulsions, <u>increased intracranial pressure</u>. **CV:** *hypertension,* hypotension, tachycardia, bradycardia, arrhythmias, <u>cardiac arrest</u>. **Eye:** diplopia, nystagmus, slight increase in intraocular pressure, temporary loss of vision, lacrimation. **GI:** anorexia, nausea, vomiting, hypersalivation. **Respiratory:** <u>respiratory depression, apnea, laryngospasm</u>. **Other:** transient erythema, skin rashes, local pain and irritation at injection site.

DRUG INTERACTIONS BARBITURATES, NARCOTICS may prolong recovery time; **halothane** decreases cardiac output, BP, and pulse; **tubocurarine** and other NONDEPOLARIZING MUSCLE RELAXANTS prolong respiratory depression; THYROID HORMONES may cause hypertension and tachycardia.

INCOMPATIBILITIES Solution/Additive: BARBITURATES, **diazepam, doxapram.**

NURSING IMPLICATIONS

Administration

- Dilute IV ketamine (100 mg/ml) with an equal volume of sterile water for injection, NS, or D5W.
- Administer direct IV slowly over 60 seconds. More rapid administration may cause respiratory depression and enhance pressor response.
- Ketamine should be administered to a patient on NPO for at least 12 h.
- Because ketamine tends to stimulate flow of saliva, an anticholinergic ("drying agent") should be included in premedication before anesthesia.
- IV thiopental, diazepam, or a narcotic may be prescribed as premedication to control severity of symptoms associated with recovery phase.
- Manufacturer cautions not to mix barbiturates in same syringe with ketamine because a precipitate will form.

- Store at 15–30C (59–86F) unless otherwise directed. Protect from heat and light.

Assessment & Drug Effects

- Recovery from ketamine anesthesia is frequently prolonged and may be accompanied by hallucinations, vivid imagery, delirium, and "dissociative anesthesia" (the feeling of separation from surroundings).
- Severity of recovery symptoms may be reduced by allowing patient to awaken quietly with minimal amount of stimulation.
- Reactions during recovery occur most commonly in patients between the ages of 16–65 y receiving IV ketamine.
- Monitor BP and vital signs. BP may rise 10–50% or higher above preanesthetic level and may remain elevated for ≥ 15 min. Ketamine tends to increase BP, cardiac output, and pulse rate and can cause respiratory depression and apnea. These effects are more likely to occur with high doses or when IV is administered too rapidly.
- Patients with history of convulsive disorders should be closely observed for signs of apparent loss of seizure control.
- Monitor airway. Aspiration is a possibility as hypersalivation occurs commonly and laryngeal and pharyngeal reflexes may be depressed. Resuscitative equipment should be immediately available. Because nausea and vomiting are not usually severe, most patients can tolerate liquids PO shortly after consciousness is regained.
- If used in ambulatory services, patient should not be released until completely recovered from anesthesia and unless accompanied by a responsible adult. Patient should be warned to avoid driving and other potentially hazardous activities for 24 h or more after anesthesia.

K

Prototype: amphotericin B, p 56

KETOCONAZOLE
(ke-to-con´a-zol)
Trade name: Nizoral
Classifications: ANTIINFECTIVE; ANTIBIOTIC; ANTIFUNGAL
Pregnancy: Category C

ACTIONS/PHARMACODYNAMICS Synthetic imidazole derivative and broad-spectrum antifungal agent closely related to miconazole. Usually

Common side effects in *italic*; life-threatening effects <u>underlined</u>; generic names in **bold**; classifications in SMALL CAPS

693

fungistatic but may be fungicidal in high concentrations. Studies suggest mode of action involves interference with synthesis of ergosterol (an essential sterol of fungal cell membrane) with resultant increase in cell membrane permeability and ultimately inhibition of fungal growth. Ketoconazole, even in conventional doses, can cause transient blockade of testosterone synthesis and may depress adrenocortical function.

USES Orally: severe systemic fungal infections including candidiasis (e.g., oral thrush, candiduria), chronic mucocutaneous candidiasis, pulmonary and disseminated coccidioidomycosis, histoplasmosis, paracoccidioidomycosis, blastomycosis, and chromomycosis. **Unlabeled oral uses:** onychomycosis, vaginal candidiasis, Cushing's syndrome associated with adrenal or pituitary adenoma; precocious puberty, dysfunctional hirsutism, and as swish and swallow preparation for prophylaxis against fungal infections in patients with neutropenia induced by cancer chemotherapy and in patients with AIDS. **Topically:** tinea corporis and tinea cruris (caused by *Epidermophyton floccosum, Trichophyton mentagrophytes,* and *Trichophyton rubrum*) and in treatment of tinea versicolor (pityriasis) caused by *Malassezia furfur (Pityrosporum obiculare)*. **Unlabeled topical uses:** tinea pedis, tinea manum, cutaneous candidiasis, seborrheic dermatitis, psoriasis.

ROUTE & DOSAGE

Fungal Infections

Adult	PO	200–400 mg once/d
	Topical	Apply 1–2 times/d to affected area and surrounding skin
Child	PO	> 2 y: 3.3–6.6 mg/kg/d as single dose

PHARMACOKINETICS Absorption: erratically absorbed from GI tract (needs an acid pH); minimal absorption topically. **Peak:** 1–2 h. **Distribution:** distributed to saliva, urine, sebum, and cerumen; CSF levels unpredictable; distributed into breast milk. **Metabolism:** metabolized in liver. **Elimination:** half-life: 8 h; primarily excreted in feces, 13% in urine.

CONTRAINDICATIONS & PRECAUTIONS Contraindicated in: hypersensitivity to ketoconazole or to any component in the formulation; chronic alcoholism, fungal meningitis. Safe use during pregnancy (category C), in nursing mothers, and in children < 2 y not determined. **Cautious use in:** achlorhydria, history of hepatic disease.

ADVERSE/SIDE EFFECTS Systemic (PO): CNS: headache, dizziness, lethargy, drowsiness, insomnia, abnormal dreams, paresthesias, confusion, nervousness, weakness (asthenia). **GI:** *nausea, vomiting,* anorexia, epigastric or abdominal pain, constipation, diarrhea, flatulence, GI bleeding. **Hematologic:** mild leukocytopenia, thrombocytopenia, thrombocytosis; with high doses: lowering of serum testosterone and ACTH-induced corticosteroid serum levels; hyponatremia (rare), transient decreases in serum cholesterol and triglycerides. **Hepatic:** transient elevation in serum liver enzymes, hepatotoxicity, <u>fatal hepatic necrosis</u> (rare). **Hypersensitivity:** skin rash, erythema, urticaria, pruritus, angioedema, <u>anaphylaxis</u>. **Reproductive:** gynecomastia (males), breast pain; uterine bleeding, loss of libido, impotence, oligospermia, hair loss. **Other:** muscle and joint pain, fever, chills, photophobia, tinnitus, change in sweat pattern, hypothyroidism (weight gain, sluggishness, fatigue, muscle cramps); <u>acute hypoadrenalism (reduction of adrenal stress syndrome)</u>, renal hypofunction. **Topical:** mild transient erythema, severe irritation, pruritus, stinging; hypersensitivity reactions (rare): swelling, contact dermatitis.

DRUG INTERACTIONS Alcohol may cause sunburnlike reaction; ANTACIDS, ANTICHOLINERGICS, H₂-RECEPTOR ANTAGONISTS decrease ketoconazole absorption; **isoniazid, rifampin** increase ketoconazole metabolism, thus decreasing its activity; levels of **phenytoin** and ketoconazole decreased; may increase **cyclosporine** levels and toxicity; **warfarin** may potentiate hypoprothrombinemia.

NURSING IMPLICATIONS

Administration

- Nausea and vomiting occur frequently during early therapy. Measures that may help to reduce GI effects include taking ketoconazole with food and dividing daily dosage into 2 doses. Discuss with physician. Do not take with antacids.
- Give drug with water, fruit juice, coffee, or tea. However, if patient has achlorhydria or reduced gastric acidity (as with surgical intervention or in the elderly) the physician may prescribe drug to be given with diluted hydrochloric acid (HCl). Ketoconazole requires an acid medium for dissolution and absorption.
- If diluted HCl is prescribed, instruct patient to dissolve each tablet in 4 ml of 0.2N HCl solution. Add this mixture to 1–2 tsp water in glass. Sip the solution through a glass or plastic straw placed as far back of teeth as possible to avoid contact of acid

with teeth surfaces. Follow immediately with about 1/2 glass of tap water; swish solution around in mouth and swallow.

- Discuss with physician procedure for washing skin before applying topical medication.
- Store in tightly covered container at 15–30C (59–86F) unless otherwise directed.

Assessment & Drug Effects

- Report promptly to physician any seizures or symptoms suggestive of hepatotoxicity (see chap 3). Immediate discontinuation of ketoconazole is essential to prevent irreversible liver damage.
- Advise patient to refrain from driving a car or using hazardous equipment until response to the drug is known. Drowsiness and dizziness are early and time-limited side effects.
- Liver function tests—AST, ALT, alkaline phosphatase, and bilirubin—should be performed before treatment is initiated and at least monthly throughout therapy.

Patient & Family Education

- Treatment is continued until all clinical and laboratory tests indicate that fungal infection has subsided.
- Usual treatment period for candidiasis is 1–4 wk.
- Instruct patient to avoid OTC drugs for gastric distress, such as Rolaids, Tums, Alka-Seltzer and to check with physician before taking any nonprescribed medicines.
- Caution patient not to alter the dose or dose interval and not to stop taking ketoconazole before consulting the physician.
- Instruct patient to notify physician if condition fails to respond to topical medication therapy or worsens or if signs of irritation or sensitivity occur.

Prototype: ibuprofen, p 160

KETOPROFEN
(kee-toe-proe'fen)
Trade name: Orudis
Classifications: CNS AGENT; ANALGESIC; ANTIPYRETIC; NSAID
Pregnancy: Category B

ACTIONS/PHARMACODYNAMICS Nonsteroidal antiinflammatory drug structurally related to ibuprofen. Blocks prostaglandin synthesis by inhibiting cyclooxygenase, the enzyme that converts arachidonic acid to precursors of prostaglandins (cyclic endoperoxidases). Ketoprofen activity also includes modulation of T cell function, inhibition of inflammatory cell chemotaxis, and decreased release of superoxide radicals or increased scavanging of these compounds at inflammatory sites. Analgesic potency matches that of indomethacin and is stronger than that of aspirin. Inhibits platelet aggregation (returns to normal in 24–36 h after drug is discontinued) and prolongs bleeding time. Has fewer adverse GI effects than aspirin. Not associated with physical dependence, addiction, or tolerance.

USES Acute or long-term treatment of rheumatoid arthritis and osteoarthritis; primary dysmenorrhea; symptomatic relief of postoperative, dental, and postpartum pain; visceral pain associated with cancer. **Unlabeled uses:** Reiter's syndrome, juvenile arthritis, acute gouty arthritis, biliary pain, renal colic.

ROUTE & DOSAGE

Inflammatory Disease

Adult PO 75 mg t.i.d. or 50 mg q.i.d. (max 300 mg/d)

Mild to Moderate Pain, Dysmenorrhea

Adult PO 25–50 mg q6–8h

PHARMACOKINETICS Absorption: readily absorbed from GI tract. **Onset:** 1–2 h. **Peak:** 1–2 h. **Duration:** 4–6 h. **Metabolism:** metabolized in liver. **Elimination:** half-life: 1.1–4 h; excreted primarily in urine, with some biliary excretion.

CONTRAINDICATIONS & PRECAUTIONS Contraindicated in: patient in whom aspirin or other NSAID induces asthma, urticaria, bronchospasm, severe rhinitis, shock. Safe use during pregnancy (category B), in nursing mothers, or in children < 12 y not established. **Cautious use in:** history of GI disease, GI bleeding, active ulcer; renal or hepatic impairment, patient who may be adversely affected by prolongation of bleeding time; heart failure, hypertension; patient receiving diuretics; geriatric patient; myasthenia gravis.

ADVERSE/SIDE EFFECTS CNS: trouble in sleeping, nervousness, *headache, CNS excitation,* dizziness; CNS depression (drowsiness, fatigue, difficulty in concentration); amnesia, nightmares, migraine, paresthesias, vertigo. **CV:** peripheral edema, palpitations, hypertension, tachycardia, facial edema, va-

K

Common side effects in *italic*; life-threatening effects <u>underlined</u>; generic names in **bold**; classifications in SMALL CAPS

695

sodilation, postural hypotension. **Eye/ENT:** visual disturbances, conjunctivitis, eye pain, retinal hemorrhage, pigmentation changes; dry nose or throat, tinnitus, hearing impairment. **GI:** *dyspepsia,* drug-induced peptic ulcer, GI bleeding, nausea, vomiting, diarrhea, constipation, flatulence, stomach pain, anorexia, dry mouth, stomatitis, sore tongue, gingivitis, increased or excessive salivation, rectal burning and hemorrhage, melena. **Hematologic:** prolonged bleeding time, anemia, purpura, agranulocytosis, thrombocytosis. **Hepatic:** jaundice, elevated ALT, AST. **Skin:** rash, pruritus, urticaria, erythema, alopecia (infrequent), photosensitivity, sweating. **Other:** gynecomastia, changes in libido, aggravation of diabetes mellitus, laryngospasm, bronchospasm, laryngeal edema, pharyngitis, urinary tract irritation (dysuria, frequency/urgency), renal impairment.

DRUG INTERACTIONS ORAL ANTICOAGULANTS, **heparin** may prolong bleeding time; may increase **lithium** toxicity; may increase **methotrexate** toxicity.

NURSING IMPLICATIONS

Administration

- Administer capsules 30 min before or at least 2 h after meals. To reduce GI irritation, give with food, milk, or prescribed antacid.
- Store drug at 15–30C (59–86F) in tightly closed, light-resistant container unless otherwise directed.

Assessment & Drug Effects

- Both baseline and periodic evaluations of hemoglobin, renal and hepatic function, and auditory and ophthalmologic status are recommended during prolonged or high-dose therapy.
- As with other NSAIDs, the antipyretic and antiinflammatory effects of ketoprofen may mask usual signs and symptoms of infection.
- Monitor for signs and symptoms of GI ulceration (e.g., stool for occult blood, persistent indigestion).

Patient & Family Education

- Ketoprofen provides palliation not cure for rheumatoid arthritis or osteoarthritis. May be used concomitantly with gold compounds, antimalarials, or corticosteroids.
- Advise patient to report promptly signs of jaundice (see chap 3) and the following symptoms: blurred vision, tinnitus, urinary urgency or frequency, unexplained bleeding, weight gain with edema.
- Inform patient about possible CNS effects (lightheadedness, dizziness, drowsiness) and caution

against dangerous activities until reaction to the drug has been determined.
- Inform patients that alcohol and aspirin may increase risk of GI ulceration and bleeding tendencies and therefore should be avoided.
- Advise patients to tell dentist or surgeon that they are taking ketoprofen.

Prototype: ibuprofen, p 160

KETOROLAC TROMETHAMINE
(ke-tor´o-lac)
Trade name: Toradol
Classifications: CNS AGENT; ANALGESIC; ANTIPYRETIC; NSAID
Pregnancy: Category B

ACTIONS/PHARMACODYNAMICS Ketorolac exhibits analgesic, antiinflammatory, and antipyretic activity. It inhibits synthesis of prostaglandins and is a peripherally acting analgesic. Ketorolac does not have any known effects on opiate receptors.

USES Short-term management of pain.

ROUTE & DOSAGE

Adult	IM	30–60 mg loading dose, then 15–30 mg q6h; maximum recommended daily dose is 150 mg first day and 120 mg subsequent days; the lower doses (30 mg load, then 15 mg q6h) are recommended for elderly patients and patients weighing < 50 kg (110 lb)

PHARMACOKINETICS Peak: 45–60 min. **Distribution:** distributed into breast milk. **Metabolism:** metabolized in liver. **Elimination:** half-life: 4–6 h; excreted in urine.

CONTRAINDICATIONS & PRECAUTIONS Contraindicated in: hypersensitivity to ketorolac; individuals with complete or partial syndrome of nasal polyps, angioedema, and bronchiospastic reaction to aspirin or other NSAIDs; during labor and delivery. **Cautious use in:** history of peptic ulcers; impaired renal or hepatic function; elderly; pregnancy (category B) and nursing mothers. Safety and effectiveness in children has not been established.

ADVERSE/SIDE EFFECTS CNS: *drowsiness,* dizziness, headache. **GI:** *nausea,* dyspepsia, GI pain, hemorrhage. **Other:** edema, sweating, pain at injection site.

DRUG INTERACTIONS May increase **methotrexate** levels and toxicity; may increase **lithium** levels and toxicity.

NURSING IMPLICATIONS

Administration

- Reduced dosages are necessary with the elderly because of renal effects of NSAIDs.
- Injection site pain has been reported in some patients receiving multiple doses. Rotate injection sites.
- Store at 15–30C (59–86F).

Assessment & Drug Effects

- Obtain a detailed drug history before initiating therapy.
- Monitor urinalysis results. Hematuria and proteinuria have been observed with long-term use.
- Monitor urine output, which may be decreased by ketorolac in the elderly, patients with a history of renal impairment, heart failure, or liver dysfunction or who are taking diuretics. Discontinuation of drug will return urine output to pretreatment level.
- Monitor for changes in liver function studies.
- Monitor for signs and symptoms of bleeding. Ketorolac decreases platelet aggregation and thus may prolong bleeding time.
- Monitor for signs and symptoms of GI distress or bleeding including nausea, GI pain, diarrhea, melena, or hematemesis.
- Patients with a history of cardiac decompensation should be observed closely for evidence of fluid retention and edema.

Patient & Family Education

- Inform patients on long-term therapy to watch for the signs and symptoms of GI ulceration and bleeding (e.g., bloody emesis, black tarry stools).
- Inform patients about possible CNS effects (dizziness, drowsiness) and caution them to avoid dangerous activities until reaction to the drug is known.

Prototype: propranolol, p 109

LABETALOL HYDROCHLORIDE
(la-bet´a-lole)
Trade names: Normodyne, Trandate
Classifications: AUTONOMIC NERVOUS SYSTEM AGENT; ALPHA- AND BETA-ADRENERGIC ANTAGONIST (SYMPATHOLYTIC); ANTIHYPERTENSIVE
Pregnancy: Category C

ACTIONS/PHARMACODYNAMICS Adrenergic receptor blocking agent that combines selective alpha activity and nonselective beta adrenergic blocking actions. Both activities contribute to blood pressure reduction. Alpha blockade results in vasodilation, decreased peripheral resistance, and orthostatic hypotension and only slightly affects cardiac output and coronary artery blood flow. Beta blocking effects on sinus node, AV node, and ventricular muscle lead to bradycardia, delay in AV conduction, and depression of cardiac contractility. Similar to propranolol and other nonselective beta blockers in ability to decrease resting and exercise-induced heart rate but generally less than produced by those agents. Depresses plasma renin activity both at rest and during exercise. Also has weak membrane stabilizing properties at recommended doses. Does not abolish digitalis-induced inotropic action on heart muscle.

USES Mild, moderate, and severe hypertension, primarily as a step-2 drug. May be used alone or in combination with other antihypertensive agents, especially thiazide diuretics.

ROUTE & DOSAGE

Hypertension

Adult	PO	100 mg b.i.d.; may gradually increase to 200–400 mg b.i.d. (max 1200–2400 mg/d)
	IV	20 mg slowly over 2 min, with 40–80 mg q10min if needed up to 300 mg total, *or* 2 mg/min continuous infusion up to 300 mg total dose

PHARMACOKINETICS Absorption: readily absorbed from GI tract, but only 25% reaches systemic circulation because of first pass metabolism. **Onset:** 20 min–2 h PO; 2–5 min IV. **Peak:** 1–4 h PO; 5–15 min IV. **Duration:** 8–24 h PO; 2–4 h IV. **Distribution:** crosses

L

Common side effects in *italic*; life-threatening effects underlined;
generic names in **bold**; classifications in SMALL CAPS

697

placenta; distributed into breast milk. **Metabolism:** metabolized in liver. **Elimination:** half-life: 3–8 h; 60% excreted in urine, 40% in bile.

CONTRAINDICATIONS & PRECAUTIONS Contraindicated in: bronchial asthma; uncontrolled cardiac failure, heart block (greater than first degree), cardiogenic shock, severe bradycardia. Safe use during pregnancy (category C), in nursing women, and in children not established. **Cautious use in:** nonallergic bronchospastic disease (COPD), well-compensated patients with history of heart failure; pheochromocytoma; impaired hepatic function, jaundice; diabetes mellitus; peripheral vascular disease.

ADVERSE/SIDE EFFECTS CNS: dizziness, fatigue/malaise (asthenia), headache, tremors, transient paresthesias (especially scalp tingling), hypoesthesia (numbness) following IV, mental depression, drowsiness, sleep disturbances, nightmares. **CV:** *postural hypotension,* lightheadedness, angina pectoris, palpitation, bradycardia, syncope, pedal or peripheral edema, pulmonary edema, CHF, flushing, cold extremities, arrhythmias (following IV), paradoxical hypertension (patients with pheochromocytoma). **Eye:** dry eyes, vision disturbances. **GI:** nausea, vomiting, dyspepsia, constipation, diarrhea, taste disturbances, cholestasis with or without jaundice, increases in serum transaminases, dry mouth. **GU:** acute urinary retention, difficult micturition, impotence, ejaculation failure, loss of libido, Peyronie's disease. **Renal:** transient rises in BUN and serum creatinine (associated with drops in BP in patients with renal disease). **Respiratory:** dyspnea, bronchospasm. **Skin:** rashes of various types, transient scalp tingling, reversible alopecia, increased sweating, pruritus. **Other:** nasal stuffiness, rhinorrhea, myalgia, muscle cramps, toxic myopathy, antimitochondrial antibodies, positive antinuclear antibodies (ANA), SLE syndrome, pain at IV injection site.

DIAGNOSTIC TEST INTERFERENCES False increases in *urinary catecholamines* when measured by *nonspecific trihydroxyindole (THI) reaction* (due to labetalol metabolites) but not with specific radioenzymatic or high performance liquid chromatography assay techniques.

DRUG INTERACTIONS Cimetidine may increase effects of labetalol; **glutethimide** decreases effects of labetalol; **halothane** adds to hypotensive effects; may mask symptoms of hypoglycemia caused by ORAL SULFONYLUREAS, **insulin;** BETA-AGONISTS antagonize effects of labetalol.

NURSING IMPLICATIONS

Administration

- Administer PO preparation preferably with or immediately after food. Food increases drug bioavailability. Advise consistency.
- Patient should be supine when receiving labetalol IV. Take BP immediately before administration.
- Drug may be given undiluted by direct IV or further diluted in most IV solutions and administered as a continuous infusion.
- *Administration by direct IV injection:* Give a 20 mg dose slowly over 2 min. Maximum hypotensive effect occurs 5–15 min after each administration.
- *Administration by continuous IV infusion:* Rate is adjusted according to BP response. Normal rate is 2 mg/min. Once the desired BP is attained, labetalol is discontinued.
- Controlled infusion pump device is recommended for maintaining accurate flow rate during IV infusion. Physician should prescribe precise flow rate and should specify adjustments to be made according to BP response. (Usually administered at rate of 2 mg/min.)
- Store at 2–30C (36–86F) unless otherwise advised. Do not freeze. Protect tablets from moisture.

Assessment & Drug Effects

- Baseline BP readings are generally taken with patient supine after standing, and immediately after exercise. Discuss with physician.
- Monitor BP and pulse during dosage adjustment period. Standing BP is used as indicator for making dosage adjustments and for assessing patient's tolerance of dosage increases. Generally taken after patient stands for 10 min. Clarify with physician.
- *After IV administration:* (1) monitor BP at 5 min intervals for 30 min; (2) then at 30 min intervals for 2 h; (3) then hourly for about 6 h, and as indicated thereafter. PO therapy is usually started when supine diastolic pressure rises about 10 mm Hg.
- Supine position should be maintained for at least 3 h after IV administration. At the end of this time, determine patient's ability to tolerate elevated and upright positions before allowing ambulation. Manage this slowly.

Patient & Family Education

- Caution patient that postural hypotension is most likely to occur during peak plasma levels, i.e., 2–4 h after drug administration.
- Instruct patient to adopt the habit of making all position changes slowly and in stages, particularly from recumbent to upright position. Bear in mind

that elderly patients are especially sensitive to hypotensive effects (lightheadedness, dizziness). Inform patient of other measures that may help to prevent postural hypotension: (1) Lie or sit down immediately if lightheadedness occurs. (2) Use a commode or urinal at night. Suggest that men sit down to urinate. (3) Avoid extremes of environmental heat; take warm rather than hot showers or baths; avoid sunbathing. Consult physician about use of support hose.

- Since labetalol can cause dizziness and lightheadedness, advise patient to avoid potentially hazardous activities until reaction to drug is known.
- Diabetic patients should be closely monitored. Inform patient that labetalol may mask usual cardiovascular response to acute hypoglycemia, e.g., tachycardia.
- Reassure patient that most adverse effects (e.g., scalp tingling) are mild, transient, and dose related and occur early in therapy.
- Stress importance of keeping follow-up appointments. Tests of liver and renal function should be performed periodically during therapy.
- Discontinuation of labetalol after chronic administration should be done by gradual reduction of dosage over a 1–2 wk period. Patient should be closely monitored and advised to restrict physical activity during this time. Patients with coronary artery disease should be told beforehand by physician what to do if anginal pain is experienced. (Generally, labetalol is reinstituted promptly.) In addition to angina, abrupt discontinuation of labetalol can result in acute MI.

LACTULOSE

(lak´tyoo-lose)

Trade name: Cephulac, Chronulac
Classifications: GI AGENT; HYPEROSMOTIC LAXATIVE
Pregnancy: Category C

ACTIONS/PHARMACODYNAMICS Synthetic disaccharide derivative of lactose. Commercially available preparations contain galactose (< 2.2 g/15 ml), lactose (< 1.2 g/15 ml), and other sugars (1.2 g). Action in reducing blood ammonia appears to involve metabolism of lactose to organic acids by resident intestinal bacteria. The result is acidification of colon contents, which retards diffusion of nonionic ammonia (NH_3) from colon to blood while promoting its migration from blood to colon. In the acidic colon, NH_3 is converted to nonabsorbable ammonia ions (NH_4) and is then expelled in feces by laxative action. Osmotic effect of organic acids causes laxative action, which moves water from plasma to intestines, softens stools, and stimulates peristalsis by pressure from stool water content.

USES Prevention and treatment of portal-systemic encephalopathy (PSE), including stages of hepatic precoma and coma, and by prescription for relief of chronic constipation. **Unlabeled uses:** to restore regular bowel habit posthemorrhoidectomy; to evacuate bowel in elderly patients with severe constipation after barium studies; and for treatment of chronic constipation in children.

ROUTE & DOSAGE

Prevention and Treatment of Portal-Systemic Encephalopathy

Adult	PO	30–45 ml t.i.d. or q.i.d. adjusted to produce 2 or 3 soft stools/d
Child	PO	Infant: 2.5–10 ml/d in divided doses adjusted to produce 2–3 soft stools/d
		Child/Adolescent: 40–90 ml/d in divided doses adjusted to produce 2–3 soft stools/d

Management of Acute Portal-Systemic Encephalopathy

Adult	PO	30–45 ml q1–2h until laxation is achieved, then adjusted to produce 2–3 soft stools/d
	Rectal	300 ml diluted with 700 ml water given via rectal balloon catheter, and retained for 30–60 min; may repeat in 4–6 h if necessary or until patient can take PO

Chronic Constipation

Adult	PO	30–60 ml/d prn
Child	PO	7.5 ml/d after breakfast

PHARMACOKINETICS Absorption: poorly absorbed from GI tract. **Metabolism:** metabolized in gut by intestinal bacteria.

CONTRAINDICATIONS & PRECAUTIONS Contraindicated in: low galactose diet. Safe use during pregnancy (category C), in nursing mothers, and in children not established. **Cautious use in:** diabetes mellitus; concomitant use with electrocautery procedures (proctoscopy, colonoscopy); elderly and debilitated patients; pediatric use.

Common side effects in *italic*; life-threatening effects underlined; generic names in **bold**; classifications in SMALL CAPS

699

ADVERSE/SIDE EFFECTS Initial dose: flatulence, borborygmi, belching, abdominal cramps, pain, and distension; *diarrhea* (excessive dose), nausea, vomiting, colon accumulation of hydrogen gas; hypernatremia.

DRUG INTERACTIONS LAXATIVES may incorrectly suggest therapeutic action of lactulose.

NURSING IMPLICATIONS

Administration
- Administer with fruit juice, water, or milk (if not contraindicated) to increase palatability. Laxative effect is enhanced by taking lactulose with ample liquids. Avoid meal times.
- When endoscopic examination or intubation procedures are necessary or danger of aspiration exists, lactulose may be administered as a retention enema via a rectal balloon catheter. If solution is evacuated too soon, instillation may be promptly repeated.
- If solution is refrigerated, it will be too viscous to pour. Storing at room temperature will reduce viscosity; do not freeze. Avoid prolonged exposure to temperatures above 30C (86F) or to direct light. Normal darkening does not affect action, but discard solution that is very dark or cloudy.

Assessment & Drug Effects
- Any factor that slows gastric or small intestine transit time may extend initial response time to PO lactulose therapy (e.g., food, constipation, hypercatabolic states, infection).
- If the initial dose for children causes diarrhea, the dose is reduced immediately. If diarrhea persists, lactulose is discontinued.
- Maintaining a fecal pH of 5–5.5 is essential for ammonia elimination (usually achieved when patient has 2 or 3 soft stools daily).
- Therapeutic response (decreased blood ammonia) in patient with hepatic encephalopathy is marked by improved EEG patterns and mental state: clearing of confusion, apathy, and irritation. (**Normal blood ammonia:** 12–55 µmol/L)
- Changes associated with aging retard and reduce capacity of the elderly to adjust to electrolyte imbalance. Lactulose-induced osmotic changes in the bowel support intestinal water loss and potential hypernatremia. Fluid intake (often self-limited by the elderly) should be actively promoted (≤ 1500–2000 ml/d) during drug therapy for constipation. Discuss with physician.
- A potential therapeutic hazard with lactulose therapy is the accumulation of intestinal gas (hydrogen) from bacterial degradation of the drug. Preparation for colonoscopy or proctoscopy requires thorough bowel cleansing with nonfermentable or nonfoaming solution (i.e., avoid alkaline or soapsuds solution).

Patient & Family Education
- Laxative action is not instituted until drug reaches the colon; therefore transit time before reaching the colon and during passage through colon affects response time. About 24–48 h is needed.
- Warn patient who may be discouraged by slow onset of drug action not to self-medicate with another laxative.
- Advise patient on prolonged therapy to report to the physician if diarrhea (i.e., more than 2 or 3 soft stools/d) persists more than 24–48 h. Diarrhea is a sign of overdosage. Dose adjustment is indicated.

LEUCOVORIN CALCIUM

(loo-koe-vor´in)
Trade names: Calcium Folinate, Citrovorum Factor, Folinic Acid, Wellcovorin
Classifications: BLOOD FORMER; ANTIANEMIC AGENT; ANTIDOTE
Pregnancy: Category C

ACTIONS/PHARMACODYNAMICS Tetrahydrofolic acid derivative and reduced form of folic acid. Unlike folic acid, it does not require enzymatic reduction and therefore is readily available to participate in reactions. Functions as an essential cell growth factor. When given during antineoplastic therapy, leucovorin prevents serious toxicity by protecting cells from the action of folic acid antagonists such as methotrexate. This process is called "leucovorin or folinic acid rescue." Reportedly it is superior to folic acid in this respect because folic acid antagonists interfere with conversion of folic acid to leucovorin but do not affect action of leucovorin itself.

USES Folate-deficient megaloblastic anemias due to sprue, pregnancy, and nutritional deficiency when oral therapy is not feasible. Also to prevent or diminish toxicity of antineoplastic folic acid antagonists, particularly methotrexate; and as adjunct with antifols (e.g., pyrimethamine) in pneumocystosis or toxoplasmosis to prevent significant bone marrow toxicity.

L

ROUTE & DOSAGE

Megaloblastic Anemia

Adult	IM/IV	no more than 1 mg/d
Child	IM/IV	Same as for adult

Leucovorin Rescue for Methotrexate Toxicity

Adult	PO/IM/IV	10 mg/m² followed by 10 mg/m² q6h for 72 h; further doses based on serum methotrexate concentrations
Child	PO/IM/IV	Same as for adult

Leucovorin Rescue for Other Folate Antagonist Toxicity

Adult	PO/IM/IV	5–15 mg/d
Child	PO/IM/IV	Same as for adult

Adjunct for Treatment of Pneumocystosis or Toxoplasmosis

Adult	PO/IM/IV	3–6 mg t.i.d.
Child	PO/IM/IV	Same as for adult

PHARMACOKINETICS Onset: within 30 min. **Duration:** 3–6 h. **Distribution:** crosses placenta; distributed into breast milk. **Metabolism:** metabolized in liver and intestinal mucosa to tetrahydrofolic acid derivatives. **Elimination:** 80–90% excreted in urine, 5–8% in feces.

CONTRAINDICATIONS & PRECAUTIONS Contraindicated in: undiagnosed anemia, pernicious anemia, or other megaloblastic anemias secondary to vitamin B_{12} deficiency. Safe use during pregnancy (category C) and in nursing mothers not established. **Cautious use in:** renal dysfunction.

ADVERSE/SIDE EFFECTS Allergic sensitization (*urticaria, pruritus, rash, wheezing*); thrombocytosis.

INCOMPATIBILITIES Solution/Additive: droperidol. Y-Site: droperidol.

NURSING IMPLICATIONS

Administration

- For reconstitution, manufacturer recommends using 5 ml bacteriostatic water for injection, which contains benzyl alcohol, for each 50 mg vial. (Leucovorin calcium contains no preservatives.) When reconstituted as directed, solution must be used within 7 d. If reconstituted with sterile water for injection, use immediately.
- Reconstituted leucovorin is further diluted in 100–500 ml of most IV solutions.

- IV leucovorin solution is infused over 15–60 min, depending on the volume of solution.
- To be effective as antidote for overdosage of folic acid antagonists, leucovorin must be administered within 1 h if possible; usually ineffective if delayed more than 4 h. Duration of treatment depends on hematologic response to leucovorin.
- Store at 15–30C (59–86F) unless otherwise directed. Protect from light.

Assessment & Drug Effects

- Use of leucovorin alone in treatment of pernicious anemia or other megaloblastic anemias associated with vitamin B_{12} deficiency can result in an apparent hematological remission while allowing already present neurologic damage to progress.
- Plasma methotrexate levels may be used to determine dosage and duration of leucovorin rescue therapy. Creatinine clearance determinations prior to initiation of leucovorin rescue, urine pH prior to and about every 6 h throughout leucovorin rescue, and daily serum creatinine levels are recommended to detect onset of renal function impairment.

Patient & Family Education

- Instruct patient to report signs and symptoms of a hypersensitivity reaction immediately (see chap 3).

LEUPROLIDE ACETATE

(loo-proe´lide)

Trade names: Lupron, Lupron Depot
Classifications: ANTINEOPLASTIC, HORMONE SUBSTITUTE
Pregnancy: Category NR

L

ACTIONS/PHARMACODYNAMICS Synthetic analog of naturally occurring porcine or bovine gonadotropin releasing hormone (GnRH); a new approach to manipulation of androgen-sensitive carcinoma. Leuprolide occupies and desensitizes pituitary GnRH receptors, resulting initially (for short-term) in release of gonadotropins (luteinizing hormone [LH] and follicle-stimulating hormone [FSH]) and stimulation of ovarian and testicular steroidogenesis. During long-term administration, both gonadotropin secretion and steroidogenesis are suppressed, leading to prostatic and testicular atrophy. **Contraceptive effect:** by inhibiting gonadotropin release, ovulation or spermatogenesis is suppressed. **Antitumor effect:** may inhibit growth of hormone-dependent tumors. Leuprolide is therapeutically equivalent to diethyl-

Common side effects in *italic*; life-threatening effects <u>underlined</u>; generic names in **bold**; classifications in SMALL CAPS

701

stilbestrol (DES) in medical castration palliation but has fewer side effects.

USES Palliative treatment of advanced prostatic carcinoma as alternative to orchiectomy or estrogen administration. **Unlabeled uses:** breast cancer; male contraceptive; endometriosis; delayed puberty.

ROUTE & DOSAGE

Palliative Treatment for Prostate Cancer

Adult	SC	1 mg/d
	IM	7.5 mg/mo (depot preparation)

PHARMACOKINETICS Absorption: readily absorbed from SC or IM sites. **Metabolism:** metabolized by enzymes in hypothalamus and anterior pituitary. **Elimination:** half-life: 3 h.

CONTRAINDICATIONS & PRECAUTIONS Contraindicated in: following orchiectomy or estrogen therapy. **Cautious use in:** life-threatening carcinoma in which rapid symptomatic relief is necessary; known hypersensitivity to benzyl alcohol.

ADVERSE/SIDE EFFECTS *Disease flare (worsening of signs and symptoms of carcinoma).* **CNS:** dizziness, pain, headache, paresthesia. *Rare:* blurred vision, insomnia, memory disorders, numbness. **CV:** *peripheral edema,* cardiac arrhythmias, MI; *Causal relationships not established:* thrombophlebitis, pulmonary embolism, CHF. **Endocrine:** *hot flushes, impotence, decreased libido,* gynecomastia, breast tenderness, amenorrhea, vaginal bleeding, thyroid enlargement, hypoglycemia. **GI:** nausea, vomiting, constipation, anorexia, sour taste, GI bleeding, diarrhea. **Musculoskeletal:** increased bone pain, myalgia. **Renal:** increased hematuria, dysuria, flank pain. *Rare:* polyuria, increased BUN. **Other:** injection site irritation, pleural rub, pulmonary fibrosis flare; decreased Hct, Hgb; asthenia, fatigue, fever, facial swelling, pruritus, rash, hair loss.

NURSING IMPLICATIONS

Administration

- Do not administer drug formulation if particulate matter or discoloration is present.
- Refrigerate unopened vials at 2–8C (36–46F). Store vial in use at 15–30C (59–86F) for several months with minimal loss of potency. Protect from light and freezing.

Assessment & Drug Effects

- Inspect injection site daily. If local hypersensitivity reactions occur (erythema, induration), suspect sensitivity to benzyl alcohol. Report to physician.
- Monitor I&O ratio and pattern. Report hematuria and decreased output. Carefully monitor voiding problems. Advise patient to discuss these symptoms with physician.
- *Laboratory evidence of therapeutic response:* reduction in concentrations of serum prostatic acid phosphatase and serum testosterone to levels equal to or less than pretreatment levels. A gradual rise in values after their decrease may signify treatment failure.

Patient & Family Education

- Patient may be instructed to self-medicate with leuprolide. Review package information insert with patient. Caution patient to use only the syringes provided with medication kit. If it becomes absolutely necessary, the only acceptable substitute is a 0.5 ml disposable, low-dose U-100 insulin syringe (BD #8461). Instruct patient to fill this syringe to the 20-unit mark.
- Inform patient that bone pain and voiding problems (i.e., symptoms of tumor obstruction) usually increase during first several weeks of continuous treatment but are transient. Hot flushes may be experienced also.
- Caution patient to report worsening of neurologic signs and symptoms (paresthesia and weakness in lower limbs). Evaluate safety and capability to ambulate unassisted.
- Inform female patient that continuous treatment may cause amenorrhea and other menstrual irregularities.

Prototype: pilocarpine, p 209

LEVOBUNOLOL

(lee-voe-byoo´noe-lole)
Trade name: Betagan
Classifications: EYE PREPARATION; AUTONOMIC NERVOUS SYSTEM AGENT; BETA-ADRENERGIC ANTAGONIST (SYMPATHOLYTIC)
Pregnancy: Category C

ACTIONS/PHARMACODYNAMICS Nonselective ophthalmic beta-adrenergic blocking agent, similar to timolol. Exact mechanism of action not determined but appears to lower intraocular pressure (IOP) by decreasing formation of aqueous humor. Reduces IOP whether elevated or normal, with or without glaucoma. Has little or no effect on pupil size, accommodation, visual acuity, or tear secretion. Mean decrease in IOP may exceed that produced by timolol, and there is some evidence that IOP of untreated eye may also be reduced to some extent. Lacks significant membrane-stabilizing (local anesthetic) action and intrinsic sympathetic activity. Like timolol, systemic absorption can cause beta-adrenergic blocking actions on bronchi, bronchioles, and heart. Reportedly, tolerance to IOP-lowering effect can develop with long-term use.

USES To lower IOP in chronic open-angle glaucoma and ocular hypertension. **Unlabeled use:** as adjunct with a topical miotic for treatment of acute and chronic angle-closure glaucoma.

ROUTE & DOSAGE

Glaucoma

Adult	Topical (Ophthalmic)	1–2 drops 1–2 times/d

PHARMACOKINETICS Absorption: some systemic absorption from topical administration. **Onset:** 0.5–1 h. **Peak:** 2–6 h. **Duration:** 24 h.

CONTRAINDICATIONS & PRECAUTIONS Contraindicated in: hypersensitivity to levobunolol or to any component of the formulation (e.g., bisulfite); bronchial asthma (or history of), severe COPD; sinus bradycardia, second and third degree AV block, overt cardiac failure, cardiogenic shock. Safe use during pregnancy (category C) and in nursing mothers not established. **Cautious use in:** diminished pulmonary or cardiac function, nonallergic bronchospasm, history of allergies; myasthenia gravis (may potentiate muscle weakness); diabetes mellitus; hyperthyroidism; patients undergoing surgery (including dental); elderly patients.

ADVERSE/SIDE EFFECTS Because levobunolol may be absorbed systemically, the same reactions associated with beta blockers in general apply. **CNS:** transient ataxia, dizziness, lethargy, depression, insomnia, headache, asthenia (weakness), fatigue, cerebral ischemia. **CV:** chest pain; irregular slow or pounding heartbeat; bradycardia, arrhythmias, syncope, hypotension, edema of feet, ankle, legs; CHF (prolonged use). **Eye:** erythema, conjunctivitis, *transient burning, stinging,* itching sensation. *Rare:* blepharitis, blepharoptosis, iridocyclitis, band keratopathy, visual disturbances including refraction changes, diplopia, lacrimation, decreased corneal sensitivity (prolonged use). **GI:** nausea, vomiting, anorexia, heartburn, diarrhea. **Hypersensitivity (rare):** skin rash, urticaria, pruritus, anaphylaxis. **Respiratory:** dyspnea, shortness of breath, exacerbation of asthma, bronchospasm.

DRUG INTERACTIONS Reserpine and other CATECHOLAMINE-DEPLETING AGENTS may compound hypotensive effects or cause bradycardia.

NURSING IMPLICATIONS

Administration

- To prevent systemic absorption, immediately after instilling eye drops, apply gentle finger pressure to nasolacrimal drainage system for 1–2 min.
- Store at 15–30C (59–86F) in light-resistant container unless otherwise directed.

Assessment & Drug Effects

- Tonometric readings of IOP should be taken before and at regular intervals during therapy. *Normal IOP:* 12–20 mm Hg. Because IOP varies during the day, it should be measured at different times to determine adequacy of response. IOP tends to be higher on awakening and lowest in the evening.
- Patients with impaired cardiac function and the elderly should report to physician signs and symptoms of CHF (see chap 3). Establish baseline pulse and BP in these patients and check at regular intervals.

Patient & Family Education

- Instruct patient in proper administration of eyedrops to reduce potential systemic side effects.
- Advise patient not to take OTC medications containing sympathomimetic agents (i.e., ephedrine, epinephrine, phenylephrine), such as remedies for colds, sinus problems, hay fever, without consulting the physician.
- Caution diabetic patient that levobunolol may mask some of the usual symptoms of acute hypoglycemia.
- Caution patients to inform physician and dentist that they are taking levobunolol, particularly if a surgical procedure is to be performed.

L

Common side effects in *italic*; life-threatening effects underlined; generic names in **bold**; classifications in SMALL CAPS

703

LEVOCARNITINE (L-CARNITINE)

(lev-o-car´-ni-teen)
Trade names: Carnitor, VitaCarn
Classifications: VITAMIN; NUTRITIONAL SUPPLEMENT
Pregnancy: Category B

ACTIONS/PHARMACODYNAMICS Levocarnitine is a naturally occurring amino acid derivative required in energy metabolism. It facilitates long-chain fatty acid entry into cellular mitochondria, where it is used during oxidation and energy production. Deficiency of levocarnitine may lead to elevated triglyceride and free fatty acid concentrations, reduced ketogenesis, and lipid infiltration of liver and muscle. Severe chronic deficiency may lead to hypoglycemia, progressive myasthenia, hypotonia, lethargy, hepatomegaly, hepatic encephalopathy, hepatic coma, cardiomegaly, CHF, cardiac arrest, neurologic disturbances, and impaired infant growth and development.

USES Inborn systemic carnitine deficiency, a genetic impairment of normal biosynthesis or use of levocarnitine from dietary sources. **Unlabeled use:** modifying abnormal plasma lipoprotein patterns associated with hemodialysis.

ROUTE & DOSAGE

L-Carnitine Deficiency

Adult	PO	1–3 g/d for patients weighing > 50 kg (110 lb)
		weighing < 50 kg (110 lb): 50–100 mg/kg/d (max 3 g)
Child	PO	weighing < 50 kg (110 lb): 50–100 mg/kg/d (max 3 g)

PHARMACOKINETICS Elimination: excreted in urine and feces. Approximately 53–73% of L-carnitine is removed by hemodialysis.

CONTRAINDICATIONS & PRECAUTIONS Contraindications: none known. **Cautious use in:** pregnancy (category B) and nursing mothers.

ADVERSE/SIDE EFFECTS GI: *nausea,* vomiting, abdominal cramps, diarrhea.

NURSING IMPLICATIONS

Administration

- Scheduling the medication at evenly spaced intervals will increase tolerance to the drug.

- Doses should be spaced every 3 to 4 hours, preferable during or following meals. No more than 1 gram (10 ml) can be taken at each dose.
- The oral solution may be consumed alone or dissolved in other liquid food.
- Medication should be consumed slowly in order to maximize tolerance and decrease gastrointestinal upset.
- Store at room temperature between 15–30C (59–86F) away from heat, light, and moisture.

Assessment & Drug Effects

- Monitor tolerance closely during first week and after any dosage increase. Drug has caused transient GI complaints including nausea, vomiting, abdominal cramps, and diarrhea.
- Monitor plasma carnitine, free fatty acid, and triglyceride levels. Determination of these values is recommended at periodic intervals to assess the efficacy of levocarnitine.

Patient & Family Education

- Advise patient not to use the D,L-carnitine sold in health food stores. Its use can lower carnitine plasma level.
- The dietary source of levocarnitine is food of animal origin, such as meat and dairy products.
- If a dose is missed, patient should omit the dose since dosage intervals are relatively short (e.g., q3–4h).

LEVODOPA

See AUTONOMIC NERVOUS SYSTEM AGENTS, ANTICHOLINERGIC (PARASYMPATHOLYTIC), ANTIPARKINSONISM AGENT prototype, p 114.

Prototype: morphine sulfate, p 156

LEVORPHANOL TARTRATE

(lee-vor´fa-nole)
Trade name: Levo-Dromoran
Classifications: CNS AGENT; ANALGESIC; ANTIPYRETIC; NARCOTIC (OPIATE) AGONIST
Pregnancy: Category B
Controlled substance: Schedule II

L

ACTIONS/PHARMACODYNAMICS Synthetic morphinan derivative with agonist activity only. Actions, uses, contraindications, precautions, and adverse reactions similar to those of morphine. More potent as an analgesic and has somewhat longer duration of action than morphine. Reported to cause less nausea, vomiting, and constipation than equivalent doses of morphine but may produce more sedation, smooth-muscle stimulation, and respiratory depression.

USES To relieve moderate to severe pain. Also preoperatively to allay apprehension.

ROUTE & DOSAGE

Moderate to Severe Pain

Adult   PO/SC   2–3 mg q6–8h prn

PHARMACOKINETICS Peak: 60–90 min. **Duration:** 6–8 h. **Distribution:** crosses placenta; distributed into breast milk. **Metabolism:** metabolized in liver. **Elimination:** half-life: 1.2 h; excreted in urine.

ADVERSE/SIDE EFFECTS CNS: euphoria, *sedation, drowsiness,* nervousness, confusion. **CV:** hypotension, fast, slow, or pounding heartbeat. **GI:** *nausea,* vomiting, dry mouth, cramps, *constipation.* **GU:** urinary frequency, urinary retention, sedation. **Other:** blurred vision; respiratory depression, physical dependence.

DRUG INTERACTIONS Alcohol and other CNS DEPRESSANTS compound sedation and CNS depression.

INCOMPATIBILITIES Solution/Additive: aminophylline, ammonium chloride, BARBITURATES, **chlorothiazide, heparin, methacillin, phenytoin, sodium bicarbonate.**

NURSING IMPLICATIONS

Administration

- Levorphanol should be given in the smallest effective dose to minimize the possibility of tolerance and physical dependence.
- Store tablets and injection at 15–30C (59–86F) unless otherwise directed. Tablets should be stored in tightly-covered, light-resistant containers.

Assessment & Drug Effects

- Assess degree of pain relief. Drug is most effective when peaks and valleys of pain relief are avoided.

- Monitor bowel function.
- Monitor ambulation, especially in elderly patients.

Patient & Family Education

- Advise patient to avoid alcohol and other CNS depressants unless approved by physician.
- Caution patient to avoid driving and other potentially hazardous activities.
- Advise patient that ambulation may increase frequency of nausea and vomiting.
- Instruct patient to increase fluid and fiber intake to off-set constipating effects of the drug.

LEVOTHYROXINE SODIUM

See HORMONES & SYNTHETIC SUBSTITUTES, THYROID prototype, p 244.

Prototype: procainamide hydrochloride, p 140

LIDOCAINE HYDROCHLORIDE
(lye´doe-kane)

Trade names: Anestacon, Baylocaine, BayCaine, Delcaine, Dilocaine, L-Caine, Lida-Mantle, Lidoject-1, LidoPen Auto Injector, Nervocaine, Nulicaine, Octocaine, Ultracaine, Xylocaine, Xylocard

Classifications: CARDIOVASCULAR AGENT; ANTIARRHYTHMIC; CNS AGENT; LOCAL ANESTHETIC

Pregnancy: Category B

ACTIONS/PHARMACODYNAMICS Aminoacyl amide with anesthetic and antiarrhythmic (class Ib) properties. Cardiac actions similar to those of procainamide and quinidine but has little effect on myocardial contractility, A-V and intraventricular conduction, cardiac output, and systolic arterial pressure in equivalent doses. Exerts antiarrhythmic action by suppressing automaticity in His-Purkinje system and by elevating electrical stimulation threshold of ventricle during diastole. Progressive depression of CNS occurs with increasing blood concentrations; produces anticonvulsant, sedative, and analgesic effects. Action as local anesthetic is more prompt, more intense, and longer lasting than that of procaine. Suppresses cough and gag reflexes.

USES Rapid control of ventricular arrhythmias occurring during acute MI, cardiac surgery, and cardiac catheterization and those caused by digitalis intoxication. Also as surface and infiltration anesthesia and for nerve block, including caudal and spinal block anesthesia and to relieve local discomfort of skin and mucous membranes. **Unlabeled use:** refractory status epilepticus.

ROUTE & DOSAGE

Ventricular Arrhythmias

Adult	IV	50–100 mg bolus at a rate of 20–50 mg/min; may repeat in 5 min, then start infusion of 20–50 µg/kg/min (1–4 mg/min) immediately after first bolus
	IM/SC	200–300 mg IM; may repeat once after 60–90 min
Child	IV	0.5–1 mg/kg bolus dose, then 10–50 µg/kg/min infusion

Anesthetic Uses

Adult	Infiltration	0.5–1% solution
	Nerve block	1–2% solution
	Epidural	1–2% solution
	Caudal	1–1.5% solution
	Spinal	5% with glucose
	Saddle block	1.5% with dextrose
	Topical	2.5–5% jelly, ointment, cream, or solution

PHARMACOKINETICS Onset: 45–90 s IV; 5–15 min IM; 2–5 min topical. **Duration:** 10–20 min IV; 60–90 min IM; 30–60 min topical; > 100 min injected for anesthesia. **Distribution:** crosses blood-brain barrier and placenta; distributed into breast milk. **Metabolism:** metabolized in liver. **Elimination:** half-life: 1.5–2 h; excreted in urine.

CONTRAINDICATIONS & PRECAUTIONS Con-

traindicated in: history of hypersensitivity to amide-type local anesthetics; application or injection of lidocaine anesthetic in presence of severe trauma or sepsis, blood dyscrasias, supraventricular arrhythmias, Stokes-Adams syndrome, untreated sinus bradycardia, severe degrees of sinoatrial, atrioventricular, and intraventricular heart block. Safe use during pregnancy (category B), in nursing mothers, and in children not established. **Cautious use in:** liver or renal disease, CHF, marked hypoxia, respiratory depression, hypovolemia, shock; myasthenia gravis;

debilitated patients, the elderly; family history of malignant hyperthermia (fulminant hypermetabolism). Topical use in eyes, over large body areas, over prolonged periods, in severe or extensive trauma or skin disorders.

ADVERSE/SIDE EFFECTS CNS: drowsiness, dizziness, lightheadedness, restlessness, confusion, disorientation, irritability, apprehension, euphoria, wild excitement, numbness of lips or tongue and other paresthesias including sensations of heat and cold, chest heaviness, difficulty in speaking, difficulty in breathing or swallowing, muscular twitching, tremors, psychosis. With high doses: convulsions, respiratory depression and arrest. **CV:** (with high doses): hypotension, bradycardia, conduction disorders including heart block, cardiovascular collapse, cardiac arrest. **Ears:** tinnitus, decreased hearing. **Eye:** blurred or double vision, impaired color perception. **Other:** anorexia, nausea, vomiting, excessive perspiration, soreness at IM site, local thrombophlebitis (with prolonged IV infusion), hypersensitivity reactions (urticaria, rash, edema, anaphylactoid reactions).

DIAGNOSTIC TEST INTERFERENCES Increases in *creatine phosphokinase* (CPK) level may occur for 48 h after IM dose and may interfere with test for presence of MI.

DRUG INTERACTIONS BARBITURATES decrease lidocaine activity; **cimetidine,** BETA-BLOCKERS, **quinidine** increase pharmacologic effects of lidocaine; **phenytoin** increases cardiac depressant effects; **procainamide** compounds neurologic and cardiac effects.

INCOMPATIBILITIES Solution/Additive: phenytoin, cefazolin. Y-Site: phenytoin.

NURSING IMPLICATIONS

Administration

- Only lidocaine hydrochloride injection without preservatives or epinephrine that is specifically labeled for IV use should be used for IV injection or infusion.
- Bolus dose of lidocaine may be given undiluted by direct IV at a rate of 50 mg or fraction thereof over 1 min.
- Lidocaine may be added to D5W for infusion. For adults, add 1 g to 250–500 ml; for children, add 120 mg to 100 ml.
- For IV infusion, use microdropper and infusion pump. Physician will prescribe specific rate of

Common side effects in *italic*; life-threatening effects underlined; generic names in **bold**; classifications in SMALL CAPS

flow, usually no more than 4 mg/min. Rate must be closely monitored.

- Lidocaine should not be added to transfusion assemblies.
- IV infusion should be terminated as soon as patient's basic cardiac rhythm stabilizes or at earliest signs and symptoms of toxicity (infusions are rarely continued beyond 24 h). An oral antiarrhythmic is used for maintenance therapy.
- Deltoid muscle is recommended as the preferred IM site, because faster and higher peak blood levels are produced than by injection into gluteus or lateral thigh. Carefully aspirate to avoid inadvertent intravascular administration.
- Topical lidocaine should not be applied to large areas of skin or to broken or abraded surfaces. Consult physician about duration of treatment and whether area being treated can be covered with a dressing.
- Avoid contacting eyes with topical preparation.
- **Anesthetic use:** Lidocaine solutions containing preservatives should not be used for spinal or epidural (including caudal) block.
- Partially used solutions of lidocaine without preservatives should be discarded after initial use.
- Inspect solutions for particulate matter and discoloration prior to administration and discard if either is present.
- Store all preparations at 15–30C (59–86F) unless otherwise directed.

Assessment & Drug Effects

- If ECG signs of excessive cardiac depression occur, such as prolongation of PR interval or QRS complex and the appearance or aggravation of arrhythmias, infusion should be stopped immediately.
- Constant ECG monitoring and frequent determinations of BP, respirations, and CNS status are essential to avoid potential overdosage and toxicity.
- Auscultate lungs for basilar rales, especially in patients who tend to metabolize the drug slowly (e.g., CHF, cardiogenic shock, hepatic dysfunction).
- In patients receiving IV infusions of lidocaine or those with high lidocaine blood levels watch for **neurotoxic effects:** drowsiness, dizziness, confusion, paresthesias, visual disturbances, excitement, behavioral changes.
- Lidocaine blood levels of approximately 1.5 to 6 μg/ml are reported to provide "usually effective" antiarrhythmic activity. Blood levels greater than 7 μg/ml are potentially toxic.

Patient & Family Education

- Instruct patient using lidocaine solution for relief of

mouth discomfort to swish and spit it out. For use in pharnyx, lidocaine solution should be gargled and may be swallowed (as prescribed).

- Patient should know that oral topical anesthetics, e.g., Xylocaine Viscous, may interfere with swallowing reflex. Food should not be ingested within 60 min after drug application, especially in pediatric, elderly, or debilitated patients. Also, warn patient against chewing gum while buccal and throat membranes are anesthetized to prevent biting trauma.

Prototype: clindamycin, p 64

LINCOMYCIN HYDROCHLORIDE
(lin-koe-mye´sin)

Trade name: Lincocin
Classifications: ANTIINFECTIVE; ANTIBIOTIC
Pregnancy: Category B

ACTIONS/PHARMACODYNAMICS Derived from *Streptomyces lincolnensis*. Bacteriostatic or bactericidal depending on concentration used and sensitivity of organism. Acts by binding selectively to 50S subunits of bacterial ribosomes, thus suppressing protein synthesis. Similar to clindamycin in antibacterial activity and demonstrates some cross-resistance with it. Effective against most of the common gram-positive pathogens, particularly streptococci, pneumococci, and staphylococci. Also effective against *Bacteroides* and other anaerobes; however, little activity against most gram-negative organisms and ineffective against viruses, yeasts, or fungi. Resistance by *Staphylococcus* is acquired in stepwise manner. Lincomycin is reported to have neuromuscular blocking properties.

USES Reserved for treatment of serious infections caused by susceptible bacteria in penicillin-allergic patients or patients for whom penicillin is inappropriate.

PHARMACOKINETICS Absorption: partially absorbed from GI tract (20–30%). **Peak:** 2–4 h PO; 30 min IM. **Duration:** 6–8 h PO; 12–14 h IM; 14 h IV. **Distribution:** high concentrations in bone, aqueous humor, bile, and peritoneal, pleural, and synovial fluids; crosses placenta; distributed into breast milk. **Metabolism:** partially metabolized in liver. **Elimination:** half-life: 5 h; excreted in urine and feces.

L

Common side effects in *italic*; life-threatening effects underlined; generic names in **bold**; classifications in SMALL CAPS

707

ROUTE & DOSAGE

Infections

Adult	PO	500 mg q6–8h (max 8 g/d)
	IM	600 mg q12–24h
	IV	600 mg–1 g q8–12h
Child	PO	> 1 mo: 30–60 mg/kg in 3–4 divided doses
	IM	10 mg/kg q12–24h
	IV	10–20 mg/kg/d in 2–3 divided doses

CONTRAINDICATIONS & PRECAUTIONS Contraindicated in: previous hypersensitivity to lincomycin and clindamycin; impaired hepatic function, known monilial infections (unless treated concurrently); use in newborns. Safe use in pregnancy (category B) and nursing mothers not established. **Cautious use in:** impaired renal function; history of GI disease, particularly colitis; history of liver, endocrine, or metabolic diseases; history of asthma, hay fever, eczema, drug or other allergies; elderly patients.

ADVERSE/SIDE EFFECTS CV: hypotension, syncope, <u>cardiopulmonary arrest</u> (particularly after rapid IV). **GI:** glossitis, stomatitis, *nausea, vomiting,* anorexia, decreased taste acuity, unpleasant or altered taste, abdominal cramps, *diarrhea,* acute enterocolitis, <u>pseudomembranous colitis (potentially fatal)</u>. **Hematologic:** neutropenia, leukopenia, <u>agranulocytosis</u>, thrombocytopenic purpura, <u>aplastic anemia</u>, pancytopenia (rare). **Hypersensitivity:** pruritus, urticaria, skin rashes, exfoliative and vesiculobullous dermatitis, erythema multiforme resembling Stevens-Johnson syndrome (rare), angioedema, photosensitivity, <u>anaphylactoid reaction</u>, serum sickness. **Other:** superinfections (proctitis, pruritus ani, vaginitis), tinnitus, vertigo, dizziness, headache, generalized myalgia, thrombophlebitis following IV use (infrequent); pain at IM injection site (infrequent); jaundice and abnormal liver function tests (direct relationship to lincomycin not established), serum triglycerides, CPK.

DRUG INTERACTIONS kaolin pectin decreases lincomycin absorption; **tubocurarine, pancuronium** may enhance neuromuscular blockade.

INCOMPATIBILITIES Solution/Additive: penicillin G, phenytoin, ampicillin, carbenicillin, methicillin.

NURSING IMPLICATIONS

Administration

- Absorption is reduced and delayed by presence of food in stomach. Administer oral drug with a full glass (240 ml [8 oz]) of water at least 1–2 h before or 2–3 h after meals.
- Administer IM injection deep into large muscle mass; inject slowly to minimize pain. Rotate injection sites.
- For IV administration, 1 g of lincomycin is diluted in at least 100 ml of D5W, NS, or other compatible solution. Rate of infusion should not exceed 1 g/h.
- Follow manufacturer's directions for further information on reconstitution, storage time, compatible IV fluids, and IV administration rates.
- Store unopened vials and oral drug at 15–30C (59–86F) unless otherwise directed.

Assessment & Drug Effects

- Culture and susceptibility tests should be performed initially and during therapy to determine continued microbial susceptibility.
- A careful history should be taken of previous sensitivities to drugs or other allergens.
- Monitor BP and pulse in patients receiving parenteral drug. Have patient remain recumbent following drug administration until BP stability is assured.
- Relatively high incidence of diarrhea (20%) is associated with use of lincomycin. Monitor patients closely and report changes in bowel frequency. If significant diarrhea occurs, drug should be discontinued.
- Examine IM and IV injection sites daily for signs of inflammation.
- Diarrhea, acute colitis, or pseudomembranous colitis (see Signs & Symptoms, chap 3) may occur up to several weeks after cessation of therapy. Advise patients to report promptly the onset of perianal irritation, diarrhea, or blood and mucus in stools.
- Serum drug levels should be monitored closely in patients with severe impairment of renal function (levels tend to be higher). Recommended dosage for these patients is 25–30% of that for patients with normal renal function.
- Periodic hepatic and renal function studies and complete blood cell counts are indicated during prolonged drug therapy.
- Superinfections by nonsusceptible organisms are most likely to occur when duration of therapy exceeds 10 d. (See Signs & Symptoms, chap 3.)

Patient & Family Education

- Antiperistaltic agents may prolong and worsen diarrhea by delaying removal of toxins from colon.
- Advise patients to report immediately symptoms of hypersensitivity (see chap 3). Drug should be discontinued.
- Instruct patient to take drug for full course of therapy as prescribed.

LINDANE

See SKIN & MUCOUS MEMBRANE AGENTS, SCABICIDE prototype, p 263.

Prototype: levothyroxine, p 244

LIOTHYRONINE SODIUM

(lye-oh-thye´roe-neen)
Trade names: Cytomel, Tertroxin, T_3
Classifications: SYNTHETIC HORMONE; THYROID
Pregnancy: Category A

ACTIONS/PHARMACODYNAMICS Synthetic form of natural thyroid hormone. Shares actions and uses of thyroid but has more rapid action and more rapid disappearance of effect, permitting quick dosage adjustment if necessary; 25 µg are equivalent to approximately 65 mg of thyroid or thyroglobulin. May be used in T_3 suppression test to differentiate suspected hyperthyroidism from euthyroidism. See thyroid for contraindications and precautions.

USES Replacement or supplemental therapy for cretinism, myxedema, goiter, secondary (pituitary) or tertiary (hypothalamic) hypothyroidism, and T_3 suppression test.

PHARMACOKINETICS Absorption: completely absorbed from GI tract. **Peak:** 24–72 h. **Duration:** up to 72 h. **Distribution:** gradually released into tissue cells. **Elimination:** half-life: 6–7 d.

ADVERSE/SIDE EFFECTS Result from overdosage; evidenced as signs and symptoms of hyperthyroidism (see chap 3). *Children:* accelerated rate of bone maturation.

ROUTE & DOSAGE

Thyroid Replacement

Adult	PO	25–75 µg/d
Child	PO	5 µg/d gradually increased by 5 µg/d q3–4d until desired response

Myxedema

Adult	PO	5–100 µg/d

Goiter

Adult	PO	5–75 µg/d

T_3 Suppression Test

Adult	PO	75–100 µg/d for 7 d

DRUG INTERACTIONS Cholestyramine, colestipol decrease absorption; **epinephrine, norepinephrine** increase risk of cardiac insufficiency; ORAL ANTICOAGULANTS may potentiate hypoprothrombinemia.

NURSING IMPLICATIONS

Administration

- When changing to liothyronine from thyroid, levothyroxine, or thyroglobulin, discontinue other medication, initiate liothyronine at low dosage, with gradual increases according to patient's response.
- *T_3 suppression test:* 75–100 µg liothyronine daily is given for 7 d. Radioactive iodine (RAI) (I 131) uptake tests are performed before and after the 7 d course of liothyronine. In hyperthyroidism, 24 h RAI uptake will not be significantly affected; in euthyroid patient, 24 h RAI uptake will decrease to less than 20% of base line value.
- Store tablets in heat-, light-, and moisture-proof container at 15–30C (59–86F).

Assessment & Drug Effects

- Note that metabolic effects persist a few days after drug withdrawal.
- Infants with thyroid dysfunction (mother provides little or no thyroid hormone to fetus) are started on replacement therapy as soon as possible to prevent permanent mental and physical changes.
- Residual actions of other thyroid preparations may persist for weeks; therefore, during early period of liothyronine substitution for another preparation, watch for possible additive effects, particularly if the patient is elderly, has cardiovascular disease, or is a child.
- With onset of overdosage symptoms (hyperthy-

Common side effects in *italic*; life-threatening effects <u>underlined</u>; generic names in **bold**; classifications in SMALL CAPS

709

roidism; see chap 3), drug is withheld for 1 or 2 d; usually therapy can be resumed with lower dosage.

Patient & Family Education
- Instruct patient to take medication exactly as ordered.
- Teach patient the signs and symptoms of hyperthyroidism (see chap 3) and advise patient to report their appearance to physician promptly.

Prototype: levothyroxine, p 244

LIOTRIX
(lye´oh-trix)

Trade names: Euthroid, Thyrolar, T_3/T_4
Classifications: SYNTHETIC HORMONE; THYROID
Pregnancy: Category A

ACTIONS/PHARMACODYNAMICS A mixture of synthetic levothyroxine (T_4) and liothyronine (T_3) combined in a constant 4:1 ratio by weight. Actions and pharmacokinetics as for thyroid. Products by different manufacturers differ in total amounts of each drug included in the formulation.

USES Replacement or supplemental therapy for cretinism, myxedema, goiter, and secondary (pituitary) or tertiary (hypothalamic) hypothyroidism. Also with antithyroid agents in thyrotoxicosis and to prevent goitrogenesis and hypothyroidism.

ROUTE & DOSAGE

Thyroid Replacement

Adult	PO	12.5–30 µg/d gradually increased to desired response
Child	PO	Same as for adult

CONTRAINDICATIONS & PRECAUTIONS Contraindicated in: thyrotoxicosis, acute MI, morphologic hypogonadism, nephrosis, adrenal deficiency due to hypopituitarism. **Cautious use in:** concomitant anticoagulant therapy; myxedema; angina pectoris, hypertension, arteriosclerosis; renal dysfunction.

ADVERSE/SIDE EFFECTS CNS: nervousness, headache, tremors, insomnia. **CV:** palpitation, tachycardia, angina pectoris, cardiac arrhythmias, hypertension, CHF. **GI:** nausea, abdominal cramps, diarrhea. **Other:** weight loss, heat intolerance, fever,

sweating, menstrual irregularities. *Infants, children:* accelerated rate of bone maturation.

DRUG INTERACTIONS Cholestyramine, colestipol decrease absorption; **epinephrine, norepinephrine** increase risk of cardiac insufficiency; ORAL ANTICOAGULANTS may potentiate hypoprothrombinemia.

NURSING IMPLICATIONS

Administration
- Usually administered as a single daily dose, preferably before breakfast.
- Changeover from another thyroid preparation can be made by direct substitution of liotrix for current dose of the other product, with gradual dose increase every 1 or 2 wk.
- Store in heat-, light-, and moisture-proof container at 15–30C (59–86F). Shelf-life: 2 y.

Assessment & Drug Effects
- Note that metabolic effects persist a few days after drug withdrawal.
- Infants with thyroid dysfunction (mother provides little or no thyroid hormone to fetus) are started on replacement therapy as soon as possible to prevent permanent mental and physical changes.
- Residual actions of other thyroid preparations may persist for weeks; therefore, during early period of liotrix substitution for another preparation, watch for possible additive effects, particularly if the patient is elderly, has cardiovascular disease, or is a child.
- With onset of overdosage symptoms (hyperthyroidism; see chap 3), drug is withheld for 1 or 2 d; usually therapy can be resumed with lower dosage.

Patient & Family Education
- Diabetic patients may require an increase in insulin or oral hypoglycemic dosage while taking liotrix. Decrease in dosage of antidiabetic drug may then be necessary if liotrix dosage is reduced or if drug is withdrawn.
- Euthyroid patient should report headache, since this may indicate need for dosage adjustment or change to another thyroid preparation.
- Available liotrix preparations contain variable amounts of T_3 and T_4. Instruct patients to have their prescriptions filled with the same brand currently being taken.
- Instruct patient to take medication exactly as ordered.

L

- Teach patient the signs and symptoms of hyperthyroidism (see chap 3) and advise patient to report their appearance to physician promptly.

Prototype: captopril, p 138

LISINOPRIL

(ly-sin´-o-pril)
Trade names: Prinivil, Zestril
Classifications: CARDIOVASCULAR AGENT;
ANGIOTENSIN-CONVERTING ENZYME INHIBITOR;
ANTIHYPERTENSIVE; VASODILATOR
Pregnancy: Category C

ACTIONS/PHARMACODYNAMICS Lowers BP by specific inhibition of the angiotensin-converting enzyme (ACE). This interrupts conversion sequences initiated by renin that form angiotensin II, a potent vasoconstrictor. ACE inhibition alters hemodynamics without compensatory reflex tachycardia or changes in cardiac output (except in patients with CHF). Inhibition of ACE also decreases circulating aldosterone, which is normally released in response to angiotensin II stimulation. Reduced aldosterone is associated with a potassium-sparing effect. Lisinopril decreases peripheral resistance (afterload) and pulmonary vascular resistance. There is improved cardiac output and exercise tolerance.

USES Hypertension. It may be given alone or concomitantly with other classes of antihypertensive agents. **Unlabeled use:** CHF in combination with diuretics and digitalis therapy.

ROUTE & DOSAGE

Hypertension

Adult PO 10 mg once/d; may increase up to 20–40 mg 1–2 times/d (max 80 mg/d)

PHARMACOKINETICS Absorption: 25% absorbed from GI tract. **Onset:** 1 h. **Peak:** 6–8 h. **Duration:** 24 h. **Distribution:** limited amount crosses blood-brain barrier; crosses placenta; small amount distributed in breast milk. **Metabolism:** is not metabolized. **Elimination:** half-life: 12 h; excreted primarily in urine.

CONTRAINDICATIONS & PRECAUTIONS Contraindicated in: patients with a history of angioedema related to treatment with an angiotensin converting enzyme inhibitor. **Cautious use in:** impaired renal function, hyperkalemia, patients on diuretic therapy; pregnancy (category C), nursing mothers; autoimmune diseases especially systemic lupus erythematosus (SLE).

ADVERSE/SIDE EFFECTS CNS: headache, dizziness, fatigue. **CV:** hypotension, chest pain. **GI:** nausea, vomiting, diarrhea, anorexia, constipation. **Other:** dyspnea, cough, rash, azotemia, hyperkalemia, increased BUN and creatinine levels.

DRUG INTERACTIONS Indomethacin and other NSAIDS may decrease antihypertensive activity; POTASSIUM SUPPLEMENTS, POTASSIUM-SPARING DIURETICS may cause hyperkalemia; may increase **lithium** levels and toxicity.

NURSING IMPLICATIONS

Administration

- For diuretic-treated patients an initial dose of 5 mg is given. Monitor drug effect for 2 h or until the BP is stabilized for at least 1 additional hour.
- Absorption of drug is not affected by food; therefore it can be given without regard to meals.
- It is recommended that previous diuretic therapy be withdrawn 2 to 3 d before therapy is initiated, except in patients with accelerated or malignant hypertension.
- Lisinopril is removed from blood by hemodialysis; therefore, administer following dialysis.
- Concurrent administration with a diuretic may compound hypotensive effect.
- Concurrent administration of salt substitute containing potassium may result in hyperkalemia since the drug is potassium sparing.

Assessment & Drug Effects

- Sudden and severe hypotension may occur within the first 1–5 h after the initial dose, particularly in patients who are sodium- or volume-depleted because of diuretic therapy. Withdrawal of diuretic therapy or increase in salt intake 2 to 3 d before start of therapy or use of a lower dose will minimize the hypotensive reaction.
- It is usually effective in once daily dosing. However, if the antihypertensive effect is diminished in less than 24 h, an increase in dosage may be necessary.
- Evaluate effect of drug by measuring BP just prior to dosing to determine whether satisfactory control is being maintained for 24 h.
- BP measurements are recommended at periodic in-

Common side effects in *italic*; life-threatening effects underlined; generic names in **bold**; classifications in SMALL CAPS

711

tervals. If excessive hypotension occurs, place patient in supine position and notify physician.

- Closely monitor for angioedema of extremities, face, lips, tongue, glottis, and larynx. Promptly discontinue drug and notify physician. Carefully monitor for airway obstruction until swelling is relieved.
- Monitor serum sodium and serum potassium levels for hyponatremia and hyperkalemia.
- Renal function studies are recommended at periodic intervals, especially in patients with severe volume or sodium replacement or those with severe CHF.
- Leukocyte count determination should be made prior to initiation of treatment, every month for the first 3–6 mo of therapy, and at periodic intervals for 1 y. Therapy should be discontinued if neutropenia (neutrophil count <1000/mm^3) develops.

Patient & Family Education

- Instruct patient that severe hypersensitivity reaction to any ACE inhibitor may include hoarseness, swelling of the face, mouth, hands, or feet or sudden trouble breathing. If these occur, discontinue drug and contact physician immediately.
- Discuss the importance of proper diet, including sodium and potassium restrictions. Advise patient not to use salt substitute containing potassium.
- Discuss importance of continued compliance with high BP medication. If a dose is missed, instruct patient to take it as soon as possible but not if it is too close to the time of the next dose in order to avoid double dosing.
- Since the drug may cause dizziness and lightheadedness, instruct patient to avoid driving or other potential hazardous activity until reaction to the drug is known.
- Advise patients on lithium that lisinopril increases the risk of lithium toxicity.
- Promptly notify physician of any indication of infection (e.g., sore throat, fever).
- Instruct patients to check with physician before they use any new medicine (prescription or nonprescription) or if any new medical problem develops while they are using this medicine.
- Advise patient not to store drug in a moist area. Heat and moisture may cause the medicine to break down.

LITHIUM

See CENTRAL NERVOUS SYSTEM AGENTS, PSYCHOTHERAPEUTIC, ANTIMANIC prototype, p 187.

Prototype: cyclophosphamide, p 91

LOMUSTINE

(loe-mus´teen)
Trade names: CeeNU, CCNU
Classifications: ANTINEOPLASTIC; ALKYLATING AGENT
Pregnancy: Category D

ACTIONS/PHARMACODYNAMICS Lipid-soluble alkylating nitrosourea with actions like those of carmustine. Inhibits synthesis of both DNA and RNA; has myelosuppressive effect.

USES Palliative therapy in addition to other modalities or with other chemotherapeutic agents in primary and metastatic brain tumors and as secondary therapy in Hodgkin's disease. **Unlabeled uses:** GI, lung, and renal carcinomas, non-Hodgkin's lymphomas, malignant melanoma, and multiple myelomas.

ROUTE & DOSAGE

Palliative Therapy

Adult	PO	130 mg/m^2 as single dose, repeated in 6 wk; subsequent doses based on hematologic response (WBC > 4000/mm^3, platelets > 100,000/mm^3)
Child	PO	Same as for adult

PHARMACOKINETICS Absorption: readily absorbed from GI tract. **Peak:** 1–6 h. **Distribution:** readily crosses blood-brain barrier; crosses placenta; distributed into breast milk. **Metabolism:** metabolized in liver to several active metabolites. **Elimination:** half-life: 16–48 h; excreted in urine.

CONTRAINDICATIONS & PRECAUTIONS Contraindicated in: immunization with live virus vaccines, viral infections. Safe use during pregnancy (category D) and in nursing mothers not established. Reported to be carcinogenic in laboratory animals. **Cautious use in:** patients with decreased circulating platelets, leukocytes, or erythrocytes; renal or hepatic function impairment; infection; previous cytotoxic or radiation therapy.

L

ADVERSE/SIDE EFFECTS CNS: lethargy, ataxia, disorientation, difficult speech (causal relationship not established). **GI:** anorexia, *nausea, vomiting,* stomatitis. **Hematologic:** delayed (cumulative) myelo-suppression; (thrombocytopenia, leukopenia); anemia. **Other:** transient elevations of liver function tests, alopecia, pulmonary toxicity (rare); nephrotoxicity, skin rash, itching.

NURSING IMPLICATIONS

Administration

- Take preferably on an empty stomach to reduce possibility of nausea. An antiemetic given before lomustine may prevent nausea.
- Store capsules away from excessive heat (over 40C).

Assessment & Drug Effects

- Since hematologic toxicity is delayed and cumulative, a repeat course is not given before 6 wk and not until platelets have returned to above 100,000/mm³ and leukocytes to above 4000/mm³.
- Blood counts should be monitored weekly for at least 6 wk after last dose. Liver and kidney function tests should be performed periodically.
- Care given should avoid IM administration of drugs and other invasive procedures during nadir of platelets.
- Thrombocytopenia occurs about 4 wk and leukopenia about 6 wk after a dose, persisting 1–2 wk.
- Inspect oral cavity daily for symptoms of superinfections (see chap 3) and for signs of stomatitis or xerostomia.

Patient & Family Education

- Nausea and vomiting may occur 3–5 h after drug administration, usually lasting less than 24 h.
- Anorexia may persist for 2 or 3 d after a dose.
- Myelosuppression reduces capacity to control infections. Advise patient to report signs of sore throat, couth, fever. It also presents dangers of thrombocytopenia. Report unexplained bleeding or easy bruising.
- Contraceptive measures are recommended during therapy.
- The possibility of hair loss should be discussed.
- Pharmacist will prepare prescribed dose by combining various capsule strengths. Explain to patient that a given dose may include capsules of different colors.

Prototype: diphenoxylate hydrochloride with atropine sulfate, p 213

LOPERAMIDE
(loe-per´a-mide)
Trade names: Imodium, Imodium AD
Classifications: GI AGENT; ANTIDIARRHEAL
Pregnancy: Category B

ACTIONS/PHARMACODYNAMICS Synthetic piperidine derivative chemically related to diphenoxylate and to meperidine. Reportedly as effective an antidiarrheal as diphenoxylate with longer duration of action. Inhibits GI peristaltic activity by direct action on circular and longitudinal intestinal muscles. Prolongs transit time of intestinal contents, increases consistency of stools, and reduces fluid and electrolyte loss.

USES Acute nonspecific diarrhea, chronic diarrhea associated with inflammatory bowel disease, and to reduce fecal volume from ileostomies.

ROUTE & DOSAGE

Acute Diarrhea

Adult	PO	4 mg followed by 2 mg after each unformed stool (max 16 mg/d)
Child	PO	2–6 y: 1 mg t.i.d.
		6–8 y: 2 mg b.i.d.
		8–12 y: 2 mg t.i.d.

Chronic Diarrhea

Adult	PO	4 mg followed by 2 mg after each unformed stool until diarrhea is controlled (max 16 mg/d)
Child	PO	0.1 mg/kg after each unformed stool (usually 1 mg)

PHARMACOKINETICS Absorption: poorly absorbed from GI tract. **Onset:** 30–60 min. **Peak:** 2.5 h solution; 4–5 h capsules. **Duration:** 4–5 h. **Metabolism:** metabolized in liver. **Elimination:** half-life: 11 h; primarily excreted in feces, <2% excreted in urine.

CONTRAINDICATIONS & PRECAUTIONS Contraindicated in: conditions in which constipation should be avoided, severe colitis, acute diarrhea caused by broad-spectrum antibiotics (pseudomembranous colitis) or associated with microorganisms that penetrate intestinal mucosa, e.g., toxigenic

Common side effects in *italic*; life-threatening effects underlined; generic names in **bold**; classifications in SMALL CAPS

713

Escherichia coli, Salmonella, or *Shigella.* Safe use during pregnancy (category B), in nursing mothers, and in children <2 y not established. **Cautious use in:** dehydration; diarrhea caused by invasive bacteria; impaired hepatic function; prostatic hypertrophy; history of narcotic dependence.

ADVERSE/SIDE EFFECTS CNS: drowsiness, fatigue, dizziness, CNS depression (overdosage). **GI:** abdominal discomfort or pain, abdominal distension, bloating, constipation, nausea, vomiting, anorexia, dry mouth. **Hypersensitivity:** skin rash. **Other:** fever, toxic megacolon (patients with ulcerative colitis).

NURSING IMPLICATIONS

Administration
- For adults, drug is usually given after each unformed stool up to a maximum of 16 mg/d.
- Store at 15–30C (59–86F) unless otherwise specified.

Assessment & Drug Effects
- In acute diarrhea, loperamide should be discontinued if there is no improvement after 48 h of therapy.
- Patients with chronic diarrhea usually respond to loperamide therapy within 10 d. If improvement does not occur within this time, it is unlikely that symptoms will be controlled by further administration. Loperamide may be continued under medical guidance if diarrhea cannot be controlled by diet or specific treatment, e.g., antibiotics.
- If the patient with ulcerative colitis develops abdominal distension or other GI symptoms, notify physician promptly (possible signs of potentially fatal toxic megacolon).

Patient & Family Education
- Advise patient to notify physician if diarrhea does not stop in a few days or if abdominal pain, distension, or fever develops.
- Instruct patient to record number and consistency of stools. Fluids and electrolytes should be monitored, especially in young children.
- Because loperamide may cause drowsiness and dizziness, caution patient to avoid driving and other potentially hazardous activities until drug response is known.
- Inform patient that alcohol and other CNS depressants may enhance drowsiness and therefore should not be taken concomitantly unless otherwise advised by physician.
- Dry mouth may be reduced by frequent rinsing

with clear warm water and by increasing fluid intake. If these measures fail, a saliva substitute, e.g., Xero-Lube, Moi-stir, may help (available OTC).

LORAZEPAM

See CNS AGENTS, ANXIOLYTIC, SEDATIVE-HYPNOTIC, BENZODIAZEPINE, prototype, p 177.

LOVASTATIN

See CARDIOVASCULAR AGENTS, ANTILIPEMIC, LIPID-LOWERING AGENT prototype, p 143.

Prototype: chlorpromazine, p 191

LOXAPINE HYDROCHLORIDE
(lox´a-peen)
Trade names: Loxitane C, Loxitane IM

LOXAPINE SUCCINATE
Trade names: Loxapac, Loxitane
Classifications: CNS AGENT; PSYCHOTHERAPEUTIC; ANTIPSYCHOTIC (TRANQUILIZER)
Pregnancy: Category C

ACTIONS/PHARMACODYNAMICS Dibenzoxazepine antipsychotic, chemically distinct from other antipsychotics. Exact mode of action not established. Stabilizes emotional component of schizophrenia by acting on subcortical level of CNS. Sedative action is less than that produced by chlorpromazine, but anticholinergic effects are comparable and extrapyramidal effects may be more intense. Also has antiemetic activity; lowers seizure threshold in patients with history of convulsive disorders.

USES Manifestations of psychotic disorders. **Unlabeled use:** anxiety associated with mental depression.

Common side effects in *italic*; life-threatening effects underlined; generic names in **bold**; classifications in SMALL CAPS

ROUTE & DOSAGE

Psychosis

Adult	PO	Start with 10 mg b.i.d. and rapidly increase to maintenance levels of 60–100 mg/d in 2–4 divided doses (max 250 mg/d)
	IM	12.5–50 mg q4–6h

PHARMACOKINETICS Absorption: readily absorbed from GI tract. **Onset:** 20–30 min. **Peak:** 1.5–3 h. **Duration:** 12 h. **Distribution:** widely distributed; crosses placenta; distributed into breast milk. **Metabolism:** metabolized in liver. **Elimination:** half-life: 19 h; 50% excreted in urine, 50% excreted in feces.

CONTRAINDICATIONS & PRECAUTIONS Contraindicated in: severe drug-induced CNS depression; comatose states, children <16 y. Safe use during pregnancy (category C) and in nursing mothers not established. **Cautious use in:** glaucoma, prostatic hypertrophy, urinary retention, history of convulsive disorders, cardiovascular disease.

ADVERSE SIDE EFFECTS CNS: *drowsiness,* sedation, dizziness, syncope, EEG changes, paresthesias, staggering gait, muscle weakness, *extrapyramidal effects,* akathisia, <u>tardive dyskinesia, neuroleptic malignant syndrome.</u> **CV:** *orthostatic hypotension,* hypertension, tachycardia. **ENT:** nasal congestion, tinnitus. **Eye:** blurred vision, ptosis. **GI:** constipation, dry mouth. **Skin:** dermatitis, facial edema, pruritus, photosensitivity. **Other:** urinary retention, polydipsia, weight gain or loss, hyperpyrexia, galactorrhea (rare); transient leukopenia, menstrual irregularities.

DRUG INTERACTIONS Alcohol and other CNS DEPRESSANTS potentiate CNS depression; will inhibit vasopressor effects of **epinephrine.**

NURSING IMPLICATIONS

Administration

- Loxapine should be taken with food, milk, or water to reduce possibility of stomach irritation.
- Dilute oral concentrate in about 2–3 oz (60–90 ml) water or orange or grapefruit juice shortly before administration (do not store diluted solution). Measured with calibrated dropper dispensed with drug.
- When therapy is to be terminated, dosage should be gradually reduced over period of several days.
- Protect medication from light. Intensification of straw color to light amber is acceptable. If solution is noticeably discolored, however, discard.
- Store at 15–30C (59–86F); protect from light and freezing.

Assessment & Drug Effects

- Determine BP pattern before and during therapy: both hypotension and hypertension have been reported as adverse reactions.
- Observe carefully for extrapyramidal effects such as acute dystonia (see Signs & Symptoms, chap 3) during early therapy with loxapine. Most symptoms disappear with dose adjustment or with antiparkinsonism drug therapy.
- If a patient is on long-term treatment with this drug, be alert to first signs of impending tardive dyskinesia: fine vermicular movements of the tongue. Discontinue therapy and report promptly.
- Monitor I&O and bowel elimination patterns and check for bladder distension. The depressed patient often fails to report urinary retention or constipation.
- Risk of seizures is increased in those with history of convulsive disorders.

Patient & Family Education

- Caution patient not to change the dosage regimen in any way unless the physician approves.
- The patient should be warned to avoid self-dosing with OTC drugs unless prescribed by the physician.
- Drowsiness usually decreases with continued therapy. If it persists and interferes with ADL, consult physician. A change in time of administration or dose may help to prevent interference with normal physical activities.
- Instruct patient not to drive a car or engage in any activity that requires mental coordination and physical skill until drug response is known.
- Dry mouth discomfort should be attended to, since deprivation of saliva fosters tissue erosion and demineralization of tooth surfaces. Frequent warm water rinses and, if there is salivary response, sugar-free gum and candy may be helpful. Avoid overuse of commercial mouth rinses, since many contain alcohol, which enhances drying and irritation.
- If patient complains of blurred or colored vision, report it to physician. Ocular toxicity is possible.
- Advise patient to withhold drug dose if the following appear: light-colored stools, bruising, unexplained bleeding, prolonged constipation, tremor, restlessness and excitement, sore throat and fever, rash.
- Caution patient to stay out of bright sun. Exposed skin area should be covered with sun-screen lotion.

L

Common side effects in *italic*; life-threatening effects <u>underlined</u>; generic names in **bold**; classifications in SMALL CAPS

715

Prototype: cyclosporine, p 248

LYMPHOCYTE IMMUNE GLOBULIN

Trade names: ATG, Atgam
Classifications: IMMUNOSUPPRESSANT; SERUM
Pregnancy: Category C

ACTIONS/PHARMACODYNAMICS Lymphocyte immune globulin (antithymocyte globulin or ATG) is an immunoglobulin (IgG) and lymphocyte-selective immunosuppressant derived from serum of healthy horses that have been immunized with human thymus lymphocytes. Action mechanism is not clear: it appears that ATG nonspecifically binds to circulating cytotoxic T lymphocytes (killer cells), alters their formation, and reduces their number. Has little effect on B cells and is not associated with severe lymphopenia. May contain antibodies to other formed elements in blood; by unknown mechanism produces a hemopoietic response in some patients with aplastic anemia. ATG therapy increases susceptibility of patient to viral infections: it may reactivate or support infection with cytomegalovirus, herpes simplex virus (especially labial infections), or with Epstein-Barr virus (EBV). Because it is given concomitantly with other immunosuppressants (cyclosporine, glucocorticoids, azathioprine), efficacy and safety of ATG alone have not been demonstrated. As with other immunosuppressant agents, carcinogenicity of this drug may be expressed; antineoplastic therapy is not recommended, however, unless the lymphoproliferative disorder does not resolve within a few months. Activity of solution may differ from lot-to-lot because precise methods for determining potency have not been established.

USES Primarily to prevent or delay onset or to reverse acute renal allograft rejection. **Unlabeled uses:** moderate and severe aplastic anemia in patients unsuitable for bone marrow transplantation, T cell malignancy, acute and chronic graft-vs-host disease, and to prevent rejection of skin allografts.

PHARMACOKINETICS Distribution: poorly distributed into lymphoid tissues (spleen, lymph nodes); probably crosses placenta and into breast milk. **Elimination:** half-life: approximately 6 d; about 1% of dose is excreted in urine.

ROUTE & DOSAGE

Renal Allotransplantation

Adult	IV	10–30 mg/kg/d by slow IV infusion
Child	IV	5–25 mg/kg/d by slow IV infusion

Prevention of Allograft Rejection

Adult	IV	15 mg/kg/d for 14 d followed by 15 mg/kg q.o.d. for 14 d

Treatment of Allograft Rejection

Adult	IV	10–15 mg/kg/d for 14 d followed by 15 mg/kg q.o.d. for 14 d if needed

Aplastic Anemia

Adult	IV	15 mg/kg/d for 14 d followed by 15 mg/kg q.o.d. for 14 d or 15 mg/kg/d for 10 d

CONTRAINDICATIONS & PRECAUTIONS Contraindicated in: hypersensitivity to thimerosal (preservative) or to other equine gamma globulin preparations; history of previous systemic reaction to ATG, hemorrhagic diatheses; use in renal transplant patient not receiving a concomitant immunosuppressant. Safe use during pregnancy (category C) or by nursing mothers not established. **Cautious use in:** children (experience limited).

ADVERSE/SIDE EFFECTS CNS: headache, paresthesia, seizures. **CV:** peripheral thrombophlebitis, hypotension; tachycardia (rare). **GI:** nausea, vomiting, diarrhea, stomatitis, hiccups, epigastric pain, abdominal distension. **Hematologic:** *leukopenia, thrombocytopenia.* **Musculoskeletal:** arthralgia, myalgias, chest or back pain. **Respiratory:** dyspnea, laryngospasm, pulmonary edema. **Skin:** *rash, pruritus,* urticaria, wheal and flare. **Other:** *chills, fever,* night sweats, pain at infusion site, hyperglycemia, hypertension, systemic infection, wound dehiscence; anaphylaxis, *serum sickness,* herpes simplex virus reactivation.

DRUG INTERACTIONS Azathioprine, CORTICOSTEROIDS, other IMMUNOSUPPRESSANTS increase degree of immunosuppression.

NURSING IMPLICATIONS

Administration

- Lymphocyte immune globulin (ATG) should be administered only by physician experienced with immunosuppressant therapy and management of renal transplant patients and only in area equipped with staff and facilities to deal with serious sensitivity reactions.

- Before first dose it is usual to do an intradermal skin test to rule out allergy to the drug. Inject 0.1 ml of a 1:1000 dilution (5 μg equine IgG in normal saline) and a saline control. If local reaction occurs (wheal or erythema more than 10 mm) or if there is pseudopod formation, itching, or local swelling, use caution during infusion. If systemic reaction develops (generalized rash, tachycardia, dyspnea, hypotension, anaphylaxis), discontinue infusion.
- **Preparation of infusion:** (ATG is available as concentrate: 50 mg/ml in 5 ml ampule): Dilute required dose of ATG concentrate with 0.45% or 0.9% NaCl injection; final concentration preferably not to exceed 1 mg equine IgG/ml. Dextrose injection or highly acidic solutions not recommended as diluents. Invert IV solution container into which ATG concentrate is added to prevent its contact with air inside container.
- Be aware that ATG concentrate may differ lot-to-lot. This means that freedom from allergy to one lot does not predict safe use of an ampule from another lot. Record lot number of concentrate in use.
- Administration of ATG into high-flow veins decreases potential for phlebitis and thrombosis.
- Visually inspect concentrate and diluted solution for particulate matter (may develop during storage) and discoloration; discard if present. Inline filters (0.2–5 μm) are generally used. Infusion should be timed to take at least 4 h (usually 4–8 h).
- Total storage time (including storage time and actual infusion time) to keep diluted solutions: no more than 12 h. Refrigerate ampules and diluted solutions (if prepared before time of infusion) at 2–8C (35–46F). Do not freeze.

Assessment & Drug Effects
- Discontinue infusion and initiate appropriate therapy promptly with onset of anaphylactic response (respiratory distress; pain in chest, flank, back; hypotension, anxiety).
- Predictive value of skin test is not proven. Observe patient carefully; allergic reaction can occur even when test is negative.
- Closely monitor BP, vital signs, and patient's complaints during entire administration period. Prompt treatment is indicated for observed and reported symptoms of anaphylaxis (incidence: 1%), serum sickness, or allergic response. Always have available at bedside equipment for assisted respiration, epinephrine, antihistamines, corticosteroid, vasopressor.
- Watch closely for **signs and symptoms of serum sickness:** fever, malaise, arthralgia, nausea, vomiting, lymphadenopathy and morbilliform eruptions on trunk and extremities. Rash begins as asymptomatic pale pink macules in periumbilical region, axilla, and groin, then rapidly becomes generalized, erythematous, and confluent. Bands of progumin erythema along the sides of hands, fingers, feet, toes, and at margins of palm or plantar skin are characteristic.
- In ATG-induced serum sickness, when platelet count is low, petechiae and purpura rapidly replace rash as distributed over the body. Petechial areas are especially noticeable on legs but also on palms and soles.
- Serum sickness may occur during drug administration or when treatment is stopped but usually occurs 6–18 d after initiation of therapy.
- Because patient is usually receiving concomitant corticosteroids and antimetabolites, monitor carefully for signs of thrombocytopenia, concurrent infection, leukopenia.
- If other immunosuppressant therapy being used concomitantly is reduced, masked reactions to ATG may emerge. Monitor patient closely.
- Monitor patient's temperature and attend to complaints of sore throat or rhinorrhea. Physician may stop ATG treatment if these symptoms occur.
- Inspect patient's mouth daily to prevent serious overgrowth problems. If patient is unable to brush and floss teeth, it should be done for him.

Patient & Family Education
- Instruct patients to immediately report pain in chest, flank, or back; chills; pruritus; night sweats; sore throat.

Prototype: vasopressin, p 239

LYPRESSIN
(lye-press´in)
Trade name: Diapid
Classification: SYNTHETIC HORMONE; PITUITARY (ANTIDIURETIC)
Pregnancy: Category B

ACTIONS/PHARMACODYNAMICS Lysine vasopressin; synthetic polypeptide with pharmacologic actions similar to those of vasopressin. Possesses antidiuretic activity, with little oxytocic and minimal cardiovascular pressor (vasopressor) activity in therapeutic doses. Promotes reabsorption of water in kidneys (antidiuretic hormone effect) by increasing permeability to water in renal distal tubule. As a result, urine increases in osmolality with concurrent reduction in water (urine) output.

USES To control or prevent complications of central diabetes insipidus due to deficiency of endogenous posterior pituitary antidiuretic hormone. Particularly useful in patients who are nonresponsive to other forms of therapy and who experience allergic or other undesirable effects from vasopressin of animal origin.

ROUTE & DOSAGE

Diabetes Insipidus

Adult	Intranasal	1–2 sprays in each nostril q.i.d.
Child	Intranasal	Same as for adult

PHARMACOKINETICS Onset: 0.5–2 h. **Duration:** 3–8 h. **Metabolism:** metabolized in kidneys and liver. **Elimination:** half-life: 15 min; excreted in urine.

CONTRAINDICATIONS & PRECAUTIONS Contraindicated in: pregnancy (category B). **Cautious use in:** patients for whom pressor effects would be undesirable, coronary artery disease, known sensitivity to antidiuretic hormone.

ADVERSE/SIDE EFFECTS Infrequent and mild: **Local:** rhinorrhea, nasal congestion and irritation, pruritus and ulceration of nasal passages. **Systemic:** headache, conjunctivitis, heartburn secondary to excessive nasal administration with postnasal drip, abdominal cramps, increased bowel movements. **Other:** with inadvertent oral inhalation: substernal tightness, coughing, and transient dyspnea; marked but transient fluid retention (overdosage); hypersensitivity.

DRUG INTERACTIONS Demeclocycline, lithium, other VASOPRESSORS may decrease antidiuretic response; **carbamazepine, chlorpropamide, clofibrate** may prolong antidiuretic response.

NURSING IMPLICATIONS

Administration

- Instruct patient to clear nasal passages well before administering the spray. Warn patient not to inhale the spray.
- A uniform, well-diffused spray will be delivered by holding bottle upright and inserting nozzle into nostril with patient's head in a vertical position.
- If more than 2 sprays for each nostril are needed

q4–6h to give relief, the frequency of administration rather than number of sprays per dose should be increased. Large doses (excess) will drain posteriorly into digestive tract, where drug will be inactivated. Warn patients not to increase dosage without physician's order.
- Have patient close eyes before actuating spray to prevent inadvertent contact of drug with conjunctiva.

Assessment & Drug Effects

- At beginning of therapy, establish baseline for BP and weight.
- Monitor I & D, urine, and serum osmololity.
- Monitor for and report symptoms of water intoxication (see chap 3). This occurs with overdose and is usually transient.

Patient & Family Education

- See instructions for use of intranasal spray under administration.
- If nocturia is a problem, physician may prescribe an additional dose at bedtime.
- If the patient develops a cold or allergy, absorption of lypressin will be diminished. Advise the patient to report to physician; adjustment of therapy may be required.
- Lypressin dosage is individualized to control **symptoms of diabetes insipidus:** frequent urination and excessive thirst.
- Skin tests may be performed for patients with history of hypersensitivity to antidiuretic hormones prior to initiation of therapy.

Prototype: sulfisoxazole, p 88

MAFENIDE ACETATE
(ma´fe-nide)
Trade name: Sulfamylon
Classifications: ANTIINFECTIVE; SULFONAMIDE DERIVATIVE
Pregnancy: Category C

ACTIONS/PHARMACODYNAMICS Topical sulfonamide derivative. Bacteriostatic against many gram-positive and gram-negative organisms, including *Pseudomonas aeruginosa,* and certain strains of anaerobes. Topical applications produce marked reduction of bacterial growth in avascular tissue. Active in presence of pus and serum and not affected by changes in pH of tissue environment. Major metabolite of mafenide inhibits carbonic anhydrase, which may result in alkaline urine and metabolic acidosis when large amounts of drug are absorbed from application sites. Cross-sensitivity with other sulfonamides not established.

USES Adjunctive therapy in second- and third-degree burns to prevent sepsis.

ROUTE & DOSAGE

Burns

Adult	Topical	Apply aseptically to burn areas to a thickness of approximately 15 mm (1/16 in) once or twice daily

PHARMACOKINETICS Absorption: rapidly absorbed from burn surface. **Peak:** 2–4 h. **Metabolism:** rapidly inactivated in blood to a weak carbonic anhydrase inhibitor. **Elimination:** eliminated through kidneys.

CONTRAINDICATIONS & PRECAUTIONS Contraindicated in: history of hypersensitivity to mafenide or to any ingredients in the formulation (e.g., metabisulfite); respiratory (inhalation) injury, pulmonary infection. Safe use during pregnancy (category C) not established. **Cautious use in:** impaired renal or pulmonary function.

ADVERSE/SIDE EFFECTS Hypersensitivity: pruritus, rash, urticaria, blisters, facial edema, eosinophilia. **Skin:** *intense pain, burning, or stinging at application sites,* bleeding of skin, excessive body water loss, delayed eschar separation, excoriation of new skin, superinfections. **Other:** metabolic acidosis, fatal hemolytic anemia (rare); bone marrow suppression (rare).

NURSING IMPLICATIONS

Administration

- Wound cleaning and removal of debris should be carried out before each reapplication of mafenide cream. Discuss with physician.
- Mafenide cream is applied aseptically to cleansed, debrided burn areas with sterile gloved hand.

- Burn areas must be covered with cream at all times. When necessary, reapplications should be made to areas from which cream has been removed (e.g., by patient's activity).
- Store in tight, light-resistant containers. Avoid extremes of temperature.

Assessment & Drug Effects

- Monitor vital signs. Report immediately changes in BP, pulse, and respiratory rate and volume.
- Monitor I&O. Report oliguria or changes in I&O ratio and pattern.
- Acid-base balance should be monitored in patients with extensive burns and in those with pulmonary or renal dysfunction. Be alert to signs and symptoms of metabolic acidosis (see chap 3).
- In patients with extensive burns, it is advisable to maintain a flow chart to monitor mental status, vital signs, I&O, weight, burn wound care, medications, and laboratory data.
- Be alert to evidence of superinfections (see Signs & Symptoms, chap 3), particularly in and below burn eschar.
- It is frequently difficult to distinguish between adverse reactions to mafenide and the effects of severe burns. Accurate observations are critical.
- Allergic reactions have reportedly occurred 10–14 d after initiation of mafenide therapy. Temporary discontinuation of drug may be necessary.
- Intensity of local pain caused by mafenide may require administration of analgesic. Report to physician.
- Mafenide therapy is usually continued until healing is progressing well (usually ≤ 60 d) or site is ready for grafting (after about 35–40 d). It is not withdrawn while there is a possibility of infection unless adverse reactions intervene.

Prototype: aluminum hydroxide, p 212

MAGALDRATE
(mag´al-drate)
Trade names: Hydromagnesium aluminate, Lowsium, Riopan
Classification: GI AGENT; ANTACID
Pregnancy: Category C

ACTIONS/PHARMACODYNAMICS Complex of aluminum and magnesium hydroxides (not just a physical mixture). Nonsystemic antacid with true

M

Common side effects in *italic*; life-threatening effects underlined; generic names in **bold**; classifications in SMALL CAPS

719

buffering action and high acid-neutralizing capacity. By reducing gastric acidity, stomach pH increases and proteolytic activity of pepsin is inhibited. Also increases lower esophageal sphincter tone. Reportedly does not produce alkalosis or acid rebound and is not as likely to produce alterations of bowel function that occur with either aluminum or magensium hydroxide alone. Low sodium content (not more than 0.3 mg of sodium per 400 mg tablet or 5 ml of suspension).

USES Symptomatic relief of hyperacidity associated with peptic ulcer, gastritis, peptic esophagitis, and hiatal hernia, particularly in patients who need to restrict sodium.

ROUTE & DOSAGE

Antacid

Adult	PO	480–1080 mg (5–10 ml suspension or 1–2 tablets) q.i.d. (max 20 tablets or 100 ml/d)

PHARMACOKINETICS Absorption: minimally absorbed from GI tract. **Duration:** buffering action may persist for 60 min.

CONTRAINDICATIONS & PRECAUTIONS Contraindicated in: sensitivity to components. Pregnancy (category C). **Cautious use in:** impaired renal function.

ADVERSE/SIDE EFFECTS Infrequent: constipation or diarrhea (with prolonged use), hypermagnesemia (in patients with impaired renal function).

NURSING IMPLICATIONS

Administration
- Shake suspension vigorously before pouring. Preferably administered between meals and at bedtime.
- Suspension should be taken with sufficient water to ensure passage of drug into stomach.
- Chewable tablet should be chewed thoroughly before it is swallowed. Tablet to be swallowed whole should be taken with enough water to ensure prompt swallowing without chewing.

Assessment & Drug Effects
- Question patient about effectiveness of medication in relieving GI distress.

- Patients on prolonged therapy should be periodically checked for electrolyte imbalance (i.e., hypermagnesemia).

Patient & Family Education
- In common with other antacids, magaldrate may cause premature dissolution and absorption of enteric-coated tablets and may interfere with the absorption of oral tetracyclines and other oral medications.
- In general it is advisable not to take other oral drugs within 1–2 h of an antacid.

Prototype: magnesium hydroxide, p 220

MAGNESIUM CITRATE

Trade names: Citrate of Magnesia, Citroma, Citro-Nesia
Classification: GI AGENT; SALINE CATHARTIC
Pregnancy: Category B

ACTIONS/PHARMACODYNAMICS Contains magnesium carbonate, citric acid, and potassium or sodium bicarbonate for added effervescence, in a lemon oil or cherry-flavored base. Promotes bowel evacuation by causing osmotic retention of fluid, which distends colon and stimulates peristaltic activity. Magnesium content approximately 140 mEq/200 ml.

USES To evacuate bowel prior to certain surgical and diagnostic procedures and to help eliminate parasites and toxic materials after treatment with a vermifuge.

ROUTE & DOSAGE

Bowel Evacuation

Adult	PO	240 ml once
Child	PO	2–6 y: 4–12 ml
		6–12 y: 50–100 ml

CONTRAINDICATIONS & PRECAUTIONS Contraindicated in: renal disease; nausea, vomiting, diarrhea, abdominal pain, acute surgical abdomen; intestinal impaction, obstruction or perforation; rectal bleeding; use of solutions containing sodium bicarbonate in patients on sodium-restricted diets.

M

ADVERSE/SIDE EFFECTS Abdominal cramps, nausea, fluid and electrolyte imbalance, hypermagnesemia (prolonged use).

NURSING IMPLICATIONS

Administration

- Most effective when taken on an empty stomach with a full (240 ml) glass of water. Time dosing so that it does not interfere with sleep. Produces a watery or semifluid evacuation in 2–6 h.
- To increase palatability manufacturer suggests chilling the solution by pouring it over ice or refrigerating it until ready to use.
- Once container is opened, magnesium citrate will lose some of its effervescence. This may affect palatability somewhat but not quality of preparation.
- Store in tightly covered containers at 2–30C (36–86F).

Assessment & Drug Effects

- Since drug may cause intense bowel evacuation, patient should be monitored for dehydration, hypokalemia, and hyponatremia (see Signs & Symptoms, chap 3).
- Patients on prolonged therapy should be periodically checked for electrolyte imbalance (i.e., hypermagnesemia).

Patient & Family Education

- Advise all patients, especially the elderly, that this drug should not be used for routine treatment of constipation.
- Advise patients that some degree of abdominal cramping is to be expected.

MAGNESIUM HYDROXIDE

See GASTROINTESTINAL AGENT, SALINE CATHARTIC prototype, p 220.

Prototype: magnesium hydroxide, p 220

MAGNESIUM OXIDE

Trade names: Mag-Ox, Maox, Par-Mag, Uro-Mag
Classifications: GI AGENT; ANTACID; SALINE CATHARTIC

ACTIONS/PHARMACODYNAMICS Nonsystemic antacid with high neutralizing capacity and relatively long duration of action. Its action is essentially the same as that of magnesium hydroxide.

Uses Essentially the same as those of magnesium hydroxide. May also be used as a magnesium supplement.

ROUTE & DOSAGE

Antacid

Adult	PO	280–1500 mg with water or milk q.i.d., p.c. and h.s.

Laxative

Adult	PO	2–4 g with water or milk h.s.

Magnesium Supplement

Adult	PO	400–1200 mg/d in divided doses

PHARMACOKINETICS Absorption: 30–50% absorbed from GI tract. **Elimination:** eliminated in urine.

ADVERSE/SIDE EFFECTS *Diarrhea,* abdominal cramps, nausea; hypermagnesemia, renal stones (chronic use).

NURSING IMPLICATIONS

Administration

- In common with other antacids, magnesium oxide can cause premature dissolution and absorption of enteric-coated and sustained release tablets and also may complex with and thus reduce absorption of PO tetracyclines and other oral drugs. In general, it is advisable not to take other oral medications within 1–2 h of an antacid.
- Store in airtight containers at 15–30C (59–86F) unless otherwise directed. On exposure to air, magnesium oxide rapidly absorbs moisture and carbon dioxide.

M

Assessment & Drug Effects

▪ Since drug may cause intense bowel evacuation, patient should be monitored for dehydration, hypokalemia, and hyponatremia (see Signs & Symptoms, chap 3).

▪ Patients on prolonged therapy should be periodically checked for electrolyte imbalance (i.e., hypermagnesemia).

Patient & Family Education

▪ As with other antacids, the liquid preparation is reportedly more effective than the tablet form.

Prototype: aspirin, p 161

MAGNESIUM SALICYLATE

Trade names: Doan's Pills, Magan, Mobidin
Classifications: CNS AGENT; ANTIPYRETIC; NONNARCOTIC ANALGESIC; SALICYLATE; NSAID
Pregnancy: Category C

ACTIONS/PHARMACODYNAMICS Sodium-free salicylate derivative with low incidence of GI irritation. In equal doses, less potent than aspirin as an analgesic and antipyretic. Unlike aspirin, not associated with asthmatic reactions and does not inhibit platelet aggregation or increase bleeding time. Magnesium salicylate 1 g is equivalent to 1 g aspirin.

USES Relief of pain and inflammation in rheumatoid arthritis, osteoarthritis, bursitis, and other musculoskeletal disorders.

ROUTE & DOSAGE

Analgesic/Antipyretic
Adult   PO   650 mg t.i.d. or q.i.d.

Arthritic Conditions
Adult   PO   Up to 9.6 g/d in divided doses

CONTRAINDICATIONS & PRECAUTIONS Contraindicated in: hypersensitivity to salicylates, erosive gastritis, peptic ulcer; advanced renal insufficiency, liver damage, bleeding disorders, before surgery. Safe use during pregnancy (category C), in nursing mothers, and in children < 12 y not established.

ADVERSE/SIDE EFFECTS Salicylism: *dizziness, drowsiness, tinnitus, hearing loss, nausea, vomiting,* hypermagnesemia (with high doses in patients with renal insufficiency).

DRUG INTERACTIONS Aminosalicylic acid increases risk of salicylate toxicity; **ammonium chloride** and other ACIDIFYING AGENTS decrease renal elimination and increase risk of salicylate toxicity; anticoagulants—added risk of bleeding with ANTICOAGULANTS; CARBONIC ANHYDRASE INHIBITORS enhance salicylate toxicity; CORTICOSTEROIDS compound ulcerogenic effects; increases **methotrexate** toxicity; low doses of salicylates may antagonize uricosuric effects of **probenecid, sulfinpyrazone.**

NURSING IMPLICATIONS

Administration

▪ Administer with a full glass of water or with food or milk to minimize gastric irritation.

Assessment & Drug Effects

▪ If used in high dosages or in patients with any degree of renal impairment, serum magnesium levels should be monitored because of risk of hypermagnesemia.

▪ Use of salicylates in children or teenagers with influenza or chicken pox may be associated with development of Reye's syndrome and is therefore not advised.

Patient & Family Education

▪ Advise patient to promptly report tinnitus, hearing loss, or dizziness.

▪ Advise patient not to take aspirin-containing drugs without consent of physician.

▪ Note: In Canada, Doan's pills contain acetaminophen plus salicylamide.

Prototype: magnesium hydroxide, p 220

MAGNESIUM SULFATE

Trade name: Epsom Salt
Classifications: GI AGENT; SALINE CATHARTIC; REPLACEMENT AGENT; ANTICONVULSANT
Pregnancy: Category A

ACTIONS/PHARMACODYNAMICS When taken PO, magnesium sulfate acts as laxative by osmotic retention of fluid, which distends colon, in-

M

creases water content of feces, and causes mechanical stimulation of bowel activity. When given parenterally, it acts as CNS depressant and also depressant of smooth, skeletal, and cardiac muscle function. Anticonvulsant properties thought to be produced by CNS depression, principally by decreasing the amount of acetylcholine liberated from motor nerve terminals, thus producing peripheral neuromuscular blockade. Believed to act on myocardium by slowing rate of S-A node impulse formation and prolonging conduction time. In excessive doses, produces vasodilation by ganglionic blockade and direct action on blood vessels.

USES PO to relieve acute constipation and to evacuate bowel in preparation for x-ray of intestines. Parenterally to control seizures in toxemia of pregnancy, epilepsy, and acute nephritis and for prophylaxis and treatment of hypomagnesemia. Topically to reduce edema, inflammation, and itching. **Unlabeled uses:** to inhibit premature labor (tocolytic action) and as adjunct in hyperalimentation.

ROUTE & DOSAGE

Laxative

Adult	PO	10–15 g once/d

Preeclampsia, Eclampsia

Adult	IM/IV	4 g in 250 ml D5W infused slowly, followed by 4–5 g IM in alternate buttocks q4h

Hypomagnesemic Seizures

Adult	IM/IV	*Mild:* 1 g q6h for 4 doses *Severe:* 250 mg/kg infused over 4 h
Child	IM/IV	100 mg/kg q4–6h

Total Parenteral Nutrition

Adult	IV	0.5–3 g/d

PHARMACOKINETICS Onset: 1–2 h PO; 1 h IM. **Duration:** 30 min IV; 3–4 h PO. **Distribution:** crosses placenta; distributed into breast milk. **Elimination:** eliminated in kidneys.

CONTRAINDICATIONS & PRECAUTIONS Contraindicated in: myocardial damage; heart block; IV administration during the 2 h preceding delivery; PO use in patients with abdominal pain, nausea, vomiting, fecal impaction, or intestinal irritation, obstruction, or perforation; pregnancy (category A). **Cautious use in:** impaired renal function, digitalized patients, concomitant use of other CNS depressants or neuromuscular blocking agents.

ADVERSE/SIDE EFFECTS Hypermagnesemia: *flushing, sweating, extreme thirst, hypotension, sedation, confusion,* depressed reflexes or no reflexes, muscle weakness, flaccid paralysis, hypothermia, depressed cardiac function, <u>complete heart block, circulatory collapse, respiratory paralysis;</u> hypocalcemia. **Repeated laxative use:** dehydration, electrolyte imbalance including hypocalcemia.

DRUG INTERACTIONS NEUROMUSCULAR BLOCKING AGENTS add to respiratory depression and apnea.

INCOMPATIBILITIES Solution/Additive: 10% fat emulsion; calcium gluceptate, clindamycin, dobutamine, polymyxin B sulfate, procaine, sodium bicarbonate.

NURSING IMPLICATIONS

Administration

- For laxative action, magnesium sulfate is best administered in the morning or midafternoon in a glass of water. Bitter, salty taste may be disguised by chilling or flavoring with lemon or orange juice.
- A 10% solution may be given by direct IV at a rate of 1.5 ml/min or 150 mg/min.
- A solution of 4 g in 250 ml of D5W may be infused at a rate not to exceed 3 ml/min.

Assessment & Drug Effects

- When magnesium sulfate is given IV, patient requires constant observation. Check BP and pulse q10–15min or more often if indicated.
- Monitoring of plasma magnesium levels is advised in patients receiving drug parenterally (**normal:** 1.8–3.0 mEq/L). Plasma levels in excess of 4 mEq/L are reflected in depressed deep tendon reflexes and other symptoms of magnesium intoxication. See adverse/side effects. Cardiac arrest occurs at levels in excess of 25 mEq/L.
- Early indicators of magnesium toxicity (hypermagnesemia) include cathartic effect, profound thirst, feeling of warmth, sedation, confusion, depressed deep tendon reflexes, and muscle weakness. Calcium and phosphorus levels should be monitored also.
- Monitor I&O (in patients receiving drug parenterally). Report oliguria and changes in I&O ratio.
- Before each repeated parenteral dose, patellar reflex should be tested. Depression or absence of reflexes is a useful index of early magnesium intoxication. Also check respiratory rate and character and urinary output, especially in patients with impaired renal function. Therapy is generally not con-

Common side effects in *italic*; life-threatening effects <u>underlined</u>; generic names in **bold**; classifications in SMALL CAPS

723

M

tinued if urinary output is less than 100 ml during the 4 h preceding each dose.

- Newborns of mothers who received parenteral magnesium sulfate within a few hours of delivery should be observed for signs of toxicity, including respiratory and neuromuscular depression.
- Patients receiving the drug for hypomagnesemia should be observed for improvement in these signs of deficiency: irritability, choreiform movements, tremors, tetany, twitching, muscle cramps, tachycardia, hypertension, psychotic behavior. (Hypomagnesemia is frequently associated with other electrolyte deficiencies, especially calcium and potassium.)

Patient & Family Education
- Sufficient water should be taken during the day when drug is administered orally to prevent net loss of body water.
- Recommended daily allowances of magnesium are obtained in a normal diet. Rich sources are wholegrain cereals, legumes, nuts, meats, seafood, milk, most green leafy vegetables, and bananas.

MANNITOL

See ELECTROLYTIC & WATER BALANCE AGENTS, DIURETIC, OSMOTIC prototype, p 200.

Prototype: imipramine, p 184

MAPROTILINE HYDROCHLORIDE

(ma-proe´ti-leen)
Trade name: Ludiomil
Classifications: CNS AGENT; PSYCHOTHERAPEUTIC; TETRACYCLIC ANTIDEPRESSANT
Pregnancy: Category B

ACTIONS/PHARMACODYNAMICS Tetracyclic antidepressant pharmacologically and therapeutically similar to the tricyclic antidepressants. Has significant sedative effect and less prominent anticholinergic action; may lower seizure threshold. Useful in depression associated with anxiety and sleep disturbances.xx

USES Treatment of depressive neurosis (dysthymic disorder) and manic-depressive illness, depressed type (major depressive disorder).

ROUTE & DOSAGE

Mild to Moderate Depression

Adult   PO   start at 75 mg/d and gradually increase q2wk up to 150 mg/d in single or divided doses

Severe Depression

Adult   PO   start at 100–150 mg/d and gradually increase up to 300 mg/d in single or divided doses if needed

---

PHARMACOKINETICS Absorption: slowly absorbed from GI tract. **Peak:** 12 h. **Distribution:** distributed chiefly to brain, lungs, liver and kidneys. **Metabolism:** metabolized in liver. **Elimination:** half-life: 51 h; 70% excreted in urine, 30% in feces.

CONTRAINDICATIONS & PRECAUTIONS Contraindicated in: patients < 18 y; history of seizure disorder.

ADVERSE/SIDE EFFECTS CNS: seizures, exacerbation of psychosis, hallucinations, tremors, excitement, confusion, dizziness, *drowsiness*. **CV:** *orthostatic hypotension,* hypertension, tachycardia. **Eye:** accommodation disturbances, blurred vision, mydriasis. **GI:** nausea, vomiting, epigastric distress, *constipation, dry mouth.* **GU:** *urinary retention,* frequency. **Hypersensitivity:** skin rash, urticaria, photosensitivity.

DRUG INTERACTIONS May decrease some response to ANTIHYPERTENSIVES; CNS DEPRESSANTS, **alcohol,** HYPNOTICS, BARBITURATES, SEDATIVES potentiate CNS depression; may increase hypoprothrombinemic effect of ORAL ANTICOAGULANTS; transient delirium with **ethchlorvynol;** with **levodopa,** SYMPATHOMIMETICS (e.g., **epinephrine, norepinephrine**) there is possibility of sympathetic hyperactivity with hypertension and hyperpyrexia; with MAO INHIBITORS there is possibility of severe reactions, toxic psychosis, cardiovascular instability; **methylphenidate** increases plasma TCA levels; THYROID DRUGS increase possibility of arrhythmias; **cimetidine** may increase plasma TCA levels.

NURSING IMPLICATIONS

Administration
- Drug may be given as single dose or in divided doses. Risk of seizures is reduced by initiating therapy with low dosages.
- Store drug at 15–30C (59–86F) unless otherwise specified.

Common side effects in *italic*; life-threatening effects underlined; generic names in **bold**; classifications in SMALL CAPS

Assessment & Drug Effects

- Therapeutic effects are sometimes seen in 3–7 d; 2–3 wk are usually necessary.
- Assess level of sedative effect. If recovering patient becomes too lethargic to care for personal hygiene or to maintain food intake and interactions with others, report to physician.
- The severely depressed patient may need assistance with personal hygiene, particularly because of excessive sweating caused by the drug.
- Monitor bowel elimination pattern and I&O ratio. Severe constipation and urinary retention are potential problems, especially in the elderly. Advise increased fluid intake (at least 1500 ml/d).
- Risk of seizures appears to be high in heavy drinkers. Observe seizure precautions.
- If patient uses excessive amounts of alcohol, it should be borne in mind that the potentiation of maprotiline effects may increase the danger of overdosage or suicide attempt.

Patient & Family Education

- Urge outpatient on high doses to report symptoms of stomatitis and dry mouth. Sore or dry mouth interferes with mastication and swallowing and can be a major cause of poor food intake, dental problems, and lack of compliance. Consult physician about use of a saliva substitute (e.g., Moi-Stir).
- Caution patient that ability to perform tasks requiring alertness and skill may be impaired during early therapy.
- Urge patient not to change dose or dose schedule without consulting physician.
- Advise patient not to use OTC drugs unless physician approves.
- The actions of both alcohol and maprotiline are potentiated when they are used together during therapy and for ≤ 2 wk after maprotiline is discontinued. Consult physician about amount of alcohol, if any, that can be taken.

Prototype: diethylpropion, p 196

MAZINDOL
(may´zin-dole)
Trade names: Mazanor, Sanorex
Classifications: CNS AGENT; RESPIRATORY AND CEREBRAL STIMULANT; ANOREXIANT
Pregnancy: Category C
Controlled substance: Schedule IV

ACTIONS/PHARMACODYNAMICS Pharmacologic properties are similar to those of amphetamines. Produces CNS and cardiac stimulation in addition to amphetamine-like effects. Appears to exert primary effects on limbic system and to alter norepinephrine metabolism by inhibiting normal neuronal uptake mechanism.

USES Short-term management of exogenous obesity.

ROUTE & DOSAGE

Obesity
Adult   PO   1 mg t.i.d. a.c. *or* 2 mg once/d 1 h before lunch

PHARMACOKINETICS Absorption: readily absorbed from GI tract. **Onset:** 30–60 min. **Duration:** 8–15 h. **Metabolism:** metabolized in liver. **Elimination:** half-life: 2.5–9 h; 95% excreted in feces, 2–5% in urine.

CONTRAINDICATIONS & PRECAUTIONS Contraindicated in: glaucoma; severe hypertension; symptomatic cardiovascular disease, including arrhythmias; agitated states; history of drug abuse; during or within 14 d after administration of MAO inhibitors; children < 12 y. Safe use during pregnancy (category C) not established. **Cautious use in:** hyperexcitability states.

ADVERSE/SIDE EFFECTS CNS: *restlessness,* dizziness, insomnia, dysphoria, depression, tremor, headache, drowsiness, weakness. **CV:** palpitation, tachycardia. **Endocrine:** impotence, changes in libido (rare). **GI:** *dry mouth,* unpleasant taste, diarrhea, constipation, nausea, vomiting. **Skin:** rash, excessive sweating, clamminess.

DRUG INTERACTIONS Acetazolamide, sodium bicarbonate decrease mazindol elimination; **ammonium chloride, ascorbic acid** increase mazindol elimination; the effects of mazindol and BARBITURATES may be antagonized; **furazolidone** may increase BP effects of mazindol, and interaction may persist for several weeks after discontinuing furazolidone; antihypertensive effects of **guanethidine, guanadryl** antagonized; MAO INHIBITORS, **selegiline** can cause hypertensive crisis—do not administer mazindol during or within 14 d of administration of these drugs; PHENOTHIAZINES may inhibit mood elevating effects of mazindol; BETA-ADRENERGIC AGONISTS increase adverse cardiovascular effects of mazindol.

M

NURSING IMPLICATIONS

Administration

- Drug is given 1 h before meals if t.i.d. or 1 h before lunch if q.d. dose.
- Drug may be taken with meals if GI discomfort occurs.

Assessment & Drug Effects

- Monitor weight periodically.
- If patient experiences excessive restlessness or insomnia, drug may have to be taken early in the day.

Patient & Family Education

- Rate of weight loss is greatest during first few weeks of therapy and tends to decrease thereafter.
- Insulin requirements of patients with diabetes may be decreased in association with use of mazindol and concomitant caloric restriction and weight loss.
- Tolerance may develop within a few weeks. When it occurs, drug should be discontinued.
- Caution patients that mazindol may impair ability to perform hazardous activities such as driving a car or operating machinery.
- Instruct patient not to take more medication than prescribed.
- Instruct patient to report excessively dry mouth or constipation.

MEBENDAZOLE

See ANTIINFECTIVES, ANTHELMINTIC prototype, p 53.

Prototype: methyldopa, p 148

MECAMYLAMINE HYDROCHLORIDE

(mek-a-mill´a-meen)
Trade name: Inversine
Classifications: CARDIOVASCULAR AGENT; CENTRAL ACTING ANTIHYPERTENSIVE

ACTIONS/PHARMACODYNAMICS Potent, long-acting secondary amine nondepolarizing ganglionic blocking agent. Blocks neurotransmission at both sympathetic and parasympathetic ganglia by competing with ACh for cholinergic receptor sites on postsynaptic membranes. Reduces BP in both normotensive and hypertensive individuals, generally with greater decrease in standing or sitting BP than in supine BPs. Tolerance rarely develops; curarelike effects may be produced by large doses.

USES Moderately severe to severe hypertension and uncomplicated malignant hypertension.

ROUTE & DOSAGE

Moderately Severe to Severe Hypertension

Adult	PO	2.5 mg b.i.d. p.c. for 2 d, increased by increments of 2.5 mg at intervals of ≥ 2 d until desired BP response is attained (2.5–25 mg/d in 2–4 divided doses)

PHARMACOKINETICS Absorption: almost completely absorbed from GI tract. **Onset:** 30 min–2 h. **Peak:** 3–5 h. **Duration:** 6–12 h. **Distribution:** crosses blood-brain barrier and placenta; distributed into breast milk. **Metabolism:** metabolized in liver. **Elimination:** primarily excreted in urine.

CONTRAINDICATIONS & PRECAUTIONS Contraindicated in: coronary insufficiency, pyloric stenosis, glaucoma, uremia, chronic pyelonephritis, recent MI; mild labile hypertension; unreliable uncooperative patients; pregnancy. **Cautious use in:** rising or elevated BUN; renal, cerebral, or coronary vascular pathology; recent CVA; prostatic hypertrophy, bladder neck obstruction, urethral stricture.

ADVERSE/SIDE EFFECTS Mostly dose-related. **CNS:** weakness, fatigue, sedation, headache, paresthesias, choreiform movements, tremor, nervousness, anxiety, insomnia, slurred speech, seizures, mental aberrations, confusion, mania, or depression. **CV:** *orthostatic hypotension,* changes in heart rate, dizziness, syncope, precipitation of angina. **EENT:** mydriasis, *blurred vision,* cyclopegia, nasal congestion, *dry mouth* with dysphagia, glossitis. **GI:** *anorexia,* glossitis, *nausea, vomiting, constipation, diarrhea,* adynamic ileus. **Other:** decreased libido, impotence, *urinary retention,* dysuria, malaise, hyperuricemia, interstitial pulmonary edema and fibrosis, anhidrosis, exacerbation of psoriasis, hyperuricemia (asymptomatic).

DRUG INTERACTIONS Alcohol, other ANTIHYPERTENSIVE AGENTS, **bethanechol,** THIAZIDE DIURETICS potentiate hypotensive effects; **acetazolamide, sodium bicarbonate** increase mecamylamine toxicity because they decrease its elimination.

Common side effects in *italic*; life-threatening effects underlined; generic names in **bold**; classifications in SMALL CAPS

NURSING IMPLICATIONS

Administration

- Administration of drug after meals may result in more gradual absorption and smoother control of BP. Timing relative to meals should be consistent.
- Because of diurnal variations in BP, physician may prescribe a relatively small dose in the morning or omission of morning dose (morning BP usually lower) and larger doses for afternoon or evening.
- Mecamylamine withdrawal should be accomplished slowly. Sudden discontinuation of drug can result in severe hypertensive rebound with CVA and acute CHF. Usually, other antihypertensive therapy must be substituted gradually, and patient must be supervised daily during period of dosage adjustment.
- Store at 15–30C (59–86F) unless otherwise directed.

Assessment & Drug Effects

- Initial regulation of dosage should be dictated by BP readings in standing position at time of maximal drug effect, as well as symptoms of orthostatic hypotension (faintness, dizziness, lightheadedness). Also note any changes in pulse rate.
- Partial tolerance may develop in some patients, necessitating dosage adjustment. Follow-up supervision is an essential part of therapy.
- Constipation, frequent loose stools with abdominal distension, or decreased bowel sounds may be the first signs of paralytic ileus (relatively frequent) and should be reported promptly. Paralytic ileus is sometimes preceded by small, frequent stools.

Patient & Family Education

- Some physicians direct their patients to check BP before taking mecamylamine and to reduce or omit a dose if reading is below a previously designated figure.
- Instruct patient to make position changes slowly and in stages, particularly from recumbent to upright posture, and to sit on edge of bed and move ankles and feet before ambulating.
- Advise patient to lie down immediately if he or she is feeling lightheaded or dizzy. Adverse reactions should be reported immediately, as drug effects may last hours to days after drug is discontinued.
- Patients should be informed of factors that may potentiate the action of mecamylamine: excessive heat, fever, infection, alcohol, vigorous exercise, salt depletion (vomiting, diarrhea, excessive sweating, diuresis). Hypotensive action may also be prominent during pregnancy, anesthesia, or surgery.
- Seasonal variations may alter the hypotensive effect, e.g., usually smaller doses are required in summer than in winter.
- Caution patient to avoid driving and other potentially hazardous activities until reaction to drug is known.
- If mouth dryness is a problem, advise patient to rinse mouth frequently with clear warm water; try sugarless gum or lemon drops. If these measures fail, a saliva substitute, e.g., Xero-Lube, Moi-stir, may help (available OTC).

MECHLORETHAMINE HYDROCHLORIDE

See ANTINEOPLASTICS, NITROGEN MUSTARD prototype, p 96.

MECLIZINE HYDROCHLORIDE

See ANTIHISTAMINES, ANTIVERTIGO AGENT prototype, p 50.

Prototype: tetracycline, p 74

MECLOCYCLINE SULFOSALICYLATE
(me-kloe-sye´kleen)
Trade name: Meclan
Classifications: ANTIINFECTIVE; ANTIBIOTIC; TETRACYCLINE
Pregnancy: Category B

ACTIONS/PHARMACODYNAMICS Synthetic derivative of oxytetracycline. Antibacterial action appears to be related to ability to suppress growth of susceptible organisms, principally *Propionibacterium acnes*, an anaerobic organism in sebaceous glands and follicles. Another proposed mechanism of action is the reduction of free fatty acids in sebum. (Free fatty acids are believed to contribute to formation of inflammatory acne lesions and comedones.) Inactive against viruses and fungi. Sensitivity and contact dermatitis have not been demonstrated by patch testing. The commercial preparation Meclan contains sodium formaldehyde sulfoxylate.

M

Common side effects in *italic*; life-threatening effects underlined; generic names in **bold**; classifications in SMALL CAPS

727

USES Inflammatory acne vulgaris.

ROUTE & DOSAGE

Inflammatory Acne Vulgaris

Adult	Topical	Apply to affected areas b.i.d., AM and PM

PHARMACOKINETICS Absorption: not absorbed systemically in measurable amounts.

CONTRAINDICATIONS & PRECAUTIONS Contraindicated in: hypersensitivity to tetracyclines or to any ingredients in the formulation, e.g., formaldehyde. Safe use during pregnancy (category B), in nursing women, and in children < 11 y not established.

ADVERSE/SIDE EFFECTS Skin irritation; stinging, burning sensation; temporary yellow staining of skin around hair follicles (with excessive applications), superinfections.

NURSING IMPLICATIONS

Administration

- Apply cream generously morning and evening over affected skin areas.
- Less frequent applications may be used depending on patient's response.

Assessment & Drug Effects

- Since significant percutaneous absorption may result with prolonged use, carefully monitor patients with renal or hepatic dysfunction.
- Monitor for signs and symptoms of superinfection (see chap 3).

Patient & Family Education

- Advise patient to apply medication as directed and to keep follow-up appointments. Overuse of tetracycline preparations can result in overgrowth of nonsusceptible organisms.
- Inform patient that excessive applications of meclocycline may cause temporary staining around hair roots and also can stain fabrics.
- Avoid use of meclocycline near or in eyes, ears, nose, mouth, or other mucous membranes.
- Advise patient to notify physician if noticeable improvement has not occurred by 6–8 wk. Maximum benefit may not be apparent for ≤ 12 wk.
- Patients should be informed that skin areas treated with meclocycline will fluoresce under ultraviolet light.
- Possibility of cumulative drying or irritant effects can occur with use of abrasive or medicated soaps

and cleaners, other topical acne preparations, alcohol-containing preparations (e.g., after-shave astringents, lotions), "cover-up" medications, peeling agents (e.g., benzoyl peroxide, resorcinol, sulfur, salicylic acid, tretinoin. These preparations should be used with caution and only under medical guidance.

- **Skin hygiene:** some clinicians advise thorough cleansing of skin with soap and water twice daily; a cosmetic scrubbing pad (e.g., Buf-Puf) facilitates removal of dry scales.

Prototype: ibuprofen, p 160

MECLOFENAMATE SODIUM
(me-kloe-fen-am´ate)
Trade name: Meclomen
Classifications: CNS AGENT; ANTIPYRETIC; NONNARCOTIC ANALGESIC; NSAID
Pregnancy: Category B (D in third trimester)

ACTIONS/PHARMACODYNAMICS Halogenated anthranilic acid derivative with pharmacologic properties similar to those of ibuprofen. Has palliative antiinflammatory, analgesic, and antipyretic activity. Action mechanism unclear, but animal studies suggest that effects may result from inhibition of prostaglandin synthesis and competition for binding at prostaglandin receptor sites. Does not appear to alter course of arthritis. Comparable to ibuprofen with respect to drug efficacy in rheumatoid arthritis and to GI side effects but produces fewer reactions involving special senses and less fecal blood loss than aspirin. Transient inhibition of platelet aggregation has been reported; platelet count and bleeding time are not apparently affected.

USES Symptomatic treatment of acute or chronic rheumatoid arthritis and osteoarthritis. Also in combination with gold salts or corticosteroids in treatment of rheumatoid arthritis. **Unlabeled uses:** management of psoriatic arthritis, mild to moderate postoperative pain, dysmenorrhea.

ROUTE & DOSAGE

Inflammatory Disease

Adult	PO	200–400 mg/d in 3–4 divided doses (max 400 mg/d)

PHARMACOKINETICS Absorption: rapidly and completely absorbed from GI tract. **Peak:** 1–2 h.

Common side effects in *italic*; life-threatening effects underlined; generic names in **bold**; classifications in SMALL CAPS

Duration: 2–4 h. **Distribution:** crosses placenta. **Metabolism:** metabolized in liver. **Elimination:** half-life: 2–3.3 h; 60% excreted in urine, 30% in feces.

CONTRAINDICATIONS & PRECAUTIONS Contraindicated in: patient in whom bronchospasm, urticaria, and allergic rhinitis are induced by aspirin or other NSAIDs, first (category B) and third trimester of pregnancy (category D), nursing mothers, children < 14 y, patient designated as functional class IV rheumatoid arthritis (incapacitated, bedridden, or confined to wheelchair, little or no self-care); active peptic ulcer. **Cautious use in:** history of upper GI tract disease; compromised cardiac and renal function, or other conditions predisposing to fluid retention.

ADVERSE/SIDE EFFECTS CNS: *dizziness,* vertigo, lack of concentration, confusion, *headache,* tinnitus, hearing loss (rare). **CV:** edema. **GI:** *severe diarrhea (dose-related),* peptic ulceration, <u>GI bleeding</u>, dyspepsia, abdominal pain, *nausea,* vomiting (may be severe), flatulence, eructation, pyrosis, anorexia, constipation, stomatitis. **Hepatic:** *abnormal liver function tests,* cholestatic jaundice. **Other:** hot flashes, blurred vision. **Renal:** elevated BUN and creatinine, renal failure, hematuria, renal calculi. **Skin:** rash, pruritus, urticaria.

DRUG INTERACTIONS ORAL ANTICOAGULANTS, **heparin** may prolong bleeding time; may increase **lithium** toxicity; increases pharmacologic and toxic activity of **phenytoin,** SULFONYLUREAS, SULFONAMIDES, **warfarin** through protein-binding displacement.

NURSING IMPLICATIONS

Administration

- If patient complains of GI distress, suggest administration with food or milk, or an aluminum and magnesium hydroxide antacid (Maalox) may be prescribed. If symptoms persist, the physician should be consulted.
- Store in airtight, light-resistant container at 15–30C (59–86F) unless otherwise directed.

Assessment & Drug Effects

- Clinical improvement in the rheumatoid patient is evidenced within 2–3 wk with reduction in number of tender joints, severity of tenderness, and duration of morning stiffness.
- Improvement in the osteoarthritic patient is reflected by reduced night pain, pain on walking, starting pain, and pain with passive motion and improved joint function.

- Diarrhea is the most frequent adverse effect and is usually dose related. Reportedly, the incidence of diarrhea is lower in patients with osteoarthritis than in those with rheumatoid arthritis.
- Check patient's self-medication habits. Many elderly persons use "soda bicarb" routinely to "settle the stomach."
- The patient with renal damage should be closely monitored and perhaps given lower doses. Incidence of adverse reactions is potentially high because the drug is excreted primarily by the kidneys. Monitor I&O ratio. Encourage fluid intake of at least 8 glasses of liquid a day.
- **Overdose treatment** includes emesis or gastric lavage and administration of activated charcoal. Support for vital functions should be readily available.

Patient & Family Education

- Instruct patient to stop taking this drug and promptly notify the physician if nausea, vomiting, severe diarrhea, and abdominal pain occur. Generally dose reduction or temporary withdrawal will control symptoms.
- Although incidence of side effects related to special senses is low, instruct patient to report without delay if blurred vision, tinnitus, or taste disturbances occur.
- Because visual disturbances have been reported with other NSAIDs, ophthalmic examinations are recommended before and periodically during treatment and whenever patient experiences visual disturbances.
- If patient becomes pregnant while on meclofenamate therapy, she should notify the physician.
- The patient should be weighed under standard conditions (similar clothing, same time of day) twice weekly. A weight gain of more than 2.5 to 3.5 kg (3–4 lb)/wk should be reported as well as signs of edema: swollen ankles, tibiae, hands, feet.
- The sodium content of meclofenamate tablets should be considered if the patient is on restricted sodium intake.
- Discourage use of OTC drugs without approval of physician. Many contain aspirin (increases potential for toxicity) and sodium (augments sodium component of the meclofenamate compound).
- Dizziness, a troublesome early side effect, frequently disappears in time. Advise patient to avoid driving a car or using hazardous equipment until response to drug is known.
- If patient is receiving a PO anticoagulant, patient should immediately report any sign of bleeding (e.g., melena, epistaxis, ecchymosis). Prothrombin times should be closely monitored.

M

- Response to therapy should be periodically evaluated. Urge patient to keep appointments for clinical evaluation of drug effectiveness and for laboratory studies.
- Advise patient to inform surgeon or dentist that patient is on meclofenamate therapy.

Prototype: progesterone, p 241

MEDROXYPROGESTERONE ACETATE

(me-drox´ee-proe-jess´te-rone)
Trade names: Amen, Curretab, Depo-Provera, Provera
Classifications: HORMONE; PROGESTIN; ANTINEOPLASTIC
Pregnancy: Category X

ACTIONS/PHARMACODYNAMICS Synthetic derivative of progesterone with prolonged, variable duration of action and androgenic and antiestrogenic activity. Has no deleterious effects on lipid metabolism. Induces and maintains endometrium, preventing uterine bleeding; inhibits production of pituitary gonadotropin, preventing ovulation; and produces thick cervical mucus resistant to passage of sperm.

USES Dysfunctional uterine bleeding; parenteral form (Depo-Provera) used in adjunctive, palliative treatment of inoperable, recurrent, and metastatic endometrial or renal carcinoma. **Unlabeled uses (Depo-Provera):** contraception, obstructive sleep apnea.

CONTRAINDICATIONS & PRECAUTIONS Contraindicated in: pregnancy (category X); history of thromboembolic disorders. **Cautious use in:** asthma, seizure disorders, migraine, cardiac or renal dysfunction, liver disease.

ADVERSE/SIDE EFFECTS CNS: <u>cerebral thrombosis or hemorrhage</u>, headache, depression. **CV:** hypertension, pulmonary embolism, edema. **GI:** nausea, vomiting, cholestatic jaundice, abdominal cramps. **Reproductive:** *breakthrough bleeding,* cervical erosion, changes in menstrual flow, dysmenorrhea, vaginal candidiasis. **Skin:** angioneurotic edema. **Other:** weight changes; *breast tenderness,* enlargement or secretion, hyperpyrexia (rare).

ROUTE & DOSAGE

Secondary Amenorrhea

Adult PO 5–10 mg/d for 5–10 d beginning anytime if endometrium is adequately estrogen primed (withdrawal bleeding occurs in 3–7 d after discontinuing therapy)

Abnormal Bleeding Due to Hormonal Imbalance

Adult PO 5–10 mg/d for 5–10 d beginning on the assumed or calculated 16th or 21st day of menstrual cycle; if bleeding is controlled, administer 2 subsequent cycles

Carcinoma

Adult IM 400–1000 mg/wk; continue at 400 mg/mo if improvement occurs and disease stabilizes

Contraceptive

Adult IM 150 mg q3mo

NURSING IMPLICATIONS

See progesterone for numerous additional nursing implications.

Administration
- Oral drug may be given with food to minimize GI distress.
- Administer IM deep into a large muscle.
- Store at 15–30C (59–86F); protect from freezing.

Assessment & Drug Effects
- IM injection may be painful. Monitor sites for evidence of sterile abscess. A residual lump and discoloration of tissue may develop.
- Monitor for signs and symptoms of thrombophlebitis (see chap 3).

Patient & Family Education
- After repeated IM injections, infertility and amenorrhea may persist for as long as 18 mo.
- Planned menstrual cycling with medroxyprogesterone may benefit the patient with a history of recurrent episodes of abnormal uterine bleeding.
- Teach patient self-breast examination (SBE).
- Discuss package insert with patient to assure complete understanding of progestin therapy.

Common side effects in *italic*; life-threatening effects <u>underlined</u>; generic names in **bold**; classifications in SMALL CAPS

Prototype: ibuprofen, p 160

MEFENAMIC ACID

(me-fe-nam´ik)

Trade names: Ponstan, Ponstel

Classifications: CNS AGENT; NONNARCOTIC ANALGESIC; ANTIPYRETIC; NSAID

Pregnancy: Category C

ACTIONS/PHARMACODYNAMICS Anthranilic acid derivative with analgesic, antiinflammatory, and antipyretic actions similar to those of ibuprofen. Like ibuprofen, inhibits prostaglandin synthesis and affects platelet function. No evidence that it is superior to aspirin. Associated with a number of serious adverse reactions, particularly when used for prolonged periods at high doses.

USES Short-term relief of mild to moderate pain including primary dysmenorrhea.

ROUTE & DOSAGE

Mild to Moderate Pain

Adult	PO	500 mg loading dose, then 250 mg q6h prn

PHARMACOKINETICS Absorption: rapidly and completely absorbed from GI tract. **Peak:** 2–4 h. **Duration:** ≤ 6 h. **Distribution:** distributed in breast milk. **Metabolism:** partially metabolized in liver. **Elimination:** half-life: 2 h; 50% excreted in urine, 50% in feces.

CONTRAINDICATIONS & PRECAUTIONS Contraindicated in: hypersensitivity to drug, GI inflammation, or ulceration. Safe use in children < 14 y, during pregnancy (category C), and in nursing mothers not established. **Cautious use in:** history of renal or hepatic disease; blood dyscrasias; asthma; diabetes mellitus; hypersensitivity to aspirin. See also drug interactions.

ADVERSE/SIDE EFFECTS CNS: drowsiness, insomnia, dizziness, vertigo, unsteady gait, nervousness, confusion, headache; status epilepticus with overdose. **GI:** *severe diarrhea*, GI inflammation, ulceration, and bleeding; *nausea, vomiting,* abdominal cramps, flatus, constipation. **Hematologic:** prolonged prothrombin time, severe autoimmune hemolytic anemia (long-term use), leukopenia, eosinophilia, agranulocytosis, thrombocytopenic purpura, megaloblastic anemia, pancytopenia, bone marrow hypoplasia. **Renal:** nephrotoxicity, dysuria, albuminuria, hematuria, elevation of BUN. **Skin:** urticaria, rash, facial edema. **Other:** eye irritation, loss of color vision (reversible), blurred vision, ear pain, perspiration, increased need for insulin in diabetic patients, hepatic toxicity, palpitation, dyspnea; acute exacerbation of asthma; bronchoconstriction (in patients sensitive to aspirin).

DIAGNOSTIC TEST INTERFERENCES False-positive reactions for ***urinary bilirubin*** (using diazo tablet test).

DRUG INTERACTIONS Mefenamic acid may prolong bleeding time with ORAL ANTICOAGULANTS, **heparin;** may increase **lithium** toxicity; increases pharmacologic and toxic activity of **phenytoin,** SULFONYLUREAS, SULFONAMIDES, **warfarin** because of protein binding displacement.

NURSING IMPLICATIONS

Administration

- Administer with meals, food, or milk to minimize GI adverse effects.
- Use of drug for a period exceeding 1 wk is not recommended (manufacturer's warning).

Assessment & Drug Effects

- Patients who develop severe diarrhea and vomiting should be assessed for dehydration and electrolyte imbalance.
- Patients on long-term therapy should have periodic blood counts, Hct and Hgb, and renal function tests.

Patient & Family Education

- Mefenamic acid should be discontinued promptly if diarrhea, dark stools, hematemesis, ecchymoses, epistaxis, or rash occur and should not be used thereafter. Advise patients to report these signs to the physician.
- Advise patient to notify physician if persistent GI discomfort, sore throat, fever, or malaise occurs.
- Since the drug may cause dizziness and drowsiness, caution patients to avoid driving a car and other potentially hazardous activities until response to drug is known.
- Diabetic patients may show increased need for insulin.

Common side effects in *italic*; life-threatening effects underlined; generic names in **bold**; classifications in SMALL CAPS

731

M

MEGESTROL ACETATE

(me-jess´trole)
Trade names: Megace, Pallace
Classifications: ANTINEOPLASTIC; HORMONE;
PROGESTIN
Pregnancy: Category X

ACTIONS/PHARMACODYNAMICS Progestational hormone with antineoplastic properties. Mechanism of action unclear; however, an antiluteinizing effect mediated via the pituitary has been postulated. Has local effect when instilled directly into the endometrial cavity.

USES Palliative agent for treatment of advanced carcinoma of breast or endometrium. **Unlabeled use:** appetite stimulant in patients with AIDS.

ROUTE & DOSAGE

Palliative Treatment for Advanced Breast Cancer
Adult   PO   40 mg q.i.d.

Palliative Treatment for Advanced Endometrial Cancer
Adult   PO   40–320 mg/d in divided doses

PHARMACOKINETICS Absorption: appears to be well absorbed from GI tract. **Onset:** onset of objective response in breast cancer in 6–8 wk. **Peak:** 1–3 h. **Duration:** 3–12 mo. **Metabolism:** completely metabolized in liver. **Elimination:** 57–78% of dose excreted in urine within 10 d.

CONTRAINDICATIONS & PRECAUTIONS Contraindicated in: diagnostic test for pregnancy; use in neoplastic diseases other than cancer of endometrium and breast; first 4 mo of pregnancy (category X).

ADVERSE/SIDE EFFECTS Carpal tunnel syndrome, alopecia, deep vein thrombophlebitis, breast tenderness, abdominal pain, nausea, vomiting, headache, allergic-type reactions (including bronchial asthma).

NURSING IMPLICATIONS

Administration

- Drug may be given without regard to meals.
- Store in tightly closed container at 15–30C (59–86F) unless otherwise specified.

Assessment & Drug Effects

- Monitor weight periodically. Drug appears to cause weight gain by increasing appetite.
- Notify physician if abdominal pain, headache, nausea, vomiting, or breast tenderness become pronounced.
- Monitor for allergic reactions, including breathing distress characteristic of asthma; rash, urticaria, anaphylaxis, tachypnea, anxiety. Stop medication if they appear and notify physician.

Patient & Family Education

- Contraception measures are recommended during therapy for carcinoma with megestrol.
- Teach patient self-breast examination (SBE).
- Teach patient signs and symptoms of thrombophlebitis (see chap 3).
- Discuss package insert with patient to assure her understanding of megestrol therapy.

MELPHALAN

(mel´fa-lan)
Trade names: Alkeran, Pam, L-Pam,
Phenylalanine Mustard
Classifications: ANTINEOPLASTIC; NITROGEN
MUSTARD; ALKYLATING AGENT
Pregnancy: Category D

ACTIONS/PHARMACODYNAMICS Nitrogen mustard chemically and pharmacologically related to mechlorethamine. Has strong immunosuppressive and myelosuppressive effects but, unlike mechlorethamine, lacks vesicant propertes. Carcinogenic potential suspected.

USES Chiefly for palliative treatment of multiple myeloma. Also many other neoplasms, including Hodgkin's disease and carcinomas of breast and ovary. **Unlabeled use:** polycythemia vera.

PHARMACOKINETICS Absorption: incompletely and variably absorbed from GI tract. **Peak:** 2 h. **Distribution:** widely distributed to all tissues. **Metabolism:** metabolized by spontaneous hydrolysis in plasma. **Elimination:** half-life: 1.5 h; 25–30% excreted in urine, 25–50% excreted in feces.

M

ROUTE & DOSAGE

Multiple Myeloma

Adult   PO   6 mg/d for 2–3 wk; drug is then withdrawn for 4–5 wk; when WBC and platelet counts start to rise, restart at 2 mg/d

Epithelial Ovarian Cancer

Adult   PO   0.2 mg/kg/d in divided doses for 5 d as single course; may repeat course q4–5wk, depending on hematologic tolerance

CONTRAINDICATIONS & PRECAUTIONS **Contraindicated in:** use during pregnancy (category D) or in men and women of childbearing age not established. **Cautious use:** recent treatment with other chemotherapeutic agent; concurrent administration with radiation therapy; severe anemia, neutropenia, or thrombocytopenia, impaired renal function.

ADVERSE/SIDE EFFECTS **Hematologic:** <u>leukopenia</u>, <u>agranulocytosis</u>, <u>thrombocytopenia</u>, anemia, acute nonlymphatic leukemia. **Other:** uremia, angioneurotic peripheral edema, minor neurologic toxicity (rare), *nausea, vomiting* (with high doses); occasional stomatitis, *diarrhea,* hypersensitivity reactions, temporary alopecia, skin rash, bronchopulmonary dysplasia (rare), pulmonary fibrosis, menstrual irregularities, hyperuricemia.

DRUG INTERACTIONS Increases risk of nephrotoxicity with **cyclosporine.**

NURSING IMPLICATIONS

Administration
- Administer PO drug with meals to reduce nausea and vomiting. An antiemetic may be ordered.
- Store in light-resistant airtight containers at 15–30C (59–86F) unless otherwise directed.

Assessment & Drug Effects
- Leukocyte and platelet counts are done 2–3 times/wk during dosage adjustment period; WBC is usually determined each week for 6–8 wk during maintenance therapy.
- Nadirs of platelets and leukocytes occur within a few weeks after therapy begins; recovery is rapid.
- Dosage adjustment is primarily based on blood counts. Usually, drug is discontinued after 2–3 wk treatment for about 4 wk. When WBC and platelet counts begin to rise, maintenance dose of 2 mg/d is instituted.

- Monitor laboratory reports to anticipate leukopenic and thrombocytopenic periods.
- A degree of myelosuppression is maintained during therapy so as to keep leukocyte count in range of 3000–3500/mm³.
- Monitor serum uric acid levels and keep physician informed. Flank and joint pains may signal onset of hyperuricemia.

Patient & Family Education
- A favorable response to oral melphalan in patients with multiple myeloma may be gradual over many months. Encourage patient not to abandon treatment too soon to receive maximum benefit.
- Instruct patient to be alert to onset of fever, profound weakness, chills, tachycardia, cough, sore throat, changes in kidney function, or prolonged infections and report them to physician.
- Inform patient that reversible alopecia is an expected side effect.

MENADIOL SODIUM DIPHOSPHATE (VITAMIN K₄)

(men-a-dye´ole)
Trade name: Synkayvite
Classification: VITAMIN K₄
Pregnancy: Category C (X near term)

ACTIONS/PHARMACODYNAMICS Synthetic, water soluble analog of vitamin K analog derived from menadione. Has same actions, uses, contraindications, precautions, and adverse reactions as menadione (p. 734) but is about one-half as potent. Like menadione, it does not counteract action of heparin. Its use as a liver function test has generally been replaced by newer methods. In combination with radiotherapy it may selectively increase radiosensitivity of tumor cells through an unknown action. Also reported to reduce adenosine triphosphate level in tumor cells.

USES Same as those of menadione (p 734).

ROUTE & DOSAGE

Prevention and Treatment of Vitamin K Deficiency

Adult   PO/SC/IM/IV   5–15 mg/d

PHARMACOKINETICS **Absorption:** readily absorbed from GI tract; converted to menadione in body. **Onset:** 1–2 h SC, IM.

M

Common side effects in *italic*; life-threatening effects <u>underlined</u>; generic names in **bold**; classifications in SMALL CAPS

733

ADVERSE/SIDE EFFECTS Nausea, vomiting, allergic reaction; pruritus, urticaria, rash.

NURSING IMPLICATIONS

Administration

- May be given IV undiluted at a rate of a single dose over 60 seconds.
- May be added to most IV infusion solutions.
- Store in tight, light-resistant containers at 15–30C (59–86F) unless otherwise directed.

Assessment & Drug Effects

- Dosage and duration of treatment are determined by prothrombin times and clinical response.
- Solutions of menadiol sodium diphosphate may be irritating to skin; monitor injection sites.

MENADIONE (VITAMIN K$_3$)

(men-a-dye´one)

Trade name: Menaphthone
Classification: VITAMIN K$_3$
Pregnancy: Category C (X near term)

ACTIONS/PHARMACODYNAMICS Synthetic, fat-soluble vitamin K analog. Similar in activity to naturally occurring vitamin K, which is essential in hepatic biosynthesis of blood coagulation factors II, VII, IX, X. Mechanism of action unknown.

USES Prevention and treatment of hypoprothrombinemia caused by vitamin K deficiency secondary to oral antiinfective therapy and salicylates. Also effective in prevention and treatment of hypothrombinemia resulting from inadequate absorption and synthesis of vitamin K, as in obstructive jaundice, biliary fistula, ulcerative colitis, celiac disease, intestinal resection, regional enteritis, cystic fibrosis of pancreas. Largely replaced by phytonadione (vitamin K$_1$) as an antidote for oral anticoagulant overdosage and in prophylaxis and treatment of hemorrhagic disease of newborns. Like other forms of vitamin K, ineffective in treatment of heparin overdosage.

ROUTE & DOSAGE

Hypoprothrombinemia

Adult	PO	5–10 mg/d
	IV/IM/SC	5–15 mg 1–2 times/d
Child	PO	50–100 µg/d
	IV/IM/SC	5–10 mg 1–2 times/d

PHARMACOKINETICS Absorption: menadione, but not menadiol sodium diphosphate, requires bile salts for absorption from GI tract. **Onset:** 1–2 h after IM. **Duration:** 8–24 h IM. **Distribution:** crosses placenta. **Elimination:** unknown.

CONTRAINDICATIONS & PRECAUTIONS Contraindicated in: severe liver disease; patients with G6PD deficiency; administration to mothers during last few weeks of pregnancy (category X) as prophylaxis against hemorrhagic disease of newborn; use in neonates. Effects on human fertility and teratogenic potential not known.

ADVERSE/SIDE EFFECTS Gastric upset, headache, allergic reactions (skin rash, urticaria); erythrocyte hemolysis (persons with G6PD deficiency and newborns). With large doses: BSP retention, prolonged prothrombin time, further depression of liver function (patients with hepatic disease). In infants, particularly prematures, or when administered to mother before delivery: hemolytic anemia, hemoglobinuria, hyperbilirubinemia, kernicterus, brain damage, death.

DRUG INTERACTIONS ORAL ANTICOAGULANTS may attenuate effects.

NURSING IMPLICATIONS

Administration

- Drug may be given by direct IV undiluted over 60 seconds or added to a compatible solution for continuous infusion.

Assessment & Drug Effects

- Prothrombin times and clinical response are used as guides for dosage and duration of treatment.
- Therapeutic response to menadione is indicated by shortening of prothrombin, bleeding, and clotting times and by a decrease in hemorrhagic tendencies.

MENOTROPINS

(men-oh-troe´pins)

Trade name: Pergonal
Classifications: HORMONE; GONADOTROPIN
Pregnancy: Category C

ACTIONS/PHARMACODYNAMICS Purified preparation of exogenous gonadotropins, extracted

M

from human menopausal urinary gonadotropin and standardized biologically for follicle-stimulating hormone (FSH) and luteinizing hormone (LH) gonadotropic activities. Promotes growth of graafian follicles in women who do not have primary anovulation. Treatment usually results only in ovarian follicular growth and maturation. With clinical proof of follicular maturation, ovulation is induced by menotropins followed by administration of human chorionic gonadotropin (HCG). Stimulates spermatogenesis in men with primary or secondary hypogonadotropic hypogonadism after pretreatment with HCG.

USES With HCG (in sequence) to induce ovulation and pregnancy in the infertile woman with functional anovulation (i.e., secondary to pituitary insufficiency). Also used in conjunction with HCG to treat male infertility.

ROUTE & DOSAGE

Induction of Ovulation

Adult   IM   1 ampul (75 IU of FSH and LH) daily for 9–12 d, followed by HCG 1 d after last dose of menotropins. If ovulation occurs without pregnancy, regimen may be repeated twice at same dosage before increasing dose to 2 ampuls daily continuing as before. If ovulation occurs without pregnancy, treatment may be repeated at monthly intervals for 2 more courses

Stimulation of Spermatogenesis

Adult   IM   Following pretreatment with HCG, 1 ampul 3 times/wk and 2000 U HCG 2 times/wk until detection of spermatozoa in the ejaculate (4–6 mo). If spermatogenesis dose not increase, continue treatments or increase to 2 ampuls 3 times/wk

PHARMACOKINETICS **Distribution:** testes in males, ovaries in females. **Elimination:** 8% excreted in urine within 24 h.

CONTRAINDICATIONS & PRECAUTIONS Contraindicated in: pregnancy, primary anovulation; thyroid and adrenal dysfunction; organic intracranial lesion; infertility caused by factors other than anovulation; abnormal bleeding of unknown origin, ovarian cysts or enlargement not due to polycystic ovary syndrome; men with normal urinary gonadotropin concentrations, or primary testicular failure.

ADVERSE/SIDE EFFECTS Dose related: mild to *moderate ovarian enlargement,* abdominal distension and pain, ovarian hyperstimulation syndrome (sudden ovarian enlargement accompanied by ascites with or without pain or pleural effusion), hemoperitoneum, fever, nausea, vomiting, diarrhea, arterial thromboembolism (rare), hypovolemia, multiple ovulations, follicular cysts, birth defects; gynecomastia (men).

NURSING IMPLICATIONS

Administration

- Drug is prepared immediately before administration by dissolving ampul contents in 1–2 ml of sterile NaCl injection. Unused portion should be discarded.
- When total estrogen excretion level is more than 100 µg/24 h, HCG is not administered because hyperstimulation syndrome is more likely to occur.

Assessment & Drug Effects

- Treatment for women is preceded by a thorough gynecologic and endocrinologic examination to rule out early pregnancy, primary ovarian failure, neoplastic lesion; husband's fertility is also evaluated.
- Treatment for men is preceded by at least 4–6 mo of HCG or until normal serum testosterone concentration is achieved.
- Most reliable index of follicular maturation (estrogenic activity) is the rate of urinary estrogen excretion. Other indirect estimates include serial examination of vaginal smears and cervical mucus specimens.
- Patient should be examined at least every other day and for 2 wk after HCG injection to detect excessive ovarian stimulation.
- Hypersensitivity syndrome, which generally occurs within 2 wk after initiation of treatment, develops rapidly over 3–4 d. This syndrome is an indication for discontinuation of treatment and hospitalization of patient.

Patient & Family Education

- Teach patient to recognize *indirect indices of progesterone production:* rise in basal body temperature (BBT), menstruation following shift in BBT, increased volume of thin and watery vaginal secretion.
- The couple should be encouraged to have intercourse daily beginning on day before administration of HCG until ovulation becomes apparent from indices of progestational activity.

M

- Warn patient to report immediately *symptoms of hyperstimulation syndrome:* abdominal distension and pain, dyspnea, vaginal bleeding.
- Advise patient to weigh herself every other day to detect sudden weight gain. Patient should understand the range of weight gain to be reported to physician.
- Mild ovarian enlargement (with or without abdominal distension and pain) usually regresses without treatment in 2–3 wk.
- Generally, pregnancy occurs within 4–6 courses of therapy.
- Patient should be aware of statistics related to multiple births after menotropin-HCG treatment.
- For the man receiving menotropin therapy, if there is no evidence of increased spermatogenesis after 4 mo, therapy can continue with increased dosage of menotropins.

Prototype: morphine, p 156

MEPERIDINE HYDROCHLORIDE

(me-per´i-deen)

Trade names: Demerol, Pethadol, Pethidine Hydrochloride

Classifications: CNS AGENT; NARCOTIC (OPIATE) AGONIST ANALGESIC; ANTIPYRETIC

Pregnancy: Category B (D at term)

Controlled substance: Schedule II

ACTIONS/PHARMACODYNAMICS Synthetic morphinelike compound. Chemically dissimilar to morphine, but in equianalgesic doses it is qualitatively comparable with regard to analgesic effects, sedation, euphoria, pupillary constriction, and respiratory depression. Reported to differ from morphine in that it has a somewhat more rapid onset and shorter duration of action and produces less depression of cough reflex, constipation, urinary retention, and smooth muscle spasm. Usual doses produce either no pupillary change or slight miosis, but overdosage results in marked miosis or mydriasis. Also, unlike morphine, has little or no antidiarrheic or antitussive action and produces CNS stimulation in toxic doses. In common with morphine, it causes sensitization of labyrinthine apparatus, stimulation of chemoreceptor trigger zone, and depression of medullary vasomotor center; it also has vagolytic and anticholinergic actions and may inhibit release of ACTH and gonadotropic hormones. Promotes release of histamine and antidiuretic hormone and elevation of blood sugar.

USES Relief of moderate to severe pain, for preoperative medication, for support of anesthesia, and for obstetric analgesia.

ROUTE & DOSAGE

Moderate to Severe Pain

Adult	PO/SC/IM/IV	50–150 mg q3–4h as needed
Child	PO/SC/IM/IV	1 mg/kg q4–6h (max ≤ 100 mg q4h)

Preoperative

Adult	IM/SC	50–150 mg 30–90 min before surgery
Child	IM/SC	1–2.2 mg/kg 30–90 min before surgery

Obstetric Analgesia

Adult	IM/SC	50–100 mg when pains become regular; may be repeated q1–3h

PHARMACOKINETICS Absorption: 50–60% absorbed from GI tract. **Onset:** 15 min PO; 10 min IM, SC; 5 min IV. **Peak:** 1 h PO, IM, SC. **Duration:** 2–4 h PO, IM, SC; 2 h IV. **Distribution:** crosses placenta; distributed into breast milk. **Metabolism:** metabolized in liver. **Elimination:** half-life: 3–5 h; excreted in urine.

CONTRAINDICATIONS & PRECAUTIONS Contraindicated in: hypersensitivity to meperidine, convulsive disorders, acute abdominal conditions prior to diagnosis, pregnancy prior to labor (category B); at term (category D), nursing mothers. **Cautious use in:** head injuries, increased intracranial pressure, asthma and other respiratory conditions, supraventricular tachycardias, prostatic hypertrophy, urethral stricture, glaucoma, elderly or debilitated patients, impaired renal or hepatic function, hypothyroidism, Addison's disease.

ADVERSE/SIDE EFFECTS Allergic: *pruritus,* urticaria, skin rashes, wheal and flare over IV site. **CNS:** *dizziness,* weakness, euphoria, dysphoria, *sedation,* headache, uncoordinated muscle movements, disorientation, decreased cough reflex, miosis, corneal anesthesia, <u>respiratory depression</u>. Toxic doses: muscle twitching, tremors, hyperactive reflexes, excitement, hypersensitivity to external stimuli, agitation, confusion, hallucinations, dilated pupils, <u>convul-</u>

sions. **CV:** facial flushing, lightheadedness, hypotension, syncope, palpitation, bradycardia, tachycardia, cardiovascular collapse, cardiac arrest (toxic doses). **GI:** dry mouth, *nausea,* vomiting, *constipation,* biliary tract spasm. **Other:** oliguria, urinary retention, profuse perspiration, respiratory depression in newborn, bronchoconstriction (large doses), phlebitis (following IV use), pain, tissue irritation and induration, particularly following subcutaneous injection; increased levels of serum amylase, BSP retention, bilirubin, AST, ALT.

DIAGNOSTIC TEST INTERFERENCES High doses of meperidine may interfere with *gastric emptying studies* by causing delay in gastric emptying.

DRUG INTERACTIONS Alcohol and other CNS DEPRESSANTS, **cimetidine** cause additive sedation and CNS DEPRESSION; amphetamines may potentiate CNS STIMULATION; MAO inhibitors, **selegiline, furazolidone** may cause excessive and prolonged CNS depression, convulsions, cardiovascular collapse; **phenytoin** may increase toxic meperidine metabolites.

INCOMPATIBILITIES Solution/Additive: aminophylline, BARBITURATES, **heparin, methicillin, morphine, phenytoin, sodium bicarbonate. Y-Site: cefoperazone, heparin, mezlocillin, minocycline, tetracycline.**

NURSING IMPLICATIONS

Administration

- Although the SC route is sometimes prescribed, it is painful and can cause local irritation. The IM route is generally preferred when repeated doses are required.
- Carefully aspirate before giving IM injection to avoid inadvertent IV administration. IV injection of undiluted drug can cause a marked increase in heart rate and syncope.
- A high incidence of severe untoward effects is associated with IV use. Facilities for administration of oxygen and control of respiration should be immediately available, as well as a narcotic antagonist.
- When meperidine is given by direct IV, dilute 50 mg in a minimum of 5 ml of NS or sterile water to yield 10 mg/ml. Inject it slowly at a rate not to exceed 25 mg/min. Slower injection preferred.

- When meperidine is given by continuous infusion, dilute it to a concentration of 1–10 mg/ml in NS, D5W, or other compatible solution. Infusion rate should not exceed 25 mg/min. Slower rate is preferred.
- The syrup formulation should be taken in half a glass of water. Undiluted syrup may cause topical anesthesia of mucous membranes.
- Preserved in tightly closed, light-resistant containers preferably between 15–30C (59–86F), unless otherwise directed by manufacturer.

Assessment & Drug Effects

- Narcotic analgesics should be given in the smallest effective dose and for the least period of time compatible with patient's needs.
- Assess patient's need for prn medication; check time of last dose and validity of physician's order. Follow agency policy regarding time limit of narcotic orders. Record time of onset, duration, and quality of pain, preferably in patient's words.
- In patients receiving repeated doses, note respiratory rate, depth, and rhythm and size of pupils. If respirations are 12/min or below and pupils are constricted or dilated (see actions and uses) or breathing is shallow, or if signs of CNS hyperactivity are present, consult physician before administering drug.
- Vital signs should be monitored closely. Heart rate may increase markedly, and hypotension may occur. Meperidine may cause severe hypotension in postoperative patients and those with depleted blood volume.
- Deep breathing, coughing (unless contraindicated), and changes in position at scheduled intervals may help to overcome the respiratory depressant effects of meperidine.
- Parenteral administration has caused corneal anesthesia and thus abolishment of corneal reflex in some patients. Be alert for this possibility.
- Chart the patient's response to meperidine and evaluate continued need for the drug. Suggest to physician a change to a milder analgesic when in your judgment it is indicated.
- Repeated use of meperidine can lead to tolerance and psychic and physical dependence of the morphine type.
- Abrupt discontinuation of meperidine following repeated use results in morphine-like withdrawal symptoms. Symptoms develop more rapidly (within 3 h, peaking in 8–12 h) and are of shorter duration than with morphine. Nausea, vomiting, diarrhea, and pupillary dilatation are less promi-

M

Common side effects in *italic*; life-threatening effects underlined; generic names in **bold**; classifications in SMALL CAPS

737

nent, but muscle twitching, restlessness, and nervousness are greater than produced by morphine.

Patient & Family Education

- Caution patient not to smoke and not to ambulate without assistance after receiving the drug. Side rails are advisable.
- Ambulatory patients are more likely than supine patients to manifest nausea, vomiting, dizziness, and faintness associated with fall in BP (these symptoms may also occur in patients without pain who are given meperidine). Symptoms are lessened by the recumbent position and aggravated by the head-up position.
- Caution ambulatory patients to avoid driving a car or engaging in other hazardous activities until any drowsiness and dizziness have passed.
- Caution patients not to take other CNS depressants or ingest alcohol because of their additive effects.

Prototype: isoproterenol, p 105

MEPHENTERMINE SULFATE

(me-fen´ter-meen)
Trade name: Wyamine
Classification: AUTONOMIC NERVOUS SYSTEM AGENT; BETA-ADRENERGIC AGONIST (SYMPATHOMIMETIC)
Pregnancy: Category D

ACTIONS/PHARMACODYNAMICS Synthetic sympathomimetic with alpha- and predominant beta-adrenergic activity. Acts directly and chiefly indirectly by releasing norepinephrine from tissue storage sites. Elevation of blood pressure results primarily from positive inotropic action and increased cardiac output, and to lesser extent from increase in peripheral resistance caused by peripheral vasoconstriction. Heart rate may be reflexly slowed. Antiarrhythmic action results from decrease in AV conduction time, atrial refractory period, and conduction time in ventricular muscle. CNS effects are usually not prominent except with large doses.

USES Mainly as pressor agent in treatment of hypotension secondary to ganglionic blockade or spinal anesthesia. Also has been used as an emergency measure in therapy of shock secondary to hemorrhage until whole blood replacement is available; as adjunct in treatment of cardiogenic shock, and to abolish certain cardiac arrhythmias.

ROUTE & DOSAGE

Hypotension

Adult	IM	10–80 mg
	IV	10–80 mg
Child	IM	0.4 mg/kg
	IV	0.4 mg/kg

Hypotensive Emergency

Adult	IV	20–60 mg as an IV infusion (1.2 mg/ml in D5W)

PHARMACOKINETICS Onset: 5–15 min IM; immediate IV. **Duration:** 1–4 h IM; 15–30 min IV. **Metabolism:** rapidly metabolized in liver. **Elimination:** excreted in urine.

CONTRAINDICATIONS & PRECAUTIONS Contraindicated in: shock secondary to hemorrhage (except in emergency). Safe use during pregnancy (category D) or lactation not established. **Cautious use in:** arteriosclerosis, cardiovascular disease, hypovolemia, hypertension, hyperthyroidism, patients with known hypersensitivities, chronically ill patients.

ADVERSE/SIDE EFFECTS CNS: euphoria, anorexia, weeping, nervousness, anxiety, tremor, seizures. **CV:** tachycardia. With large doses: cardiac arrhythmias, marked elevation of blood pressure, incoherence, drowsiness.

DRUG INTERACTIONS Mephentermine may be ineffective in patients receiving **reserpine, guanethidine**, PHENOTHIAZINES; MAO inhibitors, sympathomimetic amines, **furazolidone, isoniazid** may potentiate pressor response; **methyldopa**, TRICYCLIC ANTIDEPRESSANTS may potentiate or inhibit pressor response; **cyclopropane, halothane** may cause serious arrhythmia; may increase risk of **digoxin**-induced arrhythmias.

INCOMPATIBILITIES Solution/Additive: epinephrine, hydralazine.

NURSING IMPLICATIONS

Administration

- Mephentermine may be given by direct IV undiluted at a rate of 30 mg/min. It may be further diluted by adding 600 mg to 50 ml of D5W and infused at a rate of 1–5 mg/min. IV flow rate is usually prescribed by physician.

Common side effects in *italic*; life-threatening effects underlined; generic names in **bold**; classifications in SMALL CAPS

- Mephentermine is incompatible with epinephrine hydrochloride and hydralazine hydrochloride.
- Preserved in tightly closed, light-resistant containers preferably at 15–30C (59–86F), unless otherwise directed by manufacturer.

Assessment & Drug Effects
- Close observation of patient and monitoring of BP, heart rate, ECG, and central venous pressure (CVP) are essential.
- During IV administration, check BP and pulse q2min until stabilized at prescribed level, then q5min thereafter during therapy. Continue monitoring vital signs for at least 45–60 min and longer if indicated after therapy.

Prototype: phenytoin, p 172

MEPHENYTOIN
(me-fen´i-toyn)
Trade name: Mesantoin
Classifications: CNS AGENT; HYDANTOIN ANTICONVULSANT
Pregnancy: Category C

ACTIONS/PHARMACODYNAMICS Hydantoin derivative, with actions, contraindications, precautions, and adverse reactions similar to those of phenytoin. Reported to have lower incidence of ataxia, gingival hyperplasia, gastric distress, and hirsutism, but produces more sedative and hypnotic action than phenytoin; causes serious toxic reactions, including fatal blood dyscrasias, more frequently. Relatively ineffective for petit mal seizures.

USES Control of grand mal, focal, jacksonian, and psychomotor seizures in patients refractory to less toxic anticonvulsants. Usually used concomitantly with other antiepilepsy agents.

ROUTE & DOSAGE

Seizures

Adult	PO	50–100 mg/d during first week, increase weekly to 200–600 mg/d in 3 divided doses
Child	PO	50–100 mg/d during first week, increase weekly to 100–400 mg/d in 3 divided doses

PHARMACOKINETICS Absorption: readily absorbed from GI tract. **Onset:** 30 min. **Duration:** 24–48 h. **Metabolism:** metabolized in liver. **Elimination:** half-life: 144 h; excreted in urine.

CONTRAINDICATIONS & PRECAUTIONS Contraindicated in: use in conjunction with oxazolidinedione anticonvulsant agents, e.g., paramethadione, trimethadione (toxic synergism). Safe use during pregnancy (category D) not established. **Cautious use in:** history of drug hypersensitivities.

ADVERSE/SIDE EFFECTS CNS: drowsiness, dizziness. **Dermatologic:** skin and mucous membrane manifestations (exfoliative dermatitis, erythema multiforme, toxic epidermal necrolysis, other skin rashes). **Hematologic:** blood dyscrasias: leukopenia, neutropenia, agranulocytosis, thrombocytopenia, aplastic anemia. **Other:** hepatic damage, periarteritis nodosa, systemic lupus erythematosus syndrome.

DRUG INTERACTIONS See Phenytoin.

DIAGNOSTIC TEST INTERFERENCES See phenytoin.

NURSING IMPLICATIONS

Administration
- May be given with food to reduce GI distress.
- Dose should not be increased until it is taken for at least 1 wk.
- Change from another anticonvulsant agent to mephenytoin is accomplished gradually by increasing dose at weekly intervals and reducing dose of drug to be discontinued over 3–6 wk.

Assessment & Drug Effects
- Patients should be kept under close supervision at all times, as drug is associated with severe adverse effects. Serious blood dyscrasias have occurred 2 wk–30 mo after initiation of therapy.
- Screening tests of liver function, total white cell count, and differential count should precede initiation of therapy.
- Blood studies should be performed q2wk and should be continued until patient is on maintenance dosage for 2 wk; then they should be repeated monthly for 1 yr, and thereafter every 3 mo (unless neutrophil count drops to 2500/mm^3 or 1600/mm^3, then performed every 2 wk).
- Medication should be discontinued if neutrophil count falls to 1600/mm^3.

M

Common side effects in *italic*; life-threatening effects underlined; generic names in **bold**; classifications in SMALL CAPS

Patient & Family Education

- When mephenytoin replaces another antiepilepsy agent, the dosage of mephenytoin should be gradually increased while the drug being discontinued is gradually decreased over period of 3–6 wk.
- The most frequent side effect of mephenytoin therapy is drowsiness, usually diminished by reduction of dosage. Caution patient to avoid hazardous activities until reactions to the drug have been determined. Supervision of ambulation and side rails may be indicated for some patients during early therapy.
- Advise patients to report immediately the onset of drowsiness, ataxia, skin rash, sore throat, fever, mucous membrane bleeding, or glandular swelling. All are indications of developing toxic reaction.
- Discontinuation of mephenytoin should be accomplished gradually to minimize the risk of precipitating seizures or status epilepticus.

Prototype: phenobarbital, p 167

MEPHOBARBITAL
(me-foe-bar´bi-tal)
Trade names: Mebaral, Methylphenobarbital
Classifications: CNS AGENT; BARBITURATE; ANTICONVULSANT; SEDATIVE-HYPNOTIC
Pregnancy: Category D
Controlled substance: Schedule IV

ACTIONS/PHARMACODYNAMICS Long-acting barbiturate with pharmacologic properties similar to those of phenobarbital; however, larger doses are required to produce comparable anticonvulsant effects. Exerts strong sedative action, but relatively mild hypnotic effect. Clinical uses, contraindications, precautions, and adverse reactions are as for phenobarbital.

USES To control grand mal and petit mal epilepsy, alone or in combination with other anticonvulsant agents, and for sedative effect in management of delirium tremens and other acute agitation and anxiety states.

PHARMACOKINETICS Absorption: 50% absorbed from GI tract. **Onset:** 60 min. **Duration:** 10–12 h. **Metabolism:** metabolized in liver to phenobarbital. **Elimination:** half-life: 34 h; excreted in urine. Alkalinization of urine or increase of urinary flow significantly increases the rate of phenobarbital excretion.

ROUTE & DOSAGE

Anticonvulsant

Adult	PO	400–600 mg/d in divided doses
Child	PO	≤ 5 y: 16–32 mg t.i.d. or q.i.d.
		≥ 5 y: 32–64 mg t.i.d. or q.i.d.

Sedative

Adult	PO	32–100 mg t.i.d. or q.i.d.
Child	PO	≤ 5 y: 16–32 mg t.i.d. or q.i.d.
		≥ 5 y: 32–64 mg t.i.d. or q.i.d.

Delirium Tremens

Adult	PO	200 mg t.i.d. or q.i.d.

CONTRAINDICATIONS & PRECAUTIONS Contraindicated in: hypersensitivity to barbiturates. Safe use during pregnancy (category D) not established. **Cautious use in:** fever, hyperthyroidism, alcoholism; hepatic, renal, or cardiac dysfunction.

ADVERSE/SIDE EFFECTS CNS: *drowsiness*, dizziness, unsteadiness, hangover, paradoxical excitement. **GI:** nausea, vomiting, constipation. **Other:** hypersensitivity reactions, <u>respiratory depression</u>.

DRUG INTERACTIONS See phenobarbital.

NURSING IMPLICATIONS

Administration

- Change from other anticonvulsant to mephobarbital should be accomplished by gradually tapering off the former as mephobarbital doses are increased to maintain seizure control.
- When mephobarbital is prescribed concurrently with phenobarbital, the dose should be about one-half the amount of each used alone. When prescribed concurrently with phenytoin, the dose of phenytoin is usually reduced.
- Mephobarbital may be prescribed as a single dose at bedtime (if seizures generally occur at night) or during the day (if attacks are diurnal).
- When mephobarbital anticonvulsant therapy is to be discontinued, dosage should be reduced gradually over 4 or 5 days to avoid precipitating seizures of status epilepticus.

Assessment & Drug Effects

- Barbiturates have no analgesic action, and they may be expected to produce restlessness when they are given to patients in pain.
- The elderly or debilitated and children sometimes have a paradoxical response to barbiturate therapy,

M

Common side effects in *italic*; life-threatening effects <u>underlined</u>; generic names in **bold**; classifications in SMALL CAPS

i.e., irritability, marked excitement (aggression in children), depression, and confusion.

Patient & Family Education

- Abrupt cessation after prolonged mephobarbital therapy may result in withdrawal symptoms (tremulousness, weakness, insomnia, delirium, convulsions).
- Since mephobarbital may cause drowsiness and dizziness, caution patients to avoid hazardous activities such as driving a car until response to drug has stabilized.
- Alcohol in any amount should not be taken with a barbiturate.

MEPROBAMATE

See CENTRAL NERVOUS SYSTEM AGENTS, ANX-IOLYTIC, SEDATIVE-HYPNOTIC, CARBAMATE proto-type, p 179.

Prototype: fluorouracil, p 94

MERCAPTOPURINE (6-MP, 6-MERCAPTOPURINE)

(mer-kap-toe-pyoor´een)
Trade name: Purinethol
Classifications: ANTINEOPLASTIC; ANTIMETABOLITE; IMMUNOSUPPRESSANT
Pregnancy: Category D

ACTIONS/PHARMACODYNAMICS Antimetabolite and purine antagonist. Inhibits purine metabolism by unclear mechanism. Blocks conversion of inosinic acid to adenine and xanthine ribotides within sensitive tumor cells. Also inhibits adenine-containing coenzymes, suggesting an influence over multiple cellular reactions. Has delayed immunosuppressive properties and carcinogenic potential.

USES Primarily for acute lymphocytic and myelogenous leukemia. Response in adults is less than in children, but mercaptopurine is initial drug of choice. In chronic granulocytic leukemia, produces temporary remission. **Unlabeled uses:** prevention of transplant graft rejection; SLE; rheumatoid arthritis; Crohn's disease.

PHARMACOKINETICS Absorption: approximately 50% absorbed from GI tract. **Peak:** 2 h. **Distribution:** distributes into total body water. **Metabolism:** rapidly metabolized by xanthine oxidase in liver. **Elimination:** half-life: 20–50 min; 11% excreted in urine within 6 h.

ROUTE & DOSAGE

Leukemias

Adult	PO	2.5 mg/kg/d; may increase up to 5 mg/kg/d after 4 wk if needed; *maintenance dose:* 1.25–2.5 mg/kg/d
Child	PO	Same as for adult

CONTRAINDICATIONS & PRECAUTIONS Contraindicated in: prior resistance to mercaptopurine; first trimester of pregnancy (category D), infections. **Cautious use in:** impaired renal or hepatic function; concomitant use with allopurinol.

ADVERSE/SIDE EFFECTS GI: stomatitis, esophagitis, *anorexia, nausea, vomiting, diarrhea,* steatorrhea (rare), intestinal ulcerations. **Hematologic:** leukopenia, anemia, eosinophilia, pancytopenia, thrombocytopenia, abnormal bleeding, bone marrow hypoplasia. **Other:** impaired liver function, hyperuricemia, skin rash, oliguria, renal impairment, drug fever, hepatic necrosis.

DRUG INTERACTIONS Allopurinol may inhibit metabolism and thus increase toxicity of mercaptopurine; may potentiate or antagonize anticoagulant effects of **warfarin.**

NURSING IMPLICATIONS

Administration

- The most effective dose with optimum therapeutic effect and least toxicity varies from patient to patient. Therefore careful titration of dosage is necessary.
- The total daily dose may be given at one time.
- The dose of mercaptopurine is usually reduced by 1/3–1/4 when allopurinol in given concurrently.
- Store tablets in light- and air-resistant container.

Assessment & Drug Effects

- Drug should be discontinued at the first sign of an abnormally large or rapid fall in platelet and leukocyte count. Notify physician.
- Start flow chart at beginning of therapy to record baseline data related to I&O ratio and pattern and body weight. Dosage determination and clues to onset of renal dysfunction depend on accurate comparative data.
- Weigh patient under standard conditions once weekly and record weight.

M

Common side effects in *italic*; life-threatening effects underlined; generic names in **bold**; classifications in SMALL CAPS

741

- Monitor daily laboratory reports for suggested adaptations in nursing management. Blood picture may change dramatically in a short period, and counts may continue to decrease several days after drug is withdrawn.
- Check vital signs daily. Report febrile states promptly.
- During periods of leukopenia, protect patient from exposure to trauma, infections, or other stresses (restrict visitors and personnel who have colds).
- Nausea, vomiting, and diarrhea are uncommon during drug administration, but they may signal excessive dosage, especially in adults.
- Oral ulcerations are rare; those that occur resemble lesions of thrush (creamy white exudative patches on inflamed painful mucosa). Inspect buccal membranes if patient complains of discomfort.
- If thrombocytopenia develops, watch for signs of abnormal bleeding (ecchymoses, petechiae, melena, bleeding gums); report them immediately.
- In acute leukemia, mercaptopurine may be continued in spite of thrombocytopenia and bleeding. Often, bleeding stops and platelet count rises during treatment.
- Hepatic toxicity occurs most often when dose exceeds 2.5 mg/kg/d. Jaundice signals onset of hepatic toxicity and may necessitate terminating use. Report other signs such as clay-colored stools or frothy dark urine. In some instances, jaundice appears and subsequently disappears during mercaptopurine therapy; it may persist days after drug is discontinued.

Patient & Family Education

- Instruct patient to report any signs of bleeding (e.g., hematuria, bruising, bleeding gums).
- Instruct patient to report signs of hepatic toxicity (see chap 3).
- Increase hydration (10–12 glasses of fluid daily) to reduce risk of hyperuricemia. Consult physician about desirable volume.
- Instruct patient to notify physician of onset of chills, nausea, vomiting, flank or joint pain, swelling of legs or feet, or symptoms of anemia.

MESALAMINE

(me-sal′a-meen)

Trade name: Rowasa

Classifications: MUCOUS MEMBRANE AGENT; ANTIINFLAMMATORY

Pregnancy: Category C

ACTIONS/PHARMACODYNAMICS Mesalamine 5-aminosalicylic acid (5-ASA) provides topical antiinflammatory action in the colon of patients with ulcerative colitis. It is thought that the drug diminishes inflammation by blocking cyclooxygenase and inhibiting prostaglandin synthesis in the colon.

USES Indicated in active mild to moderate distal ulcerative colitis, proctosigmoiditis, or proctitis. **Unlabeled use:** Crohn's disease.

ROUTE & DOSAGE

Ulcerative Colitis

Adult	Rectal	4 g once/d h.s.; enema should be retained for about 8 h if possible

PHARMACOKINETICS Absorption: 5–35% absorbed from colon depending on retention time of enema. **Peak:** 3–6 h. **Distribution:** rectal administration may reach as high as the ascending colon. **Elimination:** half-life: 5–10 h; excreted primarily in feces; absorbed drug excreted in urine.

CONTRAINDICATIONS & PRECAUTIONS Contraindicated in: hypersensitivity to mesalamine. **Cautious use in:** renal impairment, pregnancy (category C). Sensitivity to sulfasalazine or salicylates. Not known if it is excreted in breast milk. Safety and efficacy in children have not been established.

ADVERSE/SIDE EFFECTS CNS: *headache,* fatigue, asthenia, malaise, weakness, dizziness. **GI:** *abdominal pain, cramps, or discomfort,* flatulence, nausea, diarrhea, constipation, hemorrhoids, rectal pain. **Other:** sensitivity reactions, rash, pruritus, alopecia, fever.

NURSING IMPLICATIONS

Administration

- Emptying bowel immediately prior to enema is important for best results.
- Shake the bottle well to make sure the suspension is homogenized.
- Mesalamine rectal suspension should be used at bed time with the objective of retaining it all night.
- Store at 15–30C (59–86F).

Assessment & Drug Effects

- The kidney is the major target organ for mesalamine toxicity. Careful monitoring of urinalysis, BUN, and creatinine is essential, especially in patients with preexisting renal disease.

M

Common side effects in *italic*; life-threatening effects underlined; generic names in **bold**; classifications in SMALL CAPS

- Suspension contains a sulfite that may cause allergic-type reaction in asthmatics and some nonasthmatic persons; assess for signs and symptoms (e.g., hives, itching, wheezing, anaphylaxis).
- Response to therapy may occur within 3–21 d, however, the usual course of therapy is from 3–6 wk, depending on symptoms and sigmoidoscopic examinations.
- Rare instances of pericarditis have been reported with this drug. Watch for chest pain or dyspnea.

Patient & Family Education

- Instruct patients to promptly report cramping, abdominal pain, or bloody diarrhea, which are indications for immediate drug withdrawal.
- Instruct patients to check with doctor if rectal irritation (e.g., bleeding, blistering, pain, burning, itching) occurs while they are using this drug.
- Advise patients to check with physician before they use any new medicine (prescription or OTC).
- Instruct patients to continue medication for full time of treatment even if they are feeling better.
- Store away from heat and light.

MESNA

(mes´na)

Trade name: Mesnex
Classification: ANTIDOTE, DETOXIFYING AGENT
Pregnancy: Category B

ACTIONS/PHARMACODYNAMICS

Mesna is a detoxifying agent used to inhibit the hemorrhagic cystitis induced by ifosfamide. It is analogous to the physiological cysteine-cystine system. In the kidney the thiol compound mesna reacts chemically with urotoxic ifosfamide metabolites, resulting in their detoxification, and thus significantly decreases the incidence of hematuria.

USES

Prophylaxis for ifosfamide-induced hemorrhagic cystitis. Not effective in preventing hematuria due to other pathologic conditions such as thrombocytopenia. **Unlabeled use:** reduces the incidence of cyclophosphamide-induced hemorrhagic cystitis.

ROUTE & DOSAGE

Use with Ifosfamide

Adult	IV	Dose = 20% of ifosfamide dose and is given at time of ifosfamide administration and 4 and 8 h after ifosfamide administration
Child		Not established

PHARMACOKINETICS

Metabolism: rapidly oxidized in liver to active metabolite dimesna; dimesna is further metabolized in kidney. **Elimination:** half-life: mesna 0.36 h, dimesna 1.17 h, 65% excreted in urine within 24 h.

CONTRAINDICATIONS & PRECAUTIONS

Contraindicated in: hypersensitivity to mesna or other thiol compounds. **Cautious use in:** pregnant women (category B) and only if the benefits clearly outweigh any possible risk to fetus.

ADVERSE/SIDE EFFECTS

GI: *bad taste in mouth, soft stools,* nausea, vomiting.

DIAGNOSTIC TEST INTERFERENCES

May produce a false-positive result in test for ***urinary ketones.***

DRUG INTERACTIONS

Not compatible with **cisplatin.** Can mix with ifosfamide.

INCOMPATIBILITIES

Solution/additive: cisplatin.

NURSING IMPLICATIONS

Administration

- To be effective, mesna must be administered with each dose of ifosfamide.
- IV solution is prepared by adding 4 ml of 5% dextrose, 5% dextrose and NS, 0.9% NaCl, or lactated Ringer's solution for each 100 mg of mesna to produce a solution containing a final mesna concentration of 20 mg/ml.
- Following dilution give a single dose by direct IV over 60 seconds.
- Parenteral drug products should be inspected visually for particulate matter and discoloration prior to administration.
- Any unused portion of the ampule of mesna should be discarded because drug oxidizes on contact with air.
- Diluted solutions of mesna are chemically and physically stable for 24 h at 25C (77F). However, it is recommended that diluted solutions be refrigerated or used within 6 h of mixing.
- Store below 40C (104F) at 15–30C (59–86F) unless otherwise specified.

Assessment & Drug Effects

- Examination of a morning specimen of urine for microscopic hematuria is recommended prior to each dose of ifosfamide or cyclophosphamide and mesna.

M

Common side effects in *italic*; life-threatening effects underlined; generic names in **bold**; classifications in SMALL CAPS

743

- A false-positive test for urinary ketones may arise in patients treated with mesna. In this test a red-violet color develops that, with the addition of glacial acetic acid, will turn to violet.
- About 6% of patients treated with mesna along with ifosfamide still develop hematuria.

Patient & Family Education

- Inform patients that mesna prevents ifosfamide-induced hemorrhagic cystitis; it will not prevent or alleviate other adverse reactions or toxicities associated with ifosfamide therapy.
- Advise patients to report any unusual or allergic reactions to mesna.
- Advise patients to check with physician before they use any new prescription or OTC medicine.

Prototype: chlorpromazine, p 191

MESORIDAZINE BESYLATE
(mez-oh-rid´a-zeen)
Trade name: Serentil
Classifications: CNS AGENT; PSYCHOTHERAPEUTIC; PHENOTHIAZINE ANTIPSYCHOTIC
Pregnancy: Category C

ACTIONS/PHARMACODYNAMICS Piperidine derivative of phenothiazine. Major tranquilizer with stronger sedative action than produced by chlorpromazine but has more antiemetic action and lower incidence of extrapyramidal side effects. Produces psychomotor slowing and reduces emotional stress.

USES Schizophrenia, behavioral problems in mental deficiency and chronic brain syndrome, acute and chronic alcoholism. Also to reduce symptoms of anxiety and tension associated with many neurotic disorders.

PHARMACOKINETICS **Absorption:** readily absorbed from GI tract. **Peak:** 2 h PO; 30 min IM. **Duration:** 4–6 h PO; 6–8 h IM. **Metabolism:** metabolized in liver. **Elimination:** half-life: 24–48 h; excreted in urine and bile.

CONTRAINDICATIONS & PRECAUTIONS Contraindicated in: known sensitivity to other phenothiazines; severely depressed (drug-induced) patient, comatose state, children < 12 y. Safe use during preg-

ROUTE & DOSAGE

Psychotic Disorders

Adult	PO	10–50 mg b.i.d. or t.i.d.; may increase as needed up to 400 mg/d
	IM	25 mg; may repeat in 30–60 min if necessary

Management of Hyperactivity

Adult	PO	25 mg t.i.d. up to 75–300 mg/d

Alcohol Dependence

Adult	PO	25 mg b.i.d. up to 50–200 mg/d

Anxiety & Tension

Adult	PO	10 mg b.i.d. up to 150 mg/d

---

nancy (category C) and in nursing mothers not established. **Cautious use in:** previously detected cancer of breast; glaucoma; prostatic hypertrophy, urinary retention; history of cardiovascular disease.

ADVERSE/SIDE EFFECTS Dizziness, *sedation,* fainting, blurred vision, xerostomia, nasal congestion, urinary retention, constipation, decreased sweating, contact dermatitis, tachycardia, *orthostatic hypotension,* extrapyramidal effects.

NURSING IMPLICATIONS

Administration

- Just before administration, dilute PO concentrate in about 1/2 glass (120 ml) of fluid. Suggested diluents: fruit juices, water, soup, carbonated beverage. Measure drug with calibrated dispenser included in original package. Explain use of dispenser and dose to patient.
- Inject IM solution slowly and deeply into upper outer quadrant of buttock. Advise patient to lie still for 20–30 min after the injection to minimize possible dizziness.
- Slight yellowing of the solution will not change potency; however, darkened solution should be discarded.
- Protect solution from light and freezing. Store below 25C (77F); refrigeration is not necessary.

Assessment & Drug Effects

- Monitor I&O and bowel elimination patterns and check bladder for distension. The depressed patient often fails to report urinary discomfort or constipation.
- If patient complains of blurred vision, report to physician. Periodic ophthalmic examinations are advisable with long-term therapy.
- Monitor BP with patient supine and standing.

Patient & Family Education

- Caution patient to avoid spilling drug on skin since it may cause contact dermatitis. Thoroughly rinse off with water if spilling occurs.
- Because of possible dizziness and drowsiness during early period of therapy, advise patient not to drive a car or engage in any dangerous activity until drug response is known.
- Drowsiness usually decreases with continued therapy. If it persists and interferes with ADL, consult physician. A change in time of administration or dose may help to prevent interference with normal physical activities.
- Warn patient of possibility of orthostatic hypotension. Advise patient to dangle legs over bedside upon arising from sleep.
- Alcohol should be avoided during mesoridazine therapy.
- Xerostomia discomfort (e.g., dry mouth) should be attended to, since deprivation of saliva fosters tissue erosion and demineralization of tooth surfaces. Frequent warm water rinses and, if there is salivary response, sugarfree gum or candy may be helpful. Avoid commercial mouth rinses.

Prototype: Isoproterenol HCl, p 105

METAPROTERENOL SULFATE

(met-a-proe-ter´e-nole)

Trade names: Alupent, Metaprel, Prometa

Classifications: AUTONOMIC NERVOUS SYSTEM AGENT; BETA-ADRENERGIC AGONIST; BRONCHODILATOR; RESPIRATORY SMOOTH MUSCLE RELAXANT

Pregnancy: Category C

ACTIONS/PHARMACODYNAMICS Potent synthetic sympathomimetic amine similar to isoproterenol in chemical structure and pharmacologic actions. Acts selectively on beta$_2$-adrenergic receptors to relax smooth muscle of bronchi, uterus, and blood vessels supplying skeletal muscles. Reportedly has less stimulant action on beta$_1$ receptors of heart than does isoproterenol.

USES Bronchodilator in symptomatic relief of asthma and reversible bronchospasm associated with bronchitis and emphysema. **Unlabeled uses:** treatment and prophylaxis of heart block and to avert progress of premature labor (tocolytic action).

ROUTE & DOSAGE

Bronchospasm

Adult	PO	20 mg q6–8h
	Metered Dose Inhaler	2–3 inhalations q3–4h (max 12 inhalations/d)
	Nebulizer	5–10 inhalations of undiluted 5% solution
	IPPB	2.5 ml of 0.4–0.6% solution q4–6h
Child	PO	> 9 y: 20 mg q6–8h
		6–9 y: 10 mg q6–8h
		< 6 y: 1.2–2.6 mg/kg/d in 3–4 divided doses

PHARMACOKINETICS Absorption: 40% of PO doses reaches systemic circulation. **Onset:** inhaled: 1 min; PO 15 min. **Peak:** 1 h all routes. **Duration:** inhaled: 1–5 h; PO 4 h. **Metabolism:** metabolized in liver. **Elimination:** excreted in urine.

CONTRAINDICATIONS & PRECAUTIONS Contraindicated in: sensitivity to other sympathomimetic agents; cardiac arrhythmias associated with tachycardia; hyperthyroidism. Safe use during pregnancy (category C); by nursing mothers, and in children < 12 y (for aerosol use) and < 6 y (for PO use) not established. **Cautious use in:** the elderly; hypertension, coronary artery disease; hyperthyroidism; diabetes.

ADVERSE/SIDE EFFECTS CNS: nervousness, weakness, drowsiness, *tremor (particularly after PO administration),* headache, fatigue. **CV:** *tachycardia,* hypertension, <u>cardiac arrest</u>, palpitation. **GI:** nausea, vomiting, bad taste. **Other:** occasional difficulty in micturition and muscle cramps, throat irritation, cough, exacerbation of asthma.

DRUG INTERACTIONS Epinephrine, other SYMPATHOMIMETIC BRONCHODILATORS may compound effects of metaproterenol; MAO INHIBITORS, TRICYCLIC ANTIDEPRESSANTS potentiate action of metaproterenol on vascular system; the effects of both metaproterenol and BETA-ADRENERGIC BLOCKERS are antagonized.

NURSING IMPLICATIONS

Administration

- Oral drug may be taken with food to reduce GI distress.

M

Common side effects in *italic*; life-threatening effects <u>underlined</u>; generic names in **bold**; classifications in SMALL CAPS

745

▪ *Metered aerosol dose:* instruct patient to shake container, exhale through nose as completely as possible, administer aerosol while inhaling deeply through mouth, and to hold breath about 10 seconds before exhaling slowly. Administer second inhalation 10 min after first.

▪ Patient may use tablets and aerosol concomitantly.

▪ Protect from light and heat. Store at 15–30C (59–86F) unless otherwise directed.

Assessment & Drug Effects

▪ Monitor respiratory status. Auscultate lungs before and after inhalation to determine efficacy of drug in decreasing airway resistance.

▪ Monitor cardiac status. Report tachycardia and hypotension.

Patient & Family Education

▪ Drug may have shorter duration of action after long-term use. Instruct patients to report failure to respond to usual dose.

▪ Warn patients not to increase dose or frequency unless ordered by physician; there is the possibility of serious adverse effects.

▪ Advise patient that tremor is an anticipated side effect.

Prototype: epinephrine, p 102

METARAMINOL BITARTRATE

(met-a-ram´i-nole)

Trade name: Aramine

Classifications: AUTONOMIC NERVOUS SYSTEM AGENT; ALPHA- AND BETA-ADRENERGIC AGONIST (SYMPATHOMIMETIC)

Pregnancy: Category D

ACTIONS/PHARMACODYNAMICS Potent synthetic sympathomimetic amine. Overall effects similar to those of norepinephrine; but metaraminol is not as potent, has more gradual onset and longer duration of action, and usually lacks CNS stimulant effects. Acts directly on α-adrenergic receptors (vasoconstriction) and also directly stimulates beta$_1$ receptors of heart (positive inotropic effect); indirectly causes release of norepinephrine from storage sites. Tachyphylaxis may occur with prolonged use by depletion of epinephrine stores in nerve endings; in addition, metaraminol may function as weak or false neurotransmitter by replacing norepinephrine

in sympathetic nerve endings, with resultant worsening of shock state. Vasoconstrictor action increases pulmonary arterial pressure, produces sustained rise in systolic and diastolic pressures, and reduces blood flow to kidneys and other vital organs and probably skin and skeletal muscles.

USES Prevention and treatment of acute hypotensive states occurring with spinal anesthesia and as adjunct in treatment of hypotension due to hemorrhage, reaction to medication, surgical complications, brain damage, cardiogenic shock, and septicemia. **Unlabeled uses:** provocative test for diagnosis of familial Mediterranean fever and to increase cardiac output in pericardial tamponade.

ROUTE & DOSAGE

Hypotension

Adult	SC/IM	2–10 mg; may repeat in 10 min if necessary
	IV	0.5–5 mg followed by IV infusion of 15–100 mg in 500 ml of D5W or NS
Child	SC/IM	0.1 mg/kg; may repeat in 10 min if necessary
	IV	0.01 mg/kg followed by IV infusion of 0.04 mg/kg (each milligram diluted in 25 ml of D5W or NS)

PHARMACOKINETICS Onset: 1–2 min IV; < 10 min IM; 5–20 min SC. **Duration:** 20–90 min. **Metabolism:** metabolized in tissues. **Elimination:** excreted in urine.

CONTRAINDICATIONS & PRECAUTIONS Contraindicated in: use with cyclopropane, halothane, within 14 d of MAO inhibitor therapy; peripheral or mesenteric thrombosis; pulmonary edema, cardiac arrest; untreated hypoxia, hypercapnia, and acidosis; as sole therapy in hypovolemia. Safe use during pregnancy (category D) not established. **Cautious use in:** digitalized patients; hypertension; thyroid disease; diabetes mellitus; cirrhosis of liver; history of malaria (may produce relapse).

ADVERSE/SIDE EFFECTS Apprehension, restlessness, headache, tremor, nausea, vomiting, weakness, flushing, pallor, sweating, precordial pain, palpitation, tachycardia, bradycardia, decreased urinary output, metabolic acidosis (hypovolemic patients), hyperglycemia. **Excessive dosage:** severe hypertension, headache, convulsions, acute pulmonary edema, arrhythmias, cardiac arrest. **Injection site reactions (especially following SC):** abscess formation, tissue necrosis, sloughing. **Prolonged use:** plasma volume de-

M

pletion with recurrence of shock state, hypotension.

DRUG INTERACTIONS ERGOT ALKALOIDS, **furazolidone, guanethidine,** MAO INHIBITORS, TRICYCLIC ANTIDEPRESSANTS may cause an excessive pressor response; **phentolamine** may decrease pressor response; increases risk of arrhythmias with **halothane, cyclopropane.**

INCOMPATIBILITIES Solution/Additive: amphotericin B, dexamethasone, erythromycin, fibrinogen, hydrocortisone, methicillin, methylprednisolone, penicillin, thiopental, warfarin.

NURSING IMPLICATIONS

Administration

- Patients receiving drug IV must be constantly attended, with infusion flow rate being closely monitored. Changes in flow rate must be made cautiously, since the drug has cumulative effect and prolonged action.
- Up to 5 mg may be given undiluted by direct IV over at least 1 min.
- *For adults:* 15–100 mg may be dissolved in 500 ml of D5W, NS, or other compatible IV fluid and titrated to maintain BP at a desired level.
- *For children:* IV infusion is prepared to yield a concentration of 1 mg for each 25 ml of solution.
- IV flow rate will be prescribed by physician (usually, systolic BP is maintained at 80–100 mm Hg for previously normotensive patients; for previously hypertensive patients it is maintained at 30–40 mm Hg below the usual pressure).
- When infusion is to be discontinued, flow rate should be reduced gradually, and abrupt withdrawal avoided. Equipment for reinstituting therapy should be immediately available.
- Care should be taken to avoid extravasation during IV infusion. Injury to local tissue and necrosis may result.
- SC injection is especially likely to cause tissue necrosis and sloughing; therefore it is generally not prescribed, particularly in shock therapy.
- Avoid exposure of drug to excessive heat, and protect it from light.

Assessment & Drug Effects

- Except in emergency situations, blood volume should be corrected as fully as possible before therapy is initiated.
- During IV infusion, check BP q5min until it is stabilized at prescribed level, then q15min thereafter throughout therapy. Also note pulse rate and qual

ity. Continue monitoring at regular intervals for several hours after infusion is complete.
- Observe I&O ratio and pattern. Keep physician informed of renal response. Urinary output may decrease initially, then increase as BP approaches normal levels. With excessive dosage, output may again decrease.
- Metaraminol may cause diuresis in patients with cirrhosis of liver. Patients should be carefully monitored for excessive losses of water, sodium, and potassium.
- Patients with diabetes should be closely monitored for loss of diabetes control.

Patient & Family Education

- Instruct patient to immediately report pain at IV insertion site or site of SC injection.
- Instruct patient to immediately report respiratory distress, chest pain, or palpitations.

Prototype: morphine, p 156

METHADONE HYDROCHLORIDE

(meth´a-done)
Trade names: Dolophine
Classifications: CNS AGENT; NARCOTIC (OPIATE) AGONIST ANALGESIC
Pregnancy: Category B (D for use of high doses at term)
Controlled Substance: Schedule II

ACTIONS/PHARMACODYNAMICS Synthetic diphenylheptane derivative with pharmacologic properties qualitatively similar to those of morphine but is orally effective and has longer duration of action. A single oral dose produces less sedation and euphoria than does morphine, but repeated doses produce marked sedation (cumulative action). Causes less constipation than morphine, but respiratory depressant effect (principal danger of overdosage) and antitussive actions are comparable. Highly addictive, with abuse potential that matches that of morphine; abstinence syndrome develops more slowly; withdrawal symptoms are less intense but more prolonged.

USES To relieve severe pain; for detoxification and temporary maintenance treatment in hospital and in federally controlled maintenance programs for ambulatory patients with narcotic abstinence syndrome.

Common side effects in *italic*; life-threatening effects <u>underlined</u>;
generic names in **bold**; classifications in SMALL CAPS

747

ROUTE & DOSAGE

Moderate to Severe Acute Pain

Adult   PO/SC/IM   2.5–10 mg q3–4h prn

Chronic Pain

Adult   PO/SC/IM   5–20 mg q6–8h

Detoxification Treatment

Adult   PO/SC/IM   15–40 mg once/d; usually maintained at 20–120 mg/d

PHARMACOKINETICS Absorption: well absorbed from GI tract. **Onset:** 30–60 min PO; 10–20 min IM/SC. **Peak:** 1–2 h. **Duration:** 6–8 h PO, IM, SC; may last 22–48 h with chronic dosing. **Distribution:** crosses placenta; distributed into breast milk. **Metabolism:** metabolized in liver. **Elimination:** half-life: 15–25 h; excreted in urine.

CONTRAINDICATIONS & PRECAUTIONS Contraindicated in: obstetric analgesia. Safe use during pregnancy (category B), (category D for use of high doses at term), in nursing mothers, and for treatment of narcotic addiction in patients < 18 y not established. **Cautious use in:** hepatic, renal, or cardiac dysfunction.

ADVERSE/SIDE EFFECTS *Drowsiness,* nausea, vomiting, dry mouth, *constipation,* lightheadedness, dizziness, transient fall in BP, bone and muscle pain, hallucinations, impotence, <u>respiratory depression</u>.

DRUG INTERACTIONS Alcohol and other CNS DEPRESSANTS, **cimetidine** add to sedation and CNS depression; AMPHETAMINES may potentiate CNS stimulation; with MAO INHIBITORS, **selegiline, furazolidone** causes excessive and prolonged CNS depression, convulsions, cardiovascular collapse.

INCOMPATIBILITIES Solution/Additive: aminophylline, ammonium chloride, BARBITURATES, **chlorothiazide, heparin, methicillin, phenytoin, sodium bicarbonate.**

NURSING IMPLICATIONS

Administration

- For analgesic effect, methadone should be administered in the smallest effective dose to minimize the possibility of tolerance and physical and psychic dependence.
- IM route is preferred when repeated parenteral administration is required (SC injections may cause local irritation and induration). Aspirate syringe carefully before injecting drug to avoid inadvertent IV administration. Rotate injection sites.
- **Detoxification treatment:** methadone is administered in decreasing doses (PO formulation is preferred) over a period not exceeding 21 d to suppress abstinence symptoms during narcotic withdrawal.
- Preserve in tight, light-resistant containers at 15–30C (59–86F) unless otherwise directed.

Assessment & Drug Effects

- Evaluate the patient's continued need for methadone for pain. Adjustment of dosage and lengthening of between-dose intervals may be possible.
- Principal danger of overdosage, as with morphine, is extreme respiratory depression.
- Because of the cumulative effects of methadone, abstinence symptoms may not appear for 36–72 h after last dose and may last 10–14 d. Symptoms are usually of mild intensity (anorexia, insomnia, anxiety, abdominal discomfort, weakness, headache, sweating, hot and cold flashes). Purposive behavior is prominent by the sixth day.
- Narcotic antagonists such as naloxone, naltrexone, and levallorphan terminate methadone intoxication by competing for narcotic binding sites. Since antagonist action is shorter (1–3 h) than that of methadone (36–48 h or more), repeated doses for 8–24 h may be required. Patient should be watched closely for recurrence of respiratory depression.

Patient & Family Education

- Orthostatic hypotension, sweating, constipation, drowsiness, GI symptoms, and other transient side effects of therapeutic doses appear to be more prominent in ambulatory patients. Most side effects disappear over a period of several weeks.
- Instruct patients to make position changes slowly, particularly from recumbent to upright position, and to sit or lie down if they feel dizzy or faint.
- Patients should be informed that methadone may impair mental and physical abilities required for performance of potentially hazardous activities, such as driving a car or operating machinery.
- **Methadone maintenance program:** consists of substituting stable doses of PO methadone to eliminate compulsive craving and euphoric effects of parenterally administered narcotics. Treatment frequently begins with daily doses at an ambulatory clinic. Later, take-home doses of methadone may be dispensed as PO liquid (dissolved in juice to discourage parenteral injection).

M

Common side effects in *italic*; life-threatening effects <u>underlined</u>; generic names in **bold**; classifications in SMALL CAPS

Prototype: amphetamine, p 194

METHAMPHETAMINE HYDROCHLORIDE

(meth-am-fet´a-meen)
Trade names: Desoxyephedrine
Hydrochloride, Desoxyn, Methampex
Classifications: CNS AGENT; RESPIRATORY AND
CEREBRAL STIMULANT; ANOREXIANT; AM-
PHETAMINE
Pregnancy: Category C
Controlled substance: Schedule II

ACTIONS/PHARMACODYNAMICS Sympathomimetic amine chemically related to amphetamine.
CNS stimulant actions (mood elevation, depression of
appetite, decreased fatigue) approximately equal to
those of amphetamine, but accompanied by less peripheral activity. However, larger doses produce increased cardiac output, possibly reflex slowing of
heart rate, and sustained increase in BP, chiefly by
cardiac stimulation. Excessive doses depress myocardium.

USES Short-term adjunct in management of exogenous obesity, as adjunctive therapy in attention
deficit disorder (ADD), narcolepsy, epilepsy, and
postencephalitic parkinsonism, and in treatment of
certain depressive reactions, especially when charac
terized by apathy and psychomotor retardation.

ROUTE & DOSAGE

Attention Deficit Disorder

Child   PO   ≥ 6 y: 2.5–5 mg 1–2 times/d; may increase by 5 mg at weekly intervals up to
20–25 mg/d

Obesity

Adult   PO   2.5–5 mg 1–3 times/d 30 min before
meals; *or* 5–15 mg of long-acting form
once/d

PHARMACOKINETICS Absorption: readily ab-
sorbed from the GI tract. **Duration:** 6–12 h. **Distribution:**
all tissues especially the CNS; excreted in breast milk.
Metabolism: metabolized in liver. **Elimination:** renal
elimination.

**CONTRAINDICATIONS & PRECAUTIONS Con-
traindicated in:** during pregnancy, especially first
trimester (category C), as anorexiant in children < 12

y; patients receiving MAO inhibitors; arteriosclerotic
parkinsonism. **Cautious use in:** mild hypertension; psy-
chopathic personalities; hyperexcitability states; history of suicide attempts; elderly or debilitated patients.

ADVERSE/SIDE EFFECTS CNS: (stimulation):
restlessness, tremor, hyperreflexia, insomnia, headache, nervousness, anxiety, dizziness, euphoria or
dysphoria. **CV:** palpitation, arrhythmias, hypertension, hypotension, <u>circulatory collapse</u>. **GI:** dry
mouth, unpleasant taste, nausea, vomiting, diarrhea,
constipation, increased intraocular pressure. **Other:**
psychotic episodes (rare), depression.

**DRUG INTERACTIONS Acetazolamide, sodium
bicarbonate** decrease amphetamine elimination;
ammonium chloride, ascorbic acid increase amphetamine elimination; effects of both methamphetamine and BARBITURATES may be antagonized;
furazolidone may increase BP effects of amphetamines—interaction may persist for several
weeks after discontinuing furazolidone; antagonizes
antihypertensive effects of **guanethidine, guanadryl;** MAO INHIBITORS, **selegiline** can cause hypertensive crisis (fatalities reported)—do not administer amphetamines during or within 14 d of
administration of these drugs; PHENOTHIAZINES may
inhibit mood elevating effects of amphetamines; TRI-
CYCLIC ANTIDEPRESSANTS enhance amphetamine effects because they increase norepinephrine release;
BETA-ADRENERGIC AGONISTS increase adverse cardiovascular effects of amphetamines.

NURSING IMPLICATIONS

Administration

- If possible, medication should be taken early in the
  day to avoid insomnia.
- When used for treatment of obesity, drug is administered 30 min before each meal. If insomnia results, advise patient to inform physician.
- Preserve in tight, light-resistant containers.

Assessment & Drug Effects

- Paradoxic increase in depression or agitation sometimes occurs in depressed patients. Report immediately; drug should be withdrawn.
- Duration of methamphetamine use in treatment of
  obesity should not exceed a few weeks.

Patient & Family Education

- Tolerance develops readily, and prolonged use
  may lead to drug dependence. High abuse poten-

Common side effects in *italic*; life-threatening effects <u>underlined</u>;
generic names in **bold**; classifications in SMALL CAPS

749

M

tial. Commonly known as "speed" or "crystal" among drug abusers.

- Withdrawal after prolonged use is frequently followed by lethargy that may persist for several weeks.
- Instruct patients to weigh themselves every other day under standard conditions and maintain a record of weight loss.

Prototype: acetazolamide, p 206

METHAZOLAMIDE

(meth-a-zoe′la-mide)

Trade name: Neptazane
Classifications: EYE PREPARATION; CARBONIC ANHYDRASE INHIBITOR; SULFONAMIDE DERIVATIVE; ANTIGLAUCOMA
Pregnancy: Category C

ACTIONS/PHARMACODYNAMICS Nonbactericidal sulfonamide derivative similar to acetazolamide but with slower onset and longer duration of action. Appears to cause more drowsiness and fatigue than acetazolamide does, and has less diuretic activity. Actions, contraindications, precautions, and adverse reactions as for acetazolamide.

USES Adjunctive treatment in chronic simple (open-angle) glaucoma and secondary glaucoma and preoperatively in acute angle-closure glaucoma when delay of surgery is desired in order to lower intraocular pressure. May be used concomitantly with miotic and osmotic agents.

ROUTE & DOSAGE

Glaucoma

Adult PO 50–100 mg b.i.d. or t.i.d.

PHARMACOKINETICS Absorption: slowly absorbed from GI tract. **Onset:** 2–4 h. **Peak:** 6–8 h. **Duration:** 10–18 h. **Distribution:** distributed throughout body, concentrating in RBCs, plasma, and kidneys; crosses placenta. **Metabolism:** partially metabolized in liver. **Elimination:** excreted primarily in urine.

CONTRAINDICATIONS & PRECAUTIONS Contraindicated in: glaucoma due to severe peripheral anterior synechiae, severe or absolute glaucoma, hemorrhagic glaucoma; hypokalemia, hyponatremia; pregnancy (category C).

ADVERSE/SIDE EFFECTS Malaise, drowsiness, fatigue, lethargy, mild GI disturbance, anorexia, headache, vertigo, paresthesias, mental confusion, depression.

DRUG INTERACTIONS Renal excretion of AMPHETAMINES, **ephedrine, flecainide, quinidine, procainamide,** TRICYCLIC ANTIDEPRESSANTS may be decreased, thereby enhancing or prolonging their effects; increases renal excretion of **lithium;** excretion of **phenobarbital** may be increased; **amphotericin B,** CORTICOSTEROIDS may add to potassium loss; hypokalemia caused by methazolamide may predispose patients on DIGITALIS GLYCOSIDES to digitalis toxicity; patients on high doses of SALICYLATES are at higher risk for salicylate toxicity.

NURSING IMPLICATIONS

Administration

- Drug may be given with meals to minimize GI distress.

Assessment & Drug Effects

- Supervise ambulation in elderly, since drug may cause vertigo.
- Since drug may cause fatigue and lethargy, assess patient's ability to perform ADL.

Patient & Family Education

- Instruct patient that drug may cause drowsiness. Advise caution with hazardous activities until reaction to drug is known.
- Brand interchange is not recommended without evidence of therapeutic equivalence.

Prototype: trimethoprim, p 90

METHENAMINE HIPPURATE

(meth-en′a-meen hip′yoo-rate)
Trade names: Hiprex, Urex

METHENAMINE MANDELATE

Trade names: Mandelamine, Mandameth, Mandelets
Classification: URINARY TRACT ANTIINFECTIVE
Pregnancy: Category C

ACTIONS/PHARMACODYNAMICS Chemical combination of methenamine with hippuric acid or with mandelic acid. In an acid medium this tertiary

M

amine liberates formaldehyde, a nonspecific antibiotic agent with bactericidal activity. (Methenamine itself has no antibacterial effect, but its salts contribute to urine acidity and also provide weak antibacterial action.) Most bacteria and fungi are susceptible to formaldehyde; however, bacteria that are urease-positive (e.g., *Proteus* sp) convert urea to ammonium hydroxide, which prevents the generation of formaldehyde from methenamine.

USES Prophylactic treatment of recurrent urinary tract infections (UTIs). Also long-term prophylaxis when residual urine is present (e.g., neurogenic bladder).

ROUTE & DOSAGE

UTI Prophylaxis

Adult	PO	Hippurate: 1 g b.i.d.
		Mandelate: 1 g q.i.d.
Child	PO	6–12 y: Hippurate: 0.5–1 g b.i.d.
		Mandelate: 500 mg q.i.d. or 50 mg/kg/d in 3 divided doses
		≤ 6 y: Mandelate: 18.4 mg/kg q.i.d.

PHARMACOKINETICS Absorption: readily absorbed from GI tract, although 10–30% of dose is hydrolyzed to formaldehyde in stomach. **Peak:** 2 h. **Duration:** up to 6 h or until patient voids. **Distribution:** crosses placenta; distributed into breast milk. **Metabolism:** hydrolyzed in acid pH to formaldehyde. **Elimination:** half-life: 4 h; excreted in urine.

CONTRAINDICATIONS & PRECAUTIONS Contraindicated in: renal insufficiency; hepatic disease; gout; severe dehydration; combined therapy with sulfonamides. Safe use during pregnancy (category C), in nursing mothers, and in children < 6 y (mandelate) not established. **Cautious use in:** PO suspension for patients susceptible to lipoid pneumonia (e.g., the elderly, debilitated patient).

ADVERSE/SIDE EFFECTS GI: nausea, vomiting, diarrhea, abdominal cramps, anorexia. **Hypersensitivity:** rash, pruritus, urticaria, stomatitis. **Renal:** bladder irritation, dysuria, frequency, albuminuria, hematuria, crystalluria. **Other:** generalized edema, head-ache, tinnitus, muscle cramps, transient elevations of serum AST, ALT.

DIAGNOSTIC TEST INTERFERENCES Methenamine (formaldehyde) may produce falsely elevated values for *urinary catecholamines* and *urinary steroids* (17-hydroxycorticosteroids) (by Reddy method). Possibility of false *urine glucose determinations* with Benedict's test. Methenamine interferes with *urobilinogen* and possibly *urinary VMA* determinations.

DRUG INTERACTIONS Sulfamethoxazole forms insoluble precipitate in acid urine; **acetazolamide, sodium bicarbonate** may prevent hydrolysis to formaldehyde.

NURSING IMPLICATIONS

Administration

▪ Administer after meals and at bedtime to minimize gastric distress.
▪ PO suspension contains a vegetable oil base; administer with caution to the elderly or the debilitated patient because of the possibility of lipid (aspiration) pneumonia.
▪ Reconstitute PO granules by dissolving 1 packet (500 mg or 1 g) in 60–120 ml water immediately before use. Solution may remain cloudy after reconstitution.
▪ Store at 15–30C (59–86F) in tightly closed container; protect from excessive heat.

Assessment & Drug Effects

▪ Monitor urine pH, since a value of 5.5 or less is required for optimum drug action.
▪ Monitor I&O ratio and pattern. Methenamine is most effective when fluid intake is maintained at 1500 or 2000 ml/d.
▪ Generally fluids are not forced, as copious amounts with this drug may increase diuresis, elevate urine pH, and dilute formaldehyde concentration to subinhibitory levels. If specific gravity goes below 1.015 (normal: 1.006–1.030) fluids will be restricted.
▪ If patient complains of gastric distress, consult physician about changing formulation to enteric-coated tablet.
▪ Supplemental acidification to maintain pH of 5.5 or below required for drug action may be necessary. This can be accomplished by drugs (ascorbic acid, ammonium chloride) or by foods.

Patient & Family Education

▪ Patient should be instructed how to read dipstick tests for pH and specific gravity and to report if required values are not attained.
▪ Caution patient not to self-medicate with OTC antacids containing sodium bicarbonate or sodium carbonate (to prevent raising urine pH).
▪ Supplementary acidification may be achieved by

M

limited intake of foods that can increase urine pH: vegetables, fruits, and fruit juice (except cranberry, plum, prune) and liberal intake of foods that can decrease urine pH: proteins, cranberry juice, plums, prunes.

Prototype: penicillin G potassium, p 71

METHICILLIN SODIUM

(meth-i-sill´in)
Trade name: Staphcillin
Classifications: ANTIINFECTIVE; β-LACTAM ANTIBIOTIC; PENICILLIN
Pregnancy: Category B

ACTIONS/PHARMACODYNAMICS Semisynthetic salt of penicillin with antimicrobial spectrum similar to that of penicillin G; differs from the latter in its high resistance to penicillinase-producing strains of staphylococci. Not as effective as penicillin G against non-penicillinase-producing staphylococci, streptococci, or pneumococci. A growing number of methicillin-resistant strains are reported to be developing.

USES Primarily in infections caused by penicillinase-producing staphylococci. May be used to initiate therapy in suspected staphylococcal infections pending results of culture and sensitivity tests.

ROUTE & DOSAGE

Staphylococcal Infections

| Adult | IM/IV | 1–2 g q4–6h up to 12 g/d |
| Child | IM/IV | 100–300 mg/kg/d divided q4–6h |

PHARMACOKINETICS Peak: 30–60 min IM; 15 min IV. **Duration:** 4 h IM; 2 h IV. **Distribution:** distributes into CNS with inflamed meninges; crosses placenta; distributed into breast milk. **Metabolism:** small amount metabolized in liver. **Elimination:** half-life: 0.4–0.5 h; 80% excreted in urine, 20% in feces.

CONTRAINDICATIONS & PRECAUTIONS Contraindicated in: hypersensitivity to penicillins or cephalosporins. IV dosage in infants not established. Safe use during pregnancy (category B) not established. **Cautious use in:** history of allergy, asthma; nursing women, pediatric use; impaired renal function.

ADVERSE/SIDE EFFECTS Hypersensitivity reactions: *skin rash,* pruritus, urticaria, eosinophilia, serum sickness, anaphylactic reaction, *acute interstitial nephritis.* Also reported: bone marrow depression (anemia, neutropenia, granulocytopenia, agranulocytosis), neuropathy, irritation at IM site, thrombophlebitis (after IV administration); oral, rectal, vaginal candidal superinfections.

INCOMPATIBILITIES Solution/Additive: amikacin, chlorpromazine, codeine, hydrocortisone, levorphanol, meperidine, metaraminol, methadone, methohexital, morphine, tetracyclines, promethazine, sodium bicarbonate, vancomycin, heparin, streptomycin.

NURSING IMPLICATIONS

Administration

- Reportedly well tolerated by deep intragluteal injection, although it may be painful. Rotate injection sites.
- Methicillin is reconstituted with sterile water for injection or NaCl injection (1.5 ml/g; 5.7 ml/4g; 8.6 ml/6g). Resulting concentration is 500 mg/ml. Shake vial vigorously before withdrawing contents.
- Each 1 ml (500 mg) is further diluted with 25 ml of sterile water or NS and given by direct IV at a rate of 10 ml/min.
- Solution may be further diluted by addition to a compatible IV infusion solution and given over 30 min–8 h.
- *Stability of diluted concentrations:* 2 mg/ml, 4 h; 10–30 mg/ml, 8 h.
- Reconstituted methicillin solutions are stable for 24 h at room temperature (59–86F) and for 4 d under refrigeration (36–46F). Solutions gradually darken to a deep orange color and acquire a distinctive hydrogen sulfide odor upon standing for prolonged periods at room temperature. Discard such solutions.
- Methicillin is reported to be incompatible with many drugs including other antibiotics. Use only solutions recommended by manufacturer.
- Drug therapy is generally continued at least 48 h, or in the case of serious systemic infections, for at least 1–2 wk after patient has become afebrile and asymptomatic and cultures are negative. Treatment of osteomyelitis may require several weeks of intensive therapy.

Assessment & Drug Effects

- Culture and susceptibility tests should be performed initially and periodically during therapy.

M

- Before starting therapy, obtain history of previous hypersensitivity reactions to penicillins, cephalosporins, or any other allergens.
- Observe all injection sites for evidence of irritation or inflammation.
- Periodic assessment of renal, hematopoietic, and hepatic function are advised during prolonged therapy.
- Frequent blood level measurements are advised in infants, as urinary excretion of drug is slower in this age group.
- Febrile reactions are reported to occur in some patients 1–2 h after IV administration.
- Monitor patients for signs and symptoms of *interstitial nephritis,* a hypersensitivity reaction that occurs 2–4 wk after initiation of therapy: spiking fever, anorexia, skin rash, oliguria, hematuria, cloudy urine (pyuria, albuminuria), eosinophilia. Usually reversible following prompt termination of drug.
- Monitor for signs and symptoms of superinfections (see chap 3).

Patient & Family Education
- Instruct patient to immediately report symptoms of a hypersensitivity reaction (see chap 3).

Prototype: propylthiouracil, p 243

METHIMAZOLE
(meth-im´a-zole)
Trade name: Tapazole
Classifications: SYNTHETIC HORMONE;
ANTITHYROID AGENT
Pregnancy: Category D

ACTIONS/PHARMACODYNAMICS Thioamide with actions and uses similar to those of propylthiouracil but 10 times as potent. Actions are less consistent, but effects appear more promptly than those of propylthiouracil. See propylthiouracil for contraindications and precautions and adverse/side effects.

USES Hyperthyroidism and prior to surgery or radiotherapy of the thyroid; may be used cautiously to treat hyperthyroidism in pregnancy.

ROUTE & DOSAGE

Hyperthyroidism

Adult	PO	5–15 mg q8h
Child	PO	0.2–0.4 mg/kg/d divided q8h

PHARMACOKINETICS Absorption: readily absorbed from GI tract. **Onset:** 30–40 min. **Peak:** 1 h. **Duration:** 2–4 h. **Distribution:** crosses placenta; distributed into breast milk. **Elimination:** half-life: 5–13 h; 12% excreted in urine within 24 h.

CONTRAINDICATIONS & PRECAUTIONS Contraindicated in: pregnancy (category D), breast feeding. **Cautious use in:** other drugs known to cause agranulocytosis.

NURSING IMPLICATIONS

Administration
- Take medication at same time each day relative to meals.
- Store drug in light-resistant container at 15–30C (59–86F).

Assessment & Drug Effects
- Periodic blood work is indicated, since agranulocytosis is a rare, but possible side effect.
- Monitor PT in patients on oral anticoagulants. Anticoagulant activity may be potentiated.

Patient & Family Education
- Instruct patient to adhere to established dosage regimen (i.e., not to double, decrease, or omit doses and not to alter the interval between doses).
- Skin rash or swelling of cervical lymph nodes indicates need to discontinue drug and change to another antithyroid agent.
- Notify physician promptly if the following symptoms appear: bruising, unexplained bleeding, sore throat, fever, jaundice.
- Dosage may be suspended about 2 wk before anticipated delivery and restored in postpartum period if required.
- Advise patient who has had drug-induced jaundice that it may persist up to 10 wk after withdrawal of methimazole.
- Methimazole does not induce hypothyroidis.

Prototype: cyclobenzaprine, p 122

METHOCARBAMOL
(meth-oh-kar´ba-mole)
Trade names: Delaxin, Marbaxin, Robaxin
Classifications: AUTONOMIC NERVOUS SYSTEM AGENT; CENTRAL ACTING SKELETAL MUSCLE RELAXANT
Pregnancy: Category C

M

Common side effects in *italic*; life-threatening effects underlined; generic names in **bold**; classifications in SMALL CAPS

753

ACTIONS/PHARMACODYNAMICS Propane-diol-derivative monocarbamate with actions similar to those of cyclobenzaprine, but it produces higher plasma levels more rapidly and for longer periods. Exerts skeletal muscle relaxant action by depressing multisynaptic pathways in spinal cord and possibly by sedative effect. Has no direct action on skeletal muscles.

USES Adjunct to physical therapy and other measures in management of discomfort associated with acute musculoskeletal disorders. Also used intravenously as adjunct in management of neuromuscular manifestations of tetanus.

ROUTE & DOSAGE

Acute Musculoskeletal Disorders

Adult	PO	1.5 g q.i.d. for 2–3 d, then 4–4.5 g/d in 3–6 divided doses
	IM	0.5–1 g q8h
	IV	1–3 g/d in divided doses given at a max rate of 300 mg/min

Tetanus

Adult	PO	Up to 24 g/d in divided doses crushed and suspended in saline, flushed down a nasogastric tube
	IV	1–2 g/d directly into IV tubing at a max rate of 300 mg/min; may be repeated q6h until nasogastric tube is possible
Child	PO	15 mg/kg repeated q6h as needed up to 1.8 g/m²/d for 3 consecutive d if necessary

PHARMACOKINETICS Absorption: readily absorbed from GI tract. **Onset:** 30 min. **Peak:** 1–2 h. **Metabolism:** metabolized in liver. **Elimination:** half-life: 1–2 h; excreted in urine.

CONTRAINDICATIONS & PRECAUTIONS Contraindicated in: comatose states, CNS depression, acidosis, renal dysfunction (injectable methocarbamol contains polyethylene glycol 300 in vehicle, which may cause urea retention and acidotic problems). Safe use during pregnancy (category C), in nursing women, and in children < 12 y (except for tetanus) not established. **Cautious use in:** epilepsy.

ADVERSE/SIDE EFFECTS Allergic (parenteral or PO use): urticaria, pruritus, rash, conjunctivitis, nasal congestion, headache, blurred vision, fever, <u>anaphylactic reaction</u>. **PO use:** *drowsiness, dizziness, lightheadedness,* syncope (rare), headache, nausea.

Parenteral use: thrombophlebitis, pain, sloughing (with extravasation), flushing, metallic taste, syncope, hypotension, bradycardia, convulsions. **Other:** slight reduction of white cell count with prolonged therapy.

DRUG INTERACTIONS Alcohol and other CNS DEPRESSANTS enhance CNS depression.

DIAGNOSTIC TEST INTERFERENCES Methocarbamol may cause false increases in ***urinary 5-HIAA*** (with nitrosonaphthol reagent) and ***VMA*** (Gitlow method).

NURSING IMPLICATIONS

Administration

- IV methocarbamol may be given by direct IV undiluted or diluted in up to 250 ml of NS or D5W and infused at a rate of 300 mg/min for adults.
- Patient should be recumbent during and for at least 15 min after IV injection in order to reduce the possibility of orthostatic hypotension and other adverse reactions. Monitor vital signs and IV flow rate.
- Care should be taken to avoid extravasation of IV solution, which may result in thrombophlebitis and sloughing.
- IM dose should not exceed 5 ml (0.5 g) into each gluteal region. Insert needle deep, and carefully aspirate. Inject drug slowly. Rotate injection sites and observe daily for evidence of irritation.
- Methocarbamol should not be administered SC.
- PO administration should replace parenteral use as soon as feasible.
- Store at 15–30C (59–86F) unless otherwise directed.

Assessment & Drug Effects

- Periodic WBC counts are advised during prolonged therapy.
- Supervise ambulation following parenteral administration.

Patient & Family Education

- Advise patient to make position changes slowly, particularly from recumbent to upright position, and to dangle legs before standing.
- Adverse reactions after PO administration are usually mild and transient and subside with dosage reduction. Caution patients regarding drowsiness and dizziness. Advise against activities requiring mental alertness and physical coordination until response to drug action is known.
- Urine may darken to brown, black, or green on standing.

M

Prototype: thiopental, p 164

METHOHEXITAL SODIUM

(meth-oh-hex′i-tal)
Trade names: Brietal, Brevital Sodium
Classifications: CNS AGENT; GENERAL ANES-
THETIC; BARBITURATE
Pregnancy: Category C
Controlled substance: Schedule IV

ACTIONS/PHARMACODYNAMICS Rapid, ultra-short-acting barbiturate anesthetic agent. More potent than thiopental but has less cumulative effect and shorter duration of action, and recovery is more rapid. Abnormal muscle movements, coughing, sneezing, and laryngospasm reportedly occur more frequently than with thiopental. See thiopental for pharmacokinetics, contraindications and precautions, and adverse/side effects.

USES Induction of anesthesia, as supplement for other anesthetics, and as general anesthetic for brief operative procedures.

ROUTE & DOSAGE

Induction of Anesthesia

Adult   IV   5–12 ml of 1% solution (50–120 mg) at a rate of 1 ml (5 mg) q5min, then 2–4 ml (20–40 mg) q4–7min prn

CONTRAINDICATIONS & PRECAUTIONS Contraindicated in: pregnancy (category C).

DRUG INTERACTIONS Alcohol and other CNS DEPRESSANTS enhance CNS depression.

INCOMPATIBILITIES Solution/Additive: atropine, chlorpromazine, glycopyrrolate, hydralazine, kanamycin, lidocaine, methicillin, methyldopa, prochlorperazine, promazine, promethazine, streptomycin, TETRACYCLINES.

NURSING IMPLICATIONS

Administration

- Patient should be recumbent during drug administration. Fall in BP may occur in susceptible patients receiving drug in upright position.
- Stable in sterile water for injection at room temperature for at least 6 wk. Solutions prepared with iso-

tonic NaCl injection or 5% dextrose injection are stable for about 24 h. Only clear, colorless solutions should be used.

- Methohexital solution is incompatible with acid solutions (e.g., atropine) and with silicone). Do not allow contact with rubber stoppers or parts of syringes treated with silicone.

Assessment & Drug Effects

- Hiccups are not uncommon, particularly with rapid injection; they sometimes persist after anesthesia.
- Facilities for assisting respiration and administration of oxygen should be readily available in the event of respiratory distress.

Prototype: fluorouracil, p 94

METHOTREXATE

(meth-oh-trex′ate)
Trade names: Amethopterin, MTX, Rheumatrex

METHOTREXATE SODIUM

Trade names: Folex, Mexate
Classifications: ANTINEOPLASTIC; ANTIMETABO-
LITE; IMMUNOSUPPRESSANT
Pregnancy: Category D

ACTIONS/PHARMACODYNAMICS Antimetabolite and folic acid antagonist. Blocks folinic acid (active principle of folic acid) participation in nucleic acid synthesis, thereby interfering with mitotic process. Rapidly proliferating tissues (malignant cells, bone marrow) are sensitive to this effect. In psoriasis, reproductive rate of epithelial cells is higher than in normal cells. Methotrexate controls the psoriatic process by its effect on mitosis. Some evidence of toxicity usually accompanies therapeutic response. Induces remission slowly; use often preceded by other antineoplastic therapies.

USES Principally in combination regimens to maintain induced remissions in neoplastic diseases. Effective in treatment of gestational choriocarcinoma and hydatidiform mole and as immunosuppressant in kidney transplantation, for acute and subacute leukemias and leukemic meningitis, especially in children. Used in lymphosarcoma, in certain inoperable tumors of head, neck, and pelvis, and in mycosis fungoides. Also used to treat severe psoriasis non-

M

Common side effects in *italic*; life-threatening effects <u>underlined</u>;
generic names in **bold**; classifications in SMALL CAPS

755

responsive to other forms of therapy, rheumatoid arthritis. **Unlabeled uses:** psoriatic arthritis, SLE, polymyositis.

ROUTE & DOSAGE

Trophoblastic neoplasm

Adult	PO	15–30 mg/d for 5 d; repeat q12wk for 3–5 courses
	IM/IV	15–30 mg/d for 5 d; repeat q12wk for 3–5 courses

Leukemia

Adult	IM/IV	Induction: 3.3 mg/m^2/d
	PO/IM/IV	Maintenance: 20–30 mg/m^2 2 times/wk

Lymphoma

Adult	PO	12–25 mg/d for 4–8 d with 7–10 d rest intervals

Psoriasis

Adult	PO	2.5–5 mg q12h for 3 doses each wk up to 25–30 mg/wk
	IM/IV	10–25 mg/wk

Rheumatoid Arthritis

Adult	PO	2.5–5 mg q12h for 3 doses each wk or 7.5 mg once/wk

PHARMACOKINETICS Absorption: readily absorbed from GI tract. **Peak:** 0.5–2 h IM/IV; 1–4 h PO. **Distribution:** widely distributed with highest concentrations in kidneys, gallbladder, spleen, liver, and skin; minimal passage across blood-brain barrier; crosses placenta; distributed into breast milk. **Metabolism:** metabolized in liver. **Elimination:** half-life: 2–4 h; excreted primarily in urine.

CONTRAINDICATIONS & PRECAUTIONS Contraindicated in: pregnancy (category D), men and women in childbearing age; hepatic and renal insufficiency; concomitant administration of hepatotoxic drugs and hematopoietic depressants; alcohol; ultraviolet exposure to psoriatic lesions; preexisting blood dyscrasias. **Cautious use in:** infections; peptic ulcer, ulcerative colitis; very young or old patients; cancer patients with preexisting bone marrow impairment, poor nutritional status.

ADVERSE/SIDE EFFECTS Dose-related and reversible. **CNS:** *headache*, drowsiness, blurred vision, dizziness, aphasia, hemiparesis; arachnoiditis, convulsions (after intrathecal administration); mental confusion, tremors, ataxia, coma. **GI:** hepatotoxicity,

GI ulcerations and hemorrhage, *ulcerative stomatitis, glossitis, gingivitis,* pharyngitis, nausea, vomiting, diarrhea, hepatic cirrhosis. **GU:** defective oogenesis or spermatogenesis, nephropathy, hematuria, menstrual dysfunction, infertility, abortion, fetal defects. **Hematologic:** *leukopenia, thrombocytopenia,* anemia, marked myelosuppression, aplastic bone marrow, telangiectasis, thrombophlebitis at intraarterial catheter site, hypogammaglobulinemia, hyperuricemia. **Skin:** erythematous rashes, pruritus, urticaria, folliculitis, vasculitis, photosensitivity, depigmentation, hyperpigmentation, alopecia. **Other:** malaise, undue fatigue, systemic toxicity (after intrathecal and intraarterial administration), chills, fever, decreased resistance to infection, septicemia, osteoporosis, metabolic changes precipitating diabetes and sudden death, pneumonitis, pulmonary fibrosis.

DIAGNOSTIC TEST INTERFERENCES Severe reactions may occur when *live vaccines* are administered because of immunosuppressive activity of methotrexate.

DRUG INTERACTIONS Alcohol increases risk of hepatotoxicity; **chloramphenicol,** SALICYLATES, NSAIDS, SULFONAMIDES, SULFONYLUREAS, **phenylbutazone, phenytoin,** TETRACYCLINES, **PABA, penicillin, probenecid** may increase methotrexate levels with increased toxicity; **folic acid** may alter response to methotrexate.

INCOMPATIBILITIES Solution/Additive: bleomycin, prednisolone, droperidol, heparin, metoclopramide, ranitidine. Y-site: droperidol, ranitidine.

NURSING IMPLICATIONS

Administration

- A test dose (5–10 mg parenterally) 1 wk before therapy precedes treatment of psoriasis.
- Avoid skin exposure and inhalation of drug particles.
- IV methotrexate is diluted by adding 5 mg to 2 ml of NS or D5W without preservatives to yield 2.5 mg/ml. Diluted drug is given by direct IV at a rate of 10 mg or fraction thereof over 60 seconds.
- Oral preparations should be given 1–2 h before or 2–3 h after meals.
- Preserve drug in tight, light-resistant container.

Assessment & Drug Effects

- Hepatic and renal function tests, blood tests, and chest x-rays should be part of the health data base.

Tests are repeated at weekly intervals during methotrexate therapy.

- Hepatic function tests may be abnormal 1–3 d after methotrexate administration.
- Prolonged treatment with small frequent doses may lead to hepatotoxicity, which is best diagnosed by liver biopsy.
- Ulcerative stomatitis with glossitis and gingivitis, often the first signs of toxicity, necessitate interruption of therapy or dosage adjustment. Inspect mouth daily; report patchy necrotic areas, bleeding and discomfort, or overgrowth (black, furry tongue).
- In presence of hyperuricemia, patient may be kept well hydrated (about 2000 ml/24 h) to dilute hyperuric fluids and given allopurinol to prevent urate deposition.
- Monitor I&O ratio and pattern. Severe nephrotoxicity (hematuria, dysuria, azotemia, oliguria) fosters drug accumulation and renal damage and requires dosage adjustment or discontinuation.
- During leukopenic periods, prevent patient exposure to personnel and visitors with infections or colds. Be alert to onset of agranulocytosis (cough, extreme fatigue, sore throat, chills, fever) and report symptoms promptly. Methotrexate therapy will be interrupted and appropriate antibiotic drugs prescribed.
- Be alert for and report *symptoms of thrombocytopenia*: ecchymoses, petechiae, epistaxis, melena, hematuria, vaginal bleeding, slow and protracted oozing following trauma.
- Bloody diarrhea necessitates interruption of therapy to prevent perforation or hemorrhagic enteritis. Report to physician.
- Diabetes may be precipitated; therefore, tests for glucosuria should be performed periodically, and significant symptoms such as polydipsia and polyuria should be reported.
- Monitor all laboratory reports daily as indicators for adaptations in nursing and drug regimens.
- If an overdosage of methotrexate is given, leucovorin may be employed as antidote (must be given within the first hour of overdosage).

Patient & Family Education
- Patient should be fully informed of dangers of this drug and warned to report promptly any abnormal symptoms.
- Leucovorin calcium given within 12 h after methotrexate protects normal tissues from lethal effects of the drug.
- Alcohol ingestion increases the incidence and severity of methotrexate hepatotoxicity.

- Fastidious mouth care prevents infection, provides comfort, and is essential to maintenance of adequate nutritional status.
- Alopecia is reversible; hair regrowth begins after drug discontinuation, but it may require several months.
- Methotrexate may precipitate gouty arthritis. Instruct the patient to report joint pains to physician.
- Warn patient not to self-medicate with vitamins. Some OTC compounds may include folic acid (or its derivatives), which alters methotrexate response.
- Contraceptive measures should be used both during and for at least 8 wk following therapy.
- Exposure to ultraviolet light and to sunlight may aggravate psoriatic lesions in patients on methotrexate therapy.
- Burning and erythema may occur in psoriatic areas after each dose of methotrexate. Instruct patient to notify physician if psoriasis worsens.
- Advise patient to adhere to dosage schedule (i.e., not to omit, increase, or decrease dose or change dose intervals).

Prototype: chlorpromazine, p 191

METHOTRIMEPRAZINE
(meth-oh-trye-mep´ra-zeen)
Trade names: Levoprome, Nozinan
Classifications: CNS AGENT; NONNARCOTIC ANALGESIC; PHENOTHIAZINE ANXIOLYTIC, SEDATIVE-HYPNOTIC
Pregnancy: Category C

ACTIONS/PHARMACODYNAMICS Aliphatic (propylamino) derivative of phenothiazine with CNS actions similar to those of chlorpromazine. In addition to tranquilizing and sedative effects, also has prominent analgesic properties. Extrapyramidal symptoms and dry mouth reportedly uncommon, but orthostatic hypotension and sedation effects are more prominent. Also exhibits antiemetic, antipruritic, weak anticholinergic, and local anesthetic properties. Raises pain threshold and may also produce amnesia. Nearly as potent as morphine in analgesic effect (15 mg of methotrimeprazine is reportedly equal to 10 mg of morphine). Unlike morphine-type analgesics, psychic and physical dependence not re-

Common side effects in *italic*; life-threatening effects <u>underlined</u>; generic names in **bold**; classifications in SMALL CAPS

757

ported with methotrimeprazine, it has no antitussive activity, and it rarely produces respiratory depression.

USES To relieve moderate to severe pain in nonambulatory patients and for analgesia and sedation when respiratory depression is to be avoided, as in obstetrics and pre- and postoperatively.

ROUTE & DOSAGE

Analgesia, Sedation
Adult   IM   10–20 mg q4–6h

Preoperative Medication
Adult   IM   2–20 mg 45 min–3 h before surgery

Postoperative Analgesia
Adult   IM   2.5–7.5 mg q4–6h as needed

PHARMACOKINETICS Onset: 20–40 min. **Peak:** 1–2 h. **Duration:** 4 h. **Distribution:** crosses CSF and placenta; distributed into breast milk. **Metabolism:** metabolized in liver. **Elimination:** slowly excreted in urine; elimination may continue for 1 wk after a single dose.

CONTRAINDICATIONS & PRECAUTIONS Contraindicated in: hypersensitivity to phenothiazines and to ingredients in the formulation, e.g., bisulfite; severe cardiac, renal, or hepatic disease; history of convulsive disorders; significant hypotension; comatose states; premature labor; children < 12 y; concomitant use with antihypertensive agents, including MAO inhibitors. **Cautious use in:** elderly and debilitated patients with heart disease; early pregnancy (category C).

ADVERSE/SIDE EFFECTS CNS: *excessive sedation, drowsiness, amnesia,* disorientation, euphoria, delirium, extrapyramidal symptoms. **CV:** *orthostatic hypotension with faintness,* weakness, dizziness; tachycardia, bradycardia, palpitation. **EENT:** blurred vision, nasal congestion. **GI:** nausea, vomiting, abdominal discomfort, dry mouth. **GU:** dysuria, hematuria. **Other:** headache, slurred speech, fever, chills, hypotonic uterine inertia (rare), injection site reactions, elevated serum bilirubin (rare), respiratory depression (infrequent). **With prolonged high dosage:** increased weight, jaundice, severe blood dyscrasias including agranulocytosis and pancytopenia.

DRUG INTERACTIONS Alcohol and other CNS DEPRESSANTS enhance CNS depression; with ANTICHOLINERGIC AGENTS, aggravation of extrapyramidal symptoms, CNS stimulation, delirium, tachycardia, and hypotension; ANTIHYPERTENSIVE AGENTS, MAO INHIBITORS add to hypotensive effects; **epinephrine** may antagonize pressor effects; SKELETAL MUSCLE RELAXANTS may prolong duration of muscle relaxation.

INCOMPATIBILITIES Solution/Additive: ranitidine. **Y-Site:** heparin.

NURSING IMPLICATIONS

Administration
- Administer IM injection deep into large muscle mass (subcutaneous injection causes severe local irritation).
- Pain at injection site and local inflammatory reaction commonly occur. Rotate injection sites and observe daily.
- The manufacturer states that methotrimeprazine may be mixed in the same syringe with either atropine or scopolamine, but not with any other drugs. (Dosage of atropine or scopolamine should be reduced.)
- Methotrimeprazine is rarely administered beyond 30 d, except when narcotic drugs are contraindicated or in terminal illness.
- Protect drug from light.

Assessment & Drug Effects
- Orthostatic hypotension with faintness, weakness, and dizziness may occur within 10–20 min after drug administration and may last 4–6 h and occasionally as long as 12 h. Ambulation should be avoided or carefully supervised for at least 6 h, but preferably 12 h. Tolerance to these effects usually develops with successive doses.
- Excessive sedation and amnesia also occur commonly during early drug therapy.
- BP and pulse should be checked frequently until dosage requirements and response are stabilized. Elderly and debilitated patients require close monitoring.
- When drug is used for prolonged periods, periodic blood studies and liver function tests are recommended.
- Injection formulation contains bisulfite, an allergen for some individuals.
- If severe hypotension occurs, treatment with epinephrine is specifically contraindicated.

Common side effects in *italic*; life-threatening effects underlined; generic names in **bold**; classifications in SMALL CAPS

METHOXAMINE HYDROCHLORIDE

See AUTONOMIC NERVOUS SYSTEM AGENTS, ALPHA ADRENERGIC AGONIST (SYMPATHOMIMETIC) prototype, p 101.

METHOXSALEN

See SKIN AND MUCOUS MEMBRANE AGENTS, PSORALEN prototype, p 261.

Prototype: atropine, p 116

METHSCOPOLAMINE BROMIDE
(meth-skoe-pol´a-meen)
Trade name: Pamine
Classifications: AUTONOMIC NERVOUS SYSTEM AGENT; ANTICHOLINERGIC (PARASYMPATHOLYTIC); ANTIMUSCARINIC, ANTISPASMODIC
Pregnancy: Category C

ACTIONS/PHARMACODYNAMICS Quaternary ammonium derivative of scopolamine but lacks scopolamine's CNS actions. Its spasmolytic and antisecretory actions are quantitatively similar to those of atropine, but they last longer. Has greater selectivity in blocking vagal impulses from GI tract than either scopolamine or atropine.

USES Adjunct in treatment of peptic ulcer, irritable bowel syndrome, and a variety of other GI conditions. Also may be used to control excessive sweating and salivation, migraine headaches, and premenstrual cramps.

ROUTE & DOSAGE

Adults　PO　2.5–5 mg 30 min a.c. and h.s.

PHARMACOKINETICS Absorption: erratic after PO administration. **Onset:** approximately 1 h. **Duration:** 4–6 h. **Elimination:** excreted primarily in urine and bile; some unchanged drug excreted in feces.

CONTRAINDICATIONS & PRECAUTIONS Contraindicated in: hypersensitivity to any of the drug's constituents, prostatic hypertrophy, pyloric obstruction, intestinal atony, tachycardia, cardiac disease. Safe use during pregnancy (category C) not established. **Cautious use in:** elderly and debilitated patients.

ADVERSE/SIDE EFFECTS Dry mouth, blurred vision, dizziness, drowsiness, constipation, flushing of skin, urinary hesitancy or retention.

NURSING IMPLICATIONS

Administration
- PO preparation is usually administered 30 min before meals and at bedtime.
- Preserve in tight, light-resistant containers.

Assessment & Drug Effects
- Incidence and severity of side effects are generally dose-related and therefore may be controlled by dosage reduction. Dosage is usually maintained at a level that produces slight dryness of mouth.
- Urinary retention may be an indication for discontinuation of the drug. Report promptly.

Patient & Family Education
- Because methscopolamine may cause dizziness and drowsiness, warn patient not to engage in activities requiring mental alertness, such as driving a car, until response to drug is known. Caution patient to make position changes slowly and in stages.
- Dryness of mouth may be relieved by sugarless chewing gum or candy or by frequent rinsing of mouth with water.

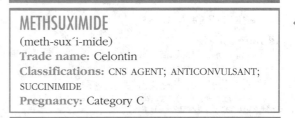

Prototype: ethosuximide, p 174

METHSUXIMIDE
(meth-sux´i-mide)
Trade name: Celontin
Classifications: CNS AGENT; ANTICONVULSANT; SUCCINIMIDE
Pregnancy: Category C

ACTIONS/PHARMACODYNAMICS Succinimide derivative with actions, contraindications, precautions, and adverse reactions similar to those of ethosuximide. Associated with high incidence of adverse effects.

USES Control of absence (petit mal) seizures refractory to other anticonvulsants. May be used in combi-

Common side effects in *italic*; life-threatening effects underlined; generic names in **bold**; classifications in SMALL CAPS

759

nation with other anticonvulsants in mixed types of epilepsy.

ROUTE & DOSAGE

Absence Seizures

Adult	PO	300 mg/d; may increase q4–7d as needed (max 1.2 g/d in divided doses)
Child	PO	Same as for adult

PHARMACOKINETICS Absorption: readily absorbed from GI tract. **Peak:** 1–3 h. **Metabolism:** metabolized in liver. **Elimination:** half-life: 3 h; excreted slowly in urine; small amounts excreted in bile and feces.

CONTRAINDICATIONS & PRECAUTIONS Contraindicated in: hypersensitivity to succinimides; drug allergies; hepatic or renal disease; blood dyscrasias; pregnancy (category C).

ADVERSE/SIDE EFFECTS CNS: *drowsiness, dizziness, ataxia;* headache, insomnia, diplopia, photophobia, severe mental depression, behavioral changes. **GI:** *nausea, vomiting, anorexia, diarrhea, constipation, epigastric* or *abdominal pain, weight loss.* **Hypersensitivity:** skin eruptions, fever, hiccups, periorbital edema and hyperemia, blood dyscrasias including aplastic anemia, SLE. **Other:** renal and hepatic damage.

DRUG INTERACTIONS Carbamazepine decreases methsuximide levels; **isoniazid** significantly increases methsuximide levels; the levels of both **phenobarbital** and methsuximide may be altered, with increased seizure frequency.

NURSING IMPLICATIONS

Administration

- Drug should be taken exactly as prescribed.
- Store capsules away from heat at 15–30C (59–86F) unless otherwise directed.

Assessment & Drug Effects

- Drug tolerance varies among patients. Patient must be closely observed when dosage is increased or decreased or when other medication is being added or eliminated.
- Observe patient closely for behavioral changes. Drug should be withdrawn (slowly) at first appearance of depression, aggression, or other unusual behavioral manifestations to prevent progression to acute psychosis.

- Periodic blood cell counts, tests of liver function, and urinalysis should be performed during therapy.
- Since drug may cause drowsiness, dizziness, and visual disturbances, caution patients to avoid potentially hazardous activities such as driving a car until drug response is known.

Patient & Family Education

- Advise patient to report immediately the onset of adverse effects (often controlled by dosage reduction). Development of a rash may herald more serious reactions.
- Advise patient to report immediately any signs of infection (e.g., sore throat, fever).
- Abrupt drug withdrawal may precipitate petit mal seizures.
- Advise patient to carry identification indicating that he or she has epilepsy and is taking medication.

Prototype: hydrochlorothiazide, p 203

METHYCLOTHIAZIDE

(meth-i-kloe-thye´a-zide)
Trade names: Aquatensen, Duretic, Enduron, Ethon
Classifications: ELECTROLYTIC & WATER BALANCE AGENT; THIAZIDE DIURETIC
Pregnancy: Category C

ACTIONS/PHARMACODYNAMICS Thiazide (benzothiadiazine) diuretic. Similar to hydrochlorothiazide in actions, uses, contraindications, adverse reactions, and interactions.

USES Primary (step 1) agent in stepped care approach to antihypertensive treatment and adjunctively in the management of edema associated with CHF, renal pathology, and hepatic cirrhosis.

ROUTE & DOSAGE

Edema

Adult	PO	2.5–10 mg once/d or 3–5 times/wk

Hypertension

Adult	PO	2.5–10 mg/d
Child	PO	0.05–0.2 mg/kg/d

PHARMACOKINETICS Absorption: incompletely absorbed. **Onset:** 2 h. **Peak:** 6 h. **Duration:** > 24 h.

Common side effects in *italic*; life-threatening effects underlined; generic names in **bold**; classifications in SMALL CAPS

Distribution: distributed throughout extracellular tissue; concentrates in kidney; crosses placenta; distributed in breast milk. **Metabolism:** does not appear to be metabolized. **Elimination:** excreted in urine.

CONTRAINDICATIONS & PRECAUTIONS Contraindicated in: hypersensitivity to thiazides, sulfonamide derivatives; anuria, hypokalemia, pregnancy (category C), nursing mothers. **Cautious use in:** impaired renal or hepatic function, gout, SLE, hypercalcemia, diabetes mellitus.

ADVERSE/SIDE EFFECTS Postural hypotension, sialadenitis, unusual fatigue, dizziness, paresthesias, photosensitivity, yellow vision, *hypokalemia,* agranulocytosis.

DRUG INTERACTIONS Amphotericin B, CORTICOSTEROIDS increase hypokalemic effects; may antagonize hypoglycemic effects of **insulin,** SULFONYLUREAS; **cholestyramine, colestipol** decrease thiazide absorption; intensifies hypoglycemic and hypotensive effects of **diazoxide;** increased potassium and magnesium loss may cause **digoxin** toxicity; decreases **lithium** excretion, increasing its toxicity; NSAIDS may attenuate diuresis, and risk of NSAID-induced renal failure increased.

NURSING IMPLICATIONS

Administration

- Administer drug early in AM after eating (to reduce gastric irritation) to prevent sleep interruption because of diuresis. If 2 doses are ordered, administer second dose no later than 3 PM.
- Store drug at 15–30C (59–86F) unless otherwise instructed.

Assessment & Drug Effects

- Antihypertensive effects may be noted in 3–4 d; maximal effects may require 3–4 wk.
- Monitor BP and I&O ratio during first phase of antihypertensive therapy. Report a sudden fall in BP, which may initiate severe postural hypotension and potentially dangerous perfusion problems, especially in the extremities.
- Monitor patient for signs of hypokalemia (see chap 3). Report promptly. Physician may change dose and institute replacement therapy.

Patient & Family Education

- Hypokalemia is rarely severe in most patients even on long-term therapy with thiazides if they eat a balanced diet. To prevent onset, urge patient to eat potassium-rich foods (potatoes, whole grain cereals, beef, fruit juices, skim milk) and to include a banana (about 370 mg potassium) and at least 180 ml (6 oz) orange juice (about 330 mg potassium) every day.

- The diabetic patient should be watched carefully for loss of diabetes control or early signs of hyperglycemia (see chap 3). The symptoms are slow to develop.
- Counsel patient to avoid use of OTC drugs unless they are approved by the physician. Many preparations contain both potassium and sodium, and electrolyte imbalance side effects may be induced.
- The elderly are more responsive to excessive diuresis; advise them that orthostatic hypotension may be a problem.
- Instruct patient with orthostatic hypotension to change from recumbency to upright positions slowly and in stages; to avoid hot baths or showers, extended exposure to sunlight, and standing still. Provide assistance as necessary to prevent falling.
- Advise patient to avoid driving a vehicle or working with dangerous equipment until adjustment to the hypotensive effects of this drug has been made.

Prototype: aspirin, p 161

METHYL SALICYLATE

Nonproprietary names: betula oil, gaultheria oil, oil of wintergreen, sweet birch oil
Classifications: SKIN AGENT; CNS AGENT; NONNARCOTIC ANALGESIC; SALICYLATE

ACTIONS/PHARMACODYNAMICS Relieves pain in muscles and joints by increasing cutaneous blood flow, thereby producing sensation of warmth and comfort. It is thought that systemic analgesic effects and toxicity can occur from local absorption.

USES Applied topically to provide temporary symptomatic relief of minor discomforts of osteoarthritis, rheumatoid arthritis, and low back pain.

ROUTE & DOSAGE

Minor Arthritis or Muscle Pain

Adult	Topical	Applied as ointment or liniment by gentle massage several times/d

---

Common side effects in *italic*; life-threatening effects <u>underlined</u>; generic names in **bold**; classifications in SMALL CAPS

761

ADVERSE/SIDE EFFECTS *Redness, rash, burning sensation,* blistering. Systemic poisoning: salicylism.

NURSING IMPLICATIONS

Patient & Family Education

- Avoid getting medication into eyes or on mucous membranes, open wounds, irritated or broken skin. Do not apply to large areas of the body.
- Do not bandage or apply heat to affected part.
- Wash hand thoroughly with soap and water after applying medication.
- Discontinue medication if excessive redness or irritation develops.
- Methyl salicylate is a common ingredient in many external analgesic preparations (e.g., Ben Gay, Heet, Musterole, Sloan's Liniment).

Prototype: psyllium hydrophilic muciloid, p 219

METHYLCELLULOSE

(meth-ill-sell´yoo-lose)
Trade names: Citrucel, Cologel, Maltsupex; artificial tears: Isopto, Moisture Drops, Tears Naturale
Classifications: GI AGENT; BULK LAXATIVE; EYE PREPARATION
Pregnancy: Category C

ACTIONS/PHARMACODYNAMICS Hydrophilic semisynthetic cellulose derivative. PO preparation swells on contact with water to form a demulcent nonabsorbable gel that facilitates passage of stool and reflexly stimulates peristalsis. Ophthalmic preparations (artificial tears) are sterile, viscous, water-soluble, nongreasy lubricant combinations of methylcellulose with buffers and preservatives.

USES Orally as adjunct in treatment of chronic constipation. Also in ophthalmic preparations for relief of dry eyes and eye irritation associated with deficient tear production, for corneal exposure from half-open eye during coma, and as ocular lubricant for artificial eyes and contact lenses.

CONTRAINDICATIONS & PRECAUTIONS Contraindicated in: nausea, vomiting, abdominal pain, intestinal obstruction, ulceration or stenosis, diarrhea; pregnancy (category C).

ROUTE & DOSAGE

Constipation

Adult	PO	5–20 ml t.i.d.
Child	PO	5–10 ml 1–2 times/d

Artificial Tears

Adult	Ophthalmic	1–2 drops in eye t.i.d. or q.i.d. prn

ADVERSE/SIDE EFFECTS PO: *diarrhea,* nausea, vomiting, fecal impaction, esophageal obstruction.

NURSING IMPLICATIONS

Administration

- Each PO dose should be taken with 1 or more glasses of water; additional fluids should be taken during the day. Fecal impaction can occur if fluid intake by mouth is insufficient.

Patient & Family Education

- Caution patient not to chew the tablet form because it may start to swell in the esophagus and cause obstruction.
- Laxation generally occurs in 12–24 h; however, some patients may require 2–3 d of medication.
- Advise patient to discontinue use of ophthalmic preparation if eye discomfort or irritation occurs and to report to physician.

METHYLDOPA

See CARDIOVASCULAR AGENTS, CENTRAL ACTING ANTIHYPERTENSIVE prototype, p 148.

METHYLENE BLUE

(meth´i-leen)
Trade name: Urolene Blue
Classifications: ANTIDOTE; DIAGNOSTIC AGENT
Pregnancy: Category C

ACTIONS/PHARMACODYNAMICS Mildly antiseptic dye with oxidation-reduction action and tissue-staining property. In relatively high concentrations, it oxidizes ferrous iron of reduced hemoglobin to the ferric form, thus producing methemoglobin, which complexes with cyanide. In contrast, low concentrations act as catalytic intermediary electron ac-

Common side effects in *italic*; life-threatening effects underlined; generic names in **bold**; classifications in SMALL CAPS

ceptor in conversion of methemoglobin to hemoglobin. Prolonged administration accelerates destruction of erythrocytes.

USES Idiopathic and drug-induced methemoglobinemia; as antidote for cyanide poisoning; as diagnostic agent, indicator dye, and for medical and surgical marking. Also oxalate phosphate urinary tract calculi. **Unlabeled uses:** cutaneous viral infections; diagnosis of gastroesophageal reflux in pediatrics.

ROUTE & DOSAGE

Urolithiasis

Adult   PO   65–130 mg b.i.d. or t.i.d. p.c.

Methhemoglobinemia, Cyanide Poisoning

Adult   IV   1–2 mg/kg of 1% solution injected slowly over several minutes

PHARMACOKINETICS Absorption: readily absorbed from GI tract. **Metabolism:** rapidly reduced in tissues to the metabolite leukomethylene blue. **Elimination:** excreted slowly in urine; some excretion in bile and feces.

CONTRAINDICATIONS & PRECAUTIONS Contraindicated in: history of allergy to methylene blue, renal insufficiency. Safe use during pregnancy (category C) not established. Methylene blue is ineffective in patients with G6PD deficiency, intrathecal injection.

ADVERSE/SIDE EFFECTS Bladder irritation, nausea, vomiting, diarrhea, abdominal pain, hemolysis (patients with G6PD deficiency). Large IV doses: fever, profuse sweating, precordial pain, methemoglobinemia, cardiovascular abnormalities. *With continued administration: marked anemia.*

DIAGNOSTIC TEST INTERFERENCES Methylene blue may interfere with tests for ***urinary pH.***

NURSING IMPLICATIONS

Administration

- Should be administered after meals with full glass of water.

Assessment & Drug Effects

- Since continued administration may cause marked anemia, frequent hemoglobin determinations are advised.

Patient & Family Education

- Encourage fluid intake to at least 2000 ml/d.
- Inform patients that drug may impart blue-green color to urine and feces.

Prototype: ergotamine, p 112

METHYLERGONOVINE MALEATE

(meth-ill-er-goe-noe´veen)

Trade name: Methergine

Classifications: AUTONOMIC NERVOUS SYSTEM AGENT; ADRENERGIC ANTAGONIST (SYMPATHOLYTIC); ERGOT ALKALOID; OXYTOCIC

ACTIONS/PHARMACODYNAMICS Ergot alkaloid that induces rapid, sustained titanic uterine contraction that shortens third stage of labor and reduces blood loss. Has minimal vasoconstrictive activity. See ergonovine maleate (p. 563) for contraindications and precautions and adverse/side effects.

USES Routine management after delivery of placenta and for postpartum atony, subinvolution, and hemorrhage. With full obstetric supervision, may be used during second stage of labor.

ROUTE & DOSAGE

Postpartum Hemorrhage

Adult   PO   0.2–0.4 mg q6–12h until danger of atony passes (2–7 d)

       IM/IV   0.2 mg q2–4h up to a max of 5 doses

PHARMACOKINETICS Absorption: readily absorbed from GI tract. **Onset:** 5–15 min PO; 2–5 min IM; immediate IV. **Duration:** 3 or more h PO; 3 h IM; 45 min IV. **Distribution:** distributed into breast milk. **Metabolism:** slowly metabolized in liver. **Elimination:** half-life: 0.5–2 h; excreted mainly in feces, small amount in urine.

DRUG INTERACTIONS PARENTERAL SYMPATHOMIMETICS, other ERGOT ALKALOIDS add to pressor effects and carry risk of hypertension.

NURSING IMPLICATIONS

Administration

- IV methylergonovine may be given by direct IV undiluted at a rate of 0.2 mg over 60 seconds.

M

Common side effects in *italic*; life-threatening effects <u>underlined</u>; generic names in **bold**; classifications in SMALL CAPS

763

- Ampules containing discolored solution or visible particles should not be used. Store at 15–30C (59–86F) unless otherwise directed. Protect from light.

Assessment & Drug Effects

- Monitor vital signs (particularly BP) and uterine response during and after parenteral administration of methylergonovine until partum period is stabilized (about 1–2 h).
- Notify physician if BP suddenly increases or if there are frequent periods of uterine relaxation.

Prototype: amphetamine, p 194

METHYLPHENIDATE HYDROCHLORIDE

(meth-ill-fen´i-date)
Trade names: Methidate, Ritalin, Ritalin-SR
Classification: CNS AGENT; RESPIRATORY AND CEREBRAL STIMULANT
Pregnancy: Category C
Controlled substance: Schedule II

ACTIONS/PHARMACODYNAMICS Piperidine derivative with pharmacologic actions and abuse potential qualitatively similar to those of amphetamine. Acts mainly on cerebral cortex. Exerts mild CNS and respiratory stimulation analeptic effect with potency intermediate between those of amphetamine and caffeine. Effects more prominent on mental than on motor activities. Also believed to have an anorexiant effect.

USES Adjunctive therapy in hyperkinetic syndromes characterized by attention deficit disorders (ADD), narcolepsy, mild depression, and apathetic or withdrawn senile behavior.

ROUTE & DOSAGE

Narcolepsy

Adult	PO	10 mg b.i.d. or t.i.d. 30–45 min p.c. (range 20–40 mg/d)

Attention Deficit Disorder

Child	PO	5–10 mg before breakfast and lunch, with a gradual increase of 5–10 mg/wk as needed (max 60 mg/d)

PHARMACOKINETICS Absorption: readily absorbed from GI tract. **Peak:** 1.9 h; 4–7 h extended release. **Duration:** 3–6 h; 8 h extended release. **Elimination:** excreted in urine.

CONTRAINDICATIONS & PRECAUTIONS Contraindicated in: hypersensitivity to drug; history of marked anxiety, agitation; motor tics, or Tourette's disease. Safe use in pregnancy (category C), by nursing mothers or children < 6 y of age not established. **Cautious use in:** the alcoholic; the emotionally unstable patient; history of drug dependence; hypertension; history of seizures.

ADVERSE/SIDE EFFECTS CNS: dizziness, drowsiness, *nervousness, insomnia.* **CV:** palpitations, changes in BP and pulse rate, angina, cardiac arrhythmias. **Eye:** difficulty with accommodation, blurred vision. **GI:** dry throat, anorexia, nausea; <u>hepatotoxicity</u>; abdominal pain. **Other:** hypersensitivity reactions (rash, fever, arthralgia, urticaria, <u>exfoliative dermatitis</u>, erythema multiforme); growth suppression.

DRUG INTERACTIONS MAO INHIBITORS may cause hypertensive crisis; antagonizes hypotensive effects of **guanethidine, bretylium.**

NURSING IMPLICATIONS

Administration

- Administer 30–45 min before meals. To avoid insomnia, last dose should be taken before 6 PM.
- *Sustained release tablets:* swallow whole; do not crush.
- Store at 15–30C (59–86F).

Assessment & Drug Effects

- BP and pulse should be monitored at appropriate intervals.
- Periodic CBC and differential and platelet counts are advised during prolonged therapy.
- Chronic abusive use can lead to tolerance, psychic dependence, and psychoses.
- Drug therapy in children should not be indefinite. If improvement is not observed after 1 mo, drug should be discontinued. During prolonged therapy, periodic drug-free periods are recommended to assess the child's condition.
- Careful supervision is required for drug withdrawal following prolonged use. Abrupt withdrawal may result in severe depression and psychotic behavior.

Patient & Family Education

- Nervousness and insomnia may diminish with time or require reduction of dosage or omission of af-

Common side effects in *italic*; life-threatening effects <u>underlined</u>; generic names in **bold**; classifications in SMALL CAPS

M

ternoon or evening dose. Advise patients to report these and other adverse effects.
- Advise patients to check weight at least 2 or 3 times weekly and to report weight loss. Height and weight should be checked in children, and failure to gain in either should be reported.

Prototype: prednisone, p 225

METHYLPREDNISOLONE
(meth-ill-pred-niss´oh-lone)
Trade name: Medrol

METHYLPREDNISOLONE ACETATE
Trade names: depMedalone, Depoject, Depo-Medrol, Depopred, Duralone, Med-Depo, Medralone, Medrone, M-Prednisol, Pre-Dep, Rep-Pred

METHYLPREDNISOLONE SODIUM SUCCINATE
Trade names: A-MethaPred, Solu-Medrol
Classifications: SYNTHETIC HORMONE; ADRENAL CORTICOSTEROID; GLUCOCORTICOID; ANTIINFLAMMATORY
Pregnancy: Category C

ACTIONS/PHARMACODYNAMICS Intermediate acting synthetic adrenal corticosteroid with similar glucocorticoid activity but considerably less sodium and water retention effects than those of hydrocortisone. On weight basis, 4 mg methylprednisolone is equivalent to 20 mg hydrocortisone and 5 mg prednisone. Acetate has longer duration of action and more rapid onset of activity than parent compound. Sodium succinate is characterized by rapid onset of action and is used for emergency therapy of short duration.

USES An antiinflammatory agent in the management of acute and chronic inflammatory diseases, for palliative management of neoplastic diseases, and for control of severe acute and chronic allergic processes. High dose, short-term therapy: management of acute bronchial asthma, prevention of fat embolism in patient with long-bone fracture. **Unlabeled uses:** acetate form used as a long-acting contraceptive and for spinal cord injury, lupus nephritis, multiple sclerosis.

ROUTE & DOSAGE

Inflammation

Adult	PO	2–60 mg/d in 1 or more divided doses
	IM	Acetate: 4–80 mg/wk for 1–4 wk
		Succinate: 10–250 mg q6h
	IV	10–250 mg q6h

Acute Spinal Cord Injury

Adult	IV	30 mg/kg over 15 min, followed in 45 min by 5.4 mg/kg/h × 23 h

PHARMACOKINETICS Absorption: readily absorbed from GI tract. **Peak:** 1–2 h PO; 4–8 d IM. **Duration:** 1.25–1.5 d PO; 1–5 wk IM. **Metabolism:** metabolized in liver. **Elimination:** half-life: > 3.5 h; HPA suppression: 18–36 h.

CONTRAINDICATIONS & PRECAUTIONS Contraindicated in: systemic fungal infections. Safe use by children and during pregnancy (category C) and lactation not established. **Cautious use in:** Cushing's syndrome; GI ulceration; hypertension; varicella, vaccinia; diabetes mellitus; emotional instability or psychotic tendencies.

ADVERSE/SIDE EFFECTS Severe hypokalemia, CHF, euphoria, insomnia, delayed wound healing, edema, leukocytosis, psychosis, confusion, osteoporosis.

DRUG INTERACTIONS Amphotericin B, furosemide, THIAZIDE DIURETICS increase potassium loss; with ATTENUATED VIRUS VACCINES, may enhance virus replication or increase vaccine side effects; **isoniazid, phenytoin, phenobarbital, rifampin** decrease effectiveness of methylprednisolone because they increase metabolism of steroids.

INCOMPATIBILITIES Solution/Additive: calcium gluconate, glycopyrrolate, metaraminol, nafcillin, penicillin G sodium, doxapram.

NURSING IMPLICATIONS

Administration
- Tablet may be crushed before administration and taken with fluid of patient's choice.
- The oral preparation will be less irritating if given with food.
- Alternate day therapy may be used when methylprednisolone is given over long period of time.
- Provided in Mix-O-Vial from which solution is

M

Common side effects in *italic*; life-threatening effects underlined; generic names in **bold**; classifications in SMALL CAPS

765

withdrawn and given by direct IV at a rate of 500 mg or fraction thereof over 60 seconds or longer.

- Methylprednisolone sodium succinate solution should be used within 48 h after preparation.
- Avoid contacting eyes with the ointment.
- Store at 15–30C (59–86F). Prevent freezing.

Assessment & Drug Effects

- Monitor urine for glucosuria. The diabetic may require increased doses of insulin or sulfonylurea.
- Monitor for and report signs and symptoms of hypokalemia (see chap 3).
- Monitor for and report signs and symptoms of Cushing's syndrome (see chap 3).

Patient & Family Education

- Instruct patient not to alter established dosage regimen (i.e., not to increase, decrease, or omit doses or change dose intervals). Withdrawal symptoms (rebound inflammation, fever) can be induced with sudden discontinuation of therapy.
- Instruct patient to report immediately onset of signs of hypocorticism adrenal insufficiency: fatigue, nausea, anorexia, joint pain, muscular weakness, dizziness, fever.

Prototype: testosterone, p 229

METHYLTESTOSTERONE

(meth-ill-tess-toss´te-rone)

Trade names: Android, Metandren, Oreton-Methyl, Testred, Virilon

Classifications: HORMONE; ANDROGEN/ANABOLIC STEROID

Pregnancy: Category X

Controlled substance: Schedule III

ACTIONS/PHARMACODYNAMICS Orally effective, short-acting steroid with androgen/anabolic activity ratio (1:1) similar to that of testosterone but less effective than its esters. Fails to produce full sexual maturation when administered to preadolescent male with complete testicular failure unless preceded by testosterone therapy.

USES Androgen replacement therapy, delayed puberty (male), palliation of female mammary cancer (1–5 y postmenopausal), postpartum breast engorgement.

ROUTE & DOSAGE

Replacement

Adult	PO	10–50 mg/d in divided doses

Breast Cancer

Adult	PO	50–200 mg/d in divided doses for duration of therapeutic response or no longer than 3 mo if no remission

Postpartum Breast Engorgement

Adult	PO	80 mg/d for 3–5 d

PHARMACOKINETICS Absorption: readily absorbed from GI tract. **Metabolism:** metabolized in liver. **Elimination:** excreted in urine.

CONTRAINDICATIONS & PRECAUTIONS Contraindicated in: hepatic dysfunction; pregnancy (category X); prostate cancer. **Cautious use in:** hepatic, renal, or cardiac dysfunction.

ADVERSE/SIDE EFFECTS <u>Cholestatic hepatitis with jaundice</u>, renal calculi (especially in immobilized patient), irritation of oral mucosa with buccal administration, *acne, gynecomastia, edema,* oligospermia, priapism, menstrual irregularities.

DRUG INTERACTIONS Increases risk of bleeding associated with ORAL ANTICOAGULANTS; possibly increases risk of **cyclosporine** toxicity; may decrease glucose level, making adjustment of doses of **insulin,** SULFONYLUREAS necessary.

NURSING IMPLICATIONS

Administration

- *Buccal tablet:* should be placed in upper or lower buccal pouch between cheek and gum. Instruct patient not to chew or swallow tablet and to avoid eating, drinking, or smoking until absorption is complete. Tablet requires 30–60 min to dissolve. Change location of absorption site with each dose.
- Store drug at 15–30C (59–86F). Avoid freezing.

Assessment & Drug Effects

- Monitor hepatic function periodically; report signs of hepatic toxicity (see chap 3).
- Monitor for flank pain, abdominal pain radiating to groin, or other symptoms of renal calculi.

Patient & Family Education

- Good oral hygiene should be stressed as a means to decrease infection of cheek membranes irritated by buccal formulation.

Common side effects in *italic*; life-threatening effects <u>underlined</u>; generic names in **bold**; classifications in SMALL CAPS

M

- Instruct patient to report inflamed or painful oral membranes. In addition to physical discomfort, absorption rate is changed by altered mucosal surface.
- Since dosage sufficient to produce remission in breast cancer is quantitatively similar to that used for androgen replacement in the male, women should be prepared for distressing and undesirable side effects of virilization.
- Advise women to report promptly if signs of virilism appear. Voice change and hirsutism may be irreversible, even after drug is withdrawn.
- Instruct men to report priapism or other signs of excess sexual stimulation. The physician will terminate methyltestosterone therapy.
- Jaundice with or without pruritus appears to be dose related. Instruct patient to report symptoms to physician. If liver function tests are altered at the same time, this drug will be withdrawn.

Prototype: secobarbital, p 175

METHYPRYLON

(meth-i-prye´lon)
Trade name: Noludar
Classification: CNS AGENT; HYPNOTIC
Pregnancy: Category B
Controlled substance: Schedule III

ACTIONS/PHARMACODYNAMICS Piperidine derivative structurally related to glutethimide. Produces CNS depressant effects similar to those of short-acting barbiturates. Hypnotic doses suppress REM sleep.

USES Hypnotic for relief of simple insomnia. Sometimes used as sedative, but value for this purpose not established.

ROUTE & DOSAGE

Hypnotic

Adult	PO	200–400 mg 15 min before retiring
Adolescent	PO	> 12 y: 50–200 mg h.s.

PHARMACOKINETICS Absorption: readily absorbed from GI tract. **Onset:** 45–60 min. **Peak:** 1 h. **Duration:** 5–8 h. **Metabolism:** metabolized in liver; some enterohepatic circulation. **Elimination:** half-life: 3–6 h; excreted in urine.

CONTRAINDICATIONS & PRECAUTIONS Contraindicated in: porphyria; known hypersensitivity to methyprylon; patient who is hallucinating or who is psychotic. Safe use during pregnancy (category B) and in nursing mothers and children < 12 y not established. **Cautious use in:** hepatic or renal impairment, addiction-prone individuals, mental depression, history of suicidal tendencies.

ADVERSE/SIDE EFFECTS *Morning drowsiness,* dizziness, nausea, vomiting, diarrhea, esophagitis, headache, paradoxic excitation, skin rash, exacerbation of intermittent porphyria. Reported, but causal relationship not established: neutropenia, thrombocytopenia. **Acute toxicity:** somnolence, confusion, constricted pupils, hyperpyrexia, hypothermia, shock, pulmonary edema, respiratory depression; occasionally during recovery: excitation, convulsions, delirium, hallucinations.

DIAGNOSTIC TEST INTERFERENCES Methyprylon may interfere with ***urinary steroid*** determinations.

DRUG INTERACTIONS Alcohol and other CNS DEPRESSANTS add to CNS depression.

NURSING IMPLICATIONS

Administration

- Hypnotic dose is administered 15 min before patient retires. Prepare patient for sleep before administering drug.
- Preserve in tightly closed, light-resistant containers.

Assessment & Drug Effects

- In some patients, suppression of REM sleep may cause irritability, tension, confusion, and tremors.
- Although tolerance develops to suppression of REM sleep, during chronic administration, REM rebound may occur when drug is withdrawn: increased dreaming, nightmares, insomnia, hallucinations.
- Tolerance may develop to hypnotic and sedative effects but not to toxic effects.
- Psychologic and physical dependence may occur, especially after prolonged use of large doses. Patient's continued need for methyprylon should be evaluated regularly.
- Periodic blood counts are advised if drug is used repeatedly or over prolonged periods.

Patient & Family Education

- Warn patient about possible additive effects with alcohol and other CNS depressants.

M

Common side effects in *italic*; life-threatening effects underlined; generic names in **bold**; classifications in SMALL CAPS

767

- Caution patient to avoid driving a car or engaging in other activities requiring mental alertness until response to drug is known.
- Gradual drug withdrawal is advised after prolonged use. Sudden discontinuation may result in *withdrawal symptoms:* confusion, marked nervousness, insomnia, sweating, polyuria, hyperreflexia, delirium, miosis, hallucinations, convulsion, death.

Prototype: ergotamine, p 112

METHYSERGIDE

(meth-i-ser´jide)
Trade name: Sansert
Classifications: AUTONOMIC NERVOUS SYSTEM AGENT; ERGOT ALKALOID
Pregnancy: Category C

ACTIONS/PHARMACODYNAMICS Ergot derivative and congener of LSD. Unlike ergotamine, has weak vasoconstrictor and oxytoxic actions. Action mechanism in migraine prevention unclear. Serotonin (a strong vasoconstrictor) levels are reduced during an attack. Methysergide replaces serotonin on cranial artery receptor sites during an attack, thereby preserving vasoconstriction afforded by serotonin. Ineffective treatment of acute attacks. Prolonged use has been known to promote fibrotic processes.

USES Prophylactic management of severe recurrent migraine, cluster, and other vascular headaches unresponsive to other antimigraine drugs. **Unlabeled uses:** diarrhea and malabsorption associated with GI hypermotility in carcinoid disease; postgastrectomy dumping syndrome.

ROUTE & DOSAGE

Headache Prophylaxis
Adult   PO   4–8 mg/d in divided doses with meals; should not be administered continuously for > 6 mo; a drug-free interval of 3–4 wk must follow each 6 mo course

Diarrhea Associated with Carcinoid Disease
Adult   PO   2–16 mg t.i.d.

PHARMACOKINETICS Absorption: readily absorbed from GI tract. **Distribution:** widely distributed, including into breast milk. **Metabolism:** metabolized in liver. **Elimination:** half-life: 10 h; excreted in urine.

CONTRAINDICATIONS & PRECAUTIONS Contraindicated in: fibrotic processes; pulmonary or collagen diseases; edema; serious infections; debilitated states. Pregnancy (category C), severe peripheral vascular disease, severe hypertension, severe arteriosclerosis, phlebitis or cellulitis of lower limbs, impaired liver or renal function.

ADVERSE/SIDE EFFECTS CNS: *insomnia,* drowsiness, vertigo, mild euphoria, confusion, excitement, feelings of unreality or depersonalization, distortions of body image, depression, anxiety, hallucinations, nightmares, ataxia, hyperesthesia, paresthesia. **CV:** peripheral edema, thrombophlebitis, claudication, impaired circulation, angina of effort, ECG changes, *postural hypotension,* tachycardia. **Fibrotic complications:** retroperitoneal fibrosis (fatigue, malaise, fever, urinary obstruction with girdle or flank pain, dysuria, oliguria, polyuria, increased BUN and sedimentation rate), pleuropulmonary fibrosis (dyspnea, chest pain and tightness, pleural friction rubs and effusion) and cardiac fibrosis (fibrotic thickening of cardiac valves with murmurs). **GI:** *nausea, vomiting, heartburn,* hyperchlorhydria, *abdominal pain, diarrhea,* constipation. **Skin:** facial flushing, telangiectasia, rash, excessive hair loss. **Other:** neutropenia, eosinophilia, weakness, arthralgia, myalgia, weight gain, scotomas, nasal stuffiness, positive direct Coombs' test.

NURSING IMPLICATIONS

Administration

- GI side effects can frequently be prevented by gradual introduction of medication and by administering drug with meals.
- Continuous administration of methysergide should not exceed 6 mo without a medication-free interval of 3–4 wk.
- Preserve in tight, light-resistant containers at 15–30C (59–86F) unless otherwise directed.

Assessment & Drug Effects

- One or 2 d of drug therapy are required before protective drug action is realized; at end of therapy, protection continues 2 d beyond last dose.
- Therapeutic trial period of 3 wk is advised to determine patient's response to methysergide. If no response occurs in this time, it is unlikely that longer administration will be of benefit.
- Pretreatment and periodic assessments of cardiac status, renal function, blood count, and sedimentation rate are advised.
- Since incidence of side effects is relatively high (usually reversible with discontinuation of drug),

M

Common side effects in *italic*; life-threatening effects <u>underlined</u>; generic names in **bold**; classifications in SMALL CAPS

patient should be examined regularly for fibrotic and vascular complications: auscultate heart and lungs; check peripheral pulses, and auscultate major vessels for bruits; observe for signs of phlebitis or venous obstruction. Also, question patient concerning presence of CNS symptoms and other adverse effects.

Patient & Family Education

- Instruct patient to report the following immediately: onset of abdominal, back, or chest pain; dyspnea; leg pains while walking; cold, numb, or painful extremities; fever; dysuria or other urinary problems; edema; weight gain.
- Counsel patient to weigh self daily and teach patient how to check extremities for edema.
- Caloric restriction and reduction of salt intake may be prescribed. Consult physician and instruct patient accordingly.
- Advise patient to make position changes slowly, particularly from recumbent to upright posture, and to dangle legs a few minutes before standing. Also instruct patient to lie down if faintness occurs.
- To avoid "headache rebound," drug should be withdrawn gradually over 2- or 3-wk period.
- Patients with migraine should be helped to identify underlying emotional and physical stresses that may precipitate attacks.

Prototype: bethanechol, p 120

METOCLOPRAMIDE HYDROCHLORIDE

(met-oh-kloe-pra´mide)

Trade names: Clopra, Emex, Maxeran, Maxolon, Octamide, Reclomide, Reglan
Classifications: AUTONOMIC NERVOUS SYSTEM AGENT; DIRECT-ACTING CHOLINERGIC (PARASYMPATHOMIMETIC); GI AGENT; ANTIEMETIC
Pregnancy: Category B

ACTIONS/PHARMACODYNAMICS Potent central dopamine receptor antagonist. Structurally related to procainamide but has little antiarrhythmic or anesthetic activity. Exact mechanism of action not clear but appears to sensitize GI smooth muscle to effects of acetylcholine by direct action. Increases resting tone of esophageal sphincter (thereby increasing lower esophageal sphincter pressure) and increases tone and amplitude of upper GI contractions. As a result, gastric emptying and intestinal transit are accel-

erated with little effect if any on gastric, biliary, or pancreatic secretions. Antiemetic action results from drug-induced elevation of CTZ threshold and enhanced gastric emptying (which blocks the gastric stasis that precedes vomiting). Has no apparent effect on seizure threshold. Inhibits central and peripheral effects of apomorphine and indirectly stimulates release of prolactin. Directly stimulates secretion of aldosterone but has no effect on plasma renin activity or plasma potassium or cortisol concentrations. High doses produce neuroleptic actions similar to those of antipsychotic agents (e.g., phenothiazines). Metoclopramide actions can be reduced or abolished by anticholinergics. Mutagenicity and carcinogenicity potential not known.

USES Management of diabetic gastric stasis (gastroparesis); to prevent nausea and vomiting associated with emetogenic cancer chemotherapy (e.g., cisplatin, dacarbazine); to facilitate intubation of small bowel; symptomatic treatment of gastroesophageal reflux.

ROUTE & DOSAGE

Gastroesophageal Reflux

Adult	PO	10–15 mg q.i.d. a.c. and h.s.

Diabetic Gastroparesis

Adult	PO	10 mg q.i.d. a.c. and h.s. for 2–8 wk

Small-bowel Intubation, Radiologic Examination

Adult	IM/IV	10 mg administered over 1–2 min
Child	IM/IV	6–14 y: 2.5–5 mg over 1–2 min
	IM/IV	< 6 y: 0.1 mg/kg over 1–2 min

Chemotherapy-induced Emesis

Adult	PO	2 mg/kg 1 h before antineoplastic administration; may repeat q2h for 3 more doses if needed
	IM/IV	2 mg/kg 30 min before antineoplastic administration; may repeat q2h for 2 doses, then q3h for 3 doses if needed

PHARMACOKINETICS Absorption: readily absorbed from GI tract. **Onset:** 30–60 min PO; 10–15 min IM; 1–3 min IV. **Peak:** 1–2 h. **Duration:** 1–3 h. **Distribution:** distributed to most body tissues including CNS; crosses placenta; distributed into breast milk. **Metabolism:** minimally metabolized in liver. **Elimination:** half-life: 2.5–6 h; 95% excreted in urine, 5% in feces.

CONTRAINDICATIONS & PRECAUTIONS Contraindicated in: sensitivity or intolerance to metoclo-

M

Common side effects in *italic*; life-threatening effects underlined; generic names in **bold**; classifications in SMALL CAPS

769

pramide; allergy to sulfiting agents; history of seizure disorders; concurrent use of drugs that can cause extrapyramidal symptoms; pheochromocytoma; mechanical GI obstruction or perforation; history of breast cancer. Safe use during pregnancy (category B), and in nursing mothers not established. **Cautious use in:** CHF, hypokalemia; renal dysfunction; GI hemorrhage; history of intermittent porphyria.

ADVERSE/SIDE EFFECTS CNS: *mild sedation* (50% of patients), *fatigue, restlessness,* agitation, headache, insomnia, disorientation, *extrapyramidal symptoms* (acute dystonic type). **CV (rare):** hypotension, supraventricular tachycardia, hypertensive crisis. **GI:** nausea, constipation, *diarrhea,* dry mouth. **Other:** urticarial or maculopapular rash, glossal or periorbital edema, methemoglobinemia, galactorrhea, gynecomastia, amenorrhea, impotence, altered drug absorption.

DIAGNOSTIC TEST INTERFERENCES Metoclopramide may interfere with gonadorelin test by increasing *serum prolactin* levels.

DRUG INTERACTIONS Alcohol and other CNS DEPRESSANTS add to sedation; ANTICHOLINERGICS, OPIATE ANALGESICS may antagonize effect on GI motility; PHENOTHIAZINES may potentiate extrapyramidal symptoms.

INCOMPATIBILITIES Solution/Additive: cisplatin, erythromycin, TETRACYCLINES, **ampicillin, calcium gluconate, cephalothin, chloramphenicol, furosemide, methotrexate, penicillin G potassium, sodium bicarbonate. Y-Site: furosemide.**

NURSING IMPLICATIONS

Administration

- Oral form is usually taken 30 min before meals and at bedtime.
- Each milliliter of the injection form contains about 0.14 mEq of sodium (sodium bisulfite and NaCl). For cancer drug–induced emesis, doses > 10 mg IV should be diluted in 50 ml of compatible parenteral solution and administered over 15 min. Doses of 10 mg or less may be given undiluted by direct IV over 1–2 min.
- Bags of metoclopramide should be protected from light during IV infusion (use of aluminum foil or a thick cotton cover).
- Discard open ampules; do not store for future use.
- The injection form contains sodium metabisulfite as antioxidant. If patient has history of allergy to sul-

fiting agents, this product should be avoided.
- Store in light-resistant bottle at 15–30C (59–86F). Tablets are stable for 3 y; solutions and injections, for 5 y.

Assessment & Drug Effects

- Extrapyramidal symptoms are most likely to occur in children, young adults and the elderly and with high-dose treatment of vomiting associated with cancer chemotherapy. Symptoms can take months to regress. Report immediately the onset of restlessness, involuntary movements, facial grimacing, rigidity, or tremors.
- Therapeutic effectiveness in patient with diabetic gastroparesis is indicated by relief of anorexia, nausea, vomiting, persistent fullness after meals.
- During early treatment period, serum aldosterone may be elevated; however, after prolonged administration periods, it returns to pretreatment level.
- Monitor for possible hypernatremia and hypokalemia (see Signs & Symptoms, chap 3), especially if patient has CHF or cirrhosis.
- Adverse reactions associated with increased serum prolactin concentration (galactorrhea, menstrual disorders, gynecomastia) usually disappear within a few weeks or months after drug treatment is stopped.

Patient & Family Education

- Caution patients to avoid driving and other potentially hazardous activities for a few hours after drug administration.
- Instruct patient to report signs of acute dystonia (see chap 3) immediately.

Prototype: tubocurarine, p 124

METOCURINE IODIDE
(met-oh-kyoo´reen)
Trade name: Metubine Iodide
Classifications: AUTONOMIC NERVOUS SYSTEM AGENT; NONDEPOLARIZING SKELETAL MUSCLE RELAXANT
Pregnancy: Category C

ACTIONS/PHARMACODYNAMICS Semisynthetic nondepolarizing neuromuscular blocking agent. Pharmacologic effects almost identical to those of tubocurarine but is reportedly 2–3 times more potent. Has a slightly shorter duration of action, less histamine-releasing effect, and produces less ganglionic blockade.

USES Adjunct to anesthesia to induce skeletal muscle relaxation. Has been used to reduce intensity of skeletal muscle contractions in drug- or electrically induced convulsions and to facilitate endotracheal intubation.

ROUTE & DOSAGE

Adjunct to General Anesthesia

Adult IV 0.1–0.3 mg/kg over 30–60 s with 0.5–1 mg q30–90min prn

Adjunct for Intubation

Adult IV 0.2–0.4 mg/kg over 30–60 s

Electroshock Therapy

Adult IV 1.75–5.5 mg/kg

PHARMACOKINETICS Onset: 1–4 min. **Peak:** 3–5 min. **Duration:** 35–90 min. **Distribution:** crosses placenta. **Elimination:** half-life: 3.6 h; primarily excreted in urine, small amount in feces.

CONTRAINDICATIONS & PRECAUTIONS Contraindicated in: hypersensitivity to metocurine or to iodides; allergy, asthma. **Cautious use in:** myasthenia gravis, renal, hepatic, or pulmonary impairment, respiratory depression, electrolyte disturbances. Pregnancy category C.

ADVERSE/SIDE EFFECTS Same toxic potential as for tubocurarine. *Hypotension,* dizziness, increased salivation, bronchospasm, respiratory depression, decreased GI motility and tone, hypersensitivity reactions.

INCOMPATIBILITIES Solution/Additive: ALKALINE SOLUTIONS. **Y-Site:** BARBITURATES, **meperidine, morphine.**

NURSING IMPLICATIONS

Administration

- Metocurine is incompatible with alkaline solutions. Do not administer in same syringe with barbiturates, meperidine, or morphine because a precipitate will form.
- Metocurine solution should be protected from prolonged exposure to heat and direct sunlight.
- Store at 15–30C (59–86F).

Assessment & Drug Effects

- Complete recovery from IV dose may require several hours.

- A peripheral nerve stimulator may be used to monitor response.

Prototype: hydrochlorothiazide, p 203

METOLAZONE
(me-tole´a-zone)
Trade names: Diulo, Mykrox, Zaroxolyn
Classifications: ELECTROLYTIC & WATER BALANCE AGENT; DIURETIC; CARDIOVASCULAR AGENT; ANTIHYPERTENSIVE
Pregnancy: Category D

ACTIONS/PHARMACODYNAMICS Quinazoline derivative diuretic structurally and pharmacologically similar to hydrochlorothiazide. Appears to be more effective as a diuretic than thiazides in patients with severe renal failure.

USES Management of hypertension as sole agent or to enhance effectiveness of other antihypertensives in severe form of hypertension; also edema associated with CHF and renal disease.

ROUTE & DOSAGE

Edema

Adult PO 5–20 mg/d

Hypertension

Adult PO 2.5–5 mg/d
           Mykrox: 0.5–1 mg/d

PHARMACOKINETICS Absorption: incompletely absorbed; Mykrox has greater absorption. **Onset:** 1 h. **Peak:** 2–8 h. **Duration:** 12–24 h. **Distribution:** distributed throughout extracellular tissue; concentrates in kidney; crosses placenta; distributed in breast milk. **Metabolism:** does not appear to be metabolized. **Elimination:** half-life: 14 h; excreted in urine.

CONTRAINDICATIONS & PRECAUTIONS Contraindicated in: anuria, hypokalemia; hepatic coma or precoma; hypersensitivity to metolazone and sulfonamides; pregnancy (category D), nursing mothers. **Cautious use in:** history of gout; allergies; concomitant use of digitalis glycosides; renal and hepatic dysfunction.

ADVERSE/SIDE EFFECTS Cholestatic jaundice, vertigo, orthostatic hypotension, venous thrombosis,

Common side effects in *italic*; life-threatening effects underlined; generic names in **bold**; classifications in SMALL CAPS

771

M

leukopenia, dehydration, *hypokalemia, hyperuricemia, hyperglycemia.*

DRUG INTERACTIONS Amphotericin B, CORTICOSTEROIDS increase hypokalemic effects; may antagonize hypoglycemic effects of SULFONYLUREAS, **insulin; cholestyramine, colestipol** decrease thiazide absorption; intensifies hypoglycemic and hypotensive effects of **diazoxide;** because of increased potassium and magnesium loss, may cause **digoxin** toxicity; decreases **lithium** excretion, increasing its toxicity; NSAIDS may attenuate diuresis—increased risk of NSAID-induced renal failure.

NURSING IMPLICATIONS

Administration

- Schedule doses to avoid nocturia and interrupted sleep. Administer PO early in AM after eating to prevent gastric irritation (if given in 2 doses, schedule second dose no later than 3 PM).
- Store tablets in tightly closed container at 15–30C (59–86F) unless otherwise specified.

Assessment & Drug Effects

- Geriatric patients may be more sensitive to effects of usual adult dose; thus overdosage and adverse reactions should be anticipated.
- When adverse reactions are moderate to severe, metolazone therapy should be terminated.
- Antihypertensive effects may be observed in 3 or 4 d, but 3–4 wk are required for maximum effect.
- Serum potassium should be determined at regular intervals. Prolonged treatment with metolazone and inadequate potassium intake increase potential for hypokalemia (see Signs & Symptoms, chap 3).

Patient & Family Education

- Warn patient not to drink alcohol, since it potentiates orthostatic hypotension.
- Antihypertensive therapy may require as adjunct a high-potassium, low-sodium, and low-calorie diet.
- Hypokalemia is rarely severe in most patients. To prevent onset, urge patient to eat a normal diet (usually includes potassium-rich foods such as potatoes, fruit juices, cereals, skim milk) and to include a banana (about 370 mg potassium) and at least 180 ml (6 oz) orange juice (about 330 mg potassium) every day.
- If hypokalemia develops, dietary potassium supplement of 1000–2000 mg (25–50 mEq) is usually an adequate treatment.

Prototype: propranolol, p 109

METOPROLOL TARTRATE

(me-toe´proe-lole)

Trade names: Apo-Metoprolol, Betaloc, Lopressor, Norometoprol

Classifications: AUTONOMIC NERVOUS SYSTEM AGENT; BETA-ADRENERGIC ANTAGONIST (SYMPATHOLYTIC); ANTIHYPERTENSIVE

Pregnancy: Category C

ACTIONS/PHARMACODYNAMICS Beta-adrenergic blocking agent with preferential effect on $beta_1$ adrenoreceptors located primarily on cardiac muscle. At higher doses, metoprolol also inhibits $beta_2$ receptors located chiefly on bronchial and vascular musculature. Reduces heart rate and cardiac output at rest and during exercise; lowers both supine and standing BP, slows sinus rate and decreases myocardial automaticity. Antihypertensive action may be due to competitive antagonism of catecholamines at cardiac adrenergic neuron sites, drug-induced reduction of sympathetic outflow to the periphery (central effect), and to suppression of renin activity. Has minimal effect on muscle glycogenolysis or on insulin release. Antianginal effect (reduction of oxygen consumption and demand by myocardial muscle) is like that of propranolol.

USES Management of mild to severe hypertension (monotherapy or in combination with a thiazide or vasodilator or both; long-term treatment of angina pectoris and prophylactic management of stable angina pectoris reduce the risk of mortality after an MI.

ROUTE & DOSAGE

Hypertension

Adult	PO	50–100 mg/d in 1–2 divided doses; may increase weekly up to 100–450 mg/d

Angina Pectoris

Adult	PO	100 mg/d in 2 divided doses; may increase weekly up to 100–400 mg/d

Myocardial Infarction

Adult	IV	5 mg q2min for 3 doses, followed by PO therapy
	PO	50 mg q6h for 48 h, then 100 mg b.i.d.

Common side effects in *italic*; life-threatening effects underlined; generic names in **bold**; classifications in SMALL CAPS

PHARMACOKINETICS Absorption: readily absorbed from GI tract; 50% of dose reaches systemic circulation. **Onset:** 15 min. **Peak:** 1.5 h. **Duration:** 13–19 h. **Distribution:** crosses blood-brain barrier and placenta, distributed into breast milk. **Metabolism:** extensively metabolized in liver. **Elimination:** half-life: 3–4 h; excreted in urine.

CONTRAINDICATIONS & PRECAUTIONS Contraindicated in: cardiogenic shock, sinus bradycardia, heart block greater than first degree, overt cardiac failure, right ventricular failure secondary to pulmonary hypertension. Safe use during pregnancy (category C), in nursing mothers, and in children not established. **Cautious use in:** impaired hepatic or renal function; cardiomegaly, CHF controlled by digitalis and diuretics; A-V conduction defects; bronchial asthma and other bronchospastic diseases; history of allergy; thyrotoxicosis; diabetes mellitus; peripheral vascular disease.

ADVERSE/SIDE EFFECTS Allergic: erythematous rash, fever, muscle aches, sore throat, <u>laryngospasm</u>, respiratory distress. **CNS:** *dizziness, fatigue,* headache, *insomnia,* nightmares, increased dreaming, hallucinations, mental depression. **CV:** *bradycardia,* palpitation, cold extremities, Raynaud's phenomenon, intermittent claudication, angina pectoris, CHF, intensification of AV block, AV dissociation, <u>complete heart block, cardiac arrest</u>. **Eye; ear:** visual disturbances, inflamed conjunctiva and eyelids, punctate keratitis, keratoconjunctivitis, corneal ulcerations, dry eyes (decreased tear production); tinnitus. **GI:** nausea, *heartburn,* gastric pain, diarrhea or constipation, flatulence. **Hematologic:** eosinophilia, agranulocytosis, thrombocytopenic and nonthrombocytopenic purpura. **Skin:** dry skin, pruritus, alopecia (reversible), skin eruptions. **Other:** dry mouth and mucous membranes, sweating, restless legs; hypoglycemia, bronchospasm (with high doses), Peyronie's disease (rare), *shortness of breath.*

DIAGNOSTIC TEST INTERFERENCES In common with other beta-blockers, metoprolol may cause elevated ***BUN*** and ***serum creatinine levels*** (patients with severe heart disease), elevated ***serum transaminase, alkaline phosphatase, lactate dehydrogenase,*** and ***serum uric acid.***

DRUG INTERACTIONS BARBITURATES, **rifampin** may decrease effects of metoprolol; **cimetidine, methimazole, propylthiouracil,** ORAL CONTRACEP- TIVES may increase effects of metoprolol; additive bradycardia with **digoxin;** effects of both metoprolol and **hydralazine** may be increased; **indomethacin** may attenuate hypotensive response, BETA AGONISTS and metoprolol mutually antagonistic, **verapamil** may increase risk of heart block and bradycardia.

NURSING IMPLICATIONS

Administration

- Ingestion with food slightly enhances absorption; however, administration with food is not essential. It is important that drug be given with or without food consistently to minimize possible variations in bioavailability.
- IV metoprolol may be given by direct IV undiluted at a rate of 5 mg over 60 seconds.
- Store at 15–30C (59–86F). Protect from heat, light, and moisture.

Assessment & Drug Effects

- Take apical pulse and BP before administering drug. Report to physician significant changes in rate, rhythm, or quality of pulse or variations in BP prior to administration.
- During IV administration, BP, heart rate, and ECG should be carefully monitored.
- For patients with hypertension, take several BP readings close to the end of a 12 h dosing interval to evaluate adequacy of dosage, particularly in patients on twice daily doses. Some patients require doses 3 times a day to maintain satisfactory control.
- Hypertensive patients with CHF controlled by digitalis and diuretics must be closely observed for impending heart failure: dyspnea on exertion, orthopnea, night cough, edema, distended neck veins. Monitor I&O, daily weight; auscultate daily for pulmonary rales.
- Maximal effect on BP is achieved usually after 1 wk of therapy.
- Drug should be withdrawn if patient presents symptoms of mental depression because it can progress to catatonia. Possible symptoms of depression: disinterest in people, surroundings, food, personal hygiene; withdrawal, apathy, sadness, difficulty in concentrating, insomnia.
- Since metoprolol masks signs of hyperthyroidism (see chap 3), patients with thyrotoxicosis must be closely monitored. Abrupt withdrawal may precipitate thyroid storm.
- Because of beta-blocking action, usual rise in pulse rate may not occur in response to stress situations such as fever or following vigorous exercise.
- Baseline and regularly scheduled evaluations

M

Common side effects in *italic*; life-threatening effects <u>underlined</u>; generic names in **bold**; classifications in SMALL CAPS

773

should be made of blood cell counts, blood glu-cose (diabetic patients), cardiac function, hepatic and renal function.

Patient & Family Education

- Patient receiving metoprolol should be instructed to take radial pulse before each dose. Advise patient to report to physician if it is slower than base rate (e.g., 60 bpm) or becomes irregular. Consult physician for parameters.
- Inform patient that most adverse effects tend to be mild and transient and that they generally disappear with continued therapy.
- Insomnia or increased dreaming may be reduced by avoiding late evening doses.
- Patients with diabetes mellitus should be monitored closely. Metroprolol may mask some symptoms of hypoglycemia (e.g., BP and heart rate changes) and may prolong hypoglycemia. Alert patient to other possible signs of hypoglycemia not affected by metoprolol that should be reported: sweating, fatigue, hunger, inability to concentrate.
- Instruct patient to protect extremities from cold and not to smoke. Advise patient to report cold, painful, or tender feet or hands or other symptoms of Raynaud's disease (intermittent pallor, cyanosis or redness, paresthesias). Physician may prescribe a vasodilator.
- Instruct patient to report immediately to physician the onset of ocular symptoms.
- If mouth dryness is bothersome, advise the following measures: rinse mouth frequently with clear warm water; increase noncalorie liquid intake if it has been inadequate; sugarless gum or lemon-drops.
- Eye dryness may be relieved by use of sterile artificial tears available OTC.
- Since metoprolol may cause dizziness, particularly during early therapy, advise patient to avoid driving and other potentially hazardous activities until drug effects are known.
- Emphasize importance of compliance and caution patient not to alter established dosage regimen.
- When metoprolol is to be discontinued, dosage should be reduced gradually over a period of 1–2 wk. Sudden withdrawal can result in increase in anginal attacks and MI in patients with angina pectoris and thyroid storm in patients with hyperthyroidism.
- Advisable for patients on prolonged therapy to wear or carry medical identification. Instruct patient to inform dentist or surgeon that he or she is taking metoprolol.

METRONIDAZOLE

See ANTIINFECTIVE, ANTITRICHOMONAL prototype, p 81.

METYROSINE

(me-tye´roe-seen)
Trade name: Demser
Classification: ENZYME INHIBITOR
Pregnancy: Category C

ACTIONS/PHARMACODYNAMICS By blocking the enzyme tyrosine hydroxylase, metyrosine inhibits the conversion of tyrosine to DOPA (dihydroxyphenylalanine), which is the initial and rate-setting step in synthesis of catecholamines (dopamine, epinephrine, norepinephrine). In patients with pheochromocytoma (adrenal tumor that causes overproduction of catecholamines, mainly epinephrine and norepinephrine), catecholamine synthesis may be reduced by as much as 80%, ameliorating hypertensive attacks and associated symptoms.

USES Short-term management of pheochromocytoma until surgery is performed, in long-term control when surgery is contraindicated, and in patients with malignant pheochromocytoma. **Unlabeled use:** has been used in selected patients with schizophrenia to potentiate antipsychotic effects of phenothiazines.

ROUTE & DOSAGE

Pheochromocytoma

Adult	PO	250 mg q.i.d.; may increase to 2–3 g/d in divided doses (max 4 g/d)

PHARMACOKINETICS Absorption: readily absorbed from GI tract. **Peak:** 2–3 d. **Duration:** 3–4 d. **Distribution:** crosses blood-brain barrier. **Elimination:** half-life: 3.4–7.2 h; excreted in urine.

CONTRAINDICATIONS & PRECAUTIONS Contraindicated in: control of essential hypertension. Safe use during pregnancy (category C), in nursing women, and in children <12 y not established. **Cautious use in:** impaired hepatic or renal function.

M

Common side effects in *italic*; life-threatening effects underlined; generic names in **bold**; classifications in SMALL CAPS

ADVERSE/SIDE EFFECTS CNS: *sedation,* fatigue; *extrapyramidal signs: drooling, difficulty in speaking (dysarthria), tremors,* jaw-stiffness (trismus); frank parkinsonism, psychic disturbances (anxiety, depression, hallucinations, disorientation, confusion), headache, muscle spasms. **GI:** *diarrhea,* nausea, vomiting, abdominal pain, dry mouth. **Hypersensitivity:** rash, urticaria. **Renal:** transient dysuria, oliguria, crystalluria, urolithiasis, hematuria, enuresis. **Reproductive:** impotence, failure of ejaculation, breast swelling, galactorrhea. **Other:** peripheral edema, nasal stuffiness, shortness of breath, eosinophilia, increased AST.

DIAGNOSTIC TEST INTERFERENCES False increases in ***urinary catecholamines*** may occur because of catechol metabolites of metyrosine.

DRUG INTERACTIONS Alcohol and other CNS DEPRESSANTS add to sedation and CNS depression; **droperidol, haloperidol,** PHENOTHIAZINES potentiate extrapyramidal effects.

NURSING IMPLICATIONS

Administration

- Advise patient to take each dose with a full glass of water and to be consistent about time medication is to be taken.
- Store at 15–30C (59–86F) unless otherwise directed.

Assessment & Drug Effects

- Monitor I&O ratio and pattern. Fluid intake must be enough (e.g., 10–12 glasses or more) to maintain urinary output of 2000 ml or more to minimize risk of crystalluria.
- Routine urinalysis should be performed; if crystals occur, fluid intake should be increased further. If crystalluria persists, metyrosine dosage should be decreased or drug discontinued.
- Baseline and regularly scheduled measurements should be made of urinary catecholamines and their metabolites (metanephrines and VMA). Metabolite excretion should decrease in patients with pheochromocytoma. Other baseline and regular determinations should include vital signs, ECG, renal and hepatic function tests (in patients with dysfunction), BMR, and blood and urine sugar tests.
- In addition to reduction of urinary metanephrines and VMA, clinical effectiveness with pheochromocytoma is determined by decrease in frequency of hypertensive attacks and associated symptoms (elevated blood pressure, headache, nausea, vomit-

ing, sweating, tachycardia), and possibly reduction of hyperglycemia, glycosuria, and BMR.

- Supervise ambulation. Sedative effects occur commonly within the first 24 h after drug is started. Maximal sedative effects in 2 or 3 d, after which time they begin to subside (usually within 1 wk). Sedation may persist in patients taking > 2 g/d.

Patient & Family Education

- Advise patient to notify physician if the following metyrosine side effects occur: diarrhea, particularly if it is severe or persists, painful urination, jaw stiffness, drooling, difficult speech, tremors, disorientation. Dosage reduction or discontinuation of drug may be indicated.
- Caution patient to avoid driving and other potentially hazardous activities until reaction to drug is determined.
- Abrupt discontinuation of metyrosine may result in psychic stimulation, feeling of increased energy, temporary changes in sleep pattern (usually insomnia). Symptoms may last for 2 or 3 d.
- Patient on prolonged therapy should be advised to carry medical identification and to notify all physicians and dentists involved in care about drug regimen.

Prototype: procainamide, p 140

MEXILETINE
(mex-il´e-teen)
Trade name: Mexitil
Classifications: CARDIOVASCULAR AGENT; ANTIARRHYTHMIC
Pregnancy: Category C

M

ACTIONS/PHARMACODYNAMICS Analog of lidocaine with potent anesthetic action and class IB electrophysiologic properties similar to those of procainamide. Shortens action potential duration and refractory period and improves resting potential. Has little or no effect on atrial tissue and produces modest suppression of sinus node automatically and AV nodal conduction. Prolongs the His to ventricular interval (HQ) only if patient has preexisting conduction disturbance (consistent with selective effect of class IB agents on abnormal tissue). It should be noted that lidocaine response is not a reliable predictor of mexiletine effectiveness. Produces modest negative inotropic and hypotensive effects.

Common side effects in *italic*; life-threatening effects underlined; generic names in **bold**; classifications in SMALL CAPS

775

USES Acute and chronic ventricular arrhythmias; prevention of recurrent cardiac arrests; suppression of PVCs due to ventricular tachyarrhythmias. **Unlabeled uses:** Wolff-Parkinson-White syndrome and supraventricular arrhythmias.

ROUTE & DOSAGE

Ventricular Arrhythmias

Adult   PO   200–300 mg q8h (max 1200 mg/d)

PHARMACOKINETICS Absorption: readily absorbed from GI tract. **Peak:** 2–3 h. **Distribution:** distributed into breast milk. **Metabolism:** metabolized in liver. **Elimination:** half-life: 10–12 h; excreted in urine; renal elimination increases with urinary acidification.

CONTRAINDICATIONS & PRECAUTIONS Contraindicated in: severe left ventricular failure, cardiogenic shock, severe bradyarrhythmias. Pregnancy category C, preexisting second- or third-degree heart block.

ADVERSE/SIDE EFFECTS CNS: *dizziness, tremor, nervousness, incoordination,* headache, blurred vision, paresthesias, numbness. **CV:** <u>exacerbated arrhythmias</u>, palpitations, chest pain, syncope, hypotension. **GI:** *nausea, vomiting, heartburn,* diarrhea, constipation, dry mouth, abdominal pain. **Other:** rash, dyspnea, edema, arthralgia, fever, impotence, malaise, urinary retention, hiccups.

DRUG INTERACTIONS Phenytoin, phenobarbital, rifampin may decrease mexiletine levels; **cimetidine** may increase mexiletine levels.

NURSING IMPLICATIONS

Administration

▪ Administered with food or milk to reduce gastric distress.

Assessment & Drug Effects

▪ Check pulse and BP before administration of mexiletine, until both are stabilized. Patient should understand that changes in pulse rate and regularity may signal decreasing clinical effectiveness of drug.
▪ Effective serum concentration: 0.5–2 µg/ml.
▪ CNS adverse reactions predominate (intention tremors, nystagmus, blurred vision, dizziness, ataxia, confusion, nausea). Supervise ambulation in the weak, debilitated patient or the elderly during drug stabilization period.

▪ Drug compliance with mexiletine is affected particularly by the distressing side effects of tremor, ataxia, and eye symptoms.
▪ Check frequently with patient about adherence to drug regimen. If side effects are increasing, consult physician. Dose adjustment or discontinuation may be needed.

Patient & Family Education

▪ Instruct patient about *pulse parameters to be reported:* changes in rhythm and rate (bradycardia = pulse below 60); symptomatic bradycardia (lightheadedness, syncope, dizziness), and postural hypotension.

Prototype: penicillin G potassium, p 71

MEZLOCILLIN SODIUM
(mez-loe-sill´in)
Trade name: Mezlin
Classifications: ANTIINFECTIVE; BETA-LACTAM ANTIBIOTIC; PENICILLIN
Pregnancy: Category B

ACTIONS/PHARMACODYNAMICS Semisynthetic acylureidopenicillin with extended spectrum. Structurally resembles ampicillin and has similar but wider antibacterial spectrum than either ampicillin, carbenicillin, or ticarcillin. In common with other penicillins, mezlocillin is bactericidal and acts by interfering with bacterial cell wall synthesis. Active against a wide variety of gram-negative and gram-positive bacteria including aerobic and anaerobic strains. Broadened spectrum of activity includes strains of pathogenic aerobic gram-negative bacteria, e.g., *Bacteroides, Enterobacter, Escherichia, Haemophilus, Klebsiella, Pseudomonas, Proteus,* and *Serratia,* and gram-positive organisms such as *Streptococcus faecalis* (enterococcus). Inactive against penicillinase-producing strains of *Staphylococcus aureus.*

USES Primarily for serious infections caused by *Pseudomonas aeruginosa* alone or in combination with an aminoglycoside or a cephalosporin. Also used to treat other infections caused by susceptible strains.

PHARMACOKINETICS Peak: 45 min IM; 5 min IV. **Distribution:** widely distributed with highest concentrations in urine and bile; adequate CSF penetration with inflamed meninges; crosses placenta; distributed into breast milk. **Metabolism:** slightly metabolized in liver. **Elimination:** half-life: 50–55 min; 75% excreted in urine, up to 25% excreted in bile.

ROUTE & DOSAGE

Uncomplicated Urinary Tract Infection

Adult   IM/IV   1.5–2 g q6h (100–125 mg/kg/d)

Moderate to Severe Infections

Adult   IM/IV   4 g q6h (150–200 mg/kg/d)

Life-threatening Infection, *Pseudomonas* Infections

Adult   IM/IV   3 g q4h (max 24 g/d)

Child   IM/IV   1 mo–12 y: 50–75 mg/kg q4h

                 < 1 mo: 75 mg/kg q8–12h

CONTRAINDICATIONS & PRECAUTIONS Contraindicated in: history of hypersensitivity to penicillins or cephalosporins. Safe use during pregnancy (category B) and in nursing mothers not established. **Cautious use in:** patients with known or suspected allergies to drugs or other substances; renal impairment, uremia; hypokalemia; bleeding tendencies.

ADVERSE/SIDE EFFECTS CNS: convulsive seizures, neuromuscular hyperirritability. **GI:** abnormal taste sensations, nausea, vomiting, *diarrhea*. **Hematologic:** neutropenia, leukopenia, eosinophilia, thrombocytopenia (infrequent), hypokalemia (rare); increases in AST, ALT, alkaline phosphatase, serum bilirubin, creatinine, BUN, decreased Hct and Hgb. **Hypersensitivity:** *rash*, pruritus, urticaria, drug fever, <u>anaphylactic reactions</u>. ***Local:*** pain (following IM), thrombophlebitis (IV injection); superinfections.

DRUG INTERACTIONS Mezlocillin increases risk of bleeding associated with ANTICOAGULANTS; **probenecid** decreases elimination of mezlocillin.

INCOMPATIBILITIES Solution/Additive: ciprofloxacin, AMINOGLYCOSIDES. **Y-Site: ciprofloxacin, meperidine, verapamil,** AMINOGLYCOSIDES.

NURSING IMPLICATIONS

Administration

- IM injections should be made into a relatively large muscle such as the gluteus maximus (upper outer quadrant). Discomfort associated with IM administration may be lessened by giving injection slowly (over 12–15 seconds) and by reconstituting solution with lidocaine 0.5–1% (lessens pain). Do not exceed 2 g per IM injection.
- Each 1 g of IV mezlocillin must be diluted with 10

ml of sterile water, D5W, or NS. Shake to dissolve. Solution may be given by direct IV over 3–5 min or further diluted to a volume of 50–100 ml and infused over 30 min. Primary infusion should be temporarily withheld during infusion of mezlocillin.

- Mezlocillin and aminoglycoside antibiotics (e.g., gentamicin) are chemically incompatible; do not mix together in IV solution. Administer them 1 h apart, especially if patient is elderly or has renal insufficiency.
- Store unopened vials and infusion bottles at or below 30C (86F) unless otherwise directed. Powder and reconstituted solutions may darken slightly, but this does not indicate loss of potency. Solutions should be clear. If a precipitate should form under refrigeration, warm solution to 37C (98.6F) in a water bath and shake well.

Assessment & Drug Effects

- Culture and susceptibility tests should be performed before and periodically during therapy.
- Before initiation of therapy a detailed history should be obtained to determine previous hypersensitivity, especially to penicillins and cephalosporins but also to other substances.
- Observe IV sites for evidence of thrombophlebitis (see Signs & Symptoms, chap 3).
- Be prepared to administer emergency therapy for anaphylactoid reaction (see Signs & Symptoms, chap 3) whenever a penicillin antibiotic is administered. Monitor patient response frequently.
- Monitor patient carefully during the first 30 min after initiation of IV therapy for signs of hypersensitivity and anaphylactoid reaction (see Signs & Symptoms, chap 3).
- Bleeding abnormalities (thrombocytopenia), although rare, are particularly likely to occur in patients with impaired renal function. Observe and report ecchymoses, petechiae, bleeding gums, nosebleeds, or any other evidence of bleeding.
- Be alert to signs of superinfections (see Signs & Symptoms, chap 3).
- Baseline and regularly scheduled studies of blood, renal, and hepatic function should be performed during long-term therapy.

Patient & Family Education

- Inform patient that therapy generally continues for at least 2 d after signs and symptoms of infection have subsided. Usual duration of therapy for serious infections is 7–10 d, but it may be longer in complicated infections.
- Inform patient that antibiotic therapy for group A beta-hemolytic streptococcal infections should

M

Common side effects in *italic*; life-threatening effects <u>underlined</u>; generic names in **bold**; classifications in SMALL CAPS

777

continue for at least 10 d to reduce risk of rheumatic fever or glomerulonephritis.
- Advise women to report onset of symptoms of *Candida* vaginitis. *Candida* vaginitis symptoms are moderate amount of white, cheesy, nonodorous vaginal discharge, vaginal inflammation, and itching.
- Instruct patient to report a skin rash or pruritus. The patient should then be assessed for other signs of hypersensitivity (see Signs & Symptoms, chap 3). Mezlocillin may need to be discontinued.

Prototype: amphotericin B, p 56

MICONAZOLE NITRATE

(mi-kon´a-zole)
Trade names: Micatin, Monistat
Classifications: ANTIINFECTIVE; ANTIBIOTIC; ANTIFUNGAL
Pregnancy: Category B

ACTIONS/PHARMACODYNAMICS Broad-spectrum agent with fungicidal activity against *Candida albicans* and other species of this genus. Inhibits growth of common dermatophytes *Trichophyton rubrum, Trichophyton mentagrophytes, Epidermophyton floccosum,* and organism responsible for tinea versicolor *(Malassezia furfur).* Mode of action unclear but appears to inhibit uptake of components essential for cell reproduction and growth and to alter cell wall structure, thus promoting cell death.

USES Vulvovaginal candidiasis, tinea pedis (athlete's foot), tinea cruris, tinea corporis, and tinea versicolor caused by dermatophytes. **Parenteral:** severe systemic infections including coccidioidomycosis, candidiasis, cryptococcosis, paracoccidioidomycosis, and chronic mucocutaneous candidiasis. IV infusion is inadequate therapy for urinary bladder infections or for fungal meningitis; these conditions require supplements of miconazole by intrathecal administration and bladder irrigation.

PHARMACOKINETICS Absorption: small amount absorbed from vagina. **Metabolism:** rapidly metabolized in liver. **Elimination:** half-life: 2.1–24 h; excreted in urine and feces.

ROUTE & DOSAGE

Fungal Infection

Adult	Intravaginal	1 applicatorful of cream or 1 100 mg suppository h.s. for 7 d or 1 200 mg suppository h.s. for 3 d
	IV	200–3600 mg/d in 3 divided doses or 20 mg intrathecally q3–7d
	Bladder Instillation	200 mg of diluted solution b.i.d. to q.i.d. or by continuous infusion
Child	IV	20–40 mg/kg/d in divided doses (max 15 mg/kg/infusion)

CONTRAINDICATIONS & PRECAUTIONS Contraindicated in: safe use in children < 1 y of age, during pregnancy after first trimester (category B), and in nursing women not established. **Cautious use in:** hepatic or renal impairment.

ADVERSE/SIDE EFFECTS Tachycardia, cardiac arrhythmias (with rapid IV injection); vulvovaginal burning, itching or irritation, pelvic cramps, hives, skin rash, and headache. **Parenteral:** phlebitis, pruritus, rash, nausea, vomiting, diarrhea, febrile reaction, drowsiness, flushing, hyponatremia (transient), decreased hematocrit; thrombocytopenia, hyperlipemia, arrhythmias, anaphylaxis.

DIAGNOSTIC TEST INTERFERENCES Possibility of false-positive *urine protein* determinations (when mezlocillin concentration in urine is high) using sulfosalicylic acid and boiling test, acetic acid test, biuret reaction, nitric acid test; bromphenol blue reagent test (Multi-stix) is not affected.

DRUG INTERACTIONS Decreased antifungal activity of both **amphotericin B** and miconazole; **warfarin** may increase prothrombin time; SULFONYLUREAS may cause severe hypoglycemia.

NURSING IMPLICATIONS

Administration

- Treatment with miconazole is preferably started in hospital to permit careful monitoring of drug response. Culture and susceptibility studies should be performed.

M

- Hypersensitivity test should be performed prior to IV administration. An initial test dose of 200 mg is administered by physician. Monitor patient for hypersensitivity reactions.
  Drug is diluted for IV injection in at least 200 ml NS or D5W solution. A 20 ml ampule contains 10 mg/ml. Following dilution, solution is stable at room temperature for 48 h. If solution darkens in color, discard it. This is a sign of deterioration.
- IV administration should be slow (over a period of 30–60 min) to prevent nausea and risk of arrhythmias or tachycardia. Physician prescribes flow rate. Rapid injection may produce arrhythmia. Have immediately available emergency drugs and resuscitation equipment.
- Ask physician about how to cleanse affected area prior to application of cream or lotion.
- Use lotion rather than cream for intertriginous areas to prevent maceration.
- Massage affected area gently until cream disappears.
- Store at 15–30C (59–86F) unless otherwise directed.

Assessment & Drug Effects
- Hgb, Hct, electrolytes, triglycerides, and cholesterol values should be determined initially and periodically during therapy.
- If nausea is a problem, the patient may be premedicated with an antiemetic or antihistamine.
- Clinical improvement from topical application should be expected in 1 or 2 wk. If no improvement in 4 wk, the diagnosis is reevaluated. Tinea pedis infection should be treated for 1 mo to assure permanent recovery.
- Pathogens causing vaginitis should be identified before treatment since miconazole is effective only against candidal vulvovaginitis.

Patient & Family Education
- The full course of treatment should be completed to assure recovery.
- Avoid contact of drug with eyes.
- Instruct patient to insert applicator of drug high into the vagina and to use a sanitary napkin to prevent staining.
- Persistent vulvovaginitis should be reevaluated if 3–4 wk does not bring relief. Advise patient to report to physician for urine and blood glucose studies, since vaginitis may be a symptom of unrecognized diabetes mellitus.
- Advise patient to avoid sexual intercourse during treatment period to prevent reinfection.

MICROFIBRILLAR COLLAGEN HEMOSTAT
Trade name: Avitene
Classification: BLOOD COAGULATOR, HEMOSTATIC
Pregnancy: Category C

ACTIONS/PHARMACODYNAMICS Absorbable topical hemostatic agent derived from purified collagen from skin of cattle. On contact with a bleeding surface, platelets adhere to its fibrils and undergo a reaction that triggers their aggregation into thrombi. Reportedly does not interfere with bone regeneration or healing. Hemostatic effect is not inhibited by heparin or aspirin. Not effective in systemic clotting disorders such as hemophilia.

USES Adjunct to hemostasis when control of bleeding by ligature is ineffective or impractical, as in superficial injuries of spleen or liver, large oozing surfaces, and anastomotic sites.

ROUTE & DOSAGE

Hemostasis

Adult	Topical	Apply dry directly to source of bleeding (site compressed with a dry sponge immediately before application) and apply pressure with dry sponge for 1–5 or more minutes, depending on severity of bleeding

CONTRAINDICATIONS & PRECAUTIONS Contraindicated in: closure of skin incisions, use in contaminated wounds. Safe use during pregnancy (category C) not established.

ADVERSE/SIDE EFFECTS Potentiation of infection, hematoma, abscess formation, wound dehiscence (separation), adhesion formation, mediastinitis, allergic reactions, foreign body reactions.

NURSING IMPLICATIONS

Administration
- Gloves and forceps used to handle product must be dry, since the drug will readily adhere to a moist surface.
- Material is inactivated by autoclaving.
- This product should not be resterilized.

M

Common side effects in *italic*; life-threatening effects underlined; generic names in **bold**; classifications in SMALL CAPS

779

> **Prototype: lorazepam, p 177**

MIDAZOLAM HYDROCHLORIDE
(mid´az-zoe-lam)
Trade name: Versed
Classifications: CNS AGENT; GENERAL
ANESTHETIC; BENZODIAZEPINE ANXIOLYTIC,
SEDATIVE-HYPNOTIC
Pregnancy: Category D
Controlled substance: Schedule IV

ACTIONS/PHARMACODYNAMICS Short-acting parenteral benzodiazepine; CNS depressant with sedative-hypnotic, anxiolytic, muscle relaxant, anticonvulsant, and anterograde amnestic effects; 3–4 times as potent as diazepam, another parenteral benzodiazepine. Mechanism of action unclear but is similar to that of other benzodiazepines. Intensifies activity of gamma-aminobenzoic acid (GABA), a major inhibitory neurotransmitter of the brain, by interfering with its reuptake and promoting its accumulation at neuronal synapses. This calms the patient, relaxes skeletal muscles, and in high doses produces sleep.

USES Sedation before general anesthesia, induction of general anesthesia; to impair memory of perioperative events (anterograde amnesia); for conscious sedation prior to short diagnostic and endoscopic procedures; and as the hypnotic supplement to nitrous oxide and oxygen (balanced anesthesia) for short surgical procedures.

ROUTE & DOSAGE

Conscious Sedation

Adult	IM	0.07–0.08 mg/kg 30–60 min before procedure
	IV	1–1.5 mg; may repeat in 2 min prn

IV Induction for General Anesthesia

Adult	IV	Premedicated: 0.15–0.25 mg/kg over 20–30 s; allow 2 min for effect
		Nonpremedicated: 0.3–0.35 mg/kg over 20–30 s; allow 2 min for effect

PHARMACOKINETICS Onset: 1–5 min IV; 5–15 min IM. **Peak:** 20–60 min. **Duration:** < 2 h IV; 1–6 h IM. **Distribution:** crosses blood-brain barrier and placenta. **Metabolism:** metabolized in liver. **Elimination:** half-life: 1–4 h; excreted in urine.

CONTRAINDICATIONS & PRECAUTIONS Contraindicated in: intolerance to benzodiazepines; acute narrow-angle glaucoma; shock; coma; acute alcohol intoxication; intraarterial injection. Safe use in pregnancy (category D), labor and delivery, by nursing mothers, or by children not established. **Cautious use in:** patient with COPD; chronic renal failure; CHF; the elderly.

ADVERSE/SIDE EFFECTS CNS: *anterograde amnesia,* headache, lightheadedness, euphoria, confusion, agitation, anxiety, emergence delirium, prolonged emergence and dreaming during emergence from anesthesia; insomnia, muscle tremor, ataxia, dizziness, dysphoria, dysphonia, slurred speech, paresthesia. **CV:** hypotension, bigeminy, PVCs, vasovagal episode, tachycardia, nodal rhythm. **Eye, ear:** blurred vision, diplopia, nystagmus, pinpoint pupils, blocked ears. **GI:** (low incidence) nausea, vomiting; retching, acid taste, excessive salivation. **Respiratory:** coughing, laryngospasm, bronchospasm, dyspnea, hyperventilation, respiratory arrest, wheezing, airway obstruction, tachypnea. **Skin:** hives, swelling, burning, pain, induration at injection site. **Other:** hiccups, lethargy, chills, yawning, weakness, toothache.

DRUG INTERACTIONS Alcohol, CNS DEPRESSANTS, ANTICONVULSANTS potentiate CNS depression; **cimetidine** increases midazolam plasma levels, increasing its toxicity; may decrease antiparkinsonism effects of **levodopa;** may increase **phenytoin** levels; **smoking** decreases sedative and antianxiety effects.

INCOMPATIBILITIES Solution/Additive: dimenhydrinate, pentobarbital, perphenazine, prochlorperazine, ranitidine. Y-Site: dimenhydrinate, pentobarbital, perphenazine, prochlorperazine, ranitidine.

NURSING IMPLICATIONS

Administration

- Water solubility of this agent makes it compatible with other preanesthetic medications (e.g., morphine, meperidine, atropine, scopolamine) and with standard diluents.
- IV midazolam is given diluted to a concentration of 0.25 mg/ml in NS or D5W. Avoid rapid injection, which may cause respiratory depression.
- Although incidence of phlebitis is rare, inspect injection site for redness, pain, swelling, and other signs of extravasation. Inject IM drug deep into a large muscle mass. Intraarterial injection should be avoided.

Common side effects in *italic*; life-threatening effects underlined; generic names in **bold**; classifications in SMALL CAPS

- If stored at 15–30C (59–86F), therapeutic activity is retained for 2 y from date of manufacture.

Assessment & Drug Effects

- If the patient is premedicated with a narcotic agonist analgesic, the conscious sedation period may be marked by hypotension. Protective supervision of ambulation will be important for several hours after recovery from the anesthetic.
- Anterograde amnesia (dose related) correlates well with degree of drowsiness and is about the same as that for lorazepam. Most patients do not recall induction.
- In the obese patient, half-life is prolonged; therefore duration of effects is prolonged (i.e., amnesia, postoperative recovery). Monitor vital signs for entire recovery period.
- **Overdose symptoms:** somnolence, confusion, sedation, diminished reflexes, coma, untoward effects on vital signs.

Patient & Family Education

- Patient may feel drowsy, weak, or tired for 1–2 d after drug has been given. Warn patient not to drive a car or perform other tasks requiring alertness and coordination until effects of midazolam disappear.
- Prepare patient for the amnesia to prevent an upsetting postoperative period. In the elderly, amnesia can have a profound effect.
- Patient teaching during amnestic period may not be remembered. Even if dose is small and depth of amnesia is unclear, provide written instructions with verbal teaching to assure future understanding and compliance.

Prototype: docusate, p 222

MINERAL OIL

Trade names: Agoral Plain, Heavy Mineral Oil, Kondremul Plain, Liquid Petrolatum, Milkinol, Neo-Cultol, Nujol, Petrogalar Pain, Zymenol
Classifications: GI AGENT; STOOL SOFTENER
Pregnancy: Category C

ACTIONS/PHARMACODYNAMICS Mixture of hydrocarbons obtained from petroleum. Lubricates and softens feces, retards water absorption from fecal content, eases passage of stool.

USES Temporary relief of constipation, when straining at stool is contraindicated (e.g., hypertension, certain cardiac disorders, following anorectal surgery), and to relieve fecal impaction. Also used as pharmaceutical solvent and vehicle.

ROUTE & DOSAGE

Constipation

Adult	PO	15–30 ml prn
	Rectal	90–120 ml
Child	PO	≥ 6 y: 5–15 ml once/d

PHARMACOKINETICS Absorption: limited absorption from GI tract. **Distribution:** distributes to mesenteric lymph nodes, intestinal mucosa, liver, and spleen. **Elimination:** eliminated in stool in 6–10 h.

CONTRAINDICATIONS & PRECAUTIONS Contraindicated in: nausea, vomiting, abdominal pain, intestinal obstruction, oral administration to dysphagic patients; use with emollients. **Cautious use in:** oral use in elderly or debilitated patients; during pregnancy (category C).

ADVERSE/SIDE EFFECTS Occasionally, pruritus ani; interference with postoperative anorectal wound healing; <u>with aspiration: pulmonary granuloma, lipid pneumonitis</u>. Prolonged use: anorexia, nausea, vomiting, nutritional deficiencies, hypoprothrombinemia.

DRUG INTERACTIONS May potentiate effects of ORAL ANTICOAGULANTS by decreasing the absorption of Vitamin K; large doses may decrease the absorption of **warfarin;** STOOL SOFTENERS may form a concretion in the GI tract.

NURSING IMPLICATIONS

Administration

- Usually administered in the evening. Digestion and passage of food from stomach may be delayed if taken within 2 h of mealtime.
- Potential of lipid pneumonia from aspiration is especially high in the elderly and debilitated patient. Administer with patient in upright position and avoid giving just before patient retires.
- Although tasteless, mineral oil consistency may be objectionable. Many patients prefer to drink orange juice or suck on slice of orange after taking oil; others prefer to mix it in orange juice.
- Emulsified preparations are reportedly more palat-

M

able; however, this form may enhance absorption of oil through intestinal mucosa.

- Administration of retention enema is generally followed by a cleansing enema in 30–60 min. Consult physician.

Patient & Family Education

- Prolonged use (> 2 wk) can reduce absorption of fat-soluble vitamins A, D, E, and K, carotene, calcium, and phosphates.
- Repeated oral use or rectal administration may result in oil seepage from rectum with soiling of clothing. Forewarn patient to be prepared for this possibility to avoid embarrassment.
- Application of mineral oil to nasal passages to relieve dryness should be avoided because of danger of migration of droplets from pharynx into lungs, with resulting lipid pneumonia. Aqueous vehicles are safer.
- Frequent or prolonged use of mineral oil may result in dependence.

Prototype: tetracycline, p 74

MINOCYCLINE HYDROCHLORIDE

(mi-noe-sye′kleen)
Trade names: Minocin, Vectrin
Classifications: ANTIINFECTIVE; TETRACYCLINE ANTIBIOTIC; ANTIACNE
Pregnancy: Category D

M

ACTIONS/PHARMACODYNAMICS Semisynthetic tetracycline derivative with actions, uses, contraindications, precautions, and adverse reactions as for tetracycline. Appears to be active against strains of staphylococci resistant to other tetracyclines, and photosensitivity occurs only rarely. Reported to be more completely absorbed than other tetracyclines because it is more lipid-soluble.

ROUTE & DOSAGE

Antiinfective

Adult	PO/IV	200 mg followed by 100 mg q12h
Child	PO/IV	> 8 y: 4.4 mg/kg followed by 2 mg/kg q12h

PHARMACOKINETICS Absorption: 90–100% absorbed from GI tract. **Peak:** 2–3 h. **Distribution:** tends to accumulate in adipose tissue; crosses placenta; dis-

tributed into breast milk. **Metabolism:** partially metabolized. **Elimination:** half-life: 11–26 h; 20–30% excreted in feces; about 12% excreted in urine.

CONTRAINDICATIONS & PRECAUTIONS Contraindicated in: hypersensitivity to tetracyclines; oral administration in meningococcal infections; children < 8 y. Safe use during pregnancy (category D) not established. **Cautious use in:** renal impairment.

ADVERSE/SIDE EFFECTS *CNS side effects (weakness, lightheadedness, ataxia, dizziness or vertigo),* nausea, cramps, diarrhea, flatulence.

DRUG INTERACTIONS ANTACIDS, **iron, calcium, magnesium, zinc, kaolin-pectin, sodium bicarbonate, bismuth subsalicylate** can significantly decrease minocycline absorption; effects of both **desmopressin** and minocycline antagonized; increases **digoxin** absorption, increasing risk of digoxin toxicity; **methoxyflurane** increases risk of renal failure. **Food-drug interactions:** dairy products significantly decrease minocycline absorption; food may also decrease its absorption.

INCOMPATIBILITIES Solution/Additive: doxapram. **Y-Site: hydromorphone, meperidine, morphine.**

NURSING IMPLICATIONS

Administration

- For *IV administration:* reconstitute 100 mg with 5 ml of sterile water for injection; may be further diluted with 500–1000 ml of compatible solutions (e.g., NaCl, dextrose, Ringer's).
- Administer diluted IV solution by intermittent infusion at a rate determined by the total volume of solution.
- Check expiration date. Outdated tetracycline can cause severe adverse side effects.
- Reconstituted solution is stable at room temperature for 24 h; further diluted solution should be used immediately.
- Absorption of oral drug does not appear to be significantly influenced by presence of food or dairy products in stomach.
- Prolonged use of this drug is not advised because of the risk of superinfection.

Assessment & Drug Effects

- Prior to administration, culture and sensitivity test should be done and repeated at regular intervals during drug therapy.

- Prior to administration, obtain history of hypersensitivity reactions; drug is contraindicated with known tetracycline hypersensitivity.
- Carefully monitor IV infusion site, since thrombophlebitis occurs relatively often. (See Signs & Symptoms, chap 3.)
- Carefully monitor for signs of hypersensitivity response (see chap 3), particularly in patients with history of allergies, especially to drugs.
- Monitor for signs of superinfection (see chap 3).
- Risk of toxic effects increases with renal and hepatic impairment; carefully assess at-risk patients.
- Serum drug level determinations are advised in patients receiving prolonged therapy.
- Supervise ambulation, since lightheadedness, dizziness, and vertigo occur frequently.

Patient & Family Education
- Advise patients to avoid hazardous activities or those requiring alertness while on minocycline.
- Instruct patients to use a sun screen when outdoors and to otherwise protect themselves from direct sunlight since photosensitivity reaction may occur.
- Advise patients to report vestibular side effects (e.g., dizziness), which usually occur during first week of therapy. Effects are reversible if drug is withdrawn.
- Instruct patient to promptly report loose stools or diarrhea or other signs of superinfection.
- Advise women to use nonhormonal methods of contraception while they are taking drug.

| Prototype: hydralazine, p 152 |

MINOXIDIL
(mi-nox´i-dill)
Trade names: Loniten, Rogaine
Classifications: CARDIOVASCULAR AGENT; NONNITRATE VASODILATOR; ANTIHYPERTENSIVE
Pregnancy: Category C

ACTIONS/PHARMACODYNAMICS Direct-acting vasodilator similar to other drugs of this class (e.g., hydralazine), but hypotensive effect is more pronounced. Appears to act by blocking calcium uptake through cell membrane. Reduces elevated systolic and diastolic blood pressures in supine and standing positions, by decreasing peripheral vascular resistance. Has little or no effect on venous system. Hypotensive action is accompanied by reflex activa-

tion of sympathetic, vagal inhibitory, and renal homeostatic mechanisms; increased sympathetic stimulation also activates the renin-angiotensin-aldosterone system. The net result is increased heart rate and cardiac output, sodium retention, and edema, which usually necessitates concomitant supportive drug therapy. Does not affect vasomotor reflexes and therefore does not produce orthostatic hypotension. Drug-induced hair growth (hypertrichosis) with systemic minoxidil usually develops after 1 y of therapy: it is nonvirilizing, involving face and limbs of the female and generalized increase in body hair in men. Topical minoxidil reverses balding to some degree. Action mechanism is uncertain. Antiandrogenic effects are absent. It is speculated that growth is the result of direct stimulation of hair follicle epithelium and possibly enhancement of cutaneous blood flow. A topical preparation of minoxidil is available: lacks systemic side effects because of minimal percutaneous absorption.

USES Step 4 agent in stepped care approach to treat severe hypertension that is symptomatic or associated with damage to target organs and is not manageable with maximum therapeutic doses of a diuretic plus two other antihypertensive drugs. Used with a diuretic to prevent fluid retention and a beta-adrenergic blocking agent (e.g., propranolol) or an alpha-adrenergic agonist (e.g., clonidine or methyldopa) to prevent tachycardia. (Topical) to treat alopecia areata and male pattern alopecia.

ROUTE & DOSAGE

Hypertension

Adult	PO	5 mg/d, increased q3–5d up to 40 mg/d in single or divided doses as needed (max 100 mg/d)
Child	PO	0.2 mg/kg/d (max 5 mg/d) initially, gradually increased to 0.25–1 mg/kg/d in divided doses (max 50 mg/d)

Male Pattern Alopecia

Adult	Topical	Apply 1 ml of 2% solution to affected area b.i.d.

PHARMACOKINETICS Absorption: readily absorbed from GI tract. **Onset:** 30 min PO; at least 4 mo topical. **Peak:** 2–8 h PO. **Duration:** 2–5 d PO; new hair growth will remain 3–4 mo after withdrawal of topical. **Distribution:** widely distributed including into breast milk. **Metabolism:** metabolized in liver. **Elimination:** half-life: 4.2 h; 97% excreted in urine and feces.

Common side effects in *italic*; life-threatening effects underlined; generic names in **bold**; classifications in SMALL CAPS

783

CONTRAINDICATIONS & PRECAUTIONS Contraindicated in: pheochromocytoma; acute MI, dissecting aortic aneurysm. Safe use during pregnancy (category C) or in nursing mothers or children not established. **Cautious use in:** severe renal impairment; recent MI (within preceding month); coronary artery disease, chronic CHF.

ADVERSE/SIDE EFFECTS CV: *tachycardia,* angina pectoris, *ECG changes,* pericardial effusion and tamponade, rebound hypertension (following drug withdrawal), pulmonary hypertension (causal relationship not established), intermittent claudication; *edema,* including pulmonary edema; *CHF (salt and water retention).* **Skin:** *hypertrichosis,* darkening of skin, transient pruritus, Stevens-Johnson syndrome, hypersensitivity rash. With topical use: itching, flushing, scaling, dermatitis, folliculitis. **Other:** nausea, headache, fatigue, breast tenderness, gynecomastia, polymenorrhea, thrombocytopenia.

DIAGNOSTIC TEST INTERFERENCES *Hematocrit, hemoglobin,* and *erythrocyte count* usually decrease (about 7%) during early therapy; *serum alkaline phosphatase, BUN,* and *creatinine* may increase during early therapy.

DRUG INTERACTIONS Epinephrine, norepinephrine cause excessive cardiac stimulation; **guanethidine** causes profound orthostatic hypotension.

NURSING IMPLICATIONS

Administration
- Minoxidil may be taken without regard to meals or food.
- Patients with malignant hypertension, particularly those receiving guanethidine, should have initial treatment in a hospital setting.
- Dose adjustment intervals are normally at least 3 d. If more rapid adjustment is necessary, adjustments can be made q6h with careful monitoring.
- For patients who develop refractory fluid retention, some clinicians withdraw drug for 1 or 2 d and then resume therapy aimed at more vigorous diuresis.
- Store in tightly covered container at 15–30C (59–86F) unless otherwise directed.

Assessment & Drug Effects
- Take BP and apical pulse before administering medication and report significant changes. Consult physician for parameters.
- Monitor BP and pulse at regular intervals during

therapy. Abrupt reduction in BP can result in CVA and MI. Keep physician informed.
- Fluid and electrolyte balance should be closely followed throughout therapy. Sodium and water retention commonly occur. Consult physician regarding sodium restriction. If patient is on diuretic therapy, potassium intake and serum potassium levels will require monitoring.
- Monitor I&O and daily weight. Report unusual changes in I&O ratio or daily weight gain ≥ 1 kg (2 lb).
- Observe patient daily for edema and auscultate lungs for rales. Be alert to signs and symptoms of CHF (see chap 3).
- Observe patient for symptoms of pericardial effusion or tamponade. Symptoms are similar to those of CHF, but additionally patient may have paradoxical pulse (normal inspiratory reduction in systolic BP may fall as much as 10–20 mm Hg).
- Rebound hypertension has followed minoxidil withdrawal. Conversion to conventional therapy must be accomplished gradually and with close observation of patient.

Patient & Family Education
- Patients on home care should be told usual pulse rate and instructed to count radial pulse for one full minute before taking drug. Advise patient to report an increase of 20 or more bpm.
- Instruct patient to notify physician promptly if the following signs or symptoms appear: increase of 20 or more bpm in resting pulse; breathing difficulty; dizziness; lightheadedness; fainting; edema (tight shoes or rings, puffiness, pitting); weight gain, chest pain, arm or shoulder pain; easy bruising or bleeding.
- Review package insert with patient (dispensed with product). Emphasize importance of taking drug as prescribed and caution patient not to skip or alter dosage and not to discontinue medication without consulting physician.
- Patient should be thoroughly informed of possibility of *hypertrichosis:* elongation, thickening, and increased pigmentation of fine body hair, especially of face, arms, and back. It develops 3–9 wk after start of therapy and occurs in approximately 80% of patients. It is not an endocrine disorder and is reversible within 1–6 mo following discontinuation of minoxidil.
- *Patient information for treatment of baldness:* A complete physical examination is advised before topical minoxidil (Rogaine) is used.
- A history of hypertension is not a contraindication to use of topical minoxidil, but coronary heart dis-

Common side effects in *italic*; life-threatening effects <u>underlined</u>; generic names in **bold**; classifications in SMALL CAPS

ease, valvular dysfunction, and heart failure are.

- Report any dermatologic adverse effects or any other adverse effect promptly. Follow-up examinations are usually scheduled for q4–6mo.
- Stress strict compliance; regular use maximizes chance of at least some hair regrowth.

Prototype: Dinoprostone, p 251

MISOPROSTOL
(my-so-prost´ole)
Trade name: Cytotec
Classification: PROSTAGLANDIN
Pregnancy: Category X

ACTIONS/PHARMACODYNAMICS Misoprostol, a synthetic prostaglandin E_1 analog, has both antisecretory (inhibiting gastric acid secretion) and mucosal protective properties. It can increase bicarbonate and mucosal protective properties. It also increases bicarbonate and mucous production. Misoprostol inhibits basal and nocturnal gastric acid secretion and acid secretion in response to a variety of stimuli, including meals, histamine, pentagastrin, and coffee. Misoprostol produces uterine contractions that may endanger pregnancy and cause a miscarriage.

USES Prevention of NSAID (including aspirin)-induced gastric ulcers in patients at high risk of complications from a gastric ulcer, e.g., the elderly and patients with a concomitant debilitating disease or a history of ulcers. The drug is taken for the duration of NSAID therapy and does not interfere with the efficacy of the NSAID. **Unlabeled use:** short-term treatment of duodenal ulcers.

ROUTE & DOSAGE

Prevention of NSAID-induced Ulcers

Adult   PO   100–200 µg q.i.d. p.c. and h.s.

PHARMACOKINETICS Absorption: readily absorbed from GI tract; extensive first pass metabolism. **Onset:** 30 min. **Peak:** 60–90 min. **Duration:** at least 3 h. **Metabolism:** metabolized in liver. **Elimination:** half-life: 20–40 min; primarily excreted in urine; small amount excreted in feces.

CONTRAINDICATIONS & PRECAUTIONS Contraindicated in: pregnant women (category X), history of allergies to prostaglandins, and nursing mothers. **Cautious use in:** renal impairment. Safety in children < 18 y has not been established.

ADVERSE/SIDE EFFECTS CNS: headache. **GI:** *diarrhea, abdominal pain,* nausea, flatulence, dyspepsia, vomiting, constipation. **GU:** spotting, cramps, dysmenorrhea, uterine contractions.

DRUG INTERACTIONS MAGNESIUM-CONTAINING ANTACIDS may increase diarrhea.

NURSING IMPLICATIONS

Administration
- Maximum plasma concentrations are diminished when misoprostol is taken with food. Because of GI side effects, however, manufacturer recommends that drug be taken with food.
- Store away from heat, light, and moisture.

Assessment & Drug Effects
- Diarrhea is a common side effect and is dose related. It is usually self-limiting (often resolving in 8 d). The incidence of diarrhea can be minimized by taking the drug after meals and at bedtime.

Patient & Family Education
- Avoid using magnesium-containing antacids because of increased incidence of diarrhea.
- Before using a new medicine (prescription or nonprescription) or if a new medical problem develops, check with doctor.
- Postmenopausal bleeding may be drug related. Report to physician.
- Advise women of childbearing potential that they must not be pregnant when misoprostol therapy is initiated, and they must use an effective contraception method while taking the drug.
- Advise of the abortifacient property of the drug. If woman becomes pregnant, the drug should be discontinued and the doctor contacted immediately. Drug-induced miscarriages may be incomplete and may lead to dangerous bleeding, surgery, infertility, or maternal or fetal death.

M

MITOMYCIN

(mye-toe-mye´sin)
Trade name: Mutamycin
Classifications: ANTINEOPLASTIC; ANTIBIOTIC
Pregnancy: Category D

ACTIONS/PHARMACODYNAMICS Potent antibiotic antineoplastic compound produced by *Streptomyces caespitosus* with wide range of antibacterial activity. Described extensively in the literature as mitomycin-C. Effective in certain tumors nonresponsive to surgery, radiation, or other chemotherapeutic agents. Action mechanism not clear but reportedly combines with DNA (attachment site unknown), thereby interfering with cellular and enzymatic RNA and protein synthesis. Mitomycin has been shown to be carcinogenic in mice and rats; thus selected patients must be aware of the inherent risk in spite of possible therapeutic benefits.

USES In combination with other chemotherapeutic agents in palliative, adjunctive treatment of disseminated adenocarcinoma of breast, pancreas, or stomach, squamous cell carcinoma of head, neck, lung, and cervix. Not recommended to replace surgery or radiotherapy or as a single primary therapeutic agent.

ROUTE & DOSAGE

Cancer

Adult	IV	20 mg/m²/d as a single dose q6–8wk; additional doses based on hematologic response

PHARMACOKINETICS Metabolism: metabolized rapidly in liver. **Elimination:** half-life: 17 min; excreted in urine.

CONTRAINDICATIONS & PRECAUTIONS Contraindicated in: hypersensitivity or idiosyncracy reaction; thrombocytopenia; coagulation disorders or bleeding tendencies; pregnancy (category D). **Cautious use in:** renal impairment; myelosuppression.

ADVERSE/SIDE EFFECTS CNS: paresthesias. **GI:** stomatitis, *nausea, vomiting,* anorexia. **Hematologic:** bone marrow toxicity *(thrombocytopenia, leukopenia* occurring 4–8 wk after treatment onset). **Respiratory:** acute bronchospasm, hemoptysis, dyspnea, nonproductive cough, pneumonia, interstitial pneumonitis. **Skin:** desquamation; induration, pain, necrosis, cellulitis at injection site; reversible alopecia, purple discoloration of nail beds. **Other:** fever (may or may not be drug induced): headache, blurred vision, drowsiness, fatigue, edema, syncope, confusion, thrombophlebitis, anemia, hematemesis, diarrhea, pain, hemolytic uremic syndrome.

INCOMPATIBILITIES Solution/Additive: DEXTROSE-CONTAINING SOLUTIONS.

NURSING IMPLICATIONS

Administration

- Patient receiving mitomycin should be hospitalized so that emergency treatment will be available.
- ***Reconstitution of IV solution:*** add sterile water for injection 10 ml to vial containing 5 mg mitomycin (and mannitol). Shake to dissolve. If product does not clear immediately, allow to stand at room temperature until solution is obtained. Reconstituted solution is purple.
- Administer reconstituted solution by direct IV over 5–10 min or longer as determined by volume of solution.
- Avoid extravasation to prevent extreme tissue reaction (cellulitis) to the toxic drug.
- Storage and stability of solutions: unreconstituted: stable for at least 4 y at room temperature. Avoid excess heat. Reconstituted with sterile water for injection (0.5 mg/ml): stable for 14 d refrigerated or 7 d at room temperature. Diluted in 5% dextrose injection (20–40 µg/ml): stable at room temperature for 3 h.

Assessment & Drug Effects

- Usually drug is not administered if serum creatinine is > 1.7 mg/dl.
- If platelet count falls below 150,000/mm³ and WBC is down to 4000/mm³ or if prothrombin or bleeding times are prolonged, treatment is suspended or modified.
- Because of cumulative myelosuppression, laboratory studies of platelet counts, prothrombin and bleeding times, differential and hemoglobin studies, serum creatinine are performed frequently during treatment and for at least 7 wk after treatment is terminated.
- Monitor I&O ratio and pattern. Any sign of impaired kidney function should be reported: change in ratio, dysuria, hematuria, oliguria, frequency, urgency. Keep patient well hydrated (at least 2000–2500 ml orally daily if tolerated). Drug is nephrotoxic.
- Observe closely for signs of infection. Monitor body temperature frequently.
- Inspect oral cavity daily for signs of stomatitis or superinfection (see chap 3).

Common side effects in *italic*; life-threatening effects underlined; generic names in **bold**; classifications in SMALL CAPS

Patient & Family Education

- Instruct patient to immediately report respiratory distress.
- Instruct patient to report immediately if signs of common cold present.
- Inform patient that alopecia is reversible with cessation of treatment.

MITOTANE

(mye´toe-tane)
Trade name: Lysodren
Classifications: ADRENOCORTICAL CYTOTOXIC; ANTINEOPLASTIC
Pregnancy: Category C

ACTIONS/PHARMACODYNAMICS Cytotoxic agent with suppressant action on the adrenal cortex. Modifies peripheral metabolism of steroids and reduces production of adrenal steroids. Extraadrenal metabolism of cortisol is altered, leading to reduction in 17-hydroxycorticosteroids (17-OHCS); however, plasma levels of corticosteroids do not fall. Apparently increases formation of 6-beta-hydroxy-cortisol.

USES Inoperable adrenal cortical carcinoma (functional and nonfunctional). **Unlabeled use:** Cushing's syndrome secondary to pituitary disorders.

ROUTE & DOSAGE

Adrenocortical Carcinoma

Adult	PO	9–10 g/d in divided doses t.i.d. or q.i.d.; tolerated doses range from 2–16 g/d

PHARMACOKINETICS Absorption: approximately 40% absorbed from GI tract. **Onset:** 2–4 wk. **Peak:** 3–5 h. **Distribution:** deposits in most body tissues, especially adipose tissue. **Metabolism:** metabolized in liver. **Elimination:** half-life: 18–159 d; small amount excreted in bile.

CONTRAINDICATIONS & PRECAUTIONS Contraindicated in: pregnancy (category C) and nursing women only after risk-benefit ratio to mother and fetus has been assessed. **Cautious use in:** hepatic disease.

ADVERSE/SIDE EFFECTS CNS: vertigo, dizziness, drowsiness, tiredness, depression, *lethargy, sedation, brain damage, impaired neurologic function.* **CV:** hypertension, hypotension, flushing. **GI:** *anorexia, nausea, vomiting, diarrhea.* **GU:** hematuria, hemorrhagic cystitis, albuminuria. **Other:** adrenocortical insufficiency, blurred vision, diplopia, lens opacity, toxic retinopathy, generalized aching, fever, cutaneous eruptions and pigmentation, muscle twitching, hypersensitivity reactions, pruritus, hyperpyrexia, *rash, hypouricemia, hypercholesterolemia.*

DIAGNOSTIC TEST INTERFERENCES Mitotane decreases *protein-bound iodine (PBI)* and *urinary 17-OHCS levels.*

DRUG INTERACTIONS Potentiates sedative effects of **alcohol** and other CNS DEPRESSANTS; may increase the metabolism of **phenytoin, phenobarbital, warfarin,** decreasing their effectiveness.

NURSING IMPLICATIONS

Administration

- Mitotane treatment is started and continued in the hospital until stable dosage regimen is established. Drug is continued at least 3 mo to determine efficacy.
- Nausea and vomiting may be reduced or alleviated by antiemetic therapy before and during drug therapy.
- If an emergency occurs, mitotane may be temporarily withdrawn, since adrenal suppression is its prime action. Exogenous steroids may be required until the already depressed adrenal starts secreting steroids.
- Store in tight, light-resistant containers at 15–30C (59–86F) unless otherwise directed.

Assessment & Drug Effects

- Monitor pulse and BP for early signs of shock (adrenal insufficiency).
- Observe for symptoms of hepatotoxicity (see chap 3). Report them promptly, since reduced hepatic capacity can increase toxicity of mitotane and because dose may have to be decreased.
- Medication causes aching muscles, fever, flushing, and muscle twitching. If these symptoms persist and become more severe, the physician should be notified.
- Monitor the obese patient for symptoms of adrenal hypofunction. Because a large portion of the drug deposits in fatty tissue, this person is particularly susceptible to prolonged side effects. A higher than average dose may be necessary.
- Long-term continuous treatment with high doses

M

may lead to brain damage. Neurologic and behavioral assessments should be made at regular intervals throughout therapy.

- If no clinical benefits are seen in 3 mo, the treatment is considered a failure. About 10% of patients have reportedly shown continued response beyond 3 mo of treatment (maintenance of clinical status or slowed growth of metastatic lesions).
- The patient frequently fails to respond to mitotane after the third or fourth course of therapy.

Patient & Family Education
- To reduce possibility of infarction and hemorrhage in a tumor due to drug action, all possible tumor tissue is surgically removed from large metastatic masses before mitotane treatment is started.
- Mitotane does not cure but reduces tumor mass; reduces pain, weakness, anorexia, and steroid symptoms.
- *Symptoms of adrenal insufficiency* (weakness, fatigue, orthostatic hypotension, pigmentation, weight loss, dehydration, anorexia, nausea, vomiting, and diarrhea) should be reported to physician.
- Advise patient to use caution when driving or performing hazardous tasks requiring alertness because of drug-induced drowsiness, tiredness, dizziness. These symptoms tend to recede with continuation in therapy.
- Contraceptive measures are advised during therapy because of teratogenic properties of the drug. If the woman suspects she is pregnant, she should notify the physician.

Prototype: chlorpromazine, p 191

MOLINDONE HYDROCHLORIDE
(moe-lin´done)
Trade name: Moban
Classifications: CNS AGENT; PSYCHOTHERAPEUTIC; PHENOTHIAZINE ANTIPSYCHOTIC (TRANQUILIZERS)
Pregnancy: Category C

ACTIONS/PHARMACODYNAMICS Dihydroindolone derivative tranquilizer, structurally unrelated but pharmacologically similar to the piperazine phenothiazines. Has less sedative but comparable anticholinergic activity and greater incidence of extrapyramidal side effects than chlorpromazine. EEG studies suggest that ascending reticular system is chief site of action. Reportedly lowers convulsive threshold and produces tranquilization without compromising alertness.

USES Management of manifestations of psychotic disorders.

ROUTE & DOSAGE

Psychotic Disorders

Adult	PO	50–75 mg/d in 3–4 divided doses; may be increased to 100 mg/d in 3–4 d; may be able to decrease to 15–60 mg/d in divided doses (max 225 mg/d)

PHARMACOKINETICS Absorption: readily absorbed from GI tract. **Peak:** 1 h. **Duration:** 24–36 h. **Distribution:** distributed into breast milk. **Metabolism:** metabolized in liver. **Elimination:** half-life: 1.5 h; excreted in urine and feces.

CONTRAINDICATIONS & PRECAUTIONS Contraindicated in: known hypersensitivity to molindone or to phenothiazines; severe CNS depression; comatose states; children < 12 y. Safe use during pregnancy (category C) and by nursing mothers has not been established. **Cautious use in:** persons who may be harmed by increase in physical activity; prostatic hypertrophy; cardiovascular disease; previously detected cancer of breast.

ADVERSE/SIDE EFFECTS *Transient drowsiness,* insomnia, *extrapyramidal symptoms* (dose related), dry mouth, tinnitus, blurred vision, nasal congestion, xerostomia, constipation, urinary retention, euphoria, mild photosensitivity, tachycardia, change in weight, SLE-like syndrome, heavy menses, amenorrhea, galactorrhea, gynecomastia, increased libido, premature ejaculation, hepatotoxicity, neuroleptic malignant syndrome.

NURSING IMPLICATIONS

Administration
- Store medication in tightly capped, light-resistant bottles. Protect from heat and moisture.

Assessment & Drug Effects
- Withhold dose and consult with physician if the following symptoms occur: tremor, involuntary

twitching, exaggerated restlessness, changes in vision, light-colored stools, sore throat, fever, rash.

- Monitor bowel pattern and urinary output. The depressed patient may not report constipation or urinary retention, both side effects of this medicine.
- Antiemetic action may mask signs of intestinal obstruction, brain disease, or drug toxicity.
- Since this drug increases motor activity, supervise ambulation and other ADL in the elderly or debilitated or patient with impaired vision to prevent injury or falling.
- In early treatment be alert to onset of parkinsonism (extrapyramidal) symptoms: rigidity, immobility, reduction of voluntary movements, tremors, fine vermicular tongue movements. Withhold dose and report promptly to physician. Usually a change in dose will interrupt progressive development of extrapyramidal side effects.

Patient & Family Education

- Counsel patient to take drug as prescribed: the patient should not alter the dose regimen or stop the medication without consulting his or her physician.
- Dizziness during early therapy usually disappears as treatment continues.
- Caution patient not to drive or engage in other activities requiring mental or physical coordination until response to the drug is known.
- Warn patient to avoid alcohol and self-medication with other depressants during therapy. Patient should receive the physician's approval before using any OTC drug.
- Xerostomia (dry mouth) may be relieved by frequent rinses with warm water and by increasing noncaloric fluid intake. Avoid use of commercial mouth rinses, which can change oral flora leading to *Candida* infection and tissue erosion. Use of a saliva substitute also helps to keep oral surfaces moist (e.g., Moi-stir, Xerolube). Discuss with physician.
- Caution patient with angina to avoid overexertion and to report increase in frequency of precordial pain.
- Conditioned avoidance behavior is suppressed by molindone, thus increasing the danger of falling and receiving burns.
- Recommend that the patient on long-term treatment have periodic ophthalmic examinations.
- Resumption of menses in previously amenorrheic patients has been reported.
- The tablet contains calcium, which may interfere with absorption of phenytoin or tetracyclines.

MONOOCTANOIN

(mon-oh-ock´ta-noyn)

Trade name: Moctanin

Classification: CHOLELITHOLYTIC

Pregnancy: Category C

ACTIONS/PHARMACODYNAMICS Semisynthetic monoglyceride detergent and cholesterol-solubilizing agent. Shrinks, softens, and dissolves cholesterol gallstones, depending on size and number. An effective alternative to removal of gallstones in some patients, superior to other solvent-type medications (e.g., chenodiol). Clinical efficacy related mainly to amount of cholesterol in the stones: i.e., degree of solubilization is more rapid and complete when cholesterol content is high; if stone is highly pigmented (bilirubinate or calcium content is high), monooctanoin is less effective. Complete dissolution is more likely when there is but one stone than when multiple stones are present; 1 ml monooctanoin can dissolve 120 mg of cholesterol.

USES To dissolve cholesterol (radiolucent) gallstones retained in the biliary tract after cholecystectomy when other means are not viable or are unsuccessful.

ROUTE & DOSAGE

Radiolucent Gallstones

Adult	Biliary Instillation	3–5 ml/h at pressure of 10 cm H$_2$O for 2–10 d (avg 5 d)

PHARMACOKINETICS Metabolism: metabolized by pancreatic lipase and other digestive enzymes to fatty acids and glycerol, which are readily absorbed by the portal vein.

CONTRAINDICATIONS & PRECAUTIONS Contraindicated in: noncholesterol gallstones; impaired hepatic function; obstructive jaundice; pancreatitis; history of intolerance of vegetable oils; recent duodenal ulcer, or jejunitis, infection. Safe use during pregnancy (category C) or by children not established. **Cautious use in:** nursing mothers, bile duct obstruction.

ADVERSE/SIDE EFFECTS CNS: drowsiness, depression. **GI:** *abdominal pain* (50%), metallic taste, epigastric burning, anorexia, *nausea* (32%), *vomiting* (20%), *diarrhea* (19%), reversible irritability of duo-

---

Common side effects in *italic*; life-threatening effects <u>underlined</u>; generic names in **bold**; classifications in SMALL CAPS

789

denal mucosa, pancreatitis (rare). **Hematologic:** leukopenia, bleeding from duodenal ulcer, hypokalemia, increase in serum amylase. **Other:** shortness of breath (acidosis from drug absorption), back pain, pruritus, fatigue, facial flushing, diaphoresis, fever.

NURSING IMPLICATIONS

Administration

- Monooctanoin is administered by continuous perfusion through a percutaneous transhepatic catheter directly inserted into the common bile duct.
- Infusion is usually administered with a positive pressure or peristaltic perfusion pump equipped with an overflow manometer. Monitor pressure to prevent exceeding 15 cm H_2O.
- Monitor flow rate carefully and adjust if necessary. If rate is too fast, incidence of GI side effects are apt to increase. Be alert to persistent nausea and diarrhea.
- Avoid extremes in room temperature during the continuous perfusion. As the temperature of monooctanoin solution drops, viscosity of the solution increases and its ability to dissolve cholesterol stones decreases. Perfusion temperature is brought to room temperature 21–27C (70–80F) before the perfusion is started and should not be allowed to drop below 18C (65F) during the treatment.
- Perfusion of monooctanoin may be interrupted for 1–2 h at mealtimes to reduce GI side effects.
- Store at room temperature.

Assessment & Drug Effects

- Discomfort from side effects may be relieved by temporary interruption of the treatment. Abdominal pain does not appear to be dose- or perfusion-rate dependent. If side effects persist, drug may have to be discontinued.
- Monitor vital signs. An elevated temperature with chills combined with severe right upper quadrant abdominal pain and jaundice suggest onset of ascending cholangitis. Report to physician.
- Correlate lab studies of WBC with patient's complaint of sore throat accompanied by fever and chills; leukopenia should be ruled out.
- Monooctanoin treatment is discontinued and alternative forms of therapy are considered if little or no gallstone dissolution occurs after 10 d of treatment (determined by repeat cholangiograms).

MORPHINE SULFATE

See CENTRAL NERVOUS SYSTEM AGENTS, ANALGESIC, ANTIPYRETIC, NARCOTIC (OPIATE) AGONIST prototype, p 156.

Prototype: cefotaxime sodium, p 62

MOXALACTAM DISODIUM
(mox′a-lak-tam)
Trade name: Moxam
Classifications: ANTIINFECTIVE; BETA-LACTAM ANTIBIOTIC; THIRD GENERATION CEPHALOSPORIN
Pregnancy: Category C

ACTIONS/PHARMACODYNAMICS Synthetic, broad-spectrum beta-lactam antibiotic with prolonged action; usually classified as third generation cephalosporin. In general, spectrum of activity resembles that of other third generation members, particularly cefotaxime. Like cefotaxime, is less active than first and second generation cephalosporins against gram-positive cocci (e.g., *Staphylococcus aureus,* group A and B streptococci, *Streptococcus pneumoniae*). Active against most gram-negative aerobes especially *Escherichia coli, Klebsiella pneumoniae,* and *Serratia marcescens.* Activity against *Pseudomonas aeruginosa* is variable, and it is usually not active against *Acinetobacter.* More highly resistant to inactivation by beta-lactamases (cephalosporinase and penicillinase) than cefotaxime and other cephalosporins. In common with other cephalosporins, acts by inhibiting cell wall synthesis and lacks activity against fungi and viruses. Moxalactam may affect vitamin K–dependent clotting factors and platelet function possibly by eliminating K-producing gut bacteria from GI tract. Unlike other cephalosporins, crosses blood-brain barrier whether or not meninges are inflamed. Contains 3.8 mEq of sodium per gram.

USES Serious infections of lower respiratory and urinary tracts, skin and skin structure, bone and joint, and for intraabdominal infections, septicemia, and meningitis. Used alone or with an aminoglycoside.

PHARMACOKINETICS Peak: 0.5–2 h after IM; 15–20 min after IV. **Distribution:** crosses blood-brain barrier and placenta. **Elimination:** half-life: 2–3.5 h;

80% excreted unchanged in urine; small amount excreted in bile.

ROUTE & DOSAGE

Moderate to Severe Infections

Adult	IV/IM	2–6 g/d divided q8–12h up to 4 g q8h
Child	IV/IM	50 mg/kg q6–8h up to 200 mg/kg or 12 g/d
Neonates	IV/IM	50 mg/kg q8–12h up to 200 mg/kg or 12 g/d

CONTRAINDICATIONS & PRECAUTIONS Contraindicated in: history of hypersensitivity to moxalactam or other cephalosporins. Safe use during pregnancy (category C) and in nursing women not established. **Cautious use in:** history of type I hypersensitivity to penicillins (urticaria, angioedema, anaphylaxis), history of other allergies, particularly to drugs; impaired renal or hepatic function; history of bleeding disorders or GI diseases, particularly colitis.

ADVERSE/SIDE EFFECTS GI: anorexia, diarrhea, nausea, vomiting, pseudomembranous colitis. **Hematologic:** *hypoprothrombinemia,* anemia, mild transient neutropenia, leukopenia, granulocytopenia, thrombocytopenia, thrombocytosis, eosinophilia, elevation of hepatic enzymes. **Hypersensitivity:** skin rash, purpura, fever, urticaria, pruritus, serum sickness–like reactions, dyspnea, angioedema. **Renal** (causal relationships not established): hematuria, pyuria, proteinuria, increases in BUN and serum creatinine. **Other:** seizures, bleeding problems including pulmonary hemorrhage. Local (site) reactions: mild burning pain (IM site); phlebitis, thrombophlebitis (following IV administration).

DIAGNOSTIC TEST INTERFERENCES Positive **direct Coombs' test** may occur (can interfere with hematologic and crossmatching procedures). Unlike other cephalosporins, moxalactam does not interfere with **urine glucose** tests.

DRUG INTERACTIONS Probenecid decreases renal elimination of moxalactam; produces disulfiram reaction with **alcohol** and ALCOHOL-CONTAINING PREPARATIONS; increases risk of bleeding with **warfarin, heparin, aspirin.**

INCOMPATIBILITIES Solution/Additive: AMINO-GLYCOSIDES. **Y-Site:** AMINOGLYCOSIDES, **labetalol, meperidine, perphenazine.**

NURSING IMPLICATIONS

Administration

- IM injections should be made deep into large muscle mass such as the upper outer quadrant of gluteus maximus. Rotate injection sites.
- For **IM administration:** moxalactam should be diluted with either sterile or bacteriostatic water, sterile or bacteriostatic 0.9% NaCl for injection, or 0.5% or 1.0% lidocaine hydrochloride injection (by prescription).
- For **direct IV administration:** dilute each 1 g in 10 ml D5W, NS, or other compatible solution; may be given by direct IV slowly over 3–5 min, or through tubing of a free-flowing compatible IV infusion solution.
- Initially diluted solution may be further diluted in 30–50 ml IV solution and given by intermittent infusion.
- Refer to manufacturer's directions for reconstitution, compatible solutions, storage, stability information, and for specific recommendations for IV administration.
- Frozen solutions of moxalactam should be allowed to thaw naturally at room temperature without warming. Do not refreeze.
- Store vials at < 26C (78F) unless otherwise directed. Protect from light.

Assessment & Drug Effects

- Culture and susceptibility tests should be performed prior to and periodically during therapy to monitor drug effectiveness and bacterial resistance. Therapy may be instituted pending test results.
- Before therapy is initiated, a careful inquiry should be made regarding previous hypersensitivity reactions to cephalosporins, penicillins, and history of previous allergies.
- Pseudomembranous colitis, a potentially life-threatening complication, should be considered a possible cause of diarrhea. Discontinuation of drug may be required.
- Monitor I&O ratio and pattern in patients with impaired renal function or who are receiving high dosages or an aminoglycoside antibiotic concomitantly. Renal status (serum creatinine, BUN, creatinine clearance) and bleeding time should be evaluated at regular intervals.
- Baseline and periodic hematologic, renal, and hepatic function tests should be performed for all patients during prolonged therapy. Patients receiving concomitant therapy with an aminoglycoside antibiotic should also have periodic audiometric tests. Bleeding time (BT), prothrombin time (PT), and partial thromboplastin time (PTT) should be moni-

M

Common side effects in *italic*; life-threatening effects underlined; generic names in **bold**; classifications in SMALL CAPS

791

tored in patients receiving > 4 g/d for more than 3 d and in patients with significantly impaired renal function.

- Prophylactic doses of vitamin K (e.g., 10 mg/wk) may be prescribed to reduce possibility of bleeding problems associated with hypoprothrombinemia. Observe patient for signs of bleeding and be alert to complaints that suggest bleeding tendencies: petechiae, ecchymoses, nosebleeds, bleeding gums, hemoptysis, bleeding from IM or IV sites, cloudy urine (possibly hematuria).
- Bleeding abnormalities associated with hypoprothrombinemia are most commonly due to low vitamin K reserves, such as occurs in the debilitated and malnourished, in postoperative patients, patients with renal or hepatic disease, or malabsorption syndromes.
- Platelet dysfunction and prolonged bleeding time are dose-dependent and usually can be avoided by limiting dosage to 4 g/d.
- If bleeding occurs because of platelet dysfunction, which may be manifested by prolonged PT, PTT, and BT, drug should be discontinued.
- Observe for and report onset of superinfections (see Signs & Symptoms, chap 3).

Patient & Family Education

- Advise patient to promptly report onset of loose stools or diarrhea.
- Advise patient to abstain from alcohol or alcohol-containing beverages during drug therapy with moxalactam and for several days after last dose. Alcohol and moxalactam may cause a disulfiram-type reaction (see chap 3).

MUPIROCIN
(mu-pi-ro´sin)
Trade name: Bactroban
Classifications: ANTIINFECTIVE; PSEUDOMONIC ACID ANTIBIOTIC
Pregnancy: Category B

ACTIONS/PHARMACODYNAMICS Mupirocin, a topical antibacterial produced by fermentation of *Pseudomonas fluorescens,* inhibits bacterial protein synthesis by binding with the bacterial transfer-RNA. Susceptible bacteria are *Staphylococcus aureus* (including methicillin-resistant and beta-lactamase-producing strains), *Staphylococcus epidermidis, Staphylococcus saprophyticus,* and *Streptococcus pyogenes.*

USES Impetigo due to *Staphylococcus aureus,* beta-hemolytic streptococci, and *Streptococcus pyogenes.*

Unlabeled uses: superficial skin infections, nasal carriage of *S. aureus.*

ROUTE & DOSAGE

Impetigo

Adult	Topical	Apply to affected area t.i.d.; if no response in 3–5 d, reevaluate; usually continue for 1–2 wk
Child	Topical	Same as for adult

Elimination of Staphylococcal Nasal Carriage

Child	Topical	Apply intranasally b.i.d. to q.i.d. for 5–14 d

PHARMACOKINETICS Absorption: not systemically absorbed.

CONTRAINDICATIONS & PRECAUTIONS Contraindicated in: hypersensitivity to any of its components and for ophthalmic use. **Cautious use in:** pregnancy (category B) and nursing mothers, burn patients.

ADVERSE/SIDE EFFECTS Burning, stinging, pain, pruritus, rash, erythema, dry skin, tenderness, swelling. **Intranasal:** local stinging, soreness, dry skin, pruritus.

DRUG INTERACTIONS Incompatible with **salicylic acid 2%;** do not mix in HYDROPHILIC VEHICLES (e.g., Aquaphor) or COAL TAR SOLUTIONS; **chloramphenicol** may interfere with bactericidal action of mupirocin.

NURSING IMPLICATIONS

Administration

- A thin layer of medication should be applied to affected area.
- The area being treated may be covered with a gauze dressing if desired.

Assessment & Drug Effects

- Prolonged or repeated therapy may result in superinfection by nonsusceptible organisms. Watch for signs and symptoms of superinfection (see chap 3).
- Patients should show a clinical response within 3–5 d; if they do not, drug use should be reevaluated.
- Discontinue the drug and notify physician if signs of contact dermatitis develop or if exudate production increases.

Patient & Family Education

- Nursing mothers should be advised to temporarily discontinue nursing while using mupirocin.

M

- If a sensitivity reaction or chemical irritation should occur (e.g., increased redness, itching, burning), discontinue drug and contact physician.

Prototype: cyclosporine, p 248

MUROMONAB-CD3

(myoo-roe-moe´nab)
Trade name: Orthoclone OKT3
Classification: IMMUNOSUPPRESSANT
Pregnancy: Category C

ACTIONS/PHARMACODYNAMICS Murine monoclonal antibody (purified $IgG_{2\alpha}$). Specifically targets the T3 (CD3) molecule in the antigenic recognition site of the human T-cell membrane. Following this antigenic challenge, CD3-positive T-cells are rapidly removed from circulation, and T-lymphocyte action leading to renal inflammation and destruction is blocked, thus reversing graft rejection. The ability of muromonab-CD3 to specifically target T-cells offers a treatment strategy in acute renal rejection that can substitute for a broad-spectrum attack on all the body's lymphocytes. Antibodies to this agent have occurred with mean time of appearance: 20 ± 2 d. When this happens, efficacy during a second challenge may be limited and serious reactions may occur. Lymphomas may follow immunosuppression therapy with muromonab-CD3; incidence is related to intensity and duration of drug-induced immunosuppression.

USES Acute allograft rejection in renal transplant patients. **Unlabeled use:** acute allograft rejection in heart and liver transplant patients.

ROUTE & DOSAGE

Transplant Rejection

Adult   IV   5 mg/d administered in < 1 min for 10–14 d

PHARMACOKINETICS Onset: the number of circulating CD3-positive T-cells decreases within minutes. **Peak:** 2–7 d. **Duration:** 7 d.

CONTRAINDICATIONS & PRECAUTIONS Contraindicated in: intolerance to any product of murine origin, patient with fluid overload; weight gain of more than 3% within week prior to treatment; infection: chickenpox (existing, recent, including recent exposure), herpes zoster. Safe use during pregnancy (category C), in children, and by nursing mothers not established. **Cautious use in:** repeated courses.

ADVERSE/SIDE EFFECTS (Especially during first 2 d of therapy): **GI:** *nausea, vomiting, diarrhea.* **Respiratory:** <u>severe pulmonary edema,</u> *dyspnea, chest pain, wheezing.* **Other:** *fever, chills,* malaise, *tremor,* tachycardia; increased susceptibility to cytomegalovirus (common), herpes simplex (common), *Pneumocystis carinii, Legionella, Cryptococcus, Serratia* organisms, and gram-negative bacteria.

NURSING IMPLICATIONS

Administration

- Muromonab-CD3 should be administered only by physician experienced with immunosuppressive therapy and management of renal transplant patients and only in area equipped with staff and facilities to deal with cardiac resuscitation.
- Drug is given by IV rapid (bolus) injection; should not be given by IV infusion or in conjunction with other drug solutions.
- *Preparation of IV solutions:* Do not shake ampule. Draw sterile solution into syringe through a low protein-binding 0.2 or 0.22 µm filter. Discard filter; attach syringe to an appropriate needle for IV bolus injection.
- Administration of IV methylprednisolone sodium succinate before and IV hydrocortisone sodium succinate 30 min after muromonab-CD3 is strongly suggested to decrease incidence of first dose reaction.
- Concomitant maintenance immunosuppressive therapy is reduced or discontinued during drug therapy with muromonab-CD3 and resumed about 3 d prior to end of therapy.
- Store at 2–8C (36–46F) unless otherwise stipulated. Avoid freezing.

Assessment & Drug Effects

- If patient has a fever exceeding 37.8C (100F) before treatment, consult physician. Immediate attempts are made to lower temperature to at least 37.8C (100F) with antipyretics before muromonab-CD3 is administered.
- The patient with pretreatment fluid overload is particularly susceptible to acute pulmonary edema (may be fatal). Should it occur, be prepared for prompt intubation, oxygenation, and corticosteroid drug administration.
- Closely monitor patient's response for 48 h for first dose reaction (occurs within 45–60 min after first dose and lasts several hours). It may occur (less se-

M

Common side effects in *italic*; life-threatening effects <u>underlined</u>; generic names in **bold**; classifications in SMALL CAPS

793

vere) after second dose; then usually does not occur with subsequent doses. Symptoms: chills, dyspnea, malaise, high fever.

- Monitor vital signs. If temperature rises above 37.8C (100F), suspect infection (commonly observed in first 45 d of therapy). Take temperature before treatment and several hours after drug administration to detect first signs of infection.

NABILONE

(na´bi-lone)
Trade name: Cesamet
Classifications: GI AGENT; ANTIEMETIC
Pregnancy: Category B
Controlled substance: Schedule II

ACTIONS/PHARMACODYNAMICS Synthetic derivative of tetrahydrocannabinol (THC), the principal psychoactive constituent of marijuana. Action mechanism not clear; inhibits vomiting control mechanism in the medulla oblongata, producing potent antiemetic activity; nontherapeutic actions are exactly like those of marijuana *(Cannabis sativa)*. Has mild anxiolytic properties that may increase its efficacy. Produces dose-dependent hypotension and minimal bronchodilatation (insufficient to produce effective bronchodilatation in the asthmatic patient).

USES Chemotherapy-induced nausea and vomiting in patient who is refractory to conventional antiemetics. Is especially effective in treatment of cisplatin-induced nausea.

ROUTE & DOSAGE

Chemotherapy-induced Nausea

Adult	PO	2 mg b.i.d. beginning 1–3 h before initiation of chemotherapy and continuing up to 48 h after chemotherapy

PHARMACOKINETICS Absorption: readily absorbed from GI tract. **Onset:** 30–60 min. **Peak:** 2 h. **Duration:** 8 h. **Metabolism:** extensively metabolized. **Elimination:** half-life: 2 h; 65% eliminated in bile, 20% in urine.

CONTRAINDICATIONS & PRECAUTIONS Contraindicated in: nausea and vomiting caused by other than chemotherapeutic agents; hypersensitivity to marijuana, sesame oil. Safe use during pregnancy (category B), by nursing mothers, or patients <18 y

not established. **Cautious use in:** first exposure especially in elderly or cardiac patient; hypertension; psychiatric illness; hepatic dysfunction; patient receiving other psychoactive drugs.

ADVERSE/SIDE EFFECTS CNS: *dizziness, drowsiness, vertigo,* ataxia, visual disturbances; *psychological high,* depression, asthenia, headache, *euphoria,* hallucinations, tremor, syncope, nightmares, confusion, seizures, toxic psychoses. **CV:** orthostatic hypotension, tachycardia. **GI:** *dry mouth (30%),* anorexia.

DRUG INTERACTIONS Alcohol and other CNS DEPRESSANTS add to CNS depression.

NURSING IMPLICATIONS

Administration

- Nabilone administration will be tailored and administered according to need.
- Prevent anticipatory or conditioned nausea and vomiting by administration of drug before the first chemotherapy treatment and by maintaining drug concentration in the body (individualize dosage). For example: administer drug 30 min before meals and 1–3 h before treatments.
- Encourage patient to sleep during expected periods of vomiting if possible. If patient awakes with nausea, give the prescribed antiemetic and urge patient to rest in bed for 30 min.

Assessment & Drug Effects

- An antiemetic can mask symptoms of overdosage from other drugs and obscure diagnosis of conditions associated with nausea (and vomiting) as primary symptoms.
- Symptoms of toxic psychosis, orthostatic hypotension, ataxia, and visual disturbances may necessitate withdrawal of drug.
- Nausea and vomiting can lead to fluid and electrolyte imbalance. Assess patient on antiemetic therapy for potential clinical problems (e.g., I&O ratio and pattern; vital signs including BP; skin turgor; urine-specific gravity; thirst; condition of oral membranes and tongue surface).

Patient & Family Education

- Relaxation techniques, positive imagery, or hypnosis may help to decrease nausea and vomiting. If patient is willing, initiate learning program with a qualified practitioner.
- Xerostomia (dry mouth) interferes with speaking and swallowing and fosters demineralization of

Common side effects in *italic*; life-threatening effects underlined; generic names in **bold**; classifications in SMALL CAPS

tooth enamel. Frequent swishing of mouth with cool water or solution of patient's choice may relieve dryness. A saliva substitute (e.g., Moi-Stir) may help.

- Effects of nabilone may persist for 72 or more hours. Alert patient and family member of possible drug-induced mood swings, behavior changes, or other neurologic side effects, which may continue for at least 3 d after last dose of nabilone.
- Caution patient to avoid driving or other potentially hazardous activities that require judgment and skills until response to nabilone is known.

Prototype: propranolol, p 109

NADOLOL
(nay-doe´lole)

Trade name: Corgard
Classifications: AUTONOMIC NERVOUS SYSTEM AGENT; BETA-ADRENERGIC ANTAGONIST (SYMPATHOLYTIC, BLOCKING AGENT); CARDIOVASCULAR AGENT; ANTIHYPERTENSIVE; ANTIANGINAL
Pregnancy: Category C

ACTIONS/PHARMACODYNAMICS Nonselective beta-adrenergic blocking agent pharmacologically and chemically similar to propranolol. Inhibits response to adrenergic stimuli by competitively blocking beta-adrenergic receptors within heart. As a result, reduces heart rate and cardiac output at rest and during exercise, and also decreases conduction velocity through AV node and myocardial automaticity. Unlike propranolol, has no membrane-stabilizing activity and little direct myocardial depressant effect. Suppression of beta$_2$-adrenergic receptors in bronchial and vascular smooth muscle can cause bronchospasm and a Raynaud's-like phenomenon. Decreases standing and supine BPs by an unknown mechanism. Reduces plasma renin activity.

USES Hypertension either alone or in combination with a diuretic. Also long-term prophylactic management of angina pectoris.

ROUTE & DOSAGE

Hypertension, Angina

Adult	PO	40 mg once/d; may increase up to 240–320 mg/d in 1–2 divided doses

PHARMACOKINETICS Absorption: 30–40% of PO dose absorbed. **Peak:** 2–4 h. **Duration:** 17–24 h. **Distribution:** widely distributed; crosses placenta; distributed in breast milk. **Metabolism:** no hepatic metabolism. **Elimination:** half-life: 10–24 h, 70% excreted in urine; also excreted in feces.

CONTRAINDICATIONS & PRECAUTIONS Contraindicated in: bronchial asthma, severe COPD, inadequate myocardial function, sinus bradycardia, greater than first-degree conduction block, overt cardiac failure, cardiogenic shock. Safe use during pregnancy (category C), in nursing mothers, and in children <18 y not established. **Cautious use in:** CHF; diabetes mellitus; hyperthyroidism; renal impairment.

ADVERSE/SIDE EFFECTS Allergic: rash, pruritus, fever, sore throat, laryngospasm, respiratory disturbances. **CNS:** *dizziness, fatigue,* sedation, headache, paresthesias, behavioral changes; rare: mental depression, hallucinations, disorientation. **CV:** *bradycardia, peripheral vascular insufficiency (Raynaud's type),* palpitation, postural hypotension, conduction or rhythm disturbances, CHF. **Eyes:** blurred vision, dry eyes. **ENT:** nasal stuffiness, tinnitus, vertigo, dry mouth. **GI:** nausea, vomiting, anorexia, diarrhea, constipation, abdominal cramps, bloating, flatulence, dry mouth. **Hematologic:** agranulocytosis, thrombocytopenia. **Other:** weight gain, sleep disturbances, dry skin, impotence.

DRUG INTERACTIONS NSAIDs may decrease hypotensive effects; may mask symptoms of a hypoglycemic reaction to **insulin,** SULFONYLUREAS; **prazosin, terazosin** may increase severe hypotensive response to first dose.

NURSING IMPLICATIONS

Administration
- May be administered without regard to food. Presence of food in GI tract does not affect rate or extent of absorption.
- If nadolol is to be discontinued, dosage should be reduced over a 1–2 wk period. Abrupt withdrawal can precipitate MI or thyroid storm in susceptible patients.
- Protect drug from light. Store at room temperature.

Assessment & Drug Effects
- Assess heart rate and BP before administration of each dose. Withhold drug and notify physician if apical pulse drops below 60 bpm or systolic BP below 90 mm Hg.

N

Common side effects in *italic*; life-threatening effects underlined; generic names in **bold**; classifications in SMALL CAPS

- Monitor weight. Advise patient to report weight gain of 1–1.5 kg (2–3 lb) in a day and any other possible signs of CHF (e.g., cough, fatigue, dyspnea, rapid pulse, edema).
- Therapeutic effectiveness for patients with angina is evaluated by reduction in frequency of anginal attacks and improved exercise tolerance. Improvement should coincide with steady state serum concentration reached within 6–9 d. Keep physician informed of drug effect.
- Patients with diabetes mellitus should be closely monitored. Beta-adrenergic blockade produced by nadolol may prevent important clinical manifestations of hypoglycemia (e.g., tachycardia, BP changes).
- Monitor I&O ratio and creatinine clearance in patients with impaired renal function or with cardiac problems. Dosage intervals will be lengthened with decreases in creatinine clearance.

Patient & Family Education

- Patient should know usual pulse rate and be taught to check it before taking each dose. Instruct patient to withhold medication and to consult physician if pulse rate drops below 60 or becomes irregular.
- Emphasize importance of compliance and caution patient not to stop medication or alter dosage without consulting physician.
- Caution patient to avoid driving and other potentially hazardous activities until reaction to drug is known.

Prototype: penicillin G potassium, p 71

NAFCILLIN SODIUM
(naf-sill´in)

Trade names: Nafcil, Nallpen, Unipen
Classifications: ANTIINFECTIVE; BETA-LACTAM ANTIBIOTIC; PENICILLIN
Pregnancy: Category B

ACTIONS/PHARMACODYNAMICS Semisynthetic, acid-stable, penicillinase-resistant penicillin. Mechanism of bactericidal action, contraindications, precautions, and adverse reactions as for penicillin G. Effective against both penicillin-sensitive and penicillin-resistant strains of *Staphylococcus aureus*. Also active against pneumococci and group A beta-hemolytic streptococci. Highly active against penicilinase-producing staphylococci but less potent than penicillin G against penicillin-sensitive microorganisms and generally ineffective against methicillin-resistant staphylococci.

USES Primarily, infections caused by penicillinase-producing staphylococci. May also be used to initiate treatment in suspected staphylococcal infections pending culture and sensitivity test results. As with other penicillins, serum concentrations are considerably enhanced by concurrent use of probenecid.

ROUTE & DOSAGE

Staphylococcal Infections

Adult	IM/IV	500 mg–2 g q4–6h up to 12 g/d
	PO	250–1000 mg q4–6h
Child	IM/IV	100–300 mg/kg/d divided q4–6h
	PO	50–100 mg/kg/d in 4 divided doses

PHARMACOKINETICS Absorption: incompletely and erratically absorbed orally. **Peak:** 30–120 min IM; 15 min IV. **Duration:** 4 h PO; 4–6 h IM. **Distribution:** distributes into CNS with inflamed meninges; crosses placenta; distributed into breast milk. **Metabolism:** enters enterohepatic circulation. **Elimination:** half-life: 1 h; primarily excreted in bile; 10–30% excreted in urine.

CONTRAINDICATIONS & PRECAUTIONS Contraindicated in: hypersensitivity to penicillins, cephalosporins, and other allergens; use of oral drug in severe infections, gastric dilatation, cardiospasm, or intestinal hypermotility; IV use in neonates and infants. Safe use during pregnancy (category B) not established. **Cautious use in:** history of or suspected atopy or allergy (eczema, hives, hay fever, asthma).

ADVERSE/SIDE EFFECTS Nausea, vomiting, *diarrhea*. **Allergic:** urticaria, pruritus, rash, eosinophilia, drug fever, <u>anaphylaxis</u> (particularly following parenteral therapy), allergic interstitial nephritis. Pain and tissue irritation and increase in serum transaminase activity (following IM); hypokalemia (with high IV doses); thrombophlebitis following IV; neutropenia (long-term therapy).

DIAGNOSTIC TEST INTERFERENCES Nafcillin in large doses can cause false-positive *urine protein* tests using sulfosalicylic acid method.

DRUG INTERACTIONS May antagonize hypoprothrombinemic effects of **warfarin.**

Common side effects in *italic*; life-threatening effects <u>underlined</u>; generic names in **bold**; classifications in SMALL CAPS

INCOMPATIBILITIES Solution/Additive: aminophylline, ascorbic acid, aztreonam, bleomycin, cytarabine, hydrocortisone, methylprednisolone, promazine. Y-Site: droperidol, Innovar, labetalol, nalbuphine, pentazocine, verapamil.

NURSING IMPLICATIONS

Administration

- Oral dose is best taken on an empty stomach (at least 1 h before or 2 h after meals), since food interferes with absorption. Additionally, GI absorption of nafcillin is erratic.
- Oral solution should be dated after reconstitution and refrigerated. Discard unused portions after 1 wk.
- For IM injection, reconstitute with sterile water for injection, 0.9% NaCl injection, or bacteriostatic water for injection (with benzyl alcohol or parabens). Follow manufacturer's directions for attaining desired concentration.
- Following reconstitution, IM solutions are stable for 7 d under refrigeration and for 3 d at room temperature. Vial should be labeled and dated.
- *IM injection in adults:* Inject deeply into gluteal muscle. Make certain solution is clear. Select site carefully. Injection into or near major peripheral nerves or local vessels can result in neurovascular damage. Rotate injection sites.
- *IM injection in children:* The preferred IM site in children <3 y is the midlateral or anterolateral thigh. Follow agency policy.
- *IV injection:* required dose should be diluted with 15–30 ml sterile water for injection or isotonic NaCl for injection and administered over 5–10 min period, either directly or into tubing of running IV infusion.
- *Continuous IV infusion:* concentration of drug should be within range of 2–40 mg/ml. Rate and volume of infusion should be adjusted so that desired dose is administered before solution loses its stability.
- Compatible IV infusion solutions include isotonic NaCl; 5% dextrose in water or in 0.4% NaCl; Ringer's injection; or sodium lactate (30 mg/ml concentration). Discard unused portions 24 h after reconstitution.

Assessment & Drug Effects

- Culture and sensitivity tests should be performed prior to initiation of therapy and periodically thereafter.
- A careful history should be obtained before therapy to determine any prior allergic reactions to penicillins, cephalosporins, and other allergens.

- IV therapy is usually not given for more than 24–48 h because of the possibility of thrombophlebitis (see Signs & Symptoms, chap 3), particularly in the elderly. Inspect IV site for inflammatory reaction. Also check IV site for leakage; in the elderly patient especially, loss of tissue elasticity with aging may promote extravasation around the needle.
- Allergic reactions, principally rash, occur most commonly. Nausea, vomiting, and diarrhea may occur with oral therapy.
- Twice weekly differential WBC counts are advised in patients receiving IV nafcillin therapy for longer than 2 wk. Nafcillin-induced neutropenia (agranulocytosis) occurs commonly during third week of therapy. It may be associated with malaise, fever, sore mouth, or throat.
- Periodic assessments of hepatic and renal functions are advised during prolonged therapy.
- Be alert for signs of bacterial or fungal superinfections (see chap 3) in patient on prolonged therapy.
- Nafcillin sodium contains approximately 3 mEq of sodium per gram. Determine IV sodium intake for patients with sodium restriction.

Patient & Family Education

- Instruct patient to promptly report signs and symptoms of neutropenia (see assessment & drug effects), superinfection, or hypokalemia (see chap 3).

Prototype: amphotericin B, p 56

NAFTIFINE HYDROCHLORIDE
(naf´ti-feen)
Trade name: Naftin
Classifications: SKIN AGENT; ANTIINFECTIVE; ANTIBIOTIC; ANTIFUNGAL
Pregnancy: Category B

N

ACTIONS/PHARMACODYNAMICS Naftifine is a broad-spectrum antifungal agent. It is fungicidal against *Trichophyton rubrum*, *Trichophyton mentagrophytes*, *Trichophyton tonsurans*, *Epidermophyton floccosum*, *Microsporum canis*, *Microsporum audouinii*, and *Microsporum gypseum* and fungistatic against *Candida* sp, including *Candida albicans*. Although the exact mechanism against fungi is not known, naftifine appears to interfere with sterol biosynthesis in the fungi.

USES Topical treatment of tinea pedis, tinea cruris, and tinea corporis.

ROUTE & DOSAGE

Tinea Infections

Adult	Topical	Apply to affected area b.i.d. in morning and evening

PHARMACOKINETICS Absorption: approximately 6% is absorbed systemically. **Duration:** retained in skin in fungistatic concentrations for 24 h. **Elimination:** half-life: 2–3 d; excreted in urine and feces.

CONTRAINDICATIONS & PRECAUTIONS Contraindicated in: hypersensitivity to naftifine. **Cautious use in:** pregnancy (category B) and nursing mothers. Safety and efficacy for use in children have not been established.

ADVERSE/SIDE EFFECTS Transient burning and stinging, dryness, erythema, pruritus, and local irritation.

NURSING IMPLICATIONS

Administration

▪ Gently massage a sufficient quantity using gloves into the affected area and surrounding skin once a day with the cream, twice a day (morning and evening) with the gel. Wash hands after application.
▪ Treatment should continue 1–2 wk after symptoms subside.

Assessment & Drug Effects

▪ Clinical improvement should be seen within 4 wk.

Patient & Family Education

▪ Advise patient to avoid use of occlusive dressings or wrappings unless directed by the physician.
▪ Advise patient to avoid contact with eyes, nose, mouth, and other mucous membranes.
▪ If no improvement is seen after 4 wks, instruct patient to consult physician.
▪ Instruct patient to use topical naftifine for the full prescribed treatment period, usually 1–2 wk after symptoms subside.
▪ If irritation or sensitivity develops, advise patient to discontinue the drug and contact physician.

Prototype: morphine, p 156

NALBUPHINE HYDROCHLORIDE
(nal´byoo-feen)
Trade name: Nubain
Classifications: CNS AGENT; ANTIPYRETIC; ANALGESIC; NARCOTIC (OPIATE) AGONIST
Pregnancy: Category B

ACTIONS/PHARMACODYNAMICS Synthetic narcotic analgesic with agonist and weak antagonist properties. Structurally similar to naloxone and oxymorphone, but pharmacologic effects are like those of pentazocine and butorphanol. Analgesic potency is about 3 or 4 times greater than that of pentazocine and approximately equal to that produced by equivalent doses of morphine. On a weight basis, produces respiratory depression about equal to that of morphine; however, in contrast to morphine, doses > 30 mg produce no further respiratory depression. Antagonistic potency is approximately one fourth that of naloxone and about 10 times greater than that of pentazocine.

USES Symptomatic relief of moderate to severe pain. Also preoperative sedation analgesia and as a supplement to surgical anesthesia.

ROUTE & DOSAGE

Moderate to Severe Pain

Adult	SC/IM/IV	10–20 mg q3–6h prn (max 160 mg/d)

PHARMACOKINETICS Onset: 2–3 min IV; 15 min IM. **Peak:** 30 min IV. **Duration:** 3–6 h. **Distribution:** crosses placenta. **Metabolism:** metabolized in liver. **Elimination:** half-life: 5 h; eliminated in urine.

CONTRAINDICATIONS & PRECAUTIONS Contraindicated in: history of hypersensitivity to drug. Safe use during pregnancy (category B) and in patients <18 y not established. **Cautious use in:** history of emotional instability or drug abuse; head injury, increased intracranial pressure; impaired respirations; impaired renal or hepatic function; MI; biliary tract surgery.

ADVERSE/SIDE EFFECTS *Sedation; sweaty, clammy skin; nausea, vomiting, dizziness,* dry mouth, vertigo. **CNS:** nervousness, depression, restlessness, crying, euphoria, dysphoria, distortion of body image, unusual dreams, confusion, hallucinations; numbness and tingling sensations, headache, miosis. **CV:** hypertension, hypotension, bradycardia, tachycardia, flushing. **GI:** abdominal cramps, bitter taste. **Hypersensitivity:** pruritus, urticaria, burning sensation. **Respiratory:** dyspnea, asthma, respiratory depression. **Other:** speech difficulty, urinary urgency, blurred vision.

DRUG INTERACTIONS Alcohol and other CNS DEPRESSANTS add to CNS depression.

INCOMPATIBILITIES Solution/Additive: diazepam, pentobarbital, promethazine, thiethylperazine. Y-Site: nafcillin.

NURSING IMPLICATIONS

Administration

- May be given by direct IV undiluted at a rate of 10 mg over 3–5 min.
- Protect nalbuphine from light and store at 15–30C (59–86F) unless otherwise directed.

Assessment & Drug Effects

- Assess respiratory rate before drug administration. Withhold drug and notify physician if respiratory rate falls below 12.
- May produce allergic response in persons with sulfite sensitivity.
- Administer with caution to patients with hepatic or renal impairment.
- May produce drowsiness. Monitor ambulatory patients.
- Use of drug during labor and delivery may cause respiratory depression of newborn.
- Abrupt termination of nalbuphine following prolonged use may result in symptoms similar to narcotic withdrawal: nausea, vomiting, abdominal cramps, lacrimation, nasal congestion, piloerection, fever, restlessness, anxiety.

Patient & Family Education

- Caution patient to avoid driving and other potentially hazardous activities until reaction to drug is determined.
- Inform patient that concurrent use of alcohol and other CNS depressants may result in additive effects.

Prototype: ciprofloxacin, p 87

NALIDIXIC ACID

(nal-i-dix´ik)
Trade name: NegGram
Classifications: URINARY TRACT ANTIINFECTIVE; ANTIBIOTIC; QUINOLONE
Pregnancy: Category B

ACTIONS/PHARMACODYNAMICS Synthetic quinolone with marked bactericidal activity against most gram-negative urinary tract pathogens with the exception of strains of *Pseudomonas*. Also effective against some strains of *Shigella* and *Salmonella*. Gram-positive bacteria are relatively resistant to drug action. Intracellular action (by unknown mechanism) inhibits microbial DNA replication and RNA synthesis. No antagonism or synergism has been reported with cephalosporins or penicillins, but bacterial resistance has been reported (2–14% of patients). Antibacterial activity is not substantially affected by pH changes in urine.

USES Urinary tract infections caused by susceptible gram-negative organisms including most *Proteus* strains, *Klebsiella*, *Enterobacter*, and *Escherichia coli*. **Unlabeled uses:** GI tract infections caused by susceptible strains of *Shigella sonnei;* prophylaxis of bacteriuria and in bladder irrigation for low-grade cystitis.

ROUTE & DOSAGE

Urinary Tract Infections

Adult	PO	Acute therapy: 1 g q.i.d.
		Chronic therapy: 500 mg q.i.d.
Child	PO	> 3 mo: Acute therapy: 55 mg/kg/d in 4 divided doses
		Chronic therapy: 33 mg/kg/d in 4 divided doses

PHARMACOKINETICS Absorption: readily absorbed from GI tract. **Peak:** urine: 3–4 h. **Distribution:** crosses placenta; distributed into breast milk. **Metabolism:** partially metabolized in liver; some metabolism in kidneys. **Elimination:** half-life: 1.1–2.5 h; excreted in urine.

CONTRAINDICATIONS & PRECAUTIONS Contraindicated in: history of convulsive disorders; first trimester of pregnancy; infants <3 mo of age. **Cautious**

use in: prepubertal child; second and third trimesters of pregnancy (category B), renal or hepatic disease; epilepsy; cerebral arteriosclerosis; respiratory insufficiency, patients with G6PD deficiency.

ADVERSE/SIDE EFFECTS CNS: drowsiness, headache, malaise, dizziness, vertigo, syncope, weakness, myalgia, peripheral neuritis, confusion, excitement, mental depression, seizures (in epilepsy), insomnia. Rare: increased intracranial pressure, acute psychoses, sixth cranial nerve palsy, paresthesia. **Eye:** visual disturbances: blurred vision, difficulty in focusing, decreased visual acuity, double vision, altered color perception; light intolerance, eye pain or burning, nystagmus. **GI:** abdominal pain, *nausea, vomiting,* diarrhea. **Hematologic:** eosinophilia, thrombocytopenia, leukopenia, hemolytic anemia (especially in G6PD deficiency). **Hypersensitivity:** photosensitivity, angioedema, pruritus, urticaria, rash, fever, chills, arthralgia, hypersensitivity pneumonitis, anaphylaxis (rare). **Other:** cholestasis, metabolic acidosis, cartilage erosions in weight-bearing joints and other signs of arthropathy, especially in prepubertal child; transient increase in AST, BUN, and serum creatinine concentrations.

DIAGNOSTIC TEST INTERFERENCE False-positive urine tests for **glucose** with cupric sulfate reagent (e.g., Benedict's or Clinitest) but not with glucose oxidase methods (e.g., Clinstix, TesTape). May cause elevation of **urinary 17-ketosteroids** (Zimmerman method) and urine **vanillymandelic acid** (VMA).

DRUG INTERACTIONS Antacids may decrease absorption of nalidixic acid; may increase hypoprothrombinemic effects of **warfarin.**

NURSING IMPLICATIONS

Administration
- Reportedly, blood concentrations are increased when drug is administered at least 1 h before meals. If patient complains of GI distress, administer with food or milk.
- Store in tight container at 15–30C (59–86F). Avoid freezing.

Assessment & Drug Effects
- Culture and susceptibility tests are advised prior to initiation of treatment and periodically thereafter. Bacterial resistance sometimes develops within 48 h after start of therapy.
- CNS reactions tend to occur 30 min after initiation of treatment or after second or third dose. Infants, children, and the elderly are especially susceptible. Report immediately the onset of marked irritability, vomiting, bulging of anterior fontanelle, headache, excitement or drowsiness, papilledema, vertigo.
- Blood counts and renal and hepatic function tests are recommended if therapy is continued longer than 2 wk.
- **Overdose symptoms:** increased intracranial pressure, toxic psychosis, convulsions, metabolic acidosis, vomiting, lethargy.

Patient & Family Education
- Caution patient to use drug exactly as prescribed and not to change dosage. Omitted doses, especially in early days of therapy, may promote development of bacterial resistance. Patient should take full amount of medication.
- Patient should be made aware of what to do when a dose of nalidixic acid is missed.
- Encourage patient to maintain adequate hydration (2000–3000 ml/d if tolerated) during treatment period. If I&O ratio or pattern changes, consult physician.
- Advise parent to observe how prepubertal child walks. If child limps or complains of joint pain, promptly report to physician.
- Caution patient to avoid exposure to direct sunlight or ultraviolet light while receiving drug. Therapy should be discontinued if photosensitivity occurs (erythema or bullae). Susceptible patients may be photosensitive up to 3 mo after termination of drug.
- Subjective visual disturbances may occur during first few days of therapy. Report to physician. Symptoms usually disappear promptly with reduction of dosage or discontinuation of therapy.

NALOXONE HYDROCHLORIDE

(nal-ox´one)
Trade name: Narcan
Classifications: CNS AGENT; NARCOTIC (OPIATE) ANTAGONIST
Pregnancy: Category B

ACTIONS/PHARMACODYNAMICS *N*-allyl analog of oxymorphone. A "pure" narcotic antagonist, essentially free of agonistic (morphinelike) properties. Thus, unlike the narcotic antagonist levallorphan, produces no significant analgesia, respiratory depression, psychotomimetic effects, or miosis when administered in the absence of narcotics and possesses more potent narcotic antagonist action. Not effective against non-opioid-induced respiratory depression. Tolerance and psychic or physical dependence not reported.

USES Narcotic overdosage and for complete or partial reversal of narcotic depression including respiratory depression induced by natural and synthetic narcotics and by pentazocine and propoxyphene. Drug of choice when nature of depressant drug is not known and for diagnosis of suspected acute opioid overdosage. **Unlabeled uses:** shock and to reverse alcohol-induced or clonidine-induced coma or respiratory depression.

ROUTE & DOSAGE

Opiate Overdose

Adult	IV	0.4–2 mg; may be repeated q2–3min up to 10 mg if necessary
Child	IV	0.01 mg/kg; may be repeated q2–3min up to 10 mg if necessary

Postoperative Opiate Depression

Adult	IV	0.1–0.2 mg; may be repeated q2–3min for up to 3 doses if necessary
Child	IV	0.005–0.01 mg/kg; may be repeated q2–3min up to 3 doses if necessary

Asphyxia Neonatorum

Child	IV	0.01 mg/kg into umbilical vein; may be repeated q2–3min up to 3 doses if necessary

PHARMACOKINETICS Onset: 2 min. **Duration:** 45 min. **Distribution:** crosses placenta. **Metabolism:** metabolized in liver. **Elimination:** half-life: 60–90 min; excreted in urine.

CONTRAINDICATIONS & PRECAUTIONS Contraindicated in: respiratory depression due to nonopioid drugs. Safe use during pregnancy (other than labor) (category B) and in nursing mothers not established. **Cautious use in:** neonates and children; known or suspected narcotic dependence; cardiac irritability.

ADVERSE/SIDE EFFECTS *Excessive dosage in narcotic depression:* reversal of analgesia, increased BP, tremors, hyperventilation, slight drowsiness, elevated partial thromboplastin time. *Too rapid reversal:* nausea, vomiting, sweating, tachycardia.

NURSING IMPLICATIONS

Administration

- May be given rapidly by direct IV in 0.1–0.2 mg increments at 2–3 min intervals until desired narcotic reversal is achieved.
- Do not mix naloxone with preparations containing a metabisulfite or bisulfite or high molecular weight anions (e.g., dextran) or with alkaline pH solutions. Compatible admixtures should be used within 24 h.
- Protect drug from excessive light. Store at 15–30C (59–86F).

Assessment & Drug Effects

- Duration of action of some narcotics may exceed that of naloxone; therefore, patient must be closely observed. Keep physician informed; repeat naloxone dose may be necessary.
- Narcotic abstinence symptoms induced by naloxone generally start to diminish 20–40 min after administration and usually disappear within 90 min.
- Monitor respirations and other vital signs. In some patients, respirations may "overshoot" to higher level than that prior to respiratory depression.
- Surgical and obstetric patients should be closely monitored for bleeding. Naloxone has been associated with abnormal coagulation test results. Also observe for reversal of analgesia, which may be manifested by nausea, vomiting, sweating, tachycardia.

NALTREXONE HYDROCHLORIDE
(nal-trex´one)
Trade name: Trexan
Classifications: CNS AGENT; NARCOTIC (OPIATE) ANTAGONIST
Pregnancy: Category C

ACTIONS/PHARMACODYNAMICS A pure opioid antagonist with prolonged pharmacologic effect; structurally and pharmacologically similar to naloxone. Weakens or completely and reversibly blocks the subjective effects (the "high") of IV opioids and analgesics possessing both agonist and antagonist activity (e.g., butorphanol). Mechanism of action not clearly delineated, but it appears that competitive binding at opioid receptor sites reduces euphoria and drug craving without supporting the addiction. Since the antagonist action is provided by competition, it is surmountable, but only with dangerously large doses of a narcotic. When administered chronically with morphine, it blocks physical dependence on morphine. In general, efficacy of this nonaddicting drug depends on its pure antagonist effect and upon a motivated, relatively opiate-free subject ("postaddict").

USES Adjunct to the maintenance of an opioid-free state in detoxified addicts who are and desire to remain narcotic free. **Unlabeled uses:** two other compulsive consumption syndromes: alcoholism and obesity.

ROUTE & DOSAGE

Treatment of Opiate Cessation

Adult	PO	25 mg followed by another 25 mg in 1 h if no withdrawal response. Maintenance regimen is individualized (up to 800 mg/d)

PHARMACOKINETICS Absorption: rapidly absorbed from GI tract; 20% reaches systemic circulation (first pass effect). **Onset:** 15–30 min. **Peak:** 1 h. **Duration:** 24–72 h. **Metabolism:** metabolized in liver to active metabolite. **Elimination:** half-life: 10–13 h; excreted in urine.

CONTRAINDICATIONS & PRECAUTIONS Contraindicated in: patient who is receiving opioid analgesics or is in acute opioid withdrawal; the opioid-dependent patient; acute hepatitis, liver failure. Also contraindicated in any individual who (1) fails naloxone challenge, (2) has a positive urine screen for opioids, or (3) has a history of sensitivity to naltrexone. Safe use during pregnancy (category C), by children <18 y, or by nursing mothers not established.

ADVERSE/SIDE EFFECTS CNS: *difficulty sleeping,* nightmares, bad dreams, *anxiety, headache, nervousness,* reduced or increased energy, irritability, dizziness, depression, fatigue, drowsiness, restlessness, confusion, hallucinations, paranoia. **CV:** epistaxis, phlebitis, edema, hypertension, palpitations, tachycardia, nonspecific ECG changes. **GI:** dry mouth, anorexia, *nausea, vomiting,* diarrhea, constipation, *abdominal cramps/pain,* excess gas, hemorrhoids, ulcer, <u>hepatotoxicity</u>. **GU:** delayed ejaculation, decreased potency; increased frequency, painful urination, changed libido. **Musculoskeletal:** *muscle and joint pains,* tremors. **Respiratory:** nasal congestion, rhinorrhea, sneezing, sore throat, excess mucus, sinus trouble, hoarseness, cough, chest pain. **Skin:** skin rash, urticaria, pruritus, oily skin, acne, alopecia. **Special senses:** blurred vision; burning, light sensitivity; swollen, aching, strained eyes; "clogged" or aching ears, tinnitus. **Other:** weight gain or loss, chills, increased thirst, yawning, fever, inguinal pain, cold feet, excessive sweating.

NURSING IMPLICATIONS

Administration

- Treatment is not started until naloxone challenge is negative, patient has been opioid free 7–10 d (as verified by urine analysis for opioids), and patient reports or manifests no withdrawal symptoms.
- Compliance may be improved by establishing a maintenance schedule of dosing q48–72h.

Assessment & Drug Effects

The naloxone challenge test (administered IV or SC) is given before starting the abstinence program with naltrexone:

- A portion of the IV dose is injected, and with the needle left in place the patient is observed for 30 seconds for *withdrawal symptoms:* stuffiness or runny nose, tearing, yawning, sweating, tremors, vomiting, gooseflesh, feeling of temperature change, bone, joint, and muscle pains, abdominal cramps. If none, remainder of dose is injected and patient is observed for the next 20 min.
- The SC dose is followed by an observation period of 45 min for symptoms of withdrawal.
- Question patient during observation periods to assist in recognition of withdrawal should it occur.
- *Interpretation:* Evidence of withdrawal symptoms indicates that the patient is a potential risk and should not enter a naltrexone program. If no signs or symptoms appear, drug therapy can begin. In case of doubt that the patient is opioid free, confirmatory rechallenge is done.
- Accidental ingestion of naltrexone by an opioid-dependent individual causes withdrawal symptoms to appear within 5 min and to remain for as long as 48 h. Fluid therapy to replace losses by vomiting and diarrhea, monitoring for respiratory and cardiac symptoms, and protective treatment measures because of changes in mental state are provided during the recovery period.
- Liver function tests are checked before the treatment is started, at monthly intervals for 6 mo, and then periodically as indicated.

Patient & Family Education

- Heroin addiction has been successively treated with methadone, although disadvantages are serious: it causes euphoria or sedation, is addictive, and is dangerous in overdosage. Transfer from methadone to naltrexone may be desirable and can

Common side effects in *italic;* life-threatening effects <u>underlined;</u>
generic names in **bold**; classifications in SMALL CAPS

be done after gradual withdrawal and final discontinuation of methadone.

- The patient should be instructed to report promptly onset of signs of hepatic toxicity (see chap 3). The drug will be discontinued.
- Advise patient not to self-dose with OTC drugs for treatment of cough, colds, diarrhea, or analgesia. Many available preparations contain small doses of an opioid. Consult physician for safe drugs if they are needed.
- A doctor or dentist who treats a naltrexone user should be informed of the drug use.
- **Opioid overdose syndrome** comprises coma, flaccid paralysis, miosis, and respiratory depression. Discuss with the patient the danger of overdosing with an opiate while on naltrexone therapy. Small doses even at frequent intervals will give no desired effects; however, a dose large enough to produce a high is dangerous and may be fatal.
- Advise patient to wear identification jewelry indicating naltrexone use.

Prototype: testosterone, p 229

NANDROLONE DECANOATE

(nan'droe-lone)

Trade names: Anabolin LA, Analone, Androlone-D, Deca-Durabolin, Hybolin Decaneate

NANDROLONE PHENPROPIONATE

Trade names: Anabolin, Androlone, Durabolin, Hybolin Improved, Nandrobolic
Classifications: SYNTHETIC HORMONE; ANABOLIC/ANDROGEN STEROID
Pregnancy: Category X
Controlled substance: Schedule III

ACTIONS/PHARMACODYNAMICS Synthetic steroid with high ratio of anabolic activity to androgenic activity. Both esters have same actions and uses but differ in action duration: decanoate actions last 3–4 wk; phenpropionate ester continues to exert anabolic effect for 1–3 wk.

USES Control of metastatic breast cancer, management of anemia of renal insufficiency.

CONTRAINDICATIONS & PRECAUTIONS Contraindicated in: pregnancy (category X); males with prostate or breast cancer, hepatic dysfunction,

nephrotic syndrome, hypercalcemia. **Cautious use in:** benign prostatic hypertrophy, history of MI.

ROUTE & DOSAGE

Anemia (Decanoate)

Adult	IM	50–200 mg/wk
Child	IM	2–13 y: 25–50 mg q3–4wk

Metastatic Breast Cancer (Phenpropionate)

Adult	IM	50–100 mg/wk

ADVERSE/SIDE EFFECTS GI: *nausea, vomiting,* diarrhea, anorexia, abdominal fullness, cholestatic jaundice, <u>hepatic necrosis, hepatocellular neoplasms</u>. **CNS:** excitation, insomnia, chills, toxic confusion. **Endocrine:** *acne, virilization.* **Metabolic:** sodium, chloride, water, potassium, phosphate, and calcium retention, ankle edema, glucose intolerance. **Other:** muscle cramps, increased cholesterol, leukopenia.

DRUG INTERACTIONS May increase hypoprothrombinemic effects of **warfarin;** may decrease **insulin** and SULFONYLUREA requirements; CORTICOSTEROIDS may increase edema.

NURSING IMPLICATIONS

Administration
- Inject drug deep IM, preferably into gluteal muscle in adult; follow agency policy regarding IM site in small child.
- Intermittent therapy is usually recommended (4 mo course of treatment followed by 6–8 wk rest period).

Assessment & Drug Effects
- Baseline and periodic liver function evaluations and electrolyte levels are recommended. Monitor for signs and symptoms of hepatic toxicity (see chap 3) and electrolyte imbalance, especially hyperkalemia and hypercalcemia (see chap 3).
- Drug may interfere with glycemic regulation in diabetics.

Patient & Family Education
- Inform women of the potential for virilization (e.g., increased facial and body hair, deepening of voice).

NAPHAZOLINE HYDROCHLORIDE

See EYE, EAR, NOSE & THROAT PREPARATIONS, VASOCONSTRICTOR, DECONGESTANT prototype, p 211.

Common side effects in *italic*; life-threatening effects <u>underlined</u>; generic names in **bold**; classifications in SMALL CAPS

803

Prototype: ibuprofen, p 160

NAPROXEN

(na-prox´en)
Trade names: Apo-Naproxen, Naprosyn, Naxen, Novonaprox

NAPROXEN SODIUM

Trade names: Anaprox, Anaprox DS
Classifications: CNS AGENT; ANTIPYRETIC; NONNARCOTIC ANALGESIC; NSAID
Pregnancy: Category B

ACTIONS/PHARMACODYNAMICS Propionic acid derivative. Nonsteroidal antiinflammatory drug (NSAID) with analgesic and antipyretic properties similar to those of other propionic acid derivatives, e.g., ibuprofen, fenoprofen, ketoprofen. Mechanism of action thought to be related to inhibition of prostaglandin synthesis. In common with other drugs of this group, inhibits platelet aggregation and prolongs bleeding time but does not alter whole blood clotting or prothrombin time or platelet count. Cross-sensitivity with other NSAIDs has been reported. Naproxen does not appear to have uricosuric activity.

USES Antiinflammatory and analgesic effects in symptomatic treatment of acute and chronic rheumatoid arthritis, juvenile arthritis (naproxen only), and for treatment of primary dysmenorrhea. Also management of ankylosing spondylitis, osteoarthritis, and gout. **Unlabeled uses:** Paget's disease of bone, Bartter's syndrome.

ROUTE & DOSAGE

275 mg naproxen sodium = 250 mg naproxen

Inflammatory Disease

Adult	PO	250–500 mg b.i.d. (max 1000 mg/d naproxen, 1100 mg/d naproxen sodium)
Child	PO	10 mg/kg/d in 2 divided doses

Mild to Moderate Pain, Dysmenorrhea

Adult	PO	500 mg followed by 250 mg q6–8h prn up to 1250 mg/d

PHARMACOKINETICS Absorption: almost completely absorbed from GI tract when taken on empty stomach. **Peak:** 2 h naproxen; 1 h naproxen sodium. **Duration:** 7 h. **Metabolism:** metabolized in liver. **Elimination:** half-life: 12–15 h; excreted primarily in urine; some biliary excretion (<1%).

CONTRAINDICATIONS & PRECAUTIONS Contraindicated in: active peptic ulcer; patients in whom asthma, rhinitis, urticaria, bronchospasm, or shock is precipitated by aspirin or other NSAIDs. Safe use during pregnancy (category B), in nursing mothers, or in children <2 y not established. **Cautious use in:** history of upper GI tract disorders; impaired renal, hepatic, or cardiac function; patients on sodium restriction (naproxen sodium); low pretreatment Hgb concentration; fluid retention, hypertension, heart failure; geriatric patients.

ADVERSE/SIDE EFFECTS CNS: *headache, drowsiness, dizziness,* lightheadedness, depression. **CV:** palpitation, dyspnea, peripheral edema. **Eye; ear:** blurred vision, tinnitus, hearing loss. **GI:** *anorexia, heartburn,* indigestion, *nausea,* vomiting, GI bleeding. **Hematologic:** agranulocytosis, thrombocytopenia. **Skin:** pruritus, rash, ecchymosis. **Other:** thirst, menstrual disturbances, nephrotoxicity, jaundice, pseudoporphyria, (photosensitivity phenomenon), pulmonary edema, elevated serum ALT, AST.

DIAGNOSTIC TEST INTERFERENCES Transient elevations in *BUN* and serum *alkaline phosphatase* may occur. Naproxen may interfere with some urinary assays of *5-HIAA* and may cause falsely high *urinary 17-KGS* levels (using *m*-dinitrobenzene reagent). Naproxen should be withdrawn 72 h before adrenal function tests.

DRUG INTERACTIONS Bleeding time effects of ORAL ANTICOAGULANTS, **heparin** may be prolonged; may increase **lithium** toxicity.

NURSING IMPLICATIONS

Administration

- May be administered with food or an antacid (if prescribed) to reduce incidence of GI upset. Food and some antacids (e.g., magnesium oxide and aluminum hydroxide) delay absorption of naproxen but apparently not total amount absorbed. Absorption is reportedly enhanced by sodium bicarbonate.
- Note that naproxen sodium should not be used concomitantly with the related drug naproxen since they both circulate in plasma as the naproxen anion.

Common side effects in *italic*; life-threatening effects underlined; generic names in **bold**; classifications in SMALL CAPS

- Store naproxen at 15–30C (59–86F) in tightly closed container. Avoid freezing.

Assessment & Drug Effects
- Take a detailed drug history prior to initiation of therapy. In those with aspirin or other NSAID sensitivity, observe for signs of allergic response.
- Baseline and periodic evaluations of hemoglobin and renal and hepatic function and auditory and ophthalmic examinations are recommended in patients receiving prolonged or high dose therapy.
- Patients with arthritis may experience symptomatic relief (reduction in joint pain, swelling, stiffness) within 24–48 h with naproxen sodium therapy and in 2–4 wk with naproxen.

Patient & Family Education
- Inform patient that full therapeutic effect of naproxen may not be experienced for 3–4 wk.
- Since naproxen may cause dizziness and drowsiness, advise patients to exercise caution when they are driving or performing other potentially hazardous activities.
- Inform patient that alcohol and aspirin may increase risk of GI ulceration and bleeding and, therefore, should be avoided unless otherwise advised by physician.
- Since naproxen may prolong bleeding time, caution patient to inform dentist or surgeon that this drug is being taken.

Prototype: amphotericin B, p 56

NATAMYCIN
(na-ta-mye´sin)
Trade name: Natacyn
Classifications: ANTIINFECTIVE; MACROLIDE ANTIBIOTIC; ANTIFUNGAL

ACTIONS/PHARMACODYNAMICS Tetraene polyene compound derived from *Streptomyces natalensis*. Effective against many yeasts and filamentous fungi including *Candida, Aspergillus, Cephalosporium, Fusarium,* and *Penicillium.* Action mechanism simulates that of amphotericin B and nystatin: by binding to sterols in the bacterial cell membrane, natamycin changes the structure and integrity of the cell, leading to loss of intracellular potassium and other essential constituents and destruction of the organism. Has some activity in vivo against *Tricho-*

monas vaginalis; is not active against gram-positive or gram-negative bacteria or viruses. Has low order of toxicity.

USES Topically to treat blepharitis, conjunctivitis, and keratitis caused by susceptible fungi. Drug of choice for *Fusarium solani* keratitis. **Unlabeled uses:** oral, cutaneous, and vaginal candidiasis; intranasal treatment of pulmonary aspergillosis.

ROUTE & DOSAGE

Fungal Keratitis

Adult	Ophthalmic Instillation	1 drop in conjunctival sac of infected eye q1–2h for 3–4 d; then decrease to 1 drop q6–8h, then gradually decrease to 1 drop q4–7d

PHARMACOKINETICS Absorption: drug adheres to ulcerated surface of the cornea and is retained in conjunctival fornices. Does not appear to be systemically absorbed.

CONTRAINDICATIONS & PRECAUTIONS Contraindicated in: concomitant administration of a corticosteroid. Safe use during pregnancy not established.

ADVERSE/SIDE EFFECTS Reports scanty. Blurred vision, photophobia, eye pain. Uneven adherence of suspension to epithelial ulcerations or in fornices.

NURSING IMPLICATIONS

Administration
- Thorough handwashing before and after treatment is imperative. Infection is easily transferred from infected to noninfected eye and to other individuals.
- Store ophthalmic suspension at 2–24C (36–75F) unless otherwise directed. Shake well before using.

Assessment & Drug Effects
- Inspect eye for response and tolerance at least twice weekly.
- Lack of improvement in keratitis within 7–10 d suggests that causative organisms may not be susceptible to natamycin. Reevaluation is indicated and possibly a change in therapy.

Patient & Family Education
- Temporary photophobia should be anticipated. Tell patient to be prepared to wear sunglasses out-

N

Common side effects in *italic*; life-threatening effects <u>underlined</u>; generic names in **bold**; classifications in SMALL CAPS

805

doors after drug administration and perhaps for a few hours indoors.

- Instruct patient to return to ophthalmologist for reevaluation of eye problem if he or she experiences *symptoms of conjunctivitis:* pain, discharge, itching, scratching "foreign body sensation," changes in vision.
- Teach appropriate technique for application of eye drops.
- Encourage patient to keep hands away from eyes, even if discomfort begs for scratching, rubbing, etc.
- Facecloths and hand towels should be used only by the patient to prevent transmission of the fungal infection.

Prototype: gentamicin, p 53

NEOMYCIN SULFATE

(nee-oh-mye´sin)

Trade names: Mycifradin, Myciguent
Classifications: ANTIINFECTIVE; AMINOGLYCO-SIDE ANTIBIOTIC

ACTIONS/PHARMACODYNAMICS Aminoglycoside antibiotic obtained from *Streptomyces fradiae;* reported to be the most potent in neuromuscular blocking action and the most toxic of this group. Broad spectrum of antibacterial activity, and actions similar to those of gentamicin.

USES Severe diarrhea caused by enteropathogenic *Escherichia coli;* preoperative intestinal antisepsis; to inhibit nitrogen-forming bacteria of GI tract in patients with cirrhosis or hepatic coma and for urinary tract infections caused by susceptible organisms. Also topically for short-term treatment of eye, ear, and skin infections. Available in a variety of creams, ointments, and sprays in combination with other antibiotics and corticosteroids.

PHARMACOKINETICS Absorption: 3% absorbed from GI tract in adults; up to 10% absorbed in neonates. **Peak:** 1–4 h. **Elimination:** half-life: 3 h; 97% excreted unchanged in feces.

CONTRAINDICATIONS & PRECAUTIONS Contraindicated in: use of oral drug in patients with intestinal obstruction; ulcerative bowel lesions; topical applications over large skin areas; parenteral use in patients with renal disease or impaired hearing;

parkinsonism; myasthenia gravis. Safe use during pregnancy not established. **Cautious use in:** topical otic applications in patients with perforated eardrum.

ROUTE & DOSAGE

Intestinal Antisepsis

Adult	PO	1 g q1h x 4 doses, then 1 g q4h x 5 doses
Child	PO	10.3 mg/kg q4–6h for 3 d

Hepatic Coma

Adult	PO	4–12 g/d in 4 divided doses for 5–6 d
Child	PO	437.5–1225 mg/m² q6h for 5–6 d

Diarrhea

Adult	PO	50 mg/kg in 4 divided doses for 2–3 d
	IM	1.3–2.6 mg/kg q6h
Child	PO	8.75 mg/kg q6h for 2–3 d

Cutaneous Infections

Adult	Topical	Apply 1–3 times/d

ADVERSE/SIDE EFFECTS Oral use: mild laxative effect, *diarrhea, nausea, vomiting;* prolonged therapy: malabsorption-like syndrome including cyanocobalamin (vitamin B_{12}) deficiency, low serum cholesterol. **Systemic absorption:** <u>nephrotoxicity, ototoxicity, neuromuscular blockade</u> with muscular and <u>respiratory paralysis,</u> hypersensitivity reactions. **Topical use:** *redness,* scaling, pruritus, dermatitis.

DRUG INTERACTIONS May decrease absorption of **cyanocobalamin.**

NURSING IMPLICATIONS

Administration

- *Patients with hepatic coma:* When neomycin therapy is initiated, protein is usually restricted from diet, and carbohydrate intake is increased. Diuretics are generally withheld. As symptoms subside and cerebral functions clear, protein intake is gradually increased.
- Neomycin retention enema is sometimes prescribed for patients with hepatic coma. Recommended dilution for adults: 200 ml/L of 1% solution or 100 ml of 2% solution to be retained for 20 min to more than 1 h, as prescribed.
- *Preoperative bowel preparation:* Saline laxative is generally given immediately before neomycin therapy is initiated.

- For applications to skin: consult physician about what to use for cleansing the part to be treated before each neomycin application.
- Topical therapy of external ear is most effective if canal is clean and dry prior to instillation of neomycin. Consult physician. Duration of treatment should be limited to 7–10 d.
- Parenteral solutions should be refrigerated (2–15C, 35–59F) to minimize possibility of contamination and discoloration and should be used as soon as possible, preferably within 1 wk after reconstitution.

Assessment & Drug Effects

- Patients with renal or hepatic dysfunction receiving IM or extended oral neomycin therapy should have audiometric studies twice weekly, daily urinalysis for albumin, casts, and cells, and BUN every other day. Baseline determinations should be done before initiation of therapy. Serum drug levels also are advised (toxic levels reportedly range from 8 to 30 µg/ml, although individual variations exist).
- Neomycin can cause irreversible damage to auditory branch of eighth cranial nerve. At first, loss of hearing most often involves high-frequency sounds, then may progress to normal hearing frequencies. Severity and persistence of ototoxic symptoms depend on dosage and duration of drug therapy. Early reporting is essential.
- Monitor I&O in patients receiving oral or parenteral therapy. Report oliguria or changes in I&O ratio. Inadequate neomycin excretion results in high serum drug levels and risk of nephrotoxicity and ototoxicity.
- **Topical use:** The possibility of systemic absorption and sensitization should be considered. High incidence of allergic dermatitis is associated with topical neomycin. Sensitivity may be manifested as persistent dermatitis. Caution patient to stop treatment and report to physician if irritation occurs.

Patient & Family Education

- Advise patient to report any unusual symptom related to ears or hearing, e.g., tinnitus, roaring sounds, loss of hearing acuity, dizziness.
- Patients who develop sensitivity should be informed that they will probably continue to be sensitive to neomycin and to other aminoglycoside antibiotics (gentamicin, kanamycin, neomycin, streptomycin).
- Caution patient not to exceed prescribed dosage or duration of therapy.

NEOSTIGMINE

See AUTONOMIC NERVOUS SYSTEM AGENTS, CHOLINERGIC (PARASYMPATHOMIMETIC), CHOLINESTERASE INHIBITOR prototype, p 118.

Prototype: gentamicin, p 53

NETILMICIN SULFATE

(ne-til-mye´sin)
Trade name: Netromycin
Classifications: ANTIINFECTIVE; AMINOGLYCOSIDE ANTIBIOTIC
Pregnancy: Category D

ACTIONS/PHARMACODYNAMICS Rapid-acting, broad-spectrum, semisynthetic aminoglycoside derivative of sisomicin. In common with other aminoglycosides, appears to act by interfering with protein synthesis of bacterial cell wall. Spectrum of activity comparable to that of gentamicin, but netilmicin is also effective against gentamicin-resistant bacteria. Not inactivated by most strains of bacteria resistant to other aminoglycosides. Bactericidal action primarily against gram-negative organisms including *Citrobacter, Enterobacter, Escherichia coli, Klebsiella, Proteus mirabilis, Pseudomonas aeruginosa, Salmonella, Serratia,* and certain gram-positive bacteria such as *Staphylococcus pyogenes* and *Streptococcus faecalis.* Like other aminoglycosides, not effective against most anaerobic bacteria (*Bacteroides* and *Clostridium* species), viruses, or fungi. Reportedly less ototoxic and nephrotoxic than other aminoglycosides but has high potential for neuromuscular blocking action.

USES Short-term treatment of serious or life-threatening infections including septicemia, peritonitis, in traabdominal abscess, lower respiratory tract infections, and complicated urinary tract infection, infections of bones and joints, skin and its structures. May be administered in conjunction with a beta-lactam antibiotic (e.g., a penicillin or cephalosporin) for synergistic effect pending results of susceptibility testing.

PHARMACOKINETICS Peak: end of IV infusion; 30–60 min IM. **Distribution:** does not cross blood-brain

N

Common side effects in *italic*; life-threatening effects underlined; generic names in **bold**; classifications in SMALL CAPS

807

barrier; accumulates in renal cortex; crosses placenta; distributed into breast milk. **Elimination:** half-life: 2–2.5 h; excreted in urine.

ROUTE & DOSAGE

Moderate to Severe Infections (all doses based on ideal body weight)

Adult	IV/IM	1.3–2.2 mg/kg q8h or 2–3.25 mg/kg q12h
Child	IV/IM	6 wk–12 y: 1.8–2.7 mg/kg q8h or 2.7–4 mg/kg q12h
		<6 wk: 2–3.5 mg/kg q12h

Complicated Urinary Tract Infection

Adult	IV/IM	1.5–2 mg/kg q12h

CONTRAINDICATIONS & PRECAUTIONS **Contraindicated in:** history of hypersensitivity or toxic reaction to netilmicin or other aminoglycosides or to bisulfites or any other ingredient in the formulation, pregnancy (category D), nursing infants, minor infections. **Cautious use in:** impaired renal function; premature infants; neonates, the elderly; patients with ascites, edema, dehydration; severe burns; cystic fibrosis; fever; anemia; myasthenia gravis, parkinsonism; history of ear disease; infant botulism.

ADVERSE/SIDE EFFECTS Low incidence in patients with normal renal function. **CNS:** headache, lethargy, drowsiness, paresthesias, tremors, muscle twitching, peripheral neuritis, disorientation, seizures, neuromuscular blockade; musculoskeletal weakness or paralysis, respiratory depression or paralysis. **CV:** palpitation, hypotension. **ENT:** ototoxicity (usually irreversible: eighth cranial nerve auditory branch: tinnitus, hearing loss, ringing, buzzing or fullness in ears; vestibular branch: vertigo, nystagmus, ataxia, nausea, and vomiting). **Eye:** blurred vision. **GI:** nausea, vomiting, diarrhea, stomatitis, proctitis, enterocolitis (possibly superinfections). **Hematologic:** increases in ALT, AST, alkaline phosphatase, bilirubin; anemia, eosinophilia, neutropenia, thrombocytopenia, thrombocytosis, prolonged PT, agranulocytosis, leukopenia, leukemoid reaction, hyperkalemia. **Hypersensitivity:** rash, pruritus. **Renal:** nephrotoxicity, increase in serum creatinine and BUN; decrease in creatinine clearance; hematuria, proteinuria, urinary frequency, oliguria, polyuria. **Other:** fever, edema, arthralgia; pain, induration, and hematoma at injection site.

DIAGNOSTIC TEST INTERFERENCES Concomitant netilmicin-cephalosporin therapy may cause false elevations of ***creatinine*** determinations. Concomitant use of beta-lactam antibiotics (cephalosporins, penicillins) may result in falsely low ***aminoglycoside levels*** (mutual inactivation may continue in body fluid specimen unless promptly assayed, or frozen, or treated with beta-lactamase).

DRUG INTERACTIONS ANESTHETICS, SKELETAL MUSCLE RELAXANTS add to neuromuscular blocking effects; **acyclovir, amphotericin B, bacitracin, capreomycin,** CEPHALOSPORINS, **colistin, cisplatin, carboplatin, methoxyflurane, polymyxin B, vancomycin, furosemide, ethacrynic acid** increase risk of ototoxicity or nephrotoxicity or both.

INCOMPATIBILITIES Solution/Additive: furosemide, heparin. Y-Site: furosemide.

NURSING IMPLICATIONS

Administration
- Netilmicin containing 100 mg/ml and preserved with benzyl alcohol should not be used for neonates, infants, or children (benzyl alcohol may be toxic to this age group). Netromycin pediatric injection 25 mg/ml and Netromycin neonatal injection 10 mg/ml do not contain benzyl alcohol. All preparations contain a metabisulfite or bisulfite to which some individuals may be allergic.
- For adults, prescribed dose for IV infusion is diluted with 50–200 ml of D5W, NS, or other compatible IV solution (see manufacturer's package insert); solution may be infused over 30–120 min, as prescribed.
- Diluted solutions retain potency for up to 72 h when stored in glass containers either at room temperature or refrigerated. Do not use solutions that are discolored or that contain particulate matter.
- Avoid mixing netilmicin with other drugs without first determining compatibility.
- Store at 2–30C (36–86F) unless otherwise directed by manufacturer. Avoid freezing.

Assessment & Drug Effects
- Culture and sensitivity tests should be done prior to initiation of therapy. Therapy may begin before test results are available.
- Obtain patient's pretreatment weight so that physician can calculate dosage. For obese patients, dosage should be based on ideal body weight (IBW): for males = 50 kg + (2.3 kg × cm over 150 cm [5 ft]); for females = 45 kg + (2.3 kg × cm over 150 cm [5 ft]).
- Renal function should be evaluated before and pe-

riodically during therapy. Close monitoring is particularly important for high-risk patients (i.e., renal function impairment, the elderly, dehydrated patients, burn patients, and patients receiving high doses or prolonged therapy).

- Monitor I&O ratio and pattern and report significant changes. Keep patient well hydrated throughout therapy to minimize possibility of chemical irritation of renal tubules and to reduce risk of toxicity. Consult physician for guidelines.
- Dosage adjustments for patients with impaired renal function are based on creatinine clearance rates, serum creatinine, or on peak and trough serum drug levels.
- To determine peak serum drug levels, blood is drawn 1 h after IM injection or IV infusion begins. To determine trough serum drug levels, blood is drawn just before next scheduled dose. Desirable peak values: 6–10 µg/ml; desirable trough values: 0.5–2 µg/ml. Peak values > 16 µg/ml and trough values > 4 µg/ml are associated with a high potential for toxicity.
- Close monitoring of serum drug concentrations is especially important for patients with fever, edema, severe burns, and anemia. Peak serum drug levels tend to be significantly reduced in these patients.
- Urinalysis may be done daily in high risk patients to determine presence of albumin, casts, white or red blood cells, and lowering of specific gravity. All represent signs of renal irritation and the need for increased hydration.
- Patients should be evaluated before and during therapy for hearing acuity and vestibular status. Notify physician promptly if patient complains of any hearing loss, tinnitus, vertigo, or ataxia.
- If therapeutic effectiveness is not evident within 3–5 d, bacterial susceptibility tests should be repeated.
- For most patients, therapy may last 7–14 d. However, carefully selected patients with complicated infections may require longer therapy.
- Watch for signs of superinfection (see chap 3), especially of upper respiratory tract. Also suspect overgrowth of opportunistic organisms if patient develops sore rectum, diarrhea, vaginal discharge, sore mouth, fever.

NIACIN (VITAMIN B₃, NICOTINIC ACID)
(nye´a sin)

Trade names: Niac, Nicobid, Nico-400, Nicolar, Nico-Span, Nicotinex, Novoniacin, Span-Niacin-150, Tega-Span, Tri-B3

NIACINAMIDE (NICOTINAMIDE)

Classifications: VITAMIN B₃; CARDIOVASCULAR AGENT; ANTILIPEMIC; LIPID-LOWERING AGENT
Pregnancy: Categories A and C

ACTIONS/PHARMACODYNAMICS Niacin is a water-soluble, heat-stable, B-complex vitamin (B₃). Functions with riboflavin as a control agent in coenzyme system that converts protein, carbohydrate, and fat to energy through oxidation-reduction. Produces vasodilation (primarily of cutaneous vessels) by direct action on vascular smooth muscles. Inhibits hepatic synthesis of VLDL, cholesterol and triglyceride, and, indirectly, LDL. Large doses effectively reduce elevated serum cholesterol and total lipid levels in hypercholesterolemia and hyperlipidemic states. Unclear whether drug-induced reduction of cholesterol and lipids has a beneficial effect on morbidity or mortality caused by atherosclerosis or coronary heart disease.

Niacinamide, an amide of niacin, is used as an alternative in the prevention and treatment of pellagra. Preferred by some clinicians to niacin because it lacks unpleasant vasodilatory action and the hypolipemic, hepatic, and GI effects of niacin.

USES In prophylaxis and treatment of pellagra, usually in combination with other B-complex vitamins, and in deficiency states accompanying carcinoid syndrome, isoniazid therapy, Hartnup's disease, and chronic alcoholism. Also in adjuvant treatment of hyperlipidemia (elevated cholesterol or triglycerides) in patient who does not respond adequately to diet or weight loss. Also as vasodilator in peripheral vascular disorders, Meniere's disease, and labyrinthine syndrome, as well as to counteract LSD toxicity and to distinguish between psychoses of dietary and nondietary origin.

PHARMACOKINETICS Absorption: readily absorbed from GI tract. **Peak:** 20–70 min. **Distribution:** distributed into breast milk. **Metabolism:** metabolized in liver. **Elimination:** half-life: 45 min; excreted primarily in urine.

N

Common side effects in *italic*; life-threatening effects <u>underlined</u>; generic names in **bold**; classifications in SMALL CAPS

809

ROUTE & DOSAGE

Niacin Deficiency

Adult	PO	10–20 mg/d
	SC/IM/Slow IV	25–100 mg 2–5 times/d

Pellagra

Adult	PO	300–500 mg/d in divided doses

Hyperlipidemia

Adult	PO	1.5–3 g/d in divided doses; may increase up to 6 g/d if necessary

CONTRAINDICATIONS & PRECAUTIONS Contraindicated in: hypersensitivity to niacin; hepatic impairment; severe hypotension; hemorrhaging or arterial bleeding; active peptic ulcer. Used during pregnancy (category A); if dose is larger than RDA, category C; in nursing women not established. **Cautious use in:** history of gallbladder disease, liver disease, and peptic ulcer; glaucoma; angina; coronary artery disease; diabetes mellitus; predisposition to gout; allergy.

ADVERSE/SIDE EFFECTS CNS: *transient headache, tingling of extremities,* syncope; with chronic use: nervousness, panic, toxic amblyopia, proptosis, blurred vision, loss of central vision. **CV:** *generalized flushing with sensation of warmth,* postural hypotension, vasovagal attacks, cardiac arrhythmias (rare). **GI:** *abnormalities of hepatic function tests; jaundice, bloating, flatulence,* hunger pains, *nausea,* vomiting, GI disorders, activation of peptic ulcer, xerostomia. **Skin:** *increased sebaceous gland activity,* dry skin, skin rash, *pruritus,* keratitis nigricans. **Other:** hyperuricemia, allergy, hyperglycemia, glycosuria, hypoprothrombinemia, hypoalbuminemia.

DIAGNOSTIC TEST INTERFERENCES Niacin causes elevated serum **bilirubin, uric acid, alkaline phosphatase, AST, ALT, LDH** levels and may cause **glucose intolerance.** Decreases **serum cholesterol** 15–30% and may cause false elevations with certain fluorometric methods of determining **urinary catecholamines.** Niacin may cause false-positive **urine glucose** tests using copper sulfate reagents, e.g., Benedict's solution.

DRUG INTERACTIONS Potentiates hypotensive effects of ANTIHYPERTENSIVE AGENTS.

NURSING IMPLICATIONS

Administration

- For treatment of niacin deficiency, small doses given frequently during the day are more effective than a single large daily dose, since a considerable amount of the latter is excreted in urine.
- In treatment of hyperlipidemia, dosage is individualized according to effect on serum lipid levels.
- IV drug may be given by direct IV undiluted at a rate of 2 mg over 60 seconds; 50–100 mg of drug may be diluted in 500 ml of NS to yield concentrations of 0.1–0.2 mg/ml and infused over 12–24 h.
- Parenteral therapy is continued until patient can take a complete well-balanced diet and oral niacin.
- Give oral drug with meals to decrease GI distress. Give with cold water (not hot beverage) if necessary to facilitate swallowing.
- Store drug at 15–30C (59–86F) in light- and moisture-proof container.

Assessment & Drug Effects

- Therapeutic response usually begins within 24 h. Note and record effect of therapy on clinical manifestations of deficiency (fiery red tongue, excessive saliva secretion and infection of oral membranes, nausea, vomiting, diarrhea, confusion).
- Baseline and periodic tests of blood glucose and liver function should be performed in patients receiving prolonged high dose therapy.
- Diabetics and patients on high doses will require close monitoring. Hyperglycemia, glycosuria, ketonuria, and increased insulin requirements have been reported.
- Observe patient closely for evidence of hepatic dysfunction (jaundice, dark urine, light-colored stools, pruritus) and hyperuricemia in patient predisposed to gout (flank, joint, or stomach pain; altered urine excretion pattern).

Patient & Family Education

- Inform patient that cutaneous warmth and flushing in face, neck, and ears may occur within first 2 h after oral ingestion and immediately after parenteral administration and may last several hours. Effects are usually transient and subside as therapy continues.
- Caution patient to sit or lie down and to avoid sudden posture changes if weakness or dizziness occurs. These symptoms and persistent flushing should be reported to the physician. Relief may be obtained by reduction of dosage, increasing subsequent doses in small increments, or by changing to sustained-action formulation.

N

Common side effects in *italic*; life-threatening effects underlined; generic names in **bold**; classifications in SMALL CAPS

- Alcohol and large doses of niacin cause increased flushing and sensation of warmth. Alcohol should be limited if patient is being treated for hyper-triglyceridemia.
- Caution patient with skin manifestations to avoid exposure to direct sunlight until lesions have entirely cleared.
- **RDA for niacin: infants:** 6–8 mg; **children 4–6:** 11 mg; **adult males:** 18 mg; **adult females:** 13 mg; additional 2 mg during pregnancy and an additional 5 mg during lactation are required.
- Rich niacin food sources: liver, kidney, lean meats, poultry, fish, brewer's yeast, wheat germ, peanuts, and other legumes.

Prototype: verapamil, p 144

NICARDIPINE HYDROCHLORIDE
(ni-car′di-peen)
Trade name: Cardene
Classifications: CARDIOVASCULAR AGENT; CALCIUM CHANNEL BLOCKER; ANTIHYPERTENSIVE
Pregnancy: Category C

ACTIONS/PHARMACODYNAMICS Nicardipine is a calcium entry blocker that inhibits the transmembrane influx of calcium ions into cardiac muscle and smooth muscle without changing calcium concentrations, thus affecting contractility, and it more selectively affects vascular smooth muscle than cardiac muscle. Thus it relaxes coronary vascular smooth muscle with little or no negative inotropic effect. It significantly decreases systemic vascular resistance. It reduces BP at rest and during isometric and dynamic exercise.

USES Either alone or with beta-blockers for chronic, stable (effort-associated) angina; either alone or with other antihypertensives for essential hypertension. **Unlabeled use:** CHF.

ROUTE & DOSAGE

Hypertension, Angina
Adult   PO   20–40 mg t.i.d.

PHARMACOKINETICS Absorption: readily absorbed from GI tract; 35% reaches systemic circulation (first pass metabolism). **Onset:** 20 min. **Peak:** 0.5–2 h. **Metabolism:** completely metabolized in liver.

Elimination: half-life: 8.6 h; 60% excreted in urine, 35% in feces.

CONTRAINDICATIONS & PRECAUTIONS Contraindicated in: hypersensitivity to nicardipine, advanced aortic stenosis, and nursing mothers. **Cautious use in:** CHF, pregnancy (category C), and renal or liver impairment.

ADVERSE/SIDE EFFECTS CNS: *fatigue,* weakness, anxiety. **CV:** *flushing, headache, peripheral edema, lightheadedness, diaphoresis, increased angina, hypotension,* palpitations, dyspnea, tachycardia, syncope. **GI:** anorexia, nausea, vomiting, dry mouth, constipation, dyspepsia. **Other:** rash.

DRUG INTERACTIONS Concomitant nicardipine and **cyclosporine** therapy resulted in significant increases in cyclosporine serum concentrations at 1–30 d after initiation of nicardipine therapy; following withdrawal of nicardipine, cyclosporine levels decreased.

NURSING IMPLICATIONS

Administration
- Dosages are individualized and titrated for each patient until desired effect is achieved. Usual initial dose is 20 mg.
- Drug dose should be increased to desired level at 3 d intervals to ensure achievement of steady state plasma levels.
- Nicardipine should be taken on empty stomach. High fat meals may decrease blood nicardipine levels.
- Dose adjustment may be necessary for patients with impaired hepatic or renal function. Plasma drug levels will increase with decreased hepatic function.
- To prevent symptoms of withdrawal, do not abruptly discontinue drug.

Assessment & Drug Effects
- Establish baseline data before treatment is started including BP, pulse, and lab evaluations of hepatic and renal function.
- Carefully monitor BP during initiation and titration of dosage. Hypotension with or without an increase in heart rate may occur, especially in patients who are hypertensive or who are already taking antihypertensive medication.
- Observe for large peak and trough differences in BP. Initially BP should be measured at peak effect (1–2 h after dosing) and at trough effect (8 h after dosing).

Common side effects in *italic*; life-threatening effects underlined; generic names in **bold**; classifications in SMALL CAPS

811

- Observe for an increase in frequency, duration, and severity of angina when initiating or increasing dosage. Record nitroglycerin use and any changes in previous anginal pattern.

Patient & Family Education

- Instruct patient to record any increase in frequency, duration, and severity of angina when initiating or increasing dosage. Instruct patient to keep a record of nitroglycerin use and to report promptly any changes in previous anginal pattern. Increased incidence and severity of angina has occurred in some patients using nicardipine.
- Stress the importance of compliance. Warn patient not to change dosage regimen without consulting physician. Instruct patient not to omit, increase, or decrease dose or to change the dose interval in order to avoid symptoms of withdrawal.
- Abrupt withdrawal may cause an increased frequency and duration of chest pain. Advise patient that drug must be gradually tapered under medical supervision.
- Warn patient to adhere to established guidelines for exercise program because nicardipine reduces anginal pain and thus can give a false interpretation of tolerance.
- Caution patient to arise slowly from a recumbent position and to avoid driving or operating dangerous equipment until response to nicardipine is established.
- Instruct patient to notify physician if any of the following occur: irregular heart beat, shortness of breath, swelling of the feet, pronounced dizziness, nausea, or drop in BP.

Prototype: mebendazole, p 53

NICLOSAMIDE

(ni-kloe´sa-mide)
Trade name: Niclocide
Classifications: ANTIINFECTIVE; ANTHELMINTIC
Pregnancy: Category B

ACTIONS/PHARMACODYNAMICS Salicylanilide derivative reportedly effective against most tapeworms that infect man. Acts by inhibiting oxidative phosphorylation in mitochondria of cestodes. On contact, kills scolex and proximal segments of tapeworm, which may then be partially or fully digested in intestines. Lacks ovicidal action and is not effective in larval or tissue encystment stage of tapeworm infections, e.g., cysticercosis.

USES Intestinal tapeworm (cestode) infections, e.g., *Taenia saginata* (beef tapeworm), *Diphyllobothrium latum* (fish tapeworm), *Hymenolepis nana* (dwarf tapeworm), *Hymenolepis diminuta* (rat tapeworm), and *Dipylidium caninum* (dog or cat tapeworm).

ROUTE & DOSAGE

Beef & Fish Tapeworms

Adult	PO	2 g as a single dose
Child	PO	> 34 kg: 1.5 g as a single dose
		11–34 kg: 1 g as a single dose

Dwarf Tapeworm

Adult	PO	2 g/d as a single dose for 7 d
Child	PO	> 34 kg: 1.5 g/d as a single dose for 6 d
		11–34 kg: 1 g as a single dose on day 1, then 500 mg once/d for the next 6 d

PHARMACOKINETICS Absorption: minimally absorbed from GI tract. **Elimination:** excreted in feces.

CONTRAINDICATIONS & PRECAUTIONS Contraindicated in: safe use during pregnancy (category B), in nursing women, and in children <2 y not established.

ADVERSE/SIDE EFFECTS CNS: drowsiness, dizziness, headache, irritability. **GI:** nausea, vomiting, abdominal discomfort, anorexia, diarrhea, constipation, oral irritation, bad taste, rectal bleeding. **Skin:** skin rash, pruritus ani, alopecia, sweating, urticaria (rare). **Other:** fever, weakness, edema of an arm, backache, palpitation. Rare: Transient rise in AST.

NURSING IMPLICATIONS

Administration

- Should be taken after a light meal. Instruct patient to chew tablet thoroughly, then swallow with a little water.
- For young children, tablet may be crushed to a fine powder and mixed with sufficient water to form a paste for ease of ingestion. Niclosamide is vanilla flavored and reportedly not unpleasant to the taste.
- Store below 30C (86F) protected from light unless otherwise directed.

Assessment & Drug Effects

- Presence of ova or segments in stool on day 7 after therapy indicates treatment failure and need for second course of therapy.

- Stool examinations may be required at 1 and 3 mo following therapy to determine cure. No patient is considered cured unless stools have been negative for at least 3 mo.

Patient & Family Education

- **Fish Tapeworm** (*Diphyllobothrium latum*): ***Source of infection:*** fresh water flea to fish to humans. *Prophylaxis:* proper disposal of excreta and avoiding ingestion of raw or undercooked fish.
- **Beef Tapeworm** (*Taenia saginata*): ***Source of infection:*** infected beef.
- **Dwarf Tapeworm** (*Hymenolepis nana*): ***Source of infection:*** fecal contamination of food. ***Prophylaxis:*** proper disposal of excreta. Instruct patient to use meticulous personal and environmental hygiene. Autoinfection occurs commonly.

NICOTINE POLACRILEX

(nik´o-teen)
Trade name: Nicorette
Classifications: CNS AND AUTONOMIC NERVOUS SYSTEM AGENT; CHOLINERGIC (PARASYMPATHOMIMETIC)
Pregnancy: Category X

ACTIONS/PHARMACODYNAMICS A chewing gum containing nicotine, available by prescription only. Nicotine resin complex is a formulation of 2 mg of nicotine bound to the cation exchange resin polacrilin, buffered to pH 8.5. Each piece of gum contains about 0.44 mEq sodium. The nicotine is a highly purified extract from dried tobacco leaves and is primarily classified as a ganglionic cholinergic receptor agonist. Its pharmacologic activity is complex and varied, resulting in both adrenergic and cholinergic effects. Thus exposure to nicotine produces widespread responses: stimulant and depressant effects on peripheral and central nervous systems, respiratory stimulation, peripheral vasoconstriction; increased heart rate, contractile force, output, and stroke volume; increased tone and motor activity of GI tract smooth muscle; and more specifically nausea, vomiting, diarrhea, hypersalivation; increase in bronchial secretion (initially), and antidiuretic activity. The heavy smoker is tolerant to most of these effects; but exposure to nicotine (as in the gum) can cause the nonsmoker to experience tachycardia,

symptoms of CNS stimulation, and increased BP. Rationale for use of nicotine resin complex is that smoking is partially due to physical dependence on nicotine as evidenced by appearance of withdrawal symptoms during nicotine deprivation. For some smokers, nicotine gum seems to relieve the desire for nicotine and reduces withdrawal symptoms, permitting the patient then to focus attention on overcoming the habit features of smoking. Success rate with nicotine gum use appears to be greatest in smokers with a high "physical" type of nicotine dependence.

USES In conjunction with a medically supervised behavior modification program, as a temporary and alternate source of nicotine by the nicotine-dependent smoker who is withdrawing from cigarette smoking.

ROUTE & DOSAGE

Smoking Cessation

Adult	PO	Chew 1 piece of gum when patient has an urge to smoke, may be repeated as needed; max 30 pieces of gum/d

PHARMACOKINETICS Absorption: approximately 90% of the nicotine in a piece of gum is released slowly over a 15–30 min period; rate of release is controlled by vigor and duration of chewing; readily absorbed from buccal mucosa. **Distribution:** crosses placenta; distributed into breast milk. **Metabolism:** metabolized principally in liver. **Elimination:** half-life: 30–120 min; excreted in urine.

CONTRAINDICATIONS & PRECAUTIONS Contraindicated in: nonsmokers, immediate post-MI period, life-threatening arrhythmias, active temporomandibular joint disease, severe angina pectoris, women with childbearing potential (unless effective contraception is used). Risk-benefit ratio associated with use during pregnancy must be carefully considered (category X). Safe use by children and adolescents not established. **Cautious use in:** vasospastic disease (e.g., Buerger's disease, Prinzmetal variant angina), cardiac arrhythmias, hyperthyroidism, type I (IDDM) diabetes mellitus, pheochromocytoma, esophagitis, oral and pharyngeal inflammation; patient with dentures, denture caps, or partial bridges; hypertension and peptic ulcer disease (active or inactive) and by mother only if benefit of a smoking cessation program outweighs risks.

ADVERSE/SIDE EFFECTS CNS: *headache, dizziness, light-headedness,* insomnia, irritability, depen-

Common side effects in *italic*; life-threatening effects <u>underlined</u>;
generic names in **bold**; classifications in SMALL CAPS

813

dence on nicotine resin complex. **CV:** arrhythmias, tachycardia, palpitations. **GU:** air swallowing, *jaw-ache, nausea,* belching, salivation, anorexia, dry mouth, laxative effects, constipation, *indigestion*. **Other:** *sore mouth or throat,* coughing, *hiccups,* hoarseness; injury to mouth, teeth, temporomandibular joint, *irritation/tingling of tongue*. Acute overdose—***nicotine intoxication:*** nausea, vomiting, sialorrhea, abdominal pain, diarrhea, perspiration, severe headache, dizziness, disturbed hearing and vision, mental confusion, severe weakness, fainting, hypotension, dyspnea, weak, rapid irregular pulse, seizures, <u>death</u> (from <u>respiratory failure</u> secondary to drug-induced <u>respiratory muscle paralysis</u>).

DRUG INTERACTIONS May increase metabolism of **caffeine, theophylline.**

NURSING IMPLICATIONS

Assessment & Drug Effects
- Nicotine is known to be one of the most toxic of all poisons. The gum must be considered a hazardous drug vehicle. Monitor for adverse effects.
- Treatment with nicotine resin gum is at first slightly aversive to most patients and may lead to non-compliance.
- Smokers that seem to benefit most from use of nicotine gum have a high "physical" type of nicotine dependence characterized by preferring cigarette brands with nicotine levels over 0.9 mg; finding the first cigarette in AM the hardest to give up; smoking the first cigarette within 15 min of arising; smoking most in the AM; smoking over 15 cigarettes/d.
- Most adverse local effects (irritation of tongue, mouth, and throat, jaw-muscle aches, dislike of taste) are transient and subside in a few days. Modification of the chewing technique may help.
- Usually a medical evaluation is done at least once a month to reinforce progress or to determine if patient should continue the cessation therapy.
- Protect from light (nicotine is photosensitive and will turn brown when exposed to light). Store at less than 30C (86F).

Patient & Family Education
- When a patient stops smoking, withdrawal symptoms can be minimized by a gradual reduction in nicotine intake.
- Nicotine polacrilex facilitates a gradual reduction in cigarette use while preventing withdrawal symptoms.
- Smoking a cigarette causes a rapid rise in serum nicotine, which peaks within 2 min after the cigarette, then rapidly decreases. Chewing nicotine gum causes a slow increase in serum nicotine over a period of 15–30 min.
- Chewing 1 piece of 2 mg gum per hour produces a nicotine level less than one half that produced by smoking 1 cigarette/h but provides relief from abstinence symptoms.
- Specific written instructions are packaged with the gum. Review these carefully with the patient to establish understanding of chewing method.
- The process of chewing controls the amount of nicotine that enters the body. The full dose of nicotine from a piece of gum is obtained through approximately 30 min of intermittent chewing.
- When urge to smoke is experienced, patient should chew one piece of gum slowly until nicotine is tasted or there is a slight tingling in the mouth (usually after 15 chews); stop chewing until taste or tingling disappears, then again chew slowly until taste reappears.
- Chew only one piece of gum at a time. Chewing gum too rapidly can cause excessive buccal absorption and lead to adverse effects: nausea, hiccups, throat irritation.
- Chewing many pieces of gum simultaneously or in rapid succession may cause an acute nicotine overdose (nicotine intoxication).
- To prevent transference of nicotine dependence from cigarette to gum, patient should be encouraged to gradually decrease number of pieces chewed in 24 h. Usually a period of 3 mo is allowed before patient is advised to taper use of gum.
- Withdrawal or abstinence symptoms (usually appear within 24 h after the last cigarette) include craving for tobacco, anxiety, difficulty in concentration, headache, GI disturbances, irritability.
- Abstinence symptoms may persist for days or weeks after the patient stops smoking. The craving to smoke may last for years.
- If patient becomes pregnant during cessation therapy, she should be informed of the potential hazard to the fetus. Nicotine resin complex has been associated with depressed fetal respirations.

N

Common side effects in *italic*; life-threatening effects <u>underlined</u>; generic names in **bold**; classifications in SMALL CAPS

Prototype: verapamil, p 144

NIFEDIPINE

(nye-fed'i-peen)
Trade names: Adalat, Procardia, Procardia XL
Classifications: CARDIOVASCULAR AGENT;
CALCIUM CHANNEL BLOCKER; ANTIARRHYTHMIC;
NONNITRATE VASODILATOR
Pregnancy: Category C

ACTIONS/PHARMACODYNAMICS
Calcium channel blocking agent similar to verapamil in actions, uses, and limitations. Selectively blocks calcium ion influx across cell membranes of cardiac muscle and vascular smooth muscle without changing serum calcium concentrations. Reduces myocardial oxygen utilization and supply and relaxes and prevents coronary artery spasm; has little or no effect on SA and AV nodal conduction with therapeutic dosing. Decreases peripheral vascular resistance and increases cardiac output. Vasodilation (hypotensive effect) of both coronary and peripheral vessels is greater than that produced by verapamil or diltiazem and frequently results in reflex tachycardia. Decreased peripheral vascular resistance also leads to a rise in peripheral blood flow, the basis for (unlabeled) use of this drug in treatment of Raynaud's phenomenon. Has minimal effect on myocardial contractility. Class IV antiarrhythmic.

USES
Vasospastic "variant" or Printzmetal's angina and chronic stable angina without vasospasm. Mild to moderate hypertension alone or in combination with a diuretic (steps 2, 3, 4 of stepped-care approach in antihypertensive therapy). **Unlabeled uses:** esophageal disorders; vascular headaches; Raynaud's phenomenon; asthma; cardiomyopathy; primary pulmonary hypertension.

ROUTE & DOSAGE

Angina

Adult	PO	10–20 mg t.i.d. up to 180 mg/d

Hypertension

Adult	PO	10–20 mg t.i.d. up to 180 mg/d or 30–90 mg sustained release once/d

Hypertensive Emergency

Adult	PO	10–20 mg q20–30min if necessary

PHARMACOKINETICS
Absorption: readily absorbed from GI tract; 45–75% reaches systemic circulation (first pass metabolism). **Onset:** 10–30 min. **Peak:** 30 min. **Distribution:** distributed into breast milk. **Metabolism:** metabolized in liver. **Elimination:** half-life: 2–5 h; 75–80% excreted in urine, 15% in feces.

CONTRAINDICATIONS & PRECAUTIONS
Contraindicated in: known hypersensitivity to nifedipine. Safe use during pregnancy (category C) and in children not established. **Cautious use in:** concomitant use with hypotensives; CHF; nursing mothers.

ADVERSE/SIDE EFFECTS
CNS: *dizziness, lightheadedness,* nervousness, mood changes, weakness, jitteriness, sleep disturbances, blurred vision, retinal ischemia, difficulty in balance, *headache.* **CV:** hypotension, *facial flushing, heat sensation,* myocardial infarction, palpitations, *peripheral edema.* **GI:** nausea, heartburn, *diarrhea,* constipation, cramps, flatulance, cholestasis (rare). **Musculoskeletal:** inflammation, joint stiffness, muscle cramps. **Other:** sore throat, weakness, dermatitis, pruritus, urticaria, gingival hyperplasia, fever, sweating, chills, febrile reaction, nasal congestion, sexual difficulties. **Overdosage:** prolonged systemic hypotension.

DIAGNOSTIC TEST INTERFERENCES
Nifedipine may cause mild to moderate increases of ***alkaline phosphatase, CPK, LDH, AST, ALT.***

DRUG INTERACTIONS
BETA BLOCKERS may increase likelihood of CHF; may increase risk of **phenytoin** toxicity.

NURSING IMPLICATIONS

Administration
- May be co-administered with SL nitroglycerin and with long-acting nitrates.
- In a hypertensive emergency, nifedipine capsule may be swallowed whole or contents may be given SL. Puncture capsule with a pin and squeeze contents under the tongue (puncture about 10 times). The punctured capsule may also be chewed.
- Discontinuation of drug should be gradual, with close medical supervision to prevent severe hypotensive and other side effects.
- Protect capsules from light and moisture; store at 15–25C (59–77F).

Assessment & Drug Effects
- Careful monitoring of BP during titration period is indicated. Severe hypotension may be produced,

N

Common side effects in *italic*; life-threatening effects underlined;
generic names in **bold**; classifications in SMALL CAPS

815

especially if patient is also taking other drugs known to lower BP. Withhold drug and notify physician if systolic BP <90.

- Monitor the blood sugar in patient who is diabetic. Nifedipine has diabetogenic properties.
- Monitor for gingival hyperplasia and report promptly. This is a rare but serious side effect (which is similar to phenytoin-induced hyperplasia).

Patient & Family Education

- Occasionally a patient has developed increased frequency, duration, and severity of angina on starting treatment with this drug or when dosage is increased. Counsel patient to keep a record of nitroglycerin use and to report promptly if changes in previous pattern occur.
- Warn patient not to change nifedipine dosage regimen without consulting physician. Withdrawal symptoms may occur with abrupt discontinuation of the drug (chest pain, increase in anginal episodes, MI, dysrhythmias).
- Instruct patient to maintain good oral hygiene (i.e., brush after eating, floss at least once daily, and have dentist check condition of gums and teeth on a routine basis).
- Patient should visually inspect gums every day. Changes in gingivae may be gradual, and bleeding may be exhibited only with probing.
- *Symptoms of hyperplasia* (easy bleeding of gingivae and gradual enlargening of gingival mass, especially on buccal side of lower anterior teeth) should be treated promptly; scaling and gingivectomy may be necessary.
- Drug will be discontinued if gingival hyperplasia occurs.
- It has been shown that smoking decreases the efficacy of nifedipine and that it has direct and adverse effects on the heart in the patient on nifedipine treatment.

N

Prototype: verapamil, p 144

NIMODIPINE
(ni-mo´di-peen)
Trade name: Nimotop
Classifications: CARDIOVASCULAR AGENT; CALCIUM CHANNEL BLOCKER
Pregnancy: Category C

ACTIONS/PHARMACODYNAMICS Nimodipine, a calcium channel blocking agent, is relatively selective for cerebral arteries compared with arteries elsewhere in the body. This may be attributed to the drug's high lipid solubility and specific binding to cerebral tissue.

USES To improve neurologic deficits due to spasm following subarachnoid hemorrhage from ruptured congenital intracranial aneurysms in patients who are in good neurologic condition postictus (e.g., Hunt and Hess Grades I–III). **Unlabeled uses:** migraine headaches, ischemic seizures.

ROUTE & DOSAGE

Subarachnoid Hemorrhage

Adult	PO	60 mg q4h for 21 d; start therapy within 96 h of subarachnoid hemorrhage

PHARMACOKINETICS Absorption: readily absorbed from GI tract; approximately 13% reaches systemic circulation (first pass metabolism). **Peak:** 1 h. **Distribution:** crosses blood-brain barrier; possibly crosses placenta; distributed into breast milk. **Metabolism:** 85% metabolized in liver; 15% metabolized in kidneys. **Elimination:** half-life: 8–9 h; > 50% excreted in urine, 32% in feces.

CONTRAINDICATIONS & PRECAUTIONS Contraindications: none known. **Cautious use in:** hepatic impairment, pregnancy (category C), and nursing mothers. Safety and effectiveness in children have not been established.

ADVERSE/SIDE EFFECTS CNS: headache. **CV:** *hypotension.* **GI:** hemorrhage, mild, transient increase in liver function tests.

DRUG INTERACTIONS Hypotensive effects may be increased when nimodipine combined with other calcium channel blockers.

NURSING IMPLICATIONS

Administration

- Therapy must begin within 96 h of the subarachnoid hemorrhage and continue q4h for 21 d.
- If patient is unable to swallow, make a hole in both ends of the capsule with an 18-gauge needle and extract the contents into a syringe. Empty the contents into an enteral (if in use) tube and wash down with 30 ml of NS.

Common side effects in *italic*; life-threatening effects underlined; generic names in **bold**; classifications in SMALL CAPS

- Store below 40C (104F), preferably at 15–30C (59–86F) in a tightly closed container. Protect from light.

Assessment & Drug Effects

- Take apical pulse prior to administering drug and hold it if pulse is below 60. Notify the physician.
- Establish baseline data before treatment is started: BP, pulse, and laboratory evaluations of hepatic and renal function.
- Monitor frequently for adverse drug effects, including hypotension, peripheral edema, tachycardia, or skin rash.
- In elderly patients, risk of hypotension is increased. Monitor frequently for dizziness or lightheadedness.

Patient & Family Education

- Advise patient to report gradual weight gain and evidence of edema (e.g., tight rings on fingers, ankle swelling).
- Instruct patient on importance of keeping followup appointments for monitoring of progress during therapy.
- Instruct patient that compliance with medication schedule is important.
- Instruct women not to breast feed while taking this drug.

Prototype: trimethoprim, p 90

NITROFURANTOIN

(nye-troe-fyoor´an-toyn)

Trade names: Apo-Nitrofurantoin, Furadantin, Furalan, Furan, Furanite, Furantoin, Nephronex, Nitrofan, Novofuran, Sarodant

NITROFURANTOIN MACROCRYSTALS

Trade name: Macrodantin
Classifications: URINARY TRACT ANTIINFECTIVE
Pregnancy: Category B

ACTIONS/PHARMACODYNAMICS Synthetic nitrofuran derivative related to nitrofurazone. Active against wide variety of gram-negative and gram-positive microorganisms, including strains of *Escherichia coli, Staphylococcus aureus, Streptococcus faecalis,* enterococci, and *Klebsiella-Aerobacter. Pseudomonas aeruginosa* and many strains of *Proteus* are resistant. Presumed to act by interfering with several bacterial enzyme systems. Highly soluble in urine and reportedly most active in acid urine. Antimicrobial concentrations in urine exceed those in blood.

USES Pyelonephritis, pyelitis, and cystitis caused by susceptible organisms.

ROUTE & DOSAGE

Pyelonephritis, Cystitis

Adult	PO	50–100 mg q.i.d.
Child	PO	1 mo–12 y: 5–7 mg/kg/d in 4 divided doses

Chronic Suppressive Therapy

Adult	PO	50–100 mg h.s.
Child	PO	1 mo–12 y: 1 mg/kg/d in 1–2 divided doses

PHARMACOKINETICS Absorption: readily absorbed from GI tract. **Peak:** urine: 30 min. **Distribution:** crosses placenta; distributed into breast milk. **Metabolism:** partially metabolized in liver. **Elimination:** half-life: 20 min; primarily excreted in urine.

CONTRAINDICATIONS & PRECAUTIONS Contraindicated in: anuria, oliguria, significant impairment of renal function (creatinine clearance <40 ml/min); G6PD deficiency; infants <3 mo. Safe use during pregnancy (category B), pregnancy at term, and in nursing mothers not established. **Cautious use in:** history of asthma, anemia, diabetes, vitamin B deficiency, electrolyte imbalance, debilitating disease.

ADVERSE/SIDE EFFECTS CNS: peripheral neuropathy, headache, nystagmus, drowsiness, vertigo. **GI:** *anorexia, nausea, vomiting,* abdominal pain, diarrhea. **Hematologic (rare):** hemolytic or megaloblastic anemia (especially in patients with G6PD deficiency), granulocytosis. **Hypersensitivity:** allergic pneumonitis, eosinophilia, skin eruptions, pruritus, urticaria, angioedema, <u>anaphylaxis</u>, asthmatic attack (patients with history of asthma), drug fever, arthralgia, cholestatic jaundice, <u>exfoliative dermatitis</u>. **Others:** transient alopecia, genitourinary superinfections (especially with *Pseudomonas*), tooth staining from direct contact with oral suspension and crushed tablets (infants), crystalluria (elderly patients); pulmonary sensitivity reactions (<u>interstitial pneumonitis or fibrosis</u>), <u>hepatic necrosis</u>, dark yellow or brown urine.

DIAGNOSTIC TEST INTERFERENCES Nitrofurantoin metabolite may produce false-positive *urine glucose* test results with Benedict's reagent.

N

Common side effects in *italic*; life-threatening effects <u>underlined</u>; generic names in **bold**; classifications in SMALL CAPS

817

DRUG INTERACTIONS ANTACIDS may decrease absorption of nitrofurantoin; **nalidixic acid,** other QUINOLONES may antagonize antimicrobial effects; **probenecid, sulfinpyrazone** increase risk of nitrofurantoin toxicity.

NURSING IMPLICATIONS

Administration

- Drug must be given at equally spaced intervals around the clock to maintain therapeutic urinary drug levels.
- Administer oral drug with food or milk to minimize gastric irritation.
- Because of the possibility of tooth staining, advise patient to avoid crushing tablets, to dilute oral suspension in milk, water, or fruit juice, and to rinse mouth thoroughly after taking drug.
- Treatment is continued for at least 3 d after sterile urines are obtained. Course of treatment for acute infections rarely exceeds 14 d.
- Dispensed in amber-colored containers; strong light darkens drug.

Assessment & Drug Effects

- Culture and sensitivity tests are performed prior to therapy and are recommended in patients with recurrent infections.
- Monitor I&O. Report oliguria and any change in I&O ratio. Drug should be discontinued if oliguria or anuria develops or creatinine clearance falls below 40 ml/min.
- Be alert to signs of urinary tract superinfections (e.g., milky urine, foul-smelling urine, perineal irritation, dysuria).
- Nausea occurs fairly frequently and may be relieved by using macrocrystalline preparation (Macrodantin) or by reduction in dosage.
- Acute pulmonary sensitivity reaction usually occurs within first week of therapy and appears to be more common in the elderly. May be manifested by mild to severe flulike syndrome. Eosinophilia generally develops in a few days. Recovery usually occurs rapidly after drug is discontinued.
- Subacute or chronic pulmonary sensitivity reaction is associated with prolonged therapy. Commonly manifested by insidious onset of malaise, cough, dyspnea on exertion, altered pulmonary function.
- Peripheral neuropathy can be severe and irreversible. Be alert for and advise the patient to report onset of muscle weakness, tingling, numbness, or other sensations. Reportedly these are most likely to occur in patients with renal impairment, anemia, diabetes, electrolyte imbalance, vitamin B deficiency, or debilitating disease. Drug should be discontinued immediately.

Patient & Family Education

- Forewarn patient that IM injection of nitrofurantoin may be painful (pain may be severe enough to warrant discontinuation of drug by this route).
- Inform patient that nitrofurantoin may impart a harmless brown color to urine.
- Advise patient to consult physician regarding fluid intake. Generally, fluids are not forced; however, intake should be adequate.

NITROFURAZONE

(nye-troe-fyoor´a-zone)
Trade names: Furacin, Nitrofural
Classifications: ANTIINFECTIVE; SKIN & MUCOUS MEMBRANE AGENT
Pregnancy: Category C

ACTIONS/PHARMACODYNAMICS Synthetic nitrofuran related to nitrofurantoin. Bactericidal against most microorganisms causing surface infections, including many that have developed antibiotic resistance. Activity against *Pseudomonas aeruginosa* and certain strains of *Proteus* is limited; has no activity against fungi or viruses. Acts by inhibiting aerobic and anaerobic cycles in bacterial carbohydrate metabolism.

USES Topically as adjunctive therapy to combat bacterial infection in second- and third-degree burns; to prevent infection of skin grafts and donor sites. Has been used orally in other countries for treatment of late stage of African trypanosomiasis.

ROUTE & DOSAGE

Bacterial Infections Associated with Burns or Skin Grafts

Adult	Topical	Apply directly to lesion or dressings; reapply dressings or solutions daily for second- or third-degree burns or q4–5d for second-degree burn with minimum exudation

CONTRAINDICATIONS & PRECAUTIONS Contraindicated in: safe use during pregnancy not established. **Cautious use in:** known or suspected renal impairment, G6PD deficiency.

ADVERSE/SIDE EFFECTS *Allergic contact dermatitis,* irritation, sensitization, superinfections.

N

NURSING IMPLICATIONS

Administration

- Confine applications of nitrofurazone to the part being treated. When wet dressings are used, normal skin surrounding the wound should be protected with an agent such as sterile petrolatum, petrolatum gauze, or zinc oxide. Consult physician.
- Dressing removal may be facilitated by flushing the gauze with sterile isotonic saline solution.
- Consult physician regarding procedure for cleaning wound following each dressing removal.
- Preserve in tight, light-resistant containers, away from heat. Drug darkens slowly on exposure to light, but reportedly this does not appreciably affect potency.

Assessment & Drug Effects

- Drug should be discontinued with onset of symptoms of sensitization or allergy (e.g., redness, itching, burning, swelling, rash, failure to heal), and superinfections (e.g., black furry tongue, thrush, malodorous vaginal discharge, anogenital itching, diarrhea).

Patient & Family Education

- Instruct patient or family in appropriate technique for application of medication to skin lesions.

NITROGLYCERIN

See CARDIOVASCULAR AGENT, NITRATE VASODILATOR prototype, p 149.

Prototype: hydralazine, p 152

NITROPRUSSIDE, SODIUM

(nye-troe-pruss´ide)
Trade names: Nipride, Nitropress
Classifications: CARDIOVASCULAR AGENT; ANTIHYPERTENSIVE; NONNITRATE VASODILATOR
Pregnancy: Category C

ACTIONS/PHARMACODYNAMICS Potent, rapid-acting hypotensive agent with effects similar to those of nitrates. Acts directly on vascular smooth muscle to produce peripheral vasodilation, with consequent marked lowering of arterial BP, associated with slight increase in heart rate, mild decrease in cardiac output, and moderate lowering of peripheral vascular resistance. Thiocyanate metabolite may inhibit uptake and binding of iodine, with prolonged therapy.

USES Short-term, rapid reduction of BP in hypertensive crises and for producing controlled hypotension during anesthesia to reduce bleeding. **Unlabeled uses:** refractory CHF or acute MI.

ROUTE & DOSAGE

Hypertensive Crisis

Adult   IV   0.5–10 µg/kg/min (average 3 µg/kg/min)

PHARMACOKINETICS Onset: within 2 min. **Duration:** 1–10 min after infusion is terminated. **Metabolism:** rapidly converted to cyanogen in erythrocytes and tissue, which is metabolized to thiocyanate in liver. **Elimination:** half-life: (thiocyanate) 2.7–7 d; excreted in urine primarily as thiocyanate.

CONTRAINDICATIONS & PRECAUTIONS Contraindicated in: compensatory hypertension, as in arteriovenous shunt or coarctation of aorta, and for control of hypotension in patients with inadequate cerebral circulation. Safe use during pregnancy (category C) and in children not established. **Cautious use in:** hepatic insufficiency, hypothyroidism, severe renal impairment, hyponatremia, elderly patients with low vitamin B_{12} plasma levels or with Leber's optic atrophy.

ADVERSE/SIDE EFFECTS Usually associated with too rapid reduction in BP: nausea, retching, abdominal pain, nasal stuffiness, diaphoresis, headache, dizziness, apprehension, restlessness, muscle twitching, retrosternal discomfort, palpitation, increase or transient lowering of pulse rate. **Other:** irritation at infusion site, hypothyroidism with prolonged therapy (rare), increase in serum creatinine, fall or rise in total plasma cobalamins. **Overdosage or Prolonged Use (> 48 h)** (thiocyanate toxicity): profound hypotension, tinnitus, blurred vision, fatigue, metabolic acidosis, pink skin color, absence of reflexes, faint heart sounds, loss of consciousness.

NURSING IMPLICATIONS

Administration

- Solutions must be freshly prepared with D5W and used no later than 4 h after reconstitution.

N

Common side effects in *italic*; life-threatening effects <u>underlined</u>; generic names in **bold**; classifications in SMALL CAPS

819

- IV nitroprusside is diluted by dissolving 50 mg in 2–3 ml of D5W and then further diluted in 250 ml D5W (200 μg/ml) or 500 ml D5W (100 μg/ml).
- No other drug should be added to sodium nitroprusside infusion.
- Following reconstitution, solutions usually have faint brownish tint; if solution is highly colored, do not use it. Promptly wrap container with aluminum foil or other opaque material to protect drug from light.
- Administered by infusion pump or similar device that will allow precise measurement of flow rate required to lower BP.
- Protect drug from light, heat, and moisture; store at 15–30C (59–86F) unless otherwise directed.

Assessment & Drug Effects
- Constant monitoring is required to titrate IV infusion rate to BP response.
- Adverse effects are usually relieved by slowing IV rate or by stopping drug; they may be minimized by keeping patient supine.
- If BP begins to rise after drug infusion rate is decreased or infusion is discontinued, notify physician immediately.
- Monitor I&O.
- Monitoring blood thiocyanate level is recommended in patients receiving prolonged treatment or in patients with severe renal dysfunction (levels usually are not allowed to exceed 10 mg/dl). Determination of plasma cyanogen level following 1 or 2 d of therapy is advised in patients with impaired hepatic function.

Prototype: cimetidine, p 216

NIZATIDINE
(ni-za´ti-deen)
Trade name: Axid
Classifications: GI AGENT; ANTISECRETORY (H₂-RECEPTOR ANTAGONIST)
Pregnancy: Category C

N

ACTIONS/PHARMACODYNAMICS
Nizatidine inhibits secretion of gastric acid by reversible, competitive blockage of histamine at the H_2 receptor, particularly those in the gastric parietal cells. Significantly reduces nocturnal gastric acid secretion for up to 12 h.

USES Active duodenal ulcers and maintenance therapy for duodenal ulcers.

ROUTE & DOSAGE

Active Duodenal Ulcer
Adult PO 150 mg b.i.d. or 300 mg h.s.

Maintenance Therapy
Adult PO 150 mg h.s.

PHARMACOKINETICS Absorption: > 90% absorbed from GI tract. **Peak:** 0.5–3 h. **Metabolism:** metabolized in liver. **Elimination:** half-life: 1–2 h; 60% excreted in urine unchanged.

CONTRAINDICATIONS & PRECAUTIONS Contraindicated in: hypersensitivity to nizatidine or other H_2 receptor antagonists. **Cautious use in:** renal impairment, pregnancy (category C). Distribution into breast milk is unknown.

ADVERSE/SIDE EFFECTS CNS: somnolence, fatigue. **Skin:** pruritus, sweating. **Other:** hyperuricemia.

NURSING IMPLICATIONS

Administration
- Drug is usually given once daily at bedtime. Dose may be divided and given twice daily.
- Antacids consisting of aluminum and magnesium hydroxides with simethicone decrease nizatidine absorption by about 10%. Administer the antacid 2 h after nizatidine.

Assessment & Drug Effects
- Monitor patient for alleviation of symptoms. Most ulcers should heal within 4 wk.
- Since asymptomatic ventricular tachycardia is a side effect of the drug, monitor cardiac patient's apical pulse.
- Monitor for persistence of ulcer symptoms in patients who continue to smoke during therapy.
- Monitor liver enzyme studies (AST, ALT) or alkaline phosphatase. Nizatidine may cause hepatocellular injury.

Patient & Family Education
- Instruct patient to take medications for the full course of therapy even though symptoms may be relieved.
- Instruct patient not to take other prescription or nonprescription medications without consulting with physician.

- Instruct patient in the importance of stopping smoking since smoking adversely affects healing of ulcers and effectiveness of the drug.

NONOXYNOL-9
(noe-nox´ee-nole)
Trade names: Conceptrol, Delfen, Gynol II, Koromex, Today
Classifications: SPERMICIDE CONTRACEPTIVE

ACTIONS/PHARMACODYNAMICS Nonionic surfactant spermicidal impregnated into a soft, pliable, and disposable polyurethane sponge or incorporated into foams, gels, jelly, or suppositories. Applied over the cervix, this agent blocks entrance to uterus by sperm, traps and absorbs seminal fluid, then releases the immediately available spermicide. Immobilizes sperm by cell membrane disruption. Nonoxynol-9 inhibits growth of certain organisms including *Staphylococcus aureus*, thought to be responsible for toxic shock syndrome (TSS). Primarily provides protection against lower genital tract infections and thus also against upper genital tract infections and their sequellae. When used correctly this vaginal spermicide is effective as a contraceptive for multiple coital encounters over a 24-h period. Clinical trials suggest that regular use of the spermicide may reduce the risk of contracting sexually transmitted diseases (STDs), including genital herpes, gonorrhea, and *Chlamydia trachomatis*, and may protect against organisms that are possible inducers of cervical cancer. Studies have failed to show teratogenic effects associated with nonoxynol-9 use as a spermicide. As with other contraceptive methods, most pregnancies result from product or user failure.

USES As barrier contraceptive alone or in conjunction with a vaginal diaphragm or with a condom.

ROUTE & DOSAGE

Contraceptive

Adult	Topical	Apply or insert 30–60 min before intercourse; sponge is effective for 24 h; other formulations should be repeated before each intercourse

PHARMACOKINETICS Onset: spermicidal action is prompt upon contact with sperm; minimal systemic absorption.

CONTRAINDICATIONS & PRECAUTIONS Contraindicated in: cystocele, prolapsed uterus, sensitivity or allergy to polyurethane or to nonoxynol-9; vaginitis; history of TSS; pregnancy; immediately after delivery or abortion; during menstruation.

ADVERSE/SIDE EFFECTS *Candidiasis;* vaginal irritation (uncommon) and dryness; increase in vaginal infections; menstrual and nonmenstrual TSS.

NURSING IMPLICATIONS

Patient & Family Education
- Patient should stop using the contraceptive sponge or other forms of nonoxynol-9 if pregnancy is suspected.
- Since nonoxynol-9 antifungal properties are weaker than its antibacterial potency, vulvovaginal candidiasis frequently occurs. Symptoms should be reported: burning, inflammation, intense vaginal and vulvar itching, cheesy, curdlike discharge, dyspareunia, dysuria.

General guidelines for use of vaginal spermicide
- Use spermicide before the first and every subsequent act of intercourse.
- *Foams, gels, jelly, cream:* fully load intravaginal applicator and insert about 2/3 of its length (7.5–10 cm [3–4 in]) into vagina.
- Coitus should not occur in a position that permits spermicide to seep out of vagina.
- Avoid douching for 6–8 h after coitus to prevent dilution or removal of spermicide.
- When a spermicide is used and intercourse takes place immediately before walking or exercising, insert a tampon.
- *Use of a diaphragm:* place 1–3 tsp spermicide formulation in dome prior to insertion. After diaphragm is in place, additional spermicide is recommended. Spermicide and diaphragm should be left in place 6 h after intercourse.

Spermicide sponge
- Use of the sponge has been associated with toxic shock syndrome (TSS). If the following symptoms develop, stop using the sponge: fever, myalgias, desquamating rash, chills, edema, nausea, vomiting, watery diarrhea. Most clinicians counsel against future use of the contraceptive sponge by the patient who has had TSS.
- Some physicians advocate use of sponge only as a back-up or interim method of contraception.
- The contraceptive sponge does not require fitting; one size fits all.

N

Common side effects in *italic*; life-threatening effects <u>underlined</u>; generic names in **bold**; classifications in SMALL CAPS

821

- Thoroughly moisten sponge with clear tap water; squeeze out excess fluid (will feel soapy and wet). Fold in half with convex side up and attached loop hanging down.
- Insertion: Slide sponge into vagina and place over external os of the cervix.
- Leave sponge in place at least 6 h after intercourse.
- Remove sponge within 24 h after its insertion.
- Vaginal irritation may be due to remnants of sponge left behind after difficult removal. Consult physician for vaginal examination and diagnosis.
- Store all forms of drug at 15–30C (59–86F) protected from moisture and light.

Prototype: epinephrine, p 102

NOREPINEPHRINE BITARTRATE
(nor-ep-i-nef´rin)

Trade names: Levarterenol, Levophed, Noradrenaline

Classifications: AUTONOMIC NERVOUS SYSTEM AGENT; ALPHA- AND BETA-ADRENERGIC AGONIST (SYMPATHOMIMETIC)

Pregnancy: Category D

ACTIONS/PHARMACODYNAMICS Direct-acting sympathomimetic amine identical to body catecholamine norepinephrine. Acts directly and predominantly on alpha-adrenergic receptors; little action on beta-receptors except in heart (beta$_1$ receptors). Main therapeutic effects are vasoconstriction and cardiac stimulation. Has powerful constrictor action on resistance and capacitance blood vessels. Reduces blood flow to kidney, other vital organs, skin, and skeletal muscle. Peripheral vasoconstriction (alpha-adrenergic action) and moderate inotropic stimulation of heart (beta-adrenergic action) result in increased systolic and diastolic blood pressure, myocardial oxygenation, coronary artery blood flow, and work of heart. Cardiac output varies reflexly with systemic BP. Reflex increase of vagal activity in response to pronounced effect on arterial BP may cause bradycardia. Causes less CNS stimulation and has less effect on metabolism than does epinephrine; however, in large doses it can increase glycogenolysis and inhibit pancreatic insulin release, with resulting hyperglycemia. May cause contraction of pregnant uterus.

USES To restore BP in certain acute hypotensive states such as shock, sympathectomy, pheochromo-

cytomectomy, spinal anesthesia, poliomyelitis, MI, septicemia, blood transfusion, and drug reactions. Also used as adjunct in treatment of cardiac arrest.

ROUTE & DOSAGE

Hypotension

Adult	IV	Initial: 8–12 μg/min; titrate to maintenance dose of 2–4 μg/min
Child	IV	Initial: 2 μg/min; titrate to maintenance dose of 0.1 μg/kg/min

PHARMACOKINETICS **Onset:** very rapid. **Duration:** 1–2 min after termination of infusion. **Distribution:** localizes in sympathetic nerve endings; crosses placenta. **Metabolism:** metabolized in liver and other tissues by catechol-o-methyl transferase and monoamine oxidase. **Elimination:** excreted in urine.

CONTRAINDICATIONS & PRECAUTIONS **Contraindicated in:** use as sole therapy in hypovolemic states, except as temporary emergency measure; mesenteric or peripheral vascular thrombosis; profound hypoxia or hypercarbia; pregnancy (category D); use during cyclopropane or halothane anesthesia. **Cautious use in:** hypertension; hyperthyroidism; severe heart disease; elderly patients; within 14 d of MAOI therapy, patients receiving tricyclic antidepressants.

ADVERSE/SIDE EFFECTS Headache, palpitation, hypertension, reflex bradycardia, <u>fatal arrhythmias</u> (large doses), respiratory difficulty, restlessness, anxiety, *tremors,* dizziness, weakness, insomnia, pallor, tissue necrosis at injection site (with extravasation), swelling of thyroid gland (rare). **With prolonged administration:** plasma volume depletion, edema, hemorrhage, intestinal, <u>hepatic,</u> and renal <u>necrosis</u>. **Overdosage or individual sensitivity:** blurred vision, photophobia, hyperglycemia, retrosternal and pharyngeal pain, profuse sweating, vomiting, severe hypertension, violent headache, <u>cerebral hemorrhage,</u> convulsions.

DRUG INTERACTIONS ALPHA AND BETA BLOCKERS antagonize pressor effects; ERGOT ALKALOIDS, **furazolidone, guanethidine, methyldopa,** TRICYCLIC ANTIDEPRESSANTS may potentiate pressor effects; **halothane, cyclopropane** increase risk of arrhythmias.

INCOMPATIBILITIES **Solution/Additive:** **aminophylline, amobarbital, whole blood, cephapirin, chlorothiazide, chlorpheniramine, pentobarbi-**

N

Common side effects in *italic*; life-threatening effects <u>underlined</u>; generic names in **bold**; classifications in SMALL CAPS

tal, phenobarbital, phenytoin, secobarbital, sodium bicarbonate, sodium iodide, strepto-mycin, thiopental.

NURSING IMPLICATIONS

Administration

- IV infusion of norepinephrine in saline alone is not recommended. Dextrose (in distilled water or saline solution) is used to prevent oxidation and thus loss of potency. Usual dilution is a 4 ml ampul in 1000 ml diluent to yield 4 μg/ml.
- Do not use solution if discoloration or precipitate is present. Protect from light.
- Initial rate of infusion is 2–3 ml/min (8–12 μg/min); then titrated to maintain BP, usually 0.5–1 ml/min (2–4 μg/min). An infusion pump is used. Consult physician for specific titration guidelines.
- In patients with severe hypotension after MI, the physician may prescribe addition of heparin to norepinephrine infusion to prevent thrombosis of infused vein and perivenous reaction.
- Risk of extravasation is reportedly reduced if infusion is administered through a plastic catheter inserted deep into vein.
- Flow rate must be constantly monitored. Check infusion site frequently (tape should not obscure injection site). Report immediately any evidence of extravasation: blanching along course of infused vein (may occur without obvious extravasation), cold, hard swelling around injection site.
- **Antidote for extravasation ischemia:** phentolamine, 5–10 mg in 10–15 ml NS injection, is infiltrated throughout affected area (using syringe with fine hypodermic needle) as soon as possible. Some physicians prefer to add phentolamine (5–10 mg) to each liter of infusion solution as a preventive against sloughing should extravasation occur.
- If therapy is to be prolonged, it is advisable to change infusion sites at intervals to allow effect of local vasoconstriction to subside.
- When therapy is to be discontinued, infusion rate is slowed gradually. Abrupt withdrawal should be avoided.

Assessment & Drug Effects

- Patient should be monitored constantly while receiving norepinephrine. Take baseline BP and pulse before start of therapy, then q2min from initiation of drug until stabilization occurs at desired level, then every 5 min during drug administration.
- In normotensive patients it is recommended that flow rate be adjusted to maintain BP at low normal (usually 80–100 mm Hg systolic). In previously hypertensive patients, systolic is generally maintained no higher than 40 mm Hg below preexisting systolic level.
- In addition to vital signs, carefully observe and record mental status (index of cerebral circulation), skin temperature of extremities, and color (especially of earlobes, lips, nail beds).
- Monitor I&O. Urinary retention and renal shutdown are possibilities, especially in hypovolemic patients. Urinary output is a sensitive indicator of the degree of renal perfusion. Report decrease in urinary output or change in I&O ratio.
- Be alert to patient's complaints of headache, vomiting, palpitation, arrhythmias, chest pain, photophobia, and blurred vision as possible symptoms of overdosage. Reflex bradycardia may occur as a result of rise in BP.
- Continue to monitor vital signs and observe patient closely after cessation of therapy for clinical sign of circulatory inadequacy.

Prototype: progesterone, p 241

NORETHINDRONE

(nor-eth-in´drone)

Trade names: Micronor, Norlutin, Nor-Q.D.

NORETHINDRONE ACETATE

Trade name: Norlutate
Classifications: SYNTHETIC HORMONE; PROGESTIN
Pregnancy: Category X

ACTIONS/PHARMACODYNAMICS Synthetic progestational hormone with androgenic, anabolic, and estrogenic properties. (The acetate form is the most potent anabolic agent available with approximately double the progestational potency of norethindrone.) May produce excess estrogenic effect. Mechanism for prevention of contraception unclear. Progestin-only contraceptives alter cervical mucus, exert progestational effect on endometrium, interfere with implantation, and, in some cases, suppress ovulation.

USES To treat amenorrhea, abnormal uterine bleeding due to hormonal imbalance in absence of organic pathology; endometriosis. Also alone or in combination with an estrogen for birth control.

N

Common side effects in *italic*; life-threatening effects <u>underlined</u>; generic names in **bold**; classifications in SMALL CAPS

823

ROUTE & DOSAGE

Amenorrhea

Adult	PO	Norethindrone: 5–20 mg on day 5 through day 25 of menstrual cycle
		Acetate: 2.5–10 mg on day 5 through day 25 of menstrual cycle

Endometriosis

Adult	PO	Norethindrone: 10 mg/d for 2 wk; increase by 5 mg/d q2wk up to 30 mg/d; dose may remain at this level for 6–9 mo or until breakthrough bleeding
		Acetate: 5 mg/d for 2 wk; increase by 2.5 mg/d q2wk up to 15 mg/d; dose may remain at this level for 6–9 mo or until breakthrough bleeding

Progestin-only Contraception

Adult	PO	Norethindrone: 0.35 mg/d starting on day 1 of menstrual flow, then continuing indefinitely

PHARMACOKINETICS Absorption: readily absorbed from GI tract. **Metabolism:** metabolized in liver. **Elimination:** excreted in urine and feces as metabolites.

CONTRAINDICATIONS & PRECAUTIONS Contraindicated in: known or suspected pregnancy (Category X), thromboembolic disorders, cerebral vascular or coronary vascular disease, carcinoma of breast, endometrium, or liver, and abnormal vaginal bleeding.

ADVERSE/SIDE EFFECTS CNS: <u>cerebral thrombosis or hemorrhage</u>, depression. **CV:** hypertension, <u>pulmonary embolism</u>, edema. **GI:** nausea, vomiting, cholestatic jaundice, abdominal cramps. **Reproductive:** *breakthrough bleeding,* cervical erosion, changes in menstrual flow, dysmenorrhea, vaginal candidiasis. **Other:** *weight changes; breast tenderness,* enlargement or secretion.

NURSING IMPLICATIONS

Administration

- Dosing schedule is based on a 28-day menstrual cycle.
- When starting the minipill regimen, the patient should use a second method of birth control for the first cycle or for 3 wk to insure full protection.
- The minipill can be started right after delivery in the nonnursing mother; however, she should be aware of an increased risk of thromboembolic disease during the postpartum period.

Assessment & Drug Effects

- Monitor for signs and symptoms of thrombophlebitis (see chap 3).
- Drug should be withheld and physician notified if any of the following occur: sudden complete or partial loss of vision, proptosis, diplopia, or migraine headache.

Patient & Family Education

Continuous regimen with progestin-only contraception (minipill), e.g., Micronor, Nor-Q.D.:

- Advise patient to wait at least 3 mo before becoming pregnant after stopping the minipill to prevent birth defects. A nonhormonal method of contraception should be employed until pregnancy is desired.
- In the event of a missed menstrual period: (1) if patient has not adhered to prescribed dosing regimen, the possibility of pregnancy should be considered after 45 d from the last menstrual period; progestin-only contraceptive should be withheld until pregnancy is ruled out; (2) if patient has adhered to prescribed regimen and misses 2 consecutive periods, pregnancy should be ruled out, and a nonhormonal method of birth control should be used before continuing the regimen.
- Review package insert with the patient to assure understanding of use of norethindrone.
- Instruct patient to report promptly prolonged vaginal bleeding or amenorrhea.
- Teach patient self-breast examination (SBE).
- Urge patient to keep appointments for physical checkups (q6–12mo) during period of hormonal birth control.
- Store at 15–30C (59–86F); protect drug from light and from freezing.

Prototype: ciprofloxacin, p 87

NORFLOXACIN

(nor-flox´a-sin)
Trade name: Noroxin
Classifications: URINARY TRACT ANTIINFECTIVE; ANTIBIOTIC; QUINOLONE
Pregnancy: Category C

ACTIONS/PHARMACODYNAMICS Fluoroquinolone derivative of nalidixic acid with potent broad-spectrum activity; more potent than the amino-

N

glycosides, cephalosporins, tetracyclines. Action (unlike that of penicillins and cephalosporins) is intracellular. Alters structure of bacterial DNA-gyrase, thus promoting double stranded DNA breakage, interfering with synthesis of bacterial protein and blocking bacterial survival. Active against virtually all bacterial urinary tract pathogens including *Escherichia coli, Klebsiella pneumoniae, Enterobacter cloacae,* indole-positive *Proteus* sp, *Pseudomonas aeruginosa, Staphylococcus aureus,* group D streptococci, *Neisseria gonorrhoeae,* and against common GI pathogens (e.g., *Salmonella, Shigella).* Generally ineffective against obligate anaerobes. Development of resistance (especially to *P. aeruginosa, K. pneumoniae, Acinetobacter* sp, and enterococci) has been reported, but drug has strong activity against many strains of multiple-antibiotic-resistant bacteria. No reported evidence of mutagenicity, carcinogenicity, or cross-allergenicity with penicillins, cephalosporins, or sulfonamides.

USES Adults with complicated and uncomplicated urinary tract infection (UTI) caused by susceptible organisms. **Unlabeled uses:** gonorrhea, gastroenteritis, and prevention of travelers' diarrhea.

ROUTE & DOSAGE

Urinary Tract Infection
Adult   PO   400 mg b.i.d.

Gonorrhea or Gonococcal Urethritis
Adult   PO   800 mg once/d

Bacterial Gastroenteritis
Adult   PO   400 mg q8–12h

PHARMACOKINETICS Absorption: 30–40% absorbed from GI tract. **Peak:** 1–2 h. **Distribution:** renal parenchyma, gallbladder, liver, prostate; crosses placenta; distributed into breast milk. **Metabolism:** metabolized in liver. **Elimination:** half-life: 3–4 h; excreted in urine and feces.

CONTRAINDICATIONS & PRECAUTIONS Contraindicated in: use in individual with known factors that predispose to seizures (effect of drug on brain function not known); history of hypersensitivity to norfloxacin and other quinolone antiinfectives. Safe use during pregnancy (category C), by nursing mothers, and by children, not established. **Cautious use in:** impaired renal function, adolescent children if skeletal growth is complete.

ADVERSE/SIDE EFFECTS (approximately 3–4% of patients). **Arthropathy:** joint swelling, cartilage erosion in weight-bearing joints, tendonitis. In immunosuppressed adult: acute ankle and hip pain followed by acute pain, tenderness, and swelling of tendon sheath of middle finger of both hands after 4 wk of therapy. **CNS:** *headache,* dizziness, lightheadedness, fatigue, drowsiness, somnolence, depression, insomnia, seizures. **GI:** *nausea,* abdominal pain, diarrhea, vomiting, anorexia, dyspepsia, dysphagia, dry mouth, bitter taste, heartburn, flatulence, pruritus ani. **Hematologic:** leukopenia, neutropenia, anemia (rare), decreased Hct. **Hepatic:** increased serum AST, ALT, alkaline phosphatase, LDH (rare). **Renal:** with high doses: crystalluria (not associated with renal toxicity). **Other:** tinnitus (rare); vulvar irritation.

DRUG INTERACTIONS ANTACIDS, **iron, sucralfate** decrease absorption; **nitrofurantoin** may antagonize antibacterial effects; may increase hypoprothrombinemic effects of **warfarin;** may cause slight increase in **theophylline** levels.

NURSING IMPLICATIONS

Administration

- Administer norfloxacin 1 h before or 2 h after meals with a full glass of water. Encourage high fluid intake (at least 2500–3000 ml/d if tolerated) to provide adequate urine output and hydration, important in the prevention of crystalluria (rare side effect).
- If patient is also taking an antacid, administer it at least 2 h after norfloxacin to prevent interference with absorption. Aluminum or magnesium ions in the antacid may bind to and form insoluble complexes with the quinolone in GI tract.
- Store at 40C (104F) or less in tightly closed container. Do not freeze.

Assessment & Drug Effects

- Urine specimens are collected before starting and during therapy for culture and susceptibility testing.
- If patient is adequately hydrated, yet I&O ratio and pattern changes are noted, or if condition does not improve within a few days, report to the physician. Dosage may need to be modified.

Patient & Family Education

- Advise patient to take drug at same time each day (e.g., if drug is prescribed for twice daily, take it 12 h apart: 8 AM and 8 PM). It should not be necessary to establish a schedule that interferes with sleep.
- Caution patient to take norfloxacin exactly as prescribed. Erratic dosing can encourage emergence

N

Common side effects in *italic*; life-threatening effects underlined; generic names in **bold**; classifications in SMALL CAPS

825

of resistant bacteria; underdosing or premature discontinuation of treatment can cause return of UTI symptoms.

- Patient should be made aware of what to do when a dose of norfloxacin is missed.
- Although dry mouth reportedly occurs in less than 1%, instruct to report to a dentist if it occurs and persists for more than 2 wk. Sugar-free gum, a saliva substitute (e.g., Moi-stir, Xero-Lube), or frequent sips of water help to hydrate oral membranes and prevent demineralization of tooth surfaces.

Prototype: progesterone, p 241

NORGESTREL
(nor-jess´trel)
Trade name: Ovrette
Classifications: HORMONE; PROGESTIN
Pregnancy: Category X

ACTIONS/PHARMACODYNAMICS Potent progestational hormone with androgenic, antiestrogenic, and anabolic properties. Induces and maintains endometrium, preventing uterine bleeding; inhibits production of pituitary gonadotropin, preventing ovulation; and produces thick cervical mucus resistant to passage of sperm.

USES A progestin-only contraceptive (minipill).

ROUTE & DOSAGE

Progestin-only Contraception

Adult PO 0.075 mg/d starting on day 1 of menstrual flow, then continuing indefinitely

PHARMACOKINETICS Absorption: readily absorbed from GI tract. **Metabolism:** metabolized in liver. **Elimination:** excreted in urine and feces as metabolites.

CONTRAINDICATIONS & PRECAUTIONS Contraindicated in: known or suspected pregnancy (Category X), thromboembolic disorders, cerebral vascular or coronary vascular disease, carcinoma of breast, endometrium, or liver, and abnormal vaginal bleeding.

ADVERSE/SIDE EFFECTS CNS: cerebral thrombosis or hemorrhage, depression. **CV:** hypertension, pulmonary embolism, edema. **GI:** nausea, vomiting, cholestatic jaundice, abdominal cramps. **Reproductive:** *breakthrough bleeding,* cervical erosion, changes in menstrual flow, dysmenorrhea, vaginal candidiasis. **Other:** *weight changes; breast tenderness,* enlargement, or secretion.

NURSING IMPLICATIONS

Administration

- When starting the mini-pill regimen, the patient should use a second method of birth control for the first cycle or for 3 wk to insure full protection.
- The minipill can be started right after delivery in the nonnursing mother; however, she should be aware of an increased risk of thromboembolic disease during the postpartum period.
- Minipill is to be taken at same time each day, even if user is menstruating.
- Store at 15–30C (59–86F) in a tightly closed container.

Assessment & Drug Effects

- Monitor for signs and symptoms of thrombophlebitis (see chap 3).
- Drug should be withheld and physician notified if any of the following occur: sudden complete or partial loss of vision, proptosis, diplopia, or migraine headache.

Patient & Family Education

- Amount and duration of flow, cycle length, breakthrough bleeding, spotting, and amenorrhea vary greatly with use of the progestin-only contraceptive.
- Advise patient to wait at least 3 mo before becoming pregnant after stopping the minipill to prevent birth defects. A nonhormonal method of contraception should be employed until pregnancy is desired.
- In the event of a missed menstrual period: (1) if patient has not adhered to prescribed dosing regimen, the possibility of pregnancy should be considered after 45 d from the last menstrual period; progestin-only contraceptive should be withheld until pregnancy is ruled out; (2) if patient has adhered to prescribed regimen and misses 2 consecutive periods, pregnancy should be ruled out and a nonhormonal method of birth control should be used before continuation of the regimen.
- Review package insert with patient to assure understanding about use of norgestrel.
- Teach patient self-breast examination (SBE).

N

NORMAL SERUM ALBUMIN, HUMAN

See BLOOD DERIVATIVE, PLASMA VOLUME
EXPANDER prototype, p 126.

Prototype: imipramine, p 184

NORTRIPTYLINE HYDROCHLORIDE
(nor-trip´ti-leen)
Trade names: Aventyl, Pamelor
Classifications: CNS AGENT; PSYCHOTHERAPEU-
TIC; TRICYCLIC ANTIDEPRESSANT
Pregnancy: Category D

ACTIONS/PHARMACODYNAMICS Secondary
amine derivative of amitriptyline. Tricyclic antidepressant (TCA) with less sedative and anticholinergic
effects than imipramine. Action mechanism unclear;
mood elevation may be due to its inhibition of reuptake of norepinephrine at the presynaptic membrane.

USES To treat endogenous depression. Similar in actions, uses, limitations, and interactions to imipramine.

ROUTE & DOSAGE

Antidepressant

Adult	PO	25 mg t.i.d. or q.i.d., gradually in-creased to 100–150 mg/d
Adolescent	PO	30–50 mg/d in divided doses

PHARMACOKINETICS Absorption: rapidly absorbed from GI tract. **Peak:** 7–8.5 h. **Distribution:**
crosses placenta; distributed in breast milk.
Metabolism: metabolized in liver. **Elimination:** half-life:
16–90 h; primarily excreted in urine.

**CONTRAINDICATIONS & PRECAUTIONS Con-
traindicated in:** children <12 y; pregnancy, lactation,
during or within 14 d of MAO inhibitor therapy; acute
recovery period after MI; pregnancy (category D).
Cautious use in: narrow-angle glaucoma, hyperthyroidism, concurrent administration of thyroid medications, concurrent use with electroshock therapy.

ADVERSE/SIDE EFFECTS *Urinary retention,* paralytic ileus, *orthostatic hypotension,* drowsiness, confusional state (especially in the elderly and with high
dosage), agranulocytosis, tremors, hyperhydrosis,
dry mouth, blurred vision, photosensitivity reaction.

DRUG INTERACTIONS May decrease some antihypertensive response to ANTIHYPERTENSIVES; CNS
DEPRESSANTS, **alcohol,** HYPNOTICS, BARBITURATES,
SEDATIVES potentiate CNS depression; may increase
hypoprothombinemic effect of ORAL ANTICOAGU-
LANTS; **ethchlorvynol** may cause transient delirium;
levodopa, SYMPATHOMIMETICS (e.g., epinephrine,
norepinephrine) pose possibility of sympathetic hyperactivity with hypertension and hyperpyrexia; MAO
INHIBITORS pose possibility of severe reactions—toxic
psychosis, cardiovascular instability; **methylphenidate** increases plasma TCA levels; THYROID
DRUGS may increase possibility of arrhythmias; **cimetidine** may increase plasma TCA levels.

NURSING IMPLICATIONS

Administration
- Administer drug with food to decrease gastric distress.
- Oral solution does not require dilution. Aventyl is
a 4% alcohol solution.
- Supervise drug ingestion to be sure patient swallows medication.
- Store drug in tightly closed container at 15–30C
(59–86F) unless otherwise specified.

Assessment & Drug Effects
- Nortriptyline has a narrow therapeutic plasma level
range, a characteristic called "therapeutic window."
Drug levels above or below the therapeutic window are associated with decreased rate of response.
- Therapeutic response may not occur for 2 wk or
more.
- Monitor BP and pulse rate during adjustment period of TCA therapy. If systolic BP falls more than
20 mm Hg or if there is a sudden increase in pulse
rate, withhold medication and notify the physician.
- If psychotic signs increase, notify physician.
Because of the therapeutic window effect of nortriptyline, a substitute TCA may be prescribed
rather than an increase in dosage.
- Inspect oral membranes daily if patient is on high
doses of TCA. Urge outpatient to report stomatitis
or dry mouth. Sore mouth can be a major cause of
poor nutrition and noncompliance. Consult physician about use of a saliva substitute (e.g., VA-
Oralube, Moi-stir).

Common side effects in *italic*; life-threatening effects underlined;
generic names in **bold**; classifications in SMALL CAPS

827

- Monitor bowel elimination pattern and I&O ratio. Urinary retention and severe constipation are potential problems, especially in the elderly. Advise increased fluid intake; consult physician about stool softener.
- Observe patient with history of glaucoma. Symptoms that may signal acute attack (severe headache, eye pain, dilated pupils, halos of light, nausea, vomiting) should be reported promptly.
- Fine tremors may be reduced or alleviated by propranolol. Report symptom to physician.
- Alcohol potentiation may increase the danger of overdosage or suicide attempt.

Patient & Family Education

- Caution patient that ability to perform tasks requiring alertness and skill may be impaired.
- Urge patient not to use OTC drugs unless physician approves.
- The actions of both alcohol and nortriptyline are potentiated when used together and for up to 2 wk after the TCA is discontinued. Consult physician about safe amount of alcohol, if any, that can be taken.
- The effects of barbiturates and other CNS depressants are enhanced by nortriptyline.

NOVOBIOCIN SODIUM

(noe-voe-bye´o-sin)
Trade name: Albamycin
Classifications: ANTIINFECTIVE; ANTIBIOTIC
Pregnancy: Category C

ACTIONS/PHARMACODYNAMICS Antibiotic obtained from cultures of *Streptomyces niveus* or *Streptomyces spheroides*. Bacteriostatic action appears to involve interference with synthesis of bacterial cell wall and inhibition of bacterial protein and nucleic acid synthesis. Cell membrane stability and integrity are also affected because of complexing of drug with magnesium within cell wall. Active in vitro against many gram-positive bacteria including *Staphylococcus aureus, Streptococcus pneumoniae,* group A streptococci, and viridans streptococci, and against some gram-positive bacilli. Enterococci are usually resistant to novobiocin. Also active against gram-negative bacteria including *Haemophilus influenzae* and *Neisseria gonorrhoeae*. Resistant strains of *S. aureus* may develop rapidly during therapy. Cross-resistance between novobiocin and other antiinfectives has not been reported.

USES Serious infections due to *S. aureus* in patients unresponsive to less toxic antiinfectives or not sensitive to other antiinfectives.

ROUTE & DOSAGE

S. aureus Infections

Adult	PO	250 mg q6h or 500 mg q12h up to 2 g/d
Child	PO	15–45 mg/kg/d in 2–4 divided doses

PHARMACOKINETICS Absorption: readily absorbed from GI tract. **Peak:** 1–4 h. **Distribution:** highest concentrations in liver, small intestine, and bile; distributed into breast milk. **Elimination:** excreted primarily in bile and feces.

CONTRAINDICATIONS & PRECAUTIONS Contraindicated in: neonates, during pregnancy (category C). **Cautious use in:** hepatic dysfunction.

ADVERSE/SIDE EFFECTS GI: *nausea, vomiting, diarrhea, anorexia, abdominal distress.* **Hematologic:** pancytopenia, agranulocytosis, anemia, thrombocytopenia, hemolytic anemia, positive direct and indirect antiglobin (Coombs') test. **Hepatic:** jaundice, elevated serum bilirubin. **Hypersensitivity:** *urticaria,* maculopapular dermatitis, swollen joints, Stevens-Johnson syndrome, erythema multiforme, pruritus, fever, eosinophilia. **Other:** dizziness, drowsiness, light-headedness. Causal relationship not established: allergic pneumonitis, myocarditis, alopecia, intestinal hemorrhage, superinfections.

DIAGNOSTIC TEST INTERFERENCES A yellow metabolite may appear if serum interferes with **serum bilirubin** determinations (Evelyn-Malloy method).

DRUG INTERACTIONS TETRACYCLINES may reduce novobiocin effectiveness.

NURSING IMPLICATIONS

Administration

- Drug must be taken at correct time intervals (i.e., q6h or q12h) to be effective.
- When novobiocin is given concurrently with tetracyclines, schedule the two drugs to be taken at least 3 h apart.

Common side effects in *italic*; life-threatening effects underlined; generic names in **bold**; classifications in SMALL CAPS

Assessment & Drug Effects

- Novobiocin is an extremely potent sensitizing agent. Side effects should be reported promptly.
- A yellow metabolite of novobiocin can cause jaundicelike skin coloration. Differentiation of drug-induced effect from frank jaundice will depend on other signs of hepatic dysfunction (i.e., dark urine, pruritus, elevated serum bilirubin). Advise patient to report symptoms promptly.
- Inspect skin for signs of thrombocyte dyscrasia: petechiae, ecchymoses, easy bruising; these signs or epistaxis or bleeding for unexplained reason should be reported promptly.

Patient & Family Education

- Drug resistance may develop rapidly. Advise patient to report if there is a reversal in prior evidence of therapeutic response to drug therapy.
- Duration of therapy depends on the infection but inform patient that it will continue about 48 h after febrile condition is past or when evidence of the infection is eradicated. Patient should not stop treatment just because he or she feels better.
- Patient should not alter regimen without consulting physician; sensitivity and adverse effects may occur as well as a loss of therapeutic effects.
- Warn patient not to use leftover novobiocin to self-medicate for another infection.
- Symptoms of superinfections (see chap 3) should receive prompt attention and thus should be reported immediately.

Prototype: isoproterenol, p 105

NYLIDRIN HYDROCHLORIDE
(nye´li-drin)

Trade names: Adrin, Arlidin, Rolidrin
Classifications: AUTONOMIC NERVOUS SYSTEM AGENT; BETA-ADRENERGIC AGONIST (SYMPATHOMIMETIC); VASODILATOR
Pregnancy: Category C

ACTIONS/PHARMACODYNAMICS Sympathomimetic amine. Acts predominantly on beta-adrenergic receptors. Increases blood flow to skeletal muscle by direct vasodilating action on arteries and arterioles; also slightly increases cerebral blood flow. Produces increase in cardiac output and some increase in heart rate; systolic BP usually rises slightly, and diastolic may fall. Effect on cutaneous blood flow is negligible. Clinical value not established.

USES Vasospastic disorders such as peripheral vascular disease, e.g., acrocyanosis, Raynaud's syndrome, frostbite, night leg cramps, thromboangiitis obliterans, ischemic ulcer, diabetic vascular disease, Ménière's disease, circulatory disturbances of inner ear.

ROUTE & DOSAGE

Vasodilator
Adult   PO   3–12 mg t.i.d. or q.i.d.

PHARMACOKINETICS Absorption: readily absorbed from GI tract. **Onset:** 10 min. **Peak:** 30 min. **Duration:** 2 h. **Metabolism:** metabolized in liver. **Elimination:** excreted slowly in urine.

CONTRAINDICATIONS & PRECAUTIONS Contraindicated in: history of recent MI, cardiac disease such as tachyarrhythmias, uncompensated heart failure, angina pectoris, thyrotoxicosis, peptic ulcer. Pregnancy category C. **Cautious use in:** hypertension, peptic ulcer, cardiac disorders.

ADVERSE/SIDE EFFECTS *Trembling, nervousness,* weakness, dizziness, palpitation, nausea, vomiting, postural hypotension.

NURSING IMPLICATIONS

Administration

- Drug is readily absorbed from GI tract and may be given without regard to meals.

Assessment & Drug Effects

- Palpitation is a prominent side effect that usually disappears with continued therapy; if it persists, reduction in dosage may be necessary.
- Observe for clinical response to therapy. For patients with peripheral vascular disease, note relief of rest pain, or intermittent claudication, and nail growth. For patients with circulatory disturbances of inner ear, note relief of dizziness, nausea, and nystagmus.

Patient & Family Education

- Inform the patient that the benefits of nylidrin may not be apparent until after several weeks of therapy.
- Hygienic care of extremities, properly fitting shoes and stockings, abstinence from smoking, avoidance of exposure to cold, and guidelines regarding acceptable activities are essential aspects of care in patients with peripheral vascular disease.

N

Prototype: amphotericin B, p 56

NYSTATIN
(nye-stat´in)
Trade names: Mycostatin, Mykinal, Nadostine, Nilstat, Nyaderm, Nystex, O-V Statin
Classifications: ANTIINFECTIVE; ANTIBIOTIC; ANTIFUNGAL
Pregnancy: Category C

ACTIONS/PHARMACODYNAMICS
Nontoxic, nonsensitizing antifungal antibiotic produced by *Streptomyces noursei*. Has both fungistatic and fungicidal activity against a variety of yeasts and fungi; not appreciably active against bacteria, viruses, or protozoa. Binds to sterols in fungal cell membrane, thereby changing membrane potential and allowing leakage of intracellular components.

USES
Local infections of skin and mucous membranes caused by *Candida* sp including *Candida albicans*: e.g., paronychia; cutaneous, oropharyngeal, vulvovaginal, and intestinal candidiasis.

ROUTE & DOSAGE

Candida Infections

Adult	PO	500,000–1,000,000 U t.i.d.
		1–4 troches 4–5 times/d
		Suspension: 400,000–600,000 U q.i.d.
	Vaginal	1–2 tablets daily for 2 wk
Child	PO	Suspension: 400,000–600,000 U q.i.d.
Infants	PO	100,000–200,000 U q.i.d.

PHARMACOKINETICS
Absorption: poorly absorbed from GI tract. **Elimination:** excreted in feces.

CONTRAINDICATIONS & PRECAUTIONS
Contraindicated in: use of vaginal tablets during pregnancy (category C); vaginal infections caused by *Gardnerella vaginalis* or *Trichomonas* sp.

ADVERSE/SIDE EFFECTS
Usually mild: nausea, vomiting, epigastric distress, diarrhea (especially with high oral doses); hypersensitivity reactions (rare).

NURSING IMPLICATIONS

Administration
- Note that nystatin vaginal tablets may be given PO for treatment of candidiasis.
- Avoid contact of drug with hands. Hypersensitivity reactions occur rarely with nystatin alone; however, preservatives in some formulations are associated with a high incidence of contact dermatitis. Advise patient to report onset of redness, swelling, or irritation. Drug should be discontinued if these symptoms occur.
- Store all formulations except vaginal tablets at 15–30C (59–86F), vaginal tablets in refrigerator below 15C (59F). Avoid freezing of any formulation. Protect from excess heat and light.

Patient & Family Education
Oral candidiasis (thrush) treatment
(after meals and at bedtime)
- *Oral suspension:* Rinse mouth with 1–2 tsp nystatin oral suspension. Keep in mouth (swish) as long as possible (at least 2 min), then expectorate. (Drug may be swallowed if patient cannot retain liquid in mouth or cannot expectorate or if ordered "swish and swallow.") Children, infants: apply drug with swab to each side of mouth. Avoid food or drink for 30 min after treatment.
- *Troche:* leave in mouth until dissolved (about 30 min). Do not chew or swallow. Avoid food and drink during period of dissolving, and for 30 min after treatment.
- *Care of dentures* (essential to effective treatment): remove dentures before each rinse with oral suspension and before use of troche. Advise patient to remove dentures at night (infection occurs more frequently in person who wears dentures 24 h a day).
- Treatment of oral candidiasis should be continued at least 48 h after disappearance of perioral symptoms and mouth cultures are normal.

Candidiasis of feet, skin, and nails
- Instruct patient to dust shoes and stockings, as well as feet, with nystatin dusting powder.
- Occlusive dressings (including tight-fitting underclothing) or applications of ointment preparation to moist, dark areas of body favor growth of yeast and therefore should be avoided.
- Cream is preferred to the ointment for intertriginous areas. For very moist lesions, powder is usually prescribed. Infected areas should be cleaned gently with tepid water before each application.
- Treatment of cutaneous candidal infections is continued for at least 2 wk and discontinued only after two negative tests for *Candida*.

Common side effects in *italic*; life-threatening effects underlined; generic names in **bold**; classifications in SMALL CAPS

Vulvovaginal candidiasis
- Inform patient that medication should be continued during menstruation. In most cases 2 wk of therapy are sufficient; however, some patients may require longer treatment.
- Vaginal tablets may be used up to 6 wk before term to prevent thrush in the newborn.

OCTREOTIDE ACETATE
(oc-tre´o-tide)
Trade name: Sandostatin
Classification: SYNTHETIC HORMONE; ANTIDIARRHEAL
Pregnancy: Category B

ACTIONS/PHARMACODYNAMICS A long-acting octapeptide that mimics the natural hormone somatastatin. Octreotide suppresses secretion of serotonin, pancreatic peptides, gastrin, vasoactive intestinal peptide, insulin, glucagon, secretin and motilin. It stimulates fluid and electrolyte absorption from the GI tract, prolongs intestinal transit time, and also inhibits the growth hormone.

USES Symptomatic treatment of severe diarrhea and flushing episodes associated with metastatic carcinoid tumors. Also watery diarrhea associated with vasoactive intestinal peptide (VIP) tumors. **Unlabeled uses:** acromegaly associated with pituitary tumors, fistula drainage, variceal bleeding.

ROUTE & DOSAGE

Carcinoid Syndrome

Adult	SC	100–600 µg/d in 2–4 divided doses; titrate to response.
Child	SC	1–10 µg/kg/d in 2–4 divided doses; titrate to response

VIPoma

Adult	SC	200–300 µg/d in 2–4 divided doses; titrate to response
Child	SC	1–10 µg/kg/d in 2–4 divided doses; titrate to response

PHARMACOKINETICS Absorption: rapidly absorbed from SC injection site. **Peak:** 0.4 h. **Duration:** up to 12 h. **Metabolism:** 68% metabolized in liver. **Elimination:** half-life: 1.5 h; excreted in urine.

CONTRAINDICATIONS & PRECAUTIONS Contraindicated in: hypersensitivity to octreotide. **Cautious use in:** cholelithiasis, renal impairment, pregnancy (category B), diabetes, and hypothyroidism. It is not known whether it is excreted in breast milk.

ADVERSE/SIDE EFFECTS CNS: headache, fatigue, dizziness. **GI:** *nausea, diarrhea,* abdominal pain and discomfort. **Metabolic:** hypoglycemia, hyperglycemia, increased liver transaminases, hypothyroidism (after long-term use). **Other:** flushing, edema, injection site pain.

DRUG INTERACTIONS May decrease **cyclosporine** levels; may alter other drug and nutrient absorption because of alterations in GI motility.

NURSING IMPLICATIONS

Administration
- Do not use solution if particulates or discoloration is observed.
- Subcutaneous injection is the recommended route of administration. However, under emergency conditions, an IV bolus may be given by direct injection over 60 seconds.
- To reduce local irritation, allow solution to reach room temperature before injection and administer slowly.
- For prolonged storage, ampules should be refrigerated at 2–8C. Ampules stored at room temperature should be used within 24 h.

Assessment & Drug Effects
- Monitor for hypoglycemia and hyperglycemia (see Signs & Symptoms, chap 3), since octreotide may alter the balance between insulin, glucagon, and growth hormone.
- Monitor fluid and electrolyte balance, as octreotide stimulates fluid and electrolyte absorption from GI tract.
- Dietary fat absorption may be altered in some clients. Monitor fecal fat and serum carotene to aid in the assessment of possible drug-induced aggravation of fat malabsorption.

Patient & Family Education
- Provide instruction on proper technique for SC injection if self-medication is required.
- Inform patient that preferred sites for SC injections of octreotide are the hip, thigh, and abdomen.
- Inform patient that multiple injections at the same SC injection site within short periods of time are not recommended. This is to avoid irritating the area.

■ To minimize GI side effects, instruct patient to give injections between meals and at bedtime.

OMEPRAZOLE

(o-me´pra-zole)
Trade name: Prilosec
Classifications: GI AGENT; ANTISECRETORY
Pregnancy: Category C

ACTIONS/PHARMACODYNAMICS Omeprazole belongs to a new class of antisecretory compounds that do not exhibit anticholinergic or H_2 histamine antagonistic properties but suppress the H^+-K^+ ATPase enzyme system of the gastric parietal cell, which is necessary in gastric acid production.

USES Gastroesophageal reflux disease including severe erosive esophagitis (4 to 8 wk treatment). Long-term treatment of pathologic hypersecretory conditions such as Zollinger-Ellison syndrome, multiple endocrine adenomas, and systemic mastocytosis. **Unlabeled use:** duodenal ulcers.

ROUTE & DOSAGE

Gastroesophageal Reflux
Adult   PO   20 mg once/d for 4–8 wk

Hypersecretory Disease
Adult   PO   60 mg once/d up to 120 mg t.i.d.

PHARMACOKINETICS **Absorption:** poorly absorbed from GI tract; 30–40% reaches systemic circulation. **Onset:** 0.5–3.5 h. **Peak:** peak inhibition of gastric acid secretion: 5 d. **Metabolism:** metabolized in liver. **Elimination:** half-life: 0.5–1.5 h; 80% excreted in urine, 20% in feces.

CONTRAINDICATIONS & PRECAUTIONS **Contraindicated in:** long-term use for gastroesophageal reflux disease, duodenal ulcers, lactation. **Cautious use in:** pregnancy (category C). Safety and effectiveness in children have not been established.

ADVERSE/SIDE EFFECTS CNS: headache, dizziness, fatigue. **GI:** *diarrhea, abdominal pain, nausea,* mild transient increases in liver function tests. **Other:** rash.

DRUG INTERACTIONS Concomitant administration of **diazepam** and omeprazole may increase diazepam concentrations. Concomitant administration of **phenytoin** and omeprazole may increase phenytoin levels. Concomitant administration of **warfarin** and omeprazole may increase warfarin levels.

DIAGNOSTIC TEST INTERFERENCES Omeprazole has been reported to significantly impair peak *cortisol* response to exogenous ACTH. This finding is undergoing further investigation.

NURSING IMPLICATIONS

Administration
■ Capsules must be swallowed whole and should be taken before eating.
■ Antacids may be administered with omeprazole.

Assessment & Drug Effects
■ Symptomatic response to therapy with omeprazole does not preclude gastric malignancy.
■ Monitor urinalysis for hematuria and proteinuria.

Patient & Family Education
■ Instruct patient to swallow capsule whole—not to open, chew, or crush—and to take drug before eating, preferably before breakfast.
■ Lactating women should discontinue nursing prior to taking the drug.
■ Instruct patient to report any changes in urinary elimination such as pain or discomfort associated with urination.
■ Instruct patient to report severe diarrhea. The drug may need to be discontinued.

ONDANSETRON HYDROCHLORIDE

(on-dan´si-tron)
Trade name: Zofran
Classifications: GI AGENT; ANTIEMETIC; ANTIVERTIGO
Pregnancy: Category B

ACTIONS/PHARMACODYNAMICS Ondansetron is a selective serotonin receptor antagonist used for prevention of nausea and vomiting associated with cancer chemotherapy. Serotonin receptors are located centrally in the chemoreceptor trigger zone (CTZ) and peripherally on the vagal nerve terminals. Serotonin is released from the wall of the small intestine and stimulates the vagal afferents through the serotonin receptors and initiates the vomiting reflex.

O

Common side effects in *italic*; life-threatening effects underlined; generic names in **bold**; classifications in SMALL CAPS

It is not known whether ondansetron antiemetic action is mediated centrally or peripherally or by both.

USES Prevention of nausea and vomiting associated with initial and repeated courses of cancer chemotherapy, including high-dose cisplatin.

ROUTE & DOSAGE

Nausea and Vomiting

Adult	IV	0.15 mg/kg infused over 15 min beginning 30 min before start of chemotherapy, followed by 0.15 mg/kg 4 and 8 h after first dose of ondansetron; may also give 8 mg bolus, then 1 mg/h by continuous infusion (max 32 mg/d)
Child	IV	4–18 y: Same as for adult

PHARMACOKINETICS Peak: 1–1.5 h. **Metabolism:** metabolized in liver. **Elimination:** half-life: 3 h; 44–60% excreted in urine within 24 h; approximately 25% excreted in feces.

CONTRAINDICATIONS & PRECAUTIONS Contraindicated in: hypersensitivity to ondansetron. **Cautious use in:** pregnancy (category B), nursing mothers, and children ≤ 3 y.

ADVERSE/SIDE EFFECTS CNS: dizziness and lightheadedness, *headache, sedation*. **GI:** *diarrhea*, constipation, dry mouth, transient increases in liver aminotransferases and bilirubin.

NURSING IMPLICATIONS

Administration

- Dilute IV injection in 50 ml of 5% dextrose or 0.9% NaCl solution before administering.
- When three separate doses are administered, infuse each over 15 min.
- The diluted solution is stable under normal lighting conditions at room temperature for 48 h.

Assessment & Drug Effects

- Monitor fluid and electrolyte status. Diarrhea, which may cause fluid and electrolyte imbalance, is a potential adverse effect of the drug.
- Monitor cardiovascular status, especially in patients with a history of coronary artery disease. Rare cases of tachycardia and angina have been reported.

Patient & Family Education

- Inform patient that headache requiring an analgesic for relief is a common adverse effect.

Prototype: morphine, p 156

OPIUM ALKALOIDS HYDROCHLORIDES
(oh´pee-um)
Trade name: Pantopon
Classifications: CNS AGENT; ANTIPYRETIC; NARCOTIC (OPIATE) AGONIST ANALGESIC
Pregnancy: Category C
Controlled substance: Schedule II

ACTIONS/PHARMACODYNAMICS A mixture of opium alkaloids in the same proportions as found in the natural opium powder. Contains about 50% anhydrous morphine or about 5 times the amount found in opium powder. The commercially available injection contains alcohol, glycerin, and parabens as preservatives. Analgesic activity results from the morphine component of the mixture; small doses have antidiarrheal effects.

USES To relieve severe pain; Pantopon, however, has been largely replaced by other narcotics.

ROUTE & DOSAGE

Severe Pain

Adult	IM/SC	5–20 mg q4–5h

PHARMACOKINETICS Peak: 50–90 min SC; 30–60 min IM. **Duration:** up to 7 h. **Distribution:** crosses placenta; distributed into breast milk. **Metabolism:** metabolized in liver. **Elimination:** excreted in urine.

ADVERSE/SIDE EFFECTS See morphine.

DRUG INTERACTIONS Alcohol and other CNS DEPRESSANTS add to CNS effects.

INCOMPATIBILITIES Solution/Additive: dimenhydrinate, pentobarbital, perphenazine, ranitidine.

NURSING IMPLICATIONS

Administration
See nursing implications for morphine.
- A dose of 20 mg opium alkaloids hydrochlorides is therapeutically equivalent to 15 mg morphine.

O

Common side effects in *italic*; life-threatening effects <u>underlined</u>; generic names in **bold**; classifications in SMALL CAPS

833

> **Prototype: morphine, p 156**

OPIUM, POWDERED

OPIUM TINCTURE (LAUDANUM)

(oh´pee-um)
Trade name: Deodorized Opium Tincture
Classifications: CNS AGENT; ANTIPYRETIC;
NARCOTIC (OPIATE) AGONIST ANALGESIC;
ANTIDIARRHEAL
Pregnancy: Category B
Controlled substance: Schedule II

ACTIONS/PHARMACODYNAMICS Opium obtained from the unripe capsules of *Papaver somniferum* or *Papaver album* contains several natural alkaloids including morphine, codeine, papaverine. Powdered opium contains 10–10.5% anhydrous morphine with added inert diluents and is light brown or yellowish-brown. Opium tincture is an alcoholic solution containing 50 mg anhydrous morphine/5 ml (19% alcohol). Antidiarrheal effects (primarily due to morphine content) result from decreased digestive secretions, increased GI smooth muscle tone, inhibition of GI motility and propulsion. These actions lead to prolonged transit of intestinal contents, dessication of feces, and constipation.

USES Symptomatic treatment of acute diarrhea and to treat severe withdrawal symptoms in neonates born to women addicted to opiates.

ROUTE & DOSAGE

Acute Diarrhea

Adult   PO   0.6 ml q.i.d. up to 1 ml q.i.d. (max 6 ml/d)

Neonatal Withdrawal

Child   PO   Make a 1:25 aqueous dilution; then give 3–6 drops q3–6h as needed or 0.2 ml q3h; dose may be increased by 0.05 ml q3h until withdrawal symptoms are controlled; gradually decrease dose after withdrawal symptoms have stabilized

PHARMACOKINETICS Absorption: variable absorption from GI tract. **Distribution:** crosses placenta; distributed into breast milk. **Metabolism:** metabolized in liver. **Elimination:** excreted in urine.

CONTRAINDICATIONS & PRECAUTIONS Contraindicated in: diarrhea caused by poisoning (until poison is completely eliminated); pregnancy (category B). **Cautious use in:** history of opiate agonist dependence; asthma, severe prostatic hypertrophy, hepatic disease.

ADVERSE/SIDE EFFECTS Nausea and other GI disturbances (infrequent). **Acute toxicity:** depression of CNS.

DRUG INTERACTIONS Alcohol and other CNS DEPRESSANTS add to CNS effects.

NURSING IMPLICATIONS

Administration

- Do not confuse this preparation with camphorated opium tincture (paregoric), which contains only 2 mg anhydrous morphine/5 ml, thus requiring a higher dose volume than that required for therapeutic dose of deodorized opium tincture.
- Give drug diluted with about one third glass of water to assure passage of entire dose into stomach.
- Preserve in tight, light-resistant containers.

Assessment & Drug Effects

- If respirations are 12/min or below or have changed in character and rate, withhold medication and report to physician.
- Note character and frequency of stools; drug should be discontinued as soon as diarrhea is controlled.
- Frequently offer small amounts of fluid but attempt to maintain 3000–4000 ml fluid total in 24 h.
- Monitor body weight, I&O ratio and pattern, and temperature. If patient develops fever of 38.8C (102F) or above, electrolyte and hydration levels may need to be evaluated. Consult physician.

Patient & Family Education

- Inform patient that constipation may be a consequence of antidiarrheal therapy but that normal habit pattern usually is reestablished with resumption of normal dietary intake.
- Addiction is possible with prolonged use or with drug abuse.

O

Common side effects in *italic*; life-threatening effects <u>underlined</u>; generic names in **bold**; classifications in SMALL CAPS

Prototypes: estradiol, p 236, and progesterone, p 241

ORAL CONTRACEPTIVES (ESTROGEN PROGESTIN COMBINATIONS)

Trade names: Brevicon, Demulen, Enovid, Loestrin, Modicon, Norinyl, Norlestrin, Ortho-Novum, Ovcon, Ovral, Tri-Norinyl, Triphasic, and others
Classifications: HORMONES; ESTROGEN-PROGESTIN COMBINATIONS
Pregnancy: Category X

ACTIONS/PHARMACODYNAMICS Fixed combination of estrogen and progestin produces contraception by preventing ovulation and rendering reproductive tract structures hostile to sperm penetration and zygote implantation. Estrogen suppresses release of gonadotropins: follicle-stimulating hormone (FSH) and luteinizing hormone (LH). Progestin causes structural and secretory changes in endometrium and inhibits ferning of cervical secretions, thus supporting an impenetrable mucoid network. Efficacy and many adverse side effects of oral contraceptives (OCs) are due largely to estrogen component, while differences between combinations are due to relative potency and dominance of either progestational or estrogenic activity. All combination products incorporate an estrogen (ethinyl estradiol or mestranol) with one of six progestins (norethynodrel, norethindrone, norethindrone acetate, ethynodiol diacetate, levonorgestrel, norgestrel). Claims are made that by supplying a varied progestin dosage in the OC cyclic regimen similar to changes in endogenous progestin levels, the risk of serious cardiovascular complications may be decreased, and breakthrough bleeding, bloating, edema and menstrual tension may be increased. Three types of estrogen-progestin combinations are available: (1) monophasic, fixed dosage of estrogen-progestin throughout the cycle; (2) biphasic, amount of estrogen remains the same throughout cycle, less progestin in first half of cycle (supports endometrial proliferation) and increased progestin in second half (allows adequate secretory development); (3) triphasic, estrogen amount is the same or varies throughout cycle, progestin amount varies.

USES To prevent conception and to treat hypermenorrhea and endometriosis. **Unlabeled use:** postcoital contraceptive or "morning after pill" (Ovral).

ROUTE & DOSAGE

Contraception

Adult   PO   1 active tablet daily for 21 d; then take placebo tablet or no tablets for 7 d; repeat cycle

Postcoital Contraception

Adult   PO   Take 2 Ovral tablets within 72 h of intercourse, then 2 tablets 12 h later

PHARMACOKINETICS Absorption: readily absorbed from GI tract. **Distribution:** widely distributed; crosses placenta; small amount distributed into breast milk. **Metabolism:** metabolized in liver. **Elimination:** half-life: 6–45 h; excreted in urine and feces.

CONTRAINDICATIONS & PRECAUTIONS Contraindicated in: pregnancy (category X), nursing mothers, missed abortion. Familial or personal history of or existence of breast or other estrogen-dependent neoplasm, recurrent chronic cystic mastitis, history of or existence of thrombophlebitis or thromboembolic disorders, cerebral vascular or coronary artery disease, MI, serious hepatic dysfunction, hepatic neoplasm, family history of hepatic porphyria, undiagnosed abnormal vaginal bleeding, women age 40 and over, adolescents with incomplete epiphyseal closure. **Cautious use in:** history of depression, preexisting hypertension, or cardiac or renal disease; impaired liver function, history of migraine, convulsive disorders, or asthma; multiparous women with grossly irregular menses, diabetes, or familial history of diabetes; gallbladder disease, lupus erythematosus, rheumatic disease, varicosities, smokers.

ADVERSE/SIDE EFFECTS CV: malignant hypertension, thrombotic and thromboembolic disorders, *mild to moderate increase in BP*, increase in size of varicosities, edema. **Eye:** unexplained loss of vision, optic neuritis, proptosis, diplopia, change in corneal curvature (steepening), intolerance to contact lenses, retinal thrombosis, papilledema. **GI:** *nausea,* cholelithiasis, gallbladder disease, cholestatic jaundice, benign hepatic adenomas; diarrhea, constipation, abdominal cramps. **GU:** ureteral dilation, increased incidence of urinary tract infection, hemolytic uremia syndrome, renal failure. **Metabolic:** *decreased glucose tolerance,* pyridoxine deficiency (see also diagnostic test interferences). **Reproductive:** increased risk of congenital anomalies, decreased quality and quantity of breast milk, dysmenorrhea, increased size of preexisting uterine fibroids, *menstrual disorders.* **Estrogen excess:** *nausea;* bloating, menstrual tension, cervical mucorrhea, polyposis,

0

Common side effects in *italic*; life-threatening effects underlined, generic names in **bold**; classifications in SMALL CAPS

835

chloasma, hypertension, migraine headache, breast fullness or tenderness, *edema.* **Estrogen deficiency:** hypomenorrhea, *early or midcycle breakthrough bleeding,* increased spotting. **Progestin excess:** hypomenorrhea, breast regression, *vaginal candidiasis,* depression, fatigue, weight gain, increased appetite, acne, oily scalp, hair loss. **Progestin deficiency:** late-cycle breakthrough bleeding, amenorrhea. **Other:** rash (allergic), paresthesias, photosensitivity (photoallergy or phototoxicity), acute intermittent porphyria.

DIAGNOSTIC TEST INTERFERENCES Oral contraceptives increase *BSP* retention, *prothrombin* and *coagulation factors II, VII, VIII, IX, X; platelet aggregability, thyroid-binding globulin, PBI, T_4; transcortin; corticosteroid, triglyceride* and *phospholipid* levels; *ceruloplasmin, aldosterone, amylase, transferrin; renin* activity, *vitamin A.* OCs decrease *antithrombin III, T_3* resin uptake, serum *folate, glucose tolerance, albumen, vitamin B_{12}* and reduce the *metyrapone* test response.

DRUG INTERACTIONS Aminocaproic acid may increase clotting factors, leading to hypercoagulable state; BARBITURATES, ANTICONVULSANTS, ANTIBIOTICS, **rifampin,** ANTIFUNGALS reduce efficacy of OCs and increase incidence of breakthrough bleeding and risk of pregnancy.

NURSING IMPLICATIONS

Administration
- Medication may be given without regard to meals.
- Intervals between one dose and the next should not exceed 24 h.

Assessment & Drug Effects
- Complete medical and family history should be taken prior to initiation of OC therapy. Baseline and periodic physical examination should include BP, breasts, abdomen, pelvis, Pap smear, and other relevant tests.
- Pregnancy should be ruled out before oral contraceptive therapy is begun.
- Check BP periodically. In some women changes in BP occur within each cycle; in others, slow increase of pressure, particularly diastolic, over several months is significant. Drug-induced BP elevation is usually reversible with cessation of OC.
- Nausea with or without vomiting occurs in approximately 10% of patients during the first cycle and is reportedly one of the major reasons for voluntary

discontinuation of therapy. Most side effects tend to disappear in third or fourth cycle of use. Instruct patient to report symptoms that persist after fourth cycle. Dose adjustment or a different product may be indicated.
- Hirsutism and loss of hair are reversible with discontinuation of OC or by change of selected combination.
- Acne may improve, worsen, or develop for first time. In women on OC for at least 1 y, postcontraceptive acne sometimes occurs 3–4 mo after stopping drug and may continue for 6–12 mo.
- Anovulation or amenorrhea following termination of OC regimen may persist more than 6 mo. The user with pretreatment oligomenorrhea or secondary amenorrhea is most apt to have oversuppression syndrome.
- Oral contraception may mask onset of climacteric. To determine if it has started, physician may advise patient to discontinue pill and to use alternate method of contraception. If menstruation occurs, the pill is indicated.

Patient & Family Education
- Tablets should be taken regularly at 24 h intervals (e.g., with a meal or at bedtime).
- In the first week of the initial cycle, patient should also use an additional method of birth control.
- If user forgets to take a tablet, she should take it as soon as she remembers or should take 2 tablets the next day. If 2 consecutive tablets are omitted, she should take 2 tablets daily for the next 2 days, then resume the regular schedule. If 3 consecutive tablets are missed, she should begin a new compact of tablets, starting 7 d after last tablet was taken.
- Use an additional form of birth control for 7 d after 2 missed doses or 14 d after 3 missed doses.
- Ovulation is unlikely with omission of 1 daily dose; however, the possibility of escaped ovulation, spotting, or breakthrough bleeding increases with each missed dose.
- If intracycle bleeding resembling menstruation occurs, patient should discontinue medication, then begin taking tablets from a new compact on day 5. If bleeding persists, advise patient to see physician.
- If 2 consecutive periods should be missed, user should see physician to rule out pregnancy before continuing on OC.
- If possible, hormone contraception should not be used until infant is weaned; alternate method of birth control should be used during this period.
- Oral contraception can be started immediately after delivery in the nonnursing mother.
- Urge patient not to skip scheduled visits for physi-

Common side effects in *italic;* life-threatening effects <u>underlined;</u> generic names in **bold;** classifications in SMALL CAPS

cal checkups while on contraceptive therapy. Teach breast self-examination and emphasize importance of doing this every month.

- Users with clinical conditions worsened by fluid retention should report exaggeration of symptoms promptly. Frequent weight checks should be recorded to permit early recognition of fluid retention.
- Inform patient of the increased risk of thromboembolic and cardiovascular problems and increased incidence of gallbladder disease with OC use.
- Teach patient how to elicit Homans' sign and to be alert to other manifestations of thrombotic or thromboembolic disorders: severe headache (especially if persistent and recurrent), dizziness, blurred vision, leg or chest pain, respiratory distress, unexplained cough. Advise patient to withhold drug if any of these symptoms appear and to report them promptly to physician.
- Sudden abdominal pain should be reported immediately to rule out ectopic pregnancy.
- Ophthalmic sequelae can occur as soon as 24 h after initiation of oral contraception. Advise patient to stop the drug and contact physician if unexplained partial or complete, sudden or gradual loss of vision, protrusion of eyeballs (proptosis), or diplopia occurs.
- Leukorrhea is an expected physical reaction to the OC; however, if OC use is accompanied by vaginal itching and irritation, candidiasis should be ruled out. Caution patient to report discomfort promptly.
- Instruct the diabetic to report positive urine or blood glucose test to physician. Adjustment of antidiabetic medication may be necessary. The potential diabetic (family history) should also be closely observed for onset of diabetes.
- Smokers who are OC users have a fivefold greater risk of fatal MI than nonsmoker OC users and a tenfold greater risk than non-OC users who are nonsmokers. The risk increases with age (marked in women >35y) and with heavy smoking (15 or more cigarettes/d).

Prototype: cyclobenzaprine, p 122

ORPHENADRINE CITRATE

(or-fen´a-dreen)
Trade names: Banflex, Disipal, Flexon, Myolin, Norflex, Ro-Orphena, X-Otag
Classifications: AUTONOMIC NERVOUS SYSTEM AGENT; ANTICHOLINERGIC (PARASYMPATHOLYTIC); CENTRAL-ACTING SKELETAL MUSCLE RELAXANT
Pregnancy: Category C

ACTIONS/PHARMACODYNAMICS Tertiary amine anticholinergic agent and central-acting skeletal muscle relaxant. Structurally similar to diphenhydramine and also closely related to chlorphenoxamine. Relaxes tense skeletal muscles indirectly, possibly by analgesic action or by atropinelike central action. Has some local anesthetic and antihistaminic activity but less than that of diphenhydramine. Also produces slight euphoria.

USES To relieve muscle spasm discomfort associated with acute musculoskeletal conditions.

ROUTE & DOSAGE

Muscle Spasm

Adult	PO	100 mg b.i.d.
	IM/IV	60 mg; may repeat in 12 h if needed

PHARMACOKINETICS Absorption: readily absorbed from GI tract. **Peak:** 2 h. **Duration:** 4–6 h. **Distribution:** rapidly distributed in tissues; crosses placenta. **Metabolism:** metabolized in liver. **Elimination:** half-life: 14 h; excreted in urine.

CONTRAINDICATIONS & PRECAUTIONS Contraindicated in: narrow-angle glaucoma; pyloric or duodenal obstruction, stenosing peptic ulcers; prostatic hypertrophy or bladder neck obstruction; myasthenia gravis; cardiospasm (megaloesophagus). Safe use during pregnancy (category C) and in the pediatric age group not established. **Cautious use in:** history of tachycardia, cardiac decompensation, arrhythmias, coronary insufficiency.

ADVERSE/SIDE EFFECTS CNS: *drowsiness,* weakness, headache, dizziness; mild CNS stimulation (high doses): restlessness, anxiety, tremors, confusion, hallucinations, agitation, tachycardia, palpitation, syncope. **Eye:** increased ocular tension, dilated pupils, blurred vision. **GI:** *dry mouth,* nausea, vomiting, abdominal cramps, constipation. **GU:** *urinary hesitancy or retention.* **Hypersensitivity:** pruritus, urticaria, rash, underlined:anaphylactic reaction (rare). **Other:** aplastic anemia (rare): causal relationship not established.

DRUG INTERACTIONS Propoxyphene may cause increased confusion, anxiety, and tremors.

NURSING IMPLICATIONS

Administration

- Orphenadrine citrate and orphenadrine hydrochloride are not interchangeable.

O

Common side effects in *italic*; life-threatening effects underlined; generic names in **bold**; classifications in SMALL CAPS

837

- IV orphenadrine may be given by direct IV undiluted at a rate of 60 mg (2 ml) over 5 min.
- Sustained release tablets must be swallowed whole.
- Protect orphenadrine from light.

Assessment & Drug Effects

- Periodic studies of blood, urine, and liver function are recommended with prolonged therapy.
- Complaints of mouth dryness, urinary hesitancy or retention, headache, tremors, GI problems, palpitation, or rapid pulse should be communicated to physician. Dosage reduction or drug withdrawal is indicated.
- The elderly patient is particularly sensitive to anticholinergic effects (urinary hesitancy, constipation) and therefore should be closely observed. Have patient void before taking drug.
- Keep physician informed of therapeutic drug effect. In the patient with parkinsonism, orphenadrine reduces muscular rigidity but has little effect on tremors. Some reduction in excessive salivation and perspiration may occur, and patient may appear mildly euphoric.

Patient & Family Education

- Mouth dryness may be relieved by frequent rinsing with clear tepid water, increasing noncaloric fluid intake, sugarless gum, or lemondrops. If these measures fail, a saliva substitute may help.
- Caution patient to avoid potentially hazardous activities until reaction to drug is known.
- Warn patient that concomitant use of alcohol and other CNS depressants may potentiate depressant effects.

Prototype: penicillin G, p 71

OXACILLIN SODIUM

(ox-a-sill´in)
Trade names: Bactocill, Prostaphlin
Classifications: ANTIINFECTIVE; BETA-LACTAM ANTIBIOTIC; PENICILLIN
Pregnancy: Category B

O

ACTIONS/PHARMACODYNAMICS Semisynthetic, acid-stable, penicillinase-resistant isoxazoyl penicillin. Mechanism of bactericidal action, contraindications, precautions, and adverse reactions as for penicillin G. In common with other isoxazoyl penicillins (cloxacillin, dicloxacillin), it is highly active against most penicillinase-producing staphylococci, is less potent than penicillin G against penicillin-sensitive microorganisms, and is generally ineffective against gram-negative bacteria and methicillin-resistant staphylococci.

USES Primarily, infections caused by penicillinase-producing staphylococci and penicillin-resistant staphylococci. May be used to initiate therapy in suspected staphylococcal infections pending culture and sensitivity test results. As with other penicillins, serum concentrations are enhanced by concurrent use of probenecid.

ROUTE & DOSAGE

Staphylococcal Infections

Adult	IM/IV	500 mg–2 g q4–6h up to 12 g/d
	PO	250–1000 mg q4–6h
Child	IM/IV	50–100 mg/kg/d divided q4–6h
	PO	50–100 mg/kg/d in 4 divided doses

PHARMACOKINETICS Absorption: incompletely and erratically absorbed orally. **Peak:** 30–120 min IM; 15 min IV. **Duration:** 4 h PO; 4–6 h IM. **Distribution:** distributes into CNS with inflamed meninges; crosses placenta; distributed into breast milk. **Metabolism:** enters enterohepatic circulation. **Elimination:** half-life: 0.5–1 h; primarily excreted in urine, some in bile.

CONTRAINDICATIONS & PRECAUTIONS Contraindicated in: hypersensitivity to penicillins or cephalosporins. Safe use during pregnancy (category B) not established. **Cautious use in:** history of or suspected atopy or allergy (hives, eczema, hay fever, asthma); premature infants, neonates.

ADVERSE/SIDE EFFECTS Nausea, vomiting, flatulence, *diarrhea*. **High-dose therapy:** interstitial nephritis, transient hematuria, albuminuria, azotemia (newborns and infants on high doses); thrombophlebitis (IV therapy), superinfections. **Hypersensitivity:** pruritus, rash, urticaria, wheezing, sneezing, fever, anaphylaxis; hepatocellular dysfunction (elevated AST, ALT, hepatitis), eosinophilia, leukopenia, thrombocytopenia, granulocytopenia, agranulocytosis; neutropenia (reported in children).

DIAGNOSTIC TEST INTERFERENCES Oxacillin in large doses can cause false-positive *urine protein tests* using sulfosalicylic acid methods.

INCOMPATIBILITIES Solution/Additive: cytarabine, TETRACYCLINES. **Y-Site: verapamil.**

NURSING IMPLICATIONS

Administration

- Oral oxacillin is best taken with a full glass of water on an empty stomach (either 1 h before meals or 2 h after meals). Food reduces absorption.
- Following reconstitution of oral solution, it is stable for 3 d at room temperature and for 14 d if refrigerated. Container should be so labeled and dated.
- For IM administration, reconstitute each 250 mg with 1.4 ml sterile water for injection and indicate date and time of reconstitution on vial. Shake vial vigorously until drug is completely dissolved. Discard unused portions after 3 d at room temperature or 7 d under refrigeration. Do not use undated vials.
- **IM administration:** administer IM to adults by deep intragluteal injection. Follow agency policy for IM site in young children and infants. Injection into or near a major peripheral nerve or blood vessel can cause neurovascular damage. Rotate injection sites.
- **IV administration:** for direct IV administration, reconstitute with sterile water for injection or isotonic NaCl by adding 1.4 ml of diluent to each 250 mg. The resulting concentration (250 mg/1.5 ml) is further diluted by adding 5 ml to each 500 mg or fraction thereof.
- Reconstituted and properly diluted solution may be given by direct IV at a rate of 1 g or fraction thereof over 10 min.
- For IV infusion the reconstituted solution is added to a compatible IV solution (e.g., isotonic NaCl, D5W, NS, lactated Ringer's injection, or others recommended by manufacturer) and infused over 6 h.
- The total sodium content (including that contributed by buffer) in each gram of oxacillin is approximately 3.1 mEq or 71 mg.

Assessment & Drug Effects

- Prior to first dose inquiry should be made concerning hypersensitivity reactions to penicillins, cephalosporins, and other allergens.
- Hepatic dysfunction (possibly a hypersensitivity reaction) has been associated with IV oxacillin; it is reversible with discontinuation of drug. Symptoms may resemble viral hepatitis or general signs of hypersensitivity and should be reported promptly: hives, rash, fever, nausea, vomiting, abdominal discomfort, anorexia, malaise, jaundice (with dark yellow to brown urine, light-colored or clay-colored stools, pruritus).
- Withhold next drug dose and report the onset of hypersensitivity reactions and superinfections (see Signs & Symptoms, chap 3).

Patient & Family Education

- Instruct patient to take the oral medication around the clock, not to miss a dose, and to continue taking it until it is all gone unless otherwise directed by physician.
- Instruct patients on prolonged therapy to report symptoms of agranulocytosis (see chap 3).

Prototype: mebendazole, p 53

OXAMINIQUINE
(ox-am′ni-kwin)
Trade name: Vansil
Classifications: ANTIINFECTIVE; ANTHELMINTIC
Pregnancy: Category C

ACTIONS/PHARMACODYNAMICS Tetrahydroquinone derivative prepared in the presence of *Aspergillus sclerotiorum*. Mechanism of action not fully explained, but it appears that drug-induced strong contractions and paralysis of worm musculature leads to immobilization of their suckers and dislodgment from their usual residence in mesenteric veins to the liver. Normal blood flow passively carries dead and dying worms to the liver, where they are retained and subsequently elicit host tissue reactions (e.g., phagocytosis). Dislodgment of schistosomes begins about 2 d after single oral dose of oxaminiquine; movement is not complete until 6 d after treatment with the drug. After treatment, surviving unpaired females return to mesenteric vessels; however, oviposition (egg laying) seems to stop in 24–48 h after drug treatment, reducing egg load and removing principal cause of pathology associated with schistosomal infection. Is not cercaricidal. Drug metabolites do not possess antischistosomal activity.

USES All stages of *Schistosoma mansoni* infection, including acute and chronic phases with hepatosplenic involvement.

ROUTE & DOSAGE

Schistosomiasis

Adult	PO	12–15 mg/kg as single dose
Child	PO	<30 kg: 10 mg/kg × 2 doses at 2–8 h intervals

PHARMACOKINETICS Absorption: readily absorbed from GI tract. **Peak:** 1–3 h. **Metabolism:** extensively metabolized in GI mucosa. **Elimination:** half-life: 1–2.5 h; excreted in urine.

O

Common side effects in *italic*; life-threatening effects underlined; generic names in **bold**; classifications in SMALL CAPS

839

CONTRAINDICATIONS & PRECAUTIONS Con-traindicated in: safe use during pregnancy (category C) and lactation or in children not established. **Cautious use in:** history of convulsant disorders.

ADVERSE/SIDE EFFECTS CNS: *transitory dizzi-ness, drowsiness, headache,* epileptic convulsions (rare); insomnia, malaise, reversible amnesia (rare); persistent fever (in patients being treated in Egypt); EEG abnormalities. **GI:** anorexia, nausea, vomiting, abdominal pain. **Hematologic:** increased erythrocyte sedimentation rate, reticulocyte count, and increased or decreased leukocyte count. **Other:** urticaria, elevated liver enzyme concentrations, convulsions, serum alkaline phosphatase, AST, ALT (not considered drug-related), red-orange urine.

FOOD-DRUG INTERACTIONS Rate and extent of absorption are decreased by food.

NURSING IMPLICATIONS

Administration
▪ Administer with food if necessary to reduce GI distress and improve tolerance.
▪ Store product in tightly closed container at controlled room temperature less than 30C (86F).

Assessment & Drug Effects
▪ Since > 30% of patients experience dizziness or drowsiness, supervision of ambulation and other safety precautions may be warranted.

Patient & Family Education
▪ Because drug can cause dizziness or drowsiness, advise patient to use caution while driving or performing other tasks requiring alertness.
▪ Inform patient that drug may change the normal urine color to a harmless orange-red.
▪ If patient has a history of seizures, the possibility of seizures is increased because of drug action. (Occur within hours of drug administration.)

Prototype: lorazepam, p 177

OXAZEPAM
(ox-a′ze-pam)
Trade names: Ox-Pam, Serax, Zapex
Classifications: CNS AGENT; ANXIOLYTIC; SEDATIVE-HYPNOTIC; BENZODIAZEPINE
Pregnancy: Category C
Controlled substance: Schedule IV

ACTIONS/PHARMACODYNAMICS Benzodia-zepine derivative related to lorazepam with which it shares actions, uses, limitations and interactions.

USES Management of anxiety and tension associated with a wide range of emotional disturbances. Also to control acute withdrawal symptoms in chronic alcoholism.

ROUTE & DOSAGE

Anxiety
Adult   PO   10–30 mg t.i.d. or q.i.d.

Acute Alcohol Withdrawal
Adult   PO   15–30 mg t.i.d. or q.i.d.

PHARMACOKINETICS Absorption: readily absorbed from GI tract. **Peak:** 2–3 h. **Distribution:** crosses placenta; distributed into breast milk. **Metabolism:** metabolized in liver. **Elimination:** half-life: 2–8 h; primarily excreted in urine, some in feces.

CONTRAINDICATIONS & PRECAUTIONS Con-traindicated in: hypersensitivity to oxazepam and other benzodiazepines; psychoses, pregnancy (category C), nursing mothers, children <12 y; acute-angle glaucoma, acute alcohol intoxication. **Cautious use in:** elderly and debilitated patients; impaired renal and hepatic function; addiction-prone patients; COPD; mental depression.

ADVERSE/SIDE EFFECTS Usually infrequent and mild. **CNS:** *drowsiness,* dizziness, mental confusion, vertigo, ataxia, headache, lethargy, syncope, tremor, slurred speech, paradoxic reaction (euphoria, excitement). **GI:** nausea, xerostomia, jaundice. **Other:** skin rash, edema, hypotension, leukopenia, altered libido, edema.

DRUG INTERACTIONS Alcohol, CNS DEPRESSANTS, ANTICONVULSANTS potentiate CNS depression; **cimetidine** increases oxazepam plasma levels, increasing its toxicity; may decrease antiparkinsonism effects of **levodopa;** may increase **phenytoin** levels; **smoking** decreases sedative and antianxiety effects.

NURSING IMPLICATIONS

Administration
▪ May be given with food if GI upset occurs.
▪ Store in tightly closed container at 15–30C (59–86F) unless otherwise specified.

Assessment & Drug Effects

- Elderly patients should be observed closely for signs of overdosage. Report to physician if daytime psychomotor function is depressed.
- Liver function tests and blood counts should be performed on a regular planned basis.
- Excessive and prolonged use may cause physical dependence.

Patient & Family Education

- Mild paradoxic stimulation of affect and excitement with sleep disturbances may occur within the first 2 wk of therapy. Report promptly. Dosage reduction is indicated.
- Instruct patients not to change dose or dose schedule and to refrain from using drug to treat a self-diagnosed condition.
- Advise patient to consult physician before self-medicating with OTC drugs.
- Caution patient against driving a car or operating dangerous machinery until response to drug has been evaluated.
- Warn patient not to drink alcoholic beverages while being treated with oxazepam. The CNS depressant effects of each agent may be intensified.
- Patient should be advised that if she becomes pregnant during therapy or intends to become pregnant she should communicate with her physician about the desirability of discontinuing the drug.
- Following prolonged therapy, drug should be withdrawn slowly to avoid precipitating withdrawal symptoms (seizures, mental confusion, nausea, vomiting, muscle and abdominal cramps, tremulousness, sleep disturbances, unusual irritability, hyperhydrosis).

Prototype: amphotericin B, p 56

OXICONAZOLE NITRATE

(ox i-con´a-zolc)
Trade name: Oxistat
Classifications: SKIN AGENT; ANTIFUNGAL
Pregnancy: Category B

ACTIONS/PHARMACODYNAMICS Oxiconazole is a synthetic antifungal agent. It presumably works by altering cellular membranes, resulting in increased membrane permeability, secondary metabolic effects, and growth inhibition.

USES Topical treatment of tinea pedis, tinea cruris, and tinea corporis due to *Trichophyton rubrum* and *Trichophyton mentagrophytes;* also used for cutaneous candidiasis caused by *Candida albicans* and *Candida tropicalis.*

ROUTE & DOSAGE

Tinea and Other Dermal Infections

Adult   Topical   Apply to affected area b.i.d. in morning and evening

PHARMACOKINETICS Absorption: <0.3% is absorbed systemically.

CONTRAINDICATIONS & PRECAUTIONS Contraindicated in: hypersensitivity to oxiconazole. **Cautious use in:** pregnancy (category B) and nursing mothers.

ADVERSE/SIDE EFFECTS Transient burning and stinging, dryness, erythema, pruritus, and local irritation.

NURSING IMPLICATIONS

Administration

- Apply cream to cover the affected areas once daily (in the evening).
- Tinea corporis and tinea cruris should be treated for 2 wk and tinea pedis should be treated for 1 mo to reduce the possibility of recurrence.
- Store at 15–30C (59–86F).

Patient & Family Education

- Medication is for external use only. Do not use intravaginally.
- If irritation or sensitivity develops, discontinue drug and contact physician.
- Avoid contact with eyes.
- If no improvement is noted after the prescribed treatment period, the physician should be consulted.

OXIDIZED CELLULOSE

Trade names: Novocell, Oxycel, Surgicel
Classifications: BLOOD COAGULATOR; HEMOSTATIC

O

Common side effects in *italic*; life-threatening effects <u>underlined</u>; generic names in **bold**; classifications in SMALL CAPS

841

ACTIONS/PHARMACODYNAMICS Sterile, absorbable hemostatic material prepared from cellulose. On contact with blood, it swells into a brownish or black gelatinous mass that acts as artificial clot. Gradually absorbed from tissue bed, usually within 2–7 d; complete absorption of large amounts may require up to 6 wk or more.

USES To control capillary, venous, and small arterial hemorrhage when suture or ligation is impractical or ineffective.

ROUTE & DOSAGE

Control Hemorrhage

Adult	Topical	Using aseptic technique, apply to bleeding surface with mild pressure until hemostasis is obtained

CONTRAINDICATIONS & PRECAUTIONS Contraindicated in: use as wadding or packing; use for implantation in bone defects, including fractures and laminectomy procedures (interferes with callus formation and may cause cysts and nerve damage); hemorrhage from large arteries or nonhemorrhagic oozing surfaces; impregnation with antiinfective materials or other hemostatic substances.

ADVERSE/SIDE EFFECTS Foreign-body reactions, burning, stinging sensations, sneezing (when used for rhinologic procedures), <u>necrosis due to tight packing</u>, prolonged drainage.

NURSING IMPLICATIONS

Administration

- Hemostatic effect is greater when material is applied dry.
- Hemostatic effect is not enhanced by thrombin (activity of thrombin is destroyed by low pH of oxidized cellulose). Absorption may be prevented by previous applications of silver nitrate or other escharotic materials.
- Only as much as necessary for hemostasis should be used; material is applied to bleeding site or held firmly in place until bleeding stops.
- Once hemostasis is achieved, oxidized cellulose is usually removed from site of application. Removal is facilitated by irrigation with sterile water or saline. Observe wound site for bleeding following removal.

- Oxidized cellulose is off-white or dusty yellow, but it may darken in its sealed container with age. Reportedly this does not affect its hemostatic action.
- Material is supplied as a sterile preparation and cannot be resterilized. Autoclaving or other forms of heat sterilization cause physical breakdown. Discard unused portions.

Prototype: theophylline, p 136

OXTRIPHYLLINE

(ox-trye´fi-lin)
Trade names: Choledyl, Choledyl-SA, Choline Theophyllinate
Classifications: BRONCHODILATOR (RESPIRATORY SMOOTH MUSCLE RELAXANT) XANTHINE
Pregnancy: Category C

ACTIONS/PHARMACODYNAMICS Choline salt of theophylline, with similar actions, uses, and limitations as other theophylline derivatives. Contains 64% theophylline. Compared to aminophylline, reportedly more stable, more soluble, and more uniformly and predictably absorbed, and produces less gastric irritation. Development of tolerance reported infrequently; therefore useful in long-term therapy.

ROUTE & DOSAGE

Asthma, COPD

Adult	PO	4.7 mg/kg (usual dose 200 mg) q8h
Child	PO	9–16 y and adult smoker: 4.7 mg/kg (usual dose 200 mg) q6h 1–9 y: 6.2 mg/kg q6h

PHARMACOKINETICS Absorption: well absorbed from GI tract. **Duration:** 4–8 h; varies with age, smoking, and liver function. **Distribution:** crosses placenta; distributed into breast milk. **Metabolism:** extensively metabolized in liver. **Elimination:** half-life: 4 h in adults; parent drug and metabolites excreted by kidneys.

CONTRAINDICATIONS & PRECAUTIONS Contraindicated in: hypersensitivity to xanthines; coronary artery disease; renal, liver impairment. Safe use during pregnancy (category C), in nursing women, and in children <2 y not established. **Cautious use in:** peptic ulcer; prostatic hypertrophy; diabetes mellitus; glaucoma.

ADVERSE/SIDE EFFECTS CNS: restlessness, dizziness, insomnia, convulsions, *muscle twitching.* **CV:** palpitation, tachycardia, flushing, hypotension. **GI:** *nausea,* vomiting, anorexia, epigastric pain, diarrhea, activation of peptic ulcer. **GU:** transient urinary frequency, kidney irritation. **Other:** urticaria, fever, dehydration.

DRUG INTERACTIONS Increases **lithium** excretion, lowering lithium levels; **cimetidine,** high dose **allopurinol** (600 mg/d), **ciprofloxacin, erythromycin, troleandomycin** can significantly increase theophylline levels.

NURSING IMPLICATIONS
See theophylline for numerous additional nursing implications.

Administration
- Preferably taken on an empty stomach (30 min to 1 h before or 2 h after meals); however, may be taken after meals and at bedtime to reduce GI distress. Sustained release tablet permits dosing q12h.
- Preserve in tightly closed containers, away from heat. Elixir should be protected from light.

Patient & Family Education
- Advise patient to report gastric distress, palpitation, and CNS stimulation (irritability, restlessness, nervousness, insomnia). Reduction in dosage may be indicated.

Prototype: atropine, p 116

OXYBUTYNIN CHLORIDE
(ox-i-byoo′ti-nin)
Trade name: Ditropan
Classifications: AUTONOMIC NERVOUS SYSTEM AGENT; ANTICHOLINERGIC (PARASYMPATHOLYTIC); ANTIMUSCARINIC; ANTISPASMODIC
Pregnancy: Category C

ACTIONS/PHARMACODYNAMICS Synthetic tertiary amine with prominent antispasmodic activity. Exerts direct antispasmodic (papaverine-like) action, and inhibits muscarinic effects of acetylcholine on smooth muscle. Animal studies have shown that anticholinergic activity is about one fifth that of atropine, but antispasmodic action is four to ten times more potent.

USES To relieve symptoms associated with voiding in patients with uninhibited neurogenic bladder and reflex neurogenic bladder. Also has been used to relieve pain of bladder spasm following transurethral surgical procedures.

PHARMACOKINETICS Onset: 0.5–1 h. **Peak:** 3–6 h. **Duration:** 6–10 h. **Metabolism:** metabolized in liver. **Elimination:** excreted primarily in urine.

ROUTE & DOSAGE

Neurogenic Bladder

Adult	PO	5 mg b.i.d. or t.i.d. (max 20 mg/d)
Child	PO	> 5 y: 5 mg b.i.d. (max 15 mg/d)

CONTRAINDICATIONS & PRECAUTIONS Contraindicated in: glaucoma, myasthenia gravis, partial or complete GI obstruction, paralytic ileus, intestinal atony (especially elderly or debilitated patients), megacolon, severe colitis, GU obstruction, unstable cardiovascular status. Safe use during pregnancy (category C) and in children <5 y not established. **Cautious use in:** the elderly; autonomic neuropathy, hiatus hernia with reflex esophagitis; hepatic or renal dysfunction; urinary infection; hyperthyroidism; CHF, coronary artery disease, hypertension; prostatic hypertrophy.

ADVERSE/SIDE EFFECTS CNS: *drowsiness,* dizziness, weakness, insomnia, restlessness, psychotic behavior (overdosage). **CV:** palpitations, tachycardia, flushing. **Eye:** mydriasis, *blurred vision,* cyclopegia, increased ocular tension. **GI:** *dry mouth,* nausea, vomiting, *constipation,* bloated feeling. **GU:** urinary hesitancy or retention, impotence. **Hypersensitivity:** severe allergic reactions including urticaria, skin rashes. **Other:** suppression of lactation, decreased sweating, fever.

NURSING IMPLICATIONS

Administration
- Note that the maximum dose is 5 mg q.i.d.
- Store in tight containers at 15–30C (59–86F).

Assessment & Drug Effects
- The diagnosis of neurogenic bladder should be confirmed before initiation of therapy.
- Periodic interruptions of therapy are recommended to determine patient's need for continued treatment. Tolerance has occurred in some patients.
- Keep physician informed of expected responses to drug therapy (e.g., effect on urinary frequency, ur-

0

Common side effects in *italic*; life-threatening effects underlined; generic names in **bold**; classifications in SMALL CAPS

843

gency, urge incontinence, nocturia, completeness of bladder emptying).

- Patients with colostomy or ileostomy should be closely monitored; abdominal distension and the onset of diarrhea in these patients may be early signs of intestinal obstruction or of toxic megacolon.

Patient & Family Education

- Since oxybutynin may cause dizziness, drowsiness, and blurred vision, caution patient to avoid driving and other potentially hazardous activities until reaction to drug is known.
- Advise patient to avoid hot environments. By suppressing sweating, oxybutynin can cause fever and heat stroke.

Prototype: morphine, p 156

OXYCODONE HYDROCHLORIDE
(ox-i-koe´done)

OXYCODONE TEREPHTHALATE

Trade name: Percocet-5, Percodan, Percodan-Demi, Roxicet, Roxicodone
Classifications: CNS AGENT; ANTIPYRETIC; NARCOTIC (OPIATE) AGONIST ANALGESIC
Pregnancy: Categories B (D for prolonged use or use of high doses at term)
Controlled substance: Schedule II

ACTIONS/PHARMACODYNAMICS Semisynthetic derivative of opium alkaloid thebaine with actions qualitatively similar to those of morphine. Most prominent actions involve CNS and organs composed of smooth muscle. Binds with stereospecific receptors in various sites of CNS to alter both perception of pain and emotional response to pain, but precise mechanism of action not clear. Appears to be more effective in relief of acute than long-standing pain. As potent as morphine and 10–12 times more potent than codeine; withdrawal symptoms match those of morphine. Produces mild sedation but has little or no effect on cough reflex.

USES Relief of moderate to moderately severe pain such as may occur with bursitis, dislocations, simple fractures and other injuries, and neuralgia. Relieves postoperative, postextractional, postpartum pain.

ROUTE & DOSAGE

Moderate to Severe Pain

Adult	PO	5–10 mg q6h prn
Child	PO	≥ 12 y: 2.5 mg q6h prn
		6–12 y: 1.25 mg q6h prn

PHARMACOKINETICS Absorption: readily absorbed from GI tract. **Onset:** 10–15 min. **Peak:** 30–60 min. **Duration:** 4–5 h. **Distribution:** crosses placenta; distributed into breast milk. **Metabolism:** metabolized in liver. **Elimination:** excreted primarily in urine.

CONTRAINDICATIONS & PRECAUTIONS Contraindicated in: hypersensitivity to oxycodone and principal drugs with which it is combined; during pregnancy (category B); for prolonged use or high doses at term: category D; nursing women, and children <6 y. **Cautious use in:** alcoholism; renal or hepatic disease; viral infections; Addison's disease; cardiac arrhythmias; chronic ulcerative colitis; history of drug abuse or dependency; gallbladder disease, acute abdominal conditions; head injury, intracranial lesions; hypothyroidism; prostatic hypertrophy; respiratory disease; urethral stricture; elderly or debilitated patients; peptic ulcer or coagulation abnormalities (combination products containing aspirin).

ADVERSE/SIDE EFFECTS Lightheadedness, dizziness, *sedation,* anorexia, *nausea,* vomiting, *constipation,* euphoria, dysphoria, shortness of breath, pruritus, skin rash, bradycardia, unusual bleeding or bruising, jaundice, dysuria, frequency of urination, urinary retention, <u>respiratory depression, hepatotoxicity</u> (combinations containing acetaminophen).

DIAGNOSTIC TEST INTERFERENCES *Serum amylase* levels may be elevated because oxycodone causes spasm of sphincter of Oddi. ***Blood glucose determinations:*** false decrease (measured by glucose oxidase-peroxidase method). ***5-HIAA determination:*** false positive with use of nitrosonaphthol reagent (quantitative test is unaffected).

DRUG INTERACTIONS Alcohol and other CNS DEPRESSANTS add to CNS depressant activity.

NURSING IMPLICATIONS

Administration

- Administer after meals or with milk to reduce gastric irritation.
- Percodan contains aspirin. Do not administer to

person with aspirin hypersensitivity. Percocet contains acetaminophen.

- Store this dangerous medication in a place inaccessible to children at 15–30C (59–86F). Protect from light.

Assessment & Drug Effect

- Nausea may occur during first few days of therapy; if it continues, consult physician.
- Lightheadedness, dizziness, sedation, or fainting appear to be more prominent in ambulatory than in nonambulatory patients and may be alleviated if patient lies down.
- Evaluate patient's continued need for oxycodone preparations. Psychic and physical dependence and tolerance may develop with repeated use. The potential for drug abuse is high.
- Laboratory studies of hepatic function and hematologic status should be checked periodically in patients on high dosage.
- The ingestion of large doses of Percodan and Percodan-Demi can result in acute salicylate intoxication. An overdose of Percocet-5 could lead to acetaminophen poisoning.
- Serious overdosage of any oxycodone preparation presents problems associated with a narcotic overdose (respiratory depression, circulatory collapse, extreme somnolence progressing to stupor or coma).

Patient & Family Education

- Warn patient not to alter dosage regimen by increasing, decreasing, or shortening intervals between doses. Habit formation and liver damage may be induced.
- Caution patient to avoid potentially hazardous activities such as driving a car or operating machinery while using oxycodone preparation.
- Caution patient that taking large amounts of alcoholic beverages while using oxycodone preparation increases risk of liver damage.
- Instruct patient to check with physician before taking OTC drugs for colds, stomach distress, allergies, insomnia, or pain while also taking oxycodone.
- Tell patient to inform surgeon or dentist that oxycodone preparation is being taken before any surgical procedure is undertaken.

Prototype: naphazoline, p 211

OXYMETAZOLINE HYDROCHLORIDE
(ox-i-met-az´oh-leen)
Trade names: Afrin, Dristan Long Lasting, Duramist Plus, Duration, Nafrine, Neo-Synephrine 12 Hour, Nostrilla, Sinex Long Lasting
Classifications: NASAL DECONGESTANT; AUTONOMIC NERVOUS SYSTEM AGENT; ALPHA-ADRENERGIC AGONIST (SYMPATHOMIMETIC)
Pregnancy: Category C

ACTIONS/PHARMACODYNAMICS Imidazoline-derivative sympathomimetic agent structurally and pharmacologically related to naphazoline. Direct action on alpha receptors of sympathetic nervous system produces constriction of smaller arterioles in nasal passages and prolonged decongestant effect. Has no effect on beta receptors.

USES Relief of nasal congestion in a variety of allergic and infectious disorders of the upper respiratory tract; used as nasal tampon to facilitate intranasal examination or before nasal surgery. Also used as adjunct in treatment and prevention of middle ear infection by decreasing congestion of eustachian ostia.

ROUTE & DOSAGE

Nasal Congestion

Adult	Topical (Intranasal)	2–3 drops or 2–3 sprays of 0.05% solution into each nostril b.i.d. for up to 3–5 d
Child	Topical (Intranasal)	> 6 y: Same as for adult 2–5y: 2–3 drops or 2–3 sprays of 0.025% solution into each nostril b.i.d. for up to 3–5 d

PHARMACOKINETICS Onset: 5–10 min. **Duration:** 6–10 h.

CONTRAINDICATIONS & PRECAUTIONS Contraindicated in: use in children <6 y. Safe use during pregnancy (category C) not established. **Cautious use in:** within 14 d of MAO inhibitors, coronary artery disease, hypertension, hyperthyroidism, diabetes mellitus.

ADVERSE/SIDE EFFECTS *Burning*, stinging, dryness of nasal mucosa, *sneezing*. With excessive

Common side effects in *italic*; life-threatening effects underlined; generic names in **bold**; classifications in SMALL CAPS

845

use: headache, lightheadedness, drowsiness, insomnia, palpitations, *rebound congestion*.

NURSING IMPLICATIONS

Patient & Family Education

- Usually administered in the morning and at bedtime. Effects appear within 30 min and last about 6–7 h.
- Nasal spray is delivered with patient in upright position. Instruct patient to place spray nozzle in nostril without occluding it and to bend head slightly forward and sniff briskly during administration.
- Lateral, head-low position is recommended for instillation of nose drops.
- Instruct patient to rinse dropper or spray tip in hot water after each use to prevent contamination of solution by nasal secretions.
- Instruct patient to wash hands carefully after handling oxymetazoline. Anisocoria (inequality of pupil size, blurred vision) can develop if eyes are rubbed with contaminated fingers.
- Caution patient not to exceed recommended dosage. Rebound congestion (chemical rhinitis) may occur with prolonged or excessive use.
- Systemic effects can result from swallowing excessive medication.

Prototype: testosterone, p 229

OXYMETHOLONE

(ox-i-meth´oh-lone)

Trade names: Anadrol, Anapolon
Classifications: HORMONE; ANDROGEN/ANABOLIC STEROID
Pregnancy: Category X
Controlled substance: Schedule III

ACTIONS/PHARMACODYNAMICS Potent steroid with androgenic:anabolic activity ratio approximately 1:3. Promotes body tissue building and inhibits tissue-depleting processes; supports nitrogen, potassium, chloride, and phosphorus conservation. Enhances weight gain and combats depression and weakness in debilitating conditions. Stimulates bone growth, aids in bone matrix reconstitution, and may support calcification of metastatic lesions of breast cancer. Prevents or reverses profound nitrogen loss associated with corticosteroid therapy without compromising antiinflammatory activity. Mechanism of action in refractory anemias is unclear but may be due to direct stimulation of bone marrow or protein anabolic activity or to androgenic stimulation of erythropoiesis. Suppresses pituitary gonadotropic functions and may exert direct effect on testes. Potentially has all the side effects of testosterone.

USES Aplastic anemia. **Unlabeled uses:** osteoporosis, catabolic conditions.

ROUTE & DOSAGE

Aplastic Anemia

Adult	PO	1–5 mg/kg/d
Child	PO	Same as for adult

PHARMACOKINETICS **Absorption:** readily absorbed from GI tract. **Metabolism:** metabolized in liver. **Elimination:** half-life: 9 h; excreted in urine.

CONTRAINDICATIONS & PRECAUTIONS **Contraindicated in:** prostatic hypertrophy with obstruction; pregnancy (category X); use in nursing mothers or children not established; prostatic or male breast cancer; cardiac, renal, hepatic decompensation; nephrosis; premature infant. **Cautious use in:** prepubertal males; geriatric male patients; diabetes mellitus; coronary disease; patient taking ACTH, corticosteroids, anticoagulants.

ADVERSE/SIDE EFFECTS Androgenic in women: suppression of ovulation, lactation, or menstruation; *hoarseness or deepening of voice* (often irreversible); *hirsutism; oily skin; acne;* clitoral enlargement; regression of breasts; male-pattern baldness (in disseminated breast cancer). Men: prepubertal: premature epiphyseal closure, phallic enlargement, priapism. Postpubertal: testicular atrophy, decreased ejaculatory volume, azoospermia, oligospermia (after prolonged administration or excessive dosage), impotence, epididymitis, gynecomastia. **CV:** *edema,* skin flush. **GI:** *nausea, vomiting, anorexia,* diarrhea, jaundice, hepatotoxicity. **GU:** bladder irritability. **Hypoestrogenic:** female: flushing, sweating; vaginitis with pruritus, drying, bleeding; menstrual irregularities. **Other:** hypercalcemia.

NURSING IMPLICATIONS

Administration

- A course of therapy for treatment of osteoporosis is 7–21 d.
- For treatment of anemias, a minimum trial period of 3–6 mo is recommended, since response tends to be slow.

Common side effects in *italic*; life-threatening effects underlined; generic names in **bold**; classifications in SMALL CAPS

- Store at 15–30C (59–86F). Protect from heat and light.

Assessment & Drug Effects
- Closely monitor patient with a history of seizures, since an increase in their frequency may be noted.
- Monitor periodically for edema that may develop with or without CHF.
- Monitor for hypercalcemia (see Signs & Symptoms, chap 3), especially in women with breast cancer.
- Periodic liver function tests are especially important for the elderly patient. Drug should be stopped with first sign of liver toxicity (jaundice).
- Optimal effects in treatment of osteoporosis are usually experienced in 4–6 wk.

Patient & Family Education
- Inform diabetic that glucose tolerance may be decreased; instruct patient to monitor blood and urine closely.
- Instruct women to notify physician of signs of virilization.

Prototype: morphine, p 156

OXYMORPHONE HYDROCHLORIDE
(ox-i-mor´fone)

Trade name: Numorphan
Classifications: CNS AGENT; ANTIPYRETIC; NARCOTIC (OPIATE) AGONIST ANALGESIC
Pregnancy: Categories B and D (D for prolonged use of high doses at term)
Controlled substance: Schedule II

ACTIONS/PHARMACODYNAMICS Semisynthetic phenanthrene derivative structurally and pharmacologically related to morphine. Analgesic action of 1 mg is reportedly equivalent to that of 10 mg of morphine. Produces mild sedation and, unlike morphine, has little antitussive action. In equianalgesic doses may cause less constipation and antitussive effect than does morphine but more nausea, vomiting, and euphoria.

USES Relief of moderate to severe pain, preoperative medication, obstetric analgesia, support of anesthesia, and relief of anxiety in patients with dyspnea associated with acute ventricular failure and pulmonary edema.

ROUTE & DOSAGE

Moderate to Severe Pain

Adult	SC/IM	1–1.5 mg q4–6h prn
	IV	0.5 mg q4–6h
	PR	5 mg q4–6h prn

PHARMACOKINETICS Onset: 5–10 min IV; 10–15 min IM; 15–30 min PR. **Peak:** 1–1.5 h. **Duration:** 3–6 h. **Distribution:** crosses placenta. **Metabolism:** metabolized in liver. **Elimination:** eliminated in urine.

CONTRAINDICATIONS & PRECAUTIONS Contraindicated in: use for pulmonary edema resulting from chemical respiratory irritants. Safe use during pregnancy (category B), for prolonged use and high doses: Category D; in nursing mothers and in children <12 y not established.

ADVERSE/SIDE EFFECTS *Nausea, vomiting,* euphoria, *dizziness,* respiratory depression (see morphine).

DRUG INTERACTIONS Alcohol and other CNS DEPRESSANTS add to CNS depression.

NURSING IMPLICATIONS

Administration
- IV oxymorphone may be given by direct IV diluted in 5 ml of sterile water or NS and injected at a rate of 0.5 mg over 2–5 min.
- Protect drug from light. Store suppositories in refrigerator (2–15C, 36–59F).

Assessment & Drug Effects
- Monitor respiratory rate. Withhold drug and notify physician if rate falls below 12 breaths per minute.
- Supervise ambulation and advise patient of possible lightheadedness.
- Evaluate patient's continued need for narcotic analgesic. Prolonged use can lead to dependence of morphine type.
- Medication contains sulfite and may precipitate a hypersensitivity reaction in susceptible patient.
- Elderly and debilitated patients are most susceptible to CNS depressant effects of drug.

Patient & Family Education
- Advise ambulatory patient to exercise caution because of potential for injury from dizziness.
- Advise patients not to consume alcohol while they are taking oxymorphone.

Common side effects in *italic*; life-threatening effects underlined; generic names in **bold**; classifications in SMALL CAPS

Prototype: atropine, p 116

OXYPHENCYCLIMINE HYDROCHLORIDE

(ox-y-fen-cy´cli-meen)
Trade name: Daricon
Classifications: AUTONOMIC NERVOUS SYSTEM
AGENT; ANTICHOLINERGIC (PARASYMPATHOLYTIC);
ANTISPASMODIC
Pregnancy: Category C

ACTIONS/PHARMACODYNAMICS Tertiary
amine compound with little or no antimuscarinic activity and therefore no significant effect on gastric acid secretion. It exhibits a nonspecific direct relaxant effect on smooth muscle to reduce tone and motility of the GI tract.

USES Indicated for irritable bowel syndrome and as adjunct for peptic ulcer disease.

ROUTE & DOSAGE

Adjunct for Peptic Ulcer Disease, Irritable Bowel Syndrome
Adult   PO   5–10 mg b.i.d. in morning and evening

PHARMACOKINETICS Absorption: rapidly absorbed from GI tract. **Onset:** 1–2 h. **Duration:** > 12 h. **Elimination:** excreted in urine; unabsorbed drug excreted in feces.

CONTRAINDICATIONS & PRECAUTIONS Contraindicated in: history of hypersensitivity to anticholinergic drugs; obstructive diseases of GI and GU tracts, paralytic ileus, intestinal atony, biliary tract disease, unstable cardiovascular status, severe ulcerative colitis, toxic megacolon, myasthenia gravis; use in infants <6 wk. Safe use during pregnancy (category C), in nursing mothers, and in children not established. **Cautious use in:** glaucoma, prostatic hypertrophy, autonomic neuropathy, ulcerative colitis, hyperthyroidism, coronary heart disease, CHF, arrhythmias, hypertension, hepatic and renal disease, hiatal hernia associated with esophageal reflux.

ADVERSE/SIDE EFFECTS CNS: headache, nervousness, drowsiness, weakness, dizziness, depression, insomnia, mental confusion or excitement, especially in geriatric patients. **CV:** *palpitations, tachycardia,* hypotension. **Eye:** blurred vision, mydriasis. **GI:** *xerostomia,* loss of taste, *constipation,* nausea, vomiting. **GU:** urinary hesitancy and retention. **Skin:** anhidrosis, <u>anaphylaxis</u>, urticaria, rash. **Over-**

dosage: curariform neuromuscular block and ganglionic blockage manifested by <u>respiratory paralysis</u>.

DRUG INTERACTIONS Amantadine, ANTIHISTAMINES, TRICYCLIC ANTIDEPRESSANTS, **quinidine, disopyramide, procainamide** add to anticholinergic effects; decreases **levodopa** effects; **methotrimeprazine** may precipitate extrapyramidal effects; decreases antipsychotic effects (decreases absorption) of PHENOTHIAZINES.

NURSING IMPLICATIONS

Administration
- Usually administered in the morning (30 min before breakfast) and at bedtime.
- Store at room temperature below 30C (86F) unless otherwise directed.

Assessment & Drug Effects
- Monitor HR for tachycardia, especially in patients with a history of cardiovascular disease.
- Monitor glycemic control in diabetics. Decreased GI motility may slow postprandial elevation of blood sugar.
- Monitor elderly and debilitated patients for excitement, agitation, drowsiness, or confusion. Report to physician.

Patient & Family Education
- Advise patient to avoid hot environments. Oxyphencycline may increase risk of heatstroke by decreasing sweating. This is a particular problem of the elderly because of age-related reduction in sweating response to heat.
- May cause drowsiness and blurred vision; caution patient to avoid activities requiring mental alertness, such as operating a motor vehicle or dangerous machinery, until reactions to drug are known.
- Instruct patient to report changes in urinary volume or voiding pattern.

Prototype: tetracycline, p 74

OXYTETRACYCLINE

(ox-i-tet-ra-sye´kleen)
Trade name: Terramycin

OXYTETRACYCLINE HYDROCHLORIDE

Trade names: E.P. Mycin, Terramycin, Uri-Tet
Classifications: ANTIINFECTIVE; ANTIBIOTIC; TETRACYCLINE
Pregnancy: Category D

Common side effects in *italic*; life-threatening effects <u>underlined</u>; generic names in **bold**; classifications in SMALL CAPS

O

ACTIONS/PHARMACODYNAMICS Broad-spectrum antibiotic with actions, uses, contraindications, precautions, and adverse reactions similar to those of tetracycline.

ROUTE & DOSAGE

Antiinfective

Adult	PO	250–500 mg q6–12h
	IM	100 mg q8–12h
	IV	250–500 mg q12h (max 500 mg q6h)
Child	PO	> 8 y: 25–50 mg/kg/d in 4 divided doses
	IM	> 8 y: 15–25 mg/kg/d in 2–3 divided doses (max 250 mg/dose)
	IV	> 8 y: 10–20 mg/kg/d in 2 divided doses

PHARMACOKINETICS Absorption: about 60% absorbed from GI tract and IM site. **Peak:** 2–4 h. **Distribution:** appears to concentrate in hepatic system; crosses placenta; distributed into breast milk. **Metabolism:** partially metabolized. **Elimination:** half-life 6–10 h; excreted in feces and urine.

CONTRAINDICATIONS & PRECAUTIONS Contraindicated in: hypersensitivity to tetracyclines; during tooth development (last half of pregnancy [category D], infancy, childhood to age 8 y). **Cautious use in:** impaired renal function.

ADVERSE/SIDE EFFECTS *Nausea, vomiting, diarrhea, stomatitis,* skin rash, superinfections, renal toxicity.

DRUG INTERACTIONS ANTACIDS, **iron, calcium, magnesium, zinc, kaolin-pectin, sodium bicarbonate, bismuth subsalicylate** can significantly decrease oxytetracycline absorption; effects of both **desmopressin** and oxytetracycline antagonized; increases **digoxin** absorption, increasing risk of digoxin toxicity; **methoxyflurane** increases risk of renal failure. **Food-Drug interactions:** dairy products significantly decrease oxytetracycline absorption; food may decrease drug absorption.

NURSING IMPLICATIONS

Administration

- Dosage is reduced in the presence of renal impairment. Normal doses may result in liver toxicity.
- Check expiration date. Degradation products of outdated tetracyclines can be highly nephrotoxic.

- Food may interfere with rate and extent of absorption of oral drug. Administer at least 1 h before or 2 h following meals. Do not give with antacids, milk, milk products, or other calcium-containing foods.
- The commercially available solution for IM use contains only 2% lidocaine. Administer by deep IM. Do not use IM solution for IV administration.
- Only oxytetracycline hydrochloride for injection can be given IV. IV solution is prepared by adding 10 ml of sterile water for injection or D5W to the 250 or 500 mg vial. Further dilute with a minimum of 100 ml D5W, NS, or Ringer's lactate. Infuse slowly over 15–30 min. A slower rate of infusion and a large amount of diluent will reduce vein irritation.
- Syrup formulation (oxytetracycline calcium) should be stored in a cool place protected from light.
- Dry powder for parenteral use is stable at room temperature. Reconstituted solutions are stable for 48 h refrigerated (2–8C, 36–46.4F).

Assessment & Drug Effects

- Monitor for signs and symptoms of superinfection (see chap 3).
- Discontinue drug and notify physician at the first sign of a hypersensitivity response (see chap 3).

Patient & Family Education

- Instruct patient to discard unused drug when course of therapy has ended.
- Caution patient to avoid excessive exposure to sunlight because of the possibility of photosensitivity.

OXYTOCIN INJECTION

See OXYTOCIC prototype, p 250.

PANCREATIN

(pan´kree-a-tin)
Trade names: Creon, Dizymes, Hi-Vegi-Lip Tablets
Classifications: ENZYME; DIGESTANT
Pregnancy: Category C

ACTIONS/PHARMACODYNAMICS Pancreatic enzyme concentrate of bovine or porcine origin containing principally lipase, protease, and amylase in

P

Common side effects in *italic*; life-threatening effects <u>underlined</u>; generic names in **bold**; classifications in SMALL CAPS

849

standardized amounts. Assists in digestion of starch, protein, and fats; decreases nitrogen and fat content of stool.

USES Digestive aid in conditions associated with exocrine pancreatic deficiency such as chronic pancreatitis, pancreatectomy or gastrectomy, and cystic fibrosis. Also has been used as a presumptive test for pancreatic function.

ROUTE & DOSAGE

Pancreatic Insufficiency

Adult	PO	8,000–24,000 USP units daily in divided doses 1–2 h before, during, or 1 h after meals, with an extra dose taken with any food eaten between meals (up to 36,000 USP units/d)

CONTRAINDICATIONS & PRECAUTIONS

Cautious use in: history of hypersensitivity reactions to beef or pork products. Safe use during pregnancy (category C) not established.

ADVERSE/SIDE EFFECTS With large doses: anorexia, nausea, vomiting, diarrhea, buccal and anal soreness (particularly in infants), hypersensitivity reactions (sneezing, lacrimation, skin rashes).

DRUG INTERACTIONS Iron absorption may be decreased.

NURSING IMPLICATIONS

Administration

- Since pancreatin is inactivated by gastric pepsin and acid pH, it may be prescribed to be taken with or after an antacid, cimetidine, ranitidine, or similar drug.
- Enteric-coated tablets are to be swallowed whole, not crushed or chewed.
- Store in tight containers at room temperature not exceeding 30C (86F).

Assessment & Drug Effects

- Monitor patient for symptoms of diabetes mellitus (polyuria, thirst, hunger, pruritus). Insulin-dependent diabetes frequently occurs in these patients.
- Monitor I&O and weight. Note appetite, quality of stools, weight loss, abdominal bloating (pancreatic insufficiency may present as diabetes mellitus, steatorrhea, bulky stools).
- Periodic measurement of fecal fat and nitrogen, serum carotene and calcium, and prothrombin activity may be made to evaluate response to drug therapy.

Patient & Family Education

- Instruct patient in the proper timing of medication in relation to meals.

PANCRELIPASE

(pan-kre-li´pase)

Trade names: Cotazym, Cotazym-S, Festal II, Ilozyme, Ku-Zyme-Hp, Pancrease, Viokase
Classifications: ENZYME; DIGESTANT
Pregnancy: Category C

ACTIONS/PHARMACODYNAMICS Pancreatic enzyme concentrate of porcine origin standardized for lipase content. Similar to pancreatin but on a weight basis has 12 times the lipolytic activity and at least 4 times the trypsin and amylase content of pancreatin.

USES Replacement therapy in symptomatic treatment of malabsorption syndrome due to cystic fibrosis and other conditions associated with exocrine pancreatic insufficiency.

ROUTE & DOSAGE

Pancreatic Insufficiency

Adult	PO	1–3 capsules or tablets or 1–2 packets of powder 1–2 h before, during, or 1 h after meals, with an extra dose taken with any food eaten between meals
Child	PO	1–2 capsules or tablets 1–2 h before, during, or 1 h after meals, with an extra dose taken with any food eaten between meals

CONTRAINDICATIONS & PRECAUTIONS

Cautious use in: history of allergy to hog protein or enzymes. Safe use during pregnancy (category C) not established.

ADVERSE/SIDE EFFECTS High doses: anorexia, nausea, vomiting, diarrhea, hyperuricosuria.

DRUG INTERACTIONS Iron absorption may be decreased.

NURSING IMPLICATIONS

Administration

- Enteric coated preparations are not to be crushed or chewed.

P

- For children powder form may be sprinkled on food.
- Cimetidine, ranitidine, or an antacid may be prescribed to be given before pancrelipase to prevent its destruction by gastric pepsin and acid pH.
- Dosage is usually determined by fat content in diet (suggested ratio: 300 mg pancrelipase for each 17 g dietary fat).

Assessment & Drug Effects
- Monitor I&O and weight. Note appetite and quality of stools, weight loss, abdominal bloating, polyuria, thirst, hunger, itching. Pancreatic insufficiency is frequently associated with steatorrhea, bulky stools, and insulin-dependent diabetes.

Patient & Family Education
- Instruct patient in the proper timing of medication in relation to meals.

Prototype: tubocurarine, p 124

PANCURONIUM BROMIDE
(pan-kyoo-roe´nee-um)

Trade name: Pavulon
Classifications: AUTONOMIC NERVOUS SYSTEM AGENT; NONDEPOLARIZING SKELETAL MUSCLE RELAXANT
Pregnancy: Category C

ACTIONS/PHARMACODYNAMICS Synthetic curariform nondepolarizing neuromuscular blocking agent. Similar to tubocurarine chloride in actions, uses, and limitations. Reported to be approximately 5 times as potent as tubocurarine but produces little or no histamine release or ganglionic blockade and thus does not cause bronchospasm or hypotension. In high doses, has direct blocking effect on acetylcholine receptors of heart and may increase heart rate, cardiac output, and arterial pressure.

USES Adjunct to anesthesia to induce skeletal muscle relaxation. Also to facilitate management of patients undergoing mechanical ventilation.

PHARMACOKINETICS Onset: 30–45 s. **Peak:** 2–3 min. **Duration:** 60 min. **Distribution:** well distributed to tissues and extracellular fluids; crosses placenta in small amounts. **Metabolism:** small amount metabolized in liver. **Elimination:** half-life: 2 h; excreted primarily in urine.

ROUTE & DOSAGE

Skeletal Muscle Relaxation

Adult	IV	0.04 0.1 mg/kg initial dose; additional doses of 0.01 mg/kg may be given at 30–60 min intervals

CONTRAINDICATIONS & PRECAUTIONS Contraindicated in: hypersensitivity to the drug or bromides; tachycardia. Safe use during pregnancy (category C) not established. **Cautious use in:** debilitated patients; myasthenia gravis; pulmonary, hepatic or renal disease; fluid or electrolyte imbalance.

ADVERSE/SIDE EFFECTS *Increased pulse rate and BP,* ventricular extrasystoles, transient acneiform rash, burning sensation along course of vein, salivation, skeletal muscle weakness, <u>respiratory depression</u>.

DIAGNOSTIC TEST INTERFERENCES Pancuronium may decrease **serum cholinesterase** concentrations.

DRUG INTERACTIONS GENERAL ANESTHETICS increase neuromuscular blocking and duration of action; AMINOGLYCOSIDES, **bacitracin, polymyxin B, clindamycin, lidocaine,** parenteral **magnesium, quinidine, quinine, trimethaphan, verapamil** increase neuromuscular blockade; DIURETICS may increase or decrease neuromuscular blockade; **lithium** prolongs duration of neuromuscular blockade; NARCOTIC ANALGESICS possibly add to respiratory depression; **succinylcholine** increases onset and depth of neuromuscular blockade; **phenytoin** may cause resistance to or reversal of neuromuscular blockade.

NURSING IMPLICATIONS

Administration
- Plastic syringe may be used for administration, but drug may adsorb to plastic with prolonged storage.
- May be given by direct IV undiluted over 30–90 seconds.
- Refrigerate at 2–8C (36–46F). Do not freeze.

Assessment & Drug Effects
- Observe patient closely for residual muscle weakness and signs of respiratory distress during recovery period. Monitor BP and vital signs.
- Peripheral nerve stimulator may be used to assess the effects of pancuronium and to monitor restoration of neuromuscular function.

P

PAPAIN
(pa-pay´in)
Trade names: Panafil, Soflens
Classification: PROTEOLYTIC ENZYME

ACTIONS/PHARMACODYNAMICS Combination of proteolytic enzymes extracted from *Carica papaya*. At recommended doses, does not affect uninjured cells or tissues.

USES Topically for enzymatic debridement, promotion of normal healing, and deodorization of surface lesions. Soflens is used as an enzymatic cleaner of contact lenses.

ROUTE & DOSAGE

Enzymatic Debridement

Adult   Topical   Apply to lesion 1–2 times/d

CONTRAINDICATIONS & PRECAUTIONS Contraindicated in: history of allergy to papaya. Safe use during pregnancy not established. **Cautious use in:** topical preparation not to be used in eyes.

ADVERSE/SIDE EFFECTS Occasional stinging or itching.

NURSING IMPLICATIONS

Administration
- Before each application of ointment, irrigate wound with mild (prescribed) cleansing solution to remove accumulated debris.
- Hydrogen peroxide inactivates topical papain and therefore should not be used as an irrigating solution.
- Topical preparations may be covered with gauze.
- Store at 15–30C (59–86F) unless otherwise directed.

Assessment & Drug Effects
- Itching or stinging sensation sometimes occurs when papain is first applied. If symptoms persist, report to physician.

Prototype: hydralazine, p 152

PAPAVERINE HYDROCHLORIDE
(pa-pav´er-een)
Trade names: Cerebid, Cerespan, Dipav, Durapav, Genabid, Myobid, Orapav, P-200, Pavabid, Pavacap, Pavacen, Pavadur, Pavagen, Pava-Par, Pavased, Pavasule, Pavatyme, Paverolan, Pavex, Paverine, Ro-Papav, Vasal, Vasospan, Vazosan
Classifications: CARDIOVASCULAR AGENT; NONNITRATE VASODILATOR
Pregnancy: Category C

ACTIONS/PHARMACODYNAMICS Benzylisoquinoline alkaloid prepared synthetically or from opium. Lacks pharmacologic properties of narcotics; reportedly does not promote tolerance or habituation and has little if any analgesic effect. Exerts nonspecific direct spasmolytic effect on smooth muscles unrelated to innervation. Action is especially pronounced on coronary, cerebral, pulmonary, and peripheral arteries when spasm is present. Like quinidine, acts directly on myocardium, depresses conduction and irritability, and prolongs refractory period. Stimulates respiration by action on carotid and aortic body chemoreceptors. Relaxes smooth muscles of bronchi, GI tract, ureters, and biliary system. Objective proof of therapeutic value is reportedly lacking.

USES Primarily for relief of cerebral and peripheral ischemia associated with arterial spasm and MI complicated by arrhythmias. Also visceral spasm as in ureteral, biliary, and GI colic. **Unlabeled uses:** impotence, cardiac bypass surgery.

ROUTE & DOSAGE

Cerebral and Peripheral Ischemia

Adult	PO	100–300 mg 3–5 times/d
		150 mg sustained release q8–12h
	IM/IV	30–120 mg q3h as needed
Child	IM/IV	6 mg/kg/24 h divided into 4 doses

Impotence

Adult	IM	0.5–37.5 mg injected into the corpus cavernosum of the penis as needed for erection

Common side effects in *italic*; life-threatening effects <u>underlined</u>; generic names in **bold**; classifications in SMALL CAPS

PHARMACOKINETICS Absorption: readily absorbed from GI tract. **Peak:** 1–2 h. **Duration:** 6 h regular tablets; 12 h sustained release. **Metabolism:** metabolized in liver. **Elimination:** half-life 90 min; excreted in urine chiefly as metabolites.

CONTRAINDICATIONS & PRECAUTIONS Contraindicated in: parenteral use in complete AV block. Safe use during pregnancy (category C), in nursing mothers, and in children not established. **Cautious use in:** glaucoma; myocardial depression; angina pectoris; recent stroke.

ADVERSE/SIDE EFFECTS PO: nausea, anorexia, constipation, diarrhea, abdominal distress, dizziness, drowsiness, headache. **Parenteral (low incidence):** general discomfort, facial flushing, sweating, dry mouth and throat, pruritus, skin rash, dizziness, headache, excessive drowsiness and sedation (large doses), slight rise in BP, increased depth of respiration, paroxysmal tachycardia, transient ventricular ectopic rhythms, hepatotoxicity (jaundice, eosinophilia, abnormal liver function tests); with rapid IV administration: respiratory depression, AV block, arrhythmias, fatal apnea; priapism. **Overdosage:** diplopia, nystagmus, weakness, drowsiness, coma, respiratory depression.

DRUG INTERACTIONS May decrease **levodopa** effectiveness; **morphine** may antagonize smooth muscle relaxation effect of papaverine.

NURSING IMPLICATIONS

Administration

- Oral formulations may be taken with or following meals; milk or prescribed antacid may be given to reduce possibility of nausea.
- Timed-release forms should be swallowed whole and must not be chewed or crushed.
- Aspirate carefully before injecting IM to avoid inadvertent entry into blood vessel, and administer slowly.
- When given IV, papaverine may be given undiluted or diluted in an equal volume of sterile water for injection; drug must be administered slowly over 1–2 min.
- Parenteral papaverine is incompatible with lactated Ringer's injection (forms precipitate).
- Preserve in tightly covered, light-resistant containers.

Assessment & Drug Effects

- Monitor pulse, respiration, and BP in patients receiving drug parenterally. If significant changes are noted, withhold medication and report promptly to physician.
- Hepatic function and blood tests should be performed periodically. Hepatotoxicity (thought to be a hypersensitivity reaction) is reversible with prompt drug withdrawal.

Patient & Family Education

- Instruct patient to notify physician if any side effect persists or if GI symptoms, jaundice, or skin rash appear. Hepatic function tests may be indicated. Because of the possibility of drowsiness and dizziness, advise patient to avoid driving and other potentially hazardous tasks until reaction to drug is known. Alcohol may increase drowsiness and dizziness.

Prototype: phenobarbital, p 167

PARALDEHYDE
(par-al´de-hyde)
Trade names: Paracetaldehyde, Paral
Classifications: CNS AGENT; ANTICONVULSANT; SEDATIVE-HYPNOTIC; BARBITURATE
Pregnancy: Category C
Controlled substance: Schedule IV

ACTIONS/PHARMACODYNAMICS Cyclic ether formed by polymerization of acetaldehyde. Potent CNS depressant with sedative and hypnotic actions similar to those of alcohol, barbiturates, and chloral hydrate.

USES Sedative and hypnotic in acute agitation due to alcohol withdrawal; used to control convulsions arising from tetanus, eclampsia, status epilepticus, and drug poisoning. Has been used rectally to induce basal anesthesia, particularly in children.

PHARMACOKINETICS Absorption: readily absorbed from GI tract. **Onset:** 10–15 min. **Duration:** 6–8 h. **Distribution:** distributed into CNS; crosses placenta. **Metabolism:** 80–90% of doses metabolized in liver. **Elimination:** half-life: 7.5 h; excreted through lungs (11–28%) and urine.

CONTRAINDICATIONS & PRECAUTIONS Contraindicated in: severe hepatic insufficiency; respiratory disease; GI inflammation or ulceration; disulfiram therapy. Pregnancy category C.

P

Common side effects in *italic*; life-threatening effects underlined; generic names in **bold**; classifications in SMALL CAPS

853

ROUTE & DOSAGE

Both oral and rectal doses must be diluted before they are administered.

Hypnotic

Adult	PO	10–30 ml prn
Child	PO	0.3 ml/kg

Sedative

Adult	PO	5–10 ml prn
Child	PO	0.15 ml/kg

Seizures Secondary to Tetanus

Adult	PO	up to 12 ml diluted 1:10 q4h prn

Seizures Secondary to Other Poisons

Adult	PR	5–15 ml diluted in 200 ml per rectal tube

Status Epilepticus

Child	PR	1 ml/y of age up to 5 ml, may repeat in 1 h if necessary, then change to PO
	PO	2–5 ml q2–4h

Alcohol Withdrawal Seizures

Adult	PO	5–10 ml q4–6h for 24 h; then q6h prn

ADVERSE/SIDE EFFECTS *Irritation of mucous membrane (oral and rectal routes),* nausea, vomiting, unpleasant taste and odor, hangover, dizziness, ataxia, *erythematous skin rash;* occasionally confusion and paradoxical excitement. **Prolonged use:** <u>toxic hepatitis</u>, nephrosis, metabolic acidosis. **Overdosage:** rapid labored breathing, <u>respiratory depression</u>, pulmonary hemorrhage and edema, hypotension, bleeding gastritis, renal and liver damage, acidosis, <u>dilation and failure of right heart, cardiovascular collapse</u>.

DIAGNOSTIC TEST INTERFERENCES Chronic use of alcohol (ethanol) and paraldehyde may cause false-positive ***serum ketones*** (nitroprusside tube dilution method) and ***urine ketones*** (Acetest) and may interfere with ***urinary steroid*** (17-OHCS) determinations by modification of Reddy, Jenkins, Thorn procedure.

DRUG INTERACTIONS Disulfiram may increase paraldehyde levels; **alcohol** and other CNS DEPRESSANTS add to CNS depressant effects—fatalities reported with alcohol.

NURSING IMPLICATIONS

Administration

- In some hospitals, physicians administer parenteral paraldehyde because of danger of circulatory collapse or pulmonary edema, sterile abscesses, nerve injury, and paralysis.
- Paraldehyde is a colorless clear liquid with a strong characteristic odor and a burning, disagreeable taste.
- On exposure to light, air, and heat, drug liberates acetaldehyde, which oxidizes to acetic acid. Do not use solution if it is colored in any way or smells of acetic acid (vinegar odor).
- Decomposed paraldehyde is extremely corrosive to tissues and can cause fatal poisoning. Discard unused contents of any container that has been open for more than 24 h.
- Do not use plastics for measuring or administering paraldehyde. Contact with plastic materials can decompose paraldehyde to toxic compounds. Parenteral preparation should be drawn into a glass syringe; use rubber catheter for rectal administration.
- Give oral drug well diluted in iced fruit juice or milk to reduce irritation of GI tract and mask odor and taste. Oral capsules are available.
- When given rectally, drug should be diluted with at least 2 volumes of olive oil or cottonseed oil or dissolved in 200 ml of 0.9% NaCl solution to prevent rectal irritation.
- IM injection should be made deep into upper outer quadrant of buttock well away from nerve trunks. Paraldehyde can cause nerve injury and paralysis. Aspirate carefully before injecting drug, and massage injection site well. Rotate injection sites. Not to exceed 5 ml per injection site.
- Rapid withdrawal after prolonged use may produce delirium tremens and hallucinations.
- Preserve in tight, light-resistant containers in amounts not exceeding 30 ml and at temperatures not over 25C (77F). Keep away from heat, open flames, and sparks.

Assessment & Drug Effects

- When paraldehyde is given by IV route (infrequently used), CNS depression may be preceded by a brief period of excitement and coughing. The coughing that sometimes occurs when paraldehyde is given IV may be due to untoward effects on pulmonary capillaries. Monitor patient closely for hypotension and respiratory depression.
- Bronchial secretions may be increased. Keep the patient turned on side to prevent aspiration. Suctioning may be necessary.
- Patient's breath will have a characteristic odor for several hours.
- Tolerance and physical and psychologic dependence can occur with prolonged use. Paraldehyde addiction resembles alcoholism.

Common side effects in *italic*; life-threatening effects <u>underlined</u>; generic names in **bold**; classifications in SMALL CAPS

Prototype: phenytoin, p 172

PARAMETHADIONE
(par-a-meth-a-dye´one)
Trade name: Paradione
Classifications: CNS AGENT; HYDANTOIN ANTICONVULSANT
Pregnancy: Category D

ACTIONS/PHARMACODYNAMICS Oxazolidinedione (dione-type) anticonvulsant agent with pharmacologic actions, uses, contraindications, precautions, and adverse reactions similar to those of trimethadione. Unlike trimethadione, chronic administration is not associated with myasthenia gravis–like syndrome, and although incidence of other toxic reactions is lower, it is reportedly less effective. Causes slightly greater sedative effect than trimethadione.

USES To control absence (petit mal) seizures refractory to other drugs.

ROUTE & DOSAGE

Absence Seizures

Adult	PO	300 mg t.i.d.; may increase by 300 mg/d at weekly intervals (max 2.4 g/d)
Child	PO	>6 y: 300 mg t.i.d. or q.i.d.
		2–6 y: 200 mg t.i.d.
		<2 y: 100 mg t.i.d.

PHARMACOKINETICS Absorption: readily absorbed from GI tract. **Metabolism:** metabolized in liver to active metabolites. **Elimination:** excreted slowly in urine.

CONTRAINDICATIONS & PRECAUTIONS Contraindicated in: hypersensitivity to oxazolidinedione anticonvulsants; severe blood dyscrasias, renal and hepatic dysfunction. Safe use during pregnancy (category D) and in nursing mothers not established. **Cautious use in:** retinal or optic nerve disease.

ADVERSE/SIDE EFFECTS *Sedation, drowsiness.* Infrequent: ataxia, headache, dizziness, paresthesias, vaginal bleeding, changes in BP, visual symptoms, GI distress, rash, alopecia, lymphadenopathy, abnormal liver function tests, albuminuria, mild neutropenia, aplastic anemia, exfoliative dermatitis, erythema multiforme, nephrotic syndrome, hepatitis, lupus.

NURSING IMPLICATIONS

Administration

- Capsule form contains an oily liquid and must be swallowed whole and not chewed or crushed.
- Oral solution contains alcohol 65% and should be diluted with water before administration.
- Drug should be withdrawn gradually to avoid precipitating seizure activity.
- Store in tightly covered containers at 15–30C (59–86F) unless otherwise directed. Solution should be stored in light-resistant container.

Assessment & Drug Effects

- Liver function tests, urinalysis, and CBC should be done prior to and at monthly intervals during therapy. If blood counts remain normal for 12 mo, intervals may be increased. Blood counts are done more frequently if neutrophil count drops to <3000/mm^3, and drug is withdrawn if count drops to 2500/mm^3 or less.

Patient & Family Education

- Advise patient to measure oral solution with graduated dropper provided by manufacturer.
- Since drug may cause drowsiness and visual symptoms, caution patient to avoid driving and other potentially hazardous activities until reaction to drug is known.
- Instruct patient to report any unusual symptom to physician. Drug should be discontinued if patient develops jaundice, swollen glands, skin rash, hair loss, unexplained fever, fatigue, tendency to bleed or bruise, or sore mouth or throat.

Prototype: prednisone, p 225

PARAMETHASONE ACETATE
(par-a-meth´a-sone)
Trade name: Haldrone
Classifications: SYNTHETIC HORMONE; ADRENAL CORTICOSTEROID; GLUCOCORTICOID; ANTIINFLAMMATORY
Pregnancy: Category C

ACTIONS/PHARMACODYNAMICS Long-acting synthetic steroid with antiinflammatory action but little sodium-retaining potency. On weight basis, 2 mg paramethasone is equivalent to 5 mg prednisone. Has no particular advantages over other cortico-

P

Common side effects in *italic*; life-threatening effects underlined; generic names in **bold**; classifications in SMALL CAPS

855

steroids. Similar to prednisone in actions, uses, absorption, and fate.

ROUTE & DOSAGE

Allergies, Inflammation

Adult	PO	2–24 mg/d in 3–4 divided doses; then decrease to lowest dose necessary
Child	PO	58–200 µg/kg/d in 1–4 divided doses

PHARMACOKINETICS Absorption: readily absorbed from GI tract. **Peak:** 1–2 h. **Duration:** 2 d. **Distribution:** crosses placenta; distributed into breast milk. **Elimination:** half-life: 3–45 h; HPA suppression: 36–54 h.

CONTRAINDICATIONS & PRECAUTIONS Contraindicated in: systemic fungal infections; ocular herpes simplex; keratitis; safe use during pregnancy (category C), lactation, and by children <6 y not established.

ADVERSE/SIDE EFFECTS Increase in appetite, growth retardation, hypocalcemia (prolonged treatment), psychic derangement. Same as those of prednisone.

DRUG INTERACTIONS Since BARBITURATES, **phenytoin, rifampin** increase steroid metabolism, may need to increase paramethasone doses; **amphotericin B,** DIURETICS add to potassium loss; **ambenonium, neostigmine, pyridostigmine** may cause severe muscle weakness in patients with myasthenia gravis; may inhibit antibody response to VACCINES, TOXOIDS.

NURSING IMPLICATIONS

See prednisone for numerous additional nursing implications.

Administration

- If drug is to be stopped after long-term therapy, it should be withdrawn gradually to prevent onset of hypocortisolism.
- Store in light-resistant container at 15–30C (59–86F).

Assessment & Drug Effects

- At high dosage (> 15 mg/d), urinary excretion of calcium and nitrogen increases significantly.
- Monitor electrolytes, creatinine, and BUN periodically.

Prototype: diphenoxylate HCl with atropine sulfate, p 213

PAREGORIC (CAMPHORATED OPIUM TINCTURE)

(par-e-gor´ik)

Classifications: GI AGENT; ANTIDIARRHEAL; CNS AGENT; ANTIPYRETIC NARCOTIC (OPIATE) AGONIST ANALGESIC

Pregnancy: Categories B and D (D for prolonged use or high doses at term)

Controlled substance: Schedule III

ACTIONS/PHARMACODYNAMICS Contains 2 mg anhydrous morphine, alcohol, benzoic acid, camphor, and anise oil. Pharmacologic activity is due to morphine content. Increases smooth muscle tone of GI tract, decreases motility and effective propulsive peristalsis, and diminishes digestive secretions. Delayed transit of intestinal contents results in desiccation of feces and constipation. Available in fixed combination as brown mixture: a 12% paregoric solution with glycyrrhiza fluid extract, antimony potassium tartrate and alcohol.

USES Short-term treatment for symptomatic relief of acute diarrhea and abdominal cramps.

ROUTE & DOSAGE

Acute Diarrhea

Adult	PO	5–10 ml after loose bowel movement; may be administered q2h up to q.i.d. if needed
Child	PO	0.25–0.5 ml/kg 1–4 times/d

PHARMACOKINETICS Absorption: readily absorbed from GI tract. **Duration:** 4–5 h. **Distribution:** crosses placenta; distributed into breast milk. **Metabolism:** metabolized in liver. **Elimination:** half-life: 2–3 h; excreted in urine.

CONTRAINDICATIONS & PRECAUTIONS Contraindicated in: hypersensitivity to opium alkaloids; diarrhea caused by poisons (until eliminated). Pregnancy category B; with prolonged use or high doses at term, category D. **Cautious use in:** asthma; hepatic disease; history of opiate agonist dependence; severe prostatic hypertrophy.

P

ADVERSE/SIDE EFFECTS GI: anorexia, nausea, vomiting, *constipation,* abdominal pain. **Other:** with high doses: dizziness, faintness, drowsiness, facial flushing, sweating, physical dependence.

DRUG INTERACTIONS Alcohol and other CNS DEPRESSANTS add to CNS effects.

NURSING IMPLICATIONS

Administration

- Not to be confused with opium tincture, deodorized, which contains 25 times more anhydrous morphine than the camphorated tincture.
- Administer paregoric in sufficient water (2 or 3 swallows) to assure its passage into the stomach (mixture will appear milky).
- Preserve in tight, light-resistant container at 15–30C (59–86F) unless otherwise directed.

Assessment & Drug Effect

- Paregoric may worsen the course of diarrhea by delaying the elimination of pathogens.
- Adverse effects are primarily due to morphine content. Paregoric abuse results because of the narcotic content of the drug.
- Assess for fluid and electrolyte imbalance until diarrhea has stopped.

Patient & Family Education

- Instruct patient to adhere strictly to prescribed dosage schedule.
- Bed rest is advisable if diarrhea is severe with a high level of fluid loss.
- Replacement of fluids and electrolytes is a vital adjunct to drug therapy for diarrhea. Instruct patient to drink warm clear liquids and to avoid dairy products, concentrated sweets, and cold drinks until diarrhea stops.
- Advise patient to observe character and frequency of stools. Drug should be discontinued as soon as diarrhea is controlled. Urge patient to report promptly to physician if diarrhea persists more than 3 d, if fever is > 38.8C (102F), abdominal pain develops, or if mucus or blood is passed.
- Inform patient that constipation is often a consequence of antidiarrheal treatment and that normal pattern is usually established as dietary intake increases.

PARGYLINE HYDROCHLORIDE
(par´gi-leen)
Trade name: Eutonyl
Classifications: CNS AGENT;
PSYCHOTHERAPEUTIC; MAO INHIBITOR
ANTIDEPRESSANT; ANTIHYPERTENSIVE
Pregnancy: Category C

ACTIONS/PHARMACODYNAMICS Nonhydrazine MAO inhibitor with pharmacologic actions similar to those of other MAO inhibitors. Like phenelzine, but reportedly less hepatotoxic. Exerts hypotensive effect and reportedly produces mood elevation. Mechanism of hypotensive activity not known but thought to be related in part to modification of ganglionic transmission. Most prominent effect is orthostatic (hypotensive).

USES Moderate to severe hypertension. May be used concurrently with other antihypertensive agents such as thiazides or rauwolfia alkaloids.

ROUTE & DOSAGE

Hypertension

Adult	PO	25 mg once/d; may be increased by 10 mg/d weekly; usual range 50–75 mg/d (max 200 mg/d)

PHARMACOKINETICS Elimination: excreted primarily in urine.

CONTRAINDICATIONS & PRECAUTIONS Contraindicated in: mild, labile, or malignant hypertension; hyperactive or excitable individuals; paranoid schizophrenia; hyperthyroidism; pheochromocytoma; advanced renal failure. Safe use during pregnancy (category C), lactation, in women of childbearing potential, and in children <12 y not established. **Cautious use in:** liver disease; arteriosclerosis, coronary artery disease; parkinsonism; diabetes mellitus.

ADVERSE/SIDE EFFECTS *Orthostatic hypotension,* sweating, dry mouth, fluid retention, CHF, increased appetite, *weight gain,* nausea, vomiting, mild constipation, headache, arthralgia, difficulty in micturition, impotence or delayed ejaculation, rash, purpura, nightmares, hyperexcitability, muscle twitching

P

and other extrapyramidal symptoms, drug fever (rare), hypoglycemia (optic atrophy not reported, although it is associated with use of other MAO inhibitors). **Overdosage:** agitation, confusion, hallucinations, mania, hyperreflexia, convulsions, hypertension or hypotension.

DRUG INTERACTIONS May increase therapeutic and toxic effects of **levodopa; meperidine** may cause cardiovascular instability, agitation, convulsions, or coma; may potentiate hypoglycemic effects of SULFONYLUREAS, **insulin;** SYMPATHOMIMETICS may cause headache, hyperpyrexia, possible hypertensive crisis; TRICYCLIC ANTIDEPRESSANTS may cause nausea, dizziness, seizures, cardiovascular instability. **Food-drug interactions:** tyramine-containing food (see phenelzine) may precipitate hypertensive crisis.

NURSING IMPLICATIONS

Administration
- If drug therapy is temporarily interrupted for any reason, it should be reinstituted at a lower dosage.
- Drug may augment hypotensive effects of anesthetic agents and therefore should be discontinued at least 2 wk prior to elective surgery.

Assessment & Drug Effects
- Dosage adjustments are based on BP in standing position.
- Actions of pargyline are cumulative. Maximal therapeutic effect may occur in 4 d, but it may not appear for 3 wk or more; action may persist for 3 wk after therapy is discontinued.
- Febrile illness can potentiate the hypotensive effect of pargyline. Temporary drug withdrawal may be necessary.
- Diabetics may require adjustment in antidiabetic medication. Severe drug-induced hypoglycemia (see Signs & Symptoms, chap 3) can occur.
- Pargyline may unmask psychotic symptoms in patients with preexisting emotional problems.
- Urinalyses, liver function tests, and CBCs should be performed periodically during therapy.
- Patients with impaired renal function should be closely observed for signs of cumulative drug effects. Monitor I&O and BUN in these patients.

Patient & Family Education
- Instruct patient to report symptoms of orthostatic hypotension (dizziness, weakness, palpitation, fainting); dosage adjustment is indicated.
- Warn patient to make position changes slowly, especially when getting out of bed, and to lie or sit down immediately if feeling dizzy or faint.
- Advise patient not to take alcohol, sedatives, tranquilizers, or other CNS depressants without prior approval of physician.
- Instruct patient to keep daily record of weight and to check ankles and tibias for edema. Pargyline tends to promote weight gain from fluid retention as well as increased appetite.
- Since drug may suppress anginal pain, warn patient not to increase physical activity in response to drug-induced sense of well-being.
- Caution patient not to add any medication to drug regimen without consulting physician. OTC preparations containing dextromethorphan or sympathomimetic amines can precipitate hypertensive crisis (e.g., appetite suppressants, nasal decongestants, cold and hay fever remedies).
- Acute hypertensive reaction (severe headache, marked hypertension, chest pain, palpitation, tachycardia, bradycardia) can result from ingestion of foods or liquids high in tyramine or tryptophan. Provide family or responsible family member with list of foods to avoid.
- Advise diabetic patient using a sulfonylurea of the potential for severe hypoglycemia.

Prototype: emetine, p 51

PAROMOMYCIN SULFATE
(par-oh-moe-mye´sin)
Trade name: Humatin
Classifications: ANTIINFECTIVE; AMEBICIDE; AMINOGLYCOSIDE ANTIBIOTIC
Pregnancy: Category C

ACTIONS/PHARMACODYNAMICS Aminoglycoside antibiotic produced by certain strains of *Streptomyces rimosus* with broad spectrum of antibacterial activity closely paralleling that of kanamycin and neomycin. Exerts direct bactericidal and amebicidal action, primarily in lumen of GI tract. Ineffective against extraintestinal amebiasis. Reportedly significantly reduces serum cholesterol.

USES Acute and chronic intestinal amebiasis and to rid bowel of nitrogen-forming bacteria in patients with hepatic coma; used preoperatively to suppress intestinal flora. Also tapeworm infestation.

PHARMACOKINETICS Absorption: poorly absorbed from intact GI tract. **Elimination:** in feces.

ROUTE & DOSAGE

Intestinal Amebiasis

Adult	PO	25–35 mg/kg divided in 3 doses for 5–10 d
Child	PO	Same as for adult

Hepatic Coma

Adult	PO	4 g/d in 2–4 divided doses for 5–6 d

CONTRAINDICATIONS & PRECAUTIONS Contraindicated in: intestinal obstruction; impaired renal function. Pregnancy category C. **Cautious use in:** GI ulceration.

ADVERSE/SIDE EFFECTS CNS: headache, vertigo. **GI:** *diarrhea, abdominal cramps,* steatorrhea, *nausea, vomiting, heartburn,* secondary enterocolitis. **Skin:** exanthema, rash, pruritus. **Other:** ototoxicity, nephrotoxicity (in patients with GI inflammation or ulcerations), eosinophilia, overgrowth of nonsusceptible organisms.

DIAGNOSTIC TEST INTERFERENCES Prolonged use of paromomycin may cause reduction in *serum cholesterol.*

NURSING IMPLICATIONS

Administration
- Usually administered after meals to prevent gastric distress.

Assessment & Drug Effects
- Be alert for appearance of a superinfection during therapy (see Signs & Symptoms, chap 3).
- Patients with history of GI ulceration must be closely monitored for nephrotoxicity and ototoxicity (see Signs & Symptoms, chap 3). Drug absorption can take place through diseased mucosa.
- Criterion of cure is absence of amebae in stool specimens examined at weekly intervals for 6 wk after completion of treatment, and thereafter at monthly intervals for 2 y.

Patient & Family Education
- Patients receiving drug for intestinal amebiasis should be excluded from preparing, processing, and serving food until treatment is complete. Isolation is not required.
- Emphasize personal hygiene, particularly handwashing after defecation and before eating food, and sanitary disposal of feces.

Prototype: amphetamine, p 194

PEMOLINE
(pem´oh-leen)
Trade name: Cylert
Classifications: CNS AGENT; RESPIRATORY AND CEREBRAL STIMULANT
Pregnancy: Category B
Controlled substance: Schedule IV

ACTIONS/PHARMACODYNAMICS Oxazolidinone derivative with pharmacologic actions qualitatively similar to those of amphetamine and methylphenidate but with weak sympathomimetic activity. Capable of producing increased motor activity, mental alertness, diminished sense of fatigue, and mild euphoria. Also thought to have anorexigenic effect.

USES Adjunctive therapy to other remedial measures (psychologic, educational, social) in minimal brain dysfunction (attention deficit disorder [ADD]) in carefully selected children. **Unlabeled use:** mild stimulant for geriatric patients.

ROUTE & DOSAGE

Attention Deficit Disorder

Child	PO	>6 y: 37.5 mg/d; may be increased by 18.75 mg at weekly intervals (max 112.5 mg/d)

PHARMACOKINETICS Absorption: readily absorbed from GI tract. **Onset:** 2–3 wk. **Peak:** 2–4 h. **Duration:** 8 h. **Metabolism:** metabolized in liver. **Elimination:** half-life: 9–14 h; excreted in urine.

CONTRAINDICATIONS & PRECAUTIONS Contraindicated in: known hypersensitivity to pemoline; children <6 y. Safe use during pregnancy (category B) and in nursing women not established. **Cautious use in:** impaired hepatic and renal function; history of drug abuse; psychosis; emotional instability.

ADVERSE/SIDE EFFECTS *Insomnia, anorexia,* abdominal discomfort, malaise, nausea, diarrhea, skin rash, irritability, fatigue, mild depression, dizziness, headache, drowsiness, dyskinetic movements of eyes or other parts of body; convulsions. **Overdosage:** nervousness, tachycardia, hallucinations, excitement, agitation, restlessness. Also reported: el-

P

Common side effects in *italic*; life-threatening effects <u>underlined</u>; generic names in **bold**; classifications in SMALL CAPS

859

evated AST, ALT, and alkaline phosphatase (after several months of therapy); jaundice, reversible hepatic damage (rare).

NURSING IMPLICATIONS

Administration

- Administer drug in morning to provide maximal effectiveness and to avoid insomnia.
- Chewable tablet may be chewed or swallowed whole.
- Store at 15–30C (59–86F) unless otherwise directed.

Assessment & Drug Effects

- Insomnia and anorexia (most frequent side effects) appear to be dose-related.
- Monitor weight and height (growth rate) throughout therapy. Anorexia is often accompanied by weight loss.
- Careful clinical evaluation and supervision of patient are essential. Patients receiving long-term therapy should have periodic liver function studies.
- Occasional interruption of drug therapy is advised to determine if behavioral symptoms recur.

Patient & Family Education

- Caution patient to avoid potentially hazardous activities until the reaction to drug is known.
- Significant benefits of drug therapy may not be evident until third or fourth wk of drug administration.
- Pemoline can produce tolerance and physical and psychologic dependence.

Prototype: propanolol, p 109

PENBUTOLOL

(pen-bu´tol-ol)

Trade name: Levatol

Classifications: AUTONOMIC NERVOUS SYSTEM AGENT; BETA ADRENERGIC ANTAGONIST (BLOCKING AGENT; SYMPATHOLYTIC); CARDIOVASCULAR AGENT; ANTIHYPERTENSIVE

Pregnancy: Category C

ACTIONS/PHARMACODYNAMICS Penbutolol is a synthetic beta$_1$ (cardiac) and beta$_2$ (bronchial) adrenergic blocking agent. It lowers both supine and standing BP in hypertensive patients. Hypotensive effect is associated with decreased cardiac output, suppressed renin activity, as well as beta-blockage.

USES Mild to moderate hypertension. May be used alone or with other antihypertensive agents.

ROUTE & DOSAGE

Hypertension

Adult   PO   10–20 mg once/d; may increase to 40–80 mg/d if needed

---

PHARMACOKINETICS Absorption: readily absorbed from GI tract. **Peak:** 2–3 h. **Duration:** 20 h. **Metabolism:** metabolized in liver. **Elimination:** half-life: 5 h; excreted in urine.

CONTRAINDICATIONS & PRECAUTIONS Contraindicated in: clients with cardiogenic shock, sinus bradycardia, second and third degree AV block, bronchial asthma, and hypersensitivity to the drug. **Cautious use in:** cardiac failure, chronic bronchitis, emphysema, diabetes, pregnancy (category C), and nursing mothers. Safety and effectiveness in children has not been established.

ADVERSE/SIDE EFFECTS CNS: dizziness, fatigue, *headache,* insomnia. **CV:** AV block, bradycardia. **GI:** nausea, diarrhea, dyspepsia. **Respiratory:** cough, dyspnea. **Other:** impotence.

DRUG INTERACTIONS DIURETICS and other HYPOTENSIVE AGENTS increase hypotensive effect; effects of **albuterol, metaproterenol, terbutaline, pirbuterol,** and penbutolol are antagonized; NSAIDS blunt hypotensive effect; decreases hypoglycemic effect of **glyburide; amiodarone** increases risk of bradycardia and sinus arrest.

NURSING IMPLICATIONS

Administration

- May be taken without regard to meals.
- Should be discontinued by reducing the dose gradually over 1 to 2 wk.

Assessment & Drug Effects

- Take apical pulse before administering drug. If pulse is below 60, hold the drug and contact physician.
- If BP is not stabilized, take a BP reading before giving drug. If systolic pressure is ≤ 90 mm Hg, hold drug and contact physician.
- Check BP near end of dosage interval or before administration of next dose to evaluate effectiveness.
- Apical pulse, respirations, BP, and circulation to extremities should be closely monitored through-

out periods of dosage adjustment. Consult physician regarding acceptable parameters.

- The full effectiveness of the drug is not seen for 4–6 wk.
- Watch for signs and symptoms of bronchial constriction. Report promptly and withhold drug.
- Diabetics should be closely monitored. Penbutolol suppresses clinical signs of hypoglycemia (e.g., BP changes, increased pulse rate) and may prolong hypoglycemic state.
- During drug withdrawal, carefully monitor for exacerbation of angina.

Patient & Family Education
- Instruct patient not to interrupt or discontinue the drug without physician's advice because of the possible exacerbation of ischemic heart disease.
- Instruct diabetics to report signs and symptoms of hypoglycemia (see chap 3).
- Since penbutolol may cause dizziness and lightheadedness due to mild hypotension, caution patient to avoid driving or other potentially hazardous activities until reaction is known.
- Advise patient to make position changes slowly and to avoid prolonged standing. Notify physician if dizziness and lightheadedness persist.
- Stress the importance of compliance and warn patient not to alter established regimen, i.e., not to omit, increase, or decrease dosage or change dosage interval.
- Caution patient to avoid prolonged exposure of extremities to cold.
- Counsel patient to avoid excesses of alcohol. Heavy alcohol consumption (i.e., > 60 ml (2 oz)/d) may elevate arterial pressure; therefore, to maintain treatment effectiveness, either avoid alcohol or drink moderately (<60 ml/d). Consult physician.

PENICILLAMINE
(pen-i-sill´a-meen)
Trade names: Cuprimine, Depen
Classification: CHELATING AGENT

ACTIONS/PHARMACODYNAMICS Thiol compound prepared by hydrolysis of penicillin but lacking antibacterial activity. Forms stable soluble chelate with copper, zinc, iron, lead, mercury, and possibly other heavy metals and promotes their excretion in urine. Also combines chemically with cystine to form a soluble disulfide complex that prevents stone formation and may even dissolve existing cystitic stones. Mechanism of action in rheumatoid arthritis

not known but appears to be related to inhibition of collagen formation. Cross-sensitivity between penicillin and penicillamine can occur.

USES To promote renal excretion of excess copper in Wilson's disease (hepatolenticular degeneration). Also active rheumatoid arthritis in patients who have failed to respond to conventional therapy; cystinuria. **Unlabeled uses:** scleroderma, primary biliary cirrhosis, porphyria cutanea tarda, lead poisoning.

ROUTE & DOSAGE

Wilson's Disease

Adult	PO	250 mg q.i.d., with 3 doses 1 h a.c. and the last dose at least 2 h after the last meal

Cystinuria

Adult	PO	250–500 mg q.i.d., with doses adjusted to limit urinary excretion of cystine to 100–200 mg/d
Child	PO	30 mg/kg/d in 4 divided doses with doses adjusted to limit urinary excretion of cystine to 100–200 mg/d

Rheumatoid Arthritis

Adult	PO	125–250 mg/d; may increase at 1–3 mo intervals up to 1–1.5 g/d

PHARMACOKINETICS Absorption: readily absorbed from GI tract. **Peak:** 1 h. **Distribution:** crosses placenta. **Metabolism:** metabolized in liver. **Elimination:** excreted in urine and feces.

CONTRAINDICATIONS & PRECAUTIONS Contraindicated in: hypersensitivity to penicillamine or to any penicillin; history of penicillamine-related aplastic anemia or agranulocytosis; patients with rheumatoid arthritis who have renal insufficiency or who are pregnant, during pregnancy in patients with cystinuria; concomitant administration with drugs that can cause severe hematologic or renal reactions, e.g., antimalarials, gold salts, immunosuppressants, oxyphenbutazone, phenylbutazone. **Cautious use in:** allergy-prone individuals.

ADVERSE/SIDE EFFECTS Allergic: *generalized pruritus, urticaria, early and late occurring rashes,* pemphiguslike rash, fever, arthralgia, lymphadenopathy, thyroiditis, SLE-like syndrome. *GI: anorexia, nausea, vomiting,* epigastric pain, diarrhea, oral lesions, *reduction or loss of taste perception (particularly salt and sweet), metallic taste,* activation of peptic ulcer. **Hematologic:** thrombocytopenia, leukopenia,

P

Common side effects in *italic*; life-threatening effects underlined; generic names in **bold**; classifications in SMALL CAPS

861

agranulocytosis, thrombotic thrombocytopenic purpura, hemolytic anemia, aplastic anemia. **Hepatic:** cholestatic jaundice. **Renal:** membranous glomerulopathy, Goodpasture's syndrome, proteinuria, hematuria. **Other:** tinnitus, optic neuritis, thrombophlebitis, hyperpyrexia, alopecia, myasthenia gravis syndrome, mammary hyperplasia, alveolitis, skin friability, excessive skin wrinkling, pancreatitis, pyridoxine deficiency, tingling of feet, ptosis, weakness.

DRUG INTERACTIONS ANTIMALARIALS, CYTOTOXICS, **gold** therapy may potentiate hematologic and renal adverse effects; **iron** may decrease penicillamine absorption.

NURSING IMPLICATIONS

Administration
- Not to be confused with penicillin.
- Taken on an empty stomach (60 min before or 2 h after meals) to avoid absorption of metals in foods by penicillamine.
- If patient cannot swallow capsules or tablets, contents may be administered in 15–30 ml of chilled fruit juice.

Assessment & Drug Effects
- Penicillamine can produce severe toxic reactions involving skin, blood, kidneys, and liver.
- Allergic reactions occur in about one third of patients receiving penicillamine. Temporary interruptions of therapy increase possibility of sensitivity reactions.
- White and differential blood cell counts, direct platelet counts, hemoglobin, and urinalyses should be done prior to initiation of therapy and every 3 d during the first month of therapy, then every 2 wk thereafter. Liver function tests and eye examinations should be performed before start of therapy and at least twice yearly thereafter.
- Clinical evidence of therapeutic effectiveness may not be apparent until 1–3 mo of drug therapy.
- Therapeutic effectiveness in **Wilson's disease** is indicated by improvement in psychiatric and neurologic symptoms, visual symptoms, and hepatic function. In some patients, neurologic symptoms become more prominent during initial therapy and then subside.
- *Rheumatoid arthritis:* record evidence of drug effectiveness such as improvement in grip strength, decrease in stiffness following immobility, reduction of pain, decrease in sedimentation rate and rheumatoid factor.

- Dosage should be reduced or drug discontinued if the patient with rheumatoid arthritis develops proteinuria >1 g (some clinicians accept ≤2 g) or if platelet count drops to <100,000/mm^3, or platelet count falls 3500–4000/mm^3, or neutropenia occurs.

Patient & Family Education
- Temperature should be taken nightly during first few months of therapy. Fever is a possible early sign of allergy.
- Instruct patient to observe skin over pressure sites: knees, elbows, shoulder blades, toes, buttocks. Penicillamine increases skin friability. Report unusual bruising or bleeding, sore mouth or throat, fever, skin rash, or any other unusual symptoms.

Prototype: penicillin G potassium, p 71

PENICILLIN G BENZATHINE
(pen-i-sill´in)
Trade names: Bicillin, Bicillin L-A, Permapen
Classifications: ANTIINFECTIVE; BETA-LACTAM ANTIBIOTIC; NATURAL PENICILLIN
Pregnancy: Category B

ACTIONS/PHARMACODYNAMICS Acid-stable, penicillinase-sensitive, repository (long-acting) form of penicillin G. Because it has extremely low water solubility, it is absorbed slowly in body. Produces lower blood concentrations than other penicillin G compounds but has the longest duration of antimicrobial activity of all other available parenteral or repository penicillins. Has local anesthetic effect comparable to that of penicillin G procaine. Like penicillin G potassium in actions, uses, contraindications, precautions, and adverse reactions.

USES Infections highly susceptible to penicillin G, such as streptococcal, pneumococcal, and staphylococcal infections, venereal disease such as syphilis (including early, late, and congenital forms), and nonvenereal diseases, e.g., yaws, bejel, and pinta. Also used in prophylaxis of rheumatic fever.

PHARMACOKINETICS **Absorption:** slowly absorbed from IM site. **Peak:** 12–24 h. **Duration:** 26 d. **Distribution:** crosses placenta; distributed into breast milk. **Metabolism:** hydrolyzed to penicillin in body. **Elimination:** excreted slowly by kidneys.

ROUTE & DOSAGE

Mild to Moderate Infections

Adult	IM	1,200,000 U once/d
Child	IM	>27 kg: 900,000 U once/d
		<27 kg: 300,000–600,000 U once/d

Syphilis

Adult	IM	<1 y duration: 2,400,000 U as single dose
		>1 y duration: 2,400,000 U/wk for 3 wk
Child	IM	Congenital: 50,000 U/kg as single dose

Prophylaxis for Rheumatic Fever

Adult	IM	1,200,000 U q4wk
Child	IM	1,200,000 U q3–4wk

CONTRAINDICATIONS & PRECAUTIONS Contraindicated in: hypersensitivity to penicillins or cephalosporins; pregnancy (category C). **Cautious use in:** history of or suspected atopy or allergy (eczema, hives, hay fever, asthma).

ADVERSE/SIDE EFFECTS *Local pain,* tenderness, and fever associated with IM injection, Jarisch-Herxheimer reaction in patients with syphilis. **Hypersensitivity:** pruritus, urticaria and other skin eruptions, chills, fever, wheezing, anaphylaxis, eosinophilia, hemolytic anemia and other blood abnormalities, neuropathy, nephrotoxicity; myocarditis (rare), superinfections.

NURSING IMPLICATIONS

See penicillin G potassium for numerous additional nursing implications.

Administration

- Not to be confused with preparations containing procaine penicillin G (e.g., Bicillin C-R).
- IM injection should be made deep into upper outer quadrant of buttock. In infants and small children the preferred site is the midlateral aspect of the thigh.
- Shake multiple-dose vial vigorously before withdrawing desired IM dose. Shake prepared cartridge unit vigorously before injecting drug. Injection form is for IM use only.
- Select IM site with care. Injection into or near a major peripheral nerve can result in nerve damage. Inadvertent IV administration has resulted in arterial occlusion and cardiac arrest.
- Injections should be made at a slow steady rate to prevent needle blockage.
- Store at 15–30C (59–86F).

Assessment & Drug Effects

- Prior to initiation of drug therapy, determine history of hypersensitivity reactions to penicillins, cephalosporins, or other allergens.
- As with other penicillins, culture and sensitivity tests should be done prior to initiation of therapy and periodically thereafter.

Patient & Family Education

- Instruct patient to take medication around the clock, not to miss a dose, and to continue taking medication until it is all gone.
- Instruct patient to report immediately to physician the onset of an allergic reaction. There is great risk of severe and prolonged reactions because drug is absorbed so slowly.

PENICILLIN G POTASSIUM

See ANTIINFECTIVE, ANTIBIOTIC, NATURAL PENICILLIN prototype, p 71.

Prototype: penicillin G potassium, p 71

PENICILLIN G PROCAINE

Trade names: Ayercillin, Crysticillin A.S., Duracillin A.S., Procaine Benzylpenicillin, Pfizerpen-AS, Wycillin
Classifications: ANTIINFECTIVE; BETA-LACTAM ANTIBIOTIC; NATURAL PENICILLIN
Pregnancy: Category B

ACTIONS/PHARMACODYNAMICS Repository (long-acting) form of penicillin G. The procaine salt has low solubility and thus creates a tissue depot from which penicillin is slowly absorbed. Accordingly, the number of injections required to maintain effective blood levels is reduced. Also, procaine exerts a local anesthetic effect. Same actions and antibacterial activity as for penicillin G and is similarly inactivated by penicillinase and gastric acids. Onset of action is slower and produces lower serum concentrations than equivalent doses of penicillin G, but has longer duration of action. Prepared in aqueous suspension.

P

Common side effects in *italic*; life-threatening effects underlined; generic names in **bold**; classifications in SMALL CAPS

863

USES Moderately severe infections due to penicillin G–sensitive microorganisms that are susceptible to low but prolonged serum penicillin concentrations. Commonly, uncomplicated pneumococcal pneumonia, 1 d treatment of uncomplicated gonorrheal infections, and all stages of syphilis. May be used concomitantly with penicillin G or probenecid when more rapid action and higher blood levels are indicated.

ROUTE & DOSAGE

Moderate to Severe Infections

Adult	IM	600,000–1,200,000 U once/d
Child	IM	300,000 U once/d

Pneumococcal Pneumonia

Adult	IM	600,000 U q12h

Uncomplicated Gonorrhea

Adult	IM	4,800,000 U divided between 2 different injection sites at one visit preceded by 1 g of probenecid 30 min before injections

Syphilis

Adult	IM	Primary, secondary, latent: 600,000 U/d for 8 d
		Late latent, tertiary, neurosyphilis: 600,000 U/d for 10–15 d
Child	IM	500,000–1,000,000 U/m² once/d

PHARMACOKINETICS Absorption: slowly absorbed from IM site. **Peak:** 1–3 h. **Duration:** 15–20 h. **Distribution:** crosses placenta; distributed into breast milk. **Metabolism:** hydrolyzed to penicillin in body. **Elimination:** excreted by kidneys within 24–36 h.

CONTRAINDICATIONS & PRECAUTIONS Contraindicated in: history of hypersensitivity to any of the penicillins, cephalosporins, or to procaine or any other "caine-type" local anesthetic; neonates. Pregnancy category B. **Cautious use in:** history of or suspected atopy or allergy.

ADVERSE/SIDE EFFECTS Hypersensitivity: *Procaine toxicity:* mental disturbances (anxiety, confusion, depression, combativeness, hallucinations), expressed fear of impending death, weakness, dizziness, headache, tinnitus, unusual tastes, palpitation, changes in pulse rate and BP, seizures.

NURSING IMPLICATIONS

Administration

- Note expiration date. Multiple-dose vial should be shaken thoroughly before withdrawing medication to ensure uniform suspension of drug.
- Administer IM deeply into upper outer quadrant of gluteus muscle; in infants and small children midlateral aspect of thigh is generally preferred. Injections are almost painless because of local anesthetic action of procaine. Select IM site carefully. Accidental injection into or near major peripheral nerves and blood vessels can cause neurovascular damage. Subcutaneous or intraarterial injection is contraindicated.
- Aspirate carefully before injecting drug to avoid entry into a blood vessel. Inadvertent IV administration reportedly has resulted in pulmonary infarcts and death. Inject drug at a slow, but steady rate to prevent needle blockage. Rotate injection sites.
- Note manufacturer's directions for storage. Generally, penicillin G procaine aqueous suspension (A.S.) is stored in refrigerator. Avoid freezing.

Assessment & Drug Effects

- Before treatment is initiated, an exact history should be obtained of patient's previous exposure and sensitivity to penicillins, cephalosporins, and to procaine, and other allergic reactions of any kind.
- If sensitivity is suspected, physician may test patient by injecting 0.1 ml of 1–2% procaine hydrochloride intradermally. The appearance of a wheal, flare, or eruption indicates procaine sensitivity.
- Be alert to the possibility of a transient toxic reaction to procaine, particularly when large single doses are administered. The reaction manifested by mental disturbance and other symptoms (see adverse/side effects) occurs almost immediately and usually subsides after 15–30 min.
- Report onset of rash, pruritus, fever, chills or other symptoms of an allergic reaction to physician. Reactions may be difficult to treat because drug action is relatively prolonged.

Common side effects in *italic*; life-threatening effects <u>underlined</u>; generic names in **bold**; classifications in SMALL CAPS

Prototype: penicillin G potassium, p 71

PENICILLIN V

PENICILLIN V POTASSIUM

Trade names: Apo-Pen-VK, Beepen VK, Betapen-VK, Ledercillin VK, Nadopen-V, Novopen-VK, Penapar VK, Penicillin VK, Pen-V, Pen-Vee K, Robicillin VK, Uticillin VK, V-Cillin K, VC-K, Veetids

Classifications: ANTIINFECTIVE; BETA-LACTAM ANTIBIOTIC; NATURAL PENICILLIN

Pregnancy: Category B

ACTIONS/PHARMACODYNAMICS Acid-stable phenoxymethyl analog of penicillin G with which it shares actions; is bactericidal, and is inactivated by penicillinase. Less active than penicillin G against gonococci and other gram-negative microorganisms.

USES Mild to moderate infections caused by susceptible streptococci, pneumococci, and staphylococci. Also Vincent's infection and as prophylaxis in rheumatic fever.

ROUTE & DOSAGE

Mild to Moderate Infections

Adult	PO	125–500 mg q6h
Child	PO	<12 y: 15–50 mg/kg/d in 3–6 divided doses

Endocarditis Prophylaxis

Adult	PO	2 g 30–60 min before procedure; then 500 mg q6h for 8 doses
Child	PO	<30 kg: 1 g 30–60 min before procedure; then 250 mg q6h for 8 doses

PHARMACOKINETICS Absorption: 60–73% absorbed from GI tract. **Peak:** 30–60 min. **Duration:** 6 h. **Distribution:** highest levels in kidneys; crosses placenta; distributed into breast milk. **Elimination:** half-life: 30 min; excreted in urine.

CONTRAINDICATIONS & PRECAUTIONS Contraindicated in: hypersensitivity to any penicillin or cephalosporin. History of or suspected atopy or allergy (hay fever, asthma, hives, eczema). Pregnancy category B.

ADVERSE/SIDE EFFECTS Nausea, vomiting, *diarrhea,* epigastric distress; *hypersensitivity reactions:* flushing, pruritus, urticaria or other skin eruptions, eosinophilia, anaphylaxis; hemolytic anemia, leukopenia, thrombocytopenia, neuropathy, superinfections.

NURSING IMPLICATIONS

See penicillin G potassium for numerous additional nursing implications.

Administration

- Drug may be better absorbed and result in higher blood levels when taken after a meal than on an empty stomach.
- Following reconstitution, oral solution is stable for 14 d under refrigeration. Date and time of reconstitution and discard date should appear on container. Shake well before pouring.
- If oral liquid preparation is not dispensed with a specially marked measuring device, question pharmacist. The average household measure is not accurate enough for this formulation.

Assessment & Drug Effects

- Culture and sensitivity tests should be obtained before initiation of therapy and at regular intervals throughout therapy.
- Before therapy begins, careful inquiry should be made concerning hypersensitivity reactions to penicillins, cephalosporins, and other allergens.
- Patients receiving prolonged therapy should have evaluations of renal, hepatic, and hematologic systems at regular intervals.

Patient & Family Education

- Inform patient that to maintain a constant blood level, penicillin V should be given around the clock at specific intervals.
- Instruct patient not to miss any doses and to continue taking medication until it is all gone unless otherwise directed by the physician.
- As with other penicillin preparations, advise patient to withhold medication and to report promptly to physician the onset of hypersensitivity reactions and superinfections (see Signs & Symptoms, chap 3).

P

Common side effects in *italic*; life-threatening effects underlined; generic names in **bold**; classifications in SMALL CAPS

865

Prototype: nitroglycerin, p 149

PENTAERYTHRITOL TETRANITRATE
(pen-ta-er-ith´ri-tole)
Trade names: Duotrate, Naptrate, Pentol, Pentritol, Pentylan, Peritrate, P.E.T.N.
Classifications: CARDIOVASCULAR AGENT; NITRATE VASODILATOR
Pregnancy: Category C

ACTIONS/PHARMACODYNAMICS Nitric acid ester of a tetrahydric alcohol. Actions, contraindications, precautions, and adverse/side effects as for nitroglycerin. Slower acting than nitroglycerin but duration of action is longer. Not effective for control of acute attacks. Tolerance can occur, and cross tolerance with other nitrites and nitrates is possible.

USES Prophylactically for long-term management of angina pectoris.

ROUTE & DOSAGE

Angina

Adult　　PO　　10–20 mg t.i.d. or q.i.d. up to 40 mg q.i.d.; *or* 80 mg sustained release q12h

PHARMACOKINETICS Absorption: 50–60% absorbed from GI tract. **Onset:** 20–60 min. **Duration:** 4–5 h; up to 12 h with sustained release. **Metabolism:** metabolized in liver. **Elimination:** half-life: 10 min; excreted primarily in urine; small amounts in feces.

NURSING IMPLICATIONS

Administration
- Not to be used to relieve an acute episode of anginal pain.
- Administered at least 30 min before or 1 h after meals and at bedtime. Sustained-release forms also taken on an empty stomach (1 dose on arising and second dose 12 h later).
- Avoid sudden discontinuation of pentaerythritol therapy; coronary vasospasm may be induced.
- Protect drug from exposure to heat and moisture to prevent loss of potency. Store at 15–30C (59–86F).

Assessment & Drug Effects
- Orthostatic hypotension can be particularly dangerous for the elderly. Evaluate incidence; if troublesome, notify physician.

Patient & Family Education
- Advise patient to report onset of skin rash or persistent headaches to physician. Discontinuation of therapy may be required.
- Inform patient that alcohol may enhance drug hypotensive effect.
- Chronic administration may produce tolerance and may impair response to nitroglycerin or other concomitantly administered nitrites or nitrates. Advise patient to report signs of decreasing therapeutic effect.
- Caution patient not to engage in activities requiring mental alertness and skill until drug response has stabilized.
- In presence of high environmental temperature, heat prostration can occur with use of this drug, especially in the elderly.

PENTAMIDINE ISOETHIONATE
(pen-tam´i-deen)
Trade names: Nebupent, Pentam 300
Classifications: ANTIINFECTIVE; ANTIPROTOZOAL
Pregnancy: Category C

ACTIONS/PHARMACODYNAMICS Aromatic diamide antiprotozoal drug effective against the sporozoan parasite *Pneumocystis carinii*. Action mechanism is unclear, but drug appears to block parasite reproduction by interfering with nucleotide (DNA, RNA), phospholipid, and protein synthesis. This parasite rarely causes infection in the general population, but if the patient is immunocompromised (e.g., AIDS) carinii pneumocystosis can be fatal. Pentamidine also has trypanosomicidal and leishmonicidal activity, but required doses for these conditions are quite toxic.

USES *P. carinii* pneumonia (PCP). **Unlabeled uses:** African trypanosomiasis and visceral leishmoniasis. (Drug supply for the latter uses is through the Centers for Disease Control, Atlanta, Ga.)

ROUTE & DOSAGE

Treatment of *Pneumocystis carinii* Pneumonia

Adult　　IM/IV　　4 mg/kg once/d for 14–21 d; infuse IV over 60 min

Child　　IM/IV　　Same as for adult

Prophylaxis of *Pneumocystis carinii* Pneumonia

Adult　　Inhaled　　300 mg per nebulizer q4wk

Common side effects in *italic*; life-threatening effects underlined; generic names in **bold**; classifications in SMALL CAPS

P

PHARMACOKINETICS Absorption: readily absorbed after IM injection. **Distribution:** leaves bloodstream rapidly to bind extensively to body tissues. **Elimination:** 50–66% excreted in urine within 6 h; small amounts found in urine for as long as 6–8 wk.

CONTRAINDICATIONS & PRECAUTIONS Contraindicated in: safe use in pregnancy (category C) not established. **Cautious use in:** hypertension, hypotension; hyperglycemia; hypoglycemia; hypocalcemia; blood dyscrasias; hepatic or renal dysfunction; diabetes mellitus.

ADVERSE/SIDE EFFECTS CNS: confusion, hallucinations, neuralgia, dizziness, sweating. **CV:** <u>sudden, severe hypotension</u>, cardiac arrhythmias, ventricular tachycardia, phlebitis. **GI:** anorexia, nausea, vomiting, pancreatitis, unpleasant taste. **Hematologic:** leukopenia, thrombocytopenia, anemia. **Metabolic:** <u>hypoglycemia</u>, hypocalcemia, *hyperkalemia.* **Respiratory:** *cough, bronchospasm,* laryngitis, shortness of breath, chest pain, <u>pneumothorax</u>. **Other:** Stevens-Johnson syndrome, <u>acute renal failure</u>, facial flush (with IV injection), *local reactions at injection site.*

DRUG INTERACTIONS AMINOGLYCOSIDES, **amphotericin B, cyclosporine, vancomycin,** other NEPHROTOXIC DRUGS increase risk of nephrotoxicity.

NURSING IMPLICATIONS

Administration

- **Preparation of pentamidine solution for administration: IM:** dissolve contents of 1 vial (300 mg) in 3 ml sterile water for injection. **IV:** dissolve contents of 1 vial in 3–5 ml sterile water for injection or 5% dextrose solution. Further dilute in 50–250 ml of D5W and infuse over 60 min.
- The IM injection is painful and frequently causes local reactions (pain, induration, swelling). Select alternate sites for daily doses and institute local treatment if indicated.
- IV solutions of 1.0–2.5 mg/ml prepared in 5% dextrose injection are stable at room temperature for up to 24 h. Dry product should be stored at 2–8C (35–46F). Protect solution and drug product from light. Discard unused portions.

Assessment & Drug Effects

- Severe sudden hypotension may develop after a single dose. The patient should be in a supine position while receiving the drug. Monitor BP continuously during the infusion, every half hour for 2 h thereafter, and then every 4 h until BP stabilizes.

- Renal, cardiac, and hepatic function may be changed by pentamidine. Monitor HR, blood glucose, and electrolyte balance.
- Measure and record I&O ratio and pattern and check patient's pulse (to detect arrhythmia) at least twice daily.
- Dosage adjustment is indicated in renal failure; therefore signs of impending dysfunction should be promptly reported (e.g., changed I&O ratio, oliguria, edema).
- Characteristics of pneumonia in the immunocompromised patient include constant fever, scanty (if any) sputum, dyspnea, tachypnea, and cyanosis.
- Fever is a constant symptom in *P. carinii* pneumonia, but it may be rapidly elevated (as high as 40C [104F]) shortly after drug infusion. Monitor temperature changes and institute measures to lower the temperature as indicated.

Patient & Family Education

- Advise patient to promptly report increasing respiratory difficulty.

Prototype: morphine, p 156

PENTAZOCINE HYDROCHLORIDE

(pen-taz´oh-seen)
Trade names: Talwin, Talwin NX
Classifications: CNS AGENT; ANTIPYRETIC; NARCOTIC (OPIATE) AGONIST-ANTAGONIST; ANALGESIC
Pregnancy: Category C
Controlled substance: Schedule IV

ACTIONS/PHARMACODYNAMICS Synthetic benzomorphan analgesic structurally related to phenazocine. On a weight basis, analgesic potency approximately one third that of morphine and somewhat greater than that of codeine. In general, adverse reactions are qualitatively similar to those of morphine. Unlike morphine, large doses may increase BP and heart rate. Also, acts as weak narcotic antagonist and has sedative properties.

USES Relief of moderate to severe pain; also used for preoperative analgesia or sedation, and as supplement to surgical anesthesia.

PHARMACOKINETICS Absorption: readily absorbed from GI tract; 20% reaches systemic circula-

P

Common side effects in *italic*; life-threatening effects <u>underlined</u>; generic names in **bold**; classifications in SMALL CAPS

867

ROUTE & DOSAGE

Moderate to Severe Pain (Excluding Patients in Labor)

Adult	PO	50–100 mg q3–4h (max 600 mg/d)
	IM/IV/SC	30 mg q3–4h (max 360 mg/d)

Women in Labor

Adult	IM	20–30 mg IM; 20 mg may be repeated 1 or 2 times at 2–3 h intervals

tion (first pass metabolism). **Onset:** 15–30 min PO, IM, SC; 2–3 min IV. **Peak:** 1–3 h PO, IM; 15 min IV. **Duration:** 3 h PO, IM; 1 h IV. **Distribution:** crosses placenta. **Metabolism:** extensively metabolized in liver. **Elimination:** half-life: 2–3 h; excreted primarily in urine; small amount in feces.

CONTRAINDICATIONS & PRECAUTIONS **Contraindicated in:** head injury, increased intracranial pressure; emotionally unstable patients, or history of drug abuse. Safe use during pregnancy (other than labor) (category B) and in children <12 y not established. **Cautious use in:** impaired renal or hepatic function; respiratory depression; biliary surgery; patients with MI who have nausea and vomiting.

ADVERSE/SIDE EFFECTS *Drowsiness,* sweating, flushing, *dizziness, lightheadedness, euphoria, nausea, vomiting,* constipation (infrequent), dry mouth, alterations of taste, urinary retention, visual disturbances, allergic reactions, injection-site reactions (induration, nodule formation, sloughing, sclerosis, cutaneous depression), rash, pruritus. **High doses:** <u>respiratory depression</u>, hypertension, palpitation, tachycardia, <u>shock</u>, psychotomimetic effects, confusion, anxiety, hallucinations, disturbed dreams, bizarre thoughts, euphoria and other mood alterations.

DRUG INTERACTIONS **Alcohol** and other CNS DEPRESSANTS add to CNS depression; NARCOTIC ANALGESICS may precipitate narcotic withdrawal syndrome.

INCOMPATIBILITIES **Solution/Additive: aminophylline,** BARBITURATES, **sodium bicarbonate, glycopyrrolate, heparin, nafcillin. Y-Site: glycopyrrolate, heparin, nafcillin.**

NURSING IMPLICATIONS

Administration

- Talwin-Nx (oral) is a combination of pentazocine and naloxone (Nx). The Nx stands for naloxone, which is added to prevent the effect of pentazocine if the oral product is misused by using it for injection.
- IM administration is preferable to SC route when frequent injections over an extended period are required. Rotation of injection sites are recommended. Observe injection sites daily for signs of irritation or inflammation.
- IV pentazocine may be given by direct IV undiluted or diluted with 1 ml sterile water for injection for each 5 mg. Give slowly at a rate of 5 mg over 60 seconds.
- Do not mix pentazocine in same syringe with soluble barbiturates, because precipitation will occur.
- Preserve in tight, light-resistant containers. Store at 15–30C (59–86F).

Assessment & Drug Effects

- Tolerance to analgesic effect sometimes occurs. Psychologic and physical dependence have been reported in patients with history of drug abuse, but rarely in patients without such history. Addiction liability matches that of codeine.
- Pentazocine may produce acute withdrawal symptoms in some patients who have been receiving opioids on a regular basis.

Patient & Family Education

- Caution ambulatory patients to avoid potentially hazardous activities such as driving a car or operating machinery until response to drug is known.
- Abrupt discontinuation of drug following extended use may result in chills, abdominal and muscle cramps, yawning, rhinorrhea, lacrimation, itching, restlessness, anxiety, drug-seeking behavior.

Prototype: secobarbital, p 175

PENTOBARBITAL
(pen-toe-bar´bi-tal)
Trade name: Nembutal

PENTOBARBITAL SODIUM

Trade names: Mase-Pent, Nembutal Sodium, Novopentobarb
Classifications: CNS AGENT; ANXIOLYTIC; BARBITURATE SEDATIVE-HYPNOTIC
Pregnancy: Category D
Controlled substance: Schedule II

P

ACTIONS/PHARMACODYNAMICS Short-acting barbiturate with actions, contraindications, precautions, and adverse reactions as for other barbiturates. Potent respiratory depressant.

USES Sedative or hypnotic for preanesthetic medication, induction of general anesthesia, adjunct in manipulative or diagnostic procedures, and emergency control of acute convulsions.

ROUTE & DOSAGE

Sedative

Adult	PO	20–30 mg b.i.d. to q.i.d.
Child	PO	2–6 mg/kg/d in 3 divided doses (max 100 mg/d)

Preoperative Sedation

Adult	PO	150–200 mg in 2 divided doses
	IM	150–200 mg in 2 divided doses
	IV	100 mg; may increase to 500 mg if necessary

Hypnotic

Adult	PO	120–200 mg
	IM	150–200 mg
Child	PO	30–120 mg
	IM	2–6 mg/kg (max 100 mg)

PHARMACOKINETICS Onset: 15–30 min PO; 10–15 min IM; 1 min IV. **Duration:** 1–4 h PO; 15 min IV. **Distribution:** crosses placenta. **Metabolism:** metabolized primarily in liver. **Elimination:** half-life: 4–50 h; excreted in urine.

CONTRAINDICATIONS & PRECAUTIONS Contraindicated in: pregnancy (category D). See secobarbital.

ADVERSE/SIDE EFFECTS With rapid IV: <u>respiratory depression</u>, <u>laryngospasm</u>, bronchospasm, <u>apnea</u>, hypotension. Also see secobarbital.

DRUG INTERACTIONS Phenmetrazine antagonizes effects of pentobarbital; CNS DEPRESSANTS, **alcohol,** SEDATIVES add to CNS depression; MAO INHIBITORS cause excessive CNS depression; **methoxyflurane** creates risk of nephrotoxicity.

INCOMPATIBILITIES Solution/additive: chlorpheniramine, codeine, ephedrine, hydrocortisone, hydroxyzine, insulin, levorphanol, methadone, norepinephrine, TETRACYCLINES, **penicillin G, pentazocine, phenytoin, promazine,** promethazine, sodium bicarbonate, streptomycin, succinylcholine, triflubromazine, vancomycin, cimetidine, benzquinamide, butorphanol, chlorpromazine, dimenhydrinate, diphenhydramine, droperidol, fentanyl, glycopyrrolate, meperidine, midazolam, morphine, nalbuphine, perphenazine, prochlorperazine, ranitidine. **Y-site:** cimetidine, butorphanol, glycopyrrolate, midazolam, nalbuphine, perphenazine, ranitidine.

NURSING IMPLICATIONS

Administration

- Do not use parenteral solutions that appear cloudy or in which a precipitate has formed.
- IV route should be used only when other routes are not feasible. May be given by direct IV undiluted or diluted (preferred) with sterile water, D5W, NS, or other compatible IV solutions.
- IV administration should be slow; rate should not exceed 50 mg/min.
- Parenteral solution is highly alkaline. Extreme care should be taken to avoid extravasation and intraarterial injection. Necrosis may result.
- IM injections should be made deep into large muscle mass, preferably upper outer quadrant of buttock. Aspirate needle carefully before injecting it to prevent inadvertent entry into blood vessel. No more than 5 ml (250 mg) should be injected in any one site because of possible tissue irritation.

Assessment & Drug Effects

- During IV administration monitor BP, pulse, and respiration q3–5min. Observe patient closely; maintain airway. Equipment for artificial respiration should be immediately available.
- After IM administration of hypnotic dose, observe patient closely for adverse effects for at least 30 min.

Patient & Family Education

- Caution ambulatory patients against operating a motor vehicle or machinery for the remainder of day after taking drug.

PENTOXIFYLLINE

(pen-tox-i´fi-leen)
Trade name: Trental
Classifications: HEMORHEOLOGIC AGENT; ANTIPLATELET AGENT
Pregnancy: Category C

P

Common side effects in *italic*; life-threatening effects <u>underlined</u>; generic names in **bold**; classifications in SMALL CAPS

869

ACTIONS/PHARMACODYNAMICS A methylxanthine with hemorheologic properties. Useful in restoration of blood flow through nutritive capillary microcirculation that has been compromised by structural and flow dynamic changes in cerebral and peripheral vascular disorders. Action mechanism is not clear but pentoxifylline administration is followed by decreased blood viscosity and improved blood flow, with consequent reduction of tissue hypoxia. *Specific effects:* (1) increased deformability (flexibility) of RBC, thereby easing their passage through microcirculatory capillaries; (2) decreased RBC hyperaggregation; (3) decreased synthesis of thromboxane A_2, leading to reduced platelet aggregation (antiplatelet action); (4) increased cell membrane permeability, which promotes nutrient exchange at tissue level; and (5) increased blood fibrinolytic activity (watchdog property that prevents intravascular coagulation). Drug action (appears to be unrelated to vasodilation) interrupts the vicious cycle of tissue hypoxia, sludging and stasis of capillary blood flow, microthrombotic activity, reduced oxygen delivery to ischemic cells. With increased blood flow to the extremities, the limiting pain and paresthesia of intermittent claudication is reduced; further, psychopathologic conditions associated with cerebral hypoxia are improved.

USES Intermittent claudication associated with occlusive peripheral vascular disease; diabetic angiopathies. **Unlabeled uses:** to improve psychopathologic symptoms in patient with cerebrovascular insufficiency and to reduce incidence of stroke in the patient with recurrent TIAs.

ROUTE & DOSAGE

Intermittent Claudication

Adult   PO   400 mg t.i.d. with meals

PHARMACOKINETICS Absorption: readily absorbed from GI tract; 10–50% reaches systemic circulation (first pass metabolism). **Peak:** 2–4 h. **Distribution:** distributed into breast milk. **Metabolism:** metabolized in liver and erythrocytes. **Elimination:** half-life: 0.4–0.8 h; excreted primarily in urine.

CONTRAINDICATIONS & PRECAUTIONS Contraindicated in: intolerance to pentoxifylline or to methylxanthines (caffeine and theophylline). Safe use in pregnancy (category C), in nursing mothers, or in children <18 y not established. **Cautious use in:** angina, hypotension, arrhythmias, cerebrovascular disease.

ADVERSE/SIDE EFFECTS CNS: agitation, nervousness, *dizziness,* drowsiness, headache, insomnia, tremor, confusion. **CV:** angina, chest pain, dyspnea, arrhythmias, palpitations, hypotension, edema, flushing. **Eye:** blurred vision, conjunctivitis, scotomas. **GI:** abdominal discomfort, belching, flatus, bloating, diarrhea, *dyspepsia, nausea, vomiting.* **Skin:** brittle fingernails, pruritus, rash, urticaria. **Other:** earache, unpleasant taste, excessive salivation, leukopenia, malaise, sore throat, swollen neck glands, weight change. (Rare, causal relationship unknown): arrhythmia, tachycardia, hepatitis, jaundice, decreased serum fibrinogen, pancytopenia, purpura, thrombocytopenia. **Overdosage:** fever, flushing, hypotension, convulsions, somnolence, loss of consciousness.

NURSING IMPLICATIONS

Administration

- When pentoxifylline is given with food, absorption is delayed, but total amount absorbed is not affected; serum levels are lowered, however. May be taken on an empty stomach or with food; be consistent with time of day and relationship to food in establishing the daily regimen.
- Store tablets at 15–30C (59–86F).

Assessment & Drug Effects

- Therapeutic effects may be evident within 2–4 wk, but treatment is continued at least 8 wk before therapeutic failure is admitted.
- Successful treatment provides relief from pain and cramping in calf muscles, buttocks, thighs, and feet during exercise and improves walking performance (time and duration).
- If patient is also on antihypertensive treatment, monitor BP. Pentoxifylline may slightly decrease an already stabilized BP, necessitating a reduced dose of the hypotensive drug.

Patient & Family Education

- Before patient reestablishes walking as exercise, the patient should be checked by the physician to determine CV status and capacity.
- Advise patient to pay particular attention to care of the feet because of arterial insufficiency (diminished perfusion to feet).
- Bleeding and prolonged prothrombin time in patient treated with pentoxifylline have been reported. Advise patient to report promptly unexplained bleeding, easy bruising, epistaxis, petechiae.
- Because of potential side effects (i.e., somnolence, blurred vision, dizziness) advise patient to avoid

Common side effects in *italic*; life-threatening effects underlined; generic names in **bold**; classifications in SMALL CAPS

driving or working with dangerous machinery until drug response has stabilized.

PERMETHRIN

See SKIN & MUCOUS MEMBRANE AGENT, PEDICULICIDE prototype, p 260.

Prototype: chlorpromazine, p 191

PERPHENAZINE

(per-fen´a-zeen)
Trade names: Phenazine, Trilafon
Classifications: CNS AGENT; PSYCHOTHERAPEU-TIC; PHENOTHIAZINE ANTIPSYCHOTIC (TRANQUIL-IZER), ANTIEMETIC

ACTIONS/PHARMACODYNAMICS Piperazine phenothiazine similar to chlorpromazine. Affects all parts of CNS, particularly the hypothalamus. Antipsychotic effect: antagonizes the neurotransmitter dopamine by action on dopaminergic receptors in brain. Antiemetic action results from direct blockade of dopamine in the chemoreceptor trigger zone (CTZ) in the medulla. Produces less sedation and hypotension, greater antiemetic effects, higher incidence of extrapyramidal effects, and lower levels of anticholinergic side effects than chlorpromazine.

USES Psychotic disorders, symptomatic control of severe nausea and vomiting, acute conditions such as violent retching during surgery, and intractable hiccups.

PHARMACOKINETICS Absorption: poorly absorbed from GI tract; 20% reaches systemic circulation. **Onset:** 10 min IM. **Peak:** 1–2 h IM; 4–8 h PO. **Duration:** 6–12 h. **Distribution:** crosses placenta. **Metabolism:** metabolized in liver with some metabolism in GI tract. **Elimination:** half-life: 9.5 h; excreted in urine and feces.

CONTRAINDICATIONS & PRECAUTIONS Contraindicated in: hypersensitivity to perphenazine and other phenothiazines; preexisting liver damage, suspected or established subcortical brain damage, comatose states; bone marrow depression. Safe use

ROUTE & DOSAGE

Psychotic Disorders

Adult	PO	4–16 mg b.i.d. to q.i.d.
		8–32 mg sustained release b.i.d. (max 64 mg/d)
	IM	5 mg q6h (max 15–30 mg/d)
	IV	Dilute to 0.5 mg/ml in NS; administer at not more than 1 mg q1–2min or 5 mg by slow infusion
Child	PO	4 mg b.i.d. to q.i.d.
		8 mg sustained release b.i.d. (max 16 mg/d)
	IM	Same as for adult
	IV	Same as for adult

Nausea

Adult	PO	8–16 mg b.i.d. to q.i.d.
	IM	5 mg q6h (max 15 mg/d)

---

during pregnancy, in nursing mothers, and in children <12 y not established. **Cautious use in:** previously diagnosed breast cancer; hepatic or renal dysfunction, cardiovascular disorders, alcohol withdrawal, epilepsy, psychic depression, patients with suicidal tendency, glaucoma, history of intestinal or GU obstruction, geriatric or debilitated patients, patients who will be exposed to extremes of heat or cold, or to phosphorous insecticides.

ADVERSE/SIDE EFFECTS CNS: *extrapyramidal effects (dystonic reactions, akathisia, parkinsonian syndrome, tardive dyskinesia), sedation,* convulsions. **CV:** *orthostatic hypotension,* tachycardia, bradycardia. **Eye:** mydriasis, blurred vision, corneal and lenticular deposits. **GI:** constipation, *dry mouth,* increased appetite, adynamic ileus. **GU:** *urinary retention,* gynecomastia, menstrual irregularities, inhibited ejaculation. **Hematologic:** <u>agranulocytosis</u>, thrombocytopenic purpura, <u>aplastic</u> or hemolytic <u>anemia</u>. **Hepatic:** abnormal liver function tests, cholestatic jaundice. **Hypersensitivity:** photosensitivity, itching, erythema, urticaria, angioneurotic edema, drug fever, <u>anaphylactoid reaction</u>. **Local:** pain at injection site, sterile abscess. **Other:** nasal congestion, decreased sweating, hyperprolactinemia, galactorrhea, weight gain.

DIAGNOSTIC TEST INTERFERENCES Perphenazine may cause falsely abnormal *thyroid function* tests because of elevations of thyroid globulin.

P

Common side effects in *italic*; life-threatening effects <u>underlined</u>; generic names in **bold**; classifications in SMALL CAPS

871

DRUG INTERACTIONS Alcohol and other CNS DEPRESSANTS enhance CNS depression; ANTACIDS, ANTIDIARRHEALS may decrease absorption of phenothiazines; ANTICHOLINERGIC AGENTS add to anticholinergic effects including fecal impaction and paralytic ileus; BARBITURATES, ANESTHETICS increase hypotension and excitation.

INCOMPATIBILITIES Solution/additive: midazolam, pentobarbital, thiethylperazine. Y-site: cefoperazone, midazolam, pentobarbital.

NURSING IMPLICATIONS

Administration

- Extended release tablet (not recommended for children) should be swallowed whole.
- Perphenazine oral concentrate is intended for hospital use only. Before administration, each 5 ml (16 mg) must be diluted with 60 ml water, milk, saline solution, 7-Up or other compatible carbonated beverages. Do not use liquids that cause color changes or precipitate.
- Administer IM injection deep into upper quadrant of the buttock, with patient in recumbent position. Advise patient to continue lying down for at least 1 h after injection. Monitor BP and pulse. Injection may be painful. Rotate injection sites; and observe daily for signs of inflammation. Usually patient can be transferred to the oral therapy (at equal or higher doses) within 24–48 h.
- IV perphenazine is given by direct IV, with each 5 mg diluted in 9 ml NS, at a rate of 0.5 mg (1 ml) over 60 seconds.
- Avoid skin contact with liquid forms of perphenazine. Contact dermatitis has been reported.
- Protect solutions from light. Do not use precipitated or darkened parenteral solution; however, slight yellowing does not alter potency or therapeutic effects.
- Store at 15–30C (59–86F) in tightly covered, light-resistant container unless otherwise specified. Protect from freezing.

Assessment & Drug Effects

- Establish baseline BP before initiation of drug therapy and check it at regular intervals, especially during early therapy.
- BP and pulse should be monitored continuously during IV administration. Keep patient supine until assured that vital signs are stable. Elderly patients in particular should be observed carefully for hypotension and extrapyramidal reactions. Have immediately available: norepinephrine (Levophed)

(epinephrine is contraindicated) and drugs for controlling extrapyramidal reactions: benztropine mesylate (Cogentin), and diphenhydramine.

- A high incidence of extrapyramidal effects accompanies use of perphenazine, particularly with high doses and parenteral administration. Report restlessness, weakness of extremities, dystonic reactions (spasms of neck and shoulder muscles, rigidity of back, difficulty swallowing or talking); motor restlessness (akathisia): inability to be still; and parkinsonian syndrome: tremors, shuffling gait, drooling (hypersalivation), slow speech.
- Patients on long-term therapy are at high risk of developing *irreversible tardive dyskinesia:* fine, worm-like (vermicular) movements or rapid protrusions of the tongue, chewing motions, lip smacking. Withhold medication and report immediately to physician. Patients (if competent) and responsible family members should be informed about tardive dyskinesia. Early reporting is essential.
- Differential blood cell counts and hepatic, and renal function studies, ECG, and ophthalmologic examination should be done before initiation of therapy and periodically during therapy.
- If jaundice appears between weeks 2 and 4, suspect hypersensitivity, withhold drug, and report to physician.
- Monitor I&O ratio and bowel elimination pattern.
- Be alert to the patient's altered tolerance to environmental temperature changes. Be cautious with external heat devices. Conditioned avoidance behavior may be depressed, and a severe burn could result.
- Antiemetic effect of this drug may obscure signs of toxicity due to overdosage of other drugs or make it more difficult to diagnose conditions with nausea as a primary symptom.

Patient & Family Education

- Caution patient to make all position changes slowly and in stages, particularly from recumbent to upright posture, and to lie down or sit down if lightheadedness or dizziness occurs.
- Caution patient to avoid potentially hazardous activities such as driving a car or operating machinery until reaction to drug is known. Perphenazine may produce hypotension (dizziness, lightheadedness), and sedation especially during early therapy.
- Photosensitivity results in skin color changes from brown to blue-gray. Caution patient to avoid long exposure to sunlight and to sunlamps.
- Review dosage regimen with patient. Advise strict adherence to it and to consult physician before changing it for any reason.
- Discontinuation of perphenazine following pro-

Common side effects in *italic*; life-threatening effects <u>underlined</u>; generic names in **bold**; classifications in SMALL CAPS

longed therapy should be accomplished gradually over a period of several weeks.

- Caution patient to avoid OTC drugs unless physician prescribes them.
- Perphenazine may discolor urine reddish brown.

Prototype: phenytoin, p 172

PHENACEMIDE
(fe-nass´e-mide)
Trade name: Phenurone
Classifications: CNS AGENT; HYDANTOIN ANTICONVULSANT
Pregnancy: Category D

ACTIONS/PHARMACODYNAMICS Potent structural analog of the hydantoins. Prevents or modifies seizure by elevating threshold for minimal convulsive activity. Found to be equal to or more effective than other antiseizure agents, but high toxicity potential removes it from first choice category.

USES Alone or with other anticonvulsants to treat severe epileptic states, especially mixed forms of psychomotor seizures refractory to other drugs.

ROUTE & DOSAGE

Seizures

Adult	PO	250–500 mg t.i.d.; may increase by 500 mg/d q1–3wk up to 1.5–5 g/d
Child	PO	5–10 y: 125–250 mg t.i.d.; may increase by 250 mg/d q1–3wk up to 750 mg–2.5 g/d

PHARMACOKINETICS Absorption: readily absorbed from GI tract. **Duration:** 5 h. **Metabolism:** metabolized in liver. **Elimination:** excreted in urine.

CONTRAINDICATIONS & PRECAUTIONS Contraindicated in: safe use during pregnancy (category D) or in nursing women not established; severe personality disorders. **Cautious use in:** liver impairment; allergies; concomitant use with another anticonvulsant.

ADVERSE/SIDE EFFECTS CNS: headache, drowsiness, insomnia, dizziness, paresthesias, personality changes, suicidal tendencies, toxic psychoses. **GI:** nausea, anorexia, weight loss, hepatitis. **Hematologic:** leukopenia, aplastic anemia, agranulocytosis.

Other: skin rash; nephritis with marked albuminuria, drowsiness, ataxia, hepatitis, and coma.

NURSING IMPLICATIONS

Administration
- Administration of drug with food may minimize GI side effects.

Assessment & Drug Effects
- Complete blood counts, liver function tests, and urine tests should be performed before and at monthly intervals during therapy. If no abnormalities appear after 12 mo, intervals may be widened.

Patient & Family Education
- Patient and responsible family members should be advised of need for close medical supervision because drug has high potential for serious toxicity.
- Personality changes, including attempts at suicide, are possible drug effects. Instruct patient and family to report changes in behavior (e.g., depression, apathy, aggressiveness, paranoia, and severe headaches).
- Advise patient and family to report immediately the onset of fever, sore mouth or throat, and malaise, skin rash or other allergic manifestations, easy bruising or unexplained bleeding (symptoms of developing blood dyscrasia), or jaundice (see Signs & Symptoms, chap 3).
- Counsel patient to be cautious about driving or engaging in any activity requiring alertness until response to phenacemide is known.

PHENAZOPYRIDINE HYDROCHLORIDE
(fen-az-oh-peer´i-deen)
Trade names: Azo-Standard, Baridium, Di-Azo, Geridium, Phenazo, Phenazodine, Pyridiate, Pyridium, Pyronium, Urodine, Urogesic
Classification: URINARY TRACT ANALGESIC
Pregnancy: Category B

ACTIONS/PHARMACODYNAMICS Azo dye with local anesthetic action on urinary tract mucosa. Precise mechanism of action not known. Imparts little or no antibacterial activity.

USES Symptomatic relief of pain, burning, frequency, and urgency arising from irritation of urinary tract mucosa, as from infection, trauma, surgery, or instrumentation.

P

Common side effects in *italic*; life-threatening effects underlined; generic names in **bold**; classifications in SMALL CAPS

873

ROUTE & DOSAGE

Cystitis

Adult	PO	200 mg t.i.d.
Child	PO	12 mg/kg/d in 3 divided doses

PHARMACOKINETICS Absorption: readily absorbed from GI tract. **Distribution:** crosses placenta in trace amounts. **Metabolism:** metabolized in liver and other tissues. **Elimination:** primarily excreted in urine.

CONTRAINDICATIONS & PRECAUTIONS Contraindicated in: renal insufficiency, glomerulonephritis, pyelonephritis during pregnancy (category B), severe hepatitis. **Cautious use in:** GI disturbances; glucose-6-phosphate dehydrogenase deficiency.

ADVERSE/SIDE EFFECTS Infrequent: headache, vertigo, mild GI disturbances; in patients with impaired renal function or with high dosage or prolonged therapy: methemoglobinemia, hemolytic anemia, skin pigmentation, renal stones, transient acute renal failure.

DIAGNOSTIC TEST INTERFERENCES Phenazopyridine may interfere with any urinary test that is based on color reactions or spectrometry: ***bromsulphalein*** and ***phenolsulfonphthalein*** excretion tests; urinary ***glucose*** test using Clinistix or TesTape (copper-reduction methods such as Clinitest and Benedict's test reportedly not affected); ***bilirubin*** using "foam test" or Ictotest; ***ketones*** using nitroprusside (e.g., Acetest, Ketostix, or Gerhardt ferric chloride); urinary ***protein*** using Albustix, Albutest, or nitric acid ring test; urinary ***steroids; urobilinogen;*** assays for ***porphyrins.***

NURSING IMPLICATIONS

Administration

- Phenazopyridine should be taken after meals.

Assessment & Drug Effects

- Patients on prolonged therapy or with impaired renal function should have periodic blood work and renal function tests.

Patient & Family Education

- Inform patient that drug will impart an orange to red color to urine and may stain fabric.
- Appearance of yellowish tinge to skin or sclerae may indicate drug accumulation due to renal impairment. Advise patient to report immediately. Drug should be discontinued.

- Phenazopyridine should be discontinued when pain and discomfort are relieved (usually 3–15 d). Instruct patient to keep physician informed.

Prototype: amphetamine, p 194

PHENDIMETRAZINE TARTRATE

(fen-dye-me´tra-zeen)

Trade names: Adphen, Bacarate, Bontril PDM, Di-Ap-Trol, Limit, Melfiat, Metra, Obalan, Obeval, Obezine, PDM, Phenzine, Plegine, Sprx I, Statobex, Trimstat, Weightrol

Classifications: CNS AGENT; RESPIRATORY AND CEREBRAL STIMULANT; ANOREXIANT

Pregnancy: Category X

Controlled substance: Schedule III

ACTIONS/PHARMACODYNAMICS Sympathomimetic amine with actions similar to those of other amphetamine-like compounds.

USES Adjunct to control endogenous obesity.

ROUTE & DOSAGE

Obesity

Adult	PO	35 mg b.i.d. or t.i.d. 30–60 min a.c.; or 105 mg sustained release once/d mid-morning

PHARMACOKINETICS Absorption: readily absorbed from GI tract. **Duration:** 4 h regular tabs; 12 h sustained release. **Elimination:** excreted in urine.

CONTRAINDICATIONS & PRECAUTIONS Contraindicated in: hypersensitivity to sympathomimetic amines, pregnancy, children <12 y, severe coronary artery disease, moderate to severe hypertension, cardiac decompensation, hyperthyroidism, glaucoma, agitated persons, history of drug abuse, concomitant use with MAO inhibitors, CNS stimulants.

ADVERSE/SIDE EFFECTS *Nervousness, insomnia,* dizziness, mouth dryness, glossitis, stomatitis, nausea, mydriasis, blurring of vision, difficulty in starting urination, cystitis, constipation, abdominal cramps, palpitation, tachycardia, elevation of BP.

DRUG INTERACTIONS Acetazolamide, sodium bicarbonate decrease phendimetrazine elimination; **ammonium chloride, ascorbic acid** increase phendimetrazine elimination; effects of both

P

Common side effects in *italic*; life-threatening effects <u>underlined</u>; generic names in **bold**; classifications in SMALL CAPS

phendimetrazine and BARBITURATES may be antagonized; **furazolidone** may increase effects of amphetamines—interaction may persist for several weeks after discontinuation of furazolidone; antagonizes antihypertensive effects of **guanethidine, guanadryl;** do not administer amphetamines during or within 14 d of MAO INHIBITORS, **selegiline**—can cause hypertensive crisis (fatalities reported); may inhibit mood elevating effects of PHENOTHIAZINES; TRICYCLIC ANTIDEPRESSANTS enhance amphetamine effects because of increased norepinephrine release; BETA-AGONISTS increase adverse cardiovascular effects.

NURSING IMPLICATIONS

Administration

- Administer 1 h before meals. Sustained-release form is administered in the morning. Give last dose at least 6 h before patient retires to avoid insomnia.

Assessment & Drug Effects

- Monitor HR and BP periodically. Report tachycardia and hypertension promptly. Discontinuation or dosage adjustment may be indicated.

Patient & Family Education

- Psychogenic dependence is a possibility, as with all amphetamine-like compounds.
- Advise patient to avoid excessive use of CNS stimulants such as coffee, tea, colas.

PHENELZINE SULFATE

See CENTRAL NERVOUS SYSTEM AGENT, PSYCHOTHERAPEUTIC, MONOAMINE OXIDASE INHIBITOR ANTIDEPRESSANT, prototype, p 182.

Prototype: amphetamine, p 194

PHENMETRAZINE HYDROCHLORIDE

(fen-met´ra-zeen)

Trade name: Preludin

Classifications: CNS AGENT; RESPIRATORY AND CEREBRAL STIMULANT; AMPHETAMINE; ANOREXIANT

Pregnancy: Category C

Controlled substance: Schedule II

ACTIONS/PHARMACODYNAMICS Sympathomimetic agent chemically and pharmacologically related to amphetamine that reportedly produces less CNS stimulation.

USES Solely for short-term management of endogenous obesity.

ROUTE & DOSAGE

Obesity

Adult	PO	75 mg once/d midmorning

PHARMACOKINETICS Absorption: readily absorbed from GI tract. **Peak:** 5–12 h. **Duration:** 12 h. **Elimination:** excreted in urine.

CONTRAINDICATIONS & PRECAUTIONS Contraindicated in: history of hypersensitivity to sympathomimetic amines, hypertension, advanced arteriosclerosis, symptomatic cardiovascular disease; hyperthyroidism; glaucoma (narrow angle), hyperexcitable or psychotic states; concomitant use of CNS stimulants during or within 2 wk of MAO inhibitors. Safe use during pregnancy (category C) and in children <12 y not established.

ADVERSE/SIDE EFFECTS CNS: *nervousness, dizziness, insomnia,* headache. **CV:** palpitation, tachycardia, elevated BP. **ENT:** blurred vision, dry mouth. **GI:** nausea, abdominal cramps, constipation. **Other:** sweating, frequent urination, urticaria, changes in libido, impotence. Large doses for prolonged periods: marked insomnia, irritability, severe dermatoses, hyperactivity, severe mental depression, personality changes, psychosis.

DRUG INTERACTIONS Acetazolamide, sodium bicarbonate decrease phenmetrazine elimination, **ammonium chloride, ascorbic acid** increase phenmetrazine elimination; may antagonize the effects of both BARBITURATES and phenmetrazine; **furazolidone** may increase BP effects of amphetamines—interaction may persist for several weeks after discontinuation of furazolidone; antagonizes antihypertensive effects of **guanethidine, guanadryl;** MAO INHIBITORS **selegiline** can cause hypertensive crisis (fatalities reported)—do not administer amphetamines during or within 14 d of these drugs; PHENOTHIAZINES may inhibit mood elevating effects;

P

TRICYCLIC ANTIDEPRESSANTS enhance amphetamine effects because of increased norepinephrine release; BETA-AGONISTS increase adverse cardiovascular effects.

NURSING IMPLICATIONS

Administration

- Conventional tablet is administered at least 1 h before meals.
- Do not administer along with or within 14 d of MAO inhibitors. Hypertensive crisis may result.
- Sustained-release form may be taken in the morning; administration time should be determined by period of day anorexiant effect is needed (generally taken at least 12 h before bedtime). Advise patient to swallow tablet whole.

Assessment & Drug Effects

- BP checks before and periodically during treatment are advised.
- Sustained-release tablets contain tartrazine, which may cause allergic type reactions including bronchial asthma in susceptible individuals. This reaction is frequently seen in patients with aspirin hypersensitivity.

Patient & Family Education

- Advise patient against excessive use of CNS stimulants such as coffee, tea, and cola drinks.
- Since drug may cause blurred vision and dizziness, caution patient to avoid potentially hazardous activities such as driving a car or operating machinery until reaction to drug is known.
- Instruct patient to notify physician if nervousness, dizziness, or palpitation occur.
- Mouth dryness may be relieved by rinsing with warm water.
- As with other amphetamines, physical and psychic dependence and tolerance may develop with prolonged use.

PHENOBARBITAL

See CNS AGENT, BARBITURATE ANTICONVULSANT prototype, p 167.

Prototype: bisacodyl, p 221

PHENOLPHTHALEIN

(fee-nol-thay´leen)

Trade names: Alophen, Correctol, Espotabs, Evac-U-Gen, Evac-U-Lax, Ex-Lax, Feen-a-Mint, Lax-Pill, Modane, Phenolax, Prulet

Classifications: GI AGENT; STIMULANT LAXATIVE

Pregnancy: Category C

ACTIONS/PHARMACODYNAMICS Diphenylmethane laxative similar to bisacodyl in pharmacologic properties. Common ingredient in several OTC fixed combination laxative drugs. Used for temporary relief of simple constipation.

ROUTE & DOSAGE

Laxative

Adult	PO	30–200 mg as directed

PHARMACOKINETICS Absorption: up to 15% of dose absorbed from GI tract. **Onset:** 6–8 h. **Metabolism:** metabolized in liver with some enterohepatic cycling. **Elimination:** 85% excreted in feces, 15% in urine.

CONTRAINDICATIONS & PRECAUTIONS Contraindicated in: hypersensitivity to phenolphthalein; abdominal pain, nausea, vomiting; fecal impaction, intestinal obstruction, or perforation.

ADVERSE/SIDE EFFECTS Allergic reactions: skin eruptions, urticaria, Stevens-Johnson syndrome, SLE-like syndrome. **Large doses or chronic use:** electrolyte imbalance, impaired glucose tolerance from potassium loss.

DIAGNOSTIC TEST INTERFERENCES Phenolphthalein may interfere with *BSP excretion* test.

NURSING IMPLICATIONS

Patient & Family Education

- Usually administered at bedtime to produce effect the next morning (approximately 6–8 h later).
- Since drug enters enterohepatic circulation, inform patient that laxative effect may persist for several days.
- Advise patient to avoid prolonged or frequent use. Dependence on drug action, as well as electrolyte imbalance, can occur.

P

- Drug may impart reddish or purplish pink discoloration to alkaline urine or feces (made alkaline by soapsuds enema). Inform patient of this possibility.
- Instruct patient to discontinue drug immediately if skin rash appears.
- Skin lesions resulting from allergic reaction may persist for months or years and may leave residual pigmentation.

Prototype: prazosin, p 108

PHENOXYBENZAMINE HYDROCHLORIDE

(fen-ox-ee-ben´za-meen)
Trade name: Dibenzyline
Classifications: AUTONOMIC NERVOUS SYSTEM AGENT; ALPHA-ADRENERGIC ANTAGONIST (BLOCKING AGENT, SYMPATHOLYTIC); ANTIHYPERTENSIVE
Pregnancy: Category C

ACTIONS/PHARMACODYNAMICS Long-acting alpha-adrenergic blocking agent. Apparently produces noncompetitive blockade ("chemical sympathectomy") of alpha-adrenergic receptor sites at postganglionic synapse. Alpha receptor sites are thus unable to react to endogenous or exogenous sympathomimetic agents. Blocks excitatory (alpha) effects of epinephrine, including vasoconstriction, but does not affect adrenergic cardiac inhibitory (beta) actions. Produces dilatation of muscular, cutaneous, and pulmonary vascular systems but does not significantly alter cardiac output or renal, hepatic, and cerebral blood flow. Causes orthostatic hypotension in both normotensive and hypertensive patients and also blocks pupillary dilation and retraction of eyelids.

USES Management of pheochromocytoma. **Unlabeled uses:** to improve circulation in peripheral vasospastic conditions such as Raynaud's acrocyanosis and frostbite sequelae, for adjunctive treatment of shock, hypertensive crisis.

PHARMACOKINETICS Absorption: variably absorbed (approximately 30%) from GI tract. **Onset:** 2 h. **Peak:** 4–6 h. **Duration:** 3–4 d. **Distribution:** accumulates in adipose tissue. **Elimination:** half-life: 24 h; 80% excreted in urine and bile within 24 h.

CONTRAINDICATIONS & PRECAUTIONS Contraindicated in: instances when fall in BP would be dangerous; compensated congestive failure. **Cautious**

ROUTE & DOSAGE

Management of Pheochromocytoma

Adult	PO	5–10 mg b.i.d.; may increase by 10 mg/d at 4 d intervals to desired response (usual range 20–60 mg/d in 2–3 divided doses)
Child	PO	0.2 mg/kg/d in 1–2 divided doses; may increase by 0.2 mg/kg/d at 4 d intervals to desired response (usual range 0.4–1.2 mg/kg/d)

use in: marked cerebral or coronary arteriosclerosis, CHF; renal insufficiency; respiratory infections. Safe use during pregnancy (category C) not established.

ADVERSE/SIDE EFFECTS *Nasal congestion,* dry mouth, *miosis,* drooping of eyelids, *postural hypotension, tachycardia,* palpitation, *dizziness,* fainting, inhibition of ejaculation, drowsiness, sedation, tiredness, weakness, lethargy, confusion, headache, GI irritation, vomiting, <u>shock</u>, CNS stimulation (large doses), allergic contact dermatitis.

NURSING IMPLICATIONS

Administration

- Giving the drug with milk or in divided doses may reduce gastric irritation.
- Preserve in airtight containers protected from light.

Assessment & Drug Effects

- During period of dosage adjustment, monitor BP and note pulse quality, rate, and rhythm in recumbent and standing positions. (Hypotension and tachycardia are most likely to occur in standing position.) Patient should be closely observed for at least 4 d from one dosage increment to the next.
- Since phenoxybenzamine has cumulative action, onset of therapeutic effects may not occur until after 2 wk of therapy, and full therapeutic effects may not be apparent for several more weeks.
- Therapeutic effectiveness with pheochromocytoma is indicated by decreases in BP, pulse, and sweating. With peripheral vasospastic problems, observe for improvement in skin color, temperature, and quality of peripheral pulses, as well as less sensitivity to cold.

Patient & Family Education

- Instruct patient to make position changes slowly, particularly from recumbent to upright posture, and to dangle legs and exercise ankles and feet for a few minutes before standing.

P

Common side effects in *italic*; life-threatening effects <u>underlined</u>; generic names in **bold**; classifications in SMALL CAPS

877

- Inform patient that postural hypotension and palpitations usually disappear with continued therapy but that they may reappear under conditions that promote vasodilation, such as strenuous exercise or ingestion of a large meal or alcohol.
- Inform patient that miosis, nasal stuffiness, and inhibition of ejaculation generally decrease with continued therapy.
- Advise patient not to take OTC medications for coughs, colds, or allergy without approval of physician. (Many contain sympathomimetic agents that cause BP elevation.)

Prototype: ethosuximide, p 174

PHENSUXIMIDE
(fen-sux´i-mide)
Trade name: Milontin
Classifications: CNS AGENT; SUCCINIMIDE ANTICONVULSANT
Pregnancy: Category D

ACTIONS/PHARMACODYNAMICS Succinimide derivative reportedly less potent and less effective than other drugs of this class. Apparently depresses the motor cortex and elevates the threshold of CNS to seizure activity.

USES Management of petit mal epilepsy (absence seizures) and with other anticonvulsants when other forms of epilepsy coexist with petit mal.

ROUTE & DOSAGE

Absence Seizures

Adult	PO	0.5–1 g b.i.d. or t.i.d.
Child	PO	Same as for adult

PHARMACOKINETICS Absorption: readily absorbed from GI tract. **Peak:** 1–4 h. **Metabolism:** metabolized in liver. **Elimination:** half-life: 5–12 h; excreted slowly in urine; small amounts excreted in bile and feces.

CONTRAINDICATIONS & PRECAUTIONS Contraindicated in: intermittent porphyria; pregnancy (category D); hepatic or renal disease.

ADVERSE/SIDE EFFECTS *Drowsiness,* dizziness, ataxia, alopecia, muscle weakness, *anorexia, nau-*

sea, vomiting, flushing, periorbital edema, pruritus, skin rash, reversible nephropathy, granulocytopenia.

DRUG INTERACTIONS Carbamazepine decreases phensuximide levels; **isoniazid** significantly increases phensuximide levels; levels of both **phenobarbital** and phensuximide may be altered with increased seizure frequency.

NURSING IMPLICATIONS

Administration
- Shake oral suspension well before pouring to assure uniform dosage.
- Protect from light and heat and store at 15–30C (59–86F) unless otherwise advised.

Assessment & Drug Effects
- Monitor weight, especially in children, since anorexic effects of drug might cause weight loss.
- Periodic renal function and blood tests should be performed, especially with long-term therapy.

Patient & Family Education
- Advise patient to report onset of skin rash or other unusual symptoms to physician.
- Inform patient that phensuximide may color urine pink, red, or red brown.
- Concomitant use of OTC drugs must be discouraged unless the physician approves; loss of seizure control can be induced by ingredients in some popular OTC drugs.
- Caution against potentially hazardous tasks such as driving a car or operating machinery until response to drug is known.

Prototype: amphetamine, p 194

PHENTERMINE HYDROCHLORIDE
(fen´ter-meen)
Trade names: Adipex-P, Fastin, Ionamin, Obe-Nix, Obephen, Obermine, Obestin, Parmine, Phentrol, Tora, Unifast, Wilpowr
Classifications: CNS AGENT; RESPIRATORY AND CEREBRAL STIMULANT; ANOREXIANT; AMPHETAMINE
Pregnancy: Category C
Controlled substance: Schedule IV

ACTIONS/PHARMACODYNAMICS Sympathomimetic amine related chemically and pharmacolog-

P

Common side effects in *italic*; life-threatening effects underlined;
generic names in **bold**; classifications in SMALL CAPS

ically to amphetamine. Cardiovascular actions and CNS stimulant effects are less prominent than those of amphetamine. Available as the hydrochloride salt and as a complex with a cationic-exchange resin of sulfonated polystyrene. Resin complex reacts with cations in GI tract and is designed to give controlled release of drug over 10–14 hr period. Effects of conventional oral tablet (hydrochloride) persist about 4 h.

USES Short-term (a few weeks) adjunct in management of exogenous obesity.

ROUTE & DOSAGE

Obesity

Adult	PO	8 mg t.i.d. 30 min a.c. or 15–30 mg sustained once/d before breakfast

CONTRAINDICATIONS & PRECAUTIONS Contraindicated in: history of hypersensitivity to sympathomimetic amines; during or within 14 d of MAO inhibitor use; glaucoma; angina; children ≤ 12 y. Safe use during pregnancy (category C) not established. **Cautious use in:** advanced arteriosclerosis, symptomatic cardiovascular disease, moderate to severe hypertension; hyperthyroidism; glaucoma; agitated states; history of drug abuse.

ADVERSE/SIDE EFFECTS *Nervousness,* dizziness, *insomnia,* dry mouth, nausea, constipation, hypertension, palpitations, tachycardia, decreased sexual desire, impotence; severe dermatoses, marked insomnia, irritability, hyperactivity, psychoses. **Abrupt cessation following prolonged high dosage:** extreme fatigue, depression, changes in sleep EEG pattern.

DRUG INTERACTIONS Acetazolamide, sodium bicarbonate decrease phentermine elimination; **ammonium chloride, ascorbic acid** increase phentermine elimination; effects of both phentermine and barbiturates may be antagonized; **furazolidone** may increase BP effects of amphetamines—interaction may persist for several weeks after discontinuation of furazolidone; antagonizes antihypertensive effects of **guanethidine, guanadryl;** MAO INHIBITOR, **selegiline** can cause hypertensive crisis (fatalities reported)—do not administer amphetamines during or within 14 d of these drugs; PHENOTHIAZINES may inhibit mood elevating effects; TRICYCLIC ANTIDEPRESSANTS enhance amphetamine effects through increased norepinephrine release; BETA-AGONISTS increase adverse cardiovascular effects.

NURSING IMPLICATIONS

Administration

- Not to be confused with chlorphentermine, also an anorexiant, but given at much higher dosages.
- To prevent insomnia, late evening medication should be avoided.

Assessment & Drug Effects

- Tolerance to anorexigenic effect usually occurs within a few weeks. Drug should be discontinued when this occurs.
- Renal excretion is enhanced by urinary acidification; reabsorption and recycling are enhanced by alkaline urine.

Patient & Family Education

- Avoid caffeine drinks, which increase amphetamine-like and related amine effects.
- Instruct patient to notify physician if palpitations, nervousness, or dizziness occur.
- Caution patient to avoid potentially hazardous activities such as driving a car or operating machinery until response to the drug is known.

Prototype: prazosin, p 108

PHENTOLAMINE MESYLATE

(fen-tole´a-meen)
Trade names: Regitine, Rogitine
Classifications: AUTONOMIC NERVOUS SYSTEM AGENT; ALPHA-ADRENERGIC ANTAGONIST (BLOCKING AGENT, SYMPATHOLYTIC); ANTIHYPERTENSIVE
Pregnancy: Category C

ACTIONS/PHARMACODYNAMICS Imidazoline alpha-adrenergic blocking agent structurally related to tolazoline but with more potent blocking effects. Competitively blocks alpha-adrenergic receptors, but action is transient and incomplete. Prevents hypertension resulting from elevated levels of circulating epinephrine or norepinephrine. Causes vasodilation and decreases general vascular resistance and pulmonary arterial pressure, primarily by direct action on vascular smooth muscle. Through stimulation of beta-adrenergic receptors, produces positive inotropic and chronotropic cardiac effects and increases cardiac output. Also has histaminelike action that stimulates gastric secretions.

P

Common side effects in *italic;* life-threatening effects <u>underlined;</u> generic names in **bold**; classifications in SMALL CAPS

879

USES Diagnosis of pheochromocytoma and to prevent or control hypertensive episodes prior to or during pheochromocytomectomy. **Unlabeled use:** prevention of dermal necrosis and sloughing following IV administration or extravasation of norepinephrine.

ROUTE & DOSAGE

To Prevent Hypertensive Episode During Surgery

Adult	IV/IM	2–5 mg as needed
Child	IV/IM	1 mg or 0.1 mg/kg

To Test for Pheochromocytoma

Adult	IV/IM	5 mg
Child	IV/IM	0.1 mg/kg

To Prevent Necrosis from Norepinephrine Infusions

Adult	IV	10 mg added to each liter of IV fluid containing norepinephrine

To Treat Catecholamine Extravasation

Adult	Intradermal	5–10 mg diluted in 10 ml of normal saline injected into affected area within 12 h of extravasation

PHARMACOKINETICS Peak: 2 min IV; 15–20 min IM. **Duration:** 10–15 min IV; 3–4 h IM. **Elimination:** half-life: 19 min; excreted in urine.

CONTRAINDICATIONS & PRECAUTIONS Contraindicated in: MI (previous or present), coronary artery disease. Safe use during pregnancy (category C) and in nursing mothers and lactation not established. **Cautious use in:** gastritis, peptic ulcer.

ADVERSE/SIDE EFFECTS Weakness, dizziness, flushing, *orthostatic hypotension,* nasal stuffiness, conjunctival infection. **GI:** *abdominal pain, nausea, vomiting, diarrhea, exacerbation of peptic ulcer.* With parenteral administration especially, *acute and prolonged hypotension, tachycardia, anginal pain,* cardiac arrhythmias, MI, cerebrovascular spasm, shocklike state.

NURSING IMPLICATIONS

Administration

- Reconstitute 5 mg vial with 1 ml of sterile water for injection. May be further diluted with up to 10 ml of sterile water and given by direct IV over 60 seconds. Manufacturer recommends that reconstituted solutions be used immediately.

- Patient should be in supine position when receiving drug parenterally. Monitor BP and pulse q2min until stabilized.
- Store in tight, light-resistant containers at 15–30C (59–86F).

Assessment & Drug Effects

- **Test for pheochromocytoma:** (1) Medications not deemed absolutely essential should be withheld at least 24 h, preferably 48–72 h; antihypertensive agents withheld until BP returns to pretreatment level (rauwolfia drugs withdrawn at least 4 wk prior to testing). (2) Keep patient at rest in supine position throughout test, preferably in quiet darkened room. (3) Take BP q10min for at least 30 min; when BP stabilizes, injection should be administered by physician. (4) **IV administration:** record BP immediately after injection and at 30-second intervals for first 3 min; then at 1 min intervals for next 7 min. **IM administration:** BP determinations at 5 min intervals for 30–45 min.
- **Test results:** Positive response (indicated by drop in systolic pressure of at least 35 mm Hg and 25 mm Hg diastolic) suggests pheochromocytoma. Presumptive negative response: BP is unchanged, elevated, or reduced less than 35 mm Hg systolic and 25 mm Hg diastolic.

Patient & Family Education

- Advise patient to avoid sudden changes in position, particularly from recumbent to upright posture and to dangle legs and exercise ankles and toes for a few minutes before ambulating.
- Instruct patient to lie down or sit down in head-low position immediately if he or she feels lightheaded or dizzy.

Prototype: ibuprofen, p 160

PHENYLBUTAZONE

(fen-ill-byoo´ta-zone)
Trade names: Azolid, Butazolidin
Classifications: CNS AGENT; ANALGESIC; ANTIPYRETIC; NSAID
Pregnancy: Category D

ACTIONS/PHARMACODYNAMICS Pyrazolone derivative with antiinflammatory, antipyretic, analgesic, and mild uricosuric properties. Specific antiinflammatory action mechanism unknown but appears

P

to be associated with prostaglandin synthesis, leukocyte migration, and release or activity of lysosomal enzymes. Inhibits platelet aggregation. Does not cure inflammatory condition but produces effective short-term symptomatic relief of pain and disability. Should not be used as a general analgesic or antipyretic.

USES Short-term treatment of acute gouty arthritis, active rheumatoid arthritis and ankylosing spondylitis, and acute attacks of degenerative joint disease of hips and knees.

ROUTE & DOSAGE

Rheumatoid Arthritis, Ankylosing Spondylitis, Osteoarthritis

Adult PO 300–600 mg/d in 3–4 divided doses

Acute Gouty Arthritis

Adult PO 400 mg initially; then 100 mg q4h until relief

PHARMACOKINETICS Absorption: rapidly and completely absorbed. **Peak:** 2.5 h. **Distribution:** widely distributed; crosses placenta; distributed into breast milk. **Metabolism:** metabolized in liver to oxyphenbutazone, an active metabolite. **Elimination:** half-life: 50–100 h; 60% excreted in urine, 30% in feces.

CONTRAINDICATIONS & PRECAUTIONS Contraindicated in: phenylbutazone or oxyphenbutazone sensitivity and idiosyncracy, history of peptic ulcer, GI inflammatory disease, pancreatitis, stomatitis; aspirin hypersensitivity; drug allergy; blood dyscrasias; renal disease; hepatic dysfunction; left ventricular failure, borderline cardiac failure, severe hypertension; edema; polymyalgia rheumatica; temporal arteritis; concomitant use with other drugs such as chemotherapeutic agents, use with long-term anticoagulant (oral) therapy, children <14 y, senile patient. Safe use during pregnancy (category D), especially during third trimester, not established. **Cautious use in:** glaucoma, patients >40 y, asthma.

ADVERSE/SIDE EFFECTS CV: hypertension, pericarditis, cardiac decompensation. **Endocrine/metabolic:** hyperglycemia, thyroid hyperplasia, toxic goiter, myxedema; sodium, chloride, and fluid retention; rapid plasma volume expansion with plasma dilution, metabolic acidosis, respiratory alkalosis. **Eye/Ear:** Optic neuritis, retinal hemorrhage and detachment, oculomotor palsy, toxic amblyopia, blurred vision, conjunctivitis, scotomas; hearing loss, tinnitus. **GI:** *recurring dyspepsia* (including heartburn and indigestion), *nausea,* vomiting, constipation, di-

arrhea, xerostomia, ulcerative stomatitis and esophagitis, salivary gland enlargement, epigastric pain, constipation, abdominal distension with flatulence, ulceration of bowel, reactivation of peptic ulcer, hepatitis (fatal and nonfatal), pancreatitis. **Hematologic:** bone marrow depression, pancytopenia, thrombocytopenia, agranulocytosis, aplastic anemia, leukopenia, leukemia. **Hypersensitivity:** asthma, urticaria, anaphylaxis, drug fever, serum sickness, Stevens-Johnson syndrome, activation of SLE, Lyell's syndrome. **Renal:** hematuria, proteinuria, glomerulonephritis, acute renal failure, nephrotic syndrome, renal calculi, azotemia. **Skin:** fixed drug eruptions, erythema nodosum and multiforme, nonthrombocytopenic purpura. **Other:** trembling, nervousness, taste disturbances, headache, confusion.

DIAGNOSTIC TEST INTERFERENCES Phenylbutazone reduces *iodine uptake* by thyroid gland.

DRUG INTERACTIONS Increases activity and toxicity of **warfarin,** ORAL HYPOGLYCEMIC AGENTS, **phenytoin,** salicylates, SULFONAMIDES; increases **digitoxin** metabolism; increases **methotrexate** toxicity.

NURSING IMPLICATIONS

Administration

- Possible GI irritation can be minimized by administering drug with meals, with full glass of milk, or with an antacid (prescribed)
- Tablet may be crushed and capsule may be emptied if patient cannot swallow it whole. Mix crushed powder or capsule contents with fluid of patient's choice or with food. Should not be swallowed dry.
- Store drug at 15–30C (59–86F) in light- and moisture-resistant container.

Assessment & Drug Effects

- Steady state therapeutic serum levels (95 µg/ml) reached in 3–4 d.
- Frequent regular blood studies are advisable when drug is given beyond 1 wk, the usual treatment period.
- Any significant change in hematology, i.e., fall in total white count, relative decrease in granulocytes, appearance of blast forms, fall in Hct, signals the necessity to stop treatment pending complete hematology studies.
- Although phenylbutazone increases action of oral anticoagulants when they are given concomitantly, it does not affect prothrombin activity when administered alone; however, the combination of an-

P

tiplatelet and ulcerogenic action of phenylbutzone contributes to the hazard of serious hemorrhage during drug therapy.

- Monitor patient with asthma, especially if patient is also sensitive to aspirin. This drug like others with prostaglandin-synthesis inhibition activity may precipitate an acute asthma attack.
- *Smoking-drug relationships:* smoking shortens half-life and increases clearance rate of phenylbutazone. It is possible that the heavy smoker may require an adjusted dosage regimen.
- *Overdose symptoms:* prompt onset of respiratory or metabolic acidosis with hyperventilation that can progress to trismus, tonic-clonic seizures, shock, coma, hypotension, oliguria. Other symptoms include: nausea, vomiting, epigastric pain, excessive perspiration, euphoria, psychoses, headache, vertigo, insomnia, tinnitus, edema, cyanosis, agitation, hallucinations, convulsions, hematuria. Buccal or GI mucosal ulcerations are late manifestations of massive overdosage.

Patient & Family Education

- Urge patient to report for all scheduled blood studies. Hematologic toxicity may occur suddenly or many days or weeks after drug use has been terminated.
- Patients should be closely followed during therapy and made fully aware of potential adverse reactions.
- Warn patient to discontinue drug therapy immediately and report to physician: fever, stomatitis, oral ulcerations, salivary gland enlargement, severe sore throat, epigastric pain, dyspepsia, unusual unexplained bleeding and bruising, tarry stools, skin rashes, edema, pruritus, jaundice.
- Any eye symptom should be investigated. Drug should be discontinued and a complete ophthalmic examination scheduled.
- Phenylbutazone may cause drowsiness; therefore, advise patient to observe caution while driving or performing tasks requiring alertness until response to drug is known.
- Instruct patient to keep a record of daily weight and to check for lower leg, ankle, or facial edema. Advise patient to report sudden weight gain (i.e., gain of 2–3 lb within 2–3 d). Edema may signify hepatic or renal dysfunction or electrolyte imbalance and may indicate necessity of stopping therapy. In the elderly a reduction of dose may suffice to reduce edema of ankles and face.
- Check with physician about alcohol ingestion. Alcohol impairs motor coordination in the patient receiving phenylbutazone (probably an additive effect).

- Urge patient not to self-dose with OTC drugs unless advised to do so by physician. Many pain relief OTC preparations contain aspirin.

Prototype: methoxamine, p 101

PHENYLEPHRINE HYDROCHLORIDE
(fen-ill-ef´rin)

Trade names: AK-Dilate Ophthalmic, Alconefrin, Isopto Frin, Mydfrin, Neo-Synephrine, Nostril, Prefrin Liquifilm, Rhinall, Sinarest Nasal, Sinex, Sinophen, Vacon

Classifications: AUTONOMIC NERVOUS SYSTEM AGENT; ALPHA-ADRENERGIC AGONIST; EYE & NOSE PREPARATION; MYDRIATIC; DECONGESTANT

Pregnancy: Category C

ACTIONS/PHARMACODYNAMICS Potent, synthetic, direct-acting sympathomimetic with strong alpha-adrenergic and weak beta-adrenergic cardiac stimulant actions. Produces little or no CNS stimulation. Elevates systolic and diastolic pressures through arteriolar constriction; also constricts capacitance vessels and increases venous return to heart. Rise in BP causes reflex bradycardia. Topical applications to eye produce vasoconstriction and prompt mydriasis of short duration, usually without causing cycloplegia. Reduces intraocular pressure by increasing outflow and decreasing rate of aqueous humor secretion. Nasal decongestant action qualitatively similar to that of epinephrine but more potent and has longer duration of action.

USES Parenterally to maintain BP during anesthesia, to treat vascular failure in shock, and to overcome paroxysmal supraventricular tachycardia. Used topically for rhinitis of common cold, allergic rhinitis, and sinusitis; in selected patients with wide-angle glaucoma; as mydriatic for ophthalmoscopic examination or surgery, and for relief of uveitis.

PHARMACOKINETICS Onset: immediate IV; 10–15 min IM/SC. **Duration:** 15–20 min IV; 30–120 min IM/SC; 3–6 h topical. **Metabolism:** metabolized in liver and tissues by monoamine oxidase.

CONTRAINDICATIONS & PRECAUTIONS Contraindicated in: severe coronary disease, severe hypertension, ventricular tachycardia; narrow-angle glaucoma (ophthalmic preparations); pregnancy (cate-

P

ROUTE & DOSAGE

Hypotension

Adult	IM/SC	1–10 mg; initial dose not to exceed 5 mg, q10–15min as needed
	IV	0.1–0.18 mg/min until BP stabilizes; then 0.04–0.06 mg/min for maintenance

Ophthalmoscopy

Adult	Ophthalmic	1 drop of 2.5% or 10% solution before examination
Child	Ophthalmic	1 drop of 2.5% solution before examination

Vasoconstrictor

Adult	Ophthalmic	2 drops of 0.12–0.15% solution q3–4h as necessary
	Intranasal	Small amount of nasal jelly placed into each nostril q3–4h as needed *or* 2–3 drops or sprays of 0.25–0.5% solution q3–4h as needed
Child:	Intranasal	<6 y: 2–3 drops or sprays of 0.125% solution q3–4h as needed
		6–12 y: 2–3 drops or sprays of 0.25% solution q3–4h as needed

gory C). **Cautious use in:** hyperthyroidism; diabetes mellitus; myocardial disease, cerebral arteriosclerosis, bradycardia; elderly patients; 21 d before or following termination of MAO inhibitor therapy. **10% ophthalmic solution:** cardiovascular disease; diabetes mellitus; hypertension; aneurysms; infants.

ADVERSE/SIDE EFFECTS Eye: *transient stinging,* lacrimation, browache, headache, blurred vision, conjunctival allergy (pigmentary deposits on lids, conjunctiva, and cornea with prolonged use), increased sensitivity to light. **Intranasal:** *rebound congestion* (hyperemia and edema of mucosa), *burning, stinging, dryness, sneezing.* **Systemic effects:** palpitation, tachycardia, bradycardia (overdosage), extrasystoles, hypertension, trembling, sweating, pallor, sense of fullness in head, tingling of extremities, sleeplessness, dizziness, lightheadedness, weakness, restlessness, anxiety, precordial pain, *tremor,* severe visceral or peripheral vasoconstriction, necrosis if IV infiltrates.

DRUG INTERACTIONS ERGOT ALKALOIDS, **guanethidine, reserpine,** TRICYCLIC ANTIDEPRESSANTS increase pressor effects of phenylephrine; **halothane, digoxin** increase risk of arrhythmias; MAO INHIBITORS cause hypertensive crisis; **oxytocin** causes persistent hypertension; ALPHA BLOCKERS, BETA BLOCKERS antagonize effects of phenylephrine.

NURSING IMPLICATIONS

Administration

- IV phenylephrine may be given by IV infusion by diluting each 10 mg in 500 ml D5W or NS (concentration: 0.2 mg/ml); titrate to maintain BP.
- **Nasal preparations:** instruct patient to blow nose gently (with both nostrils open) to clear nasal passages before administration of medication.
- *Instillation (Drops):* tilt head back while sitting or standing up, or lie on bed and hang head over side. Stay in position a few minutes to permit medication to spread through nose. *(Spray):* with head upright, squeeze bottle quickly and firmly to produce 1 or 2 sprays into each nostril; wait 3–5 min, blow nose, and repeat dose. *(Jelly):* place in each nostril and sniff it well back into nose.
- **Ophthalmic preparations:** to avoid excessive systemic absorption, instruct patient to apply pressure to lacrimal sac during and for 1–2 min after instillation of drops.
- A local anesthetic may be instilled in eyes before the phenylephrine to reduce discomfort of stinging and burning.
- Clean tips and droppers of nasal solution dispensers with hot water after use to prevent contamination of solution. Droppers of ophthalmic solution bottles should not touch any surface including the eye.
- Wash hands carefully after handling the drug. Anisocoria (inequality in pupil size, blurred vision) can be caused by rubbing the eye with phenylpropranolamine-contaminated finger.
- Solutions and jelly change color to brown, form a precipitate, and lose potency with exposure to air, strong light, or heat. Do not transfer solutions from original container to another.
- Store in original container at 15–30C (59–86F) protected from freezing, strong light, and exposure to air.

Assessment & Drug Effects

- During IV administration, monitor pulse, BP, and central venous pressure (q2–5min). IV overdoses can induce ventricular dysrhythmias. Control flow rate and dosage to prevent excessive increases.
- Instillation of 2.5–10% strength ophthalmic solution can cause burning and stinging.

P

Common side effects in *italic*; life-threatening effects underlined; generic names in **bold**; classifications in SMALL CAPS

883

- Observe for congestion or rebound miosis after topical administration to eye.

Patient & Family Education
- Caution patient not to exceed recommended dosage regardless of formulation.
- If no relief is experienced from preparation in 5 d, patient should inform the physician.
- Systemic absorption from nasal and conjunctival membranes can occur, though infrequently (see adverse/side effects). Stop the drug and report to the physician if adverse effects occur.
- Inform patient that after instillation of ophthalmic drops, pupils will be large and eyes may be more sensitive to light than usual. Advise patient to use sunglasses in bright light and to stop medication and notify physician if this sensitivity persists beyond 12 h after drug has been discontinued.
- Caution patient that some ophthalmic solutions may stain contact lenses.
- Caution patient to avoid swallowing solutions or jelly; systemic effects may be induced.

Prototype: epinephrine, p 102

PHENYLPROPANOLAMINE HYDROCHLORIDE
(fen-ill-proe-pa-nole´a-meen)
Trade names: Acutrim, Allerest Timed Release, Contac, Dex-A-Diet, Dexatrim, Diadax, Phen-Lets, Rhidecon, Westrim
Classifications: AUTONOMIC NERVOUS SYSTEM AGENT; ALPHA- AND BETA-ADRENERGIC AGONIST (SYMPATHOMIMETIC); NASAL DECONGESTANT; CNS AGENT; ANOREXIANT
Pregnancy: Category C

ACTIONS/PHARMACODYNAMICS   Indirect-acting sympathomimetic amine with prominent peripheral adrenergic effects similar to those of epinephrine, but its action is more prolonged and it causes less CNS stimulation. Acts by stimulating alpha-adrenergic (excitatory) receptors of vascular smooth muscles, causing vasoconstriction and blanching of nasal mucosa. Also depresses appetite center in CNS.

USES Symptomatic relief of nasal congestion associated with allergies, hay fever, common cold, sinusitis, nasopharyngitis. Used parenterally as vasopressor

ROUTE & DOSAGE

Appetite Suppressant

Adult	PO	25 mg t.i.d. 30 min a.c. or 75 mg sustained release once/d before breakfast (max 75 mg/d)

Decongestant

Adult	PO	25 mg q4h prn *or* 75 mg sustained release q12h prn (max 150 mg/d)
Child	PO	2–6 y: 6.25 mg q4h prn (max 37.5 mg/d)
		6–12 y: 12.5 mg q4h prn (max 75 mg/d)

---

during surgery, particularly during spinal anesthesia; exogenous obesity.

PHARMACOKINETICS Absorption: readily absorbed from GI tract. **Onset:** 15–30 min. **Peak:** 1–2 h (3.5 h sustained release). **Duration:** 3 h (12 h sustained release). **Metabolism:** small amount metabolized in liver. **Elimination:** half-life: 3–4 h; excreted in urine.

CONTRAINDICATIONS & PRECAUTIONS Contraindicated in: concomitant use with MAO inhibitors. **Cautious use in:** hypertension, cardiovascular disease, hyperthyroidism, diabetes, prostatic enlargement, tricyclic antidepressants.

ADVERSE/SIDE EFFECTS Larger doses: *hypertension,* tachycardia, *palpitation,* nervousness, restlessness, *insomnia.* **Overdosage:** tachycardia, rapid respirations, disorientation, kidney failure, dilated pupils, headache, CNS stimulation, nausea, vomiting, anorexia, seizures.

DRUG INTERACTIONS Antagonizes antihypertensive effects of **guanethidine, guanadryl, reserpine.** MAO INHIBITOR, **selegiline** can cause hypertensive crisis (fatalities reported)—do not administer phenylpropanolamine during or within 14 d of these drugs, may inhibit mood elevating effects of PHENOTHIAZINES; TRICYCLIC ANTIDEPRESSANTS enhance pressor effects of phenylpropanolamine.

NURSING IMPLICATIONS
See epinephrine for additional nursing implications.

Administration
- Preserve in tight, light-resistant containers.

Patient & Family Education
- Caution patient not to exceed recommended dosage.

Common side effects in *italic*; life-threatening effects underlined; generic names in **bold**; classifications in SMALL CAPS

P

- The use of OTC combination drugs without physician's approval while patient is receiving phenylpropanolamine should be discouraged.

PHENYTOIN

See CENTRAL NERVOUS SYSTEM AGENTS, ANTICONVULSANT, HYDANTOIN prototype, p 172.

Prototype: neostigmine, p 118

PHYSOSTIGMINE SALICYLATE

(fi-zoe-stig´meen)
Trade names: Antilirium, Isopto Eserine

PHYSOSTIGMINE SULFATE

Trade name: Eserine Sulfate
Classifications: AUTONOMIC NERVOUS SYSTEM AGENT; CHOLINERGIC (PARASYMPATHOMIMETIC); CHOLINESTERASE INHIBITOR; EYE PREPARATION; MIOTIC (ANTIGLAUCOMA AGENT); MIOTIC
Pregnancy: Category C

ACTIONS/PHARMACODYNAMICS Reversible anticholinesterase and tertiary amine. Alkaloid of West African calabar or ordeal bean, *Physostigma venenosum*. Chief effect: increases concentration of acetylcholine at cholinergic transmission sites; prolongs and exaggerates its action. Similar to neostigmine in actions and adverse effects, but produces greater secretion of glands, constriction of pupil, and effect on BP and less action on skeletal muscle. Also has direct blocking action on autonomic ganglia. Parenteral physostigmine can produce transient decrease in manic symptoms as well as precipitate mental depression. Topical application to conjunctiva produces constriction of ciliary muscle (spasm of accommodation) and iris sphincter (miosis), as result of which the iris is pulled away from anterior chamber angle, thus facilitating drainage of aqueous humor, with lowering of intraocular pressure.

USES To reverse CNS and cardiac effects of tricyclic antidepressant overdose, to reverse CNS toxic effects of atropine, scopolamine, and similar anticholinergic drugs, and to antagonize CNS depressant effects of diazepam. Applied topically to eye to reduce intraocular tension in glaucoma. **Orphan drug:** for hereditary ataxias.

ROUTE & DOSAGE

Reversal of Anticholinergic Effects

Adult IM/IV 0.5–3 mg (IV not faster than 1 mg/min); repeat as needed

Glaucoma

Adult Topical Instill ointment in conjunctival sac at bedtime or instill 1–2 drops of 0.25–0.5% solution 3–4 times/d

PHARMACOKINETICS Absorption: readily absorbed from mucous membranes, muscle, subcutaneous tissue; 10–12% absorbed from GI tract. **Onset:** 3–8 min IM/IV; 2 min ophthalmic. **Duration:** 0.5–5 h IM/IV; 12–36 h ophthalmic. **Distribution:** crosses blood-brain barrier. **Metabolism:** metabolized in plasma by cholinesterases. **Elimination:** half-life: 15–40 min; excretion not fully understood; small amounts excreted in urine.

CONTRAINDICATIONS & PRECAUTIONS Contraindicated in: asthma; diabetes mellitus; gangrene; cardiovascular disease; mechanical obstruction of intestinal or urogenital tract; any vagotonic state; secondary glaucoma; inflammatory disease of iris or ciliary body; concomitant use with choline esters (e.g., methacholine, bethanechol) or depolarizing neuromuscular blocking agents (e.g., decamethonium, succinylcholine). Safe use during pregnancy (category C) not established. **Cautious use in:** epilepsy; parkinsonism; bradycardia; hyperthyroidism; peptic ulcer; hypotension.

ADVERSE/SIDE EFFECTS Acute toxicity: <u>cholinergic crisis</u>. **CNS:** restlessness, hallucinations, twitching, tremors, *sweating,* weakness, ataxia, convulsions, <u>collapse, respiratory paralysis, pulmonary edema</u>. **With rapid IV:** bradycardia, hyperactivity, respiratory distress, convulsions. **Eye:** headache, eye and brow pain, *marked miosis,* twitching of eyelids, *lacrimation,* dimness and blurring of vision; **prolonged use:** changes in pigmented epithelium of iris, chronic conjunctivitis, follicular cysts, contact allergic dermatitis. **Systemic absorption:** *nausea, vomiting, epigastric pain, diarrhea,* involuntary urination or defecation, miosis, *salivation, sweating, lacrimation,* rhinorrhea, dyspnea, bronchospasm, irregular pulse, palpitation, bradycardia, rise in BP.

DRUG INTERACTIONS Antagonizes effects of **echothiophate, isoflurophate.**

P

Common side effects in *italic*; life-threatening effects <u>underlined</u>; generic names in **bold**; classifications in SMALL CAPS

885

NURSING IMPLICATIONS

Administration

- IV physostigmine is given by direct IV undiluted at a slow rate, no more than 1 mg/min. Rapid administration and overdosage can cause a cholinergic crisis (muscle cramps, hypertension, respiratory depression and paralysis, diaphoresis, nausea, vomiting, diarrhea, involuntary micturition, CNS stimulation, fear, agitation, restlessness).
- The patient with brown or hazel eyes may require a stronger ophthalmic solution or more frequent instillation for desired effects than the patient with blue eyes.
- Physostigmine ophthalmic ointment may be prescribed at bedtime for patients with glaucoma to prevent nocturnal rise in ocular tension.
- To reduce the possibility of systemic effects, apply gentle pressure over lacrimal sac during and for 1 or 2 min following instillation. Instruct patient to avoid squeezing lids together. Blot excess medication with clean tissue.
- Preserve in tight light-resistant container. Use only clear, colorless solutions. Red-tinted solution indicates oxidation, and such solutions should be discarded.
- Store at 15–30C (59–86F).

Assessment & Drug Effects

- Closely monitor vital signs and state of consciousness in patients receiving drug for atropine poisoning. Since physostigmine is usually rapidly destroyed, patient can lapse into delirium and coma within 1 to 2 h; repeat doses may be required.
- Monitor closely for side effects related to CNS and for signs of sensitivity to physostigmine. Have atropine sulfate readily available for clinical emergency.
- When used parenterally or orally the following symptoms indicate need to discontinue drug: excessive salivation, emesis, frequent urination, or diarrhea. Excessive sweating or nausea may be eliminated by dose reduction.
- When used as topical ophthalmic agent, be alert to symptoms of systemic absorption (see adverse/side effects). Dosage should be reduced or drug discontinued.

Patient & Family Education

- Inform patient that physostigmine ophthalmic preparations may produce annoying lid twitching, temporary blurring of vision, and difficulty in seeing in dimmed light; therefore, necessary safety precautions should be taken.
- Emphasize the need for following prescribed drug regimen for glaucoma, and urge patient to remain under medical supervision.
- Teaching plan for glaucoma should include proper administration of eyedrops and adverse symptoms to be reported.
- Patient should be advised to wear identification tag indicating the presence of glaucoma and the medication being taken.

PHYTONADIONE (VITAMIN K$_1$)

(fye-toe-na-dye´one)
Trade names: AquaMEPHYTON, Konakion, Mephyton, Phylloquinone
Classifications: SYNTHETIC VITAMIN; ANTIDOTE
Pregnancy: Category C

ACTIONS/PHARMACODYNAMICS Fat-soluble naphthoquinone derivative chemically identical to and with similar degree of activity as naturally occurring vitamin K. Vitamin K is essential for hepatic biosynthesis of blood clotting factors II (prothrombin), VII (proconvertin), IX (plasma thromboplastin component), and X (Stuart factor). Promotes liver synthesis of clotting factors by unknown mechanism. Antagonizes inhibitory effects of coumarin and indandione anticoagulants on the hepatic synthesis of these clotting factors. Does not reverse anticoagulant action of heparin. Pharmacologically more active than menadione and derivatives, and action is more prompt and prolonged. Reportedly demonstrates wide margin of safety when used in newborns.

USES Drug of choice as antidote for overdosage of coumarin and indandione oral anticoagulants. Also reverses hypoprothrombinemia secondary to administration of oral antibiotics, quinidine, quinine, salicylates, sulfonamides, excessive vitamin A, and secondary to inadequate absorption and synthesis of vitamin K (as in obstructive jaundice, biliary fistula, ulcerative colitis, intestinal resection, prolonged hyperalimentation). Also prophylaxis of and therapy for neonatal hemorrhagic disease.

PHARMACOKINETICS Absorption: readily absorbed from intestinal lymph only if bile is present. **Onset:** 6–12 h PO; 1–2 h IM/SC; 15 min IV. **Peak:** hemorrhage usually controlled within 3–8 h; normal prothrombin time may be obtained in 12–14 h after administration. **Distribution:** concentrates briefly in liver

P

ROUTE & DOSAGE

Anticoagulant Overdose

Adult	PO/SC/IM	2.5–10 mg; rarely up to 50 mg/d; may repeat parenteral dose after 6–8 h if needed; PO dose may be repeated after 12–24 h
	IV	Emergency only: 10–15 mg at a rate ≤1 mg/min; may be repeated in 4 h if bleeding continues

Hemorrhagic Disease of Newborns

Infant	IM/SC	0.5–1 mg immediately after delivery; may repeat in 6–8 h if necessary

Other Prothrombin Deficiencies

Adult	IM/SC	2–25 mg
Child	IM/SC	5–10 mg
Infant	IM/SC	1 mg

after absorption; crosses placenta; distributed into breast milk. **Metabolism:** rapidly metabolized in liver. **Elimination:** excreted in urine and bile.

CONTRAINDICATIONS & PRECAUTIONS Contraindicated in: severe liver disease. Pregnancy (category C). Effect on fertility and teratogenic potential not known.

ADVERSE/SIDE EFFECTS Gastric upset, headache (after oral dose). **Following IV:** hypersensitivity or anaphylaxis-like reaction: facial flushing, cramp-like pains, convulsive movements, chills, fever, diaphoresis, weakness, dizziness, peculiar taste sensation, *bronchospasm,* dyspnea, sensation of chest constriction, shock, cardiac arrest, respiratory arrest. **Injection site:** pain, hematoma, and nodule formation, erythematous skin eruptions (with repeated injections). Paradoxic hypoprothrombinemia (patients with severe liver disease). **Newborns (following large doses):** hyperbilirubinemia, severe hemolytic anemia, kernicterus, brain damage, death.

DIAGNOSTIC TEST INTERFERENCES Falsely elevated *urine steroids* (by modifications of Reddy, Jenkins, Thorn procedure).

DRUG INTERACTIONS Antagonizes effects of **warfarin; cholestyramine, colistipol, mineral oil** decrease absorption of oral phytonadione.

NURSING IMPLICATIONS

Administration

- Note that Konakion (which contains a phenol preservative) is intended for IM use only. AquaMEPHYTON may be given subcutaneously, IM, or IV as prescribed.
- *IM injection:* in adults and older children, IM injection should be given in upper outer quadrant of buttocks. For infants and young children, anterolateral aspect of thigh or deltoid region is preferred. Carefully aspirate to avoid intravascular injection. Apply gentle pressure to site following injection. Swelling (internal bleeding) and pain sometimes occur with SC or IM administration.
- *IV infusion:* for IV infusion, dilution may be made with 0.9% NaCl, 5% dextrose, or 5% dextrose in 0.9% NaCl injection. Other diluents should not be used. Administer solution immediately after dilution at a rate not to exceed 1 mg/min. Discard unused solution and contents in open ampul.
- Phytonadione is photosensitive. Protect infusion solution from light by wrapping container with aluminum foil or other opaque material.
- Patients with bile deficiency receiving oral phytonadione will require concomitant administration of bile salts to assure adequate absorption.
- If possible, drugs that inhibit or interfere with vitamin K activity (e.g., oral antibiotics, salicylates) may be discontinued or given at reduced dosages as an alternative or addition to phytonadione therapy.
- Store in tight, light-resistant containers in a dark place at 15–30C (59–86F). Protect from light at all times.

Assessment & Drug Effects

- Severe reactions, including fatalities, have occurred during and immediately after IV injection (see adverse/side effects). Patient should be under constant surveillance. Monitor vital signs.
- Frequency, dose, and therapy duration are guided by prothrombin times and clinical response.
- *Therapeutic responses to phytonadione:* shortened prothrombin, bleeding, and clotting times, as well as decreased hemorrhagic tendencies.
- Some patients with liver disease, especially women, develop an itchy erythematous rash at injection sites following repeated IM doses. The rash is at first localized and later may spread and corresponds to inadequate control of prothrombin time. It appears within a few days to several weeks after initiation of therapy and subsides with scaling in 2–12 wk. A change to another form of vitamin

P

Common side effects in *italic*; life-threatening effects underlined; generic names in **bold**; classifications in SMALL CAPS

887

K such as menadiol sodium diphosphate (Synkayvite) has resolved the problem.

- Patients on large doses may develop temporary resistance to coumarin- or indandione-type anticoagulants. If oral anticoagulant is reinstituted, larger than former doses of anticoagulant may be needed. Some patients may require change to heparin.
- Use of phytonadione to correct anticoagulant-induced prothrombin deficiency may promote the same clotting hazards that existed prior to anticoagulant therapy.

Patient & Family Education

- Advise patient stabilized on phytonadione to maintain consistency in diet and to avoid significant increases in daily intake of vitamin K–rich foods. *Good sources of vitamin K:* asparagus, broccoli, cabbage, lettuce, turnip greens, pork or beef liver, green tea, spinach, watercress, tomatoes.

PILOCARPINE HYDROCHLORIDE

See EYE, EAR, NOSE & THROAT PREPARATIONS, MIOTIC (ANTIGLAUCOMA AGENT) prototype, p 209.

Prototype: haloperidol, p 189

PIMOZIDE

(pi´moe-zide)
Trade name: Orap
Classifications: CNS AGENT; PSYCHOTHERAPEUTIC; BUTYROPHENONE ANTIPSYCHOTIC (TRANQUILIZER)
Pregnancy: Category C

ACTIONS/PHARMACODYNAMICS Orphan neuroleptic agent; analog of the butyrophenones and derivative of meperidine-like analgesics. A potent central dopamine antagonist that alters release and turnover of central dopamine stores; has no effect on turnover of norepinephrine. Blockade of CNS dopaminergic receptors results in suppression of the motor and phonic tics that characterize Tourette's disorder. Produces less sedation and fewer extrapyramidal reactions than haloperidol; lowers seizure threshold. Animal studies suggest that pimozide may be tumorigenic in humans.

USES To suppress severe motor and phonic tics in patient with Tourette's disorder who has failed to respond satisfactorily to standard treatment (e.g., haloperidol).

ROUTE & DOSAGE

Tourette´s Disorder

Adult	PO	1–2 mg/d in divided doses; gradually increase dose q.o.d. up to 0.2 mg/kg/d or 7–16 mg/d in divided doses, whichever is less (max 0.3 mg/kg/d or 20 mg/d)

PHARMACOKINETICS Absorption: slowly and variably absorbed from GI tract (40–50% absorbed). **Peak:** 6–8 h. **Metabolism:** metabolized in liver to 2 major metabolites. **Elimination:** half-life: 55 h; 80–85% excreted in urine, 15–20% in feces.

CONTRAINDICATIONS & PRECAUTIONS Contraindicated in: treatment of simple tics other than those associated with Tourette´s disorder; drug-induced tics; history of cardiac dysrhythmias and conditions marked by prolonged QT syndrome, patient taking drugs that may prolong QT interval (e.g., quinidine); severe toxic CNS depression. Safe use in children <12 y, during pregnancy (category C), and by nursing mothers not established. **Cautious use in:** renal and hepatic dysfunction; patients receiving anticonvulsant therapy.

ADVERSE/SIDE EFFECTS CNS: headache, *sedation, drowsiness,* insomnia, *akathisia,* speech disorder, *torticollis, tremor,* handwriting changes, *akinesia,* grand mal seizures, fainting, hyperpyrexia, persistent tardive dyskinesia, *rigidity, oculogyric crisis,* hyperreflexia; neuroleptic malignant syndrome; *extrapyramidal dysfunction,* hyperthermia, autonomic dysfunction; *tachycardia, labile BP,* diaphoresis, dyspnea, urinary incontinence; elevated CPK, WBC, liver function enzymes; respiratory failure, acute renal failure, stupor. **CV:** prolongation of QT interval, inverted or flattened T wave, appearance of U wave, *orthostatic hypotension,* palpitations. **GU:** loss of libido, impotence, nocturia, urinary frequency, amenorrhea, dysmenorrhea, mild glactorrhea. **Skin:** sweating, skin irritation. **Special senses:** visual disturbances, photosensitivity, decreased accommodation, blurred vision, cataracts. **Other:** weight changes, asthenia, chest pain, periorbital edema, increased salivation, nausea, vomiting, diarrhea, anorexia, abdominal cramps, constipation.

DRUG INTERACTIONS Alcohol and other CNS DEPRESSANTS increase CNS depression; ANTICHOLINERGIC AGENTS (e.g., TRICYCLIC ANTIDEPRESSANTS, **at-**

P

ropine) increase anticholinergic effects; PHENO-THIAZINES, TRICYCLIC ANTIDEPRESSANTS, ANTIARRHYTHMICS increase risk of arrhythmias and heart block; pimozide antagonizes effects of ANTICONVULSANTS—there is loss of seizure control.

NURSING IMPLICATIONS

See haloperidol for additional nursing implications.

Administration

- Drug dose is increased gradually, usually over 1–3 wk, until maintenance dose is reached.
- When drug is to be discontinued, the regimen should be adjusted by prescription: slow, gradual changes over a period of days or weeks (drug has a long half-life). Sudden withdrawal may cause reemergence of original symptoms (motor and phonic tics) and of neuromuscular side effects of the drug.

Assessment & Drug Effects

- ECG baseline data should be obtained at beginning of therapy and checked periodicaly, especially during period of dosage adjustment.
- One of the adverse effects is widening of the QT interval (QRS complex and T wave), representing both ventricular depolarization and repolarization. Widening or prolongation of the interval suggests developing cardiotoxicity.
- Risk of tardive dyskinesia appears to be greatest in women, in the elderly, and those on high dosage.
- Extrapyramidal reactions often appear within the first few days of therapy, are dose-related, and usually occur when dose is high.
- Anticholinergic effects (dry mouth, constipation) may increase as dose is increased.

Patient & Family Education

- Advise patient to adhere to established drug regimen (i.e., dose or intervals should not be changed and dose should be discontinued only with physician's guidance).
- Discuss measures to help patient tolerate dry mouth (frequent rinsing with water, saliva substitute, increased fluid intake) and constipation (increased dietary fiber, drink 6–8 glasses of water daily).
- Warn patient that drug-caused hand tremors, drowsiness, and blurred vision may impair alertness and ability to safely drive a car or to engage in dangerous activities.
- Pseudoparkinsonism symptoms (see chap 3) are usually mild and reversible with dose adjustment.
- Both patient and family should be alerted to the earliest symptom of tardive dyskinesia ("flycatching"—an involuntary movement of the tongue), which should be reported promptly to the physician.
- Urge patient to return for periodic assessments of therapy benefit and cardiac status.
- Moderation or abstinence from alcohol is advised to prevent augmenting CNS depressant effects of pimozide.

Prototype: propranolol, p 109

PINDOLOL

(pin´doe-lole)
Trade name: Visken
Classifications: BETA-ADRENERGIC ANTAGONIST (BLOCKING AGENT, SYMPATHOLYTIC); CARDIOVASCULAR AGENT; ANTIHYPERTENSIVE
Pregnancy: Category B

ACTIONS/PHARMACODYNAMICS Nonselective beta-adrenergic blocking agent. Possesses slight intrinsic sympathomimetic activity (ISA) or partial beta-agonist effect in therapeutic dose ranges. Thus pindolol exerts vasodilator as well as hypotensive effects. Hypotensive mechanism is similar to that of propranolol: competitively blocks beta-adrenergic receptors primarily in myocardium, and beta receptors within bronchial and smooth muscle. Membrane-stabilizing or anesthetic-like action has been demonstrated but only at plasma levels above therapeutic safety. Has negative chronotropic and inotropic properties and slows conduction in AV node (but to lesser extent than other beta-blockers). Does not consistently affect cardiac output, resting heart rate, or renin release; it does, however, decrease peripheral vascular resistance, perhaps the major factor in pindolol's hypotensive effect. The ISA can be completely reversed by other beta-antagonists.

USES Management of hypertension (in stepped-care approach: step 1) concurrently with a thiazide diuretic or as single agent. Used in patient who has failed to respond to diet, exercise, and weight reduction. **Unlabeled use:** stress and exercise-induced chronic stable angina pectoris.

PHARMACOKINETICS Absorption: rapidly absorbed from GI tract; 50–95% reaches systemic circulation (first pass metabolism). **Onset:** 3 h. **Peak:** 1–2 h. **Duration:** 24 h. **Distribution:** distributed into breast milk. **Metabolism:** 40–60% metabolized in liver. **Elimination:** half-life: 3–4 h; excreted in urine.

P

Common side effects in *italic*; life-threatening effects <u>underlined</u>; generic names in **bold**; classifications in SMALL CAPS

889

ROUTE & DOSAGE

Hypertension

Adult   PO   5 mg b.i.d.; may increase by 10 mg/d q2–3wk if needed up to max of 60 mg/d in 2–3 divided doses

Angina Pectoris

Adult   PO   15–40 mg/d in 3–4 divided doses

CONTRAINDICATIONS & PRECAUTIONS Contraindicated in: bronchospastic diseases, severe bradycardia, cardiogenic shock, cardiac failure. Safe use in pregnancy (category B), nursing mothers, and children not established. **Cautious use in:** nonallergic bronchospasm, CHF, diabetes mellitus, hyperthyroidism, impaired hepatic and renal function.

ADVERSE/SIDE EFFECTS CNS: *fatigue,* dizziness, insomnia, drowsiness, confusion, fainting, decreased libido. **CV:** *bradycardia,* hypotension, CHF. **GI:** nausea, *diarrhea, constipation,* flatulence. **Respiratory:** bronchospasm, pulmonary edema, dyspnea. **Sensitivity reactions:** antinuclear antibodies (ANA) (10–30% of patients). **Other:** back or joint pain, agranulocytosis, impotence, hypoglycemia (may mask symptoms of a hypoglycemic reaction).

DRUG INTERACTIONS DIURETICS and other HYPOTENSIVE AGENTS increase hypotensive effect; effects of **albuterol, metaproterenol, terbutaline, pirbuterol** and pindolol antagonized; NSAIDs blunt hypotensive effect; decreases hypoglycemic effect of **glyburide; amiodarone** increases risk of bradycardia and sinus arrest.

NURSING IMPLICATIONS

Administration

- Food does not decrease bioavailability but may increase rate of absorption. Give drug at same time of day each day with respect to time of food intake for most predictable results.
- Withdrawal or discontinuation of treatment is gradual over a period of 1–2 wk.

Assessment & Drug Effects

- Monitor HR and BP. Report bradycardia and hypotension. Dosage adjustment may be indicated.
- Hypotensive effect may begin within 7 d but is not therapeutically maximum until about 2 wk after beginning of treatment with pindolol.

Patient & Family Education

- Pindolol masks the dizziness and sweating premonitory symptoms of hypoglycemia.

- Abrupt withdrawal of drug might precipitate a thyroid crisis in a patient with hyperthyroidism, and angina in the patient with ischemic heart disease, leading to an MI. Warn any patient on pindolol to adhere to the prescribed drug regimen. If a change is desired, consult physician first.

Prototype: penicillin G potassium, p 71

PIPERACILLIN SODIUM

(pi-per´a-sill-in)

Trade name: Pipracil
Classifications: ANTIINFECTIVE; BETA-LACTAM ANTIBIOTIC; NATURAL PENICILLIN
Pregnancy: Category B

ACTIONS/PHARMACODYNAMICS Extended-spectrum parenteral penicillin with antibiotic activity against most gram-negative and many gram-positive anaerobic and aerobic organisms including members of *Clostridium, Bacteroides, Klebsiella, Enterobacter, Pseudomonas, Proteus,* and *Serratia* species and the anaerobic and aerobic cocci. Action is similar to that of other penicillins: by interference with bacterial cell wall synthesis, promotes loss of membrane integrity, leading to osmotic instability and death of the organism. Penicillins do not affect human cells in this way because of the differences in cell wall structure. Less active than penicillin G against pneumococci and group A streptococci but comparable to ampicillin against enterococci. Penicillinase-producing staphylococci are resistant to piperacillin. Contains less sodium and is therefore less likely to cause fluid retention than carbenicillin or ticarcillin.

USES Susceptible organisms that cause gynecologic, skin and skin structure, gonococcal, and streptococcal infections; lower respiratory tract, intraabdominal, and bone and joint infections; septicemia, urinary tract infections. Also prophylactically prior to and during surgery and as empiric antiinfective therapy in granulocytopenic patients.

PHARMACOKINETICS Peak: 45 min IM; 5 min IV. **Distribution:** widely distributed with highest concentrations in urine and bile; adequate CSF penetration with inflamed meninges; crosses placenta; distributed into breast milk. **Metabolism:** slightly metabolized in liver. **Elimination:** half-life: 0.6–1.35 h; primarily excreted in urine, partly in bile.

ROUTE & DOSAGE

Uncomplicated Urinary Tract Infection

Adult   IV/IM   8–16 g/d divided q6–8h

Moderate to Severe Infections

Adult   IV/IM   4 g q6h (150–200 mg/kg/d)

Life-threatening Infection, *Pseudomonas* Infections

Adult   IV/IM   3 g q4h (max 24 g/d)

Uncomplicated Gonococcal Infections

Adult   IM   2 g with 1 g probenecid given 30 min before piperacillin

---

CONTRAINDICATIONS & PRECAUTIONS Contraindicated in: hypersensitivity to penicillins, cephalosporins, or other drugs. Safe use in children <12 y, lactating mother, and during pregnancy (category B) not established. **Cautious use in:** hepatic and renal dysfunction, hypersensitivity to cephalosporins.

ADVERSE/SIDE EFFECTS Rare: abnormal platelet aggregation and prolonged prothrombin time (with high doses). Also see penicillin G potassium.

DRUG INTERACTIONS May increase risk of bleeding with ANTICOAGULANTS; **probenecid** decreases elimination of piperacillin.

INCOMPATIBILITIES   Solution/Additive: AMINOGLYCOSIDES. **Y-site:** AMINOGLYCOSIDES.

NURSING IMPLICATIONS

Administration

- Do not mix piperacillin with an aminoglycoside in a syringe or infusion bottle; aminoglycoside will be inactivated.
- Piperacillin for direct IV injection is reconstituted by diluting 1 g with 5 ml sterile water or NS and is given over 3–5 min. Reconstituted solution may be further diluted with 50–100 ml NS or D5W and is infused over 30 min.
- IM injections should be limited to 2 g/site. Use the gluteal muscle, preferably. The deltoid muscle should be used only if well developed. Diluents for reconstitution of drug include sterile water for injection, bacteriostatic NaCl injection, lactated Ringer's injection for IVs and sterile lidocaine HCl injection 0.5–1.0% without epinephrine for IM. When reconstituted, solution contains 1 g/2.5 ml.
- Patients undergoing hemodialysis usually receive a maximum dosage of 2 g piperacillin q8h and an additional 1 g dose after each dialysis period.
- Doses and frequency are usually modified if creatinine clearance is <40 ml/min.
- Duration of therapy depends on type and severity of infection but usually continues for at least 48–72 h after patient is asymptomatic and evidence that infection is eradicated has been obtained.
- Store reconstituted solution at room temperature for 24 h, up to 1 wk refrigerated, and up to 1 mo frozen.

Assessment & Drug Effects

- Prior to administration inquire about history of hypersensitivity to penicillins, cephalosporins, or other drugs.
- Monitor for hypersensitivity response; discontinue drug and notify physician if allergic response noted.
- Since high doses may induce coagulation abnormalities, monitor for hemorrhagic manifestations.

Prototype: mebendazole, p 53

PIPERAZINE CITRATE

(pi´per-a-zeen)
Trade names: Antepar, Bryrel, Entacyl, Pin-Tega, Pipril, Veriga, Vermazine, Vermirex
Classifications: ANTIINFECTIVE; ANTHELMINTIC
Pregnancy: Category B

ACTIONS/PHARMACODYNAMICS Appears to act by producing muscle paralysis in parasite, thus promoting elimination through intestinal peristalsis.

USES Pinworm disease (*Enterobius vermicularis*) and roundworm or ascariasis (*Ascaris lumbricoides*) infestations.

ROUTE & DOSAGE

Roundworms

Adult   PO   3.5 g once/d for 2 d
Child   PO   75 mg/kg (max 3.5 g) once/d for 2 d

Pinworms

Adult   PO   65 mg/kg (max 2.5 g) once/d for 7–8 d
Child   PO   Same as for adult

PHARMACOKINETICS   Absorption: readily absorbed from GI tract. **Elimination:** excreted in urine.

P

Common side effects in *italic*; life-threatening effects underlined; generic names in **bold**; classifications in SMALL CAPS

891

CONTRAINDICATIONS & PRECAUTIONS Con-traindicated in: impaired renal or hepatic function, convulsive disorders. Safe use during pregnancy (category B) not established. **Cautious use in:** malnutrition; anemia.

ADVERSE/SIDE EFFECTS Low toxicity. Usually with excessive dosage: **CNS:** headache, vertigo, ataxia, tremors, choreiform movements, muscular weakness, hyporeflexia, paresthesia, sense of detachment, memory defect, EEG abnormalities, convulsions. **ENT:** blurred vision, paralytic strabismus, nystagmus, cataracts, lacrimation, rhinorrhea, accommodative defects. **GI:** nausea, vomiting, abdominal cramps, diarrhea. **Hypersensitivity:** urticaria, erythema multiforme, photosensitivity, purpura, fever, productive cough, bronchospasm, arthralgia, hemolytic anemia.

DRUG INTERACTIONS PHENOTHIAZINES may exaggerate extrapyramidal effects or cause seizures.

NURSING IMPLICATIONS

Administration
- Drug may be given with food to reduce gastric distress.
- Store at controlled room temperature protected from heat and light.

Patient & Family Education
- Caution patient not to exceed recommended dosage schedule because of danger of neurotoxicity with high dosages.
- Instruct patient to withhold medication if CNS, GI, or hypersensitivity reactions occur and report them to physician.
- In severe infections, course of therapy may be repeated after 1 wk rest period.
- Pinworms and roundworms are transmitted by direct and indirect transfer of ova (e.g., by hands, food, and contaminated articles). Instruct patient and family in personal hygiene.

Prototype: cyclophosphamide, p 91

PIPOBROMAN
(pi-poe-broe´man)
Trade name: Vercyte
Classifications: ANTINEOPLASTIC; ALKYLATING AGENT
Pregnancy: Category D

P

ACTIONS/PHARMACODYNAMICS Dicarboxylic acid neutral amide of piperazine with toxic hematopoietic depressant properties. Exact mechanism of action unknown but is classified as a polyfunctional alkylating agent. Blocks DNA, RNA, and protein synthesis in rapidly proliferating cells.

USES Primarily, polycythemia. Also to produce remissions in chronic myelocytic leukemia.

ROUTE & DOSAGE

Polycythemia

Adult	PO	1 mg/kg/d for at least 30 d; may be increased to 1.5–3 mg/kg/d if no response, then reduce to 0.1–0.2 mg/kg/d

Chronic Myelocytic Leukemia

Adult	PO	1.5–2.5 mg/kg/d until optimal clinical response; maintenance dose: 7–175 mg/d

PHARMACOKINETICS Absorption: readily absorbed from GI tract. **Metabolism:** unknown. **Elimination:** unknown.

CONTRAINDICATIONS & PRECAUTIONS Con-traindicated in: children <15 y, myelosuppression from radiation or previous cytotoxic chemotherapy, pregnancy (category D).

ADVERSE/SIDE EFFECTS Nausea, vomiting, abdominal cramps, diarrhea, anorexia (transient), skin rash, thrombocytopenia, anemia, leukopenia.

NURSING IMPLICATIONS

Administration
- Since patient requires close observation, therapy is usually initiated in the hospital.

Assessment & Drug Effects
- Maintenance therapy is usually started when Hct is reduced 50–55% in polycythemia vera, or when leukocyte count approaches 10,000/mm³ in chronic myelocytic leukemia.
- Bone marrow studies should be performed prior to therapy and repeated at time of maximum hematologic response. Liver and kidney function tests should also be performed before and during therapy.
- Leukocyte and thrombocyte counts are advised every other day and CBCs weekly until desired response is obtained or toxic effects intervene.

Common side effects in *italic*; life-threatening effects underlined; generic names in **bold**; classifications in SMALL CAPS

- Therapy is interrupted when platelet count falls to 150,000/mm³ or WBC to 3,000/mm³.
- Therapy is discontinued if there is a rapid drop in hemoglobin, increased bilirubin levels, or reticulocytosis.
- Myelosuppression may not appear for 4 wk or more after treatment begins.
- Observe carefully for ecchymoses, petechiae, purpura, melena, and hemoptysis and report to physician promptly.
- If nausea, vomiting, diarrhea, and skin rash persist, therapy will be interrupted.

Prototype: ibuprofen, p 160

PIROXICAM
(peer-ox´i-kam)

Trade name: Feldene
Classifications: CNS AGENT; ANTIPYRETIC; NONNARCOTIC ANALGESIC; NSAID
Pregnancy: Category C

ACTIONS/PHARMACODYNAMICS Oxicam nonsteroidal antiinflammatory drug (NSAID) with analgesic, antipyretic, and antiinflammatory properties. Exact mechanism of action not clear. Strongly inhibits enzyme cyclooxygenase, biogenic catalyst of prostaglandin synthesis. (Prostaglandins are naturally occurring mediators of the inflammatory process, are found throughout the body, and are formed in every tissue; therefore the potential loci for NSAID action is vast.) Drug-induced reduction in prostaglandin levels is associated with decreased inflammatory processes in bone-joint disease (including crystal disorders) and with possible interference with platelet aggregation. Reportedly causes less gastric erosion and fecal blood loss than aspirin does.

USES Acute and long-term relief of mild to moderate pain and for symptomatic treatment of osteoarthritis and rheumatoid arthritis. **Unlabeled use:** acute and chronic relief of mild to moderate pain.

ROUTE & DOSAGE

Arthritis, Pain
Adult   PO   10–20 mg 1–2 times/d

PHARMACOKINETICS Absorption: well absorbed from GI tract. **Onset:** 1 h analgesia; 7 d for rheumatoid arthritis. **Peak:** 3–5 h analgesia; 2–4 wk antirheumatic. **Duration:** 48–72 h analgesia. **Distribution:** small amount distributed into breast milk. **Metabolism:** extensively metabolized in liver. **Elimination:** half-life: 30–86 h; excreted primarily in urine, some in bile (<5%).

CONTRAINDICATIONS & PRECAUTIONS Contraindicated in: hemophilia; syndrome (bronchospasm, nasal polyps, angioedema) precipitated by aspirin or other NSAID; active peptic ulcer, GI bleeding. Safe use in children, during pregnancy (category C), and in nursing mothers not established. **Cautious use in:** history of upper GI disease including ulcerative colitis; renal dysfunction; compromised cardiac function; hypertension or other conditions predisposing to fluid retention; coagulation disorders.

ADVERSE/SIDE EFFECTS CNS: somnolence, dizziness, vertigo, depression, insomnia, nervousness. Causal relationships not established: akathisia, depression, hallucinations, dream abnormalities, mental confusion, paresthesias. **CV/Respiratory:** peripheral edema, hypertension, worsening of CHF, exacerbation of angina. **ENT:** tinnitus, hearing loss. **Eye:** blurred vision, reduced visual acuity, changes in color vision, scotomas, corneal deposits, retinal disturbances. **GI:** *nausea, vomiting, dyspepsia,* GI bleeding, diarrhea, constipation, flatulence, dry mouth, peptic ulceration, anorexia, jaundice, hepatitis. **Hematologic:** anemia, decreases in Hgb, Hct; leukopenia, eosinophilia, aplastic anemia; thrombocytopenia, *prolonged bleeding time.* **Skin:** urticaria, erythema multiforme, maculopapular, vesiculobullous rash; photosensitivity, sweating, Stevens-Johnson syndrome, bruising, dermatitis. **Other:** bronchospasm, allergic rhinitis, angioedema, fever, hypoglycemia, hyperglycemia, hyperkalemia, weight gain; dysuria, dyspnea, palpitations, syncope, muscle cramps, fever, hypersensitivity reactions, acute renal failure, papillary necrosis, hematuria, proteinuria, nephrotic syndrome.

DRUG INTERACTIONS ORAL ANTICOAGULANTS, **heparin** may prolong bleeding time; may increase **lithium** toxicity; **alcohol, aspirin** increase risk of GI hemorrhage.

NURSING IMPLICATIONS

Administration
- Patient should take drug at the same time every day.
- Administration of capsule with food or fluid may help to reduce GI irritation.

Common side effects in *italic*; life-threatening effects underlined; generic names in **bold**; classifications in SMALL CAPS

893

- Concomitant administration of an antacid to reduce gastric distress does not interfere with piroxicam absorption or action.
- Dose adjustments, usually made on basis of clinical response, are made at intervals of weeks rather than days in order to prevent overdosage.
- Store in tightly closed container at 15–30C (59–86F) unless otherwise directed.

Assessment & Drug Effects

- Evaluation of antirheumatic effect cannot be made for at least 7 d.
- *Clinical evidence of benefits from drug therapy:* pain relief in motion and in rest, reduction in night pain, stiffness, and swelling; increased ROM (range of motion) in all joints.
- Appearance of adverse/side effects may be delayed for 7–10 d after start of therapy (except for an allergic reaction).
- Periodic laboratory test levels (BUN, ALT, AST) as well as cell counts, Hgb, and Hct should be evaluated in patient (especially the elderly) receiving piroxicam for an extended period.

Patient & Family Education

- If patient misses a dose, advise taking the drug when omission is discovered if it is 6–8 h before the next scheduled dose. Otherwise, omit the dose and reestablish regimen at next scheduled hour.
- Advise against self-dosing with aspirin or other OTC drug without physician's advice.
- Warn patient not to increase dosage beyond prescribed regimen. Patient should understand that long half-life of drug may cause delayed therapeutic effect. Higher than recommended doses are associated with increased incidence of GI irritation and peptic ulcer.
- Incidence of GI bleeding with this drug is relatively high. Instruct patient to promptly report symptoms of melena, hematemesis, or severe gastric pain.
- Be alert to *symptoms of drug-induced anemia:* profound fatigue, skin and mucous membrane pallor, lethargy.
- Since alcohol may increase the risk of GI bleeding, its use should be avoided or at least modified.
- If piroxicam is used concomitantly with an anticoagulant, advise patient to be alert to signs of hypoprothrombinemia during and for several days after therapy has been discontinued: ecchymoses, petechiae, unexplained bleeding, epistaxis, hematuria.
- Since side effects (i.e., blurred vision, vertigo, dizziness) may impair ability to perform activities requiring mental alertness, caution patient to avoid driving a car or engaging in hazardous activities until response to drug is known.
- Because most of drug is excreted by kidneys, impaired renal function increases danger of toxicity. Patient should drink at least 6–8 full glasses of water daily and report signs of renal insufficiency (see chap 3).

Prototype: normal human serum albumin, p 126

PLASMA PROTEIN FRACTION

Trade names: Plasmanate, Plasma-Plex; Plasmatein, PPF, Protenate
Classifications: BLOOD DERIVATIVE; PLASMA VOLUME EXPANDER
Pregnancy: Category C

ACTIONS/PHARMACODYNAMICS Five percent solution of stabilized human plasma proteins in NaCl containing approximately 88% albumin, 7% alpha-globulin, and 5% beta-globulin. Each liter contains about 145 mEq sodium, 85 mEq chloride, and 2 mEq potassium. Oncotic action approximately equivalent to that of human plasma; does not provide coagulation factors or gamma globulins. Heat-treated to minimize hazard of transmitting serum hepatitis; risk of sensitization is reduced since it lacks cellular elements. Does not require cross matching.

USES Emergency treatment of hypovolemic shock due to burns, trauma, surgery, infections; temporary measure in treatment of blood loss when whole blood is not available; to replenish plasma protein in patients with hypoproteinemia (if sodium restriction is not a problem).

ROUTE & DOSAGE

Plasma Volume Expansion

Adult	IV	250–500 ml at a max rate of 10 ml/min
Child	IV	6.6–33 ml/kg at a rate of 5–10 ml/min

Hypoproteinemia

Adult	IV	1–1.5 L/d infused at a rate not to exceed 5–8 ml/min

CONTRAINDICATIONS & PRECAUTIONS Contraindicated in: severe anemia, cardiac failure; patients undergoing cardiopulmonary bypass surgery. Pregnancy (category C). **Cautious use in:** patients with low cardiac reserve; absence of albumin deficiency; hepatic or renal failure.

P

ADVERSE/SIDE EFFECTS Low incidence: nausea, vomiting, hypersalivation, headache. **Hypersensitivity:** tingling, chills, fever, cyanosis, chest tightness, backache, urticaria, erythema, shock (systemic anaphylaxis). **With rapid IV infusion:** circulatory overload, pulmonary edema.

NURSING IMPLICATIONS

Administration

- Check expiration date on label. Solutions that show a sediment or appear turbid should not be used. Do not use solutions that have been frozen.
- Once container is opened, solution should be used within 4 h because it contains no preservatives. Discard unused portions.
- Rate of infusion and volume of total dose will depend on patient's age, diagnosis, degree of venous and pulmonary congestion, Hct, and Hgb determinations. Specific flow rate should be prescribed by physician.
- As with any oncotically active solution, infusion rate should be relatively slow. Range may vary from 1–10 ml/min.
- Plasma protein fraction is reportedly incompatible with solutions containing alcohol or norepinephrine (levarterenol bitartrate).
- Storage temperature varies with manufacturer. See package insert.

Assessment & Drug Effects

- Monitor BP and pulse. Frequency of readings will depend on patient's condition. Flow rate adjustments are made according to clinical response and BP. Slow or stop infusion if patient suddenly becomes hypotensive.
- A widening pulse pressure (difference between systolic and diastolic) correlates with increase in cardiac output and should be reported.
- Report changes in I&O ratio and pattern.
- Observe patient closely during and after infusion for signs of hypervolemia or circulatory overload (see chap 3). Report these symptoms immediately to physician.
- Make careful observations of patient who has had either injury or surgery in order to detect bleeding points that failed to bleed at lower BP.

PLICAMYCIN

(plik-a-mi´-cin)
Trade name: Mithracin
Classifications: ANTINEOPLASTIC; ANTIBIOTIC
Pregnancy: Category C

ACTIONS/PHARMACODYNAMICS Cytotoxic antibiotic produced by *Streptomyces plicatus,* with minimal immunosuppressive activity. Complexes with DNA, thus inhibiting DNA-directed RNA synthesis. May lower serum calcium levels by unclear mechanism. Appears to block hypercalcemic action of vitamin D, and may inhibit parathyroid hormone effect on osteoclasts. Interferes with synthesis of various clotting factors. High toxicity with low therapeutic index limits clinical use.

USES To treat hospitalized patients with hypercalcemia or hypercalciuria associated with advanced neoplasms and to treat testicular malignancy.

ROUTE & DOSAGE

Neoplasia

Adult	IV	25–30 μg/kg once/d for 8–10 d or until toxicity necessitates discontinuing (max 30 μg/kg/d for 10 d)

Malignant Hypercalcemia

Adult	IV	25 μg/kg once/d for 3–4 d; may repeat after 1 wk

PHARMACOKINETICS Distribution: crosses blood-brain barrier; appears to localize in areas of bone active resorption. **Elimination:** excreted in urine.

CONTRAINDICATIONS & PRECAUTIONS Contraindicated in: bleeding and coagulation disorders, myelosuppression; electrolyte imbalance (especially hypocalcemia, hypokalemia, hypophosphatemia); pregnancy (category C). **Cautious use in:** patients with prior abdominal or mediastinal radiology; liver or renal impairment.

ADVERSE/SIDE EFFECTS CNS: drowsiness, irritability, dizziness, weakness, headache, mental depression. **GI:** *stomatitis, anorexia, nausea, vomiting, diarrhea,* widespread intestinal hemorrhage. **Hematologic:** thrombocytopenia, bleeding and coagulation disorders (dose-related), leukopenia (mild). **Other:** fever, marked facial flushing, hemoptysis, nonspecific or acneiform skin rash, phlebitis, hypophosphatemia, hypokalemia, hypocalciuria, abnormal liver and renal function tests.

DRUG INTERACTIONS Concomitant administration of *vitamin D* may enhance hypercalcemia.

P

Common side effects in *italic*; life-threatening effects underlined; generic names in **bold**; classifications in SMALL CAPS

895

NURSING IMPLICATIONS

Administration

- When edema, ascites, or hydrothorax is present, drug dose is based on ideal body weight.
- Dilute each 25 mg with 4.9 ml of sterile water to yield 500 µg/ml. May be further diluted in either 1000 ml 5% dextrose or 0.9% NaCl injection and infused over a 4–6 h period.
- Carefully regulate IV flow rate (established by physician); GI side effects increase when rate is too fast.
- Terminate infusion immediately if extravasation occurs. Apply moderate heat to disperse the drug and to minimize tissue irritation.
- Unused portions of reconstituted solution should be discarded and new ones prepared daily.
- Refrigerate unreconstituted vials at 2–8C (36–46F).

Assessment & Drug Effects

- Therapy is usually interrupted if leukocyte count is <4000/mm³, if platelet count is <150,000/mm³, or if prothrombin time is > 4 seconds higher than control. (Normal: 12–14 seconds.)
- Establish flow chart at beginning of therapy, permitting continuous record of weight and I&O ratio and pattern.
- Frequent assessments of liver and hematologic (platelet count, bleeding and prothrombin times) and renal function are performed throughout therapy and for several days after last dose.
- Thrombocytopenia, frequently evidenced by a single or persistent episode of epistaxis or hematemesis, may be rapid in onset during or after a course of treatment. Report marked facial flushing, which is often an early symptom.
- Inspect skin daily for signs of purpura. Hemoptysis may occur because of bleeding into metastasis; report this immediately.
- Rebound hypercalcemia (normal: 9–10.6 mg/dl) following plicamycin-induced hypocalcemia may persist 2–4 d. See chapter 3 for signs and symptoms of *hypercalcemia*.
- The hypercalcemia patient may be dehydrated. Monitor I&O ratio to assure adequate fluid intake.
- Signs of antiblastic action on GI mucosal cells (hematemesis, melena) necessitate stopping drug use.
- Check patient's bowel function daily to prevent high fecal impaction due to diminished peristalsis.
- Consult physician about dietary calcium intake and coordinate dietary planning with dietitian, patient, and family.

PODOPHYLLUM RESIN
(pode-oh-fill´um)

Trade names: Pod-Ben-25, Podoben, Podofin
Classifications: SKIN AGENT; KERATOLYTIC AGENT

ACTIONS/PHARMACODYNAMICS Potent cytotoxic and keratolytic agent with caustic action, derived from rhizomes and roots of *Podophyllum peltatum* (mandrake, May apple). Available as a topical solution of podophyllum resin in compound benzoin tincture 10% and alcohol 70.5%. Directly affects epithelial cell metabolism, causing degeneration and arrest of mitosis. Slow disruption of cells and tissue erosion that follows (caustic action) selectively affects embryonic and tumor cells more than adult cells. Inhibits release of iodine from thyrotropin-stimulated thyroid and catecholamine release from adrenal medulla. Binds to tubulin in spindle microtubules, causing disruption of the mitotic spindle and blockade of chromosome movement. In addition, other cellular processes are impaired, leading to destruction of cells and tissues.

USES Benign growths including external genital and perianal warts, papillomas, fibroids.

ROUTE & DOSAGE

Condylomata Acuminata

Adult	Topical	Use 10% solution; repeat 1–2 times/wk for up to 4 applications

Verruca Vulgaris (Common Wart)

Adult	Topical	Use 5% solution, 1–5 applications/d

Multiple Superficial Epitheliomatosis, Keratoses

Adult	Topical	Apply daily for several days

NOTE: Use 10–25% solution for areas <10 cm² or 5% solution for areas of 10–20 cm², anal or genital warts; apply drug to dry surface; allow area to dry between drops; wash off after 1–4 h.

CONTRAINDICATIONS & PRECAUTIONS Contraindicated in: birthmarks, moles, or warts with hair growth from them; cervical, urethral, oral warts; normal skin and mucous membranes peripheral to treated areas; pregnancy; diabetes mellitus; patient with poor circulation; irritated, friable, or bleeding skin; application of drug over large area.

P

ADVERSE/SIDE EFFECTS <u>Severe systemic toxicity</u> (sometimes fatal), sensorimotor neuropathy (reversible), and <u>bone marrow suppression</u> similar to that caused by antineoplastic drug toxicity. Specifically: **CNS:** lethargy, mental confusion, disorientation, delirium, agitation, seizures, progressive stupor, polyneuritis, pyrexia, coma, visual and auditory hallucinations, acute psychotic reaction, ataxia, hypotonia, areflexia, increased CSF protein. **CV:** sinus tachycardia. **Hematologic:** leukopenia, thrombocytopenia. **GI:** *nausea, vomiting, diarrhea, abdominal pain,* hepatotoxicity. **Peripheral neuropathy:** paralytic ileus, urinary retention, symptomatic orthostatic hypotension, paresthesias and weakness of extremities, stocking-glove sensory loss, absent ankle reflexes, decreased response to painful stimuli. **Renal:** <u>renal failure.</u> **Respiratory:** decreased respirations, <u>apnea,</u> hyperventilation. **Other:** increased serum concentrations of LDH, AST, and alkaline phosphatase.

NURSING IMPLICATIONS

Administration

- This potent drug is usually applied by an experienced clinician.
- *CDC-recommended duration of therapy:* no longer than 6 h. Also recommended: 7–10 d should elapse between courses of therapy to decrease the potential for systemic toxicity.
- Podophyllum resin contact with eyes or similar mucosal surfaces should be avoided; should it occur, flush thoroughly with lukewarm water for 15 min and remove film precipitated by the water.
- Avoid application of drug to normal tissue. If it occurs, remove with alcohol. Protect surfaces surrounding area to be treated with a layer of petrolatum or flexible collodion.
- Thorough removal of drug with soap and water should follow each treatment of accessible tissue surface.
- A protective coat of talcum powder may be applied after treatment and drying of anogenital area.
- If application causes extreme pain, pruritus, or swelling, remove drug with alcohol.
- Before reapplication of the drug to a common wart, the clinician may gently remove keratinized surface with smooth surface of an emery board to enhance penetration. One manufacturer recommends that application of solution be followed by covering the wart with a nonporous, slightly elastic tape for up to 24 h. Wart is removed with tape or, if necessary, by curettage.
- Store podophyllum resin in tight, light-resistant container; avoid exposure to excessive heat.

Assessment & Drug Effects

- Treatment for external perianal warts is usually preceded by a proctologic evaluation. Podophyllin is delayed until test results are known.
- Warts become blanched, then necrotic within 24–48 h. Sloughing begins after about 72 h with no scarring. Frequently a mild topical antiinfective agent, with or without a dressing, is applied until the healing is complete.
- Sensorimotor polyneuropathy, if it occurs, appears about 2 wk after application of drug, worsens for 3 mo, and may persist for up to 9 mo. Cerebral effects may persist for 7–10 d; ataxia, hypotonia, and areflexia improve more slowly than effects on sensorium.

Patient & Family Education

- If self-administered as for treatment of verruca vulgaris (common wart), the patient should be thoroughly instructed in the proper technique of treatment. Patient should also be fully aware of the need to report treatment failure.
- As with any STD, the patient's sex partner should be examined.
- *Systemic toxicity:* may be severe and serious and is associated with application of drug to large areas, to tissue that is friable, bleeding, or recently biopsied, or for prolonged time. It may occur within hours of application. When patient is self-medicating with podophyllum resin, stress the dangers of overuse or misuse of the drug.
- Review symptoms of toxicity with patient and advise prompt reporting should they appear. (See adverse/side effects.)

Prototype: psyllium, p 219

POLYCARBOPHIL

(pol-i-kar´boe-fil)

Trade names: FiberCon, Mitrolan
Classifications: GI AGENT; BULK LAXATIVE; ANTIDIARRHEAL
Pregnancy: Category C

ACTIONS/PHARMACODYNAMICS Calcium polycarbophil is hydrophilic. Absorbs free water in intestinal tract and opposes dehydrating forces of bowel by forming a gelatinous mass, thereby restoring more normal moisture level and motility in the lower GI tract. Produces well-formed stool and re-

P

Common side effects in *italic*; life-threatening effects <u>underlined</u>; generic names in **bold**; classifications in SMALL CAPS

897

duces diarrhea. Contains negligible amount of sodium (0.02 mEq, or 0.46% sodium/tablet) and is dextrose free.

USES Constipation or diarrhea associated with acute bowel syndrome, diverticulosis, irritable bowel and in patients who should not strain during defecation. Also choleretic diarrhea, diarrhea caused by small-bowel surgery or vagotomy, and disease of terminal ileum.

ROUTE & DOSAGE

Constipation or Diarrhea

Adult	PO	1 g q.i.d. prn (max 6 g/d)
Child	PO	6–12 y: 500 mg t.i.d. prn (max 3 g/d)
		3–6 y: 500 mg b.i.d. prn (max 1.5 g/d)

PHARMACOKINETICS Absorption: not absorbed from GI tract. **Onset:** 12–24 h. **Peak:** 1–3 d.

CONTRAINDICATIONS & PRECAUTIONS Contraindicated in: partial or complete GI obstruction; fecal impaction; dysphagia; acute abdominal pain; rectal bleeding; undiagnosed abdominal pain, or other symptoms pathognomonic of appendicitis; poisonings; before radiologic bowel examination; bowel surgery. Use in children <3 y not established.

ADVERSE/SIDE EFFECTS GI: esophageal blockage, intestinal impaction, *abdominal fullness*. **Other:** low serum potassium, elevated blood glucose levels (with extended use), asthma, skin rash.

DRUG INTERACTIONS May decrease absorption and clinical effects of ANTIBIOTICS, **warfarin, digoxin, nitrofurantoin,** SALICYLATES.

NURSING IMPLICATIONS

Administration

- Crush tablets before administration or have patient chew tablets well before swallowing.
- Each dose should be administered with a full glass (240 ml [8 oz]) of water or other liquid.
- In severe diarrhea, dose may be repeated every 30 min up to the maximum dose in 24 h.
- Abdominal fullness may be prevented by taking smaller doses more frequently during the day.
- Store in tightly closed container at 15–30C (59–86F) unless otherwise directed.

Assessment & Drug Effects

- If patient is being treated for diarrhea, determine duration and severity of diarrhea before medical treatment in order to anticipate signs of fluid-electrolyte losses.
- Monitor and record number and consistency of stools per day, presence and location of abdominal discomfort (i.e., tenderness, distension), and bowel sounds.
- Monitor and record I&O ratio and pattern. Dehydration is indicated if urine specific gravity is >1,030 and if output is <30 ml/h.
- Daily weights provide a rough estimate of fluid loss.
- Dehydration from an episode of diarrhea appears rapidly in young children and the elderly. Inspect oral cavity for dryness, and be alert to systemic signs (e.g., thirst and fever).

Patient & Family Education

- If sudden changes in bowel habit persist more than 1 wk, action is minimal or ineffective for 1 wk, or if there is no antidiarrheal action within 2 d, consult physician.
- Extended use may cause dependence on the drug for normal bowel function.
- Diet and exercise as well as medication are important in a plan designed to restore a more normal bowel habit.
- If patient is also taking an oral anticoagulant, digoxin, salicylates, or nitrofurantoin, warn against discontinuing polycarbophil unless physician advises patient to do so. Established serum concentrations (and drug effects) may be altered by physical binding of any of these drugs to polycarbophil.
- This OTC medication is packaged with manufacturer's directions for use. Inform patient of this and review them with patient if necessary.

Prototype: estradiol, p 236

POLYESTRADIOL PHOSPHATE

(pol-ee-ess-tra-dye´ole)
Trade name: Estradurin
Classifications: ANTINEOPLASTIC; ESTROGEN HORMONE
Pregnancy: Category X

ACTIONS/PHARMACODYNAMICS Estrogen derivative. Provides a continuous active level of exogenous estradiol that functions to alter the hor-

P

monal milieu of a tumor originating from hormone-responsive tissue. Suppresses pituitary secretion of luteinizing or interstitial cell stimulating hormone (LH), an action that in turn depresses ("turns off") an androgen secretion by the testes (antitumor effect). Tumor growth is interrupted, but existing neoplastic cells are not killed.

USES Palliative treatment of an inoperable, progressing prostatic carcinoma.

ROUTE & DOSAGE

Prostatic Carcinoma

Adult	IM	40 mg q2–4wk or less frequently depending on response; may increase dose up to 80 mg

PHARMACOKINETICS Absorption: readily absorbed from IM site; leaves bloodstream within 24 h. **Distribution:** stored in reticuloendothelial system. **Metabolism:** metabolized in liver. **Elimination:** excreted in bile and urine.

CONTRAINDICATIONS & PRECAUTIONS Contraindicated in: men with known or suspected cancer of the breast except in appropriately selected patients being treated for metastatic disease; known or suspected estrogen-dependent neoplasm; active thromboembolic disorders. **Cautious use in:** hypertension; gallbladder disease; diabetes mellitus; heart failure; hepatic or renal dysfunction.

ADVERSE/SIDE EFFECTS CNS: headache, dizziness, depression, libido changes. **CV:** thromboembolic disorders, *hypertension.* **GI:** *nausea,* vomiting, diarrhea, anorexia, weight changes, bloating, cholestatic jaundice. **GU:** mastodynia gynecomastia, impotence, testicular atrophy. **Metabolic:** reduced carbohydrate tolerance, hypercalcemia, *fluid retention.* **Other:** leg cramps.

NURSING IMPLICATIONS

Administration

▪ Reconstitution of IM solution: introduce sterile diluent into vial of drug powder using a 20-gauge needle and 5 ml syringe. Swirl gently to produce clear solution; do not shake vigorously. Discard cloudy solution.
▪ Administer drug deeply into large muscle mass (e.g., gluteus maximus). A transitory burning sensation may occur, but this usually does not continue with subsequent doses. If it continues, there-

after the dose may be given with a local anesthetic. Consult physician.
▪ Increasing the dosage prolongs action but does not increase blood level.
▪ Store lyophilized powder and reconstituted solution at 15–30C (59–86F) away from direct light. Stability remains about 10 d, as long as solution is clear.

Patient & Family Education

▪ Clinical response should be apparent within 3 mo. Hormone is usually continued until disease is again progressive, then stopped.
▪ Teach patient how to elicit **Homans' sign:** pain in calf and popliteal region with forced dorsiflexion of foot (early sign of thrombosis).
▪ Instruct patient to report a positive Homans' sign and the following symptoms of thromboembolic disorders immediately: tenderness, swelling, and redness in extremity; sudden, severe headache or chest pain, slurring of speech; change in vision; tenderness, pain, sudden shortness of breath. If physician is not available, patient should go to the nearest hospital emergency room.

POLYMYXIN B SULFATE

(pol-i-mix´in)
Trade name: Aerosporin
Classifications: ANTIINFECTIVE; ANTIBIOTIC
Pregnancy: Category B

ACTIONS/PHARMACODYNAMICS Basic polypeptide antibiotic of the polymyxin group derived from strains of *Bacillus polymyxa.* Binds to lipid phosphates in bacterial membranes and, through cationic detergent action, changes permeability to permit leakage of cytoplasm. Bactericidal against susceptible gram negative organisms, particularly most strains of *Escherichia coli, Haemophilus influenzae, Enterobacter aerogenes,* and *Klebsiella pneumoniae.* Most species of *Proteus* and *Neisseria* are resistant, as are all gram-positive organisms and fungi. Spectrum of antibacterial activity is similar to that of colistin derivatives; both cross-resistance and cross-sensitivity reported. Neuromuscular blocking action usually associated with high serum levels, intracellular potassium deficit, or low serum calcium concentration.

USES Topically and in combination with other antiinfectives or corticosteroids for various superficial in-

P

Common side effects in *italic*; life-threatening effects <u>underlined</u>; generic names in **bold**; classifications in SMALL CAPS

899

fections of eye, ear, mucous membrane, and skin. Concurrent systemic antiinfective therapy may be required for treatment of intraocular infection and severe progressive corneal ulcer. Used parenterally only in hospitalized patients for treatment of severe acute infections of urinary tract, bloodstream, and meninges; and in combination with neosporin for continuous bladder irrigation to prevent bacteremia associated with use of indwelling catheter.

ROUTE & DOSAGE

Infections

Adult	IV	15,000–25,000 U/kg/d divided q12h
	IM	25,000–30,000 U/kg/d divided q4–6h
	GU	1 ml/L 0.9% NaCl q24h
	Topical	1–2 drops in eye q1h
Child	IV	15,000–25,000 U/kg/d divided q12h
	IM	25,000–30,000 U/kg/d divided q4–6h

PHARMACOKINETICS Absorption: not absorbed from GI tract. **Peak:** 2 h IM. **Distribution:** widely distributed except to CSF, synovial fluid, and eye; does not cross placenta. **Metabolism:** unknown. **Elimination:** half-life: 4.3–6 h; 60% excreted unchanged in urine.

CONTRAINDICATIONS & PRECAUTIONS Contraindicated in: hypersensitivity to polymyxin antibiotics; concurrent and sequential use of other nephrotoxic and neurotoxic drugs; concurrent use of skeletal muscle relaxants, ether, or sodium citrate. Safe use during pregnancy (category B) not established. **Cautious use in:** impaired renal function; myasthenia gravis.

ADVERSE/SIDE EFFECTS CNS: irritability, facial flushing, drowsiness, dizziness, vertigo, ataxia, circumoral, lingual, and peripheral paresthesias (stocking-glove distribution); blurred vision, nystagmus, slurred speech, dysphagia, ototoxicity (vestibular and auditory) with high doses; convulsions, coma; neuromuscular blockade (generalized muscle weakness, respiratory depression or arrest); meningeal irritation, increased protein and cell count in cerebrospinal fluid, fever, headache, stiff neck (intrathecal use). **Hypersensitivity:** drug fever, dermatoses, pruritus, urticaria, local irritation and burning (topical use), eosinophilia, anaphylactoid reaction (rarely). **Nephrotoxicity:** rising blood drug levels without increase in dosage; albuminuria, cylinduria, azotemia, hematuria. **Other:** GI disturbances, severe pain (IM site), thrombophlebitis (IV site), superinfections, electrolyte disturbances (prolonged use; also reported in patients with acute leukemia).

DRUG INTERACTIONS ANESTHETICS and NEUROMUSCULAR BLOCKING AGENTS may prolong skeletal muscle relaxation. AMINOGLYCOSIDES and **amphotericin B** have additive nephrotoxic potential.

INCOMPATIBILITIES Solution/Additive: amphotericin B, cephalothin, chloramphenicol, chlorothiazide, heparin, magnesium sulfate, prednisolone, sodium phosphate, tetracycline.

NURSING IMPLICATIONS

Administration

- When drug is given IM or intrathecally, it should be given only to hospitalized patients, where constant supervision can be provided by physicians.
- Routine administration by IM route not recommended because it causes intense discomfort, particularly in infants and children. Pain, described as "aching" or "drawing," radiates along peripheral nerve distribution, 40–60 min after IM injection. Addition of procaine 1% (if hospital policy permits) may prevent its occurrence. Note: procaine must not be used for IV or intrathecal administration.
- In adults, IM injection should be made deep into upper outer quadrant of buttock. Select IM site carefully to avoid injection into nerves or blood vessels. Rotate injection sites. Follow agency policy for IM site used in children.
- To reconstitute for IV administration, dissolve 500,000 U in 5 ml sterile water for injection or NS to yield 100,000 U/ml. Withdraw a single dose and then further dilute the dose in 300–500 ml of D5W. Infuse over period of 60–90 min. Inspect injection site for signs of phlebitis and irritation.
- Protect unreconstituted product and reconstituted solution from light and freezing. Store in refrigerator at 2–8C (36–46F). Parenteral solutions are stable for 1 wk when refrigerated. Discard unused portion after 72 h.

Assessment & Drug Effects

- Culture and susceptibility tests should be done prior to first dose and periodically thereafter to determine continuing sensitivity of causative organisms.
- Baseline serum electrolytes and renal function tests should be performed before parenteral therapy. Frequent monitoring of renal function and serum drug levels is advised during therapy.

P

Common side effects in *italic*; life-threatening effects underlined; generic names in **bold**; classifications in SMALL CAPS

- Electrolytes should be monitored at regular intervals during prolonged therapy. Patients with low serum calcium and low intracellular potassium are particularly prone to develop neuromuscular blockade.
- Dosage is reduced (as indicated by creatinine clearance) in the patient with renal impairment.
- Inspect tongue every day. Assess for signs and symptoms of superinfection (see Chapter 3). Polymyxin therapy supports the growth of opportunistic organisms. Report symptoms promptly.
- Some degree of renal toxicity usually occurs within first 3 or 4 d of therapy even with therapeutic doses. Monitor I & O. Fluid intake should be sufficient to maintain daily urinary output of at least 1500 ml. Consult physician.
- Decreases in urine output (change in I & O ratio), proteinuria, cellular casts, rising BUN, serum creatinine, or serum drug levels (not associated with dosage increase) can be interpreted as signs of nephrotoxicity. If any of these signs occur, withhold drug and report findings to physician.
- Nephrotoxicity is generally reversible, but it may progress even after drug is discontinued. Therefore, close monitoring of kidney function is essential, even following termination of therapy.
- Respiratory arrest has occurred with first dose and also as long as 45 d after initiation of therapy. It occurs most commonly in patients with renal failure and high plasma drug levels and is often preceded by dyspnea and restlessness.

Patient & Family Education
- Encourage to report immediately muscle weakness, shortness of breath, dyspnea, depressed respiration. These symptoms are rapidly reversible if drug is withdrawn immediately. Resuscitative equipment, oxygen, and IV $CaCl_2$ should be available at all times.
- Eyelid irritation, itching and burning with ophthalmic drops should be reported promptly to the physician. Stop drug administration immediately.
- Transient neurologic disturbances (paresthesias, numbness, dizziness) occur commonly and usually respond to dosage reduction. Report promptly.
- Warn to report promptly onset of stiff neck and headache (possible symptoms of neurotoxic reactions, including neuromuscular blockade). This response is usually associated with high serum drug levels and/or nephrotoxicity.
- Instruct patient to promptly report signs and symptoms of superinfection (see Chapter 3).

Prototype: hydrochlorothiazide, p 203

POLYTHIAZIDE
(pol-i-thye´a-zide)
Trade name: Renese
Classifications: ELECTROLYTIC & WATER BALANCE AGENT; THIAZIDE DIURETIC; ANTIHYPERTENSIVE
Pregnancy: Category D

ACTIONS/PHARMACODYNAMICS Benzothiadiazine (thiazide) derivative. Similar to hydrochlorothiazide in actions, uses, contraindications, adverse reactions, and interactions.

USES Primary agent in stepped care approach to antihypertensive treatment and adjunctively in the management of edema associated with CHF, renal pathology, and hepatic cirrhosis. Available in fixed combination with prazosin (Minizide) and with reserpine (Renese-R).

ROUTE & DOSAGE

Edema

Adult	PO	1–4 mg/d *or* q.o.d.

Hypertension

Adult	PO	2–4 mg/d
Child	PO	0.02–0.08 mg/kg/d

PHARMACOKINETICS Onset: 2 h. **Peak:** 6 h. **Duration:** 24–48 h. **Distribution:** distributed throughout extracellular tissue; concentrates in kidney; crosses placenta; distributed into breast milk. **Metabolism:** does not appear to be metabolized. **Elimination:** excreted in urine.

CONTRAINDICATIONS & PRECAUTIONS Contraindicated in: hypersensitivity to other thiazides or sulfonamides; anuria, pregnancy (category D), nursing mothers. **Cautious use in:** renal and hepatic dysfunction, SLE, gout, diabetes mellitus.

ADVERSE/SIDE EFFECTS <u>Agranulocytosis</u>, vascular thrombosis, *hyperuricemia, hypokalemia, hyperglycemia,* orthostatic hypotension, hepatic encephalopathy, photosensitivity.

P

DRUG INTERACTIONS Amphotericin B, CORTI-COSTEROIDS increase hypokalemic effects; may antagonize hypoglycemic effects of **insulin,** SUL-FONYL-UREAS; **cholestyramine, colistipol** decrease thiazide absorption; intensifies hypoglycemic and hypotensive effects of **diazoxide.** Increased potassium and magnesium loss may cause **digoxin** toxicity; decreases **lithium** excretion, increasing its toxicity; NSAIDS may attenuate diuresis and increased risk of NSAID-induced renal failure.

NURSING IMPLICATIONS

Administration

- Administer drug early in AM after eating (to reduce gastric irritation) and to prevent interrupted sleep because of diuresis.
- Store drug in tightly closed container at 15–30C (59–86F) unless otherwise instructed.

Assessment & Drug Effects

- Elderly patients may be more sensitive to the average adult therapeutic dose. Excessive diuresis may induce sudden hypotension and serious electrolyte imbalance.
- Antihypertensive effects may be noted in 3–4 d; maximal effects may require 3–4 wk. Effects persist for at least 1 wk after drug is discontinued.
- Monitor for signs and symptoms of hypokalemia and hyperglycemia (see chap 3).
- Monitor serum electrolytes and blood glucose periodically.

Patient & Family Education

- If orthostatic hypotension is a clinical problem, instruct patient to change from recumbency to upright positions slowly and in stages; to avoid hot baths or showers, extended exposure to sunlight, and standing still.
- Urge patient to include specific sources of potassium in daily diet such as a banana (about 370 mg potassium) and at least 180 ml (6 oz) orange juice (about 330 mg potassium).
- Advise patient to maintain prescribed dosage regimen.
- Warn patient about the possibility of photosensitivity reaction and instruct him or her to notify physician if it occurs. Thiazide-related photosensitivity is considered a photoallergy (ultraviolet radiation changes drug structure and makes it allergenic for some individuals) and occurs 10–14 d after initial sun exposure. Advise use of a sunscreen lotion with a high SPF (12–15).
- Counsel patient to avoid OTC drugs unless approved by the physician. Many preparations contain both potassium and sodium and if misused or if patient overdoses, electrolyte side effects could be induced.

POTASSIUM CHLORIDE
(poe-tass´ee-um)
Trade names: Apo-K, K-10, Kalium Durules Kaochlor, Kaochlor-20 Concentrate, Kaon-Cl, Kato, Kay Ciel, KCl 5% and 20%, K-Long, K-Lor, Klor-10%, KLOR-Con, Kloride, Klorvess, Klotrix, K-DUR, K-Lyte/Cl, K-tab, Micro-K Extentabs, Novolente K, Pan-Kloride, Roychlor 10% and 20%, Rum-K, SK-Potassium Chloride, Slo-Pot, Slow-K

POTASSIUM GLUCONATE

Trade names: Kalinate, Kaon, Kao-Nor, Kaylixir, K-G Elixir, Potassium Rougier, Royonate
Classifications: ELECTROLYTIC & WATER BALANCE AGENT; REPLACEMENT SOLUTION
Pregnancy: Category A

ACTIONS/PHARMACODYNAMICS Potassium, the principal intracellular cation, is essential for maintenance of intracellular isotonicity, transmission of nerve impulses, contraction of cardiac, skeletal, and smooth muscles, maintenance of normal renal function, and for enzyme activity. In the steady state, potassium movement is physiologically coupled with that of sodium; entry of potassium into cells is associated with energy-driven extrusion of sodium from cell; potassium secretion-excretion in distal convoluted tubule is accompanied by sodium resorption. Normally, intracellular concentration is about 150 mEq/L; plasma concentration (adult) is 3.5–5 mEq/L (neonate, 7.7 mEq/L). Plays a prominent role in both genesis and correction of imbalances in acid-base metabolism; thus, potassium salts assume special importance as therapeutic agents but are also dangerous if improperly prescribed and administered.

USES To prevent and treat potassium deficit secondary to diuretic or corticosteroid therapy. Also indicated when potassium is depleted by severe vomiting, diarrhea; intestinal drainage, fistulas, or malabsorption; prolonged diuresis, diabetic acidosis.

Effective in the treatment of hypokalemic alkalosis (chloride, not the gluconate).

ROUTE & DOSAGE

Hypokalemia

Adult	PO	10–100 mEq/d in divided doses
	IV	10–40 mEq/h diluted to at least 10–20 mEq/100 ml of solution to a max of 200–400 mEq/d; monitor higher doses carefully
Child	PO	1–3 mEq/kg/d in divided doses; extended release tablets not recommended in children
	IV	up to 3 mEq/kg/24 h at a rate ≤ 0.02 mEq/kg/min

PHARMACOKINETICS Absorption: readily absorbed from upper GI tract. **Elimination:** 90% excreted in urine, 10% in feces.

CONTRAINDICATIONS & PRECAUTIONS Contraindicated in: severe renal impairment; severe hemolytic reactions; untreated Addison's disease; crush syndrome; early postoperative oliguria (except during GI drainage); adynamic ileus; acute dehydration; heat cramps, hyperkalemia, patients receiving potassium-sparing diuretics, digitalis intoxication with AV conduction disturbance. **Cautious use in:** cardiac or renal disease; systemic acidosis; slow-release potassium preparations in presence of delayed GI transit or Meckel's diverticulum; extensive tissue breakdown (such as severe burns); pregnancy (category A).

ADVERSE/SIDE EFFECTS *Nausea, vomiting,* diarrhea, abdominal distension and pain, skin rash (rare), oliguria. Hyperkalemia (serum potassium > 5.5 mEq/L): mental confusion, irritability, listlessness, paresthesias of extremities, muscle weakness and heaviness of limbs, difficulty in swallowing, <u>flaccid paralysis</u>, anuria, <u>respiratory distress</u>, hypotension, bradycardia; <u>cardiac depression, arrhythmias, or arrest</u>; altered sensitivity to digitalis glycosides. *ECG changes in hyperkalemia:* tenting (peaking) of T wave (especially in right precordial leads), lowering of R with deepening of S waves and depression of RST; prolonged P-R interval, widened QRS complex, decreased amplitude and disappearance of P waves, prolonged Q-T interval, signs of right and left bundle block, <u>deterioration of QRS contour and finally ventricular fibrillation and death.</u>

DRUG INTERACTIONS POTASSIUM-SPARING DIURETICS, ANGIOTENSIN-CONVERTING ENZYME (ACE) INHIBITORS may cause hyperkalemia.

INCOMPATIBILITIES Solution/additive: amphotericin B, dobutamine (potassium phosphate only). **Y-site: diazepam, ergotamine, methylprednisolone, phenytoin, promethazine.**

NURSING IMPLICATIONS

Administration

- Some patients find it difficult to swallow the large sized KCl tablet. Administer while patient is sitting up or standing (never in recumbent position) to prevent drug-induced esophagitis.
- No potassium salt tablets should be crushed and then taken dry or chewed. Be certain patient does not suck tablet (oral ulcerations have been reported if tablet is allowed to dissolve in mouth). Whole tablet should be swallowed with large glass of water or fruit juice (if allowed) to wash drug down and to start esophageal peristalsis.
- Follow instructions regarding dilution. In general, each 20 mEq potassium (chloride, gluconate) should be diluted in at least 90 ml water or juice. Liquids, powders, and effervescent tablets must be completely dissolved in a large glass of water or fruit juice before administration. Allow "fizzing" to stop before giving to patient to sip slowly with meal or immediately after eating over 5–10 min. Dilution minimizes saline cathartic effect, gastric distress, and unpleasant taste.
- Dilute elixir as directed before giving it through nasogastric tube.
- An antacid may improve the tolerance of KCl by decreasing its irritating effect on GI mucosa; 10 ml KCl flavored syrup mixed with 15 ml antacid has given relief. Consult physician.
- If potassium supplement is given in conjunction with a diuretic, it may be preferable to give the potassium on days other than when diuretic is given.
- KCl is never administered by IV "push" or IM or in concentrated amounts by any route. Add the drug to infusion fluid with plastic bag in upright (noninfusion) position to prevent delivery of excessive amount of KCl in first few minutes of the treatment.
- For IV infusion add desired amount to 100–1000 ml IV solution (compatible with all standard solutions). Usual maximum is 40 mEq/1000 ml. When IV concentration is 40 mEq/L or more, there is danger of irritation to veins.

P

Common side effects in *italic*; life-threatening effects <u>underlined</u>; generic names in **bold**; classifications in SMALL CAPS

903

- Infuse IV KCl at rate not to exceed 20 mEq/h.
- Potassium infusion should be administered slowly to prevent fatal hyperkalemia. Flow rate will be prescribed according to serial ECG and serum electrolyte determinations.
- Discontinue KCl and notify physician if oliguria develops.
- Extreme care should be taken to prevent extravasation and infiltration. Palpate entry site occasionally to confirm needle position. At first sign, discontinue infusion and immediately remove needle or catheter.
- *Treatment of potassium intoxication:* eliminate all potassium-containing foods and medications. Have available parenteral calcium to overcome cardiotoxicity (not used in patient receiving digitalis); parenteral sodium bicarbonate, glucose infusion with regular insulin (facilitates shift of potassium into cell), cation exchange resins (hasten potassium elimination). Hemodialysis and peritoneal dialysis may be required.
- Color in some commercial oral solutions fades with exposure to light, but drug effectiveness is reportedly not altered.
- Unless manufacturer advises otherwise, store all preparations of KCl at 15–30C (59–86F). Protect from light, and do not freeze.

Assessment & Drug Effects

- Monitor I&O ratio and pattern in patients receiving the parenteral drug. If oliguria occurs, stop infusion promptly and notify physician.
- Use of extended-release tablets reduces the danger of bowel ulcerations and potential compliance problems. However, esophageal and gastric ulceration in cardiac patients with esophageal compression from left atrial enlargement have been reported with use of this formulation. Report signs (esophageal or epigastric pain or hematemesis). A liquid preparation in such a patient could be more tolerable.
- Irregular heartbeat is usually the earliest clinical indication of hyperkalemia. Care of patient receiving parenteral potassium demands close surveillance of the cardiac monitor.
- The risk of hyperkalemia with potassium supplement increases (1) in the elderly because of decremental changes in kidney function associated with aging, (2) when dietary intake of potassium suddenly increases, and (3) when renal function is significantly compromised.
- Potassium intoxication (hyperkalemia, see Signs & Symptoms, chap 3) may result from any therapeutic dosage, and the patient may be asymptomatic. Monitoring of potassium is of extreme importance.

Patient & Family Education

- The extended-release tablet (e.g., Slow-K) utilizes a wax matrix as carrier for KCl crystals. After absorption of drug, the tablet carcass appears in the stool. Inform the patient that this is no cause for alarm.
- When potassium supplement is prescribed, compliance may be a problem because of unpalatability, gastric distress following ingestion of drug, or mental confusion (associated with hypokalemia). Teach patient and family importance of this drug and adherence to established dose regimen.
- Before discharge from medical supervision, help patient to design an acceptable, feasible dosing schedule for KCl and other drugs being taken concomitantly (e.g., digitalis, diuretics).
- Patient should be well informed about sources of potassium with special reference to foods and OTC drugs.
- Avoid licorice; large amounts can cause both hypokalemia and sodium retention.
- Salt substitutes contain a substantial amount of potassium and electrolytes other than sodium. Instruct patient not to use any substitute unless it is specifically ordered by the physician.
- Caution patient not to self-prescribe laxatives. Chronic laxative use has been associated with diarrhea-induced potassium loss.
- Large losses of potassium can also occur because of persistent vomiting. If this occurs, notify physician.
- Urge patient on long-term replacement therapy to report continuing signs of potassium deficit: weakness, fatigue, polyuria, polydipsia.
- Counsel patient to assume responsibility for informing dentist or new physician that a potassium drug has been prescribed as maintenance therapy.
- Foil-wrapped powders and tablets should not be opened before use.

Prototype: Guaifenesin, p 99

POTASSIUM IODIDE

Trade names: Iosat, Pima, SSKI
Classifications: EXPECTORANT; ANTITHYROID AGENT
Pregnancy: Category D

Common side effects in *italic*; life-threatening effects underlined; generic names in **bold**; classifications in SMALL CAPS

ACTIONS/PHARMACODYNAMICS Pharmacologic use primarily related to iodide portion of molecule. Exact mechanism not clear but it is believed that by direct action on bronchial tissue, potassium iodide (KI) increases secretion of respiratory fluids, thereby decreasing mucus viscosity. If patient is euthyroid, excess iodide (i.e., beyond dietary intake) causes minimal change in thyroid gland mass. Conversely, when thyroid is hyperplastic, excess iodide temporarily inhibits secretion of thyroid hormone, fosters colloid accumulation in thyroid follicles, and decreases vascularity of gland. "Escape" from temporary effects (i.e., return of thyrotoxic symptoms) may occur after 10–14 d continuous treatment; consequently iodide administration for hyperthyroidism is limited to short-term therapy. KI oral solution is an aqueous solution of the drug: a clear liquid with a characteristic strong, salty taste (97–103 g KI/100 ml). Strong iodine solution (Lugol's solution) is an aqueous solution containing 4.5–5.5 g iodine and 9.5–10.5 g of KI/100 ml. This solution is transparent, dark brown and has an odor of iodine. KI saturated solution (SSKI): 1 g/ml. KI contains 6 mEq (234 mg) of potassium per gram.

USES To facilitate bronchial drainage and cough in emphysema, asthma, chronic bronchitis, bronchiectasis, and respiratory tract allergies characterized by difficult-to-raise sputum. Also used alone for hyperthyroidism or in conjunction with antithyroid drugs and propranolol in treatment of thyrotoxic crisis; in immediate preoperative period for thyroidectomy to decrease vascularity, fragility, and size of thyroid gland and for treatment of persistent or recurring hyperthyroidism that occurs in Graves' disease patients. Used as a radiation protectant in patients receiving radioactive iodine and to shield the thyroid from radiation in the wake of a serious nuclear plant accident. (Use as an expectorant has been largely replaced by other agents.)

PHARMACOKINETICS Absorption: adequately absorbed from GI tract. **Distribution:** crosses placenta. **Elimination:** cleared from plasma by renal excretion or thyroid uptake.

CONTRAINDICATIONS & PRECAUTIONS Contraindicated in: hypersensitivity or idiosyncrasy to iodine; hyperthyroidism; hyperkalemia; acute bronchitis. Safe use during pregnancy (category D) and in nursing mothers and children not established. **Cautious use in:** renal impairment; cardiac disease; pulmonary tuberculosis; Addison's disease.

ROUTE & DOSAGE

To Reduce Thyroid Vascularity

Adult	PO	50–250 mg t.i.d. for 10–14 d before surgery
Child	PO	Same as for adult

Expectorant

Adult	PO	300–650 mg p.c. b.i.d. or t.i.d.
Child	PO	60–250 mg p.c. b.i.d. or t.i.d.

Thyroid Blocking in Radiation Emergency

Adult	PO	130 mg/d for 10 d
Child	PO	>1 y: 130 mg/d for 10 d
		<1 y: 65 mg/d for 10 d

Adjunct to Management of Thyroid Crisis

Adult	IV	500 mg q4h

ADVERSE/SIDE EFFECTS GI: *diarrhea, nausea, vomiting, stomach pain,* nonspecific small bowel lesions (associated with enteric coated tablets). **Hypersensitivity:** angioneurotic edema, cutaneous and mucosal hemorrhage, fever, arthralgias, lymph node enlargement, eosinophilia. **Iodine poisoning (iodism):** metallic taste, stomatitis, salivation, coryza, sneezing; swollen and tender salivary glands (sialadenitis), frontal headache, vomiting (blue vomitus if stomach contained starches, otherwise yellow vomitus), bloody diarrhea. **Metabolic:** hyperthyroid adenoma, goiter, hypothyroidism, collagen disease–like syndromes. **Other:** irregular heart beat, mental confusion, acneiform skin lesions (prolonged use), weakness, paresthesias, productive cough, pulmonary edema, periorbital edema, flare-up of adolescent acne.

DIAGNOSTIC TEST INTERFERENCES Potassium iodide may alter *thyroid function* test results and may interfere with *urinary 17-OHCS* determinations.

DRUG INTERACTIONS ANTITHYROID DRUGS, **lithium** may potentiate hypothyroid and goitrogenic actions; POTASSIUM-SPARING DIURETICS, POTASSIUM SUPPLEMENTS, ACE INHIBITORS increase risk of hyperkalemia.

NURSING IMPLICATIONS

Administration

- To disguise salty taste and to minimize gastric distress, drug is taken with meals in a full glass (240 ml) of water or fruit juice and at bedtime with food or juice.

Common side effects in *italic*; life-threatening effects underlined; generic names in **bold**; classifications in SMALL CAPS

905

- Enteric-coated tablets are not commonly used because they reportedly cause small-bowel lesions and possibly obstruction, perforation, and hemorrhage. If patient is using this form, instruct him or her to swallow tablet whole and not to crush or chew it. Precede swallowing with a swallow of fluid; then take tablet with a full glass of water (or other fluid).
- Avoid giving KI with milk; absorption of the drug may be decreased by dairy products.
- When iodide is administered to prepare thyroid gland for surgery, strict adherence to schedule and accurate dose measurements are essential, particularly at end of treatment period when possibility of "escape" (from iodide) effect on thyroid gland increases.
- If crystals form in the solution, they may be dissolved by placing container in warm water and gently agitating it.
- Solutions may turn brownish yellow on standing, especially if exposed to light, because of liberated trace of free iodine. Discard such solutions.
- Store in airtight, light-resistant container at 15–30C (59–86F) unless otherwise directed.

Assessment & Drug Effects

- Serum potassium levels should be determined before and periodically during therapy. **(Normal serum potassium:** 3.6–5.5 mEq/L.)
- Keep physician informed about characteristics of sputum: quantity, consistency, color.

Patient & Family Education

- Advise patient to report promptly the occurrence of GI bleeding, abdominal pain, distension, nausea, or vomiting.
- Instruct patient to report clinical signs of iodism (see adverse/side effects). Usually symptoms will subside with dose reduction and lengthened intervals between doses.
- Foods rich in iodine to be avoided if patient develops iodism are vegetables growing near seacoast, seafoods, fish liver oils, iodized salt.
- Sudden withdrawal following prolonged use may precipitate thyroid storm.
- Warn patient to avoid use of OTC drugs without consulting physician. Many preparations contain iodides and could augment prescribed dose, e.g., cough syrups, gargles, asthma medication, salt substitutes, cod liver oil, multiple vitamins (often suspended in iodide solutions).
- Impress on the patient taking KI as an expectorant that optimum hydration is the best expectorant. Encourage increased daily fluid intake.

POVIDONE-IODINE

(poe´vi-done eye´oh-din)

Trade names: Acu-dyne, Betadine, Biodine, Bridine, Efodine, Frepp, Iodex, Isodine, Operand, Proviodine

Classifications: SKIN & MUCOUS MEMBRANE AGENT; ANTIINFECTIVE

Pregnancy: Category D

ACTIONS/PHARMACODYNAMICS Water-soluble iodine complex (iodophor) with nonselective broad microbiocidal spectrum that includes gram-positive, gram-negative, and antibiotic-resistant organisms, fungi, viruses, protozoa, and yeast. On contact with skin, liberates free iodine; maintains germicidal action in presence of blood, serum, and pus. Unlike iodine, it is virtually nonstinging and nonirritating to skin and mucous membrane and nonstaining to skin and clothing. Reportedly not as effective as aqueous solutions or tincture of iodine.

USES Prevention and treatment of surface infections, as antiseptic for burns, lacerations, abrasions, and other minor wounds, and in management of vaginitis (monilial, trichomonas vaginalis, and nonspecific forms).

ROUTE & DOSAGE

Prevention and Treatment of Surface Infections

Adult	Topical	Apply to area as needed

CONTRAINDICATIONS & PRECAUTIONS Contraindicated in: sensitivity to iodine; use as vaginal antiseptic during pregnancy (category D). **Cautious use in:** extensive burns; particularly in patients with metabolic acidosis or renal dysfunction.

ADVERSE/SIDE EFFECTS Systemic absorption can occur with extensive burns: ioderma, metabolic acidosis, renal impairment.

DIAGNOSTIC TEST INTERFERENCES Urine contaminated with povidone-iodine (as might occur following surgical skin prep or vaginal use) can cause false-positive test for **occult blood.** There is possibility of interference with **PBI** levels (study results are conflicting).

NURSING IMPLICATIONS

Administration

- Treated areas can be bandaged.
- Avoid contact with eyes.

P

Assessment & Drug Effects

- Question patient about iodine hypersensitivity before application. Do not use with history of iodine sensitivity.
- Use should be discontinued if irritation, redness, or swelling develops.

PRALIDOXIME CHLORIDE
(pra-li-dox´eem)
Trade names: PAM, Protopam Chloride
Classification: ANTIDOTE
Pregnancy: Category C

ACTIONS/PHARMACODYNAMICS Quaternary ammonium oxime. Reactivates cholinesterase inhibited by phosphate esters (e.g., organophosphorous insecticides and related compounds) by displacing the enzyme from its receptor sites; the free enzyme then can resume its function of degrading accumulated acetylcholine, thereby restoring normal neuromuscular transmission. Less effective against carbamate anticholinesterases (ambenonium, neostigmine, pyridostigmine). More active against effects of anticholinesterases at skeletal neuromuscular junction than at autonomic effector sites or in CNS respiratory center; therefore, atropine must be given concomitantly to block effects of acetylcholine and accumulation in these sites. Effective against nicotinic effects of anticholinesterase poisoning (muscle twitching, fasciculations, cramps, weakness), but action against muscarinic effects (bronchoconstriction, increased secretions, diarrhea) is less striking than that of atropine.

USES As antidote in treatment of poisoning by organophosphate insecticides and pesticides with anticholinesterase activity (e.g., parathion, TEPP, sarin) and to control overdosage by anticholinesterase drugs used in treatment of myasthenia gravis (cholinergic crisis). **Unlabeled use:** to reverse toxicity of echothiophate ophthalmic solution.

PHARMACOKINETICS Peak: 5–15 min IV; 10–20 min IM. **Distribution:** distributed throughout extracellular fluids; crosses blood-brain barrier slowly if at all. **Metabolism:** probably metabolized in liver. **Elimination:** half-life: 0.8–2.7 h; rapidly excreted in urine.

CONTRAINDICATIONS & PRECAUTIONS Contraindicated in: use in poisoning by carbamate insecticide Sevin, inorganic phosphates, or organophosphates having no anticholinesterase activity; asthma, peptic ulcer, severe cardiac disease, patients receiving aminophylline, theophylline, morphine, succinyl choline, reserpine, or phenothiazines. Safe use during pregnancy (category C) not established. **Cautious use in:** myasthenia gravis; renal insufficiency; concomitant use of barbiturates in organophosphorous poisoning.

ROUTE & DOSAGE

Organophosphate Poisoning

Adult	IV	1–2 g in 100 ml NS infused over 15–30 min; or 1–2 g as 5% solution in sterile water over not less than 5 min; may repeat after 1 h if muscle weakness not relieved
	IM/SC	1–2 g if IV route is not feasible
Child	IV	20–40 mg/kg as for adult

Anticholinesterase Overdose In Myasthenia Gravis

Adult	IV	1–2 g in 100 ml NS infused over 15–30 min, followed by increments of 250 mg q5min prn

---

ADVERSE/SIDE EFFECTS Most commonly following IV use (usually mild and transient): *dizziness, nausea, blurred vision, diplopia, impaired accommodation, tachycardia, hypertension* (dose-related), *hyperventilation, headache, drowsiness, muscular weakness.* **With rapid IV:** tachycardia, <u>laryngospasm</u>, muscle rigidity.

NURSING IMPLICATIONS

Administration

- Generally used only in hospitalized patients. Have on hand respirator, suction apparatus, tracheostomy set, oxygen, IV sodium thiopental (2.5% solution) for control of convulsions, atropine, gastric lavage equipment for ingested poison.
- Treatment is most effective if started within a few hours after organophosphate poisoning has occurred. If exposure to poison was through skin, initial measures should include removal of contaminated clothing and washing skin thoroughly with sodium bicarbonate solution or alcohol.
- Pralidoxime is started at the same time as atropine. Atropine sulfate 2–4 mg (adults) or 0.5–1 mg (children) is given IV (given IM if cyanosis is present) at 5–10-min intervals until signs of atropinism appear: flushing, dry mouth and throat, dilated pupils, rapid pulse, restlessness, disorientation.

P

Common side effects in *italic*; life-threatening effects <u>underlined</u>; generic names in **bold**; classifications in SMALL CAPS

907

Some degree of atropinism is usually maintained for at least 48 h.

- Reconstitute 1 g vial by adding 20 ml NS to produce a concentration of 50 mg/ml (a 5% solution). If pulmonary edema is present, give without further dilution slowly by direct IV over at least 5 min.
- Reconstituted solution may be further diluted in 100 ml NS and infused over 15–30 min (preferred).
- Infusion should be stopped or IV rate reduced if hypertension occurs.

Assessment & Drug Effects

- Monitor BP, vital signs, and I&O. Report oliguria or changes in I&O ratio.
- It is difficult to differentiate toxic effects of organophosphates or atropine from toxic effects of pralidoxime. Be alert for these signs and report them immediately: reduction in muscle strength, onset of muscle twitching, changes in respiratory pattern, altered level of consciousness, increases or changes in heart rate and rhythm.
- Excitement and manic behavior reportedly may occur following recovery of consciousness. Observe necessary safety precautions.
- Patient should be kept under close observation for 48–72 h, particularly when poison was ingested, because of likelihood of continued absorption of organophosphate from lower bowel.
- Pralidoxime is relatively short-acting. In patients with myasthenia gravis, overdosage with pralidoxime may convert cholinergic crisis into myasthenic crisis.

Prototype: procaine, p 166

PRAMOXINE HYDROCHLORIDE

(pra-mox´een)
Trade names: Fleet Relief Anesthetic Hemorrhoidal, Prax, ProctoFoam, Tronolane, Tronothane
Classifications: CNS AGENT; LOCAL ANESTHETIC (MUCOSAL); ANTIPRURITIC
Pregnancy: Category C

ACTIONS/PHARMACODYNAMICS Morpholine derivative; differs chemically from the amide- or ester-type anesthetics; therefore can be used in patient sensitive to these classes of drugs. Produces anesthesia by blocking conduction and propagation of sensory nerve impulses in skin and mucous membranes. Potency matches that of benzocaine as a topical anesthetic. Does not abolish gag reflex.

USES To relieve pain caused by minor burns and wounds; for temporary relief of pruritus secondary to dermatoses, hemorrhoids, and anal fissures; and to facilitate sigmoidoscopic examination.

ROUTE & DOSAGE

Relief of Minor Pain and Itching		
Adult	Topical	Apply t.i.d. or q.i.d.
Child	Topical	≥ 2 y: Same as for adult

PHARMACOKINETICS Onset: 3–5 min. **Duration:** up to 5 h.

CONTRAINDICATIONS & PRECAUTIONS Contraindicated in: application to large areas of skin; prolonged use; preparation for laryngopharyngeal examination; bronchoscopy, or gastroscopy. Safe use in children <2 y or during pregnancy (category C) not established. **Cautious use in:** extensive skin disorders.

ADVERSE/SIDE EFFECTS Local: burning, stinging, sensitization.

NURSING IMPLICATIONS

Administration

- Before use for temporary relief of hemorrhoidal pain and itching, thoroughly clean and dry rectal area. Administer rectal preparations in the morning and evening and after bowel movement or as directed by physician.
- Apply lotion or cream to affected surfaces with a gloved hand. Wash hands thoroughly before and after treatment.
- Do not apply to eyes or nasal membranes.
- Store at 15–30C (59–86F); protect from light; avoid freezing.

Patient & Family Education

- Advise patient to discontinue use of drug if condition being treated does not improve within 2–3 wk or if it worsens, or if rash or condition not present before treatment appears, or if treated area becomes inflamed or infected.
- If rectal bleeding and pain occur during hemorrhoid treatment, drug should be discontinued and physician consulted.

P

Prototype: lorazepam, p 177

PRAZEPAM

(pra´ze-pam)
Trade name: Centrax
Classifications: CNS AGENT; BENZODIAZEPINE
ANXIOLYTIC, SEDATIVE-HYPNOTIC
Pregnancy: Category C

ACTIONS/PHARMACODYNAMICS Benzodiaz-epine derivative structurally and pharmacologically related to lorazepam. Has hypnotic and sedative effects.

USES Anxiety disorders or for short-term relief of symptoms of anxiety.

ROUTE & DOSAGE

Hypnotic
Adult   PO   20–40 mg h.s.

Sedative
Adult   PO   10–20 mg t.i.d.

PHARMACOKINETICS Absorption: readily absorbed from GI tract. **Peak:** 6 h. **Duration:** 48 h. **Distribution:** crosses placenta; distributed into breast milk. **Metabolism:** metabolized in liver to active form. **Elimination:** half-life: 30–100 h (active metabolite); excreted in urine.

CONTRAINDICATIONS & PRECAUTIONS Con-traindicated in: hypersensitivity to prazepam and other benzodiazepines; psychoses, concomitant use during or within 14 d of MAO inhibitors, age <18 y; acute narrow-angle glaucoma; acute alcohol intoxication; pregnancy (category C), nursing mothers. **Cautious use in:** elderly and debilitated patients; impaired renal and hepatic function; addiction-prone patients; mental depression.

ADVERSE/SIDE EFFECTS Usually mild. **CNS:** blurred vision, *drowsiness,* fatigue, dizziness, mental confusion, vertigo, ataxia, headache, lethargy, syncope, slurred speech, tremor, paradoxic reaction (excitement, euphoria). **GI:** nausea, vomiting, xerostomia, gastric pain, diarrhea, constipation, jaundice. **Other:** skin rash, edema, hypotension, leukopenia, weight gain, altered libido.

DRUG INTERACTIONS Cimetidine, disulfiram, ORAL CONTRACEPTIVES may increase effects of prazepam; **alcohol** adds to CNS depression.

NURSING IMPLICATIONS

Administration
- Dose is individualized and is gradually adjusted to a range of 20–60 mg/d to minimize adverse effects.
- Following prolonged therapy drug should be withdrawn slowly to avoid precipitating withdrawal symptoms (seizures, mental confusion, nausea, vomiting, muscle and abdominal cramps, tremulousness, unusual irritability, hyperhydrosis).
- Store in tightly closed container at 15–30C (59–86F) unless otherwise specified.

Assessment & Drug Effects
- Liver function tests and blood counts should be performed on a regularly planned basis.
- Elderly patients should be observed closely for signs of overdosage. Report to physician if daytime psychomotor function is depressed.

Patient & Family Education
- Continued effectiveness of response to prazepam should be reassessed at end of 4 mo. Urge patient to keep appointments with physician.
- Instruct patient not to change dose or dose schedule. Furthermore, patient should refrain from using it to treat a self-diagnosed condition.
- Advise patient to consult physician before self-medicating with OTC drugs.
- Caution patient against driving a car or operating dangerous machinery until response to drug has been evaluated.
- Warn patient not to drink alcoholic beverages while being treated with prazepam. The CNS depressant effects of each agent are intensified.
- Patient should be advised that if she becomes pregnant during therapy or intends to become pregnant, she should communicate with her physician about the desirability of discontinuing the drug.

Prototype: mebendazole, p 53

PRAZIQUANTEL

(pray-zi-kwon´tel)
Trade name: Biltricide
Classifications: ANTIINFECTIVE; ANTHELMINTIC
Pregnancy: Category B

P

Common side effects in *italic*; life-threatening effects underlined; generic names in **bold**; classifications in SMALL CAPS

ACTIONS/PHARMACODYNAMICS Synthetic agent with broad spectrum of anthelmintic activity against all developmental stages of schistosomes and other trematodes (flukes) and against cestodes (tapeworm). Increases permeability of parasite cell membrane to calcium. Drug-induced influx of calcium ions induces strong contractions and paralysis of worm musculature, leading to immobilization of their suckers and dislodgment from their residence in blood vessel walls. Normal blood flow passively carries dead and dying worms to the liver, where they are retained and subsequently elicit host tissue reactions (e.g., phagocytosis). Praziquantel is active against all developmental stages of schistosomes, including cercaria (free-swimming larvae that emerge from the intermediate snail host). Activity against other trematodes (flukes) not fully understood; activity against cestodes (tapeworms) not clear but may be similar to that against schistosomes.

USES All stages of schistosomiasis (bilharziasis) caused by all schistosoma species pathogenic to humans. Other trematode infections caused by Chinese liver fluke: **Unlabeled uses:** lung, intestinal, sheep liver, and intestinal flukes and tapeworm infections.

ROUTE & DOSAGE

Schistosomiasis

Adult	PO	60 mg/kg in 3 equally divided doses at 4–6 h intervals on the same day; may repeat in 2–3 mo after exposure
Child	PO	> 4 y: Same as for adult

Other Trematodes

Adult	PO	75 mg/kg in 3 equally divided doses at 4–6 h intervals on the same day
Child	PO	> 4 y: Same as for adult

Cestodiasis (Adult or Intestinal Stage)

Adult	PO	10–20 mg/kg as single dose

Cestodiasis (Larval or Tissue Stage)

Adult	PO	50 mg/kg in 3 divided doses/d for 14 d

PHARMACOKINETICS Absorption: approximately 80% absorbed from GI tract. **Peak:** 1–3 h. **Distribution:** crosses blood-brain barrier; distributed into breast milk. **Metabolism:** extensively metabolized in liver, including first pass metabolism. **Elimination:** half-life: 0.8–1.5 h, metabolites 4–5 h; excreted in urine.

CONTRAINDICATIONS & PRECAUTIONS Contraindicated in: hypersensitivity to drug; ocular cysticercosis. Safe use in children <4 y not established; use during pregnancy (category B) only when clearly needed. Women should not nurse on day of praziquantel therapy or for 72 h after last dose of drug.

ADVERSE/SIDE EFFECTS CNS: *dizziness, headache, malaise,* drowsiness, lassitude, giddiness, CSF reaction syndrome (exacerbation of neurologic signs and symptoms such as seizures, increased CSF protein concentration, increased anticysticercal IgG levels, hyperthermia, intracranial hypertension) in patient treated for cerebral cysticercosis. **GI:** *abdominal pain or discomfort with or without nausea;* vomiting, anorexia, diarrhea. **Hepatic:** *increased AST, ALT (slight).* **Other:** pruritus, urticaria, fever, sweating, symptoms of host-mediated immunologic response to antigen release from worms (fever, eosinophilia).

DIAGNOSTIC TEST INTERFERENCES Be mindful that selected drugs may interfere with stool studies for ova and parasites: ***iron, bismuth, oil (mineral*** or ***castor), metamucil*** (if ingested within 1 wk of test), ***barium, antibiotics, antiamebic*** and ***antimalarial drugs,*** and ***gallbladder dye*** (if administered within 3 wk of test).

NURSING IMPLICATIONS

Administration

- Scored tablets are easily subdivided. If 1/4 tablet is required, break the segment from the outer end.
- Administer oral dose preferably with food and fluids. Tablets can be broken into quarters but should not be chewed. Advise patient to take sufficient fluid to wash down the medication. Tablets are soluble in water; gagging or vomiting because of bitter taste may result if tablets are retained in the mouth.
- Treatment for cestodiasis (tapeworm) may be followed by gentle purgation 2 h after drug administration to facilitate rapid removal of tapeworms and ova. The patient should be reexamined in 2 or 3 mo to ensure complete eradication of the infections.
- Store tablets in tight containers at <30C (86F).

Patient & Family Education

- Because of potential drug-induced dizziness and drowsiness, the patient should be warned not to drive a car or operate hazardous machinery on day of praziquantel treatment or the following day.
- Schistosomiasis can be acquired by swimming in cercaria-infested freshwater in many parts of the world, especially Africa and the Middle East (larvae

Common side effects in *italic;* life-threatening effects underlined; generic names in **bold;** classifications in SMALL CAPS enter the body through the skin). Diarrhea, urinary disturbances, hematuria, hepatic cirrhosis, chronic dysentery are the most common symptoms. Ova in urine, stool, and rectal and liver biopsy confirm the diagnosis.

- Usually all schistosomal worms are dead 7 d following treatment with praziquantel.
- Cure rates are generally lower in children and in patients with the heavy worm burden characteristic of massive infection.
- Instruct patient being treated for cestode infection to contact physician if patient develops a sustained headache or high fever. Conjunctive treatment with corticosteroids may be employed for treatment of cerebral cysticercosis (caused by pork tapeworm) to hasten recovery and reduce symptoms of CSF reaction syndrome (see adverse/side effects).

PRAZOSIN HYDROCHLORIDE

See AUTONOMIC NERVOUS SYSTEM AGENT, ALPHA ADRENERGIC ANTAGONIST (BLOCKING AGENT, SYMPATHOLYTIC) prototype, p 108.

Prototype: prednisone, p 225

PREDNISOLONE

(pred-niss´oh-lone)
Trade names: Delta-Cortef, Inflamase Forte, Nova-Pred, Novoprednisolone, Prelone

PREDNISOLONE ACETATE

Trade names: Ak-Tate, Econopred, Key-Pred, Pred Forte, Predcor

PREDNISOLONE SODIUM PHOSPHATE

Trade names: AK-Pred, Hydeltrasol, Inflamase, Inflamase Mild, Pred Mild, PSP-IV

PREDNISOLONE TEBUTATE

Trade names: Hydeltra-T.B.A., Nor-Pred T.B.A., Predcor-TBA, Prednisol TBA
Classifications: SYNTHETIC HORMONE; ADRENAL CORTICOSTEROID; GLUCOCORTICOID; ANTIINFLAMMATORY
Pregnancy: Category C

ACTIONS/PHARMACODYNAMICS Intermediate-acting synthetic dehydrogenated analog of hydrocortisone with 3–5 times greater potency. Mineralocorticoid properties are minimal, and potential for sodium and water retention and potassium loss is reduced. **HPA suppression:** 24–36 h. Side effects minimal.

USES Principally as an antiinflammatory and immunosuppressant agent.

ROUTE & DOSAGE

Antiinflammatory

Adult	PO	5–60 mg/d in single or divided doses
	IM	Acetate/Phosphate: 6–60 mg/d
		Tebutate: 2–60 mg q wk
	IV	Phosphate: 4–60 mg/d
	Ophthalmic	1–2 drops in conjunctival sac q.h. during the day; then q 2 h at night; may decrease to 1 drop t.i.d. or q.i.d.
Child	PO	0.14–2 mg/kg/d in single or divided doses
	IM	Acetate/Phosphate: 0.04–0.25 mg/kg 1–2 times/d
	IV	Phosphate: 0.04–0.25 mg/kg 1–2 times/d

PHARMACOKINETICS Absorption: readily absorbed from GI tract. **Peak:** 1–2 h. **Duration:** 1–1.5 d. **Distribution:** crosses placenta; distributed into breast milk. **Metabolism:** metabolized in liver. **Elimination:** half-life: 3.5 h; HPA suppression: 24–36 h; excreted in urine.

ADVERSE/SIDE EFFECTS Hirsutism (occasional); perforation of cornea (with topical drug); sensitivity to heat; fat embolism, adverse effects on growth and development of the individual and on sperm; hypotension and shocklike reactions; insomnia; gastric irritation or ulceration; ecchymotic skin lesions; vasomotor symptoms. Also see prednisone. Safe use during pregnancy (category C), by lactating women, or children not established.

DRUG INTERACTIONS BARBITURATES, **phenytoin, rifampin** increase steroid metabolism—may need increased doses of prednisolone; **amphotericin B,** DIURETICS add to potassium loss; **ambenonium, neostigmine, pyridostigmine** may

Common side effects in *italic*; life-threatening effects underlined; generic names in **bold**; classifications in SMALL CAPS

911

P

cause severe muscle weakness in patients with myasthenia gravis; VACCINES, TOXOIDS may inhibit antibody response.

INCOMPATIBILITIES Solution/additive: calcium gluceptate, metaraminol, methotrexate, polymyxin B.

NURSING IMPLICATIONS

Administration

- Administer with meals to reduce gastric irritation. If distress continues, consult physician about possible adjunctive antacid therapy.
- IV prednisolone sodium phosphate may be given by direct IV undiluted at a rate of 10 mg or fraction thereof over 60 seconds.
- IV prednisolone may be added to IV infusions of NS or D5W (50–1000 ml) and infused at ordered rate.
- Store in airtight containers protected from light at 15–30C (59–86F); do not freeze.

Assessment & Drug Effects

- Since ophthalmic corticosteroid treatment may increase intraocular pressure in susceptible individuals, it is usual to have frequent tonometric examinations during prolonged therapy.
- In diseases caused by microorganisms, infection may be masked, activated, or enhanced by corticosteroids. Be alert to subclinical signs of lack of improvement such as continued drainage, low-grade fever, and interrupted healing. Observe and report exacerbation of symptoms after short period of therapeutic response.
- Temporary local discomfort may follow injection of prednisolone into bursa or joint.

Patient & Family Education

- Advise patient to adhere to established dosage regimen, i.e., should not increase, decrease, or omit doses or change dose intervals.

Alternate Day Therapy (ADT) for Patient on Long-term Therapy

- With ADT the 48 h requirement for steroids is administered as a single dose every other morning.
- ADT minimizes adverse/side effects associated with long-term treatment while maintaining the desired therapeutic effect.
- If patient becomes symptomatic during period of switching to dose consolidation on the off or drugless day, a single small dose of glucocorticoid should be given on the off day and gradually reduced.
- If an acute flare is precipitated (high fever, reactivation of inflammatory condition being treated), ADT may have to be abandoned.

See prednisone for numerous additional nursing implications.

PREDNISONE

See HORMONES, ADRENAL CORTICOSTEROID, GLUCOCORTICOID prototype, p 225.

Prototype: chloroquine, p 79

PRIMAQUINE PHOSPHATE

(prim´a-kween)
Classifications: ANTIINFECTIVE; ANTIMALARIAL
Pregnancy: Category C

ACTIONS/PHARMACODYNAMICS Synthetic 8-aminoquinoline that acts on primary exoerythrocytic forms of *Plasmodium vivax* and *Plasmodium falciparum* by an incompletely known mechanism. Destroys late tissue forms of *P. vivax* and thus effects radical cure (prevents relapse). Also has gametocidal activity against all species of plasmodia that infect man and thus can interrupt transmission of malaria. For treatment of acute attacks, always used in conjunction with a 4-aminoquinoline antimalarial such as chloroquine, which destroys erythrocytic parasites.

USES To prevent relapse ("radical" or "clinical" cure) of *P. vivax* and *P. ovale* malarias and to prevent attacks after departure from areas where *P. vivax* and *P. ovale* malarias are endemic.

PHARMACOKINETICS Absorption: readily absorbed from GI tract. **Peak:** 6 h. **Metabolism:** rapidly metabolized in liver to active metabolites. **Elimination:** half-life: 3.7–9.6 h; excreted in urine.

CONTRAINDICATIONS & PRECAUTIONS Contraindicated in: rheumatoid arthritis; lupus erythematosus; hemolytic drugs, concomitant or recent use of agents capable of bone marrow depression, e.g.,

ROUTE & DOSAGE

Malaria Relapse Prevention

Adult	PO	15 mg once/d for 14 d concomitantly or consecutively with chloroquine or hydroxychloroquine on first 3 d of acute attack
Child	PO	0.3 mg/kg once/d for 14 d concomitantly or consecutively with chloroquine or hydroxychloroquine on first 3 d of acute attack

Malaria Prophylaxis

Adult	PO	15 mg once/d for 14 d beginning immediately after leaving malarious area
Child	PO	0.3 mg/kg once/d for 14 d beginning immediately after leaving malarious area

quinacrine; patients with G6PD deficiency. NADH methemoglobin reductase deficiency, pregnancy (category C).

ADVERSE/SIDE EFFECTS <u>Hematologic reactions including granulocytopenia and acute hemolytic anemia in patients with G6PD deficiency</u>. **Overdosage:** nausea, vomiting, epigastric distress, abdominal cramps, pruritus, methemoglobinemia (cyanosis): headache, confusion, mental depression, hypertension, arrhythmias (rare), moderate leukocytosis or leukopenia, anemia, granulocytopenia, <u>agranulocytosis</u>, disturbances of visual accommodation.

DRUG INTERACTIONS Toxicity of both **quinacrine** and primaquine increased.

NURSING IMPLICATIONS

Administration

- Administration of drug at mealtime or with an antacid (prescribed) may prevent or relieve gastric irritation. Notify physician if GI symptoms persist.
- Preserve in tight, light-resistant containers.

Assessment & Drug Effects

- Primaquine may precipitate acute hemolytic anemia in persons with G6PD deficiency, an inherited error of metabolism carried on the X chromosome, present in about 10% of American black males and certain white ethnic groups: Sardinians, Sephardic Jews, Greeks, and Iranians. Whites manifest more intense expression of hemolytic reaction than do blacks.

- Patients whose ethnic origin indicates the possibility of G6PD deficiency should be screened prior to initiation of therapy.
- Repeated hematologic studies (particularly blood cell counts and hemoglobin) and urinalyses should be performed during therapy.

Patient & Family Education

- Advise all patients to examine urine after each voiding and to report darkening of urine, red-tinged urine, and decrease in urine volume. Also report chills, fever, precordial pain, cyanosis (all suggest a hemolytic reaction). Sudden reductions in hemoglobin or erythrocyte count suggest an impending hemolytic reaction.

Prototype: phenobarbital, p 167

PRIMIDONE
(pri′mi-done)

Trade names: Apo-Primidone, Myidone, Mysoline, Sertan

Classifications: CNS AGENT; BARBITURATE ANTICONVULSANT

Pregnancy: Category D

ACTIONS/PHARMACODYNAMICS Not a true barbiturate but closely related chemically and with similar mechanism of action. Converted in body to phenobarbital and phenylethylmalonamide (PEMA). Appears to increase metabolism of vitamin D so that more is needed to fulfill normal requirements. May also impair calcium, folic acid, and vitamin B_{12} metabolism and utilization.

USES Alone or concomitantly with other anticonvulsant agents in the prophylactic management of complex partial (psychomotor) and generalized tonic-clonic (grand mal) seizures. **Unlabeled use:** essential tremor.

ROUTE & DOSAGE

Seizures

Adult	PO	250 mg/d, increased by 250 mg/wk up to a max of 2 g in 2–4 divided doses
Child	PO	8–12 y: Same as for adult
		<8 y: 125 mg/d, increased by 125 mg/wk up to a max of 1 g in 2–4 divided doses

PHARMACOKINETICS Absorption: approximately 60–80% absorbed from GI tract. **Peak:** 4 h. **Distribution:** distributed into breast milk. **Metabolism:** metabolized in liver to phenobarbital and PEMA. **Elimination:** half-life: Primidone 3–24 h; PEMA 24–48 h; phenobarbital 72–144 h; excreted in urine.

CONTRAINDICATIONS & PRECAUTIONS Contraindicated in: safe use during pregnancy (category D) and in nursing mothers not established. Hypersensitivity to barbiturates, porphyria. **Cautious use in:** chronic lung disease; hepatic or renal disease; hyperactive children.

ADVERSE/SIDE EFFECTS CNS: *drowsiness, sedation, vertigo, ataxia, headache,* excitement (children), confusion, unusual fatigue, hyperirritability, emotional disturbances, acute psychoses (usually patients with psychomotor epilepsy). **Eye:** diplopia, nystagmus, swelling of eyelids. **GI:** *nausea, vomiting, anorexia.* **Hematologic:** leukopenia, thrombocytopenia, eosinophilia, decreased serum folate levels, megaloblastic anemia (rare). **Other:** alopecia, impotence, maculopapular or morbilliform rash, edema, lupus erythematosus–like syndrome, lymphadenopathy, osteomalacia.

DRUG INTERACTIONS See phenobarbital.

NURSING IMPLICATIONS

Administration
- Tablet may be crushed before administration and taken with fluid of patient's choice.
- If drug causes GI distress, it may be taken with food.
- Transition from another anticonvulsant to primidone should not be completed in <2 mo.

Assessment & Drug Effects
- Baseline and periodic studies should be made of CBC, SMA-12 (q6mo), and primidone and phenobarbital blood levels. (***Therapeutic blood level for primidone:*** 5–10 µg/ml; ***for phenobarbital:*** 15–40 µg/ml.)
- Dosage may be adjusted with reference to primidone or phenobarbital metabolite plasma levels (concentrations of primidone > 10 µg/ml are usually associated with significant ataxia and lethargy).
- Therapeutic response may not be evident for several weeks.
- Observe for signs and symptoms of folic acid deficiency: mental dysfunction, psychiatric disorders, neuropathy, megaloblastic anemia. When indicated, serum folate levels should be determined.
- Neonatal hemorrhage has been reported in newborns whose mothers were taking primidone. Monitor closely for bleeding.
- Presence of unusual drowsiness in nursing newborns of primidone-treated mothers is an indication to discontinue nursing.

Patient & Family Education
- Because drowsiness, dizziness, and ataxia may be severe at beginning of treatment, advise patient to avoid driving and other potentially hazardous activities. Symptoms tend to disappear with continued therapy; if they persist, dosage reduction or drug withdrawal may be necessary.
- Advise patient to avoid alcohol and other CNS depressants unless otherwise directed by physician.
- Caution patient not to take OTC medications unless approved by physician.
- Pregnant women should receive prophylactic vitamin K therapy for 1 mo prior to and during delivery to prevent neonatal hemorrhage.
- Primidone withdrawal should be done gradually to avoid precipitating status epilepticus.
- Advise patient to carry medical information card or jewelry with name of drug, physician's name, and telephone number.

Prototype: colchicine, p 46

PROBENECID
(proe-ben´e-sid)
Trade names: Benemid, Benuryl, Probalan, SK-Probenecid
Classifications: ANTIGOUT AGENT; SULFONAMIDE

ACTIONS/PHARMACODYNAMICS   Sulfonamide-derivative renal tubular blocking agent. In sufficiently high doses, competitively inhibits renal tubular reabsorption of uric acid, thereby promoting its excretion and reducing serum urate levels (subtherapeutic doses may depress uric acid excretion). Prevents formation of new tophaceous deposits, and causes gradual shrinking of old tophi. Since it has no analgesic or antiinflammatory activity, it is of no value in acute gout and may exacerbate and prolong

P

Common side effects in *italic*; life-threatening effects <u>underlined</u>; generic names in **bold**; classifications in SMALL CAPS

acute phase. Increases plasma levels of weak organic acids, including beta-lactam antibiotics, by competitively inhibiting their renal tubular secretion.

USES Hyperuricemia in chronic gouty arthritis and tophaceous gout. **Unlabeled uses:** adjuvant to therapy with penicillin G and penicillin analogs to elevate and prolong plasma concentrations of these antibiotics; to promote uric acid excretion in hyperuricemia secondary to administration of thiazides and related diuretics, furosemide, ethacrynic acid, pyrazinamide.

ROUTE & DOSAGE

Gout

Adult	PO	250 mg b.i.d. for 1 wk, then 500 mg b.i.d. (max 3 g/d)

Adjunct for Penicillin or Cephalosporin Therapy

Adult	PO	500 mg q.i.d. or 1 g with single dose therapy (e.g., gonorrhea)
Child	PO	2–14 y or <50 kg: 25–40 mg/kg/d in 4 divided doses

PHARMACOKINETICS Absorption: readily absorbed from GI tract. **Onset:** 30 min. **Peak:** 2–4 h. **Duration:** 8 h. **Distribution:** crosses placenta. **Metabolism:** metabolized in liver. **Elimination:** half-life: 4–17 h; excreted in urine.

CONTRAINDICATIONS & PRECAUTIONS Contraindicated in: blood dyscrasias; uric acid kidney stones; during or within 2–3 wk of acute gouty attack; overexcretion of uric acid (> 1000 mg/d), patients with creatinine clearance <50 mg/min; use with penicillin in presence of known renal impairment, use for hyperuricemia secondary to cancer chemotherapy. Safe use during pregnancy (category B), in nursing mothers, and in children <2 y not established. **Cautious use in:** history of peptic ulcer.

ADVERSE/SIDE EFFECTS *Headache, nausea, vomiting, anorexia,* sore gums, urinary frequency, flushing, dizziness, anemia, hemolytic anemia (possibly related to G6PD deficiency). Nephrotic syndrome, hepatic necrosis, and aplastic anemia (rare). Exacerbations of gout, uric acid kidney stones. **Hypersensitivity:** dermatitis, pruritus, fever, anaphylaxis. **Overdosage:** CNS stimulation, convulsions, respiratory depression.

DIAGNOSTIC TEST INTERFERENCES False-positive results ***urine glucose*** tests are possible with Benedict's solution or Clinitest (glucose oxidase methods not affected, e.g., Clinistix, TesTape).

DRUG INTERACTIONS SALICYLATES may decrease uricosuric activity; may decrease **methotrexate** elimination, causing increased toxicity; decreases **nitrofurantoin** efficacy and increases its toxicity.

NURSING IMPLICATIONS

Administration

- GI side effects minimized by taking drug after meals, with food, milk, or with antacid (prescribed). If symptoms persist, dosage reduction may be required.
- PO sodium bicarbonate (3–7.5 g/d) or potassium citrate (7.5 g/d) may be prescribed to alkalinize urine until serum uric acid levels return to normal range (3–7 mg/dl).
- Because frequency of acute gouty attacks may increase during first 6–12 mo of therapy, physician may prescribe concurrent prophylactic doses of colchicine for first 3–6 mo of probenecid therapy (probenecid alone aggravates acute gout). Probenecid is available in combination with colchicine, e.g., ColBenemid.
- Tablets should be stored in tightly closed containers at 15–30C (59–86F). Expiration date is 3–5 y after date of manufacture.

Assessment & Drug Effects

- When gouty attacks have been absent for 6 mo or more and serum urate levels are controlled, daily dosage may be cautiously decreased by 0.5 g q6mo to lowest effective dosage that maintains stable serum urate levels.
- When urinary alkalinizers are used, periodic determinations of acid-base balance are advised. Some physicians prescribe acetazolamide at bedtime to keep urine alkaline and dilute throughout night.
- Patients taking sulfonylureas may require dosage adjustment. Probenecid enhances hypoglycemic actions of these drugs. See also diagnostic test interferences.
- Urate tophaceous deposits should decrease in size with probenecid therapy. Classic locations are in cartilage of ear pinna and big toe, but they can occur in bursae, tendons, skin, kidneys, and other tissues.

P

Patient & Family Education

- Increased uric acid excretion promoted by probenecid predisposes to renal calculi. Therefore, during early therapy, high fluid intake (approximately 3000 ml/d) is recommended to maintain daily urinary output of at least 2000 ml or more.
- Physician may advise restriction of high-purine foods during early therapy until uric acid level stabilizes. *Foods high in purine:* organ meats (sweetbreads, liver, kidney), meat extracts, meat soups, gravy, anchovies, sardines. Moderate amounts are present in other meats, fish, seafood, asparagus, spinach, peas, dried legumes, wild game.
- Alcohol may increase serum urate levels and therefore should be avoided.
- Caution patient not to stop taking drug without consulting physician. Irregular dosage schedule may sharply elevate serum urate level and precipitate acute gout.
- Lifelong therapy is usually required in patients with symptomatic hyperuricemia. Advise patient to keep scheduled appointments with physician and appointments for studies of renal function and hematology.
- Instruct patient to report symptoms of hypersensitivity to physician. Discontinuation of drug is indicated.
- Advise patient not to take aspirin or other OTC medications without consulting physician. If a mild analgesic is required, acetaminophen is usually allowed.

Prototype: lovastatin, p 143

PROBUCOL

(proe´byoo-kole)
Trade name: Lorelco
Classifications: CARDIOVASCULAR AGENT; ANTILIPEMIC; LIPID-LOWERING AGENT
Pregnancy: Category C

ACTIONS/PHARMACODYNAMICS Lowers serum cholesterol levels by reducing low density lipoprotein (LDL) concentrations. Therapeutic action thought to be due to inhibition of early stages of cholesterol synthesis, to increased bile acid excretion in feces, and inhibition (minimal) of dietary cholesterol absorption. Serum triglyceride (VLDL) levels are not appreciably lowered by this agent. It is not known whether a cholesterol-lowering drug has an effect, no effect, or a detrimental effect on morbidity or mortality related to atherosclerosis or coronary heart disease.

USES To lower elevated cholesterol concentrations in patients with type II hyperlipoproteinemia, especially type IIa and type III. Use is adjunctive to diet and is indicated for patients who fail to respond adequately to diet, weight reduction, and control of diabetes mellitus.

ROUTE & DOSAGE

Hypercholesterolemia		
Adult	PO	500 mg b.i.d.

PHARMACOKINETICS Absorption: <10% absorbed from GI tract. **Peak:** 1–3 mo. **Distribution:** accumulates in adipose tissue; may remain in fat 6 mo or longer. **Elimination:** half-life: 20 d; excreted in bile and feces.

CONTRAINDICATIONS & PRECAUTIONS Contraindicated in: hypersensitivity to probucol; pregnancy (category C), nursing mothers, children; patient with unresponsive CHF; frequent multifocal or paired ventricular extrasystoles; primary biliary cirrhosis. **Cautious use in:** patients behaviorally incapable of strict adherence to diet therapy; impaired hepatic function, cholelithiasis.

ADVERSE/SIDE EFFECTS CNS: headache, dizziness, paresthesias, peripheral neuritis, decreased sense of taste and smell. **CV:** palpitations, chest pain, prolonged QT interval, syncope, ventricular arrhythmias, sudden death. **ENT:** blurred vision, tinnitus, conjunctivitis, tearing. **GI:** nausea, vomiting, anorexia, heartburn, GI bleeding, *diarrhea,* flatulence, abdominal pain. **Hematologic:** eosinophilia, low Hgb, Hct, thrombocytopenia. **Other:** rash, pruritus, impotence, enlargement of multinodal goiter, nocturia, hyperhidrosis, fetid sweat, angioneurotic edema.

DRUG INTERACTIONS TRICYCLIC ANTIDEPRESSANTS, **quinidine,** PHENOTHIAZINES, BETA-BLOCKERS, **digoxin** increase risk of ventricular arrhythmias.

DIAGNOSTIC TEST INTERFERENCES Probucol therapy is accompanied by transient elevations in serum transaminases *(AST, ALT), bilirubin, alkaline phosphatase, creatine, phosphokinase, uric acid, BUN,* and *blood glucose. Hematocrit, hemoglobin* and *eosinophil values* may be decreased.

P

Common side effects in *italic*; life-threatening effects underlined; generic names in **bold**; classifications in SMALL CAPS

NURSING IMPLICATIONS

Administration

- Administer drug with morning and evening meals to enhance its action.
- Store in light- and moisture-proof container at 15–30C (59–86F) unless otherwise specified.

Assessment & Drug Effects

- Baseline data to be established before treatment begins include existing serum cholesterol and triglyceride levels.
- *Normal serum cholesterol levels* (150–280 mg/dl) should be checked frequently during first month of therapy. Usually a favorable decline in levels is observed within 2 mo of probucol therapy. If improvement not observed within 4 mo, drug is discontinued.
- If there is a sustained rise in *serum triglycerides (normal:* 40–150 mg/dl), investigate degree of compliance with special diet, carbohydrate and caloric intake, and alcohol intake. Reinforce and emphasize importance of strict adherance to dietary regimen. Probucol will be withdrawn if hypertriglyceridemia persists.
- Monitor pulse during early therapy. Irregularity in rhythm and strength should be evaluated by ECG. (If patient has history of or existing myocardial damage or dysrhythmia, periodic ECG evaluations should accompany therapy with probucol.) Drug is discontinued if pronounced QT interval prolongation or arrhythmias are observed.
- Xanthelasma and xanthomas may disappear or reduce in size during probucol therapy. Keep physician informed.

Patient & Family Education

- The patient should fully understand that this drug does not reduce necessity to adhere to special diet.
- The dosage of oral anticoagulant or oral hypoglycemic agents is not altered when they are used concomitantly with probucol.
- Any unexplained bleeding (ecchymoses, petechiae, epistaxis, black stools) must be reported to physician as soon as observed.
- Counsel patient not to change dose intervals of probucol. Patient should not increase or decrease doses or discontinue taking the drug without the physician's approval.
- Instruct patient to check with the physician before self-dosing with OTC medications.
- Alcohol intake is usually not allowed during probucol therapy.
- Swelling of face, oral membranes, hands, or feet and symptoms of angioneurotic edema should be reported; drug will be discontinued.
- GI side effects are generally transient and seldom require treatment or discontinuation of drug therapy. If GI side effects are persistent, patient should report to the physician because of danger of fluid and electrolyte imbalance and dehydration.
- Strict birth control measures should be used by women in childbearing years during probucol therapy. If pregnancy is desired, it is recommended that birth control be practiced at least 6 mo after the drug is withdrawn to insure its complete elimination before conception.

PROCAINAMIDE HYDROCHLORIDE

See CARDIOVASCULAR AGENT, ANTIARRHYTHMIC prototype, p 140.

PROCAINE HYDROCHLORIDE

See CNS AGENT, LOCAL ANESTHETIC prototype, p 166.

Prototype: fluorouracil, p 94

PROCARBAZINE HYDROCHLORIDE

(proe-kar´ba-zeen)
Trade names: Matulane, Natulan
Classifications: ANTINEOPLASTIC; ANTIMETABOLITE
Pregnancy: Category D

ACTIONS/PHARMACODYNAMICS Hydrazine derivative with antimetabolite properties; cell cycle–specific for the S phase of cell division. Precise mechanism of action unknown. Suppresses mitosis at interphase, and causes chromatin derangement. Highly toxic to rapidly proliferating tissue. Has immunosuppressive properties and exhibits monamine oxidase (MAO) inhibition activity. May delay myelosuppression. No cross-resistance with radiotherapy, steroids, or other antineoplastics has been demonstrated. Reportedly does not affect survival time but may produce remissions of at least 1 mo duration.

P

Common side effects in *italic*; life-threatening effects <u>underlined</u>; generic names in **bold**; classifications in SMALL CAPS

917

USES Adjunct in palliative treatment of Hodgkin's disease. **Unlabeled use:** solid tumors.

ROUTE & DOSAGE

Adjunct for Hodgkin's Disease

Adult	PO	2–4 mg/kg/d in single or divided doses for 1 wk, then 4–6 mg/kg/d until WBC <4000/mm³ or platelets are <100,000/mm³ or maximum response obtained; drug is then discontinued until bone marrow recovery is satisfactory; treatment is started again at 1–2 mg/kg/d
Child	PO	50 mg/m²/d in single or divided doses for 1 wk, then 100 mg/m²/d until WBC <4000/mm³ or platelets are <100,000/mm³ or maximum response obtained; drug is then discontinued until bone marrow recovery is satisfactory; treatment is started again at 50 mg/m²/d

PHARMACOKINETICS Absorption: readily absorbed from GI tract. **Peak:** 1 h. **Distribution:** widely distributed with high concentrations in liver, kidneys, intestinal wall, and skin. **Metabolism:** metabolized in liver. **Elimination:** half-life: 1 h; excreted in urine.

CONTRAINDICATIONS & PRECAUTIONS Contraindicated in: myelosuppression; alcohol ingestion; foods high in tyramine content; sympathomimetic drugs. MAO inhibitors should be discontinued 14 d prior to therapy; tricyclic antidepressants, 7 d before therapy. Safe use during pregnancy (category D) and lactation not established. **Cautious use in:** concomitant administration with CNS depressants; hepatic or kidney impairment; following radiation or chemotherapy before at least 1 mo has elapsed; hepatic and renal impairment; infection; diabetes mellitus.

ADVERSE/SIDE EFFECTS CNS: myalgia, arthralgia, paresthesias, weakness, fatigue, lethargy, drowsiness, neuropathies, mental depression, acute psychosis, hallucinations, dizziness, headache, ataxia, nervousness, insomnia, <u>coma</u>, confusion, seizures. **GI:** *severe nausea and vomiting*, anorexia, stomatitis, dry mouth, dysphagia, diarrhea, constipation, jaundice. **Hematologic:** <u>bone marrow suppression (leukopenia, anemia, thrombocytopenia)</u>, hemolysis, bleeding tendencies. **Infrequent:** apprehension, nightmares, slurred speech, footdrop, decreased reflexes, tremors. **Skin:** dermatitis, pruritus, herpes, hyperpigmentation, flushing, alopecia. **Other:** ascites, *pleural effusion, cough,* hoarseness, hypotension, tachycardia, chills, fever, sweating, gynecomastia, depressed spermatogenesis, atrophy of testes; rare: edema, nystagmus, photophobia, retinal hemorrhage, diplopia, papilledema; altered hearing; photosensitivity; <u>intercurrent infections</u>.

DIAGNOSTIC TEST INTERFERENCES Procarbazine may enhance the effects of **CNS depressants.** A disulfiram-like reaction may occur following ingestion of **alcohol.**

DRUG INTERACTIONS Alcohol, PHENOTHIAZINES, and other **CNS depressants** add to CNS depression; TRICYCLIC ANTIDEPRESSANTS, MAO INHIBITORS, SYMPATHOMIMETICS, **ephedrine, phenylpropanolamine** may precipitate hypertensive crisis, hyperpyrexia; seizures, or death. **Food-Drug interactions:** tyramine-containing foods may precipitate hypertensive crisis (see phenelzine sulfate (MAO inhibitor), p 182.

NURSING IMPLICATIONS

Administration

- Toxicity is a serious problem and demands that patient be hospitalized and under close medical and nursing supervision during treatment induction period.
- Store at 15–30C (59–86F). Protect from freezing, moisture, and light.

Assessment & Drug Effects

- Start flow sheet and record baseline BP, weight, temperature, pulse, and I&O ratio and pattern.
- Hematologic status (Hgb, Hct, WBC, differential, reticulocyte and platelet counts) should be determined initially and at least q3–4d. Hepatic and renal studies (transaminase, alkaline phosphatase, BUN, urinalysis) are also indicated initially and at least weekly during therapy.
- Patient's hematologic status should be monitored carefully for indicators that suggest special nursing interventions and need for dosage adjustment or drug withdrawal.
- As patient approaches nadir of leukopenia (<4000/mm³), protect patient from exposure to infection and trauma. Alert patient to report any sign of impending infection. Note and report changes in voiding pattern, hematuria, and dysuria (possible signs of urinary tract infection). I&O ratio and temperature should be closely monitored.
- Prompt cessation of therapy is usual with appearance of CNS signs and symptoms (paresthesias, neuropathies, confusion), leukopenia (WBC count

Common side effects in *italic*; life-threatening effects <u>underlined</u>; generic names in **bold**; classifications in SMALL CAPS

<4000/mm^3), thrombocytopenia (platelet count <100,000/mm^3), hypersensitivity reaction, the first small ulceration or persistent spot soreness of oral cavity, diarrhea, and bleeding. Patient should be warned to report promptly any signs and symptoms of toxicity.

- Symptoms of pleural effusion, an allergic reaction to procarbazine (chills, fever, weakness, shortness of breath, productive cough) should be reported promptly. Drug will be discontinued.
- Be alert to signs of hepatic dysfunction: jaundice (yellow skin, sclerae, and soft palate), frothy or dark urine, clay-colored stools.
- Tolerance to nausea and vomiting (most common side effects) usually develops by end of first week of treatment. Doses are kept at a minimum during this time. If vomiting persists, therapy will be interrupted.

Patient & Family Education

- Since procarbazine has MAO inhibitory activity, OTC nose drops, cough medicines, and antiobesity preparations containing sympathomimetic drugs (e.g., ephedrine, amphetamine, epinephrine) and tricyclic antidepressants should be avoided because they may cause hypertensive crises. Warn patient not to use OTC preparations without physician's approval.
- Intake of foods high in tyramine content should be avoided.
- Warn patient that ingestion of any form of alcohol may precipitate a disulfiram-type reaction (see Signs & Symptoms, chap 3).
- Instruct patient to report immediately signs of hemorrhagic tendencies: bleeding into skin and mucosa, epistaxis, hemoptysis, hematemesis, hematuria, melena, ecchymoses, petechiae. Bone marrow depression often occurs 2–8 wk after start of therapy.
- Advise patient to avoid excessive exposure to the sun because of potential photosensitivity reaction: cover as much skin area as possible with clothing, and use sunscreen lotion (SPF > 12) on all exposed skin surfaces.
- Since drowsiness, dizziness, and blurred vision are possible side effects, warn patient to use caution while driving or performing hazardous tasks until response to drug is known.
- Advise use of contraceptive measures during procarbazine therapy.

PROCHLORPERAZINE

See GI AGENT, ANTIEMETIC prototype, p 215.

Prototype: atropine, p 116

PROCYCLIDINE HYDROCHLORIDE

(proe-sye´kli-deen)
Trade names: Kemadrin, Procyclid
Classifications: AUTONOMIC NERVOUS SYSTEM AGENT; ANTICHOLINERGIC (PARASYMPATHOLYTIC); ANTIMUSCARINIC, ANTISPASMODIC; ANTIPARKINSONISM AGENT
Pregnancy: Category C

ACTIONS/PHARMACODYNAMICS Centrally acting synthetic anticholinergic agent with actions similar to those of atropine; closely related to trihexyphenidyl.

USES To relieve symptoms of parkinsonism syndrome (postencephalitic, arteriosclerotic, and idiopathic), and drug-induced extrapyramidal symptoms.

ROUTE & DOSAGE

Parkinsonism Symptoms

Adult	PO	2.5 mg t.i.d. p.c.; may be gradually increased to 5 mg t.i.d. if tolerated with an additional 5 mg h.s. (max 45–60 mg/d)

PHARMACOKINETICS Onset: 35–40 min. **Duration:** 4–6 h.

CONTRAINDICATIONS & PRECAUTIONS Contraindicated in: angle-closure glaucoma. Safe use during pregnancy (category C), in nursing mothers, and in children not established. **Cautious use:** hypotension; mental disorders; tachycardia; prostatic hypertrophy.

ADVERSE/SIDE EFFECTS *Dry mouth,* blurred vision, mydriasis, photophobia, palpitation, tachycardia, flushing of skin, decreased sweating, headache, *hypotension,* lightheadedness, nausea, vomiting, epigastric distress, dizziness, urinary retention, feeling of muscle weakness, constipation, <u>paralytic ileus</u>, acute suppurative parotitis, skin eruptions; (occasionally): mental confusion, psychotic-like symptoms.

P

Common side effects in *italic*; life-threatening effects <u>underlined</u>; generic names in **bold**; classifications in SMALL CAPS

919

NURSING IMPLICATIONS

Administration

- Side effects may be minimized by administration of drug during or after meals.
- Store in tightly closed containers at 15–30C (59–86F) unless otherwise directed.

Assessment & Drug Effects

- Monitor heart rate and rhythm and BP. Report palpitations, tachycardia, paradoxical bradycardia or decreasing BP. Dosage adjustment or discontinuation of drug may be indicated.
- Procyclidine is usually more effective in controlling rigidity than tremors. Tremors may temporarily appear to be exaggerated as rigidity is relieved, especially in patients with severe spasticity.
- Drug occasionally causes mental confusion, disorientation, agitation, and psychoticlike symptoms, particularly in elderly patients who have low BP. Observe for and report these symptoms to physician.
- Check for constipation and abdominal distension and provide information for preventing constipation.
- Since dosage is guided by clinical response, observe and record improvement (or lack of it) that accompanies therapy.

Patient & Family Education

- If urinary hesitancy or retention is a problem, advise the patient to void before taking drug.
- Since procyclidine may cause blurred vision and dizziness, caution the patient to avoid potentially hazardous activities until reaction to drug is known.
- Drug-induced dryness of mouth may be relieved by sugarless gum or hard candy and by frequent rinses with warm water or by increasing noncaloric fluid intake. If these measures fail, a saliva substitute, available OTC, may help (e.g., Orex, Xero-Lube).
- Advise patient to avoid alcohol and not to take other CNS depressants unless otherwise advised by physician.

PROGESTERONE

See HORMONE, PROGESTIN prototype, p 241.

Prototype: chlorpromazine, p 191

PROMAZINE HYDROCHLORIDE

(proe´ma-zeen)
Trade names: Promanyl, Prozine, Sparine
Classifications: CNS AGENT; PSYCHOTHERAPEUTIC; PHENOTHIAZINE ANTIPSYCHOTIC (TRANQUILIZER)
Pregnancy: Category C

ACTIONS/PHARMACODYNAMICS   Aliphatic (ethylamino) derivative of phenothiazine. Compared with chlorpromazine has weak antipsychotic activity and extrapyramidal effects occur less frequently. Although drug-induced agranulocytosis is rare, it occurs more often than with other phenothiazines.

USES Manifestations of psychotic disorders and for reducing agitation and paranoia associated with alcohol withdrawal.

ROUTE & DOSAGE

Psychotic Disorders

Adult	PO/IM	10–200 mg q4–6h up to 1000 mg/d
Adolescent	PO/IM	> 12 y: 10–25 mg q4–6h

CONTRAINDICATIONS & PRECAUTIONS Contraindicated in: hypersensitivity to phenothiazines; myelosuppression; CNS depression; children <12 y of age, Reye's syndrome. Safe use during pregnancy (category C) and by nursing mothers not established. **Cautious use in:** prostatic hypertrophy; cardiovascular or hepatic disease; paralytic ileus; xerostomia; angle closure glaucoma; persons exposed to extremes in temperature or to organophosphorous insecticides; convulsive disorders.

ADVERSE/SIDE EFFECTS *Drowsiness, orthostatic hypotension.* Also, blurred vision, photosensitivity, constipation, epileptic seizures in susceptible individuals, leukopenia, <u>agranulocytosis (rare)</u>.

NURSING IMPLICATIONS

Administration

- Oral route should be used whenever possible. Parenteral administration is reserved for acutely disturbed or uncooperative patients or those who cannot tolerate an oral preparation.

P

Common side effects in *italic*; life-threatening effects <u>underlined</u>; generic names in **bold**; classifications in SMALL CAPS

- Absorption is inhibited by antacids; therefore administer promazine 1 h before or 1 h after antacid.
- Syrup (10 mg/5ml) or oral concentrate (30 mg/ml) may be prescribed when tablet is unsuitable or refused. Dilute the concentrate immediately before administration with fruit juice, chocolate-flavored drinks, carbonated drinks, or soup. (For best taste, 10 ml of diluent for each 25 mg of drug.) Avoid coffee or tea ingestion near time of taking oral preparation. Explain dosage and dilution to patient if drug is to be self-administered.
- Parenteral administration is seldom given to the ambulatory patient except to treat an acute psychotic condition.
- IM injection is made deep into upper outer quadrant of buttock. Tissue irritation can occur if given SC. Carefully aspirate before injecting drug slowly. Intraarterial injection can cause arterial or arteriolar spasm and consequent impairment of local circulation. Rotate injection sites.
- IV route is reserved only for hospitalized patients; routine use not recommended. Localized cellulitis, thrombophlebitis, and gangrene have occurred because of improper drug dilution, extravasation, or injections made into previously damaged blood vessels.
- IV promazine in concentrations of 25 mg/ml or less may be given by direct IV undiluted at a rate of 25 mg over 60 seconds. More concentrated preparations should be diluted in NS to yield no more than 25 mg/ml
- Store in light-resistant container at 15–30C (59–86F) unless otherwise directed.

Assessment & Drug Effects

- Incidence of postural hypotension and drowsiness is particularly high after parenteral administration. Monitor BP and pulse before administration and between doses. Keep patient recumbent for about 1 h after dose is given.
- Monitor I&O ratio and bowel elimination pattern. Check for abdominal distension and pain. Encourage adequate fluid intake as prophylaxis for constipation and xerostomia. The depressed patient may not seek help for either symptom or for urinary retention.
- Symptoms suggesting agranulocytosis should be reported promptly (see chap 3).

Patient & Family Education

- Warn patient that dizziness or faintness may occur on arising. Advise making all position changes slowly, particularly from recumbent to upright position.

- Warn patient to avoid alcohol during therapy.
- Promazine may cause contact dermatitis. Caution patient to avoid spilling oral solutions on hands or clothing. Wash exposed skin well with soap and water.
- Promazine may color urine pink to red to reddish brown.
- OTC drugs should be approved by physician during antipsychotic therapy.

Prototype: prochlorperazine, p 215

PROMETHAZINE HYDROCHLORIDE
(proe-meth´a-zeen)

Trade names: Ganphen, Histantil, K-Phen, Pentazine, Phenazine, Phencen, Phenergan, Phenoject-50, Prometh, Promine, Prorex, Prothazine, Provigan, Remsed, V-Gan
Classifications: GI AGENT; ANTIEMETIC; ANTIVERTIGO AGENT; PHENOTHIAZINE
Pregnancy: Category C

ACTIONS/PHARMACODYNAMICS Long-acting ethylamino derivative of phenothiazine with marked antihistaminic activity and prominent sedative, amnesic, antiemetic, and anti-motion-sickness actions. Unlike other phenothiazine derivatives, it is relatively free of extrapyramidal side effects; however, in high doses it carries same potential for toxicity. In common with other antihistamines, exerts antiserotonin, anticholinergic, and local anesthetic action. Prevents most actions of histamine by competing with it for H_1-receptor sites on effector cells. Antiemetic action thought to be due to depression of CTZ in medulla. Reported to have slight antitussive activity, but this may be due to anticholinergic and CNS depressant effects.

USES Symptomatic relief of various allergic conditions, to ameliorate and prevent reactions to blood and plasma, and in prophylaxis and treatment of motion sickness, nausea, and vomiting. Preoperative, postoperative, and obstetric sedation and as adjunct to analgesics for control of pain.

PHARMACOKINETICS Absorption: readily absorbed from GI tract. **Onset:** 20 min PO/PR/IM; 5 min IV. **Duration:** 2–8 h. **Distribution:** crosses placenta. **Metabolism:** metabolized in liver. **Elimination:** slowly excreted in urine and feces.

Common side effects in *italic*; life-threatening effects underlined; generic names in **bold**; classifications in SMALL CAPS

P

ROUTE & DOSAGE

Motion Sickness

Adult	PO/PR/IM/IV	25 mg b.i.d.
Child	PO/PR/IM/IV	12.5–25 mg b.i.d.

Nausea

Adult	PO/PR/IM/IV	12.5–25 mg q4–6h prn
Child	PO/PR/IM/IV	0.25–0.5 mg/kg q4–6h prn

Allergies

Adult	PO/PR/IM/IV	12.5 mg q.i.d. *or* 25 mg h.s.
Child	PO/PR/IM/IV	6.25–12.5 mg q.i.d. *or* 25 mg h.s.

Sedation

Adult	PO/PR/IM/IV	25–50 mg preoperatively *or* h.s.
Child	PO/PR/IM/IV	12.5–25 mg preoperatively *or* h.s.

CONTRAINDICATIONS & PRECAUTIONS Contraindicated in: hypersensitivity to phenothiazines; narrow-angle glaucoma; stenosing peptic ulcer, pyloroduodenal obstruction; prostatic hypertrophy; bladder neck obstruction; epilepsy; bone marrow depression; comatose or severely depressed states; pregnancy (category C), nursing mothers, newborn or premature infants, acutely ill or dehydrated children. **Cautious use in:** impaired hepatic function; cardiovascular disease; asthma; acute or chronic respiratory impairment (particularly in children), hypertension; elderly or debilitated patients.

ADVERSE/SIDE EFFECTS Acute toxicity: deep sleep, coma, convulsions, cardiorespiratory symptoms, extrapyramidal reactions, nightmares (in children), CNS stimulation, abnormal movements, <u>respiratory depression</u>. Toxic potential as for other phenothiazines. **CNS:** sedation *drowsiness,* confusion, dizziness, disturbed coordination, restlessness, tremors. **CV:** transient mild hypotension or hypertension. **GI:** anorexia, nausea, vomiting, constipation. **Hematologic:** leukopenia, <u>agranulocytosis</u>. **Other:** photosensitivity, irregular respiration, *blurred vision,* urinary retention; *dry mouth,* nose, or throat.

DIAGNOSTIC TEST INTERFERENCES Promethazine may interfere with **blood grouping** in ABO system and may produce false results with **urinary pregnancy tests** (Gravindex, false-positive; Prepurex and Dap tests, false-negative). Promethazine can cause significant alterations of flare response in **intradermal allergen tests** if performed within 4 d of patient's receiving promethazine.

DRUG INTERACTIONS Alcohol and other CNS DEPRESSANTS add to CNS depression and anticholinergic effects.

INCOMPATIBILITIES Solution/additive: **aminophphylline, carbenicillin, chloramphenicol, chlo-rothiazide, heparin, hydrocortisone, methicillin, methohexital, penicillin G sodium, pentobarbital, phenobarbital, thiopental, diatrizoate, dimenhydrinate, iodipamide, iothalamate, nalbuphine. Y-site: heparin, carbenicillin.**

NURSING IMPLICATIONS

Administration

- Administration of oral medication with food, milk or a full glass of water may minimize GI distress.
- Tablet may be crushed and mixed with water or food before swallowing.
- Oral doses for allergy are generally prescribed before meals and on retiring or as single dose at bedtime.
- Inspect parenteral drug before preparation. Discard if it is darkened or contains precipitate.
- **IM injection** is made deep into large muscle mass. Aspirate carefully before injecting drug. Intra-arterial injection can cause arterial or arteriolar spasm, with resultant gangrene. Subcutaneous injection (also contraindicated) can cause chemical irritation and necrosis. Rotate injection sites and observe daily.
- IV promethazine in concentrations of 25 mg/ml or less may be given by direct IV undiluted over 2 min. More concentrated preparations should be diluted in NS to yield no more than 25 mg/ml.
- When promethazine is administered by IV infusion, wrap IV bottle with aluminum foil to protect drug from light.
- Promethazine injection is incompatible with a number of drugs, especially those with alkaline pH (see incompatibilities).
- Store in tight, light-resistant container at 15–30C (59–86F) unless otherwise directed.

Assessment & Drug Effects

- Promethazine sometimes produces marked sedation and dizziness. Side rails and supervision of ambulation may be advisable.
- Antiemetic action may mask symptoms of unrecognized disease and signs of drug overdosage as well as dizziness, vertigo, or tinnitus associated with toxic doses of aspirin or other ototoxic drugs.
- Patients in pain may develop involuntary (athetoid) movements of upper extremities following par-

enteral administration. These symptoms usually disappear after pain is controlled.

- Respiratory function should be monitored in patients with respiratory problems, particularly children. Promethazine may suppress cough reflex and cause thickening of bronchial secretions.
- Dry mouth may be relieved by frequent rinses with warm water or by increasing noncaloric fluid intake (if allowed) or by sugarless gum or lemon drops. If these measures fail, a saliva substitute may help (e.g., Moi-Stir, Orex, Xero-Lube.)

Patient & Family Education

- When administered as prophylaxis against motion sickness, initial dose should be taken 30–60 min before anticipated travel and repeated at 8–12 h intervals if necessary. For duration of journey, repeat dose on arising and again at evening meal.
- Advise ambulatory patient to avoid driving a car or engaging in other activities requiring mental alertness and normal reaction time until response to drug is known.
- Promethazine may cause photosensitivity. Advise patient to avoid sunlamps or prolonged exposure to sunlight. A sunscreen lotion may be advisable during initial drug therapy.
- Advise patient not to take OTC medications without physician's approval, and caution against alcohol and other CNS depressants.

Prototype: atropine, p 116

PROPANTHELINE BROMIDE

(proe-pan´the-leen)
Trade names: Banlin, Norpanth, Noropropanthil, Pro-Banthine, Propanthel
Classifications: ANTISPASMODIC; ANTICHOLINERGIC
Pregnancy: Category C

ACTIONS/PHARMACODYNAMICS Synthetic quaternary ammonium compound. Similar to atropine in peripheral effects, contraindications, precautions, and adverse reactions. Potent in antimuscarinic activity and in nondepolarizing ganglionic blocking action. Very high doses block neurotransmission at myoneural junction.

USES Adjunct in treatment of peptic ulcer, irritable bowel syndrome, pancreatitis, ureteral and urinary

bladder spasm. Also used prior to radiologic diagnostic procedures to reduce duodenal motility.

ROUTE & DOSAGE

Irritable Bowel Syndrome

Adult PO 15 mg 30 min a.c. and 30 mg h.s. (max 120 mg/d)

PHARMACOKINETICS Absorption: incompletely absorbed from GI tract. **Onset:** 30–45 min. **Duration:** 4–6 h. **Metabolism:** 50% metabolized in GI tract before absorption; 50% metabolized in liver. **Elimination:** half-life: 9 h; excreted primarily in urine; some excreted in bile.

CONTRAINDICATIONS & PRECAUTIONS Contraindicated in: pregnancy (category C).

ADVERSE/SIDE EFFECTS *Constipation,* difficult urination, *dry mouth,* blurred vision, mydriasis, increased intraocular pressure, drowsiness, decreased sexual activity.

NURSING IMPLICATIONS

Administration

- Oral preparation is generally administered 30–60 min before meals and at bedtime. Advise the patient not to chew tablet; drug is bitter.
- Sustained-release tablets should not be crushed or chewed. Regular tablets may be crushed and mixed with fluid or food before swallowing.
- If patient is also receiving an antacid (or antidiarrheal agent), propantheline should be taken at least 1 h before or 1 h after the other drug.
- Store dry powder and tablets at 15–30C (59–86F), protected from freezing and moisture.

Assessment & Drug Effects

- Assess bowel sounds, especially in presence of ulcerative colitis, since paralytic ileus may develop, predisposing to toxic megacolon.
- The elderly or debilitated patient may respond to a usual dose with agitation, excitement, confusion, drowsiness. If these symptoms are observed, stop the drug and report to physician.
- Patients with cardiac disease should have periodic checks of BP and heart sounds and rhythm.

Patient & Family Education

- Alcoholic beverages should be avoided while patient is receiving propantheline.
- Urinary hesitancy or retention (especially likely to

P

Common side effects in *italic*; life-threatening effects underlined; generic names in **bold**; classifications in SMALL CAPS

923

occur in elderly patients) may be avoided by advising patient to void just prior to each dose. Instruct the patient to note daily urinary volume and to report voiding problems to physician.
- Dry mouth may be relieved by frequent rinsing with warm tap water, by sugar-free gum or hard candy. If symptoms persist, report to physician.
- Caution patient to maintain adequate fluid and high-fiber food intake to prevent constipation.
- Postural hypotension and tachycardia may occur during early therapy. Instruct the patient to make all position changes slowly and to lie down immediately if faintness, weakness, or palpitations occur. Advise the patient to report these symptoms to the physician.
- Caution the patient to avoid potentially hazardous activities such as driving a car or operating machinery until response to drug is known.

Prototype: morphine, p 156

PROPOXYPHENE HYDROCHLORIDE

(proe-pox´i-feen)
Trade names: 642, Darvon, Doxaphene, Novopropoxyn, Profene

PROPOXYPHENE NAPSYLATE

Trade names: Darvon-N
Classifications: CNS AGENT; NARCOTIC (OPIATE) AGONIST ANALGESIC
Pregnancy: Categories C (D for prolonged use)
Controlled substance: Schedule IV

ACTIONS/PHARMACODYNAMICS Centrally acting opioid structurally related to methadone. Analgesic potency about 1/2–2/3 that of codeine. Unlike codeine, propoxyphene has little or no antitussive effect, and abuse liability is somewhat lower. Has no significant antiinflammatory or antipyretic actions. The hydrochloride is freely soluble in water and is more rapidly and completely absorbed than the napsylate, which is only slightly water soluble. Lower incidence of GI side effects reported with the napsylate salt.

USES Relief of mild to moderate pain. **Unlabeled use:** to suppress narcotic withdrawal symptoms.

ROUTE & DOSAGE

Mild to Moderate Pain*

Adult	PO	65 mg HCl or 100 mg napsylate q4h prn (max: 390 mg HCl/d, 600 mg napsylate/d)

*100 mg napsylate = 65 mg HCl

PHARMACOKINETICS Absorption: readily absorbed from upper part of small intestine. **Onset:** 15–60 min. **Peak:** 2–3 h. **Duration:** 4–6 h. **Distribution:** crosses placenta; distributed into breast milk. **Metabolism:** metabolized in liver. **Elimination:** half-life: 6–12 h, 30–36 h for metabolite; excreted in urine.

CONTRAINDICATIONS & PRECAUTIONS Contraindicated in: hypersensitivity to drug; suicidal individuals; alcoholism; dependence on opiates. Safe use during pregnancy (category C); for prolonged use (category D); and in children not established. **Cautious use in:** renal or hepatic disease.

ADVERSE/SIDE EFFECTS CNS: dizziness, lightheadedness, *drowsiness,* sedation, unusual fatigue or weakness, restlessness, tremor, euphoria, dysphoria, headache, paradoxic excitement. **GI:** nausea, vomiting, abdominal pain, constipation. **Other:** minor visual disturbances, headache, skin eruptions (hypersensitivity), hypoglycemia (patients with impaired renal function); liver dysfunction. **Overdosage:** mental confusion, toxic psychosis, coma, convulsions, respiratory depression, pulmonary edema, acidosis, pinpoint pupils (dilate with advancing hypoxia), circulatory collapse, ECG abnormalities, nephrogenic diabetes insipidus.

DRUG INTERACTIONS Alcohol and other CNS DEPRESSANTS add to CNS depression—fatalities reported with alcohol; may increase hypoprothrombinemic effects of **warfarin;** may increase **carbamazepine** toxicity through decreased metabolism; **orphenadrine** increases CNS stimulation, anxiety, tremors, confusion.

NURSING IMPLICATIONS

Administration

- Capsules may be emptied and contents mixed with water or food before they are swallowed.
- Absorption may be somewhat delayed by presence of food in stomach.
- Store at 15–30C (59–86F) unless otherwise directed.

P

Assessment & Drug Effects

- Evaluate patient's need for continued use of this drug. Propoxyphene is commonly abused. **Overdose:** Fatalities occur commonly within first hour following overdosage; therefore prompt action is required.
- Effectiveness of propoxyphene may be reduced in smokers. Smoking induces liver enzymes responsible for metabolizing propoxyphene.
- When propoxyphene is included in combination products, precautions relative to each drug ingredient must be considered.
- Tremulousness, restlessness ("speeding"), and mild euphoria occur frequently.
- Dizziness, lightheadedness, drowsiness, nausea, and vomiting appear to be more prominent in the ambulatory patient. Symptoms may be relieved if patient lies down.

Patient & Family Education

- Caution ambulatory patients not to drive a car and to avoid other potentially hazardous activities.
- Caution patient not to exceed recommended dose and to avoid alcohol and other CNS depressants.
- Tolerance and physical and psychic dependence of the morphine type can occur with excessive use.

PROPRANOLOL HYDROCHLORIDE

See AUTONOMIC NERVOUS SYSTEM AGENT, BETA ADRENERGIC ANTAGONIST (BLOCKING AGENT, SYMPATHOLYTIC) prototype, p 109.

PROPYLTHIOURACIL

See HORMONES, ANTITHYROID AGENT prototype, p 243.

PROTAMINE SULFATE

(proe´ta-meen)
Classification: ANTIDOTE
Pregnancy: Category C

ACTIONS/PHARMACODYNAMICS Purified mixture of simple, low-molecular-weight proteins obtained from sperm or testes of suitable fish species. When used alone, has anticoagulant effect. Because it is strongly basic, protamine combines with strongly acidic heparin to produce a stable complex, and thus anticoagulant effect of both drugs is neutralized.

USES Antidote for heparin calcium or heparin sodium overdosage (after heparin has been discontinued). **Unlabeled use:** antidote for heparin administration during extracorporeal circulation.

ROUTE & DOSAGE

Antidote for Heparin Overdose

Adult	IV	Each milligram of protamine will neutralize 90 U of beef-lung heparin, 115 U of intestinal mucosa–derived heparin, and 100 U of calcium heparin; calculate approximate dose and give the first 25–50 mg by slow IV push followed by the rest by continuous infusion over 8–16 h

PHARMACOKINETICS Onset: 5 min. **Duration:** 2 h.

CONTRAINDICATIONS & PRECAUTIONS Contraindicated in: hemorrhage not induced by heparin overdosage. Pregnancy category C. **Cautious use in:** cardiovascular disease, history of allergy to fish, vasectomized or infertile males, patients who have received protamine-containing insulin.

ADVERSE/SIDE EFFECTS _Abrupt drop in BP_ (with rapid IV infusion), bradycardia, dyspnea, nausea, vomiting, lassitude; transient flushing and feeling of warmth. **Bleeding:** protamine overdose or "heparin rebound" (hyperheparinemia). **Hypersensitivity reactions:** urticaria, angioedema, pulmonary edema, <u>anaphylaxis</u>.

NURSING IMPLICATIONS

Administration

- Since protamine has a longer half-life than heparin and also has some anticoagulant effect of its own, dose must be carefully titrated to prevent excess anticoagulation.
- Reconstitute each 50 mg with 5 ml of sterile water for injection. Shake until dissolved. May be given by direct IV over 1–3 min without further dilution.
- Reconstituted solution may be further diluted in NS or D5W and infused at a rate not to exceed 50 mg over 10 min.

P

Common side effects in _italic_; life-threatening effects <u>underlined</u>;
generic names in **bold**; classifications in SMALL CAPS

925

- Protamine sulfate injection should be stored at 2–8C (36–46F); protamine powder for injection and reconstituted solution at 15–30C (59–86F). Avoid freezing. Solutions are stable for 72 h at this temperature.

Assessment & Drug Effects

- Protamine is not used if only minor bleeding occurs during heparin therapy because withdrawal of heparin will usually correct minor bleeding within a few hours.
- Monitor BP and pulse q15–30min, or more often if indicated. Continue for at least 2–3 h after each dose, or longer as dictated by patient's condition. Be prepared to treat patient for shock as well as hemorrhage.
- The effect of protamine in neutralizing heparin is monitored by APTT or ACT values. Coagulation tests are usually performed 5–15 min after administration of protamine, and again in 2–8 h if desirable.
- Patients undergoing extracorporeal dialysis or patients who have had cardiac surgery must be observed carefully for bleeding (heparin rebound). Even with apparent adequate neutralization of heparin by protamine, bleeding may occur 30 min to 18 h after surgery. Monitor vital signs closely. Additional protamine may be required in these patients.

Prototype: imipramine, p 184

PROTRIPTYLINE HYDROCHLORIDE

(proe-trip´te-leen)
Trade names: Triptil, Vivactil
Classifications: CNS AGENT; PSYCHOTHERAPEUTIC; TRICYCLIC ANTIDEPRESSANT; AUTONOMIC NERVOUS SYSTEM AGENT
Pregnancy: Category C

ACTIONS/PHARMACODYNAMICS Tricyclic antidepressant (TCA) with more rapid onset of action than imipramine. Has little if any sedative properties characteristic of most other TCAs but causes tachycardia, CNS stimulation, and strong anticholinergic activity; orthostatic hypotension occurs frequently. Actions, limitations, and interactions are similar to those of imipramine.

USES Symptomatic treatment of endogenous depression in patient under close medical supervision.

Particularly effective for depression manifested by psychomotor retardation, apathy, and fatigue.

ROUTE & DOSAGE

Antidepressant

Adult	PO	15–40 mg/d in 3–4 divided doses (max 60 mg/d)
Adolescent	PO	15 mg/d in divided doses

PHARMACOKINETICS Absorption: rapidly absorbed from GI tract. **Peak levels:** 24–30 h. **Distribution:** crosses placenta; distributed into breast milk. **Metabolism:** metabolized in liver. **Elimination:** half-life: 54–98 h; primarily excreted in urine.

CONTRAINDICATIONS & PRECAUTIONS Contraindicated in: use in children; concurrent use of MAO inhibitors; during acute recovery phase following MI; pregnancy (category C). **Cautious use in:** hepatic, cardiovascular, or renal dysfunction; diabetes mellitus; hyperthyroidism; patients with insomnia.

ADVERSE/SIDE EFFECTS Allergic: photosensitivity, edema (general or of face and tongue). **Anticholinergic:** *xerostomia,* blurred vision, *constipation,* paralytic ileus, *urinary retention,* confusional states. **CNS:** insomnia, headache, confusion. **CV:** change in heat or cold tolerance; *orthostatic hypotension, tachycardia.*

DRUG INTERACTIONS May decrease some response to ANTIHYPERTENSIVES; CNS DEPRESSANTS, **alcohol,** HYPNOTICS, BARBITURATES, SEDATIVES potentiate CNS depression; ORAL ANTICOAGULANTS may increase hypoprothombinemic effects; **ethchlorvynol** causes transient delirium; **levodopa,** SYMPATHOMIMETICS (e.g., **epinephrine, norepinephrine**) increase possibility of sympathetic hyperactivity with hypertension and hyperpyrexia; MAO INHIBITORS present possibility of severe reactions—toxic psychosis, cardiovascular instability; **methylphenidiate** increases plasma TCA levels; THYROID DRUGS may increase possibility of arrhythmias; **cimetidine** may increase plasma TCA levels.

NURSING IMPLICATIONS

Administration

- Tablet may be crushed before administration and taken with fluid or mixed with food.
- Increase in dosage should be made in the morning dose to prevent sleep interference and because this TCA has psychic energizing action.

P

- Last dose of day should be taken no later than midafternoon; insomnia rather than drowsiness is a frequent side effect.
- To reduce possibility of relapse, maintenance therapy is generally continued at least 3 mo after satisfactory improvement is noted.
- Store drug in tightly closed container at 15–30C (59–86F) unless otherwise directed.

Assessment & Drug Effects

- Has fairly rapid onset of initial effect characterized by increased activity and energy, usually within 1 wk after therapy is initiated.
- If the elderly patient has a dose higher than 20 mg/d, monitor CV system responses closely.
- Maximum antidepressant effect may not occur for 2 wk or more after therapy begins.
- Monitor vital signs closely during early therapy, particularly in patients with cardiovascular disorders and in elderly patients receiving daily doses in excess of 20 mg. If BP falls more than 20 mm Hg and if there is a sudden increase in pulse rate, withhold drug and inform physician.
- During early therapy and when patient is on large doses, monitor I&O ratio and question patient about bowel regularity.
- Anticholinergic effects are prominent (xerostomia, blurred vision, constipation, paralytic ileus, urinary retention, delayed micturition). Assess and advise physician as indicated.
- Xerostomia can interfere with appetite, fluid intake, and integrity of tooth surfaces. Assess condition of oral membranes frequently; institute symptomatic treatment if necessary.
- Suicide is an inherent risk with any depressed patient and may remain until there is significant improvement. Supervise patient closely during early treatment period.
- If a patient uses excessive amounts of alcohol it should be borne in mind that the potentiation of TCA effects may increase the danger of overdosage or suicide attempt.
- Patients receiving large doses for prolonged periods or in combination with other drugs should have periodic determinations of liver function and blood cell counts.

Patient & Family Education

- The actions of both alcohol and protriptyline are potentiated when used together during therapy and for up to 2 wk after the TCA is discontinued. Consult physician about safe amount of alcohol, if any, that can be taken.
- Smoking increases the metabolism of TCAs and therefore reduces its effectiveness. Urge patient to stop or to reduce smoking. Apparent treatment failure may be due to the nicotine effect.
- Advise patient to consult physician before taking any OTC medications.
- The effects of barbiturates and other CNS depressants are enhanced by TCAs.
- Caution patient to avoid hazardous activities requiring alertness and skill until response to drug is known.
- Photosensitivity reactions may occur. Until this possibility is ruled out, advise patient to avoid exposure to the sun without protecting skin with sunscreen lotion (SPF ≥ 12), if allowed, and to avoid sun between the hours of 10 and 3 when sun's rays are nearest.

Prototype: epinephrine, p 102

PSEUDOEPHEDRINE HYDROCHLORIDE
(soo-doe-e-fed´rin)

Trade names: Cenafed, Decongestant Syrup, Dorcol Children's Decongestant, Eltor, Eltor 120, Halofed, Neofed, Novafed, PediaCare, Pseudofrin, Robidrine, Sudafed, Sudrin
Classifications: AUTONOMIC NERVOUS SYSTEM AGENT; ALPHA- AND BETA-ADRENERGIC AGONIST (SYMPATHOMIMETIC); DECONGESTANT
Pregnancy: Category C

ACTIONS/PHARMACODYNAMICS Sympathomimetic amine that, like ephedrine, produces decongestion of respiratory tract mucosa by action on sympathetic nerve endings. Unlike ephedrine, also acts directly on smooth muscle and constricts renal and vertebral arteries. Has fewer side effects, less pressor action and longer duration of effects than ephedrine. Produces little, if any, congestive rebound or irritation that occur with nasal sprays and solutions.

USES Symptomatic relief of nasal congestion associated with rhinitis, coryza, and sinusitis and for eustachian tube congestion.

ROUTE & DOSAGE

Nasal Congestion

Adult	PO	60 mg q4–6h or 120 mg sustained release q12h
Child	PO	6–11 y: 30 mg q4–6h (max 120 mg/d)
		2–6 y: 15 mg q4–6h (max 60 mg/d)

P

PHARMACOKINETICS Absorption: readily absorbed from GI tract. **Onset:** 15–30 min. **Duration:** 4–6 h (8–12 h sustained release). **Distribution:** crosses placenta; distributed into breast milk. **Metabolism:** partially metabolized in liver. **Elimination:** excreted in urine.

CONTRAINDICATIONS & PRECAUTIONS Contraindicated in: hypersensitivity to sympathomimetic amines; severe hypertension; coronary artery disease; use within 14 d of MAO inhibitors; glaucoma; hyperthyroidism; prostatic hypertrophy. Safe use during pregnancy (category C), in nursing mothers, and in children <6 y not established. **Cautious use in:** hypertension, heart disease.

ADVERSE/SIDE EFFECTS *Transient stimulation,* tremulousness, difficulty in voiding, arrhythmias, palpitation, *tachycardia, nervousness,* dizziness, headache, sleeplessness, numbness of extremities, anorexia, dry mouth, nausea, vomiting.

DRUG INTERACTIONS Other SYMPATHOMIMETICS increase pressor effects and toxicity; MAO INHIBITORS may precipitate hypertensive crisis; BETA-BLOCKERS may increase pressor effects; may decrease antihypertensive effects of **guanethidine, methyldopa, reserpine.**

NURSING IMPLICATIONS

Administration

▪ Tablet may be crushed before administration and taken with fluid of patient's choice.

Asssessment & Drug Effects

▪ Monitor HR and BP, especially in those with a history of cardiac disease. Report tachycardia or hypertension.

Patient & Family Education

▪ Since drug may act as a stimulant, advise patient to avoid taking it within 2 h of bedtime.
▪ Advise patient to withhold medication if extreme restlessness or signs of sensitivity occur and to consult physician.
▪ Warn patient against concomitant use of OTC medications; many contain ephedrine or other sympathomimetic amines and might intensify action of pseudoephedrine. Consult physician.

PSYLLIUM HYDROPHILIC MUCILOID

See GI AGENT, BULK LAXATIVE prototype, p 219.

Prototype: mebendazole, p 53

PYRANTEL PAMOATE
(pi-ran´tel)
Trade names: Antiminth, Combantriln
Classifications: ANTIINFECTIVE; ANTHELMINTIC
Pregnancy: Category C

ACTIONS/PHARMACODYNAMICS Exerts selective depolarizing neuromuscular blocking action, which results in spastic paralysis of worm; also inhibits cholinesterases.

USES *Enterobius vermicularis* (pinworm) and *Ascaris lumbricoides* (roundworm) infestations. **Unlabeled uses:** hookworm infestations; trichostrongylosis.

ROUTE & DOSAGE

Pinworm or Roundworm

Adult	PO	11 mg/kg as a single dose (max 1 g)
Child	PO	Same as for adult

PHARMACOKINETICS Absorption: poorly absorbed from GI tract. **Peak:** 1–3 h. **Metabolism:** metabolized in liver. **Elimination:** > 50% excreted in feces, 7% in urine.

CONTRAINDICATIONS & PRECAUTIONS Contraindicated in: safe use during pregnancy (category C) and in children <2 y not established. **Cautious use in:** liver dysfunction; malnutrition; dehydration; anemia.

ADVERSE/SIDE EFFECTS CNS: dizziness, headache, drowsiness, insomnia. **GI:** anorexia, *nausea,* vomiting, abdominal distension, diarrhea, *tenesmus,* transient elevation of AST. **Other:** skin rashes.

DRUG INTERACTIONS Piperazine and pyrantel may be mutually antagonistic.

NURSING IMPLICATIONS

Administration

▪ Shake suspension well before pouring it to assure accurate dosage.
▪ May be taken with milk or fruit juices and without regard to prior ingestion of food or time of day.
▪ Purging is not necessary before, during, or after therapy.
▪ Store below 30C (86F). Protect from light.

Prototype: isoniazid, p 83

PYRAZINAMIDE

(peer-a-zin´a-mide)
Trade names: Tebrazid
Classifications: ANTIINFECTIVE; ANTITUBECULO-
SIS AGENT
Pregnancy: Category C

ACTIONS/PHARMACODYNAMICS Pyrazinoic
acid amide, analog of nicotinamide and bacteriostatic
against *Mycobacterium tuberculosis*. When employed alone, resistance may develop in 6–7 wk;
therefore, administration with other effective agents
is recommended. Appears to interfere with renal capacity to concentrate and excrete uric acid; thus may
cause hyperuricemia.

USES Short-term therapy of advanced tuberculosis
before surgery and to treat patients unresponsive to
primary agents (e.g., isoniazid, streptomycin).

ROUTE & DOSAGE

Tuberculosis

Adult	PO	20–35 mg/kg/d in 3–4 divided doses (max 3 g/d)

PHARMACOKINETICS Absorption: readily ab-
sorbed from GI tract. **Peak:** 2 h. **Distribution:** crosses
blood-brain barrier. **Metabolism:** metabolized in liver.
Elimination: half-life: 9–10 h; excreted slowly in urine.

**CONTRAINDICATIONS & PRECAUTIONS Con-
traindicated in:** severe hepatic damage. Safe use during pregnancy (category C) and in children not established. **Cautious use in:** presence or family history of
gout or diabetes mellitus; impaired renal function;
history of peptic ulcer; acute intermittent porphyria.

ADVERSE/SIDE EFFECTS Arthralgia, *active gout,*
difficulty in urination, headache, photosensitivity, urticaria, skin rash (rare), sideroblastic or hemolytic
anemia, splenomegaly, lymphadenopathy, <u>fatal
hemoptysis</u>, aggravation of peptic ulcer, *rise in serum
uric acid, hepatotoxicity, abnormal liver function
tests,* acute yellow atrophy of liver, decreased plasma
prothrombin.

DIAGNOSTIC TEST INTERFERENCES Pyrazinamide may produce a temporary decrease in *17-*

keto-steroids and an increase in ***protein-bound
iodine.***

NURSING IMPLICATIONS

Administration

- Drug should be discontinued if hepatic reactions
  (jaundice, pruritis, icteric sclerae, yellow skin) or
  hyperuricemia with acute gout (severe pain in great
  toe and other joints) occur.
- Store tightly closed container at 15–30C (59–86F).

Assessment & Drug Effect

- The patient receiving pyrazinamide requires close
  observation and medical supervision. He or she
  should receive at least one other effective antituberculosis agent concurrently.
- Patients should be examined at regular intervals
  and questioned about possible signs of toxicity:
  liver enlargement or tenderness, jaundice, fever,
  anorexia, malaise, impaired vascular integrity (ecchymoses, petechiae, abnormal bleeding).
- Hepatic reactions appear to occur more frequently
  in patients receiving high doses.
- Liver function tests (especially AST, ALT, serum
  bilirubin) should be done prior to and at 2–4 wk intervals during therapy. Blood uric acid determinations are advised before, during, and following
  therapy.

Patient & Family Education

- Report to physician the onset of difficulty in voiding. Patient should be urged to keep fluid intake at
  a 2000 ml/d level if possible.
- Patients with diabetes should be closely monitored
  and advised of possible loss of glycemic control.

Prototype: permethrin, p 260

PYRETHRINS

(peer´e-thrins)
Trade names: A-200 Pyrinate, Barc, Blue,
Pyrinate, Pyrinyl, R & C, RID, TISIT, Triple X
Classifications: SKIN AGENT; PEDICULICIDE
ANTIINFECTIVE
Pregnancy: Category C

ACTIONS/PHARMACODYNAMICS Pedicul-
icide solution comprised of pyrethrins and piperonyl
butoxide in deodorized kerosene. Acts as a contact

P

Common side effects in *italic*; life-threatening effects <u>underlined</u>;
generic names in **bold**; classifications in SMALL CAPS

929

poison affecting the parasite's nervous system, causing paralysis and death. Controls head lice, pubic (crab) lice, and body lice and their eggs (nits).

USES External treatment of *Pediculus humanus* infestations.

ROUTE & DOSAGE

Pediculus humanus Infestations

Adult	Topical	See nursing implications for appropriate application

CONTRAINDICATIONS & PRECAUTIONS Contraindicated in: sensitivity to solution components; skin infections and abrasions; pregnancy (category C). **Cautious use in:** ragweed-sensitized patient, infants, children.

ADVERSE/SIDE EFFECTS Irritation with repeated use.

NURSING IMPLICATIONS

Administration
Application of Drug
▪ Apply enough solution to completely wet infested area, including hair.
▪ Allow to remain on area for 10 min.
▪ Wash and rinse with large amounts of warm water.
▪ Use fine-toothed comb to remove lice and eggs from hair.
▪ Shampoo hair to restore body and luster.
▪ Treatment may be repeated if necessary once in 24 h.
▪ Repeat treatment in 7–10 d to kill newly hatched lice.
▪ Do not apply to eyebrows or eyelashes without consulting physician.
▪ In accidental contact of eyes, flush with copious amounts of warm water.

Patient & Family Education
▪ Pyrethrins should not be swallowed, inhaled, or allowed to contact mucosal surfaces or the eyes.
▪ If treated area becomes irritated, discontinue use and consult physician.
▪ Each family member should be examined carefully; if infested, he or she should also be treated immediately to prevent spread or reinfestation of previously treated patient.
▪ Dry clean, boil, or otherwise treat contaminated clothing. Sterilize (soak in pyrethrins) comb and brushes used by patient.

▪ Teach patient not to share comb, brush, or headgear with another person.

Prototype: neostigmine, p 118

PYRIDOSTIGMINE BROMIDE
(peer-id-oh-stig´meen)
Trade names: Mestinon, Regonol
Classifications: AUTONOMIC NERVOUS SYSTEM AGENT; CHOLINERGIC (PARASYMPATHOMIMETIC); CHOLINESTERASE INHIBITOR
Pregnancy: Category C

ACTIONS/PHARMACODYNAMICS Analog of neostigmine; indirect-acting cholinergic with anticholinesterase activity. By blocking the destruction of acetylcholine (a neurotransmitter), drug facilitates transmission of impulses across myoneural junctions. Has fewer side effects and longer duration of action than neostigmine.

USES Myasthenia gravis and as an antagonist to nondepolarizing skeletal muscle relaxants (e.g., curariform drugs).

ROUTE & DOSAGE

Myasthenia Gravis

Adult	PO	60 mg–1.5 g/d spaced according to requirements and response of individual patient
		Sustained release: 180–540 mg 1–2 times/d at intervals of at least 6 h
	IM/IV	Approximately 1/30th of PO dose
Child	PO	7 mg/kg/d divided into 5–6 doses
Neonates	PO	5 mg q4–6h
	IM/IV	0.05–0.15 mg/kg q4–6h

Reversal of Muscle Relaxants

Adult	IV	10–20 mg immediately preceded by IV atropine

PHARMACOKINETICS Absorption: poorly absorbed from GI tract. **Onset:** 30–45 min PO; 15 min IM; 2–5 min IV. **Duration:** 3–6 h. **Distribution:** crosses placenta. **Metabolism:** metabolized in liver and in serum and tissue by cholinesterases. **Elimination:** excreted in urine.

P

CONTRAINDICATIONS & PRECAUTIONS Contraindicated in: hypersensitivity to anticholinesterase agents or to bromides. Mechanical obstruction of urinary or intestinal tract; bradycardia, hypotension. Safe use during pregnancy (category C) or in nursing mothers not established. **Cautious use in:** bronchial asthma; epilepsy; vagotonia; hyperthyroidism; peptic ulcer; cardiac dysrhythmias.

ADVERSE/SIDE EFFECTS Acneiform (bromide) rash, thrombophlebitis (following IV administration). **With large doses:** Muscarinic effects: *nausea, vomiting, diarrhea, miosis, excessive salivation and sweating,* increased bronchial secretion, <u>bronchoconstriction</u>, bradycardia, weakness, fasciculation and hypotension.

DRUG INTERACTIONS Atropine NONDEPOLARIZING MUSCLE RELAXANTS antagonize effects of pyridostigmine.

NURSING IMPLICATIONS

Administration
- Administer drug with food or fluid.
- Swallow sustained-release tablet whole.
- A syrup is available. Some patients may not like it because it is sweet; try to make it more palatable by giving it over ice chips. The syrup formulation contains 5% alcohol.
- Sustained-release tablets are generally prescribed only at bedtime for patients who complain of weakness on awakening.
- Pyridostigmine syrup should be protected from light.
- IV pyridostigmine is given by direct IV undiluted at a rate of 0.5 mg over 1 min for myasthenia gravis; 5 mg over 1 min for reversal of muscle relaxants. Do not add to IV solutions.
- Store at 15–30C (59–86F). Protect from light and moisture.

Assessment & Drug Effects
- Failure of patient to show improvement may reflect either underdosage or overdosage. Report increasing muscular weakness, cramps, or fasciculations.
- Atropine may be used to abolish GI side effects or other muscarinic side effects. Observe patient closely because atropine may mask signs of overdosage (cholinergic crisis): increasing muscle weakness, which through involvement of respiratory muscles can lead to death.
- Monitor vital signs frequently, especially respiratory rate.

- Observe for signs of cholinergic reactions (see chap 3), particularly when drug is administered IV.
- Neonates of myasthenic mothers who have received pyridostigmine should be closely observed for difficulty in breathing, swallowing, or sucking.
- When used as muscle relaxant antagonist, patient should be continuously observed. Airway and respiratory assistance must be maintained until full recovery of voluntary respiration and neuromuscular transmission is assured. Complete recovery usually occurs within 30 min.

Patient & Family Education
- Duration of drug action reportedly may vary with physical and emotional stress, as well as with severity of disease.
- Report onset of rash. Drug discontinuation may be indicated.
- Sustained-release tablets may become mottled in appearance; this does not affect their potency.

PYRIDOXINE HYDROCHLORIDE (VITAMIN B$_6$)
(peer-i-dox´een)
Trade names: Beesix, Hexa-Betalin, NesTrex, Pyroxine
Classification: VITAMIN
Pregnancy: Categories A (C if > RDA)

ACTIONS/PHARMACODYNAMICS Water-soluble complex of three closely related compounds (pyridoxine and its active derivatives pyridoxamine and pyridoxal) with B$_6$ activity. Considered essential to human nutrition, although a deficiency syndrome is not well defined. Converted in body to pyridoxal, a coenzyme that functions in protein, fat, and carbohydrate metabolism and in facilitating release of glycogen from liver and muscle. In protein metabolism, participates in many enzymatic transformations of amino acids and conversion of tryptophan to niacin and serotonin. Aids in energy transformation in brain and nerve cells, and is thought to stimulate heme production.

USES Prophylaxis and treatment of pyridoxine deficiency, as seen with inadequate dietary intake, drug-induced deficiency (e.g., isoniazid, oral contraceptives), and inborn errors of metabolism (vitamin B$_6$–dependent convulsions or anemia). Also to prevent chloramphenicol-induced optic neuritis, to treat acute toxicity caused by overdosage of cycloserine, hydralzine, isoniazid (INH); alcoholic polyneuritis;

P

sideroblastic anemia associated with high serum iron concentration. Has been used for management of many other conditions ranging from nausea and vomiting in radiation sickness and pregnancy to suppression of postpartum lactation.

ROUTE & DOSAGE

Dietary Deficiency

Adult	PO/IM/IV	2.5–10 mg/d for 3 wk, then may reduce to 2.5–5 mg/d

Pyridoxine Deficiency Syndrome

Adult	PO/IM/IV	Initial: up to 600 mg/d may be required
		Maintenance: up to 50 mg/d

Isoniazid-induced Deficiency

Adult	PO/IM/IV	100–200 mg/d for 3 wk, then 25–100 mg/d

PHARMACOKINETICS Absorption: readily absorbed from GI tract. **Distribution:** stored in liver; crosses placenta. **Metabolism:** metabolized in liver. **Elimination:** excreted in urine.

CONTRAINDICATIONS & PRECAUTIONS Contraindicated in: safe use of large doses in pregnancy (category A) or category C if more than RDA, in nursing mothers, and in children not established.

ADVERSE/SIDE EFFECTS Rarely: paresthesias, somnolence seizures (particularly following large parenteral doses), slight flushing or feeling of warmth, low folic acid levels, temporary burning or stinging pain in injection site.

DRUG INTERACTIONS Isoniazid, cycloserine, penicillamine, hydralazine, and ORAL CONTRACEPTIVES may increase pyridoxine requirements; may reverse or antagonize therapeutic effects of **levodopa.**

NURSING IMPLICATIONS

Administration

- May be given without regard to food.
- IV pyridoxine may be given by direct IV undiluted at a rate of 50 mg or fraction thereof over 60 seconds. May also be added to most IV infusions.
- Preserve in tight, light-resistant containers at 15–30C (59–86F). Avoid freezing.

Assessment & Drug Effects

- Therapeutic effectiveness of vitamin B_6 therapy is evaluated by improvement of B_6 *deficiency manifes-*

tations: nausea, vomiting, skin lesions resembling those of riboflavin and niacin deficiency (seborrhea-like lesions about eyes, nose, and mouth, glossitis, stomatitis), edema, CNS symptoms (depression, irritability, peripheral neuritis, convulsions), hypochromic microcytic anemia.

- A complete dietary history should be recorded so that poor eating habits can be identified and corrected (a single vitamin deficiency is rare; patient can be expected to have multiple vitamin deficiencies).

Patient & Family Education

- Recommended dietary allowance (RDA) of pyridoxine: 2.2 mg for adults; 2.6 mg during pregnancy and lactation. Need for pyridoxine increases with amount of protein in diet.
- Rich dietary sources of vitamin B_6 include yeast, wheat germ, whole grain cereals, muscle and glandular meats (especially liver), legumes, green vegetables, bananas.
- Advise patient not to self-medicate with vitamin combinations (OTC) without first consulting physician.

Prototype: chloroquine, p 79

PYRIMETHAMINE

(peer-i-meth´a-meen)
Trade name: Daraprim
Classifications: ANTIINFECTIVE; ANTIMALARIAL
Pregnancy: Category C

ACTIONS/PHARMACODYNAMICS Long-acting folic acid antagonist chemically related to metabolite of chloroguanide. Selectively inhibits action of dehydrofolic reductate in parasite with resulting blockade of folic acid metabolism. Has no gametocidal activity but prevents development of fertilized gametes in mosquito and thus helps to prevent transmission of malaria. Because action against blood-borne schizonts is slow in onset, has little value as single agent in treatment of acute primary malarial attack. Cross-resistance with chloroguanide may occur.

USES Prophylaxis of malaria due to susceptible strains of plasmodia. May be used conjointly with fast-acting antimalarial (e.g., chloroquine, quinacrine, quinine) to initiate transmission control and suppressive cure. Used with a sulfonamide to provide synergistic action in treatment of toxoplasmosis.

ROUTE & DOSAGE

Malaria Chemoprophylaxis

Adult   PO   25 mg once/wk

Child   PO   > 10 y: 25 mg once/wk
          4–10 y: 12.5 mg once/wk
          <4 y: 6.25 mg once/wk

Toxoplasmosis

Adult   PO   50–75 mg/d with a sulfonamide for 1–3 wk; then decrease dose by half and continue for 1 mo

Child   PO   1 mg/kg/d divided into 2 doses with a sulfonamide for 1–3 wk; then decrease to 0.5 mg/kg/d for 1 mo (max 25 mg/d)

PHARMACOKINETICS Absorption: readily absorbed from GI tract. **Peak:** 2 h. **Distribution:** concentrates in kidneys, lungs, liver, and spleen; distributed into breast milk. **Elimination:** half-life: 54–148 h; excreted slowly in urine; excretion may extend over 30 d or longer.

CONTRAINDICATIONS & PRECAUTIONS Contraindicated in: chloroguanide-resistant malaria, megaloblastic anemia caused by folate deficiency. Safe use during pregnancy (category C) not established. **Cautious use in:** patients with convulsive disorders receiving high doses of an anticonvulsant (e.g., phenytoin).

ADVERSE/SIDE EFFECTS With *large doses or prolonged therapy:* anorexia, vomiting, atrophic glossitis, abdominal cramps, skin rashes, *folic acid deficiency (megaloblastic anemia, leukopenia, thrombocytopenia, pancytopenia,* diarrhea). *Acute toxicity:* CNS stimulation including convulsions, respiratory failure.

DRUG INTERACTIONS Folic acid, para-aminobenzoic acid (PABA) may decrease effectiveness against toxoplasmosis.

NURSING IMPLICATIONS

Administration

- GI distress may be minimized by taking drug with meals. If symptoms persist, dosage reduction may be necessary.
- For malaria prophylaxis, drug should be taken on same day each week. Administration should begin when individual enters malarious area and should continue for 10 wk after leaving the area.
- Some physicians prescribe leucovorin concurrently for patients on high-dosage therapy to prevent the hematologic complications of folic acid deficiency.

Assessment & Drug Effects

- Dosages required for treatment of toxoplasmosis approach toxic levels. Blood counts, including platelets, should be performed twice weekly during therapy. If hematologic abnormalities appear, dosage should be reduced or drug discontinued; parenteral leucovorin (folinic acid) (leucovorin rescue) will be administered until blood counts return to normal.

Patient & Family Education

- Folic acid deficiency may occur with long-term use of pyrimethamine. Instruct patient to report symptoms: weakness, and pallor (from anemia), ulcerations of oral mucosa, superinfections, glossitis; GI disturbances such as diarrhea and poor fat absorption, fever. Folate (folinic acid) replacement may be prescribed. Encourage patient to increase food sources of folates (if allowed) in diet.

Prototype: lorazepam, p 177

QUAZEPAM

(qua´ze-pam)
Trade name: Doral
Classifications: CNS AGENT; BENZODIAZEPINE ANXIOLYTIC, SEDATIVE-HYPNOTIC
Pregnancy: Category X

ACTIONS/PHARMACODYNAMICS Quazepam is believed to potentiate gamma aminobutyric acid (GABA) neuronal inhibition in the limbic, neocortical, and mesencephalic reticular systems. It significantly decreases sleep latency and total wake time and significantly increases sleep time. REM sleep is essentially unchanged. No transient sleep disturbance such as "rebound insomnia" was observed after withdrawal of the drug.

USES Insomnia characterized by difficulty in falling asleep, frequent nocturnal awakenings, or early morning awakenings.

ROUTE & DOSAGE

Insomnia

Adult   PO   7.5–15 mg h.s.

Q

Common side effects in *italic*; life-threatening effects underlined; generic names in **bold**; classifications in SMALL CAPS

933

PHARMACOKINETICS Absorption: readily absorbed from GI tract. **Onset:** 30 min. **Peak:** 2 h. **Distribution:** crosses placenta; distributed into breast milk. **Metabolism:** metabolized in liver to active metabolites. **Elimination:** half-life: 39 h; excreted in urine and feces.

CONTRAINDICATIONS & PRECAUTIONS Contraindicated in: hypersensitivity to quazepam or benzodiazepines; sleep apnea; pregnancy (category X). **Cautious use in:** impaired hepatic and renal function. Not recommended for nursing mothers. Safety and effectiveness in children < 18 y not established.

ADVERSE/SIDE EFFECTS CNS: *drowsiness, headache,* fatigue, dizziness, dry mouth. **GI:** dyspepsia.

DRUG INTERACTIONS Alcohol, CNS DEPRESSANTS, ANTICONVULSANTS potentiate CNS depression; **cimetidine** increases quazepam plasma levels, increasing its toxicity; may decrease antiparkinsonism effects of **levodopa;** may increase **phenytoin** levels; **smoking** decreases sedative effects of quazepam.

NURSING IMPLICATIONS

Administration
- Initial dose is usually 15 mg but can often be effectively reduced after several nights of therapy.
- In the elderly, dose should be reduced to lowest effective dose as soon as possible.

Assessment & Drug Effects
- Monitor for respiratory depression in patients with chronic respiratory insufficiency.
- Monitor for suicidal tendencies in previously depressed clients.
- Daytime drowsiness is more likely to occur with the elderly client.

Patient & Family Education
- Instruct patient to inform physician about any alcohol consumption and prescription or nonprescription medication being taken. Alcohol generally should not be used since it potentiates CNS depressant effects.
- Instruct patient to inform physician if she is to become pregnant or if pregnancy occurs while she is taking this medicine. The drug causes birth defects.
- Until reaction to the drug is known, advise patient not to drive a car or operate potentially dangerous machinery.
- Instruct patient not to increase the dose and to inform the doctor if the drug "no longer works."
- Advise patient that drug may cause daytime sedation, which may persist for several days even after drug is discontinued.

Prototype: mebendazole, p 53

QUINACRINE HYDROCHLORIDE

(kwin´a-kreen)
Trade name: Atabrine
Classifications: ANTIINFECTIVE; ANTHELMINTIC; ORPHAN DRUG
Pregnancy: Category C

ACTIONS/PHARMACODYNAMICS Acridine dye derivative. Eradicates beef, pork, dwarf, and fish tapeworm and *Giardia lamblia* by causing worm scolex to detach from intestinal tract. Acts as suppressive agent and controls clinical attacks of malaria but is not a true prophylactic agent and does not produce a radical cure.

USES Tapeworm infestations and giardiasis. Use as antimalarial has been largely superseded by more effective and less toxic drugs.

PHARMACOKINETICS Absorption: readily absorbed from GI tract. **Peak:** 8 h. **Duration:** detected in plasma for 4–6 wk. **Distribution:** concentrates in liver, lungs, pancreas, and erythrocytes; crosses placenta; distributed into breast milk. **Elimination:** slowly excreted in urine.

CONTRAINDICATIONS & PRECAUTIONS Contraindicated in: psoriasis, porphyria; pregnancy (category C); concomitant use of primaquine; intracavitary use in pneumothorax. **Cautious use in:** adults > 60 y, children < 1 y, history of psychosis; hepatic disease; alcoholism; concomitant use with hepatotoxic drugs; G6PD deficiency.

ADVERSE/SIDE EFFECTS CNS: *headache,* dizziness, vertigo, restlessness, confusion, irritability, emotional changes, insomnia, nightmares, psychotic reactions, convulsions (large doses). **GI:** *nausea, vomiting,* anorexia, *diarrhea, abdominal cramps.* **Skin:** *yellow pigmentation,* urticaria, <u>exfoliative dermatitis</u>, contact dermatitis, lichen planus–like eruptions. **Other:** (usually with prolonged therapy): <u>aplastic anemia, agranulocytosis</u>, hepatitis, corneal edema or deposits (reversible), retinopathy (rare), fever.

Common side effects in *italic*; life-threatening effects <u>underlined</u>; generic names in **bold**; classifications in SMALL CAPS

P

ROUTE & DOSAGE

Beef, Pork, or Fish Tapeworm

Adult	PO	200 mg with 600 mg sodium bicarbonate q10min for 4 doses
Child	PO	11–14 y: 200 mg with 300 mg sodium bicarbonate q10min for 3 doses
		5–10 y: 200 mg with 300 mg sodium bicarbonate q10min for 2 doses

Dwarf Tapeworm

Adult	PO	300 mg q20min for 3 doses, then 100 mg 3 times daily for 3 d
Child	PO	11–14 y: 400 mg initially, then 100 mg t.i.d. for 3 d
		8–10 y: 300 mg initially, then 100 mg b.i.d. for 3 d
		4–8 y: 200 mg initially, then 100 mg after breakfast for 3 d

Giardiasis

Adult	PO	100 mg t.i.d. for 5 d
Child	PO	2 mg/kg t.i.d. for 5 d (max 300 mg/d)

Malaria Supression

Adult	PO	100 mg once/d
Child	PO	50 mg once/d

DIAGNOSTIC TEST INTERFERENCES Possibility of false-positive *adrenal function tests* using Mattingly method (quinacrine is fluorescent in aqueous media).

DRUG INTERACTIONS Alcohol may cause disulfiram-like reaction; increased toxicity with **primaquine.**

NURSING IMPLICATIONS

Administration
Tapeworm Infestations

- Patient is given a bland liquid or no-residue semisolid, nonfat diet for 24–48 h before start of drug therapy, with fasting after evening meal before and on morning of treatment.
- Generally a saline purge and cleansing enema are given before treatment to reduce amount of stool that must be examined for scolex. Saline purge is repeated 1–2 h after quinacrine is administered. Sodium bicarbonate is prescribed with each dose of quinacrine to reduce tendency to nausea and vomiting.
- For pork tapeworm (*Taenia solium*), drug is ad-

ministered by duodenal tube to prevent vomiting. Vomiting may cause passage of worm segments (proglottids) into stomach, with subsequent release of ova and invasion of tissue (cysticercosis).

Giardiasis

- Administer quinacrine after meals; stools are examined 2 wk after last dose. Repeat course may be given, if indicated.

Malarial

- Quinacrine should be taken after meals with a full glass of water, tea, or fruit juice.
- For suppression of malaria, medication should be taken for 1–3 mo.

Assessment & Drug Effects

- CBCs and ophthalmoscopic examinations should be done periodically in patients on prolonged drug therapy.
- Be alert for symptoms of drug-induced behavioral changes and psychosis. Psychotic reactions may last 2–4 wk after drug is stopped.

Patient & Family Education

- Inform patients that drug colors skin a reversible yellow (not jaundice) and sometimes may give a grayish blue tinge resembling cyanosis to ears, nasal cartilage, and fingernail beds. Skin discoloration usually disappears in about 2 wk after drug is discontinued.
- Advise patients to report immediately the onset of skin eruptions or visual disturbances (e.g., halos of light, focusing difficulties, blurred vision).
- With tapeworm, entire stool specimen is collected for 48 h to find the scolex (worm head). Worm is usually passed within 4–10 h. Cure is presumed if scolex is found; dwarf tapeworm infestations are usually multiple and require more persistent treatment.
- If scolex is not found, stools should be examined periodically for tapeworm; stools must be free of worm eggs or segments for 3–6 mo to be certain of cure.

Prototype: estradiol, p 236

QUINESTROL

(kwin-ess'trole)
Trade name: Estrovis
Classifications: HORMONE; ESTROGEN
Pregnancy: Category X

P

Common side effects in *italic*; life-threatening effects underlined; generic names in **bold**; classifications in SMALL CAPS

935

ACTIONS/PHARMACODYNAMICS Long-lasting orally effective estrogen with actions and uses similar to those of estradiol.

USES Moderate to severe vasomotor symptoms associated with menopause, atrophic vaginitis, kraurosis vulvae, female hypogonadism, female castration, primary ovarian failure.

ROUTE & DOSAGE

Menopause, Female Hypogonadism, Primary Ovarian Failure

Adult   PO   100 µg/d for 7 d; then 100 µg/wk beginning 2 wk after initiation of therapy; may be increased to 200 µg/wk if necessary

PHARMACOKINETICS Absorption: readily absorbed from GI tract. **Peak:** peak relief 4–8 wk. **Distribution:** stored in adipose tissue. **Metabolism:** metabolized in liver. **Elimination:** half-life: 120 h; slowly excreted in bile and urine.

CONTRAINDICATIONS & PRECAUTIONS Contraindicated in: breast cancer, known or suspected pregnancy (category X). **Cautious use in:** hypertension; gallbladder disease; diabetes mellitus; heart failure; hepatic or renal dysfunction.

ADVERSE/SIDE EFFECTS CV: thromboembolic disorders, *hypertension.* **GI:** *nausea,* vomiting, diarrhea, anorexia, weight changes, bloating, cholestatic jaundice. **Metabolic:** reduced carbohydrate tolerance, hypercalcemia, *fluid retention.* **Reproductive:** mastodynia, breakthrough bleeding, changes in menstrual flow, dysmenorrhea, amenorrhea. **Other:** leg cramps.

DRUG INTERACTIONS Carbamazepine, phenytoin, rifampin decrease estrogen levels through increased metabolism; CORTICOSTEROIDS may enhance steroid effects; ORAL ANTICOAGULANTS may decrease anticoagulant effects.

NURSING IMPLICATIONS

Administration

- Tablet may be taken with food or fluid of patient's choice.
- Store at 15–30C (59–86F) in a tightly capped container.

Assessment & Drug Effects

- Patients with conditions that may be influenced by fluid retention (migraine, cardiac or renal dysfunction, asthma, epilepsy, hypertension) should be monitored carefully. Check BP on a regular basis.

Patient & Family Education

- Advise the diabetic to report altered blood and urine glucose tests. Estrogen activity may increase requirement for hypoglycemic medication.
- Advise patient to determine weight under standard conditions 1 or 2 times/wk and to report sudden weight gain or other signs of fluid retention.
- Inform patient that fluid retention may precipitate migraine and hypertension.
- Estrogen stimulation in women sterilized because of endometriosis may cause serious bleeding in remaining foci of endometrial tissues. Report unexplained and sudden pain.
- Advise patient to report severe abdominal pain and tenderness, an abdominal mass, and possible symptoms of hepatic adenoma or hepatic hemorrhage.
- If user suspects she is pregnant, she should stop taking the estrogen immediately and inform the physician. She should be apprised of the potential risk of masculinization of female fetus.
- Symptoms of vaginal candidiasis (thick, white, curdlike secretions and inflamed congested introitus) should be reported to permit appropriate treatment.
- Explain to patient receiving quinestrol for postmenopausal symptoms that menstruallike bleeding may occur but does not indicate return of fertility. (Estrogen suppresses ovulation.)
- Teach or reinforce previous teaching of self-examination of the breast.
- Attempts to discontinue or taper medication should be made at 3–6 mo intervals.
- Urge patient to read package insert to assure understanding of estrogen therapy.

Prototype: Procainamide, p 140

QUINIDINE GLUCONATE

(kwin′i-deen)
Trade names: Duraquin, Quinaglute Duratabs, Quinate, Quinatime, Quin-Release
Classifications: CARDIOVASCULAR AGENT; ANTIARRHYTHMIC
Pregnancy: Category C

ACTIONS/PHARMACODYNAMICS Dextro isomer of quinine; class I-A antiarrhythmic agent. Similar to quinidine sulfate in actions, uses, contraindications, and adverse reactions. Parenteral form used

Common side effects in *italic*; life-threatening effects underlined; generic names in **bold**; classifications in SMALL CAPS

when oral therapy not feasible or when rapid effects are required. Contains 62.3% anhydrous quinidine alkaloid base. **Unlabeled use:** IV form, severe malaria.

ROUTE & DOSAGE

Acute Tachycardia

Adult	PO	324–660 mg q8–12h
	IM	600 mg, then 400 mg q2h prn
	IV	200–750 mg at a rate of 16 mg/min

PHARMACOKINETICS Absorption: well absorbed from GI tract. **Onset:** 1–3 h PO; 15 min IM. **Peak:** 0.5–1 h. **Duration:** 6–8 h. **Distribution:** widely distributed to most body tissues except the brain; crosses placenta; distributed into breast milk. **Metabolism:** metabolized in liver. **Elimination:** half-life: 6–8 h; > 95% excreted in urine, < 5% in feces.

CONTRAINDICATIONS & PRECAUTIONS Contraindicated in: safe use during pregnancy (category C), during lactation, and by children not established. See quinidine sulfate.

ADVERSE/SIDE EFFECTS Particularly with IV use: *nausea, vomiting, abdominal cramps,* urge to defecate or urinate, cold sweat, apprehension, severe hypotension. Also see quinidine sulfate.

DRUG INTERACTIONS May increase **digoxin** levels by 50%; **amiodarone** may increase quinidine levels, increasing risk of heart block; other ANTIARRHYTHMICS, PHENOTHIAZINES, **reserpine** add to cardiac depressant effects; ANTICHOLINERGIC AGENTS add to vagolytic effects; CHOLINERGIC AGENTS may antagonize cardiac effects; ANTICONVULSANTS, BARBITURATES, **rifampin** increase the metabolism of quinidine, causing decreased efficacy; CARBONIC ANHYDRASE INHIBITORS, **sodium bicarbonate,** CHRONIC ANTACIDS decrease renal elimination of quinidine, increasing its toxicity; **verapamil** causes significant hypotension; may increase hypoprothrombinemic effects of **warfarin.**

NURSING IMPLICATIONS

Administration

- Examine parenteral solution before preparation; use only if clear and colorless.
- When administering drug IM, aspirate syringe carefully before injection to avoid inadvertent entry into blood vessel.
- IV quinidine is prepared by diluting 800 mg (10 ml)

in at least 40 ml D5W to yield a maximum concentration of 16 mg/ml. Administer via infusion pump at a rate not to exceed 16 mg (1 ml)/min.

- Severe hypotension is most likely to occur in patients receiving drug IV. Supine position during drug administration is advisable.
- Instruct patient not to crush or chew tablet before he or she swallows it.
- Extended-action tablet is used only for maintenance and prophylactic therapy. Advise patient to swallow tablet whole.
- Quinidine plasma levels are generally higher when oral dose is taken on an empty stomach (i.e., 1 h before or 2 h after meals). GI distress may be minimized by administration of oral drug with food, however.
- Protect solutions from light and heat to prevent brownish discoloration and possibly precipitation.

Assessment & Drug Effects

- Some physicians give an initial test dose (50–200 mg IM) or 1 tablet PO to determine sensitivity. If positive, patient will display symptoms of cinchonism: tinnitus, headache, nausea, visual disturbances.
- Continuous monitoring of ECG and BP and frequent determinations of plasma quinidine levels are advised when drug is administered intravenously.
- Report to the physician immediately the following *indications to stop quinidine:* (1) worsening of minor side effects, (2) restoration of sinus rhythm, (3) prolongation of QRS complex (beyond 25%), (4) changes in QT or refractory period, (5) disappearance of P waves, (6) sudden onset of or increase in PVCs, and (7) decrease in heart rate to 120 bpm.
- Observe patient closely following each parenteral dose. Amount of subsequent dose is gauged by response to preceding dose.

See quinidine sulfate for additional nursing implications.

Prototype: procainamide, p 140

QUINIDINE POLYGALACTURONATE
(kwin´i-deen)
Trade name: Cardioquin
Classifications: CARDIOVASCULAR AGENT; ANTIARRHYTHMIC
Pregnancy: Category X

Q

Common side effects in *italic*; life-threatening effects <u>underlined</u>; generic names in **bold**; classifications in SMALL CAPS

937

Similar to quinidine sulfate in actions/pharmacodynamics, contraindications & precautions, and adverse/side effects. Reportedly has a lower incidence of associated GI irritation than quinidine sulfate has. Polygalacturonate slows the ionization of quinidine.

ROUTE & DOSAGE

Atrial Fibrillation or Flutter

Adult	PO	275–825 mg q3–4h for 4 or more doses until arrhythmia terminates; then 137.5–275 mg b.i.d. or t.i.d.

PHARMACOKINETICS Absorption: slowly dissociates in GI tract and is absorbed as free quinidine. **Onset:** 1–3 h. **Peak:** 0.5–1 h. **Duration:** 6–8 h. **Distribution:** widely distributed to most body tissues except the brain; crosses placenta; distributed into breast milk. **Metabolism:** metabolized in liver. **Elimination:** half-life: 6–8 h; > 95% excreted in urine, < 5% in feces.

DRUG INTERACTIONS May increase **digoxin** levels by 50%; **amiodarone** may increase quinidine levels, thus increasing risk of heart block; other ANTIARRHYTHMICS, PHENOTHIAZINES, **reserpine** add to cardiac depressant effects; ANTICHOLINERGIC AGENTS add to vagolytic effects; CHOLINERGIC AGENTS may antagonize cardiac effects; ANTICONVULSANTS, BARBITURATES, **rifampin** increase the metabolism of quinidine, decreasing its efficacy; CARBONIC ANHYDRASE INHIBITORS, **sodium bicarbonate,** CHRONIC ANTACIDS decreases renal elimination of quinidine, thus increasing its toxicity; **verapamil** causes significant hypotension; may increase hypoprothrombinemic effects of **warfarin.**

NURSING IMPLICATIONS
See quinidine sulfate.

Prototype: procainamide, p 140

QUINIDINE SULFATE
(kwin´i-deen sul-fate)
Trade names: Apo-Quinidine, Cin-Quin, Novoquinidin, Quinidex Extentabs, Quinora, SK-Quinidine Sulfate
Classifications: CARDIOVASCULAR AGENT; ANTIARRHYTHMIC
Pregnancy: Category C

ACTIONS/PHARMACODYNAMICS Dextro isomer of quinine and alkaloid of *Cinchona*. Class I-A antiarrhythmic. Like quinine, exhibits some antimalarial, antipyretic, and oxytocic properties. Contains 83% anhydrous quinidine alkaloid. Cardiac actions similar to those of procainamide. At the cellular level, decreases sodium influx during depolarization and potassium efflux in repolarization; also reduces calcium transport across cell membrane. Depresses myocardial excitability, contractility, automaticity, and conduction velocity, and prolongs effective refractory period. Anticholinergic action blocks vagal stimulation of AV node, thus tending to increase ventricular rate, particularly in larger doses. Also exerts muscle relaxant action by decreasing effective transmission across neuromuscular junction. Hypotensive effect is produced primarily by peripheral vasodilation and in part by alpha-adrenergic blockade.

USES Premature atrial, AV junctional, and ventricular contraction; paroxysmal atrial tachycardia, chronic ventricular tachycardia (when not associated with complete heart block); maintenance therapy after electrical conversion of atrial fibrillation or flutter.

ROUTE & DOSAGE

Ectopic Beats

Adult	PO	200–300 mg t.i.d. or q.i.d.
Child	PO	6 mg/kg 5 times/d

Ventricular Arrhythmias

Adult	PO	400–600 mg q2–3h until arrhythmia terminates, then 200–300 mg 3–4 times/d

Atrial Fibrillation or Flutter

Adult	PO	200 mg q2–3h for 5–8 doses until sinus rhythm restored or toxicity occurs (max 3–4 g); then 200–300 mg t.i.d. or q.i.d.

PHARMACOKINETICS Absorption: almost completely absorbed from GI tract. **Onset:** 1–3 h. **Peak:** 0.5–1 h. **Duration:** 6–8 h. **Distribution:** widely distributed to most body tissues except the brain; crosses placenta; distributed into breast milk. **Metabolism:** metabolized in liver. **Elimination:** half-life: 6–8 h; > 95% excreted in urine, < 5% in feces.

CONTRAINDICATIONS & PRECAUTIONS Contraindicated in: hypersensitivity or idiosyncrasy to quinine or *Cinchona* derivatives; safe use during pregnancy (category C), during lactation, or in children

Q

not established. Thrombocytopenic purpura resulting from prior use of quinidine, intraventricular conduction defects, complete AV block, ectopic impulses and rhythms due to escape mechanisms; thyrotoxicosis, acute rheumatic fever, subacute bacterial endocarditis, extensive myocardial damage, frank CHF, hypotensive states; myasthenia gravis; digitalis intoxication. **Cautious use in:** incomplete heart block; impaired renal or hepatic function; bronchial asthma or other respiratory disorders; myasthenia gravis; potassium imbalance.

ADVERSE/SIDE EFFECTS CNS: headache, fever, tremors, apprehension, delirium, syncope with sudden loss of consciousness, and ventricular arrhythmias, disturbed hearing (tinnitus, auditory acuity). **CV:** hypotension, CHF, widened QRS complex, bradycardia, heart block, atrial flutter, ventricular flutter, fibrillation or tachycardia; quinidine syncope, torsades de pointes. **Eye:** mydriasis, blurred vision, disturbed color perception, reduced visual field, photophobia, diplopia, night blindness, scotomas, optic neuritis. **GI:** *nausea, vomiting, diarrhea, abdominal pain,* hepatic dysfunction. **Hematologic:** acute hemolytic anemia, hypoprothrombinemia, thrombocytopenic purpura (rare), leukopenia, agranulocytosis (rare). **Hypersensitivity:** may include symptoms of cinchonism plus angioedema, acute asthma, respiratory depression, vasculitis (rare), vascular collapse. **Skin:** rash, urticaria, cutaneous flushing with intense pruritus, photosensitivity. **Other:** SLE; Cinchonism: nausea, vomiting, headache, dizziness, fever, tremors, vertigo, tinnitus, visual disturbances. **Overdosage:** hypokalemia, cinchonism, tachyarrhythmias, seizures.

DRUG INTERACTIONS May increase **digoxin** levels by 50%; **amiodarone** may increase quinidine levels, thus increasing its risk of heart block; other ANTIARRHYTHMICS, PHENOTHIAZINES, **RESERPINE** add to cardiac depressant effects; ANTICHOLINERGIC AGENTS add to vagolytic effects; CHOLINERGIC AGENTS may antagonize cardiac effects; ANTICONVULSANTS, BARBITURATES, **rifampin** increase the metabolism of quinidine, thus decreasing its efficacy; CARBONIC ANHYDRASE INHIBITORS, **sodium bicarbonate,** CHRONIC ANTACIDS decrease renal elimination of quinidine, thus increasing its toxicity; **verapamil** causes significant hypotension; may increase hypoprothrombinemic effects of **warfarin.**

NURSING IMPLICATIONS

Administration

- Test dose is used by some physicians to determine idiosyncrasy before establishing full dosage schedule.
- For optimum absorption, quinidine is taken with a full glass of water on an empty stomach (i.e., 1 h before or 2 h after meals). If GI symptoms occur (nausea, vomiting, diarrhea are most common), administer drug with food.
- Sustained release tablet is usually reserved for maintenance and prophylactic therapy.
- Dosage is adjusted to maintain plasma concentration between 2 and 5 µg/ml. Levels of 8 µg/L or more are associated with myocardial toxicity.
- Preserve in tight, light-resistant containers away from excessive heat.

Assessment & Drug Effects

- Observe cardiac monitor and report immediately the following *indications for stopping quinidine:* (1) sinus rhythm, (2) widening QRS complex in excess of 25% (i.e., > 0.12 seconds), (3) changes in QT interval or refractory period, (4) disappearance of P waves, (5) sudden onset of or increase in ectopic ventricular beats (extrasystoles, PVCs), (6) decrease in heart rate to 120 bpm. Also report immediately any worsening of minor side effects.
- Continuous monitoring of ECG and BP is required. Close observation of patient (check sensorium and be alert for any sign of toxicity) and frequent determinations of plasma quinidine concentrations are indicated when large doses (more than 2 g/d) are used or when quinidine is given parenterally (e.g., quinidine gluconate).
- During acute treatment, monitor vital signs q1–2h or more often as needed. Count apical pulse for a full minute. Report any change in pulse rate, rhythm, or quality or any fall in BP.
- Severe hypotension is most likely to occur in patients receiving high oral doses or parenteral quinidine, i.e., quinidine gluconate.
- Reversion to sinus rhythm in long-standing fibrillation or when fibrillation is complicated by CHF involves some risk of embolization from dislodgment of atrial mural emboli.
- Quinidine can cause unpredictable rhythm abnormalities in the digitalized heart. Patients with atrial flutter or fibrillation may be pretreated with digitalis (until ventricular rate is 100 bpm) to increase AV nodal block and thus reduce possibility of paradoxic tachycardia.
- Monitor I&O. Diarrhea occurs commonly during

Q

early therapy; most patients become tolerant to this side effect. If symptoms become severe, serum electrolytes and acid-base and fluid balance should be evaluated. Dosage adjustment may be required.

▪ During long-term therapy, periodic blood counts, serum electrolyte determinations, and kidney and liver function tests are advised.

Patient & Family Education

▪ Instruct patient to report feeling of faintness ("quinidine syncope") caused by quinidine-induced changes in ventricular rhythm resulting in decreased cardiac output and syncope.

▪ Hypersensitivity reactions usually appear 3–20 d after drug is started. Fever occurs commonly and may or may not be accompanied by other symptoms. Advise patient to inform physician if they occur.

▪ A diet high in alkaline ash foods (vegetables, citrus fruit, milk) may prolong half-life of quinidine by decreasing its excretion and increasing danger of toxicity. Advise patient to eat a balanced diet: no excesses in fruit or fruit juices, milk, or a vegetarian diet.

▪ Advise patient not to self-medicate with OTC drugs without advice from physician.

▪ Discuss medication schedule with patient. Advise patient not to increase, decrease, skip, or discontinue doses without consulting physician.

▪ Advise patient to notify physician immediately of disturbances in vision, ringing in ears, sense of breathlessness, onset of palpitations, and unpleasant sensation in chest and to note time of occurrence and duration of chest symptoms.

Prototype: chloroquine, p 79

QUININE SULFATE
(kwye´nine)
Trade names: Novoquinine, Quin-260, Quinamm, Quine, Quinite, Quiphile, Strema
Classifications: ANTIINFECTIVE; ANTIMALARIAL
Pregnancy: Category X

ACTIONS/PHARMACODYNAMICS Chief alkaloid from bark of cinchona tree. Exact mechanism of antimalarial action uncertain. Inhibits protein synthesis and depresses many enzyme systems in malaria parasite. has schizonticidal action and is gametocidal with *Plasmodium vivax* and *Plasmodium malariae*

but not *Plasmodium falciparum.* Resembles salicylates in analgesic and antipyretic properties and exerts curare-like skeletal-muscle relaxant effect. Also has oxytocic action and hypoprothrombinemic effect. Qualitatively similar to quinidine in cardiovascular effects. Generally replaced by less toxic and more effective agents in treatment of malaria.

USES Chloroquine-resistant falciparum malaria and in combination with other antimalarials for radical cure of relapsing vivax malaria; also relief of nocturnal recumbency leg cramps.

ROUTE & DOSAGE

Acute Malaria

Adult	PO	650 mg q8h for 3 d
Child	PO	25 mg/kg/d in three divided doses q8h for 3 d

Malaria Chemoprophylaxis

Adult	PO	325 mg b.i.d. for 6 wk

Nocturnal Leg Cramps

Adult	PO	260–300 mg h.s.

PHARMACOKINETICS Absorption: well absorbed from GI tract. **Peak:** 1–3 h. **Duration:** 6–8 h. **Distribution:** widely distributed to most body tissues except the brain; crosses placenta; distributed into breast milk. **Metabolism:** metabolized in liver. **Elimination:** half-life: 8–21 h; > 95% excreted in urine, < 5% in feces.

CONTRAINDICATIONS & PRECAUTIONS Contraindicated in: tinnitus, optic neuritis; myasthenia gravis; G6PD deficiency; pregnancy (category X). **Cautious use in:** cardiac arrhythmias. Same precautions as for quinidine sulfate when used in patients with cardiovascular conditions.

ADVERSE/SIDE EFFECTS Cinchonism: tinnitus, decreased auditory acuity, dizziness, vertigo, headache, visual impairment, *nausea, vomiting, diarrhea,* fever. **CNS:** confusion, excitement, apprehension, syncope, delirium. **CV:** angina. **Hematologic:** leukopenia, thrombocytopenia, <u>agranulocytosis</u>, hypoprothrombinemia, hemolytic anemia. **Hypersensitivity:** cutaneous flushing, visual impairment, pruritus, skin rash, fever, gastric distress, dyspnea, tinnitus. **Toxicity:** decrease in BP and respiration, tachycardia, <u>hypothermia</u>, convulsions, <u>cardiovascular collapse</u>, <u>coma</u>, blackwater fever (extensive intravascular hemolysis with renal failure), <u>death</u>. **Other:** urticaria, acute asthma.

Q

DIAGNOSTIC TEST INTERFERENCES Quinine may interfere with determinations of *urinary cate-cholamines* (Sobel and Henry modification procedure) and *urinary steroids* (17 hydroxycorticosteroids) (modification of Reddy, Jenkins, Thorn method).

DRUG INTERACTIONS May increase **digoxin** levels; ANTICHOLINERGIC AGENTS add to vagolytic effects; CHOLINERGIC AGENTS may antagonize cardiac effects; ANTICONVULSANTS, BARBITURATES, **rifampin** increase the metabolism of quinine, thus decreasing its efficacy; CARBONIC ANHYDRASE INHIBITORS, **sodium bicarbonate,** CHRONIC ANTACIDS decrease renal elimination of quinine, thus increasing its toxicity; **warfarin** may increase hypoprothrombinemic effects.

NURSING IMPLICATIONS

Administration
- Administer drug with or after meals or a snack to minimize gastric irritation. Quinine has potent local irritant effect on gastric mucosa. Advise patients not to crush capsule; drug is not only irritating but also extremely bitter.
- Preserve in tight, light-resistant containers.

Assessment & Drug Effects
- Be alert to signs of *rising plasma concentration of quinine:* tinnitus and hearing impairment, which usually do not occur until concentration is 10 µg/ml or more.
- In patients with atrial fibrillation, follow the same precautions with quinine as are used with quinidine, since quinine may produce cardiotoxicity in these patients.

Patient & Family Education
- Patients should be informed about possible adverse reactions and advised to report promptly the onset of any unusual symptom.

Prototype: cimetidine, p 216

RANITIDINE HYDROCHLORIDE
(ra-nye´te-deen)
Trade name: Zantac
CLASSIFICATIONS: GI AGENT; ANTISECRETORY (H₂-RECEPTOR ANTAGONIST)
Pregnancy: Category B

ACTIONS/PHARMACODYNAMICS A potent antiulcer drug that competitively and reversibly inhibits histamine action at H₂-receptor sites on parietal cells. Blocks daytime and nocturnal basal gastric acid secretion stimulated by histamine and reduces gastric acid release in response to food, pentogastrin, and insulin. Indirectly reduces pepsin secretion but appears to have minimal effect on fasting and postprandial serum gastrin concentrations or secretion of gastric intrinsic factor or mucus. Increases gastric bacterial flora (nitrate-reducing organisms), reduces hepatic blood flow, and delays gastric emptying, but clinical significance of these actions is unclear. Lacks antiandrogenic activity and does not appear to alter mean daily insulin requirement in patients with type I (IDDM) diabetes mellitus. Does not interact with hepatic cytochrome P450 (microsomal) enzyme system; therefore drug interaction potential is minimal; can be given with drugs metabolized by oxidation in the liver without concern for interference with their clearance, e.g., phenytoin, warfarin, theophylline, diazepam, propranolol.

USES Short-term treatment of active duodenal ulcer; maintenance therapy for duodenal ulcer patient after healing of acute ulcer; treatment of gastroesophageal reflux disease; short-term treatment of active, benign gastric ulcer; and treatment of pathologic GI hypersecretory conditions (e.g., Zollinger-Ellison syndrome, systemic mastocytosis, and postoperative hypersecretion).

ROUTE & DOSAGE

Duodenal Ulcer, Gastric Ulcer, Gastroesophageal Reflux

Adult	PO	150 mg b.i.d. *or* 300 mg h.s.
	IV	50 mg q6–8h; 150–300 mg/24 h by continuous infusion

Duodenal Ulcer, Maintenance Therapy

Adult	PO	150 mg h.s.

Pathologic Hypersecretory Conditions

Adult	PO	150 mg b.i.d. up to 6.3 g/d
	IV	50 mg q6–8h

PHARMACOKINETICS Absorption: incompletely absorbed from GI tract (50% reaches systemic circulation). **Peak:** 2–3 h PO. **Duration:** 8–12 h. **Distribution:** distributed into breast milk. **Metabolism:** metabolized in liver. **Elimination:** half-life: 2–3 h; excreted in urine, with some excreted in feces.

R

Common side effects in *italic*; life-threatening effects <u>underlined</u>; generic names in **bold**; classifications in SMALL CAPS

941

CONTRAINDICATIONS & PRECAUTIONS Contraindicated in: safe use during pregnancy (category B), in nursing mothers, and in children < 12 y not established. **Cautious use in:** hepatic and renal dysfunction.

ADVERSE/SIDE EFFECTS Generally infrequent. **CNS:** headache, malaise, dizziness, somnolence, insomnia, vertigo. Rare: mental confusion, agitation, depression, hallucinations in elderly patients; increased intraocular pressure (ocular pain, blurred vision). **CV** (rare)**:** tachycardia, bradycardia, PVCs. **GI:** constipation, nausea, abdominal pain, diarrhea; hepatotoxicity (rare). **Reproductive** (rare)**:** gynecomastia, impotence. **Other:** rash, reversible decreases in WBC and platelet counts (clinically unimportant); hypersensitivity reactions, anaphylaxis (rare).

DIAGNOSTIC TEST INTERFERENCES Ranitidine may produce slight elevations in **serum creatinine** (without concurrent increase in BUN); (rare) increases in **AST, ALT, alkaline phosphatase, LDH** and total **bilirubin.** Produces false-positive tests for **urine protein** with Multistix (use sulphosalicylic acid instead).

INCOMPATIBILITIES Solution/additive: amphotericin B, clindamycin, chlorpromazine, diazepam, hydroxyzine, methotrimeprazine, midazolam, nalbuphine, OPIUM ALKALOIDS, **phenobarbital. Y-site: methotrimeprazine, midazolam,** OPIUM ALKALOIDS, **phenobarbital.**

NURSING IMPLICATIONS

Administration

- Simultaneous administration of food does not appear to reduce ranitidine absorption or serum concentrations.
- Adjunctive antacid treatment of pain may be necessary and can be given without affecting action of ranitidine. Administer the antacid 2 h before or after ranitidine.
- IV ranitidine must be diluted prior to use; 50 mg ranitidine injection is diluted in 0.9% NaCl injection or other compatible IV solution to a total volume of 20 ml. Give by direct IV at a rate of 4 ml/min or 20 ml over not less than 5 min.
- For intermittent IV infusion, dilute 50 mg in 50–100 ml of NS, D5W, or other compatible IV solution and infuse over 15–30 min.
- IM ranitidine does not need to be diluted.
- If patient is having hemodialysis treatments, the scheduled ranitidine dose should coincide with the end of hemodialysis.
- Store tablets in light-resistant, tightly capped container at 15–30C (59–86F) in a dry place.

Assessment & Drug Effects

- It has been shown that to inhibit 50% of the stimulated gastric acid secretion, serum concentrations of ranitidine need to be 36–94 ng/ml. Concentrations in this range are maintained after a 150 mg dose for up to 12 h.
- The potential for toxicity resulting from decreased clearance (elimination) and therefore prolonged action is greatest in the elderly patient or the patient with hepatic or renal dysfunction.
- Creatinine clearance is monitored if renal dysfunction is present or suspected. When clearance is < 50 ml/min, manufacturer recommends reduction of the dose to 150 mg once q24h with cautious and gradual reduction of the interval to q12h or less, if necessary.
- The incidence of hepatotoxicity is low (and is thought to be a hypersensitivity reaction), but be alert to early signs: jaundice (dark urine, pruritus, yellow sclera and skin), elevated transaminases (especially ALT) and LDH.
- Long-term ranitidine therapy may lead to vitamin B_{12} deficiency.

Patient & Family Education

- Long duration of action provides ulcer pain relief that is maintained through the night as well as the day.
- Endoscopic examination is usually performed at end of 2 wk of therapy because about 37% of patients have been completely healed in that time.
- Most patients have healed ulcers by 4 wk; however, if healing cannot be confirmed endoscopically, treatment may be continued for up to 8 wk.
- Even if symptomatic relief is provided by ranitidine, this should not be interpreted as absence of gastric malignancy. Follow-up examinations will be scheduled after therapy is discontinued.
- Since a family member ordinarily recognizes jaundice from hepatotoxicity sooner than the patient does, discuss these possible symptoms with patient and family. Urge adherence to scheduled periodic laboratory checkups during ranitidine treatment.
- Instruct patient not to supplement therapy with OTC remedies for gastric distress or pain without physician's advice (e.g., Mylanta II reduces ranitidine absorption).
- Smoking has been shown to decrease ranitidine efficacy and adversely affect ulcer healing. Urge patient to stop smoking, informing him or her that

Common side effects in *italic*; life-threatening effects underlined; generic names in **bold**; classifications in SMALL CAPS

giving it up may be more important in preventing ulcer recurrence than the medication.

Prototype: reserpine, p 154

RESCINNAMINE
(res-cin´na-meen)
Trade name: Moderil
Classifications: CARDIOVASCULAR AGENT; RAUWOLFIA ALKALOID; ANTIHYPERTENSIVE; AUTONOMIC NERVOUS SYSTEM AGENT; ADRENERGIC ANTAGONIST (SYMPATHOLYTIC)
Pregnancy: Category C

ACTIONS/PHARMACODYNAMICS Rescinnamine probably exerts its antihypertensive effect through the depletion of tissue stores of catecholamines (epinephrine and norepinephrine) from peripheral sites. Depression of the sympathetic nerve function decreases heart rate and lowers arterial BP.

USES Mild essential hypertension.

ROUTE & DOSAGE

Hypertension
Adult　PO　0.25–1 mg/d

PHARMACOKINETICS Absorption: readily absorbed from GI tract. **Onset:** 2–3 wk. **Peak:** 2 h. **Duration:** > 24 h. **Distribution:** crosses blood-brain barrier and placenta; distributed into breast milk. **Metabolism:** metabolized in liver. **Elimination:** up to 60% excreted in feces; approximately 10% excreted unchanged in urine.

CONTRAINDICATIONS & PRECAUTIONS Contraindicated in: hypersensitivity to rauwolfia derivatives, mental depression (especially if suicidal); active peptic ulcer, ulcerative colitis; electroconvulsive therapy; and nursing mothers. **Cautious use in:** history of mental depression; history of breast cancer; pregnancy (category C); history of peptic ulcer, ulcerative colitis or gall stones; renal impairment; bronchial asthma; allergy to aspirin.

ADVERSE/SIDE EFFECTS CV: *bradycardia, hypotension,* chest pain, arrhythmias. **CNS:** *drowsiness,* depression, nervousness, paradoxical anxiety, nightmares, *fatigue, lethargy.* **GI:** abdominal cramps, diarrhea, nausea, vomiting, anorexia, peptic ulcers, dry mouth. **ENT:** epistaxis, blurred vision, lacrimation, miosis, glucoma, uveitis, optic atrophy, nasal congestion. **Hematologic:** thrombocytopenia anemia. **Skin:** rash pruritus. **Other:** dysuria, dyspnea, impotence, gynecomastia, galactorrhea, edema.

DRUG INTERACTIONS Alcohol and other CNS DEPRESSANTS add to depression; **digoxin** may increase risk of arrhythmias; MAO INHIBITORS may cause excitation or hypertension; may decrease effects of **levodopa.**

NURSING IMPLICATIONS

Administration
- Administer with meals or food to minimize possibility of gastric irritation (drug increases gastric secretions).
- Dosage adjustments should be made at 7–14 d intervals to allow full effects of dosage to occur.
- Administer high doses cautiously because serious mental depression and other side effects may be considerably increased.

Assessment & Drug Effects
- Take BP and pulse at frequent intervals and compare them to baseline determinations. (Note: drop in BP may be accompanied by bradycardia rather than tachycardia.)
- Drug should be withheld and physician notified if despondency, early morning insomnia, loss of appetite, or impotence occur.
- Monitor for dizziness, drowsiness, or faintness. Take appropriate safety precautions.
- Drug may induce depression, which may persist for several months after drug withdrawal and may be severe enough to result in suicide.
- Both cardiovascular effects (antihypertensive effect and bradycardia) and CNS effects (sedative, tranquilizer) may persist following withdrawal of this drug.

Patient & Family Education
- Advise patient to take drug at the same time each day, not to skip or double doses, and not to stop therapy without advice of physician.
- Since drowsiness, sedation, and dizziness are possible side effects, instruct patient to avoid driving and other potentially hazardous activities until reaction to drug is known.
- Instruct patient to check for edema and to record weight daily. Distinction must be made between weight gain from edema and that from increased

R

Common side effects in *italic*; life-threatening effects <u>underlined</u>; generic names in **bold**; classifications in SMALL CAPS

943

appetite. Consult physician about gain of 6–10 kg (3–5 lb) in 1 wk.

- Because of severe adverse effects to infants of nursing mothers, either the drug or nursing by the mother must be discontinued.

RESERPINE

See CARDIOVASCULAR AGENT, RAUWOLFIA ALKALOID prototype, p 154.

Rh₀(D) IMMUNE GLOBULIN

Trade names: Gamulin Rh, HypRho-D, Rhesonativ, RhoGAM, Win Rho

Rh₀(D) IMMUNE GLOBULIN MICRO-DOSE

ACTIONS/PHARMACODYNAMICS Sterile nonpyrogenic gamma globulin solution containing immunoglobulins (IgG). Prepared from a human plasma or serum pool with high titer of anti-Rh₀(D) antibody (anti-Rh antibody) and confirmed nonreactivity for hepatitis B surface antigen (HBsAg). The solution is at least 90% IgG; thimerosal (a mercury derivative) is the preservative. The globulin provides passive immunity by suppressing active antibody response and formation of anti-Rh₀(D) (isoimmunization) in Rh-negative (Rh₀(D)-negative, Dᵘ-negative) individuals previously exposed to Rh-positive (Rh₀(D)-positive, Dᵘ-positive) blood. Such exposure occurs in Rh-negative women when Rh-positive fetal RBCs enter maternal circulation: during third stage of labor, fetal-maternal hemorrhage (as early as second trimester), amniocentesis, or other trauma during pregnancy, termination of pregnancy, and following transfusion with Rh-positive RBC, whole blood, or components (platelets, WBC) prepared from Rh-positive blood. Although the mechanism of action is unclear, it is hypothesized that anti-Rh antibody in the immune globulin solution binds to the Rh antigen on fetal RBC that have entered maternal circulation, thus suppressing a maternal primary immune response with its production of anti-Rh₀(D).

USES To prevent isoimmunization in Rh-negative individuals exposed to Rh-positive RBC (see above). Rh₀(D) immune globulin micro-dose is for use only

after spontaneous or induced abortion or termination of ectopic pregnancy up to and including 12 wk of gestation.

ROUTE & DOSAGE

Antepartum Prophylaxis

Adult	IM	1 vial at approximately 28 wk; followed by 1 vial within 72 h of delivery if infant is Rh-positive

Postpartum Prophylaxis

Adult	IM	1 vial within 72 h of delivery if infant is Rh-positive

Following Amniocentesis, Miscarriage, Abortion, Ectopic Pregnancy

Adult	IM	1 vial of the microdose, preferably within 3 h but at least within 72 h

Transfusion Accident

Adult	IM	1 vial for each volume of RBCs infused divided by 15, given at least within 72 h of accident

CONTRAINDICATIONS & PRECAUTIONS Contraindicated in: Rh₀(D)-positive or Dᵘ-positive patient; person previously immunized against Rh₀(D) factor, hypersensitivity for thimerosal (in commercial preparations), thrombocytopenia, or bleeding disorders.

ADVERSE/SIDE EFFECTS Infrequent: injection site irritation, slight fever, myalgia, lethargy, splenomegaly (causal relationship not confirmed).

DRUG INTERACTIONS May interfere with immune response to **live virus vaccine;** should delay use of live virus vaccines for 3 mo after administration of Rh₀(D) immune globulin.

NURSING IMPLICATIONS

Administration

- Lot numbers of drug used for the cross-match and the drug to be administered must be the same.
- Rh₀(D) immune globulin is administered IM only to the mothers and not to the infant.
- Use the deltoid muscle. The IM may be given in divided doses at different sites, all at once or at intervals, as long as the entire dose is given within 72 h after delivery or termination of pregnancy.
- Follow manufacturer's directions for reconstitution and use supplied sterile water diluent. Administer immediately. Commercially prepared solutions should be refrigerated, although they may be stable up to 30 d at room temperature according to man-

ufacturers. Solutions that have been frozen should be discarded.

- Each vial of Rh₀(D) immune globulin contains enough anti-Rh₀(D) to suppress the immunizing potential of 15 ml Rh-positive packed RBC. Each vial of micro-dose contains enough anti-Rh₀(D) to suppress the immune response to 2.5 ml of Rh-positive packed RBC.
- Although systemic allergic reactions occur rarely, epinephrine should be immediately available.
- Store powder at 2–8C (36–46F) unless otherwise directed. Avoid freezing.

Assessment & Drug Effects

- Obtain history of systemic allergic reactions to human immune globulin preparations prior to drug administration.
- Before administration of Rh₀(D) immune globulin and immediately after delivery, send sample of newborn's cord blood to laboratory for cross-match and typing. Confirm that mother is Rh₀(D) and Dᵘ-negative. Infant must be Rh-positive.

Patient & Family Education

- Approximately 13% of white Americans lack Rh₀(D) completely and therefore are Rh-negative. About 7–10% of black Americans are Rh-negative. About 1% of American Indians and Asian Americans are Rh-negative.
- Administration of Rh₀(D) immune globulin (antibody) prevents hemolytic disease of the newborn in a subsequent pregnancy.

Prototype: acyclovir, p 85

RIBAVIRIN

(rye-ba-vye´rin)

Trade names: Tribavirin, Vilona, Viramid, Virazole

Classifications: ANTIINFECTIVE; ANTIVIRAL

Pregnancy: Category X

ACTIONS/PHARMACODYNAMICS Synthetic nucleoside (analog of guanosine) with broad-spectrum antiviral activity against DNA and RNA viruses. Exact mode of virostatic action not fully understood but is believed to involve multiple mechanisms. Appears to exert selective antiviral action by interfering with viral ribonucleic protein synthesis, ultimately leading to inhibition of viral replication. It does not

influence interferon synthesis. Active against many RNA and DNA viruses, including respiratory syncytial virus (RSV), influenza A and B, parainfluenza, measles, mumps, Lassa fever enterovirus 72 (formerly called hepatitis A), yellow fever, HIV, herpes simplex virus (HSV-1 and HSV-2), and vaccinia. Other activities of ribavirin such as immunosuppression and tumor suppression are being investigated. Immune responses appear to depend on cellular drug concentrations: low concentrations seem to stimulate and high concentrations appear to inhibit immune responses. Generally not active against poliovirus and coxsackieviruses. Unlike other antiviral agents, virus resistance to ribavirin does not appear to develop.

USES Only for aerosol treatment of carefully selected hospitalized infants and young children with severe lower respiratory tract infection caused by respiratory syncytial virus (RSV). **Unlabeled uses:** prophylaxis and treatment of influenza A and B; pneumonia caused by adenovirus; Lassa fever, measles, HSV-1, HSV-2, hepatitis A, herpes zoster, and for carefully selected patients with AIDS and AIDS-related complex (ARC).

ROUTE & DOSAGE

Respiratory Syncytial Virus

Child	Inhalation	20 mg via SPAG nebulizer administered over 12–18 h/d for a minimum of 3 d and a max of 7 d

PHARMACOKINETICS Absorption: rapidly absorbed systemically from lungs. **Peak:** 60–90 min. **Distribution:** crosses placenta; distributed into breast milk. **Metabolism:** metabolized in cells to an active metabolite. **Elimination:** half-life: 24 h in plasma, 16–40 d in RBCs; 85% excreted in urine, 15% in feces.

CONTRAINDICATIONS & PRECAUTIONS Contraindicated in: mild RSV infections of lower respiratory tract; infants requiring simultaneous assisted ventilation; severe cardiopulmonary disease; prolonged or multiple courses of ribavirin inhalation therapy. Safe use during pregnancy (category X), and in nursing mothers not established. **Cautious use in:** COPD, asthma.

ADVERSE/SIDE EFFECTS Causal relationships not conclusive.* (Aerosol therapy is generally well tolerated.) **CV:*** hypotension (faintness, lightheadedness, unusual fatigue), <u>cardiac arrest</u>. **Eye:** blurred vision, conjunctivitis, erythema of eyelids, itching,

R

Common side effects in *italic*; life-threatening effects <u>underlined</u>; generic names in **bold**; classifications in SMALL CAPS

945

sensation of foreign body in eye, increased sensitivity to light. **Hematologic:** reticulocytosis, anemia.* **Respiratory:*** deterioration of respiratory function, dyspnea, apnea, chest soreness, pneumothorax, bacterial pneumonia, ventilator dependence. **Skin:*** rash. **Other:** transient increases in AST, ALT, bilirubin; abdominal cramps.

DRUG INTERACTIONS Ribavirin may antagonize the antiviral effects of **zidovudine** (formerly AZT) against HIV.

NURSING IMPLICATIONS

Administration

- Note that aerosol solution is prepared with either sterile water for injection or sterile water for inhalation, without preservatives or any other added substance. See manufacturer's package insert for preparation directions.
- Inspect solution for discoloration or presence of particulate matter. Discard discolored or cloudy solutions.
- Ribavirin for inhalation is administered only by SPAG-2 aerosol generator. No other aerosol medication is to be given concomitantly with ribavirin.
- The solution in the SPAG-2 reservoir should be discarded at least q24h and whenever liquid level is low before fresh reconstituted solution is added.
- Following reconstitution, solution may be stored at 20–30C (68–86F) for 24 h.
- Store unopened vial in a dry place at 15–25C (59–78F) unless otherwise directed.

Assessment & Drug Effects

- Specimens should be obtained for rapid diagnosis of RSV infection before therapy is initiated or at least during the first 24 h of ribavirin therapy. Ribavirin should not be continued without laboratory confirmation of RSV infection.
- Efficacy of ribavirin in RSV infections appears to be greatest if treatment is initiated within the first 3 d.
- Respiratory function and fluid status must be closely monitored during therapy. Note rate and character of respirations and pulse before treatment begins and at frequent intervals during therapy. Observe for signs of labored breathing: dyspnea, apnea; rapid, shallow respirations, intercostal and substernal retraction, nasal flaring, limited excursion of lungs, cyanosis. Auscultate lungs for abnormal breath sounds.
- Patients requiring simultaneous assisted ventilation should be closely observed for signs of worsening pulmonary function. Every 2 h check equipment carefully, including endotracheal tube, for malfunctioning. Precipitation of ribavirin and accumulation of fluid in tubing can obstruct the apparatus and cause inadequate ventilation and gas exchange.
- Consult physician about management of fluid and food intake and keep an accurate record of I&O.

RIBOFLAVIN (VITAMIN B$_2$)

(rye´boo-flay-vin)
Classification: VITAMIN
Pregnancy: Category A (C if > RDA)

ACTIONS/PHARMACODYNAMICS Water-soluble vitamin and component of the flavoprotein enzymes that work together with a wide variety of proteins to catalyze many cellular respiratory reactions by which the body derives its energy.

USES To prevent riboflavin deficiency and to treat ariboflavinosis; also to treat microcytic anemia and as a supplement to other B vitamins in treatment of pellagra and beriberi.

ROUTE & DOSAGE

Nutritional Supplement

Adult	PO	5–10 mg/d
Child	PO	1–4 mg/d

Nutritional Deficiency

Adult	PO	5–30 mg/d in divided doses
Child	PO	3–10 mg/d

PHARMACOKINETICS Absorption: readily absorbed from GI tract. **Distribution:** little is stored; excess amounts are excreted in urine. **Elimination:** half-life: 66–84 min; excreted in urine.

CONTRAINDICATIONS & PRECAUTIONS Cautious use in: pregnancy (category A).

ADVERSE/SIDE EFFECTS Apparently nontoxic.

DIAGNOSTIC TEST INTERFERENCES In large doses, riboflavin may produce yellow-green fluorescence in **urine** and thus cause false elevations in certain fluorometric determinations of **urinary catecholamines.**

NURSING IMPLICATIONS

Administration

- Administer oral preparation with food to enhance absorption.
- Preserve in airtight containers protected from light.

Assessment & Drug Effects

- Therapeutic effectiveness of vitamin B_2 therapy is evaluated by improvement of clinical manifestations of deficiency: digestive disturbances, headache, burning sensation of skin (especially "burning" feet), cracking at corners of mouth (cheilosis), glossitis, seborrheic dermatitis (often at angle of nose and anogenital region) and other skin lesions, mental depression, corneal vascularization (with photophobia, burning and itchy eyes, lacrimation, roughness of eyelids), anemia, neuropathy.
- Collaborate with physician, dietitian, patient, and responsible family member in planning for diet teaching. A complete dietary history is an essential part of vitamin replacement so that poor eating habits can be identified and corrected. Deficiency in one vitamin is usually associated with other vitamin deficiencies.

Patient & Family Education

- Inform patient receiving large doses that an intense yellow discoloration of urine may occur.
- *Rich dietary sources of riboflavin:* liver, kidney, beef, pork, heart, eggs, milk and milk products, yeast, whole-grain cereals, vitamin A–enriched breakfast cereals, and green vegetables, mushrooms.

Prototype: isoniazid, p 83

RIFAMPIN

(rif´am-pin)
Trade names: Rifadin, Rimactane, Rofact
Classifications: ANTIINFECTIVE; ANTIBIOTIC; ANTILEPROSY (SULFONE) AGENT; ANTITUBERCULOSIS AGENT

ACTIONS/PHARMACODYNAMICS Semisynthetic derivative of rifamycin B, an antibiotic derived from *Streptococcus mediterranei,* with bacteriostatic and bactericidal actions. Inhibits DNA-dependent RNA polymerase activity in susceptible bacterial cells, thereby suppressing RNA synthesis. Active against *Mycobacterium tuberculosis, Mycobacterium leprae,* *Neisseria meningitidis,* and a wide range of gram-negative and gram-positive organisms. Since resistant strains emerge rapidly when it is employed alone, it is used in conjunction with other antitubercular agents in treatment of tuberculosis.

USES Primarily as adjuvant with other antituberculosis agents in initial treatment and retreatment of clinical tuberculosis; as short-term therapy to eliminate meningococci from nasopharynx of asymptomatic carriers of *N. meningitidis* when risk of meningococcal meningitis is high. **Unlabeled uses:** chemoprophylaxis in contacts of patients with *Haemophilus influenzae* type B infection; alone or in combination with dapsone and other antiinfectives in treatment of leprosy (especially dapsone-resistant leprosy). Also infections caused by susceptible gram-negative and gram-positive bacteria that fail to respond to other antiinfectives; in combination with erythromycin or tetracycline for treatment of Legionnaire's disease.

ROUTE & DOSAGE

Pulmonary Tuberculosis

Adult	PO/IV	600 mg once/d in conjunction with other antituberculosis agents
Child	PO	10–20 mg/kg/d (max 600 mg/d)

Meningococcal Carriers

Adult	PO	600 mg b.i.d. for 2 consecutive d
Child	PO	10–20 mg/kg twice daily for 2 consecutive days (max 600 mg/d)

Prophylaxis for *H. influenzae* Type b

Adult	PO	600 mg/d for 4 d
Child	PO	10–20 mg/kg/d for 4 d (max 600 mg/d)

Dapsone-sensitive Multibacillary Leprosy

Adult	PO	600 mg once/mo with clofazimine and dapsone for a minimum of 2 y

---

PHARMACOKINETICS **Absorption:** readily absorbed from GI tract. **Peak:** 2–4 h. **Distribution:** widely distributed, including CSF; crosses placenta; distributed into breast milk. **Metabolism:** metabolized in liver to active and inactive metabolites; is enterohepatically cycled. **Elimination:** half-life: 3 h; up to 30% excreted in urine, 60–65% in feces.

CONTRAINDICATIONS & PRECAUTIONS Contraindicated in: obstructive biliary disease; intermittent rifampin therapy. Safe use during pregnancy and in

R

children > 5 y not established. **Cautious use in:** hepatic disease; history of alcoholism; concomitant use of other hepatotoxic agents.

ADVERSE/SIDE EFFECTS CNS: fatigue, drowsiness, headache, ataxia, confusion, dizziness, inability to concentrate, generalized numbness, pain in extremities, muscular weakness, visual disturbances, transient low-frequency hearing loss (infrequent), conjunctivitis. **GI:** *heartburn, epigastric distress, nausea, vomiting, anorexia, flatulence, cramps, diarrhea,* pseudomembranous colitis. **Hematologic:** thrombocytopenia, transient leukopenia, anemia, including hemolytic anemia. **Hypersensitivity:** fever, pruritus, urticaria, skin eruptions, soreness of mouth and tongue, eosinophilia, hemolysis. **Renal:** hemoglobinuria, hematuria, acute renal failure. **Other:** hemoptysis, light-chain proteinuria, flulike syndrome, menstrual disorders, hepatorenal syndrome (with intermittent therapy), *transient elevations in liver function tests* (bilirubin, BSP, alkaline phosphatase, ALT, AST), pancreatitis (infrequent). **Overdosage:** GI symptoms, increasing lethargy, liver enlargement and tenderness, jaundice, brownish-red or orange discoloration of skin, sweat, saliva, tears, and feces; unconsciousness.

DIAGNOSTIC TEST INTERFERENCES Rifampin interferes with contrast media used for *gallbladder study;* therefore test should precede daily dose of rifampin. May also cause retention of *BSP.* Inhibits standard assays for *serum folate* and *vitamin B$_{12}$.*

DRUG INTERACTIONS Alcohol, isoniazid increase risk of hepatotoxicity; *p-aminosalicylic acid (PAS)* decreases concentrations of rifampin; decreases concentrations of BARBITURATES, BENZODIAZEPINES, **clofibrate,** CORTICOSTEROIDS, **dapsone, digitoxin, methadone, metoprolol, warfarin,** SULFONYLUREAS, ORAL CONTRACEPTIVES, PROGESTINS, **propranolol, quinidine, ketoconazole, fluconazole,** leading to potential therapeutic failure.

NURSING IMPLICATIONS

Administration

▪ Capsule may be emptied and contents swallowed with fluid or mixed with food.
▪ An oral suspension can be prepared from capsules for use in pediatric patients. Consult pharmacist for specific preparation directions.
▪ Administer 1 h before or 2 h after a meal. Peak serum levels are delayed and may be slightly lower when given with food.

▪ A desiccant should be kept in bottle containing capsules; they become unstable with moisture.
▪ IV rifampin is diluted by adding 10 ml of sterile water for injection to each 600 mg vial to yield 60 mg/ml. The ordered dose is withdrawn and further diluted in 100–500 ml of D5W. Infuse over 30 min to 3 h, depending on volume of solution. A less concentrated solution infused over a longer period is preferred.

Assessment & Drug Effects

▪ Serology and susceptibility testing should be performed prior to and in the event of positive cultures.
▪ Periodic hepatic function tests are advised. Patients with hepatic disease must be closely monitored.
▪ If patient is also receiving an anticoagulant, prothrombin times should be performed daily or as necessary to establish and maintain required anticoagulant activity.

Patient & Family Education

▪ Caution patient not to interrupt prescribed dosage regimen. Hepatorenal reaction with flulike syndrome has occurred when therapy has been resumed following interruption.
▪ Inform patients that drug may impart a harmless red-orange color to urine, feces, sputum, sweat, and tears. Soft contact lens may be permanently stained.
▪ Instruct patients to report onset of jaundice, hypersensitivity reactions, and persistence of GI adverse effects.
▪ Patients taking oral contraceptives (OC) should consider alternative methods of contraception. Concomitant use of rifampin and OC leads to decreased effectiveness of the contraceptive and to menstrual disturbances (spotting, breakthrough bleeding).
▪ Caution patient to keep drug out of reach of children.

Prototype: isoproterenol, p 105

RITODRINE HYDROCHLORIDE

(ri´toe-dreen)
Trade name: Yutopar
Classifications: AUTONOMIC NERVOUS SYSTEM AGENT; BETA-ADRENERGIC AGONIST
Pregnancy: Category C

Common side effects in *italic*; life-threatening effects underlined; generic names in **bold**; classifications in SMALL CAPS

ACTIONS/PHARMACODYNAMICS Beta$_2$-adrenergic agonist clinically effective in preventing or delaying of preterm labor (tocolytic effect). Preferentially stimulates beta$_2$-receptors in uterine smooth muscle, reducing intensity and frequency of uterine contractions and lengthening gestation period. (Actions may be eliminated by beta-adrenergic antagonists.) Beta$_2$-receptor stimulation also results in bronchial relaxation and slight effect on vascular smooth muscles. Transitory cardiovascular effects including increased cardiac output, increased maternal and fetal heart rates, and widening of maternal pulse pressure (beta$_1$-stimulation) are common. Administered parenterally in individualized doses with beginning of contractions and continued until they are inhibited. Oral medication then given until delivery of a mature infant is assured. Safety and effectiveness during advanced labor has not been established. Animal studies have shown no teratogenic or carcinogenic effects, but drug is used only when clearly warranted by clinical condition.

USES To manage premature labor in selected patients.

ROUTE & DOSAGE

Premature Labor

Adult	PO	Start 30 min before terminating infusion; 10 mg q2h for first 24 h, then 10–20 mg q4–6h (max 120 mg/d)
	IV	50–100 µg/min; may increase by 50 µg/min q10min until uterine relaxation is achieved; may continue for up to 12 h after contractions have ceased

PHARMACOKINETICS Absorption: 30% absorbed from GI tract. **Peak:** 30–60 min. **Distribution:** crosses placenta. **Metabolism:** metabolized in liver. **Elimination:** half-life: 1.7–2.6 h; excreted in urine.

CONTRAINDICATIONS & PRECAUTIONS Contraindicated in: mild to moderate preeclampsia or eclampsia, intrauterine infection, cervix dilated 4 cm or more (in a singleton pregnancy); pregnancy (category C); hypertension; diabetes mellitus; prior to 20th wk or after 36th wk of pregnancy or if continuation of pregnancy would be hazardous to mother and fetus (e.g., antepartum hemorrhage, eclampsia, intrauterine fetal death, maternal cardiac disease, pulmonary hypertension, maternal hyperthyroidism, severe diabetes mellitus). Also hypovolemia, cardiac arrhythmias associated with tachycardia or digitalis intoxication, uncontrolled hypertension; thyrotoxicosis; bronchial asthma being treated with betamimetics or steroids. **Cautious use in:** concomitant use of potassium-depleting diuretics, cardiac disease.

ADVERSE/SIDE EFFECTS More pronounced and frequent following IV infusion: *altered maternal and fetal heart rates and maternal BP* (dose related); *temporary hyperglycemia, palpitations,* arrhythmias, tremor, nausea, vomiting, headache, erythema; *nervousness,* restlessness, anxiety, malaise, chest pain, pulmonary edema. Infrequent: <u>anaphylactic shock</u>, rash, epigastric distress, ileus, bloating, constipation, diarrhea, dyspnea, hyperventilation, glycosuria, hemolytic icterus, sweating, chills, drowsiness, weakness, myotonic and muscular dystrophies.

DIAGNOSTIC TEST INTERFERENCES Ritodrine (IV route) may produce an increase in **serum** levels of **glucose, insulin,** and **free fatty acids,** and a decrease in **serum potassium.** It temporarily elevates results of **glucose tolerance test.**

DRUG INTERACTIONS CORTICOSTEROIDS may precipitate pulmonary edema; BETA-AGONISTS add to cardiovascular adverse effects; effects of both ritodrine and BETA-BLOCKERS antagonized.

NURSING IMPLICATIONS

Administration

- Preparation of IV solution: 150 mg ritodrine is added to 500 ml 5% dextrose or NS solution, giving a final concentration of 0.3 mg/ml (300 µg/ml).
- IV solution should be clear and should not be administered if it is cloudy or if a precipitate is present.
- Monitor IV infusion flow rate to prevent circulation overload. Use a microdrip and infusion pump.
- Place patient in left lateral recumbent position throughout the infusion period to reduce risk of hypotension.
- Store drug below 30C (86F). Do not freeze.

Assessment & Drug Effects

- Uterine contractions will decrease in frequency and intensity during treatment.
- Pronounced dose-related side effects require continuous monitoring of maternal and fetal heart rates and maternal BP while infusion is running.
- Occult cardiac disease has been unmasked by use of ritodrine.
- If patient is also on steroid therapy, hospitalization for treatment with ritodrine is advised. Be alert to signs and symptoms of pulmonary edema (see chap 3).

R

Common side effects in *italic*; life-threatening effects <u>underlined</u>; generic names in **bold**; classifications in SMALL CAPS

949

S

Prototype: aspirin, p 161

SALICYLIC ACID

Trade names: Calicylic, Compound W, Freezone, Hydrisalic, Keralyt, Occlusal, Salacid, Saligel, Salonil

Classifications: SKIN AGENT; KERATOLYTIC; ANTIACNE; SALICYLATE

Pregnancy: Category C

ACTIONS/PHARMACODYNAMICS   Causes swelling and softening of keratin, cornified epithelium, and scales, thereby facilitating their removal. Has weak bacteriostatic and fungistatic actions. May be destructive to tissues in concentrations above 6%.

USES Topical aid in hyperkeratotic skin disorders such as psoriasis and various ichthyoses, calluses, and warts and to produce exfoliation in superficial fungal infections, acne, and seborrheic dermatitis. Available in plaster form or as ether-alcohol solution (with 20% salicylic acid and collodion) for removal of warts, corns, and calluses.

ROUTE & DOSAGE

Seborrheic Dermatitis, Psoriasis, Dandruff

Adult	Topical	1.8–3% solution: apply to body 1–2 times/d or shampoo 2 times/wk

Warts

Adult	Topical	5–17% solution: soak wart and dry thoroughly; apply solution 1–2 times/d for 1 wk

Acne

Adult	Topical	0.5–2% solution: apply solution 1–3 times/d

CONTRAINDICATIONS & PRECAUTIONS Contraindicated in: sensitivity to salicylates; applications over large areas or for prolonged periods. Use of high concentrations or collodion preparations on moles, birthmarks, warts with hairs, inflamed or infected skin, patients with diabetes mellitus or peripheral vascular disease. Concurrent use of other keratolytic agents (acne preparations) or peeling agents. Pregnancy (category C). **Cautious use in:** children <12 y.

ADVERSE/SIDE EFFECTS *Irritation, burning of skin.* **Systemic absorption (salicylism):** dizziness, tinnitus, impaired hearing, mental confusion, headache, hyperventilation.

NURSING IMPLICATIONS

Administration

- Physician should prescribe specific dosage form, strength, and details of application.
- Avoid contact of medication with eyes and mucous membranes.

Patient & Family Education

- Advise patients to wash hands thoroughly following use of cream, gel, lotion, or ointment forms unless hands are also being treated.
- Caution patient to use drug as directed. Systemic absorption has been reported. Also application to normal skin can cause irritation and burning.
- Physician may prescribe hydration of part (wet packs, soaks, or baths) before or after application and an occlusive dressing at night to enhance drug effect. Use medication only as directed.

For implications of possible systemic effects, see aspirin, p 161.

Prototype: aspirin, p 161

SALSALATE

Trade names: Artha-G, Disalcid, Mono-Gesic

Classifications: CNS AGENT; SALICYLATE ANALGESIC, ANTIPYRETIC; NSAID

Pregnancy: Category C

ACTIONS/PHARMACODYNAMICS   Actions similar to those of other salicylates. Clinical studies suggest that salsalate does not produce significant gastric irritation, and it has not been associated with reactions causing asthmatic attacks in susceptible individuals. The incidence of side effects in general appears to be lower than that of other salicylates. Unlike aspirin it does not appear to inhibit platelet aggregation.

USES Symptomatic treatment, rheumatoid arthritis, osteoarthritis, and related rheumatic disorders.

ROUTE & DOSAGE

Arthritis

Adult	PO	325–3000 mg/d in divided doses (max 4 g/d)

Common side effects in *italic*; life-threatening effects <u>underlined</u>; generic names in **bold**; classifications in SMALL CAPS

PHARMACOKINETICS Absorption: readily absorbed from small intestine. **Peak:** 1.5–4 h. **Metabolism:** hydrolyzed in liver, GI mucosa, plasma, whole blood, and other tissues. **Elimination:** half-life: 1 h. excreted in urine.

CONTRAINDICATIONS & PRECAUTIONS Contraindicated in: hypersensitivity to salicylates, chronic renal insufficiency, peptic ulcer, pregnancy (category C), children < 12 y.

ADVERSE/SIDE EFFECTS Occasionally, nausea, dyspepsia, heartburn. **Overdosage** (salicylism): tinnitus, hearing loss (reversible), vertigo, flushing, headache, confusion, drowsiness, hyperventilation, sweating, vomiting, diarrhea.

NURSING IMPLICATIONS

Administration

▪ Administer with a full glass of water or with food or milk to reduce GI side effects.

Assessment & Drug Effects

▪ Symptom relief is gradual (may require 3–4 d to establish steady-state salicylate level).
▪ Monitor for adverse GI effects, especially in patient with a history of peptic ulcer disease.

Patient & Family Education

▪ Warn patient not to take another salicylate (e.g., aspirin) while on salsalate therapy.
▪ Inform diabetic patient that drug may induce hypoglycemia when it is used with sulfonylureas.
▪ Instruct patient to report tinnitus, hearing loss, vertigo, rash, or nausea.

Prototype: epoetin alfa, p 130

SARGRAMOSTIM

(sar-gra´mos-tim)
Trade names: Leukine, Prokine
Classification: HEMATOPOIETIC GROWTH FACTOR
Pregnancy: Category C

ACTIONS/PHARMACODYNAMICS Sargramostim is a recombinant human granulocytemacrophage colony stimulating factor (GM-CSF) produced by recombinant DNA technology in a yeast.

GM-CSF is a hematopoietic growth factor that stimulates proliferation and differentiation of hematopoietic progenitor cells in the granulocyte-macrophage pathways. Sargramostim increases the cytotoxity of monocytes to certain neoplastic cell lines and activates polymorphonuclear neutrophils (PMNs) to inhibit the growth of tumor cells.

USES Myeloid reconstitution after autologous bone marrow transplantation for patients with non-Hodgkin's lymphoma (NHL), acute lymphoblastic leukemia (ALL), and Hodgkin's disease. **Unlabeled uses:** to increase WBC counts in AIDS patients; to decrease leukopenia secondary to myelosuppressive chemotherapy; to correct neutropenia in aplastic anemia and in liver and kidney transplantations.

ROUTE & DOSAGE

Autologous Bone Marrow Transplant

Adult	IV	250 µg/m²/d infused over 2 h for 21 d; begin 2–4 h after bone marrow transfusion and not less than 24 h after last dose of chemotherapy or 12 h after last radiation therapy

Neutropenia

Adult	SC	3–15 µg/kg/d

PHARMACOKINETICS Absorption: readily absorbed from SC site. **Onset:** 3–6 h. **Peak:** 1–2 h. **Duration:** 5–10 d SC. **Elimination:** half-life: 80–150 min; probably excreted in urine.

CONTRAINDICATIONS & PRECAUTIONS Contraindicated in: excessive leukemic myeloid blasts in bone marrow or blood; known hypersensitivity to GM-CSF or yeast products. **Cautious use in:** history of cardiac arrhythmias, preexisting cardiac disease, hypoxia, CHF, pulmonary infiltrates; renal and hepatic dysfunction; pregnancy (category C), and nursing mothers. Safety and efficacy in children not established; however, adverse side effects have been comparable to those in adults.

ADVERSE/SIDE EFFECTS CNS: lethargy, malaise, headache, fatigue. **CV:** abnormal ST segment depression, supraventricular arrhythmias, edema, *hypotension, tachycardia,* underline pericardial effusion, pericarditis. **Hematologic:** anemia, *thrombocytopenia.* **GI:** nausea, vomiting, diarrhea, anorexia. **Other:** *bone pain, myalgia, arthralgias,* weight gain, hyperuricemia, *fever,* pleural effusion, *rash, pruritus,* **first-dose reaction:** some or all of the following symptoms: hypotension, tachycardia, fever, rigors, flushing, nausea, vomiting, diaphoresis, back pain, leg spasms, and dyspnea.

Common side effects in *italic*; life-threatening effects underlined; generic names in **bold**; classifications in SMALL CAPS

951

DRUG INTERACTIONS CORTICOSTEROIDS should be used cautiously with sargramostim because the myeloproliferative effects may be potentiated. **Lithium** should be used with caution with sargramostim because it may potentiate the myeloproliferative effects.

NURSING IMPLICATIONS

Administration

- Sargramostim should not be administered within 24 h preceding or following chemotherapy or within 12 h preceding or following radiotherapy.
- Reconstitute each 250 or 500 µg vial with 1 ml of sterile water for injection (without preservative). Direct sterile water against side of vial and swirl gently. Avoid excessive or vigorous agitation. Do not shake.
- To dilute for IV infusion use 0.9% NaCl. If the final concentration is < 10 µg/ml, add albumin (human) to NS before addition of sargramostim. Use 1 mg albumin per 1 ml of 0.9% NaCl to give a final concentration of 0.1% albumin.
- Administer as soon as possible and within 6 h of reconstitution or dilution for IV infusion. After 6 h, discard it.
- Sargramostim vials are single-dose vials. Discard unused portion.
- If the absolute neutrophil count exceeds 20,000/mm^3 or if platelet count exceeds 500,000/mm^3, interrupt administration and reduce the dose by 50%. Notify the physician.
- If the patient experiences dyspnea during administration, reduce the IV rate 50%. If respiratory symptoms worsen, discontinue infusion. Notify physician.
- ***Administration after autologous bone marrow transplantation:*** ordered dose (usually 250 µg/m^2/d) for 21 d and give IV over 2 h. Begin IV 2–4 h after bone marrow infusion and at least 24 h after last dose of chemotherapy and at least 12 h after last dose of radiation.
- Refrigerate the sterile powder, the reconstituted solution, and the diluted solution at 2–8C (36–46F). Do not freeze or shake.

Assessment & Drug Effects

- Obtain a CBC and platelet count prior to initiation of therapy.
- Treatment should be discontinued if WBC ≥ 50,000 /mm^3. Notify the physician.
- Notify physician of any severe adverse reaction immediately.
- Occasional transient supraventricular arrhythmias

have occurred during administration, particularly in those with a history of cardiac arrhythmias. Arrhythmias are reversed with discontinuation of drug.
- Give special attention to respiratory symptoms (dyspnea) during and immediately following infusion, especially in patients with preexisting pulmonary disease.
- Peripheral edema, pleural or pericardial effusion has occurred after administration. It is reversible with dose reduction. Use drug with caution in patients with preexisting fluid retention, pulmonary infiltrates, or CHF.
- Biweekly monitoring of renal and hepatic function is necessary in patients with renal or hepatic dysfunction prior to the initiation of therapy.
- Monitor serum creatinine, bilirubin, and liver enzymes.
- Biweekly monitoring of CBC with differential should be continued during therapy.
- Potentially sargramostim can act as a growth factor for myeloid malignancies. Should disease progression be detected, discontinue therapy and notify physician.

Patient & Family Education

- Instruct patient to notify nurse or physician immediately of any adverse effect (e.g., dyspnea, palpitations) experienced during or after drug administration.

Prototype: atropine, p 116

SCOPOLAMINE

(skoe-pol´a-meen)
Trade names: Transderm-Scōp, Transderm-V

SCOPOLAMINE HYDROBROMIDE

Trade names: Hyoscine, Isopto-Hyoscine, Murocoll, Triptone
Classifications: AUTONOMIC NERVOUS SYSTEM AGENT; ANTICHOLINERGIC (PARASYMPATHOLYTIC); ANTIMUSCARINIC, ANTISPASMODIC
Pregnancy: Category C

ACTIONS/PHARMACODYNAMICS Alkaloid of belladonna with peripheral actions resembling those of atropine. In contrast to atropine, produces CNS depression, with marked sedative and tranquilizing effects, and is less effective in preventing reflex bradycardia during anesthesia (tends to slow heart even in large doses). More potent in mydriatic and cycloplegic actions and in inhibiting secretions of salivary, bronchial, and sweat glands, but has less prominent effect on heart, intestines, and bronchial muscles.

USES In obstetrics with morphine to produce amnesia and sedation ("twilight sleep") and as preanesthetic medication. To control spasticity (and drooling) in postencephalitic parkinsonism, paralysis agitans, and other spastic states, as prophylactic agent for motion sickness and as mydriatic and cycloplegic in ophthalmology. Therapeutic system (Transderm-Scōp) is used to prevent nausea and vomiting associated with motion sickness.

ROUTE & DOSAGE

Preanesthetic

Adult	PO	0.5–1 mg
	IM/SC/IV	0.3–0.6 mg
Child	PO	0.006 mg/kg
	IM/SC/IV	0.006 mg/kg

Motion Sickness

Adult	PO	0.25–0.6 mg 1 h before anticipated travel
	Topical	1 patch q72h starting 12 h before anticipated travel
Child	PO	0.006 mg/kg 1 h before anticipated travel

Refraction

Adult	Ophthalmic	1–2 drops in eye 1 h before refraction

Uveitis

Adult	Ophthalmic	1–2 drops in eye up to q.i.d.

PHARMACOKINETICS Absorption: readily absorbed from GI tract and percutaneously. **Peak:** 20–60 min. **Duration:** 5–7 d. **Distribution:** crosses placenta; distributed to CNS. **Metabolism:** metabolized in liver. **Elimination:** excreted in urine.

CONTRAINDICATIONS & PRECAUTIONS Contraindicated in: asthma; hepatitis; toxemia of pregnancy; pregnancy (category C). **Cautious use in:** cardiac disease; patients over 40 y, pyloric obstruction, urinary bladder neck obstruction, angle-closure glaucoma, thyrotoxicosis, paralytic ileus.

ADVERSE/SIDE EFFECTS Sense of fatigue, dizziness, *drowsiness, dry mouth and throat, constipation,* urinary retention, disorientation, decreased heart rate, dilated pupils, photophobia, depressed respiration, restlessness, hallucinations, toxic psychosis. **Eye:** blurred vision, *local irritation,* follicular conjunctivitis. **Skin:** local irritation from patch adhesive, rash.

DRUG INTERACTIONS Amantadine, ANTIHISTAMINES, TRICYCLIC ANTIDEPRESSANTS, **quinidine, disopyramide, procainamide** add to anticholinergic effects; decreases **levodopa** effects; **methotrimeprazine** may precipitate extrapyramidal effects; decreases antipsychotic effects (decreased absorption) of PHENOTHIAZINES.

NURSING IMPLICATIONS

Administration

- May be given by direct IV diluted in sterile water for injection. Inject diluted solution slowly.
- To minimize possibility of systemic absorption, apply pressure against lacrimal sac during and for 1 or 2 min following instillation of eye drops.

Therapeutic system (transderm-scōp) (a controlled release system):

- Transdermal disc system should be applied to dry surface behind the ear.
- If disc system becomes dislodged, it can be replaced by another on another site behind the ear.
- Preserve in tight, light-resistant containers.

Assessment & Drug Effects

- Some patients manifest excitement, delirium, disorientation, and garrulousness shortly after drug is administered until sedative effect takes hold. Observe patient closely for these effects.
- Side rails are advisable, particularly for the elderly, because of amnesic effect of scopolamine.
- In the presence of pain, scopolamine may cause delirium, restlessness, and excitement unless given with an analgesic.
- Tolerance may develop with prolonged use.
- Ophthalmic use should be terminated if local irritation, edema, or conjunctivitis occur.

Patient & Family Education

- When used as mydriatic or cycloplegic, caution the patient that vision will be blurred; instruct patient to avoid potentially hazardous activities such as driving a car or operating machinery until vision clears.
- Disc system is effective if applied as soon as 2–3 h before anticipated motion; however, therapeutic effect is best with 12 h of application.
- Advise patient to place disc on skin site the night before an expected trip.

Common side effects in *italic*; life-threatening effects underlined; generic names in **bold**; classifications in SMALL CAPS

953

- Advise patient to wash hands carefully after handling scopolamine. Anisocoria (unequal size of pupils, blurred vision can develop by rubbing eye with drug-contaminated finger).

SECOBARBITAL SODIUM

See CENTRAL NERVOUS SYSTEM AGENT, ANXIOLYTIC, SEDATIVE-HYPNOTIC, BARBITURATE, prototype, p 175.

SELENIUM SULFIDE

(se-lee'nee-um)
Trade names: Exsel, Selsun, Selsun Blue
Classifications: SKIN AGENT; ANTIINFECTIVE; ANTIBIOTIC; ANTIFUNGAL
Pregnancy: Category C

ACTIONS/PHARMACODYNAMICS Aqueous solution containing 52–55.5% selenium; has antibacterial and mild antifungal activity. Mechanism of action and causal relationships have not been established, but drug is active against *Pityrosporum ovale,* a yeast-like fungus found in the normal flora of the scalp. Absorption of selenium sulfide into epithelial tissue cells is followed by degradation of compound to selenium and sulfide ions. Selenium ions block enzyme systems involved in epithelial cell growth (cell turnover). As a result, rate of turnover in cells with normal or higher than normal turnover rates is reduced (cytostatic or antimitotic effects). Selenium sulfide has a pH 2–6, a slight odor, and a local irritant effect.

USES Itching and flaking of the scalp associated with dandruff, seborrheic dermatitis of the scalp, and tinea versicolor.

PHARMACOKINETICS Absorption: no percutaneous absorption if skin is intact.

CONTRAINDICATIONS & PRECAUTIONS Contraindicated in: application to damaged or inflamed skin surfaces; as treatment of tinea versicolor during pregnancy. Use during pregnancy (category C) as antiseborrheic only when clearly needed. Safe use in children not established. **Cautious use in:** prolonged skin contact; use in genital area or skin folds.

ROUTE & DOSAGE

Dandruff Control, Seborrheic Dermatitis

Adult	Topical	Massage 5–10 ml of a 1–2.5% solution into wet scalp and leave on for 2–3 min; rinse thoroughly; then repeat application and rinse well again; initially, shampoo 2 times/wk for 2 wk; then decrease to once q1–4wk prn

Tinea Versicolor

Adult	Topical	Apply a 2.5% solution to affected area with a small amount of water to form a lather; leave on for 10 min; then rinse thoroughly; repeat once/d for 7 d

ADVERSE/SIDE EFFECTS *Skin irritation (stinging),* rebound oiliness of scalp, hair discoloration, diffuse hair loss (reversible), systemic toxicity (if applied to abraded, infected skin).

NURSING IMPLICATIONS

Administration

- Wash hands thoroughly after application of selenium sulfide to affected areas. Advise removing jewelry before treatment; drug will damage it.
- Genital areas and skin folds should be rinsed well with water and dried after treatment for tinea versicolor to prevent irritation.
- Store in tight container, protected from heat, at 15–30C (59–86F). Avoid freezing.

Patient & Family Education

- If lotion contacts the eyes, thoroughly rinse with water to prevent chemical conjunctivitis.
- Caution patient not to use this drug more frequently than required to maintain control of dandruff.
- Hair loss is reversible, usually within 2–3 wk after treatment is discontinued.
- Systemic toxicity may result from application of lotion to damaged skin (percutaneous absorption), from prolonged use (overdosage), and from accidental ingestion. Warn patient to discontinue use if skin is irritated or if treatment fails. ***Toxicity symptoms:*** tremors, anorexia, occasional vomiting, lethargy, weakness, severe perspiration, garlicky breath, lower abdominal pain. Symptoms disappear 10–12 d after treatment is stopped.

Common side effects in *italic*; life-threatening effects underlined; generic names in **bold**; classifications in SMALL CAPS

Prototype: bisacodyl, p 221

SENNA

Trade names: Black Draught, Genna, Gentlax B, Senexon, Senokot, Senolax
Classifications: GI AGENT; STIMULANT LAXATIVE
Pregnancy: Category C

ACTIONS/PHARMACODYNAMICS Anthraquinone derivative prepared from dried leaflet of *Cassia acutifolia* or *Cassia angustifolia*. Similar to cascara sagrada but with more potent action. Senna glycosides are converted in colon to active aglycones, which stimulate Auerbach's plexus to induce peristalsis. Available as crude drug (e.g., Black Draught) crystalline senna glycosides (sennosides A and B) and as standardized senna concentrate (e.g., Senokot). Standardized concentrate is purified and standardized for uniform action and is claimed to produce less colic than crude form.

USES Acute constipation and preoperative and pre radiographic bowel evacuation.

ROUTE & DOSAGE

Constipation

Adult	PO	Standard senna concentrate: 1–2 tablets or 1/2–1 tsp h.s. (max 4 tablets or 2 tsp b.i.d.)
		Syrup, Liquid: 10–15 ml at h.s.
Child	PO	Standard senna concentrate: >27 kg: 1 tablet or 1/2 tsp h.s.
		Syrup, Liquid: 5–15 y: 5–10 ml h.s.
		1–5 y: 2.5–5 ml h.s.
		1 mo-1 y: 1.25–2.5 ml h.s.

PHARMACOKINETICS Onset: 6–10 h; may take up to 24 h. **Metabolism:** metabolized in liver. **Elimination:** excreted in feces.

CONTRAINDICATIONS & PRECAUTIONS Contraindicated in: irritable colon, nausea, vomiting, abdominal pain, intestinal obstruction, pregnancy (category C), nursing mothers.

ADVERSE/SIDE EFFECTS Abdominal cramps, flatulence, nausea. *Prolonged use:* watery diarrhea, excessive loss of water and electrolytes, weight loss, melanotic segmentation of colonic mucosa (reversible).

NURSING IMPLICATIONS

Administration
- Generally administered at bedtime for relief of constipation.
- When given for preoperative or prediagnostic bowel preparation, usually given between 2 and 4 PM on day prior to procedure. Diet is then confined to clear liquids.
- Avoid exposure of drug to excessive heat; fluid extracts should be protected from light.

Assessment & Drug Effects
- Some patients may experience considerable abdominal cramping; if medication is to be repeated, dose reduction may be indicated.

Patient & Family Education
- Inform patient that drug may color urine yellowish brown (acid urine) or reddish brown (alkaline urine). Feces may be similarly colored.
- Caution patient that continued use may lead to dependence. If constipation persists, consult physician.

See bisacodyl for additional nursing implications.

SILVER NITRATE (AgNO₃)

Trade names: Dey Drops Silver Nitrate

SILVER NITRATE, TOUGHENED

Trade names: Lunar Caustic, Silver Nitrate Pencil
Classifications: ANTIINFECTIVE; EYE PREPARATION; SKIN & MUCOUS MEMBRANE AGENT
Pregnancy: Category C

ACTIONS/PHARMACODYNAMICS Has bactericidal, astringent, and caustic properties. Contact of silver ion with chloride in tissue results in precipitation to silver chloride, which limits its effectiveness and penetrating ability. Its bactericidal action is thought to be due to its ability to interfere with essential metabolic actions of microbial cells. Degree of action depends on concentration used and period of time drug is allowed to remain in contact with tissue.

USES Silver nitrate ophthalmic solution is used to prevent and treat ophthalmia neonatorum. Weak solutions are also used to irrigate bladder and urethra. Strong concentrations and toughened silver nitrate

---

Common side effects in *italic*; life-threatening effects <u>underlined</u>; generic names in **bold**; classifications in SMALL CAPS

955

S

are used to cauterize mucous membranes, wounds, granulomatous tissue, and warts. **Unlabeled use:** (0.1–0.5% solution) wet dressings in burns and on lesions.

ROUTE & DOSAGE

Ophthalmia Neonatorum

Child	Topical	2 drops of 1% solution instilled into eye; eyelids are first cleaned with sterile cotton and sterile water to remove blood, mucus, or meconium; Drug should remain in contact with whole conjunctival sac for ≥30 s

Cauterization

Adult	Topical	Use 10%, 25% or 50% solution

ADVERSE/SIDE EFFECTS *Transient chemical irritation of eyes (redness, edema, discharge)* is expected reaction following eye instillations. Argyria (silver discoloration of tissue) with prolonged use.

NURSING IMPLICATIONS

Administration

- Use only silver nitrate ophthalmic solution for the eyes.
- For wound cauterization, area to be treated should first be cleaned to remove organic matter (may interfere with drug action). If toughened silver nitrate (silver nitrate pencil) is used, it should be dipped in water and applied to area for period of time according to degree of action desired. Treated area will appear grayish black (silver stain).
- Medication should be confined to specific area to be treated. If healthy skin is accidentally touched, it may be washed with physiologic salt solution (the chloride in salt solution forms insoluble precipitate with silver nitrate and thus cancels its action).
- Handle silver nitrate with care. Solutions leave gray or black stain on skin, clothing, and utensils. Skin stains (argyria) usually persist indefinitely or disappear only slowly. Argyria may be exaggerated by exposure to sunlight. Concentrations of silver nitrate 5% and higher are caustic.
- Preserve in tight, light-resistant containers.

SILVER PROTEIN, MILD

Trade name: Argyrol S.S.
Classifications: ANTIINFECTIVE; EYE PREPARATION; SKIN & MUCOUS MEMBRANE AGENT
Pregnancy: Category C

ACTIONS/PHARMACODYNAMICS Colloidal compound of silver and a protein derivative. Contains less concentration of ionized silver than silver nitrate does and consequently is less irritating to tissues. Has antimicrobial activity against both gram-negative and gram-positive organism. See silver nitrate for actions and adverse reactions.

USES Preoperatively in eye surgery to stain and coagulate mucus, which can then be removed by irrigation, and for mild inflammatory conditions of eye, nose, and throat.

ROUTE & DOSAGE

Preoperatively in Eye Surgery

Adult	Topical	2–3 drops of 10–20% solution; then rinsed with sterile irrigating solution

Mild Inflammatory Conditions

Adult	Topical	1–3 drops into eye q3–4h for several days

NURSING IMPLICATIONS

Administration

- Store in tightly covered light-resistant containers. See silver nitrate for nursing implications.

Prototype: sulfisoxazole, p 88

SILVER SULFADIAZINE

(sul-fa-dye´a-zeen)
Trade name: Silvadene
Classifications: ANTIINFECTIVE; SULFONAMIDE
Pregnancy: Category C

ACTIONS/PHARMACODYNAMICS Produced by reaction of silver nitrate with sulfadiazine. Mechanism of action differs from that of either component. Silver salt is released slowly and exerts bactericidal effect only on bacterial cell membrane and wall, rather than by inhibiting folic acid synthesis; antibacterial activity is not inhibited by *p*-aminobenzoic acid (PABA). Contact with sodium chloride in body tissues and fluids results in slow release of sulfadiazine, which may be systemically absorbed from application site. Has broad antimicrobial activity including many gram-negative and gram-positive bacteria and yeast. Does not affect electrolyte balance and reportedly does not alter acid-base balance.

Common side effects in *italic*; life-threatening effects underlined; generic names in **bold**; classifications in SMALL CAPS

USES Prevention and treatment of sepsis in second- and third-degree burns.

ROUTE & DOSAGE

Burn Wound Treatment

Adult	Topical	Apply 1% cream 1–2 times/d to thickness of approximately 1.5 mm (1/16 in)

CONTRAINDICATIONS & PRECAUTIONS Contraindicated in: hypersensitivity to other sulfonamides; G6PD deficiency; pregnancy (category C), pregnant women at term, premature and newborn infants < 2 mo. **Cautious use in:** impaired renal or hepatic function.

ADVERSE/SIDE EFFECTS Pain (occasionally), burning, itching, rash, reversible leukopenia. Potential for toxicity as for other sulfonamides if applied to extensive areas of the body surface.

DRUG INTERACTIONS PROTEOLYTIC ENZYMES are inactivated by silver in cream.

NURSING IMPLICATIONS

Administration

- Silver sulfadiazine cream is water soluble and white; if it darkens, do not use.
- Applied with sterile, gloved hands to cleansed, debrided burned areas. Cream should be reapplied to areas where it has been removed by patient activity; burn wounds should be covered with medication at all times.
- If possible, patient should be bathed daily (in whirlpool or shower or in bed) as aid to debridement. Drug should then be reapplied.
- Dressings are not required but may be used if necessary. Silver sulfadiazine does not stain clothing.
- Preserve at room temperature away from heat.

Assessment & Drug Effects

- Observe for and report hypersensitivity reaction manifested by rash, itching, or burning sensation in unburned areas.
- When drug is applied to extensive areas, serum sulfa concentrations, urinalysis, and kidney function tests should be monitored, since significant quantities of drug may be absorbed. Observe patient for reactions attributed to sulfonamides.
- Occasionally, pain is experienced on application; intensity and duration depend on depth of burn. Analgesic may be required.

- Unless adverse reactions occur, treatment should continue until satisfactory healing or until burn site is ready for grafting.

SIMETHICONE

(si-meth′i-kone)
Trade names: Gas-x, Mylicon, Phazyme, Silain
Classifications: GI AGENT; ANTIFLATULENT

ACTIONS/PHARMACODYNAMICS A surfactant (surface-active agent) claimed to defoam gastric juice by causing small gas bubbles to break up and coalesce so they can be more easily removed by belching or passing flatus.

USES To relieve flatulence and functional gastric bloating.

ROUTE & DOSAGE

Gas

Adult	PO	40–125 mg after meals and at bedtime as needed (max 500 mg/d)

NURSING IMPLICATIONS

Administration

- Shake suspension well before pouring.
- Instruct patients to chew tablet form thoroughly before they swallow it.

SODIUM BICARBONATE (NaHCO₃)

Classifications: GI AGENT; ANTACID; ELECTROLYTIC BALANCE AGENT
Pregnancy: Category C

ACTIONS/PHARMACODYNAMICS Short-acting, potent systemic antacid. Rapidly neutralizes gastric acid to form sodium chloride, carbon dioxide, and water. After absorption of sodium bicarbonate (baking soda), plasma alkali reserve is increased and excess sodium and bicarbonate ions are excreted in urine, thus rendering urine less acid. Not suitable for treatment of peptic ulcer because it is short-acting, high in sodium, and may cause gastric distension (from CO_2 release), systemic alkalosis, and possibly acid-rebound. In the presence of acidosis, replaces

Common side effects in *italic*; life-threatening effects <u>underlined</u>; generic names in **bold**; classifications in SMALL CAPS

957

bicarbonate ions and thus restores buffering capacity of body. Each gram of sodium bicarbonate contains approximately 12 mEq of sodium.

USES Systemic alkalinizer to correct metabolic acidosis (as occurs in diabetes mellitus, shock, cardiac arrest, or vascular collapse), to minimize uric acid crystallization associated with uricosuric agents, to increase the solubility of sulfonamides, and to enhance renal excretion of barbiturate and salicylate overdosage. Commonly used as home remedy for relief of occasional heartburn, indigestion, or sour stomach. Used topically as paste, bath, or soak to relieve itching and minor skin irritations such as sunburn, insect bites, prickly heat, poison ivy, sumac, or oak. Sterile solutions are used to buffer acidic parenteral solutions to prevent acidosis. Also as a buffering agent in many commercial products (e.g., mouthwashes, douches, enemas, ophthalmic solutions).

ROUTE & DOSAGE

Antacid

Adult	PO	0.3–2 g 1–4 times/d or 1/2 tsp of powder in glass of water

Urinary Alkalinizer

Adult	PO	4 g initially; then 1–2 g q4h
Child	PO	84–840 mg/kg/d in divided doses

Cardiac Arrest

Adult	IV	1 mEq/kg of a 7.5% or 8.4% solution initially; then 0.5 mEq/kg q10min depending on arterial blood gas determinations (8.4% solutions contain 50mEq/50 ml); give over 1–2 min
Child	IV	0.5–1 mEq/kg of a 4.2% solution q10min depending on arterial blood gas determinations; give over 1–2 min

Metabolic Acidosis

Adult	IV	2–5 mEq/kg by IV infusion over a 4–8 h period
Infant	IV	2–3 mEq/kg/d of a 4.2% solution over a 4–8 h period

PHARMACOKINETICS Absorption: readily absorbed from GI tract. **Onset:** 15 min. **Duration:** 1–2 h. **Elimination:** excreted in urine within 3–4 h.

CONTRAINDICATIONS & PRECAUTIONS Contraindicated in: prolonged therapy with sodium bicarbonate; patients losing chlorides (as from vomiting, GI suction, diuresis); heart disease, hypertension; renal insufficiency; peptic ulcer; pregnancy (category

C). **Cautious use in:** edema, sodium-retaining disorders; elderly patients.

ADVERSE/SIDE EFFECTS GI: *belching, gastric distension,* flatulence. **Metabolic:** metabolic alkalosis; electrolyte imbalance: sodium overload (pulmonary edema), hypocalcemia (tetany), hypokalemia. **Rapid IV in neonates:** hypernatremia, reduction in CSF pressure, intracranial hemorrhage. **Other:** milk-alkali syndrome, severe tissue damage following extravasation of IV solution, dehydration, renal calculi or crystals, impaired renal function, renal calculi.

DIAGNOSTIC TEST INTERFERENCES Small increase in **blood lactate** levels (following IV infusion of sodium bicarbonate); false-positive **urinary protein** determinations (using Ames reagent, sulfoacetic acid, heat and acetic acid or nitric acid ring method); elevated **urinary urobilinogen** levels (urobilinogen excretion increases in alkaline urine).

INCOMPATIBILITIES Solution/Additive: alcohol, 5% lactated Ringers, ascorbic acid, carmustine, cisplatin, codeine, corticotropin, dobutamine, dopamine, epinephrine, glycopyrrolate, hydromorphone, imipenem-cilastatin, insulin, isoproterenol, labetalol, levorphanol, magnesium sulfate, meperidine, methadone, methicillin, metoclopramide, morphine, norepinephrine, oxytetracycline, pentazocine, phenobarbital, procaine, secobarbital, streptomycin, succinylcholine, tetracycline, thiopental, vancomycin, vitamin B complex with C. Y-Site: amrinone, verapamil.

NURSING IMPLICATIONS

Administration

- Infusion should be stopped immediately if extravasation occurs. Severe tissue damage has followed tissue infiltration.
- Avoid adding sodium bicarbonate to infusion solutions containing other drugs without consulting pharmacist.
- *Topical use* (manufacturer's directions): Bath or soak: 1/2 cup or more into tub of warm water. Footsoak: 4 tbsp/L(qt) warm water; soak 5–10 min. Paste: 3 parts sodium bicarbonate to 1 part water. Solutions in water slowly decompose: decomposition is accelerated by agitating or warming the solution.
- Store in airtight containers. Note expiration date.

Common side effects in *italic*; life-threatening effects underlined; generic names in **bold**; classifications in SMALL CAPS

Assessment & Drug Effects

- Long-term use of oral preparation with milk or calcium can cause *milk-alkali syndrome:* anorexia, nausea, vomiting, headache, mental confusion, hypercalcemia, hypophosphatemia, soft tissue calcification, renal and ureteral calculi, renal insufficiency, metabolic alkalosis.
- *Urinary alkalinization:* urinary pH should be monitored as a guide to dosage (pH testing with nitrazine paper may be done at intervals throughout the day and dosage adjustments made accordingly).
- *Metabolic acidosis:* patient should be closely monitored by observations of clinical condition; measurements of acid-base status (blood pH, Po_2, Pco_2, HCO_3, and other electrolytes, are usually made several times daily during acute period). Observe for signs of alkalosis (overtreatment), (see chap 3).
- Observe for and report improvement or reversal in signs and symptoms, of metabolic acidosis (see chap 3).

Patient & Family Education

- Discourage use of sodium bicarbonate as antacid. A nonabsorbable alternative (OTC) for repeated use is safer.
- Caution patient who self-medicates that routine doses of sodium bicarbonate or soda mints may be sufficient to cause sodium retention and alkalosis, especially when renal function is impaired. Antacids should not be taken longer than 2 wk except under advice and supervision of a physician.
- Commonly used OTC antacid products containing sodium bicarbonate: Alka-Seltzer, Bromo-Seltzer, Gaviscon.

SODIUM CHLORIDE 20%

Classification: ABORTIFACIENT
Pregnancy: Category X

ACTIONS/PHARMACODYNAMICS Hypertonic saline instillation into the amniotic sac induces abortion and fetal death. Mechanism is unclear, but abortifacient activity may be a response to prostaglandins released by hypertonic NaCl-damaged decidual cells. Uterine contractions, induced by the saline solution are sufficient to cause evacuation of fetus and placenta; however, in 25–40% of the patients, abortion may be incomplete.

USES To induce abortion late in the second trimester of pregnancy. Oxytocin may be used as an adjunct (concurrent) uterine stimulant.

ROUTE & DOSAGE

Induce Abortion

Adult	Intraamniotic	Instill 20% solution in volumes equal to amount of amniotic fluid removed or a max of 200–250 ml, administered slowly over 20–30 min; repeated in 48 h if uterine contractility, cervical effacement, or cervical dilation is inadequate or if labor has not begun

---

PHARMACOKINETICS Absorption: some drug diffuses into maternal blood. **Onset:** within 51 h. **Distribution:** sodium concentration in amniotic fluid must be at least 2.2 mEq/ml to induce abortion; most of drug concentrates in decidua and fetal part of placenta.

CONTRAINDICATIONS & PRECAUTIONS Contraindicated in: pregnancy of less than 15 wk or more than 24 wk, prior uterine surgery (including cervix), pelvic adhesions, sickle cell disease, diabetes mellitus, increased intraamniotic pressure (as in contracting or hypertonic uterus), poor health, blood disorders, coagulation factor deficiencies. **Cautious use in:** malignant hypertension, cardiovascular and renal disease, thrombocytopenia, fibrinolytic defects.

ADVERSE/SIDE EFFECTS Within first 12–24 h after instillation: coagulation changes; increased plasma volume, fibrin levels, thrombin, prothrombin, and partial thromboplastin times. **With overdistension of amniotic cavity by excess NaCl:** ascites, hypervolemia, <u>circulation failure, uterine necrosis</u>, severe electrolyte disturbances. **With delayed abortion:** retained placenta, hemorrhagic fever, infection, sepsis. **Other:** mild self-limiting form of disseminated intravascular coagulation, cervical lacerations and perforation, uterine rupture, <u>pulmonary embolism</u>, fever, flushing, <u>cortical necrosis of kidneys</u>.

DRUG INTERACTIONS Indomethacin may delay onset time of abortion; **terbutaline, ritodrine** inhibit uterine activity induced by hypertonic NaCl.

Common side effects in *italic*; life-threatening effects <u>underlined</u>; generic names in **bold**; classifications in SMALL CAPS

959

S

NURSING IMPLICATIONS

Administration

- Preparatory to procedure, skin is surgically prepared. By transabdominal tap, about 1 ml amniotic fluid is withdrawn to confirm location of needle (amniotic fluid has pH 7.4 and ability to fern). If blood is present or if no amniotic fluid is withdrawn, needle is repositioned. Some clinicians then remove all amniotic fluid (30–250 ml); others prefer not to before NaCl instillation.
- Instillation is through a 3-way stopcock with needle and polyethylene catheter inserted into amniotic cavity.
- Within 1–2 h after hypertonic solution instillation and after uterine response to the solution has ceased, IV infusion of dilute solution of oxytocin may be administered; rate, 20–100 mU/min Oxytocin action as an adjunctive uterine stimulant shortens the abortifacient-abortion interval.
- *Treatment of extraamniotic injection:* procedure stopped promptly; IV infusion of D5W, additional support for hypernatremic shock.

Assessment & Drug Effects

- Observe patient for at least 30 min after instillation procedure. Be available for complaints and to check vital signs (temperature, pulse rate, BP).
- Intraamniotic instillation is a painless procedure. No anesthetic or sedative is needed or given so that patient is able to report early signs of extraamniotic injection: mental confusion, hypotension, severe headache, vague distress, extreme nervousness, pain, sensation of heat, thirst, fingertip numbness, dry mouth, salty taste, tinnitus.
- Suspect accidental intraperitoneal, intravascular, or myometrial injection if patient begins vomiting. Cardiovascular collapse, seizures, and maternal death may follow.

Patient & Family Education

- Instruct patient to drink at least 2 L water on day of procedure to promote NaCl excretion.
- With onset of labor, signs of rupture of fetal membrane, vaginal bleeding, fever, or any other untoward symptom, patient should return promptly to treatment center.
- If labor has not begun within 48 h after hypertonic saline instillation, patient should return to physician for evaluation and treatment.

SODIUM FLUORIDE

Trade names: Fluor-A-Day, Fluorinse, Fluoritabs, Flura-Drops, Karidium, Pediaflor, Point-Two, Thera-Flur-N
Classification: PROPHYLACTIC: DENTAL
Pregnancy: Category C

ACTIONS/PHARMACODYNAMICS Source of the fluorine ion, a trace element. Its incorporation into developing tooth enamel hardens surfaces and increases resistance to cariogenic microbial processes. Topical application reduces acid production by bacteria in dental plaque and promotes remineralization of acid-damaged enamel. Application to exposed root surfaces supports formation of insoluble materials within dentinal tubules, thereby blocking transport of offending stimuli. Arrests rapid dental decay associated with drug-, radiation-, or age-related xerostomia. One of the few agents known that stimulates osteoblastic activity, leading to increased bone mass.

USES When fluoride ion concentration in drinking water is 0.7 ppm or less, to prevent periodontal disease and dental caries, to treat dental cervical hypersensitivity, and to control dental caries associated with xerostomia. **Unlabeled uses:** adjunctive treatment of osteoporosis; management of bone lesions in multiple myeloma; to reduce bone pain in patient with metastatic prostatic carcinoma; to stabilize progression of hearing loss in a limited number of patients with otosclerosis.

PHARMACOKINETICS Absorption: readily absorbed from GI tract. **Distribution:** fluoride is stored in bones and teeth; crosses placenta; distributed into breast milk. **Elimination:** rapidly excreted, primarily in urine with small amounts in feces.

CONTRAINDICATIONS & PRECAUTIONS Contraindicated in: when daily intake of fluoride from drinking water exceeds 0.7 ppm, low-sodium or sodium-free diets, hypersensitivity to fluoride, gels or dental rinses by children < 6 y, 1 mg tablet or rinse in children < 3 y, or 1 mg rinse in children < 6 y, pregnancy (category C).

ADVERSE/SIDE EFFECTS Topical application: rash, atopic dermatitis, urticaria, stomatitis, GI and respiratory allergic reactions. Acute toxicity: salty or soapy taste, dehydration, thirst, excessive salivation,

Common side effects in *italic*; life-threatening effects underlined; generic names in **bold**; classifications in SMALL CAPS

muscle weakness, rash, tremors, <u>shock,</u> <u>death from cardiac and respiratory failure</u>. **Chronic overdose:** dental fluorosis (brown or white mottling of tooth enamel), osseous fluorosis (patchy mineralization and possible decrease in bone strength). **Fatal dose:** 500 mg in children; 5–10 g in untreated adults.

ROUTE & DOSAGE

Prevent Periodontal Disease (Drinking Water Concentration < 0.3 ppm)

Child	PO	birth–2 y: 0.25 mg/d
		2–3 y: 0.5 mg/d
		3–13 y: 1 mg/d

Prevent Periodontal Disease (Drinking Water Concentration 0.3–0.7 ppm)

Child	PO	birth–2 y: 0.125 mg/d
		2–3 y: 0.25 mg/d
		3–13 y: 0.5 mg/d

Prevent Dental Caries

Child	Topical	6–12 y: 5 ml of 0.2% solution daily
		> 12 y: 10 ml of 0.2% solution daily

Desensitization of Exposed Root Surfaces

Child	Topical	0.2% rinsing solution once nightly after brushing and flossing

NURSING IMPLICATIONS

Administration

- All fluorine preparations should be applied or taken after thorough brushing and flossing and preferably at bedtime.
- Avoid giving sodium fluoride with milk or dairy products. Calcium from these products combines with fluorine, decreasing its absorption.
- Drops or tablets are taken preferably after meals. Drops may be taken undiluted or mixed with fluids or foods.
- Tablets should be dissolved in the mouth or chewed before they are swallowed. Administer at bedtime (after brushing the teeth).
- If patient's mouth is sore, the neutral preparation (Thera-Flur N) is better tolerated.
- *Treatment for dental cervical hypersensitivity:* thoroughly brush teeth; then swish PO solution around and between teeth for 1 min; expectorate. If gel is used, apply a few drops to toothbrush and brush gently onto affected surfaces.
- Gel-drops may also be applied with applicators supplied by the dentist. Spread gel on inner surfaces of applicators, which are then placed over lower and upper teeth at the same time. Instruct user to bite down lightly for 6 min and to then remove applicators and rinse mouth thoroughly. Applicators are cleaned with cold water.
- Store in tight plastic or paraffin-lined glass containers (sodium fluoride reacts with ordinary glass at a slow but appreciable rate) at 15–30C (59–86F). Avoid freezing.

Patient & Family Education

- Topically applied or rinse preparations are not to be swallowed.
- Do not eat, drink, or rinse mouth for at least 30 min after using the rinsing solution.
- Advise patient not to exceed recommended dosage. If mottling of teeth occurs, notify dentist.

Prophylactic Fluorine Regimen

- Sodium fluoride gel or solution used in orthodontic treatment regimen is applied immediately before attachment or reattachment of the tooth-encircling bands.
- To be effective, fluorine supplementation must be consistent and continuous from infancy until 12–14 y.
- A high fluorine content in drinking water and water used in food processing in addition to prescribed fluoride therapy may be a cause of dental fluorosis.
- If the family moves or if there is a change in water supply, consult dentist about continuation of fluoride therapy. (Mottling may occur if drinking water has fluorine content >1.5 ppm.)
- Dental fluorosis occurs only during tooth development but remains throughout life. If mild, it appears as opaque paper-white areas on tooth surfaces; if moderate, as brown stains with pitting.
- Pregnant or lactating women should consult physician about continuing fluorine therapy.

SODIUM IODIDE I 131

Trade name: Iodotope I-131
Classifications: ANTINEOPLASTIC; RADIOPHARMACEUTICAL
Pregnancy: Category X

ACTIONS/PHARMACODYNAMICS   Radiopharmaceutical with relatively long half-life (8.06 d). Processed in form of sodium iodide from products of uranium fission or neutron bombardment of tellurium. Chemically and physiologically identical to stable, naturally occurring iodide. Affords relatively

Common side effects in *italic*; life-threatening effects <u>underlined</u>; generic names in **bold**; classifications in SMALL CAPS

961

simple, effective, economic means of treating hyper-thyroidism (Graves' disease) by ablation without surgery. Therapeutic doses of radioactive iodine (RAI) deliver ionizing radiation to follicular cells, thereby damaging and destroying thyroid and neo-plastic tissues. About 10% of oral radiation is caused by gamma radiation and 90% by beta radiation.

USES Hyperthyroidism and thyrotoxicosis and to suppress neoplastic disease of thyroid. As a diagnos-tic aid, tracer doses are used in thyroid function stud-ies and imaging to evaluate suspected hyperthy-roidism and to visualize thyroid malignancy and metastasis.

ROUTE & DOSAGE

Hyperthyroidism

Adult	PO	4–10 mCi as a single dose; second dose, if necessary, after 6 wk

Carcinoma of Thyroid

Adult	PO	50 mCi as a single dose; subsequent doses of 100–150 mCi if necessary

PHARMACOKINETICS Absorption: readily ab-sorbed from GI tract. **Onset:** evident in blood within 3–6 min. **Distribution:** concentrates in thyroid gland; iodide secretion from this gland permits radioactivity detection in nasal secretion, oral cavity, trachea, fe-male breast, gallbladder, liver, and intestines; crosses placenta; distributed into breast milk. **Metabolism:** dis-integrates by beta and gamma emission. **Elimination:** half-life: 8.06 d; excreted primarily by kidneys, with small amounts in sweat and feces; radiation of thera-peutic dose is expended within 56 d.

CONTRAINDICATIONS & PRECAUTIONS Con-traindicated in: acute hyperthyroidism; large nodular goiter; preexisting vomiting or diarrhea; use of an-tithyroid, thyroid hormone, or iodine-containing preparations within 15 d, recent MI, pregnancy (cat-egory X), nursing mothers, lactation; sensitivity to io-dine; patients <30 y unless indications are excep-tional. **Cautious use in:** impaired renal and cardiac function.

ADVERSE/SIDE EFFECTS Primary *hypothy-roidism, thyroid nodules,* thyroid cancer (in chil-dren), *angioedema, petechiae,* transient thyroiditis (marked thyroid tenderness with swelling, feeling of fullness, fever, malaise, aching of teeth, headache, transient decrease in erythrocyte sedimentation rate, pain referred to ear, chest, or throat), alopecia (re-

versible), genetically transmissible chromosomal ab-normalities, myelosuppression, blood dyscrasias.

NURSING IMPLICATIONS

Administration

- All antithyroid, thyroid, or iodine-containing medi-cations are stopped 5–7 d before iodine-131 dose. After treatment, antithyroid drugs are not resumed, but other drugs taken to treat hyperthyroidism symptoms (e.g., propranolol) can be resumed until onset of full therapeutic effect of [131]I (normally 5–6 wk).
- Presence of food may delay absorption; therefore patient should fast overnight prior to RAI adminis-tration.
- When administering oral liquid ^{131}I, rinse container 2 or 3 times to ensure delivery of total dose. Glass or plastic cups are preferable to wax cups or paper cups.
- Given only during or 10 d after menstruation.
- Solution is clear and colorless; however, on stand-ing, bottle and solution may darken (without inter-fering with efficacy).

Assessment & Drug Effects

- Expected pattern of response to therapy: first 2 wk, minimal chemical or clinical change in thyrotoxi-cosis; next 4–8 wk, decrease in thyroid function, which reaches nadir (acute effects of radiation) be-tween 8–12 wk after treatment.
- If patient is hyperthyroid following treatment, RAI is repeated in 16 wk and q3–4mo thereafter until euthyroid state is achieved.

Patient & Family Education

- Urge patient to empty bladder frequently after ther-apeutic dosages of ^{131}I to reduce gonadal radiation.
- Urge patient to force fluids for first 48 h after treat-ment to aid in flushing out the radiopharmaceu-tical.
- Emphasize need for rest following RAI therapy. Consult physician for activity guides.
- Frequently, thyroxine replacement is instituted after patient achieves euthyroid state as prophy-laxis against myxedema. Patient should understand that this will be lifelong medication and that patient will need to return to physician at least once a year for medical surveillance. Consult physician about when to discuss this with the patient and family.
- Teach the patient the symptoms of hypothy-roidism.
- Transient thyroiditis (see adverse/side effects) may occur within 1 wk after RAI treatment. Patient

Common side effects in *italic*; life-threatening effects underlined; generic names in **bold**; classifications in SMALL CAPS

should report symptoms promptly to permit treatment.

- Temporary thinning of hair may begin 2 or 3 mo after treatment.
- Urine is slightly radioactive for 24 h but may be flushed down toilet. Saliva and vomiting is highly radioactive for 6–8 h. Urge patient to refrain from expectorating for 24 h if possible. Urine, saliva, and perspiration remain radioactive for 3 d.
- Instruct visitors to remain several feet away from the patient who is on therapeutic RAI. Usually visiting is restricted the first day after treatment with > 30 mCi.
- Avoid extended contact with small children (do not cuddle or hold on lap) until 7 d after treatment with ^{131}I.
- Avoid sleeping in same room with another person 7 d after the treatment date.

SODIUM POLYSTYRENE SULFONATE
(pol-ee-stye´reen)

Trade names: Kayexalate, SPS Suspension
Classification: RESIN EXCHANGE AGENT, CATION
Pregnancy: Category C

ACTIONS/PHARMACODYNAMICS Sulfonic cation-exchange resin. Removes potassium from body by exchanging sodium ion for potassium, particularly in large intestine; potassium-containing resin is then excreted. Small amounts of other cations such as calcium and magnesium may be lost during treatment.

USES Hyperkalemia.

ROUTE & DOSAGE

Hyperkalemia

Adult	PO	15 g suspended in 70% sorbitol or 20–100 ml of other fluid 1–4 times/d
	PR	30–50 g/100 ml 70% sorbitol q6h as warm emulsion high into sigmoid colon
Child	PO	Calculate appropriate amount on exchange rate of 1 mEq of potassium per gram of resin and suspend in 70% sorbitol or other appropriate solution

---

CONTRAINDICATIONS & PRECAUTIONS Cautious use in: The elderly, acute or chronic renal failure; patients receiving digitalis preparations; patients who cannot tolerate even a small increase in sodium load,

e.g., CHF, severe hypertension, and marked edema; pregnancy (category C).

ADVERSE/SIDE EFFECTS GI: *constipation, fecal impaction (in the elderly);* anorexia, gastric irritation, nausea, vomiting, diarrhea (with sorbitol emulsions). **Other:** sodium retention, hypocalcemia, hypokalemia, hypomagnesemia.

DRUG INTERACTIONS ANTACIDS, LAXATIVES containing **calcium** or **magnesium** may decrease potassium exchange capability of the resin.

NURSING IMPLICATIONS

Administration

- Oral dose should be given as a suspension in a small quantity of water or in syrup. Usual amount of fluid ranges from 20–100 ml or approximately 3–4 ml/g of drug.

Administration of Drug in Enema Form

- Use warm fluid (as prescribed) to prepare the emulsion.
- Administer at body temperature and introduce by gravity, keeping suspension particles in solution by stirring. Flush suspension with 50–100 ml of fluid; then clamp tube and leave it in place.
- Urge patient to retain enema at least 30–60 min but as long as several hours if possible.
- Irrigate colon (after enema solution has been expelled) with 1 or 2 quarts flushing solution (should be nonsodium containing). Drain returns constantly through a Y-tube connection.
- Store remainder of prepared solution for 24 h; then discard.

Assessment & Drug Effects

- Serum potassium levels should be determined daily throughout therapy. Acid-base balance, electrolytes, and minerals should also be monitored in patients receiving repeated doses.
- Serum potassium levels do not always reflect intracellular potassium deficiency. Therefore, observe patient closely for early clinical signs of severe hypokalemia (see chap 3). ECGs are also recommended.
- Usually a mild laxative is prescribed to prevent constipation (common side effect) and fecal impaction. Check bowel function daily. Elderly patients are particularly prone to fecal impaction.
- Since drug contains approximately 100 mg (4.1 mEq) of sodium per gram (1 tsp, 15 mEq sodium), sodium content from dietary and other sources may be restricted. Consult physician.

Common side effects in *italic*; life-threatening effects underlined;
generic names in **bold**; classifications in SMALL CAPS

963

Prototype: aspirin, p 161

SODIUM SALICYLATE

Trade name: Uracel-5
Classifications: CNS AGENT; SALICYLATE
ANALGESIC, ANTIPYRETIC; NSAID
Pregnancy: Category C

ACTIONS/PHARMACODYNAMICS Properties similar to those of aspirin but less effective. Liberates free salicylic acid in the stomach and therefore tends to cause gastric irritation. Unlike aspirin, does not inhibit platelet aggregation. Increases prothrombin time, like aspirin, but reportedly is associated with less occult blood loss.

USES Primarily in treatment of acute pain, rheumatoid arthritis, osteoarthritis. May be used as an alternative in individuals with GI intolerance to aspirin.

ROUTE & DOSAGE

Analgesia, Antipyresis

Adult	PO	325–650 mg q4h prn
	IV	500 mg diluted in 1 L NS or lactated Ringer's and infused over 4–8 h; may repeat x 1
Child	PO	2–11 y: 25–50 mg/kg/d in 4–6 divided doses

Arthritis

Adult	PO	3.6–5.4 g/d divided q4–6h
Child	PO	80–100 mg/kg/d divide q4–6h (max 130 mg/kg/d)

PHARMACOKINETICS Absorption: 80–100% absorbed. **Peak:** 0.25–2 h. **Distribution:** widely distributed in most body tissues; crosses placenta. **Metabolism:** metabolized in liver. **Elimination:** half-life: 2–18 h (dose dependent); 50% of dose is eliminated in urine in 2–4 h (low doses) or 15–30 h (high doses); excreted in breast milk.

CONTRAINDICATIONS & PRECAUTIONS Contraindicated in: hypersensitivity to other salicylates, severe renal disease, heart failure, patients on low-sodium diets; pregnancy (category C).

ADVERSE/SIDE EFFECTS *Tinnitus,* diminished hearing, nausea, vomiting, hypersensitivity reactions, *thrombophlebitis (with rapid infusion),* sloughing of soft tissues (with extravasation), pulmonary edema in patients with rheumatic fever.

DRUG INTERACTIONS Aminosalicylic acid increases risk of salicylate toxicity; **ammonium chloride** and other ACIDIFYING AGENTS decrease renal elimination and thus increase risk of salicylate toxicity; ANTICOAGULANTS add to risk of bleeding; aspirin doses >2 g/d increase hypoglycemic activity of SULFONYLUREAS; carbonic anhydrase inhibitors enhance salicylate toxicity; CORTICOSTEROIDS add to ulcerogenic effects of salicylates; increases **methotrexate** toxicity; low doses of salicylates may antagonize uricosuric effects of **probenecid, sulfinpyrazone.**

NURSING IMPLICATIONS

Administration

- Administer with food, milk, or a full glass (240 ml) of water to minimize risk of gastric irritation. Caution patient not to chew or crush tablet.
- Some physicians prescribe concurrent administration of sodium bicarbonate or other antacid to prevent gastric irritation, although it may increase urinary excretion of salicylate and thus lower blood salicylate levels.
- In the symptomatic treatment of rheumatic fever the dosage of sodium salicylate is the same as that employed with aspirin.
- For patients receiving sodium salicylate IV, frequent checks of infusion site for extravasation and prescribed infusion rate (should be slow) are advised.
- Sodium salicylate is incompatible with mineral acids and ferric salts.
- Store in light-resistant containers. Turns pink on exposure to light.

Assessment & Drug Effects

- Serum salicylate levels may be required as a guide for adequate dosing of patients on long-term therapy.
- There are 2 mEq (46 mg) of sodium in each 325 mg tablet of sodium salicylate.
- Monitor for adverse GI effects, especially in patients with a history of peptic ulcer disease.

Patient & Family Education

- Warn patient not to self-dose with aspirin or any other OTC drug during sodium salicylate therapy.
- Instruct patient to report tinnitus, hearing loss, vertigo, rash, or nausea.

Common side effects in *italic*; life-threatening effects underlined; generic names in **bold**; classifications in SMALL CAPS

Prototype: aspirin, p 161

SODIUM THIOSALICYLATE

Trade names: Arthrolate, Thiocyl, Thiosal, Tusal
Classifications: CNS AGENT; SALICYLATE
ANALGESIC, ANTIPYRETIC
Pregnancy: Category C

ACTIONS/PHARMACODYNAMICS Sodium salt of thiosalicylic acid with analgesic activity that may be due to interference with transmission of peripheral pain impulse reaching cerebral level.

USES To ameliorate moderate pain in arthritis; also used in rheumatic fever. Has been used for acute gout, but other agents are more effective.

ROUTE & DOSAGE

Acute Gout
Adult IM 100 mg q3–4h; then 100 mg/d

Analgesia
Adult IM 50–100 mg/d or on alternate days

Rheumatic Fever
Adult IM 100–150 mg q4–6h for 3 d; then 100 mg b.i.d.

CONTRAINDICATIONS & PRECAUTIONS Contraindicated in: pregnancy (category C).

ADVERSE/SIDE EFFECTS See aspirin.

DRUG INTERACTIONS Aminosalicylic acid increases risk of salicylate toxicity; **ammonium chloride** and other ACIDIFYING AGENTS decrease renal elimination, thus increasing risk of salicylate toxicity; ANTICOAGULANTS add to risk of bleeding; aspirin doses >2 g/d increase hypoglycemic activity of SULFONYLUREAS; CARBONIC ANHYDRASE INHIBITORS enhance salicylate toxicity; CORTICOSTEROIDS add to ulcerogenic effects of salicylates; increases **methotrexate** toxicity; low doses of salicylates may antagonize uricosuric effects of **probenecid, sulfinpyrazone.**

NURSING IMPLICATIONS
See aspirin for numerous nursing implications.

SOMATREM

(soe´ma-trem)
Trade name: Protropin
Classification: HORMONE
Pregnancy: Category C

ACTIONS/PHARMACODYNAMICS Biosynthetic product of recombinant DNA technology. The second genetically engineered pharmaceutical to be approved by the FDA (first: human insulin). Contains exact sequence of 191 amino acids in pituitary-derived human growth hormone (GH) plus an amino terminal methionyl group not found in natural GH. Therapeutically equivalent to natural GH (somatropin) of pituitary origin, a product removed from the market by the FDA in 1987. Somatrem affects metabolism and growth of most body tissues including red cell mass, with possible exception of eye and brain. In presence of GH deficiency, promotes skeletal growth at epiphyseal plates of long bones by increasing levels of the mediator somatomedin-C and by increasing synthesis of protein, chondroitin sulfate, and collagen. Increases number and size of muscle cells. Promotes renal retention of potassium, phosphates, and sodium; also increases renal excretion of calcium with simultaneous increase in intestinal absorption of calcium. Synergistic with insulin in its anabolic effects but antagonistic to insulin in regulation of serum glucose. In patient with diabetes mellitus especially, may impair glucose tolerance, decrease sensitivity to exogenous insulin and increase serum glucose levels. Inhibits lipogenesis and promotes mobilization of stored lipids, resulting in reduced body fat stores and elevation of circulating fatty acids. May induce GH antibody formation (IgG), but effect of antibodies on endogenous GH activity is unknown. Safety of using any form of GH to increase adult stature in short children with normal GH levels has not been established.

USES Long-term treatment of children with growth failure due to deficiency of endogenous GH.

ROUTE & DOSAGE

Growth Hormone Deficiency
Child IM/SC Doses up to 0.1 mg/kg (0.2 U/kg) 3 times/wk with a minimum of 48 h between doses; may be increased in older children if epiphyses have not closed

---

Common side effects in *italic*; life-threatening effects <u>underlined</u>; generic names in **bold**; classifications in SMALL CAPS

965

S

PHARMACOKINETICS Metabolism: metabolized in liver. **Elimination:** half-life: 20–30 min; excreted in urine.

CONTRAINDICATIONS & PRECAUTIONS Contraindicated in: patient with closed epiphyses; underlying progressive intracranial tumor; pregnancy (Category C). **Cautious use in:** diabetes mellitus or family history of the disease; concomitant use of glucocorticoids; concomitant or prior use of thyroid or androgens in prepubertal male; hypothyroidism. Patient with known sensitivity to benzyl alcohol.

ADVERSE/SIDE EFFECTS Allergic reaction (systemic): peripheral edema, headache, myalgia, weakness. **Excess dosage:** diabetes mellitus, atherosclerosis, organ enlargement, hypertension, acromegalic features in children. **Metabolic:** glucose intolerance, ACTH deficiency, hypothyroidism. **Other:** recurrent intracranial tumor growth, persistent antibodies to GH; pain, swelling at injection site.

DIAGNOSTIC TEST INTERFERENCES Somatrem may reduce *glucose tolerance, serum T_4* (thyroxin) concentration, *RAI uptake,* and *thyroxine-binding capacity.*

DRUG INTERACTIONS ANABOLIC STEROIDS, **thyroid hormone,** ANDROGENS, ESTROGENS may accelerate epiphyseal closure; **ACTH,** CORTICOSTEROIDS may inhibit growth response to somatrem.

NURSING IMPLICATIONS

Administration

- Reconstitute each vial (containing 5 ml lyophilized powder) with 1–5 ml bacteriostatic water for injection, aiming stream of water against vial wall. Swirl vial gently to mix contents. Do not shake. If reconstituted solution is cloudy or has crystals, do not administer. Refrigeration may cause cloudiness. pH of reconstituted solution: about 7.8.
- Use disposable syringe small enough to administer prescribed doses with accuracy and needle long enough to insure injection into muscle layer.
- Benzyl alcohol is the preservative in bacteriostatic water for injection and may be toxic to the newborn. Water for injection USP is the preferred diluent for this age group.
- Discard unused reconstituted solution within 7 d.
- Refrigerate lyophilized powder and reconstituted solution at 2–8C (36–46F). Do not freeze. Expiration dates are on labels.

Assessment & Drug Effects

- Before treatment is begun, careful documentation is made of growth rate for at least 6–12 mo. Thyroid, adrenal, and gonadal functions are also evaluated to rule out multiple pituitary hormone deficiency.
- Annual bone age assessments are advised in all patients and especially those also receiving thyroid, androgen, or estrogen replacement therapy, since concurrent use of these agents may precipitate early epiphyseal closure. Urge parent to take child for growth assessment on appointed annual dates.
- Thyroid status should also be evaluated at regular intervals. Untreated hypothyroidism may interfere with response to somatrem.
- Diabetic patients or those with family history of diabetes should be observed closely. Blood or urine glucose determinations should be evaluated regularly to recognize glucose intolerance.
- Patient with GH deficiency secondary to intracranial lesion should be examined frequently for progression or recurrence of underlying disease. Somatrem should not be used if tumor has been active during the previous 12 mo.

Patient & Family Education

- First year growth of 17.5 cm (7 in) with somatrem has been reported, but average expectations are 7.5–12.5 cm (3–5 in) in first year, slightly less in second year, and after that, normal growth rate. Additionally, subcutaneous fat diminishes but returns to pretreatment level later.
- Instruct parent to record accurate height measurements at regular intervals and to report to physician if rate is less than expected.
- Instruct parent to report child's complaints of hip or knee pain or a limp. Slipped capital femoral epiphysis may occur in patient with endocrine disorders.

SOMATROPIN

(soe-ma-troe´pin)
Trade name: Humatrope
Classification: HORMONE

ACTIONS/PHARMACODYNAMICS New recombinant growth hormone with the natural sequence of 191 amino acids characteristic of endogenous growth hormone (GH). Differs from somatrem by absence of an extra methionyl group in its structure. Somatropin appears to be less likely to produce serum antibodies to endogenous GH than somatrem is (perhaps related to the manufacturing process), but it is not clear whether lack of antigenicity is of clinical importance. Induces growth responses similar to those produced in children treated with recombinant methionyl GH (somatrem) or with GH obtained from human pituitary glands (removed from market in 1987 by FDA). (See somatrem for other pharmacodynamics and for nursing implications.)

USES Growth failure due to GH deficiency; as replacement therapy prior to epiphyseal closure in patients with idiopathic GH deficiency. Also GH deficiency secondary to intracranial tumors or panhypopituitarism.

ROUTE & DOSAGE

Growth Hormone Deficiency

Child	IM/SC	Doses up to 0.06 mg/kg (0.16 IU/kg) 3 times/wk with a minimum of 48 h between doses

PHARMACOKINETICS Metabolism: metabolized in liver. **Elimination:** half-life: 15–50 min; excreted in urine.

CONTRAINDICATIONS & PRECAUTIONS Contraindicated in: patient with closed epiphyses; underlying progressive intracranial tumor. **Cautious use in:** diabetes mellitus or family history of the disease; concomitant or prior use of thyroid or androgens in prepubertal male; hypothyroidism.

ADVERSE/SIDE EFFECTS Pain, swelling at injection site; myalgia, *hypercalciuria;* oversaturation of bile with cholesterol, high circulating GH antibodies with resulting treatment failure, hyperglycemia, ketosis, accelerated growth of intracranial tumor.

DRUG INTERACTIONS ANABOLIC STEROIDS, **thyroid hormone**, ANDROGENS, ESTROGENS may accelerate epiphyseal closure; ACTH, CORTICOSTEROIDS may inhibit growth response to somatropin.

NURSING IMPLICATIONS

Administration

- Reconstitute each vial (containing 10 IU of drug) with 5 ml bacteriostatic water for injection only. Record date of reconstitution on vial.
- Rotate IM sites to prevent tissue damage. Use needle long enough to ensure injection into muscle layer.
- Refrigerate drug at 2–8C (36–46F). Discard after 1 mo.

Assessment & Drug Effects

- Before initiating treatment, careful documentation is made of growth rate for at least 6–12 mo. In addition, GH deficiency may be confirmed by demonstrating failure of plasma GH levels to exceed 5–7 ng/ml in response to standard stimuli. Thyroid, adrenal, and gonadal functions are also evaluated to rule out multiple pituitary hormone deficiency.
- Annual bone age assessments are advised in all patients and especially those also receiving concurrent thyroid or androgen treatment, since these drugs may precipitate early epiphyseal closure. Urge parent to take child for bone age assessment on appointed annual dates.
- Hypercalciuria, a frequent side effect in the first 2–3 mo of therapy, may be symptomless; however, it may be accompanied by renal calculi, with these reportable symptoms: flank pain and colic, GI symptoms, urinary frequency, chills, fever, hematuria.
- In patients who respond initially but who later fail to respond to somatropin therapy, test for circulating GH antibodies (antisomatropin antibodies) should be performed.
- Diabetic patients or those with family history of diabetes should be observed closely. Regular testing of urine for glycosuria or fasting blood glucose levels is recommended.
- Patient with GH deficiency secondary to intracranial lesion should be examined frequently for progression or recurrence of underlying disease process.

Patient & Family Education

- During first 6 mo of successful treatment, linear growth rates may be increased 8–16 cm or more per year (average about 7 cm/y). Additionally, SC fat diminishes but returns to pretreatment value later.
- Instruct parent of child under treatment to record accurate height measurements at regular intervals and to report to physician if rate is less than expected.
- In general, growth response to somatropin is inversely proportional to duration of treatment. Somatropin should be discontinued when patient has reached satisfactory adult height, when epiphyses have fused, or when patient fails to exhibit growth response.

Common side effects in *italic*; life-threatening effects underlined; generic names in **bold**; classifications in SMALL CAPS

967

SPECTINOMYCIN HYDROCHLORIDE
(spek-ti-noe-mye′sin)
Trade name: Trobicin
Classifications: ANTIINFECTIVE; ANTIBIOTIC
Pregnancy: Category B

ACTIONS/PHARMACODYNAMICS Aminocyclitol antibiotic produced by *Streptomyces spectabilis*. Action is usually bacteriostatic. Appears to act by selectively binding to 30S subunits of bacterial ribosomes, thereby inhibiting protein synthesis. Variable activity against a wide variety of gram-negative and gram-positive organisms. Inhibits majority of *Neisseria gonorrhoeae* strains; effective for urethral and anorectal infections, but not pharyngeal. Not active against syphilis or chlamydial and mycoplasmal infections.

USES Only for treatment of uncomplicated gonorrhea in patients sensitized or resistant to penicillin or other effective drugs approved by US Centers for Disease Control. **Unlabeled uses:** disseminated gonococcal infections caused by penicillinase-producing strains of *N. gonorrhoeae* (PPNG) and sexually transmitted epididymoorchitis.

ROUTE & DOSAGE

Uncomplicated Gonorrhea

Adult	IM	2 g as single dose
Child	IM	40 mg/kg as single dose

Disseminated Gonorrhea

Adult	IM	2 g q12h

PHARMACOKINETICS Absorption: readily absorbed from IM site. **Peak:** 1 hr. **Metabolism:** metabolized in liver. **Eliminations:** half-life: 1.2–2.8 h; excreted in urine.

CONTRAINDICATIONS & PRECAUTIONS Contraindicated in: safe use during pregnancy (category B), in nursing mothers, and in infants and children not definitely established. **Cautious use in:** history of allergies.

ADVERSE/SIDE EFFECTS *Pain and soreness at injection site,* urticaria, pruritus, transient rash, headache, dizziness, nausea, vomiting, chills, fever, insomnia, nervousness. **Following multiple doses:** decrease in Hgb, Hct, Cl$_{cr}$, elevated serum alkaline phosphatase, ALT, BUN; decrease in urine output (rare).

NURSING IMPLICATIONS

Administration
- For IM use only. Administer IM injection deep into upper outer quadrant of gluteus. No more than 5 ml should be injected into single site (20-gauge needle is recommeded). Injection may be painful.
- Reconstitute with supplied diluent (bacteriostatic water for injection with 0.9% benzyl alcohol). Shake vial vigorously immediately after adding diluent and before withdrawing drug. Solution should be used within 24 h of reconstitution.
- Store at 15–30C (59–86F) unless otherwise directed.

Assessment & Drug Effects
- Observe patient for 45–60 min after injection. Systemic anaphylaxis has been reported (apprehension, pruritus, hypertension, abdominal pain, collapse).
- Patients with gonorrhea should have serologic tests for syphilis at time of diagnosis and again after 3 mo.
- Clinical effectiveness of drug should be monitored to detect antibiotic resistance.
- All gonococcal infection sites should be cultured 3–7 d after spectinomycin therapy is completed to verify eradication of infection.

SPIRONOLACTONE

See ELECTROLYTIC & WATER BALANCE AGENTS, DIURETIC, POTASSIUM-SPARING, prototype, p 202.

Prototype: testosterone, p 229

STANOZOLOL
(stan-oh′zoe-lole)
Trade name: Winstrol
Classifications: SYNTHETIC HORMONE; ANDROGEN/ANABOLIC STEROID
Pregnancy: Category X
Controlled substance: Schedule III

ACTIONS/PHARMACODYNAMICS Synthetic steroid with relatively strong anabolic and weak androgenic activity. Pharmacokinetics, contraindications, adverse effects similar to those for testosterone.

USES Primarily to increase hemoglobin in selected cases of aplastic anemia, prophylaxis to decrease the frequency and severity of hereditary angioedema.

ROUTE & DOSAGE

Anemia

Adult	PO	2 mg t.i.d. Young women: 2 mg 1-2 times/d
Child	PO	<6 y: 1 mg b.i.d. 6–12 y: 2 mg t.i.d.

NURSING IMPLICATIONS

Administration

- Administer just before or with meals to reduce incidence of gastric distress.
- Smaller dose for young women is given to prevent virilizing effects of the drug. If such effects appear (early sign: change of voice), physician should be notified.

Assessment & Drug Effects

- Monitor Hct & Hgb periodically to determine efficacy of drug.
- Patient may need to be on a restricted salt intake. Check with the physician.
- Be alert to symptoms of hypercalcemia (see chap 3).

Patient & Family Education

- Used with high caloric, high protein diet unless contraindicated.
- Stanozolol does not enhance athletic ability.

STREPTOKINASE

See BLOOD FORMERS & COAGULATORS, THROMBOLYTIC ENZYME prototype, p 134.

Prototype: gentamicin, p 53

STREPTOMYCIN SULFATE
(strep-toe-mye´sin)
Classifications: ANTIINFECTIVE; AMINOGLYCOSIDE ANTIBIOTIC; ANTITUBERCULOSIS AGENT
Pregnancy: Category C

ACTIONS/PHARMACODYNAMICS Aminoglycoside antibiotic derived from *Streptomyces griseus,* with bactericidal and bacteriostatic actions. Appears to act by interfering with normal protein synthesis in susceptible bacteria by binding to 30S subunits of ribosomes. Active against a variety of gram-positive, gram-negative, and acid-fast organisms. Because of rapid emergence of resistant strains when streptomycin sulfate is used alone, it most commonly is used concurrently with other antimicrobial agents. Reportedly, it is the least nephrotoxic of the aminoglycosides. In common with other aminoglycosides, it has a weak neuromuscular blocking effect.

USES Only in combination with other antitubercular drugs in treatment of all forms of active tuberculosis caused by susceptible organisms. Used alone or in conjunction with tetracycline for tularemia, plague, and brucellosis. Also used with other antibiotics in treatment of subacute bacterial endocarditis due to enterococci and streptococci (viridans group) and *Haemophilus influenzae* and in treatment of peritonitis, respiratory tract infections, granuloma inguinale, and chancroid when other drugs have failed.

ROUTE & DOSAGE

Tuberculosis

Adult	IM	15 mg/kg up to 1 g/d as single dose
Child	IM	20–40 mg/kg/d up to 1 g/d as single dose

Tularemia

Adult	IM	1–2 mg/d in 1–2 divided doses for 7–10 d

Plague

Adult	IM	2–4 mg/d in 2–4 divided doses

PHARMACOKINETICS Peak: 1–2 h. **Distribution:** diffuses into most body tissues and extracellular fluids; crosses placenta; distributed into breast milk. **Elimination:** half-life: 2–3 h adults, 4–10 h newborns; excreted in urine.

CONTRAINDICATIONS & PRECAUTIONS Contraindicated in: history of toxic reaction or hypersensitivity to aminoglycosides; labyrinthine disease; during pregnancy or lactation; myasthenia gravis; concurrent or sequential use of other neurotoxic or nephrotoxic agents. **Cautious use in:** impaired renal function (given in reduced dosages); use in the elderly and in prematures, neonates, and children.

Common side effects in *italic*; life-threatening effects underlined; generic names in **bold**; classifications in SMALL CAPS

969

ADVERSE/SIDE EFFECTS CNS: paresthesias (peripheral, facial). **Hypersensitivity:** skin rashes, pruritus, angioedema, <u>drug fever</u>, eosinophilia, <u>exfoliative dermatitis</u>, stomatitis, enlarged lymph nodes, <u>anaphylactic shock</u>, blood dyscrasias: leukopenia, neutropenia, pancytopenia, hemolytic or aplastic anemia. **Ototoxicity:** *labyrinthine damage,* auditory damage. **Other:** nephrotoxicity, hepatotoxicity, transient bleeding (due to inhibition of factor V and especially circumoral), headache, inability to concentrate, lassitude, muscular weakness, optic nerve toxicity (scotomas), SLE, *pain and irritation at IM site,* superinfections, neuromuscular blockade, arachnoiditis, encephalopathy, **_CNS depression syndrome (infants):_** <u>stupor, flaccidity, coma, paralysis, cardiac arrest); respiratory depression.</u>

DIAGNOSTIC TEST INTERFERENCES Streptomycin reportedly produces false-positive **urinary glucose** tests using copper sulfate methods (Benedict's solution, Clinitest) but not with glucose oxidase methods (e.g., Clinistix, TesTape). False increases in protein content in **urine** and **CSF** using Folin-Ciocalteu reaction and decreased **BUN** readings with Berthelot reaction may occur from test interferences. **Culture and sensitivity** tests may be affected if patient is taking salts such as sodium and potassium chloride, sodium sulfate and tartrate, ammonium acetate, calcium and magnesium ions.

DRUG INTERACTIONS May potentiate anticoagulant effects of **warfarin.**

NURSING IMPLICATIONS

Administration

- Administer IM deep into large muscle mass to minimize possibility of irritation. Injections are painful.
- Avoid direct contact with drug; sensitization can occur. Rubber or plastic gloves are advised during preparation of drug.
- Except for tuberculosis and subacute bacterial endocarditis, streptomycin is rarely administered for more than 7–10 d.
- Commercially prepared IM solution is intended only for IM injection (contains a preservative, and therefore is not suitable for other routes). Stable at room temperature; expiration date 1–2 y depending on manufacturer.
- Solutions made from streptomycin sulfate powder are preferably used immediately after reconstitution. See specific manufacturer's recommendations.
- Exposure to light may slightly darken solution, with no apparent loss of potency.

Assessment & Drug Effects

- Culture and sensitivity tests are done prior to and periodically during course of therapy.
- Caloric stimulation and audiometric tests should be performed before, during, and 6 mo after discontinuation of streptomycin. Periodic renal and hepatic function tests are also recommended.
- Be alert for and report immediately symptoms of ototoxicity (see chap 3). Symptoms are most likely to occur in patients with impaired renal function, patients receiving high doses (1.8–2 g/d) or other ototoxic or neurotoxic drugs, and the elderly. If drug is not discontinued promptly, irreversible damage may occur.
- **_Damage to vestibular portion of eighth cranial nerve_** (higher incidence than auditory toxicity) appears to occur in three stages. **_Acute stage:_** may be preceded for 1 or 2 d by moderately severe headache, then by nausea, vomiting, vertigo in upright position, difficulty in reading, unsteadiness, and positive Romberg sign; lasts 1–2 wk and ends abruptly. **_Chronic stage:_** characterized by difficulty in walking or in making sudden movements and ataxia; lasts approximately 2 mo. **_Compensatory stage:_** symptoms are latent and appear only when eyes are closed. Full recovery may take 12–18 mo; residual damage is permanent in some patients.
- Auditory nerve damage is usually preceded by vestibular symptoms and high-pitched tinnitus, roaring noises, impaired hearing (especially to high-pitched sounds), sense of fullness in ears. Audiometric test should be done if these symptoms appear, and drug should be discontinued. Hearing loss can be permanent if damage is extensive. Tinnitus may persist several days to weeks after drug is stopped.
- In patients with impaired renal function, drug accumulation reportedly occurs if administered more frequently than q8–12h. Frequent determinations of serum drug concentrations and periodic renal and hepatic function tests are advised (serum concentrations should not exceed 25 μg/ml in these patients).
- Although drug fever is uncommon, it is life threatening. Monitor temperature and BP. If either is altered, report to physician.
- Monitor I&O. Report oliguria or changes in I&O ratio (possible signs of diminishing renal function). Sufficient fluids to maintain urinary output of 1500 ml/24 h are generally advised. Consult physician.

Patient & Family Education

- Patient should be instructed to report any unusual symptom. Adverse reactions should be reviewed

periodically, especially in patients on prolonged therapy. Inform patient of possibility of ototoxicity.
- Instruct patient to report immediately any of the following, nausea, vomiting, vertigo, tinnitus, fullness in ears, impaired hearing.

STREPTOZOCIN
(strep-toe-zoe´sin)
Trade name: Zanosar
Classifications: NITROSOUREA; ANTINEOPLASTIC; ALKYLATING AGENT; ANTIBIOTIC
Pregnancy: Category C

ACTIONS/PHARMACODYNAMICS Antineoplastic antibiotic (produced naturally by *Streptomyces achromogenes).* Therapeutic product is synthetic and is similar to other nitrosourea antineoplastics (e.g., carmustine) but with weaker alkylating effects. Not used therapeutically as an antibiotic because of its potent cytotoxic properties. In general this drug is highly toxic and has a low therapeutic index; thus a clinically effective response is likely to be accompanied by some evidence of toxicity. Inhibits DNA synthesis in both bacterial and mammalian cells and prevents progression of cells into mitosis, affecting all phases of the cell cycle (cell-cycle nonspecific). Appears to have minimal effects on RNA or protein synthesis. Delays repair of DNA damaged by nitrosurea-induced alkylation. Unlike other nitrosoureas has markedly significant specificity for pancreas beta and exocrine cells; however, it does not appear to have clinically important diabetogenic properties. Has mild to moderate myelosuppressive activity, is mutagenic, and potentially carcinogenic. Use is limited by high incidence of nephrotoxicity (more than 50%) and strong emetogenic potential.

USES Metastatic functional and nonfunctional islet cell carcinoma of pancreas, as single agent or in combination with fluorouracil. **Unlabeled uses;** a variety of other malignant neoplasms including metastatic carcinoid tumor or carcinoid syndrome, refractory advanced Hodgkin's disease, and metastatic colorectal cancer.

ROUTE & DOSAGE

Islet Cell Carcinoma of Pancreas

Adult	IV	500 mg/m²/d for 5 consecutive days q6wk or 1 g/m²/wk for 2 wk; then increase to 1.5 g/m²/wk; infuse dose over 15 min to 6 h

PHARMACOKINETICS Absorption: undetectable in plasma within 3 h. **Distribution:** metabolite enters CSF. **Metabolism:** metabolized in liver and kidneys. **Elimination:** half life: 35–40 min, 70–80% of dose excreted in urine, 1% in feces, and 5% in expired air.

CONTRAINDICATIONS & PRECAUTIONS Contraindicated in: safe use in pregnancy (category C), during lactation, and in children has not been established; hepatic and renal dysfunction.

ADVERSE/SIDE EFFECTS CNS: confusion, lethargy, depression. **GI:** *nausea, vomiting,* diarrhea, duodenal ulcer (rare). **Hematologic:** *mild* to moderate myelosuppression *(leukopenia, thrombocytopenia, anemia);* asymptomatic eosinophilia. **Hepatic:** transient increase in AST, ALT, or alkaline phosphatase; hypoalbuminemia; severe liver dysfunction. **Metabolic:** glucose tolerance abnormalities (moderate and reversible); insulin shock with hypoglycemia, glycosuria without hyperglycemia; fever. **Renal:** nephrotoxicity: azotemia, anuria, proteinuria, hypophosphatemia, hyperchloremia; *Fanconi-like syndrome* (proximal renal tubular reabsorption defects, alkaline pH of urine, glucosuria, acetonuria, aminoaciduria); hypokalemia, hypocalcemia. **Other:** local necrosis following extravasation.

DRUG INTERACTIONS MYELOSUPPRESSIVE AGENTS add to hematologic toxicity; nephrotoxic agents (e.g., AMINOGLYCOSIDES, **vancomycin, amphotericin B, cisplatin**) increase risk of nephrotoxicity; **phenytoin** may reduce cytotoxic effect on pancreatic beta cells.

NURSING IMPLICATIONS

Administration
- Used only under constant supervision by physician experienced in therapy with cytotoxic agents and only when the benefit : risk ratio is fully and thoroughly understood by patient and family.
- Dosage adjustment may be made on basis of creatinine clearance. If it is 10–50 ml/min, 75% of usual dose is given; if clearance is less than 10 ml/min, usual dose is reduced to 50%.
- Persons handling streptozocin should wear gloves to protect against topical exposure, which may pose a carcinogen hazard. If solution or powder comes in contact with skin or mucosa, promptly flush the area thoroughly with soap and water.
- Reconstitute streptozocin powder for injection with 9.5% ml dextrose injection or 0.9% NaCl injection; resulting solution will contain 100 mg/ml strepto-

Common side effects in *italic*; life-threatening effects underlined; generic names in **bold**; classifications in SMALL CAPS

971

zocin and will be pale gold. Dilute solution further with 10–200 ml if desired with the same diluents and administer over 15 min.

- Inspect injection site frequently for **signs of extravasation:** patient complaints of stinging or burning at site, swelling around site, no blood return or questionable blood return.
- If extravasation occurs, area requires immediate attention to prevent necrosis. Remove needle, apply ice, and contact physician regarding further treatment to infiltrated tissue. Teach patient to inspect site at weekly intervals and to report changes in tissue appearance.
- An antiemetic given routinely every 4 or 6 h and prophylactically 30 min before a treatment may provide sufficient control to maintain the treatment regimen (even if it is reduction but not complete elimination of nausea and vomiting).
- Protect reconstituted solution and vials of drug from light. Reconstituted solutions should be discarded after 12 h (contains no preservative and not intended for multidose use).

Assessment & Drug Effects

- When patient is receiving medication on a weekly dosing regimen, onset of therapeutic response usually occurs about 17 d after start of therapy, reaching maximum response in about 35 d.
- Response to therapy is evidenced by reduction in organomegaly, lymph nodes, or masses.
- Functional islet cell tumors produce and secrete a variety of hormones including glucagon, insulin, calcitonin, serotonin, and others. Successful therapy with streptozocin (alone or in combination) produces a biochemical response evidenced by decreased secretion of hormones as well as measurable tumor regression. Thus, serial fasting insulin levels during treatment indicate response to the antineoplastic.
- Renal function must be adequate to prevent drug toxicity. Serial urinalyses and determinations of BUN, creatinine clearance, and serum electrolytes are obtained prior to and weekly during therapy, then for 4 wk after termination of therapy.
- Evidence of drug-induced declining renal function should be reported promptly; changes are dose related and cumulative.
- **Early laboratory evidence of renal dysfunction:** hypophosphatemia, mild proteinurea. Changes in I&O ratio and pattern.
- Mild adverse renal effects may be reversible following discontinuation of streptozocin, but nephrotoxicity may be irreversible, severe, or fatal.
- CBC should be performed at least weekly, and liver function tests at least prior to each course of therapy. Dosage adjustment or discontinuation may be required if there is evidence of decreased hepatic or bone marrow function.
- Myelosuppression is severe in 10–20% of patients and may be cumulative and more severe if patient has had prior exposure to radiation or to other antineoplastics. Be alert to symptoms of sepsis and superinfections (leukopenia) or increased tendency to bleed (thrombocytopenia).
- Platelet and leukocyte nadirs generally occur 1–2 wk after beginning therapy with streptozocin.
- Superinfection in the oral cavity is evidenced by black furry tongue (fungal overgrowth) or by white, round to irregularly shaped patches that adhere to underlying epithelium (candidiasis). Inspect mouth daily during therapy.
- Monitor and record temperature pattern to promptly recognize impending sepsis.
- Of patients receiving this antineoplastic drug 90% experience severe nausea and vomiting within 1–4 h after drug therapy begins. It may last up to 24 h and occasionally necessitates discontinuation of treatment.
- Repeat courses of streptozocin treatment are not given until patient's hepatic, renal, and hematologic functions are within acceptable limits.

Patient & Family Education

- Although this drug has minimal, if any, diabetogenic action, advise patient to report symptoms of hypoglycemia (see chap 3).
- Encourage adeqate fluid intake (2000–3000 ml/d). Hydration may protect against drug toxicity effects.
- Instruct patient to report signs of nephrotoxicity (see chap 3).
- Instruct patient not to use aspirin without consulting physician. Advise patient to promptly report **signs of bleeding:** hematuria, epistaxis, ecchymoses, petechial.
- Instruct patient to report **symptoms that suggest anemia:** shortness of breath, pale mucous membranes and nail beds, exhaustion, rapid pulse.

SUCCINYLCHOLINE

See AUTONOMIC NERVOUS SYSTEM AGENTS, SKELETAL MUSCLE RELAXANT, DEPOLARIZING, prototype, p 123.

SUCRALFATE

(soo-kral´fate)

Trade name: Carafate

Classifications: GI AGENT; ANTIULCER

Pregnancy: Category B

ACTIONS/PHARMACODYNAMICS A complex of aluminum hydroxide and sulfated sucrose structurally related to heparin but lacks its anticoagulant activity. Its action is chemically unlike any other drug used for antiulcer therapy. Following oral administration, sucralfate and gastric acid react to form a viscous, adhesive, pastelike substance that is resistant to further reaction with acid. This "paste" adheres to the GI mucosa with a major portion binding electrostatically to the positively charged protein molecules in the damaged mucosa of an ulcer crater or an acute gastric erosion caused by alcohol or other drugs. Sucralfate absorbs bile, inhibits (inactivates) the enzyme pepsin, and blocks back diffusion of H^+ ions (acid). These actions plus adherence of the pastelike complex protect damaged mucosa against further destruction from ulcerogenic secretions and drugs. The aluminum ions released as sucralfate reacts with HCl are partly responsible for sucralfate-poor absorption from GI tract. May decrease rate of gastric emptying; has no effect on activity of trypsin or pancreatic amylase.

USES Short-term (up to 8 wk) treatment of duodenal ulcer. **Unlabeled uses:** short-term treatment of gastric ulcer, aspirin-induced erosions, suspension for chemotherapy-induced mucositis.

ROUTE & DOSAGE

Duodenal Ulcer

Adult   PO   1 q.i.d. 1 h a.c. and at h.s.

PHARMACOKINETICS Absorption: minimally absorbed from GI tract (<5%). **Duration:** up to 6 h (depends on contact time with ulcer crater). **Elimination:** 90% excreted in feces.

CONTRAINDICATIONS & PRECAUTIONS Contraindicated in: safe use during pregnancy (category B), by nursing mothers, or by children has not been established.

ADVERSE/SIDE EFFECTS GI: nausea, gastric discomfort, *constipation,* diarrhea.

DRUG INTERACTIONS May decrease absorption of quinolones (e.g., **ciprofloxacin, norfloxacin**), **digoxin, phenytoin, tetracycline.**

NURSING IMPLICATIONS

Administration

- If drug is to be administered through nasogastric tube, it should be solubilized in an appropriate diluent by a pharmacist.
- Antacids may be prescribed for pain relief if needed. Administer 30 min before or after sucralfate.
- Sucralfate apparently binds to certain compounds in the intestinal tract, thereby reducing their bioavailability. To prevent this action, separate administration of these agents from that of sucralfate by 2 h.
- Store in tight container at room temperature. Stable for 2 y after manufacture.

Assessment & Drug Effects

- Successful short-term course of sucralfate therapy does not seem to alter the tendency of the duodenal ulcer to heal and then to recur.

Patient & Family Education

- Although healing has occurred within the first 2 wk of therapy, treatment is usually continued 4–8 wk (in absence of healing as demonstrated by x-ray or endoscopic examination).
- If constipation is a drug-related problem, advise patient to use the following measures (unless contraindicated): increase water intake to 8–10 glasses per day; increase physical exercise, increase dietary bulk. Consult physician: a suppository or bulk laxative (e.g., Metamucil) may be prescribed.
- Emphasize need to adhere to sucralfate regimen: patient should not omit, increase, or decrease dosage or change administration times.
- Advise patient to stop smoking. Smoking is a major factor in recurrence of duodenal ulcer. Giving up smoking may be more important in prevention of recurrence of the ulcer than medication.

Common side effects in *italic*; life-threatening effects underlined; generic names in **bold**; classifications in SMALL CAPS

973

S

| Prototype: morphine, p 156 |

SUFENTANIL CITRATE
(soo-fen´ta-nil)
Trade name: Sufenta
Classifications: CNS AGENT; NARCOTIC (OPIATE)
AGONIST ANALGESIC; GENERAL ANESTHETIC
Pregnancy: Category C
Controlled substance: Schedule II

ACTIONS/PHARMACODYNAMICS Potent synthetic opioid related to fentanyl and with similar pharmacologic actions, but about 7 times more potent. Onset of action and recovery from anesthesia occur more rapidly with sufentanil than with fentanyl. Does not appear to have significant effect on histamine release (believed to be responsible in part for peripheral vasodilation and hypotension induced by opiate agonists). In common with other opiate agonists, sufentanil can cause respiratory depression and suppression of cough reflex.

USES Analgesic supplement in maintenance of balanced general anesthesia and also as a primary anesthetic.

ROUTE & DOSAGE

Adjunct to General Anesthesia

Adult   IV   1–8 µg/kg, depending on duration of surgery; may give additional doses of 10–25 µg if needed

As Primary Anesthetic

Adult   IV   1–30 µg/kg administered with 100% oxygen and a muscle relaxant; may give additional doses of 10–25 µg if needed

Child   IV   < 12 y: 10–25 µg/kg administered with 100% oxygen and a muscle relaxant; may give additional doses of 25–50 µg up to 1–2 µg/kg/dose if needed

PHARMACOKINETICS Onset: 1.5–3 min. **Duration:** 40 min. **Distribution:** crosses blood-brain barrier. **Metabolism:** metabolized in liver and small intestine. **Elimination:** half-life: 2–3 h; excreted in urine and feces.

CONTRAINDICATIONS & PRECAUTIONS Contraindicated in: safe use during pregnancy (category C) and in nursing women not established. **Cautious use in:** pulmonary disease, reduced respiratory reserve; impaired hepatic or renal function.

ADVERSE/SIDE EFFECTS CV: bradycardia, tachycardia, hypotension, hypertension, arrhythmias. **GI:** nausea, vomiting, constipation. **Respiratory:** bronchospasm, respiratory depression (common), apnea. **Other:** skeletal muscle rigidity (especially of trunk), chills, itching, spasms of sphincter of Oddi, urinary retention.

DRUG INTERACTIONS BETA-ADRENERGIC ANTAGONISTS increase incidence of bradycardia; **alcohol** and other CNS DEPRESSANTS such as BARBITURATES, TRANQUILIZERS, OPIATES and INHALATION GENERAL ANESTHETICS add to CNS depression; **cimetidine** increases risk of respiratory depression.

NURSING IMPLICATIONS

Administration
- Sufentanil is administered only by qualified personnel, specifically prepared in the use of IV anesthesia and in the management of respiratory depression.
- Have available a narcotic antagonist (e.g., naloxone) to reverse respiratory depression.
- Because sufentanil is an opioid, the need for preoperative analgesia is generally reduced.
- Store at 15–30C (59–86F) unless otherwise directed. Protect from light during storage. Examine solution for particulate matter and discoloration (solution should be clear) before administration.

Assessment & Drug Effects
- Monitor vital signs. Observe for skeletal muscle rigidity, especially of chest wall, and respiratory depression, particularly in the elderly, and in patients who are obese, debilitated, or who have received high doses.
- If naloxone is given to reverse respiratory depression, bear in mind that the duration of sufentanil-induced respiratory depression may exceed the duration of naloxone.
- Sufentanil can produce morphinelike dependence and is frequently abused. Tolerance can occur with prolonged use.

Common side effects in *italic*; life-threatening effects underlined; generic names in **bold**; classifications in SMALL CAPS

Prototype: sulfisoxazole, p 88

SULFACETAMIDE SODIUM

(sul-fa-see´ta-mide)

Trade names: AK-Sulf, Bleph 10, Cetamide, Isopto Cetamide, Ophthacet, Sebizon, Sodium Sulamyd, Sulf-10

Classifications: ANTIINFECTIVE; SULFONAMIDE

Pregnancy: Category C

ACTIONS/PHARMACODYNAMICS Highly soluble sulfonamide effective against a wide range of gram-positive and gram-negative microorganisms. Exerts bacteriostatic effect by interfering with bacterial utilization of paraaminobenzoic acid (PABA), thereby inhibiting folic acid biosynthesis required for bacterial growth.

USES Ophthalmic preparations are used for conjunctivitis, corneal ulcers, and other superficial ocular infections and as adjunct to systemic sulfonamide therapy for trachoma. The topical lotion is used for scaly dermatoses, seborrheic dermatitis, seborrhea sicca, and other bacterial skin infections.

ROUTE & DOSAGE

Conjunctivitis

Adult	Ophthalmic	1–3 drops of 10%, 15%, or 30% solution into lower conjunctival sac q2–3h; may increase interval as patient responds; or use 1.5–2.5 cm (1/2–1 in) of 10% ointment q6h and at h.s.

CONTRAINDICATIONS & PRECAUTIONS Contraindicated in: hypersensitivity to sulfonamides or to any ingredients in the formulation. Pregnancy category C. **Cautious use in:** application of lotion to denuded or debrided skin.

ADVERSE/SIDE EFFECTS *Temporary stinging or burning sensation,* retardation of corneal healing associated with long-term use of ophthalmic ointment; hypersensitivity reactions: Stevens-Johnson syndrome, lupuslike syndrome; superinfections with nonsusceptible organisms.

DRUG INTERACTIONS Tetracaine and other LOCAL ANESTHETICS DERIVED FROM PABA may antagonize the antibacterial effects of sulfonamides; SILVER PREPARATIONS may precipitate sulfacetamide from solution.

NURSING IMPLICATIONS

Administration

- Note strength of medication prescribed and also note that ophthalmic preparations and skin lotion are not interchangeable.
- See patient instructions for instilling eye drops.
- Store in tightly closed containers at 8–15C (46–59F) unless otherwise directed. Solutions left standing for a long time may darken. If this occurs, medication should be discarded.

Assessment & Drug Effects

- Drug should be discontinued if symptoms of hypersensitivity appear (erythema, skin rash, pruritus, urticaria).

Patient & Family Education

- Wash hands thoroughly with soap and running water (before and after instillation).
- Patient should be sitting or lying down if another person is to administer medication. If patient is to instill own medication, have patient stand in front of mirror.
- Examine eye medication; discard if cloudy or dark in color. Avoid contaminating any part of eye dropper that is inserted in bottle.
- With head tilted back, pull down lower lid. At the same time, have patient look up while drop is being instilled into conjunctival sac.
- Immediately apply gentle pressure to punctum (inner canthus next to nose) for 1 min.
- As soon as pressure is applied to punctum, patient should close eyes gently, so as not to squeeze out medication.
- Report purulent eye discharge. Sulfacetamide sodium is inactivated by purulent exudates.

Prototype: sulfisoxazole, p 88

SULFADIAZINE

(sul-fa-dye´a-zeen)

Trade name: Microsulfon

Classifications: ANTIINFECTIVE; SULFONAMIDE

Pregnancy: Category B

Common side effects in *italic*; life-threatening effects underlined; generic names in **bold**; classifications in SMALL CAPS

975

S

ACTIONS/PHARMACODYNAMICS Short-acting sulfonamide, slightly less soluble than sulfisoxazole. Shares actions, uses, contraindications, precautions, and adverse reactions of other sulfonamides.

ROUTE & DOSAGE

Mild to Moderate Infections

Adult	PO	2–4 g loading dose; then 2–4 g/d in 4–6 divided doses
Child	PO	> 2 mo: 75 mg/kg loading dose; then 150 mg/kg/d in 4–6 divided doses (max 6 g/d)

Rheumatic Fever Prophylaxis

Adult	PO	> 30 kg: 1 g/d
		< 30 kg: 500 mg/d

Toxoplasmosis

Adult	PO	2–8 g/d divided q6h
Child	PO	> 2 mo: 100-200 mg/kg/d divided q6h

PHARMACOKINETICS Absorption: readily absorbed from GI tract. **Peak:** 3–6 h. **Distribution:** distributed to most tissues, including CSF; crosses placenta. **Metabolism:** metabolized in liver. **Elimination:** excreted in urine.

NURSING IMPLICATIONS

Administration

- Fluid intake must be sufficient to support urinary output of at least 1500 ml/d. If this cannot be accomplished, urinary alkalinizer such as sodium bicarbonate may be prescribed to reduce risk of crystalluria and stone formation.
- Preserve in tight, light-resistant containers.

Patient & Family Education

- Urge patient to take drug exactly as prescribed. Patient should not alter the schedule or dose and should take all that is prescribed unless physician changes the regimen.
- Early signs of blood dyscrasias (sore throat, pallor, fever) should be reported promptly to the physician.

Prototype: sulfisoxazole, p 88

SULFAMETHOXAZOLE
(sul-fa-meth-ox´a-zole)
Trade names: Gamazole, Gatanol, Urobak
Classifications: ANTIINFECTIVE; SULFONAMIDE
Pregnancy: Category B

ACTIONS/PHARMACODYNAMICS Intermediate-acting sulfonamide closely related chemically to sulfisoxazole and similar to it in actions, uses, contraindications, precautions, and adverse reactions. Intestinal absorption and urinary excretion are somewhat slower than those of sulfisoxazole, and thus it is given less frequently to avoid excessive blood levels.

USES Acute, recurrent, or chronic urinary tract infections, lymphogranuloma venereum, and other infections caused by susceptible organisms.

ROUTE & DOSAGE

Mild to Moderate Infections

Adult	PO	2 g loading dose; then 1 g q8–12h
Child	PO	> 2 mo: 50–60 mg/kg loading dose; then 25–30 mg/kg q12h (max 75 mg/kg/d)

PHARMACOKINETICS Absorption: incompletely absorbed from GI tract. **Peak:** 3–4 h. **Distribution:** distributed to most tissues, including CSF; crosses placenta. **Metabolism:** metabolized in liver. **Elimination:** half-life: 7–12 h; excreted in urine.

NURSING IMPLICATIONS

Administration

- Tablet may be crushed before administration and taken with fluid of patient's choice.
- Fluid intake must be sufficient to produce urinary output of at least 1500 ml/24 h (between 3000 and 4000 ml/24 h for adults). Concomitant administration of urinary alkalinizer may be prescribed to reduce possibility of crystalluria and stone formation.
- Preserve in tight, light-resistant containers at 15–30C (59–86F). Do not freeze.

Patient & Family Education

- Urge patient to take drug exactly as prescribed. Patient should not alter the schedule or dose and

Common side effects in *italic*; life-threatening effects underlined; generic names in **bold**; classifications in SMALL CAPS

should take all that is prescribed unless physician changes the regimen.

- Early signs of blood dyscrasias (sore throat, pallor, fever) should be reported promptly to the physician.

Prototype: sulfisoxazole, p 88

SULFASALAZINE

(sul-fa-sal´a-zeen)

Trade names: Azaline, Azulfidine, PMS Sulfasalazine, PMS Sulfasalazine E.C., Salazopyrin, SAS-Enema, SAS Enteric-500, S.A.S.-500

Classifications: ANTIINFECTIVE; SULFONAMIDE

Pregnancy: Categories B (D if near term)

ACTIONS/PHARMACODYNAMICS Locally acting sulfonamide. Believed to be converted by intestinal microflora to sulfapyridine (which has antibacterial action) and 5-aminosalicylic acid or mesalamine which may exert antiinflammatory effect. Other proposed mechanisms of action include inhibition of prostaglandins known to cause diarrhea and affect mucosal transport, interference with absorption of fluids and electrolytes from colon, and reduction in *Clostridium* and *Escherichia coli* in the stools. Contraindications, precautions, and adverse/side effects are as for other sulfonamides.

USES Ulcerative colitis and relatively mild regional enteritis. **Unlabeled uses:** granulomatous colitis, Crohn's disease, scleroderma, rheumatoid arthritis.

ROUTE & DOSAGE

Ulcerative Colitis

Adult	PO	1–2 g/d in 4 divided doses; may increase up to 8 g/d if needed
Child	PO	40–50 mg/kg/d in 4 divided doses

PHARMACOKINETICS Absorption: 10–15% absorbed from GI tract unchanged; remaining drug is hydrolyzed in colon to sulfapyridine (most of which is absorbed) and 5-aminosalicylic acid (30% of which is absorbed). **Peak:** 1.5–6 h sulfasalazine; 6–24 h sulfapyridine. **Distribution:** crosses placenta; distributed into breast milk. **Metabolism:** metabolized in intestines and liver. **Elimination:** half-life: 5–10 h; all metabolites are excreted in urine.

CONTRAINDICATIONS & PRECAUTIONS Contraindicated in: sensitivity to sulfasalazine and other sulfonamides; agranulocytosis; children <2 y; intestinal and urinary tract obstruction; pregnancy (category B), category D near term.

ADVERSE/SIDE EFFECTS *Nausea, vomiting, bloody diarrhea; anorexia,* arthralgia, rash, anemia, infertility (reversible), blood dyscrasias, hepatic injury, infectious mononucleosis–like reaction, *allergic reactions.*

DRUG INTERACTIONS Iron, ANTIBIOTICS may alter absorption of sulfasalazine.

NURSING IMPLICATIONS

Administration

- If possible, drug should be taken after eating to provide longer intestine transit time for the drug.
- Sulfasalazine should be given in evenly divided doses over each 24 h period. Intervals between nighttime doses should not exceed 8 h.
- If GI intolerance occurs after first few doses, symptoms are probably due to irritation of stomach mucosa. Symptoms may be relieved by spacing total daily dose more evenly over the day or by administration of enteric–coated tablets. Consult physician.
- Preserve in tight, light-resistant containers; store at 15–30C (59–86F).

Assessment & Drug Effects

- GI symptoms that develop after a few days of therapy may indicate need for dosage adjustment. If symptoms persist, physician may withhold drug for 5–7 d and restart it at a lower dosage level.
- Desensitization of patient who has an allergic reaction to sulfasalazine can be accomplished safely to permit continued use of the drug. Usually the process is started with one-eighth tablet daily; dose is doubled q3–7d.
- Adverse reactions generally occur within a few days to 12 wk after start of therapy and are most likely to occur in patients receiving high doses (4 g or more).
- High doses (more than 2 g/d) reduce tissue folate stores as shown by measurement of RBC folate. A daily supplement may be prescribed.

Patient & Family Education

- Some patients pass enteric-coated tablets intact in feces, possibly because they lack enzymes capable

---

Common side effects in *italic;* life-threatening effects underlined; generic names in **bold**; classifications in SMALL CAPS

977

S

of dissolving them. Advise patient to examine stools and report to physician if tablet is intact. Conventional tablet will be ordered.

▪ Forewarn patient that drug may color alkaline urine and skin orange-yellow.

▪ Advise patient to remain under close medical supervision. Relapses occur in about 40% of patients after initial satisfactory response. Response to therapy and duration of treatment are governed by endoscopic examinations.

Prototype: colchicine, p 46

SULFINPYRAZONE

(sul-fin-peer´a-zone)
Trade names: Antazone, Anturan, Anturane, Apo-Sulfinpyrazone, Aprazone, Novopyrazone, Salazopyrin, Zynol
Classifications: ANTIGOUT AGENT; URICOSURIC
Pregnancy: Category C

ACTIONS/PHARMACODYNAMICS Potent pyrazolone-derivative renal tubular blocking agent structurally related to phenylbutazone. At therapeutic doses, promotes urinary excretion of uric acid and reduces serum urate levels by competitively inhibiting tubular reabsorption of uric acid. Like all uricosurics, low doses may inhibit tubular secretion of uric acid and cause urate retention. Inhibits release of adenosine diphosphate and 5-hydroxytryptophan, and thus decreases platelet adhesiveness and increases platelet survival time; has no effect on prothrombin or blood clotting time. May cause slight but significant decrease in serum cholesterol. Since it has no apparent analgesic or antiinflammatory activity, it is not used for relief of acute gout. Reportedly not associated with cumulative effects, development of tolerance, or electrolyte imbalance.

USES Maintenance therapy in chronic gouty arthritis and tophaceous gout. **Unlabeled uses:** drug-induced hyperuricemia, to decrease platelet aggregation and increase their survival in prevention of TIAs and stroke.

PHARMACOKINETICS Absorption: readily absorbed from GI tract. **Peak:** 1–2 h. **Duration:** 4–6 h; may persist up to 10 h. **Metabolism:** metabolized in liver to active and inactive metabolites. **Elimination:** half-life: 3 h; slowly excreted in urine; 5% excreted in feces.

ROUTE & DOSAGE

Gout

Adult	PO	100–200 mg b.i.d. for 1 wk; then increase to 200–400 mg b.i.d.; may reduce to 200 mg/d after serum urate levels are controlled (max 800 mg/d)

Inhibition of Platelet Aggregation

Adult	PO	200 mg t.i.d. or q.i.d.

CONTRAINDICATIONS & PRECAUTIONS Contraindicated in: known hypersensitivity to pyrazoline derivatives; active peptic ulcer; concurrent administration of salicylates; patients with creatinine clearance less than 50 mg/min, treatment of hyperuricemia secondary to neoplastic disease or cancer chemotherapy. **Cautious use in:** impaired renal function; pregnancy (category C); history of healed peptic ulcer, use in conjunction with sulfonamides and sulfonylureas.

ADVERSE/SIDE EFFECTS GI: *nausea,* vomiting, diarrhea, *epigastric pain, blood loss, reactivation or aggravation of peptic ulcer,* ataxia, dizziness, vertigo, tinnitus; edema, labored respirations, convulsions, coma, hypersensitivity, reactions (skin rashes, fever), jaundice, precipitation of acute gout, urolithiasis, renal colic.

DRUG INTERACTIONS may decrease efficacy of **nitrofurantoin** for UTI and increase its systemic toxicity. May displace SULFONYLUREAS from protein binding and increase risk of hypoglycemia; may augment prothrombin time increased by **warfarin**; **cholestyramine** decreases absorption of sulfinpyrazone; **aspirin** may inhibit uriscouric effects of sulfinpyrazone.

DIAGNOSTIC TEST INTERFERENCES Sulfinpyrazone decreases urinary excretion of *aminohippuric acid* and *phenolsulfonphthalein.*

NURSING IMPLICATIONS

Administration

▪ Administered with meals, milk, or antacid (prescribed) to prevent local drug irritant effect. Severity and frequency of symptoms increase with dosage. Persistence of GI symptoms may require discontinuation of drug.

▪ During early therapy, fluid intake should be sufficient to support urinary output of at least 2000–3000 ml/d (consult physician), and urine should be alkalinized (e.g., with large doses vitamin C) to increase solubility of uric acid and minimize risk of uric acid stones.

Assessment & Drug Effects

- Serum urate levels are used to monitor therapy. Aim of therapy is to lower serum urate levels to about 6 mg/dl and thus to reduce joint changes, tophi formation, and frequency of acute attacks and to improve renal function.
- Periodic blood cell counts are advised during prolonged therapy. Patients with impaired renal function should have periodic assessments of renal function.
- Sulfinpyrazone may increase the frequency of acute gouty attacks during first 6–12 mo of therapy, even when serum urate levels appear to be controlled. Physician may prescribe prophylactic doses of colchicine concurrently during first 3–6 mo of treatment to prevent or at least lessen severity of attacks.

Patient & Family Education

- Patient must remain under close medical supervision while taking sulfinpyrazone. Therapy is continued indefinitely.
- Caution patient to avoid experimentation with dosage, since subtherapeutic doses may enhance urate retention, and large doses may increase risk of toxicity.
- Sulfinpyrazone therapy should be continued without interruption even when patient has an acute gouty attack, which may be treated with full therapeutic doses of colchicine or other antiinflammatory agent.
- Caution patient to avoid aspirin-containing medications. If an analgesic is required (in patients with normal renal function), generally acetaminophen is recommended.

SULFISOXAZOLE

See ANTIINFECTIVES, SULFONAMIDE prototype, p 88.

Prototype: ibuprofen, p 160

SULINDAC
(sul-in´dak)
Trade name: Clinoril
Classifications: CNS AGENT; NONNARCOTIC ANALGESIC, ANTIPYRETIC; NSAID
Pregnancy: Categories B (D in third trimester)

ACTIONS/PHARMACODYNAMICS Acetic acid derivative structurally and pharmacologically related to indomethacin. Pharmacologic properties are similar to those of aspirin but is chemically unrelated. In common with these drugs, exhibits antiinflammatory, analgesic, and antipyretic properties. Exact mechanism of antiinflammatory action not known but is thought to result from inhibition of prostaglandin synthesis. Sulindac is an inactive prodrug converted to an active sulfide metabolite in the liver. Comparable to aspirin in antiinflammatory activity but has longer half-life, lower incidence of GI intolerance and tinnitus, and less effect on bleeding time and platelet function. May prolong bleeding time, but prothrombin time, whole blood clotting time, and platelet count are not affected. Serum uric acid lowering effect is less than that of aspirin. Cross-sensitivity to other nonsteroidal antiinflammatory drugs (NSAIDs) has been reported

USES Acute and long-term symptomatic treatment of osteoarthritis, rheumatoid arthritis, ankylosing spondylitis; for acute painful shoulder (acute subacromial bursitis or supraspinatus tendinitis), and acute gouty arthritis.

ROUTE & DOSAGE

Arthritis, Ankylosing Spondylitis, Acute Gouty Arthritis

Adult PO 150–200 mg b.i.d. (max 400 mg/d)

PHARMACOKINETICS Absorption: 90% absorbed from GI tract. **Peak:** 2 h without food, 3–4 h with food. **Duration:** 10–12 h. **Distribution:** Minimal passage across placenta; distributed into breast milk. **Metabolism:** metabolized in liver to active sulfide metabolite. **Elimination:** half-life: 7.8 h sulindac, 16.4 h sulfide metabolite; 75% excreated in urine, 25% in feces.

CONTRAINDICATIONS & PRECAUTIONS Contraindicated in: hypersensitivity to sulindac; hypersen-

Common side effects in *italic*; life-threatening effects underlined; generic names in **bold**; classifications in SMALL CAPS

979

S

sitivity to aspirin (patients with "aspirin triad": acute asthma, rhinitis, nasal polyps) or to other NSAIDs; significant renal or hepatic dysfunction. Safe use during pregnancy (category B; category D in third trimester); in nursing mothers, and in children not established. **Cautious use in:** history of upper GI tract disorders, compromised cardiac function, hypertension, hemophilia or other bleeding tendencies.

ADVERSE/SIDE EFFECTS CNS: drowsiness, *dizziness, headache,* anxiety, nervousness. **CV:** palpitation, peripheral edema, CHF, (patients with marginal cardiac function). **ENT:** blurred vision, amblyopia, vertigo, tinnitus, decreased hearing. **GI:** *abdominal pain, dyspepsia, nausea, vomiting, constipation,* diarrhea, ulceration, flatulence, anorexia; stomatitis, sore or dry mucous membranes, dry mouth; rarely: gastritis, gastroenteritis, peptic ulcer, *GI bleeding.* **Hematologic:** prolonged bleeding time, aplastic anemia, thrombocytopenia. **Hypersensitivity:** angioneurotic edema, rash, pruritus, fever, chills, leukopenia, eosinophilia, anaphylaxis. **Other:** Stevens-Johnson syndrome, toxic epidermal necrolysis syndrome, rash, renal impairment.

DIAGNOSTIC TEST INTERFERENCES Abnormalities in ***liver function tests*** may occur.

DRUG INTERACTIONS Heparin, ORAL ANTICOAGULANTS may prolong bleeding time; may increase **lithium** toxicity; **aspirin**, other NSAIDS add to ulcerogenic effects; may increase **methotrexate** toxicity; **dimethylsulfoxide (DMSO)** may decrease effects of sulindac.

NURSING IMPLICATIONS

Administration
- If patient cannot swallow tablet, it may be crushed prior to administration.
- May be administered with food, milk, or antacid (if prescribed) to reduce possibility of GI upset. However, food retards absorption and delays and lowers peak concentrations.

Assessment & Drug Effects
- A detailed drug history should be elicited before initiation of therapy. See contraindications & precautions.
- Baseline and periodic evaluations of hemoglobin, renal and hepatic function, and auditory and ophthalmic examinations are recommended in patients receiving prolonged or high-dose therapy.

- Recommend an ophthalmoscopic examination if patient has eye complaints.

Patient & Family Education
- Because sulindac may cause dizziness, drowsiness, and blurred vision, advise patient to exercise caution when he or she is driving or performing other potentially hazardous activities.
- Advise patient to report the onset of skin rash, itching, hives, jaundice, black stools, swelling of feet or hands, sore throat or mouth, unusual bleeding or bruising, shortness of breath or night cough.
- Inform patient that adverse GI effects are relatively common. Instruct him or her to report abdominal pain, nausea, dyspepsia, diarrhea, or constipation.
- Therapeutic effectiveness of sulindac may not be evidenced for up to 7 d; peak effect is usually experienced in 2–3 wk (relief of joint pain and stiffness, reduction in joint swelling, increase in grip strength, and improved mobility).
- Inform patient that alcohol and aspirin may increase risk of GI ulceration and bleeding tendencies and, therefore, should be avoided while taking sulindac.
- Because sulindac may prolong bleeding time, advise patient to inform dentist or surgeon that patient is taking this drug.

SUTILAINS
(soo´ti-lains)
Trade name: Travase
Classification: ENZYME DEBRIDING AGENT
Pregnancy: Category C

ACTIONS/PHARMACODYNAMICS Concentrate of proteolytic enzymes produced by *Bacillus subtilis;* available as ointment (white petrolatum and polyethylene base). As a result of enzymatic activity sutilains selectively digests necrotic soft tissue, hemoglogin, and purulent exudate. Moisture and a pH of 6–6.8 must be present to support proteolytic activity. Action is unaffected by presence in site of topical bacitracin, gentamicin, mafenide, neomycin, penicillin, silver sulfadiazine, or streptomycin, nor is it affected by appropriate systemic antiinfectives. Action, however, is adversely affected by detergents, compounds with metallic ions, and certain antiseptics (see drug interactions). There is no consensus about efficacy of sutilains ointment in burn therapy (to remove eschar), although it is used in some medical centers to shorten preparation time for skin grafting.

USES Biochemical debridement of decubitus ulcers, second and third degree burns, pyogenic incisional or traumatic wounds, ulcers secondary to peripheral vascular disease, also used adjunctively with other measures to debride necrotic tissue (e.g., mechanical debridement).

ROUTE & DOSAGE

Ulcer and Burn Debridement

Adult   Topical   Apply t.i.d. or q.i.d.

PHARMACOKINETICS Onset: 1 h. **Peak:** 6 h. **Duration:** 8–12 h.

CONTRAINDICATIONS & PRECAUTIONS Contraindicated in: Wounds communicating with major body cavities; wound containing exposed major nerves or nervous tissue; fungating neoplastic ulcers; bleeding; dermatitis; compromised cardiac or pulmonary reserves. Safe use in wounds during pregnancy (category C) or in woman who may become pregnant not established.

ADVERSE/SIDE EFFECTS Pain, *paresthesia, bleeding, transient dermatitis.*

DRUG INTERACTIONS Benzalkonium chloride, hexachlorophene, nitrofurazone, hydrogen peroxide, IODINE COMPOUNDS, **silver nitrate, thimerosal** will inactivate sutilains.

NURSING IMPLICATIONS

Administration
Treatment Protocol
- Wear gloves. Thoroughly cleanse and irrigate wound area with sterile water or 0.9% saline solution. Gently wipe away dissolved material. Be sure all medication has been removed. Thoroughly moisten wound area.
- Change gloves and apply ointment in very thin layer (a small dab will cover an area as large as back of hand). Cover every crevice and crack in wound and extend ointment 0.5–1cm (1/4–1/2 in) beyond areas being debrided. Cover area with loose, wet dressings (not occlusive) to maintain constant moisture.
- Repeat entire protocol 3 or 4 times a day or as ordered.
- If hydrogen peroxide is used to cleanse the wound, it should be used before application of sutilains (not concomitantly).
- If used in treatment of burns, it is most effective be-

fore eschar becomes hard and dry.
- Drug-induced eschar digestion leads to increased fluid and blood loss in treated area; therefore no more than 10–15% of a burned area is treated with sutilains at one time.
- Proteolytic action produces a warm, moist, and nutritious environment for bacteria. Topical antiinfectives may be used concomitantly to prevent sepsis.
- If ointment gets into the patient's eyes, irrigate promptly and copiously with normal saline or with sterile water.
- Store at 2–8C (35–46F).

Assessment & Drug Effects
- Maximum effect is usually achieved in 5–7 d for burns and wounds and in 8–12 d for ulcers.
- Inspect wound for bleeding. If it occurs or if pain persists during interval between treatments, sutilains therapy will be discontinued.

TAMOXIFEN CITRATE

(ta-mox´i-fen)
Trade names: Nolvadex, Nolvadex-D, Tamofen
Classifications: ANTINEOPLASTIC; HORMONE
Pregnancy: Category C

ACTIONS/PHARMACODYNAMICS Nonsteroidal gonad-stimulating principle with potent antiestrogenic activity. Competes with estradiol at estrogen receptor sites in target tissues such as breast, uterus, vagina, anterior pituitary, tumor with high concentration of estrogen receptors. Tamoxifen-receptor complexes move into nucleus, decreasing DNA synthesis and estrogen responses. Ovulation may be induced by stimulation of the release of hypothalamic gonadotropic-releasing factor.

USES Palliative treatment of advanced breast cancer in postmenopausal women, adjunctively with surgery in the treatment of breast carcinoma with positive lymph nodes. **Unlabeled use:** investigationally to stimulate ovulation in selected anovulatory women desiring pregnancy.

PHARMACOKINETICS Absorption: slowly absorbed from GI tract. **Peak:** 3–6 h. **Metabolism:** metabolized in liver, enterohepatically cycled. **Elimination:** half-life: 7 d; excreted primarily in feces.

Common side effects in *italic*; life-threatening effects underlined; generic names in **bold**; classifications in SMALL CAPS

981

ROUTE & DOSAGE

Breast Carcinoma

Adult　PO　10–20 mg 1–2 times/d (morning and evening)

Stimulation of Ovulation

Adult　PO　5–40 mg b.i.d. for 4 d

CONTRAINDICATIONS & PRECAUTIONS Con-
traindicated in: pregnancy (category C), especially during first trimester. **Cautious use in:** lactation; vision disturbances; cataracts; leukopenia; thrombocytopenia.

ADVERSE/SIDE EFFECTS CNS: depression, light-headedness, dizziness, headache, mental confusion, sleepiness. **CV:** thrombosis. **Eye:** retinopathy, decreased visual acuity, blurred vision. **GI:** *nausea and vomiting (about 25% of patients),* distaste for food, anorexia. **Hematologic:** leukopenia, thrombocytopenia. **Reproductive:** changes in menstrual period, milk production and leaking from breasts, vaginal discharge and bleeding, pruritus vulvae. **Other:** skin rash or dryness, increased bone pain, and transient local disease flair; loss of hair, weight gain, shortness of breath, photosensitivity, *hot flashes,* hypercalcemia.

DIAGNOSTIC TEST INTERFERENCES Tam-
oxifen may produce transient increase in **serum calcium.**

DRUG INTERACTIONS May enhance hypopro-
thrombinemic effects of **warfarin.**

NURSING IMPLICATIONS

Administration

- If side effects are severe, sometimes a simple reduction in dosage gives sufficient relief without losing control of disease. Consult physician.
- Store at 15–30C (59–86F) in container that protects drug from light.

Assessment & Drug Effects

- An objective response may require 4–10 wk of therapy, longer if there is bone metastasis.
- Bone and tumor pain and local disease flair often necessitate administration of analgesics for pain relief. Reassure patient that this discomfort frequently signals a good tumor response.
- Soft-tissue-disease response to tamoxifen may be local swelling and marked erythema over preexisting lesions or the development of new lesions. These symptoms rapidly subside after tamoxifen treatment is initiated.

- CBCs including platelet counts are periodically assessed. Transient leukopenia and thrombocytopenia (50,000–100,000/mm³) without hemorrhagic tendency have been reported.

Patient & Family Education

- Report to physician if marked weakness, sleepiness, mental confusion, edema, dyspnea, and blurred vision occur.
- Discuss the possibility of drug-induced menstrual irregularities with patient before starting treatment.
- Avoid prolonged sun exposure, especially if skin is unprotected. Sun-screen lotions (SPF ≥12) and should be applied to all exposed skin surfaces.
- Caution patient not to change established dose schedule.
- OTC drugs should be avoided unless specifically prescribed by the physician. Discuss with patient, particularly with respect to OTC analgesics.
- Report onset of tenderness or redness in an extremity.
- Urge patient to adhere to scheduled appointments for clinical evaluation. Medical supervision is necessary during tamoxifen therapy.

Prototype: lorazepam, p 177

TEMAZEPAM

(te-maz´e-pam)
Trade name: Restoril
Classifications: CNS AGENT; BENZODIAZEPINE ANXIOLYTIC, SEDATIVE-HYPNOTIC
Pregnancy: Category X

ACTIONS/PHARMACODYNAMICS Benzodi-
azepine derivative with hypnotic, anxiolytic, sedative effects. Principal effect is significant improvement in sleep parameters as evidenced by reduced night awakenings and early morning awakenings, increased total sleep times, and absence of rebound effects. Sleep latency is not reduced, and there is minimal change in REM sleep.

USES To relieve insomnia associated with frequent nocturnal awakenings or early morning awakenings.

ROUTE & DOSAGE

Insomnia

Adult　PO　15–30 mg h.s.

Common side effects in *italic*; life-threatening effects underlined; generic names in **bold**; classifications in SMALL CAPS

PHARMACOKINETICS Absorption: readily absorbed from GI tract. **Onset:** 30–50 min. **Peak:** 2–3 h. **Duration:** 10–12 h. **Distribution:** crosses placenta; distributed into breast milk. **Metabolism:** metabolized in liver to oxazepam. **Elimination:** half-life: 8–24 h; excreted in urine.

CONTRAINDICATIONS & PRECAUTIONS Contraindicated in: pregnancy (category X); safe use in children < 18 y not established; narrow-angle glaucoma; psychoses. **Cautious use in:** nursing mother, severely depressed patient or one with suicidal ideation, history of drug abuse or dependence, acute intoxication, hepatic or renal dysfunction, elderly patients, sleep apnea.

ADVERSE/SIDE EFFECTS Usually mild and transient. **CNS:** *drowsiness,* dizziness, lethargy, confusion, headache, euphoria, relaxed feeling, weakness. **GI:** anorexia, diarrhea. **Other:** palpitations.

DRUG INTERACTIONS Alcohol, CNS DEPRESSANTS, ANTICONVULSANTS potentiate CNS depression; **cimetidine** increases temazepam plasma levels, thus increasing its toxicity; may decrease antiparkinsonism effects of **levodopa;** may increase **phenytoin** levels; smoking decreases sedative effects.

NURSING IMPLICATIONS

Administration
- Administer 20–30 min before patient retires.
- Store at 15–30C (59–86F) in tight container unless otherwise specified by manufacturer.

Assessment & Drug Effects
- Psychoactive drugs are the most frequent cause of acute confusion in the elderly. Be alert to signs of paradoxical reaction (excitement, hyperactivity, and disorientation) in this age group.
- CNS side effects are more apt to occur in the patient with hypoalbuminemia, liver disease, and the elderly patient. Report promptly incidence of bradycardia, drowsiness, dizziness, clumsiness, lack of coordination. Supervise ambulation, especially at night.
- With long-term use of this drug, hepatic and renal function tests are advised.
- *Signs of overdose:* weakness, bradycardia, somnolence, confusion, slurred speech, ataxia, coma with reduced or absent reflexes, hypertension, respiratory depression.

Patient & Family Education
- Patient should be advised that improvement in sleep will not occur until after 2 or 3 doses of drug.
- If dreams or nightmares interfere with rest, notify physician. An alternate drug or reduced dose may be prescribed.
- Inform patient that difficulty getting to sleep may continue. Drug effect is evidenced by the increased amount of rest once asleep.
- Instruct patient to avoid use of alcohol as a sedative.
- Advise patient to take a warm beverage (e.g., milk) or light snack before bedtime.
- If patient is elderly, suggest avoiding daytime "catnaps."
- If insomnia continues in spite of medication, physician should be consulted.
- Smoking should be discontinued after medication is taken.
- Use by nursing mothers may cause sedation and possibly feeding problems and weight loss in the infant.
- Warn patient not to use OTC drugs (especially for insomnia) during temazepam therapy without advice of physician.
- Advise patient to consult physician before discontinuing drug especially after long-term use. Gradual reduction of dose may be necessary to avoid withdrawal symptoms.
- Use of alcohol and other CNS depressants should be avoided.
- Patient should use extreme caution when operating machinery or driving a car because this drug may depress psychomotor skills and causes sedation.

Prototype: prazosin, p 108

TERAZOSIN
(ter-ay´zoe-sin)
Trade name: Hytrin
Classifications: AUTONOMIC NERVOUS SYSTEM AGENT; ALPHA-ADRENERGIC ANTAGONIST (SYMPATHOLYTIC, BLOCKING AGENT); CARDIOVASCULAR AGENT; ANTIHYPERTENSIVE; VASODILATOR
Pregnancy: Category C

ACTIONS/PHARMACODYNAMICS Quinazoline antihypertensive and vasodilator chemically similar to prazosin. Selectively blocks alpha$_1$–adrenergic receptors in vascular smooth muscle producing re-

Common side effects in *italic*; life-threatening effects <u>underlined</u>; generic names in **bold**; classifications in SMALL CAPS

983

T

laxation that leads to reduction of peripheral vascular resistance and lowered BP. Vasodilation is accompanied by minimal reflex increase in heart rate. By an unknown mechanism the drug frequently causes a significant decrease in mean serum cholesterol, low-density lipoprotein (LDL), and very-low-density (VLDL) cholesterol fractions. Considered a step 2 drug in the stepped-care approach to antihypertensive drug therapy reserved for the patient who has failed to respond to diet, exercise, and weight reduction and therapy with a step 1 drug. Effective when used with a beta-adrenergic blocking agent and a thiazide diuretic.

USES To treat hypertension alone or in combination with other antihypertensive agents (beta-adrenergic blocking agents, diuretics). **Unlabeled uses:** benign prostatic hypertrophy, urinary outflow obstruction.

ROUTE & DOSAGE

Hypertension, Benign Prostatic Hypertrophy, Urinary Obstruction

Adult	PO	Start with 1 mg h.s.; then 1–5 mg/d (max 20 mg/d)

PHARMACOKINETICS Absorption: readily absorbed from GI tract. **Peak:** 1–2 h. **Metabolism:** metabolized in liver. **Elimination:** half-life: 9–12 h; 60% excreted in feces, 40% in urine.

CONTRAINDICATIONS & PRECAUTIONS Contraindicated in: safe use during pregnancy (category C), in nursing mothers, and children not established.

ADVERSE/SIDE EFFECTS CNS: *asthenia (weakness), dizziness, headache,* drowsiness, weakness. **CV:** postural hypotension, palpitation, *first-dose phenomenon.* **Eye/ear:** blurred vision. **GI:** nausea. **Other:** weight gain, pain in extremities, nasal congestion, sinusitis, impotence, dyspnea, peripheral edema.

DRUG INTERACTIONS Antihypertensive effects may be attenuated by NSAIDs.

NURSING IMPLICATIONS

Administration

- Food has little or no effect on bioavailability of terazosin; administer tablet with food or fluid of patient's choice.
- The initial dose of terazosin is given at bedtime to reduce the potential for severe hypotensive effect. This may occur with first few doses. After the

initial dose, most patients take the drug in the morning.
- Store at 15–30C (59–86F) in tightly closed container away from heat and strong light. Do not freeze.

Assessment & Drug Effects

- First-dose phenomenon (precipitous decline in BP with consciousness disturbance) is rare; occurs within 90–120 min of initial dose.
- Advise patient to avoid situations that would result in injury should syncope occur after first dose. If it does develop, patient should lie down promptly and be treated symptomatically.
- Monitor BP at end of dosing interval (just before next dose) to determine level of antihypertensive control. Check BP also 2–3 h after the dose to determine if maximum and minimal responses are similar.
- Drug-induced decrease in BP appears to be more position dependent (i.e., greater in the erect position) during the first few hours after dosing than at end of 24 h.
- A greatly diminished hypotensive response at end of 24 h indicates need for change in dosage (increased dose or twice daily regimen).

Patient & Family Education

- Orthostatic hypotension can pose a problem with ambulation. Advise patient to make position changes slowly (i.e., change in direction or from recumbent to upright posture). Dangle legs and move ankles a minute or so before standing when arising. The orthostatic effect of terazosin is greatest shortly after dosing.
- Caution patient not to drive or engage in hazardous activity for at least 12 h after first dose, after dosage increase, or when treatment is resumed after interruption of therapy. Twelve hours should be sufficient time for serious side effects (orthostatic hypotension, syncope, lightheadedness, dizziness) to appear if they are going to do so.
- Instruct patient to monitor weight: a sudden gain of more than 0.5–1 kg (1–2 lb) accompanied by edema in extremities should be reported to physician. Dose adjustment may be indicated.
- Emphasize importance of uninterrupted maintenance of established drug regimen. If drug is omitted for several days, consult physician. Drug will be started with the initial dosing regimen.
- Patient should keep scheduled appointments for assessment of BP control and other clinically significant tests.
- Encourage patient who has been taught to monitor own BP to keep a daily record noting BP and time

Common side effects in *italic*; life-threatening effects <u>underlined</u>; generic names in **bold**; classifications in SMALL CAPS

taken, when medication was taken, which arm was used, position (i.e., standing, sitting) and time of day and to take this record to physician for reference at checkup appointment.

- Advise patient not to take OTC medications, particularly those that may contain an adrenergic agent (e.g., remedies for coughs, colds, allergy) without first consulting physician.

Prototype: isoproterenol, p 105

TERBUTALINE SULFATE
(ter-byoo´te-leen)
Trade names: Brethaire, Brethine, Bricanyl
Classifications: AUTONOMIC NERVOUS SYSTEM AGENT; BETA-ADRENERGIC AGONIST; BRONCHODILATOR (RESPIRATORY SMOOTH MUSCLE RELAXANT)
Pregnancy: Category B

ACTIONS/PHARMACODYNAMICS Synthetic adrenergic stimulant with selective beta$_2$- and negligible beta$_1$-agonist (cardiac) activity. Exerts preferential effect on beta$_2$-receptors in bronchial smooth muscles, inhibits histamine release from mast cells, and increases ciliary motility. These effects lead to relief of bronchospasm in chronic obstructive pulmonary disease (COPD) and significant increase in vital capacity. Other adrenergic effects include relaxation of vascular smooth muscle, contraction of GI and urinary sphincters, increase in renin, in pancreatic beta-cell secretion, and in serum HDL-cholesterol concentration. Increases uterine relaxation (thereby preventing or abolishing high intrauterine pressure).

USES Orally or subcutaneously as a bronchodilator in bronchial asthma and for reversible airway obstruction associated with bronchitis and emphysema. **Unlabeled use:** (PO and IV infusion) to delay delivery in preterm labor.

PHARMACOKINETICS Absorption: 33–50% absorbed from GI tract. **Onset:** 30 min PO; < 15 min SC; 5–30 min inhaled. **Peak:** 2–3 h PO; 30–60 min SC; 1–2 h inhaled. **Duration:** 4–8 h PO; 1.5–4 h SC; 3–4 h inhaled. **Distribution:** distributed into breast milk. **Metabolism:** metabolized in liver. **Elimination:** half-life: 3–4 h; excreted primarily in urine, 3% in feces.

ROUTE & DOSAGE

Bronchodilator

Adult	PO	2.5–5 mg t.i.d. at 6 h intervals (max 15 mg/d)
	SC	0.25 mg q15–30min up to 0.5 mg in 4 h
	Inhaled	2 inhalations separated by 60 s q4–6h
Adolescent	PO	12–15 y: 2.5 mg t.i.d. at 6 h intervals (max 7.5 mg/d)
	SC	0.25 mg q15–30min up to 0.5 mg in 4 h
	Inhaled	2 inhalations separated by 60 s q4–6h

Premature Labor

Adult	IV	10 µg/min titrated up to a max of 80 µg/min; continue at minimum effective dose for 4 h; then switch to PO
	PO	2.5 mg q4–6h

CONTRAINDICATIONS & PRECAUTIONS Contraindicated in: known hypersensitivity to sympathomimetic amines, severe hypertension and coronary artery disease, tachycardia with digitalis intoxication, within 14 d of MAO inhibitor therapy, children < 12 y, angle-closure glaucoma. Used only after evaluation of risk-benefit ratio in pregnancy (category B) and lactation. **Cautious use in:** angina, stroke, hypertension; diabetes mellitus; thyrotoxicosis; history of seizure disorders; cardiac arrhythmias; the elderly patient; renal and hepatic dysfunction.

ADVERSE/SIDE EFFECTS Dose related. **CNS:** *nervousness, tremor,* headache, *lightheadedness,* drowsiness, fatigue, seizures. **CV:** *tachycardia,* hypotension or hypertension, *palpitation,* maternal and fetal tachycardia. **GI:** nausea, vomiting. **Other:** sweating, muscle cramps.

DIAGNOSTIC TEST INTERFERENCES Terbutaline may increase *blood glucose* and free *fatty acids.*

DRUG INTERACTIONS Epinephrine, other SYMPATHOMIMETIC BRONCHODILATORS may add to effects; MAO INHIBITORS, TRICYCLIC ANTIDEPRESSANTS potentiate action on vascular system; effects of both BETA-ADRENERGIC BLOCKERS and terbutaline antagonized.

Common side effects in *italic*; life-threatening effects underlined; generic names in **bold**; classifications in SMALL CAPS

985

NURSING IMPLICATIONS

Administration

- Tablet may be crushed before administration and taken with fluid of patient's choice.
- Be certain about recommended doses: PO preparation: 2.5 mg; SC: 0.25 mg. A decimal point error can be fatal.
- SC injection is usually administered into lateral deltoid area.
- If GI symptoms occur, advise patient to take the tablets with food.
- IV terbutaline is diluted by adding each 5 mg to 1000 ml D5W or NS (for diabetics) to yield a concentration of 5 μg/ml. Infuse with microdrip and infusion pump.
- Store at 15–30C (59–86F). Protect from light and freezing.

Assessment & Drug Effects

- Cardiovascular side effects are more apt to occur when drug is given by SC route and when it is used by a patient with cardiac arrhythmia. Check pulse and BP before each dose. If perceptively altered from baseline level, consult physician.
- Most side effects are transient. However, rapid heart rate may persist for a relatively long time.
- Onset and degree of effect and incidence and severity of side effects of the SC formulation resemble those of epinephrine. Oral terbutaline appears to be equally as effective as ephedrine; however, onset of action is more rapid, and its effects last longer.
- Aerosolized terbutaline produces little cardiac stimulation or tremors.
- Muscle tremor is a fairly common side effect that appears to subside with continued use.
- The neonate born of a mother who used terbutaline during pregnancy may have hypoglycemia. Monitor for symptoms if there is reason to suspect this condition.
- **Treatment for premature labor:** Monitor patient for CV signs and symptoms for 12 h after drug is discontinued. Report tachycardia promptly. Monitor I&O ratio. Fluid restriction may be necessary. Consult physician.

Patient & Family Education

- **Inhalator therapy:** review and discuss with the patient the instructions for use of inhalator (included in the package).
- Teach the ambulatory patient on oral terbutaline how to take his or her own pulse and the limits of change that indicate need to notify the physician.

- Instruct patient to consult the physician if breathing difficulty is not relieved or if it becomes worse within 30 min after an oral dose of terbutaline.
- Terbutaline appears to have a short clinical period for sustained effectiveness. Advise patient to keep appointments with physician for evaluation of continued drug effectiveness and clinical condition.
- Tolerance can develop with chronic use of terbutaline. Advise patient to consult physician if symptomatic relief wanes. Usually a substitute agent will be prescribed.
- Instruct patient to adhere to established dosage regimen (i.e., not to change dose intervals or omit, increase, or decrease the dose).
- Be alert to the pattern of self-dosing established by the patient on long-term therapy. Caution patient that in the face of waning response, increasing the dose may cause overdosage and will not improve the clinical condition. The patient should understand that decreasing relief with continued treatment indicates need for another bronchodilator, not an increase in dose.
- Contents of the aerosol (inhalator) are under pressure. Warn patient not to puncture container, not to use or store it near heat or open flame, and not to expose it to temperatures above 49C (120F), which may cause bursting.
- No other aerosol bronchodilator should be used while the patient is being controlled by aerosol terbutaline. Warn patient not to self-medicate with an OTC aerosol.
- Warn the patient not to use OTC drugs unless the physician approves. Many cold and allergy remedies, for example, contain a sympathomimetic agent that when combined with terbutaline may be deleterious to the patient.

Prototype: diphenhydramine, p 47

TERFENADINE

(ter-fen´a-deen)
Trade names: Seldane, Teldane
Classification: ANTIHISTAMINE (H₁-RECEPTOR ANTAGONIST)
Pregnancy: Category C

ACTIONS/PHARMACODYNAMICS   Antihistamines competitively antagonize histamine at the H₁ receptor site but do not bind with histamine to inactivate it. Terfenadine binds preferentially to peripheral rather than central H_1 receptors. It antagonizes most of the pharmacologic effects of histamine. It has few or no anticholinergic and sedative effects.

USES Symptomatic relief of symptoms associated with perennial and seasonal allergic rhinitis such as sneezing, rhinorrhea, pruritus, and lacrimation.

ROUTE & DOSAGE

Allergic Rhinitis

Adult	PO	60 mg q12h
Child	PO	7–12 y: 30 mg q12h
		3–6 y: 15 mg q12h

PHARMACOKINETICS Absorption: readily absorbed from GI tract; extensive first pass metabolism. **Onset:** 1–2 h. **Peak:** 1–2 h. **Duration:** > 12 h. **Metabolism:** metabolized in liver. **Elimination:** half-life: 16–23 h; 60% excreted in bile, 40% in urine.

CONTRAINDICATIONS & PRECAUTIONS Contraindicated in: patients with known hypersensitivity to terfenadine. **Cautious use in:** pregnancy (category C) and nursing mothers. Safety and effectiveness of terfenadine in children < 12 y has not been established.

ADVERSE/SIDE EFFECTS CNS: sedation, *headache,* dizziness, weakness, fatigue. **CV:** arrhythmias. **GI:** nausea, vomiting, abdominal distress, constipation, diarrhea, dry mouth, nose, or throat, cough, epistaxis. **Other:** rash, pruritus.

NURSING IMPLICATIONS

Administration

- Safety in children <12 y has not been established.
- Store below 40C (104F), preferably between 15 and 30C (59–86F) in a light-resistant container unless otherwise specified.

Assessment & Drug Effects

- Sedative and anticholinergic effects are not as likely with terfenadine as with other antihistamines.
- Use with caution in patients with lower airway disease (including asthma), since anticholinergic effects may cause airway drying and respiratory distress.
- Geriatric patients may be more sensitive to the effects of the usual adult dose.

Patient & Family Education

- Instruct patient to take terfenadine only as needed and to not exceed the prescribed dose.

- Instruct patient to store drug in a tightly closed container in a cool, dry place, away from heat or direct sunlight.

Prototype: guaifenesin, p 99

TERPIN HYDRATE ELIXIR
(ter´pin)

TERPIN HYDRATE AND CODEINE ELIXIR

Classifications: ANTITUSSIVE; EXPECTORANT
Pregnancy: Category C
Controlled substance: Schedule V

ACTIONS/PHARMACODYNAMICS Terpin hydrate is a volatile oil derivative claimed to exert direct action on bronchial secretory cells, thereby increasing respiratory tract fluid production and facilitating expectoration. Also see codeine (p 464) for adverse/side effects and drug interactions.

USES Commonly used as a vehicle for other cough medications, e.g., terpin hydrate and codeine elixir contains 10 mg codeine in each 5 ml (added for antitussive effect).

ROUTE & DOSAGE

Cough

Adult	PO	5–10 ml q3–4h; with codeine, 5 ml t.i.d. or q.i.d.

CONTRAINDICATIONS & PRECAUTIONS Contraindicated in: severe diabetes mellitus, peptic ulcer (for self-medication); children < 12 y; pregnancy (category C). **Cautious use in:** history of alcohol dependence (contains 25–45% alcohol).

DRUG INTERACTIONS Disulfiram, metronidazole may cause disulfiram-type reaction (has a high alcohol content).

NURSING IMPLICATIONS

Administration

- Some patients experience epigastric pain if they take it on an empty stomach. If this occurs, it should be taken with food.
- Soothing, local effect of the syrup is enhanced if it is administered undiluted and not immediately followed by water.

Common side effects in *italic*; life-threatening effects underlined; generic names in **bold**; classifications in SMALL CAPS

987

Patient & Family Education

- Adequate fluid intake and humidification of air will help to liquefy sputum and relieve bronchial irritation.
- Because of the high alcoholic content (42.5%) of terpin hydrate elixir, it is undesirable to administer larger doses than recommended.
- Warn patient not to exceed recommended dose.

TESTOLACTONE

(tess-toe-lak´tone)
Trade name: Teslac
Classifications: ANTINEOPLASTIC; HORMONE
Pregnancy: Category C

ACTIONS/PHARMACODYNAMICS Chemotherapeutic agent with chemical configuration similar to that of certain androgens but devoid of androgenic activity in therapeutic doses. Exact mechanism of antineoplastic action unknown. Action simulates that of androgens without producing virilization in recommended dosage. In breast cancer, effect may result from depression of ovarian function by inhibition of synthesis of pituitary gonadotropin.

USES Adjunctive treatment in palliation of breast carcinoma in postmenopausal women when hormone therapy is indicated. Also effective in women diagnosed before menopause in whom ovarian function has been subsequently terminated.

ROUTE & DOSAGE

Adjunctive Therapy for Breast Cancer
Adult   PO   250 mg q.i.d.

PHARMACOKINETICS Absorption: readily absorbed from GI tract. **Metabolism:** metabolized in liver. **Elimination:** excreted in urine.

CONTRAINDICATIONS & PRECAUTIONS Contraindicated in: pregnancy (category C), premenopausal women, breast cancer in males. **Cautious use in:** hypercalcemia, cardiorenal disease.

ADVERSE/SIDE EFFECTS CNS: paresthesias. **Endocrine:** deepening of the voice, acne, facial hair growth, clitoral enlargement. **GI:** glossitis, anorexia; nausea, vomiting. **Other:** hypertension, edema in extremities.

DIAGNOSTIC TEST INTERFERENCES *Urinary 17-OHCS* determinations may be elevated.

DRUG INTERACTIONS May enhance hypoprothrombinemic effects of ORAL ANTICOAGULANTS.

NURSING IMPLICATIONS

Administration
- Drug may be administered without regard to food.
- Store at 15–30C (59–86F) unless otherwise directed. Protect from freezing.

Assessment & Drug Effects
- Clinical response usually occurs in 6–12 wk and is measured according to the following criteria; decrease in size of tumor; more than 50% of nonosseous lesions decrease in size even though all bone lesions remain static.
- Plasma calcium levels are checked routinely and periodically. (**Normal serum calcium:** 8.5–10.6 mg/dl.)
- Report signs that may suggest impending hypercalcemia (see chap 3).
- Note I&O ratio and pattern.
- Encourage patient mobility if feasible; if not, assist with passive exercises.

Patient & Family Education
- Testalactone treatment is usually continued for a minimum of 3 mo (unless there is active progression of the disease) to evaluate response.
- Hypercalcemia represents active remission of bone metastasis; if it occurs, appropriate therapy is instituted.

TESTOSTERONE

See HORMONES, ANDROGEN/ANABOLIC STEROID prototype, p 229.

Prototype: testosterone, p 229

TESTOSTERONE CYPIONATE

Trade names: Andro-Cyp, Andronate, depAndro, Depo-Testosterone, Depotest, Duratest, Testa-C, Testoject-L.A., and others

TESTOSTERONE ENANTHATE

Trade names: Andro L.A., Andryl, Delatest, Delatestryl, Everone, Malogex, Testone L.A., Testrin PA, and others

TESTOSTERONE PROPIONATE

Trade names: Androlan, Malogen in oil, Textex

Classifications: HORMONE; ANDROGEN/AN-ABOLIC STEROID; ANTINEOPLASTIC

Pregnancy: Category X

ACTIONS/PHARMACODYNAMICS Esters of testosterone with similar actions, androgenic/anabolic activity (1:1), and contraindications as parent compound. Duration of action of cypionate and enanthate is longer than that of testosterone. The propionate is more intense in action but has somewhat shorter duration than testosterone; parenteral route is not suited to long-term treatment.

USES Androgen replacement therapy, for delayed puberty (male), palliation of female mammary cancer (1–5 y postmenopausal), and to treat postpartum breast engorgement. Available in fixed combination with estrogens in many preparations.

ROUTE & DOSAGE

Replacement Therapy

Adult	IM	Propionate: 10–25 mg 3 times/wk; cypionate, enanthate: 50–400 mg q2–4wk

Delayed Puberty

Adult	IM	Cypionate, enanthate: 50–200 mg q2–4 wk

Postpartum Breast Engorgement

Adult	IM	Propionate: 25–50 mg/d for 3–4 d

Metastatic Breast Cancer

Adult	IM	Propionate: 100 mg 3 times/wk; cypionate, enanthate: 200–400 mg q2–4 wk

ADVERSE/SIDE EFFECTS Urticaria at injection site, postinjection induration, furunculosis, virilism. See also testosterone.

NURSING IMPLICATIONS

Administration
- Inject intramuscular preparation deep into gluteal muscle.
- Store at 15–30C (59–86F); do not freeze.

Patient and Family Education
- Advise patient to report soreness at injection site, since postinjection furunculosis may be an associated adverse reaction.
- Priapism (persistent erection) and virilization are signs of overdosage and indicate necessity for temporary drug withdrawal. Advise patient to report to physician.

Prototype: procaine, p 166

TETRACAINE HYDROCHLORIDE

(tet´ra-kane)

Trade name: Pontocaine

Classifications: CNS AGENT; LOCAL ANESTHETIC (ESTER TYPE)

Pregnancy: Category A

ACTIONS/PHARMACODYNAMICS Aminobenzoic ester; local anesthetic approximately 10 times more potent and toxic than procaine. Depresses the initial depolarization phase of the action potential, thus preventing propagation and conduction of the nerve impulse. This results in loss of sensation and motor activity in circumscribed body areas close to injection or application site.

USES Spinal anesthesia (high, low, saddle block) and topically to produce surface anesthesia: *eye:* to anesthetize conjunctiva and cornea prior to superficial procedures (including tonometry, gonioscopy, removal of foreign bodies or sutures, corneal scraping); *nose and throat:* to abolish laryngeal and esophageal reflexes prior to bronchoscopy, esophagoscopy; *skin:* to relieve pruritus, pain, burning.

PHARMACOKINETICS Onset: 1 min eye; 3 min mucosal surface; 3 min spinal. **Duration:** up to 15 min eye; 30–60 min mucosal surface; 1.5–3 h spinal. **Metabolism:** metabolized in liver and plasma. **Elimination:** excreted in urine.

Common side effects in *italic*; life-threatening effects <u>underlined</u>; generic names in **bold**; classifications in SMALL CAPS

ROUTE & DOSAGE

Local Anesthesia

Adult	Topical	1–2 drops of 0.5% solution or 1.25–2.5 cm of ointment in lower conjunctival fornix before procedure; or 0.5% solution or ointment to nose or throat before procedure
	Spinal	1% solution diluted with equal volume of 10% dextrose injected in subarachnoid space

CONTRAINDICATIONS & PRECAUTIONS Contraindicated in: elderly and debilitated patient; prolonged use of ophthalmic preparations; known hypersensitivity to tetracaine or other local anesthetics of ester type (e.g., procaine, chloroprocaine, cocaine) or to PABA or its derivatives; infection at application or injection site. Safe use during pregnancy (category C) or in children not established. **Cautious use in:** shock, in nursing mothers, cachexia, cardiac decompensation.

ADVERSE/SIDE EFFECTS <u>Anaphylactic reactions</u>, convulsions, faintness, syncope, hypotention. **CNS:** postspinal headache, headache, spinal nerve paralysis, anxiety, nervousness, seizures. **CV:** bradycardia, arrhythmias, hypotension. **Eye:** *stinging*. *Prolonged use:* corneal erosion, retardation or prevention of healing of corneal abrasion, transient pitting and sloughing of corneal surface, dry corneal epithelium. **Nose/throat:** dry membranes, prolonged depression of cough reflex.

NURSING IMPLICATIONS

Administration

- Avoid use of solutions that are cloudy, discolored, or crystallized.
- When tetracaine is used on mucosa of larynx, trachea, or esophagus, the manufacturer recommends adding 0.06 ml of a 0.1% epinephrine solution to each ml tetracaine solution to slow absorption of the anesthetic.
- Storage temperatures: ophthalmic solution and ointment: 15–30C (59–86F); topical: refrigeration. Avoid freezing. Store in tight, light-resistant containers.

Assessment & Drug Effects

- Recovery from anesthesia to the pharyngeal area is complete when patient has feeling in the hard and soft palates and when muscles in the faucial (tonsillar) pillars contract with stimulation. To test: (1)

Ask patient if he or she can feel hard palate with tongue. (2) Gently stroke soft palate with moistened cotton swab and ask patient if he or she can feel it. (3) Gently stroke soft palate with a cotton swab moistened with iced lemon water and observe whether or not pharyngeal muscles contract.

- Do not administer food or liquids until these normal pharyngeal responses are present (usually about 1 h after anesthetic administration). The first small amount of liquid (water) should be administered under supervision of the care provider.
- Increased blood concentration of the drug may result from excess application of tetracaine to the skin (to relieve pruritus or burning), application to debrided or infected skin surfaces, or too rapid injection rate.
- High blood concentrations of tetracaine can lead to adverse systemic effects involving CNS and CV systems: convulsions, respiratory arrest, dysrhythmias, cardiac arrest.

Patient & Family Education

- Caution patient not to use ophthalmic tetracaine longer than prescribed period. Prolonged use to eye surface may cause corneal epithelial erosions and retard healing of corneal surface.
- Natural barriers to eye infection and injury are removed by the anesthesia. Warn patient not to rub eye after tetracaine instillation until anesthetic effect has dissipated (evidenced by return of blink reflex). Patching for temporary protection of the corneal epithelium may be ordered.
- Instruct patient who self-medicates to wash or disinfect hands before and after administration of solutions or ointment. Review procedure for administration of eye medication.

TETRACYCLINE HYDROCHLORIDE

See ANTIINFECTIVES, TETRACYCLINE ANTIBIOTIC, prototype, p 74.

Prototype: tetracycline, p 74

TETRACYCLINE HYDROCHLORIDE, OPHTHALMIC

Trade name: Achromycin Ophthalmic
Classifications: ANTIINFECTIVE; TETRACYCLINE ANTIBIOTIC

Common side effects in *italic*; life-threatening effects <u>underlined</u>; generic names in **bold**; classifications in SMALL CAPS

ACTIONS/PHARMACODYNAMICS Broad-spectrum antimicrobial agent with bacteriostatic action. Acts by inhibiting protein synthesis in susceptible organisms. Evidence suggests that tetracycline ophthalmic may be less effective than erythromycin for prophylaxis of neonatal chlamydial conjunctivitis.

USES Superficial ocular infections caused by susceptible organisms; used as adjunct with oral tetracycline for treatment of chlamydial eye infections (trachoma; inclusion conjunctivitis). Also used for prophylaxis of ophthalmia neonatorum due to *Chlamydia trachomatis*. The U.S. Centers for Disease Control (CDC) and the American Academy of Pediatrics approve of the use of tetracycline ophthalmic (or erythromycin) as an alternative to silver nitrate 1% for prophylaxis of ophthalmia neonatorum due to *Neisseria gonorrhoeae*.

ROUTE & DOSAGE

Bacterial Ophthalmic Infections

Adult	Ophthalmic	1 cm of ointment or 1–2 drops of suspension b.i.d. to q.i.d.

Chlamydial Ophthalmic Infections

Adult	Ophthalmic	1 cm of ointment or 1–2 drops of suspension b.i.d. to q.i.d. for 1–2 mo

Prophylaxis of Chlamydial or Gonococcal Ophthalmia Neonatorum

Child	Ophthalmic	1 cm of ointment or 1–2 drops of suspension shortly after delivery

PHARMACOKINETICS Duration: 6 h ointment; 2 h suspension.

CONTRAINDICATIONS & PRECAUTIONS Contraindicated in: hypersensitivity to any of the tetracyclines; use for common eye problems.

ADVERSE/SIDE EFFECTS Hypersensitivity: itching, dermatitis, lacrimation; *transient stinging,* burning or foreign body sensation; temporary blurring of vision; pigmentation of conjunctivae; superinfection (with frequent intermittent or prolonged use).

DRUG INTERACTIONS TOPICAL CORTICOSTEROIDS may suppress or mask hypersensitivity reactions or clinical signs of superinfection.

NURSING IMPLICATIONS

Administration

- Shake ophthalmic suspension well before using to assure uniform distribution of drug.
- Tetracycline ophthalmic preparations exhibit a bright yellow fluorescence under ultraviolet light. This effect does not appear to interfere with the use of fluorescein in eye examinations.
- *Treatment for Chlamydial infections* (for children > 8 y and adults): tetracycline ophthalmic and oral; (children < 8 y generally treated with oral erythromycin or sulfisoxazole). Can resolve spontaneously within several weeks or months, but treatment shortens its course.

Prophylaxis of Gonorrheal or Chlamydial Ophthalmia Neonatorum

- Ophthalmia neonatorum is a general term that refers to any infection of the newborn conjunctiva. Preferably prophylaxis should be performed immediately after delivery or no later than 1 h after delivery.
- Gently wipe each eye with separate sterile cotton ball lightly moistened with sterile water to remove blood and vernix. Wipe from the nasal side toward outer corner of eye.
- Carefully separate eyelids and place thin strip of ointment in lower conjunctival sac of each eye. Use separate single dose dispenser for each neonate. If ophthalmic ointment is used, massage eyelids gently to facilitate spread of ointment.
- After 1 min, gently wipe away excess medication with sterile cotton. Do not flush medication from eyes following administration.
- Store at 15–30C (59–86F) in light-resistant container in a dry environment unless otherwise directed. Tetracyclines darken on exposure to sunlight in moist air.

Assessment & Drug Effects

- Culture and susceptibility tests should be initiated prior to start of therapy to determine sensitivity of infecting organism to tetracycline.
- Mild infections generally respond to therapy within 48 h. Severe infections may require several days of treatment. Keep physician informed.

Patient & Family Education

- Caution patient that vision will be blurred temporarily following administration of either ophthalmic ointment or ophthalmic suspension (contains light mineral oil).
- Advise patient to report to physician the onset of pronounced burning, stinging, itching, or other un-

Common side effects in *italic*; life-threatening effects <u>underlined</u>; generic names in **bold**; classifications in SMALL CAPS

991

usual sensations or if infection shows no improvement or appears to be worsening.

- Instruct patient to use medication for the full course of therapy as prescribed and to discard medication when no longer needed or if outdated.

Prototype: naphazoline, p 211

TETRAHYDROZOLINE HYDROCHLORIDE
(tet-ra-hye-drozz´a-leen)

Trade names: Collyrium, Malazine, Murine Plus, Optigene, Soothe, Tetraclear, Tetrasine, Tyzine, Visine

Classifications: EYE, EAR, NOSE & THROAT PREPARATION; VASOCONSTRICTOR, DECONGESTANT

Pregnancy: Category C

ACTIONS/PHARMACODYNAMICS Imidazole derivative structurally and chemically related to naphazoline. In common with naphazoline, has more marked alpha-adrenergic than beta-adrenergic activity; large doses cause CNS depression rather than the stimulation produced by other sympathomimetic amines.

USES Symptomatic relief of minor eye irritation and allergies and for nasopharyngeal congestion of allergic or inflammatory origin.

ROUTE & DOSAGE

Decongestant

Adult	Ophthalmic	1–2 drops of 0.05% solution in eye b.i.d. or t.i.d.
	Nasal	2–4 drops of 0.1% solution or spray in each nostril q3h prn
Child	Nasal	≥ 6 y: same as for adult
		2–6 y: 2–4 drops of 0.05% solution or spray in each nostril q3h prn

CONTRAINDICATIONS & PRECAUTIONS Contraindicated in: hypersensitivity to any component; use of ophthalmic preparation in glaucoma or other serious eye diseases; use of drug in children < 2 y, use of 0.1% or higher strengths in children < 6 y, use within 14 d of MAO inhibitor therapy. Safe use during pregnancy (category C) not established. **Cautious use in:** hypertension, cardiovascular disease; hyperthyroidism; diabetes mellitus; young children.

ADVERSE/SIDE EFFECTS *Transient stinging,* irritation, *sneezing,* dryness, headache, tremors, drowsiness, lightheadedness, insomnia, palpitation. **Overdosage:** CNS depression (marked drowsiness, sweating, <u>coma</u>, hypotension, <u>shock</u>, bradycardia).

NURSING IMPLICATIONS

Administration

- Since drug action lasts 4–8 h, interval between doses is at least 4–6 h.
- When using squeeze bottle, patient should be in upright position. When patient is reclining, a stream rather than a spray may be ejected, with consequent overdosage.
- Nasal drops are usually administered in lateral, head-low position.

Patient & Family Education

- Instruct patient to discontinue medication and to consult physician if relief is not obtained within 48 h or if symptoms for which drug was given persist or increase.
- Caution patient not to exceed recommended dosage. Rebound congestion and rhinitis may occur with frequent or prolonged use of nasal preparation.

THEOPHYLLINE

See BRONCHODILATOR (RESPIRATORY SMOOTH MUSCLE RELAXANT) prototype, p 136.

Prototype: mebendazole, p 53

THIABENDAZOLE
(thye-a-ben´da-zole)

Trade name: Mintezol

Classifications: ANTIINFECTIVE; ANTHELMINTIC

Pregnancy: Category C

ACTIONS/PHARMACODYNAMICS Benzimidazole with vermicidal properties; structurally related to mebendazole. Precise action mechanism not clear but has wide spectrum of anthelmintic activity. Has been shown to inhibit helminth-specific enzyme fumarate reductase. Demonstrates antiinflammatory, antipyretic, and analgesic effects in animals. Sup-

Common side effects in *italic*; life-threatening effects <u>underlined</u>; generic names in **bold**; classifications in SMALL CAPS

presses production of eggs or larvae by some parasites and may inhibit subsequent development of eggs or larvae passed in feces.

USES Enterobiasis (pinworm infestation), ascariasis (roundworm), strongyloidiasis (threadworm), cutaneous larva migrans (creeping eruption), and hookworm infestations caused by *Ancylostoma duodenale* or *Necator americanus*. Used during invasive stage of trichinosis to relieve symptoms and for mixed helminthic infestations.

ROUTE & DOSAGE

Enterobiasis, Ascariasis, Strongyloidiasis, Hookworm

Adult	PO	< 70 kg: 25 mg/kg b.i.d. x 2 d
		> 70 kg: 1.5 g b.i.d. (max 3 g/d) x 2 d
Child	PO	14–70 kg: 25 mg/kg b.i.d. x 2 d

PHARMACOKINETICS Absorption: readily absorbed from GI tract. **Peak:** 1–2 h. **Metabolism:** metabolized in liver. **Elimination:** > 90% excreted in urine; 5% in feces.

CONTRAINDICATIONS & PRECAUTIONS Contraindicated in: safe use during pregnancy (category C) and in nursing mothers not established. **Cautious use in:** hepatic or renal dysfunction, when vomiting can be dangerous, severe dehydration or malnutrition, anemia, children weighing < 15 kg.

ADVERSE/SIDE EFFECTS CNS: weariness, *dizziness*, drowsiness, headache. **CV:** hypotension, bradycardia. **GI:** *anorexia, nausea, vomiting,* epigastric distress, jaundice, cholestasis, parenchymal liver damage, diarrhea, perianal rash. **Renal:** malodor of urine, crystalluria, hematuria, nephrotoxicity, enuresis. **Other:** transient rise in cephalin flocculation and AST, transient leukopenia, hypersensitivity, hyperglycemia, pruritus.

NURSING IMPLICATIONS

Administration

- Administer drug after meals. Tablets should be chewed before they are swallowed. Shake suspension well before pouring.

Assessment & Drug Effects

- If patient is anemic, dehydrated, or malnourished, supportive treatment is indicated prior to start of thiabendazole therapy.

- Adverse/side effects generally occur 3–4 h after administration, are mild, and last for 2–8 h. Incidence tends to be related to dose and duration of treatment.
- Drug should be discontinued immediately if there are symptoms of hypersensitivity: fever, facial flush, chills, conjunctival infection, skin rashes, erythema multiforme (including Stevens-Johnson syndrome), which can be fatal.

Patient & Family Education

- CNS side effects occur frequently and may prevent the patient from driving a car or engaging in activities requiring mental alertness. Warn patient of the possibility.

THIAMINE HYDROCHLORIDE (VITAMIN B₁)

(thye´a-min)
Trade names: Apatate Drops, Bewon, Revitonus, Thio
Classifications: VITAMIN B
Pregnancy: Category A

ACTIONS/PHARMACODYNAMICS Water-soluble vitamin and member of B-complex group. Functions as an essential coenzyme in carbohydrate metabolism. Also has role in conversion of tryptophan to nicotinamide.

USES Treatment and prophylaxis of beriberi, to correct anorexia due to thiamine deficiency states, and in treatment of neuritis associated with pregnancy, pellagra, and alcoholism, including Wernicke-Korsakoff syndrome. Therapy generally includes other members of vitamin B complex, since thiamine deficiency rarely occurs alone.

ROUTE & DOSAGE

Thiamine Deficiency

Adult	IV/IM	50–100 mg t.i.d.
Child	IV/IM	10–25 mg t.i.d.

Beriberi

Adult	IV/IM	10–500 mg t.i.d. for 2 wk
Child	IV/IM	10–50 mg t.i.d.

Dietary Supplement

Adult	PO	15–30 mg/d
Child	PO	10–50 mg/d

Common side effects in *italic*; life-threatening effects <u>underlined</u>; generic names in **bold**; classifications in SMALL CAPS

993

PHARMACOKINETICS Absorption: limited absorption from GI tract. **Distribution:** widely distributed, including into breast milk. **Elimination:** excreted in urine.

ADVERSE/SIDE EFFECTS Feeling of warmth, weakness, urticaria, pruritus, sweating, nausea, restlessness, tightness of throat, angioneurotic edema, cyanosis, pulmonary edema, GI hemorrhage, cardiovascular collapse, anaphylaxis. Following rapid IV administration: slight fall in BP.

NURSING IMPLICATIONS

Administration

- IM injections may be painful. Rotate sites and apply cold compresses to area if necessary for relief of discomfort.
- IV thiamine may be given by direct IV undiluted at a rate of 100 mg over 5 min. May also be added to IV solutions and infused at ordered rate.
- Preserve in tight, light-resistant, nonmetallic containers. Thiamine is unstable in alkaline solutions (e.g., solutions of acetates, barbiturates, bicarbonates, carbonates, citrates) and neutral solutions.

Assessment & Drug Effects

- Intradermal test dose is recommended prior to administration in suspected thiamine sensitivity. Deaths have occurred following IV use.
- Careful recording of patient's dietary history is an essential part of vitamin replacement therapy. Collaborate with physician, dietitian, patient, and responsible family member in developing a diet teaching plan that can be sustained by patient.
- Therapeutic effectiveness is evaluated by improvement of **clinical manifestations of thiamine deficiency:** anorexia, gastric distress, depression, irritability, insomnia, palpitations, tachycardia, loss of memory, paresthesias, muscle weakness and pain, elevated blood pyruvic acid level (diagnostic test for thiamine deficiency), elevated lactic acid level. **Severe deficiency:** ophthalmoplegia, polyneuropathy, muscle wasting ("dry" beriberi), edema, serous effusions, CHF ("wet" beriberi).
- Body requirement of thiamine is directly proportional to carbohydrate intake and metabolic rate; thus, requirement increases when diet consists predominantly of carbohydrates. Total absence of dietary thiamine can produce a deficiency state in about 3 wk.

Patient & Family Education

- **Recommended daily allowance (RDA):** children 4–6 yr of age, 0.9 mg; adult males, 1.4 mg; adult females, 1 mg; pregnancy and lactation, 1.4 mg.
- **Food-drug relationships:** Instruct patient on **rich dietary sources of thiamine:** yeast, pork, beef, liver, wheat and other whole grains, nutrient added breakfast cereals, fresh vegetables, especially peas and dried beans.

Prototype: thiopental, p 164

THIAMYLAL SODIUM

(thye-am′i-lal)
Trade name: Surital
Classifications: CNS AGENT; GENERAL ANESTHETIC; BARBITURATE
Pregnancy: Category C
Controlled substance: Schedule III

ACTIONS/PHARMACODYNAMICS Rapid ultrashort-acting barbiturate. By depressing CNS, produces hypnosis; produces loss of anesthesia. Has poor analgesic effect and may increase sensitivity to pain if anesthetic dose is inadequate. Depresses respiratory and circulatory functions and diminishes eyelash and tendon reflexes; skeletal muscle relaxation is transient, occurring only at onset of anesthesia.

USES Induction of anesthesia, for maintenance of anesthesia by intermittent IV injection during brief operative procedures, or as an agent for inducing a hypnotic state.

ROUTE & DOSAGE

Induction and Maintenance of Anesthesia

Adult	IV	Test dose of 2 ml of 2.5% solution; if no problems, then 1 ml q5s of 2.5% solution or 0.3% solution by continuous infusion titrated to response

PHARMACOKINETICS Onset: 10–20 s. **Duration:** 20–30 min after end of infusion. **Distribution:** crosses placenta. **Metabolism:** metabolized in liver. **Elimination:** half-life: up to 9 h; excreted in urine.

CONTRAINDICATIONS & PRECAUTIONS Contraindicated in: hypersensitivity to barbiturates; latent or manifest porphyria. Safe use during pregnancy (category C) and in young children not established.

Common side effects in *italic;* life-threatening effects underlined; generic names in **bold**; classifications in SMALL CAPS

Cautious use in: coronary artery disease, impaired hepatic or renal function, status asthmaticus, hypotension, pain, shock.

ADVERSE/SIDE EFFECTS CNS: <u>respiratory depression</u>, emergence delirium, retrograde amnesia, headache. **CV:** thrombophlebitis, myocardial depression. **GI:** nausea, emesis. **Skin:** pain, swelling, sloughing at injection site. **Other:** <u>anaphylactic reaction</u>, hypothermia, hiccups, salivation, <u>laryngospasm</u>, bronchospasm.

NURSING IMPLICATIONS

Administration

- Reconstitute solution for IV injection with sterile water for injection. Do not use Ringer's solution or solutions containing bacteriostatic or buffer agents since they tend to cause precipitation. If drug is to be given by intermittent drip, isotonic NaCl is the preferred diluent; water for injection may cause extreme hypotonicity; 5% Dextrose may be used, but its acidity may be sufficient to cause precipitation.
- Avoid injection of air into solution; cloudiness may result. Discard precipitated or cloudy solutions.
- **Recommended rate of injection:** 1 ml of 2.5% solution q3s. Initially short periods of anesthesia can be produced by 3–6 ml of 2.5% solution.
- Adjunctive drugs (e.g., atropine, tubocurarine, succinylcholine) may be given concurrently, but do not mix prior to administration of the anesthetic.
- Refrigerate for up to 6 d; then discard. If drug is stored at 15–30C (59–86F), use within 24 h. Refrigeration helps to keep solutions clear.

Prototype: prochlorperazine, p 215

THIETHYLPERAZINE MALEATE
(thye-eth-il-per´a-zeen)
Trade name: Torecan
Classifications: GI AGENT; ANTIEMETIC
Pregnancy: Category X

ACTIONS/PHARMACODYNAMICS Piperazine phenothiazine derivative with contraindications, precautions, and toxic effects similar to those of prochlorperazine. Reported to have higher ratio of antiemetic action to tranquilizing action than other phenothiazines. Acts directly on chemoreceptor trigger zone as well as the vomiting center.

USES To control nausea and vomiting. **Unlabeled use:** treatment of vertigo.

ROUTE & DOSAGE

Nausea and Vomiting

Adult	PO/PR/IM	10 mg 1–3 times/d

PHARMACOKINETICS Onset: 1 h PO, PR; 30 min IM.

CONTRAINDICATIONS & PRECAUTIONS Contraindicated in: hypersensitivity to phenothiazines, CNS depression or comatose states, pregnancy (category X), IV administration. Safe use in children < 12 y, in nursing mothers, or following intracardiac or intracranial surgery not established. **Cautious use in:** renal or hepatic disease.

ADVERSE/SIDE EFFECTS *Drowsiness,* dizziness, headache, *dry mouth and nose,* blurred vision, tinnitus, restlessness, fever, orthostatic hypotension. Occasionally: extrapyramidal symptoms including convulsions; sialorrhea with altered taste sensations, cholestatic jaundice.

NURSING IMPLICATIONS

Administration

- Examine parenteral solution and administer only if it is clear and colorless.
- Patient should be recumbent when drug is being administered IM. Postural hypotension (manifested by weakness, lightheadedness, faintness) and drowsiness may occur, particularly after initial injection. Advise patient to remain in bed for about 1 h or longer, if indicated, and supervise ambulation. If vasopressor agent is required, levarterenol or phenylephrine is used. Epinephrine is contraindicated.
- Administer IM deep into large muscle mass and aspirate hypodermic carefully before injecting drug to avoid inadvertent entry into a blood vessel. IV administration is specifically contraindicated because it can cause severe hypotension.
- Store at room temperature, away from heat, in light-resistant containers. Suppositories should be stored below 25C (77F).

Assessment & Drug Effects

- Patients who have received drug preoperatively may manifest restlessness or depression during anesthesia recovery.
- Report immediately the onset of *extrapyramidal ef-*

Common side effects in *italic*; life-threatening effects <u>underlined</u>; generic names in **bold**; classifications in SMALL CAPS

995

fects: gait disturbances, difficulty in speaking, muscle spasms, torticollis, deviations in eye movements. Reduction in dosage or discontinuation of medication is indicated.

Patient & Family Education

▪ Caution patient to avoid potentially hazardous activities such as driving a car or operating machinery because of possibility of drowsiness and dizziness.

THIMEROSAL

(thye-mer´oh-sal)
Trade names: Mersol, Merthiolate
Classifications: SKIN & MUCOUS MEMBRANE AGENT; ANTIINFECTIVE
Pregnancy: Category C

ACTIONS/PHARMACODYNAMICS Topical organic mercurial with sustained bacteriostatic and fungistatic activity. Ineffective against spore-forming organisms.

USES First-aid treatment of contaminated wounds, in antisepsis of intact skin, before surgery, and in pustular dermatosis; as antifungal agent in athlete's foot for wound irrigations. Ophthalmic preparation is used to treat conjunctivitis and corneal ulcer and for prevention of infection following removal of foreign bodies. Used as preservative in most solutions sold for cleaning, wetting, soaking, and storage of contact lenses; also used as preservative for biologic and pharmaceutical products.

ROUTE & DOSAGE

Antiseptic

Adult	Topical	1:1000 solution—apply locally 1–3 times/d

CONTRAINDICATIONS & PRECAUTIONS **Contraindicated in:** history of sensitivity to thio or mercurial compounds, prolonged use, pregnancy (category C).

ADVERSE/SIDE EFFECTS **Hypersensitivity:** itching erythema, papular or vesicular eruptions. **Prolonged use:** mercury poisoning (metallic taste, salivation, stomatitis, lethargy, peripheral neuropathy).

NURSING IMPLICATIONS

Administration

▪ For first-aid treatment: appropriate cleansing should precede application of antiseptic.
▪ To prevent skin irritation, do not apply bandage or other occlusive dressing until tincture application has completely dried.
▪ Thimerosal is antagonized by whole blood and is incompatible when used concurrently or following applications of boric acid, iodine, strong acids, aluminum, silver, or other salts of heavy metals. It is compatible with sulfonamides.
▪ Preserve in tightly covered, light-resistant containers. Avoid exposure to excessive heat.

Assessment & Drug Effects

▪ Aqueous Merthiolate contains thimerosal and borate (0.14%). Both are toxic if absorbed systemically.
▪ Long-term use, especially as treatment of otitis media, may lead to potentially fatal toxicity due to inadvertent swallowing of solution.

Prototype: fluorouracil, p 94

THIOGUANINE (TG, 6-THIOGUANINE)

(thye-oh-gwah´neen)
Trade name: Lanvis
Classifications: ANTINEOPLASTIC; ANTIMETABOLITE
Pregnancy: Category X

ACTIONS/PHARMACODYNAMICS Antimetabolite and purine antagonist with immunosuppressive activity. Qualitatively and quantitatively similar to mercaptopurine. A highly toxic drug with a low therapeutic index; therapeutic response is normally accompanied by evidence of toxicity. Delays myelosuppression; has potential mutagenic and carcinogenic properties. Cross-resistance exists between mercaptopurine and thioguanine.

USES In combination with other antineoplastics for remission induction in acute myelogenous leukemia and as treatment of chronic myelogenous leukemia. Has little advantage over mercaptopurine.

PHARMACOKINETICS **Absorption:** variable and incomplete absorption from GI tract. **Peak:** 8 h.

Distribution: crosses placenta. **Metabolism:** metabolized in liver. **Elimination:** half-life: 11 h; excreted in urine.

ROUTE & DOSAGE

Leukemia

Adult	PO	2 mg/kg/d; may increase to 3 mg/kg/d if no response after 4 wk

---

ADVERSE/SIDE EFFECTS **Hematologic:** <u>leukopenia, thombocytopenia</u>, anemia. **Hepatic:** jaundice. **Other:** *hyperuricemia,* nausea, vomiting, anorexia, stomatitis, diarrhea.

NURSING IMPLICATIONS

Administration

- Because there is no known antagonist to thioguanine, prompt discontinuation of the drug is essential in avoiding irreversible myelosuppression when toxicity develops.
- Store in airtight container at 15–30C (59–86F).

Assessment & Drug Effects

- Blood counts are determined weekly; monitor reports as indicators for adaptations in drug regimens.
- Patient receiving this drug experiences an increased incidence of infections and possibly hemorrhage complications. Therapy should be discontinued at first sign of altered blood cell counts.
- Monitor I&O ratio and report oliguria.
- Observe patient's skin and sclera for jaundice. It is thought to be a reversible clinical sign, but it should be reported promptly as a symptom of toxicity; drug will be discontinued promptly.
- Expect that the leukocyte count descent may be slow over a period of 2–4 wk. Treatment is interrupted if there is a rapid fall within a few days.

Patient & Family Education

- Maintenance doses are continued throughout remissions.

THIOPENTAL SODIUM

See CENTRAL NERVOUS SYSTEM AGENT, GENERAL ANESTHETIC prototype, p 164.

Prototype: chlorpromazine, p 191

THIORIDAZINE HYDROCHLORIDE
(thye-or-rid´a-zeen)
Trade names: Mellaril, Millazine, Novoridazine, Thioril
Classifications: CNS AGENT; PSYCHOTHERAPEUTIC; PHENOTHIAZINE ANTIPSYCHOTIC (TRANQUILIZER)
Pregnancy: Category C

ACTIONS/PHARMACODYNAMICS Piperidine phenothiazine with actions, uses, limitations and interactions similar to those of chlorpromazine. Rarely produces extrapyramidal effects. Has weak antiemetic but strong anticholinergic and alpha-adrenergic agonist activity and potent sedative action.

USES Management of nonpsychotic behavioral disturbances of senility, manifestations of psychotic disorders, alcohol withdrawal; symptomatic treatment of organic brain disease. Short-term treatment of moderate to marked depression and for management of hyperkinetic behavior syndrome (attention deficit disorder).

ROUTE & DOSAGE

Psychotic Disorders

Adult	PO	50–100 mg t.i.d.; may increase up to 800 mg/d as needed or tolerated
Elderly	PO	10 mg t.i.d.; may increase up to 200 mg/d
Child	PO	> 2 y: 0.5–3 mg/kg/d in divided doses; if hospitalized, may start at 25 mg t.i.d.

Moderate to Marked Depression

Adult	PO	25 mg t.i.d.; may increase up to 200 mg/d in divided doses

---

PHARMACOKINETICS **Absorption:** well absorbed from GI tract. **Onset:** days to weeks. **Distribution:** crosses placenta; distributed into breast milk. **Metabolism:** metabolized in liver. **Elimination:** half-life: 26–36 h; excreted in urine.

CONTRAINDICATIONS & PRECAUTIONS **Contraindicated in:** hypersensitivity to phenothiazines. Severe CNS depression, CV disease, children < 2 y. Safe use during pregnancy (category C) and in nurs-

T

ing mothers not established. **Cautious use in:** premature ventricular contractions; previously diagnosed breast cancer; patients exposed to extremes in heat or to organophosphorous insecticides; respiratory disorders.

ADVERSE/SIDE EFFECTS *Sedation,* dizziness, drowsiness, lethargy, nasal congestion, blurred vision, pigmentary retinopathy; xerostomia, *constipation,* paralytic ileus; amenorrhea, breast engorgement, gynecomastia, galactorrhea, ventricular dysrhythmias, *urinary retention,* hypotension. Infrequent: extrapyramidal syndrome, nocturnal confusion, hyperactivity.

DRUG INTERACTIONS Alcohol and other CNS DEPRESSANTS add to CNS depression.

NURSING IMPLICATIONS

Administration
- Tablet may be crushed before administration and taken with fluid of patient's choice.
- If the patient is also receiving antacid or antidiarrheal medication, schedule the phenothiazine to be taken at least 1 h before or 1 h after the other medication.
- Liquid concentrate should be diluted just prior to administration with 1/2 glass of fruit juice, milk, water, carbonated beverage, or soup. Preparation and storage of bulk dilutions are not recommended.
- Increases in dose should be added to the first dose of the day to prevent sleep disturbance.
- Preserve in tightly covered, light-resistant containers at 15–30C (59–86F) unless otherwise indicated.

Assessment & Drug Effects
- Orthostatic hypotension may occur in early therapy. Female patients appear to be more susceptible than male patients.
- The patient may be unable to adjust to extremes of temperature because of drug effect on the heat regulatory center in the hypothalamus. Patient may complain of being cold even at average room temperature. The elderly patient is particularly susceptible to this modified regulatory function.
- If patient has been exposed to extremes in heat or has had an elevated temperature for several hours, be alert to the *signs of heat stroke:* red, dry, hot skin, full bounding pulse, dilated pupils, temperature above 40.6C (105F), dyspnea. Report them to physician and be prepared to institute measures to reduce temperature rapidly.

- Monitor I&O ratio and bowel elimination pattern. Check for abdominal distension and pain. Encourage adequate fluid intake as prophylaxis for constipation and xerostomia. The depressed patient may not seek help for either symptom or for urinary retention.
- Periodic blood and hepatic function tests are advised during therapy.
- Suicide is an inherent risk with any depressed patient and may remain a problem until there is significant clinical improvement. Supervise patient closely during early course of therapy. Do not permit access to more than one dose of medication and watch to see that the dose is not hoarded.

Patient & Family Education
- Explain dosage and dilution to patient if he or she is responsible for administration.
- Warn the patient against spilling drug on skin or clothing because of danger of contact dermatitis. Wash skin well in soap and water if liquid drug is spilled.
- Counsel patient to take drug as prescribed and not to alter dosing regimen or stop medication without consulting physician.
- Alcohol should be avoided during phenothiazine therapy. Concomitant use enhances CNS depression effects.
- Marked drowsiness generally subsides with continued therapy or reduction in dosage.
- Caution patient to avoid potentially hazardous activities such as driving a car or operating machinery until reaction to drug is known.
- Advise patient to make position changes slowly, particularly from recumbent to upright posture, and to dangle legs a few minutes before standing. Also inform patient that vasodilation produced by hot showers or baths or by long exposure to environmental heat may accentuate hypotensive effect.
- Do not apply heating pad or hot water bottles to the body for external heat. Because of depressed conditioned avoidance behaviors a severe burn may result.
- Instruct patient to report to physician the onset of any change in visual acuity, brownish coloring of vision, or impairment of night vision. These symptoms suggest pigmentary retinopathy (observed primarily in patients receiving extremely high doses). An ophthalmic consultation may be indicated.
- May color urine pink-red to reddish brown.
- Warn patient to avoid use of all OTC drugs unless they are approved by the physician.

Common side effects in *italic*; life-threatening effects underlined; generic names in **bold**; classifications in SMALL CAPS

Prototype: cyclophosphamide, p 91

THIOTEPA
(thye-oh-tep´a)
Trade name: TSPA
Classifications: ANTINEOPLASTIC; ALKYLATING AGENT
Pregnancy: Category D

ACTIONS/PHARMACODYNAMICS Ethylenimine cell cycle nonspecific alkylating agent that selectively reacts with DNA phosphate groups to produce chromosome cross-linkage and consequent blocking of nucleoprotein synthesis. Nonvesicant, highly toxic hematopoietic agent with a low therapeutic index. Myelosuppression is cumulative and unpredictable and may be delayed. Has some immunosuppressive activity. Like all alkylating agents thiotepa is carcinogenic and potentially mutagenic.

USES To produce remissions in malignant lymphomas, including Hodgkin's disease, and adenocarcinoma of breast and ovary. Also in chronic granulocytic and lymphocytic leukemia, superficial papillary carcinoma of urinary bladder, bronchogenic carcinoma, and in malignant effusions secondary to neoplastic disease of serosal cavities. **Unlabeled uses:** prevention of pterygium recurrences following postoperative beta-irridiation; leukemia, malignant meningeal neoplasms.

ROUTE & DOSAGE

Malignant Lymphomas

Adult	IV	0.3–0.4 mg/kg q1–4wk
	Intratumor	0.6–0.8 mg/kg directly into tumor q1–4wk
	Intracavitary	0.6–0.8 mg/kg instilled through same tubing used for paracentesis at intervals of at least 1 wk
	Intravesicular	60 mg in 30–60 ml of distilled water instilled into bladder to be retained for 2 h once/wk for 4 wk
	Intrathecal	1–10 mg/m² 1–2 times/wk

PHARMACOKINETICS Absorption: rapidly cleared from plasma. **Onset:** gradual response over several wk. **Metabolism:** metabolized in liver. **Elimination:** 60% of IV dose excreted in urine within 24–72 h.

CONTRAINDICATIONS & PRECAUTIONS Contraindicated in: hypersensitivity to drug; acute leukemia, pregnancy (category D). **Cautious use in** (if at all) chronic lymphocytic leukemia; myelosuppression produced by radiation; with other antineoplastics; bone marrow invasion by tumor cells; impaired renal or hepatic function.

ADVERSE/SIDE EFFECTS GI: anorexia, nausea, vomiting, stomatitis, ulceration of intestinal mucosa. **Hematologic:** leukopenia, thrombocytopenia, anemia, pancytopenia. **Hypersensitivity:** hives, rash, pruritus. **Reproductive:** amenorrhea, interference with spermatogenesis. **Other:** headache, febrile reactions, pain and weeping of injection site, hyperuricemia, slowed or lessened response in heavily irradiated area, sensation of throat tightness. Reported *with intravesical administration:* lower abdominal pain, hematuria, hemorrhagic chemical cystitis, vesical irritability.

NURSING IMPLICATIONS

Administration

- Use only under constant supervision by physicians experienced in therapy with cytotoxic agents.
- Avoid exposure of skin and respiratory tract to particles of thiotepa during solution preparation.
- Reconstitute with sterile water for injection. Usual dilution: 1.5 ml of diluent to vial containing 15 mg of drug (resultant solution: 10 mg/ml). Other diluents may result in hypertonic solutions which can cause irritation on injection.
- Following reconstitution, solution may be clear to slightly opaque. (If markedly opaque or contains a precipitate, do not use.) May be administered over 1–3 min without further dilution.
- Reconstituted solutions may be further diluted with 50–100 ml NaCl, dextrose, dextrose and sodium chloride, Ringer's or lactated Ringer's injection for IV infusion, or for intracavitary or perfusion therapy.
- Thiotepa may be mixed with procaine 2% and epinephrine 1:1000 for local administration.
- *Treatment of bladder tumor:* patient is dehydrated 8–12 h prior to treatment; following instillation, order may be given to reposition patient q15min for maximal area contact. Usual course of treatment is once a week for 4 wk; repeated beyond this with caution, because bone marrow depression may increase.
- Powder for injection and reconstituted solutions should be refrigerated at 2–8C (35–46F) and protected from light. Reconstituted solutions are stable for 5 d under refrigeration.

Common side effects in *italic;* life-threatening effects <u>underlined;</u>
generic names in **bold;** classifications in SMALL CAPS

999

Assessment & Drug Effects

- Most patients will manifest some evidence of toxicity; therefore close monitoring is essential.
- Because of cumulative effects, maximum myelosuppression may be delayed 3 or 4 wk after termination of therapy.
- Manufacturer recommends discontinuing therapy if leukocyte count falls to 3000/mm³ or below or if platelet count falls below 150,000/mm³.
- Hemoglobin level and leukocyte and thrombocyte counts should be determined at least weekly during therapy and for at least 3 wk after therapy is discontinued.
- Monitor leukocyte and thrombocyte counts as indicators for adaptations in nursing and drug regimens.

Patient & Family Education

- Discuss possibility of amenorrhea with patient (usually reversible in 6–8 mo).
- Warn patient to report onset of fever, bleeding, a cold or illness, no matter how mild; medical supervision may be necessary.

Prototype: chlorpromazine, p 191

THIOTHIXENE HYDROCHLORIDE

(thye-oh-thix´een)

Trade name: Navane
Classifications: CNS AGENT; PSYCHOTHERAPEUTIC; PHENOTHIAZINE ANTIPSYCHOTIC (TRANQUILIZER)
Pregnancy: Category C

ACTIONS/PHARMACODYNAMICS Thioxanthene derivative chemically and pharmacologically similar to chlorprothixene and the piperazine phenothiazines. Possesses sedative, adrenolytic, antiemetic, and weak anticholinergic activity.

USES Manifestations of psychotic disorders. **Unlabeled use:** antidepressant.

ROUTE & DOSAGE

Psychotic Disorders

Adult	PO	2 mg t.i.d.; may increase up to 15 mg/d as needed or tolerated (max 60 mg/d)
	IM	4 mg b.i.d. to q.i.d. (max 30 mg/d)

PHARMACOKINETICS **Absorption:** slowly absorbed from GI tract. **Onset:** days to weeks PO; 1–6 h IM. **Duration:** up to 12 h. **Distribution:** may remain in body for several weeks; crosses placenta. **Metabolism:** metabolized in liver. **Elimination:** half-life: 34 h; excreted in bile and feces.

CONTRAINDICATIONS & PRECAUTIONS **Contraindicated in:** hypersensitivity to thioxanthenes and phenothiazines, children < 12 y; comatose states; CNS depression; circulatory collapse; blood dyscrasias. Safe use during pregnancy (category C) not established. **Cautious use in:** history of convulsive disorders; alcohol withdrawal; glaucoma; prostatic hypertrophy; cardiovascular disease; patients who might be exposed to organophosphorous insecticides or to extreme heat; concomitant use of atropine or related drugs or ototoxic medications (especially ototoxic antibiotics); previously diagnosed breast cancer.

ADVERSE/SIDE EFFECTS *Drowsiness,* insomnia, dizziness, cerebral edema, convulsions, *extrapyramidal symptoms (dose related),* paradoxical exaggeration of psychotic symptoms; depressed cough reflex; xerostomia, constipation, tachycardia, *orthostatic hypotension* (especially with IM), impotence, gynecomastia, galactorrhea, amenorrhea, rash, contact dermatitis, photosensitivity, blurred vision, pigmentary retinopathy, decreased serum uric acid levels; sudden death, neuroleptic malignant syndrome, tardive dyskinesia.

DRUG INTERACTIONS **Alcohol** and other CNS DEPRESSANTS add to CNS depression.

NURSING IMPLICATIONS

Administration

- Oral concentrate contains 7% alcohol; it must be diluted just before administration in a cupful of water, fruit juice, carbonated beverage, milk, or soup.
- Capsule may be emptied and contents swallowed with water or mixed with food if patient prefers or if he or she is unable or unwilling to swallow the capsule.
- Administer IM injection deep into upper outer quadrant of buttock. Aspirate hypodermic carefully before injection. Rotate injection sites.
- If patient has suicidal tendency, do not permit access to more than one dose of medication; supervise its ingestion to prevent hoarding.
- Avoid contact of oral concentrate with skin and

Common side effects in *italic*; life-threatening effects underlined; generic names in **bold**; classifications in SMALL CAPS

clothing to prevent contact dermatitis. If concentrate spills, wash skin promptly with water.

- Store medication in light-resistant containers at 15–30C (56–89F) unless otherwise indicated.

Assessment & Drug Effects

- Although therapeutic response can be observed 1–6h following IM injection, it may be days or several weeks before there is a response with the oral preparation.
- Because of the possibility of orthostatic hypotension, patient receiving IM drug should be recumbent for at least 1 h following injection. Periodically check BP during this time.
- When thiothixene is added to the drug regimen of a patient on hypertensive treatment, monitor BP for excessive hypotensive response until drug therapy has been stabilized.
- Dosage adjustment may be necessary when patient is changed from IM to PO forms (capsules, concentrate).
- Hyperreflexia has been reported in infants delivered from mothers having received thiothixene.
- Periodic ophthalmic examinations and blood and hepatic function tests are advisable with prolonged therapy.
- Extrapyramidal effects (pseudoparkinsonism, akathisia, dystonia) may occur during early therapy. Report them to physician; dose adjustment or short-term therapy with an antiparkinsonism agent may provide relief.
- Be alert to first symptoms of tardive dyskinesia (see chap 3). Discontinue drug immediately and inform physician.

Patient & Family Education

- Because of danger of lightheadedness, advise patient to make position changes slowly, particularly from recumbent to upright, and to sit a few minutes before ambulation. Supervise ambulation if necessary.
- Mild drowsiness, common during first few days of drug therapy, usually subsides with continued treatment. Caution patient to avoid potentially hazardous activities until response to drug is known.
- Warn patient to avoid alcohol and other depressants during therapy.
- Counsel patient to take drug as prescribed and not to alter dosing regimen or stop medication without consulting physician. Abrupt discontinuation can cause delirium.
- Advise patient that use of all OTC drugs should be approved by the physician during therapy with this drug.

- Inform patient that although hyperhydrosis is an uncomfortable side effect, it does not indicate need to terminate therapy.
- Advise patient to avoid excessive exposure to sunlight to prevent a photosensitivity reaction. If sun exposure is expected, protect skin with sunscreen lotion (SPF 12 or above).

THROMBIN

Trade names: Fibrindex, Thrombinar, Thrombostat
Classifications: BLOOD FORMER & COAGULATOR; HEMOSTATIC
Pregnancy: Category C

ACTIONS/PHARMACODYNAMICS   Sterile plasma protein prepared from prothrombin of bovine origin. Induces clotting of whole blood or a fibrinogen solution without addition of other substances. Converts fibrinogen to thrombin. Potency standardized and expressed in terms of NIH units (1 NIH unit is amount required to clot 1 ml of standardized fibrinogen solution in 15 seconds).

USES When oozing of blood from capillaries and small venules is accessible, as in dental extraction, plastic surgery, grafting procedures, and epistaxis; also to shorten bleeding time at puncture sites in heparinized patient (i.e., following hemodialysis).

ROUTE & DOSAGE

Oozing Blood

Adult	Topical	100–2000 NIH U/ml, depending on extent of bleeding; may be used as solution, in dry form, by mixing thrombin with blood plasma to form a fibrin "glue," or in conjunction with absorbable gelatin sponge.

CONTRAINDICATIONS & PRECAUTIONS Contraindicated in: known hypersensitivity to any of drug components or to material of bovine origin, parenteral use, entry or infiltration into large blood vessels, pregnancy (category C).

ADVERSE/SIDE EFFECTS Sensitivity, allergic and febrile reactions, intravascular clotting and death when thrombin is allowed to enter large blood vessels.

Common side effects in *italic*; life-threatening effects underlined; generic names in **bold**; classifications in SMALL CAPS

1001

NURSING IMPLICATIONS

Administration

- Sponge recipient area free of blood before applying thrombin.
- Solutions may be prepared in sterile distilled water or isotonic saline.
- Solutions should be used within a few hours of preparation. If several hours are to elapse between time of preparation and use, solution should be refrigerated, or preferably frozen, and used within 48 h.
- Store lyophilized preparation at 2–8C (36–46F).

Prototype: levothyroxine sodium, p 244

THYROGLOBULIN

(thye-roe-glob´yoo-lin)
Trade name: Proloid
Classifications: HORMONE; THYROID AGENT
Pregnancy: Category A

ACTIONS/PHARMACODYNAMICS Obtained from purified extract of hog thyroid; contains levothyroxine (T_4) and liothyronine (T_3) in approximate ratio of 2.5:1. Clinical effects similar to those of thyroid.

USES Thyroid replacement therapy of all forms of hypothyroidism. Has no clinical advantage over thyroid.

ROUTE & DOSAGE

Hypothyroidism

Adult	PO	32–200 mg/d, starting with lower doses and gradually increasing at 1–2 wk intervals
Child	PO	> 4 mo: 60–180 mg/d
		1–4 mo: 30–45 mg/d

CONTRAINDICATIONS & PRECAUTIONS Contraindicated in: MI. **Cautious use in:** myxedema (such patients are extremely sensitive to thyroid), uncorrected adrenal insufficiency, pregnancy (category A).

ADVERSE/SIDE EFFECTS Signs and symptoms of hyperthyroidism (see chap 3).

DRUG INTERACTIONS Cholestyramine, colistipol decrease absorption of thyroglobulin; **epinephrine, norepinephrine** increase risk of cardiac

insufficiency; ORAL ANTICOAGULANTS may potentiate hypoprothrombinemia.

NURSING IMPLICATIONS

Administration

- Tablet may be crushed before administration and taken with fluid or mixed with food.
- Dosage highly individualized according to thyroid status.
- ***Transfer from thyroglobulin to liothyronine:*** thyroglobulin is discontinued and therapy initiated with low daily dose of liothyronine; in the reverse situation, thyroglobulin replacement precedes complete withdrawal of liothyronine by several days to prevent relapse.
- Drug is stable when stored at room temperature.

Assessment & Drug Effects

- Thyroid status may be assessed by thyroid function tests.
- Dosage is adjusted to maintain protein-bound iodine at 4–8 μg/dl.

Prototype: levothyroxine, p 244

THYROID

(thye´roid)
Trade names: Armour Thyroid, Thyrar, Westthroid
Classifications: HORMONE; THYROID AGENT
Pregnancy: Category A

ACTIONS/PHARMACODYNAMICS Preparation of desiccated animal thyroid gland containing active thyroid hormones, *l*-thyroxine (T_4) and *l*-triiodothyronine (T_3); total iodine content 0.17–0.23%. Action mechanism unknown; T_4 is largely converted to T_3, which exerts principal effects. Influences growth and maturation of various tissues (including skeletal and CNS) at critical periods. Promotes a generalized increase in metabolic rate of body tissues, producing increases in the rate of carbohydrate, protein, and fat metabolism, enzyme system activity, oxygen consumption, respiratory rate, body temperature, cardiac output, heart rate, blood volume. Thyroid affects water and ion transport and directly promotes synthesis and transcription of nuclear RNA. Potentiates actions of catecholamines; e.g., many prominent features of hyperthyroidism (tachycardia, lid lag and tremor) represent increased catecholamine effects.

Therapeutic effects are slow to be realized and prolonged.

USES Replacement or substitution therapy in primary hypothyroidism (cretinism, myxedema, simple goiter, deficiency states in pregnancy and in the elderly) and secondary hypothyroidism caused by surgery, excess radiation, or antithyroid drug therapy. May be given as adjunct to antithyroid agents when it is desirable to limit release of thyrotropic hormones and to prevent goitrogenesis and hypothyroidism.

ROUTE & DOSAGE

Mild to Moderate Hypothyroidism

Adult	PO	60 mg/d; may increase q30d to 60–180 mg/d

Severe Hypothyroidism

Adult	PO	15 mg/d; increased q2wk to 60 mg/d; then may increase q30d if needed
Child	PO	15 mg/d; may increase by 15 mg q2wk if needed

PHARMACOKINETICS Absorption: variably absorbed from GI tract. **Peak:** 1–3 wk. **Distribution:** does not readily cross placenta; minimal amounts in breast milk. **Metabolism:** deiodinated in thyroid gland. **Elimination:** half-life: T_3, 1–2 d; T_4, 6–7 d; excreted in urine and feces.

CONTRAINDICATIONS & PRECAUTIONS Contraindicated in: thyrotoxicosis; acute MI uncomplicated by hypothyroidism, cardiovascular disease; morphologic hypogonadism; nephrosis; uncorrected hypoadrenalism. **Cautious use in:** angina pectoris, hypertension, elderly patients who may have occult cardiac disease; renal insufficiency; pregnancy (category A); concomitant administration of catecholamines; diabetes mellitus; hyperthyroidism (history of); malabsorption states.

ADVERSE/SIDE EFFECTS Chronic overdosage: hyperthyroidism. **Massive overdosage:** thyroid storm: high temperature (as high as 41C [106F]), tachycardia, vomiting, shock, coma. **Overdosage** (thyrotoxicosis): staring expression in eyes, CHF, angina, cardiac arrhythmias, palpitation, tachycardia; weight loss, tremors, headache, nervousness, fever, diarrhea or abdominal cramps, insomnia, warm and moist skin, heat intolerance, leg cramps, menstrual irregularities, shock, changes in appetite, hyperglycemia (usually offset by increased tissue oxidation of sugar).

DIAGNOSTIC TEST INTERFERENCES Thyroid increases *basal metabolic rate;* may increase *blood glucose levels, creatine phosphokinase, AST, LDH, PBI.* It may decrease *serum uric acid, cholesterol, thyroid stimulating hormone (TSH), iodine 131* uptake. Many medications may produce false results in thyroid function tests.

DRUG INTERACTIONS ORAL ANTICOAGULANTS potentiate hypoprothrombinemia; may increase requirements for **insulin,** SULFONYLUREAS; **epinephrine** may precipitate coronary insufficiency; **cholestyramine** may decrease thyroid absorption.

NURSING IMPLICATIONS

Administration

- Take as a single dose, preferably on an empty stomach.
- *Transfer from thyroid treatment to liothyronine:* discontinue thyroid and initiate treatment with low daily dose of liothyronine; transfer in reverse direction: therapy initiated with replacement several days before complete withdrawal of liothyronine to avoid collapse.
- Generally dosage is initiated at low level and systematically increased in small increments to desired maintenance dose.
- Store in dark bottle to minimize spontaneous deiodination. Keep desiccated thyroid dry. Potency in this form reportedly persists for as long as 17 y.

Assessment & Drug Effects

- During institution of treatment, observe patient carefully for untoward reactions such as angina, palpitations, cardiac pain.
- Be alert for symptoms of overdosage (see adverse/side effects) that may occur 1–3 wk after therapy is started. If they develop, treatment should be interrupted for several days and restarted with reduced dosage.
- Hypothyroidism is common in the elderly. Women generally require less thyroxine replacement than men. Monitor response until regimen is stabilized to prevent iatrogenic hyperthyroidism. In drug-induced hyperthyroidism, there may also be increased bone loss. Such a patient is vulnerable to pathologic fractures.
- Earliest clinical response to thyroid (adult) is diuresis, accompanied by loss of weight and puffiness, followed by sense of well-being, increased pulse rate, increased pulse pressure, increased appetite, increased psychomotor activity, loss of constipa-

tion, normalization of skin texture and hair, and increased T_3 and T_4 serum levels.

- Pulse rate is an important clue to drug effectiveness. Count pulse before each dose during period of dosage adjustment. Consult physician if rate is 100 or more or if there has been a marked change in rate or rhythm.
- Free thyroxine index (FTI) and total serum thyroxine concentration (RT_3U) q3mo are usual during dose adjustment period.
- If patient has taken hormone during pregnancy, dose is frequently discontinued in the postpartum period, with evaluation of thyroid function 6 wk later.
- Toxic effects of thyroid develop slowly and disappear gradually. T_4 effects require up to 3–6 wk to dissipate; T_3 effects last 6–14 d after drug withdrawal.

Patient & Family Education

- Instruct patient to adhere to established dosage regimen; the dose intervals should not be changed without approval of the physician.
- Emphasize that replacement therapy for hypothyroidism is life-long; therefore, continued follow-up surveillance is important.
- The patient should not change brands of thyroid unless physician approves. Hormone content varies among brands.
- When patient is euthyroid, teach him or her to take own pulse and to record it periodically. If rate begins to increase or if rhythm changes, patient should notify physician.
- Onset of chest pain or other signs of aggravated CV disease (dyspnea, tachycardia) should be reported promptly.
- If patient is receiving anticoagulant therapy, a decrease in the requirement usually develops within 1–4 wk after starting treatment with thyroid. Close monitoring of prothrombin time (*normal:* 9–11 seconds) is necessary. Warn patient to report evidence of excess anticoagulant, evidenced by ecchymoses, petechiae, purpura, unexplained bleeding.
- Serial height measurement of the juvenile being treated with thyroid is an important means of monitoring influence of thyroid on growth.
- Prepare parent and juvenile hypothyroid patient for a dramatic response to therapy, e.g., initial rapid weight loss and catch-up growth.

THYROTROPIN

(thye-roe-troe´pin)
Trade name: Thytropar
Classifications: HORMONE; THYROID AGENT; DIAGNOSTIC AGENT; ANTINEOPLASTIC
Pregnancy: Category C

ACTIONS/PHARMACODYNAMICS Highly purified thyrotropic hormone (TSH) isolated from bovine anterior pituitary. Increases iodine uptake by the thyroid and stimulates formation and secretion of thyroid hormone. May cause hyperplasia of thyroid cells, a rapidly reversible effect.

USES Diagnostic tool to determine subclinical hypothyroidism or low thyroid reserve, to assess need for continued thyroid medication, to differentiate primary and secondary hypothyroidism, and to detect remnants and metastases of thyroid carcinoma. Also used therapeutically in management of selected types of thyroid carcinoma and adjunctively with iodine 131 to promote uptake of the radioactive substance by the thyroid.

ROUTE & DOSAGE

Diagnosis: Subclinical Hypothyroidism
Adult   IM/SC   10 IU

Differential Diagnosis: Primary and Secondary Hypothyroidism
Adult   IM/SC   10 IU/d for 1–3 d

Diagnosis: Thyroid Cancer Remnant After Surgery
Adult   IM/SC   10 IU/d for 3–7 d

Therapy of Thyroid Cancer With Metastasis
Adult   IM/SC   10 IU/d for 3–8 d

PHARMACOKINETICS Elimination: half-life: 35 min in euthyroid; rapidly cleared by kidney.

CONTRAINDICATIONS & PRECAUTIONS Contraindicated in: coronary thrombosis, pregnancy (category C). **Cautious use in:** angina pectoris, cardiac failure; hypopituitarism; adrenocortical suppression.

ADVERSE/SIDE EFFECTS Menstrual irregularities, fever, headache, nausea, vomiting, urticaria, transient hypotension, tachycardia, atrial fibrillation, thyroid swelling (especially with large doses), postinjection flare, anaphylactic reactions, induced or exaggerated angina pectoris or CHF. **Overdosage:** fever, tachycardia, vomiting, shock, coma.

NURSING IMPLICATIONS

Administration

- Ten international units lyophilized powder are dis-
  ~~solved in 2 ml sterile physiologic saline solution for~~
  injection.
- Thyrotropin is stable at room temperature when
  kept dry. Retains potency in solution at least 2 wk
  if refrigerated.

Assessment & Drug Effects

- Diagnostic tests may be made even though patient
  is receiving thyroid hormone therapy.
- *Diagnostic use:* in presence of normal thyroid tissue,
  stimulation provided by daily doses of 10 IU thyrotropin for 1–3 d causes an elevated serum thyroxine level and increased radioactive iodine uptake (RAI) by thyroid gland. If hypothyroidism is
  primary, there will be no change in RAI uptake following several days of thyrotropin stimulation.
  Conversely, there will be a significant increase in
  RAI uptake if hypothyroidism is secondary to hypopituitarism.

Prototype: penicillin G potassium, p 71

TICARCILLIN DISODIUM

(ti-car-sill´in)
Trade name: Ticar
Classifications: ANTIINFECTIVE; PENICILLIN
ANTIBIOTIC
Pregnancy: Category C

ACTIONS/PHARMACODYNAMICS Ticarcillin
disodium is a semisynthetic injectable penicillin. It is
bactericidal against gram-positive and gram-negative
organisms. Susceptible organisms include *Pseudomonas aeruginosa, Escherichia coli, Proteus mirabilis, Proteus vulgaris, Enterobacter* species,
*Haemophilus influenzae, Staphylococcus pneumo-
niae.*

USES Primarily for gram-negative bacterial infections, Bacterial septicemia, skin and soft-tissue infections, acute and chronic respiratory infections, genitourinary tract infection by susceptible organisms,
intraabdominal infections and infections of the female pelvis and reproductive system.

PHARMACOKINETICS Peak: 1–2 h IM. **Distribution:** low concentrations in CSF unless meninges are

inflamed; crosses placenta; distributed into breast
milk. **Elimination:** half-life: 67 min; 80–90% excreted
unchanged in urine within 24 h.

ROUTE & DOSAGE

Urinary Tract Infections

Adult	IM/IV	200 mg/kg/d in 4 divided doses or 1–2 g q6h
Child	IM/IV	50–200 mg/kg/d in 4 divided doses

Systemic Infections

Adult	IM/IV	15–40 g/d in 6 divided doses (max 40 g/d)
Child	IM/IV	250–500 mg/kg/d in 6 divided doses (max 40 g/d)

**CONTRAINDICATIONS & PRECAUTIONS Con-
traindicated in:** history of allergic reaction to any penicillin. **Cautious use in:** allergy to cephalosporins, pregnancy (category C).

ADVERSE/SIDE EFFECTS Hypersensitivity reactions. **CNS:** headache, blurred vision, mental deterioration, convulsions, hallucinations, seizures, giddiness, neuromuscular hyperirritability. **GI:** *diarrhea,
nausea,* vomiting, disturbances of taste or smell,
stomatitis, flatulence. **Hematologic:** eosinophilia,
thrombocytopenia, leukopenia, neutropenia, hemolytic anemia. **Other:** pain, burning, swelling at injection site; phlebitis, thrombophlebitis; superinfections,
hypernatremia, transient increases in serum AST,
ALT, BUN, and alkaline phosphatase; increases in
serum LDH, bilirubin, and creatinine and decreased
serum uric acid.

INCOMPATIBILITIES Solution/Additive: AMINO-
GLYCOSIDES, **amphotericin B, bleomycin, chloramphenicol, cytarabine, doxapram, lincomycin,** TETRACYCLINES, **vitamin B complex with C.
Y-Site:** AMINOGLYCOSIDES, **promethazine.**

NURSING IMPLICATIONS

Administration

- Intramuscular injections should not exceed 2 g/per
  injection.
- In children weighing less than 40 kg, data is insufficient to recommend an optimum dose.
- *IM injection:* reconstitute each 1 g of ticarcillin with
  2 ml of sterile water for injection, or NaCl injection
  and use promptly. Resulting concentration is 1
  g/2.6 ml.

Common side effects in *italic*; life-threatening effects <u>underlined</u>;
generic names in **bold**; classifications in SMALL CAPS

1005

- **IV administration:** reconstitute each 1 g of ticarcillin with 4 ml of sterile water for injection. Dilute reconstituted solution further with at least 20 ml of D5W, NS, or other compatible IV solution.
- Give direct IV as slowly as possible to avoid vein irritation. A dilution of 1 g/20 ml or more solution will reduce the incidence of vein irritation.
- Administer intermittent IV solutions over 30–120 min in equally divided doses.
- Solutions refrigerated longer than 72 h should **not** be used for multidose purposes.
- Store dry powder at room temperature or below.

Assessment & Drug Effects

- Culture and susceptibility tests should be done before initiating therapy; ticarcillin may be started pending results.
- Frequently assess IV access site for vein irritation and phlebitis.
- Some patients receiving high doses of ticarcillin may develop hemorrhagic manifestations associated with abnormalities of coagulation tests, such as bleeding time and platelet aggregation. If bleeding manifestations occur, ticarcillin should be discontinued.
- During prolonged treatment with ticarcillin, renal and hepatic functions studies should be monitored.
- Electrolyte and cardiac status should be monitored because of the high sodium content in ticarcillin.
- Monitor for hypokalemia (see Signs & Symptoms, chap 3). Serum potassium levels should be determined periodically.
- Serious and sometimes fatal anaphylactoid reactions have been reported in patients with penicillin hypersensitivity or with history of sensitivity to multiple allergens.

Patient & Family Education

- Frequent bacteriologic tests and clinical evaluation are necessary during treatment for chronic urinary tract infections and may be required for several months after therapy has been discontinued. Urge patients to keep all appointments.
- Instruct patient to immediately report urticaria, rashes, or pruritus.
- Instruct patient to report frequent loose stools, diarrhea, or other possible signs of pseudomembranous colitis (see chap 3).

Prototype: penicillin G potassium, p 71

TICARCILLIN DISODIUM/CLAVULANATE POTASSIUM

(tye-kar-sill´in/clav-yoo´la-nate)
Trade name: Timentin
Classifications: ANTIINFECTIVE; PENICILLIN ANTIBIOTIC
Pregnancy: Category B

ACTIONS/PHARMACODYNAMICS Injectable extended spectrum penicillin and fixed combination of ticarcillin disodium with the potassium salt of clavulanic acid, a beta-lactamase inhibitor produced by fermentation of *Streptomyces clavuligerus.* Used alone, clavulanic acid antibacterial activity is weak but in combination with ticarcillin prevents degradation by beta-lactamase and extends ticarcillin spectrum of activity against many strains of beta-lactamase-producing bacteria (synergistic effect). Synergism between the two drugs does not occur against organisms susceptible to ticarcillin alone. Susceptible strains of organisms include beta-lactamase strains of *Klebsiella* sp, *Escherichia coli, Staphylococcus aureus, Pseudomonas aeruginosa, Haemophilus influenzae, Citrobacter* sp, *Enterobacter cloacae, Serratia marcescens.* May be effectively combined with aminoglycoside antibiotics to treat certain strains of *P. aeruginosa* in patients with impaired host defenses.

USES Infections of lower respiratory tract and urinary tract and skin and skin structures, infections of bone and joint, and septicemia caused by susceptible organisms. Also mixed infections and as presumptive therapy before identification of causative organism.

ROUTE & DOSAGE

Moderate to Severe Infections

Adult	IV/IM	> 60 kg: 3.1 g q4–6h
Child	IV/IM	200–300 mg/kg/d divided q4–6h

PHARMACOKINETICS Distribution: widely distributed with highest concentrations in urine and bile; crosses placenta; distributed into breast milk. **Metabolism:** slightly metabolized in liver. **Elimination:** half-life: 1.1–1.2 h ticarcillin, 1.1–1.5 h clavulanate; excreted in urine.

CONTRAINDICATIONS & PRECAUTIONS Contraindicated in: hypersensitivity to penicillins or to cephalosporins. Safe use during pregnancy (category B) and in children < 12 y not established. **Cautious use in:** nursing women.

ADVERSE/SIDE EFFECTS See ticarcillin disodium, p 1005.

DIAGNOSTIC TEST INTERFERENCES May interfere with test methods used to determine *urinary proteins* except for tests for urinary protein that use bromphenol blue. Positive direct *antiglobulin (Coombs')* test results, apparently caused by clavulanic acid, have been reported. This test may interfere with transfusion cross-matching procedures.

DRUG INTERACTIONS May increase risk of bleeding with ANTICOAGULANTS; **probenecid** decreases elimination of ticarcillin.

INCOMPATIBILITIES Solution/Additive: AMINOGLYCOSIDES, **doxapram. Y-Site:** AMINOGLYCOSIDES.

NURSING IMPLICATIONS

Administration

- Reconstitute IV solution by adding to 3.1 g of powder 13 ml sterile water for injection or NaCl injection; shake until drug is dissolved. Resulting concentration: 200 mg/ml ticarcillin with 6.7 mg/ml clavulanic acid. Further dilute solution with NaCl injection, 5% dextrose injection, or lactated Ringer's injection. Inspect reconstituted and diluted solution: do not use if discoloration or particulate matter is present.
- Administer IV infusion over 30 min by direct infusion or through Y-type IV infusion set already in place.
- IV solutions of ticarcillin and clavulanate potassium are incompatible with sodium bicarbonate.
- Oral probenecid administered shortly before or concomitantly with ticarcillin and clavulanate potassium slows renal tubular secretion rate, resulting in higher and prolonged serum concentration of ticarcillin.
- Store vial with sterile powder: 21–24C (69–75F) or colder. If exposed to higher temperature, powder will darken, indicating degradation of clavulanate potassium and loss of potency. Discard vial. See package insert for information about storage and stability of reconstituted and diluted IV solutions of drug.

Assessment & Drug Effects

- Culture and susceptibility tests should be done before therapy is begun; however, ticarcillin/clavu-

lanate potassium may be started pending laboratory results.

- Serious and sometimes fatal anaphylactoid reactions have been reported in patient with penicillin hypersensitivity or with history of sensitivity to multiple allergens. Reported incidence is low with this combination drug.
- Generally, treatment is continued for at least 2 d after signs and symptoms have disappeared (usually 10–14 d).
- Frequent bacteriologic tests and clinical evaluation are necessary during treatment for chronic urinary tract infections and may be required for several months after therapy has been discontinued. Urge patient to keep all appointments.
- *Overdose symptoms:* may cause neuromuscular hyperirritability or seizures.

See ticarcillin disodium for Patient & Family Education, p 1006.

Prototype: propranolol, p 109

TIMOLOL MALEATE

(tye´moe-lole)

Trade names: Blocadren, Timoptic

Classifications: AUTONOMIC NERVOUS SYSTEM AGENT; BETA-ADRENERGIC ANTAGONIST (SYMPATHOLYTIC, BLOCKING AGENT); ANTIHYPERTENSIVE; EYE PREPARATION, MIOTIC (ANTIGLAUCOMA AGENT)

Pregnancy: Category C

ACTIONS/PHARMACODYNAMICS Nonselective beta-adrenergic blocking agent similar to propranolol in actions but approximately 5–10 times as potent. Demonstrates antihypertensive, antiarrhythmic, and antianginal properties, and suppresses plasma renin activity. Unlike propranolol, appears to lack quinidinelike (local anesthetic or membrane-stabilizing) effects. The first beta-adrenergic blocking agent to be approved for treatment of the post-MI patient. When applied topically, lowers elevated and normal intraocular pressure (IOP) by unknown mechanism but appears to act by reducing formation of aqueous humor and possibly by increasing outflow. In contrast to pilocarpine and other miotics, timolol does not constrict pupil and therefore does not cause night blindness, and it does not affect accommodation or visual acuity. Reportedly as effective as pilocarpine or epinephrine in reducing IOP and produces fewer and less severe adverse effects.

Common side effects in *italic*; life-threatening effects underlined; generic names in **bold**; classifications in SMALL CAPS

1007

USES Topically (ophthalmic solution) to reduce elevated IOP in chronic, open-angle glaucoma, aphakic glaucoma, secondary glaucoma, and ocular hypertension. May be used alone or in conjunction with epinephrine, pilocarpine, or a carbonic anhydrase inhibitor such as acetazolamide. Oral preparation is used as step 1 antihypertensive agent in monotherapy or in combination with a thiazide diuretic to prevent reinfarction after MI and to treat mild hypertension. **Unlabeled uses:** prophylactic management of stable, uncomplicated angina pectoris and migraine headaches.

ROUTE & DOSAGE

Glaucoma

Adult	Topical	1 drop of 0.25–0.5% solution b.i.d.; may be able to decrease to once/d

Hypertension

Adult	PO	10 mg b.i.d.; may increase to 60 mg/d in 2 divided doses

Angina

Adult	PO	15–45 mg in 3 divided doses

PHARMACOKINETICS Absorption: 90% absorbed from GI tract; 50% reaches systemic circulation; some systemic absorption from topical application. **Peak:** 1–2 h PO; 1–5 h topical. **Distribution:** distributed into breast milk. **Metabolism:** 80% metabolized in liver to inactive metabolites. **Elimination:** excreted in urine.

CONTRAINDICATIONS & PRECAUTIONS Contraindicated in: Bronchospasm, severe COPD, bronchial asthma, heart failure. Safe use during pregnancy (category C), in nursing mothers, and in children not established. **Cautious use in:** bronchitis, patients subject to bronchospasm; sinus bradycardia, greater than first degree heart block, cardiogenic shock, right ventricular failure secondary to pulmonary hypertension; myasthenia gravis; concomitant use with adrenergic augmenting drugs, e.g., MAO inhibitors.

ADVERSE/SIDE EFFECTS CNS: fatigue, lethargy, weakness, somnolence, anxiety, headache, dizziness, confusion, psychic dissociation, depression. **CV:** palpitation, bradycardia, hypotension, syncope, AV conduction disturbances, CHF. **Eye:** *eye irritation* including conjunctivitis, blepharitis, keratitis, blurred vision (rare), superficial punctate keratopathy. **GI:** anorexia, dyspepsia, nausea. **Hypersensitivity:** rash, urticaria. **Other:** difficulty in breathing, fever, bronchospasm, hypoglycemia, hypokalemia, aggravation of peripheral vascular insufficiency.

DRUG INTERACTIONS ANTIHYPERTENSIVE AGENTS, DIURETICS potentiate hypotensive effects; NSAIDs may antagonize hypotensive effects.

NURSING IMPLICATIONS

Administration

- Tablet may be crushed before administration and taken with fluid of patient's choice.
- Apply gentle pressure to lacrimal sac during and immediately following drug instillation for about 1 min to lessen possibility of systemic absorption.
- Solution can be applied safely in glaucoma patient who wears conventional hard contact lenses.
- Store at 15–30C (59–86F) in tight, light-resistant container unless otherwise directed.

Assessment & Drug Effects

- Check pulse before administering timolol, topical or oral. If there are extremes (rate or rhythm), withhold medication and call the physician.
- Monitor pulse rate and BP at regular intervals in patients with severe heart disease.
- When drug is instilled in one eye only, IOP in opposite eye may be reduced slightly also.
- Some patients develop tolerance during long-term therapy.

Patient & Family Education

- Inform patient that drug may cause slight reduction in resting heart rate. Patient should be informed about usual pulse rate and should be instructed to report significant changes. Consult physician for parameters.
- IOP must be monitored throughout ophthalmic therapy.
- Emphasize importance of adhering to regimen exactly as prescribed. Drug should not be withdrawn abruptly; angina may be exacerbated. Dosage is reduced over a period of 1 or 2 wk.
- Advise patient to report difficulty in breathing promptly. Drug withdrawal may be indicated.

Prototype: gentamicin, p 53

TOBRAMYCIN SULFATE
(toe-bra-mye´sin)
Trade names: Nebcin, Tobrex
Classifications: ANTIINFECTIVE; AMINOGLYCOSIDE ANTIBIOTIC
Pregnancy: Category D

ACTIONS/PHARMACODYNAMICS Broad-spectrum, aminoglycoside antibiotic derived from *Streptomyces tenebrarius*. Closely related to gentamicin in spectrum of antibacterial activity and pharmacologic properties. Reportedly causes less nephrotoxicity than gentamicin, but incidence of ototoxicity is similar. Cross-allergenicity and some cross-resistance among aminoglycosides have been demonstrated. Has greater antibiotic activity against *Pseudomonas aeruginosa* than other aminoglycosides.

USES Treatment of severe infections caused by susceptible organisms.

ROUTE & DOSAGE

Moderate to Severe Infections (All Doses Based on Ideal Body Weight)

Adult	IV	3 mg/kg/d divided q8h up to 5 mg/kg/d infused over 20–60 min
	IM	3 mg/kg/d divided q8h up to 5 mg/kg/d
	Topical	1–2 drops in affected eye q1–4h
Child	IV	3 mg/kg/d divided q8h up to 5 mg/kg/d infused over 20–60 min
		≤1 wk: up to 4 mg/kg/d divided q18–24h infused over 20–60 min
	IM	3 mg/kg/d divided q8h up to 5 mg/kg/d

PHARMACOKINETICS Peak: 30–90 min IM. **Duration:** up to 8 h. **Distribution:** crosses placenta; accumulates in renal cortex. **Elimination:** half-life: 2–3 h in adults; excreted in urine.

CONTRAINDICATIONS & PRECAUTIONS Contraindicated in: history of hypersensitivity to tobramycin and other aminoglycoside antibiotics. Safe use during pregnancy (category D) and in nursing mothers not established. **Cautious use in:** impaired renal function; premature and neonatal infants; concurrent use with other neurotoxic or nephrotoxic agents or potent diuretics.

ADVERSE/SIDE EFFECTS Neurotoxicity (including ototoxicity), *nephrotoxicity,* increased AST, ALT, LDH, serum bilirubin; anemia, fever, rash, pruritus, urticaria, nausea, vomiting, headache, lethargy, superinfections; hypersensitivity. Eye: *burning, stinging of eye after drug instillation;* lid itching and edema.

DRUG INTERACTIONS ANESTHETICS, SKELETAL MUSCLE RELAXANTS add to neuromuscular blocking effects; **acyclovir, amphotericin B, bacitracin,** capreomycin, CEPHALOSPORINS, **colistin, cisplatin, carboplatin, methoxyflurane, polymyxin B, vancomycin, furosemide, ethacrynic acid** increased risk of ototoxicity, nephrotoxicity.

INCOMPATIBILITIES Solution/Additive: alcohol 5% in dextrose, CEPHALOSPORINS, PENICILLINS, **clindamycin, heparin. Y-Site:** CEPHALOSPORINS, **clindamycin, penicillins, heparin.**

NURSING IMPLICATIONS

Administration

- Each IV dose is diluted in 50–100 ml or more of D5W, 0.9% NaCl, or D5/0.9% NaCl. Concentration should not exceed 1 mg/ml.
- Infuse diluted solution over 20–60 min.
- Tobramycin should not be mixed with other drugs.
- Wash hands before and after instillation of eye medication.
- Apply gentle finger pressure to lacrimal sac for 1 min after drug has been instilled in eye.
- Prior to reconstitution, store vial at 15–30C (59–86F). After reconstitution, solution may be refrigerated and used within 96 h. If kept at room temperature, use within 24 h.

Assessment & Drug Effects

- Weigh patient before treatment for calculation of dosage (by physician).
- Bacterial culture and susceptibility tests are advised prior to and during tobramycin therapy.
- As with other aminoglycosides, patient receiving tobramycin must remain under close clinical observation because of the high potential for toxicity, even in conventional doses.
- Monitoring of serum drug concentrations is advised to minimize rise of toxicity. Prolonged serum concentrations above 12 µg/ml are not recommended.
- Renal, auditory, and vestibular functions should also be closely monitored, particularly in patients with known or suspected renal impairment and patients receiving high doses.
- Drug-induced auditory changes are irreversible (may be partial or total); usually bilateral. In cochlear damage the patient may be asymptomatic, and partial or bilateral deafness may continue to develop even after therapy has been discontinued.
- Evidence of renal insufficiency or ototoxicity (see Signs & Symptoms, chap 3) or vestibular damage indicates need for discontinuation of drug or dosage adjustment.
- Monitor I&O. Report oliguria, changes in I&O ratio, and cloudy or frothy urine (may indicate protein-

Common side effects in *italic;* life-threatening effects underlined; generic names in **bold**; classifications in SMALL CAPS

1009

uria). The elderly patient is especially susceptible to renal toxicity. Patient is usually kept well hydrated to prevent chemical irritation in renal tubules. Consult physician.

- Therapy is generally continued for 7–10 d. Complicated infection may require longer course of therapy, in which case close monitoring of renal, auditory, and vestibular function and serum drug concentrations is essential.
- Monitor patient with neuromuscular disorder (e.g., myasthenia gravis) for muscular weakness. Observe ambulation and assist if necessary.
- *Ophthalmic:* prolonged use of ophthalmic solution may encourage superinfection with nonsusceptible organisms including fungi.
- *Overdose symptoms for eye medication:* increased lacrimation, keratitis, edema and itching of eye lids. Report symptoms to physician.

Patient & Family Education
- Advise patient to report symptoms of superinfections (see chap 3). Prompt treatment with an antibiotic or antifungal medication may be necessary.
- Instruct to report signs & symptoms of hearing loss, tinnitus, or vertigo.

Prototype: procainamide, p 140

TOCAINIDE HYDROCHLORIDE
(toe-kay′nide)
Trade name: Tonocard
Classifications: CARDIOVASCULAR AGENT; ANTIARRHYTHMIC
Pregnancy: Category C

ACTIONS/PHARMACODYNAMICS
Antiarrhythmic agent (class IB) and analog of lidocaine, with similar electrophysiologic characteristics and hemodynamic properties. Effective orally. Suppresses PVCs and may have particular use in arrhythmias associated with a prolonged QT interval that do not respond to quinidine-like antiarrhythmics (class IA). Decreases active potential duration in Purkinje fibers and slightly decreases resting membrane potential. Shortens effective refractory periods of atria, AV node, and ventricles without affecting AV conduction. QRS and QT intervals do not change. Exerts slight negative inotropic effect and slightly increases pulmonary and peripheral vascular resistance. Chronic oral therapy rarely precipitates cardiac decompensation; however, it has not been shown to prevent sudden death in patients with serious ventricular ectopic activity.

USES Refractory ventricular arrhythmia. To increase effectiveness, it may be combined with a class IA antiarrhythmic (e.g., quinidine, disopyramide) or with propranolol. Also used to prevent ventricular tachyarrhythmia after acute MI.

ROUTE & DOSAGE

Ventricular Arrhythmias

Adult	PO	1.2–1.8 g/d in 3 divided doses; may increase up to 2.4 g/d

PHARMACOKINETICS **Absorption:** rapidly and completely absorbed from GI tract. **Peak:** 0.5–2 h. **Distribution:** not fully known; does distribute into CNS. **Metabolism:** metabolized in liver. **Elimination:** half-life: 10–17 h; 70–80% excreted in urine within 72 h.

CONTRAINDICATIONS & PRECAUTIONS Contraindicated in: hypersensitivity to tocainide and to local anesthetics of the amide type; second- or third-degree AV block (in absence of artificial ventricular pacemaker), hypokalemia; myasthenia gravis; pregnancy (category C), nursing mothers. Safe use in children not established. **Cautious use in:** multiple drug therapy, known heart failure patient with minimum cardiac reserve; renal or hepatic disease.

ADVERSE/SIDE EFFECTS CNS: *tremors, dizziness, lightheadedness, visual disturbances, vertigo, tinnitus,* hearing loss, ataxia, paresthesia. **Rare:** agitation, memory loss, confusion, convulsions. **CV:** cardiac toxicity (rare): exacerbation of arrhythmias, complete heart block, sinus node slowing (in patient with preexisting conduction system disease); hypotension, palpitations, bradycardia, chest pain, left ventricular failure, PVCs, hot flashes. **GI:** nausea, vomiting, anorexia, abdominal pain, diarrhea, hepatitis (rare). **Respiratory:** pulmonary fibrosis, edema, embolism and alveolitis; pneumonia, dyspnea. **Skin:** (rare): rash, LE syndrome. **Other:** alopecia, sweating, night sweats, tiredness/drowsiness, sleepiness, hot/cold feelings, hematologic disorders (leukopenia, agranulocytosis, thrombocytopenia, hypoplastic anemia), claudication, cold extremities, leg cramps, urinary retention, polyuria, metallic or menthol taste, hiccups.

DRUG INTERACTIONS Lidocaine may increase risk of CNS toxicity, including seizures. BETA-BLOCKERS may lead to paranoia.

NURSING IMPLICATIONS

Administration

- Administer with food to decrease GI distress. This also protects against high peak concentration and toxicity because absorption rate is slowed. Bioavailability is not affected by food.
- When switching a patient from IV lidocaine to oral tocainide, give 600 mg oral dose of tocainide 6 h before stopping lidocaine and repeat 6 h later; then proceed to maintain therapy with tocainide.

Assessment & Drug Effects

- *Effective serum concentration:* 3.5–10 μg/ml.
- When steady-state drug level is attained (usually in about 70 h), plasma level monitoring is recommended, especially if patient has renal or hepatic dysfunction.
- Onset of tremors is a good clinical indicator that maximum dose is being approached.
- In patient with kidney or hepatic dysfunction, drug elimination is significantly decreased. Monitor I&O ratio and pattern. Instruct patient to report to physician if symptoms of renal dysfunction occur.
- Anticipate and report evidence of blood dyscrasia (see Signs & Symptoms, chap 3).
- Blood counts may be monitored during first 6 mo of treatment; abnormal counts usually stabilize within 1 mo after discontinuation of treatment.

Patient & Family Education

- The patient should fully understand what an irregular pulse signifies and how often it should be checked.
- Since drug may cause dizziness and drowsiness, warn to avoid driving and other potentially hazardous activities until drug response is known.
- Symptomatic bradycardia should be reported. Dose adjustment or discontinuation will follow.
- Advise to report promptly chest pain, exertional dyspnea, wheezing, and cough even if no fever is present. Pulmonary fibrosis is a serious side effect and should be ruled out. Drug is discontinued if pulmonary symptoms persist or if pulmonary disorder is diagnosed.

Prototype: tolbutamide, p 234

TOLAZAMIDE

(tole-az´a-mide)
Trade name: Tolinase
Classifications: HORMONE; SULFONYLUREA ANTIDIABETIC
Pregnancy: Category C

ACTIONS/PHARMACODYNAMICS Orally effective sulfonylurea hypoglycemic structurally and pharmacologically related to tolbutamide but about 5 times more potent (potency is about equal to that of chlorpropamide). Lowers blood glucose primarily by stimulating pancreatic beta cells to secrete insulin. As with other sulfonylureas, is ineffective in the absence of functioning beta cells. Contraindications, precautions, pharmacokinetics, and adverse effects as for tolbutamide.

USES Mild to moderately severe type II non-insulin-dependent diabetes mellitus (NIDDM) that cannot be controlled by diet and weight reduction and that is uncomplicated by acidosis, ketosis, coma. Effective in primary or secondary failures to other sulfonylurea.

ROUTE & DOSAGE

Non-insulin-Dependent Diabetes Mellitus

Adult	PO	100 mg–1 g q.d. to b.i.d. a.c.; may adjust dose by 100–250 mg/d at weekly intervals (max 1 g/d)

PHARMACOKINETICS Absorption: slowly absorbed from GI tract. **Onset:** 60 min. **Peak:** 4–6 h. **Duration:** 10–15 h (up to 20 h in some patients). **Distribution:** distributed in highest concentrations in liver, kidneys, and intestines; crosses placenta; distributed into breast milk. **Metabolism:** metabolized extensively in liver. **Elimination:** half-life: 7 h; 85% excreted in urine, 15% in feces.

CONTRAINDICATIONS & PRECAUTIONS Contraindicated in: known sensitivity to sulfonylureas and to sulfonamides, type I (IDDM) insulin-dependent diabetes, diabetes complicated by ketoacidosis; infection; trauma; pregnancy (category C); safe use in nursing mothers and in children not established.

Common side effects in *italic*; life-threatening effects <u>underlined</u>; generic names in **bold**; classifications in SMALL CAPS

1011

ADVERSE/SIDE EFFECTS Nausea, vomiting, hypoglycemia, vertigo, photosensitivity, agranulocytosis, cholestatic jaundice.

DRUG INTERACTIONS Alcohol elicits disulfiram–type reaction in some patients; ORAL ANTICOAGULANTS, **chloramphenicol, clofibrate, phenylbutazone,** MAO INHIBITORS, SALICYLATES, **probenecid,** SULFONAMIDES may potentiate hypoglycemic actions; THIAZIDES may antagonize hypoglycemic effects; **cimetidine** may increase tolazamide levels, causing hypoglycemia.

NURSING IMPLICATIONS

Administration

▪ Tablet may be crushed if patient is unable to swallow it whole. Be sure it is swallowed with an allowable fluid, not dry.
▪ When patient is newly diagnosed, dosage is guided by fasting blood sugar values: if less than 200 mg/dl, therapy is started with 100 mg/d before breakfast; if greater than 200 mg/dl, with 250 mg/d.
▪ *For conversion from insulin:* Patients receiving < 20 U of insulin can be placed directly on tolazamide 100 mg daily. Patients receiving < 40 U but > 20 U can be placed directly on 250 mg daily. For patients receiving > 40 U of insulin, dosage is reduced 50%, and patient is started on 250 mg of tolazamide. Dosage is then adjusted weekly or more often in patients who had received 40 U of insulin. Instruct patient to check urine 3 times daily for glucose and acetone and to report results to physician.
▪ Store at 15–30C (59–86F) in a tightly closed container unless otherwise directed. Keep drug out of the reach of children.

Assessment & Drug Effect

▪ Reduction of dose frequently alleviates most of the mild to moderately severe hypoglycemic symptoms.
▪ Unlike tolbutamide, tolazamide is effective in some patients with a history of ketoacidosis or coma; close observation of these patients is especially important during the early adjustment period.

Patient & Family Education

▪ Patient must be under close medical supervision for first 6 wk of treatment; should check urine daily for sugar and acetone.
▪ Doses > 1000 mg/d rarely provide improvement in diabetic control: patient then usually is maintained on insulin therapy only.

▪ Caution patient not to self-dose with OTC preparations unless approved or prescribed by physician.
▪ Be certain that patient understands that alcohol can precipitate a disulfiram-type reaction.

Prototype: prazosin, p 108

TOLAZOLINE HYDROCHLORIDE
(toe-laz´a-leen)
Trade name: Priscoline
Classifications: AUTONOMIC NERVOUS SYSTEM AGENT; ALPHA-ADRENERGIC ANTAGONIST (SYMPATHOLYTIC, BLOCKING AGENT); VASODILATOR
Pregnancy: Category C

ACTIONS/PHARMACODYNAMICS Imidazoline derivative structurally related to phentolamine. In addition to weak alpha-adrenergic blocking activity, beta-adrenergic action increases cardiac output and rate, cholinergic effect increases GI motility, and histaminelike activity stimulates gastric secretions and peripheral vasodilation. Vasodilation is primarily due to direct relaxant effect on vascular smooth muscle. Inhibits aldehyde dehydrogenase, and may increase or decrease pulmonary artery pressure and total pulmonary resistance.

USES Persistent pulmonary hypertension of the newborn. **Unlabeled uses:** To improve blood flow in thromboangiitis obliterans (Buerger's disease), diabetic arteriosclerosis gangrene, Raynaud's disease, causalgia, scleroderma, postthrombotic conditions, frostbite sequelae, and other peripheral vasospastic disorders; to improve visualization of vasculature during arteriography, treatment of neonatal hypoxemia, as diagnostic agent to differentiate vasospastic and obstruction components in occlusive peripheral vascular disease, and as a provocative test for glaucoma.

PHARMACOKINETICS Absorption: well absorbed from all routes. **Peak:** 30–60 min IM, SC. **Duration:** 3–4 h. **Elimination:** half-life: 1.5–41 h; excreted in urine.

CONTRAINDICATIONS & PRECAUTIONS Contraindicated in: following cerebrovascular accident; coronary artery disease; alcohol ingestion. Safe use during pregnancy (category C) and in nursing mothers not established. **Cautious use in:** gastritis, peptic ulcer (previous or current); mitral stenosis.

Common side effects in *italic*; life-threatening effects underlined; generic names in **bold**; classifications in SMALL CAPS

ROUTE & DOSAGE

Vasospastic Disorders

Adult	SC/IV/IM	10–50 mg q.i.d.
	Intraarterial	25 mg test dose infused slowly; then 50–75 mg 1–2 times/d Maintenance: 50–75 mg 2–3 times/wk

Improve Visualization of Vasculature

Adult	Intraarterial	12.5–50 mg prior to arteriography

Persistent Pulmonary Hypertension

Neonate	IV	1–2 mg/kg via scalp needle over 10 min followed by infusion of 1–2 mg/kg/h for 36–48 h

ADVERSE/SIDE EFFECTS CV: tachycardia, arrhythmias, anginal pain, postural hypotension, BP changes, marked hypertension (particularly following parenteral use). **GI:** nausea, vomiting, diarrhea, epigastric discomfort, *abdominal pain,* exacerbation of peptic ulcer. **Hematologic:** <u>agranulocytosis</u>, leukopenia, thrombocytopenia, pancytopenia. **Intraarterial administration:** *feeling of warmth or burning at injection site,* transient weakness, postural vertigo, palpitation, formication, apprehension, transient paradoxic impairment of blood supply, peripheral vasodilation. **Skin:** profuse, sweating, flushing, increased pilomotor activity with tingling and chilliness, rash. **Other:** mydriasis, edema, headache. **Severe overdosage:** hypotension progressing to shock.

DRUG INTERACTIONS Alcohol may elicit disulfiram-type reaction; **epinephrine, norepinephrine** may cause paradoxic fall in BP followed by rebound increase.

INCOMPATIBILITIES Solution/additive: ethacrynic acid.

NURSING IMPLICATIONS

Administration

- With neonate, administer initial dose of 1–2 mg/kg over 10–15 min via scalp vein using an infusion pump.
- With neonate, administer maintenance infusion of 1–2 mg/kg/h by infusion over 36–48 h.
- Drug may be diluted in D5W, 0.45–0.9% NaCl, Ringer's or any combination thereof.
- Infant may be pretreated with antacids to minimize risk of GI bleeding.

Assessment & Drug Effects

- Closely monitor cardiovascular status for hypotension or hypertension and arrhythmias. Ask physician for BP parameters.
- Assess for **signs of bleeding:** hematuria, bloody or tarry stools, hematemesis, bruising, or petechiae.
- Monitor electrolytes and arterial blood gases (ABGs) for signs of hypochloremic metabolic acidosis.
- Monitor pulmonary artery pressure (PAP) and pulmonary capillary wedge pressure (PCWP) during drug administration. A drop in PAP should be seen in 30 min of the initial dose.

TOLBUTAMIDE

See HORMONES, ANTIDIABETIC SULFONYLUREA prototype, p 234.

Prototype: ibuprofen, p 160

TOLMETIN SODIUM

(tole´met-in)
Trade names: Tolectin, Tolectin DS
Classifications: CNS AGENT; NONNARCOTIC ANALGESIC, ANTIPYRETIC; NSAID
Pregnancy: Categories B (D in 3rd trimester)

ACTIONS/PHARMACODYNAMICS Pyrrole acetic acid derivative, nonsteroidal antiinflammatory drug (NSAID) structurally and pharmacologically related to indomethacin. Possesses analgesic, antiinflammatory, and antipyretic activity. Exact mode of antiinflammatory action not known. Inhibits prostaglandin synthesis, thus decreasing plasma levels of prostaglandin E, the possible basis for antiinflammatory action. Inhibition of platelet aggregation is less than that produced by equal therapeutic doses of aspirin. Comparable to aspirin and indomethacin in antirheumatic activity, but incidence of GI symptoms and tinnitus is less than in aspirin-treated patients, and CNS effects are less than in patients receiving indomethacin. Each tablet contains 18 mg (0.784 mEq)

Common side effects in *italic*; life-threatening effects <u>underlined</u>; generic names in **bold**; classifications in SMALL CAPS

1013

of sodium. Relieves symptomatology but does not seem to alter the course of the disease.

USES In acute flares and management of chronic rheumatoid arthritis. May be used alone or in combination with gold or corticosteroids.

ROUTE & DOSAGE

Arthritis

Adult	PO	400 mg t.i.d. (max 2 g/d)
Child	PO	≥2 y: 20 mg/kg/d in 3–4 divided doses (max 30 mg/kg/d)

PHARMACOKINETICS Absorption: rapidly absorbed from GI tract. **Peak:** 30–60 min. **Distribution:** crosses blood-brain barrier and placenta; distributed into breast milk. **Metabolism:** metabolized in liver. **Elimination:** half-life: 60–90 min; excreted in urine.

CONTRAINDICATIONS & PRECAUTIONS Contraindicated in: history of intolerance or hypersensitivity to tolmetin, aspirin, and other NSAIDs; active peptic ulcer, patients with asthma, nasal polyps, rhinitis ("aspirin triad"), in patients with functional class IV rheumatoid arthritis (severely incapacitated, bedridden, or confined to a wheelchair). Safe use not established during pregnancy (category B), in third trimester (category D), in nursing mothers, and in children < 2 y. **Cautious use in:** history of upper GI tract disease; impaired renal function; compromised cardiac function.

ADVERSE/SIDE EFFECTS CNS: *headache, dizziness, vertigo, lightheadedness,* mood elevation or depression, tension, nervousness, weakness, drowsiness, insomnia, tinnitus. **CV:** mild edema (about 7% patients), sodium and water retention, mild to moderate hypertension. **GI:** epigastric or abdominal pain, dyspepsia, *nausea,* vomiting, heartburn, constipation, peptic ulcer, GI bleeding. **Hematologic:** transient and small decreases in hemoglobin and hematocrit, purpura, petechiae, granulocytopenia, leukopenia. **Renal:** hematuria, proteinuria, increased BUN. **Skin:** <u>toxic epidermal necrolysis</u>, morbilliform eruptions, urticaria, pruritus. **Other:** <u>anaphylaxis</u> (especially after drug is discontinued and then reinstituted).

DIAGNOSTIC TEST INTERFERENCES Tolmetin prolongs *bleeding time,* inhibits *platelet aggregation,* elevates *BUN, alkaline phosphatase,* and *AST* levels; may decrease *hemoglobin* and *hematocrit* values. Metabolites may produce false-positive results for *proteinuria* (with tests that rely on acid precipitation, e.g., sulfosalicylic acid).

DRUG INTERACTIONS ORAL ANTICOAGULANTS, **heparin** may prolong bleeding time; may increase **lithium** toxicity; **aspirin,** other NSAIDs add to ulcerogenic effects; may increase **methotrexate** toxicity.

NURSING IMPLICATIONS

Administration

- Treatment is preferably scheduled to include a morning dose (on arising) and a bedtime dose.
- Tablet may be crushed before administration and taken with fluid of patient's choice; capsule may be emptied and contents swallowed with water or mixed with food.
- Food delays absorption but does not affect total amount absorbed.
- Store drug in tightly capped light-resistant container at 15–30C (59–86F) unless otherwise instructed.

Assessment & Drug Effects

- The patient with renal damage should be closely monitored and perhaps given lower doses. I&O ratio should be evaluated and the patient encouraged to increase fluid intake to at least 8 full glasses of fluid per day.
- Periodic renal function tests (routine urinalysis, creatinine clearance, and serum creatinine) are recommended for patient on long-term therapy.
- Sodium bicarbonate alkalizes the urine, which increases urinary excretion of tolmetin. Thus, degree and duration of effectiveness may be reduced. Check self-medicating habits of the patient.
- Therapeutic response in patient during treatment for rheumatoid arthritis or osteoarthritis generally occurs within 1 wk with progressive improvement in succeeding week: reduced joint pain and swelling, reduction in duration of morning stiffness, improved functional capacity (increase in grip strength, delayed onset of fatigue).

Patient & Family Education

- If GI disturbances occur, instruct patient to take drug with meals or milk. Advise patient to notify physician if symptoms persist; dosage reduction may be necessary, or an antacid may be prescribed.
- Instruct patient with impaired renal or cardiac function to monitor weight (an increase of more than 2 kg [4 lb]/wk should be reported) and to check for swelling in ankles, tibiae, hands, and feet.

Common side effects in *italic*; life-threatening effects <u>underlined</u>; generic names in **bold**; classifications in SMALL CAPS

- Because of possible enhanced bleeding, warn patient to inform surgeon or dentist before treatment that patient is taking tolmetin.
- Warn patient to report promptly signs of abnormal bleeding (ecchymosis, epistaxis, melena, petechiae), itching, skin rash, persistent headache, edema.
- Dizziness and drowsiness are common side effects; therefore, caution the patient to avoid potentially hazardous activities until response to the drug is known.

Prototype: amphotericin B, p 56

TOLNAFTATE

(tole-naf´tate)
Trade names: Aftate, Pitrex, Tinactin
Classification: SKIN & MUCOUS MEMBRANE AGENT; ANTIINFECTIVE; ANTIFUNGAL ANTIBIOTIC
Pregnancy: Category C

ACTIONS/PHARMACODYNAMICS Synthetic topical antifungal agent. Action mechanism not clear, but it has been shown that tolnaftate distorts hyphae and stunts mycelial growth on susceptible fungi. Toxicity and susceptibility rates are low. Fungistatic or fungicidal to *Microsporum*, specifically *M. gypseum, M. canis, M. audouinii, M. japonicum, Trichophyton, T rubrum, T. schoenleinii, T. tonsurans*, and *Epidermophyton floccosum*, but ineffective against *Candida albicans, Cryptococcus neoformans, Aspergillus fumigatus*, bacteria, protozoa, and viruses.

USES Tinea pedis (athlete's foot), tinea cruris (jock itch), tinea corporis (body ringworm); also tinea capitis and tinea unguium if infection is superficial, plantar or palmar lesions adjunctively with keratolytic agents, and tinea versicolor (caused by *Malassezia furfur*).

ROUTE & DOSAGE

Tinea Infestations

Adult	Topical	Apply 0.5–1 cm (1/4–1/2 in) of cream or 3 drops of solution b.i.d. in morning and evening; Powder may be used prophylactically in normally moist areas

CONTRAINDICATIONS & PRECAUTIONS Contraindicated in: skin irritations prior to therapy, nail and scalp infections; safe use during pregnancy (category C) and lactation or by children < 2 y not established. **Cautious use in:** excoriated skin.

ADVERSE/SIDE EFFECTS Local irritation, stinging of skin from aerosol formulation.

NURSING IMPLICATIONS

Administration

- Thoroughly cleanse site with water and dry completely before applying tolnaftate. Massage a thin layer of drug gently into skin. Area should not be wet from excess drug after application.
- Shake aerosol powder container well before use.
- The cream and powder are not recommended for nail or scalp infection.
- Liquids (solutions) are recommended for scalp infection or to treat hairy areas.
- Store cream, gel, powder, and topical solution in light-resistant containers at 15–30C (59–86F); store aerosol container at 2–30C (38–86F). Avoid freezing and exposure to light.

Patient & Family Education

- Tolnaftate does not stain skin or clothing.
- Emphasize importance of personal cleanliness. Daily bathing, thorough rinsing, and complete drying of skin destroys the kind of environment conducive to growth of fungi.
- If hair follicles or nail beds are involved, a systemic antifungal (e.g., griseofulvin) will be necessary concomitant treatment.
- Powder and powder aerosol are effective in treatment of athlete's foot and in daily hygiene to reduce natural moisture in groin and intertriginous areas.
- If patient has athlete's foot, patient should put socks on before putting on underclothes to avoid spread of infection to groin area (jock itch).
- Pruritus, soreness, burning should be relieved within 24–72 h after start of treatment.
- Explain to patient that treatment should be continued for 2–3 wk after disappearance of all symptoms to prevent recurrence.
- In the absence of improvement within 4 wk, patient should return to physician for reevaluation of prescribed treatment.
- If skin has thickened as a result of the infection, desired clinical response may be delayed for 4–6 wk.
- Avoid contact of all drug forms with eyes.
- If solution solidifies, place container in warm water

Common side effects in *italic*; life-threatening effects underlined; generic names in **bold**; classifications in SMALL CAPS

1015

to liquefy contents. Potency is unaffected.
▪ Do not puncture or store aerosol near heat or an open flame or expose to temperature above 49C (120F). Do not place aerosol container in fire or incinerator for disposal.

Prototype: phenelzine, p 182

TRANYLCYPROMINE SULFATE
(tran-ill-sip´roe-meen)
Trade name: Parnate
Classifications: CNS AGENT; PSYCHOTHERAPEUTIC; MAO INHIBITOR ANTIDEPRESSANT
Pregnancy: Category C

ACTIONS/PHARMACODYNAMICS Potent nonhydrazine MAO inhibitor structurally similar to amphetamine. Actions and toxicity similar to those of hydrazine MAO inhibitors but also has rapid and direct amphetamine-like CNS stimulatory action, is less likely to cause hepatotoxicity, and does not produce prolonged MAO inhibition.

USES Owing to its toxic potential, use is reserved for treatment of severe mental depression in hospitalized patients who have not responded to other antidepressant therapy.

ROUTE & DOSAGE

Severe Depression

Adult   PO   30 mg/d in 2 divided doses (20 mg in AM, 10 mg in PM); may increase by 10 mg/d at 3 wk intervals up to max of 60 mg/d

CONTRAINDICATIONS & PRECAUTIONS Contraindicated in: pregnancy (category C), patients > 60 y, confirmed or suspected cerebrovascular defect, cardiovascular disease, hypertension, pheochromocytoma, history of severe or recurrent headaches.

ADVERSE/SIDE EFFECTS CNS: vertigo, dizziness, tremors, muscle twitching, headache, blurred vision. **CV:** *orthostatic hypotension,* arrhythmias, <u>hypertensive crisis</u>. **GI:** dry mouth, anorexia, constipation, diarrhea, abdominal discomfort. **Other:** rash, impotence, peripheral edema, sweating.

DRUG INTERACTIONS TRICYCLIC ANTIDEPRESSANTS, **fluoxetine**, AMPHETAMINES, **ephedrine, phenylpropanolamine, reserpine, guanethidine, buspirone, methyldopa, dopamine, levodopa, tryptophan** may precipitate hypertensive crisis, headache, or hyperexcitability; **alcohol** and other CNS DEPRESSANTS add to CNS depressant effects; **meperidine** can cause fatal cardiovascular collapse; ANESTHETICS exaggerate hypotensive and CNS depressant effects; **metrizamide** increases risk of seizures; DIURETICS and other ANTIHYPERTENSIVE AGENTS add to hypotensive effects. **Food/Drug interactions:** tyramine-containing foods—aged cheeses, processed cheeses, sour cream, wine, champagne, beer, pickled herring, anchovies, caviar, shrimp, liver, dry sausage, figs, raisins, overripe bananas or avocados, chocolate, soy sauce, bean curd, yeast extracts, yogurt, papaya products, meat tenderizers, broad beans—may precipitate hypertensive crisis.

NURSING IMPLICATIONS

Administration
▪ Tablet may be crushed before administration and taken with fluid or mixed with food if patient has difficulty swallowing a pill.
▪ Because of possibility of insomnia, usually not given in the evening.

Assessment & Drug Effects
▪ Incidence of severe hypertensive reactions appears to be greater with tranylcypromine than with other MAO inhibitors.
▪ Usually produces therapeutic response within 3 d, but full antidepressant effects may not be obtained until 2 or 3 wk of drug therapy.

Patient & Family Education
▪ Emphasize importance of avoiding tyramine-containing foods (see food-drug interactions).
▪ Inform patient that excessive use of caffeine-containing beverages (chocolate, coffee, tea, cola) can contribute to development of rapid heartbeat, arrhythmias, and hypertension.
▪ Instruct patient to make position changes slowly, particularly from recumbent to upright posture.
▪ Instruct patient to avoid hazardous activities until reaction to drug is known.
▪ Advise patient to avoid alcohol or other CNS depressants because of their possible additive effects.

Common side effects in *italic*; life-threatening effects <u>underlined</u>; generic names in **bold**; classifications in SMALL CAPS

TRAZODONE HYDROCHLORIDE

(tray´zoe-done)
Trade names: Desyrel, Desyrel Dividose
Classifications: CNS AGENT; PSYCHOTHERAPEU-
TIC; ANTIDEPRESSANT
Pregnancy: Category C

ACTIONS/PHARMACODYNAMICS Centrally
acting triazolepyridine derivative antidepressant
chemically and structurally unrelated to tricyclic,
tetracyclic, or other antidepressants. Potentiates serotonin (5–HT) effects by selectively blocking its reuptake at presynaptic membranes in CNS. Has little effect on dopamine or norepinephrine, which may
explain low incidence of cardiovascular toxicity and
minimal effect on BP with its use. Does not stimulate
CNS and causes fewer anticholinergic genitourinary
and neurologic effects as compared with other antidepressants. Produces varying degrees of sedation
in normal and mentally depressed patient, increases
total sleep time, deceases number and duration of
awakenings in depressed patient, and decreases REM
sleep. Has anxiolytic effect in severely depressed patient and exhibits mild analgesic, antihistaminic, and
skeletal muscular relaxant action. Has no anticonvulsant action.

USES Both inpatient and outpatient with major depression with or without prominent anxiety.
Unlabeled uses: adjunctive treatment of alcohol dependence, anxiety neuroses, drug-induced dyskinesias.

ROUTE & DOSAGE

Depression

Adult   PO   150 mg/d in divided doses; may increase by 50 mg/d q3–4d (max
400–600 mg/d)

PHARMACOKINETICS Absorption: readily absorbed from GI tract. **Onset:** 1–2 wk. **Peak:** 1–2 h.
Distribution: distributed into breast milk. **Metabolism:**
metabolized in liver. **Elimination:** half-life: 5–9 h; 75%
excreted in urine, 25% in feces.

**CONTRAINDICATIONS & PRECAUTIONS Con-
traindicated in:** initial recovery phase of MI, ventricular ectopy; electroshock therapy. Safe use in children

< 18 y not established; pregnancy (category C).
Cautious use in: patient with suicidal ideation, cardiac
arrhythmias or disease; nursing mother.

ADVERSE/SIDE EFFECTS Appears to be dose-related. **CNS:** *drowsiness,* lightheadedness, tiredness,
dizziness, insomnia, headache, agitation, impaired
memory and speech, disorientation. **CV:** *hypotension
(including orthostatic hypotension),* hypertension,
syncope, shortness of breath, chest pain, tachycardia,
palpitations, bradycardia, PVCs, ventricular tachycardia (short episodes of 3–4 beats). **ENT:** nasal and sinus
congestion, blurred vision, eye irritation, sweating or
clamminess, tinnitus. **GI:** *dry mouth,* anorexia, constipation, abdominal distress, nausea, vomiting, dysgeusia, flatulence, diarrhea. **GU:** hematuria, increased
frequency, delayed urine flow, early or absent
menses, male priapism, ejaculation inhibition.
Hematologic: anemia. **Musculoskeletal:** skeletal aches
and pains, muscle twitches. **Skin:** skin eruptions, rash,
pruritus, acne, photosensitivity. **Other:** weight gain or
loss.

DRUG INTERACTIONS ANTIHYPERTENSIVE AG-
ENTS may potentiate hypotensive effects; **alcohol**
and other CNS DEPRESSANTS add to depressant effects;
may increase **digoxin** or **phenytoin** levels; MAO IN-
HIBITORS may precipitate hypertensive crisis.

NURSING IMPLICATIONS

Administration

▪ Drug taken with food increases amount of absorption by 20% and appears to decrease incidence of
dizziness or lightheadedness. Urge patient to maintain the same schedule for food-drug intake
throughout treatment period to prevent variations
in serum concentration.

▪ Therapy is usually continued on minimum dosage
several months beyond optimum clinical response
to prevent recurrence of depression.

▪ Store in tightly closed, light-resistant container at
15–30C (59–86F).

Assessment & Drug Effects

▪ If patient has preexisting cardiac disease, monitor
pulse rate and regularity before administration of
drug.

▪ When trazodone is given at the same time as an
MAO inhibitor, therapy is initiated cautiously, and
dose is adjusted according to clinical response. No
interaction has been documented, but the potential
for hypertensive crisis is recognized until ruled out.

▪ Adverse/side effects generally are mild and tend to

Common side effects in *italic*; life-threatening effects <u>underlined</u>;
generic names in **bold**; classifications in SMALL CAPS

1017

decrease and disappear after the first few weeks of treatment.

- Observe patient's level of activity. If it appears to be increasing toward sleeplessness and agitation with changes in reality orientation, report to physician. Manic episodes have been reported.
- Check patient for symptoms of hypotension. If orthostatic hypotension is troublesome, suggest measures to reduce danger of falling and to help patient to tolerate the effects. Discuss with physician; a reduction of dose or discontinuation of the drug may be prescribed.
- Ask male patient if he is having inappropriate or prolonged penile erections. If he is, the drug should be discontinued and physician consulted.
- **Overdose symptoms:** extension of common adverse/side effects: vomiting, lethargy, drowsiness, and exaggerated anticholinergic effects. Seizures or arrhythmias are unusual. Death rarely occurs except when other drugs are being taken concomitantly (such as alcohol, meprobamate).

Patient & Family Education

- Therapeutic effects usually begin in 1 wk but may require 2–4 wk to reach maximum levels. Teach patient importance of adhering to regimen and have family member reenforce this teaching with patient in the home.
- Urge patient not to alter dose or intervals between doses.
- If drowsiness becomes a distressing side effect, patient should consult physician. Dose regimen may be adjusted so that largest dose is at bedtime.
- Advise patient to limit or abstain from alcohol use. The depressant effects of CNS depressants and alcohol may be potentiated by this drug.
- Warn patient not to self-medicate with OTC drugs for colds, allergy, or insomnia treatment without advice of physician. Many of these drugs contain CNS depressants.
- Adherence to follow-up appointment is important to permit dose adjustment or discontinuation, as indicated.
- Alert dentist, surgeon, or emergency personnel that drug is being used. Trazodone is discontinued as long as possible prior to elective surgery.

Prototype: Isotretinoin, p 253

TRETINOIN

(tret´i-noyn)
Trade names: Retin-A, Retinoic Acid, Vitamin A Acid
Classifications: SKIN & MUCOUS MEMBRANE AGENT; ANTIACNE (RETINOID); ANTIPSORIATIC; ORPHAN DRUG
Pregnancy: Category B

ACTIONS/PHARMACODYNAMICS A contact irritant containing retinoic acid and vitamin A acid. Reverses retention hyperkeratosis and comedone formation, primary events in acne pathology. Exact action mechanism unknown, but it is suggested that keratinocytes in the sebaceous follicle become less adherent, and turnover of follicular epithelial cells is increased (by stimulated mitosis). These two processes promote easy extrusion of the comedone and prevent it from reformation (comedolytic action). Tretinoin also increases permeability of skin and support conversion of follicular epithelium into less sturdy and almost fragile condition. Unlike benzoyl peroxide and topical antibiotics, does not reduce surface free fatty acids or bacterial colonization (principally *Propionibacterium acnes*) of skin. Although studies in albino mice suggest that the carcinogenic potential of ultraviolet radiation may be accelerated by tretinoin, the significance to humans is not clear. Long-term animal studies have not been performed.

USES Topical treatment of acne vulgaris grades I–III, especially during early stages when number of comedones is greatest; also used adjunctively in management of associated comedones and in treatment of flat warts. **Unlabeled uses:** psoriasis, senile keratosis, ichthyosis vulgaris, keratosis palmaris and plantaris, basal cell carcinoma, photodamaged skin (photoaging), and other skin conditions. **Orphan drug:** for squamous metaplasia of conjunctiva or cornea with mucous deficiency and keratinization.

ROUTE & DOSAGE

Acne
Adult	Topical	Apply once/d h.s.

PHARMACOKINETICS Absorption: minimally absorbed from intact skin. **Elimination:** about 0.1% of dose is excreted in urine within 24 h.

Common side effects in *italic*; life-threatening effects <u>underlined</u>; generic names in **bold**; classifications in SMALL CAPS

CONTRAINDICATIONS & PRECAUTIONS Contraindicated in: eczema, exposure to sunlight or ultraviolet rays (as with sunlamp); sunburn, pregnancy (category B). **Cautious use in:** patient in an occupation necessitating considerable sun exposure or weather extremes; nursing mothers.

ADVERSE/SIDE EFFECTS All reversible with discontinuation of medication. Local inflammatory reactions, transient stinging or warmth on site, redness, scaling, severe erythema, blistering, crusting and peeling, temporary hypopigmentation or hyperpigmentation.

DRUG INTERACTIONS TOPICAL ACNE MEDICATIONS (including **sulfur**, **resorcinol**, **benzoyl peroxide**, and **salicylic acid**) may increase inflammation and peeling; topical products containing **alcohol** or **menthol** may cause stinging.

NURSING IMPLICATIONS

Administration

- If patient has been using a desquamative agent, a waiting period long enough for recovery from its action should intervene before starting treatment with tretinoin.
- Cleanse, using a mild bland soap, and thoroughly dry areas being treated before applying drug. Avoid use of medicated, drying or abrasive soaps and cleansers.
- Wash hands before and after treatment. Do not apply to nonaffected skin area.
- Avoid contact of drug with eyes, mouth, angles of nose, open wounds, mucous membranes.
- Store gel and liquid formulations below 30C (86F) and solution below 27C (80F).

Assessment & Drug Effects

- Tretinoin treatment to black individuals may cause unsightly postinflammatory hyperpigmentation; dark-complexioned whites may have a mild hypopigmentary effect. Both are reversible with termination of drug treatment.
- Clinical response to tretinoin should be evident in 2 or 3 wk, but a complete and satisfactory response (in 75% of the patients) may require a period of 3 or 4 mo. Once achieved, control is maintained by less frequent applications or a change in formulation or dosage.

Patient & Family Education

- Inform patient that erythema and desquamation during the first 1–3 wk of treatment do not represent exacerbation of the skin problem but a probable response to the drug from deep previously unseen lesions.
- Urge compliance with therapy.
- As treatment is continued, lesions gradually disappear, leaving an inflammatory background; scaling and redness decrease after 8–10 wk of therapy.
- Instruct the patient to wash face no more often than 2–3 times daily.
- Topical preparations with high concentrations of alcohol, astringents, spices or lime, perfumes and shaving lotions, should not be used during treatment period.
- Inform patient that the drug is not curative; relapses commonly occur within 3–6 wk after treatment has been discontinued.
- Nonmedicated cosmetics may be used during therapy, but they should be removed thoroughly before drug is applied.
- If exposure to sun cannot be avoided, it is advisable to use a sunscreen product with SPF 15 or higher.
- Warn patient against self-medication with additional acne treatment because of danger of drug interactions.
- Inform physician if even the mildest side effects occur rather than terminating the treatment prematurely. Keep appointments for assessment of progress to permit regimen adjustment when needed.

Common side effects in *italic*; life-threatening effects underlined; generic names in **bold**; classifications in SMALL CAPS

1019

Prototype: hydrocortisone, p 255

TRIAMCINOLONE

(trye-am-sin´oh-lone)

Trade names: Aristocort, Atolone, Kenacort, Kenalog-E, Triaderm, Triamalone, Triamcort, Trianide

TRIAMCINOLONE ACETONIDE

Trade names: Acetospan, Azmacort, Cenocort A$_2$, Kenalog, Tramacort, Triam-A, Triamonide, Tri-kort, Trilog

TRIAMCINOLONE DIACETATE

Trade names: Amcort, Aristocort Forte, Articulose LA, Cenocort Forte, Clinalone-40, Kenacort, Tac-D, Tracilon, Triacort, Triam-Forte, Triamolone, Trilone, Tristoject

TRIAMCINOLONE HEXACETONIDE

Trade name: Aristospan

Classifications: HORMONE; ADRENAL CORTICO-STEROID; GLUCOCORTICOID; ANTIINFLAMMATORY

Pregnancy: Category C

ACTIONS/PHARMACODYNAMICS Immediate acting synthetic fluorinated adrenal corticosteroid with glucocorticoid and antirheumatic activity 7–13 times more potent than that of hydrocortisone. Possesses minimal sodium and water retention properties in therapeutic doses. Administered orally, 4 mg triamcinolone is equivalent to 20 mg hydrocortisone on a weight basis. Acetonide formulation has longer duration of action than parent compound; when acetonide administered into joint or bursa, pharmacologic activity begins within few hours and may persist a number of weeks. Triamcinolone differs from other corticosteriods in that it does not increase appetite.

USES An inflammatory or immunosuppressant agent. Orally inhaled: bronchial asthma in patient who has not responded to conventional inhalation treatment. Therapeutic doses do not appear to suppress HPA (hypothalamic-pituitary-adrenal) axis.

ROUTE & DOSAGE

Inflammation, Immunosuppression

Adult	PO/IM/SC	4–48 mg/d in divided doses
	Intraarticular/Intradermal	4–48 mg/d
	Inhaled	2–4 inhalations q.i.d.
	Topical	Apply sparingly b.i.d. or t.i.d.
Child	PO/IM/SC	3.3–50 mg/m^2/d in divided doses
	Intraarticular/Intradermal	3.3–50 mg/m^2/d

Acetonide

Adult	IM	60 mg; may repeat with 20–100 mg q6wk
	Intradermal	1 mg per injection site (max 30 mg total)
	Intraarticular	2.5–4.0 mg
	Inhalation	2 puffs 3–4 times/d (max 16 puffs/d)
Child	IM	6–12 y: 0.03–0.2 mg q1–7d
	Inhalation	6–12 y: 1–2 sprays t.i.d. or q.i.d. (max 12 sprays/d)

Diacetate

Adult	PO	4–48 mg/d in 1–4 divided doses
	IM	40 mg once/wk
	Intradermal	5–48 mg (max 75 mg/wk) may repeat q1–2wk if needed
	Intraarticular	2–40 mg q1–8wk
Child	PO	0.117–1.66 mg/kg/d

Hexacetonide

Adult	Intralesional	up to 0.5 mg/in^2 of skin
	Intraarticular	2–20 mg q3–4wk

PHARMACOKINETICS Absorption: readily absorbed from all routes. **Onset:** 24–48 h PO, IM. **Peak:** 1–2 h PO; 8–10 h IM. **Duration:** 2.25 d PO; 1–6 wk IM. **Metabolism:** metabolized in liver. **Elimination:** half-life: 2–5 h; HPA suppression: 18–36 h; excreted in urine.

CONTRAINDICATIONS & PRECAUTIONS Contraindicated in: safe use during pregnancy (category C), by lactating women, and by children < 6y not established. Renal dysfunction. Also see hydrocortisone.

ADVERSE/SIDE EFFECTS Muscle weakness and loss of tissue mass. **Local:** burning, itching, folliculitis, hypertrichosis, hypopigmentation. Also see hydrocortisone.

DRUG INTERACTIONS BARBITURATES, **phenytoin, rifampin** increase steroid metabolism —may need increased doses of triamcinolone; **amphotericin B**, DIURETICS add to potassium loss; **ambenonium, neostigmine, pyridostigmine** may cause severe muscle weakness in patients with myasthenia gravis; may inhibit antibody response to VACCINES, TOXOIDS.

NURSING IMPLICATIONS

Administration

- Tablet may be crushed before administration and taken with fluid of patient's choice.
- Protect drug from light. Store at 15–30C (59–86F). See hydrocortisone for numerous additional nursing implications.

Assessment & Drug Effects

- This preparation may cause natriuresis, negative nitrogen balance, with weight loss in most patients (along with headache, fatigue, and dizziness) and sodium retention with weight gain and moon facies in others. Adequate diet to counter these effects should be designed. Plan with dietitian, patient, and physician. High protein, high potassium diet is often needed.
- If a local infection develops at site of application, occlusive dressing should be discontinued and appropriate antimicrobial treatment started.
- Systemic absorption may occur after topical application, especially in children and if used over extensive areas for prolonged periods or if occlusive dressings are used. Reportable symptoms include hypercortisolism or Cushing's syndrome (see chap 3), hyperglycemia (see chap 3), glucosuria.

Patient & Family Education

- Warn patient that postural hypotension may accompany sodium loss and weight loss.
- Caution patient to adhere to drug regimen, i.e., not to increase or decrease established regimen and not to abruptly discontinue taking or using the drug.

Prototype: spironolactone, p 202

TRIAMTERENE
(trye-am´ter-een)
Trade name: Dyrenium
Classifications: WATER BALANCE AGENT; POTASSIUM-SPARING DIURETIC
Pregnancy: Category B

ACTIONS/PHARMACODYNAMICS Pteridine derivative structurally related to folic acid. Like spironolactone, has weak diuretic action and a potassium-sparing effect. Promotes excretion of sodium, chloride (to lesser extent), and carbonate, with no excretion or slight excretion of potassium ion. Unlike spironolactone, blocks potassium secretion by direct action on distal renal tubule rather than by inhibiting aldosterone; activity is independent of aldosterone levels. May decrease alkali reserve and slightly increase urinary pH. Does not appear to inhibit excretion of uric acid, but serum uric acid levels may increase in predisposed individuals. Decreased glomerular filtration rate and elevated BUN are associated with daily administration but seldom with intermittent (every other day) therapy. Has mild hypotensive effect and is a weak competitive inhibitor of dihydrofolate reductase.

USES Adjunct in the management of edema associated with CHF, hepatic cirrhosis, nephrotic syndrome, idiopathic edema, steroid-induced edema, and edema due to secondary hyperaldosteronism. Also alone or in conjunction with a thiazide or loop diuretic in patients with hypertension because of its potassium-sparing activity.

ROUTE & DOSAGE

Edema

Adult	PO	100 mg b.i.d. (max 300 mg/d); may be able to decrease to 100 mg/d or q.o.d.
Child	PO	2–4 mg/kg/d in divided doses or q.o.d. (max 300 mg/d)

PHARMACOKINETICS Absorption: rapidly but variably absorbed from GI tract. **Onset:** 2–4 h. **Duration:** 7–9 h. **Metabolism:** metabolized in liver to active and inactive metabolites. **Elimination:** half-life: 100–150 min; excreted in urine.

Common side effects in *italic*; life-threatening effects underlined; generic names in **bold**; classifications in SMALL CAPS

1021

CONTRAINDICATIONS & PRECAUTIONS Contraindicated in: hypersensitivity to drug; anuria, severe or progressive kidney disease or dysfunction; severe hepatic disease; elevated serum potassium. Safe use during pregnancy (category B) and in nursing mothers not established. **Cautious use in:** impaired renal or hepatic function; history of gouty arthritis; diabetes mellitus, history of kidney stones.

ADVERSE/SIDE EFFECTS Diarrhea, nausea, vomiting, and other GI disturbances; dizziness, headache, dry mouth, pruritus, rash, <u>anaphylaxis</u>, photosensitivity, weakness and hypotension (large doses), muscle cramps, *hyperkalemia* and other electrolyte imbalances, elevated BUN, elevated uric acid (patients predisposed to gouty arthritis), hyperchloremic acidosis, blood dyscrasias: granulocytopenia, eosinophilia, megaloblastic anemia, patients with reduced folic acid stores (e.g., hepatic cirrhosis).

DIAGNOSTIC TEST INTERFERENCES Pale blue fluorescence in urine interferes with fluorometric assay of **quinidine** and **lactic dehydrogenase activity.** Triamterene may cause increases in **blood glucose** levels (diabetic patients), **BUN, serum potassium, magnesium,** and **uric acid** and **urinary calcium excretion.**

DRUG INTERACTIONS May increase **lithium** levels, thus increasing its toxicity; **indomethacin** may decrease renal elimination of triamterene; ANGIOTENSIN-CONVERTING ENZYME (ACE) INHIBITORS, other POTASSIUM-SPARING DIURETICS may cause hyperkalemia.

NURSING IMPLICATIONS

Administration

- If patient cannot swallow capsule, it may be emptied and contents swallowed with fluid or mixed with food.
- Give drug with or after meals to prevent or minimize nausea.
- Schedule doses to prevent interruption of sleep from diuresis, e.g., with or after breakfast if a single dose is taken, or no later than 6 PM if more than one dose is prescribed. Consult physician.
- Drug should be withdrawn gradually in patients on prolonged therapy or in patients who have received high doses, in order to prevent rebound increased urinary excretion of potassium.
- Preserve in tight, light-resistant containers at 15–30C (59–86F) unless otherwise directed.

Assessment & Drug Effect

- Monitor BP during period of dosage adjustment. Hypotensive reactions, although rare, have been reported. Implications for ambulation should be noted, particularly for elderly patients.
- Weigh patient under standard conditions, prior to drug initiation and daily during therapy.
- Diuretic response usually occurs on first day of therapy, but maximum effect may not occur for several days.
- Monitor and report oliguria and unusual changes in I&O ratio. Consult physician regarding allowable fluid intake.
- Renal stone formation has been reported in patients taking high doses or who have low urine volume and increased urine acidity.
- Observe for signs and symptoms of hyperkalemia (see chap 3), particularly in patients with renal insufficiency, in patients on high-dose or prolonged therapy, in the elderly, and in patients with diabetes. Baseline and periodic determinations of serum potassium and other electrolytes should be done.
- Periodic evaluations of renal function (BUN, serum creatinine) are advised in patients with known or suspected renal insufficiency.
- Patients with cirrhosis are usually hospitalized during triamterene therapy because rapid alterations in fluid and electrolyte balance can precipitate **hepatic coma or precoma:** irritability, restlessness, confusion, stupor, liver flap (asterixis), coma.
- Periodic blood studies are advised in patients on prolonged therapy and in patients with cirrhosis since they are prone to develop megaloblastic anemia.
- Triamterene may increase blood glucose; therefore it should not be given to a diabetic patient unless blood glucose is controlled. Patients should be closely monitored.

Patient & Family Education

- Unlike most diuretics, triamterene promotes potassium retention. Therefore, potassium supplements, potassium-rich diet, and salt substitutes are usually not prescribed.
- Generally salt restriction is not stressed because of the possibility of low-salt syndrome (hyponatremia). Consult physician.
- Instruct patient to report overpowering fatigue or weakness, malaise, fever, sore throat, or mouth (possible symptoms of granulocytopenia) and unusual bleeding or bruising (thrombocytopenia).
- Warn patient that triamterene may cause photosen-

Common side effects in *italic*; life-threatening effects <u>underlined</u>; generic names in **bold**; classifications in SMALL CAPS

sitivity and therefore to avoid exposure to sun and sunlamps.

- Inform patient that triamterene may impart a harmless pale blue fluorescence to urine.

Prototype: lorazepam, p 177

TRIAZOLAM

(trye-ay´zoe-lam)
Trade name: Halcion
Classifications: CNS AGENT; BENZODIAZEPINE ANXIOLYTIC, SEDATIVE-HYPNOTIC
Pregnancy: Category X
Controlled substance: Schedule IV

ACTIONS/PHARMACODYNAMICS Benzodiazepine derivative with hypnotic effects similar to those of flurazepam but with fewer residual daytime effects. Enhances inhibitory effects of the neurotransmitter gamma aminobutyric acid (GABA) on presynaptic and postsynaptic receptors in all CNS regions but particularly in the brainstem reticular formation. Blockade of cortical and limbic arousal results in hypnotic activity. Drug-induced effects on sleep include decreased sleep latency and number of nocturnal awakenings, decreased total nocturnal wake time, and increased duration of sleep. Reduction of daytime anxiety and carry-over CNS depression is minimal.

USES Short-term management of insomnia characterized by difficulty in falling asleep, frequent wakeful periods. Following long-term use, tolerance or adaptation may develop.

ROUTE & DOSAGE

Insomnia

Adult	PO	0.125–0.25 mg h.s. (max 0.5 mg/d)

PHARMACOKINETICS Absorption: readily absorbed from GI tract. **Onset:** 15–30 min. **Peak:** 1–2 h. **Duration:** 6–8 h. **Distribution:** crosses placenta; distributed into breast milk. **Metabolism:** metabolized in liver to active metabolites. **Elimination:** half-life: 2–3 h; excreted in urine.

CONTRAINDICATIONS & PRECAUTIONS Contraindicated in: hypersensitivity to triazolam and benzodiazepines; pregnancy (category X). **Cautious use in:** depression; elderly and debilitated patients; patients with suicidal tendency, impaired renal or hepatic function; chronic pulmonary insufficiency.

ADVERSE/SIDE EFFECTS CNS: *drowsiness*, light headedness, headache, dizziness, ataxia, visual disturbances, confusional states, *memory impairment, "rebound insomnia," anterograde amnesia.* **GI:** nausea, vomiting, constipation. **Other:** paradoxical reactions, minor changes in EEG patterns.

DRUG INTERACTIONS Alcohol, CNS DEPRESSANTS, ANTICONVULSANTS potentiate CNS depression; **cimetidine** increases triazolam plasma levels, thus increasing its toxicity; may decrease antiparkinsonism effects of **levodopa.**

NURSING IMPLICATIONS

Administration

- Patient should take triazolam immediately before retiring; onset of drug action is rapid.
- Recommended doses should not be exceeded.
- Store at 15–30C (59–86F).

Assessment & Drug Effects

- Because of short half-life, under normal circumstances dose is usually cleared before next bedtime dose; therefore "morning after" grogginess rarely occurs.
- Signs of developing tolerance or adaptation (with long-term use) include increased daytime anxiety, increased wakefulness during last one third of the night.
- Periodic blood counts, urinalysis, and blood chemistries are advised during long-term use of triazolam.
- Although the drug has minimum abuse potential, it should not be used by addiction-prone patients (drug addicts, alcoholics) unless careful surveillance by health personnel is available. Habituation and dependence can occur.
- As with other benzodiazepines, smoking may decrease hypnotic effects of triazolam.
- Overdosage (accidental or by intent) will develop with 4 times the maximum recommended therapeutic dose (0.5 mg), or 2 mg.
- *Overdose symptoms:* slurred speech, somnolence, confusion, impaired coordination, coma.

Patient & Family Education

- Engaging in hazardous activities (driving a car, use of machinery) until drug response has been defined should be avoided.
- Advise patient that use of alcohol or other CNS de-

Common side effects in *italic*; life-threatening effects underlined; generic names in **bold**; classifications in SMALL CAPS

1023

pressants while on this drug increases sedative effects.

- Warn patient not to stop taking drug suddenly, especially if patient is subject to seizures. Withdrawal symptoms may occur. These range from mild dysphoria to more serious symptoms such as tremors, abdominal and muscle cramps, convulsions. Consult physician about schedule for discontinuing therapy.
- Caution patient not to increase dose without physician's advice because of toxic potential of drug.

Prototype: hydrochlorothiazide, p 203

TRICHLORMETHIAZIDE
(trye-klor-meth-eye´a-zide)
Trade names: Aquazide, Diurese, Metahydrin, Mono-Press, Naqua, Niazide, Trichlorex
Classifications: WATER BALANCE AGENT; THIAZIDE DIURETIC; ANTIHYPERTENSIVE
Pregnancy: Category B

ACTIONS/PHARMACODYNAMICS Benzothiadiazine (thiazide) derivative. Similar to hydrochlorothiazide in pharmacologic actions, uses, contraindications, precautions, adverse effects, and interactions.

USES To treat hypertension as sole agent or to enhance the effects of another antihypertensive when given in combination. Also to treat edema associated with CHF, renal decompensation, and hepatic cirrhosis.

ROUTE & DOSAGE

Edema

Adult	PO	1–4 mg 1–2 times/d

Hypertension

Adult	PO	2–4 mg/d in 1–2 divided doses
Child	PO	0.07 mg/kg/d in 1–2 divided doses

PHARMACOKINETICS Onset: 2 h. **Peak:** 6 h. **Duration:** 24 h. **Distribution:** crosses placenta; distributed into breast milk. **Elimination:** excreted in urine.

CONTRAINDICATIONS & PRECAUTIONS Contraindicated in: anuria; hypersensitivity to thiazides, sulfonamides; pregnancy (category B), lactation.

Cautious use in: history of allergy; renal and hepatic disease; gout; diabetes mellitus.

ADVERSE/SIDE EFFECTS Anorexia, paresthesias, photosensitivity, vasculitis; exacerbation of gout, SLE. Also see hydrochlorothiazide.

DRUG INTERACTIONS Amphotericin B, CORTICOSTEROIDS increase hypokalemic effects; may antagonize hypoglycemic effects of SULFONYLUREAS, insulin; **cholestyramine, colistipol** decrease thiazide absorption; intensifies hypoglycemic and hypotensive effects of **diazoxide**; increased potassium and magnesium loss with **digoxin**—may cause digoxin toxicity; decreases **lithium** excretion, thus increasing its toxicity; NSAIDs may attenuate diuresis—risk of NSAID-induced renal failure increased.

NURSING IMPLICATIONS

Administration

- Drug should be taken early in AM after breakfast to reduce gastric irritation and to prevent interruption of sleep because of diuresis. If 2 doses are ordered, schedule second dose no later than 3 PM.
- Store in tightly closed container at 15–30C (59–86F) unless otherwise instructed.

Assessment & Drug Effects

- Monitor BP and I&O ratio during first phase of antihypertensive therapy. Report a sudden fall in BP, which may initiate severe postural hypotension and potentially dangerous perfusion problems, especially in the extremities.
- Antihypertensive effects may be noted in 3–4 d; maximal effects may require 3–4 wk.
- Older patients may be more sensitive to the average adult dose. Monitor them closely.
- Monitor patient for signs of hypokalemia (see chap 3). Report them promptly. Hypokalemia is rarely severe in most patients even on long-term therapy, but the elderly are especially susceptible.
- The prediabetic or diabetic patient should be watched carefully for loss of control of diabetes or early signs of hyperglycemia: drowsiness, polyuria, anorexia, polydipsia. These symptoms are slow to develop and to recognize. Check urine for glycosuria.

Patient & Family Education

- To prevent onset of hypokalemia, urge patient to eat a balanced diet (usually includes potassium-rich foods such as fruits and fruit juices).
- Counsel patient to avoid use of OTC drugs unless

Common side effects in *italic*; life-threatening effects <u>underlined</u>; generic names in **bold**; classifications in SMALL CAPS

they are approved by the physician. Many preparations contain both potassium and sodium and if misused, or if patient overdoses, electrolyte imbalance side effects may be induced.

- Advise patient to maintain prescribed dosage regimen, not to skip, reduce, or double doses or change dose intervals.

Prototype: atropine, p 116

TRIDIHEXETHYL CHLORIDE
(trye-dye-hex-eth´ill)
Trade name: Pathilon
Classifications: AUTONOMIC NERVOUS SYSTEM AGENT; ANTICHOLINERGIC (PARASYMPATHOLYTIC); ANTIMUSCARINIC, ANTISPASMODIC
Pregnancy: Category C

ACTIONS/PHARMACODYNAMICS Synthetic (amine) quaternary ammonium compound pharmacologically related to the belladonna alkaloids. Exhibits selected anticholinergic actions similar to those of atropine. Exerts antimuscarinic activity by binding competitively with acetylcholine at postganglionic cholinergic effector sites. Decreases spasm of smooth muscle of GI tract, an action said to be responsible for relief of pain associated with peptic ulcer disease. However, there are no conclusive data that recommended doses aid in healing, prevent complications, or reduce recurrence rate of peptic ulcers.

USES Adjunct in the treatment of peptic ulcer disease and irritable bowel syndrome.

ROUTE & DOSAGE

Adult	PO	25 mg t.i.d. and 50 mg h.s. up to 25–50 mg t.i.d. or q.i.d.

PHARMACOKINETICS Absorption: incompletely absorbed from GI tract. **Elimination:** excreted in urine and feces as unchanged drug.

CONTRAINDICATIONS & PRECAUTIONS Contraindicated in: glaucoma; obstructive uropathy; obstructive disease of GI tract, ulcerative colitis; biliary tract disease; intestinal atony in the elderly or debilitated patient; unstable CV status; myasthenia gravis. Safe use during pregnancy (category C), in nursing mothers, and in children not established. **Cautious use in:** hiatal hernia, diarrhea; patient with nonobstructive prostatic hypertrophy; ileostomy, or colostomy; hyperthyroidism.

ADVERSE/SIDE EFFECTS CNS: *confusion, excitement (especially in elderly),* loss of taste, blurred vision, cycloplegia, increased ocular tension, headache, decreased sweating. **GI:** *xerostomia,* nausea, vomiting, antral stasis, *constipation.* **GU:** *urinary hesitancy and retention;* impotence. **Other:** severe allergic reaction, urticaria, tachycardia, palpitations, suppression of lactation.

DRUG INTERACTIONS Amantadine, ANTIHISTAMINES, TRICYCLIC ANTIDEPRESSANTS, **quinidine, disopyramide, procainamide** - add to anticholinergic effects; decreases **levodopa** effects; may decrease effects of **cimetidine;** decreases antipsychotic effects (decreased absorption) of PHENOTHIAZINES.

NURSING IMPLICATIONS

Administration

- Since delayed emptying (drug-induced) affects the transit of medications and food, space administration intervals in multidrug therapy to avoid drug interaction. Take tridihexethyl chloride 1 h before or 2 h after meals and other medications unless otherwise advised.

Assessment & Drug Effects

- Check pulse before drug administration. If tachycardia is present, withhold dose and consult physician.
- Decreased GI motility, and expected change in aging, may increase the hazard of drug-induced antral stasis in the elderly patient. A "full" sensation, anorexia, regurgitation, or nausea may be symptomatic of stasis and should be reported. Drug use may be discontinued.
- Decreased sweating may lead to heat prostration (fever, tachycardia, heat stroke) in an extremely warm environment, especially if patient is elderly or debilitated. Check the debilitated or otherwise threatened patient's temperature and pulse daily.
- Anticipate exaggerated anticholinergic effects in the elderly: vision and accommodation changes, confusion, excitement, or agitation, as well as constipation and urination problems, especially in the elderly age group. Drug dose adjustment or discontinuation may be prescribed.

Common side effects in *italic*; life-threatening effects underlined; generic names in **bold**; classifications in SMALL CAPS

1025

Patient & Family Education

- Because of the possibility of drug-induced drowsiness and blurred vision, patient should be warned not to drive a car or engage in dangerous activity until drug response has stabilized without such symptoms.

Prototype: chlorpromazine, p 191

TRIFLUOPERAZINE HYDROCHLORIDE

(trye-floo-oh-per′a-zeen)

Trade names: Novoflurazine, Solazine, Stelazine, Suprazine, Terfluzine, Triflurin

Classifications: CNS AGENT; PSYCHOTHERAPEUTIC; PHENOTHIAZINE ANTIPSYCHOTIC (TRANQUILIZER)

Pregnancy: Category C

ACTIONS/PHARMACODYNAMICS Piperazine phenothiazine similar to chlorpromazine in most actions, uses, limitations, and interactions. Produces less sedative, cardiovascular, and anticholinergic effects and more prominent antiemetic and extrapyramidal effects than other phenothiazines do. Total pharmacologic effects are more prolonged than those of chlorpromazine. Lowers convulsive threshold.

USES Management of manifestations of psychotic disorders; "possibly effective" control of excessive anxiety and tension associated with neuroses or somatic conditions.

ROUTE & DOSAGE

Psychotic Disorders

Adult	PO	1–2 mg b.i.d.; may increase up to 20 mg/d in hospitalized patients
	IM	1–2 mg q4–6h (max 10 mg/d)
Child	PO	6–12 y: 1 mg 1–2 times/d; may increase up to 15 mg/d in hospitalized patients
	IM	6–12 y: 1 mg 1–2 times/d; may increase up to 15 mg/d

PHARMACOKINETICS Absorption: well absorbed from GI tract. **Onset:** rapid onset. **Peak** 2–3 h. **Duration:** up to 12 h. **Metabolism:** metabolized in liver. **Elimination:** excreted in bile and feces.

CONTRAINDICATIONS & PRECAUTIONS Contraindicated in: hypersensitivity to phenothiazines; comatose states, CNS depression; blood dyscrasias; children < 6 y; bone marrow depression; preexisting hepatic disease; pregnancy (category C). **Cautious use in:** previously detected breast cancer; compromised respiratory function; seizure disorders.

ADVERSE/SIDE EFFECTS Nasal congestion, *dry mouth*, sweating, blurred vision, *drowsiness*, insomnia, dizziness, agitation, *extrapyramidal effects*, agranulocytosis, photosensitivity, skin rash, constipation, tachycardia, *hypotension*, pigmentary retinopathy, depressed cough reflex, gynecomastia, galactorrhea.

DRUG INTERACTIONS Alcohol and other CNS DEPRESSANTS add to CNS depression.

NURSING IMPLICATIONS

Administration

- Separate antacid and phenothiazine doses by at least 2 h.
- Dilute oral concentrate just before administration with about 60–120 ml suitable diluent (e.g., water, fruit juices, carbonated beverage, milk, soups, puddings). Avoid coffee or tea near time of taking oral preparation. Explain dosage and dilution to patient if drug is to be self-administered.
- Tablet may be crushed before administration and taken with fluid or mixed with food if patient will not or cannot swallow a pill.
- Monitor ingestion of tablet to see that patient does not hoard medication.
- Administer IM injection deep into upper outer quadrant of buttock. Unlike other phenothiazines, this drug apparently causes little if any pain and irritation at injection site. Rotate sites.
- Intervals between injections should be no less than 4 h because of possible cumulative effects. Oral therapy is substituted for IM treatment as soon as feasible.
- Slight yellow discoloration of injectable drug reportedly does not alter potency. If color is markedly changed, discard solution.
- Wash hands if undiluted concentrate is spilled on skin to prevent contact dermatosis.
- Store in light-resistant container at 15–30C (59–86F) unless otherwise directed.

Assessment & Drug Effects

- Hypotension and extrapyramidal effects (especially akathisia and dystonia) are most likely to occur in

---

Common side effects in *italic*; life-threatening effects underlined; generic names in **bold**; classifications in SMALL CAPS

patients receiving high doses or parenteral administration and in the elderly patient. Stop drug if patient has dysphagia, neck muscle spasm, or if tongue protrusion occurs.

Reduction in dosage or temporary discontinuation of drug usually reverses extrapyramidal symptoms.

- Monitor I&O ratio and bowel elimination pattern. Check for abdominal distension and pain. Encourage adequate fluid intake as prophylaxis for constipation and xerostomia. The depressed patient may not seek help for either symptom or for urinary retention.
- Since trifluoperazine potentiates analgesics, its use may reduce amount of narcotic required in painful long-term illness such as cancer.
- Agitation, jitteriness, and sometimes insomnia may simulate original neurotic or psychotic symptoms. (They may disappear spontaneously.) Dosage should not be increased until side effects have subsided.
- Maximum therapeutic response generally occurs within 2 or 3 wk after initiation of therapy.

Patient & Family Education

- Counsel patient to take drug as prescribed and not to alter dosing regimen or stop medication without consulting physician.
- Advise patient to consult physician about use of any OTC drugs during therapy.
- Alcohol and other depressants should not be taken during phenothiazine therapy.
- Caution patient to avoid potentially hazardous activities such as driving a car or operating machinery, especially during first days of therapy. (Drowsiness and dizziness may be prominent during this time.)
- Increase in mental and physical activity is an expected result of therapy. Caution patients with angina to avoid overexertion and to report increase in frequency of original pain.
- Patient may be unable to adjust to temperature extremes because of drug effect on thermoregulatory center. Advise patient not to apply heating pad or hot water bottles; because of depressed conditioned avoidance behaviors, a severe burn may result.
- Advise patient to cover as much skin surface as possible with clothing when he or she must be in direct sunlight. A sun screen lotion (SPF > 12) should be applied to exposed skin.
- Inform patient that urine may be discolored or reddish brown and that this is harmless.

Prototype: chlorpromazine, p 191

TRIFLUPROMAZINE
(tri-flu-pro′ma-zeen)
Trade name: Vesprin
Classifications: CNS AGENT; PSYCHOTHERAPEUTIC; PHENOTHIAZINE ANTIPSYCHOTIC; ANTIEMETIC
Pregnancy: Category C

ACTIONS/PHARMACODYNAMICS Triflupromazine has effects similar to those of chlorpromazine. Mechanism that produces strong antipsychotic effects is unclear but is thought to be related to blockade of postsynaptic dopamine receptors in the brain. It has strong anticholinergic effects and moderate to strong sedative and extrapyramidal effects. Triflupromazine has strong antiemetic activity.

USES Psychotic disorders (excluding psychotic depressive reactions). Also severe postoperative nausea and vomiting.

ROUTE & DOSAGE

Psychotic Disorders

Adult	IM	60 mg/d in divided doses (max 150 mg/d)
Child	IM	0.2–0.25 mg/kg/d in divided doses (max 10 mg/d)

Nausea and Vomiting

Adult	IM	5–15 mg q4h prn (max 60 mg/d)
Child	IM	> 2.5 y: 0.2–0.25 mg/kg/d in divided doses (max 10 mg/d)

CONTRAINDICATIONS & PRECAUTIONS Contraindicated in: subcortical brain damage, comatose or severely depressed state; hypersensitivity to phenothiazines; presence of large amounts of other CNS depressants; blood dyscrasias; liver damage. **Cautious use in:** pregnancy (category C) and in children and adolescents whose signs and symptoms suggest Reye's syndrome or encephalopathy.

ADVERSE/SIDE EFFECTS CNS: extrapyramidal symptoms, drowsiness, *dry mouth, blurred vision.* **CV:** hypotension, tachycardia. **GI:** anorexia, *constipation,* ileus, *urinary retention.* **Other:** rash.

DRUG INTERACTIONS Alcohol and other CNS DEPRESSANTS add to CNS depression.

Common side effects in *italic*; life-threatening effects underlined; generic names in **bold**; classifications in SMALL CAPS

1027

T

NURSING IMPLICATIONS

Administration

- Dosage should be increased gradually in elderly, debilitated, or emaciated patients.
- Avoid drug contact with skin, eyes, and clothing because of its potential for causing contact dermatitis.
- Inject triflupromazine IM slowly and deep into the dorsal gluteal muscle. Massage site well. Avoid SC injection. Rotate injection sites.
- Triflupromazine may be incompatible when mixed with other medications. Consult pharmacist or package literature before mixing with other medications.

Assessment & Drug Effects

- Prior to initiating therapy, assess and document client's physical and mental status. Record vital signs. Check BP standing and recumbent. Hypotension may occur especially with large doses.
- Monitor pulse since drug increases heart rate in most patients.
- Observe for signs and symptoms of tardive dyskinesia (see chap 3), which is a potentially irreversible condition. Notify physician immediately; drug may need to be discontinued.
- Observe for signs and symptoms of urinary retention.
- Observe for signs and symptoms of diminished visual acuity, reduced night vision, photophobia, and a perceived brownish discoloration of objects.
- Carefully monitor patient with respiratory disorder, since drug may lead to decreased pulmonary ventilation.
- **_Signs of overdose:_** CNS depression, somnolence, deep sleep, coma, hypotension, and extrapyramidal symptoms.

Patient & Family Education

- Instruct patient to notify physician immediately if tremors, involuntary muscle twitching, high temperature, jaundice, or changes in vision occur.
- Warn patient that medication may cause drowsiness and to use caution while driving or performing other tasks requiring alertness.
- Instruct patient to avoid alcohol and other CNS depressants because of possible additive effects.
- Instruct patient that medication may discolor the urine pink or reddish-brown.
- Warn patient that hypotension may occur. Instruct him or her to arise slowly from a recumbent position and to avoid sudden changes in posture.

- Instruct patient to avoid exposure to sunlight, as it may cause a photosensitivity reaction.
- Instruct patient to use caution in hot weather, as this medication increases susceptibility to heat stroke.

Prototype: acyclovir, p 85

TRIFLURIDINE
(trye-flure´i-deen)
Trade name: Viroptic
Classifications: ANTIINFECTIVE; ANTIVIRAL
Pregnancy: Category C

ACTIONS/PHARMACODYNAMICS Pyrimidine nucleoside structurally related to idoxuridine and an analog of thymidine. Active against herpes simplex virus (HSV) types 1 and 2, vaccinia virus, and certain strains of *Adenovirus.* Mechanism of antiviral action not completely known but appears to involve inhibition of viral DNA synthesis and viral repli-cation. Not effective against bacteria, fungi, or *Chlamydia.*

USES Topically to eyes for treatment of primary keratoconjunctivitis and recurring epithelial keratitis caused by herpes simplex virus types 1 and 2. Also for other herpetic ophthalmic infections including stromal keratitis, uveitis, and for infections caused by vaccinia and *Adenovirus,* but clinical effectiveness has not been established.

ROUTE & DOSAGE

Viral Infections of Eye

Adult	Topical	Ophthalmic solution 1%: 1 drop into affected eye q2h during waking hours until healing (reepithelialization) has occurred, (max 9 drops/d); when healing appears to be complete, dosage reduced to 1 drop q4h during waking hours for an additional 7 d (max 5 drops/d); continuous administration beyond 21 d not recommended.

PHARMACOKINETICS Absorption: Following topical application to eye, trifluridine penetrates cornea and aqueous humor (inflammation enhances penetration). Systemic absorption does not appear to be significant.

CONTRAINDICATIONS & PRECAUTIONS Contraindicated in: safe use during pregnancy (category C) and in nursing women not established. **Cautious use in:** dry eye syndrome.

ADVERSE/SIDE EFFECTS Mild transient burning or stinging, mild irritation of conjunctiva or cornea, photophobia, edema of eyelids and cornea, punctal occlusion, superficial punctate keratopathy, epithelial keratopathy, stromal edema, keratitis sicca, hyperemia, increased intraocular pressure, hypersensitivity reactions (rare).

NURSING IMPLICATIONS

Administration

- Consult pharmacist regarding concurrent use with other topical ophthalmic preparations.
- Refrigerate at 2–8C (36–46F) unless otherwise directed.

Assessment & Drug Effects

- Epithelial eye infections usually respond to therapy within 2–7 d, with complete healing occurring in 1–2 wk.
- If improvement has not occurred after 7 d of treatment or if healing has not taken place after 14 d, other therapy should be considered.

Patient & Family Education

- Urge patient to keep physician informed of progress and to keep follow-up appointments. Herpetic eye infections have a tendency to recur and can lead to corneal damage if not adequately treated.

Prototype: atropine, p 116

TRIHEXYPHENIDYL HYDROCHLORIDE
(trye-hex-ee-fen i-dill)

Trade names: Aparkane, Aphen, Apo-Trihex, Artane, Novohexidyl, Tremin, Trihexane, Trihexidyl, Trihexy

Classifications: AUTONOMIC NERVOUS SYSTEM AGENT; ANTICHOLINERGIC (PARASYMPATHOLYTIC); ANTIPARKINSONISM AGENT; ANTIMUSCARINIC, ANTISPASMODIC

Pregnancy: Category C

ACTIONS/PHARMACODYNAMICS Synthetic tertiary amine anticholinergic agent with actions, contraindications, precautions, and adverse reactions similar to those of atropine. Thought to act by blocking excess of acetylcholine at certain cerebral synaptic sites. Relaxes smooth muscle by direct effect and by atropinelike blocking action on parasympathetic nervous system. Small doses cause CNS depression; larger doses produce CNS stimulation. Antispasmodic action appears to be one-half that of atropine, and side effects are usually less frequent and less severe.

USES Symptomatic treatment of all forms of parkinsonism (arteriosclerotic, idiopathic, postencephalitic). Also to prevent or control drug-induced extrapyramidal disorders. **Unlabeled uses:** Huntington's chorea, spasmodic torticollis.

ROUTE & DOSAGE

Parkinsonism

Adult	PO	1 mg day 1, 2 mg day 2, then increase by 2 mg q3–5d up to 6–10 mg/d in 3 or more divided doses (max 15 mg/d)

Extrapyramidal Effects

Adult	PO	5–15 mg/d in divided doses

PHARMACOKINETICS Absorption: readily absorbed from GI tract. **Onset:** within 1 h. **Peak:** 2–3 h. **Duration:** 6–12 h. **Elimination:** excreted in urine.

CONTRAINDICATIONS & PRECAUTIONS Contraindicated in: narrow-angle glaucoma. Safe use during pregnancy (category C), in nursing mothers, and children not established. **Cautious use in:** history of drug hypersensitivities; arteriosclerosis; hypertension; cardiac disease, renal or hepatic disorders; obstructive diseases of GI or genitourinary tracts; elderly patients with prostatic hypertrophy.

ADVERSE/SIDE EFFECTS *Dry mouth, dizziness, blurred vision,* mydriasis, photophobia, *nausea, nervousness,* insomnia, constipation, drowsiness, urinary hesitancy or retention. **CNS:** stimulation (usually with high doses): confusion, agitation, delirium, psychotic manifestations, euphoria. **CV:** tachycardia, palpitations, hypotension, orthostatic hypotension. **Other:** hypersensitivity reactions, angle-closure glaucoma.

DRUG INTERACTIONS Reduces therapeutic effects of **chlorpromazine, haloperidol,** PHENOTHIAZINES; increases bioavailability of **digoxin;** MAO INHIBITORS potentiate actions of trihexyphenidyl.

Common side effects in *italic*; life-threatening effects underlined; generic names in **bold**; classifications in SMALL CAPS

1029

NURSING IMPLICATIONS

Administration

- May be taken before or after meals, depending on how patient reacts. Elderly patients and patients prone to excessive salivation (e.g., postencephalitic parkinsonism) may prefer to take drug after meals. If drug causes excessive mouth dryness, it may be better taken before meals, unless it causes nausea.
- Once stabilized on conventional dosage forms, patient may be switched to sustained-release capsules to permit once-a-day or twice-a-day dosing.
- Store at 15–30C (59–86F) in tight container unless otherwise directed.

Assessment & Drug Effects

- Incidence and severity of side effects are usually dose related and may be minimized by dosage reduction. Elderly patients appear to be more sensitive to usual adult doses.
- Monitor vital signs. Pulse is a particularly sensitive indicator of patient's response to drug. Report tachycardia, palpitations, paradoxical bradycardia, or fall in BP.
- CNS stimulation (see adverse/side effects) may occur with high doses and in patients with arteriosclerosis or history of hypersensitivity to other drugs. If severe, drug may be discontinued for a few days and then resumed at lower dosage.
- In patients with severe rigidity, tremors may appear to be accentuated during therapy as rigidity diminishes.
- Monitor daily I&O if patient develops urinary hesitancy or retention. Voiding before taking drug may relieve problem.
- If constipation is a problem, check for abdominal distension and bowel sounds.
- Close monitoring of intraocular pressure at regular intervals is advised.
- Close follow-up care is advisable. Tolerance may develop, necessitating dosage adjustment or use of combination therapy. Patients > 60 y frequently develop sensitivity to trihexyphenidyl action.

Patient & Family Education

- Drug-induced mouth dryness may be relieved by ice chips, sugarless gum or hard candy, by frequent sips of water, and by maintaining adequate total daily fluid intake.
- Warn patient to avoid excessive heat because drug suppresses perspiration and, therefore, heat loss.
- Caution patient not to engage in activities requiring alertness and skill, as drug causes dizziness, drowsiness, and blurred vision. Supervision of ambulation may be indicated.

Prototype: hydroxyzine, p 49

TRIMEPRAZINE TARTRATE
(trye-mep´ra-zeen)
Trade names: Panectyl, Temaril
Classifications: ANTIHISTAMINE; ANTIPRURITIC
Pregnancy: Category C

ACTIONS/PHARMACODYNAMICS Structural analog of the phenothiazines. Similar to hydroxyzine, with prominent antipruritic activity. Also shares sedative and antihistaminic effects of hydroxyzine. In common with antihistamines, exerts both anticholinergic and antiserotonin action. Suppresses the cough reflex; may exert ulcerogenic effect.

USES Primarily for symptomatic relief of pruritic symptoms in a variety of dermatologic and nondermatologic conditions. **Unlabeled use:** preoperative sedation in children.

ROUTE & DOSAGE

Pruritus

Adult	PO	2.5 mg q.i.d. or 5 mg sustained-release q12h
Child	PO	> 6 y: 5 mg sustained-release once/d
		> 3 y: 2.5 mg h.s. or t.i.d.
		6 mo–3 y: 1.25 mg h.s. or t.i.d.

CONTRAINDICATIONS & PRECAUTIONS Contraindicated in: hypersensitivity to phenothiazines; acute asthma attack; sleep apnea; pregnancy (category C), premature or full-term infants < 6 mo; use of extended-release form in children ≤ 6 y. **Cautious use in:** hepatic disease; history of GI ulceration; history of convulsive disorders in the elderly or debilitated patient; upper respiratory tract infection.

ADVERSE/SIDE EFFECTS *Drowsiness,* dizziness, *dry mucous membranes,* GI upset, allergic skin reactions, cholestatic jaundice, extrapyramidal reactions, leukopenia. In some children: paradoxic hyperactivity, irritability, insomnia, hallucinations. **Acute poisoning:** CNS depression with hypotension, hypothermia. Toxic potential as for other phenothiazines.

Common side effects in *italic*; life-threatening effects underlined; generic names in **bold**; classifications in SMALL CAPS

NURSING IMPLICATIONS

Administration

- Usually administered after each meal and at bedtime
- Preserve in tight, light-resistant containers.

Assessment & Drug Effects

- Incidence and severity of adverse effects are generally dose-related; however, in some patients individual sensitivity is involved.
- Toxic manifestations of phenothiazine derivatives are most likely to occur between 4 and 10 wk of therapy.
- If child or elderly patient has a severe upper respiratory tract infection, this drug should be used only with caution because it suppresses the cough reflex.

Patient & Family Education

- Caution parents not to administer more than the prescribed dose to children.
- Drowsiness occurs frequently, but it generally disappears after a few days of medication. If it persists, dosage adjustment is indicated.
- Patient should know that sedative action of trimeprazine is additive to that of alcohol, barbiturates, narcotics, analgesics, and other CNS depressants.
- Warn patient to avoid activities requiring mental alertness and normal reaction time, such as operating a car or other hazardous activities, until drug response is known.

TRIMETHADIONE

(trye-meth-a-dye´ one)

Trade name: Tridione
Classifications: CNS AGENT; ANTICONVULSANT
Pregnancy: Category D

ACTIONS/PHARMACODYNAMICS Oxazolidinedione derivative similar to paramethadione in pharmacologic properties. Elevates seizure threshold in cortex and basal ganglia and reduces synaptic response to repetitive low-frequency impulses. Has high potential for toxicity. Increases solubility of calcium carbonate, the principal constituent of pancreatic stones.

USES Control of absence (petit mal) seizures refractory to other anticonvulsant drugs. May be adminis-

tered concomitantly with other anticonvulsants when other forms of epilepsy coexist with petit mal.

ROUTE & DOSAGE

Absence Seizures

Adult	PO	300 mg t.i.d.; may increase by 300 mg/d q wk as needed up to max of 2.4 g/d in 3–4 divided doses
Child	PO	300–900 mg/d in 3–4 divided doses (max 1 g/m²/d)

PHARMACOKINETICS Absorption: readily absorbed from GI tract. **Peak:** 0.5–2 h. **Distribution:** crosses placenta. **Metabolism:** metabolized in liver to active metabolites. **Elimination:** half-life: 5–10 d; excreted slowly in urine.

CONTRAINDICATIONS & PRECAUTIONS Contraindicated in: hypersensitivity to oxazolidinediones, as single agent in treatment of patient with history of grand mal seizures; severe hepatic or renal impairment; blood dyscrasias. Safe use during pregnancy (category D) not established. **Cautious use in:** diseases of retina and optic nerve; renal dysfunction.

ADVERSE/SIDE EFFECTS CNS: *hemeralopia, photophobia, diplopia,* vertigo, ataxia, *drowsiness,* insomnia, headache, fatigue, malaise, paresthesias, irritability, personality changes. **GI:** hiccups, nausea, vomiting, abdominal pain, gastric distress, anorexia, weight loss. **Hematologic:** <u>severe blood dyscrasias</u>: leukopenia, neutropenia, thrombocytopenia, pancytopenia, <u>agranulocytosis, aplastic anemia</u>. **Hypersensitivity:** lymphadenopathy with splenomegaly, hepatomegaly, pruritus, morbilliform rash. **Renal:** albuminuria, nephrosis, <u>hepatotoxicity</u>, precipitation of grand mal seizures. **Skin:** <u>exfoliative dermatitis</u>, erythema multiforme, acneiform dermatitis. **Other:** bleeding gums, epistaxis, retinal and petechial hemorrhages, vaginal bleeding, SLE syndrome, myasthenia gravis–like syndrome, changes in BP.

NURSING IMPLICATIONS

Administration

- Drug may be taken with food or milk to minimize GI distress.
- Following prolonged use, withdrawal should be accomplished gradually to avoid precipitating petit mal status or seizures.
- Preserve in tightly closed containers in a dry place below 25C (77F).

Common side effects in *italic*; life-threatening effects <u>underlined</u>; generic names in **bold**; classifications in SMALL CAPS

1031

Assessment & Drug Effects

- Complete blood and differential counts and urinalyses are recommended at monthly intervals or more frequently if indicated. Therapy should be discontinued if neutrophil count drops to 2500/mm³ or below or if albuminuria persists or increases.
- Plasma concentrations of dimethadione, active metabolite of trimethadione, may be used as guide to dosage adjustment (usually maintained at about 700 μg/ml for effective seizure control).
- Because of potential for toxicity, close medical supervision, especially during first year of therapy, is essential.

Patient & Family Education

- A transitory increase in number of obscure seizures may occur at beginning of therapy. Instruct patient and responsible family member to keep a record of number, duration, and time of attacks. Clinical improvement usually occurs 1–4 wk after start of therapy.
- Visual disturbances are usually controlled by reduction in dosage.
- Drowsiness tends to diminish with continued therapy, or it can be controlled by dosage reduction. Caution patient to avoid potentially hazardous activities such as driving a car or operating machinery until this side effect is controlled.
- Instruct patient to report immediately to physician symptoms of agranulocytosis, hepatotoxicity, and thrombocytopenia (see chap 3) and hair loss or other unusual symptoms.
- Advise patient to follow prescribed regimen precisely, without interruption, changes in dosage, or abrupt discontinuation.
- Stress the importance of keeping follow-up appointments. Advise patient to wear medical identification jewelry or card at all times.

Prototype: hydralazine, p 152

TRIMETHAPHAN CAMSYLATE

(trye-meth´a-fan)

Trade name: Arfonad
Classifications: CARDIOVASCULAR AGENT; NONNITRATE VASODILATOR; ANTIHYPERTENSIVE; AUTONOMIC NERVOUS SYSTEM AGENT
Pregnancy: Category X

ACTIONS/PHARMACODYNAMICS Potent, short-acting nondepolarizing ganglionic blocking agent. Blocks transmission in both adrenergic and cholinergic ganglia by competing with acetylcholine for receptor sites on postganglionic membranes. Adrenergic blockade results in vasodilation, improved peripheral blood flow, and thus decrease in BP. Also has direct peripheral vasodilation action and thus can produce marked hypotension. BP is significantly lower in head-up position because venous dilation and peripheral pooling reduce cardiac output. Capable of causing histamine release.

USES To produce controlled hypotension for certain surgical procedures (e.g., neurologic, ophthalmic, and plastic surgery) and for short-term treatment of hypertensive crises associated with pulmonary edema. **Unlabeled uses:** acute dissecting aneurysm of aorta and ischemic heart disease.

ROUTE & DOSAGE

Controlled Hypotension, Short-term Treatment of Hypertensive Crisis

Adult	IV	Dilute 500 mg in 500 ml of 5% dextrose; infuse at 0.5–1 mg/min with gradual increase until BP control is achieved
Child	IV	50–150 μg/kg/min at a rate of 0.3–6 mg/min

PHARMACOKINETICS Onset: immediate. **Duration:** 10 min. **Distribution:** crosses placenta. **Metabolism:** metabolized by pseudocholinesterases in plasma. **Elimination:** excreted in urine.

CONTRAINDICATIONS & PRECAUTIONS Contraindicated in: Anemia, hypovolemia, shock; asphyxia, respiratory insufficiency; glaucoma; during pregnancy. **Cautious use in:** history of allergy; elderly and debilitated patients, children; cardiac disease, arteriosclerosis; hepatic or renal disease; degenerative CNS disease; Addison's disease; diabetes mellitus; patients receiving steroids, antihypertensives, anesthetics (especially spinal), and diuretics.

ADVERSE/SIDE EFFECTS CV: tachycardia or decrease in heart rate, orthostatic hypotension, angina. **GI:** nausea, vomiting, anorexia. **Hypersensitivity:** urticaria, pruritus, histaminelike reaction along course of vein. Symptoms resulting from cholinergic blockade: atony of urinary bladder or GI tract, cycloplegia, mydriasis, dry mouth, suppression of perspiration. **Other:** restlessness, extreme weakness; <u>respiratory depression</u>, <u>respiratory arrest (following large doses)</u>.

DIAGNOSTIC TEST INTERFERENCES Trimethaphan may decrease **serum potassium** and may prevent elevation of **blood glucose** that usually occurs during postoperative period.

DRUG INTERACTIONS DIURETICS, ANESTHETICS, procainamide add to hypotensive effects.

INCOMPATIBILITIES Solution/Additive: **tubocurarine.**

NURSING IMPLICATIONS

Administration

- Dilute one 10 ml ampule of Arfonad (50 mg/ml) to 500 ml with D5W, 0.9% NaCl, or Ringer's injection.
- IV infusion is started at 3–4 ml (3–4 mg)/min; then adjusted to maintain desired effect.
- IV flow rate is prescribed by physician to maintain desired BP level. Rate of infusion should be monitored constantly. Individuals vary considerably in response to drug.
- Use of an infusion pump, microdrip regulator, or similar device is recommended for precise measurement of flow rate.
- Infusion should be terminated gradually while BP is closely monitored. It is stopped before wound closure in surgery to allow BP to return to normal.
- Do not use trimethaphan infusion as a vehicle for administration of any other drugs.
- Trimethaphan is stable under refrigeration, but freezing should be avoided. The diluted solution (500 mg/500 ml) is stable at room temperature for 24 h. Store at 15–30C (59–86F).

Assessment & Drug Effects

- Take vital signs prior to initiation of therapy as a baseline for comparison during drug administration.
- Patient must be observed continuously while receiving infusion. BP should be checked q2min until stabilized at desired level, then q5min for duration of treatment. Pulse and respiration should also be monitored closely.
- Intensity of hypotensive effect is largely dependent on positioning. Decrease in BP is most marked in sitting or standing position. Excessive hypotension can be reversed by having patient assume head-low position or elevate legs.
- Continue to monitor vital signs at regular intervals after completion of treatment. Since BP returns to pretreatment level within 10 min after the infusion is terminated, an oral antihypertensive is usually initiated in patients with hypertension as soon as desired BP level is achieved with trimethaphan.
- Monitor I&O. Ganglionic blockade may reduce

renal blood flow initially as well as voiding contractions and urge to void. Check lower abdomen for bladder distension.

- Some patients become refractory to trimethaphan (tachyphylaxis) within 48 h after initiation of therapy. Notify physician promptly if BP fails to respond.

Prototype: prochlorperazine, p 215

TRIMETHOBENZAMIDE HYDROCHLORIDE
(trye-meth-oh-ben´za-mide)
Trade names: Arrestin, Hymetic, Tegamide, Ticon, Tigan, Tiject, T-Gen
Classifications: GI AGENT; ANTIEMETIC
Pregnancy: Category C

ACTIONS/PHARMACODYNAMICS Structurally related to ethanolamine antihistamines, but in therapeutic doses antihistamine activity is weak. Has sedative and antiemetic actions. Less effective than phenothiazine antiemetics but produces fewer side effects. Must be used with other agents when vomiting is severe. Primary locus of action is thought to be the chemoreceptor trigger zone (CTZ) in medulla.

USES Control of nausea and vomiting.

ROUTE & DOSAGE

Nausea and Vomiting		
Adult	PO	250 mg t.i.d. or q.i.d.
	Rectal/IM	200 mg t.i.d. or q.i.d.
Child	PO/Rectal	15–45 kg: 100–200 mg t.i.d. or q.i.d.
	Rectal	< 15 kg: 100 mg t.i.d. or q.i.d.

PHARMACOKINETICS Onset: 10–40 min PO; 15 min IM. **Duration:** 3–4 h PO; 2–3 h IM. **Elimination:** 30–50% of dose excreted unchanged in urine within 48–72 h.

CONTRAINDICATIONS & PRECAUTIONS Contraindicated in: uncomplicated vomiting in viral illness, parenteral use in children, rectal administration in prematures and newborns; known sensitivity to benzocaine (in suppository) or to similar local anesthetics. Safe use during pregnancy (category C) and in nursing mothers not established. **Cautious use in:** patients who have recently received other centrally act-

Common side effects in *italic*; life-threatening effects underlined; generic names in **bold**; classifications in SMALL CAPS

1033

ing drugs; in presence of high fever, dehydration, electrolyte imbalance.

ADVERSE/SIDE EFFECTS Hypersensitivity reactions (including allergic skin eruptions), hypotension, dizziness, drowsiness, headache, diarrhea, exaggeration of nausea, acute hepatitis, jaundice, muscle cramps. **Other:** pain, stinging, burning, redness, irritation at IM site; local irritation following rectal administration.

DRUG INTERACTIONS Alcohol and other CNS DEPRESSANTS add to depressant activity; BELLADONNA ALKALOIDS may intensify anticholinergic effects; PHENOTHIAZINES may precipitate extrapyramidal syndrome.

NURSING IMPLICATIONS

Administration
- Capsule may be emptied and contents swallowed with water or mixed with food (if patient has difficulty swallowing capsule).
- Administer IM deep into upper outer quadrant of buttock. To minimize possibility of irritation and pain, avoid escape of solution along needle track. This can be accomplished by Z-track injection or by drawing a small bubble of air into syringe after drug is measured; when medication is injected, air bubble will clear needle of drug.

Assessment & Drug Effects
- Hypotension is reported, particularly in surgical patients receiving drug parenterally. Monitor BP.
- If an acute febrile illness accompanies or begins during therapy with trimethobenzamide, report promptly and stop drug therapy.
- The antiemetic effect of drug may obscure diagnoses of GI or other pathologic conditions or signs of toxicity from other drugs.

Patient & Family Education
- Advise patient to report promptly to physician the onset of rash or other signs of hypersensitivity (see chap 3). Drug should be discontinued immediately.
- Since drug may cause drowsiness and dizziness, caution patient to avoid driving a car or other potentially hazardous activities.
- Advise patient not to drink alcohol or alcoholic beverages during therapy with this drug.

TRIMETHOPRIM

See ANTIINFECTIVE, URINARY TRACT, prototype, p 90.

Prototype: trimethoprim, p 90

TRIMETHOPRIM-SULFAMETHOXAZOLE (TMP-SMZ)

Trade names: Bactrim, Co-Trimoxazole, Septra
Classifications: URINARY TRACT ANTIINFECTIVE; SULFONAMIDE
Pregnancy: Category C

ACTIONS/PHARMACODYNAMICS Fixed combination of sulfamethoxazole (SMZ) an intermediate acting antiinfective sulfonamide, and trimethoprim (TMP), a synthetic antiinfective. Both components of the combination (5 : 1 ratio of SMZ to TMP) are synthetic folate antagonist antiinfectives. Mechanism of action is principally enzyme inhibition, which prevents bacterial synthesis of essential nucleic acid and proteins. Bacterial resistance to the combined drugs develops more slowly than to either of the drugs alone. Antibacterial activity includes most common urinary tract infection (UTI) pathogens except *Pseudomonas aeruginosa.*

USES *Pneumocystis carinii* pneumonitis, shigellosis enteritis, and severe complicated UTIs due to most strains of the Enterobacteriaceae. Also children with acute otitis media due to susceptible strains of *Haemophilus influenzae,* and acute episodes of chronic bronchitis in adults. **Unlabeled uses:** isosporiasis; prevention of traveler's diarrhea; cholera; treatment of infections caused by *Nocardia, Legionella micdadei,* and *Legionella pneumophila* and genital ulcers caused by *Haemophilus ducreyi;* prophylaxis in granulocytopenic patients.

PHARMACOKINETICS Absorption: readily absorbed from GI tract. **Peak:** 1–4 h PO. **Distribution:** widely distributed, including CNS; crosses placenta; distributed into breast milk. **Metabolism:** metabolized

Common side effects in *italic*; life-threatening effects underlined; generic names in **bold**; classifications in SMALL CAPS

in liver. **Elimination:** half-life: 8–10 h TMP, 10–13 h SMZ; excreted in urine.

ROUTE & DOSAGE

Systemic Infections

Adult	PO	160 mg TMP/800 mg SMZ (1 double strength [DS] tablet) q12h
	IV	8–10 mg/kg/d TMP divided q6–12h infused over 60–90 min
Child	PO	> 2 mo, <40 kg: 4 mg/kg/d TMP q12h
		> 40 kg: 160 mg TMP/800 mg SMZ (1 DS tablet) q12h
	IV	> 2 mo: 8–10 mg/kg/d TMP divided q6–12h infused over 60–90 min

Pneumocystis Carinii Pneumonia

Adult	IV	20 mg/kg/d TMP divided q6h infused over 60–90 min

CONTRAINDICATIONS & PRECAUTIONS Contraindicated in: hypersensitivity to TMP, SMZ, sulfonamides, or bisulfites; group A beta-hemolytic streptococcal pharyngitis; megaloblastic anemia due to folate deficiency; creatinine clearance <15 ml/min; pregnancy (category C), lactation. **Cautious use in:** impaired renal or hepatic function; possible folate deficiency; severe allergy or bronchial asthma; G6PD deficiency, hypersensitivity to sulfonamide derivative drugs (e.g., acetazolamide, thiazides, tolbutamide). Not recommended for infants <2 mo.

ADVERSE/SIDE EFFECTS *Mild to moderate rashes (including fixed drug eruptions).* **GI:** *nausea, vomiting,* diarrhea, *anorexia,* hepatitis, pseudomembranous enterocolitis, stomatitis, glossitis, abdominal pain. **GU:** renal failure, oliguria, anuria, crystalluria. **Hematologic:** agranulocytosis, aplastic anemia, megaloblastic anemia, hypoprothrombinemia. **Other:** weakness, arthralgia, myalgia, photosensitivity, toxic epidermal necrolysis, allergic myocarditis.

DIAGNOSTIC TEST INTERFERENCES May elevate levels of serum creatinine, transaminase, bilirubin, alkaline phosphatase.

DRUG INTERACTIONS may enhance hypoprothrombinemic effects of ORAL ANTICOAGULANTS; may increase **methotrexate** toxicity.

INCOMPATIBILITIES Solution/Additive: stability in dextrose and normal saline is concentration dependent; **verapamil.**

NURSING IMPLICATIONS

Administration

- Advise patient to take PO medication with a full glass of desired fluid and to maintain adequate fluid intake (at least 1500 ml/d) during therapy.
- Dosage may be adjusted in patient with renal dysfunction on basis of creatinine clearance tests. (Some clinicians reduce adult daily dose by 50% if creatinine clearance is between 15 and 30 ml/min).
- *IV infusion:* Must be diluted: add contents of 5 ml ampule to 125 ml D5W. Use within 6 h. If a dilution of 5 ml/100 ml D5W is desired, use solution within 4 h. Do not refrigerate. Administer solution over 60–90 min, avoiding bolus or rapid injection.
- Do not mix other drugs or solutions with IV infusion. Discard solution if cloudy or if crystallization appears after mixing.
- *Prophylaxis for traveler's diarrhea:* is usually reserved for the medically compromised patient: 160 mg/800 mg as a single dose. Nondrug prevention is preferable.
- Store at 15–30C (59–86F) in dry place protected from light. Avoid freezing.

Assessment & Drug Effects

- IV Septra contains sodium metabisulfite, which produces allergic-type reactions in susceptible patients: hives, itching, wheezing, anaphylaxis. Susceptibility (low in general population) is seen most frequently in asthmatics or atopic nonasthmatic persons.
- Monitor coagulation tests and prothrombin times in patient also receiving warfarin. Change in warfarin dosage may be indicated.
- Monitor I&O volume and pattern. Significant changes should be reported to forestall renal calculi formation. Also, failure of treatment (i.e., continued UTI symptoms) should be reported.
- Frequent urinalysis with macroscopic examination during therapy is advised.
- The elderly patient is at risk for severe adverse reactions, especially if liver or renal function is compromised or if certain other drugs are given. Most frequently observed: thrombocytopenia (with concurrent thiazide diuretics); severe decrease in platelets (with or without purpura); bone marrow suppression; severe skin reactions.
- *Overdose symptoms:* (no extensive experience has been reported): nausea, vomiting, anorexia, headache, dizziness, mental depression, confusion, bone marrow depression.

Common side effects in *italic*; life-threatening effects underlined; generic names in **bold**; classifications in SMALL CAPS

1035

Patient & Family Education

▪ Urge patient to report stat if rash appears. Other reportable symptoms are sore throat, fever, purpura, jaundice (early signs of serious reactions).

▪ This drug can cause fixed eruptions at the same sites each time the drug is administered. Every contact with drug may not result in eruptions; therefore patient may overlook the relationship. Instruct patient to monitor for and report fixed eruptions.

Prototype: imipramine, p 184

TRIMIPRAMINE MALEATE

(tri-mip´ra-meen)
Trade name: Surmontil
Classifications: CNS AGENT; PSYCHOTHERAPEUTIC; TRICYCLIC ANTIDEPRESSANT
Pregnancy: Category C

ACTIONS/PHARMACODYNAMICS Tricyclic antidepressant (TCA) pharmacologically similar to imipramine in actions, uses, pharmacokinetics, limitations, and interactions. Has moderate anticholinergic and strong sedative effects; therefore is useful in depression associated with anxiety and sleep disturbances. More effective in alleviation of endogenous depression than other depressive states. Recent studies suggest strong, active H_2-receptor antagonism is a characteristic of TCAs.

USES Similar to those for imipramine. **Unlabeled use:** peptic ulcer disease.

ROUTE & DOSAGE

Depression

Adult	PO	75–100 mg/d in divided doses; may increase gradually up to 300 mg/d if needed; maintenance dose usually 50–150 mg/d

PHARMACOKINETICS Absorption: rapidly absorbed from GI tract. **Peak:** 2 h. **Metabolism:** metabolized in liver. **Elimination:** half-life 9.1 h; excreted in urine and feces.

CONTRAINDICATIONS & PRECAUTIONS Contraindicated in: prostatic hypertrophy; during recovery period after MI. Safe use during pregnancy (category C) and by nursing mothers not established. **Cautious**

use in: schizophrenia, with electroshock therapy, suicidal tendency; cardiovascular, hepatic, thyroid, renal disease.

ADVERSE/SIDE EFFECTS CNS: seizures, tremor, confusion, *sedation*, blurred vision. **CV:** tachycardia, *orthostatic hypotension,* hypertension. **GI:** *xerostomia, constipation,* paralytic ileus. **Other:** *urinary retention,* photosensitivity, sweating.

DRUG INTERACTIONS May decrease some antihypertensive response to ANTIHYPERTENSIVES; CNS DEPRESSANTS, **alcohol,** HYPNOTICS, BARBITURATES, SEDATIVES potentiate CNS depression; may increase hypoprothombinemic effect of ORAL ANTICOAGULANTS; **ethchlorvynol** may cause transient delirium; with **levodopa,** SYMPATHOMIMETICS (e.g., **epinephrine, norepinephrine**), possibility of sympathetic hyperactivity with hypertension and hyperpyrexia; with MAO INHIBITORS, possibility of severe reactions, toxic psychosis, cardiovascular instability; **methylphenidiate** increases plasma TCA levels; THYROID AGENTS may increase possibility of arrhythmias; **cimetidine** may increase plasma TCA levels.

NURSING IMPLICATIONS

Administration

▪ Administer drug with food to decrease gastric distress.

▪ Supervise drug ingestion to be sure patient does not "hoard" the drug.

▪ Store in tightly closed container at 15–30C (59–86F) unless otherwise specified.

Assessment & Drug Effects

▪ Monitor BP and pulse rate during adjustment period of tricyclic antidepressant (TCA) therapy. If BP falls more than 20 mm Hg or if there is a sudden increase in pulse rate, withhold medication, and notify physician.

▪ Orthostatic hypotension may be sufficiently severe to require protective assistance when patient is ambulating. Instruct patient to change position from recumbency to standing slowly and in stages.

▪ Report signs of hepatic dysfunction: yellow skin and sclerae, light-colored stools, pruritus, abdominal discomfort.

▪ Fine tremors, a distressing extrapyramidal side effect, should be reported to the physician.

▪ Monitor bowel elimination pattern and I&O ratio. Severe constipation and urinary retention are potential problems, especially in the elderly. Advise increased fluid intake to at least 1500 ml/d (if allowed).

Common side effects in *italic*; life-threatening effects underlined; generic names in **bold**; classifications in SMALL CAPS

- Inspect oral membranes daily if patient is on high doses. Urge outpatient to report symptoms of stomatitis or xerostomia.
- If xerostomia is a problem, institute symptomatic therapy. Sore or dry mouth can be a major cause of poor food intake and noncompliance. Consult physician about use of a saliva substitute (e.g., Moistir).
- Drug may cause intolerance to heat or cold. Regulate environmental temperature and patient's clothing accordingly.
- The severely depressed patient may need assistance with personal hygiene, particularly because of excessive sweating caused by the drug.
- If a patient uses excessive amounts of alcohol, it should be borne in mind that the potentiation of TCA effects may increase the danger of overdosage or suicide attempt.

Patient & Family Education
- Caution patient that ability to perform tasks requiring alertness and skill may be impaired.
- Urge patient not to use OTC drugs unless physician approves.
- The actions of both alcohol and trimipramine are potentiated when used together during therapy and for up to 2 wk after the TCA is discontinued. Consult physician about safe amount of alcohol, if any, that can be taken.
- Advise patient that the effects of barbiturates and other CNS depressants may also be enhanced by trimipramine.
- Alert patient to the fact that because TCAs have a "lag period" of 2–4 wk, therapeutic response will be delayed. (Increased dosage does not shorten period but rather increases incidence of adverse reactions.) This period is one that fosters noncompliance. Monitor drug intake to see that therapy is not interrupted.

Prototype: methoxsalen, p 261

TRIOXSALEN
(trye-ox´sa-len)
Trade name: Trisoralen
Classifications: SKIN AGENT; PSORALEN

ACTIONS/PHARMACODYNAMICS Systemic psoralen derivative structurally and pharmacologically related to methoxsalen but that produces less intense melanogenic and erythemic responses. Produces resistance to solar damage in persons particularly susceptible to painful reactions with exposure to sunlight (e.g., blond persons or persons with fair complexions). This response appears to be related to drug-induced thickening of the horny layer of skin, with retention of melanin, resulting in formation of a stratum lucidum. Accelerates pigmentation only when followed by exposure of skin to sunlight or ultraviolet irradiation, and may reach equivalence of a full summer of sun exposure. Use to produce a cosmetic tan, however, is not advised by some clinicians because of its high potential for toxicity.

USES In conjunction with controlled exposure to ultraviolet light or sunlight to repigment vitiliginous skin, to improve tolerance to sunlight in patients with albinism, and to enhance pigmentation.

ROUTE & DOSAGE

Repigment Vitiliginous Skin

Adult	PO	10 mg/d as single dose 2–4 h before controlled exposure to ultraviolet-A (UVA) or sunlight

CONTRAINDICATIONS & PRECAUTIONS Contraindicated in: see methoxsalen.

ADVERSE/SIDE EFFECTS Skin: severe edema and erythema, painful blisters, burning and peeling of skin. **GI:** GI distress, nausea, vomiting. **CNS:** nervousness, vertigo, mental depression or excitation.

DRUG INTERACTIONS Coal tar, griseofulvin, SULFONAMIDES, PHENOTHIAZINES, THIAZIDES may increase photosensitivity reactions.

NURSING IMPLICATIONS

Administration
- Administer with milk or after a meal to reduce gastric distress.
- If trioxsalen is used to increase tolerance of skin to sunlight, treatment is continued no longer than 14 d, with dosage not exceeding 140 mg.
- Store in tightly closed, light-resistant container at 15–30C (59–86F).

Assessment & Drug Effects
- Repigmentation of idiopathic vitiligo may begin a few weeks after start of treatment, but significant effects require 6–9 mo of therapy.

Common side effects in *italic*; life-threatening effects underlined; generic names in **bold**; classifications in SMALL CAPS

1037

■ If repigmentation is not apparent after 3 mo of treatment, drug is discontinued.

Patient & Family Education
■ Following successful repigmentation with PUVA (P-psoralen, UVA) therapy, pigmentation can be maintained by periodic exposure to sunlight and trioxsalen.
■ Concomitant ingestion of furocoumarin-containing foods may intensify adverse reactions. Warn patient to avoid the following foods: figs, limes, parsley, parsnips, mustard, carrots, celery.
■ Urge patient to adhere to dosage and exposure time prescribed by physician. Severe burning may occur with overdosage.

Prototype: diphenhydramine, p 47

TRIPELENNAMINE HYDROCHLORIDE

(tri-pel-enn´a-meen)
Trade names: PBZ-SR, Pelamine, Pyribenzamine, Ro-Hist
Classifications: ANTIHISTAMINE (H_1-RECEPTOR ANTAGONIST)
Pregnancy: Category B

ACTIONS/PHARMACODYNAMICS Ethylenediamine antihistamine with mild CNS depressant effects and relatively high incidence of GI side effects. Antagonizes histamine action (i.e., increased capillary permeability, edema formation, itching, and constriction of respiratory, GI, and vascular smooth muscle). Does not inhibit gastric secretion. Has antiemetic, antitussive, anticholinergic, and local anesthetic action.

USES To relieve symptoms of various allergic conditions, to ameliorate reactions to blood or plasma, and in anaphylaxis as adjunct to epinephrine and other standard measures after acute symptoms have been controlled. Also to provide oral mucous membrane analgesia in young children with herpetic gingivostomatitis.

PHARMACOKINETICS Absorption: readily absorbed from GI tract. **Onset:** 15–30 min. **Peak:** 2–3 h. **Duration:** 4–6 h (up to 8 h with sustained-release). **Distribution:** crosses placenta; distributed into breast milk. **Metabolism:** metabolized in liver. **Elimination:** excreted in urine.

ROUTE & DOSAGE

Allergic Conditions

Adult	PO	25–50 mg q4–6h; or 100 mg sustained-release q8–12h (max 600 mg/d)
Child	PO	5 mg/kg/d in 4–6 divided doses (max 300 mg/d) (each 5 ml of tripelennamine citrate elixir is equal to 25 mg HCl)

CONTRAINDICATIONS & PRECAUTIONS Contraindicated in: narrow-angle glaucoma; symptomatic prostatic hypertrophy; bladder neck obstruction; GI obstruction or stenosis; lower respiratory tract symptoms, including asthma; within 14 d of MAO inhibitor therapy. Safe use during pregnancy (category B), in nursing mothers, and in neonates and prematures not established. **Cautious use in:** history of asthma; convulsive disorders; increased intraocular pressure; hyperthyroidism; cardiovascular disease; hypertension; diabetes mellitus.

ADVERSE/SIDE EFFECTS Atropinelike effects: *dry mouth, nose, and throat;* thickened bronchial secretions, wheezing, sensation of chest tightness, blurred vision, diplopia, headache; urinary hesitancy or retention; dysuria; palpitation, tachycardia, mild hypotension or hypertension. **CNS:** *drowsiness,* dizziness, tinnitus, vertigo, fatigue, disturbed coordination, tingling, tremors, euphoria, nervousness, restlessness, insomnia. **GI:** *epigastric distress, anorexia, nausea, vomiting, constipation* or diarrhea. **Hematologic:** leukopenia, hemolytic anemia. **Other:** skin rash, urticaria, photosensitivity, anaphylactic shock. **Overdosage:** (especially in children): hallucinations, excitement, fever, ataxia, athetosis, convulsions, coma, cardiovascular collapse.

DRUG INTERACTIONS Alcohol and other CNS DEPRESSANTS add to CNS depression; MAO INHIBITORS may intensify anticholinergic effects.

NURSING IMPLICATIONS

Administration
■ GI side effects may be lessened by administration of drug with or immediately after meals or food or with a glass of milk or water.
■ Note that the sustained-release formulation (100 mg) is not intended for use in children of any age.
■ Patients taking the sustained-release tablet should be instructed to swallow tablet whole and not to crush, break, or chew it.
■ Preserve in tight, light-resistant containers.

Common side effects in *italic*; life-threatening effects <u>underlined</u>; generic names in **bold**; classifications in SMALL CAPS

Assessment & Drug Effects

- Dizziness, sedation, and hypotension are more likely to occur in the elderly. Assistance during ambulation may be necessary.
- Patients receiving long-term therapy with antihistamines should have periodic blood cell counts.

Patient & Family Education

- Urinary hesitancy can be reduced if patient voids just before taking drug.
- Mild to moderate drowsiness, blurred vision, and dizziness occur in some patients. Caution against operating motor vehicle or engaging in hazardous activities until drug response has been determined.
- Patient should know that the effects of antihistamines may be augmented by alcohol ingestion and by use of other CNS depressants.
- Caution patient not to take OTC preparations without consulting physician.
- Antihistamines should be discontinued within 4 d before skin testing procedure for allergy because they may obscure otherwise positive reactions.

Prototype: diphenhydramine, p 47

TRIPROLIDINE HYDROCHLORIDE

(trye-proe´li-deen)
Trade names: Actidil, Bayidyl
Classifications: ANTIHISTAMINE (H$_1$-RECEPTOR ANTAGONIST)
Pregnancy: Category B

ACTIONS/PHARMACODYNAMICS Long-acting, potent propylamine (alkylamine) antihistamine, similar to diphenhydramine in actions, uses, contraindications, precautions, and adverse effects. Has rapid onset of action, with maximum effect in about 3.5 h and duration up to 12 h. Low incidence of drowsiness and other side effects. See diphenhydramine for contraindications and precautions and adverse/side effects.

ROUTE & DOSAGE

Allergies, Colds

Adult	PO	2.5 mg b.i.d. or t.i.d. (max 10 mg/d)
Child	PO	6–12 y: 1.25 mg b.i.d. or t.i.d. (max mg/d)
		2–5 y: 0.6 mg t.i.d. or q.i.d. (max 2.5 mg/d)
		4 mo–2 y: 0.3 mg t.i.d. or q.i.d. (max 1.25 mg/d)

NURSING IMPLICATIONS

- The product Actifed combines the antihistaminic action of triprolidine and the decongestant effect of pseudoephedrine.
- Preserve in tight, light-resistant containers.

See diphenhydramine for numerous additional nursing implications.

Prototype: erythromycin, p 65

TROLEANDOMYCIN

(troe-lee-an-doe-mye´sin)
Trade name: Tao
Classifications: ANTIINFECTIVE; ERYTHROMYCIN ANTIBIOTIC

ACTIONS/PHARMACODYNAMICS Derivative of oleandomycin, a macrolide antibiotic prepared from cultures of *Streptomyces antibioticus*. Chemically related to erythromycin and has similar range of antibacterial activity, but reportedly less effective; has high potential for toxicity. Cross-sensitivity with erythromycin reported.

USES Acute, severe infections of upper respiratory tract caused by susceptible strains of pneumococci and group A beta-hemolytic streptococci.

ROUTE & DOSAGE

Upper Respiratory Tract Infections

Adult	PO	250–500 mg q6h
Child	PO	6.6–11 mg/kg (125–250 mg) q6h

PHARMACOKINETICS Absorption: incompletely absorbed from GI tract. **Peak:** 2 h. **Distribution:** distributed throughout body fluids; diffusion into CSF is poor unless meninges are inflamed. **Metabolism:** metabolized in liver. **Elimination:** excreted in bile and urine.

CONTRAINDICATIONS & PRECAUTIONS Contraindicated in: use for prophylaxis or for minor infections. Safe use during pregnancy not established. **Cautious use in:** impaired hepatic function.

ADVERSE/SIDE EFFECTS *Abdominal cramps and discomfort, nausea,* vomiting, diarrhea; allergic reactions (urticaria, skin rash, <u>anaphylaxis</u>); cholestatic jaundice, superinfections.

Common side effects in *italic*; life-threatening effects <u>underlined</u>; generic names in **bold**; classifications in SMALL CAPS

1039

DIAGNOSTIC TEST INTERFERENCES Troleandomycin may cause false elevations of *urinary 17–ketosteroids* (Drekter), and *17–hydroxycorticosteroids* (Porter-Silver method).

DRUG INTERACTIONS May increase levels of **carbamazepine**, CYCLOSPORINES, and **theophylline** and their toxicity; ORAL CONTRACEPTIVES may cause cholestatic jaundice; **warfarin** may increase prothrombin time (PT); **ergotamine** may induce ischemia and peripheral vasospasm.

NURSING IMPLICATIONS

Administration
- Advise patient to take drug on an empty stomach (1 h before or 2 h after meals).
- To maintain effective blood levels, drug should be taken at evenly spaced intervals throughout the day, preferably around the clock.
- Generally, drug therapy does not exceed 10 d. For streptococcal infections, therapy should continue for 10 d to prevent development of rheumatic fever or glomerulonephritis.

Assessment & Drug Effects
- Periodic liver function tests are advised in patients receiving drug longer than 10 d or in repeated courses.
- Some patients develop an allergic type of hepatitis with right upper quadrant pain, fever, nausea, vomiting, jaundice, eosinophilia, and leukocytosis. Liver changes are reversible if drug is discontinued immediately.
- Superinfections are most likely to occur in patients on prolonged or repeated therapy. Drug should be discontinued if symptoms present (see chap 3), and appropriate therapy should be started.

Patient & Family Education
- Instruct patient to report signs of jaundice: acholic stools, pruritus, icteric sclerae.
- Instruct patient not to stop drug before full course of therapy is completed. Patient should not interrupt then restart therapy or increase or decrease dose or interval.

TROMETHAMINE
(troe-meth´a-meen)
Trade names: Tham, Tham-E
Classifications: ELECTROLYTIC BALANCE AGENT; SYSTEMIC ALKALINIZER
Pregnancy: Category C

ACTIONS/PHARMACODYNAMICS Sodium-free organic amine that acts as a proton acceptor in the body buffering system, thereby preventing or correcting acidosis. As a weak base it combines with hydrogen ions from carbonic, lactic, pyruvic, and other metabolic acids and penetrates the cell membrane to combine with intracellular acid. Also acts as a weak osmotic diuretic increasing urine pH and excretion of fixed acids, CO_2, and electrolytes. May be preferable to sodium bicarbonate in treatment of severe metabolic acidosis when sodium or CO_2 elimination is restricted.

USES To prevent or correct metabolic acidosis associated with cardiac bypass surgery and cardiac arrest and to correct excess acidity of stored blood (preserved with acid citrate dextrose [ACD]) and used in cardiac bypass surgery. (Stored blood has a pH range of 6.8–6.22.) **Unlabeled uses:** metabolic acidosis of status asthmaticus and neonatal respiratory distress syndrome.

ROUTE & DOSAGE

Dosage may be estimated from buffer base deficit of extracellular fluid using the following formula as a guide: Tromethamine ml of 0.3 M solution = Body weight (kg) × Base deficit (mEq/L)

Metabolic Acidosis Associated with Cardiac Arrest
Adult IV 3.5–6 ml/kg (126–216 mg/kg) of a 0.3 M solution into large peripheral vein; if chest is open, 55–165 ml (2–6 g) 0.3 M solution into ventricular cavity

Systemic Acidosis During Cardiac Bypass Surgery
Adult IV 9 ml/kg or approximately 500 ml (18 g) 0.3 M solution; a single dose of up to 1000 ml (36 g) may be necessary in severe acidosis

Excess Acidity of ACD Priming Blood
Adult IV 14–70 ml (0.5–2.5 g) 0.3 M solution added to each 500 ml blood

PHARMACOKINETICS Metabolism: no appreciable metabolism. **Elimination:** rapidly and preferentially excreted by kidneys; 75% excreted within 8 h.

CONTRAINDICATIONS & PRECAUTIONS Contraindicated in: anuria, uremia; chronic respiratory acidosis; pregnancy (category C), children, neonates. **Cautious use in:** > 1 d of therapy.

ADVERSE/SIDE EFFECTS Injection site: *local irritation*, tissue inflammation, *chemical phlebitis*, extravasation. **Respiratory:** respiratory depression. **Other:** increased blood coagulation time (possible); transient decrease in blood glucose, hypervolemia, hyperkalemia (with depressed renal function).

NURSING IMPLICATIONS

Administration

- Maximum allowable concentration for IV infusion is 0.3 M. Available as a 0.3 M solution or may be prepared by adding 36 g to 1 L of sterile water.
- A large antecubital vein should be selected for drug administration by slow IV infusion or via pump-oxygenator. Usually an IV catheter is used. The limb should be elevated.
- Drug administration is usually over a period of no less than 1 h. Except in life-threatening situations, drug administration is limited to 1 d.
- Observe entry site carefully. Perivascular infiltration of the highly alkaline solution may lead to vasospasm, necrosis, and tissue sloughing. Stop infusion if extravasation occurs.
- Extravasation may be treated with a procaine and hyaluronidase infiltration to reduce vasospasm and to dilute tromethamine remaining in tissues. If necessary, local infiltration of an alpha-adrenergic blocking agent (e.g., phentolamine) into the area may be ordered.
- Tromethamine solution is highly alkaline and can erode glass; discard solution 24 h after reconstitution.
- Protect drug (available as solution or powder) from freezing or extreme heat.

Assessment & Drug Effects

- Hypoxia and hypoventilation may result from drug-induced reduction of CO_2 tension (a potent stimulus to breathing), particularly if respiratory acidosis is also present. Watch for signs of hypoxia (see chap 3).
- Drug-induced hypoxia is a particular risk for the patient who is on other respiratory depressants or who has COPD or impaired renal function.
- Blood pH, Pco_2, Po_2, bicarbonate, glucose and electrolytes should be monitored before, during, and after treatment. Dosage is controlled to raise blood pH to normal limits (arterial: 7.35–7.45) and to correct acid-base imbalance.
- Monitor ECG and serum potassium if drug is given to patient with imparied renal function (reduced drug elimination). Since hyperkalemia is often associated with metabolic acidosis, be alert to early signs (see chap 3).
- *Overdose symptoms:* (total drug or too rapid administration): alkalosis, overhydration, prolonged hypoglycemia, solute overload.

Prototype: homatropine, p 210

TROPICAMIDE
(troe-pik´a-mide)
Trade name: Mydriacyl
Classifications: EYE PREPARATION; MYDRIATIC; CYCLOPLEGIC
Pregnancy: Category C

ACTIONS/PHARMACODYNAMICS Derivative of tropic acid, with pharmacologic properties similar to those of homatropine, but mydriatic and cycloplegic effects occur more rapidly and are less prolonged.

USES To induce mydriasis and cycloplegia for ophthalmologic diagnostic procedures.

ROUTE & DOSAGE

For Refraction

Adult	Ophthalmic	1–2 drops of 1% solution in each eye, repeat in 5 min; if patient is not seen within 20–30 min, an additional drop may be instilled.

Examination of Fundus

Adult	Ophthalmic	1–2 drops of 0.5% solution in each eye 15–20 min prior to examination; may repeat q30min if necessary

PHARMACOKINETICS Peak: maximal mydriasis: 20–40 min; maximal cycloplegia: 20–35 min. **Duration:** mydriasis: 6–7 h; cycloplegia: 50 min–6 h.

CONTRAINDICATIONS & PRECAUTIONS Contraindicated in: known or suspected angle-closure glaucoma. Safe use during pregnancy (category C) not established. **Cautious use in:** infants, children with brain damage or spastic paralysis, Down's syndrome.

ADVERSE/SIDE EFFECTS CNS: psychotic reactions, behavioral disturbances in children, unusual drowsiness or weakness, headache. **CV:** tachycardia. **Eye:** transient stinging, photophobia, blurred vision,

---

Common side effects in *italic*; life-threatening effects underlined;
generic names in **bold**; classifications in SMALL CAPS

1041

slight increase in intraocular pressure. **Other:** Sweating, flushing, allergic reactions.

NURSING IMPLICATIONS

Administration

▪ Possibility of systemic absorption may be minimized by applying pressure against lacrimal sac during and for 1 or 2 min following instillation.

Assessment & Drug Effects

▪ Monitor heart rate periodically and report onset of tachycardia.

Patient & Family Education

▪ Forewarn patient that transient stinging may occur on instillation.
▪ Photophobia may disappear as early as 2 h after application; if troublesome, advise patient to wear dark glasses.
▪ Caution patient to avoid potentially hazardous activities such as driving a car if vision is blurred.

TUBOCURARINE CHLORIDE

See AUTONOMIC NERVOUS SYSTEM AGENT, NONDE-POLARIZING SKELETAL MUSCLE RELAXANT prototype, p 124.

Prototype: mechlorethamine, p 96

URACIL MUSTARD

(yoor´a-sill)
Classifications: ANTINEOPLASTIC; NITROGEN MUSTARD; ALKYLATING AGENT
Pregnancy: Category X

ACTIONS/PHARMACODYNAMICS Nitrogen mustard agent thought to react selectively with phosphate groups of DNA, causing chromosomal crosslinkage and interference with normal mitosis. Lacks vesicant properties; ineffective in treatment of acute leukemia or acute blastic crisis. Has cumulative hematopoietic depressive properties at therapeutic dosage levels. Maximum bone marrow depression may not occur until 2–4 wk after uracil has been dis-

continued. Like other alkylating agents, uracil may be carcinogenic.

USES Chronic lymphocytic and myelocytic leukemia, non-Hodgkin's lymphomas, reticulum cell cancer. **Unlabeled uses:** carcinoma of lung, cervix, or ovary. Beneficial in early stages of polycythemia vera and in therapy of mycosis fungoides.

ROUTE & DOSAGE

Antineoplastic

Adult	PO	0.15 mg/kg q wk for 4 wk
Child	PO	0.30 mg/kg q wk for 4 wk

Thrombocytosis

Adult	PO	1–2 mg/d for 14 d

PHARMACOKINETICS Absorption: incompletely absorbed from GI tract. **Elimination:** plasma concentrations decrease rapidly with no evidence after 2 h; <1% recovered unchanged in urine.

CONTRAINDICATIONS & PRECAUTIONS Contraindicated in: severe leukopenia, thrombocytopenia, aplastic anemia, pregnancy (category X). **Cautious use in:** history of gout or urate renal stones; leukopenia, thrombocytopenia.

ADVERSE/SIDE EFFECTS CNS: irritability, nervousness, mental confusion, depression (rare). **GI:** *anorexia, epigastric distress, nausea, vomiting, diarrhea, oral ulcerations.* **Hematologic:** *leukopenia, thrombocytopenia,* bone marrow depression (sometimes irreversible). **Skin:** pruritus, dermatitis, pigmentation. **Other:** hepatotoxicity, hyperuricemia, amenorrhea, azoospermia.

NURSING IMPLICATIONS

Administration

▪ Administered at least 2 or 3 wk after maximum effect of previous antineoplastic or radiation has been achieved.
▪ Usually administered at bedtime to alleviate GI side effects. Severe nausea and vomiting may necessitate discontinuation of drug.

Assessment & Drug Effects

▪ As total cumulative dose of uracil approaches 1 mg/kg body weight, irreversible bone marrow damage may occur.
▪ Depression of platelets is apt to be more serious than that of leukocytes; watch carefully for begin-

Common side effects in *italic*; life-threatening effects underlined; generic names in **bold**; classifications in SMALL CAPS

ning signs of bleeding into skin and mucosa and gingival bleeding with tooth brushing. Report immediately.

- CBCs, including platelets, are advised 1 or 2 times weekly during and at least 1 mo after end of therapy. (Maximum bone marrow depression may not occur until 2–4 wk after discontinuation of therapy.)
- If possible avoid invasive procedures that could lead to bleeding during thrombocytopenic period (IM, SC, rectal temperatures).
- In some patients, drug appears to act slowly, and response may not be apparent for 2–3 mo after drug therapy is initiated.

Patient & Family Education

- Urge patient to increase fluid intake so that renal flushing occurs. Changes in I&O ratio and pattern and flank, stomach, or joint pain should be reported promptly.
- Notify physician of the following symptoms: fever, chills, oral ulcerations, sore throat, bleeding and bruising, swelling of lower legs and feet.
- Frank alopecia is not a usual side effect as with other nitrogen mustards.

Prototype: mannitol, p 200

UREA

(yoor-ee´a)

Trade names: Aquacare, Carbamex, Carbamide, Carmol, Dermaflex, Elaqua, Nutraplus, Rea Lo, Ureacin, Ureaphil

Classifications: WATER BALANCE AGENT; OSMOTIC DIURETIC; OXYTOCIC

Pregnancy: Category C

ACTIONS/PHARMACODYNAMICS Diamide salt of carbonic acid. When present in high concentrations in blood, induces diuresis by elevating osmotic pressure of glomerular filtrate, with subsequent decrease in sodium and water reabsorption and promotion of chloride and (to a lesser extent) potassium excretion. Volume and rate of urine flow is increased. Increased blood toxicity results in transudation of fluid from tissue, including brain, cerebrospinal, and intraocular fluid, into the blood. When used as an abortifacient, urea (in dextrose) is injected into amniotic sac, followed by IV oxytocin about 400 mU/min or by prostaglandin F_2. Mechanism of action is not

clear, but it is suggested that decidual damage due to the hyperosmotic drug may induce the formation of prostaglandins, which cause uterine contractions and cervical dilatation. The fetus is usually killed. Topical applications increase water binding capacity of stratum corneum and thus may soften dry scaly skin conditions.

USES To reduce or prevent intracranial pressure (cerebral edema) and intraocular pressure and to prevent acute renal failure during prolonged surgery or trauma. Also transabdominally for aborting second trimester of pregnancy. Topical preparation promotes hydration and removal of excess keratin in dry skin and hyperkeratotic conditions. **Unlabeled uses:** severe migraine attacks; acute sickle cell crisis.

ROUTE & DOSAGE

Reduction of Intracranial or Intraocular Pressure, Diuresis

Adult	IV	1–1.5 g/kg of 30% solution infused slowly over 1–2.5 h at a rate not to exceed 4 ml/min (max 120 g/24 h)
Child	IV	> 2 y: 0.5–1.5 g/kg of 30% solution infused slowly over 1–2.5 h at a rate not to exceed 4 ml/min
		< 2 y: 0.1–0.5 g/kg of 30% solution infused slowly over 1–2.5 h at a rate not to exceed 4 ml/min

Hydration of Dry Skin

Adult	Topical	Apply 2–40% cream or lotion to affected area 1–3 times/d

Second Trimester Abortion

Adult	Intraamniotic	Instill 40–50% urea solution in 5% dextrose in volumes equal to amount of amniotic fluid removed to a max of 200–250 ml

PHARMACOKINETICS Peak: 1–2 h. **Duration:** 3–10 h for diuresis and intracranial pressure reduction; 5–6 h for intraocular pressure. **Distribution:** 10% of intraamniotic instillation diffuses into maternal blood; distributed widely; good ocular penetration; crosses placenta; distributed into breast milk. **Elimination:** half-life: 1 h; excreted in urine; 50% may be reabsorbed.

CONTRAINDICATIONS & PRECAUTIONS Contraindicated in: severely impaired renal or hepatic function; CHF; active intracranial bleeding; marked

Common side effects in *italic*; life-threatening effects underlined; generic names in **bold**; classifications in SMALL CAPS

1043

dehydration; IV injection into lower extremities, especially in elderly patients; topical use for viral skin diseases or impaired circulation. Safe use in pregnancy (category C), lactation, or in children not established. (Contraindications for intraamniotic urea: impaired renal function, frank liver failure, active intracranial bleeding; marked dehydration, diabetes mellitus, sickle cell anemia.) **Cautious use in:** use on face or broken skin.

ADVERSE/SIDE EFFECTS CNS: somnolence (prolonged use in patients with renal dysfunction), *headache,* acute psychosis, confusion, disorientation, nervousness. **CV:** tachycardia, hypotension, syncope. **GI:** *nausea, vomiting,* increased thirst. **Metabolic:** fluid and electrolyte imbalance, dehydration. **Other:** intraocular hemorrhage (rapid IV), pain, irritation, sloughing, venous thrombosis, chemical phlebitis at injection site (infrequent); hyperthermia, skin rash, hemolysis (rapid IV).

DRUG INTERACTIONS May increase rate of **lithium** excretion, decreasing its effectiveness.

NURSING IMPLICATIONS

Administration

- The parenteral solution may be used orally. To improve palatability, pour medication over iced fruit juice (unsweetened) or mix with lemon juice or cola flavoring and have patient sip through a straw.
- Solution should be freshly prepared for each patient; discard unused portion. May be reconstituted with 5% or 10% dextrose injection or 10% invert sugar in water.
- Reconstituted solution should be used within a few hours if stored at room temperature. If refrigerated at 2–8C (36–46F), solution should be used within 48 h; prolonged storage leads to ammonia formation. Discard unused portions.
- Infusion flow rate will be prescribed by physician. Rapid administration may be associated with increased capillary bleeding and hemolysis.
- Urea should not be administered by same IV set through which blood is being infused.
- Urea has the potential for causing tissue damage because of its osmotic properties. Extreme care must be taken to avoid extravasation; thrombosis and tissue necrosis can occur. Inspect injection site frequently. If extravasation is suspected, discontinue the IV line stat. Consult physician about removal of needle or cannula. Institute local treatment (according to institution protocol or

physician's instructions); elevate part even if extravasation is minor.

- Dosage is individualized on basis of water and electrolyte balance, urinary volume, clinical signs.
- Action of topical preparation is enhanced by applying it to skin that is still moist following washing or bathing.

Assessment & Drug Effects

- Monitor I&O. If diuresis does not occur within 6–12 h following administration or if BUN exceeds 75 mg/dl, drug should be withheld until renal function is evaluated.
- Monitor vital signs and mental status; promptly report any changes.
- Observe postoperative patients closely for signs of hemorrhage. Urea reportedly may increase prothrombin time and promote internal oozing at suture sites.
- Patient should be encouraged to drink fluids so as to hasten excretion of urea. However, if patient complains of a headache, do not allow him or her to drink as this will counteract the osmotic effects of the drug. Consult physician about fluid volume parameters.
- Determinations of serum and urinary sodium should be performed q12h. Frequent BUN and kidney function studies are advised, particularly in patients suspected of having renal dysfunction.
- Be alert for signs of hyponatremia, hypokalemia, dehydration, or transient overhydration (due to hyperosmotic activity) (see chap 3).
- There is minimal systemic absorption of intraamniotic-instilled drug when given in the intraamniotic sac and minimal systemic effects. If patient complains of lower abdominal pain, it may be that drug is going into abdomen rather than into the amniotic sac.

See mannitol for additional nursing implications.

Prototype: streptokinase, p 134

UROKINASE

(yoor-oh-kin´ase)
Trade names: Abbokinase, Open-Cath
Classifications: BLOOD FORMER; THROMBOLYTIC ENZYME
Pregnancy: Category B

ACTIONS/PHARMACODYNAMICS   Enzyme produced by kidneys and isolated from human kidney tissue cultures. Promotes thrombolysis by acting directly on the endogenous fibrinolytic system to convert plasminogen to the enzyme plasmin, an action that occurs within as well as on the surface of a thrombus or embolus. (Plasmin degrades fibrin, fibrinogen, and other procoagulant plasma proteins.) Urokinase also has an anticoagulant effect because its action leads to high plasma levels of fibrin and fibrinogen degradation products. Activity expressed in international units (IU): i.e., ability to lyse a fibrin clot via the in vivo plasmin system. Most effective action is on fresh, recently formed thrombi.

USES Lysis of acute massive pulmonary emboli and peripheral emboli and restoration of patency in occluded IV catheters (including central venous catheter); acute MI, retinal vessel occlusion, lysis of clot-occluded arteriovenous cannulas, and various other conditions associated with thromboembolization phenomenon.

ROUTE & DOSAGE

Pulmonary Embolis

Adult	IV	4400 IU/kg diluted in 0.9% NaCl or 5% dextrose infused over 10 min, followed by continuous infusion of 4400 IU/kg/h for 12 h; administer through in-line 0.22 or 0.45 µm filter using a constant infusion pump

Occluded Coronary Artery

Adult	IV	Precede urokinase with bolus of heparin (2500–10,000 U IV); then instill urokinase 6000 IU/min for periods up to 2 h; continue until artery is maximally opened (usually 15–30 min using about 500,000 IU); administer through in-line 0.22 or 0.45 µm filter using a constant infusion pump

Central Venous Catheter Clearance

Adult	IV	Instill 5000 IU/ml solution into catheter port; after 5 min attempt to aspirate urokinase and clot, if no success after 30 min, cap port and wait 30–60 min and try again; instruct patient to exhale and hold breath any time catheter is disconnected from syringe or IV tubing; avoid excessive pressure of instillation to prevent rupture of catheter or forcing clot into circulation

PHARMACOKINETICS Absorption: rapidly cleared from circulation. **Peak:** 3–4 h. **Elimination:** half-life: 10–20 min; small amount excreted in urine and bile.

CONTRAINDICATIONS & PRECAUTIONS Contraindicated in: pregnancy (category B), during lactation, and in children. See streptokinase for additional contraindications, adverse/side effects, diagnostic test interferences, and drug interactions.

NURSING IMPLICATIONS
See streptokinase for additional nursing implications.

- Reconstituted by adding 5.2 ml sterile water for injection to vial containing 250,000 IU (resulting solution contains 50,000 IU/ml). Roll or tilt vial to mix; avoid agitating or shaking to prevent foaming and filament formation. Prepare further dilutions by adding 190 ml of 0.9% NaCl or D5W.
- Urokinase should be reconstituted immediately before use. Since the product contains no preservatives, discard unused portion. Total volume of administered fluid should not exceed 200 ml.
- Avoid adding other medication to urokinase solution.
- Store vials at 2–8C (36–46F).

Assessment & Drug Effects
- Measurable signs of clinical response may not occur for 6–8 h after therapy is started.
- Anticoagulant therapy with heparin is reinstituted at end of urokinase therapy and when TT has decreased to less than twice normal control value (usually within 3–4 h).
- Severe spontaneous bleeding, including fatality from cerebral hemorrhage, has occurred during urokinase treatment. Risk is estimated to be twice that associated with heparin therapy.

VALPROIC ACID

(val-proe´ic)
Trade names: Dalpro, Depakene, Depakote, Depakote Sprinkle, Divalproex Sodium, Myproic Acid, Valproate Sodium
Classification: ANTICONVULSANT
Pregnancy: Category D

ACTIONS/PHARMACODYNAMICS Anticonvulsant unrelated chemically to other drugs used to treat seizure disorders. Mechanism of action unknown; may be related to increased bioavailability of the inhibitory neurotransmitter gamma-aminobutyric acid (GABA) to brain neurones. Inhibits secondary phase of platelet aggregation.

Common side effects in *italic*; life-threatening effects <u>underlined</u>; generic names in **bold**; classifications in SMALL CAPS

1045

USES Alone or with other anticonvulsants in management of absence (petit mal) and mixed seizures. **Unlabeled uses:** Status epilepticus refractory to IV diazepam, petit mal variant seizures, febrile seizures in children, other types of seizures including psychomotor (temporal lobe), myoclonic, akinetic and tonic-clonic seizures, photosensitivity seizures, and those refractory to other anticonvulsants.

ROUTE & DOSAGE

Management of Seizures

Adult	PO	15 mg/kg/d in divided doses when total daily dose > 250 mg; increase at 1 wk intervals by 5–10 mg/kg/d until seizures are controlled or side effects develop (max 60 mg/kg/d)
Child	PO	Same as for adult

PHARMACOKINETICS Absorption: readily absorbed from GI tract. **Peak:** 1–4 h valproic acid; 3–5 h divalproex. **Therapeutic range:** 50–100 µg/ml. **Distribution:** crosses placenta; distributed into breast milk. **Metabolism:** metabolized in liver. **Elimination:** half-life: 5–20 h; excreted primarily in urine; small amount excreted in feces and expired air.

CONTRAINDICATIONS & PRECAUTIONS Contraindicated in: patient with bleeding disorders or hepatic dysfunction or disease. **Cautious use in:** pregnancy (category D), nursing mothers; history of renal disease; adjunctive treatment with other anticonvulsants.

ADVERSE/SIDE EFFECTS CNS: breakthrough seizures *sedation, drowsiness,* dizziness, decreased alertness. **GI:** *nausea, vomiting, indigestion (transient),* hypersalivation, anorexia with weight loss, increased appetite with weight gain, abdominal cramps, diarrhea, constipation, hepatic failure. **Hematologic:** *prolonged bleeding time,* leukopenia, lymphocytosis, thrombocytopenia, hypofibrinogenemia, bone marrow depression, anemia. **Psychiatric:** depression, hallucinations, hyperactivity, behavioral deterioration in children, aggression, emotional upset. **Other:** skin rash, transient hair loss, curliness or waviness of hair, irregular menses, secondary amenorrhea, photosensitivity; hyperammonemia (usually asymptomatic). **Overdosage:** deep coma, pulmonary edema, death.

DIAGNOSTIC TEST INTERFERENCES Valproic acid produces false-positive results for **urine ketones,** elevated **AST, ALT, LDH,** and **serum alka-** *line phosphatase,* prolonged **bleeding time,** altered **thyroid function** tests.

DRUG INTERACTIONS Alcohol and other CNS DEPRESSANTS potentiate depressant effects; other ANTICONVULSANTS, BARBITURATES increase anticonvulsant and barbiturate levels and toxicity; **aspirin, dipyridamole, warfarin** increase risk of spontaneous bleed and decrease clotting; **clonazepam** may precipitate absence seizures; SALICYLATES may increase valproic acid levels and toxicity.

NURSING IMPLICATIONS

Administration

- Tablets and capsules should not be chewed. Medication should be swallowed whole. Patient should avoid using a carbonated drink as diluent for the syrup because it will release drug from delivery vehicle. Free drug painfully irritates oral and pharyngeal membranes.
- Serious GI side effects can lead to discontinuation of therapy with valproic acid. To reduce gastric irritation, administer drug with food. Enteric-coated tablet or syrup formulation is usually well tolerated.
- Abrupt discontinuation of therapy can lead to loss of seizure control. Warn patient not to stop or alter dosage regimen without consulting physician.

Assessment & Drug Effects

- Effective *therapeutic serum levels of valproic acid:* 50–100 µg/ml.
- Monitor alertness in patient on multiple drug therapy for seizure control. Plasma levels of the adjunctive anticonvulsants should be evaluated periodically as indicators for possible neurologic toxicity.
- Increased dosage increases frequency of adverse effects. Monitor patient carefully when dose adjustments are being made and report promptly if side effects persist.
- Platelet counts and bleeding time determinations are recommended prior to initiating treatment and at periodic intervals. Liver function tests, including serum ammonia, should be performed initially and at least q2mo, especially during the first 6 mo of therapy.

Patient & Family Education

- Inform the diabetic patient that this drug may cause a false-positive test for urine ketones. Should that occur, notify the physician; a differential diagnostic blood test may be indicated.
- If spontaneous bleeding or bruising (petechiae, ec-

chymotic areas, otorrhagia, epistaxis, melena) occurs, notify physician promptly.

- Instruct patient to withhold dose and report to the physician if the following symptoms appear: visual disturbances, rash, jaundice, light-colored stools, protracted vomiting, diarrhea. Fatal hepatic failure has occurred in patients receiving this drug.
- Warn patient to avoid alcohol and self-medicating with other depressants during therapy. The use of all OTC drugs should be approved by the physician during anticonvulsant therapy. Particularly unsafe are combination drugs containing aspirin, sedatives, and medications for hay fever or other allergies.
- Advise patient not to drive a car or engage in other activities requiring mental alertness and physical coordination until reaction to drug is known.
- Patients on multiple drug therapy are at risk from hyperammonemia (lethargy, anorexia, asterixis, increased seizure frequency, vomiting). These symptoms should be reported promptly. If they persist with decreased dosage, the drug will be discontinued.
- Before any kind of surgery (including dental surgery), the patient should inform the doctor or dentist of taking valproic acid.
- Advise patient to carry medical identification card or jewelry bearing information about medication in use and the epilepsy diagnosis.

VANCOMYCIN HYDROCHLORIDE

(van-koe-mye´sin)
Trade names: Vancocin, Vancoled
Classifications: ANTIINFECTIVE; ANTIBIOTIC
Pregnancy: Category C

ACTIONS/PHARMACODYNAMICS Glucopeptide antibiotic prepared from *Streptomyces orientalis,* with bactericidal and bacteriostatic actions. Action interferes with cell membrane synthesis in multiplying organisms. Active against many gram-positive organisms, including group A beta-hemolytic streptococci, staphylococci, pneumococci, enterococci, clostridia, and corynebacteria. Gram-negative organisms, mycobacteria, and fungi are highly resistant. Cross-resistance with other antibiotics or resistance to vancomycin has not been reported.

USES Parenterally for potentially life-threatening infections in patients allergic, nonsensitive, or resistant to other less toxic antimicrobial drugs. Used orally only in *Clostridium difficile* colitis (not effective by oral route for treatment of systemic infections).

ROUTE & DOSAGE

Systemic Infections

Adult	IV	500 mg q6h or 1 g q12h; infuse over 60–90 min
Child	IV	40 mg/kg/d divided q6h; infuse over 60–90 min
Neonate	IV	10 mg/kg/d divided q8–12h; infuse over 60–90 min

C. difficile Colitis

Adult	PO	125–500 mg q6h
Child	PO	40 mg/kg/d divided q6h (max 2 g/d)

PHARMACOKINETICS Absorption: not absorbed from GI tract. **Peak:** 30 min after end of infusion. **Distribution:** diffuses into pleural, ascitic, pericardial and synovial fluids; small amount penetrates CSF if meninges are inflamed; crosses placenta. **Elimination:** half-life: 4–8 h; 80–90% of IV dose excreted in urine within 24 h; PO dose excreted in feces.

CONTRAINDICATIONS & PRECAUTIONS Contraindicated in: known hypersensitivity to vancomycin, previous hearing loss, concurrent or sequential use of other ototoxic or nephrotoxic agents, IM administration. Safe use during pregnancy (category C) not established. **Cautious use in:** neonates; impaired renal function.

ADVERSE/SIDE EFFECTS Ototoxicity (auditory portion of eighth cranial nerve), nephrotoxicity leading to uremia, hypersensitivity reactions (chills, fever, skin rash, urticaria, shocklike state); transient leukopenia, eosinophilia, anaphylactoid reaction with vascular collapse; superinfections, severe pain, thrombophlebitis at injection site; nausea, warmth, and generalized tingling following rapid IV infusion, *hypotension accompanied by flushing and erythematous rash on face and upper body* ("red-neck syndrome") following rapid IV infusion.

DRUG INTERACTIONS Adds to toxicity of OTOTOXIC AND NEPHROTOXIC DRUGS (AMINOGLYCOSIDES, **amphotericin B, colistin, polymyxin B**).

INCOMPATIBILITIES Solution/Additive: Aminophylline, BARBITURATES, **chloramphenicol, chlorothiazide, dexamethasone, heparin, methicillin, sodium bicarbonate, warfarin. Y-Site: heparin.**

NURSING IMPLICATIONS

Administration

- For oral administration, contents of vial (500 mg) may be diluted in 30 ml of water. It may also be administered at this dilution via nasogastric tube.
- *Preparation of parenteral drug:* reconstitute with 10 ml sterile water for injection for concentration of 500 mg/100 ml; Further dilute with 100–200 ml of D5W, 0.9% NaCl, or Ringer's lactate.
- Administer a single dose of 500 mg over 60–90 min.
- May be given as a continuous infusion over 24 h (1–2 g/24h).
- Rapid infusion may cause sudden hypotension.
- Extravasation of IV infusion must be avoided; severe irritation and necrosis can result.
- Oral and parenteral solution: stable for 14 d in refrigerator; after further dilution, parenteral solution is stable 24 h at room temperature.

Assessment & Drug Effects

- Monitor BP and heart rate continuously through period of drug administration.
- Periodic urinalyses, renal and hepatic function tests, and hematologic studies are advised in all patients.
- Serial tests of vancomycin blood levels are recommended in patients with borderline renal function and in patients > 60 y (target range is peak of 20–30 mg/ml and trough of < 15 mg/ml).
- Assess hearing, as vancomycin may cause damage to auditory branch (not vestibular branch) of eighth cranial nerve, with consequent deafness, which may be permanent.
- Serum levels of 60–80 µg/ml are associated with ototoxicity. Tinnitus and high tone hearing loss may precede deafness, which may progress even after drug is withdrawn. The elderly and those on high doses are especially susceptible
- Monitor I&O; report changes in I&O ratio and pattern. Oliguria or cloudy or pink urine may be a sign of nephrotoxicity (also manifested by transient elevations in BUN, albumin, and hyaline and granular casts in urine).

Patient & Family Education

- Warn patient to report ringing in ears promptly.
- Instruct patient to adhere to drug regimen, i.e., not to increase, decrease, or interrupt dosage. The full course of prescribed drug therapy should be completed.

VASOPRESSIN

See HORMONES, PITUITARY (ANTIDIURETIC) prototype, p 239.

Prototype: tubocurarine, p 124

VECURONIUM

(vek-yoo-roe´-nee-um)
Trade name: Norcuron
Classifications: AUTONOMIC NERVOUS SYSTEM AGENT; NONDEPOLARIZING SKELETAL MUSCLE RELAXANT
Pregnancy: Category C

ACTIONS/PHARMACODYNAMICS Intermediate-acting nondepolarizing skeletal muscle relaxant structurally similar to pancuronium but about 1–1 1/2 times more potent and has shorter duration of action. Unlike older neuromuscular blocking agents, demonstrates negligible histamine release and therefore has minimal direct effect on cardiovascular system. Similar to atracurium in having unique metabolic and excretion pathways (independent of renal function). However, since it relies heavily on biliary excretion, patients with hepatic disease may require dosage adjustment. Although it is 4 times more potent than atracurium it is like atracurium in having negligible cumulative tendencies with subsequent doses, provided recovery begins before dose is repeated. In common with other drugs of this class, inhibits neuromuscular transmission by competitive binding with acetylcholine to motor endplate receptors. Lacks analgesic action and has no apparent effect on pain threshold, consciousness, or cerebration; given only after induction of general anesthesia.

USES Adjunct for general anesthesia to produce skeletal muscle relaxation during surgery. Especially useful for patients with severe renal disease, limited cardiac reserve, and history of asthma or allergy. Also to facilitate endotracheal intubation. **Unlabeled use:** continuous infusion for facilitation of mechanical ventilation.

PHARMACOKINETICS Onset: <1 min. **Peak:** 3–5 min. **Duration:** 25–40 min. **Distribution:** well distributed

V

to tissues and extracellular fluids; crosses placenta; distribution into breast milk unknown. **Metabolism:** rapid nonenzymatic degradation in bloodstream. **Elimination:** half-life: 30–80 min; 30–35% excreted in urine, 30–35% in bile.

ROUTE & DOSAGE

Skeletal Muscle Relaxation

Adult	IV	0.04–0.1 mg/kg initially; then after 25–40 min, 0.01–0.15 mg/kg q12–15min or 0.001 mg/kg/min by continuous infusion
Child	IV	≥ 10 y: same as for adult

CONTRAINDICATIONS & PRECAUTIONS Contraindicated in: safe use during pregnancy (category C), in nursing mother, and in neonate not established. **Cautious use in:** severe hepatic disease; impaired acid-base, fluid, and electrolyte balance; severe obesity; adrenal or neuromuscular disease (myasthenia gravis, Eaton-Lambert syndrome); patients with slow circulation time (cardiovascular disease, old age, edematous states); malignant hyperthermia.

ADVERSE/SIDE EFFECTS Generally well tolerated. Skeletal muscle weakness, <u>respiratory depression</u>, hyperthermia.

DRUG INTERACTIONS GENERAL ANESTHETICS increase neuromuscular blockade and duration of action; AMINOGLYCOSIDES, **bacitracin, polymyxin B, clindamycin, lidocaine, parenteral magnesium, quinidine, quinine, trimethaphan, verapamil** increase neuromuscular blockade; DIURETICS may increase or decrease neuromuscular blockade; **lithium** prolongs duration of neuromuscular blockade; NARCOTIC ANALGESICS increase possibility of additive respiratory depression; **succinylcholine** increases onset and depth of neuromuscular blockade; **phenytoin** may cause resistance to or reversal of neuromuscular blockade.

NURSING IMPLICATIONS

Administration

- Administered only by qualified clinicians.
- Following reconstitution, refrigerate or store solution below 30C (86F) unless otherwise directed. Discard solution after 24 h.

Assessment & Drug Effects

- Baseline determinations of serum electrolytes, acid-base balance, renal and hepatic function are gen-

erally done as part of preanesthetic assessment.
- Peripheral nerve stimulator may be used during and following drug administration to avoid risk of overdosage and to identify residual paralysis during recovery period. It is especially indicated when cautious use of vecuronium is specified.
- Monitor vital signs at least q15min until stable, then every 30 min for the next 2 h. Also monitor airway patency until assured that patient has fully recovered from drug effects. Note rate, depth, and pattern of respirations. Obese patients and patients with myasthenia gravis or other neuromuscular disease may pose ventilation problems.
- Evaluate patients for recovery from neuromuscular blocking (curarelike) effects as evidenced by ability to breathe naturally or to take deep breaths and cough, keep eyes open, lift head keeping mouth closed, adequacy of hand grip strength. Notify physician if recovery is delayed.
- Note that recovery time may be delayed in patients with cardiovascular disease, edematous states, and in the elderly.

VERAPAMIL HYDROCHLORIDE

See CARDIOVASCULAR AGENTS, CALCIUM CHANNEL BLOCKING AGENT prototype p 144.

Prototype: acyclovir, p 85

VIDARABINE

(vye-dare´a-been)
Trade names: Adenine Arabinoside, ARA-A, Vira-A
Classifications: ANTIINFECTIVE; ANTIVIRAL
Pregnancy: Category C

ACTIONS/PHARMACODYNAMICS Pyrimidine nucleoside obtained from fermentation cultures of *Streptomyces antibioticus*. Mechanism of action not known but appears to block early stages of DNA synthesis by inhibiting DNA polymerase. Has antiviral activity against herpes simplex virus types 1 and 2, varicella zoster, vaccinia, cytomegalovirus, hepatitis B virus, and Epstein-Barr virus. Not active against smallpox, adenovirus, DNA or RNA viruses (except rhabdovirus and oncornavirus), bacteria, and fungi. A

Common side effects in *italic*; life-threatening effects <u>underlined</u>; generic names in **bold**; classifications in SMALL CAPS

1049

degree of immunocompetence must be present if drug is to be effective. Potentially mutagenic and oncogenic.

USES Systemically for treatment of herpes simplex encephalitis and herpes zoster infections in patients with suppressed immunologic responses. Used topically (ophthalmic) for treatment of acute keratoconjunctivitis and recurrent epithelial keratitis caused by herpes simplex virus types 1 and 2. Topical antibiotics and topical corticosteroids may be used concurrently.

ROUTE & DOSAGE

Herpes Simplex Encephalitis, Herpes Zoster

Adult	IV	15 mg/kg/d infused over 12–24 h

Herpes Keratitis

Adult	Ophthalmic	Instill 1 cm (1/2 in) ribbon of ointment into lower conjunctival sac q3h 5 times/d

PHARMACOKINETICS Distribution: widely distributed in body tissues and fluid; crosses blood-brain barrier; trace amounts of ophthalmic application found in aqueous humor; crosses placenta. **Metabolism:** rapidly deaminated to ara-hypoxanthine (Ara-Hx), a less active metabolite. **Elimination:** half-life: 1.5 h vidarabine, 3.3 h Ara-Hx; excreted primarily in urine.

CONTRAINDICATIONS & PRECAUTIONS Contraindicated in: safe use during pregnancy (category C) and breast feeding not established. **Cautious use in:** impaired renal or hepatic function, patients susceptible to fluid overload or cerebral edema.

ADVERSE/SIDE EFFECTS IV: CNS: (with high doses): hallucinations, confusion, psychosis, dizziness, ataxia, weakness, tremor, <u>fatal metabolic encephalopathy</u>. **GI:** (usually transient): *nausea, vomiting, anorexia, diarrhea, weight loss*. **Hematologic:** anemia, thrombocytopenia, neutropenia, decrease in WBC, Hgb, Hct. **Hepatic:** *elevated bilirubin and AST*. **Other:** malaise, pruritus, painful injection site. **Ophthalmic:** burning, itching, mild irritation, lacrimation, foreign body sensation, pain, photophobia, punctal occlusion, superficial punctate keratitis.

DRUG INTERACTIONS Allopurinol may increase potential for CNS side effects.

NURSING IMPLICATIONS

Administration
Intravenous Administration

- Dilute the vidarabine just before administration and use within 48 h.
- Shake vial well before withdrawing dose, and transfer it to appropriate IV fluid. Most IV infusion fluids are suitable. Blood products, protein, or other colloidal fluids should not be used. Follow manufacturer's directions.
- A large volume of fluid is required to dissolve vidarabine as it is only slightly soluble (1 L of IV infusion fluid will solubilize a maximum of 450 mg of vidarabine, or 1 mg of drug to 2.22 ml of IV fluid). Agitate thoroughly until drug is completely dissolved. Prewarming the IV infusion fluid to 35–40C (95–100F) will facilitate dissolution. Once dissolved, subsequent shaking is unnecessary. Do not refrigerate the dilution.
- Final dilution is administered through an in-line membrane filter (pore size of 0.45 μm or smaller).
- Infusion should be administered at a constant rate over 12–24h.

Assessment & Drug Effects

- Diagnosis of meningitis should be established before initiation of IV vidarabine therapy by studies of CSF, brain scan, EEG, or CAT. Vidarabine therapy is reportedly most effective when started before patient becomes semicomatose or comatose.
- Periodic hematologic tests are recommended during IV vidarabine therapy: Hgb, Hct, WBC, platelets.

Patient & Family Education
Ophthalmic Use

- Instruct patient to wash hands before and after treatment.
- Caution patient that vision may be temporarily hazy following instillation and to avoid potentially hazardous activities until vision clears.
- Advise patient that drug may cause sensitivity to bright light and to use sunglasses if necessary.
- Caution patient not to exceed recommended dose, frequency, and duration of treatment.

VINBLASTINE SULFATE

(vin-blast´een)
Trade names: Velban, Velbe, VLB
Classifications: ANTINEOPLASTIC
Pregnancy: Category D

Common side effects in *italic*; life-threatening effects <u>underlined</u>; generic names in **bold**; classifications in SMALL CAPS

ACTIONS/PHARMACODYNAMICS Cell cycle–specific alkaloid, extracted from periwinkle plant *Vinca rosea.* Arrests mitosis in metaphase by combination with microtubule proteins; may also interfere with other microtubular functions such as phagocytosis and cell mobility. In contrast to vincristine, has potent myelosuppressive and immunosuppressive properties but produces less neurotoxicity. Spectrum of activity not completely established.

USES Palliative treatment of Hodgkin's disease and non-Hodgkin's lymphomas, choriocarcinoma, lymphosarcoma, neuroblastoma, mycosis fungoides, advanced testicular germinal cell cancer, histiocytosis, and other malignancies resistant to other chemotherapy. Used singly or in combination with other chemotherapeutic drugs.

ROUTE & DOSAGE

Antineoplastic

Adult	IV	3.7 mg/m^2 infused over 1 min q wk; dose may be increased up to 18.5 mg/m^2 if tolerated
Child	IV	2.5 mg/m^2 infused over 1 min q wk; dose may be increased up to 12.5 mg/m^2 if tolerated

PHARMACOKINETICS Distribution: concentrates in liver, platelets, and leukocytes; poor penetration of blood-brain barrier. **Metabolism:** partially metabolized in liver. **Elimination:** half-life: 24 h; excreted in feces and urine.

CONTRAINDICATIONS & PRECAUTIONS Contraindicated in: leukopenia, bacterial infection, pregnancy (category D), men and women of childbearing potential, elderly patients with cachexia or skin ulcers. **Cautious use in:** malignant cell infiltration of bone marrow; obstructive jaundice, hepatic impairment; history of gout; use of small amount of drug for long periods; use in eyes.

ADVERSE/SIDE EFFECTS Generally dose related and short lived. **CNS:** (uncommon): mental depression, peripheral neuritis, numbness and paresthesias of tongue and extremities, loss of deep tendon reflexes, headache, convulsions. **GI:** vesiculation of mouth, stomatitis, pharyngitis, anorexia, *nausea, vomiting,* diarrhea, ileus, abdominal pain, constipation, rectal bleeding, hemorrhagic enterocolitis, bleeding of old peptic ulcer. **Hematologic:** leukopenia, thrombocytopenia and anemia. **Skin:** *alopecia (reversible),* vesiculation. **Other:** phlebitis, cellulitis, and sloughing following extravasation (at injection site); fever, weight loss, muscular pains, weakness, urinary retention, *hyperuricemia,* parotid gland pain and tenderness, tumor site pain, aspermia, Raynaud's phenomenon, photosensitivity, bronchospasm.

INCOMPATIBILITIES Solution/Additive: furosemide, heparin. Y-Site: furosemide.

NURSING IMPLICATIONS

Administration

- To prepare solution, add 10 ml NaCl injection to 10 mg of drug (yields 1 mg/ml). Other diluents not advised.
- Drug is usually injected into tubing of running IV infusion of NS or D5W over period of 1 min. If vinblastine is given directly into vein, fresh, dry needle is used. To ensure no spillage into extravascular tissue, needle and syringe should be rinsed with venous blood before withdrawal from vein.
- If extravasation occurs, stop infusion promptly; applications of moderate heat and local injection of hyaluronidase are advised to help disperse extravasated drug. Infusion should be restarted in another vein. Observe injection site; sloughing may occur.
- Avoid contact with eyes. Severe irritation and persisting corneal changes may occur. Copious amounts of water should be applied immediately and thoroughly. Wash both eyes; do not assume one eye escaped contamination.
- An antiemetic agent given before the injection may help to control nausea and vomiting.
- Reconstituted solution may be refrigerated in tight, light-resistant containers up to 30 d without loss of potency.

Assessment & Drug Effects

- Recovery from leukopenic nadir follows rapidly, usually within 7–14 d. With high doses, total leukocyte count may not return to normal for 3 wk.
- Even if 7 d have passed, drug is not administered unless WBC count has not returned to at least 4000/mm^3.
- Thrombocyte reduction seldom occurs unless patient has had prior treatment with other antineoplastics. However, be alert for unexplained bruising or bleeding, which should be promptly reported.
- With exception of epilation, leukopenia, and neurologic side effects, adverse reactions seldom persist beyond 24 h.
- Monitor bowel elimination pattern and bowel

Common side effects in *italic*; life-threatening effects underlined; generic names in **bold**; classifications in SMALL CAPS

1051

sounds to recognize severe constipation or paralytic ileus. A stool softener may be necessary.

▪ Skin surfaces over pressure areas should be inspected daily if patient is not ambulating. Note condition of skin of the elderly especially.

▪ Drug should be stopped if oral tissues break down.

Patient & Family Education

▪ Course of therapy may be continued 12 wk or more for adequate clinical trial. Encourage community-based patient to keep all appointments so that course of treatment is not interrupted.

▪ Temporary mental depression sometimes occurs on second or third day after treatment begins.

▪ Instruct patient to avoid exposure to infection, injury to skin or mucous membranes, and excessive physical stress, especially during leukocyte nadir period.

▪ Alopecia is frequently not total; in some patients, regrowth begins during maintenance therapy period.

▪ Instruct patient to report promptly onset of symptoms of agranulocytosis (see chap 3). Appropriate treatment should not be delayed.

▪ Avoid exposure to sunlight unless protected with sunscreen lotion (SPF > 12) and clothing.

VINCRISTINE SULFATE

(vin-kris′teen)
Trade names: LCR, Oncovin, VCR
Classification: ANTINEOPLASTIC
Pregnancy: Category D

ACTIONS/PHARMACODYNAMICS Cell cycle–specific vinca alkaloid (obtained from periwinkle plant *Vinca rosea*); analog of vinblastine. Antineoplastic mechanism unclear; arrests mitosis at metaphase, thereby inhibiting cell division. In contrast to vinblastine, has relatively low toxic effect on normal cells and thus produces minimal myelosuppression; however, neurologic and neuromuscular effects are more severe.

USES Acute lymphoblastic and other leukemias, Hodgkin's disease, lymphosarcoma, neuroblastoma, Wilms' tumor, lung and breast cancer, reticular cell carcinoma, and osteogenic and other sarcomas. **Unlabeled use:** for idiopathic thrombocytopenic purpura, alone or adjunctively with other antineoplastics.

ROUTE & DOSAGE

Antineoplastic

Adult	IV	1.4 mg/m² (max 2 mg/m²) at weekly intervals
Child	IV	2 mg/m² at weekly intervals

PHARMACOKINETICS Distribution: concentrates in liver, platelets, and leukocytes; poor penetration of blood-brain barrier. **Metabolism:** partially metabolized in liver. **Elimination:** half-life: 10–155 h; excreted primarily in feces.

CONTRAINDICATIONS & PRECAUTIONS Contraindicated in: obstructive jaundice; pregnancy (category D), men and women of childbearing age; patient with demyelinating form of Charcot-Marie-Tooth syndrome. **Cautious use in:** leukopenia; preexisting neuromuscular disease; hypertension; infection; patients receiving drugs with neurotoxic potential.

ADVERSE/SIDE EFFECTS Usually dose-related and reversible. **CNS:** *peripheral neuropathy,* neuritic pain, *paresthesias, especially of hands and feet;* foot and hand drop, sensory loss, athetosis, ataxia, loss of deep tendon reflexes, muscle atrophy, dysphagia, weakness in larynx and extrinsic eye muscles, ptosis, diplopia, mental depression. **Eye:** optic atrophy with blindness; transient cortical blindness, ptosis, diplopia, photophobia. **GI:** stomatitis, pharyngitis, anorexia, nausea, vomiting, diarrhea, abdominal cramps, *severe constipation (upper-colon impaction), paralytic ileus, (especially in children),* rectal bleeding; hepatotoxicity. **GU:** urinary retention, polyuria, dysuria, SIADH (high urinary sodium excretion, hyponatremia, dehydration, hypotension); uric acid nephropathy. **Skin:** urticaria, rash, *alopecia,* cellulitis and phlebitis following extravasation (at injection site). **Other:** convulsions with hypertension, malaise, fever, headache, pain in parotid gland area, hyperuricemia, hyperkalemia, weight loss, hypertension, hypotension, bronchospasm.

INCOMPATIBILITIES Solution/Additive: furosemide. Y-Site: furosemide.

NURSING IMPLICATIONS

Administration

▪ Reconstitute with provided solution (bacteriostatic NaCl) or with sterile water or physiologic saline to concentrations of 0.01 to 1.0 mg/ml.

▪ Administration directly into vein or into running in-

---

fusion should be over a 1 min period. Syringe and needle should be rinsed with venous blood before needle is withdrawn.

- If extravasation occurs, drug administration is discontinued immediately and restarted in another vein. Hyaluronidase should be injected locally into surrounding tissue. Apply moderate heat to the area to disperse drug and to minimize danger of sloughing. Be cautious because of possible sensory loss. Check agency policy or consult physician.
- Vincristine is available in solution form and does not require reconstitution. Vincristine solution must be stored in the refrigerator.

Assessment & Drug Effects

- Monitor I&O ratio and pattern, BP, and temperature daily. Record on flow chart as indicators for adaptations in nursing and drug regimen.
- Weigh patient under standard conditions weekly or more often if ordered. In the presence of edema or ascites, patient's ideal weight is used to determine dosage. Report a steady gain or sudden weight change to physician.
- Complete bone marrow remission in leukemia varies widely and may not occur for as long as 100 d after therapy is started.
- Neuromuscular side effects, most apt to appear in the patient with preexisting neuromuscular disease, usually disappear after 6 wk of treatment. Children are especially susceptible to neuromuscular side effects.
- Grasp hands of patient each day to detect onset of hand muscular weakness, and check deep tendon reflexes (depression of Achilles reflex is the earliest sign of neuropathy). Also observe for and report promptly: mental depression, ptosis, double vision, hoarseness, paresthesias, neuritic pain, and motor difficulties.
- Leukopenia occurs in a significant number of patients; leukocyte count in children usually reaches nadir on fourth day and begins to rise on fifth day after drug administration. Provide special protection against infection or injury during leukopenic days.
- To prevent injury to rectal mucosa, use of rectal thermometer or intrusive tubing should be avoided if possible.
- Walking may be impaired; check patient's ability to ambulate, and supply support if necessary.
- Care should be taken to distinguish between the depression associated with realization of neoplastic disease and that which is drug-induced.
- Dental caries or periodontal disease should be

treated, since patient is highly susceptible to superinfections.

Patient & Family Education

- Advise patient to report promptly stomach, bone or joint pain, and swelling of lower legs and ankles.
- A prophylactic regimen against constipation and paralytic ileus (adequate fluids, high-fiber diet, laxatives) is usually started at beginning of treatment with vincristine. Encourage patient to report changes in bowel habit as soon as manifested. Paralytic ileus is most likely to occur in young children.
- Alopecia (reversible) (up to 70% of patients) is reportedly the most common adverse reaction and may persist for the duration of therapy. However, regrowth of hair may start before end of treatment. Before therapy begins, discuss this side effect with patient. Inform patient that scalp hair will drop out in large clumps on pillow at night. This is a distressing side effect.

VITAMIN A

(vye´ta-min)
Trade names: Aquasol A, Del-Vi-A
Classification: VITAMIN A
Pregnancy: Categories A (X if >RDA)

ACTIONS/PHARMACODYNAMICS Synthetic fat-soluble vitamin available for clinical use as retinol or retinol esters. Obtained from seawater fish liver oils or prepared synthetically. Formulation includes vitamin A as well as its precursors, alpha, beta, and gamma carotene, and crystoxanthin. Expressed in terms of international units (IU). One IU (equivalent to 1 USP U) is equal to 0.3 µg of retinol, 0.34 µg of vitamin A acetate, or 0.6 µg of beta carotene (provitamin A). Vitamin A is essential for normal growth and development of bones and teeth, for integrity of epithelial and mucosal surfaces, and for synthesis of rhodopsin (visual purple) necessary for visual dark adaptation. Also, thought to act as cofactor in biosynthesis of adrenal steroids, mucopolysaccharides, cholesterol, and RNA. Stimulates healing of cortisone-retarded wounds when applied topically.

USES Vitamin A deficiency and as dietary supplement during periods of increased requirements, such as pregnancy, lactation, infancy, and infections. Used as replacement therapy in conditions that affect absorption, mobilization, or storage of vitamin A, e.g.,

Common side effects in *italic*; life-threatening effects <u>underlined</u>; generic names in **bold**; classifications in SMALL CAPS

1053

steatorrhea, severe biliary obstruction, hepatic cirrhosis, total gastrectomy. Used in skin disorders [e.g., folliculosis keratosis (Darier's disease), psoriasis]; however, other retinoids are being preferentially selected. Also used as a screening test for fat malabsorption.

ROUTE & DOSAGE

Severe Deficiency

Adult	PO	500,000 IU/d for 3 d followed by 50,000 IU/d for 2 wk, then 10,000–20,000 IU/d for 2 mo
	IM	100,000 IU/d for 3 d followed by 50,000 IU/d for 2 wk
Child	PO/IM	> 8 y: same as for adult
		1–8 y: 10,000 IU/kg/d for 3 d followed by 17,000–35,000 IU/d for 2 wk
		< 1 y: 10,000 IU/kg/d for 3 d followed by 7500–15,000 IU/d for 10 d

Dietary Supplement

Child	PO	4–8 y: 15,000 IU/d
		< 4 y: 10,000 IU/d

PHARMACOKINETICS Absorption: readily absorbed from GI tract in presence of bile salts, pancreatic lipase, and dietary fat. **Distribution:** stored mainly in liver; small amounts also found in kidney and body fat; distributed into breast milk. **Metabolism:** metabolized in liver. **Elimination:** excreted in feces and urine.

CONTRAINDICATIONS & PRECAUTIONS Contraindicated in: history of sensitivity to vitamin A or to any ingredient in formulation, hypervitaminosis A, oral administration to patients with malabsorption syndrome. Safe use in amounts exceeding 6000 IU during pregnancy (category A [category X if >RDA]) not established. **Cautious use in:** women on oral contraceptives, high doses in nursing mothers.

ADVERSE/SIDE EFFECTS CNS irritability, headache, intracranial hypertension (pseudotumor cerebri), increased intracranial pressure, bulging fontanelles, papilledema, exophthalmos, miosis, nystagmus. **Hypervitaminosis A syndrome:** (general manifestations): malaise, lethargy, abdominal discomfort, anorexia, vomiting. **Skeletal:** slow growth; deep tender hard lumps (subperiosteal thickening) over radius, tibia, occiput; migratory arthralgia; retarded growth; premature closure of epiphyses. **Skin:** gingivitis, lip fissures, excessive sweating, drying or cracking of skin, pruritus, increase in skin pigmentation, massive desquamation, brittle nails, alopecia. **Other:** hypomenorrhea, hepatosplenomegaly, hypercalcemia, polydipsia, polyurea, jaundice, leukopenia, hypoplastic anemias, vitamin A plasma levels > 1200 IU/dl, elevations of sedimentation rate and prothrombin time; anaphylaxis, death after IV use.

DIAGNOSTIC TEST INTERFERENCES Vitamin A may falsely increase **serum cholesterol** determinations (Zlatkis-Zak reaction); may falsely elevate **bilirubin** determination (with Ehrlich's reagent).

DRUG INTERACTIONS Mineral oil, cholestyramine may decrease absorption of vitamin A.

NURSING IMPLICATIONS

Administration

- Should be taken on empty stomach or following food or milk if GI upset occurs.
- Preserve in tight, light-resistant containers.

Assessment & Drug Effects

- Evaluation of dosage is made with consideration of patient's average daily intake of vitamin A. Dietary and drug history is advisable, e.g., intake of fortified foods, dietary supplements, self-administration or prescription drug sources. Women taking oral contraceptives tend to have significantly high plasma vitamin A levels.
- Vitamin A deficiency is often associated with protein malnutrition as well as other vitamin deficiencies. May be manifested by night blindness, retardation of growth and development, epithelial alterations, susceptibility to infection, abnormal dryness of skin, mouth, and eyes (xerophthalmia) progressing to keratomalacia (ulceration and necrosis of cornea and conjunctiva), urinary tract calculi.

Patient & Family Education

- **Recommended daily allowance (RDA):** adult females 4000 IU, adult males 5000 IU, lactating women 6000 IU, children 4–6 y 2500 IU, infants 2100 IU.
- Avoid use of mineral oil while on vitamin A therapy.
- Instruct patient to report to physician symptoms of overdosage: nausea, vomiting, anorexia, drying and cracking of skin or lips, headache, loss of hair.
- Patients receiving therapeutic doses should be closely supervised. Inform patient and family that self-medication with vitamin A is potentially harmful.

VITAMIN B₁

See **thiamine hydrochloride**, p 993.

VITAMIN B₂

See **riboflavin**, p 946.

VITAMIN B₃

See **niacin**, p 809.

VITAMIN B₆

See **pyridoxine**, p 931.

VITAMIN B₉

See **folic acid**, p 618.

VITAMIN B₁₂

See **cyanocobalamin**, p 474.

VITAMIN B₁₂ₐ

See **hydroxycobalamin**, p 656.

VITAMIN C

See **ascorbic acid**, p 317.

VITAMIN E

Trade names: Aquasol E, CEN-E, E-Ferol, E-Vital, Gordo-Vite E, Tocopherol, Vita-Plus E, Vitec
Classification: VITAMIN
Pregnancy: Category A

ACTIONS/PHARMACODYNAMICS Vitamin E refers to a group of naturally occurring fat-soluble substances known as tocopherols (alpha, beta, gamma, and delta). Alpha tocopherol, comprising 90% of the tocopherols, is the most biologically potent and has been synthesized. It prevents peroxidation, a process that adds oxygen to molecules in a way that gives rise to free radicals, highly reactive chemical structures that damage cell membranes and alter nuclear proteins. Some researchers hypothesize that this protective function may be a deterrent to the constant free radical damage thought to be a factor in the initiation and promotion of many cancers. Vitamin E is essential to the digestion and metabolism of polyunsaturated fats; it maintains the integrity of cell membranes, protects against blood clot formation by decreasing platelet aggregation, enhances vitamin A utilization, and promotes normal growth, development, and tone of muscles. Vitamin E deficiency causes no specific disease in humans but has been associated with increased susceptibility of RBC to hemolysis by biologic oxidizing agents and with edema, irritability, and hemolytic anemia in premature neonates. Low serum tocopherol in adults and children appears to be associated with creatinuria, muscle weakness, and decreased RBC survival, conditions that are completely reversed by the administration of vitamin E. Although vitamin E has not been shown to have any therapeutic value, it is prescribed for a number of clinical problems: anemia associated with protein caloric malnutrition (kwashiorkor), infertility, impotence, habitual abortion, menopausal syndrome, chronic cystic mastitis, peptic ulcer, burns, cancer prevention, skin disorders, heart diseases.

USES To treat and prevent hemolytic anemia due to vitamin E deficiency in premature neonates; to prevent retrolental fibroplasia secondary to oxygen treatment in neonates, and in treatment of diseases with secondary erythrocyte membrane abnormalities, e.g., sickle cell anemia, and G6PD deficiency and as supplement in malabsorption syndromes. Used in patients on diets containing large amounts of polyunsaturated fats for long periods and in the patient who abruptly discontinues such a diet. Also used topically for dry or chapped skin and minor skin disorders. **Unlabeled uses:** muscular dystrophy and a number of other conditions with no conclusive evidence of value. A component of many multivitamin formulations and of topical deodorant preparations as an antioxidant.

Common side effects in *italic*; life-threatening effects underlined; generic names in **bold**; classifications in SMALL CAPS

1055

ROUTE & DOSAGE

Vitamin E Deficiency

Adult	PO/IM	60–75 IU/d
Child	PO	1 IU/kg/d

Prophylaxis for Vitamin E Deficiency

Adult	PO	12–15 IU/d
Child	PO	7–10 IU/d
Neonate	PO	5 IU/d

PHARMACOKINETICS Absorption: 20–60% absorbed from GI tract if fat absorption is normal; enters blood via lymph. **Distribution:** stored mainly in adipose tissue; crosses placenta. **Metabolism:** metabolized in liver. **Elimination:** excreted primarily in bile.

ADVERSE/SIDE EFFECTS Appears to be nontoxic at therapeutic dosage range. With excessive doses for prolonged periods: skeletal muscle weakness, headache, blurred vision, fatigue, nausea, diarrhea, intestinal cramps, gonadal dysfunction; increased serum creatine kinase, cholesterol, triglycerides; decreased serum thyroxine and triiodothyronine; increased urinary estrogens, androgens; creatinuria; sterile abscess, thrombophlebitis, contact dermatitis.

DRUG INTERACTIONS Mineral oil, cholestyramine may decrease absorption of vitamin E; may enhance anticoagulant activity of **warfarin.**

NURSING IMPLICATIONS

Administration
- Should be taken on empty stomach or following food or milk if GI upset occurs.
- Preserve in tight containers protected from light.

Patient & Family Education
- The estimated daily requirement is usually provided by the normal adult diet, but requirements are higher with increased intake of unsaturated fats.
- RDA of vitamin E may be increased if patient is also taking a large dose of iron.
- In sufficient doses, may induce vitamin K deficiency.
- Wheat germ is the richest source of vitamin E; also found in vegetable oils (sunflower, corn, soybean, cottonseed); green leafy vegetables, nuts, dairy products, eggs, cereals, meat, liver.

VITAMIN K

See **menadione**, p 734.

VITAMIN K$_1$

See **phytonadione**, p 886.

VITAMIN K$_3$

See **menadione**, p 734.

VITAMIN K$_4$

See **menadiol sodium diphosphate**, p 733.

WARFARIN SODIUM

See BLOOD FORMERS, ANTICOAGULANT, p 127.

Prototype: naphazoline, p 211

XYLOMETAZOLINE HYDROCHLORIDE

(zye-loe-met-az´oh-leen)
Trade names: Neosynephrine II, Otrivin
Classifications: NASAL DECONGESTANT, VASOCONSTRICTOR
Pregnancy: Category C

ACTIONS/PHARMACODYNAMICS Imidazoline derivative with marked alpha-adrenergic activity (vasoconstriction) on dilated arterioles of nasal membrane. Has little or no beta-adrenergic activity. Structurally related to naphazoline. Decreases fluid exudate and mucosal engorgement associated with rhinitis and may open up obstructed eustachian ostia in patient with ear inflammation.

USES Temporary relief of nasal congestion associated with common cold, sinusitis, acute and chronic rhinitis, and hay fever and other allergies.

PHARMACOKINETICS Onset: 5–10 min. **Duration:** 5–6 h.

Common side effects in *italic*; life-threatening effects underlined; generic names in **bold**; classifications in SMALL CAPS

CONTRAINDICATIONS & PRECAUTIONS Contraindicated in: sensitivity to adrenergic substances; angle-closure glaucoma; concurrent therapy with MAO inhibitors or tricyclic antidepressants. Safe use during pregnancy (category C) not established. **Cautious use in:** hypertension; hyperthyroidism; heart disease, including angina; advanced arteriosclerosis, the elderly, and children.

ROUTE & DOSAGE

Nasal Congestion

Adult	Topical	1–2 sprays or 1–2 drops of 0.1% solution in each nostril q8–10h (max 3 doses/d)
Child	Topical	6 mo–12 y: 1 spray or 2–3 drops of 0.05% solution in each nostril q8–10h (max 3 doses/d)
		< 6 mo: 1 drop of 0.05% solution in each nostril q6h (max 3 doses/d)

ADVERSE/SIDE EFFECTS Usually mild and infrequent: local stinging, burning, dryness and ulceration, sneezing, headache, insomnia, drowsiness. **With excessive use:** *rebound nasal congestion* and vasodilation, tremulousness, hypertension, palpitations, tachycardia, arrhythmia, somnolence, sedation, coma.

NURSING IMPLICATIONS

Administration

- Instruct patient to clear each nostril gently before administering spray or drops.

Application of Drug

- **Spray:** Do not shake container. Hold tube vertically (spray end up) so that solution is delivered in a fine spray. Head should be erect; spray into each nostril; 3–5 min later, clear (blow) nose thoroughly.
- **Drops:** Patient should be in a lateral, head-low position to permit application of drops to lower nostril surface. Have patient remain in this position for 5 min, then apply drops to opposite nostril surface in same manner; or drops may be instilled with patient in reclining position with head tilted back as far as possible.
- Preserve in tight, light-resistant containers at 15–30C (59–86F).

Patient & Family Education

- To prevent contamination of nasal solution and to prevent spread of infection, rinse dropper and tip of nasal spray in hot water after each use and restrict use to the individual patient.

- Prolonged use may cause rebound congestion and chemical rhinitis. Caution patient not to exceed prescribed dosage and to report to physician if drug fails to provide relief within 3 or 4 d.
- Warn patient not to self-medicate with OTC drugs, sprays, or drops without physician's approval.
- Excessive use by child may lead to CNS depression.

> **Prototype: acyclovir, p 85**

ZIDOVUDINE (AZIDOTHYMIDINE, AZT)

(zye-doe´-vyoo deen)
Trade name: Retrovir
Classifications: ANTIINFECTIVE; ANTIVIRAL
Pregnancy: Category C

Z

ACTIONS/PHARMACODYNAMICS Analog of thymidine (a major nucleoside in DNA). On entering host cell, zidovudine is converted to a triphosphate (the active form) by endogenous thymidine kinase and other cellular enzymes. Appears to act by being incorporated into growing DNA chains by viral reverse transcriptase, thereby terminating viral replication. Zidovudine has antiviral action against HIV (human immunodeficiency virus), the causative agent of AIDS (acquired immune deficiency syndrome), formerly referred to as HTLV III (human T-cell lymphotropic virus, type III), LAV (lymphadenopathy-associated virus), and ARV (AIDS-associated retrovirus).

USES Patients who are HIV positive and have a CD4 count ≤ 500/mm³, asymptomatic HIV infection, early and late symptomatic HIV disease. **Unlabeled uses:** pediatric patients, postexposure chemoprophylaxis.

ROUTE & DOSAGE

Symptomatic HIV Infection

Adult	PO	200 mg q4h (1200 mg/d); after 1 mo may reduce to 100 mg q4h (600 mg/d)
	IV	1–2 mg/kg q4h (1200 mg/d)
Child	PO/IV	3 mo–13 y: 100–180 mg/m² q6h

Asymptomatic HIV Infection, Postexposure Prophylaxis

Adult	PO	100 mg q4h while awake, 5 times/d

PHARMACOKINETICS Absorption: readily absorbed from GI tract; 60–70% reaches systemic circulation (first pass metabolism). **Peak:** 0.5–1.5 h.

Common side effects in *italic*; life-threatening effects underlined; generic names in **bold**; classifications in SMALL CAPS

1057

Distribution: crosses blood-brain barrier and placenta. **Metabolism:** metabolized in liver. **Elimination:** half-life: 1 h; 63–95% excreted in urine.

CONTRAINDICATIONS & PRECAUTIONS Contraindicated in: life-threatening allergic reactions to any of the drug components. Safe use during pregnancy (category C), in nursing mothers, and in children ≤ 13 y not established. **Cautious use in:** impaired renal or hepatic function, bone marrow depression.

ADVERSE/SIDE EFFECTS CNS: headache, insomnia, dizziness, paresthesias, mild confusion, anxiety, restlessness, agitation. **GI:** *nausea,* diarrhea, vomiting, *anorexia,* GI pain. **Hematologic:** *bone marrow depression (25% of patients):* granulocytopenia, anemia. **Skin:** rash, itching, diaphoresis. **Other:** fever, dyspnea, *malaise,* weakness, *myalgia.*

DRUG INTERACTIONS Acetaminophen may enhance bone marrow suppression; **amphotericin B** increases risk of AZT toxicity; **aspirin, dapsone, doxorubicin, flucytosine indomethacin, interferon alfa, pentamidine, vincristine** may increase risk of AZT toxicity; **probenecid** will decrease AZT elimination, resulting in increased serum levels and thus toxicity.

NURSING IMPLICATIONS

Administration
- This drug is to be taken q4h around the clock.
- For IV administration withdraw required dose from vial and dilute with D5W to a concentration not to exceed 4 mg/ml. Administer over 60 min; avoid rapid infusion.

- Store at 15–25C (59–77F) protected from light unless otherwise directed.

Assessment & Drug Effects
- During the first month of therapy, patient should be evaluated at least weekly.
- Baseline and frequent (at least q2wk) blood counts should be performed. CD_4 (T_4) lymphocyte number, Hgb, granulocyte count are strongly recommended to detect hematologic toxicity.
- Myelosuppression results in anemia, which commonly occurs after 4–6 wk of therapy, and granulocytopenia in 6–8 wk. Frequently both respond to dosage adjustment. Significant anemia (Hgb <7.5 g/dl or reduction > 25% of baseline value), or granulocyte count < 750/mm^3 (or reduction > 50% of baseline) may require temporary interruption of therapy and transfusions.
- Monitor for common adverse effects, especially severe headache, nausea, insomnia, and myalgia.

Patient & Family Education
- Advise patient to contact physician promptly if health status changes for the worse or any unusual symptoms develop.
- Patients should be told that the drug is not a cure for HIV infection and that they continue to be at risk for opportunistic infections.
- Advise patients not to share drug and to take it exactly as prescribed.
- Inform patient that the drug does not reduce the risk of transmission of HIV infection through body fluids.
- It is not known if the drug is excreted in human milk. Nursing mothers should, therefore, be instructed to discontinue nursing.

Common side effects in *italic*; life-threatening effects underlined; generic names in **bold**; classifications in SMALL CAPS

APPENDIXES

◆APPENDIX A   U.S. SCHEDULES OF CONTROLLED SUBSTANCES

Schedule I

High potential for abuse and of no currently accepted medical use. Examples: heroin, LSD, marijuana, mescaline, peyote. Not obtainable by prescription, but may be legally procured for research, study, or instructional use.

Schedule II

High abuse potential and high liability for severe psychic or physical dependence. Prescription required and cannot be renewed. Includes opium derivatives, other opioids, and short-acting barbiturates. Examples: amphetamine, cocaine, meperidine, morphine, secobarbital.

Schedule III

Potential for abuse is less than for drugs in Schedules I and II. Moderate to low physical dependence and high psychological dependence. Includes certain stimulants and depressants not included in the above schedules, and preparations containing limited quantities of certain opioids. Examples: chlorphentermine, glutethimide, mazindol, paregoric, phendimetrazine. Prescription required.[a]

Schedule IV

Lower potential for abuse than Schedule III drugs. Examples: certain psychotropics (tranquilizers), chloral hydrate, chlordiazepoxide, diazepam, meprobamate, phenobarbital. Prescription required.[a]

Schedule V

Abuse potential is less than for Schedule IV drugs. Preparations contain limited quantities of certain narcotic drugs; generally intended for antitussive and antidiarrheal purposes and may be distributed without a prescription provided that:

1. Such distribution is made only by a pharmacist.
2. Not more than 240 ml or not more than 48 solid dosage units of any substance containing opium, nor more than 120 ml or not more than 24 solid dosage units of any other controlled substance may be distributed at retail to the same purchaser in any given 48-hour period without a valid prescription order.
3. The purchaser is at least 18 years old.
4. The pharmacist knows the purchaser or requests suitable identification.
5. The pharmacist keeps an official written record of: name and address of purchaser, name and quantity of controlled substance purchased, date of sale, initials of dispensing pharmacist. This record is to be made available for inspection and copying by U.S. officers authorized by the Attorney General.
6. Other federal, state or local law does not require a prescription order.

Under jurisdiction of the Federal Controlled Substances Act.
[a]Refillable up to 5 times within 6 mo, but only if so indicated by physician.

◆APPENDIX B   CANADIAN CONTROLLED SUBSTANCE CLASSIFICATIONS

Narcotics (N)

Includes products containing a narcotic. Within this broad classification are several levels of regulatory control. These levels range from strict controls for the most abusable of the substances (for example, single-entity narcotics; products containing a narcotic with one active nonnarcotic ingredient; any preparation containing heroin, hydrocodone, or oxycodone) to lesser controls for preparations containing one narcotic and two active nonnarcotic ingredients and exempt codeine preparations (those containing a limited amount of codeine plus two active nonnarcotic ingredients).

Controlled Drugs (C)

Includes nonnarcotic preparations with abuse potential. As with narcotics, different regulations apply, depending on specific content. C drugs include drugs such as amphetamines and barbiturates.

The specific drugs listed under any given controlled substance level within each classification are determined by the individual provinces.

◆APPENDIX C   A NOMOGRAM ESTIMATING BODY SURFACE AREA IN CHILDREN

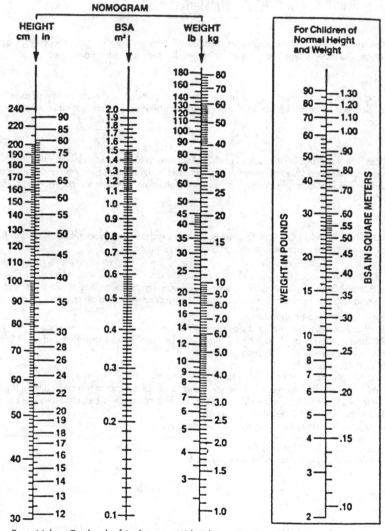

From Nelson Textbook of Pediatrics, *13th Edition. Courtesy W.B. Saunders Co.,*
Philadelphia, PA, with permission.

METRIC UNITS AND CONVERSION FACTORS

Units of Measurement	Terminology of Prefixes
Length	kilo- 1000 times greater
m = meter	centi- 100 times smaller
cm = centimeter	milli- 1000 times smaller
mm = millimeter	micro- 1,000,000 times smaller
Volume	**Conversion Factors/Equivalents**
L = liter	1 m = 100 cm = 1000 mm
ml = milliliter*	1 L = 1000 ml = 1000 cc*
cc = cubic centimeter*	1 kg = 1000 g
Weight	1 g = 1000 mg
kg = kilogram	1 mg = 1000 µg
g = gram	1 ml = 1 cc
mg = milligram	
µg (mcg) = microgram	*Note: cubic centimeter and milliliter are equivalent.

THE HOUSEHOLD SYSTEM OF MEASUREMENT

Abbreviations		Equivalents/Conversion Factors	
Volume			
Drop(s)	= gtt(s)	1 teaspoon	= 60 drops
Teaspoon	= tsp or t	1 tablespoon	= 3 teaspoons
Tablespoon	= tbsp or T	2 tablespoons	= 1 ounce
Ounce	= oz	1 cup	= 8 ounces
Pint	= pt	2 cups	= 1 pint
Quart	= qt	2 pints	= 1 quart
Gallon	= gal	4 quarts	= 1 gallon
Weight			
Pound	= lb	1 pound	= 16 ounces
Ounce	= oz		
Length			
Inch	= in	1 foot	= 12 inches
Foot	= ft		

COMMONLY USED CONVERSION FACTORS

Volume	Weight
1 ml = 15 or 16 minims	1 grain = 60 or 64 mg
5 ml = 1 fl dr (ʒ) = 1 tsp	1 mg = 1000 µg (mcg)
15 ml = 4 fl dr (ʒ) = 1 tbsp	1 g = 1000 mg = 15 grain
30 ml = 8 fl dr (ʒ) = 1 oz (ʒ)	1 kg = 1000 g = 2.2 lb

THE APOTHECARY SYSTEM OF MEASUREMENT

Abbreviations		Equivalents/Conversion Factors	
Volume			
Minim	= ɱ	1 minim	= 1 drop
Fluid dram	= fl dr (ʒ)	1 fluid dram	= 60 minims
Fluid ounce	= fl oz (ʒ)	1 fluid ounce	= 8 fluid drams
Weight			
Grain	= gr	1 dram	= 60 grains
Dram	= dr		

CONVERSION FACTORS/EQUIVALENTS

Household		Apothecary		Metric
Volume				
—	=	15–16 minims	=	1 milliliter
1 teaspoon	=	1 fluid dram	=	4–5 milliliters
1 tablespoon	=	3–4 fluid drams	=	15–16 milliliters
2 tablespoons	=	1 fluid ounce	=	30–32 milliliters
1 cup	=	8 fluid ounces	=	240 milliliters
1 pint	=	16 fluid ounces	=	500ᵃ milliliters
1 quart	=	32 fluid ounces	=	1000ᵃ milliliters
Weight				
—	=	1 grain	=	60–65 milligrams
—	=	15–16 grains	=	1 gram
—	=	1 dram	=	4 grams
2.2 pounds	=	—	=	1 kilogram
Length				
1 inch	=	—	=	2.54 centimeters
39.37 inches	=	—	=	1 meter

ᵃIn common practice these *approximate* equivalents are used.

◆APPENDIX E   FDA PREGNANCY CATEGORIES

The FDA requires that all prescription drugs absorbed systemically or known to be potentially harmful to the fetus be classified according to one of five pregnancy categories (A, B, C, D, X). The identifying letter signifies the level of risk to the fetus and is to appear in the precautions section of the package insert. The categories described by the FDA are as follows:

Category A

Controlled studies in women fail to demonstrate a risk to the fetus in the first trimester (and there is no evidence of risk in later trimesters), and the possibility of fetal harm appears remote.

Category B

Either animal-reproduction studies have not demonstrated a fetal risk but there are no controlled studies in pregnant women, or animal-reproduction studies have shown an adverse effect (other than a decrease in fertility) that was not confirmed in controlled studies in women in the first trimester (and there is no evidence of a risk in later trimesters).

Category C

Either studies in animals have revealed adverse effects on the fetus (teratogenic or embryocidal effects or other) and there are no controlled studies in women, or studies in women and animals are not available. Drugs should be given only if the potential benefit justifies the potential risk to the fetus.

Category D

There is positive evidence of human fetal risk, but the benefits from use in pregnant women may be acceptable despite the risk (e.g., if the drug is needed in a life-threatening situation or for a serious disease for which safer drugs cannot be used or are ineffective). There will be an appropriate statement in the "warnings" section of the labeling.

Category X

Studies in animals or human beings have demonstrated fetal abnormalities or there is evidence of fetal risk based on human experience, or both, and the risk of the use of the drug in pregnant women clearly outweighs any possible benefit. The drug is contraindicated in women who are or may become pregnant. There will be an appropriate statement in the "contraindications" section of the labeling.

A.P.C.	aspirin, phenacetin, caffeine
Actifed	pseudoephedrine hydrochloride, triprolidine hydrochloride
Aladrine	ephedrine sulfate, secobarbital sodium
Alazide	spironolactone, hydrochlorothiazide
Aldactazide	spironolactone, hydrochlorothiazide
Aldoclor	chlorothiazide, methyldopa
Aldopa H	hydrochlorothiazide, methyldopa
Aldoril	hydrochlorothiazide, methyldopa
Alka Seltzer (without Aspirin)	sodium bicarbonate, citric acid, potassium bicarbonate
Alka Seltzer with Aspirin	aspirin, sodium bicarbonate, citric acid
Allerest Tablets	phenylpropanolamine, chlorpheniramine
Alma-Mag Improved	aluminum hydroxide, magnesium hydroxide, simethicone
Alphaderm	hydrocortisone, urea
Aludrox	aluminum hydroxide, magnesium hydroxide
Amacodone C	hydrocodone, acetaminophen
Amaphen	acetaminophen, caffeine, butalbital
Amaphen with Codeine	codeine phosphate, acetaminophen, caffeine, butalbital
Ambenyl Cough Syrup	codeine, bromodiphenhydramine
Amesec	ephedrine, theophylline
Anacin	aspirin, caffeine
Anatuss	guaifenesin, dextromethorphan, phenylpropanolamine
Anbesol	benzocaine, phenol, alcohol
Anexsia	hydrocodone, acetaminophen
Anodynos-DHC	hydrocodone, acetaminophen
Anoquan	acetaminophen, caffeine, butalbital

Antrocol	atropine sulfate, phenobarbital
Apresazide	hydralazine hydrochloride, hydrochlorothiazide
Apresoline-Esidrex	hydralazine hydrochloride, hydrochlorothiazide
Aprodine Syrup	pseudoephedrine, triprolidine
Aprozide	hydralazine, hydrochlorothiazide
Ascriptin	aspirin, magnesium hydroxide, aluminum hydroxide
Axotal	aspirin, butalbital
B-A-C	aspirin, butalbital, caffeine, buffers
Bacticort Ophthalmic	hydrocortisone, neomycin, polymyxin B
Bancap	acetaminophen, butalbital
Bancap HC	hydrocodone bitartrate, acetaminophen
BC Tablets	aspirin, salicylamide, caffeine
Bellafoline	levorotatory alkaloids of belladonna
Bellergal-S	l-alkaloids of belladonna, phenobarbital, ergotamine, tartrazine
Biphetamine	dextroamphetamine, amphetamine
Blephamide	prednisolone acetate, sodium sulfacetamide
Brevicon	ethinyl estradiol, norethindrone
Bromfed	pseudoephedrine hydrochloride, brompheniramine maleate
Bronchial Capsules	theophylline, guaifenesin
Bronkaid Tablets	ephedrine sulfate, theophylline, guaifenesin
Bufferin	aspirin, magnesium carbonate, aluminum glycinate
Butace	acetaminophen, caffeine, butalbital
Butibel	belladonna extract, butabarbital
Cafergot	ergotamine tartrate, caffeine

Cafergot P-B	ergotamine tartrate, caffeine, belladonna, sodium pentobarbital
Caladryl	diphenhydramine, calamine, camphor, alcohol
Calcet	calcium lactate, calcium gluconate, calcium carbonate, vitamin D
Calcidrine Syrup	codeine, calcium iodide
Cam-ap-es	hydrochlorothiazide, reserpine, hydralazine hydrochloride
Capozide	captopril, hydrochlorothiazide
Carmol HC	hydrocortisone acetate, urea
Celestone-Soluspan	betamethasone acetate, betamethasone sodium phosphate
Cetacaine	benzocaine, tetracaine, butamben, benzalkonium chloride
Cetapred	prednisolone acetate, sodium sulfacetamide
Chardonna-2	belladonna, phenobarbital
Chlor-trimeton Decongestant	pseudoephedrine sulfate, chlorpheniramine maleate
Chloromycetin Hydrocortisone	hydrocortisone acetate, chloramphenicol
Chloroserpine	chlorothiazide, reserpine
Chlorzoxazone with APAP	chlorzoxazone, acetaminophen
Clindex	chlordiazepoxide, clidinium
Clinoxide	chlordiazepoxide, clidinium
Clipoxide	chlordiazepoxide, clidinium
Co-Apap	pseudoephedrine, chlorpheniramine, dextromethorphan, acetaminophen
Co-Gesic	acetaminophen, hydrocodone
Codamine	hydrocodone, phenylpropanolamine
Codiclear DH Syrup	hydrocodone, guaifenesin
Codimal DH	phenylephrine hydrochloride, pyrilamine maleate, hydrocodone bitartrate
Codimal LA	chlorpheniramine, pseudoephedrine
Col-Probenecid	probenecid, colchicine
Colabid	probenecid, colchicine
ColBenemid	probenecid, colchicine
Coldrine	pseudoephedrine, acetaminophen
Coly-Mycin S Otic	hydrocortisone acetate, neomycin sulfate, colistin sulfate, thonzonium bromide
Combipres	chlorthalidone, clonidine hydrochloride
Comtrex	chlorpheniramine, acetaminophen, pseudoephedrine
Condrin-LA	phenylpropanolamine hydrochloride, chlorpheniramine maleate
Contac	phenylpropanolamine hydrochloride, chlorpheniramine maleate
Cope	aspirin, caffeine, magnesium hydroxide, aluminum hydroxide
Cordran-N	neomycin sulfate, flurandrenolide
Correctol	docusate sodium, phenolphthalein
Corticaine	hydrocortisone acetate, dibucaine
Cortisporin	hydrocortisone, neomycin sulfate, polymyxin B
Cortisporin Ointment	hydrocortisone, neomycin sulfate, bacitracin, polymyxin B, white petrolatum
Corzide	Nadolol, bendroflumethiazide
Cotrim	trimethoprim, sulfamethoxazole
Cyclomydril	ophthalmic, cyclopentolate hydrochloride, phenylephrine hydrochloride
D.S.S. Plus	docusate sodium, casanthrol
Damason-P	hydrocodone, aspirin, caffeine
Darvocet-N	propoxyphene napsylate, acetaminophen
Darvon Compound	aspirin, caffeine, propoxyphene hydrochloride
Darvon-N with A.S.A.	propoxyphene napsylate, aspirin

Decadron with Xylocaine	dexamethasone sodium phosphate, lidocaine hydrochloride
Deconamine	pseudoephedrine hydrochloride chlorpheniramine maleate
Demerol APAP	meperidine hydrochloride, acetaminophen
Demi-Regroton	chlorthalidone, reserpine
Demulen	ethinyl estradiol, ethynodiol diacetate
Depo-Testadiol	estradiol cypionate, testosterone cypionate, chloroputanol
Deprol	meprobamate, benactyzine hydrochloride, tartrazine
Dialose Plus	docusate potassium, casanthrol
DiGel	magnesium hydroxide, aluminum hydroxide, magnesium carbonate, simethicone
Dilantin with Phenobarbital	phenytoin, phenobarbital
Dilaudid Cough Syrup	guaifenesin, hydromorphone
Dilor G	dyphylline, guaifenesin
Dimetane Decongestant	brompheniramine, phenylephrine
Dimetapp Extentabs	phenylpropanolamine hydrochloride, brompheniramine maleate
Diupres	chlorothiazide, reserpine
Diurese-R	trichlormethiazide, reserpine
Diurigen with Reserpine	reserpine, chlorothiazide
Diutensin-R	methyclothiazide, reserpine
Dolacet	hydrocodone bitartrate, acetaminophen
Dolene	propoxyphene hydrochloride, acetaminophen
Donnagel	kaolin, pectin, hyoscyamine sulfate, atropine sulfate, scopolamine hydrobromide
Donnagel-PG	opium, kaolin, pectin, hyoscyamine sulfate, atropine sulfate, scopolamine hydrobromide
Donnatal	atropine sulfate, scopolamine hydrobromide, hyoscyamine hydrobromide or sulfate, phenobarbital
Doxidan	docusate calcium, phenolphthalein
Dristan	phenylephrine hydrochloride, pheniramine maleate
Drixoral	pseudoephedrine sulfate, dexbrompheniramine maleate
Drize	phenylpropanolamine hydrochloride, chlorpheniramine maleate
Duo-Medihaler	isoproterenol hydrochloride, phenylephrine bitartrate
Duradyne	acetaminophen, aspirin, caffeine
Duradyne DHC	hydrocodone bitartrate, acetaminophen
Dyazide	triamterene, hydrochlorothiazide
Dyflex-G	dyphylline, guaifenesin
Dyline-GG	dyphylline, guaifenesin
E-Pilo	epinephrine bitartrate, pilocarpine
Elase	fibrinolysin, desoxyribonuclease
Elase-Chloromycetin	chloramphenicol, fibrinolysin, desoxyribonuclease
Elixophyllin-GG	guaifenesin, theophylline
Emprin with Codeine	codeine phosphate, aspirin
Endolor	acetaminophen, caffeine, butalbital
Enduronyl	methyclothiazide, deserpidine
Enduronyl Forte	methyclothiazide, deserpidine
Entozyme	pepsin, pancreatin, bile salts
Equagesic	aspirin, meprobamate
Equazine-M	aspirin, meprobamate
Ergo Caff	ergotamine tartrate, caffeine
Esgic	acetaminophen, caffeine, butalbital
Esimil	hydrochlorothiazide, guanethidine monosulfate
Estratest	esterified estrogens, methyltestosterone
Etrafon	perphenazine, amitriptyline
Etrafon-A	perphenazine, amitriptyline

Etrafon-Forte	perphenazine, amitriptyline
Excedrin	acetaminophen, aspirin, caffeine
Excedrin P.M.	acetaminophen, diphenhydramine citrate
Fansidar	sulfadoxine, pyrimethamine
Femcet	acetaminophen, caffeine, butalbital
Feosol Plus	ferrous sulfate, folic acid, ascorbic acid
Fergon Plus	ferrous gluconate, ascorbic acid
Ferro-Sequels	ferrous fumarate, docusate sodium
Fioricet	acetaminophen, butalbital, caffeine
Fiorinal	aspirin, butalbital, caffeine
Fiorinal with Codeine	codeine phosphate, aspirin, caffeine, butalbital
Flexaphen	chlorzoxazone, acetaminophen
Fluress	benoxinate hydrochloride, fluorescein sodium with povidone, chlorobutanol
Gaviscon	alginic acid, sodium bicarbonate, magnesium trisilicate
Gelusil	aluminum hydroxide, magnesium hydroxide, simethicone
Gemnisyn	acetaminophen, aspirin
Genora	ethinyl estradiol, norethindrone
Glyceryl-T	theophylline, guaifenesin
Granulex	trypsin, balsam Peru, castor oil
Gynex	ethinyl estradiol, norethindrone
Halotussin-DM	guaifenesin, dextromethorphan
Hexalol	methenamine, phenysalicylate, atropine sulfate, hyoscyamine, benzoic acid, methylene blue
Hycodan	hydrocodone bitartrate, homatropine methylbromide
Hycomine Compound	phenylephrine hydrochloride, chlorpheniramine maleate, hydrocodone bitartrate, acetaminophen, caffeine
Hycomine Syrup	phenlypropanolamine hydrochloride, hydrocodone bitartrate
Hycotuss Expectorant	guaifenesin, hydrocodone
Hydrazide	hydralazine, hydrochlorothiazide
Hydro-Serp	hydrochlorothiazide, reserpine
Hydrocet	hydrocodone, acetaminophen
Hydrogesic	hydrocodone, acetaminophen
Hydromox R	quinethazone, reserpine
Hydrophed	theophylline, ephedrine sulfate, hydroxyzine hydrochloride
Hydropres	hydrochlorothiazide, reserpine
Hydroserpine	hydrochlorothiazide, reserpine
Hydrosine	hydrochlorothiazide, reserpine
Ilopan-Choline	dexpanthenol, choline bitartrate
Inderide	propranolol hydrochloride, hydrochlorothiazide
Innovar	fentanyl (citrate), droperidol
Isollyl Improved	aspirin, caffeine, butalbital
Isopto P-ES	pilocarpine hydrochloride, physostigmine salicylate
Kapectolin PG	kaolin, pectin, atropine, hyoscyamine, scopolamine, powdered opium, alcohol
Kinesed	atropine sulfate, scopolamine hydrobromide, hyoscyamine hydrobromide, phenobarbital
Kondremul with Cascara	mineral oil, cascara extract, Irish moss as an emulsifier
Kondremul with Phenolphthalein	mineral oil, phenolphthalein, Irish moss as an emulsifier
Lanophyllin-GG	theophylline, guaifenesin
Levlen	ethinyl estradiol, levonorgestrel
Librax	clidinium bromide, chlordiazepoxide hydrochloride
Lidox	chlordiazepoxide, clidinium
Limbitrol	chlordiazepoxide, amitriptyline
Lo/Ovral	ethinyl estradiol, norgestrel
Lobac	chlorzoxazone, acetaminophen

Loestrin	ethinyl estradiol, norethindrone acetate
Lopressor HCT	metoprolol tartrate, hydrochlorothiazide
Lorcet	acetaminophen, propoxyphene hydrochloride
Lorcet HD	acetaminophen, hydrocodone
Lotrisone	betamethasone, clotrimazole
Lufyllin-EPG	ephedrine, dyphylline, guaifenesin, phenobarbital
Lufyllin-GG	dyphylline, guaifenesin
Maalox	aluminum hydroxide, magnesium hydroxide
Maalox Plus	aluminum hydroxide, magnesium hydroxide, simethicone
Marax	theophylline, ephedrine sulfate, hydroxyzine hydrochloride
Marnal	aspirin, caffeine, butalbital
Maxitrol	dexamethasone, neomycin sulfate
Maxzide	triamterene, hydrochlorothiazide
Medigesic	acetaminophen, caffeine, butalbital
Menrium	chlordiazepoxide, esterified estrogens
Mepergan	meperidine, promethazine
Metatensin	trichlormethiazide, reserpine
Micrainin	aspirin, meprobamate
Minizide	polythiazide, prazosin hydrochloride
Modane Plus	docusate sodium, phenolphthalin
Modicon	ethinyl estradiol, norethindrone
Moduretic	amiloride hydrochloride, hydrochlorothiazide
Murocoll-2	scopolamine hydrobromide, phenylephrine hydrochloride
Mus-Lax	chlorzoxazone, acetaminophen
Mycitracin	polymyxin B sulfate, neomycin sulfate, bacitracin
Mycolog II	triamcinolone acetonide, nystatin
Mylanta	aluminum hydroxide,

	magnesium hydroxide, simethicone
Naldecon	phenylpropanolamine hydrochloride, phenylephrine hydrochloride, chlorpheniramine maleate, phenyltoloxamine citrate
Naldecon DX Syrup	guaifenesin, dextromethorphan, phenylpropanolamine
Naldecon EX Syrup	guaifenesin, phenylpropanolamine
Nelova	ethinyl estradiol, norethindrone
Neo-Cortef	hydrocortisone acetate, neomycin sulfate
NeoDecadron	dexamethasone phosphate, neomycin sulfate
Neosporin	polymyxin B sulfate, neomycin sulfate, gramicidin
Neotal	polymyxin B, neomycin sulfate, bacitracin zinc
Neothylline-GG	dyphylline, guaifenesin
Nolamine	phenylpropanolamine hydrochloride, chlorpheniramine maleate, phenindamine tartrate
Norcet	hydrocodone, acetaminophen
Nordette	ethinyl estradiol, levonorgestrel
Norethin	ethinyl estradiol, norethindrone
Norgesic	orphenadrine citrate, aspirin, caffeine
Norgesic Forte	orphenadrine citrate, aspirin, caffeine
Norinyl	ethinyl estradiol, norethindrone
Norlestrin	ethinyl estradiol, norethindrone acetate
Normozide	labetalol, hydrochlorothiazide
Novafed A	pseudoephedrine hydrochloride, chlorpheniramine maleate
Novahistine DH	codeine phosphate, pseudoephedrine

	hydrochloride,
	chlorpheniramine maleate
Novahistine DMX	dextromethorphan
	hydrobromide, guaifenesin,
	pseudoephedrine
	hydrochloride
Novahistine Elixir	chlorphineramine maleate,
	phenylephrine
	hydrochloride
Novahistine Expectorant	codeine phosphate,
	pseudoephedrine
	hydrochloride, guaifenesin
Ophtha P/S	prednisolone acetate, sodium
	sulfacetamide
Ophthocort	hydrocortisone acetate,
	chloramphenicol, polymyxin
	B sulfate
Optimyd	prednisolone sodium
	phosphate, sodium
	sulfacetamide
Optised	phenylephrine, zinc sulfate
Oreticyl	hydrochlorothiazide,
	deserpidine
Oreticyl Forte	hydrochlorothiazide,
	deserpidine
Ornade Spansules	phenylpropanolamine
	hydrochloride,
	chlorpheniramine maleate
Ornex	phenylpropanolamine
	hydrochloride,
	acetaminophen
Oxycet	oxycodone, acetaminophen
PAC	aspirin, caffeine
Percocet	oxycodone
	hydrochloride,
	acetaminophen
Percodan	oxycodone
	hydrochloride,
	oxycodone
	terephthalate,
	aspirin
Perdiem Granules	senna, psyllium
Peri-Colace	docusate sodium,
	casanthrol
Phenaphen with Codeine	codeine phosphate,
	acetaminophen
Phenergan-C	pseudoephedrine,
	promethazine, codeine
Phenergan-D	pseudoephedrine

	hydrochloride,
	promethazine
	hydrochloride
Phrenilin	acetaminophen,
	butalbital
Phrenilin Forte	acetaminophen,
	butalbital
PMB	conjugated estrogens,
	meprobamate
Polaramine Expectorant	pseudoephedrine
	sulfate, dexchlor-
	pheniramine
	maleate, guaifenesin
Poly-Histine D	brompheniramine,
	pseudoephedrine
Polycillin-PRB	ampicillin trihydrate,
	probenecid
Polyflex	chlorzoxazone,
	acetaminophen
Polysporin	polymyxin B sulfate,
	bacitracin zinc
Prefrin-A	phenylephrine
	hydrochloride,
	pyrilamine maleate,
	antipyrine
Premarin with Methyltestosterone	conjugated estrogens,
	methyltestosterone
Probampacin	ampicillin trihydrate,
	probenecid
Proben-C	probenecid, colchicine
Pseudo-Chlor	pseudoephedrine,
	chlorpheniramine
Quadrinal	theophylline calcium
	salicylate, ephedrine
	hydrochloride, potassium
	iodide, phenobarbital
Quibron	theophylline, guaifenesin
Quibron Plus	ephedrine, theophylline,
	guaifenesin, butabarbital
Rauzide	bendroflumethiazide,
	rauwolfia serpentina
Regroton	chlorthalidone, reserpine
Renese-R	polythiazide, reserpine
Repan	acetaminophen, butalbital,
	caffeine
Rifamate	isoniazid, rifampin
Riopan Plus	magaldrate, simethicone
Robaxisal	methocarbamol, aspirin

Robitussin AC	codeine phosphate, guaifenesin
Robitussin-CF	phenylpropanolamine hydrochloride, dextromethorphan hydrobromide, guaifenesin
Robitussin-DAC	phenylpropanolamine hydrochloride, codeine phosphate, guaifenesin
Robitussin-DM	dextromethorphan hydrobromide, guaifenesin
Rondec	pseudoephedrine hydrochloride, carbinoxamine maleate
Roxicet	acetaminophen, oxycodone
Roxiprin	aspirin, oxycodone
Salazide	reserpine, hydroflumethiazide
Salutensin	reserpine, hydroflumethiazide
Sedapap	acetaminophen, butalbital, codeine
Senokot S	docusate sodium, senna concentrate
Ser-A-Gen	hydrochlorothiazide, reserpine, hydralazine hydrochloride
Ser-Ap-Es	hydrochlorothiazide, reserpine, hydralazine hydrochloride
Seralazide	hydrochlorothiazide, reserpine, hydralazine hydrochloride
Serpasil-Apresoline	reserpine, hydralazine hydrochloride
Serpasil-Esidrex	hydrochlorothiazide, reserpine
Serpazide	hydralazine, hydrochlorothiazide, reserpine
Simron Plus	elemental iron, vitamins B_6, B_{12}, C
Sinutab	pseudoephedrine hydrochloride, chlorpheniramine maleate, acetaminophen
Soma Compound	carisoprodol, aspirin
Soma Compound with Codeine	carisoprodol, aspirin, codeine phosphate, sodium metabisulfite
Spastosed	calcium carbonate, magnesium carbonate
Spironazide	spironolactone, hydrochlorothiazide
Splrozlde	spironolactone, hydrochlorothiazide
Statrol	polymyxin B sulfate, neomycin sulfate
Sudafed Plus	pseudoephedrine hydrochloride, chlorpheniramine maleate
Sulfamide	prednisolone acetate, sulfacetamide
Sulfoxyl	benzoyl peroxide, sulfur
Synalgos DC	aspirin, caffeine, dihydrocodeine
T-Gesic	hydrocodone, acetaminophen, butalbital, caffeine
Talacen	pentazocine hydrochloride, acetaminophen
Talwin Compound	aspirin, pentazocine
Tavist-D	phenylpropanolamine hydrochloride, clemastine fumarate
Tedral	theophylline, ephedrine hydrochloride, phenobarbital
Tedral SA	(sustained action) theophylline, ephedrine hydrochloride, phenobarbital
Tedrigen	ephedrine, theophylline, phenobarbital
Teebaconin and Vitamin B_6	isoniazid, pyridoxine hydrochloride
Tega-Tussin Syrup	hydrocodone, chlorpheniramine, phenylephrine
Tenoretic	chlorthalidone, atenolol
Terra-Cortril Suspension	hydrocortisone acetate, oxytetracycline
Theodrine	ephedrine, theophylline, phenobarbital
Timolide	hydrochlorothiazide, timolol maleate
Trandate HCT	hydrochlorothiazide, labetalol
Tri-Barbs	phenobarbital, butabarbital sodium, secobarbital sodium
Tri-Hydroserpine	hydrochlorothiazide, reserpine, hydralazine hydrochloride

Tri-Levlen	ethinyl estradiol, levonorgestrel
Tri-Norinyl	ethinyl estradiol, norethindrone
Triacin-C Cough Syrup	codeine, pseudoephedrine, triprolidine
Triad	acetaminophen, butalbital, caffeine
Triaminic Allergy	phenylpropanolamine hydrochloride, chlorpheniramine maleate
Triaminic Expectorant DH	phenylpropanolamine hydrochloride, pyrilamine maleate, pheniramine maleate, hydrocodone bitartrate, guaifenesin
Triaminic Expectorant with Codeine	phenylpropanolamine hydrochloride, codeine phosphate, guaifenesin
Triaprin	acetaminophen, butalbital
Triavil	perphenazine, amitriptyline
Trigesic	acetaminophen, aspirin, caffeine
Trinalin Repetabs	pseudoephedrine sulfate, azatadine maleate
Triple Antibiotic	neomycin sulfate, bacitracin zinc, polymyxin B sulfate
Triple Sulfa	sulfadiazine, sulfamerazine, sulfamethazine
Tuinal Pulvules	amobarbital sodium, secobarbital sodium
Tussionex	chlorpheniramine, hydrocodone
Ty-Tab	codeine phosphate, acetaminophen
Tylenol with Codeine	acetaminophen, codeine phosphate

Tylox	oxycodone hydrochloride, acetaminophen
Unipres	hydrochlorothiazide, reserpine, hydralazine hydrochloride
Uro-Phosphate	methenamine, sodium biphosphate
Urobiotic	oxytetracycline hydrochloride, sulfamethizole, phenazopyridine hydrochloride
Vanoxide-HC	benzoyl peroxide, hydrocortisone
Vaseretic	enalapril, hydrochlorothiazide
Vasocidin	prednisolone sodium phosphate, sodium sulfacetamide
Vasocon-A	naphazoline hydrochloride, antazoline phosphate
Vasosulf	sodium sulfacetamide, phenylephrine hydrochloride
Veltap	brompheniramine, phenylephrine, phenylpropanolamine
Vicodin	hydrocodone bitartrate, acetaminophen
Wigraine	ergotamine tartrate, caffeine, tartaric acid
WinGel	aluminum hydroxide, magnesium hydroxide
Wygesic	propoxyphene hydrochloride, acetaminophen
Zincfrin	phenylephrine hydrochloride, zinc sulfate
Zydone	hydrocodone bitartrate, acetaminophen

ABBREVIATIONS

ABGs	arterial blood gases		BUN	blood urea nitrogen
a.c.	before meals (*ante cibum*)		C	centigrade, Celsius
ACD	acid-citrate-dextrose		cAMP	cyclic adenosine monophosphate
ACE	angiotensin-converting enzyme		CBC	complete blood count
ACh	acetylcholine		cc	cubic centimeter
ACIP	Advisory Committee on Immunization Practices		Cl$_{cr}$	creatinine clearance
			CDC	Centers for Disease Control
ACLS	advanced cardiac life support		CHF	congestive heart failure
ACT	activated clotting time		cm	centimeter
ACTH	adrenocorticotropic hormone		CNS	central nervous system
ADD	attention deficit disorder		Coll	collyrium (eye wash)
ADH	antidiuretic hormone		COMT	catecholamine-*o*-methyl transferase
ADL	activities of daily living		COPD	chronic obstructive pulmonary disease
ad lib	as desired (*ad libitum*)		CPK	creatinine phosphokinase
ADT	alternate day drug (administration)		CPR	cardiopulmonary resuscitation
AIDS	acquired immunodeficiency syndrome		CRF	chronic renal failure
ALT	alanine aminotransferase (formerly SGPT)		CSF	cerebrospinal fluid
			CSP	cellulose sodium phosphate
AMP	adenosine monophosphate		CT	clotting time
ANA	antinuclear antibody		CTZ	chemoreceptor trigger zone
ANC	acid neutralizing capacity		CV	cardiovascular
APTT	activated partial thromboplastin time		CVA	cerebrovascular accident
ARC	AIDS related complex		CVP	central venous pressure
ARDS	adult respiratory distress syndrome		d	day
ASHD	arteriosclerotic heart disease		D5W	5% dextrose in water
AST	aspartate aminotransferase (formerly SGOT)		D&C	dilation and curettage
			DIC	disseminated intravascular coagulation
ATP	adenosine triphosphate		dl	deciliter (100 ml or 0.1 liter)
AV	atrioventricular		DNA	deoxyribonucleic acid
b.i.d.	two times a day (*bis in die*)		DTRs	deep tendon reflexes
BMR	basal metabolic rate		ECG	electrocardiogram
BP	blood pressure		ECT	electroconvulsive therapy
bpm	beats per minute		EEG	electroencephalogram
BSP	bromsulphalein		EENT	eye, ear, nose, throat
BT	bleeding time		e.g.	for example (*exempli gratia*)

ENT	ear, nose, throat	IOP	intraocular pressure
EPS	extrapyramidal symptoms (or syndrome)	IPPB	intermittent positive pressure breathing
ER	estrogen receptor	IU	international unit
ESR	erythrocyte sedimentation rate	IV	intravenous
F	Fahrenheit	kg	kilogram
FBS	fasting blood sugar	17-KGS	17-ketogenic steroids
FDA	Food and Drug Administration	17-KS	17-ketosteroids
FSH	follicle stimulating hormone	KVO	keep vein open
FTI	free thyroxine index	L	liter
FUO	fever of unknown origin	LDH	lactic dehydrogenase
g	gram	LDL	low density lipoprotein
G6PD	glucose-6-phosphate dehydrogenase	LE	lupus erythematosus
GABA	gamma-aminobutyric acid	LH	leuteinizing hormone
G-CSF	granulocyte colony stimulating factor	LSD	lysergic acid diethylamide
GFR	glomerular filtration rate	M	molar (strength of a solution)
GH	growth hormone	m^2	square meter (of body surface area)
GI	gastrointestinal	MAO	monamine oxidase
GU	genitourinary	MAOI	monamine oxidase inhibitor
h	hour	MBD	minimal brain dysfunction
HCG	human chorionic gonadotropin	MCH	mean corpuscular hemoglobin
Hct	hematocrit	MCHC	mean corpuscular hemoglobin concentration
HDL	high density lipoprotein		
Hgb	hemoglobin	mCi	millicurie
5-HIAA	5-hydroxyindoleacetic acid	μg	microgram (1/1000 of a milligram)
HIV	human immunodeficiency virus	μm	micrometer
HPA	hypothalamic-pituitary-adrenocortical (axis)	MDI	metered dose inhaler
		MDR	minimum daily requirements
HPV	human papilloma virus	mEq	milliequivalent
HR	heart rate	mg	milligram
h.s.	nightly or at bedtime (*hora somni*)	min	minute
I&O	intake and output	MI	myocardial infarction
IBW	ideal body weight	MIC	minimum inhibitory concentration
IC	intracoronary	ml	milliliter (1/1000 of a liter)
ICP	intracranial pressure	mm	millimeter
ICU	intensive care unit	mo	month
IDDM	insulin-dependent diabetes mellitus	N	normal (strength of a solution)
IFN	interferon	NADH	reduced form of nicotine, adenine, dinucleotide
Ig	immunoglobulin		
IM	intramuscular	NAPA	N-acetyl procainamide

nb	note well (*nota bene*)		RAI	radioactive iodine
ng	nanogram (1/1000 of a microgram)		RAST	radioallergosorbent test
NIDDM	non-insulin-dependent diabetes mellitus		RBC	red blood (cell) count
NMS	neuroleptic malignant syndrome		RDA	recommended (daily) dietary allowance
NPN	nonprotein nitrogen		REM	rapid eye movement
NPO	nothing by mouth		rem	*radiation equivalent man*
NS	normal saline		RIA	radioimmunoassay
NSAID	nonsteroidal antiinflammatory drug		RNA	ribonucleic acid
NSR	normal sinus rhythm		ROM	range of motion
OC	oral contraceptive		RT$_3$U	total serum thyroxine concentration
17-OHCS	17-hydroxycorticosteroids		s	second
OTC	over the counter (nonprescription)		SA	sinoatrial
PABA	para-aminobenzoic acid		SBE	self-breast examination; subacute bacterial endocarditis
PAS	para-aminosalicylic acid			
PAWP	pulmonary artery wedge pressure		SC	subcutaneous
PBI	protein-bound iodine		SGGT	serum gamma glutamyl transferase
PBP	penicillin-binding protein		SGOT	serum glutamic-oxaloacetic transaminase (*see* AST)
p.c.	aftermeals (*post cibum*)			
PERLA	pupils equal, react to light and accommodation		SGPT	serum glutamic-pyruvic transaminase (*see* ALT)
PG	prostaglandin		SIADH	syndrome of inappropriate antidiuretic hormone
pH	hydrogen ion concentration			
PKU	phenylketonuria		SI Units	International System of Units
PND	paroxysmal nocturnal dyspnea		SK	streptokinase
PO	by mouth or orally (*per os*)		SL	sublingual
PPM	parts per million		SLE	systemic lupus erythematosus
PR	per rectum		SMA	sequential multiple analysis
prn	when required (*pro re nata*)		SOS	if necessary (*si opus cit*)
PSP	phenolsulfonphthalein		sp	species
PSVT	paroxysmal supraventricular tachycardia		SPF	sun protection factor
PT	prothrombin time		sq	square
PTH	parathyroid hormone		SR	sedimentation rate
PTT	partial thromboplastin time		SRS-A	slow-reactive substance of anaphylaxis
PVC	premature ventricular contraction		stat	immediately
PVD	peripheral vascular disease		STD	sexually transmitted disease
PZI	protamine zinc insulin		t$\frac{1}{2}$	half-life
q	every		T$_3$	triiodothyronine
q.i.d.	four times daily		T$_4$	thyroxine
q.o.d.	every other day		TCA	tricyclic antidepressant

TIA	transient ischemic attack		UV-A	ultraviolet A wave
t.i.d.	three times a day (*ter in die*)		VDRL	venereal disease research laboratory
TPN	total parenteral nutrition		VLDL	very low density lipoprotein
TPR	temperature, pulse, respirations		VMA	vanillylmandelic acid
TSH	thyroid-stimulating hormone		VS	vital signs
TT	thrombin time		wk	week
URI	upper respiratory infection		WBC	white blood (cell) count
USP	United States Pharmacopeia		WBCT	whole blood clotting time
USPHS	United States Public Health Service		y	year
UTI	urinary tract infection			

GLOSSARY

Acid-neutralizing capacity: amount of hydrochloric acid in mEq required to keep an antacid of pH 3 for 2 hours (in vitro).

Acid rebound: hypersecretion of hydrochloric acid induced by excessive buffering of stomach as with antacid therapy.

Adverse effect: an unintended, unpredictable, and nontherapeutic response to drug action. Adverse effects occur at doses used therapeutically or for prophylaxis or diagnose. They generally result from drug toxicity, idiosyncrasies, or hypersensitivity reactions caused by the drug itself or by ingredients added during manufacture, e.g., preservatives, dyes, or vehicles.

Afterload: resistance that ventricles must work against to eject blood into the aorta during systole.

Allergic response: an abnormal and individual hypersensitivity response following exposure to a particular allergen.

Analeptic: a restorative medication that enhances excitation of the CNS without affecting inhibitory impulses.

Anaphylactoid reaction: physiologically similar to anaphylactic reaction; however, release of mediators is initiated by nonimmunologic mechanisms.

Anaphylaxis: an acute systemic response to chemical mediators (e.g., histamine and SRS-A) released chiefly from basophils and mast cells after an immune event (i.e., exposure to an antigen). An anaphylactic reaction is life threatening and is the most severe form of an immediate hypersensitivity response.

Antiarrhythmic drug classification (based on presumed mechanism of action, and effect on duration of action potential of cardiac cells):

Class I: Sodium channel blocker; depresses phase 0 (depolarization). E.g.: quinidine, procainamide, phenytoin, tocainide

Class II: Beta-adrenergic blocking agent: depresses phase 4 (resting period). E.g.: propranolol, metoprolol

Class III: Adrenergic blocking agent: prolongs phase 3 (repolarization). E.g.: bretylium, amiodarone

Class IV: Calcium channel blocking agent: depresses phase 4 (resting period) and lengthens phases 2 and 3 (repolarization). E.g.: verapamil, diltiazem

Bioavailability: fraction of active drug that reaches its action sites after administration by any route. Following an IV dose, bioavailability is 100%; however, such factors as first-pass effect, enterohepatic cycling, or biotransformation reduce bioavailability of an orally administered drug.

Biotransformation: metabolic alterations occurring at some point between absorption and renal elimination and directed toward converting drugs into more polar molecules, hence more readily excretable products. The metabolites produced by enzyme-mediated reactions (oxidation-reduction, hydrolysis, and/or conjugation) are often less active than the parent drug, may be inactive, or may acquire toxic properties including teratogenicity, carcinogenicity or mutagenicity.

Caplet: capsule shaped tablet. (Trademark of Winthrop Pharmaceuticals).

Chronotab: sustained action capsule. (Trademark of Schering).

Cumulative effect: increase in drug effect that results when intake of repeated doses exceeds the rate of drug elimination from the body.

Drug abuse: self-administered drug use that deviates from sanctioned medical, social, or cultural patterns. Alternatively, drug abuse in the nonmedical use of a substance for attaining a psychic effect, or for sustaining dependence, or for attempting suicide. Implicit in the definition is the notion of social disapproval, and compulsive behavior.

Drug dependence: psychic or physical dependence on the effects of an agent with a compulsion to continue and/or to increase its use. *Psychic dependence:* characterized by compulsive drug-seeking behavior that is maintained by its consequences: i.e., personal satisfaction from the effects of the drug. *Physical dependence:* altered physiological state resulting from repeated drug use such that withdrawal symptoms appear with dose reduction or when drug is discontinued.

Drug interaction: modification (increase, decrease, elimination or generation) of the therapeutic, preventive or diagnostic action of a drug by another drug (drug-drug interaction); by food or nutrient (food-drug interaction); or by an environmental factor (smoking-drug interaction). The interaction may produce adverse, beneficial, planned or unplanned, unexpected, clinically significant or insignificant drug actions and effects.

Drug receptor: macromolecule on the cell surface or in the cytoplasm that interacts with a drug thereby initiating the chain of biochemical events interpreted as drug effects. Because of an affinity for binding a drug, receptors determine quantitative relations between drug dose and effects, direct selectivity of drug action, and mediate action of antagonists.

Drop-Tainer: ophthalmic dropper dispenser (Alcon trademark).

Duracap: timed release capsule (Glaxco trademark).

Enterohepatic circulation: describes the recycling of a drug or metabolite which is secreted into bile and carried into the duodenum. A portion of this drug may then be reabsorbed from the intestinal lumen to appear unchanged in the blood; the remainder is excreted in feces.

Excipient: an inert substance (e.g., starch) used as a vehicle for a drug.

Enzyme induction: stimulation of microsomal enzymes by a drug resulting in its accelerated metabolism and decreased activity. If reactive intermediates are formed, drug-mediated toxicity may be exacerbated.

Filmseal: film coated tablet (Parke-Davis trademark).

Filmtab: film coated tablet (Abbott trademark).

First-pass effect: reduced bioavailability of an orally administered drug due to metabolism in GI epithelial cells and liver, or to biliary excretion. Effect may be avoided by use of sublingual tablets or rectal suppositories.

Fixed drug eruption: a drug-induced circumscribed skin lesion that persists or recurs in the same site. Residual pigmentaion may remain following drug withdrawal.

Gradumes: controlled release tablet (Abbott trademark).

Gyrocap: timed release capsule (Rores trademark).

Half-life ($t^{1/2}$): time required for concentration of a drug in the body to decrease by 50%. Half-life also represents the time necessary to reach steady state or to decline from steady state after a change (i.e., starting or stopping) in the dosing regimen. Half-life may be affected by a disease state and age of the drug user.

Hypersensitivity: exaggerated immune response to the presence of a foreign agent (antigen). *Immediate hypersensitivity response:* mediated by antibodies (immunoglobulins) and characterized by the release of SRS-A and histamine. The reaction usually occurs within minutes of exposure to the antigen. *Delayed hypersensitivity response:* mediated by sensitized T cells; occurs 12 to 48 hours after exposure to the antigen.

Immunomodulation: favorable adjustment of the immune system to combat foreign invasion of antigens and viruses

Kapseal: banded (sealed) capsule. (Parke-Davis trademark).

Loading dose: increased initial dose used to achieve steady-state promptly. A loading dose is generally indicated when time to reach steady-state is long, as when drug has a long half-life.

Microsomal enzymes: drug metabolizing enzymes located in the endoplasmic reticulum of the liver and other tissues chiefly responsible for oxidative drug metabolism, e.g., cytochrome P–450.

Nadir: lowest value or point. For example, thrombocytes and leukocytes reach a nadir in response to cytotoxic drug effects on hematopoietic tissues.

Neuroleptic malignant syndrome: Potentially fatal adverse drug effect manifested by hyperpyrexia, altered mental status, muscle rigidity, irregular pulse, fluctuating BP, diaphoresis, and tachycardia.

Orphan drug (as defined by the Orphan Drug Act, an amendment of the Federal Food, Drug and Cosmetic Act which took effect in January 1983): a drug or biological product used in the treatment, diagnosis or prevention of a rare disease. A rare disease or condition is one which affects less than 200,000 persons in the U.S., or affects more than 200,000 persons, but for which there is no reasonable expectation that drug research and development costs can be recovered from sales within the U.S. (Tatro, 1988).

Pharmacodynamics: study of mechanisms of action, biochemistry, and physiological effects of drugs.

Pharmacokinetics: study of how a drug reaches its sites of action and is removed from the body through processes of absorption, distribution, biotransformation and elimination.

Photosensitivity: drug-induced skin changes resulting in unusual susceptability to effects of sunlight or ultraviolet light.

Preload: ventricular filling pressure at the end of diastole.

Pro-drug: inactive drug form that becomes pharmacologically active through biotransformation.

Protein binding: a reversible interaction between protein and drug resulting in a drug-protein complex (bound drug) which is in equilibrium with free (active) drug in plasma and tissues. Since only free drug can diffuse to action sites, factors that influence drug-binding (e.g., displacement of bound drug by another drug, or decreased albumin concentration) may potentiate pharmacological effect.

Recall phenomenon: skin reaction due to prior radiotherapy.

Side effect: an expected, mild adverse effect (such as dry mouth or constipation associated with atropinelike drugs) caused by the pharmacologic action of a drug.

Softab: soft, chewable tablet. (Stuart trademark).

Somogyi effect: a rebound phenomenon clinically manifested by fasting hyperglycemia and worsening of diabetic control in the presence of unnecessarily large insulin doses. Hormonal response to unrecognized hypoglycemia (i.e., release of epinephrine, glucagon, growth hormone, cortisol) causes insensitivity to insulin. Increasing the amount of insulin required to treat the hyperglycemia intensifies the hypoglycemia.

Spansule: sustained release capsule. (Smith Kline & French trademark).

Steady-state plasma concentration: a state reached when the amount of drug absorbed is equivalent to the amount of drug being eliminated; plasma concentration will then fluctuate around a mean or plateau concentration. Full benefit of the drug can be expected when steady-state is reached. Drug form, elimination half-life, renal failure are factors that qualify steady-state concentration.

Tachyphylaxis: rapid decrease in response to a drug after administration of a few doses. Initial drug response cannot be restored by an increase in dose.

Therapeutic window: range of drug concentration level within which a particular drug has its safest and optimal therapeutic effect. That is, the limits between therapeutic and toxic response to a drug.

Tolerance: decreased responsiveness to pharmacodynamic action of a drug that occur during repeated administration of constant drug doses. Larger or more frequent doses or both are required to achieve the same effects observed with initial dosing.

Trade name (also called brand or proprietary name): a registered name used exclusively by the drug manufacturer who is the legal owner of the name.

Tubex: cartridge-needle unit. (Wyeth trademark).

Vaporale: cloth-covered crushable ampule for inhalation. (Burroughs Wellcome trademark).

Withdrawal symptoms: generally classed as rebound effects in the physiological systems initially modified by the drug.

INDEX

Prototype drugs in **bold**; classifications in SMALL CAPS.

Prototype drugs in **bold**; classifications in SMALL CAPS.

Prototype drugs in **bold**; classifications in SMALL CAPS.

Prototype drugs in **bold**; classifications in SMALL CAPS.

Prototype drugs in **bold**; classifications in SMALL CAPS.

Prototype drugs in **bold**; classifications in SMALL CAPS.

Prototype drugs in **bold**; classifications in SMALL CAPS.

Prototype drugs in **bold**; classifications in SMALL CAPS.

Prototype drugs in **bold**; classifications in SMALL CAPS.

Prototype drugs in **bold**; classifications in SMALL CAPS.

Prototype drugs in **bold**; classifications in SMALL CAPS.

Prototype drugs in **bold**; classifications in SMALL CAPS.

Prototype drugs in **bold**; classifications in SMALL CAPS.

Prototype drugs in **bold**; classifications in SMALL CAPS.

Prototype drugs in **bold**; classifications in SMALL CAPS.

Prototype drugs in **bold**; classifications in SMALL CAPS.

Prototype drugs in **bold**; classifications in SMALL CAPS.

Prototype drugs in **bold**; classifications in SMALL CAPS.

Prototype drugs in **bold**; classifications in SMALL CAPS.

Prototype drugs in **bold**; classifications in SMALL CAPS.

Prototype drugs in **bold**; classifications in SMALL CAPS.

Prototype drugs in **bold**; classifications in SMALL CAPS.

Prototype drugs in **bold**; classifications in SMALL CAPS.

BIBLIOGRAPHY

ARTICLES

Abate MA (1986): Medical management of cholesterol gallstones. *Drug Intell Clin Pharm* 20(2)(Feb):106-115.

Abrams J (1987): Nitrate therapy: Part 1. Current indications and rationale for its employment. *Consultant* 27(6): 154-162.

Ahmed ME, Branch RA (1986): Ribavarin (Virazole): A novel antiviral agent against viral respiratory tract infections. *Rational Drug Therapy* 20(11):1-3.

Amendola MA, Spera TD (1985): Doxycycline-induced esophagitis. *JAMA* 253(7):1009-1011.

Anderson JB (1987): The calcium-osteoporosis question addressed (letter). *Consultant* 27(1):15-16.

Bennett WR, et al (1987): Activation of the complement system by recombinant tissue plasminogen activator. *J & Am Coll Cardiology* 10(3)(Sept): 627-632.

Boldy DA, Heath A, Ruddock S, et al (1987): Activated charcoal for carbamazepine poisoning (letter). *Lancet* 1(8540):1027.

Burckart GJ, Canafax DM, Yee GC (1986): Cyclosporine monitoring. *Drug Intell Clin Pharm* 20(9):649-652.

Candella FJ (1987): Inhibitors of cholesterol synthesis and cataracts (letter). *JAMA* 257(2)(March 27):1602.

Carruthers SG (1986): Severe coughing during captopril and enalapril therapy. *Can Med Asso J* 135(3):217-218.

Covinsky JO (1987): Esmolol: A novel cardioselective, titratable, intravenous beta-blocker with ultrashort half-life. *Drug Intell Clin Pharm* 21(4)(April):316-321.

Eisendrath S, Sweeney M (1987): Toxic neuropsychiatric effects of digoxin at therapeutic serum concentrations. *Amer J Psych* 144(4):506-507.

Ferguson RK, Vlasses PH, Riley LJ Jr (1984): Captopril and enalapril: Angiotensin converting enzyme (ACE) inhibitors. *Rational Drug Therapy* 18(3):1-5.

Fisher AA (1987): Allergic contact dermatitis and conjunctivitis from benazlkonium chloride. *Cutis* 39(5):381-383.

Foulke GE, Albertson TE (1987): QRS interval in tricyclic anti-depressant overdosage; Inaccuracy as a toxicity indicator in emergency settings. *Ann Emerg Med* 16(2): 160-163.

Fraunfelder F, (1988): Ocular examination before initiation of lovastatin (Mevacor) therapy (letter). *Amer J Ophthal* 105 (Jan):91-92.

Firedman LS, Dienstao JL, Nelson PW, Russell PS, Cosimi AB (1985): Anaphylactic reaction and cardiopulmonary arrest following intravenous cyclosporin. *AJM* 78(2):343-345.

Frick M, Heikki et al (1987): Helsinki heart study: Primary-prevention trial with gemfibrozil in middle-aged men with dyslipidemia. *N Engl J Med* 317(Nov 12):1237-1245.

Frommer DA, Kulig KW, Marx JA, Rumack B (1987): Tricyclic antidepressant overdose. A review. *JAMA* 257(4):521-526.

Garden JM, Freinkel RK (1986): Systemic absorption of topical steroids. Metabolic effects as an index of mild hypercortisolism. *Arch Dermatol* 122(9):1007-1010.

Gonzales ER, et al (1987): Cimetidine versus ranitidine: Single dose, oral regimen for reducing gastric acidity and volume in ambulatory surgery patients. *Drug Intell Clin Pharm* 21(2):192-195.

Griffin MJJ, Morris JS (1987): MAOI-like reaction associated with cimetidine. *Drug Intell Clin Pharm* 21(2)(Feb):219.

Gross NJ (1987): Ipratropium bromide: First of a new class of bronchodilators. *IM* 8(6); 242-259.

Hodsman GP, et al (1986): Factors related to first dose hypotensive effect of captopril: predication and treatment. *Brit Med J* 286(6328):832-834.

Inman WH, Rawson NS (1987): Deafness with enalapril and prescription event monitoring (letter). *Lancet* 1(853):872.

Isaacsohn JL (1988): HMG-CoA reductase inhibitors: A new class of lipid-lowering drugs. *Choices in Cardiology* 2(1): (Jan/Feb):39, 44, 45.

Kaatz GW, Fekety R(1986): Combating colonization of *Clostridium difficile*. *Consultant* 26:45-58.

Kappa JR, Fisher CA, Berkowitz HD, Cottrell ED, Addoniziol VP Jr (1987): Heparin-induced platelet activation in sixteen surgical patients: Diagnosis and management. *J Vasc Surg* 5(1):101-109.

Knight KM, Doucet HJ (1987): Gastric rupture and death caused by ipecac syrup. *South Med J* 80(6):786-787.

Koegel L Jr (1985): Ototoxicity: A contemporary review of aminoglycosides, loop diuretics, acetylsalicylic acid, guinine, erythromycin, and cisplatin. *AM J Otology* 6(2): 190-199.

Kreisberg RA (1987): Hypercholesterolemia: Dietary and pharmacotherapy. *Hosp Pract* 22(4):197-232.

Lin MS, Hsieh WJ (1987): Prazosin-induced first-dose phenomenon possibly associated with hemorrhagic stroke: A report of three cases. *Drug Intell Clin Pharm* 21(9): 723-726.

Ludbrook PA (1986): Thrombolytic therapy with t-PA. *Cardiovasc Med* 11(2):37-44.

Marcus FI (1986): Amiodarone in antiarrhythmic therapy. *Cardiovasc Med* 11(2):25-36.

Mauro VF, Mauro LS (1986): Use of intermittant dobutamine infusion in congestive heart failure. *Drug Intell Clin Pharm* 20(12):919-924.

McMurray J, Matthews DM (1985): Effect of diarrhoea on a patient taking captopril. *Lancet* 1(8428):581.

Metz S, et al (1987): Rebound hypertension after discontinuation of transdermal clonidine therapy. *Am J Med* 82(1):17-19.

Morgan JP, Zappa M (1987): Topical minoxidil for hair loss. *Rational Drug Therapy* 21(5):1-4.

Murphy S, Kelly HW (1987): Cromolyn sodium: Review of mechanisms and clinical use in asthma. *Drug Intell Clin Pharm* 21(1Pt1):22-35.

Packer M, Lee WH, Yushak M, Medina N (1986): Comparison of captopril and enalapril in patients with severe chronic heart failure. *N Engl J Med* 315(14):847-853.

Packer M, et al (1987): Functional renal insufficiency during long-term therapy with captopril and enalapril in severe chronic heart failure. *Ann Int Med* 106(3):346-354.

Pont A, et al (1987): High-dose ketoconazole therapy and adrenal and testicular function in humans. *Arch Intern Med* 144(11):2150-2153.

Powers BJ, Cattau EL Jr, Zimmerman HJ (1986): Chlorzoxazone hepatotoxic reactions. An analysis of 21 identified or presumed cases. *Arc Intern Med* 146(6):1183-1186.

Pruessner HT, Hansel NK, Griffiths M (1986): Diagnosis and treatment of chlamydial infections. *Am Fam Physician* 34(1):81-92.

Re R (1987): The diagnostic and therapeutic promise of monoclonal antibodies. *Modern Medicine* 55(4):21-24.

Reitz JA (1986): Alfentanil in anesthesia and analgesia. *Drug Intell Clin Pharm* 20(5):335-341.

Roberts WN, Liang MH, Stern SH (1987): Colchicine in acute gout. Reassessment of risks and benefits. *JAMA* 257 (14):1920-1922.

Rosenberg MJ, Rojanapithayakorn W, Feldblum PJ, Higgings JE (1987): Effect of the contraceptive sponges on chlamydial infections, gonorrhea, and ondidiasis. *JAMA* 257(17):2308-2312.

Scheinberg IH, Jaffe ME, Sternlieb I (1987): The use of Trientine in preventing the effects of interrupting penicillamine therapy in Wilson's disease. *N Engl J Med* 317 (4):209-213.

Schumock G, Baker DE (1987): Pepsid, a new H_2 antagonist. *Pract Gastroent* (March/April):43-53.

Shaftic AA, et al (1986): Nifedipine-induced gingival hyperplasia. *Drug Intell Clin Pharm* 20(7-8):602-605.

Semple PF, Herd GW (1986): Cough and wheeze caused by inhibitors of angiotensin-converting enzyme (letter). *N Engl J Med* 314(1):61.

Sherman R, et al (1986): Cefoxitin-induced pseudo acute renal failure. *Clin Ther* 4:114-117.

Sternberg DE (1986): Neuroleptic malignant syndrome: The pendulum swings (editorial). *Am J Psych* 143(10):1273-1275.

Stuart GJ, Davey EB, Wight SE (1986): Continuous intravenous morphine infusions for terminal pain control: A retrospective review. *Drug Intell Clin Pharm* 20(12):968-972.

Synthetic marijuana for nausea and vomiting due to cancer chemotherapy. (1987) *Medical Letter* 29(748)(Sept. 11):83-86.

Thadani U, Whitsett TL (1987): Nitrate Therapy: Continuous or pulse dosing. *Rational Drug Ther* 21(7):1-6.

Topol EJ, et al (1987): A randomized trial of immediate versus delayed elective angioplasty after intravenous tissue plasminogen activator in acute myocardial infarction. *N Engl J Med* 317(Sept 3):581-588.

Tse CST, et al (1987): Seizure-like activity associated with impenemcilastatin. *Drug Intell Clin Pharm* 21 (7/8) (July/Aug):659-660.

Vega GL, Grundy SM (1987): Treatment of primary moderate hypercholesterolemia with lovastatin (Mevinolin) and colestipol. *JAMA* 257(1):33-38.

Wamboldt FS, Jefferson JW, Wamboldt MZ (1986): Digitalis intoxication misdiagnosed as depression by primary care physicians. *Am J Psych* 143(2):219-221.

Watson WA: Factors influencing the clinical efficacy of activated charcoal. *Drug Intell Clin Pharm* 21(2):160-166.

Weber MA (1986): Clinical experience with transdermal antihypertensive therapy. *Pract Cardiol* 12(5):104-120.

Wingo PA, Layde PM, Lee NC, Rubin G, Ory HW (1987): The risk of breast cancer in postmenopausal woman who have used estrogen replacement therapy. *JAMA* 257(2):209-215.

Wiser TH, et al (1987): Transdermal clonidine: An association with recurrent herpes simplex and hyperpigmentation. *J Am Acad Dermatol* 17(7):143-144.

BOOKS

Barnhart ER (Publisher): 1991 *Physicians' Desk Reference*, 45th ed. Oradell, NJ, Medical Economics Co, Inc.

Ganong WF (1987): *Review of Medical Physiology*, 13th ed. Norwalk, CT, Appleton & Lange.

Gilman AG, Goodman LS, Rall TW, Murad F (eds): (1985): *Goodman and Gilman's The Pharmacological Basis of Therapeutics*, 7th ed. New York, Macmillan.

Kastrup EK (ed) 1991: *Facts and Comparisons*. St. Louis, MO, JB Lippincott.

Katzung BG (ed) (1987): *Basic and Clinical Pharmacology*, 3rd ed. Norwalk, CT, Appleton & Lange.

McEvoy GK (ed) (1991): *American Hospital Formulory Service (AFHS) Drug Information 88*. Bethesda, MD, American Society of Hospital Pharmacists.

USP DI Advice for the Patient, Vol II 1991: Rockville, MD, The United States Pharmacopeial Convention, Inc.

USP DI Drug Information for the Health Care Professional, Vol I-A & B (1991): Rockville, MD, The United States Pharmacopeial Convention, Inc.